MW01091703

Withrow & MacEwen's

Small Animal Clinical Oncology

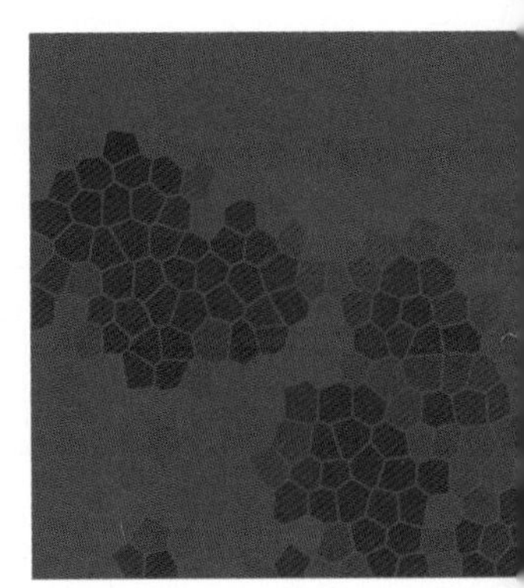

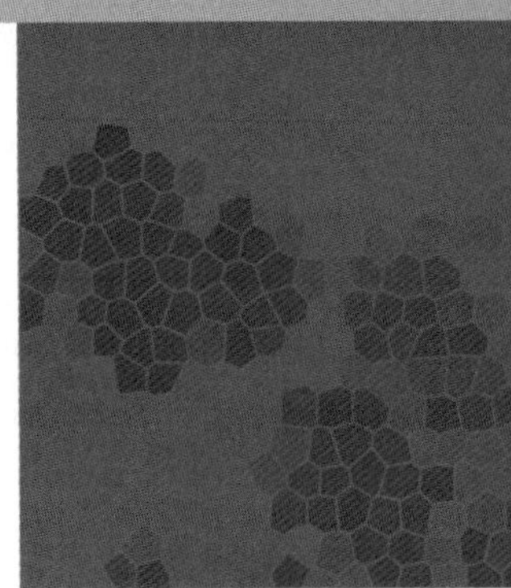

Withrow & MacEwen's

Small Animal Clinical Oncology

5th edition

Stephen J. Withrow, DVM, DACVS, DACVIM (Oncology)
Associate Director and Founder
Animal Cancer Center
Colorado State University
Fort Collins, Colorado

David M. Vail, DVM, DACVIM (Oncology)
Professor of Oncology
Barbara A. Suran Chair in Comparative Oncology
Director, Center for Clinical Trials and Research
School of Veterinary Medicine
University of Wisconsin-Madison
Madison, Wisconsin

Rodney L. Page, DVM, DACVIM (Internal Med/Oncology)
Director, Flint Animal Cancer Center
Professor of Medical Oncology
Department of Clinical Sciences
College of Veterinary Medicine & Biomedical Sciences
Colorado State University
Fort Collins, Colorado

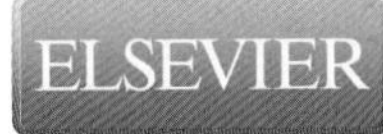

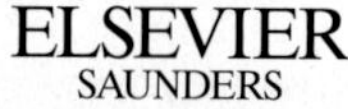

3251 Riverport Lane
St. Louis, Missouri 63043

WITHROW AND MACEWEN'S SMALL ANIMAL CLINICAL ONCOLOGY ISBN: 978-1-4377-2362-5

Notices

International Standard Book Number: 978-1-4377-2362-5

Vice President and Publisher: Linda Duncan
Content Strategy Director: Penny Rudolph
Content Development Specialist: Brandi Graham
Publishing Services Manager: Catherine Jackson
Project Manager: David Stein
Design Direction: Brian Salisbury

Printed in China

Last digit is the print number: 9 8 7 6 5 4 3 2 1

Contributors

David J. Argyle, BVMS, PhD, DECVIM-CA (Oncology), MRCVS
William Dick Professor of Clinical Studies and Dean of School
Royal (Dick) School of Veterinary Studies and Roslin Institute
The University of Edinburgh
Easter Bush
Roslin, Midlothian, United Kingdom
Tumor Biology and Metastasis
Molecular/Targeted Therapy of Cancer: Gene Therapy for Cancer
Molecular/Targeted Therapy of Cancer: Novel and Emerging Therapeutic Targets

Anne C. Avery, VMD, PhD
Associate Professor of Immunology
College of Veterinary Medicine & Biomedical Sciences
Colorado State University
Fort Collins, Colorado
Molecular Diagnostics

Philip J. Bergman, DVM, MS, PhD, DACVIM (Oncology)
Director, Clinical Studies, VCA Antech Inc.
Medical Director, Katonah-Bedford Veterinary Center
Bedford Hills, New York;
Adjunct Associate
Memorial Sloan-Kettering Cancer Center
New York, New York
Paraneoplastic Syndromes
Melanoma

Brenda N. Bonnett, BSc, DVM, PhD
Consulting Epidemiologist
B Bonnett Consulting
Wiarton, Ontario, Canada
Epidemiology and the Evidence-Based Medicine Approach

Lesley M. Butler, PhD
Assistant Professor
Environmental and Radiological Health Sciences
Colorado State University
Fort Collins, Colorado
Epidemiology and the Evidence-Based Medicine Approach

Craig A. Clifford, DVM, MS, DACVIM (Oncology)
Staff Oncologist and Director of Clinical Research
Hope Veterinary Specialists
Malvern, Pennsylvania
Miscellaneous Tumors: Histiocytic Diseases

William T.N. Culp, VMD, DACVS
Assistant Professor
Department of Surgical and Radiological Sciences
University of California-Davis
School of Veterinary Medicine
Davis, California
Tumors of the Respiratory System: Pulmonary Neoplasia

Curtis W. Dewey, DVM, MS, DACVIM (Neurology), DACVS
Associate Professor, Neurology/Neurosurgery
Chief, Section of Neurology
Department of Clinical Sciences
College of Veterinary Medicine
Cornell University
Ithaca, New York
Tumors of the Nervous System

Steven Dow, DVM, MS, PhD, DACVIM (Internal Medicine)
Professor of Immunology
Department of Clinical Sciences
Department of Microbiology, Immunology, Pathology
Colorado State University
Fort Collins, Colorado
Cancer Immunotherapy

Richard R. Dubielzig, DVM, DACVP, DACVO (hon)
Professor of Pathology
Department of Pathobiological Sciences
University of Wisconsin
Madison, Wisconsin
Ocular Tumors

E.J. Ehrhart, DVM, PhD, DACVP
Associate Professor
Department of Microbiology, Immunology and Pathology
CSU Animal Cancer Center
CSU Veterinary Diagnostic Laboratories
Colorado State University
Fort Collins, Colorado
The Pathology of Neoplasia

Nicole P. Ehrhart, VMD, MS, DACVS
Professor, Surgical Oncology
Animal Cancer Center
Colorado State University
Fort Collins, Colorado
Biopsy Principles
Tumors of the Skeletal System

Timothy M. Fan, DVM, PhD, DACVIM (Oncology, Internal Medicine)
Associate Professor
Veterinary Clinical Medicine
University of Illinois at Urbana-Champaign
Urbana, Illinois
Tumors of the Skeletal System

James P. Farese, DVM, DACVS
Associate Professor
Small Animal Clinical Sciences
University of Florida
Gainesville, Florida
Surgical Oncology
Melanoma

Lisa J. Forrest, VMD, DACVR (Radiology, Radiation Oncology)
Professor, Radiation Oncology Section Head
Surgical Sciences
School of Veterinary Medicine
University of Wisconsin-Madison
Madison, Wisconsin
Imaging in Oncology
Soft Tissue Sarcomas

Kristen R. Friedrichs, DVM, DACVP (Clinical Pathology)
Clinical Assistant Professor
Department of Pathobiological Sciences
School of Veterinary Medicine
University of Wisconsin-Madison
Madison, Wisconsin
Diagnostic Cytopathology in Clinical Oncology

Laura D. Garrett, DVM, DACVIM (Oncology)
Clinical Associate Professor, Oncology
Department of Veterinary Clinical Medicine
College of Veterinary Medicine
University of Illinois
Urbana, Illinois
Miscellaneous Tumors: Mesothelioma

Michael H. Goldschmidt, MSc, BVMS, MRCVS, DACVP
Professor, Veterinary Pathology
Department of Pathobiology
Chief, Surgical Pathology
Laboratory of Pathology and Toxicology
School of Veterinary Medicine
University of Pennsylvania
Philadelphia, Pennsylvania
Tumors of the Mammary Gland

Ira K. Gordon, DVM, DACVR
Postdoctoral Fellow
Radiation Oncology Branch
National Cancer Institute, National Institutes of Health
Bethesda, Maryland;
Radiation Oncologist
The Oncology Service, LLC
Washington, DC;
VetPrep Corp
Solana Beach, California
Radiation Therapy

Daniel L. Gustafson, BS, PhD
Associate Professor, Clinical Sciences
Director of Research, Animal Cancer Center
Colorado State University
Fort Collins, Colorado;
Director, Pharmacology Core
University of Colorado Cancer Center
Anschutz Medical Campus
University of Colorado-Denver,
Aurora, Colorado
Cancer Chemotherapy

Amanda M. Guth, DVM, PhD
Research Scientist, Animal Cancer Center
Department of Clinical Sciences
Colorado State University
Fort Collins, Colorado
Cancer Immunotherapy

Marlene L. Hauck, DVM, PhD, DACVIM (Oncology)
Professor of Oncology
Department of Clinical Sciences
College of Veterinary Medicine
North Carolina State University
Raleigh, North Carolina
Tumors of the Skin and Subcutaneous Tissues

Carolyn J. Henry, DVM, MS, DACVIM (Oncology)
Professor of Oncology
Department of Veterinary Medicine and Surgery
College of Veterinary Medicine
Division of Hematology/Oncology
School of Medicine
Interim Associate Director of Research
Ellis Fischel Cancer Center
University of Missouri
Columbia, Missouri
The Etiology of Cancer: Chemical, Physical, and Hormonal Factors
The Etiology of Cancer: Cancer-Causing Viruses

Debra A. Kamstock, DVM, PhD, DACVP
KamPath Diagnostics & Investigation;
Affiliate Faculty
Department of Clinical Sciences
Colorado State University
Fort Collins, Colorado
The Pathology of Neoplasia

Michael S. Kent, MAS, DVM, DACVIM (Oncology), DACVR (Radiation Oncology)
Associate Professor
Department of Surgical and Radiological Sciences
University of California-Davis
Davis, California
Melanoma

Chand Khanna, DVM, PhD, DACVIM (Oncology)
Senior Scientist
Head, Tumor and Metastasis Biology Section
Center for Cancer Research
National Cancer Institute
Bethesda, Maryland
Tumor Biology and Metastasis
Molecular Diagnostics

William C. Kisseberth, DVM, PhD, DACVIM (Oncology)
Associate Professor
Department of Veterinary Clinical Sciences
College of Veterinary Medicine
The Ohio State University
Columbus, Ohio
Miscellaneous Tumors: Neoplasia of the Heart

Deborah W. Knapp, DVM, MS, DACVIM (Oncology)
Dolores L. McCall Professor of Comparative Oncology
Veterinary Clinical Sciences
Purdue University
West Lafayette, Indiana
Tumors of the Urinary System

Susan L. Kraft, DVM, PhD, DACVR (Diagnostic Imaging), DACVR (Radiation Oncology)
Professor, Veterinary Radiology
Environmental and Radiological Health Sciences
Colorado State University
James L. Voss Veterinary Teaching Hospital
Fort Collins Colorado
Imaging in Oncology

Susan E. Lana, DVM, MS, DACVIM (Oncology)
Associate Professor
Animal Cancer Center
Department of Clinical Sciences
Colorado State University
Fort Collins, Colorado
Tumors of the Respiratory System: Nasosinal Tumors

Susan M. LaRue, DVM, PhD, DACVS, DACVR (Radiation Oncology)
Professor of Radiation Oncology
Environmental and Radiological Health Sciences
Colorado State University
James L. Voss Veterinary Teaching Hospital
Animal Cancer Center
Fort Collins, Colorado
Radiation Therapy

B. Duncan X. Lascelles, BSc, BVSc, PhD, CertVA, DSAS (ST), DECVS, DACVS
Professor, Small Animal Surgery and Pain Management
Department of Clinical Sciences
Comparative Pain Research Laboratory and Center for Comparative Medicine and Translational Research
College of Veterinary Medicine
North Carolina State University
Raleigh, North Carolina
Supportive Care for the Cancer Patient: Management of Chronic Cancer Pain

Jessica A. Lawrence, DVM, DACVIM (Oncology), DACVR (Radiation Oncology)
Assistant Professor of Medical Oncology
Department of Small Animal Medicine and Surgery
University of Georgia
College of Veterinary Medicine
Athens, Georgia
Tumors of the Female Reproductive System
Tumors of the Male Reproductive System

Julius M. Liptak, BVSc, MVetClinStud, FACVSc, DECVS, DACVS
Alta Vista Animal Hospital
Ottawa, Ontario, Canada
Soft Tissue Sarcomas
Cancer of the Gastrointestinal Tract: Oral Tumors
Cancer of the Gastrointestinal Tract: Hepatobiliary Tumors

Cheryl A. London, DVM, PhD, DACVIM (Oncology)
Associate Professor
Shackelford Professor of Veterinary Medicine
Department of Veterinary Biosciences
College of Veterinary Medicine
The Ohio State University
Columbus, Ohio
Molecular/Targeted Therapy of Cancer: Signal Transduction and Cancer
Mast Cell Tumors

Katharine F. Lunn, BVMS, MS, PhD, MRCVS, DACVIM (Small Animal Internal Medicine)
Associate Professor
Department of Clinical Sciences
College of Veterinary Medicine
North Carolina State University
Raleigh, North Carolina
Tumors of the Endocrine System

Dennis W. Macy, DM, MS, DACVIM (Internal Medicine/Oncology)
Professor Emeritus
Department of Clinical Sciences
College of Veterinary Medicine
Colorado State University
Fort Collins, Colorado;
Chief
Department of Medical Oncology
Desert Veterinary Specialist
Palm Desert, California;
Owner and Chief of Staff
Cancer Care Specialist
West Flamingo Animal Hospital
Las Vegas, Nevada
The Etiology of Cancer: Cancer-Causing Viruses

Margaret C. McEntee, DVM, DACVIM, DACVR(RO)
Professor and Alexander de Lahunta Chair
Department of Clinical Sciences
College of Veterinary Medicine
Cornell University
Ithaca, New York
Tumors of the Nervous System

Sarah K. McMillan, DVM
Department of Veterinary Clinical Sciences
Purdue University
West Lafayette, Indiana
Tumors of the Urinary System

Paul E. Miller, DVM, DACVO
Clinical Professor of Comparative Ophthalmology
Department of Surgical Sciences
School of Veterinary Medicine
University of Wisconsin-Madison
Madison, Wisconsin
Ocular Tumors

Jaime F. Modiano, VMD, PhD
Al and June Perlman Endowed Professor of Animal Oncology
Department of Veterinary Clinical Sciences
College of Veterinary Medicine
Masonic Cancer Center
University of Minnesota
Minneapolis, Minnesota
The Etiology of Cancer: The Genetic Basis of Cancer

Peter F. Moore, BVSc, PhD
Professor of Pathology
School of Veterinary Medicine
University of California-Davis
Davis, California
Miscellaneous Tumors: Histiocytic Diseases

Anthony J. Mutsaers, DVM, PhD, DACVIM (Oncology)
Assistant Professor
Department of Clinical Studies
Department of Biomedical Sciences
Ontario Veterinary College
University of Guelph
Guelph, Ontario, Canada
Molecular/Targeted Therapy of Cancer: Antiangiogenic and Metronomic Therapy

Christine Olver, DVM, PhD, DACVP
Associate Professor of Clinical Pathology
College of Veterinary Medicine & Biomedical Sciences
Colorado State University
Fort Collins, Colorado
Molecular Diagnostics

Rodney L. Page, DVM, DACVIM (Internal Med/Oncology)
Director, Flint Animal Cancer Center
Professor of Medical Oncology
Department of Clinical Sciences
College of Veterinary Medicine & Biomedical Sciences
Colorado State University
Fort Collins, Colorado
Epidemiology and the Evidence-Based Medicine Approach
Cancer Chemotherapy
Tumors of the Endocrine System

Melissa C. Paoloni, DVM, DACVIM (Oncology)
Director, Comparative Oncology Trials Consortium
Comparative Oncology Program
Center for Cancer Research
National Cancer Institute
Bethesda, Maryland
Molecular Diagnostics
Clinical Trials and Developmental Therapeutics

Marie E. Pinkerton, DVM, DACVP
Clinical Assistant Professor of Anatomic Pathology
Pathology Section Head
Department of Pathobiological Sciences
School of Veterinary Medicine
University of Wisconsin-Madison
Madison, Wisconsin
Hematopoietic Tumors: Canine Lymphoma and Lymphoid Leukemias

Barbara E. Powers, BS, DVM, MS, PhD, DACVP
Director of Veterinary Diagnostic Laboratory
College of Veterinary Medicine & Biomedical Sciences
Colorado State University
Fort Collins, Colorado
The Pathology of Neoplasia

Robert B. Rebhun, DVM, PhD, DACVIM (Oncology)
Assistant Professor
Department of Surgical and Radiological Sciences
School of Veterinary Medicine
University of California-Davis
Davis, California
Tumors of the Respiratory System: Pulmonary Neoplasia

Narda G. Robinson, DO, DVM, MS, FAAMA
Director
CSU Center for Comparative and Integrative Pain Medicine
Department of Clinical Sciences
Colorado State University
College of Veterinary Medicine & Biomedical Sciences
Fort Collins, Colorado
Complementary and Alternative Medicine for Cancer: The Good, the Bad, and the Dangerous

Stewart D. Ryan, BVSc(Hons), MS, DACVS
Affiliate Faculty
Colorado State University
Fort Collins, Colorado;
Director
Surgical Consultancy Services Pty. Ltd.
Hawthorn, Victoria, Australia
Tumors of the Skeletal System

Corey F. Saba, DVM, DACVIM (Oncology)
Associate Professor
Department of Medicine and Surgery
University of Georgia
College of Veterinary Medicine
Athens, Georgia
Tumors of the Female Reproductive System
Tumors of the Male Reproductive System

Kim A. Selting, DVM, MS, DACVIM (Oncology)
Associate Teaching Professor
Department of Veterinary Medicine and Surgery
University of Missouri
Columbia, Missouri
Cancer of the Gastrointestinal Tract: Intestinal Tumors

Jane R. Shaw, DVM, PhD
Assistant Professor and Director of the Argus Institute
Department of Clinical Sciences
Veterinary Teaching Hospital
Colorado State University
Fort Collins, Colorado
Supportive Care for the Cancer Patient: Relationship-Centered Approach to Cancer Communication

Katherine A. Skorupski, DVM, DACVIM (Oncology)
Associate Professor of Clinical Medical Oncology
Department of Veterinary Surgical and Radiological Sciences
University of California-Davis
Davis, California
Miscellaneous Tumors: Histiocytic Diseases

Karin U. Sorenmo, DVM, DACVIM, ECVIM-CA (Oncology)
Associate Professor of Oncology
Section Chief of Oncology
Department of Clinical Studies
School of Veterinary Medicine
University of Pennsylvania
Philadelphia, Pennsylvania
Tumors of the Mammary Gland

Carlos Henrique de Mello Souza, Med vet, MS, DACVIM (Oncology), DACVS
Surgical and Medical Oncologist, Relief
Veterinary Medical Teaching Hospital
Oklahoma State University
Stillwater, Oklahoma
Miscellaneous Tumors: Thymoma

Douglas H. Thamm, VMD, DACVIM (Oncology)
Associate Professor, Oncology
Barbara Cox Anthony Chair, Oncology
Animal Cancer Center
Department of Clinical Sciences
College of Veterinary Medicine and Biomedical Sciences
Colorado State University
Fort Collins, Colorado
Molecular/Targeted Therapy of Cancer: Novel and Emerging Therapeutic Targets
Mast Cell Tumors
Miscellaneous Tumors: Hemangiosarcoma

Michelle M. Turek, DVM, DACVIM (Oncology), DACVR (Radiation Oncology)
Assistant Professor of Radiation Oncology
College of Veterinary Medicine
The University of Georgia
Athens, Georgia
Cancer of the Gastrointestinal Tract: Perianal Tumors
Tumors of the Respiratory System: Nasosinal Tumors

David M. Vail, DVM, DACVIM (Oncology)
Professor of Oncology
Barbara A. Suran Chair in Comparative Oncology
Director, Center for Clinical Trials and Research
School of Veterinary Medicine
University of Wisconsin-Madison
Madison, Wisconsin
Clinical Trials and Developmental Therapeutics
Hematopoietic Tumors: Canine Lymphoma and Lymphoid Leukemias
Hematopoietic Tumors: Feline Lymphoma and Leukemia
Hematopoietic Tumors: Canine Acute Myeloid Leukemia, Myeloproliferative Neoplasms, and Myelodysplasia
Hematopoietic Tumors: Myeloma-Related Disorders

Joseph J. Wakshlag, DVM, PhD, DACVN, DACVSMR
Assistant Professor
Department of Clinical Sciences
Cornell University
Ithaca, New York
Supportive Care for the Cancer Patient: Nutritional Management of the Cancer Patient

Stephen J. Withrow, DVM, DACVS, DACVIM (Oncology)
Associate Director and Founder
Animal Cancer Center
Colorado State University
Fort Collins, Colorado
Biopsy Principles
Surgical Oncology
Cancer of the Gastrointestinal Tract: OralTumors
Cancer of the Gastrointestinal Tract: Salivary Gland Cancer
Cancer of the Gastrointestinal Tract: Esophageal Cancer
Cancer of the Gastrointestinal Tract: Exocrine Pancreatic Cancer
Cancer of the Gastrointestinal Tract: Gastric Cancer
Cancer of the Gastrointestinal Tract: Perianal Tumors
Tumors of the Respiratory System: Cancer of the Nasal Planum
Tumors of the Respiratory System: Cancer of the Larynx and Trachea

J. Paul Woods, DVM, MS, DACVIM (Internal Medicine, Oncology)
Co-Director, Institute for Comparative Cancer Investigation
Professor of Small Animal Medicine
Department of Clinical Studies
Ontario Veterinary College
University of Guelph
Guelph, Ontario, Canada
Miscellaneous Tumors: Canine Transmissible Venereal Tumor

Deanna R. Worley, DVM, DACVS
Assistant Professor, Surgical Oncology
Department of Clinical Sciences
Colorado State University;
Assistant Professor, Surgical Oncology
Animal Cancer Center
Colorado State University
Fort Collins, Colorado
Tumors of the Mammary Gland

Karen M. Young, VMD, PhD
Clinical Professor of Clinical Pathology
Chief of Diagnostic Services
Department of Pathobiological Sciences
School of Veterinary Medicine
University of Wisconsin–Madison
Madison, Wisconsin
Diagnostic Cytopathology in Clinical Oncology
Hematopoietic Tumors: Canine Lymphoma and Lymphoid Leukemias
Hematopoietic Tumors: Canine Acute Myeloid Leukemia, Myeloproliferative Neoplasms, and Myelodysplasia

Preface

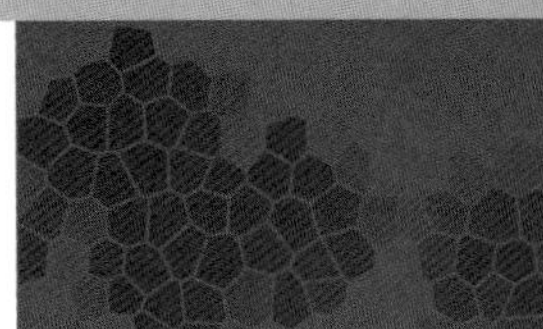

The fifth edition of *Small Animal Clinical Oncology* continues to chronicle significant advancement in the field of comparative clinical oncology. Since the first edition in 1989 this text has expanded all segments of the book to keep current with the profound changes in cancer biology and technology; in fact, each edition could be considered a milestone in the development of this specialty. The intent of this text continues to be production of a relevant summary of the field of comparative cancer biology and management for those engaged in all aspects of the veterinary profession. Approximately 20% of this edition has been substantially changed with new authors and both new additions and deletions of entire chapters to reflect an appropriate emphasis on the current state of the profession.

This text, in all its editions, parallels the expansion and maturity of comparative oncology during the last 25 years. The Specialty of Oncology was formalized under the American College of Veterinary Internal Medicine (ACVIM) in 1989 and has grown steadily, particularly in the last 10 to 15 years. Likewise, the European College of Veterinary Internal Medicine (ECVIM)–Oncology Specialty is now a robust and dynamic organization providing important resources to students and practitioners in Europe. The American College of Veterinary Surgeons (ACVS) has formally authorized the Fellowship Training Programs in Veterinary Surgical Oncology, which will promote the expansion of new centers of surgical excellence in this field. Equally important has been the growth of the Veterinary Cancer Society (VCS) and the European Society of Veterinary Oncology (ESVONC), as well as other like-minded associations in Japan (JVCS), Brazil (ABROVET) and others to develop soon. The globalization of the interest and desire for high-quality cancer care for pets is a remarkable and welcome occurrence.

During the last decade and particularly over the last 5 to 7 years, the formalization of clinical trials in companion animals for investigation of animal and human health has matured significantly. The Comparative Oncology Program at the National Cancer Institute (NCI) continues to lead the effort to promote the benefits of companion animals in human cancer control and has currently completed or initiated 18 multicenter trials through the Comparative Oncology Trials Consortium. Other clinical trial organizations and centers, within both the public and private sector, have emerged that have established a more formal infrastructure for cooperative clinical research. No better evidence of this exists than the recent Food and Drug Administration (FDA) and U.S. Department of Agriculture (USDA) approvals for products licensed for use specifically in canine cancer that occurred due to a clinician-animal health industry partnership.

Examples of marked advances in the field of cancer biology, etiology, and staging reflected in this text include a complete rewrite of the role of genetics in cancer development (Chapter 1, Section A), cancer epidemiology (Chapter 4), tumor imaging technology (Chapter 6), and the reliance on more sophisticated molecular diagnostics (Chapter 8). The rapid change in therapeutic areas include the developing indications for stereotactic radiotherapy in Chapter 12 and the increasing understanding of metronomic and antiangiogenic therapy in Chapter 14, Section C. An entire chapter has been added on clinical trials (Chapter 17) for the interested clinician scientist. All chapters devoted to specific cancer types have been updated; however, due to remarkable changes in the clinical management of certain cancers there has been a large expansion or a complete rewrite of chapters for melanoma, mast cell tumors, tumors of the skeletal system, tumors of the endocrine system, tumors of the mammary gland, urinary cancers, nervous system cancers, lymphoma, and histiocytic diseases.

There is still much to be done and future advances should continue to be a focus for expansion in subsequent editions of this text. Advancing the use and application of evidence-based medicine still remains a challenge in veterinary oncology. The desire to increase evidence-based decision making in clinical practice is being considered throughout the veterinary profession as a whole, and appropriate reporting guidelines for manuscript submission will soon be implemented in the leading veterinary journals. Such guidelines will permit sorting of high or low levels of evidence and an opportunity to engage in formal postpublication data analysis for systematic reviews. We look forward to the next edition of the text that includes therapeutic recommendations based on strong evidence. We also continue to hope that the next edition will see a quantum leap in satisfying several critical needs in the field. We urgently need improved control outcomes for canine lymphoma, hemangiosarcoma, and osteosarcoma and validated biomarkers to assist with prognostic and predictive estimates for all cancers—but in particular, those highly lethal disease processes mentioned above that have frustrated all of us for decades.

It is also important to consider potential operational impacts and solutions to the continued development of comparative oncology. The inconsistent availability of chemotherapy often now rises to levels of serious concern for continuity of care and will require innovative business solutions to ensure robust coverage of the expanding market need. It is obvious that the cost of care for companion animals will continue to rise, and the role that companion animal healthcare insurance will play in this dynamic could have far-reaching effects on the profession in the next decade. Likewise, the potential changes in the profession from increasing liability issues related to emotional pain and suffering litigation could create new operating paradigms.

The authors and editors have created the following text, which both describes the phenomenal strides made during the last 5 to 6 years and sets the standard to measure future growth and understanding of comparative oncology. We hope that it will be a useful resource for those engaged in animal and human oncology and for the ultimate improvement of the quality and length of life for our patients.

We dedicate this edition to these fine men, each of whom pioneered his particular branch of veterinary oncology:

Dr. E. Gregory MacEwen
1943-2001
The father of veterinary medical oncology,
Greg was personally responsible for educating and inspiring the current generation of medical oncologists, both as clinicians and clinician scientists.

Dr. Robert S. Brodey
1927-1979
The father of veterinary surgical oncology,
Bob will be remembered for his tireless effort to advance the field of oncology, to teach principles of surgery, and, most importantly, to preserve nature.

Dr. Edward L. Gillette
1932-2006
The father of veterinary radiation oncology,
Ed was a leader in comparative oncology. His vision and leadership have created a new and contemporary breed of oncologists in all disciplines.

Contents

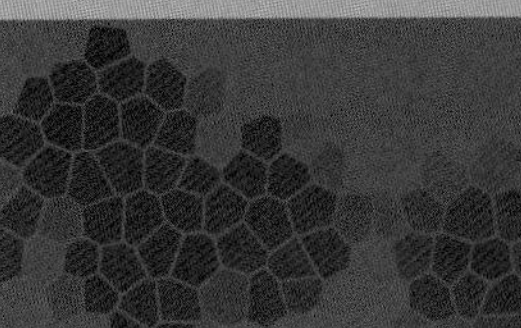

Why Worry About Cancer in Companion Animals?

Introduction

STEPHEN J. WITHROW, DAVID M. VAIL, AND RODNEY L. PAGE

Why should veterinarians be concerned about cancer in companion animals? Several compelling motivations and opportunities exist for the profession as a whole to continue, and indeed expand on, the significant role we play in the understanding, prevention, and elimination or control of this devastating constellation of disease processes. Although our prime directive is to ensure the health and quality of life of the companions under our care, the needs of our client caregivers during the difficult times of cancer diagnosis, treatment, and outcome (whether optimistic or pessimistic) should be of nearly equal importance. Because cancer is a disease that knows no species boundaries, our profession has considerable opportunity to play a key role in comparative oncologic investigations, with the ultimate goal of effecting cure or, in the absence of cure, transforming cancer from an acute life-threatening disorder into a manageable chronic condition (much like diabetes).

The sheer numbers involved highlight the magnitude of the problem of cancer in companion species. The prevalence of cancer in companion animals continues to rise and is increasing for a variety of reasons, not the least of which is related to animals living longer thanks to the increasing care offered by caregivers and the advanced veterinary care they seek. There are approximately 165 million dogs and cats at risk in the United States,[1] and cancer remains a major cause of companion animal morbidity and mortality (see Chapter 4), with at least 4 million dogs and 4 million cats developing cancer each year.[2-6] Although the true incidence or prevalence of companion animal cancer is currently not known, based on necropsy surveys describing proportional mortality, 45% of dogs that live to 10 years or older die of cancer.[4] With no age adjustment, 23% of patients presenting for necropsy died of cancer. In a 1998 Morris Animal Foundation Animal Health Survey, more than 2000 respondents stated that cancer was the leading cause of disease-related death in both dogs (47%) and cats (32%).[3] Another Morris survey performed in 2005 revealed that cancer was by far the largest health concern among dog owners (41%), with heart disease the number two concern at 7%. Regardless of the exact numbers, both the reality and the perception support the clients' point of view that cancer remains the number one concern in their minds with respect to the health and quality of life of their companions—the so called "Emperor of all maladies."[7] Furthermore, breakthroughs in the management of human cancers have received a great deal of exposure through the Internet, news media, and popular press, which further serves to educate companion caregivers and raise the level of expectations as to therapeutic possibilities and promotes an atmosphere of optimism and a demand for similar care for their animals. Increased longevity of companion animals, the increasing prevalence, and enhanced caregiver expectations require that the veterinary profession be prepared to meet these challenges and opportunities.

Because cancer is a common and serious disease for human beings, many owners have had or will have a personal experience with cancer in themselves, a family member, or a close friend. Realizing the importance of companion animals to our clients, it must be appreciated that they value the veterinarian's ability to care as much as his or her ability to cure. Keeping this in mind, the veterinarian should approach the patient with cancer in a positive, compassionate, and knowledgeable manner. Frequently the veterinary profession has taken a pessimistic approach to cancer. This attitude is not only a detriment to the companion but may also negatively reinforce unfounded fears in the client about the disease in humans. We owe it to our companion animal patients and their caregivers to be well informed and up-to-date on current treatment methods to prevent imparting unnecessary feelings of hopelessness.

Perhaps the greatest opportunity presented to our profession, beyond the immediate care of our patients' and clients' needs, is the more global role (and responsibility) we play in advancing the understanding of cancer biology, prevention, and treatment from a comparative oncology standpoint. Companion animals with spontaneously developing cancer provide an excellent opportunity to investigate many aspects of cancer from etiology to treatment. One of the most exciting achievements in veterinary oncology over the last decade has been the development of successful and collaborative consortia groups that are purposed to perform multicenter clinical trials and prospective tumor biospecimen repository collections. These include the Comparative Oncology Trials Consortium (COTC; https://ccrod.cancer.gov/confluence/display/CCRCOPWeb/Comparative+Oncology+Trials+Consortium) and the Canine Comparative Oncology and Genomics Consortium (CCOGC, www.ccogc.net) centrally managed by the National Institutes of Health (NIH)-National Cancer Institute's Comparative Oncology Program (NCI-COP) and discussed in Chapter 17. Their infrastructure allows larger scale clinical trials and provides the voice for collective advocacy in veterinary and comparative oncology. Their success is an example of the growing importance of the study of comparative tumor biology and clinical investigations. Access to novel drugs and biologics will speed clinical applications for both veterinary species and humans. Ultimately, including companion animal populations in clinical trials assessing novel drugs and biologics of interest to the National Cancer Institute, the Food and Drug Administration, and the pharmaceutical industry will both advance veterinary-based practice and inform future human clinical trials that may follow. Some of the aspects of companion animal cancer that enable attractive comparative models include the following:

1. Companion dogs and cats are genetically outbred and immunologically intact animals (like humans) as opposed to many experimental models of rodents and other animals.
2. The cancers seen in practice are spontaneously developing as opposed to experimentally induced and better recapitulate the natural human and veterinary condition.
3. Companion species share the same environment as their caregivers and may serve as epidemiologic or etiologic sentinels for the changing patterns of cancer development seen in humans.
4. Companion species have a higher incidence of some cancers (e.g., osteosarcoma, non-Hodgkin's lymphoma) than humans.
5. Most animal cancers will progress at a more rapid rate than will the human counterpart. This permits more rapid and less costly outcome determinations such as time to metastasis, local recurrence, and survival.
6. Because fewer established "gold standard" treatments exist in veterinary medicine compared to human medicine, it is ethically acceptable to attempt new forms of therapy (especially single-agent trials) on an untreated cancer rather than wait to initiate new treatments until all "known" treatments have failed, as is common in the human condition. It is important to recognize that this latitude in clinical trials can be misused to permit diverse and poorly characterized or even unethical treatments to be attempted as well. We have an obligation to ensure that our patients are not denied known effective treatment while at the same time planning well-designed prospective clinical trials of newer, scientifically sound treatment methods.
7. Companion species' cancers are more akin to human cancers than are rodent tumors in terms of patient size and cell kinetics. Dogs and cats also share similar characteristics of physiology and metabolism for most organ systems and drugs. Such correspondence allows better and safer comparison of treatment modalities such as surgery, radiation, and chemotherapy between animals and humans to be made.
8. Dogs and cats have intact immune systems as opposed to many rodent model systems, which allows immunologic assays and treatment approaches to be explored.
9. Companion animal trials are generally more economical to perform than human trials.
10. Companion animals live long enough to determine the potential late effects of treatment.
11. Regional referral centers exist to concentrate case accrual and facilitate clinical trials.
12. Clients are often willing to allow a necropsy, which is a crucial end point for not only tumor control but also treatment-related toxicity.
13. Dogs and cats are large enough for high-resolution imaging studies and multiple sampling opportunities, as well as for surgical intervention.
14. The recent elucidation of the canine genome and its resemblance and relevance to the human genome open unique and unparalleled opportunities to study comparative oncology from a genetic perspective.[8]

Clients who seek treatment for their companion animals with cancer are a devoted and compassionate subset of the population. Working with these caregivers can be a very satisfying aspect of a frequently frustrating specialty. Clients are almost always satisfied with an honest and aggressive attempt to cure, control, or palliate the disease of their companion, making the experience satisfying for the veterinarian, for the client, and, most important, for the companion.

Oncology also offers the inquisitive veterinarian a complex and challenging area for both clinical and basic research. The challenges and accomplishments in oncology have been and continue to be very impressive. Oncology offers unlimited opportunity for the pursuit of knowledge for the benefit of animals and humankind. "Cancer, unlike politics and religion, is not a topic of controversy. No one is for it. Cancer is not another word for death. Neither is it a single disease for which there is one cure. Instead, it takes many forms, and each form responds differently to treatment."[9]

Clinical and comparative oncology continues to be a rapidly advancing field of study. More training programs are developed each year that allow a wider distribution of experienced veterinarians into practice, research, industry, government, and the academic setting. Through the continued investigation of tumor biology and treatment and the inclusion of veterinary species in well-designed, rigorous, and humane clinical trials, the veterinary profession will play a key role in advancing the diagnosis, treatment, and prevention of cancer for all species.

REFERENCES

1. American Pet Products Association 2011-2012 National Pet Owners Survey. Available at http://www.americanpetproducts.org/press_industrytrends.asp. Accessed December 28th, 2011.
2. Dorn CR: Epidemiology of canine and feline tumors, *Compend Contin Educ Pract Vet* 12:307–312, 1976.
3. Animal Health Survey. In *Companion animal news*, Englewood, Colorado, 1998 and 2005, Morris Animal Foundation.
4. Bronson RT: Variation in age at death of dogs of different sexes and breeds, *Am J Vet Res* 43:2057–2059, 1982.
5. Gobar GM, Case JT, Kass PH: Program for surveillance of causes of death of dogs, using the Internet to survey small animal veterinarians, *J Am Vet Med Assoc* 213(2):251–256, 1998.
6. Hansen K, Khanna C: Spontaneous and genetically engineered animal models: use in preclinical cancer drug development, *Eur J Cancer* 40:858-880, 2004.
7. Mukherjee S: *The emperor of all maladies: a biography of cancer*, New York, 2010, Scribner.
8. Linblad-Toh K, Wade CM, Mikkelsen TS, et al: Genome sequence, comparative analysis and haplotype structure of the domestic dog, *Nature* 438:803–819, 2005.
9. Mooney S: *A snowflake in my hand*, New York, 1989, Dell Publishing, Bantam Doubleday.

The Etiology of Cancer

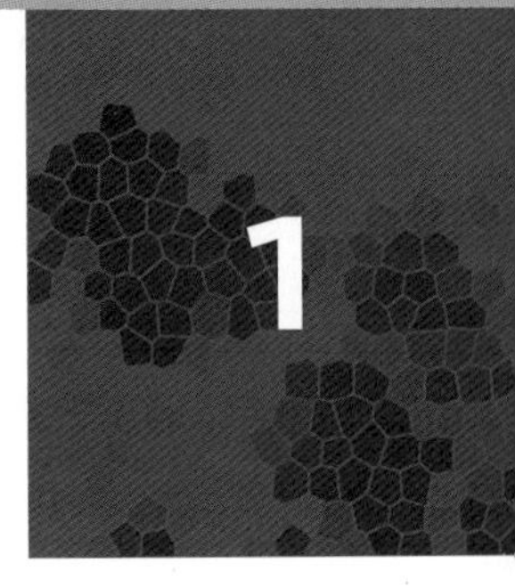

SECTION A
The Genetic Basis of Cancer

Jaime F. Modiano

This is an exciting and rapidly evolving time in the field of cancer genetics. Although it has been clear for several decades that cancer is a disease driven by the accumulation of genetic abnormalities,[1,2] new technologies are rapidly unraveling nuances in how heritable traits influence epigenetics and the tumor environment. Meticulous reductionist research done since the early 1960s helped identify hundreds of genetic abnormalities that are peculiarly associated with specific cancers, and more recent advances allowed for full sequencing of tumor genomes.[3-6] The information from these experiments has reinforced current concepts and provided insight into new areas of research. This chapter will focus on contemporary information to provide context for the genetic basis of cancer and how interactions between genes and environment impact the origin, progression, and response to therapy of hematopoietic tumors. It is probably reasonable to say that the next decade will represent a new "golden age" of discovery in cancer genetics, when many of the apparent conflicts from our traditional (reductionist) experimental approaches will be resolved by integration of data from epidemiologic, molecular, and clinical studies into a more holistic understanding of the biology of cancer.

Genes and Cancer Risk

To understand cancer, one must first realize that cancer is neither a single nor a simple disease. Rather, the term *cancer* describes a large number of diseases whose only common feature is uncontrolled cell growth and proliferation. An important concept that is universally accepted is that cancer is a genetic disease, although it is not always heritable. Tumors arise from the accumulation of mutations that eliminate normal constraints of proliferation and genetic integrity in a somatic cell. Among other causes, mutations can arise following exposure to environmental mutagens such as cigarette smoke, ultraviolet irradiation, and others. In fact, changes in cancer incidence over the course of the twentieth century, many reflecting behavior patterns (e.g., lung cancer in smokers), infectious diseases (e.g., stomach cancer in people infected with *Helicobacter pylori*), or exposure to special cultural factors such as urbanization or diet (e.g., increasing breast cancer rates in the second and subsequent generations of Asian-American women), underscore the significant influence that the environment exerts on the genetic make-up of any individual. Nevertheless, it would be incorrect to assume that the environment is wholly responsible for most tumors; most associations of cancer and exposure to potential environmental carcinogens other than tobacco products and ultraviolet or gamma irradiation are relatively weak.

Rigorous experimental evidence now supports a number of "intrinsic mutagens" that interact in complex and sometimes unpredictable ways with environmental triggers to promote cancer. For example, it is clear now that oxygen free radicals that result from chronic inflammation can act as procarcinogenic mutagens. An equally important and perhaps less well-recognized "mutagen" is the inherent error rate of enzymes that control DNA replication, which introduces from 1 in 10,000,000 to 1 in 1,000,000 mutations for each base that is replicated during each round of cell division. Most mammalian genomes comprise 2 to 3 billion base pairs, so every time a cell divides, each daughter cell is likely to carry at least a few hundred mutations in its DNA. Most mutations, whether caused by extrinsic or intrinsic factors, are silent; that is, they do not hinder the cell's ability to function. However, others can disable tumor suppressor genes or activate proto-oncogenes that respectively inhibit or promote cell division and survival. Thus it can be said that "being alive" is the single largest risk factor for cancer.

Heritable Cancer Syndromes

The existence of genetic predisposition to cancer is illustrated by well-defined heritable cancer syndromes.[7] Over 200 such syndromes have now been defined.[8] Even though they account for only 5% to 10% of all human cancers, studies of families with these syndromes provided many of the initial clues to understanding the genetic basis of sporadic (nonheritable) cancers. Although inheritance is recessive, these familial cancer syndromes show dominant patterns of inheritance and many have high penetrance.[8] All but two of the known familial cancer syndromes are due to mutations that inactivate tumor suppressor genes. As originally proposed by Knudson in his "two-hit" hypothesis from studies in children with retinoblastoma,[9] individuals at risk are obligate heterozygotes (they inherit a mutant allele and a wild-type allele). As it happens, homozygous mutations in critical growth regulatory genes usually cause embryonic lethality; however, in the case in which a single allele is affected, the mutation is present in every cell in the body. Given the rate of spontaneous mutation as described, the probability that the second, wild-type allele will be inactivated in at least one cell is extremely high, therefore facilitating tumorigenesis. This process is called *loss of heterozygosity* (LOH).

A curious observation worth noting is that different mutations in a single gene can predispose individuals to distinct cancer syndromes, whereas independent, single mutations of different genes can result in virtually the same disease, or at least diseases with indistinguishable phenotypes.[7] This is not surprising when we consider that commonly affected genes are multifunctional and parts

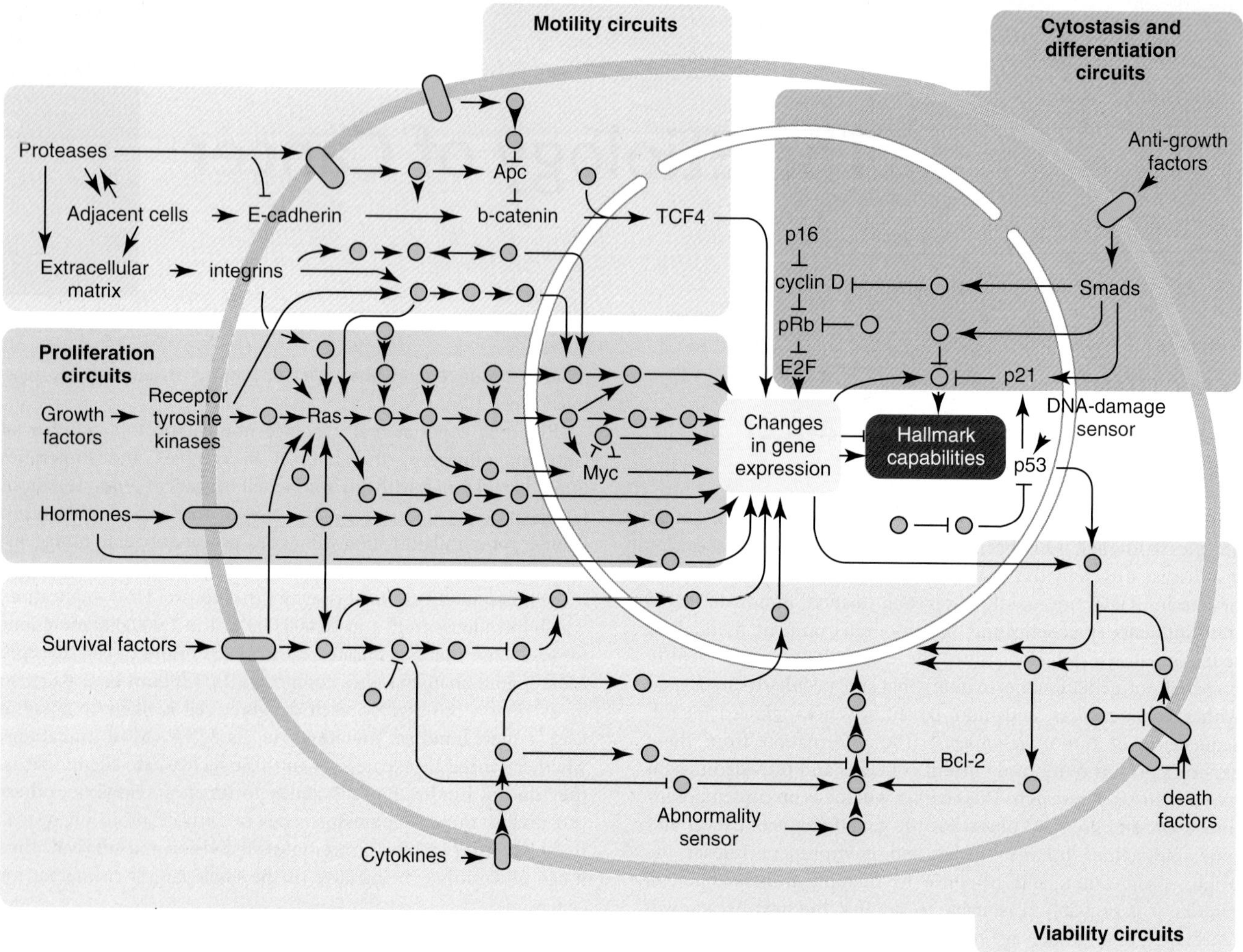

FIGURE 1-1 Intracellular signaling networks regulate the operations of the cancer cell. An elaborate integrated circuit operates within normal cells and is reprogrammed to regulate hallmark capabilities within cancer cells. Separate subcircuits, depicted here in differently colored fields, are specialized to orchestrate the various capabilities. At one level, this depiction is simplistic because there is considerable crosstalk between such subcircuits. In addition, because each cancer cell is exposed to a complex mixture of signals from its microenvironment, each of these subcircuits is connected with signals originating from other cells in the tumor microenvironment. *(Redrawn from Hanahan D, Weinberg RA: Hallmarks of cancer: The next generation,* Cell *144:646–674, 2011, with permission.)*

of complex, interactive networks or circuits[10,11] (Figure 1-1). Thus a mutation may only alter gene function along one biochemical pathway, leaving its interactions with other pathways intact. Moreover, mutations that contribute to most sporadic cancers are restricted to a small subset of genes,[12] many of which also are associated with heritable cancer syndromes. These observations have given rise to competing contemporary theories on the origins of cancer, which are addressed later in this chapter.

At least one heritable cancer syndrome (renal carcinoma and nodular dermatofibrosis [RCND] of German shepherd dogs) has been described in dogs.[13] The heritable factor (or *RCND* gene) for this syndrome maps to dog chromosome 5 (CFA 5) and specifically to the folliculin gene, which was recently described as the heritable factor for the corresponding human disease (Birt-Hogg-Dube syndrome).[14] It is probable that other syndromes comparable to those that are described in humans will eventually be identified in companion and laboratory animals, but it is unlikely that these will account for more than 5% to 10% of all cancer cases.

Genetic Influence in Sporadic Cancers

Unlike diseases due to single gene defects, cancer is a complex, multigenic disease. The "initiation, promotion, and progression" model was among the first to propose a sequential progression of mutations that could account for cancer.[15,16] In this model, a genetic event would endow a somatic cell with limitless replicative potential or another growth or survival advantage from other cells in its environment (initiation). Alone, this would not be sufficient to give rise to a tumor, as the cell would remain constrained by environmental factors. A second event would further add to the cell's ability to outcompete its neighbors in this environment, leading to its potential expansion into a recognizable tumor mass (promotion). Finally, a third event would reinforce the cell's malignant potential (invasion, tissue destruction, and metastasis), leading to clinical disease (progression). It is important to note that an "event" is not equivalent to a single mutation but rather is more likely to represent a series of mutations that act in concert to alter the cell's functional and morphologic phenotype. Although this model is overly simplistic and technically flawed (experimental evidence clearly shows that mutations are stochastic and do not occur in step-wise fashion),[17] it is nevertheless useful to convey the events that lead to carcinogenesis and it remains the foundation for our current understanding of cancer genetics and cancer evolution.

Both the environment and the individual's peculiar genetic background influence cancer risk and the natural history of tumors. This is especially clear in mice, in which the relative rate of spontaneous cancers and the susceptibility to chemically induced cancers differ according to the genetic background of various inbred strains.[18] Similar evidence exists for humans; for example, the risk of habitual smokers to develop lung cancer was found to be tightly linked to a unique allele encoding the alpha-3 subunit of the high affinity nicotinic receptor[19-21] and was later extended to this and other loci where additional nicotinic receptor subunits are encoded.[22] An association between lung cancer arising from habitual tobacco use and activity of cytochrome P450 enzymes also had been observed repeatedly for many years, and there are indeed P450 alleles (e.g., CYP1B1[23]) that also are associated with lung cancer. Together, these findings illustrate the complex relationship between genetics, environmental exposures, and probability to define cancer risk, prevention, and treatment. Specifically, alleles encoding "higher risk" nicotine receptors appear to modulate nicotine signaling, which in turn is responsible for embedding smoking behaviors and consequently exposure to dozens of potent carcinogens.[22,24] Nicotine metabolism itself by P450 enzymes also influences tobacco use; however, conversion of tobacco-specific nitrosamines to mutagenic forms by highly active P450 enzymes modulates risk of transformation.[25] Each component of risk is incremental and their interactions are not predictable. It is likely that similar relationships will be operative for many, if not most, common cancers of humans and domestic animals; defining these interactions will be a major emphasis of research during the coming decades.

There also is evidence to suggest that in some cases mutations are "directed" due to the presence of a "mutator phenotype," in which the factors that control DNA replication and repair are prone to more errors than would be expected by simple random events. This leads to different rates of cancer predisposition, which would be higher than the mean in individuals bearing this "mutator phenotype," and might explain why not all people or animals exposed to similar environmental carcinogens develop the same forms of cancer at the same rate.[26] Recent information obtained from massive parallel full genome sequencing of tumor/normal pairs in diffuse large B-cell lymphoma suggests that the mutator phenotypes may be acquired and may involve genes that mediate both DNA repair and chromatin organization.[5,6] It is important to note, however, that this does not exclude the possibility that mutator phenotypes also might be heritable.

In dogs and other domestic animals, the coexistence of genetic isolates in closed populations we call "breeds," along with animals of mixed breeding, lends itself to study how a relatively homogeneous background influences cancer in out-bred populations. Preliminary data from whole genome association studies suggest there are distinct heritable traits that segregate with common cancer phenotypes in dogs.[27,28] One common finding—and a pervasive obstacle for the completion of these studies—has been the observation of "fixed" risk alleles, making an association between individuals in the breed and disease challenging. Nevertheless, even though at the time of this writing none of these studies were yet published in the peer-reviewed literature, the reader should be alert for upcoming studies that will likely document specific risk genes for histiocytic sarcoma, transitional cell carcinoma, osteosarcoma, hemangiosarcoma, lymphoma, mammary cancer, and melanoma, among others, in susceptible dog breeds, and with the recent advent of the feline genome sequence,[29] possibly in specific cat breeds as well.[30] It remains to be seen if these traits will be shared between closely related breeds or whether they contribute to risk independently among different breeds.[31]

Perhaps as important, dogs are the first species in which genetic background has been shown to mold tumor genomes and tumor gene expression profiles.[32-35] This knowledge, together with the demonstration that causal, pathognomonic genetic abnormalities are conserved in homologous human and canine cancers,[36] opens a new area in which the precise contribution of heritable traits to sporadic cancers can be identified by using comparative systems approaches. These observations also indicate that we must assess "risk" far beyond the conventional idea of "tumor development," as heritable traits might influence risk by modulating the probability of initiating events, the probability of promoting events, or the probability of progression through the interactions between the tumor and its microenvironment.[34] A useful illustration of this concept is the occurrence of prostate cancers in men: virtually all men over 60 years of age will die *with* prostate cancer, but only a minority will die *from* prostate cancer, indicating that the major factors that influence the disease are not those that mediate transformation (at least as defined by morphologic appearance and anatomic organization), but instead those that dictate the biologic behavior of the transformed cells in the host.

Another important conceptual advance in this regard was the identification that spontaneous canine tumors had highly conserved (homologous) aberrations that had been previously characterized in human tumors. The prototypical example is a structural aberration resulting from a balanced chromosomal translocation that creates a fusion gene comprised of most of the *BCR* gene (located on chromosome 22 in humans and on chromosome 26 in dogs) and a truncated form of the *ABL* gene (coincidentally located on chromosome 9 in both humans and dogs) in chronic myelogenous leukemia (CML).[36] Both translocations give rise to a derivative chromosome, the Philadelphia (Ph) chromosome in humans and the Raleigh chromosome in dogs, as illustrated by the canine form in Figure 1-2. Numeric aberrations (changes in DNA copy number) are similarly conserved among species, as illustrated by deletions of the *RB1* locus, including the associated tumor-suppressing microRNAs in chronic lymphoid leukemias[36] and the *INK4* locus in T-cell malignancies,[37] as well as copy number gains such as *Runx2* amplification in osteosarcoma.[38]

The development of these specific tumors from cells harboring such mutations may not be at all surprising, but why would *homologous*, highly conserved pathologic rearrangements, deletions, or amplifications occur in cells from organisms separated by more than 40 million years of evolution? Is it possible they are evolutionarily related on a mechanistic basis? For example, rearrangements of the immunoglobulin heavy chain locus and the *MYC* locus are thought to be due to recognition of *MYC* flanking sequences by the recombinase enzyme system.[36] No such mechanism is known to be operative for other defined sites, so these other mutational events could occur stochastically, with their recurrent characterization across multiple species being the result of the selective advantage provided by the acquired gene to a cell of a highly specific lineage under highly specific conditions. This notion fits with Duesberg's hypothesis that aneuploidy precedes genetic instability.[39,40] Although

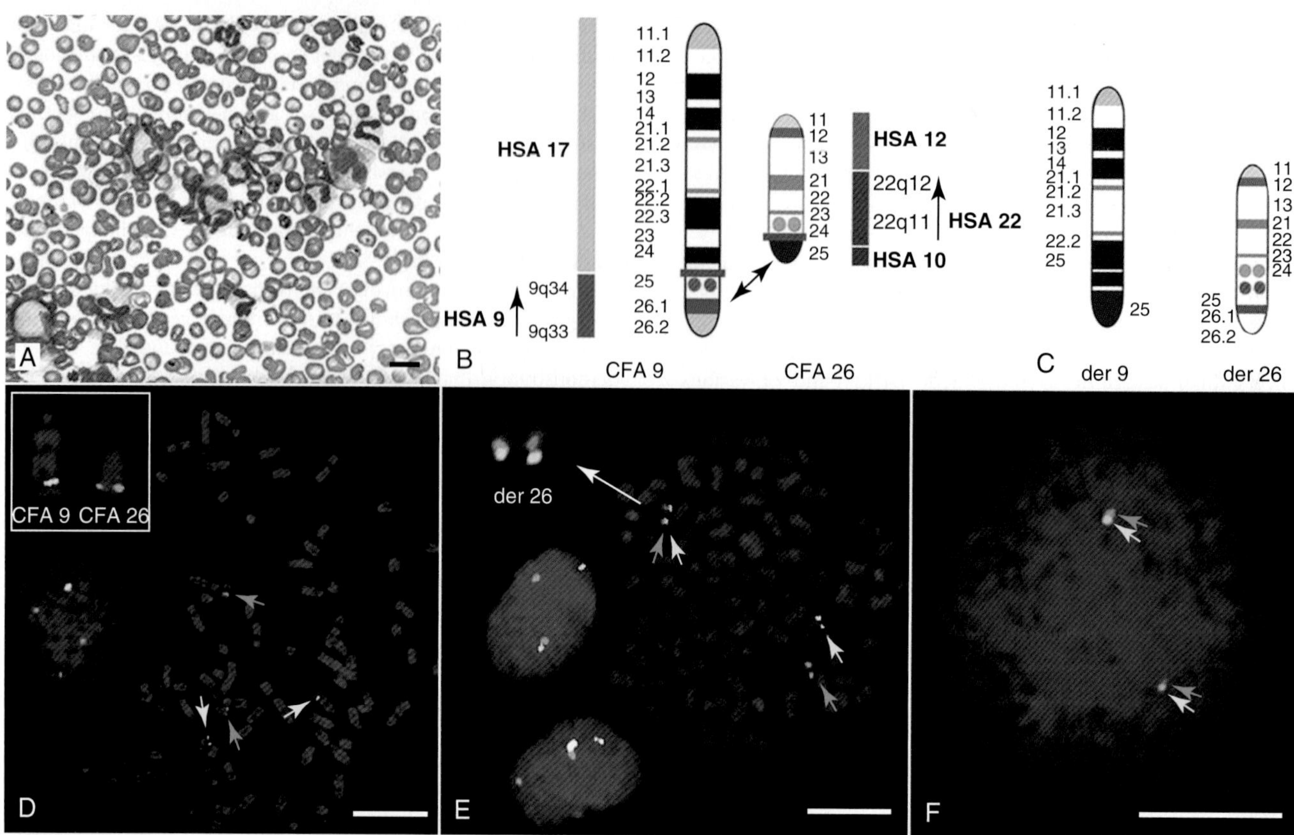

FIGURE 1-2 Conserved cytogenetic rearrangement in canine chronic myelogenous leukemia (CML). **A,** Photomicrograph of a peripheral blood smear from a dog with CML (Diff-Quik stain; original magnification ×1600). Scale bar = 10 μm. **B,** Comparative ideograms showing corresponding regions for HSA 9q34 and HSA 22q11 on canine chromosomes 9 and 26. Orange and green spots indicate the location of canine ABL and BCR. A horizontal blue line on each ideogram identifies the location of the predicted breakpoints on CFA 9 and CFA 26, below which the two regions would be exchanged to form the aberrant derivative chromosomes. **C,** Schematic representation of the predicted derivative CFA 9 and derivative CFA 26 that would be produced by such a reciprocal translocation, with the derivative 26 *(der 26)* showing co-localized signals from ABL and BCR. **D,** Fluorescence in situ hybridization (FISH) analysis of metaphase preparations and interphase nuclei in normal canine leukocytes using canine BAC clones representing canine ABL and BCR on CFA 9 *(orange spots)* and CFA 26 *(green spots),* respectively. Inset shows enlarged, single metaphase chromosomes for CFA 9 and 26 correctly oriented. **E,** Hybridization of the same two BAC probes to metaphase chromosomes and interphase nuclei of a canine CML. Heterozygous co-localization of these two BAC clones to the derivative chromosome 26 is evident in the metaphase preparation and co-localization of one green and one yellow spot is also evident in the two interphase nuclei. Inset shows the derivative CFA 26 enlarged and correctly oriented (compare to predicted der 26 in **C. F,** Interphase nucleus from the same case of CML showing the presence of an apparent homozygous 9/26 translocation event, with both yellow and green spots showing close association. Scale bars = 8 μm. *(Redrawn from Breen M, Modiano JF: Evolutionarily conserved cytogenetic changes in hematological malignancies of dogs and humans—man and his best friend share more than companionship,* Chromosome Res *16:145–154, 2008, with permission.)*

it is impossible to rule out this argument, the implication would be that such mutational events are phenomenally common, and since they are not otherwise observed frequently in other cells where their occurrence was neutral makes this highly unlikely. Another possibility is that they are related to the nuclear anatomy of the cell and specifically caused by proximity of chromosomal regions, cellular stress, inappropriate DNA repair (or as mentioned previously, recombination), and DNA sequence and chromatin features.[41] A third most intriguing possibility is that cellular genomes are reverting to a conformation that was found in a common ancestor (thus the high affinity and specificity between the rearranged chromosomal segments leads to the same recurrent event in many patients) but lost during the process of chromosomal reorganization in evolution, or that these sites represent targets for gene deletions or duplications that have been repeatedly advantageous to species under conditions of natural selection and so have become embedded in their contemporary descendants.

The clinical relevance of shared evolutionary and genetic origins should not be lost on physicians, veterinarians, or scientists. Shared origins mean shared biologic behaviors, thus supporting the rationale to apply the same therapies that have been developed for human patients to treat companion animals and vice versa. The best evidence for shared biologic behaviors comes from four recent studies of osteosarcoma, in which gene expression profiling documented overlapping characteristics of this disease in humans and in dogs.[35,42-44] Specifically, the use of biased breed cohorts and isolated tumor explants allowed our group to filter genetic noise and stromal signatures to achieve pathologic stratification of osteosarcomas from three independent dog cohorts and five independent human cohorts into prognostically significant groups.[35]

The Hallmarks of Cancer

Thirty years of research culminated in the year 2000 in an insightful and thorough review paper by Douglas Hanahan and Robert Weinberg that synthesized our knowledge into six essential, acquired characteristics necessary for cellular transformation.[45] These characteristics included (1) self-sufficiency in growth signals, (2) insensitivity to antigrowth signals, (3) the ability to evade apoptosis, (4) limitless replicative potential, (5) sustained angiogenesis, and (6) the capacity to invade tissues and metastasize. The importance of this paper was less in describing a list of events and more in the synthesis of these events because the concepts proposed by Hanahan and Weinberg created a paradigm shift in our understanding of cancer. Some of the important concepts that were clarified include: No single gene is universally responsible for transformation; five or six mutations are the minimum probable number required to endow the cancer phenotype (an observation that has since been confirmed experimentally[3]); each step is regulated by multiple interactive biochemical pathways,[10] and thus mutations of different genes along a pathway can result in equivalent phenotypes and, conversely, mutations of the same gene can result in different cancers with distinct biology; tumors behave as tissues; and the interactions between the tumor and its microenvironment are major drivers of cancer behavior.

In early 2011, Hanahan and Weinberg updated the hallmarks of cancer in a new review that will likely be even more influential than the first.[11] In this "next generation," the hallmarks of cancer were refined and reassessed, and new "enabling characteristics" (genome instability and mutation and tumor-promoting inflammation) and "emerging" hallmarks (deregulating cellular energetics and avoiding immune destruction) were added to the paradigm. The impact of this unifying conceptualization of cancer genetics and this level of understanding are clearly evident when we consider how they have influenced the design, development, implementation, and success of new cancer therapies (Figure 1-3). A summary of the information with added refinements is provided later, and the reader is referred to the original manuscripts for details, since space constraints preclude an extensive review herein.

Self-Sufficiency of Growth Signals

Arguably, the most important event in neoplastic transformation is the capability of cells to sustain chronic proliferation. Under normal conditions, cells communicate with each other and integrate environmental signals by sensing cues and gradients. For example,

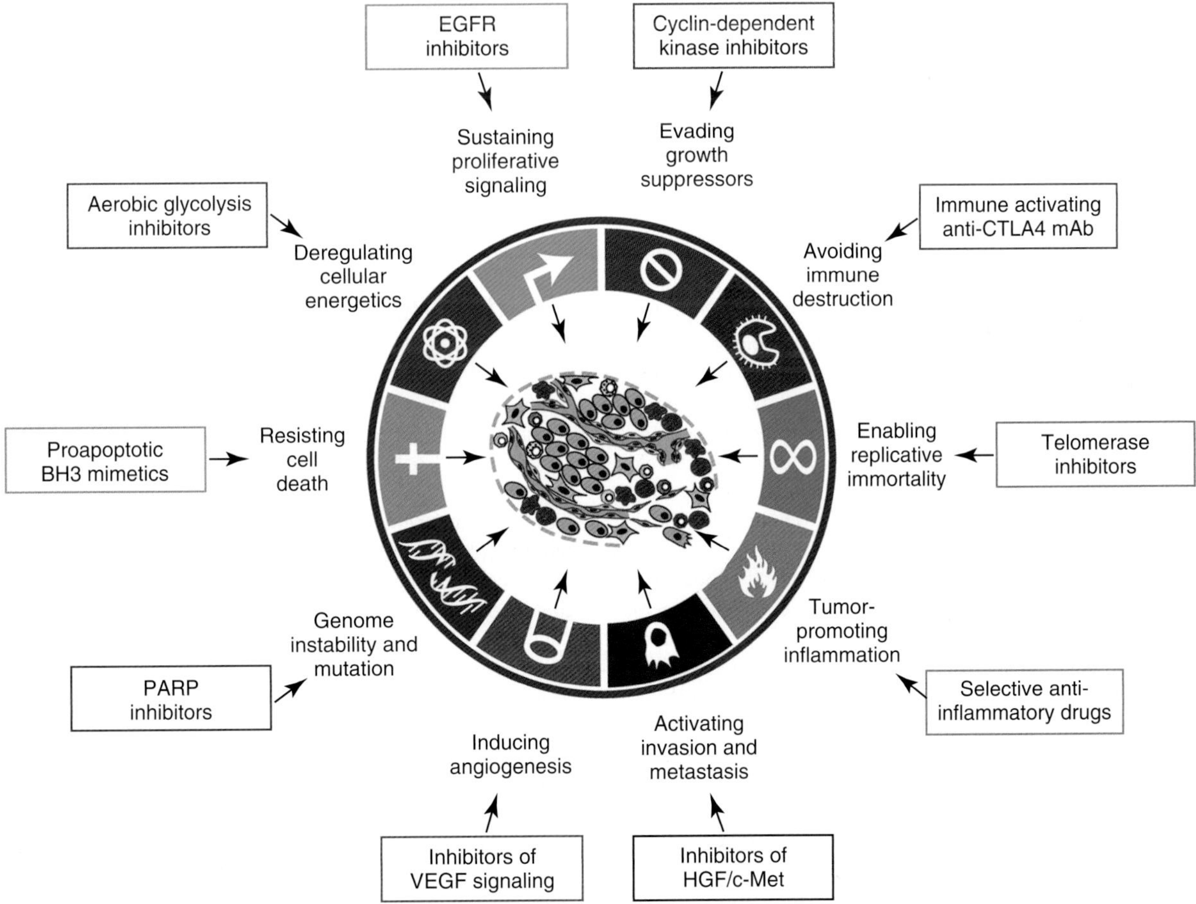

FIGURE 1-3 Therapeutic targeting of the hallmarks of cancer. Drugs that interfere with each of the acquired capabilities necessary for tumor growth and progression have been developed and are in clinical trials or in some cases approved for clinical use in treating certain forms of human cancer. Additionally, investigational drugs are being developed to target each of the enabling characteristics and emerging hallmarks, which also hold promise as cancer therapeutics. The drugs listed are but illustrative examples; there is a deep pipeline of candidate drugs with different molecular targets and modes of action in development for most of these hallmarks. *EGFR*, Epidermal growth factor receptor; *PARP*, poly ADP ribose polymerase; *VEGF*, vascular endothelial growth factor; *HGF*, hepatocyte growth factor. *(Redrawn from Hanahan D, Weinberg RA: Hallmarks of cancer: The next generation,* Cell *144:646–674, 2011, with permission.)*

migration, metabolism, and proliferation of mature hematopoietic cells are regulated in autocrine and paracrine fashions by locally secreted cytokines. The same cytokines may travel systemically and act in an endocrine fashion. Generally, the cytokines work by binding transmembrane receptors, which in turn initiate signaling cascades that culminate in transcriptional changes that allow the cell to adapt its behavior to match the environmental signal. The activity of these cytokines, their receptors, and the corresponding signaling molecules are finely tuned. The system can be shut down when the concentration of the cytokine falls below a threshold that can stably bind the receptor, when the receptor ceases to be expressed, or when signaling molecules are downregulated or otherwise inactivated. However, mutations in even one of the molecules involved in regulating these pathways can provide sustained growth signals in the absence of the initiating cytokine. Among many examples, there is a translocation between chromosome 2 and chromosome 5 (t(2;5)) that is present in almost half of human anaplastic lymphomas. The translocation creates a fusion protein between the nucleophosmin gene *(NPM1)* and the anaplastic lymphoma kinase gene *(ALK),* which aberrantly activates the Jak2/STAT5 signaling pathway[46] that is normally responsive to various interleukins (IL), including IL 2, IL-3, and IL-6. The genes that encode the normal growth-promoting proteins (such as ALK, Jak2, and STAT5) are called *proto-oncogenes;* the mutated versions that allow cells to gain self-sufficiency from the environmental signals are called *oncogenes.* It is important to note that not all growth-promoting genes have the capacity to become oncogenes and that the outcomes of oncogenic activation are most commonly senescence or apoptosis, unless there are additional events that promote stable transformation and survival.

Insensitivity to Antigrowth Signals

In addition to the hallmark capability of inducing and sustaining positively acting growth-stimulatory signals, cancer cells must also circumvent powerful programs that negatively regulate cell proliferation; many of these programs depend on the actions of tumor suppressor genes. To maintain homeostasis, cells also must integrate antigrowth signals from the environment. Quiescence in nonhematopoietic cells is enforced by signals delivered by contact inhibition.[47] Hematopoietic cells, on the other hand, utilize cell-cell contacts to maintain interactions within the niche and to regulate the timing and intensity of hematopoiesis, inflammation, and immunity.[48]

"Stop" signals are usually delivered and integrated by the products of tumor suppressor genes, which derive their name largely from the observation that their inactivation facilitates tumor formation. Tumor suppressor genes balance the activity of growth-promoting proto-oncogenes and tend to act in tandem with these in most biochemical pathways. Loss of function of one or more tumor suppressor genes occurs in virtually every cancer, with inactivation of *p53, RB1, PTEN,* or *CDKN2A* each seen in more than 50% of all tumors. Each of these pathways may contribute to the pathogenesis of bone marrow–derived tumors in companion animals, and their dysfunction also may be predictive for outcomes.[49-52]

Evasion of Cell Death

Apoptosis, or programmed cell death, is the imprinted outcome for every cell in multicellular organisms. Survival requires support from extrinsic (environmental) factors, as well as precise balance of cellular energetics and metabolism. Bone marrow–derived cells normally undergo apoptosis when concentrations of survival factors (e.g., stem cell factor, IL-3, IL-7) or nutrients are limiting or when there are severe disruptions to cellular bioenergetics.[53]

Evasion of apoptosis is an essential acquired feature of all cancers, and it can result from loss of proapoptotic tumor suppressor genes such as *p53* or *PTEN* or by gain of function of antiapoptotic genes, such as *BCL2.* Gain of function of *BCL2* in humans is generally associated with indolent, follicular lymphomas that carry t(14:18) translocations that juxtapose *BCL2* and the immunoglobulin heavy enhancer locus *(IGH).* These tumors are seen rarely in domestic animals, but evasion of apoptosis may be an important mechanism in the pathogenesis of indolent tumors seen more commonly in these species.

A more recent concept in the cell death field is autophagy—a process that tumor cells have efficiently coopted as a means to survive under adverse conditions.[54] As part of the autophagy program, intracellular vesicles termed *autophagosomes* surround intracellular organelles and fuse with lysosomes. There, the organelles are broken down and then are channeled to form new molecules that support the energy-producing machinery of the cell, allowing it to survive in the stressed, nutrient-limited environment that defines most cancers.

Tumor cells also must avoid death by anoikis or loss of integral cell-to-cell or cell-to-matrix contacts.[47] Absent these physiologic death pathways, the body often reacts to the anatomic and physiologic disruptions caused by cancer cells by targeting these cells for destruction through inflammatory pathways. This is but one pathway that leads to necrosis, since it appears that the process of necrosis also might be regulated genetically, providing another mechanism that favors survival of the whole (organism or tumor) over survival of the one. We are probably on the edge of an explosion of new findings that will further nuance our perception of how evasion (or inciting) of these cell death mechanisms contributes to neoplastic transformation and tumor progression.

Limitless Replicative Potential

Immortalization is another essential feature of cancer. The genetic program limits the number of times a cell is able to replicate, the so-called *Hayflick limit,* and when this limit is reached, replicative senescence is induced. Induction of replicative senescence does not induce death; cells maintain energetic homeostasis and remain functional, but they undergo significant genetic changes characterized by telomere erosion. Cells that are able to replicate must maintain the integrity of telomeres, which are "caps" made of repetitive DNA sequence that protect chromosomes from destruction. Solid tumors acquire immortalization predominantly by activation of the telomerase enzyme system and the consequent maintenance of telomere integrity. In hematopoietic cells, telomerase activity seems to be retained longer than in other somatic cells, so it is possible this facilitates immortalization in lymphoma and leukemia.[55] The role of immortalization and the importance of telomerase (both to maintain telomere length and to maintain other biochemical functions that are essential for cell survival) are well established; however, the role of replicative senescence has recently been questioned because improved technology has allowed researchers to circumvent this process in normal cells.[11] Mouse models complicate the story due to significant differences in telomere length between rodents and humans, so this is an area in which other models such as companion animals might provide clarity in the future.[56]

Sustained Angiogenesis

The process of angiogenesis requires the coordinated action of a variety of growth factors and cell-adhesion molecules in endothelial and stromal cells. So far, vascular endothelial growth factor-A (VEGF) and its receptors comprise the best-characterized signaling pathway in tumor angiogenesis.[57] VEGF binds several receptor tyrosine kinases, including VEGF receptor-1 (VEGFR-1 [Flt-1]) and VEGFR-2 (KDR, Flk-1). VEGFR-2 is the major mediator of the angiogenic effects of VEGF. However, VEGFR-1 is expressed by some tumor cells and may mediate chemotactic signals, thus potentially having a role in cancer growth. The expression of VEGF is upregulated by hypoxia and inflammation. The transcription factor hypoxia-inducible factor-1α (HIF), which is part of a pathway that also includes regulation by the von Hippel-Lindau (VHL) tumor suppressor gene, is a major regulator of VEGF expression. Under conditions of normal oxygen tension, VHL protein targets HIF for degradation; under low oxygen conditions, HIF increases as VHL-mediated degradation is reduced, allowing for upregulation of VEGF. Other signaling molecules also contribute to angiogenesis, including platelet-derived growth factor-β (PDGF-β) and its receptor (PDGFR), and the angiopoietins. PDGF-β is required for recruitment of pericytes and maturation of new capillaries. Recent studies also document the importance of tumor-derived PDGF in recruitment of stroma that produces VEGF and other angiogenic factors (Figure 1-4).

Folkman proposed a role for angiogenesis in cancer more than 30 years ago,[58,59] but this idea took time to gain traction in the scientific community. Even after the importance of angiogenesis was recognized, the prediction was that this process would impact solid tumors but would be relatively unimportant for tumors of the blood and lymph (lymphoma, leukemia, and multiple myeloma). The first clues that this notion was mistaken came from unexpected benefits of patients with chronic lymphocytic leukemia (CLL) treated with antiangiogenic compounds,[60-62] followed by similar success for some patients with multiple myeloma.[63,64] More recently, a European study showed that different histologic types of human non-Hodgkin's lymphoma show different patterns of angiogenesis, and these can predict outcomes for some of the most aggressive tumors, such as peripheral T-cell lymphomas.[65] One study has shown that microvessel density is similarly correlated with the aggressive behavior of canine lymphoma,[66] and similar findings have been reported for other blood-derived and solid tumors of dogs, such as mast cell cancer and mammary cancer.[67,68]

The concepts of how neoangiogenesis contributes to cancer also are undergoing refinement. For example, it is apparent now that clinical trials of antiangiogenic drugs have largely failed because their design was based on incomplete knowledge and thus incorrect assumptions. Perhaps the most informative example is the history of Bevacizumab (a humanized anti-VEGF antibody), which received approval to treat various cancers between 2004 and 2010 after it was shown to confer improved quality of life, albeit with modest survival benefits for patients. On December 6, 2010, the Federal Drug Administration (FDA) issued a press release (http://www.fda.gov/newsevents/newsroom/pressannouncements/ucm237172.htm) that announced the withdrawal of the indication for bevacizumab in treatment of metastatic breast cancer, stating that "... the drug has not been shown to be safe and effective for that use." The FDA press release also stated, "The agency is making this recommendation after reviewing the results of four clinical studies of Avastin (bevacizumab) in women with breast cancer and determining that the data indicate that the drug does not prolong overall survival in breast cancer patients or provide a sufficient benefit in slowing disease progression to outweigh the significant risk to patients. These risks include severe high blood pressure; bleeding and hemorrhage; the development of perforations (or 'holes') in the body, including in the nose, stomach, and intestines; and heart attack or heart failure."

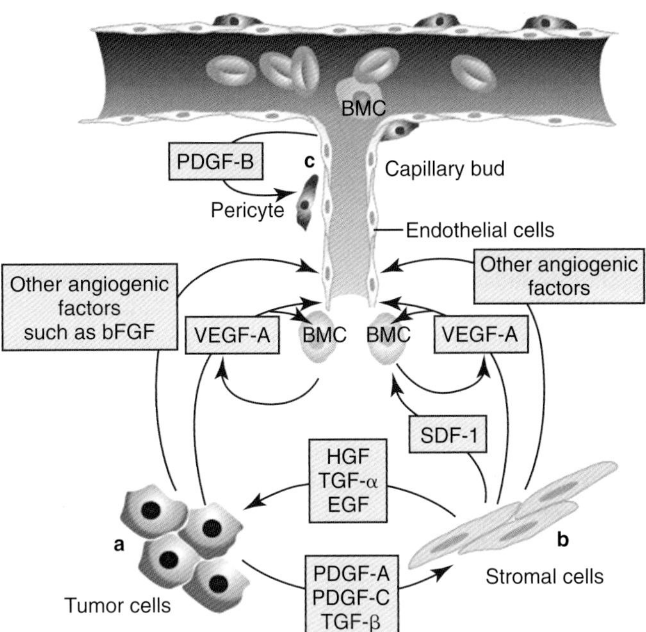

FIGURE 1-4 A few of the molecular and cellular players in the tumor/microvascular microenvironment. **A,** Tumor cells produce VEGF-A and other angiogenic factors, such as bFGF, angiopoietins, interleukin-8 (IL-8), placenta growth factor (PlGF), and VEGF-C. These stimulate resident endothelial cells to proliferate and migrate. **B,** An additional source of angiogenic factors is the stroma, which is a heterogeneous compartment, comprising fibroblastic, inflammatory, and immune cells. Recent studies indicate that tumor-associated fibroblasts produce chemokines such as SDF-1, which may recruit bone marrow–derived angiogenic cells *(BMC)*. VEGF-A or PlGF may also recruit BMC. Tumor cells may also release stromal cell-recruitment factors, such as PDGF-A, PDGF-C, or transforming growth factor *(TGF-α, TGF-β)*. A well-established function of tumor-associated fibroblasts is the production of growth/survival factor for tumor cells such as EGFR ligands, HGF, and heregulin. **C,** Endothelial cells produce PDGF-β, which promotes recruitment of pericytes in the microvasculature after activation of PDGF receptor-β (PDGFR-β) factor. *VEGF-A,* Vascular endothelial growth factor-A; *bFGF,* basic fibroblast growth factor; *SDF-1,* stromal cell–derived factor-1; *HGF,* hepatocyte growth factor; *PDGF,* platelet-derived growth factor; *EGFR,* epidermal growth factor receptor. *(Redrawn from Ferrara N, Kerbel RS: Angiogenesis as a therapeutic target,* Nature *438:967–974, 2005, with permission.)*

Indeed, the preponderance of data suggest that antiangiogenic therapies will benefit cancer patients by promoting vessel normalization, reversing the anatomic and hemodynamic dysfunction created by the tumor microenvironment, disabling some of the intrinsic advantages that this provides for cancer cells, and allowing better penetration of drugs. Vascular normalization relies on restoring the balance among all the blood vessel–forming constituents from the bone marrow and the stroma, including pericytes, myeloid-derived cells, and endothelial progenitors, all of which contribute—and respond to—the "angiogenic switch," whereby previously quiescent tissues trigger formation of new blood vessels associated with tumor growth.

Invasion and Metastasis

The role of genetic events in invasion and metastasis is still incompletely understood. The classic model of metastasis proposed by Fidler suggests a step-wise acquisition of assets that enables cells to leave the primary tumor site, travel through blood or lymph, invade stroma in favorable locations, and thus become reestablished at distant sites.[69] More recent work suggests that most tumors possess the ability to dislodge cells that travel to distant sites, and the ability of such cells to survive in capillary beds may be the most important step in the metastatic process.[70-74]

Bone marrow–derived cells have intrinsic properties that allow them to travel throughout the body, traffic through all major organs, and home to areas of inflammation. Thus bone marrow–derived tumors are inherently metastatic. Nevertheless, hematopoietic tumors that are cytologically indistinguishable can have distinct and preferential tissue distribution. We do not fully understand what events make leukemic cells stay in the peripheral circulation, while cells from corresponding lymphomas (or myeloid sarcomas) with virtually identical molecular signatures stay confined to lymphoid or visceral organs.

In epithelial neoplasms that account for the majority of tumors in humans, the epithelial-to-mesenchymal transition (EMT) has received increasing attention for its role in metastasis. EMT is a developmental program that progenitor stem cells use during morphogenesis and can be physiologically reactivated during wound healing. It remains unclear whether EMT is equally (or less) important in sarcomas more commonly seen in domestic animals, in which the cells of origin seem to retain EMT capabilities to a greater extent. Similarly, there is increasing evidence of interactions between cancer cells, the "initiating" population in the tumor (cancer stem cells [CSCs]), mesenchymal stem cells (MSCs), tumor-associated fibroblasts, inflammatory cells, and angiogenic cells, which may be responsible for invasive behaviors and possibly for survival in hostile environments that exist at distant sites (Figure 1-5).

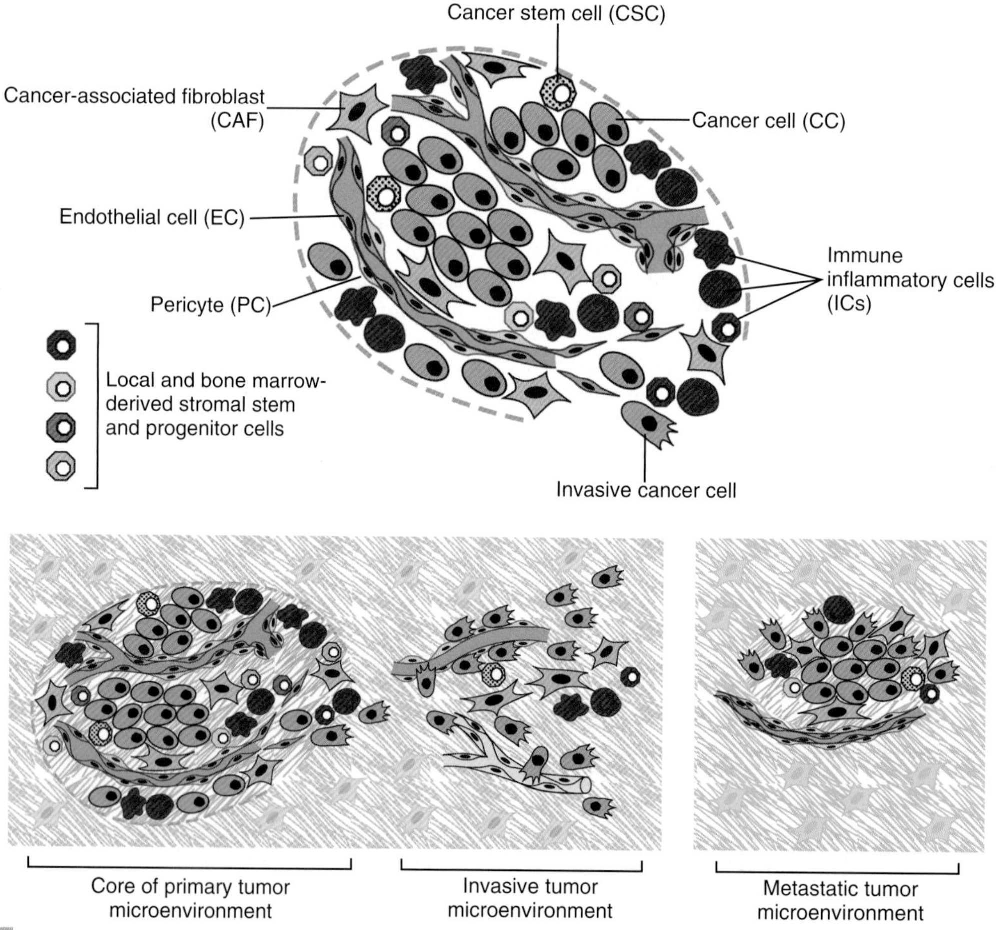

FIGURE 1-5 The cells of the tumor microenvironment. *Upper,* An assemblage of distinct cell types constitutes most solid tumors. Both the parenchyma and stroma of tumors contain distinct cell types and subtypes that collectively enable tumor growth and progression. Notably, the immune inflammatory cells present in tumors can include both tumor-promoting, as well as tumor-killing, subclasses. *Lower,* The distinctive microenvironments of tumors. The multiple stromal cell types create a succession of tumor microenvironments that change as tumors invade normal tissue and thereafter seed and colonize distant tissues. The abundance, histologic organization, and phenotypic characteristics of the stromal cell types, as well as of the extracellular matrix *(hatched background),* evolve during progression, thereby enabling primary, invasive, and then metastatic growth. The surrounding normal cells of the primary and metastatic sites, shown only schematically, likely also affect the character of the various neoplastic microenvironments. (Not shown are the premalignant stages in tumorigenesis, which also have distinctive microenvironments that are created by the abundance and characteristics of the assembled cells.) *(Redrawn from Hanahan D, Weinberg RA: Hallmarks of cancer: The next generation,* Cell *144:646–674, 2011, with permission.)*

Adaptive Evolution and the Tumor Microenvironment

There is a bidirectional flow of information between the tumor and the microenvironment, with each helping to mold the other into functional growing tissue that can evade or withstand attack by the host.[75] Our previous reference to a "selective growth advantage" that is reminiscent of Darwinian selection is not accidental. The clonal evolution theory[76] addresses the significance of sequential genetic changes providing growth and survival advantages, but to this we must add the fact that, in addition to these self-sufficient events that influence growth and survival, tumor cells must also evade "predators" (e.g., inflammation and the immune system[77,78]). In essence, the interaction of the tumor with its microenvironment and ultimately with the host is in fact subject to Darwinian laws of evolution, albeit in an accelerated time scale.[79] This is evident in the ability of tumors to modulate stromal cells to support their own growth by providing a suitable matrix and an abundance of nutrients, while maintaining antitumor responses at bay.

As is true for other selective environments, tumors that outgrow the capability of their immediate surroundings to support their growth must alter that environment to suit their needs or identify other favorable locations where they can become established. The tumor microenvironment was recently shown to exert a significant effect on the complement of genes expressed by incipient tumor cells.[80] In this case, the microenvironment was modified by gamma irradiation and the tumor was derived from orthotopic implants of chimeric Trp53-deficient mammary epithelial cells. The magnitude of change was not unlike that observed by our group when comparing the influence of breed on gene expression by canine hemangiosarcoma cells, although in our case the expression profile was maintained in a cell-autonomous fashion (i.e., ex vivo).[34] Again, the behavior of carcinomas and sarcomas may differ, and for the latter, recent experiments from our group using canine hemangiosarcoma xenotransplantation models suggest that alterations in the microenvironment might favor not only the efficiency of tumor implantation but also the extent to which the microenvironment contributes to the composition of the tumor as a whole. Incipient sarcoma cells, in turn, can reside as quiescent inhabitants of distant microenvironments themselves modulating growth, morphology, and behavior of microenvironment constituents in the process of metastatic dissemination (Figure 1-6).

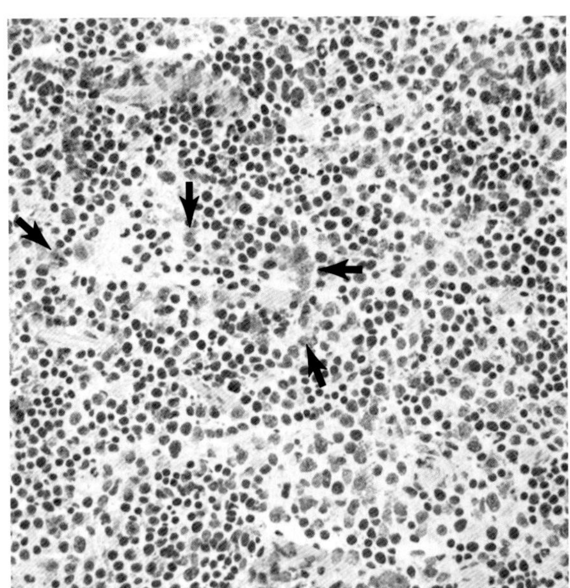

FIGURE 1-6 Incipient canine hemangiosarcoma cells in the spleen of a mouse after subcutaneous tumor xenotransplantation. SB canine hemangiosarcoma cells (5 × 104) harboring a firefly luciferase gene were injected subcutaneously in the flank of immunocompromised mice. Tumors were detectable at the local site within 14 days of injection. After 48 days, the mice were humanely sacrificed and systemic tissues were examined for the presence of luciferase-expressing (tumor) cells. The photomicrograph shows immunohistochemical staining for luciferase in a frozen section of spleen from a representative mouse. Cells with red staining in the cytoplasm represent luciferase-positive canine hemangiosarcoma cells *(arrows)*. Similar events were seen in other organs both by immunohistochemistry and by in vivo imaging. These incipient cells did not show evidence of organization into a tumor, suggesting a critical mass had not yet been reached, or possibly, that the primary subcutaneous tumor suppressed metastatic growth. In other mice, however, the incipient cells appeared to "instruct" organization of the resident spleen microenvironment into fulminant hematopoietic tumors. Magnification 200× with hematoxylin counterstain. *(Experiment, staining, and image courtesy AM Frantz, EB Dickerson, TD O'Brien, and JW Wojcieszyn.)*

Emerging and Enabling Hallmarks

Genomic Instability

The concept of genomic instability is not new but was incorporated as an "enabling hallmark" into the updated Hanahan and Weinberg model. Step-wise clonal evolution is satisfying because it can be correlated with discrete pathologic changes in tumor progression, especially for epithelial tumors where such progression can be seen in lesions that go through stages of hyperplasia, atypical hyperplasia (dysplasia), adenoma, carcinoma in situ, invasive carcinoma, and metastatic carcinoma (Figure 1-7). However, analysis of tumor genomes even in early stages usually shows aneuploidy (abnormal DNA copy number), as well as chaotic changes indicative of multiple numeric and structural DNA abnormalities. Similar abnormalities first noticed by Boveri more than 100 years ago in studies of sea urchin cells led him to formulate the "aneuploidy theory" of cancer.[81] We know now that aneuploidy is especially evident in solid tumors; based on this, Loeb proposed the existence of the "mutator phenotype" in which cells are predisposed to undergo multiple mutations, some of which inevitably lead to cancer (see earlier).[26] Some tenets of his hypothesis appear to be correct, although perhaps in different circumstances than Loeb originally envisioned, because they might relate to increased activity of polymerases with low fidelity under conditions in which the rate of DNA damage (and consequently mutations) is higher than the expected background from normal DNA replication (e.g., in lung epithelial cells from heavy smokers). However, direct measurements of mutation rates of sporadic tumors are much lower than those predicted if a "mutator phenotype" was operative in these tumors.[12] Indeed, the minimum number of mutations that are required for clinical onset of cancer in solid tumors based on sequencing of solid tumor genomes is 15 to 25,[4] but this may apply to tumors with chaotic karyotypes, as the number of mutations identified in a cytogenetically stable leukemia was significantly smaller.[3]

Still, genetic instability is a hallmark of most tumors, and while it can be partly explained by increased errors in DNA replication and chromosomal segregation in cells that are rapidly dividing, other mechanisms are clearly operative, involving telomeres and

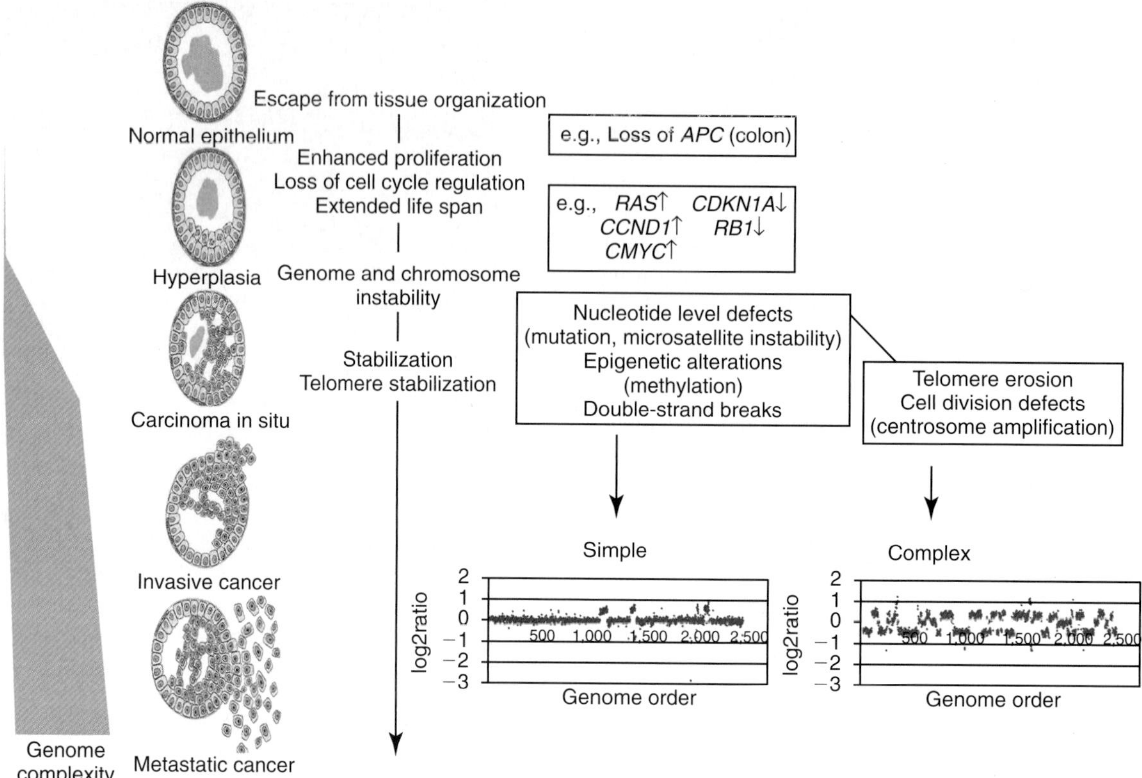

FIGURE 1-7 Schematic representation of chromosomal evolution in human solid tumor progression. The stages of progression are arranged with the earlier lesions at the top. Cells may begin to proliferate excessively owing to the loss of tissue architecture, abrogation of checkpoints, and other factors. In general, relatively few aberrations occur before the development of in situ cancer. As indicated, a sharp increase in genome complexity (the number of independent chromosomal aberrations) in many (but not all) tumors coincides with the development of in situ disease. The types and range in aberration number varies markedly between tumors, probably owing to the specific failures in checkpoint or damage surveillance that are present, as illustrated by the whole-genome array comparative genomic hybridization (CGH) profiles of HCT116, a mismatch repair-defective cell line, and T47D, a mismatch repair-proficient cell line. The copy number profiles of HCT116 and T47D are labeled as "simple" and "complex," respectively, to distinguish between tumor genomes with few or many copy number changes. The spectrum of aberrations in in situ lesions is similar to those found in more advanced malignancies. Thus an early increase in chromosomal aberration composition is followed by more modest chromosomal evolution. *(Redrawn from Albertson DG, Collins C, McCormick F, et al: Chromosome aberrations in solid tumors,* Nat Genet *34:369–376, 2003, with permission.)*

telomerase.[12,79,82-85] Although many of these changes are not "recurrent" and appear to be random products of instability, some may in fact contribute to proliferative crisis.[86] It is possible that the initiation events for many tumors occur early in life during highly proliferative stages of tissue growth and remodeling (e.g., prior to closure of the growth plates in bone cancer), but they become evident later in life when a last series of mutations allows the transformed cell to reach this crisis stage. As we alluded earlier, hematopoietic tumors seem to avoid the chaotic chromosomal instability associated with solid tumors. We do not fully understand the reasons for this, although it may be partly due to intrinsic protective mechanisms associated with the proliferative rate of bone marrow precursor cells.

Tumor-Promoting Inflammation

The role of inflammation in cancer has received considerable attention in the past 10 years. Although our understanding of this phenomenon remains incomplete, it clearly met the criteria for inclusion as an "enabling hallmark" into the updated Hanahan and Weinberg model. The importance of inflammation was inferred from the earliest microscopic studies of cancer, but it was a seminal paper by Dvorak in 1986, in which he described tumors as "wounds that never heal,"[87] that provided synthesis for the recurrent observation that tumors were often infiltrated by inflammatory cells of the innate (granulocytes, histiocytes, and macrophages) and the adaptive (lymphocytes) immune systems. Mechanistic distinctions remain to be defined between inflammation that favors tumor growth and inflammation that retards growth or eliminates the tumor,[88-90] but we can say confidently that inflammation contributes to tumor growth and survival by supplying factors that sustain proliferation; factors that limit cell death; proangiogenic factors; extracellular matrix-modifying enzymes that facilitate angiogenesis, invasion, and metastasis; and other signals that lead to activation of EMT and other hallmark-facilitating programs.[11] As noted earlier, inflammatory cells also release notably reactive oxygen species that are actively mutagenic for nearby cancer cells, accelerating their genetic evolution toward states of heightened malignancy.[91]

Reprogramming Energy Metabolism

In the early years of the twentieth century, Otto Warburg observed that cancer cells preferentially utilized glycolytic (anaerobic) rather than oxidative (aerobic) pathways to generate energy even under conditions of normal or high oxygen. This metabolic peculiarity of cancer cells, called the *Warburg effect,* seems to be driven by activated oncogenes and/or by loss of tumor suppressor genes that provide cancer cells with selective growth and survival advantages by conferring the hallmark capabilities of cell proliferation, avoidance of cytostatic controls, and attenuation of apoptosis. The reliance of cancer cells on glycolysis can be further accentuated under the hypoxic conditions. In fact, Warburg-like metabolism seems to be present in rapidly dividing embryonic tissues, suggesting a role in supporting large-scale biosynthetic programs that are required for active cell proliferation.

Cancer cells do not seem to enable the Warburg effect universally. Rather, much like other cells with high energetic demands, they seem to sort out into lactate-secreting (Warburg) and lactate-consuming cells, providing an efficient, albeit homeostatically disturbed, energy environment. Furthermore, it seems that oxygenation is not static in tumors but instead fluctuates temporally and regionally due to the instability and chaotic organization of tumor-associated neovasculature. Altered energy metabolism is proving to be as widespread in cancer cells as many of the other cancer-associated traits that have been accepted as hallmarks of cancer. This realization raises the question of whether deregulating cellular energy metabolism is therefore a core hallmark capability of cancer cells that is as fundamental as the six well-established core hallmarks. In fact, the redirection of energy metabolism is largely orchestrated by proteins that are involved in one way or another in programming the core hallmarks of cancer. When viewed in this way, aerobic glycolysis is simply another phenotype that is programmed by proliferation-inducing oncogenes and the designation of reprogrammed energy metabolism as an emerging hallmark seems most appropriate.

It is worth noting that this characteristic of tumor cells provides at least one important diagnostic advantage. Upregulation of the major glucose transporter, GLUT-1, is seen in virtually all tumors, making the cells efficient glucose scavengers. This can be exploited to image tumor cells noninvasively with precision by visualizing glucose uptake using positron-emission tomography (PET) with a radiolabeled analog of glucose (^{18}F-fluorodeoxyglucose [^{18}F-FDG]) as a reporter. The combination of PET with computed tomography (PET-CT) is now one of the most robust means to evaluate composition of tumors, minimal residual disease, and tumor-specific objective responses in patients receiving conventional and experimental therapies.

Evading Immune Destruction

Burnet and Thomas proposed the concept that the immune system can recognize and destroy incipient tumors (cancer immunosurveillance) in the 1950s.[78] However, the hypothesis was far ahead of its time, and technologic obstacles impeded proof, so the theory fell into disfavor. In recent years, the immunosurveillance theory has gained traction anew because data strongly suggest that the immune system helps to maintain tumors at bay, and thus tumors must evade the immune response to survive. In its recent incarnation, the theory has been refined to incorporate the concept of immunoediting, in which the immune system destroys strongly antigenic tumor cells, providing weakly antigenic cells a survival advantage.[78] Experimental evidence for this concept includes differences between tumors grown in immunocompetent (only weakly antigenic tumors survive) and immunocompromised mice (no selection against strongly antigenic tumors is observed), but it is unknown if immunoediting is operative in spontaneous cancers.

That the tumor microenvironment forms and maintains an immunosuppressive barrier provides more compelling evidence for the role of the immune system to limit tumor growth and metastasis. This immunosuppressive barrier includes cellular factors such as regulatory T cells (Tregs), myeloid-derived suppressor cells (MDSCs), and MSCs. Tregs, MDSCs, and MSCs can attack distinct and complementary antigen-specific (Tregs) and nonspecific (MDSCs and MSCs) facets of immune effector cell activation and function. Soluble factors, including transforming growth factor-β (TGF-β) and immunoglobulins, also contribute to the immunosuppressive barrier directly by disabling immune effector cells and indirectly by "educating" tumor-associated stromal cells, which in turn promotes secretion of stromal-derived factors that recruit additional inflammatory cells (tumor macrophages) and endothelial cells that further accelerate tumor growth.[92] This is an active area of basic and clinical research in which companion animal oncology has been at the forefront, for example, through the generation and approval of the first active gene-based therapeutic cancer vaccine for canine melanoma.[93]

Epigenetic Events

Another observation is that events leading to cancer need not necessarily be caused by mutational events but instead can be caused by epigenetic changes. Epigenetic events are those that can alter phenotype without changing the genotype. Two well-characterized epigenetic mechanisms regulate gene expression. Gene silencing can occur by methylation of CpG residues in promoter regions, as well as by histone deacetylation. Both of these events interfere with the transcriptional machinery and repress gene expression. The effects of global changes in methylation or deacetylation (e.g., by inactivation of DNA methylases or histone deacetylases) remain incompletely understood, but silencing of specific genes by methylation is implicated in numerous cancers of humans and animals.[2,94-96] One important observation is that most (or all) genes that are subject to silencing by methylation in specific cancers (e.g., *CDKN2A* in T-cell leukemia) are commonly inactivated by mutation or deletion in other cancers (e.g., *CDKN2A* in melanoma).

As is true for mutations, gene regulation by epigenetic methylation can occur sporadically or it can be heritable. Silencing of some tumor suppressor genes in sporadic cancers occurs more frequently by epigenetic methylation than by mutation or deletion. These different mechanisms of gene silencing are not equivalent, as they each result in specific tumor phenotypes. For example, data from our laboratories indicate that loss of canine chromosome 11, with resultant deletion of the *INK4* tumor suppressor locus containing the *CDKN2A, CDKN2B,* and *ARF* genes, and methylation of *CDKN2A* are each associated with morphologically distinct types of T-cell lymphoma that have a different clinical presentation and prognosis.[37,51]

Genomic imprinting presents a unique example in which heritable epigenetic changes influence cancer predisposition. Genomic imprinting refers to a pattern of gene expression that is determined by the parental origin of the gene; in other words, unlike most genes in which both parental alleles are expressed, only one allele (specifically derived from the mother or from the father, depending on the gene) of an imprinted gene is expressed and the other one is permanently repressed. Epigenetic changes in Wilms' tumor and in heritable colon cancer (among others) alter the expression of the imprinted allele, leading to loss of imprinting that causes *overexpression* of the insulin growth factor-2 *(IGF2)* gene.[2,97]

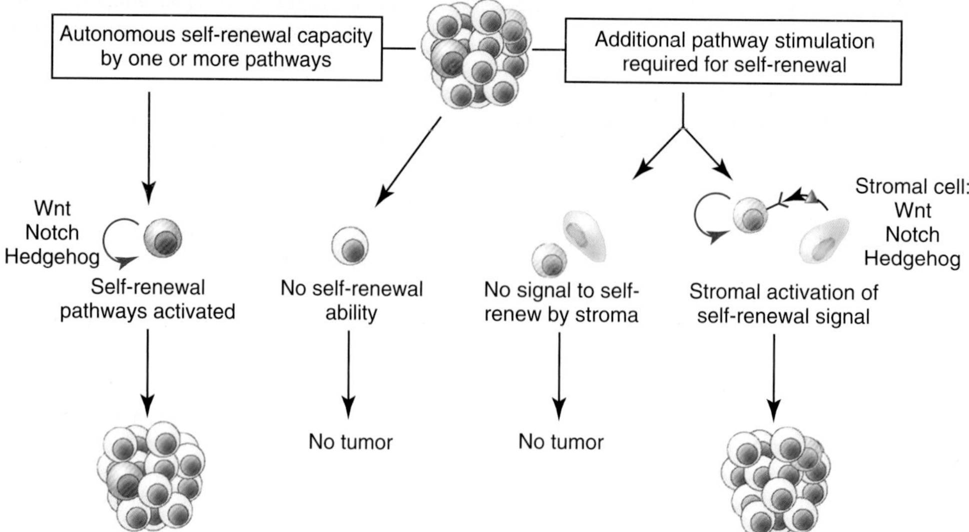

FIGURE 1-8 Multiple facets to cancer stem cell (CSC) self-renewal. Increasing evidence is emerging to support the notion that CSC self-renewal decisions can be guided by the activation of several pathways, including Wnt, Notch, Hedgehog, and others. A CSC may autonomously trigger the appropriate signaling cascade to maintain self-renewal with minimal niche support. It is likely that some CSCs need the appropriate microenvironment to provide the stimuli for uncontrolled self-renewal. Finally, some cancer cells have lost the capacity to self-renew regardless of stimulating molecules and hence cannot initiate a tumor. *(Reprinted from O'Brien CA, Kreso A, Jamieson CHM: Cancer stem cells and self-renewal,* Clin Cancer Res *16(12):3113–3120, 2010, with permission.)*

Cancer Stem Cells

The paradoxic nature of some cancers gave rise to the notion of a "cancer progenitor" or a CSC as far back as the 1960s. The best illustration for this concept was CML, where the bulk of the tumor consists of terminally differentiated neutrophils that are incapable of recreating the malignancy. However, it was apparent that there were multipotent stem cells in this tumor population. In 1994, Dick's group proved conclusively that another type of leukemia, acute myelogenous leukemia (AML), was a hierarchically organized disease in which a small number of cells that were undetectable by conventional methods could be isolated from patients and made to recapitulate the full spectrum of the disease in an animal model.[98] This gave rise to the CSC or "tumor-initiating cell" hypothesis, which is based on the concept that tumors are hierarchically organized into a subpopulation of cells that retain or acquire the capacity for self renewal and are capable and responsible for initiating and maintaining the tumor (Figure 1-8).[99] Another subpopulation of cells that consists of the CSC progeny undergo partial to complete differentiation and lose the capability to support the tumor, albeit they still contribute to the morbidity of cancer. This hypothesis fundamentally altered the way we understand cancer but also gave rise to a debate regarding how widely this model applies. The competing hypothesis is based on a model where all the cells in a tumor possess an equal capacity for self-renewal and is commonly referred to as the *stochastic model.* According to this model, the process of cancer is driven entirely (or almost entirely) by environmental selection of favorable mutations; this model would necessarily predict that cancer is an inevitable outcome for multicellular organisms, and few, if any, long-lived animals would reach reproductive age.[100] Thus this model must, by necessity, invoke the existence of protective mechanisms that are independent of cancer risk (e.g., efficient DNA repair mechanisms and immune surveillance).

It is possible that the two models represent a continuum dependent on the extent to which CSCs undergo asymmetric versus symmetric divisions. Under conditions in which CSC divisions are primarily asymmetric, few CSCs would be apparent and the population would achieve a hierarchical organization, whereas under conditions in which CSCs underwent symmetric divisions, virtually every cell in the tumor would have CSC-like properties and the organization would be more consistent with a stochastic model. The prevailing opinion is that CSCs exist and are characterized both by peculiar phenotypes and defined sets of mutations of a small number of genes.[101-103] Other mutations then endow their progeny with limited or extensive capacity to undergo programmed differentiation, thus resulting in the distinct clinical phenotypes that characterize acute and chronic leukemias or high-grade and low-grade solid tumors. The origin of CSCs is among the most important contemporary topics of investigation. CSCs may arise from mutations that occur in bona fide stem cells, they may arise by "de-differentiation" of somatic cells that acquire mutations that endow them with stem cell–like properties, or they may develop by fusion of a transformed cell and a bone marrow–derived stem cell.[104] In companion animals, putative CSCs have been identified in hemangiosarcoma, osteosarcoma, brain tumors, and possibly lymphoma.[105-108]

As is true for the rest of cancer genetics, information in this field is rapidly evolving. Large-scale bioinformatics and conceptual advances are integrating the CSC theory into the mainstream of cancer research and biology, as well as into the design for new diagnostic and therapeutic strategies. For example, it appears that much like hematopoietic stem cells, the CSC niche favors oligoclonality and some genetic diversity. Thus clonal competition can ensue, giving rise to heterogeneous tumors and maintaining a reservoir of cells that can reestablish the tumor when a therapy effectively kills the predominant CSC clone and its progeny. Similarly, clonal competition can facilitate distant spread by selection of cells with different capabilities. An extreme example may be the potential for a single tumor cell (or a small population of oligoclonal cells in a tumor) to give rise to histologically distinct tumors—an event we have observed in xenotransplanted sarcomas.

Summary

The genetic basis of cancer is now beyond question. It is estimated that at least five to seven mutational events are required for overt malignant transformation, and genomic instability seems to be necessary to establish a self-renewing population of cells (possibly CSCs) whose progeny expand to cause clinical disease. Ultimately, a subpopulation endowed with metastatic properties that is drug resistant leads to death of the cancer patient. The rate and the flow of information is such that we predict the coming decade will see transformational changes in our perception of how genes interact with the macroenvironment at the organismal level and with the microenvironment in tumors. Although it is possible that cancer in higher vertebrates is an inevitable consequence of evolution,[109] improvements in our understanding of fundamental mechanisms that account for malignant transformation and tumor progression will allow us to design strategies to improve quality of life and outcomes for cancer patients.

REFERENCES

1. Vogelstein B, Kinzler KW: Cancer genes and the pathways they control, *Nat Med* 10:789–799, 2004.
2. Ponder BA: Cancer genetics, *Nature* 411:336–341, 2001.
3. Ley TJ, et al: DNA sequencing of a cytogenetically normal acute myeloid leukaemia genome, *Nature* 456:66–72, 2008.
4. Sjoblom T, et al: The consensus coding sequences of human breast and colorectal cancers, *Science* 314:268–274, 2006.
5. Morin RD, et al: Frequent mutation of histone-modifying genes in non-Hodgkin lymphoma, *Nature* 476:298–303, 2011.
6. Pasqualucci L, et al: Analysis of the coding genome of diffuse large B-cell lymphoma, *Nat Genet* 43:830–837, 2011.
7. Fearon ER: Human cancer syndromes: clues to the origin and nature of cancer, *Science* 278:1043–1050, 1997.
8. Nagy R, Sweet K, Eng C: Highly penetrant hereditary cancer syndromes, *Oncogene* 23:6445–6470, 2004.
9. Knudson AG: Mutation and cancer: Statistical study of retinoblastoma, *Proc Natl Acad Sci U S A* 68:820–823, 1971.
10. Hahn WC, Weinberg RA: Modelling the molecular circuitry of cancer, *Nat Rev Cancer* 2:331–341, 2002.
11. Hanahan D, Weinberg RA: Hallmarks of cancer: The next generation, *Cell* 144:646–674, 2011.
12. Pihan G, Doxsey SJ: Mutations and aneuploidy: Co-conspirators in cancer? *Cancer Cell* 4:89–94, 2003.
13. Lingaas F, et al: A mutation in the canine BHD gene is associated with hereditary multifocal renal cystadenocarcinoma and nodular dermatofibrosis in the German Shepherd dog, *Hum Mol Genet* 12:3043–3053, 2003.
14. Nickerson ML, et al: Mutations in a novel gene lead to kidney tumors, lung wall defects, and benign tumors of the hair follicle in patients with the Birt-Hogg-Dube syndrome, *Cancer Cell* 2:157–164, 2002.
15. Trosko JE: Commentary: Is the concept of "tumor promotion" a useful paradigm? *Mol Carcinog* 30:131–137, 2001.
16. Kopelovich L: Hereditary adenomatosis of the colon and rectum: relevance to cancer promotion and cancer control in humans, *Cancer Genet Cytogenet* 5:333–352, 1982.
17. Heng HH: Cancer genome sequencing: the challenges ahead, *Bioessays* 29:783–794, 2007.
18. Balmain A: Cancer as a complex genetic trait: tumor susceptibility in humans and mouse models, *Cell* 108:145–152, 2002.
19. Amos CI, et al: Genome-wide association scan of tag SNPs identifies a susceptibility locus for lung cancer at 15q25.1, *Nat Genet* 40:616–622, 2008.
20. Hung RJ, et al: A susceptibility locus for lung cancer maps to nicotinic acetylcholine receptor subunit genes on 15q25, *Nature* 452:633–637, 2008.
21. Thorgeirsson TE, et al: A variant associated with nicotine dependence, lung cancer and peripheral arterial disease, *Nature* 452:638–642, 2008.
22. Liu JZ, et al: Meta-analysis and imputation refines the association of 15q25 with smoking quantity, *Nat Genet* 42:436–440, 2010.
23. Shah PP, et al: Association of functionally important polymorphisms in cytochrome P4501B1 with lung cancer, *Mutat Res* 643:4–10, 2008.
24. Hecht SS, Kassie F, Hatsukami DK: Chemoprevention of lung carcinogenesis in addicted smokers and ex-smokers, *Nat Rev Cancer* 9:476–488, 2009.
25. Jalas JR, Hecht SS, Murphy SE: Cytochrome P450 enzymes as catalysts of metabolism of 4-(methylnitrosamino)-1-(3-pyridyl)-1-butanone, a tobacco specific carcinogen, *Chem Res Toxicol* 18:95–110, 2005.
26. Loeb LA: Mutator phenotype may be required for multistage carcinogenesis, *Cancer Res* 51:3075–3079, 1991.
27. Lindblad-Toh K, et al: In Breen M, et al, editor: Genes, dogs and cancer: Fifth Canine Cancer Conference, vol 5, Orlando, 2009, IVIS.
28. Ostrander EA: In Breen M, et al, editor: Genes, dogs and cancer: Fifth Canine Cancer Conference, vol 5, Orlando, 2009, IVIS.
29. Pontius JU, et al: Initial sequence and comparative analysis of the cat genome, *Genome Res* 17:1675–1689, 2007.
30. Thomas R, et al: Microarray-based cytogenetic profiling reveals recurrent and subtype-associated genomic copy number aberrations in feline sarcomas, *Chromosome Res* 17:987–1000, 2009.
31. Hedan B, et al: Molecular cytogenetic characterization of canine histiocytic sarcoma: A spontaneous model for human histiocytic cancer identifies deletion of tumor suppressor genes and highlights influence of genetic background on tumor behavior, *BMC Cancer* 11:201, 2011.
32. Thomas R, et al: Influence of genetic background on tumor karyotypes: Evidence for breed-associated cytogenetic aberrations in canine appendicular osteosarcoma, *Chromosome Res* 17:365–377, 2009.
33. Modiano JF, et al: Distinct B-cell and T-cell lymphoproliferative disease prevalence among dog breeds indicates heritable risk, *Cancer Res* 65:5654–5661, 2005.
34. Tamburini BA, et al: Gene expression profiles of sporadic canine hemangiosarcoma are uniquely associated with breed, *PLoS ONE* 4:e5549, 2009.
35. Scott MC, et al: Molecular subtypes of osteosarcoma identified by reducing tumor heterogeneity through an interspecies comparative approach, *Bone* 49:356–367, 2011.
36. Breen M, Modiano JF: Evolutionarily conserved cytogenetic changes in hematological malignancies of dogs and humans—man and his best friend share more than companionship, *Chromosome Res* 16:145–154, 2008.
37. Fosmire SP, et al: Inactivation of the p16 cyclin-dependent kinase inhibitor in high-grade canine non-Hodgkin's T-cell lymphoma, *Vet Pathol* 44:467–478, 2007.
38. Angstadt AY, et al: Characterization of canine osteosarcoma by array comparative genomic hybridization and RT-qPCR: Signatures of genomic imbalance in canine osteosarcoma parallel the human counterpart, *Genes Chromosomes Cancer* 50(11):859–874, 2011.
39. Duesberg P, Li R: Multistep carcinogenesis: A chain reaction of aneuploidizations, *Cell Cycle* 2:202–210, 2003.
40. Duesberg P, Rausch C, Rasnick D, et al: Genetic instability of cancer cells is proportional to their degree of aneuploidy, *Proc Natl Acad Sci U S A* 95:13692–13697, 1998.
41. Mani RS, Chinnaiyan AM: Triggers for genomic rearrangements: insights into genomic, cellular and environmental influences, *Nat Rev Genet* 11:819–829, 2010.
42. O'Donoghue LE et al: Expression profiling in canine osteosarcoma: identification of biomarkers and pathways associated with outcome, *BMC Cancer* 10: 506, 2010.
43. Paoloni M, et al: Canine tumor cross-species genomics uncovers targets linked to osteosarcoma progression, *BMC Genomics* 10:625, 2009.

44. Selvarajah GT, et al: Gene expression profiling of canine osteosarcoma reveals genes associated with short and long survival times, *Mol Cancer* 8:72, 2009.
45. Hanahan D, Weinberg RA: The hallmarks of cancer. *Cell* 100:57–70, 2000.
46. Ruchatz H, Coluccia AM, Stano P, et al: Constitutive activation of Jak2 contributes to proliferation and resistance to apoptosis in NPM/ALK-transformed cells, *Exp Hematol* 31:309–315, 2003.
47. Modiano JF, Ritt MG, Wojcieszyn J, et al: Growth arrest of melanoma cells is differentially regulated by contact inhibition and serum deprivation, *DNA Cell Biol* 18:357–367, 1999.
48. Modiano JF, Johnson LD, Bellgrau D: Negative regulators in homeostasis of naive peripheral T cells, *Immunol Res* 41:137–153, 2008.
49. Levine RA, Fleischli MA: Inactivation of p53 and retinoblastoma family pathways in canine osteosarcoma cell lines, *Vet Pathol* 37:54–61, 2000.
50. Levine RA, Forest T, Smith C: Tumor suppressor PTEN is mutated in canine osteosarcoma cell lines and tumors, *Vet Pathol* 39:372–378, 2002.
51. Modiano JF, Breen M, Valli VE, et al: Predictive value of p16 or Rb inactivation in a model of naturally occurring canine non-Hodgkin's lymphoma, *Leukemia* 21:184–187, 2007.
52. Dickerson EB, et al: Mutations of phosphatase and tensin homolog deleted from chromosome 10 in canine hemangiosarcoma, *Vet Pathol* 42:618–632, 2005.
53. Hammerman PS, Fox CJ, Thompson CB: Beginnings of a signal-transduction pathway for bioenergetic control of cell survival, *Trends Biochem Sci* 29:586–592, 2004.
54. White E, DiPaola RS: The double-edged sword of autophagy modulation in cancer, *Clin Cancer Res* 15:5308–5316, 2009.
55. Ohyashiki JH, Sashida G, Tauchi T, et al: Telomeres and telomerase in hematologic neoplasia, *Oncogene* 21:680–687, 2002.
56. Pang LY, Argyle DJ: Using naturally occurring tumours in dogs and cats to study telomerase and cancer stem cell biology, *Biochim Biophys Acta* 1792:380–391, 2009.
57. Ferrara N, Kerbel RS: Angiogenesis as a therapeutic target, *Nature* 438:967–974, 2005.
58. Folkman J: The role of angiogenesis in tumor growth, *Semin Cancer Biol* 3:65–71, 1992.
59. Folkman J: Tumor angiogenesis: therapeutic implications, *N Engl J Med* 285:1182–1186, 1971.
60. Chen H, et al: In vitro and in vivo production of vascular endothelial growth factor by chronic lymphocytic leukemia cells, *Blood* 96:3181–3187, 2000.
61. Kini AR, Kay NE, Peterson LC: Increased bone marrow angiogenesis in B cell chronic lymphocytic leukemia, *Leukemia* 14:1414–1418, 2000.
62. Molica S, et al: Prognostic value of enhanced bone marrow angiogenesis in early B-cell chronic lymphocytic leukemia, *Blood* 100:3344–3351, 2002.
63. Juliusson G, et al: Frequent good partial remissions from thalidomide including best response ever in patients with advanced refractory and relapsed myeloma, *Br J Haematol* 109:89–96, 2000.
64. Tosi P, et al: Salvage therapy with thalidomide in multiple myeloma patients relapsing after autologous peripheral blood stem cell transplantation, *Haematologica* 86:409–413, 2001.
65. Jorgensen JM: The role of angiogenesis in non-Hodgkin lymphoma, *Dan Med Bull* 52:254, 2005.
66. Ranieri G, et al: Endothelial area and microvascular density in a canine non-Hodgkin's lymphoma: an interspecies model of tumor angiogenesis, *Leuk Lymphoma* 46:1639–1643, 2005.
67. Preziosi R, Sarli G, Paltrinieri M: Prognostic value of intratumoral vessel density in cutaneous mast cell tumors of the dog, *J Comp Pathol* 130:143–151, 2004.
68. Restucci B, et al: Expression of vascular endothelial growth factor receptor Flk-1 in canine mammary tumours, *J Comp Pathol* 130:99–104, 2004.
69. Fidler IJ: The pathogenesis of cancer metastasis: the 'seed and soil' hypothesis revisited, *Nat Rev Cancer* 3:453–458, 2003.
70. Kim JW, et al: Rapid apoptosis in the pulmonary vasculature distinguishes non-metastatic from metastatic melanoma cells, *Cancer Lett* 213:203–212, 2004.
71. Wong CW, et al: Intravascular location of breast cancer cells after spontaneous metastasis to the lung, *Am J Pathol* 161:749–753, 2002.
72. Wong CW, et al: Apoptosis: an early event in metastatic inefficiency, *Cancer Res* 61:333–338, 2001.
73. Koshkina NV, et al: Fas-negative osteosarcoma tumor cells are selected during metastasis to the lungs: the role of the Fas pathway in the metastatic process of osteosarcoma, *Mol Cancer Res* 5: 991–999, 2007.
74. Krishnan K, et al: Ezrin mediates growth and survival in Ewing's sarcoma through the AKT/mTOR, but not the MAPK, signaling pathway, *Clin Exp Metastasis* 23:227–236, 2006.
75. Mueller MM, Fusenig NE: Friends or foes—bipolar effects of the tumour stroma in cancer, *Nat Rev Cancer* 4:839–849, 2004.
76. Nowell PC: Mechanisms of tumor progression, *Cancer Res* 46: 2203–2207, 1986.
77. Modiano JF, et al: Fas ligand gene transfer for cancer therapy, *Cancer Ther* 2:561–570, 2004.
78. Dunn GP, Bruce AT, Ikeda H, et al: Cancer immunoediting: from immunosurveillance to tumor escape, *Nat Immunol* 3:991–998, 2002.
79. Breivik J: The evolutionary origin of genetic instability in cancer development, *Semin Cancer Biol* 15:51–60, 2005.
80. Nguyen DH, et al: Radiation acts on the microenvironment to affect breast carcinogenesis by distinct mechanisms that decrease cancer latency and affect tumor type, *Cancer Cell* 19:640–651, 2011.
81. Boveri T: Concerning the origin of malignant tumors, *J Cell Sci* 121:1–84, 2008.
82. Albertson DG, Collins C, McCormick F, et al: Chromosome aberrations in solid tumors, *Nat Genet* 34:369–376, 2003.
83. Teixeira MR, Heim S: Multiple numerical chromosome aberrations in cancer: what are their causes and what are their consequences? *Semin Cancer Biol* 15:3–12, 2005.
84. Gollin SM: Mechanisms leading to chromosomal instability, *Semin Cancer Biol* 15:33–42, 2005.
85. Rajagopalan H, Lengauer C: Aneuploidy and cancer, *Nature* 432:338–341, 2004.
86. Maser RS, DePinho RA: Connecting chromosomes, crisis, and cancer, *Science* 297:565–569, 2002.
87. Dvorak HF: Tumors: wounds that do not heal. Similarities between tumor stroma generation and wound healing, *N Engl J Med* 315:1650–1659, 1986.
88. Lin WW, Karin M: A cytokine-mediated link between innate immunity, inflammation, and cancer, *J Clin Invest* 117:1175–1183, 2007.
89. Mantovani A, Allavena P, Sica A, et al: Cancer-related inflammation, *Nature* 454:436–444, 2008.
90. Bhatia R, McGlave PB, Dewald GW, et al: Abnormal function of the bone marrow microenvironment in chronic myelogenous leukemia: role of malignant stromal macrophages, *Blood* 85:3636–3645, 1995.
91. Grivennikov SI, Greten FR, Karin M: Immunity, inflammation, and cancer, *Cell* 140:883–899, 2010.
92. Erez N, Truitt M, Olson P, et al: Cancer-associated fibroblasts are activated in incipient neoplasia to orchestrate tumor-promoting inflammation in an NF-kappaB-dependent manner, *Cancer Cell* 17:135–147, 2010.
93. Bergman PJ: Anticancer vaccines, *Vet Clin North Am Small Anim Pract* 37:1111–1119; vi-ii, 2007.
94. Wolffe AP, Matzke MA: Epigenetics: regulation through repression, *Science* 286:481–486, 1999.
95. Costello JF: Comparative epigenomics of leukemia, *Nat Genet* 37:211–212, 2005.
96. Yu L, et al: Global assessment of promoter methylation in a mouse model of cancer identifies ID4 as a putative tumor-suppressor gene in human leukemia. *Nat Genet* 37:265–274, 2005.

97. Cui H, et al: Loss of IGF2 imprinting: a potential marker of colorectal cancer risk, *Science* 299:1753–1755, 2003.
98. Lapidot T, et al: A cell initiating human acute myeloid leukaemia after transplantation into SCID mice, *Nature* 367:645–648, 1994.
99. O'Brien CA, Kreso A, Jamieson CHM: Cancer stem cells and self-renewal, *Clin Cancer Res* 16(12):3113–3120, 2010.
100. Clarke MF, Fuller M: Stem cells and cancer: two faces of eve, *Cell* 124:1111–1115, 2006.
101. Huntly BJ, Gilliland DG: Leukaemia stem cells and the evolution of cancer-stem-cell research, *Nat Rev Cancer* 5:311–321, 2005.
102. Singh SK, et al: Identification of human brain tumour initiating cells, *Nature* 432:396–401, 2004.
103. Smith GH: Mammary cancer and epithelial stem cells: a problem or a solution? *Breast Cancer Res* 4:47–50, 2002.
104. Bjerkvig R, Tysnes BB, Aboody KS, et al: Opinion: the origin of the cancer stem cell: current controversies and new insights, *Nat Rev Cancer* 5:899–904, 2005.
105. Lamerato-Kozicki AR, Helm KM, Jubala CM, et al: Canine hemangiosarcoma originates from hematopoietic precursors with potential for endothelial differentiation, *Exp Hematol* 34:870–878, 2006.
106. Wilson H, et al: Isolation and characterisation of cancer stem cells from canine osteosarcoma, *Vet J* 175(1):69–75, 2007.
107. Stoica G, et al: Identification of cancer stem cells in dog glioblastoma, *Vet Pathol* 46(3):391–406, 2009.
108. Ito D, et al: A tumor-related lymphoid progenitor population supports hierarchical tumor organization in canine B-cell lymphoma, *J Vet Intern Med* 25:890–896, 2011.
109. Modiano JF, Breen M: Shared pathogenesis of human and canine tumors—an inextricable link between cancer and evolution, *Cancer Ther* 6:239–246, 2008.

SECTION B
Chemical, Physical, and Hormonal Factors

CAROLYN J. HENRY

In 1978, the United States Congress ordered development of the first Report on Carcinogens (RoC), a document designed to educate the public and health professionals on potential cancer hazards. The document is now required by law to be released every 2 years by the Secretary of the Department of Health and Human Services. The twelfth edition of the RoC, released in 2011, lists 240 potential carcinogens, of which 54 are categorized as *known to be human carcinogens* and 186 are categorized as *reasonably anticipated to be human carcinogens.*[1] Although no such report exists for companion animals, one could reasonably assume that there would be considerable overlap between such a list and the potential carcinogens found in the RoC. The 2005 RoC was the first to include neutrons, x- and gamma-radiation, and viruses (human papillomavirus, hepatitis B virus, and hepatitis C virus). Although the list of carcinogens reportedly associated with cancer in companion animals is less extensive, this section will address chemical, physical, and hormonal factors that have been linked to carcinogenesis in pet animals. Viral carcinogenesis will be addressed in a separate section (see Section C below).

Chemical Factors

Environmental Tobacco Smoke

Despite ample evidence that secondhand smoke increases the risk of lung cancer in people,[2,3] the data for this effect in companion animals are less compelling. One case-control study involving dogs with lung cancer from two veterinary hospitals showed only a weak relationship between living with a smoker and development of lung cancer, and the risk did not increase with an increased smoke exposure index.[4] However, evidence for a relationship between exposure to environmental tobacco smoke (ETS) and development of other malignancies in companion animals is mounting.

Based on human data suggesting that smoking may increase the risk of non-Hodgkin's lymphoma,[5,6] Bertone et al examined the relationship between ETS exposure and development of feline lymphoma.[7] In a case-control study of 80 cats with malignant lymphoma and 114 control cats with renal disease that presented to Tufts University School of Veterinary Medicine (TUSVM) between 1993 and 2000, the relative risk of lymphoma for cats with any household ETS exposure was 2.4. As has been reported for male smokers,[8] the risk of lymphoma increased with increases in either duration or quantity of exposure. More recently, an Italian study of environmental risk factors for development of cancer in domestic animals demonstrated that ETS exposure increased the risk of lymphoma in dogs.[9]

Hypothesizing that inhalation and ingestion of carcinogenic compounds in ETS during grooming might also predispose cats in smoking households to development of oral squamous cell carcinoma (SCC), Bertone et al examined ETS and other environmental and lifestyle risk factors in cats with SCC.[10] The study examined a population of 36 cats with histologically confirmed oral SCC and a control population of 112 cats with renal disease, all presenting to TUSVM between 1994 and 2000. Exposure to ETS was associated with a twofold but statistically insignificant increased risk of oral SCC.[10] Interestingly, in a separate report, the investigators showed that SCC tissue from cats exposed to any ETS were 4.5 more likely to overexpress p53 and those from cats with 5 years or more of ETS exposure were 7 times more likely to overexpress p53.[11] Although the findings did not reach statistical significance, the collective work of this group provides an intriguing suggestion that both ETS and mutations in the p53 gene may play a role in the etiology of feline oral SCC.

Pesticides, Herbicides, and Insecticides

In 1991, investigators at the National Cancer Institute (NCI) completed a case-control study to examine the relationship between exposure of dogs to the herbicide, 2,4-dichlorophenoxyacetic acid (2,4-D), and development of lymphoma.[12] Dogs with a histologically confirmed diagnosis of lymphoma during a 4-year period were identified through the computerized medical record information from three veterinary teaching hospitals. Each case animal was age-matched with two control animals. The first control group consisted of dogs diagnosed with tumors other than lymphoma during the same time period and the second control group was a nontumor group, selected from all other dogs presenting to the hospital for conditions deemed unrelated to chemical exposure. Owners were questioned about household use of and potential pet exposure to commercial lawn care and owner-applied herbicides. A positive association was found between exposure to owner-applied 2,4-D or the use of commercial lawn care services and the development of canine lymphoma. The risk of lymphoma development doubled when owners applied 2,4-D liquid or granules to the lawn four or more times a year. After these findings were reported, an independent review panel was convened to assess the validity of the NCI study.[13] This panel voiced concerns about the original study design, data analysis, and interpretation, concluding that a relationship between 2,4-D exposure and the development of canine lymphoma could not be established based on the reported data. In response, the original investigators reanalyzed their data, addressing many of the concerns raised by the scientific review panel.[14] In their second study, Hayes et al used a more stringent definition of exposure to 2,4-D, including only cases in which the owner applied 2,4-D as the sole herbicide and did not use other lawn chemicals or lawn care services. Their second report did not show a statistically significant association between exposure to 2,4-D and development of lymphoma.[14] However, they concluded that their results did indicate a dose-response relationship between disease incidence and number of yearly 2,4-D applications by dog owners. In a subsequent study conducted by researchers at Michigan State University, the original 1991 data was again reanalyzed using the more stringent definition of exposure and completing a dose-response analysis. The study, which was funded by a chemical industry task force, showed no dose-response relationship between number of 2,4-D applications and the occurrence of canine lymphoma.[15] Although increased urinary excretion of 2,4-D has been demonstrated in dogs exposed to herbicide-treated lawns, a direct link between such exposure and development of lymphoma has not been shown.[16] A 2011 case-control study conducted in Italy was designed to assess the effect of residential exposure to environmental pollutants on the risk of developing lymphoma.[17] The investigators were unable to demonstrate an association between exposure to pesticides (which by their definition included herbicides) and development of lymphoma. They did, however, find that living in industrial areas and owner use of chemicals such as paints and solvents were significantly and independently associated with lymphoma.

Canine transitional cell carcinoma (TCC) of the urinary bladder is another malignancy that has been linked to environmental carcinogens including insecticides and herbicides. In a case-control study of 59 dogs with TCC and 71 age-matched and breed size–matched control dogs with other neoplasms or chronic disease, investigators compared the two populations to assess the effect of obesity, exposure to sidestream cigarette smoke and chemicals, and use of topical insecticides on risk of TCC.[18] They reported an increased risk of TCC in dogs treated with topical insecticides, with an enhancement of this risk in overweight or obese dogs. In the aforementioned study of risk factors for oral SCC in cats, Bertone et al reported a significantly increased risk of oral SCC in cats that wore flea collars.[10] However, newer topical spot-on flea and tick products have been evaluated in Scottish terrier populations due to the breed's predisposition for development of TCC of the urinary bladder and have not been shown to increase the risk of TCC.[19] Other studies of Scottish terriers have suggested that exposure to lawn and garden care products containing phenoxy herbicides, including 2,4-D, 4-chloro-2-methylphenoxy acetic acid (MCPA), and 2-(4-chloro-2-methylphenoxyl) propionic acid (MCPP), is associated with an increased risk of TCC.[20] Although it has been difficult to prove a link between phenoxy herbicides and development of lymphoma or TCC, attempts to limit exposure of pets to these products is advised.

Cyclophosphamide

The cytotoxic alkylating agent, cyclophosphamide, has been implicated in the development of urinary bladder cancer in people and dogs.[21-23] A known potential side effect of cyclophosphamide therapy is sterile hemorrhagic cystitis, which may develop due to the irritating effects of the drug's metabolite, acrolein, on the bladder mucosa. Although the specific etiology is unknown, it is speculated that chronic inflammation secondary to acrolein exposure is the underlying event that leads to bladder cancer in some patients that have undergone cyclophosphamide therapy. The author has had the experience of treating a dog for lymphoma that was found to have concurrent but clinically occult TCC of the bladder prior to initiation of cyclophosphamide chemotherapy. If an abdominal ultrasound had not been performed on this dog as part of the initial staging procedures prior to chemotherapy, the bladder TCC may have been diagnosed at a later date and incorrectly attributed to administration of cyclophosphamide. This exemplifies the danger of assuming a causal relationship for potential carcinogens, especially in animals that have a prior malignancy.

Rural versus Urban Environment

Although several reports have identified differences in cancer incidence between companion animals living in urban versus rural settings, the underlying cause for these differences is unclear. An increased incidence of some canine cancers, including lymphoma, tonsillar SCC, and nasal carcinoma,[17,18,24,25] has been reported in urban/industrial settings as compared with rural settings. However, the coexistence of multiple environmental carcinogens in the same setting makes discerning the "smoking gun" a difficult task. Nonetheless, the study of animals as sentinels of environmental health hazards has been recommended and provides supportive evidence for carcinogenic risk assessment across species.[26-29] Results of a hospital-based case-control study conducted in Naples, Italy and nearby cities with known high levels of illegal waste dumping suggest that living in these sites of waste emission increases the risk of cancer development in dogs but not cats. This may relate to reduced exposure of cats to environmental carcinogens, as they are often exclusively indoor pets.[9]

Physical Factors

Sunlight

The relationship between sunlight exposure or ultraviolet irradiation and subsequent development of skin cancer is one of the better known examples of physical carcinogenesis. Recognized for its role in human SCC induction, sunlight has also been implicated as a cause of SCC in domestic animals and livestock—an implication that is strengthened by a clear dose-response relationship shown in both epidemiologic and experimental studies.[28-31] In particular, light skin pigmentation and chronic sun exposure are associated with the development of facial, aural, and nasal planum SCC in white or partially white cats and may also play a similar role in some cutaneous SCC lesions in dogs. The portion of the ultraviolet spectrum most likely to be responsible for nonmelanotic skin lesions in people and animals is ultraviolet B (UV-B), which is in the range of 280 to 320 nm.[28] Cumulative long-term exposure to UV-B may induce skin tumors directly through genetic mutations, including mutations in p53, and indirectly by impairing the response of the immune system to tumor antigens.[28,32,33] Pets are at greatest risk of exposure to UV-B during the midday hours and should be protected from this exposure, especially if they are a lightly pigmented breed.

Trauma/Chronic Inflammation

Chronic inflammation may lead to cellular mutations that in turn cause neoplastic transformation. In four dogs with chronic pigmentary keratitis, neoplastic lesions of the cornea, including three SCC and one squamous papilloma, were reported.[34] Although the underlying etiology of the keratitis could not be confirmed, the neoplastic transformation was likely related to chronic inflammation. Earlier reports have linked feline eye tumors to ocular trauma that induces secondary uveitis and lens rupture (see Chapter 31).[35] Unlike the corneal tumors reported in dogs with pigmentary keratitis, the ocular lesions in cats were intraocular sarcomas. Despite the varied histology, the underlying etiology in all cases was thought to be related to inflammatory changes. Another companion animal malignancy thought to be associated with inflammation is vaccine-associated feline sarcoma (VAFS). This tumor type and its etiology are discussed in detail in Chapter 21.

Magnetic Fields

More than a quarter century ago, a potential link between chronic low-dose exposure to magnetic fields and development of childhood cancer was proposed.[36] Since then, multiple studies have been conducted in an attempt to discern links between magnetic fields and a variety of human cancers ranging from hematopoietic malignancies to breast cancer. The extremely low frequency (<60 Hz) magnetic fields in question are ubiquitous in today's society and are generated by household appliances, industrial machinery, and electrical power lines. Since pets share our environment and have similar exposure to magnetic fields, a similar risk of cancer development has been presumed for companion animals. In a 1995 study, the risk for development of lymphoma was found to be highest in dogs from households with the highest measured exposure to magnetic fields.[37] The risk was related to both duration and intensity of exposure and was highest for dogs that spent more than 25% of the day outdoors. In the following year at the request of Congress, a report was published by the National Research Council (NRC) that reviewed over 500 studies on the subject of cancer risk and exposure to electromagnetic fields.[38] The report concluded that, although a weak association has been shown between development of childhood leukemia and exposure to electromagnetic fields, no clear evidence exists to suggest that exposure to electromagnetic fields is a true threat to human health. To the author's knowledge, no reports on the possible link between magnetic fields and cancer in companion animals have been published since the 1995 report, although the magnetic field debate continues in the human literature. The NRC report suggested that other factors, including air quality and proximity to high traffic density, may be more likely environmental causes of cancer than low frequency magnetic fields.

Radiation

The first report of cancer development after therapeutic irradiation in a dog dates back over 25 years, when orthovoltage radiation was considered state-of-the-art.[39] At that time, the term *malignant transformation* was used to describe the development of epithelial malignancies at the site of prior irradiation for acanthomatous epulides in four dogs. Following a review of more recent cases with megavoltage irradiation, the author of the original report has since suggested that the concept of malignant transformation should be discarded, in that the occurrence of second tumors was not likely due to a true transformation of epulides into carcinomas.[40] Rather, the relatively high rate of carcinomas at previously irradiated sites for epulides is a result of less effective forms of irradiation or misclassification of the tumor type. Radiation carcinogenesis is considered the cause of second tumors arising in radiation fields. In human oncology, most tumors occurring in heavily irradiated treatment fields are mesenchymal, rather than epithelial, in origin.[41-43] Several reports of sarcomas occurring in sites of prior radiation can be found in the veterinary literature, as well,[39,44-46] with the most recent being a retrospective review of 57 dogs undergoing definitive megavoltage radiation therapy with ^{60}Cobalt photons for acanthomatous epulis.[40] In the latter report, McEntee et al describe the development of a second tumor (one sarcoma and one osteosarcoma) in 2 of the 57 irradiated dogs, occurring 5.2 and 8.7 years after the initial treatment, respectively. The overall incidence of second tumors was lower in their study than in previous reports (3.5% versus up to 18%).[39,47] The fact that no epithelial tumors were reported may indicate a more efficient targeting of a subpopulation of malignant epithelial cells by megavoltage radiotherapy, as compared to orthovoltage. The report suggests that the risk of second tumors at sites of radiation therapy is primarily of clinical concern for young dogs expected to enjoy long-term survival. Second tumors have also been reported in at least six people who have undergone stereotactic radiosurgery.[48] As this radiation technique becomes more commonplace in veterinary medicine, the possibility of second tumors may need to be considered in companion animals undergoing stereotactic radiosurgery.

Surgery and Implanted Devices

The development of sarcomas at the site of metallic implants has been reported in people, dogs, and laboratory animal models.[49,50] However, it is often difficult to discern if sarcoma development is related to fracture fixation devices or to other factors, including wound healing complications and osteomyelitis. The largest veterinary study examining the relationship between metallic implants and tumor development in dogs was published in 1993 by Li et al.[50] The authors reported on 222 dogs that developed tumors of any kind after fracture fixation, compared to 1635 dogs that underwent fracture fixation without subsequent tumor development. They concluded that use of metallic implants was not a risk factor for bone tumor development. Other types of implants and foreign materials related to surgery are sporadically implicated in carcinogenesis in human and veterinary case reports. Published examples include one dog that developed a myxoma at the site of a subcutaneous pacemaker and another that developed a jejunal osteosarcoma associated with a surgical sponge presumably not retrieved during an abdominal surgery 6 years prior.[51,52]

Asbestos

Asbestos exposure is a known risk factor for development of mesothelioma in people.[53] In fact, an estimated 60% to 88% of all cases of human mesothelioma are attributable to asbestos exposure.[53] A similar association has been found for dogs whose owners have an asbestos-related occupation or hobby.[54] This association was further supported by a study in which significantly more asbestos bodies were found in dogs with mesothelioma than in control dogs.[55] Pericardial mesothelioma was reported in five golden retrievers with histories of chronic idiopathic hemorrhagic pericardial effusion, suggesting that other factors, including breed predispositions and chronic inflammation unrelated to asbestos exposure, may be involved in the etiology of mesothelioma affecting the pericardium.[56]

Hormonal Factors

Estrogen and Progesterone

Canine Mammary Cancer

Canine mammary cancer is a well-established model of hormonal carcinogenesis in domestic animals (see Chapter 27). The most common neoplasm of female intact dogs, mammary tumors affect approximately 260/100,000 dogs in the United States each year.[57,58] Dogs spayed before their first estrous cycle have a greatly reduced risk of developing breast cancer, with the risk rising to 26% for dogs that are spayed after their second estrus.[59,60] Mammary tumors primarily affect late middle-aged (9 to 11 years) female intact dogs, with an increased incidence beginning at approximately 6 years of age.[61] Sexual steroid hormones likely have their primary effect on target cells during the very early stages of mammary carcinogenesis in dogs; thus, the protective effect of spaying is lost with time.[62-68] In addition to the influence of ovarian hormones on breast cancer development, the use of medroxyprogesterone acetate (progestin and estrogen combination) products to prevent estrus or to treat pseudopregnancy has been linked to an increased incidence of mammary tumor development in dogs.[69-71]

Progestin-induced growth hormone (GH) excess in dogs originates in the mammary gland. Within the mammary gland, the gene encoding GH may act in an autocrine/paracrine fashion, effecting cyclic epithelial changes and, perhaps, carcinogenesis. Research to determine the mechanism of progestin-induced mammary GH expression in dogs has led to the cloning and cellular localization of the canine progesterone receptor (PR).[72] The investigators concluded that within the same mammary gland cell, the activated PR may transactivate GH expression and function as a prerequisite transcription factor. However, this regulation may be lost during malignant transformation. Mammary GH expression has been reported in people as well, suggesting that evaluation of links between this hormone and mammary carcinogenesis may have implications for both species.[73,74]

Feline Mammary Cancer

Both estrogen and progesterone are thought to play important roles in feline mammary carcinogenesis, although the underlying mechanisms are less clear than for dogs. Prior studies have shown that intact female cats and those cats that are exposed regularly to progestin are at an increased risk for mammary cancer development. The literature also suggests that, as is the case in dogs, ovariectomy may be protective against feline mammary gland tumor development in cats.[57,75-77] In one study, cats ovariectomized at 6 months of age had an approximate sevenfold reduction in risk of mammary tumor development compared to intact cats.[57] What has been lacking in the veterinary literature is an epidemiologic study of cats with age-matched controls for comparison to specifically investigate the effects that spaying and age of spay have on the risk of feline mammary carcinoma development. Overley et al attempted to address these issues in a retrospective study that compared a population of 308 cats with biopsy-proven mammary carcinoma diagnosed between 2000 and 2001 and a control population of 400 female cats not diagnosed with mammary tumors but from the same biopsy service population as the affected cats. Cats from the two groups were frequency-matched by age and year of diagnosis.[77] The study reported a 91% reduction in risk for those spayed prior to 6 months of age and an 86% reduction in risk for those spayed prior to 1 year of age, compared to intact cats. Although the study was retrospective in nature and relied on questionnaire data from a survey with a 58% response rate, the manuscript is the first published report attempting to age-match controls and evaluate age at time of spay as a risk factor for mammary tumor development in cats. Although further epidemiologic evaluation and prospective assessment are needed to confirm these findings, the reported results provide some justification for recommending ovariohysterectomy prior to 1 year of age in cats.

Lymphoma

Surveillance, Epidemiology and End Results (SEER) data indicate that non-Hodgkin's lymphoma is approximately 50% more common among men than women.[78] Although a similar male predisposition is reported for canine lymphoma, the underlying role of gender in lymphoma etiology remains elusive. The author and others undertook a population-based study using the Veterinary Medical Database (VMDB) to determine the relationship between gender and development of canine lymphoma.[79] Data from 1980 to 2000 were retrieved from the VMDB and sorted by gender and reproductive status. In the statistical analysis, spayed or neutered dogs diagnosed with lymphoma were compared to intact dogs seen each year in each gender category. The VMDB included nearly 15,000 lymphoma cases in a population of over 1.2 million dogs. These data suggest that intact females were significantly less likely to develop lymphoma than were other gender groups. Based on this initial data, we propose that further examination of the role of estrogen in the development or prevention of canine lymphoma is warranted.

Androgens/Testosterone

Perianal Adenoma

Perianal adenoma is androgen dependent and occurs primarily in intact male dogs, whereas perianal adenocarcinoma occurs in both intact and castrated males. Perianal adenomas may also develop in female dogs secondary to testosterone secretion from the adrenal gland.[80] The majority of these tumors in male dogs resolve after castration, a fact that lends further support to the assertion that androgens are involved in the etiology of this tumor (see Chapter 22).[81]

Prostate Cancer

Although there is a well-established link between presence of testosterone and development of benign prostatic hyperplasia (BPH) in dogs and man, prostatic cancer risk is not higher in intact dogs compared to those that are castrated.[82] To the contrary, neutered dogs have been shown to be at increased risk. Castration is likely not an initiating event, but is thought to favor tumor progression.[83-86] A clear relationship between age at castration and risk of prostate cancer development is yet to be determined (see Chapter 28).

REFERENCES

1. Report on Carcinogens: ed 12, 2011; available at http://ntp.niehs.nih.gov.
2. Leonard CT, Sachs DPL: Environmental tobacco smoke and lung cancer incidence, *Curr Opin Pulm Med* 5:189, 1999.
3. Hackshaw AK, Law MR, Wald NJ: The accumulated evidence on lung cancer and environmental tobacco smoke, *Br Med J* 315:980, 1997.
4. Reif JS, Dunn K, Ogilvie GK, et al: Passive smoking and canine lung cancer risk, *Am J Epidemiol* 135:234, 1992.
5. Herrinton LJ, Friedman GD: Cigarette smoking and risk of non-Hodgkin's lymphoma subtypes, *Cancer Epidemiol Biomarkers Prev* 7:25, 1998.
6. Linet MS, McLaughlin JK, Hsing AW, et al: Is cigarette smoking a risk factor for non-Hodgkin's lymphoma or multiple myeloma? Results from the Lutheran Brotherhood Cohort Study, *Leuk Res* 16:621, 1992.
7. Bertone ER, Snyder LA, Moore AS: Environmental tobacco smoke and risk of malignant lymphoma in pet cats, *Am J Epidemiol* 156:268, 2002.
8. Freedman DS, Tolbert PE, Coates R: Relation of cigarette smoking to non-Hodgkin's lymphoma among middle-aged men, *Am J Epidemiol* 148:833, 1998.
9. Marconato L, Leo C, Girelli R, et al: Association between waste management and cancer in companion animals, *J Vet Intern Med* 23:564, 2009.

10. Bertone ER, Snyder LA, Moore AS: Environmental and lifestyle risk factors for oral squamous cell carcinoma in domestic cats, *J Vet Intern Med* 17:557, 2003.
11. Snyder LA, Bertone ER, Jakowski RM, et al: p53 expression and environmental tobacco smoke exposure in feline oral squamous cell carcinoma, *Vet Pathol* 41:209, 2004.
12. Hayes HM, Tarone RE, Cantor KP, et al: Case-control study of canine malignant lymphoma: Positive association with dog owner's use of 2,4-dichlorophenoxyacetic acid herbicides, *J Natl Cancer Inst* 83:1226, 1991.
13. Carlo GL, Cole P, Miller AM, et al: Review of a study reporting an association between 2,4-dichlorophenoxyacetic acid and canine malignant lymphoma: Report of an expert panel, *Reg Toxicol Pharmacol* 10:245, 1992.
14. Hayes HM, Tarone RE, Cantor KP: On the association between canine malignant lymphoma and opportunity for exposure to 2,4-dichlorophenoxyacetic acid, *Environ Res* 70:119, 1995.
15. Kaneene JB, Miller R: Re-analysis of 2,4-D use and the occurrence of canine malignant lymphoma, *Vet Hum Toxicol* 41:164, 1999.
16. Reynolds PM, Reif JS, Ramsdell HS: Canine exposure to herbicide-treated lawns and urinary excretion of 2,4-dichlorophenoxyacetic acid, *Cancer Epidemiol Biomarkers Prev* 3:233, 1994.
17. Gavazza A, Presciuttini S, Barale R, et al: Association between canine malignant lymphoma, living in industrial areas, and use of chemical by dog owners, *J Vet Intern Med* 15:190, 2001.
18. Glickman LT, Schofer FS, McKee LJ, et al: Epidemiologic study of insecticide exposures, obesity, and risk of bladder cancer in household dogs, *J Toxicol Environ Health* 28:407, 1989.
19. Raghavan M, Knapp DW, Dawson MH, et al: Topical flea and tick pesticides and the risk of transitional cell carcinoma of the urinary bladder in Scottish Terriers, *J Am Vet Med Assoc* 225:389, 2004.
20. Glickman LT, Raghavan M, Knapp DW, et al: Herbicide exposure and the risk of transitional cell carcinoma of the urinary bladder in Scottish Terriers, *J Am Vet Med Assoc* 224:1290, 2004.
21. Baker GL, Kahl LE, Zee BC, et al: Malignancy following treatment of rheumatoid arthritis with cyclophosphamide. Long-term case-control follow-up study, *Am J Med* 83:1, 1987.
22. Weller RE, Wolf AM, Oyejide A: Transitional cell carcinoma of the bladder associated with Cyclophosphamide administration, *J Am Anim Hosp Assoc* 15:733, 1979.
23. Macy DW, Withrow SJ, Hoopes J: Transitional cell carcinoma of the bladder associated with Cyclophosphamide administration, *J Am Anim Hosp Assoc* 19:965, 1983.
24. Reif JS, Bruns C, Lower KS: Cancer of the nasal cavity and paranasal sinuses and exposure to environmental tobacco smoke in pet dogs, *Am J Epidemiol* 147:488, 1998.
25. Reif JS, Cohen D: The environmental distribution of canine respiratory tract neoplasms, *Arch Environ Health* 22:136, 1971.
26. Hayes HM, Hoover R, Tarone RE: Bladder cancer in pet dogs: A sentinel for environmental cancer? *Am J Epidemiol* 114:229, 1981.
27. van der Schalie WH, Gardner HS Jr, Bantle JA, et al: Animals as sentinels of human health hazards of environmental chemicals, *Environ Health Perspect* 107:309, 1999.
28. Bukowski JA, Wartenberg D, Goldschmidt M: Environmental causes for sinonasal cancers in pet dogs, and their usefulness as sentinels of indoor cancer risk, *J Toxicol Environ Health A* 54(7):579, 1998.
29. Buckowski JA, Wartenberg D: An alternative approach for investigating the carcinogenicity of indoor air pollution: Pets as sentinels of environmental cancer risk, *Environ Health Perspect* 105:1312, 1997.
30. Fu W, Cockerell CJ: The actinic (solar) keratosis: A 21st-century perspective, *Arch Dermatol* 139:66, 2003.
31. Kahn SG, Bicker DR, Mukhtar H, et al: Ras p21 farnesylation in ultraviolet B radiation-induced tumors in the skin of SKH-1 hairless mice, *J Invest Dermatol* 102:754, 1994.
32. Lowe NJ, Weingarten D, Wortzman M: Sunscreens and phototesting, *Clin Derm* 6:40, 1988.
33. Hargis AM: A review of solar-induced lesions in domestic animals, *Comp Cont Edu* 3:287, 1981.
34. Bernays ME, Flemming D, Peiffer RL Jr: Primary corneal papilloma and squamous cell carcinoma associated with pigmentary keratitis in four dogs, *J Am Vet Med Assoc* 214:215, 1999.
35. Hakanson N, Shively JN, Reed RE: Intraocular spindle cell sarcoma following ocular trauma in a cat: Case report and literature review, *J Am Anim Hosp Assoc* 26:63, 1990.
36. Wertheimer N, Leeper E: Electrical wiring configurations and childhood cancer, *Am J Epidemiol* 109:273, 1979.
37. Reif JS, Lower KS, Ogilvie GK: Residential exposure to magnetic fields and risk of canine lymphoma, *Am J Epidemiol* 141:352, 1995.
38. National Research Council Report: *Possible health effects of exposure to residential electric and magnetic fields*, Washington, DC, 1996, National Academy Press.
39. Thrall DE: Orthovoltage radiotherapy of acanthomatous epulides in 39 dogs, *J Am Vet Med Assoc* 184:826, 1984.
40. McEntee MC, Page RL, Theon A, et al: Malignant tumor formation in dogs previously irradiated for acanthomatous epulis, *Vet Radiol Ultrasound* 45:357, 2004.
41. Kuttesch JF, Wexler LH, Marcus RB, et al: Second malignancies after Ewing's sarcoma: radiation dose-dependency of secondary sarcomas, *J Clin Oncol* 14:2818, 1996.
42. Hall EJ, Wuu CS: Radiation-induced second cancers: the impact of 3D-CRT and IMRT, *Int J Radiat Oncol Biol Phys* 56:83, 2003.
43. Suit H, Goldberg S, Niemierko A, et al: Secondary carcinogenesis in patients treated with radiation: A review of data on radiation-induced cancers in human, non-human primate, canine, and rodent subjects, *Radiation Res* 167(1):12, 2007.
44. White RAS, Jefferies AR, Gorman NT, et al: Sarcoma development following irradiation of acanthomatous epulis in two dogs, *Vet Rec* 118:668, 1986.
45. McChesney SL, Withrow SJ, Gillette EL, et al: Radiotherapy in soft tissue sarcomas in dogs, *J Am Vet Med Assoc* 194:60, 1989.
46. Gillette SM, Gillette EL, Powers BE, et al: Radiation-induced osteosarcoma in dogs after external beam or intraoperative radiation therapy, *Cancer Res* 50:54, 1990.
47. Theon AP, Rodriquez C, Griffey S, et al: Analysis of prognostic factors and patterns of failure in dogs with periodontal tumors treated with megavoltage irradiation, *J Am Vet Med Assoc* 210:785, 1997.
48. Loeffler JS, Niemierko A, Chapman P: Second tumors after radiosurgery: Tip of the iceberg or a bump in the road? *Neurosurgery* 52:1436, 2003.
49. Lewis CG, Sunderman FW Jr: Metal carcinogenesis in total joint arthroplasty: animal models, *Clin Orthop* 329S:S264, 1996.
50. Li XQ, Hom DL, Black J, et al: Relationship between metallic implants and cancer: A case control study in a canine population, *Vet Comp Orthop Traumatol* 6:70, 1993.
51. Rowland PH, Moise NS, Severson D: Myxoma at the site of a subcutaneous pacemaker in a dog, *J Am Anim Hosp Assoc* 27:649, 1991.
52. Pardo AD, Adams WH, McCracken D, et al: Primary jejunal osteosarcoma associated with a surgical sponge, *J Am Vet Med Assoc* 196:935, 1990.
53. Orenstein MR, Schenker MB: Environmental asbestos exposure and mesothelioma, *Curr Opin Pulm Med* 6:371, 2000.
54. Glickman LT, Domanski LM, Maguire TG, et al: Mesothelioma in pet dogs associated with exposure of their owners to asbestos, *Environ Res* 32:305, 1983.
55. Harbison ML, Godleski JJ: Malignant mesothelioma in urban dogs, *Vet Pathol* 20:531, 1983.
56. Machida N, Tanaka R, Takemura N, et al: Development of pericardial mesothelioma in golden retrievers with a long-term history of idiopathic haemorrhagic pericardial effusion, *J Comp Pathol* 131:166, 2004.
57. Dorn CA, Taylor DON, Schneider R: Survey of animal neoplasms in Alameda and Contra Costa Counties, California II. Cancer morbidity in dogs and cats from Alameda County, *J Natl Cancer Inst* 40:307, 1968.

58. Moulton JE: Tumors of the mammary gland, In Moulton JE, editor: *Tumours in domestic animals*, ed 3, Berkeley, 1990, University of California Press.
59. Schneider R, Dorn CR, Taylor DON: Factors influencing canine mammary tumor development and postsurgical survival, *J Natl Cancer Inst* 43:1249, 1969.
60. Brodey RS, Goldschmidt MH, Roszel JR: Canine mammary neoplasms, *J Am Anim Hosp Assoc* 19:61, 1983.
61. Perez Alenza MD, Pena L, del Castillo N, et al: Factors influencing the incidence and prognosis of canine mammary tumours, *J Small Anim Pract* 41:287, 2000.
62. MacEwen EG, Patnaik AK, Harvey HJ, et al: Estrogen receptors in canine mammary tumors, *Cancer Res* 42:2255, 1982.
63. Mialot JP, Andre F, Martin PM, et al: Etude de receptors des hormones steroids dans les tumeurs mammaries de la chienne II: correlations avec quelques caracteristiques cliniques, *Recueil Medicine Veterinaire* 158:513, 1982.
64. Monson KR, Malbica JO, Hubben K: Determination of estrogen receptors in canine mammary tumors, *Am J Vet Res* 38:1937, 1987.
65. Donnay I, Rauis J, Devleeschower N, et al: Comparison of estrogen and progesterone receptor expression in normal and mammary tissues from dogs, *Am J Vet Res* 56:1188, 1995.
66. Elling H, Ungemach FR: Simultaneous occurrence for receptors of estradiol, progesterone and dihydrotestosterone in canine mammary tumors, *J Cancer Res Clin Oncol* 105:231, 1983.
67. Sartan EA, Barnes S, Kwapien R, et al: Estrogen and progesterone receptor status of mammary carcinomas and correlations with clinical outcome in the dog, *Am J Vet Res* 53:2196, 1992.
68. Rutteman GR, Misdorp W, Blankenstein NMA, et al: Oestrogen and progestin receptors in mammary tissue of the female dog: different receptor profile in nonmalignant and malignant states, *Breast Cancer* 58:594, 1988.
69. Rutteman GR: Hormones and mammary tumour disease in the female dog: An update, *In Vivo* 4:33, 1990.
70. Stovring M, Moe L, Glattre E: A population-based case-control study of canine mammary tumors and clinical use of medroxyprogesterone acetate, *Acta Pathologica Microbiologica Immunologica Scandinavica* 105:590, 1997.
71. Zanninovic P, Simcic V: Epidemiology of mammary tumors in dogs, *Eur J Comp Anim Pract* IV:67, 1994.
72. Lantinga-van Leeuwen IS, van Garderen E, Rutteman GR, et al: Cloning and cellular localization of the canine progesterone receptor: Co-localization with growth hormone in the mammary gland, *J Steroid Biochem Molec Biol* 75:219, 2000.
73. Mol JA, Lantinga-van Leeuwen I, van Garderen E, et al: Progestin-induced mammary growth hormone (GH) production, *Adv Exp Med Biol* 480:71, 2000.
74. Rijnberk A, Kooistra HS, Mol JA: Endocrine diseases in dogs and cats: Similarities and differences with endocrine diseases in humans, *Growth Horm IGF Res* 13(suppl A):S158, 2003.
75. Hayes HM, Milne KL, Mandell CP: Epidemiological features of feline mammary carcinoma, *Vet Rec* 108:476, 1981.
76. Misdorp W, Romijin A, Hart AAM: Feline mammary tumors: A case-control study of hormonal factors, *Anticancer Res* 11:1793, 1991.
77. Overley B, Shofer FS, Goldschmidt MH, et al: Association between ovarihysterectomy and feline mammary carcinoma, *J Vet Intern Med* 19:560, 2005.
78. National Cancer Institute: *Surveillance, epidemiology and end results program public use data (1973-2000)*, Bethesda, 2003, The Institute.
79. Villamil JA, Henry CJ, Hahn AW, et al: Hormonal and sex impact on the epidemiology of canine lymphoma, *J Cancer Epidemiol* 591753, 2009. Epub 2010 Mar 14.
80. Dow SW, Olson PN, Rosychuk RAW, et al: Perianal adenomas and hypertestosteronemia in a spayed bitch with pituitary-dependent hyperadrenocorticism, *J Am Vet Med Assoc* 192:1439, 1988.
81. Wilson GP, Hayes HM: Castration for treatment of perianal gland neoplasms in the dog, *J Am Vet Med Assoc* 174:1301, 1979.
82. Waters DJ, Sakr WA, Hayden DW, et al: Workgroup 4: Spontaneous prostate carcinoma in dogs and nonhuman primates, *Prostate* 36:64, 1998.
83. Madewell BR, Gandour-Edwards R, White RWD, et al: Canine prostatic intraepithelial neoplasia: Is the comparative model relevant? *Prostate* 58:314, 2004.
84. Teske E, Naan EC, von Dijk EM, et al: Canine prostate carcinoma: epidemiological evidence of an increased risk in castrated dogs, *Mol Cell Endocrinol* 197:251, 2002.
85. Sorenmo KU, Goldschmidt M, Shofer F, et al: Immunohistochemical characteristics of canine prostatic carcinoma and correlation with castration status and castration time, *Vet Comp Oncol* 1:48, 2003.
86. Bryan JN, Keeler MR, Henry CJ, et al: A population study of neutering status as a risk factor for canine prostate cancer, *Prostate* 67:1174, 2007.

SECTION C

Cancer-Causing Viruses

DENNIS W. MACY AND CAROLYN J. HENRY

Both DNA- and RNA-containing viruses are known to cause cancer. An initial step in malignant transformation of normal cells by most tumor viruses is integration of all or part of the viral DNA (or DNA copy of retroviral RNA) into the host cell genome. For some viruses, specific viral genes (oncogenes) have been identified that lead to malignant transformation when expressed in normal cells. Other viruses, through the process of integration, activate the expression of normal cellular genes, leading to overexpression or inactivation of genes, resulting in cellular transformation or uncontrolled growth.[1]

Tumor-Causing Viruses of Dogs

Papillomaviruses

Papillomaviruses are oncogenic, contagious, and infectious and have been described in several animal species.[2] Papillomaviruses are considered species specific, and isolates of humans, cattle, and dogs lack serologic cross-reactivity.[2] However, cross-infection with other species can occur. For example, the coyote can be infected with dog isolates, and bovine papillomaviruses type 1 and type 2 have been reported to infect horses.[3] In addition, bovine papillomaviruses have been isolated from tumors in cats, indicating a unique cross-species infection in a dead-end host.[4]

Four or possibly more papillomaviruses infect dogs and are responsible for a wide spectrum of clinical syndromes. Papillomaviruses of the family Papovaviridae produce benign, mucocutaneous, and cutaneous canine papillomas and in rare cases transform into SCCs.[5,6]

The canine papillomaviruses are naked DNA viruses; they are larger than the canine parvoviruses but similar in structure. Electron microscopy has been used to detect the virus in infected tissues. Like other papillomaviruses, canine papillomaviruses are resistant, acid stable, and relatively thermostable.[7] Only a limited sequence homology exists between the DNA sequences of papillomaviruses of different species, but substantial sequence homology exists between isolates from any given species.[2]

Pathogenesis

Papillomas develop subsequent to introduction of papillomavirus through breaks in the epithelium. Different viruses derived from the same species are believed to correlate with the type of clinical

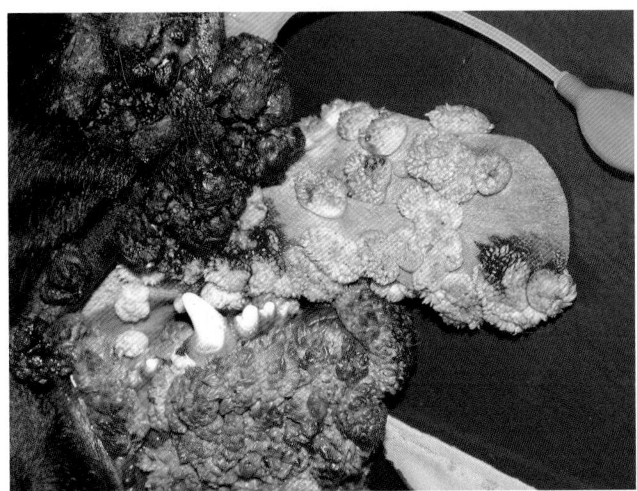

FIGURE 1-9 Multiple papillomatosis in the oral cavity of the dog.

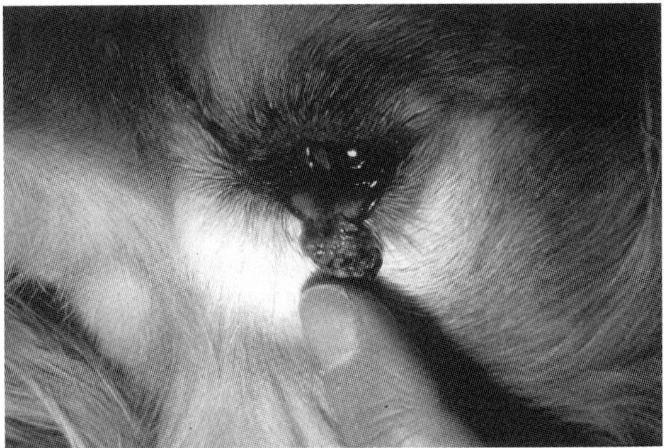

FIGURE 1-10 Solitary ocular papilloma in a dog.

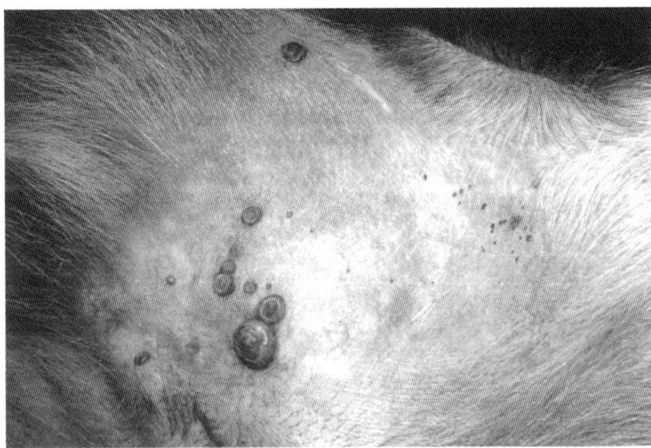

FIGURE 1-11 Multiple cutaneous papillomatosis in the inguinal region of a dog.

disease produced by the virus (i.e., oral versus cutaneous isolates). However, this feature of papillomaviruses has yet to be proven for the dog, and experimentally, ocular isolates have produced oral papillomas.[8-12] The presence and location of mature, complete viruses on the surface of papillomas are believed to aid its transmission to adjacent epithelial tissues.[2] In contrast to other oncogenic or transforming DNA viruses, papillomaviruses rarely integrate into the cellular genome and remain episomal.[2]

Infection of epithelial cells results in a marked increase in cellular mitosis and hyperplasia of cells with a strand of spongiosum, with subsequent degeneration and hyperkeratinization.[13] Clinical evidence of hyperplasia and hyperkeratinization usually manifests 4 to 6 weeks after infection.[13] Canine papillomas generally persist for 4 to 6 months in the mouth and 6 months to 1 year on the skin before undergoing spontaneous regression, and multiple warts generally regress simultaneously.[13] Although antibodies are produced against the papillomavirus, antibody levels do not appear to correlate with either growth or regression of the papilloma; the mechanism of induction or regression remains unknown, although it is thought in most cases to be associated with cellular immunity.[14] The development of multiple papillomavirus-associated epidermal hematomas and SCC in situ in a dog after treatment with prednisone and cyclosporine has been reported.[15]

Clinical Features

Papillomas may be referred to as warts, verruca vulgaris, squamous cell papillomas, or cutaneous papillomatosis. Papillomas caused by the papillomavirus usually are multiple and frequently infect young dogs. In the dog, multiple papillomatosis most frequently is seen in the oral cavity, involving the labial margins, tongue, pharyngeal mucosa, hard palate, and epiglottis (Figure 1-9).[14] Four to 8 weeks after infection, small, pale, smooth, elevated lesions appear; these quickly develop a cauliflower-like appearance, with fine, white frons extending from the surface of the lesions. Multiple sites of susceptible tissue in the oral cavity appear to be affected early in the course of the disease; as many as 50 to 100 tumors may be present at the time of diagnosis.[14] The primary complaints of owners of infected dogs are halitosis, ptyalism, hemorrhage, and difficulty eating. Most oral cavity papillomas start regressing after 4 to 8 weeks. However, some oral lesions may show incomplete regression, and some have been known to persist up to 24 months.[14]

Ocular papillomas, which are less numerous than the oral type, appear on the conjunctiva, cornea, and eyelid margins (Figure 1-10). Ocular papillomas also occur less often than oral lesions.[14] Experimentally, viruses isolated from ocular lesions can produce oral papillomatosis, although whether this occurs in nature is unknown.[8] Ocular papillomatosis most frequently occurs in dogs 6 months to 4 years of age, but it occasionally is reported in older dogs.

Multiple cutaneous papillomatosis is thought to be of viral origin (Figure 1-11); however, evidence suggests that it is not the same strain of papillomavirus that produces oral papillomatosis in the dog.[8] Multiple skin papillomatosis affects a much broader age range of canine patients, and regression of the lesion is prolonged, sometimes taking years.[14] A rare form of cutaneous papillomatosis, in which the lesion appears in the interdigital areas of the pad, has been described in greyhounds, particularly young ones (12 to 18 months of age).[12] Canine pigmented plaques have been associated with papillomaviruses in miniature schnauzers and pugs.[16] The lesions may or may not regress and are considered premalignant.

Although papillomatosis should be considered a benign disease, in rare cases, oral and corneal papillomas have transformed into SCCs.[5,6]

Treatment

Most clinicians elect not to treat papillomatosis because of the lack of proven efficacy of recommended treatments and the expected spontaneous regression of these tumors. However, if the number of papillomas increases or if the animal has significant difficulty eating, owners often request treatment. Surgical excision, cryosurgery, laser surgery, or electrosurgery for just a few lesions has resulted in regression of the remaining papillomas, presumably through immunologic mechanisms.[14,17,18] The exact mechanism by which regression of papillomas occurs is unknown. Serum from dogs in which papillomas have undergone spontaneous regression not only fails to produce tumor regression when administered to infected animals, it actually enhances existing tumor growth. However, administration of immune lymphocytes from dogs in which tumors have regressed has been shown to enhance regression.[7] This effect may be a result of induction of blocking antigen-antibody factors, which may impede cytotoxic lymphocyte action on target cells. CD4 lymphocytes activate macrophages and have been shown to inhibit the virus in dogs.[7] Interferon also has been tried, with some success (1 to 3 million IU/m^2 given subcutaneously three times a week [Monday-Wednesday-Friday]), and chemotherapy of resistant lesions has produced variable results.[19] Corticosteroids should be avoided because they are thought to contribute to the dissemination of papillomas.[20]

Most systemic chemotherapeutic agents (e.g., bleomycin, vincristine, cyclophosphamide, and doxorubicin) have failed to cause regression of papillomas. However, etretinate (1 mg/kg given orally daily) has been effective in some dogs with persistent papillomas.[21,22] Topical or intralesional compounds containing 5-fluorouracil (5-FU) have been used in both humans and dogs to treat papillomas. In the past, autogenous wart vaccines have been recommended but have proved of little value in the treatment of resistant papillomatosis of the dog.[14] In at least one study, papillomavirus vaccines have been shown to prevent the development of oral papillomas in the dog; however, cutaneous neoplasms at the injection sites have been attributed to administration of the vaccines.[11,23,24]

Tumor-Causing Viruses of the Cat

Papillomaviruses

Feline viral papillomatosis is a rarely recognized condition caused by a papillomavirus specific to the cat. The feline isolates *Felis domesticus* papillomavirus type 1 (FdPV-1), FdPV-JM, and FdPV-MY are genomically very similar to canine isolates but are considered species specific.[25] Papillomavirus-associated lesions have been reported in six species of felids besides the domestic cat: the mountain lion, Florida panther, bobcat, Asian lion, snow leopard, and clouded leopard.[26,27] Unlike in the domestic cat, in which the lesions commonly affect areas of haired skin, papillomas in exotic species most often are found in the oral cavity, similar to those in the dog.[26,27] Despite the clinical similarities, genetic and antigenic studies indicate that each species of felid is infected by a unique papillomavirus.

Pathogenesis

In cats, as in other species, papillomas are believed to develop after the virus is introduced through lesions or abrasions in the skin. Unlike in the dog, most feline case reports involve older cats (6 to 13 years of age), although papillomavirus lesions have been reported in kittens 6 to 7 months old.[28,29] As in other species, impaired T-cell function likely plays a significant role in lesion formation. Papillomas in cats that are receiving immunosuppressive therapy or are infected with the feline immunodeficiency virus (FIV) support this hypothesis.

Although papillomas most frequently are benign lesions, recent studies have associated the papillomavirus with SCCs and other malignant neoplasms in cats[30]; specifically, papillomavirus has been isolated from 30 of 63 squamous cell carcinoma in situ skin lesions. Through the use of polymerase chain reaction (PCR) techniques, papillomaviruses have been found in 17 of 19 and 9 of 12 fibropapillomas in cats.[31,32] Although a cause-and-effect relationship has yet to be proved for carcinoma in situ, Bowen's disease, fibropapillomas, and papillomaviruses, the evidence is compelling.[30-32] Over 100 papillomaviruses occur in humans and are believed responsible for cervical cancer, between 25% and 60% of SCCs of the oral cavity, and rarely even some that occur on the skin surface.[33]

Bovine papillomaviruses may also play a role in the pathogenesis of feline cutaneous fibropapillomas. In a study of 20 cats with fibropapillomas, more than half were known to have exposure to cattle, and all were within an area with dairy farms.[31] In one isolate, the nucleotide sequence was similar to that of the bovine papillomavirus. Injection of that isolate back into bovine skin resulted in asymptomatic infection. Also, although papillomaviruses generally are species specific, an association between bovine papillomavirus types 1 and 2 has been suggested as causes of equine sarcoids.[34]

Clinical Features

Lesions in the cat differ from those in the dog because they are more like plaques than warts. The plaques are several millimeters in diameter, may be white or pigmented, and are scaly or greasy. Also, lesions in the cat usually affect haired skin rather than the mucous membrane locations common for oral and ocular papillomas of the dog and wild felids.[26,27]

Diagnosis

Definitive diagnosis depends on histopathologic, immunohistochemical, or electron microscope (EM) examination of excised lesions. Histologic features include proliferation of all cell layers with little or no inflammation. Typically the epidermal hyperplasia is accompanied by acanthosis, hypergranulosis, hyperkeratosis, and ballooning degeneration of cells of the stratum spinosum and stratum granulosum. Amphophilic cytoplasmic inclusion structures may be present in cells of the upper stratum granulosum. EM findings in the lesions include intranuclear particles within keratinized cells in the superficial epithelial strata of the plaques. Immunohistology can be performed on sections using band-reactive, genus-specific antiserum. Interestingly, the histologic features of the feline fibropapilloma are very similar to those of equine sarcoids, with characteristic fibroblastic proliferation, hyperplasia of epidermis, and rete ridges.[31] PCR also has demonstrated papillomavirus DNA in the lesions.

Treatment

Surgical excision is generally used; however, parenteral alpha interferon has been suggested as an alternative. *Medications containing 5-FU that are used in humans and dogs should NOT be used in cats.* Imiquimod 5% cream (Aldara) is a novel immune-response modifier (IRM) that has been used in humans with Bowen's disease and has recently been used in cats with the same disease. Although 41% of cats treated with imiquimod developed some level of toxicity, most adverse events were manageable.[35]

Retroviruses

Retroviral infections are considered the number one infectious cause of morbidity and mortality in the domestic cat. Before the vaccine was developed and routine testing and control measures became widespread, the feline leukemia virus (FeLV) was associated with one-third of deaths in cats.[36,37] The cat is believed to be affected by the largest number of retroviruses of any companion animal, and these viruses produce a wide spectrum of diseases, including cancer.[38-40]

The cat has both endogenous and exogenous retroviruses. The endogenous retroviruses generally are considered nonpathogenic, are present in the host DNA, and are passed from generation to generation genetically, as are other chromosomal genes. The exogenous retroviruses include both pathogenic and nonpathogenic viruses and are passed horizontally and vertically between cats. Pathogenic exogenous retroviruses include FeLV and FIV.[41] The exogenous RNA sequences of FeLV play the most important role in tumorigenesis in the cat.[40] Another pathogenic retrovirus, the feline sarcoma virus (FeSV), arises from the combination of exogenous FeLV and proto-oncogenes in the cat's genome.[42] Feline syncytium-forming virus (FeSFV), also called the *feline foamy virus,* is a nonpathogenic exogenous retrovirus.[36]

FeLV is believed to have been contracted from the ancestral rat approximately 10 million years ago.[43] The ancestral source of other retroviruses is unknown. The three pathogenic retroviruses of clinical importance are FeLV, FIV, and, in rare cases, FeSV.

Feline Leukemia Virus

The retrovirus FeLV belongs to the subfamily oncornavirus, or tumor-producing RNA viruses. Like other retroviruses, it has a single strand of RNA and an enzyme, reverse transcriptase (RT), that synthesizes DNA from the virus RNA template. Nondomestic felids, including the cheetah and bobcat, can be infected by FeLV; however, it is not considered enzootic in wild felids except for European wild cats in France and Scotland.[44,45]

The basic FeLV proteins include the envelope proteins and the core proteins, several of which are important clinically. Two envelope proteins, the P15E and the GP70 glycoproteins, have particular clinical significance.[46-48] P15E is thought to be one of the mediators of immunosuppression in FeLV-infected cats.[49] The glycoprotein of the envelope GP70 may contain three subgroup antigens, A, B, and C.[50,51] An individual cat may have combinations of viruses with these subgroup viral antigens. Considerable antigenic variation exists within subgroups, which can affect the biologic properties of the individual isolates or strains of FeLV.[40,50] These subgroup antigens bind the virion to receptors on the surface of cells. The specific characters of these proteins also predict the pathogenicity, host range, infectivity, and other biologic properties of the virus.[40,50] The antibodies produced against envelope proteins can be neutralizing and thus can prevent infection. Envelope proteins are very important components of FeLV vaccines.

Core proteins (capsids) include P15C, P12, P10, and P27. P27 is quite soluble and can be found in large amounts in the cytoplasm of cells and bodily fluids, such as tears and serum.[46-48] P27 is the antigen that is detected in immunofluorescent assay (IFA) tests and enzyme-linked immunosorbent assays (ELISAs), which are commonly used in the diagnosis of FeLV infection.[51]

Transmission

FeLV is an enveloped virus and is considered very fragile. Desiccation rapidly reduces the amount of viable virus in saliva, and inactivation occurs in 1 to 2 hours. In exudates or blood, the virus may be viable for only 48 hours (at 37° C) or 1 to 2 weeks (at 22° C).[52] Like most retroviruses, FeLV is rapidly inactivated by heating and most disinfectants.[47] Given these characteristics, environmental contamination (e.g., examination tables, cages, and waiting rooms) is unlikely to be a potential source of FeLV infection.[40] Although saliva may contain up to 100,000 virus particles per milliliter, prolonged, intimate contact with infected cats usually is required for transmission. The factors most frequently incriminated in the transmission of FeLV are licking, biting, grooming, and sharing of litter pans, food bowls, and water dishes. Intimate contact is enhanced in catteries and multiple-cat households, where infection rates may be very high.[49]

Although cats may be infected with FeLV subgroups A, B, or C or other recombinants, only subgroup A has been found in cell-free fluids and is thought to be associated with natural transmission of FeLV. Subgroups B and C and other recombinants are more cell associated and are not thought to be transmitted in nature.[53-56]

Before vaccines and routine testing became available, the overall prevalence of FeLV infection in the United States was estimated at 1% to 3% of the population.[38,39] The prevalence of FeLV infection was less than 1% in single-cat households and as high as 30% in multiple-cat households.[57] The incidence of FeLV-positive test results in sick cats in the United States was approximately 11.5%.[58] Several studies have reported a decline in the prevalence of FeLV by as much as 50% over the past 20 years.[37,59,60]

The FeLV subgroups are characterized by their cross-interference with homologous but not heterologous subgroups of FeLV and by their host range and other factors. All naturally infected FeLV cats have subgroup A, 50% of infected cats have a combination of subgroups A and B, and 1% of infected cats in nature have a mixture of subgroup C either as AC or ABC.[38,58,61]

The relevance of subgroups in strains is essential to an understanding of the biodiversity of the clinical disease caused by FeLV infection. Although subgroups A, B, and C maintain 85% genomic homology, cats infected with various combinations of these subgroups may manifest vastly different diseases.

Subgroup A has a variety of strains that range from nonpathogenic to very pathogenic.[62] Although most strains of subgroup A have limited pathogenicity, their pathogenicity increases dramatically if they are present with other subgroups.

Subgroup B is created when subgroup A recombines with endogenous FeLV envelopes at sequences already in the feline genome.[63-65] Each recombination is unique, resulting in many strains of FeLV-B. The combination of subgroups A and B is more contagious and pathogenic than subgroup A alone.[58,61,62] Cats infected with subgroups A and B often develop thymic lymphoma and myeloproliferative disease.[63]

Subgroup C arises from the mutation of subgroup A.[66] Cats may be infected with a combination of C and other subgroups, although these combinations are uncommon and are found in only about 1% of naturally infected cats. FeLV-C is antigenically similar to the associated membrane antigen (feline oncornavirus-associated cell membrane antigen [FOCMA]), and cats carrying FeLV-C have developed severe erythroid hypoplasia and anemia and usually die within 1 to 2 months.[53] Further complicating the biodiversity of subgroups and strains is the fact that subgroups A and B can recombine with proto-oncogenes such as MYC or TCR, producing FeLV-MYC or FeLV-TCR.[36] Both of these recombinants are considered more potent tumor producers than their nonrecombinant FeLV parent. Another subgroup, T, is highly cytolytic for T lymphocytes and causes severe immunosuppression.[54-56]

The Rickard strain of FeLV (FeLV-R), although similar to MYC-containing recombinant strains in its ability to produce mediastinal lymphoma rapidly, does not recombine with the *MYC* gene.[36,67] Instead, it obtains some of the biologic effects by integrating adjacent to the *C-MYC* gene, causing its overexpression.[36]

Feline Oncornavirus-Associated Cell Membrane Antigen

FOCMA is a protein found on the surface of FeLV and FeLV-induced neoplasms but not on nonneoplastic feline cells.[68,69] FOCMA is detected serologically when cells expressing it react to immunoglobulins produced in cats that have regressed FeSV-induced fibrosarcoma or FeLV infection. The presence of FOCMA antibody is determined by the ability of the serum to react with FL74 cells, a transformed infected feline lymphocyte line.[70] Antibodies to FOCMA protect against neoplastic and myeloproliferative disease. Some FeLV vaccines contain FOCMA and elicit an anti-FOCMA response.[71] The relative importance of this in preventing disease in vaccinates is unknown.

Neoplastic Diseases Caused by Feline Leukemia Virus

We have much to learn about the genetic basis for the vast diversity of tumor types produced by FeLV and its recombinants. We now know that FeLV, through one or another of its recombinants, may cause virtually any hematopoietic neoplasm in the cat. The only hematopoietic neoplasms not yet associated with FeLV in nature are mast cell leukemia, eosinophilic leukemia, plasma cell tumors, and polycythemia vera.[36]

Although FeLV infection is considered the most significant infectious cause of morbidity and mortality in cats, only 20% of cats persistently infected with FeLV develop lymphoid cancer.[72,73] The cat has the highest incidence of hematopoietic neoplasms of domestic animals, and the prevalence of lymphoma ranges from 44 to 200 cases per 100,000 cats, six times the rate of this disease in humans.[36] Twenty years ago, 70% of lymphomas in cats were believed to be caused by FeLV.

Some cancers are more commonly associated with FeLV infection than others. Large, granular lymphoma and globular leukocyte tumors usually test negative for FeLV,[74,75] whereas 70% to 90% of cats with nonlymphoid hematopoietic neoplasia (myeloproliferative disease) test positive for FeLV.[36] The percentage of lymphomas that test positive for FeLV also varies, depending on the anatomic location of the tumor.[76-78] Cats with spinal, mediastinal, ocular, and renal lymphoma frequently tested positive for FeLV prior to routine vaccination (more than 70%).[79] Extranodal sites such as lymphomas of the nasal cavity and the alimentary form of lymphoma frequently test negative for FeLV infection.[36] Over the past 20 years, the multicentric FeLV-positive form has declined in young cats, and the FeLV-negative alimentary form in older cats has increased.[80-82] Although the alimentary form most often is FeLV negative, as assessed by IFA and ELISA testing, some of these lesions have been shown by PCR to be FeLV positive, which suggests that the disease may be related to previous FeLV exposure.

Although not all lymphomas are caused by FeLV, the relative risk of developing lymphoma is 62 times higher in FeLV-positive cats, and cats that are FeLV negative but that have had previous exposure to FeLV have a fortyfold increase in the risk of developing lymphoma.[83] Most spontaneous lymphomas of cats that test positive for FeLV arise from T cells, whereas FeLV-negative lymphoma frequently is of alimentary or B-cell origin.[84,85] The time from infection to tumor development varies and may depend on the age at which the cat is infected or on other factors, such as strain, anatomic location, and viral subgroup.[36] The range from the time of experimental infection to tumor production is 1 to 23 months (mean, 5.3 months).[86,87] The younger the cat when infected with FeLV, the shorter the time to the development of neoplastic disease. Some cats infected with FeLV die of immunosuppressive disease before tumors have a chance to develop.

Treatment of Feline Leukemia Virus Infections

Although no effective treatment exists to eliminate established FeLV infection in cats, a variety of antiviral and biologic response modifiers have been used to manage retroviral infections in cats and humans. The mainstay of therapy for cats infected with FeLV or other retroviruses is supportive care.[88-90] Maintaining hydration and nutritional status not only prolongs life but also enhances the patient's quality of life. The cat should be kept in a humid environment to reduce the chance of water loss. Appetite stimulants and placement of gastrostomy tubes may facilitate nutritional therapy. The cat's requirement for B vitamins is eight times that of the dog, and dietary concentrations must be maintained to maintain appetite. Semimoist cat foods often contain propylene glycol, which can shorten red blood cell survival. These foods, although often quite palatable, should not be used for the nutritional management of cats infected with FeLV.[89] Many cats with FeLV are anemic, but administering erythropoietin is not helpful because endogenous erythropoietin levels usually are 20 times normal.[91]

Biologic-Response Modifiers

A variety of biologic-response modifiers (BRMs) has been used in cats infected with FeLV,[92-100] but none has shown benefit in controlled trials. A few of the most popular are discussed here.

Interferons have been studied extensively for the management of FeLV infection, but the results have been mixed. In one study, oral and parenteral doses of either human recombinant interferon-α or bovine interferon failed to alter the viremia or result in clinical improvement. However, some uncontrolled studies have shown improvement in the clinical status of cats treated with oral interferon-α.[99] Controlled trials are needed to establish the true efficacy of these products. Orally administered interferon probably is inactivated by gastric acid in the stomach. Parenterally administered interferons from other species (i.e., bovine and human) are likely to have temporary activity because of the production of neutralizing antibodies.

Carrisyn (Acemannan) is a BRM designed to enhance macrophage phagocytosis and cell killing. Viremic cats treated with carrisyn have been reported to improve clinically; however, the studies reporting these results have not been well controlled, and the observed benefit may be due to the natural waxing and waning clinical course commonly observed in FeLV-positive cats.[100]

Lymphocyte T-cell immunomodulator (LTCI) has recently become commercially available for the treatment of cats infected with FeLV and FIV. The true efficacy of this product, if any, awaits the results of controlled trials in cats.[101]

The apparent positive effect of many of the BRMs, which, in fact, may be due to the anabolic effect observed with some of these cytokines, is thought to be based on endorphin release rather than a direct effect on the viral infection.

Reverse Transcriptase Inhibitors

Drugs that inhibit RT and retrovirus integration into the host cell have been evaluated for their potential use in the treatment of FeLV-positive cats. The drugs evaluated include suramin (a polyionic dye used to treat filariasis in humans), nucleoside analogs (AZT, DDC, DDA, and PNEA), glucose homopolymers, dextran sulfate, phosphonate, and others.[102-105] More detailed descriptions of these therapies are provided elsewhere.[102,105] In general, most of these agents have shown efficacy in vitro against FeLV, the human immunodeficiency virus (HIV), and in some cases, FIV. Most of these drugs result in some reduction in viremia in vivo, but none are capable of reversing established viremia, although some may prevent viremia if administered prophylactically. Most of these drugs cause significant toxicities at the dosages needed to produce antiviral effects and therefore have not gained popularity in clinical practice. AZT (zidovudine) is the most widely studied RT inhibitor.[106] AZT inhibits FeLV reverse transcriptase when administered at a dosage of 10 to 20 mg/kg in daily divided doses. AZT prevents viremia if given within 72 hours of exposure to FeLV. The antiviral effects of AZT appear to be synergistic with interferon.[107,108] Reversal of established experimental FeLV viremia through adoption transfer of lectin/IL-2–activated lymphocytes, interferon-α, and AZT has been reported.

Prevention and Control

The most effective means of preventing FeLV infection is to eliminate contact with viremic cats. The test and removal program is the most effective means of controlling FeLV in multiple-cat households.[109] The program consists of closing the household or cattery to new cats, testing the remaining cats every 3 months, and removing all animals that test positive. When all cats test negative for two consecutive sessions, the facility is determined to be FeLV free. New cats may enter the household or facility only after a 3-month quarantine and two negative FeLV tests. The test and removal system has been shown to reduce the incidence of FeLV in a variety of settings and geographic locations.[109]

Prevention by Vaccination

Vaccinations help control or eliminate many infectious diseases in veterinary medicine. The first commercial FeLV vaccine was introduced in 1985. Since then, seven FeLV vaccine products from six companies have been licensed for sale to veterinarians in the United States. Despite the fact that FeLV vaccines have been available for a decade, a survey of US veterinary teaching hospitals in 1991 found that only two of the 22 teaching hospitals considered FeLV vaccination to be part of their routine feline preventive medicine program.[110] The principal concern has been the perceived lack of efficacy of the FeLV vaccines. Some studies of available vaccines have reported efficacies ranging from 0 to 100%.[111] In addition to efficacy questions, it has been established that soft tissue sarcomas may develop after FeLV and rabies vaccination.[112]

FeLV vaccination issues are discussed elsewhere.[71] However, several comments regarding FeLV vaccines should help practitioners decide whether to use FeLV vaccines in their practice. FeLV vaccines may contain two or three subgroup antigens. Because only subgroup A is transmitted contagiously between cats, vaccines need only to contain subgroup A. Their primary means of protecting against tumor development is preventing persistent viremia. If a vaccine protects against persistent FeLV infection, it need not contain FOCMA. The value of FOCMA in FeLV vaccines has yet to be proved. Vaccines should protect against a variety of strains of subgroup A, and none of the available vaccines contain more than one strain of subgroup A. Differences in published comparative studies of vaccine efficacy probably are related to differences in vaccine strains and to the challenge strains used. Vaccines that contain adjuvants enhance immunity but at the expense of producing local inflammatory reactions at the injection site.[113] These local reactions may lead to the development of soft tissue sarcomas. However, the development of soft tissue sarcomas after vaccination, either with rabies or FeLV vaccines, is thought to occur in only 1 in 1000 to 1 in 10,000 vaccinates.[112] Nonadjuvanted FeLV vaccines have shown little or no inflammatory reaction 21 days after administration.[113] A canarypox-vectored FeLV nonadjuvanted vaccine is available that stimulates both cellular and humoral immunity without significant injection site inflammation. Clinical discretion should be used when recommending FeLV vaccines.

The American Association of Feline Practitioners (AAFP) does not consider FeLV vaccine a core vaccine, and only cats at significant risk should be vaccinated. Cats under 12 weeks of age have an 85% chance of becoming persistently infected, whereas cats over 6 months of age have only a 15% chance of becoming persistently infected after challenge. Age-acquired immunity of adult cats is associated with improved macrophage function and reduced viral receptors on target tissues. Annual vaccination of adult cats also appears to be a questionable practice, given age-acquired immunity and the risk of vaccine-associated sarcomas.

Feline Sarcoma Virus

FeSVs are true hybrids that result from the rare recombination of FeLV DNA provirus with cat proto-oncogenes. Cats have at least 30 proto-oncogenes.[36,114,115] Proto-oncogenes have many biologic functions; when they are altered and activated inappropriately, they are called *oncogenes,* which can play a key role in the development of cancerous phenotypes. Proto-oncogenes can be activated by mutations that produce chromosomal translocations such as those that may be associated with inflammation and vaccine-associated sarcomas, or by incorporation into a retrovirus, such as FeLV.[114-116] When FeLV-derived DNA inserts near a proto-oncogene and takes up the proto-oncogene into the FeLV provirus, formation of FeSV results. In the process, part of the FeLV GAG gene, most of the FeLV envelope gene, and all of the pole genes are lost.[115] The loss of these vital components makes FeSV dependent on FeLV as a helper virus for replication. Cats that have FeSV always test FeLV positive. Because several different recombinations may recur with several different proto-oncogenes, each recombination is a unique event, and each isolate is distinct.[116] Despite this phenotypic heterogeneity, the recombinations transform fibroblasts, and all produce fibrosarcomas.

Natural transmission of FeSV between cats has not been described, and as with other FeLV recombinants (e.g., FeLV-B), transmission of the recombinant product is not thought to occur in nature. Some cats are capable of rejecting transformed cells and producing FOCMA antibody.[90,91] FOCMA is important in the experimental response of cats to FeSV because it has been associated with tumor regression and failure to develop tumors.[117,118] Cats that fail to develop antibodies against FOCMA die quickly of fast-growing sarcomas.[119]

Clinical Features of Feline Sarcoma Virus and Induced Fibrosarcomas

Only 2% of fibrosarcomas of cats are virally induced.[42] In contrast to the solitary, slow-growing, nonvirally induced sarcomas seen in older cats, FeSV-induced tumors are multicentric and are found most frequently in young cats.[120] They are characterized by rapid growth, including doubling times as short as 12 to 72 hours.[36] This rapid growth often is accompanied by superficial ulceration. Lesions frequently occur at sites of previous bite wounds.[36] Metastasis to the lungs or other organs occurs with approximately 30% of virally induced fibrosarcomas in cats. Hypercalcemia was observed in association with multicentric fibrosarcomas in one cat with FeSV.[36] Virally induced fibrosarcomas are always FeLV positive; this helps differentiate them from vaccine-associated sarcomas, which have growth characteristics similar to those of virally induced tumors. Cats with multicentric FeSV-induced tumors have a very poor prognosis. Doxorubicin, vincristine, vinblastine, lomustine (CCNU), and radiotherapy have been used to treat vaccine-associated sarcomas in the cat.[121] Although radiotherapy often is used in combination with surgery, recurrence both within and outside the treatment fields is common.

Feline Immunodeficiency Virus

FIV, which is classified as a retrovirus in the subfamily Lentivirinae, is distinct from other retroviruses that infect cats. Like other retroviruses, FIV is an enveloped, single-stranded RNA virus in which the RNA is copied into the DNA in the infected host by RT in the virus.

The nucleotide sequence of several FIV isolates has been determined, and genetic homology falls between 36% and 97%. Despite this homology, significant differences in pathogenicity and infectivity exists between FIV strains.[122,123] Although lentiviruses are known to infect wild felids, they are antigenically distinct from domestic cat isolates; they also are well adapted to their host and seldom cause clinical disease.

Transmission

FIV is present in all bodily fluids of infected cats, similar to FeLV, but at much lower concentrations. FIV is mainly cell associated and is present in relatively low concentrations in the blood, although high amounts can be found in the saliva.[124,125] FIV is not thought to be very infectious and is mainly transmitted through biting during cat fights.[126,127]

Feline Immunodeficiency Virus–Associated Neoplasms

The prevalence of neoplasms in FIV-positive cats ranges from 1% to 62%.[83,128,129] Lymphomas and myeloid tumors (myelogenous leukemia, myeloproliferative disease) and a few carcinomas and sarcomas are the neoplasms most commonly linked to FIV infection. One study found that cats infected with FIV and FeLV are 5.6 times more likely to develop lymphoma or leukemia than if they had been infected with either virus alone. Cats with combined infections had a 77.3% greater likelihood of developing lymphoma or leukemia than noninfected cats.[83] Lymphoreticular neoplasms have been linked to HIV infection in humans and simian immunodeficiency virus (SIV) infection in nonhuman primates. In contrast to FeLV-associated lymphomas, FIV-associated lymphomas most often develop in extranodal sites and occur in older cats (mean age, 8.7 years).[83] Myeloproliferative disease also has been observed in cats naturally and in cats experimentally infected with FIV.[83,130,131]

Although lentiviruses such as FIV have not been thought to be oncogenic in themselves, they are markedly immunosuppressive and affect normal immunosurveillance of cancerous cells. FIV-positive cats with lymphoma have extremely low CD4 lymphocyte counts.[121] SCCs of the skin have been linked to FIV infection in two geographic areas, California and Colorado, but this association is believed to be due to a co-risk behavior (outdoor cats) rather than to any direct viral contribution to tumor development.[132,133] Other reports have linked FIV infection to oral SCC, mammary carcinoma, fibrosarcoma, myeloproliferative disease, and histiocytic mast cell disease.[128,134,135] The nature of these associations awaits further investigation.

Treatment

The same treatment considerations in the management of cats with FeLV can be applied to the treatment of FIV-positive cats. The most widely applied treatments have been the RT inhibitors and interferon (see the earlier discussion on the treatment of FeLV). As in the treatment of FeLV, FIV-positive cats remain positive despite these therapies. A single inactivated FIV vaccine has been licensed for use in domestic cats. However, this is an adjuvanted vaccine, and it may be associated with an increased risk of vaccine-associated sarcoma. The primary concern with the vaccine is that it generates antibodies that cross-react with the currently recommended antibody-based diagnostic test for FIV infection. PCR-based tests are not currently considered reliable for diagnosis of FIV, and antibody-based testing remains the gold standard. It is important to note that the AAFP does not recommend the use of an FIV vaccine in domestic cats.

Comparative Aspects

The association between human viruses and certain cancers has been established on the basis of epidemiologic, clinical, and molecular studies.[1] Human T-cell leukemia virus (HTLV-1) has been linked to adult T-cell leukemia. The human papillomavirus (HPV) is associated with cervical cancer. The Epstein-Barr virus (EBV) is related to the development of Burkitt's lymphoma and nasopharyngeal carcinoma, and human hepatitis B and C viruses are associated with hepatocellular carcinoma. The human herpes virus (HHV) is implicated in the development of Kaposi's sarcoma.

REFERENCES

1. Benchimol S, Minden MD: Viruses, oncogenes, and tumor suppressor genes. In Tannock IF, Hill RP, editors: *The basis science of oncology*, ed 3, New York, 1998, McGraw-Hill.
2. Pfister HH: Biology and biochemistry of papillomaviruses, *Rev Physiol Biochem Pharmacol* 99:111–181, 1984.
3. Sundberg JP, Reszler AA, Williams ES, et al: An oral papillomavirus that infected one coyote and three dogs, *Vet Pathol* 28:87–88, 1991.
4. Munday JS, Knight CG: Amplification of feline sarcoid-associated papillomaviruses DNA sequences from bovine skin, *Vet Dermatol* 21:341, 2010.
5. Belkin PV: Ocular lesions in canine oral papillomatosis, *Vet Med Small Anim Clin* 74:1520–1524, 1979.
6. Watrach AM, Small E, Case MT: Canine papilloma: progression of oral papilloma to carcinoma, *J Natl Cancer Inst* 45:915–920, 1970.
7. Nicholls PE, Starley MA: The immunology of animal papillomaviruses, *Vet Immunol Immunopathol* 73:101–127, 2000.
8. Tokita H, Konishi S: Studies on canine oral papillomatosis. II. Oncogenicity of canine oral papilloma virus to various tissues of dog with special reference to eye tumor, *Jpn J Vet Sci* 37:109–120, 1975.
9. Hare CL, Howard EB: Canine conjunctiva-corneal papillomatosis, *J Am Anim Hosp Assoc* 13:688–690, 1977.
10. Bonney CH, Koch SA, Conter AW, et al: Case report: A conjunctivocorneal papilloma with evidence of a viral etiology, *J Small Anim Pract* 21:183–188, 1980.
11. Bregman CL, Hirth RS, Sundberg JP, et al: Cutaneous neoplasms in dogs associated with canine oral papillomavirus, *Vet Pathol* 24:477–487, 1987.
12. Davis PE, Huxtable CRR, Sabcine M: Dermal papillomas in the racing greyhound, *Aust J Dermatol* 17:13–16, 1976.
13. Theilen GH, Madewell BR: Papillomatosis and fibromatosis. In Theilen GH, Madewell BR, editors: *Veterinary cancer medicine*, Philadelphia, 1987, Lea & Febiger.
14. Calvert CA: Canine viral papillomatosis. In Greene GE, editor: *Infectious diseases of the dog and cat*, Philadelphia, 1991, WB Saunders.
15. Callan MB, Preziosi D, Mauldin E: Multiple papillomavirus-associated epidermal hamartomas and squamous cell carcinomas in

situ in a dog following treatment with prednisone and cyclosporine, *Vet Dermatol* 16:338, 2005.
16. Nagata M: Canine papillomatosis. In Bonagura JD, editor: *Kirk's current veterinary therapy XIII*, Philadelphia, 2000, WB Saunders.
17. Bonney CH, Koch SA, Dice PF, et al: Papillomatosis of conjunctiva and adnexa in dogs, *J Am Vet Med Assoc* 176:48, 1980.
18. Kuntsi-Vaattovaara H, Verstraete FJM, Newsome JT, et al: Resolution of persistent oral papillomatosis in a dog after treatment with a recombinant canine oral papillomavirus vaccine, *Vet Comp Oncol* 1:57, 2003.
19. Bomholt A: Interferon therapy for laryngeal papillomatosis in adults, *Arch Otolaryngol* 109:550–552, 1983.
20. Sundberg JP, Smith EK, Herron AJ, et al: Cutaneous verrucosis in a Chinese Shar pei dog, *Vet Pathol* 31:183, 1994.
21. Nagata M: Canine papillomatosis. In Bonagura JD, editor: *Kirk's current veterinary therapy XIII*, Philadelphia, 2000, WB Saunders.
22. Nagata M, Nanko H, Moriyana A, et al: Pigmented plaques associated with papillomavirus infection in dogs: is this epidermodysplasia verruciformis? *Vet Dermatol* 6:179, 1995.
23. Bregman CL, Hinth RS, Sundberg JP, et al: Cutaneous neoplasms in dogs associated with canine oral papillomavirus vaccine, *Vet Pathol* 24:477, 1987.
24. Meunier LD: Squamous cell carcinoma in beagles subsequent to canine oral papillomavirus vaccine, *Lab Anim Sci* 40:568, 1990.
25. Munday JS, Willis KA, Kiupel M, et al: Amplification of three different papillomaviral DNA sequences from a cat with viral plaques, *Vet Dermatol* 19:400, 2008.
26. Schulman FY, Krafft AE, Janczewski T, et al: Cutaneous fibropapilloma in a mountain lion *(Felis concolor)*, *J Zoo Wildl Med* 34:179, 2003.
27. Sundberg JP, Van Ranst M, Montali R, et al: Feline papillomas and papillomaviruses, *Vet Pathol* 37:1, 2000.
28. Egberink HF, Horzinek MC: Feline viral papillomatosis. In Greene CE, editor: *Infectious diseases of the dog and cat*, ed 2, Philadelphia, 1998, WB Saunders.
29. Lozano-Alarcon F, Lewis TP, Clark EG, et al: Persistent papillomavirus infection in a cat, *J Am Anim Hosp Assoc* 32:392, 1996.
30. LeClerc SM, Clark EG, Haines DM: Papillomavirus infection in association with feline cutaneous squamous cell carcinoma *in situ*, *Proc Am Assoc Vet Derm/Am Coll Vet Derm* 13:125, 1997.
31. Schulman FY, Krafft AE, Janczewski T: Feline cutaneous fibropapillomas: clinicopathologic findings and association with papillomavirus infection, *Vet Pathol* 38:291, 2001.
32. Teifke JP, Kidney BA, Lohr CV, et al: Detection of papillomavirus DNA in mesenchymal tumour cells and not in the hyperplastic epithelium of feline sarcoids, *Vet Dermatol* 14:1, 47, 2003.
33. Munday JS, Kiuppel M: Papillomavirus-associated cutaneous neoplasia in mammals, *Vet Pathol* 47:254, 2010.
34. Angelos JA, Marti E, Lazary S, et al: Characterization of BPV-like DNA in equine sarcoids, *Arch Virol* 119:95, 1991.
35. Gill VL, Bergman PJ, Baer KE, et al: Use of Imiquimod cream (Aldara) in cats with multicentric squamous cell carcinoma in situ: 12 cases (2002-2005), *Vet Compar Oncol* 16:55, 2008.
36. Rojko JL, Hardy WD Jr: Feline leukemia virus and other retroviruses. In Sherding RG, editor: *The cat: Diseases and clinical management*, ed 2, New York, 1994, Churchill Livingstone.
37. Cotter SM: Feline viral neoplasia. In Greene CE, editor: *Infectious diseases of the dog and cat*, ed 2, Philadelphia, 1998, WB Saunders.
38. Hardy WD Jr, Hess PW, MacEwen EG, et al: Biology of feline leukemia virus in the natural environment, *Cancer Res* 36:582, 1976.
39. Essex M: Feline leukemia and sarcoma viruses. In Klein G, editor: *Viral oncology*, New York, 1980, Raven Press.
40. Hardy WD Jr: The feline leukemia virus, *J Am Anim Hosp Assoc* 17:951, 1981.
41. Pedersen NC: Feline immunodeficiency virus. In Schellekens LT, Horzinek MC, editors: *Animal models in AIDS*, Amsterdam, 1990, Elsevier.
42. Hardy WD Jr: The feline sarcoma viruses, *J Am Anim Hosp Assoc* 17:981, 1981.
43. Benveniste RE, Sherr CJ, Todaro GJ: Evolution of type C viral genes: origin of feline leukemia virus, *Science* 190:886, 1975.
44. Daniels MJ, Golder MC, Jarrett O, et al: Feline viruses in wildcats from Scotland, *J Wildl Dis* 35:121, 1999.
45. Marker L, Munson L, Basson PA, et al: Multicentric T-cell lymphoma associated with feline leukemia virus infection in a captive Namibian cheetah *(Acinonyx jubatus)*, *J Wildl Dis* 39:690, 2003.
46. Schafer W, Bolognesi DP: Mammalian type C oncornaviruses: relationships between viral structure and cell surface antigens and their possible significance in immunological defense mechanisms, *Contemp Top Immunobiol* 6:127, 1977.
47. Bolognesi DP, Montelaro RC, Frank H, et al: Assembly of type C oncornaviruses: A model, *Science* 199:183, 1978.
48. Hardy WD Jr: Immunology of oncornaviruses, *Vet Clin North Am Small Anim Pract* 4:133, 1974.
49. Sarma PS, Log T: Subgroup classification of feline leukemia and sarcoma viruses by viral interference and neutralization tests, *Virology* 54:160, 1973.
50. Sarma PS, Log T, Jain D, et al: Differential host range of viruses of feline leukemia-sarcoma complex, *Virology* 64:438, 1975.
51. Hardy WD Jr, Hirshaut Y, Hess P: Detection of the feline leukemia virus and other mammalian oncornaviruses by immunofluorescence. In Dutcher RM, Chieco-Bianchi L, editors: *Unifying concepts of leukemia*, Basel, 1973, S Karger.
52. Francis DP, Essex M, Gayzagian D: Feline leukemia virus: Survival under home and laboratory conditions, *J Clin Microbiol* 9:154, 1979.
53. Dornsife RE, Gasper PW, Mullins JI: Induction of aplastic anemia by intrabone marrow inoculation of a molecularly cloned feline retrovirus, *Leuk Res* 13:745, 1989.
54. Hartmann K, Werner RM, Egberink H, et al: Comparison of six in-house tests for the rapid diagnosis of feline immunodeficiency and feline leukaemia virus infections, *Vet Rec* 149:317, 2001.
55. Lauring AS, Anderson MM, Overbaugh J: Specificity in receptor usage by T-cell–tropic feline leukemia viruses: implications for the in vivo tropism of immunodeficiency-inducing variants, *J Virol* 75:8888, 2001.
56. Lauring AS, Cheng HH, Eiden MV, et al: Genetic and biochemical analyses of receptor and cofactor determinants for T-cell–tropic feline leukemia virus infection, *J Virol* 76:8069, 2002.
57. Essex M, Cotter SM, Sliski AH, et al: Horizontal transmission of feline leukaemia under natural conditions in a feline leukaemia cluster household, *Int J Cancer* 19:90, 1977.
58. Vail DM, Moore AS, Ogilvie GK, et al: Feline lymphoma (145 cases): proliferation indices, CD3 immunoreactivity and their association with prognosis in 90 cats receiving therapy, *J Vet Intern Med* 12:349, 1998.
59. Louwerens M, London CA, Pedersen NC, et al: Feline lymphoma in the post-feline leukemia virus era, *J Vet Intern Med* 19:329, 2005.
60. Jarrett O, Hardy WD Jr, Golder MC, et al: The frequency of occurrence of feline leukaemia virus subgroups in cats, *Int J Cancer* 21:334, 1978.
61. Jarrett O, Russell PH: Differential growth and transmission in cats of feline leukaemia viruses of subgroups A and B, *Int J Cancer* 21:466, 1978.
62. Rosenburg Z, Pederson FF, Haseltine WA: Comparative analysis of the genome of feline leukemia virus, *J Virol* 35:542, 1980.
63. Tzavaras T, Stewart M, McDougall A, et al: Molecular cloning and characterization of a defective recombinant feline leukaemia virus associated with myeloid leukaemia, *J Gen Virol* 71:343, 1990.
64. Stewart MA, Warnock M, Wheeler A, et al: Nucleotide sequences of a feline leukemia virus subgroup: A envelope gene and long terminal repeat and evidence for the recombinational origin of subgroup B viruses, *J Virol* 58:825, 1986.
65. Elder JM, Mullins JI: Nucleotide sequence of the envelope gene of Gardner-Arnstein feline leukemia virus B reveals unique sequence

homologies with a murine mink cell focus-forming virus, *J Virol* 46:871, 1983.
66. Rigby MA, Rojko JL, Stewart MA, et al: Partial dissociation of subgroup C phenotype and in vivo behaviour in feline leukaemia viruses with chimeric envelope genes, *J Gen Virol* 73:2839, 1992.
67. Heding LD, Schaller JP, Blakeslee JR, et al: Inactivation of tumor cell–associated feline oncornavirus for preparation of an infectious virus–free tumor cell immunogen, *Cancer Res* 36:1647, 1976.
68. Essex M, Klein G, Snyder SP, et al: Feline sarcoma virus (FSV)–induced tumors: correlation between humoral antibody and tumor regression, *Nature* 233:195, 1971.
69. Vedbrat S, Rasheed S, Lutz H, et al: Feline oncornavirus–associated cell membrane antigen: a viral and not a cellularly coded transformation-specific antigen of cat lymphomas, *Virology* 124:445, 1983.
70. Snyder HW, Singhal MC, Zuckerman EE, et al: The feline oncornavirus associated cell membrane antigen (FOCMA) is related to, but distinguishable from, FeLV-C gp70, *Virology* 131:315, 1983.
71. Macy DW: Vaccination against feline retroviruses. In August J, editor: *Consultations in feline internal medicine*, Philadelphia, 1994, WB Saunders.
72. Dorn CR, Taylor DON, Schneider R, et al: Survey of animal neoplasms in Alameda and Contra Costa counties, California. II. Cancer morbidity in dogs and cats from Alameda county, *J Natl Cancer Inst* 40:307, 1968.
73. Schneider R: Comparison and age- and sex-specific incidence rate patterns of the leukemia complex in the cat and the dog, *J Natl Cancer Inst* 70:971, 1983.
74. Goitsuka R, Tsuji M, Matsumoto Y, et al: A case of feline large granular lymphoma, *Jpn J Vet Sci* 50:593, 1988.
75. Finn JP, Schwartz LW: A neoplasm of globule leukocytes in the intestine of a cat, *J Comp Pathol* 82:323, 1972.
76. Hardy WD Jr, McClelland AJ, Zuckerman EE, et al: Development of virus non-producer lymphosarcomas in pet cats exposed to FeLV, *Nature* 288:90, 1980.
77. Hardy WD Jr, Zuckerman EE, McClelland AJ, et al: The immunology and epidemiology of FeLV-nonproducer feline lymphosarcomas, *Cold Spring Harbor Conf Cell Prolif* 7:677, 1980.
78. Hardy WD Jr: Hematopoietic tumors of cats. *J Am Anim Hosp Assoc* 17:921, 1981.
79. Spodnick GJ, Berg J, Moore FM, et al: Spinal lymphoma in cats: 21 cases (1976-1989), *J Am Vet Med Assoc* 200:373, 1992.
80. Hartmann K, Gerle K, Leutenegger C, et al: Feline leukemia virus: Most important oncogene in cats? Abstracts from the Fourth International Feline Retrovirus Research Symposium, Glasgow, 1998.
81. Cotter SM: Feline viral neoplasia. In Greene CE, editor: *Infectious diseases of the dog and cat*, Philadelphia, 1990, WB Saunders.
82. Teske E, van Straten G, van Noort R, et al: Chemotherapy with cyclophosphamide, vincristine, and prednisolone (COP) in cats with malignant lymphoma: New results with an old protocol, *J Vet Intern Med* 16:179, 2002.
83. Shelton GH, Grant CK, Cotter SM, et al: Feline immunodeficiency virus and feline leukemia virus infections and their relationships to lymphoid malignancies in cats: A retrospective study (1968-1988), *J Acquir Immune Defic Syndr* 3:623, 1990.
84. Hardy WD Jr, Zuckerman BE, MacEwen EG, et al: A feline leukemia and sarcoma virus–induced tumor-specific antigen, *Nature* 270:249, 1977.
85. Hardy WD Jr, Zuckerman EE, Essex M, et al: Feline oncornavirus–associated cell membrane antigen: an FeLV- and FeSV-induced tumor-specific antigen. In Clarkson B, Marks PA, Till JE, editors: *Differentiation of normal and neoplastic hematopoietic cells*, Cold Spring Harbor, New York, 1978, Cold Spring Harbor Laboratory Press.
86. Francis DP, Cotter SM, Hardy WD Jr, et al: Comparison of virus-positive and virus-negative cases of feline leukemia and lymphoma, *Cancer Res* 39:3866, 1979.
87. McClelland AJ, Hardy WD Jr, Zuckerman EE: Prognosis of healthy feline leukemia virus infected cats, *Dev Cancer Res* 4:121, 1980.
88. Cotter SM: Feline leukemia virus: pathophysiology, prevention and treatment, *Cancer Invest* 10:173, 1992.
89. Cotter SM: Management of healthy feline leukemia virus–positive cats, *J Am Vet Med Assoc* 199:1470, 1991.
90. August JR: Husbandry practices for cats infected with feline leukemia virus or feline immunodeficiency virus, *J Am Vet Med Assoc* 199:1474, 1991.
91. Kociba GJ, Lange RD, Dunn CD, et al: Serum erythropoietin changes in cats with feline leukemia virus–induced erythroid aplasia, *Vet Pathol* 20:548, 1983.
92. Snyder HW Jr, Singhal MC, Hardy WD Jr, et al: Clearance of feline leukemia virus from persistently infected pet cats treated by extracorporeal immunoadsorption is correlated with an enhanced antibody response to FeLV gp70, *J Immunol* 132:1538, 1984.
93. MacEwen EG: *Current immunotherapeutic approaches in small animals, Proceedings of the Kal Kan Symposium on Oncology*, Columbus, 1986.
94. Kitchen LW, Mather FJ: Hematologic effects of short-term oral diethylcarbamazine treatment given to chronically feline leukemia virus infected cats, *Cancer Lett* 45:183, 1989.
95. Kitchen LW, Cotter SM: Effect of diethylcarbamazine on serum antibody to feline oncornavirus–associated cell membrane antigen in feline leukemia virus–infected cats, *J Clin Lab Immunol* 25:101, 1988.
96. Barta O: Immunoadjuvant therapy. In Kirk RW, Bonagura JD, editors: *Kirk's current veterinary therapy XI: Small animal practice*, Philadelphia, 1992, WB Saunders.
97. Elmslie RE, Ogilvie GK, Dow SW, et al: Evaluation of a biologic response modifier derived from *Serratia marcescens:* effects on feline macrophages and usefulness for the prevention and treatment of viremia in feline leukemia virus–infected cats, *Mol Biother* 3:231, 1991.
98. Gasper PW, Fulton R, Thrall MA: Bone marrow transplantation: Update and current considerations. In Kirk RW, Bonagura JD, editors: *Kirk's current veterinary therapy XI: Small animal practice*, Philadelphia, 1992, WB Saunders.
99. Tompkins MB, Cummins JM: Response of feline leukemia virus–induced nonregenerative anemia to oral administration of an interferon-containing preparation, *Feline Pract* 12:6, 1982.
100. Tizard I: Use of immunomodulators as an aid to clinical management of feline leukemia virus–infected cats, *J Am Vet Med Assoc* 199:1482, 1991.
101. Gingerich DA: Lymphocyte T-cell immunomodulator (LTCI): Review of the immunopharmacology of a new veterinary biologic, *Intern J Applied Res Vet Med* 6:61, 2008.
102. Polas PV, Swenson CL, Sams R, et al: In vitro and in vivo evidence that the antiviral activity of 2-3-dideoxycytidine is target cell–dependent in a feline retrovirus animal model, *Antimicrob Agents Chemother* 34:1414, 1990.
103. Zeidner NS, Strobel JD, Perigo NA, et al: Treatment of FeLV-induced immunodeficiency syndrome (FeLV-FAIDS) with controlled release capsular implantation of 2′,3′-dideoxycytidine, *Antiviral Res* 11:147, 1989.
104. DeClerq E, Sakuma T, Baba M, et al: Antiviral activity of phosphonymethoxyalkyl derivatives of purines and pyrimidines. *Antiviral Res* 8:261, 1987.
105. Hoover EA, Ebner JP, Zeidner NS, et al: Early therapy of feline leukemia virus infection (FeLV-FAIDS) with 9-(2-phosphonylmethoxyethyl) adenine (PMEA), *Antiviral Res* 16:77, 1991.
106. Hoover EA, Zeidner NS, Mullins JI: Therapy of presymptomatic FeLV-induced immunodeficiency syndrome with AZT in combination with α-interferon, *Ann NY Acad Sci* 616:258, 1990.
107. Zeidner NS, Myles MH, Mathiason-DuBard CK, et al: α-Interferon (2b) in combination with zidovudine for the treatment of

presymptomatic feline leukemia virus–induced immunodeficiency syndrome, *Antimicrob Agents Chemother* 34:1749, 1990.
108. Zeidner NS, Mathiason-DuBard CK, Hoover EA: Reversal of feline leukemia virus infection by adoptive transfer of lectin/interleukin-2–activated lymphocytes, interferon-α and zidovudine, *J Immunother* 14:22, 1993.
109. Hardy WD Jr, McClelland AJ, Zuckerman EE, et al: Prevention of the contagious spread of feline leukaemia virus and the development of leukaemia in pet cats, *Nature* 263:326, 1976.
110. Macy DW: Unpublished data. 1992.
111. Legendre AM, Hawks DM, Sebring R: Comparison of the efficacy of three commercial FeLV vaccines in a natural challenge, *J Am Vet Med Assoc* 199:1446, 1991.
112. Hendrick WH, Kass PH, McGill LD, et al: Postvaccinal sarcomas in cats, *J Natl Cancer Inst* 86:5, 341, 1994.
113. Macy DW: Unpublished data, 1994.
114. Varmus HE: Form and function of retroviral proviruses, *Science* 216:812, 1982.
115. Coffin JM: Structure, replication and recombination of retrovirus genomes: some unifying hypotheses, *J Gen Virol* 42:1, 1979.
116. Besmer P: Acute transforming feline retroviruses, *Contemp Top Microbiol Immunol* 107:1, 1993.
117. Essex M, Klein G, Snyder SP, et al: Feline sarcoma virus (FSV)–induced tumors: correlation between humoral antibody and tumor regression, *Nature* 233:195, 1971.
118. Essex M, Klein G, Synder SP, et al: Antibody to feline oncornavirus–associated cell membrane antigen in neonatal cats, *Int J Cancer* 8:384, 1971.
119. Essex M, Cotter SM, Hardy WD Jr, et al: Feline oncornavirus–associated cell membrane antigen. IV. Antibody titers in cats with naturally occurring leukemia, lymphoma, and other diseases, *J Natl Cancer Inst* 55:463, 1975.
120. Patnaik AK, Liu SK, Hurvitz AI, et al: Nonhematopoietic neoplasms in cats, *J Natl Cancer Inst* 54:855, 1975.
121. Macy DW: Unpublished data, 1992.
122. Sieblink HJ, Chu I, Rimmelzwaan GF, et al: Isolation and partial characterization of infectious molecular clones of feline immunodeficiency virus directly obtained from bone marrow DNA of a naturally infected cat. Paper presented at the First International Conference of Feline Immunodeficiency Virus Researchers, 1990, Davis, CA.
123. Hoise MJ, Jarrett O: Serological responses of cats to feline immunodeficiency virus, *AIDS* 4:215, 1990.
124. Yamamoto JK, Sparger E, Ho EW, et al: Pathogenesis of experimentally-induced feline immunodeficiency virus infection in cats, *Am J Vet Res* 49:1246, 1988.
125. Yamamoto JK, Hansen H, Ho EW, et al: Epidemiologic and clinical aspects of feline immunodeficiency virus infection in cats from the continental United States and Canada and possible mode of transmission, *J Am Vet Med Assoc* 194:213, 1989.
126. North TW, North GLT, Pedersen NC: Feline immunodeficiency virus: A model for reverse transcriptase–targeted chemotherapy for acquired immune deficiency syndrome, *Antimicrob Agents Chemother* 33:915, 1989.
127. Fleming EJ, McCaw DL, Smith JA, et al: Clinical hematologic and survival data from cats infected with feline immunodeficiency virus: 42 cases (1983-1988), *J Am Vet Med Assoc* 199:913, 1991.
128. Ishida T, Wahiza T, Toriyabe K, et al: Feline immunodeficiency virus infection in cats in Japan, *J Am Vet Med Assoc* 194:221, 1989.
129. Sabine M, Michelsen J, Thomas F, et al: Feline AIDS, *Aust Vet Pract* 18:105, 1988.
130. Pedersen NC, Ho EW, Brown ML, et al: Isolation of a T-lymphotropic virus from domestic cats with an immunodeficiency-like syndrome, *Science* 235:790, 1987.
131. Swinney GR, Pauli JV, Hones BE, et al: Feline T-lymphotrophic virus (FTLV) in cats in New Zealand, *N Z Vet J* 37:41, 1989.
132. Hutson CA, Rideout BA, Pedersen NC: Neoplasia associated with feline immunodeficiency virus infection in cats of Southern California, *J Am Vet Med Assoc* 199:1357, 1991.
133. Macy DW, Podolsiki CL, Collins J: Prevalence of FeLV and FIV high risk cats in northeastern Colorado. Paper presented at the Tenth Annual Conference of the Veterinary Cancer Society, 1990, Auburn, AL.
134. Pedersen WC, Barlough JE: Clinical overview of feline immunodeficiency virus, *J Am Vet Med Assoc* 199:1298, 1991.
135. Neu H: FIV (FTLV)–Infektion der Katze: II Falle Beitrag zur epidemiologic, klinischen Symptomatologie undzum Krankheitsverlauf, *Kleintierpraxis* 34:373, 1989.

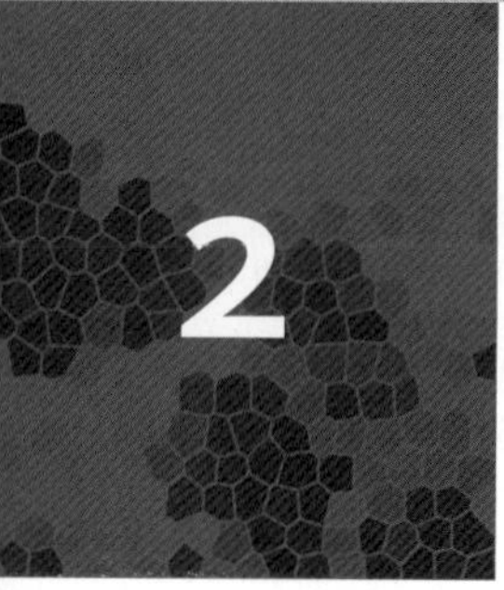

2 Tumor Biology and Metastasis

David J. Argyle and Chand Khanna

Cells of multicellular organisms form part of a specialized society that cooperate to promote survival of the organism. In this society, cell division, proliferation, and differentiation are strictly controlled and a balance exists between normal cell birth and the natural cell death rate.[1] Derangement of these normal homeostatic mechanisms can lead to uncontrolled proliferation or loss of the ability to die, leading to a normal cell taking on a malignant phenotype.

Cancer in animals is well documented throughout history but has taken on significance over the past hundred years for a number of reasons. Studies on chicken, feline, and bovine retroviruses have made significant contributions to our overall understanding of carcinogenesis through the discovery of oncogenes and tumor suppressor genes.[2] Further contributions to our understanding of viral oncogenesis have come from studies of the DNA papilloma viruses in cattle and horses, complementing research into cervical cancer in women.[3-10] This complementary cancer research has paved the way for the development of programs of research in comparative medicine that has benefits for both humans and the veterinary species. In this chapter we summarize the current understanding of the molecular mechanisms of cancer development and metastasis.

Normal Cell Division

Within an animal, all cells are subject to wear and tear, making cellular reproduction a necessity for maintenance of the individual. Reproduction of the gametes occurs by the process of meiosis, whereas reproduction of somatic cells involves two sequential phases known as *mitosis* and *cytokinesis.* Mitosis is nuclear division, and cytokinesis involves the division of the cytoplasm, the two occurring in close succession. Nuclear division is preceded by a doubling of the genetic material of the cell during a period known as interphase. As well as a copying of the chromosomes, this period is characterized by marked cellular activity in terms of RNA, protein and lipid production. The alternation between mitosis and interphase in all tissues is often referred to as the *cell cycle.* The phases of the cell cycle are shown in Figure 2-1.

Interphase (G1, G2, and S phases) is the longest phase of the cell cycle. During interphase, the chromatin is very long and slender; however, it shortens and thickens as interphase progresses. The first phase of mitosis is referred to as *prophase* and sees the first appearance of the chromosomes. As the phase progresses, the chromosomes appear as two identical sister chromatids joined at the centromere. As the nuclear membrane disappears, spindle fibers form and radiate from the two centrioles, each located at opposite poles of the cell. The spindle fibers serve to pull the chromosomes to opposite sides of the cell.

During *metaphase,* the spindle fibers pull the centromeres of the chromosomes, which become aligned to the middle of the spindle, often referred to as the *equatorial plate.* During *anaphase,* the centromeres split and the sister chromatids are pulled apart by the contraction of the spindle fibers. The final stage of cell division is *telophase,* characterized by the formation of a nuclear membrane around each group of chromosomes, is followed by cytokinesis or separation of the cytoplasm to produce two identical diploid cells. Progression through the cell cycle lasts approximately 12 to 24 hours.

The Cell Cycle

The cell cycle comprises four phases (M phase, S phase, G1, and G2) (see Figure 2-1). Nonproliferating cells are usually arrested between the M (mitosis) and S (DNA synthesis) phases and are referred to as G0 cells. The majority of cells in normal tissues are in G0. Cells are stimulated to enter the cell cycle in response to external factors including growth factors and cell adhesion. During the G1 phase of the cell cycle, cells are responsive to mitogenic signals. Once the cell cycle has traversed the restriction point (R) in the G1 phase, cell cycle transitions become autonomous.

Progression through the cell cycle is mediated by the sequential activation and inactivation of a class of proteins called *cyclin-dependent kinases* (CDKs).[11,12] CDKs consist of an inactive conserved catalytic core and are regulated at the following three levels:

1. CDK activity requires the association with regulatory subunits known as *cyclins.* The level of CDK remains constant throughout the cell cycle; however, the concentration of cyclins varies in a phase-specific manner during the cell cycle. The periodic synthesis and destruction of cyclins provides the primary level of cell cycle control (see Figure 2-1).
2. The activity of cyclin/CDK complexes is also regulated by phosphorylation. Activation of CDK/cyclin complexes requires phosphorylation by CDK-activating kinases (CAK); meanwhile the phosphorylation at threonine and serine residues suppresses activity.
3. CDKs are also tightly regulated by a class of inhibitory proteins known as CDK inhibitors (CDKI). CDKIs can block G1/S progression by binding CDKs/cyclin complexes and can be classified into the following two groups:
   a. INK4A family ($p15^{INK4b}$, $p16^{INK4a}$, $p18^{INK4c}$ and $p19^{INK4d}$). These act primarily on cdk4 and cdk6 complexes and prevent the association with cyclin D (see later discussion).
   b. CIP/KIP family ($p21^{Cip1}$, $p27^{Kip1}$, and $p57^{Kip2}$). These are less specific and can inactivate various cyclin/CDK complexes.

The first class of proteins induced in G1 following mitogenic stimulation of the cell cycle is the class D cyclins, which in turn activate CDK4 and CDK6. Cyclin D-CDK complexes cause phosphorylation of the substrate retinoblastoma protein (Rb), which results in dissociation of the transcription factor E2F from the Rb protein. The phosphorylation status of Rb plays a critical role in

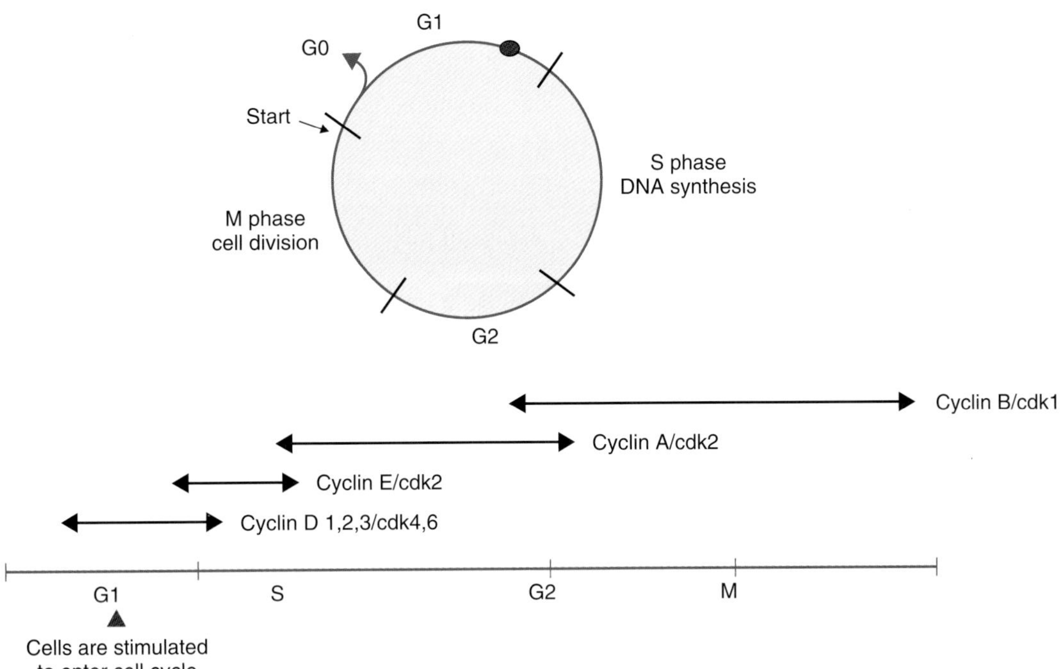

FIGURE 2-1 The cell cycle and its control. The cell cycle is divided into four phases (G1, S, G2, and M) and G0, which represents cycle-arrested cells. Cells are stimulated to enter the cell cycle in response to external factors, including growth factors and cell adhesion molecules. During G1, cells are responsive to mitogenic signals. Once the cell cycle has traversed the restriction point (R) in the G1 phase, the cell-cycle transitions become autonomous. Progression through the cell cycle is mediated by the sequential activation and inactivation of the cyclin-dependent kinases (CDKs). Control of CDK activity is through their interaction with specific cyclins (D, E, A, B) and with specific CDK inhibitors.

regulating G1 progression, and Rb is the molecular device that serves as the R point switch. Phosphorylated Rb releases E2F enabling transcription of numerous E2 responsive genes involved in DNA synthesis, and unphosphorylated RB remains associated with E2F, thereby inhibiting cell cycle progression. During G1 progression, activation of E2F also leads to induction of cyclin E. Cyclin E associates with CDK2 and the cyclin E-CDK2 complex maintains Rb in the phosphorylated state and is essential for cells to enter the S phase of cell cycle. At the G1/S phase transition, E2F induces cyclin A. During early S phase, cyclin D and E are degraded and cyclin A associates with CDK2 and CDK1; this kinase activity is essential for entry into S phase, completion of S phase, and entry into M phase. Mitosis is regulated by CDK1 in association with cyclins A and B causing phosphorylation of cytoskeletal proteins, including histones and lamins. This tight regulation on cell cycle progression prevents uncontrolled passage of normal cells through the cell cycle. The corollary of this is that loss of these control mechanisms can be a driving event in the development of cancer.

Cellular Responses to DNA Damage

When normal cells are subjected to stress signals, radiation, DNA damage, or oxygen depletion, the majority of cells have the ability to cause cell cycle arrest in G1, S, and G2 or enter programmed cell death (apoptosis) or both. Within cells, numerous surveillance systems called *checkpoints* function to recognize and respond to DNA damage. Cell cycle checkpoints occur in the G1 phase in response to DNA damage, during S phase to monitor the quality of DNA replication and the occurrence of DNA damage, and during the G2/M phase to examine the status of the spindle. The DNA damage–induced checkpoint mediated by the tumor suppressor protein p53 is the most well studied. The p53 protein plays an important role in maintaining genomic stability and forms part of a stress response pathway to various exogenous and endogenous DNA damage signals, including gamma irradiation, ultraviolet (UV) irradiation, chemicals, and oxidative stress.

p53 Functions as a Genomic Guardian

The p53 response to stress may be mediated by DNA-dependent protein kinase (DNA-PK) or by the ATM kinase and leads to phosphorylation of the N terminus of p53. In normal cells, p53 is short lived; however, phosphorylated p53 is stabilized and can then function as a transcriptional regulator binding to sequences and transactivating a number of genes, including p21.[13,14] p21 has a high affinity for G1 CDK/cyclin complexes and acts as a CDKI inhibiting kinase activity, thereby arresting cells in G1. By holding cells in G1, the replication of damaged DNA is prevented, and the cell's own DNA repair machinery has the opportunity to repair damage prior to reentering the active growth cycle (Figure 2-2).

The cellular levels of p53 protein are regulated by the product of another gene MDM2 (mouse double minute 2 oncogene).[15] The principal role of MDM2 is to act as a negative regulator of p53 function. One mechanism for MDM2 to downregulate p53 is to target p53 for degradation. The p53 protein is maintained in normal cells as an unstable protein, and its interaction with MDM2 can target p53 for degradation via a ubiquitin proteosome pathway. MDM2 can also control p53 function by suppressing p53 transcriptional activity. MDM2 is a transcriptional target of p53, and expression is induced by the binding of p53 to an internal promoter within the *mdm2* gene. MDM2 can in turn bind to a domain within the

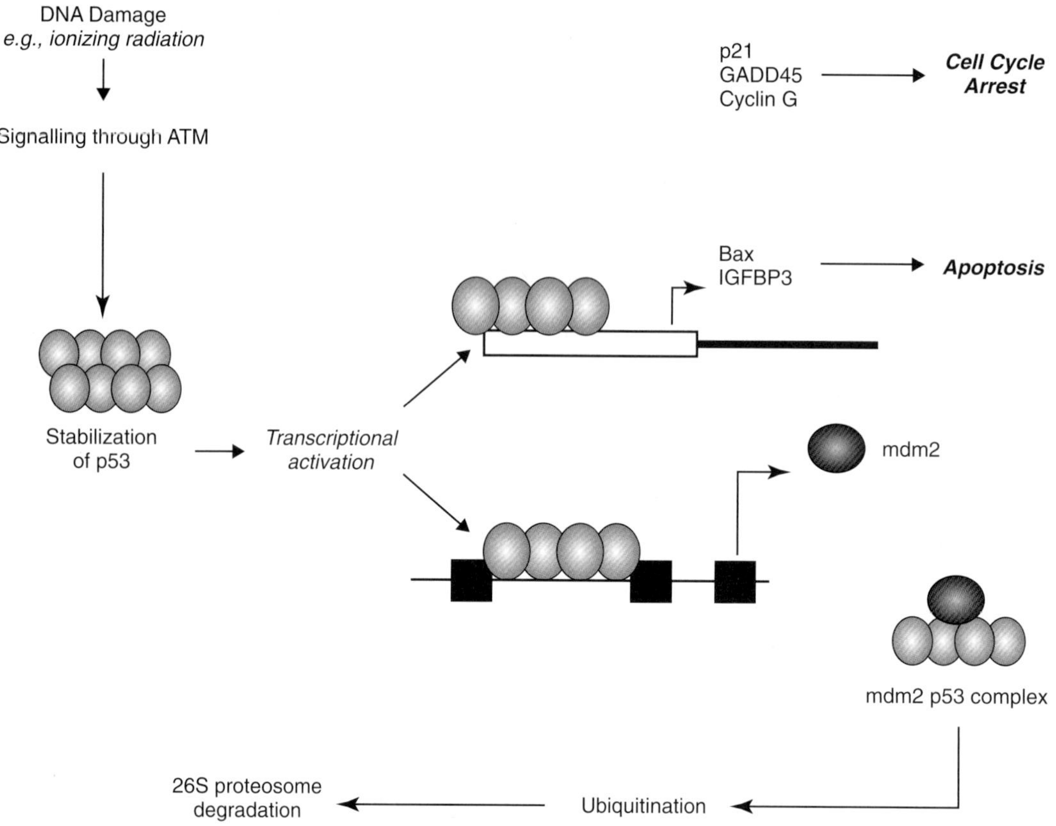

FIGURE 2-2 p53 is involved in cell cycle control. The p53 response to stress may be mediated by DNA-dependent protein kinase (DNA-PK) or by the ATM kinase and leads to phosphorylation of the N terminus of p53. In normal cells, p53 is short lived; however, phosphorylated p53 is stabilized and can then function as a transcriptional regulator binding to sequences and transactivating a number of genes, including p21 and Bax. Consequently, the cell cycle is arrested or the cell undergoes programmed cell death (apoptosis). This is a defense mechanism that allows for repair or death (if the cell is irreversibly damaged). The cellular levels of p53 protein are regulated by the product of another gene mouse double minute 2 oncogene (MDM2). The principal role of MDM2 is to act as a negative regulator of p53 function. One mechanism for MDM2 to downregulate p53 is to target p53 for degradation. The p53 protein is maintained in normal cells as an unstable protein, and its interaction with p53 can target p53 for degradation via a ubiquitin proteosome pathway. MDM2 can also control p53 function by suppressing p53 transcriptional activity. MDM2 is a transcriptional target of p53, and expression is induced by the binding of p53 to an internal promoter within the MDM2 gene. MDM2 can in turn bind to a domain within the amino terminus of p53, thereby inhibiting the transcriptional activity and G1 arrest function of p53 by masking access to the transcriptional machinery.

amino terminus of p53, thereby inhibiting the transcriptional activity and G_1 arrest function of p53 by masking access to the transcriptional machinery (see Figure 2-2).[16]

Cell Death

In contrast to necrosis, apoptosis is a distinct type of cell death most often characterized as the "programmed" self-destruction of cells that occurs in disease states, as well as part of the normal physiologic cell turnover. Whereas necrosis is characterized by swelling of the cell and lysis, in apoptosis there is cellular and nuclear shrinkage followed by fragmentation and subsequent phagocytosis. These morphologic features of apoptosis result from a number of apoptosis effectors (i.e., caspases) and regulators (particularly the Bcl-2 protein family). The molecular mechanisms involved in apoptosis are shown in Figure 2-3.[17,18] Apoptosis provides a controlled mechanism for eliminating cells that are irreversibly damaged and involves an adenosine triphosphate (ATP)-dependent activation of cellular pathways, which move calcium from the endoplasmic reticulum to the cytoplasm and activation of endonucleases. As noted previously, some of these pathways are mediated through caspases. However, a wide variety of signals can initiate an apoptotic response, including Fas ligand (CD95 or FasL) and its interaction with the Fas receptor, tumor necrosis factor (TNF) and its receptor interaction, and certain oncogenes. The Fas and TNF receptors are members of the death receptor family. These transmembrane proteins with cysteine rich extracellular domains and intracellular regions share a common structure termed the "death domain." The proapoptotic ligands for these receptors are homotrimeric peptides that are either soluble or expressed at the surface of the adjacent cell. Ligand-induced receptor clustering promotes the binding of a soluble cytosolic adapter protein called *Fas-associated death domain* (FADD), which itself contains a death domain as well as a caspase binding site, to the clustered death domains of the receptors. This leads to activation of caspase 8 and downstream activation of effector caspases for apoptosis.

Where cells are damaged and are unable to repair DNA, p53 expression can upregulate p21 and cause cell cycle arrest or can aid in directing the cell into programmed death or apoptosis through upregulation and expression of Bax (a proapoptotic Bcl-2 family protein) and also through priming of caspases. In this, the

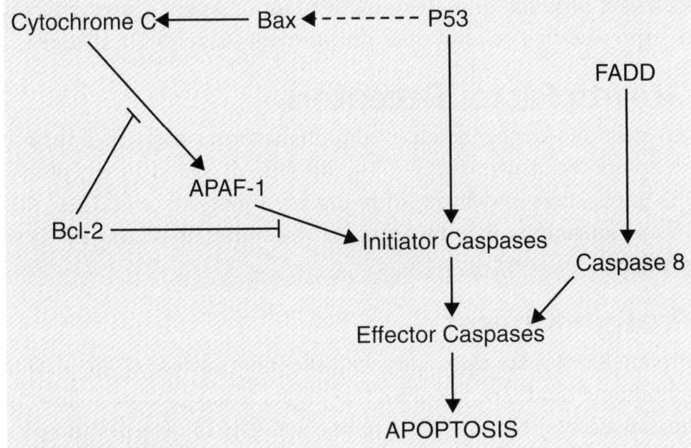

FIGURE 2-3 The mediators of apoptosis. A wide variety of signals can initiate an apoptotic response, including Fas ligand (CD95 or FasL) and its interaction with the Fas receptor, tumor necrosis factor (TNF) and its receptor interaction, and certain oncogenes. The Fas and TNF receptors are members of the death receptor family. These are transmembrane proteins with cysteine rich extracellular domains and intracellular regions that share a common structure termed the *death domain.* The proapoptotic ligands for these receptors are homotrimeric peptides that are either soluble or expressed at the surface of the adjacent cell. Ligand-induced receptor clustering promotes the binding of a soluble cytosolic adapter protein called *Fas-associated death domain* (FADD), which itself contains a death domain, as well as a caspase binding site, to the clustered death domains of the receptors. This leads to activation of caspase 8 and downstream activation of effector caspases for apoptosis.

expression of p53 can also downregulate expression of the Bcl2 gene itself (a prosurvival, negative regulator of apoptosis).

Summary

The cell cycle ensures a regulated process so that each cell can complete DNA replication before cell division occurs. The cell responds to growth and environmental signals through the cell cycle. Components of the cell cycle that have a stimulatory effect include the cyclins and the CDKs. The negative influences come from a series of checkpoints that respond to external stimuli. These include tumor suppressor genes such as p53 and Rb and also genes involved in DNA repair. The process of DNA replication is also subject to the introduction of errors, and this is closely monitored by a class of enzymes called *DNA repair enzymes.* Consequently, there are a number of safeguards within the cell cycle to ensure that normal cells are produced during division and that the DNA is accurately replicated. The next section will describe how these systems are overcome to produce a malignant cancer cell.

From Normal Cell to Cancer Cell

It is difficult to define a cancer cell in absolute terms. Tumors are usually phenotypically recognized by the fact that their cells show abnormal growth patterns and are no longer under the control of normal homeostatic growth controlling mechanisms, including apoptosis. Although the range of mechanisms involved in the development of tumors and the spectrum of tissues from which tumors are derived is diverse, they can be classified into the following three broad types:

- Benign tumors: Broadly speaking, these tumors arise in any of the tissues of the body and grow locally. Their clinical significance is the ability to cause local pressure, cause obstruction, or form a space-occupying lesion, such as a benign brain tumor. Benign tumors do not metastasize.
- In-situ tumors: These are often small tumors that arise in the epithelium. Histologically, the lesion appears to contain cancer cells, but the tumor remains in the epithelial layer and does not invade the basement membrane or the supporting mesenchyme. A typical example of this is preinvasive squamous cell carcinoma (SCC) affecting the skin of cats, which is often referred to as *Bowen's disease.*
- Cancer: This refers to a malignant tumor that has the capacity for both local invasion and distant spread by the process of metastasis.

Multistep Carcinogenesis

Cancer is the phenotypic end result of a whole series of changes that may have taken a long period of time to develop. Indeed, recent studies that have sequenced the genome of pancreatic and brain tumors have identified 63 and 60 genetic alterations on average in each cancer, respectively. From this large list of genetic alterations, there are a small number of commonly mutated genes that are "drivers" of the cancer phenotype.[19,20]

The application of a cancer-producing agent (carcinogen) to tissues does not lead to the immediate production of a cancer cell. After the initiation step produced by the agent, there follows a period of tumor promotion. This promotion may be caused by the same initiating agent or by other substances, such as normal growth promoters or hormones. The initiating step is a rapid step and affects the genetic material of the cell. If the cell does not repair this damage, then promoting factors may progress the cell toward a malignant phenotype. In contrast to initiation, progression may be a very slow process and may not even manifest in the lifetime of the animal. Each stage of multistep carcinogenesis reflects genetic changes in the cell with a selection advantage that drives the progression toward a highly malignant cell. The age-dependent incidence of cancer suggests a requirement for between four and seven rate-limiting, stochastic events to produce the malignant phenotype.[21]

These sequential events in tumor formation are a consequence of changes at the genetic level. Over the past 25 years, cancer research has generated a rich and complex body of information revealing that cancer is a disease involving dynamic changes in the genome. Seminal to our understanding of cancer biology has been the discovery of the so-called *cancer genes* or *oncogenes* and *tumor suppressor genes.* Mutations that produce oncogenes with dominant gain of function and tumor suppressor genes with recessive loss of function have been identified through their alteration in human and animal cancer cells and by their elicitation of cancer phenotypes in experimental models.

Oncogenes

The RNA tumor viruses (retroviruses) provided the first evidence that genetic factors play a role in the development of cancer. The initial observation came in 1910 when Rous demonstrated that a filterable agent (later classified as a retrovirus and termed *avian leukosis virus*) was capable of producing lymphoid tumors in chickens.[22] Retroviruses have three core genes (*gag, pol,* and *env*) and an additional gene that gives the virus the ability to transform cells. Retroviral sequences that are responsible for transforming properties are called *viral oncogenes* (v-onc). The names of these genes are

TABLE 2-1 Functional Classification of Tumor Oncogenes

ONCOGENE	NAME	ABBREVIATION
Growth factors	Platelet-derived growth factor	PDGF
	Epidermal growth factor	EGF
	Insulin-like growth factor-1	ILGF-1
	Vascular endothelial growth factor	VEGF
	Transforming growth factor-β	TGF-β
	Interleukin-2	IL-2
Growth factor receptors	PDGF receptor	PDGFR
	EGF receptor	EGFR, erbB-1
	ILGF-1 receptor	ILGF-1R
	VEGF receptor	VEGFR
	IL-2 receptor	IL-2R
	Hepatocyte growth factor receptor	met
	Heregulin receptor	neu/erbB-2
	Stem cell factor receptor	Kit
Protein kinases	Tyrosine kinase	bcr-abl
	Tyrosine kinase	src
	Serine-threonine kinase	raf/mil
	Serine-threonine kinase	mos
G-protein signal transducers	GTPase	H-*ras*
	GTPase	K-*ras*
	GTPase	N-*ras*
Nuclear proteins	Transcription factor	ets
	Transcription factor	fos
	Transcription factor	jun
	Transcription factor	myb
	Transcription factor	myc
	Transcription factor	rel

GTPase, Guanosine triphosphatase.

derived from the tumors in which they were first described (e.g., *v-ras* from rat sarcoma virus).

Viral oncogenes were subsequently shown to have cellular homologues called *cellular oncogenes* (c-onc). Later, the term *proto-oncogene* was used to describe cellular oncogenes that do not have transforming potential to form tumors in their native state but can be altered to lead to malignancy.[23] Most proto-oncogenes are key genes involved in the control of cell growth and proliferation and their roles are complex. For simplicity, their sites and modes of action in the normal cell can be divided as follows (Table 2-1):

- Growth factors
- Growth factor receptors
- Protein kinases
- Signal transducers
- Nuclear proteins and transcription factors

Growth Factors

Growth factors are molecules that act on the cell via cell surface receptors. Their contribution to carcinogenesis may be through excessive production of the growth factor or where a growth factor is expressed in a cell but does not normally function in that cell.

Growth Factor Receptors

Several proto-oncogene–derived proteins form a part of cell surface receptors for growth factors. The binding of ligand to receptor is the initial stage of delivery of mitogenic signals to cells. Their role in carcinogenesis may be through structural alterations in these proteins.

Protein Kinases

Protein kinases are associated with the inner surface of the plasma membrane and are involved in signal transduction following ligand-receptor binding. Structural changes in these genes and proteins lead to increased kinase activity that can have profound effects on signal transduction pathways.

Signal Transduction

The binding of an extracellular growth factor to the membrane receptor leads to a series of events by which the mitogenic signal is transduced to the nucleus of the cell. Essential to this signaling is the successive phosphorylation of signaling intermediaries or the second messengers such as guanosine triphosphate (GTP) and proteins that bind GTP (G-proteins). During signal transduction, GTP is converted to guanosine diphosphate (GDP) by the guanosine triphosphatase (GTPase) activity of G-proteins. A group of proto-oncogenes called *Ras* encode proteins with GTPase and GTP-binding activity and, in the normal cell, help to modulate cellular proliferation. Mutations in the Ras proto-oncogene can contribute to uncontrolled cellular proliferation.

Nuclear Proteins and Transcription Factors

Nuclear proteins and transcription factors encode proteins that control gene expression. These proto-oncogenes may have a role in cellular proliferation. Not surprisingly, changes in transcription factor activity may contribute to the development of the malignant genotype.

Mechanisms by which Oncogenes Become Activated

The advent of recombinant DNA technology has allowed scientists to unravel a number of mechanisms by which the normal products of proto-oncogenes can be disrupted to produce uncontrolled cell division. The conversion of a proto-oncogene to an oncogene is a result of somatic events in the genetic material of the target tissue. The activated allele of the oncogene dominates the wild-type allele and results in a *dominant gain of function.* This means that only one allele needs to be affected to obtain phenotypic change; this is in contrast to tumor suppressor genes in which both alleles have to be lost for phenotypic change. The mechanisms of oncogene activation are outlined in the following list and are shown in Figure 2-4.[23-30]

- *Chromosomal translocation.* Where proto-oncogenes are translocated within the genome (i.e., from one chromosome to another), their function can be greatly altered. The classic example in human medicine is the chromosomal breakpoint that produces the Philadelphia chromosome found in chronic myelogenous leukemia (CML). This involves the translocation of the c-abl oncogene on chromosome 9 to a gene on chromosome 22 (bcr). The point at which two genes come together is referred to as a *chromosomal breakpoint* (or *translocation breakpoint*). The BCR/

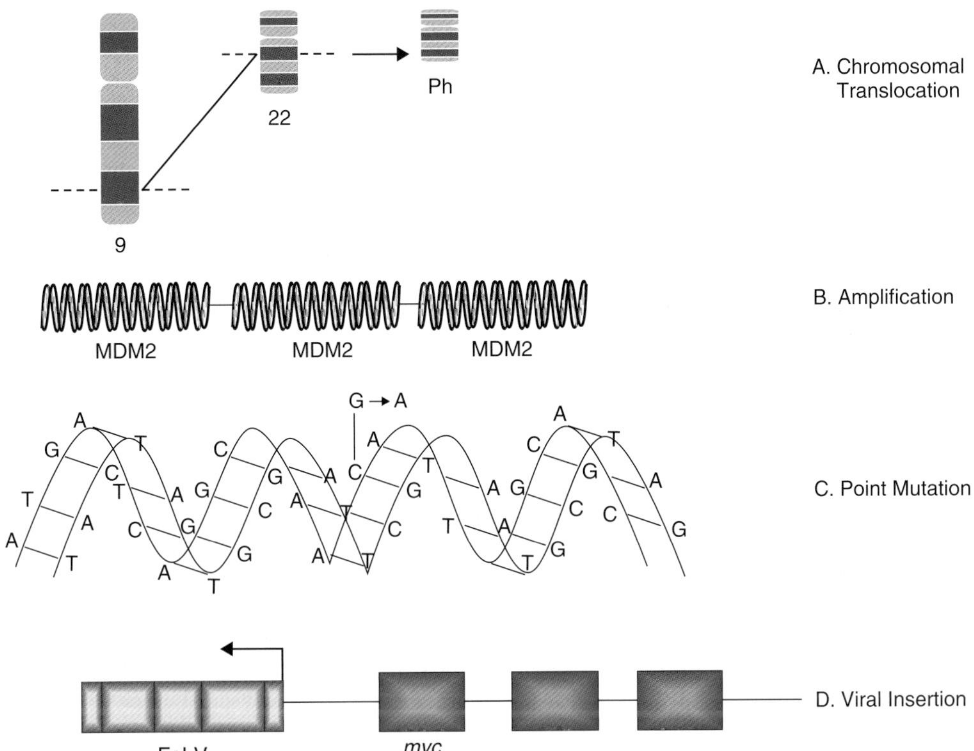

FIGURE 2-4 Methods of oncogene activation. Oncogenes can be activated by chromosomal rearrangements (e.g., BCR/ABL–induced leukemia), gene amplification (e.g., amplification of MDM2 in some sarcomas), point mutations (e.g., changes in nucleotide sequence that alters protein production), or by viral insertions (e.g., the insertion of feline leukemia virus [FeLV] at the *myc* locus in FeLV-induced lymphomas).

ABL hybrid gene produces a novel transcript whose protein product has elevated tyrosine kinase activity and can contribute to uncontrolled cellular proliferation. Transgenic mice for this chimeric gene develop lymphoblastic leukemia and lymphoma. Since this gene product is directly linked to CML formation, it is a logical target for tyrosine kinase inhibitors in the treatment of chronic myeloid leukemia in humans (CML).

- *Gene amplification.* Quantitation of gene copy number is possible by a number of molecular techniques, including comparative genomic hybridization, genotyping arrays, and Southern hybridization. Amplification of oncogenes can occur in a number of tumor types and has been demonstrated in childhood neuroblastoma, where the myc proto-oncogene (nuclear transcription factor) is amplified up to 300 times. Gene amplification is possibly the most common mechanism of proto-oncogene activation. A further example is the MDM2 proto-oncogene, which has been identified in dogs and horses, and has recently shown to be amplified in a proportion of canine soft tissue sarcomas.[31]
- *Point mutations.* These are single base changes in the DNA sequence of proto-oncogenes leading to the production of abnormal proteins. Point mutations can arise through the actions of ionizing radiation, chemical carcinogens, or errors in DNA replication and repair. A mutation in a proto-oncogene or the transcriptional machinery that controls its expression may disrupt homeostasis and result in sustained proliferation signals or a failure to respond to negative feedback signals. A classical example is the Ras proto-oncogene in which point mutations are a consistent finding in a number of human tumors. K-ras mutations have also been identified in canine lung tumors. Mutations in the Erb-B (epidermal growth factor receptor) gene have been shown in a number of human cancers to lead to ligand-independent activation. Erb-2 mutations have been identified in canine mammary tumors.
- *Viral insertions.* The discovery of oncogenes was a direct result of studies on tumor-causing viruses. In some circumstances, proto-oncogene function can be damaged by the insertion of viral elements. Occasionally, novel retroviruses are isolated from leukemias or sarcomas in animals that have been viremic with a leukemia virus for some time. These viruses induce tumors very rapidly when inoculated into members of the species of origin and are referred to as *acutely transforming oncoviruses.* The prototype of the acutely transforming virus is the Rous sarcoma virus (RSV) isolated from a fowl in 1911. Subsequently, many more have been isolated from animals infected with avian, feline, murine, or simian oncoviruses. These viruses are generated by a rare recombinatorial event between the leukemia virus with which the animal was originally infected and a cellular proto-oncogene. In this, part of the viral genome is deleted and replaced with the cellular oncogene. The virus then becomes acutely transforming because this oncogene is now under the transcriptional control of very efficient viral promoters. This then allows infection of a cell and insertion of this continuously expressed oncogene into the cellular genome leading toward rapid progression and malignancy. Evidence suggests that these acutely transforming viruses are not transmitted naturally, but all events occur in the individual animal. Because the virus has itself lost some of its own genetic material, it is defective for replication. However, they are spread throughout an animal by the provision of help from the normal leukemia virus, which provides the missing proteins in co-infected cells.

In addition to acutely transforming mechanisms, retroviruses can activate cellular oncogenes by integrating adjacent to them. A good example of this is the *myc* gene, which is frequently activated in feline T-cell lymphomas. In one mode, the virus integrates adjacent to the oncogene and transcription initiation in the viral long terminal repeat (LTR) proceeds into the adjacent oncogene, producing a hybrid mRNA. In a second form, the enhancer of the virus overrides the regulation of the c-*myc* transcription from its normal promoter.

Tumor Suppressor Genes

Changes in genes can lead to either stimulatory or inhibitory effects on cell growth and proliferation. The stimulatory effects are provided by the proto-oncogenes as described. Mutations or translocations of these genes produce positive signals leading to uncontrolled growth. In contrast, tumor formation can result from a loss of inhibitory functions associated with another class of cellular genes called the *tumor suppressor genes.* The discovery of these genes began by observations of inherited cancer syndromes in children, in particular studies of retinoblastoma. In the early 1970s, epidemiologic studies of both retinoblastoma and Wilms' tumor led Knudson to propose his "two hit" theory of tumorigenesis.

Retinoblastoma Forms the First Clues to the Existence of Tumor Suppressor Genes

Retinoblastoma occurs in two forms, a sporadic form and an inherited form (accounting for 40% of cases).[32] In the inherited form, the mode of inheritance is autosomal dominant and about half the children are affected by the condition. Knudson's model required the retinoblastoma tumor cells (in either sporadic or inherited forms) to acquire two separate genetic changes in the DNA before tumor development. The first or predisposing event could be inherited through the germ line (familial retinoblastoma) or it could arise de novo in somatic cells (sporadic form). The second event occurred in somatic cells. Thus, in sporadic retinoblastoma, both events arose in the retinal cells. However, in familial retinoblastoma, the individual had already inherited one mutant gene and only required a second hit in the remaining normal gene in somatic cells.

The mode of inheritance of retinoblastoma is dominant with incomplete penetrance. However, at the cellular level, loss or inactivation of both alleles is required to change the cells' phenotype. The retinoblastoma gene codes for Rb, which was previously described as a normal cellular gene involved in control of the cell cycle. Rb is described as a tumor suppressor and, in a cell with only one normal allele, that allele usually produces enough tumor suppressor product to remain normal. Generically, mutations in tumor suppressor genes behave very differently from oncogene mutations. Whereas activating oncogene mutations are dominant to wild type (they emit their proliferating signals regardless of the wild-type gene product), suppressor mutations are recessive. Mutation in one gene copy usually has no effect, as long as a reasonable amount of wild-type protein remains. Consequently, some texts refer to tumor suppressor genes as recessive oncogenes.

More recently, Knudson's hypothesis was confirmed when the Rb gene was cloned and characterized. The retinoblastoma tumor suppressor Rb is the principal member of a family of proteins that also encompass pRb2/p130 and p107. Rb plays a central role in regulating cell cycle progression in G1. Indeed, disruption of Rb function has been found to be a common feature of many human cancers not only retinoblastoma. Rb function can be abrogated by point mutations, deletions, or by complex formation with viral oncoproteins such as SV40 large T antigen and adenoviral E1a protein. The function of additional proteins associated with the Rb pathway are also subjected to deregulation in human cancers, including overexpression of D type cyclins, overexpression of CDK4, and downregulation of the CDKI cell cycle inhibitor p16.

Although loss of cell cycle control via the Rb pathway occurs commonly in many human tumors, little is known about the role of Rb, cyclin D, CDK4, and p16 in domesticated animal tumors.

The p53 Tumor Suppressor Gene

P53 is a gene whose product is intimately involved in cell cycle control. Its discovery by Sir David Lane in 1979 marked a major milestone in cancer research and has allowed greater understanding of molecular mechanisms of cancer and identified potential targets for therapeutic intervention.

The p53 protein has been described as the guardian of the genome by virtue of its ability to push cells into arrest or apoptosis, depending on the degree of DNA damage. Thus the p53 tumor suppressor gene plays an important role in cell cycle progression, regulation of gene expression, and the cellular response mechanisms to DNA damage. Under normal physiologic conditions, wild-type p53 can bind specific DNA sequences and regulate transcription of a number of genes involved in cell cycle progression and apoptotic pathways including $p21^{waf1/cip1}$ and bax (see Figure 2-2). The p53-mediated mechanisms are responsible for tumor suppression and prevent accumulation of potentially oncogenic mutations and genomic instability. Failure by p53 to activate such cellular functions may ultimately result in abnormal uncontrolled cell growth leading to tumorigenic transformation.[33-36]

p53 is the most frequently inactivated gene in human neoplasia, with functional loss commonly occurring through gene mutational events, including nonsense, missense and splice site mutations, allelic loss, rearrangements, and deletions. However, p53 function can also be abrogated by several nonmutational mechanisms, including nuclear exclusion, complex formation with a number of viral proteins, and through overexpression of the cellular oncogene MDM2.

The homologs of p53 and MDM2 have both been identified in domestic animal species and a number of studies indicate that this gene also has a central role in the progression of veterinary cancers.[37-41]

Cancer Arises through Multiple Molecular Mechanisms

The advances in our understanding of normal cell biology and the processes that lead to malignancy have increased dramatically over the past 30 years. The last decade has shown us that transformation of a normal cell into a malignant cell requires very few molecular, biochemical, and cellular changes that can be considered as acquired capabilities.[42,43] Further, despite the wide diversity of cancer types, these acquired capabilities appear to be common to all types of cancer. An optimistic view of increasing simplicity in cancer biology is further endorsed by the fact that all normal cells, irrespective of origin and phenotype, carry similar molecular machineries that regulate cell proliferation, differentiation, aging, and cell death.

We have discussed that tumorigenesis is a multistep process and that these steps reflect genetic alterations that drive the progression of a normal cell into a highly malignant cancer cell. This is supported by the finding that genomes of tumor cells are invariably altered at multiple sites. The spectrum of changes range from subtle point mutations in growth regulatory genes to obvious changes in chromosomal complement.

Cancer cells have defects in regulatory circuits that govern cellular proliferation and homeostasis and survival. A model has been proposed that suggests that the vast array of genetic abnormalities associated with cancer are a manifestation of eight alterations in cellular physiology that collectively contribute to malignant growth. First proposed in 2000 and updated in 2011, these "hallmarks" of cancer constitute an organizing principle for rationalizing the complexities of cancer and are underpinned by two overarching themes: *genome instability* and *chronic inflammation.*[42,43] The eight acquired characteristics can be summarized under the following headings (see Figure 1-3):

- Self-sufficient growth
- Insensitivity to antigrowth signals
- Evasion of programmed cell death (apoptosis)
- Limitless replicative potential
- Sustained angiogenesis
- Reprogramming energy metabolism
- Evading immune destruction
- Tissue invasion and metastasis

In addition, cancer exhibits another dimension of complexity in that they contain an array of "normal" cells that contribute to the acquisition and maintenance of the cancer hallmarks by creating the tumor microenvironment. The next section is an overview of these traits and the strategies by which they are acquired in cancer cells. The process of metastasis requires angiogenesis and invasion, as such the traits of sustained angiogenesis, and tissue invasion and metastasis will be collectively reviewed under a final section on metastasis.

The Hallmarks of Cancer

In the preceding section, we have described the normal cell and the role of oncogenes and tumor suppressor genes in cell cycle control and regulation. In one sense, cancer is a very common disease in animals and humans, but in fact the development of cancer is a rare event. When one considers the number of cells in the body, the proliferation and regulation of these cells and the potential for malignant transformation, then the development of a single cancer is rare. This is because of the cell's own natural defenses against progression toward the malignant phenotype. The ability of the cell to effect DNA repair or initiate cell death is a defense mechanism against malignant transformation and serves to maintain cellular homeostasis. Each of the acquired capabilities described previously represents a breach in a cell's homeostatic mechanisms. However, the biology of cancer cannot be understood by simply considering the phenotypic traits of the cancer cell. Rather the cancer phenotype is defined by the interactions between the cancer cell, the tumor microenvironment, and the enabling effects of fundamental genomic instability and chronic inflammation.

Self-Sufficiency in Growth Signals

Normal cells require mitogenic stimuli for growth and proliferation. These signals are transmitted to the nucleus by the binding of signaling molecules to specific receptors, the diffusion of growth factors into the cell, extracellular matrix components, or cell-to-cell adhesions or interactions. As previously discussed, many oncogenes act by mimicking normal growth signals. Tumor cells are not dependent on external mitogenic stimuli for proliferation and sustained growth but are self-sufficient. The liberation from dependency on exogenous signals severely disrupts normal cellular homeostasis. Arguably, the most fundamental trait of cancer cells is their ability to sustain chronic proliferation. By deregulating these signals, cancer cells become masters of their own destinies, promoting signaling (typically through intracellular kinase domains) to promote progression through the cell cycle, increases in cell size, increases in cell survival, and changes in energy metabolism.

The cancer cell can acquire this capability in the following ways:

- They may produce growth factor ligands themselves.
- They may induce stromal cells to produce such ligands.
- There may be an increase in receptor concentration on the cell surface that leads to receptor homodimerization or heterodimerization, making the cell hyperresponsive to ligands.
- There may be structural alterations in the receptor to support ligand-independent firing.
- Constitutive activation of the signaling pathway (downstream of the receptor). A good example of this is the constitutive activation of the PI3-AKT pathway, through mutations in the catalytic subunit of the PI3 kinase.
- Disruptions in negative-feedback mechanisms that attenuate proliferative signaling, such as the following:
    - Mutations in the *Ras* gene compromise the Ras GTPase activity, which acts as a negative-feedback mechanism to ensure the effects of *Ras* are only transitory.
    - *PTEN* is a tumor suppressor protein that counteracts PI3 signaling. *PTEN* loss has a similar effect to constitutive PI3 activation and promotes tumorigenesis.

Although the acquisition of growth signaling autonomy by cancer cells is conceptually satisfying, it is in fact too simplistic. One of the major problems of cancer research is to focus on the cancer cell in isolation. It is now apparent that we must also consider the contribution of the tumor microenvironment to the survival of cancer cells. Within normal tissues, paracrine and endocrine signals contribute greatly to growth and proliferation. Cell-to cell growth signaling is also likely to operate in cancer cells and may be as important as some of the autonomous mechanisms of tumor growth. It has recently been suggested that growth signals for the proliferation of carcinoma cells are derived from the tumor stromal elements (e.g., cancer or carcinoma-associated fibroblasts [CAFs]). It is therefore possible that the survival of tumor cells not only relies on the acquisition of growth signal autonomy but may also require the recruitment or modulation of stromal cells to provide these growth signals.

Insensitivity to Antigrowth Signals or Evading Growth Suppressors

Within the normal cell, multiple antiproliferative signals operate to maintain cellular quiescence and homeostasis. These signals include soluble growth inhibitors that act via cell surface receptors and immobilized inhibitors that are embedded in the extracellular matrix and on the surface of nearby cells. The signals operate to push the cell either into G0 or into a postmitotic state (usually associated with the acquisition of specific differentiation–associated characteristics) and are thus intimately associated with cell cycle control mechanisms. Cells monitor their external environment during the progression through G1 and, on the basis of external stimuli, decide whether to proliferate, become quiescent, or enter into a postmitotic state.

Most cellular programs that negatively regulate cell growth and proliferation depend on the actions of tumor suppressor genes. At the basic level, most of the antiproliferative signals are funneled through the Rb protein and its close relatives. Disruption of Rb allows cell proliferation and renders the cell insensitive to antiproliferative signals such as that provided by the well-characterized transforming growth factor-β (TGF-β).[32] The Rb protein integrates signals from diverse extracellular and intracellular sources and can control cell cycle progression. The other major tumor suppressor is p53, which integrates intracellular signals and can promote either cell cycle arrest or apoptosis (depending on the degree of cellular stress or damage). However, the effects of p53 expression are highly context dependent. Loss of Rb or p53 is associated with the malignant phenotype through the cell's ability to evade antigrowth signals.

In addition to tumor suppressor gene loss, cells can also evade antigrowth signals by the following alternative cellular programs:

- Another characteristic of the cancer cell is the evasion of contact inhibition. Cell-to-cell contact in most normal cells results in an inhibitory signal against further cell proliferation. The role of this mechanism in vivo has been thought to be to maintain tissue homeostasis. In cell culture, contact inhibition is abrogated in cancer cell monolayers, leading to their indefinite expansion. NF2 and LKB1 genes are considered tumor suppressor genes that are involved in this process and loss of these genes in vivo may promote loss of contact inhibition that contributes to the progression of cancers.
- Although TGF-β has antiproliferative effects in cancer, it is now, however, appreciated that the TGF-β pathway can be corrupted in the later stages of malignancy and can contribute to cancer progression. In this late effect, TGF-β is found to activate a cellular program termed *epithelial-to-mesenchymal transition* (EMT) that promotes invasion and metastasis (see later).

Evading Cell Death: The Roles of Apoptosis, Autophagy, and Necrosis

The growth of any tumor depends not only on the rate of cell division but also the rate of cellular attrition (mainly provided by apoptotic mechanisms). Basic molecular and pathologic studies of tumors have confirmed that acquired resistance toward apoptosis and other types of death is a hallmark of all types of cancer.

Cancer cells, through a variety of strategies, can acquire resistance to cell death and apoptosis. One of the most common ways is through loss of function of the tumor suppressor protein p53. Loss of p53 protein function occurs most often through mutation but can also be via sequestration or inactivation of the protein by viral proteins or by amplification of other oncogenes such as MDM2. Removal of normal p53 function leads to failure of the cells' sensor mechanism for DNA damage. When the cell suffers an insult such as UV radiation, hypoxia, or exposure to DNA-damaging agents, signals are funneled through p53 to cause either cell cycle arrest or apoptosis. Failure of this mechanism can contribute to the progression of the cell toward malignancy and promoting the accumulation of additional genetic defects that are not corrected at defined checkpoints in cell cycle progression.[35]

The mechanisms involved in apoptosis are now well established, as are the strategies by which cancer cells evade its actions. However, recently there have been conceptual advances involving other forms of "programmed cell death" as a barrier to cancer development. A notable example is the emerging role that autophagy plays in cancer development. *Autophagy* is a normal cellular response that operates at low basal levels in cells but can be induced in states of cellular stress such as nutrient deficiency. In autophagy, there is controlled breakdown of cellular organelles that yields energy and cellular substrates that can be used for a variety of cellular functions. Recent evidence suggests that autophagy may be involved in both tumor cell survival and, paradoxically, tumor cell death, depending on the cellular state. The link between apoptosis and autophagy suggests that autophagy may represent another barrier for cells to overcome before they can attain malignancy. In contrast, it has also been shown that irradiation or cytotoxic drug treatment in late-stage tumors may promote autophagy, leading to cells attaining a state of reversible dormancy. The situation seems to suggest that autophagy is a barrier to tumor development in early disease but, in late stage disease, may allow cancer cells to survive severe cellular stress.[44]

In both autophagy and apoptosis, the process does not lead to the release of any "proinflammatory" signals. In contrast, the process of necrosis, observed in larger tumors, causes release of signals that support an influx of inflammatory cells. For many years, this has been considered to be a positive event, helping to expose the immune system to tumor antigens and promote immune destruction. However, recent evidence suggests that some phenotypes of inflammatory macrophages can actually support tumor growth through fostering of angiogenesis, cancer cell proliferation, and invasion. Consequently, our understanding of macrophage phenotypes in cancer progression is an area of active research.

Limitless Replicative Capacity

Over 30 years ago the pioneering observations of Hayflick established that when normal human or animal cells are grown in culture, they demonstrate a finite replicative lifespan. That is, they are capable of a finite number of cell divisions, after which they undergo what has been termed *replicative senescence* and are incapable of any further cell division. The mechanism underlying the replicative clock that monitors this process has been the subject of intense research. This process has further evoked considerable interest as it is also one of the mechanisms that must be overcome to establish the immortal phenotype that is characteristic of the cancer cell.[45-47]

In mammalian cells, the DNA is organized into chromosomes within the nucleus and these are capped by specialized DNA-protein structures known as *telomeres.* The major function of these structures is protection, but they are progressively eroded at each cell division because of the inability of DNA to completely replicate itself. The result is that there is progressive telomeric attrition as cell populations double. After an estimated 50 cell divisions, cells enter an irreversible (and prolonged) state of cellular senescence (sometimes referred to as *mortality stage 1* [M1]). This period is characterized by arrest of proliferation without loss of biochemical function or viability. At the end of this period, cells exhibit altered morphology and chromosomal instability, a state often referred to as *crisis* (mortality stage 2 [M2]) (Figures 2-5 and 2-6). Thus telomeric attrition is intimately involved with the aging of cells. Cancer cells must overcome replicative senescence and take on an immortal phenotype.

It has now been demonstrated in human tumors and, more recently, tumors of the dog, that telomere maintenance is a feature of virtually all cancer types.[46-53] Tumor cells succeed in telomeric maintenance by the expression of the enzyme telomerase. From studies on cellular senescence, expression of the enzyme telomerase has emerged as a central unifying mechanism underlying the immortal phenotype of cancer cells and has thus become the most common marker of malignant cells. Telomerase is a ribonucleoprotein enzyme that maintains the protective structures at the ends of eukaryotic chromosomes, at the telomeres. In humans, telomerase expression is repressed in most somatic tissues, and telomeres shorten with each progressive cell division. In contrast, telomerase

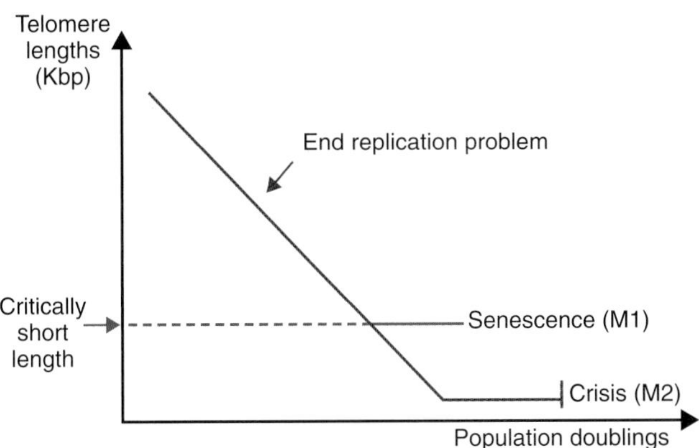

FIGURE 2-5 Telomeric attrition in cultured cells. In mammalian cells the DNA is organized into chromosomes within the nucleus, and these are capped by specialized DNA-protein structures known as *telomeres*. The major function of these structures is protection, but they are progressively eroded at each cell division because of the inability of DNA to completely replicate itself. The result is that there is progressive telomeric attrition as cell populations double. After an estimated 50 cell divisions, cells enter an irreversible (and prolonged) state of cellular senescence (sometimes referred to as *mortality stage 1* [M1]). This period is characterized by arrest of proliferation without loss of biochemical function or viability. At the end of this period, cells exhibit altered morphology and chromosomal instability, a state often referred to as *crisis* (mortality stage 2 [M2]).

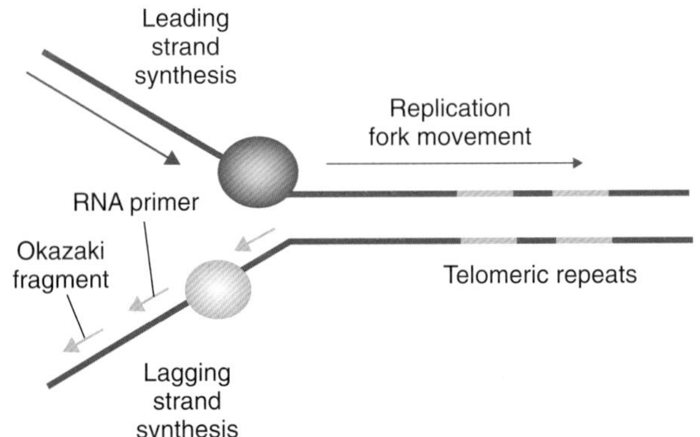

FIGURE 2-6 The end replication problem. Telomeric attrition arises because of the inability of chromosomes to completely replicate their extreme 5′ ends (end replication problem).

activity is a common finding in many human malignancies, resulting in stabilized telomere length. The telomerase complex consists of an RNA subunit that contains a domain complementary to the telomeric repeat sequence TTAGGG and a catalytic protein component. The catalytic protein component acts as a reverse transcriptase and can catalyze the addition of telomeric repeats onto the ends of chromosomes, using the RNA subunit as a template. It is now well documented that the level of telomerase in malignant tissue compared to normal tissue is much higher, and this differential is greater than that for classic enzymatic targets such as thymidylate synthase, dihydrofolate reductase, or topoisomerase II.

Telomerase biology is complex, and the mechanisms by which telomerase becomes reactivated in tumor cells is the subject of intense research. However, this represents an exciting opportunity for further understanding the complex biology of cancer and also the identification of completely novel targets for therapy.

Reprogramming Energy Metabolism

The sustained growth and proliferation of a cancer requires a corresponding adjustment of energy metabolism to ensure this growth can be fueled. Under normal conditions, cells respire aerobically in that they metabolize glucose to pyruvate with a net gain in energy as ATP.[43] Cancer cells can undergo a "metabolic switch" so that glucose is metabolized to lactate, in the presence or absence of oxygen, causing a net energy deficit. There is a corresponding upregulation of glucose transporters (e.g., GLUT-1), which increases uptake of glucose into the cytoplasm. This process is exploited in positron-emission tomography (PET) imaging as tumors will preferentially uptake a radiolabeled analog of glucose (^{18}F-fluorodeoxyglucose [FDG]). This metabolic switch is sometimes referred to as the *Warburg effect* (Figure 2-7).[54]

It is difficult to appreciate the survival advantage of this mechanism. One hypothesis is that the switch allows the diversion of glycolytic intermediates into other biosynthetic pathways that support the production of new cells. This is supported by the observation that the Warburg effect can also be detected in growing cells in the embryo. An expansion of the theory of reprogramming of energy metabolism in cancer suggests that cancer cells are advantaged by a flexibility in their ability to derive ATP. This may come from a number of metabolic pathways that derive ATP from glucose metabolism under aerobic and anaerobic conditions but may also include efficiencies in metabolizing amino acids and lipids toward ATP and other biomolecule synthesis. Such metabolic flexibility may be necessary during primary tumor development but even more so during metastatic progression (see next section).

Metastasis

Metastasis is defined as the dissemination of neoplastic cells to discontinuous secondary (or higher order) sites, where they proliferate to form a macroscopic mass. Implicit in this process is the presence of a primary tumor. Metastases are not a direct extension of the primary tumor and are not dependent on the route of spread (i.e., hematogenous versus lymphatic versus peritoneal dissemination). The process of metastasis is believed to occur through the completion of a series of step-wise events. In order for this process to occur, a cancer cell must leave the site of the primary tumor, pass through the tumor basement membrane, and then through or between endothelial cells to enter the circulation (extravasation). While in the circulation, tumor cells must be able to resist anoikis (programmed cell death associated with loss of cellular contact), evade immune recognition and physical stress, and eventually arrest at distant organs. At that distant site the cell must leave the circulation and survive in the hostile microenvironment of the foreign tissue. These secondary sites are believed to be primed to receive metastatic cells through effects that are directed and mediated by the primary tumor itself (premetastatic niche). This distant site may be the eventual target organ for metastasis or may be a temporary (sanctuary) site. In either case, the cancer cell is thought to lie dormant for a variable and often protracted period of time before moving to its final location. Following a break in dormancy, cells receive signals to proliferate, create new blood vessels (angiogenesis) or co-opt existing blood vessels, and then successfully grow into a measurable metastatic lesion. It is likely that further progression is associated with the repetition of this process resulting in the development of metastases from metastases. As such, the steps outlined here continue not only after the detection of the primary tumor but also after the detection of metastases. From a therapeutic perspective, it is therefore never too late to target the biologic steps

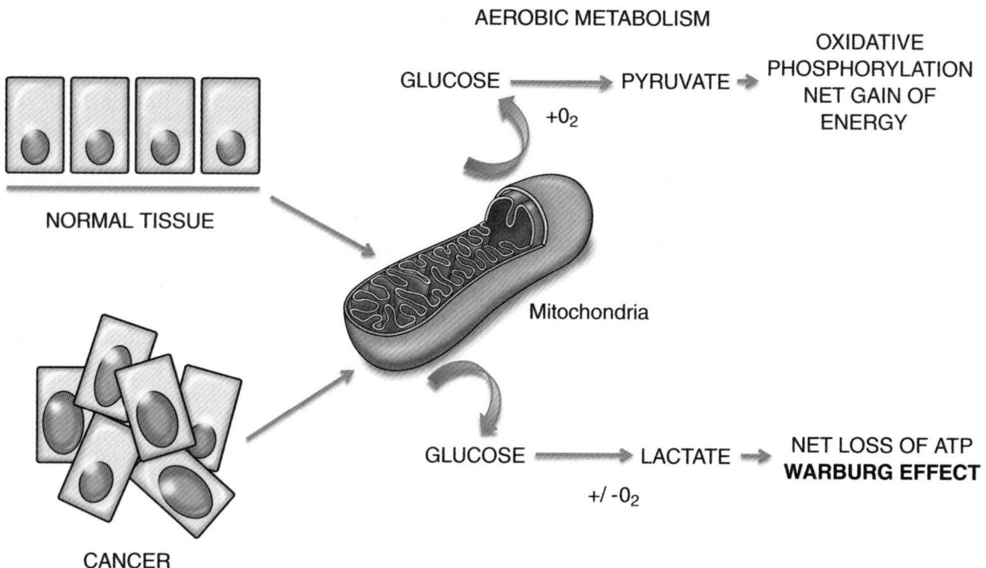

FIGURE 2-7 In normal tissues, cellular respiration in the presence of oxygen allows the production of a net gain in energy through metabolism of glucose to pyruvate. The *Warburg effect* in cancer cells refers to a metabolic switch that causes cancer cells to preferentially metabolize glucose to lactate irrespective of oxygen status, leading to a net loss of energy in the form of adenosine triphosphate (ATP).

associated with metastatic progression as a means to improve outcomes for patients. The basic tenets of this model of metastasis have been intact for over 40 years; however, a greater understanding of biologic principles associated with each metastasis process is emerging.[55]

Metastasis-Associated Genes and Metastasis Suppressor Genes

Cancer cells are not unique in their ability to complete the individual steps required for metastasis (Figure 2-8). For example, leukocytes and neuronal cells have the ability to invade tissue planes and cross vascular barriers. Several types of leukocytes demonstrate the phenotype of intermittent adherence to vascular endothelium and are able to resist anoikis. It is also true that stem cells of various phases of differentiation are able to perform many of these steps during development and in the adult.[56] What is unique about metastatic cells is that each must be able to perform all the steps required for successful metastasis. An extension of this argument is that the genetic changes that permit the metastatic process are not unique to a metastatic cancer cell; however, the metastatic cancer cell must have the appropriate set of genetic changes available to complete all the steps of the metastatic cascade.

Literally hundreds of genes and their resultant proteins have been suggested to contribute to the development of cancers and to their eventual ability to metastasize. It is possible for a single genetic change in cancer to contribute many of the metastasis-associated processes or for several genes to work together toward a single metastasis-associated process. Metastatic cancers may achieve the metastatic phenotype through distinct constellations of genetic and "epigenetic" events that in their respective sums complete the list of necessary metastasis-associated processes needed for successful metastasis. Two classes of genes have been broadly defined as contributing to the metastatic phenotype. These include metastasis promoting genes[57,58] and metastasis suppressors.[59,60] These genes have functions in normal development and physiology (i.e., cell migration, tissue invasion, and angiogenesis discussed earlier) that are subverted by the cancer cell in the acquisition of the metastatic phenotype.

The use of high through-put and genome-wide investigations has uncovered many putative metastasis-associated genes in cancer. It should be noted that many metastasis-associated genes have functions that also contribute to tumor formation and progression. Several of these metastasis-associated genes have been validated in canine and feline cancers.[61,62] For example, the metastasis-associated gene ezrin was identified using genomic approaches in murine and human studies of metastasis.[63] Ezrin is a membrane-cytoskeleton linker protein that functionally and physically connects the actin cytoskeleton to the cell membrane. The degree of ezrin expression in the primary tumor of dogs with osteosarcoma was shown to predict a more aggressive course of disease, defined by metastasis to the lung. Furthermore, recent studies have confirmed the connection between ezrin and protein kinase C (PKC) signaling in murine, canine, and human osteosarcoma cells.[64,65]

Metastasis suppressor genes have been identified in several human cancers. These genes are thought to also have normal functions in the regulation of motility, invasion, and angiogenesis. The loss of these genes is not thought to be associated with the formation of tumors; however, their loss is thought to contribute to specific steps in the metastatic cascade. The characterization, biology, and clinical impact of metastasis suppressor genes have been recently reviewed elsewhere.[66] The loss of reduced expression of metastasis suppressors has not been documented in canine or feline cancers at this time.

The following sections provide descriptions of the critical metastasis-associated processes (see Figure 2-8). Examples of genetic changes or resulting protein changes that contribute to each process is highlighted in each section, with particular emphasis on those with demonstrated associations with veterinary malignancies.

Intravasation

Following the successful growth of the primary tumor, intravasation of a cancer cell into the vascular or lymphatic circulation is the first step required during the metastatic cascade. The process of

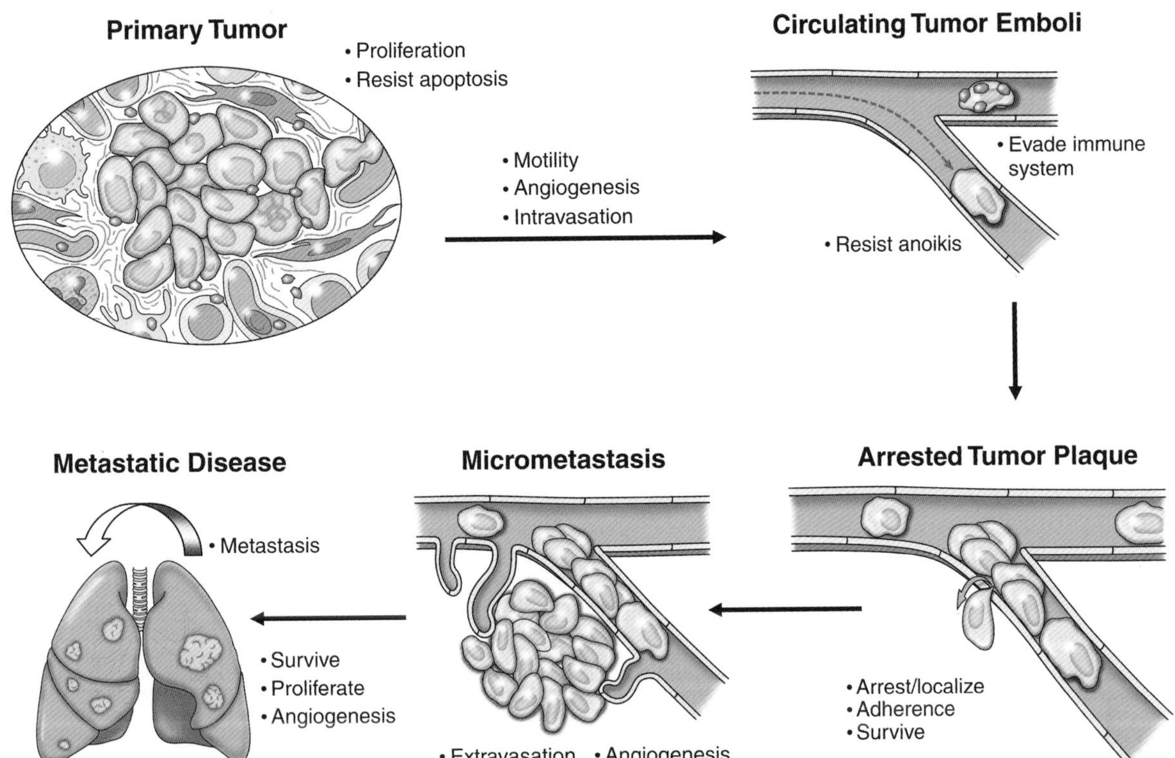

FIGURE 2-8 The metastatic cascade. The metastatic cascade describes a set of discrete steps that cells must move through as a part of the process of metastasis. This complexity begins with the recognized complexity associated with primary tumor development in which tumor cells must proliferate, resist apoptosis, and develop interactions with many host cells in the microenvironment. Subsequent steps then allow metastatic cancer cells to enter and survive in the circulation. Cells then arrest at distant locations, extravasate, and survive in the microenvironment of the distant locations. Arrest of cells may be at the eventual secondary organ where metastasis becomes clinically evident or cells may initially arrest at a "sanctuary site" where they may lie dormant before moving on to the eventual secondary site. The cellular programs that result in a break of dormancy are not well understood. Survival of cells at these sites of dormancy or the eventual secondary site is a significant hurdle for metastatic cells to overcome. Indeed, the majority of cells that arrive at distant locations are unable to survive in these distant locations. At secondary sites, tumor cells may proliferate and progress following the development of the angiogenic phenotype. It is likely that successful metastatic lesions at secondary sites are then the source of subsequent metastases within these secondary sites.

intravasation requires that a tumor cell be motile and able to digest, modulate, or escape the extracellular matrix.[67-69] The specific mechanisms used by cancer cells to invade and intravasate include the classical model of enzymatic degradation of the extracellular matrix referred to as *mesenchymal invasion* (see later discussion on epithelial-mesenchymal transition). Unlike mesenchymal invasion, tumor cells may also develop so-called *amoeboid invasion,* in which they individually slip between fibers of the extracellular matrix without evidence or a need for enzymatic degradation.[70] Finally, a distinct method termed *collective invasion* refers to the en masse regional extension of a tumor into surrounding tissues.[71] Such collective invasion is observed clinically in dogs with oral SCC and biologically high-grade/histologically low-grade fibrosarcoma. The low rate of distant metastasis associated with collective invasion suggests a lack of functional attributes necessary for true distant metastasis. It is likely that individual metastatic tumors may utilize distinct invasion programs at distinct points during metastatic progression. Not surprisingly, studies with intravital imaging (single cell imaging of cancer cells in animals) have demonstrated that only a minority of the cells in the primary tumor develop any of these forms of invasion.[72,73] Efforts are underway to define the genetic features of this minority population.[74,75]

In the classic mesenchymal form of invasion, matrix proteases and metalloproteases (MMPs) are believed to be necessary for the invasive phenotype. Expression of members of this enzyme family have been found in most human and several canine and feline malignancies, including canine osteosarcoma.[76-79] The activity of MMPs in osteosarcoma and mast cell cancers has been correlated with grade and metastatic propensity.[79,80] Similar correlative studies have been undertaken in human patients.[81] The importance of MMP activity during this early step in metastasis prompted the development of pharmacological inhibitors of MMPs. Anticancer activity of these agents in preclinical animal models and in sporadic human patients was evident; however, in randomized trials, the activity of MMPs was not observed.[82,83] The failure of these clinical trials may be explained at many levels and does not refute the importance of invasion as a critical step for a metastatic cell. Rather, these results suggest potential redundancy in the types of invasion (mesenchymal versus amoeboid) that may exist within a given cancer.[84,85] Recent evidence also suggests that the expression of matrix-degrading enzymes and other growth factors may not be necessary in the tumor cells themselves but may be provided by inflammatory cells (i.e., macrophages) recruited by the growing tumor.[86]

Epithelial-Mesenchymal Transition

Observed primarily in the context of epithelial malignancies, the ability of tumor cells to engage in the early steps in the metastatic cascade has been linked to a transcriptional program referred to as *epithelial-mesenchymal transition* (EMT).[87] This transcriptional program has been largely ascribed to the effects of a family of transcription factors, including twist, snail, and slug.[88] Activation of these and other EMT transcription factors is not necessarily associated with a morphologic change in the cancer cell but may be associated with a loss of polarity (apicobasal) in epithelial cells, a greater proportion of cells losing cell-to-cell contacts similar to mesenchymal cells (observed *in vitro*), cell motility, and invasion. In the "mesenchymal" state, suggested by EMT, epithelial cancer cells (similar to cells involved in embryogenesis) develop the phenotypic ability to undergo invasion, migration, and intravasation.[89] Interestingly, cells that are able to take on these "mesenchymal" features share signaling programs and other phenotypes with tumor-initiating cell populations.[90] Opponents of the EMT hypothesis are most critical of the use of the term *transition,* which suggests a switch in the phenotype of individual cells from an epithelial to a mesenchymal form. It is, however, reasonable and generally agreed that the effects of EMT transcription factors contribute to the early phenotypes needed for metastatic progression. Limited data also exist that suggest a need for mesenchymal cells to take on attributes of epithelial cells (likely later during metastatic progression) for successful metastasis, the so-called *mesenchymal-epithelial transition* (MET). For epithelial cancers, MET is also understood to be a final step in EMT, in which following the activation an invasive phenotype and colonization of a distant site cells will revert to their original epithelial phenotypes.

The process of intravasation concludes when a cancer cell successfully enters the vascular or lymphatic circulations. Tumor cells may enter the circulation through established blood vessels, small arterioles, venules, lymphatics, or though tumor-associated (or lined) blood vessels, in a process referred to as *vasculogenic mimicry.*[91] For larger vascular structures, the process of intravasation requires penetration of adventitial cells, including pericytes; digestion of the vascular basement membrane; and penetration between or through endothelial cells.[92] Penetration of the tumor-associated vasculature may be easier than invasion through normal vessels and may only require transit from the extracellular environment between endothelial cells into the circulation.

Survival in the Circulation (Resisting Anoikis)

Frisch and Francis reported the induction of apoptosis after disruption of the interaction between epithelial cells and the extracellular matrix.[93] This phenomenon was termed *anoikis,* from the Greek word for homelessness. In normal tissues, anoikis is a mechanism for maintaining tissue homeostasis and integrity.[94] For the metastatic cancer cell, survival during dissemination requires resistance to anoikis. In normal tissues, anoikis is prevented by two systems: cell-matrix anchorage and cell-cell interactions.[95] Anchorage of cells to the extracellular matrix is mediated primarily by transmembrane receptors referred to as *integrins.* Formation of active heterodimers trigger an intracellular cascade resulting in activation of effectors of growth and survival.[96] Integrin family members have been identified in canine sarcomas and lymphomas.[97-102] Cell-cell anchorage in many epithelial tissues is mediated by cadherins, a family of calcium-binding glycoproteins. Intracellularly, cadherins form complexes with members of the catenin protein family that link them to the actin cytoskeleton, as well as survival-promoting signal transduction cascades.[103] Loss of either cell-cell or cell-matrix interaction in normal cells triggers the activation of the caspase proteases, the hallmark of apoptotic cell death. Metastatic cancer must resist this contact-dependent death in order to be successful and do so through two nonmutually exclusive mechanisms. The first is by maintaining cell-cell contacts with other tumor cells (homotypic interactions) or with host cells such as platelets and inflammatory cells (heterotypic interactions) during metastatic progression. Both homotypic and heterotypic interactions generate intracellular signals that prevent the initiation of anoikis. Additionally, cancer cells may overexpress proteins that directly inhibit anoikis. For example, the integrin pair $\alpha_v\beta_3$ is frequently overexpressed in malignancy, including prostate cancer and melanoma.[104,105] This overexpression subverts the need for ligand binding and results in the generation of survival signals.[106] Proteins reported to be involved in resistance to anoikis include Trk B, focal adhesion kinase (FAK, the immediate effector of integrin signaling), galectin-3, and TGF-β, among others. Certainly more molecular mediators of anoikis resistance have been identified and reviewed elsewhere.[107] These molecules may be valuable antimetastasis targets for novel therapy.

Evasion of the Immune System

At all stages of metastatic progression, metastatic tumor cells must evade detection and destruction by the immune system. The ability of the host immune system to recognize and destroy tumor cells (immunosurveillance) was first proposed by Paul Ehrlich in 1909. Molecular support of the theory of immunosurveillance has come with studies of mice deficient in immunomodulatory and proinflammatory molecules such as interferon-γ (IFN-γ), interleukin-12 (IL-12), and perforin. Mice deficient in these molecules are known to develop tumors more readily than wild-type mice. Clinical evidence for immunosurveillance against cancer was first reported by Coley over 100 years ago. Through the administration of bacteria, Coley's toxin, Coley was able to induce fever and tumor regression in patients with cancer. Evidence in dogs with osteosarcoma further supports the potential value of cancer immunotherapy.[108] Indeed, survival times in dogs who develop bacterial infection at the site of a limb salvage surgery are significantly longer than in dogs who do not develop infection. Interestingly similar parallels may be seen in human osteosarcoma patients. In immunocompetent hosts, it is believed that immunosurveillance removes a large number of cancer cells from the primary tumor, from the circulation, and at distant metastatic sites. Cancer cells employ a wide variety of mechanisms to effect this evasion. The mechanisms for immunosurveillance and evasion from immunosurveillance by cancer are reviewed elsewhere and are summarized in Chapter 13 of this text.[109]

Modification of the immune system to treat cancer continues to be an attractive therapeutic strategy.[110-112] Clinical trials based on this concept have been reported throughout the veterinary literature in dogs with melanoma, soft tissue sarcoma, hemangiosarcoma, osteosarcoma, and others, using a variety of immune-based therapies.[113] Indeed, this principle has been the basis for the development and approval of a therapeutic vaccine directed against a melanoma antigen in dogs with melanoma.[114]

Arrest in Target Tissues

The arrest of circulating tumor cells at distant sites is thought to occur by two distinct but potentially overlapping mechanisms. These include size-dependent "trapping" of tumor cells within the lumen of small vessels (capillaries and veins) in the target organ, and/or receptor mediated interaction involving the tumor cell and the host vasculature.[115] Data supporting the "trapping" phenomenon comes from single-cell imaging studies in which metastatic cancer cells were observed to primarily arrest at distant vascular beds as a result of size-dependent restrictions of large tumor cells in small blood vessels.[116,117] This work was primarily conducted for metastasis to the liver and more recently metastasis to the brain.[118] This trapping phenomenon suggests that the site for metastasis from a primary tumor is largely guided by the location of the first (small vessel) vascular bed encountered by a tumor cell. Alternatively, several groups have suggested the role of specific adhesion molecules as being necessary for initial tumor arrest in the microenvironment of the secondary metastatic sites.[119-121] It is likely that both of the mechanisms play a role in the initial seeding of distant metastatic target organs. The dominant mechanism of arrest may be primarily defined by tumor type or target organ.

Early Survival at Distant Sites

Once the cancer cell or cancer embolus has arrested at its distant sites, it may immediately move out of the circulation into the target organ or may stay within the circulation.[122] In either location, the cancer cell must survive in a new microenvironment. Early survival of metastatic cells at secondary sites is a significant hurdle for the cancer cell. Several studies have shown the ability of cancer cells to arrest at multiple organs in the body. Within hours, the number of remaining cells is dramatically reduced and within days, the number of viable cells may be as low as 0.1% of the original number of cells, even for the most aggressive cancer models.[63,123] The organ selectivity for cancers is to a large extent defined by the organs in which a cancer cell can survive following initial arrest. The "seed and soil" hypothesis first articulated by Paget and then more recently by Fidler et al suggests that the success of a cancer, or metastasis, is defined by interactions between the seed (tumor cell) and the soil (the tumor microenvironment). Arrest of tumor cells in target organs may or may not be receptor mediated (discussed earlier); however, adhesion requires receptor-ligand interactions. Contributors to these steps include the cell adhesion molecules (CAMs). Multiple CAMs have been identified and are named based on their cell specificity (e.g., N-CAM for neural and L-CAM for liver). CD44 is a specific adhesion molecule (H-CAM for homing), initially identified as the receptor for the matrix component hyaluronic acid on hematopoietic cells. Expression of splice variants of CD44 on tumor cells has been demonstrated to correlate with poor prognosis in a wide variety of human tumors from acute myelogenous leukemia (AML) and Hodgkin's disease to breast and colon cancer and osteosarcoma.[124] Chemokines are a class of chemotactic cytokines that function in leukocyte trafficking and function. In metastasis, chemokines may also contribute to the metastatic process through enhanced metastatic cell survival.[125] Chemokines may be active in the recruitment of a leukocytic infiltrate to intravasated, circulating tumor cells, therein creating an embolus that can better resist shearing stress associated with circulation or through the generation of matrix degrading proteins at the distant metastatic site.

The Premetastatic Niche and Modulation of the Microenvironment

It is increasingly clear that the sites (microenvironments) of successful secondary metastasis are modulated by the presence of a primary tumor and then by the arrival of metastatic cells at the secondary site. The concept of the premetastatic niche suggests that a primary tumor modulates the microenvironment of a secondary site before the arrival of most metastatic cells.[126] The modulation of the premetastatic niche appears to be accomplished by primary tumor-induced mobilization and recruitment of specific primarily bone marrow–derived cells (bone marrow niche) to the secondary microenvironment.[127] These bone marrow–derived cells are myeloid in origin and express the vascular endothelial growth factor receptor (VEGFR). Interestingly, the sites of metastatic tumor arrest appear to preferentially include sites in which these myeloid-derived cells were first recruited. Furthermore, targeting these VEGFR-positive cells using pharmacologic and genetic tools has effectively prevented metastatic development in murine models.[127] Ongoing studies will likely uncover greater complexity of the populations of cells recruited to the premetastatic niche and potentially therapeutic targets for antimetastatic therapy (see Figure 1-5).

Following survival at the distant site, the tumor cell must proliferate and modulate its new environment. In most cases, it is believed that cancer cells extravasate from the circulation and then proliferate in the new organ. However, it is also possible for proliferation to occur within blood vessels, in a process referred to as *intravascular metastases,* and then expand out into the local tissue before further proliferation occurs.[128] In both situations, modulation of the new environment is necessary for appropriate growth and progression of the metastatic lesions. It is now recognized that part of this modulation is based on tumor-induced changes in the stroma.[129,130] These stromal changes may result in the production of growth factors or signals that are used by the tumor for further growth. These stromal cell–derived growth factors provide important signals for tumor cell proliferation and progression, including angiogenesis. The importance of tumor-stromal interaction has suggested that the "induced" tumor-stroma may be a credible target for novel cancer therapeutics.[131]

Angiogenesis

It is now well accepted that the development of new blood vessels from endothelial progenitors (vasculogenesis) or from existing blood vessels (angiogenesis) is required for cancer progression and metastasis.[132,133] Endothelial cells or endothelial progenitors are activated by tumor-derived growth factors and result in new capillaries at the tumor site.[134] In healthy tissue, endothelial cell proliferation is controlled by a balance between protein factors that activate endothelial cells and those that antagonize activation. Malignant tumors provide signals that result in endothelial cell survival, motility, invasion, differentiation, and organization. These steps are required to create a supportive vasculature for the tumor. In many ways, these required endothelial processes share parallel features with the processes required for the success of a metastatic cancer cell itself. The creation of new blood vessels requires the tumors to recruit circulating endothelial cells to their site, presumably through the release of growth factors such as vascular endothelial growth factor (VEGF). Circulating endothelial cells must survive at their new site with the help of survival signals (e.g., thrombospondin-I [TSP-I]) and form vascular tubes that then reorganize to sustain blood flow. The resulting vasculature of cancers is typically aberrant with often poorly organized and chaotic vascular structures that are leaky, with limited adventitial development and excessive branching.[135] Once developed, this angiogenic phenotype (the result of the angiogenic switch) is associated with a diverse pattern of ongoing angiogenesis and neovascularization. This ongoing process is likely complex and involves a wide variety of tumor and microenvironmental-derived growth factors and signaling molecules. Adding to this complexity, it is likely that certain phases of cancer progression are associated with and require periods of antiangiogenesis. Indeed, these hypovascularized states may directly contribute to the progression of certain cancers.[136]

Many lines of evidence support the importance of angiogenesis in the biology of metastasis. The vascularity of a primary tumor (measured by microvessel density) has been correlated with metastatic behavior for most human and many veterinary tumors. The expression of angiogenesis-associated growth or survival factors and their receptors (i.e., VEGFR) in serum and in tumors, respectively, has also been correlated with outcome; more recently, functional imaging studies using magnetic resonance imaging (MRI) and other means has provided correlates of vascularity with poor outcome.[137,138] The strength of this biologic argument has supported the development of a number of novel therapeutic agents with antiangiogenic activities. These agents have moved through discovery and development and are now approved drugs for cancer (see Section C in Chapter 14).

Metastasis from Metastases

For most solid tumors the appearance of a single metastatic nodule is followed shortly by the development of additional metastases within the same target organ and tertiary sites. It is unlikely that these metastatic sites all emerge from distinct and unique clones within the primary tumor and nearly simultaneously progress through the metastatic cascade to yield synchronous metastases at the distant site. It is reasonable and perhaps more likely that metastases develop from other metastatic sites. In this hypothesis a small number of successful clones colonize distant sites. As these clones move through progression to become successful metastases, the process of metastasis continues, resulting in metastasis from metastases. Although data supporting this hypothesis are limited, the implication for the treatment and management of cancer patients is substantial. If true, the process of metastasis from metastases would suggest that all steps in the metastatic cascade occur continuously, both before and after detection of metastases in patients. As such, all of the steps in the metastatic cascade may be targets for future therapeutic intervention.

Ongoing Controversies and Areas of Research in the Field of Metastasis

Does the Metastatic Propensity for Tumors Emerge Early or Late in the Biology of Cancer?

The development of the metastatic phenotype has been traditionally believed to be a process that happens late in carcinogenesis. In this model, referred to as the *progression model,* the genetic changes responsible for primary tumor development are in most cases distinct and precede those steps that result in the metastatic phenotype.[139,140] The progression model argues that the metastatic phenotype is acquired within a small fraction of cells within the heterogeneous primary tumor. Support for the progression model came from work by Fidler and others, who demonstrated the ability to select for rodent cancers with greater metastatic potential, through the serial passage of metastatic tumor nodules back to naïve mice. This selection phenomenon suggested that a minority of tumor cell clones within a primary tumor were endowed with the metastatic phenotype and that this small proportion were enriched in the metastases compared to the primary tumor. Application of the progression model would suggest that a period of time exists between primary tumor development and acquisition of the full metastatic phenotype. This model was thought to be the basis of the improved outcome associated with early detection of cancers and the belief that effective and definitive therapy was most likely if a diagnosis was made early. Work from Ramaswamy et al provided data to support an alternative model,[57] "the early oncogenic model" for metastasis. This alternative suggests that the genetic events that contribute to initial primary tumor development are the same or emerge at the same time as the events that contribute to the metastatic phenotype. As such, the early oncogenic model suggests that the biology of a cancer is defined early and may not be something that can be reduced through the early identification of a cancer. This is not to say that early detection of a cancer is not helpful for a patient, but rather that bad cancers may be "born" bad. This model may explain the phenomenon of the unknown primary tumor, wherein metastatic disease is detected without an apparent primary tumor.

To add complexity to the question of emergence of the metastatic phenotype, there is increasing evidence that host (genomic) differences can influence metastatic behavior of cancers, without necessarily influencing primary tumor growth.[141,142] Using a genetically engineered mouse model of mammary cancer, Hunter et al have been able to identify specific host genes that influence metastatic behavior of tumors.[141,143,144] These findings have several important implications. First, they suggest that individuals might be predisposed to aggressive metastatic progression before the development of a tumor. In addition, it suggests that there may be families in the population that are at high risk, not necessarily for tumor development, but for aggressive metastatic course once a tumor develops. Most importantly, if a significant part of a patient's metastatic risk is encoded within the patient's constitutional genome rather than within the mutated tumor genome, it may be feasible to identify those individuals at high risk for metastatic disease at the time of diagnosis of the primary tumor, or potentially before. This finding may be particularly relevant in the field of veterinary oncology, in which breed-associated genomic differences may explain the more aggressive course of disease seen in some dogs compared to others. Taken together, the risk for metastatic progression is in part defined by the genetics of the patient, genetic changes that develop early in the process of tumor development, and the subsequent and incremental emergence of aggressive metastatic cells.

Where Is the Inefficiency in Metastatic Inefficiency?

As devastating as the metastatic process is, it is equally inefficient. Estimates of this inefficiency in animal models suggest that less than 1% of cancer cells that successfully enter the circulation are able to survive at distant sites.[145] The true metastatic inefficiency of human cancers is likely to be much lower. In most studies to date, it does not seem that entry of cancer cells into the circulation is the major barrier for successful metastases. Recent studies have identified high numbers of circulating tumor cells in cancer patients who are free of metastatic disease. The clinical importance of high circulating tumor cell numbers is not clear[146]; however, it appears that for some cancers, high circulating numbers of cancer cells do not necessarily correlate with risk for metastasis. Butler and Gullino estimated that between 1 to 4×10^6 cells/g of tumor enter the systemic circulation each day in human cancers.[147] These data suggest that, although intravasation is necessary for metastasis, it is not sufficient nor is it process limiting. After removal of the primary tumor, these circulating cell counts drop and in many cases, no gross metastases develop. Although arrest at target organs may be a limitation for some cancers, the successful early survival of cancer cells at distant sites appears to be a major hurdle for successful metastases and therefore is a significant contributor to metastatic inefficiency. Metastatic cancer cells appear to be highly vulnerable to death (metastatic inefficiency) early after their arrival at a secondary site. The microenvironment of the secondary site is distinct from that of the primary tumor site and the initial tissues of origin of the cancer cell. These differences include changes in oxygen tension, pH, growth factor availability, and cellular binding partners. Collectively, these changes represent unique stresses to metastatic cancer cells. Successful metastatic cells must recognize, adapt, and endure these stresses in order to survive. Furthermore, appropriate modulation of the secondary microenvironment before the cancer cells arrive (premetastatic niche) and as a result of early and effective interaction with stromal and inflammatory cells within the new environment allow select populations of cells to survive and proliferate. The duration of this initial vulnerable state during metastatic progression may extend for the entire period of dormancy (see later). It is also likely that metastatic cells must successfully pass through additional vulnerable states later during metastatic progression. Targeting metastatic cancer cells during these vulnerable states may be an effective treatment strategy for cancer metastasis.[148]

What Is Dormancy and Where Do Dormant Cells Reside?

In spite of effective control of the primary tumor and aggressive multiagent and multimodality adjuvant therapy, the risk for metastases to distant sites remains high for several cancer histologies. Since most patients are free of gross metastases at the time of diagnosis, the development of metastases is presumed to emerge from microscopic cells that are not identifiable at the time of initial patient presentation.[149] The location, size, angiogenic state, and proliferative/apoptotic state of these microscopic cells are largely unknown. Indeed, these dormant cells may exist as single cancer cells or microscopic clusters, they may exist in a quiescent (outside the cell cycle) or in a balanced state of proliferation and apoptosis, they may lie dormant in the eventual secondary metastatic tissue site (i.e., the lung) or persist in sanctuary sites (i.e., the bone marrow). Recent insights gleaned from the tumor-initiating (cancer stem cell) model may provide further support for the hypothesis that metastatic cells are capable of residence in transient sites like the bone marrow, where they may rest in a dormant state before being recruited into the metastatic cascade. The signals that induce these presumed small populations of cells to break dormancy and emerge into gross metastases likely also involve tumor cell microenvironment interaction.[150,151]

The Enabling Characteristics

As previously suggested, the hallmarks of cancer have been defined as functional capabilities that allow cancer cells to survive, proliferate, and disseminate. The fact that these critical hallmarks can be attained within a single cancer is explained by two key enabling characteristics of cancer: genome instability and tumor-promoting inflammation.

Genome Instability

The majority of the acquired hallmarks of cancer require changes in the genome through mutation, amplification, or chromosomal translocation. However, the process of random mutation is inefficient because of the complex and fastidious maintenance mechanisms of the normal cell that monitor DNA damage and regulate repair enzymes. As such, it is actually difficult to explain why cancers arise in animals at all because the acquisition of all traits would seem an impossible task. To explain this, it may be argued that genomes must attain increased mutability or genome instability in order to overcome the redundant homeostatic mechanisms that ordinarily prevent the emergence of a cancer cell.[1,2]

The following mechanisms have been suggested that may support the development of genomic instability[43]:

- Defects affecting various components of the DNA-maintenance machinery (caretakers of the genome), which may involve mutations in caretaker genes.
- The loss of telomeric DNA, which may cause karyotypic instability and chromosomal changes (amplification/deletion).
- Inactivation of tumor suppressor genes through genetic (mutation) or epigenetic (DNA methylation/histone modifications) mechanisms.

Tumor-Promoting Inflammation

For decades it has been recognized that tumors contain inflammatory and immune cell infiltrates that have classically been considered to be an attempt by the immune system to eradicate the tumor. However, recent evidence suggests that tumor-associated inflammation may paradoxically have a tumor-promoting effect. Inflammation can contribute to neoplastic progression through one of the following various mechanisms.[43,152,153]

- The supply of growth factors and growth signals to the microenvironment that promote angiogenesis, cell proliferation, and invasion.
- Induction signals that support the process of EMT.
- Fostering the progression of premalignant lesions to fully blown cancer.
- The production of reactive oxygen species that are mutagenic.

Many of the cells that contribute to this are components of the innate immune system, particularly macrophages with a specific, cancer-promoting phenotype. Specifically, they form part of the tumor microenvironment that supports the maintenance of the cancer phenotype (see Figure 1-5).

The Pathway to Cancer

The eight acquired capabilities of cancer cells and the two overarching enabling characteristics of genome instability and tumor inflammation have been outlined. It is important to stress that the pathways by which cells become malignant are highly variable. Mutations in certain oncogenes can occur early in the progression of some tumors and late in others. As a consequence, the acquisition of the essential cancer characteristics may appear at different times in the progression of different cancers. Furthermore, in certain tumors, a specific genetic event may, on its own, contribute only partially to the acquisition of a single capability, while in others it may contribute to the simultaneous acquisition of multiple capabilities. However, irrespective of the path taken, the hallmark capabilities of cancer will remain common for multiple cancer types and will help clarify mechanisms, prognosis, and the development of new treatments.

The Tumor Microenvironment

Over the past 10 years, tumors have been increasingly considered as organ systems similar to the tissues from which they derive. This is in contrast to a reductionist view of cancer biology, which considers the tumor as just a mass of tumor cells. In reality, the tumor is a complex system containing cancer cells and supporting cells, which all contribute to the maintenance of the malignant population and support ultimate dissemination and metastasis.

Consequently, the major players in the cancer "organ system" are as follows:

- Cancer cells and cancer stem cells (CSCs)
- Endothelial cells
- Pericytes
- Immune cells
- Tumor-associated fibroblasts

Cancer Cells and Cancer Stem Cells

The concept that a cancer can arise from any cell in the body, along with the stochastic model of tumorigenesis, has recently been challenged.[154,155] Although tumor heterogeneity is a well-established concept, a new dimension to heterogeneity has been established that suggests that a tumor may contain a hierarchical structure similar to many normal organ systems. Recent evidence suggests the existence of CSCs (sometimes termed *tumor-initiating cells*), which form the founder cell population for a tumor (see Figure 1-8). It was first extensively documented for leukemia and multiple myeloma that only a small subset of cancer cells are capable of extensive proliferation. For example, when mouse myeloma cells were obtained from mouse ascites, separated from normal hematopoietic cells, and put in clonal in vitro colony-forming assays, only 1 in 10,000 to 1 in 100 cancer cells were able to form colonies. Even when leukemic cells were transplanted in vivo, only 1% to 4% of cells could form spleen colonies.[156-161] Because the differences in clonogenicity among the leukemia cells mirrored the differences in clonogenicity among normal hematopoietic cells, the clonogenic leukemic cells were described as leukemic stem cells. It has also been shown for solid cancers that the cells are phenotypically heterogeneous and that only a small proportion of cells are clonogenic in culture and in vivo.[162-165] For example, only 1 in 1000 to 1 in 5000 lung cancer, ovarian cancer, or neuroblastoma cells were found to form colonies in soft agar. Just as in the context of leukemic stem cells, these observations led to the hypothesis that only a few cancer cells are actually tumorigenic and that these tumorigenic cells could be considered as CSCs. Although the field and concept of CSCs is a controversial one, CSCs may prove to be a common constituent of many, if not all, cancer types. Features of the CSC model also fit well with a view of metastasis in which only a small number of cells within a tumor have the ability (and plasticity) to endure the stresses of metastatic progression, survive during a dormant period, and then progress, proliferate, and differentiate into the complex heterogenous metastatic lesion.

If tumor growth and metastasis are driven by a small population of CSCs, this might explain the failure to develop therapies that are consistently able to eradicate solid tumors.[154,155] Although currently available drugs can shrink metastatic tumors, these effects are usually transient and often do not appreciably extend the life of patients. One reason for the failure of these treatments is the acquisition of drug resistance by the cancer cells as they evolve; another possibility is that existing therapies fail to kill CSCs effectively.

Stem cell populations in human cancers have been identified in breast, bone, brain, colon, pancreas, liver, ovary, and skin.[154,155] The actual origin of CSCs within solid tumors has not been clarified and may actually vary between tumor types. In some tumors, it may be that the resident adult or somatic stem cell may serve as the tumor-initiating cell, and in other tumors, the initiating cell may be the resident progenitor or transit-amplifying cell. A characteristic of the CSCs is that they undergo asymmetric division and self-renew, providing a continual resident population of highly resistant cancer cells.

Existing cancer therapies have been largely developed against the bulk population of tumor cells because they are often identified by their ability to shrink tumors. Because most cells with a cancer have limited proliferative potential, an ability to shrink a tumor mainly reflects an ability to kill these cells. It seems that normal stem cells from various tissues tend to be more resistant to chemotherapeutics than mature cell types from the same tissues. If the same is true of CSCs, then one would predict that these cells would be more resistant to chemotherapeutics than tumor cells with limited proliferative potential. Even therapies that cause complete regression of tumors might spare enough CSCs to allow regrowth of the tumors. Therapies that are more specifically directed against CSCs might result in much more durable responses and even cures of metastatic tumors. In veterinary oncology, putative stem cell populations have been identified for breast, bone, brain, and liver.[154,155,166-168] Interestingly, stem cell populations appear to have altered DNA repair pathways, which may explain their resistance to conventional drugs. Identification of these populations, coupled with the availability of microarray and microRNA array technology, is allowing the identification of potential therapeutic targets.

Recent research has linked the acquisition of CSC characteristics with the EMT program, described previously in the section on metastasis.[168] Cells that undergo EMT also take on characteristics reminiscent of the CSC phenotype. For example, they have the ability to self-renew and may support the ability of cells to colonize outside of the primary tumor. One may speculate that the signaling processes that support EMT may also serve to maintain the CSC population within a tumor and may also suggest plasticity in CSC populations.

Endothelial Cells

Much of the heterogeneity in tumors is found in the stromal compartment, and many of these cells are endothelial cells, which form the tumor-associated vasculature. VEGF and fibroblast growth factor are prominent signaling pathways in formation of these vessels. More modern sequencing techniques have also identified new pathways that may represent important signaling systems for neoangiogenesis and may represent therapeutic targets (e.g., notch signaling).

Pericytes

Pericytes are mesenchymal cells that wrap around the endothelial tubing of the blood vessels. Pericytes are considered a major cell type supporting the tumor vasculature.

Immune Inflammatory Cells

As described previously, an environment of chronic inflammation is an important enabling characteristic that supports the acquisition of cancer-related traits. Cells of the innate immune system are particularly crucial for the maintenance of the tumor environment. In particular, tumor macrophages with a specific pro-tumor phenotype can enhance cellular proliferation, invasion, and neoangiogenesis.

Cancer-Associated Fibroblasts

Cancer-associated fibroblasts comprise the supporting structure for many tumors but can also promote invasion, cell proliferation, and neoangiogenesis.[43] The importance of the various cell types that make up the tumor microenvironment cannot be overstated. Although there is a complex signaling network between and within cancer cells that maintains the cancer phenotype, superimposed on top of this are the complex signaling networks between stromal components and stromal cells and cancer cells. Although we have considered earlier the potential evolution of cancer cells as they evolve from early disease to late-stage disease, it is quite possible that there is a similar evolution in the supporting structures that is dictated by the cancer itself. For example, incipient tumors may recruit stromal elements, which in turn reciprocate by promoting cell proliferation and angiogenesis. Evolution of the cancer population may then in turn feed back on the stromal population to further reprogram them to support the growing tumor. This of course could be extended to show the role of the stroma in promoting invasion and metastasis. These mechanisms underpin the complexity of understanding cancer pathogenesis as the process is highly dynamic and context dependent.

Summary and Future Directions

In this chapter we have sought to simplify as far as possible the mechanisms of carcinogenesis. It is clear that genomic instability and an environment of chronic inflammation support and provide a basis for the acquisition of the eight fundamental cancer characteristics. The identification of these pathways is providing excellent clues to the underlying mechanisms in cancer and the identification of potential therapeutic targets. However, despite our ability to make small molecules or antibodies, which aim at key targets in cancer survival, we are still a long way from a cure. The reasons for this are many but include the inherent tumor heterogeneity (in part supplied by the existence of tumor stem cells), the continual tumor evolution, and the immense and underestimated contribution of the tumor microenvironment. It is clear that multiple approaches will be required to maximize any possibility of therapeutic benefit.

REFERENCES

1. McCance KL, Roberts LK: Cellular biology. In McCance KL, Huether SE, editors: *Pathophysiology: The biological basis of disease in adults and children*, ed 3, St. Louis, 1997, Mosby.
2. Wyke J: Viruses and cancer. In Franks LM, Teich NM, editors: *The molecular and cellular biology of cancer*, ed 3, Oxford, 1997, Oxford University Press.
3. Vousden KH: Cell transformation by human papillomaviruses. In Minsen AC, Neil JC, McCrae MA, editors: *Viruses and cancer*, Cambridge, 1994, Cambridge University Press.
4. Campo MS, O'Neil BW, Barron RJ, et al: Experimental reproduction of the papilloma-carcinoma complex of the alimentary canal in cattle, *Carcinogenesis* 15(8):1597–1601, 1994.
5. Campo MS, Jarrett WF, Barron R, et al: Association of bovine papillomavirus type 2 and bracken fern with bladder cancer in cattle, *Cancer Res* 52(24):6898–6904, 1992.
6. Donner P, Greiser-Wilkie I, Moelling K: Nuclear localization and DNA binding of the transforming gene product of avian myelocytomatosis virus, *Nature* 296:262–266, 1982.
7. Reid SW, Smith KT, Jarrett WF: Detection, cloning and characterisation of papillomaviral DNA present in sarcoid tumours of Equus asinus, *Vet Rec* 135(18):430–432, 1994.
8. Gaukroger JM, Bradley A, Chandrachud L, et al: Interaction between bovine papillomavirus type 4 and cocarcinogens in the production of malignant tumours, *J Gen Virol* (Pt 10): 2275–2280, 1993.
9. Jarrett WF: Bovine papilloma viruses, *Clin Dermatol* 3(4):8–19, 1985.
10. Lancaster WD, Olson C, Meinke W: Bovine papillomavirus: presence of virus-specific DNA sequences in naturally occurring equine tumours, *Proc Nat Acad Sci U S A* 74:524–528, 1977.
11. Golias CH, Charalabopoulos A, Charalabopoulos K: Cell proliferation and cell cycle control: a mini review, *Int J Clin Prac* 58(12):1134–1141, 2004.
12. Kong N, Fotouhi N, Wovkulich PM, et al: Cell cycle inhibitors for the treatment of cancer, *Drugs of the future* 28(9):881–896, 2003.
13. Lane DP: P53: Guardian of the genome, *Nature* 358:15–16, 1992.
14. Levine AJ: P53, the cellular gatekeeper for growth and division, *Cell* 88:323–331, 1997.
15. Wu X, Bayle JH, Olson D, et al: The p53-mdm2 autoregulatory loop, *Genes Dev* 7:1126–1132, 1993.
16. Haupt Y, Maya R, Kazaz A, et al: Mdm2 promotes the rapid degradation of p53, *Nature* 387:296–299, 1997.
17. Wyllie AH, Kerr JF, Currie AR: Cell death: the significance of apoptosis, *Int Rev Cytol* 68:251–306, 1980.
18. Strasser A, Cory S, Adams JM: Deciphering the rules of programmed cell death to improve therapy of cancer and other diseases, *EMBO J* 30(18):3667–3683, 2011.
19. Jones S, Zhang X, Parsons DW, et al: Core signaling pathways in human pancreatic cancers revealed by global genomic analyses, *Science* 321(5897):1801–1806, 2008.
20. Parsons DW, Jones S, Zhang X, et al: An integrated genomic analysis of human glioblastoma Multiforme, *Science* 321(5897):1807–1812 2008.
21. McCance KL, Roberts LK: The biology of cancer. In McCance KL, Huether SE, editors: *Pathophysiology: The biological basis of disease in adults and children*, ed 3, St. Louis, 1997, Mosby.
22. Jarrett O, Onions D: Leukaemogenic viruses. In Whittaker JA, editor: *Leukaemia*, ed 2, Oxford, 1992, Blackwell Scientific Publications.
23. Balmain A, Brown K: Oncogene activation in chemical carcinogenesis, *Adv Cancer Res* 51:147–182, 1988.
24. Adams GE, Cox R: Radiation carcinogenesis. In Franks LM, Teich NM, editors: *The molecular and cellular biology of cancer*, ed 3, New York, 1997, Oxford University Press.
25. Neil JC, Hughs D, McFarlane R, et al: Transduction and rearrangement of the *myc* gene by feline leukemia virus in naturally occurring T cell leukemias, *Nature* 308:814–820, 1984.
26. Onions DE, Lees G, Forrest D, et al: Recombinant feline viruses containing the *myc* gene rapidly produce clonal tumours expressing T-cell antigen receptor gene transcripts, *Intern J Cancer* 40:40–45, 1987.
27. Teich NM: Oncogenes and cancer. In Franks LM, Teich NM, editors: *The molecular and cellular biology of cancer*, ed 3, New York, 1997, Oxford University Press.
28. Tennent R, Wigley C, Balmain A: Chemical carcinogenesis. In Franks LM, Teich NM, editors: *The molecular and cellular biology of cancer*, ed 3, New York, 1997, Oxford University Press.
29. Huret JL, Senon S, Bernheim A, et al: An atlas on genes and chromosomes in oncology and haematology, *Cell Mol Biol* 50(7):805–807, 2004.
30. Soto AM, Sonnenschein C: The somatic mutation theory of cancer: Growing problems with the paradigm? *Bioessays* 26(10):1097–1107, 2004.
31. Nasir L, Rutteman GR, Reid SWJ, et al: Analysis of p53 mutational events and MM2 amplification in canine soft-tissue sarcomas, *Cancer Lett* 174(1):83–89, 2001.
32. Weinberg RA: The retinoblastoma protein and cell cycle control, *Cell* 81:323–330, 1995.
33. Oliner JD, Kinzler KW, Meltzer PS, et al: Amplification of a gene encoding a p53 associated protein in human sarcomas, *Nature* 358:80–83, 1992.
34. Vogelstein B, Kinzler KW: P53 function and dysfunction, *Cell* 70:525–526, 1992.
35. Sluss HK, Jones SN: Analysing p53 tumour suppressor functions in mice, *Expert Opin Ther Targets* 7(1):89–99, 2003.
36. Harris CC: P53 tumor suppressor gene: from the basic research laboratory to the clinic—an abridged historical perspective, *Carcinogenesis* 17:1187–1198, 1996.
37. Nasir L, Rutteman GR, Reid SW, et al: Analysis of p53 mutational events and MDM2 amplification in canine soft-tissue sarcomas, *Cancer Lett* 174(1):83–89, 2001.

38. Nasir L, Burr P, Mcfarlane S, et al: Cloning, sequence analysis and expression of the cDNA's encoding the canine and equine homologues of the Mouse double minute two proto-oncogene, *Cancer Lett* 152:9–13, 2000.
39. Nasir L, Krasner H, Argyle DJ, et al: A Study of p53 tumour suppressor gene immunoreactivity in feline neoplasia, *Cancer Lett* 155:1–7, 2000.
40. Nasir L, Argyle DJ: Mutational analysis of p53 in two cases of Bull Mastiff lymphosarcoma, *Vet Rec* 145(1):23–24, 1999.
41. Nasir L, Argyle DJ, McFarlane ST, et al: Nucleotide sequence of a highly conserved region of the canine p53 tumour suppressor gene, *DNA Sequence* 8(1–2):83–86, 1998.
42. Hanahan D, Weinberg RA: The hallmarks of cancer, *Cell* 100(1):57–70, 2000.
43. Hanahan D, Weinberg RA: Hallmarks of cancer: The next generation, *Cell* 144(5):646–674, 2011.
44. Kimmelman AC: The dynamic nature of autophagy in cancer, *Genes Dev* 25(19):1999–2010, 2011.
45. Blasco MA, Funk W, Villeponteau B, et al: Functional characterization and developmental regulation of mouse telomerase RNA, *Science* 269:1267–1270, 1995.
46. Blasco MA, Lee H-W, Hande MP, et al: Telomere shortening and tumour formation by mouse cells lacking telomerase RNA, *Cell* 91:25–34, 1997.
47. Hayflick L: Mortality and immortality at the cellular level. A review, *Biochemistry* 62:1180–1190, 1997.
48. Biller BJ, Kitchel B, Casey D, et al: Evaluation of an assay for detecting telomerase activity in neoplastic tissues of dogs, *Am J Vet Res* 59(12):1526–1528, 1998.
49. McKenzie K, Umbricht CB, Sukumar S: Applications of telomerase research in the fight against cancer, *Mol Med Today* 5(3):114–122, 1999.
50. Nasir L, Devlin P, Mckevitt T, et al: Telomere lengths and telomerase activity in dog tissues: a potential model system to study human telomere and telomerase biology, *Neoplasia* 3(4):351–359, 2001.
51. Shay JW, Wright WE: Telomerase activity in human cancer, *Curr Opin Oncol* 8:66–71, 1996.
52. Yazawa M, Okuda M, Setoguchi A, et al: Measurement of telomerase activity in dog tumours, *J Vet Med Sci* 61(10):1125–1129, 1999.
53. Zhu J, Wang H, Bishop JM, et al: Telomerase extends the life-span of virus-transformed human cells without net telomere lengthening, *Proc Natl Acad Sci U S A* 96:3723–3728, 1999.
54. Shanmugam M, McBrayer SK, et al: Targeting the Warburg effect in hematological malignancies: from PET to therapy, *Curr Opin Oncol* 21(6):531–536, 2009.
55. Mendoza M, Khanna C: Revisiting the seed and soil in cancer metastasis, *Int J Biochem Cell Biol* 41(7):1452–1462, 2009.
56. Sell S: Stem cell origin of cancer and differentiation therapy, *Crit Rev Oncol Hematol* 51(1):1–28, 2004.
57. Ramaswamy S, et al: A molecular signature of metastasis in primary solid tumors, *Nat Genet* 33(1):49–54, 2003.
58. Clark, EA, et al: Genomic analysis of metastasis reveals an essential role for RhoC [In Process Citation], *Nature* 406(6795): 532–535, 2000.
59. Shevde LA, Welch DR: Metastasis suppressor pathways–an evolving paradigm, *Cancer Lett* 198(1):1–20, 2003.
60. Steeg PS, Perspectives on classic article: metastasis suppressor genes, *J Natl Cancer Inst* 96(6):E4, 2004.
61. Paoloni M, et al: Canine tumor cross-species genomics uncovers targets linked to osteosarcoma progression, *BMC Genom* 10:625, 2009.
62. Mayr B, Brem G, Reifinger M: Absence of S100A4 (mts1) gene mutations in various canine and feline tumours. Detection of a polymorphism in feline S100A4 (mts1), *J Vet Med A Physiol Pathol Clin Med* 47(2):123–128, 2000.
63. Khanna C, et al: The membrane-cytoskeleton linker ezrin is necessary for osteosarcoma metastasis, *Nat Med* 10(2):182–186, 2004.
64. Ren L, et al: Dysregulation of Ezrin phosphorylation prevents metastasis and alters cellular metabolism in osteosarcoma, *Cancer Res* 72(4):1001–1012, 2012.
65. Hong SH, et al: Protein kinase C regulates ezrin-radixin-moesin phosphorylation in canine osteosarcoma cells, *Vet Comp Oncol* 9(3):207–218, 2011.
66. Shoushtari AN, Szmulewitz RZ, Rinker-Schaeffer CW: Metastasis-suppressor genes in clinical practice: lost in translation? *Nat Rev Clin Oncol* 8(6):333–342, 2011.
67. Liotta LA, Kohn EC: The microenvironment of the tumour-host interface, *Nature* 411(6835):375–379, 2001.
68. Friedl P, Wolf K, Lammerding J: Nuclear mechanics during cell migration, *Curr Opin Cell Biol* 23(1):55–64, 2011.
69. Friedl P, Wolf K: Plasticity of cell migration: a multiscale tuning model, *J Cell Biol* 188(1):11–19, 2010.
70. Sabeh, F, Shimizu-Hirota R, Weiss SJ: Protease-dependent versus -independent cancer cell invasion programs: three-dimensional amoeboid movement revisited, *J Cell Biol* 185(1): 11–19, 2009.
71. Scott RW, Crighton D, Olson MF: Modeling and imaging 3-dimensional collective cell invasion. *J Vis Exp* (58):2011.
72. Condeelis J, Segall JE: Intravital imaging of cell movement in tumours, *Nat Rev Cancer* 3(12):921–930, 2003.
73. Condeelis J, Singer RH, Segall JE: The great escape: when cancer cells hijack the genes for chemotaxis and motility, *Annu Rev Cell Dev Biol* 21:695–718, 2005.
74. Wang W, et al: Single cell behavior in metastatic primary mammary tumors correlated with gene expression patterns revealed by molecular profiling, *Cancer Res* 62(21):6278–6288, 2002.
75. Wyckoff JB, Segall JE, Condeelis JS: The collection of the motile population of cells from a living tumor, *Cancer Res* 60(19):5401–5404, 2000.
76. Jankowski MK, et al: Matrix metalloproteinase activity in tumor, stromal tissue, and serum from cats with malignancies, *J Vet Intern Med* 16(1):105–108, 2002.
77. Loukopoulos P, O'Brien T, Ghoddusi M, et al: Characterisation of three novel canine osteosarcoma cell lines producing high levels of matrix metalloproteinases, *Res Vet Sci* 77:131–141, 2004.
78. Hirayama K, et al: Detection of matrix metalloproteinases in canine mammary tumours: analysis by immunohistochemistry and zymography, *J Comp Pathol* 127(4):249–256, 2002.
79. Lana SE, et al: Identification of matrix metalloproteinases in canine neoplastic tissue, *Am J Vet Res* 61(2):111–114, 2000.
80. Leibman NF, Lana SE, Hansen RA, et al: Identification of matrix metalloproteinases in canine cutaneous mast cell tumors, *J Vet Intern Med* 14:583–586, 2000.
81. Coussens LM, Fingleton B, Matrisian LM: Matrix metalloproteinase inhibitors and cancer: trials and tribulations, *Science* 295:2387–2392, 2002.
82. Coussens LM, Fingleton B, Matrisian LM: Matrix metalloproteinase inhibitors and cancer: trials and tribulations, *Science* 295(5564):2387–2392, 2002.
83. Moore AS, et al: Doxorubicin and BAY 12–9566 for the treatment of osteosarcoma in dogs: a randomized, double-blind, placebo-controlled study, *J Vet Intern Med* 21(4):783–790, 2007.
84. Ramnath N, Creaven PJ: Matrix metalloproteinase inhibitors, *Curr Oncol Rep* 6(2):96–102, 2004.
85. Rucci N, Sanita P, Angelucci A: Roles of metalloproteases in metastatic niche, *Curr Mol Med* 11(8):609–622, 2011.
86. Qian BZ, Pollard JW: Macrophage diversity enhances tumor progression and metastasis, *Cell* 141(1):39–51, 2010.
87. Foroni C, et al: Epithelial-mesenchymal transition and breast cancer: Role, molecular mechanisms and clinical impact, *Cancer Treat Rev* Epub November 25, 2011.
88. Peinado H, Olmeda D, Cano A: Snail, Zeb and bHLH factors in tumour progression: an alliance against the epithelial phenotype? *Nat Rev Cancer* 7(6):415–428, 2007.

89. Moreno-Bueno G, et al: The morphological and molecular features of the epithelial-to-mesenchymal transition, *Nat Protoc* 4(11):1591–1613, 2009.
90. Floor S, et al: Cancer cells in epithelial-to-mesenchymal transition and tumor-propagating-cancer stem cells: distinct, overlapping or same populations, *Oncogene* 30(46):4609–4621, 2011.
91. Hendrix MJ, et al: Vasculogenic mimicry and tumour-cell plasticity: lessons from melanoma, *Nat Rev Cancer* 3(6):411–421, 2003.
92. Kalluri R: Basement membranes: structure, assembly and role in tumour angiogenesis, *Nat Rev Cancer* 3(6): 422–433, 2003.
93. Frisch SM, Francis H: Disruption of epithelial cell-matrix interactions induces apoptosis, *J Cell Biol* 124(4):619–626, 1994.
94. Taddei ML, et al: Anoikis: an emerging hallmark in health and diseases, *J Pathol* 226(2):380–393, 2012.
95. Grossmann J: Molecular mechanisms of "detachment-induced apoptosis–Anoikis", *Apoptosis* 7(3):247–260, 2002.
96. Guo W, Giancotti FG: Integrin signalling during tumour progression, *Nat Rev Mol Cell Biol* 5(10):816–826, 2004.
97. Fosmire SP, Dickerson EB, Scott AM, et al: Canine malignant hemangiosarcoma as a model of primitive angiogenic endothelium, *Lab Invest* 84:562–572, 2004.
98. Akhtari M, et al: Biology of breast cancer bone metastasis, *Cancer Biol Ther* 7(1):3–9, 2008.
99. Restucci B, De Vico G, Maiolino P: Expression of beta 1 integrin in normal, dysplastic and neoplastic canine mammary gland, *J Comp Pathol* 113(2):165–173, 1995.
100. Olivry T, et al: Investigation of epidermotropism in canine mycosis fungoides: Expression of intercellular adhesion molecule-1 (ICAM-1) and beta-2 integrins, *Arch Dermatol Res* 287(2):186–192, 1995.
101. Moore PF, Rossitto PV, Danilenko DM: Canine leukocyte integrins: characterization of a CD18 homologue, *Tissue Antigens* 36(5):211–220, 1990.
102. Selvarajah GT, et al: Gene expression profiling of canine osteosarcoma reveals genes associated with short and long survival times, *Mol Cancer* 8:72, 2009.
103. Fukata M, Kaibuchi K: Rho-family GTPases in cadherin-mediated cell-cell adhesion, *Nat Rev Mol Cell Biol* 2(12):887–897, 2001.
104. Seftor RE, et al: Role of the alpha v beta 3 integrin in human melanoma cell invasion, *Proc Natl Acad Sci U S A* 89(5):1557–1561, 1992.
105. Zheng DQ, et al: Prostatic carcinoma cell migration via alpha(v) beta3 integrin is modulated by a focal adhesion kinase pathway, *Cancer Res* 59(7):1655–1664, 1999.
106. Ruoslahti E, Reed JC: Anchorage dependence, integrins, and apoptosis, *Cell* 77(4):477–478, 1994.
107. Nagaprashantha LD, et al: The sensors and regulators of cell-matrix surveillance in anoikis resistance of tumors, *Int J Cancer* 128(4):743–752, 2011.
108. Lascelles BD, et al: Improved survival associated with postoperative wound infection in dogs treated with limb-salvage surgery for osteosarcoma, *Ann Surg Oncol* 12(12):1073–1083, 2005.
109. Smyth MJ, et al: New aspects of natural-killer-cell surveillance and therapy of cancer, *Nat Rev Cancer* 2(11):850–861, 2002.
110. Mocellin S, et al: Colorectal cancer vaccines: principles, results, and perspectives, *Gastroenterology* 127(6):1821–1837, 2004.
111. Mocellin S, Rossi CR, Nitti D: Cancer vaccine development: on the way to break immune tolerance to malignant cells, *Exp Cell Res* 299(2):267–278, 2004.
112. Rao B, et al: Clinical outcomes of active specific immunotherapy in advanced colorectal cancer and suspected minimal residual colorectal cancer: a meta-analysis and system review, *J Transl Med* 9:17, 2011.
113. Bergman PJ: Cancer immunotherapy, *Vet Clin North Am Small Anim Pract* 40(3):507–518, 2010.
114. Grosenbaugh DA, et al: Safety and efficacy of a xenogeneic DNA vaccine encoding for human tyrosinase as adjunctive treatment for oral malignant melanoma in dogs following surgical excision of the primary tumor, *Am J Vet Res* 72(12):1631–1638, 2011.
115. Bagge U, Skolnik G, Ericson LE: The arrest of circulating tumor cells in the liver microcirculation. A vital fluorescence microscopic, electron microscopic and isotope study in the rat, *J Cancer Res Clin Oncol* 105(2):134–140, 1983.
116. Chambers AF, et al: Steps in tumor metastasis: new concepts from intravital videomicroscopy, *Cancer Metastasis Rev* 14(4):279–301, 1995.
117. Chambers AF, et al: Critical steps in hematogenous metastasis: an overview, *Surg Oncol Clin N Am* 10(2):243–255, vii, 2001.
118. Kienast Y, et al: Real-time imaging reveals the single steps of brain metastasis formation, *Nat Med* 16(1):116–122, 2010.
119. Li DM, Feng YM: Signaling mechanism of cell adhesion molecules in breast cancer metastasis: potential therapeutic targets, *Breast Cancer Res Treat* 128(1):7–21, 2011.
120. Zigler M, et al: PAR-1 and thrombin: the ties that bind the microenvironment to melanoma metastasis, *Cancer Res* 71(21):6561–6566, 2011.
121. Villares GJ, Zigler M, Bar-Eli M: The emerging role of the thrombin receptor (PAR-1) in melanoma metastasis–a possible therapeutic target, *Oncotarget* 2(1–2):8–17, 2011.
122. Groom AC, et al: Tumour metastasis to the liver, and the roles of proteinases and adhesion molecules: new concepts from in vivo videomicroscopy, *Can J Gastroenterol* 13(9):733–743, 1999.
123. Chambers AF: The metastatic process: basic research and clinical implications, *Oncol Res* 11(4):161–168, 1999.
124. Martin TA, et al: The role of the CD44/ezrin complex in cancer metastasis, *Crit Rev Oncol Hematol* 46(2):165–186, 2003.
125. Balkwill F: Chemokine biology in cancer, *Semin Immunol* 15(1):49–55, 2003.
126. Kaplan RN, Rafii S, Lyden D: Preparing the "soil": the premetastatic niche, *Cancer Res* 66(23):11089–11093, 2006.
127. Kaplan RN, et al: VEGFR1-positive haematopoietic bone marrow progenitors initiate the pre-metastatic niche, *Nature* 438(7069):820–827, 2005.
128. Al-Mehdi AB, et al: Intravascular origin of metastasis from the proliferation of endothelium-attached tumor cells: a new model for metastasis, *Nat Med* 6(1):100–102, 2000.
129. Cooper CR, et al: Stromal factors involved in prostate carcinoma metastasis to bone, *Cancer* 97(suppl 3):739–747, 2003.
130. De Wever O, Mareel M: Role of tissue stroma in cancer cell invasion, *J Pathol* 200(4):429–447, 2003.
131. Engels B, Rowley DA, Schreiber H: Targeting stroma to treat cancers, *Semin Cancer Biol* 22(1):41–49, 2011.
132. Folkman J: Tumor angiogenesis and tissue factor, *Nat Med* 2:167–168, 1996.
133. Folkman J: Angiogenesis: an organizing principle for drug discovery? *Nat Rev Drug Discov* 6:273–286, 2007.
134. Kerbel RS: Tumor angiogenesis: past, present and the near future, *Carcinogenesis* 21(3):505–515, 2000.
135. Nagy JA, et al: Heterogeneity of the tumor vasculature, *Semin Thromb Hemost* 36(3):321–331, 2010.
136. Olive KP, et al: Inhibition of Hedgehog signaling enhances delivery of chemotherapy in a mouse model of pancreatic cancer, *Science* 324(5933):1457–1461, 2009.
137. Pircher A, et al: Biomarkers in tumor angiogenesis and anti-angiogenic therapy, *Int J Mol Sci* 12(10):7077–7099, 2011.
138. Keara Boss M, Muradyan N, Thrall DE: DCE-MRI: A review and applications in veterinary oncology, *Vet Comp Oncol* Epub December 8, 2011.
139. Fidler IJ, Kripke ML: Metastasis results from preexisting variant cells within a malignant tumor, *Science* 197(4306):893–895, 1977.
140. Fidler IJ: The pathogenesis of cancer metastasis: the 'seed and soil' hypothesis revisited, *Nat Rev Cancer* 3(6):453–458, 2003.
141. Hunter K, Welch DR, Liu ET: Genetic background is an important determinant of metastatic potential, *Nat Genet* 34(1):23–24, author reply 25, 2003.

142. Hunter KW: Allelic diversity in the host genetic background may be an important determinant in tumor metastatic dissemination, *Cancer Lett* 200(2):97–105, 2003.
143. Hunter KW: Host genetics and tumour metastasis, *Br J Cancer* 90(4):752–755, 2004.
144. Khanna C, Hunter K: Modeling metastasis in vivo, *Carcinogenesis* 26(3):513–523, 2005.
145. Luzzi KJ, et al: Multistep nature of metastatic inefficiency: Dormancy of solitary cells after successful extravasation and limited survival of early micrometastases, *Am J Pathol* 153(3):865–873, 1998.
146. Loberg RD, et al: Detection and isolation of circulating tumor cells in urologic cancers: a review, *Neoplasia* 6(4):302–309, 2004.
147. Butler TP, Gullino PM: Quantitation of cell shedding into efferent blood of mammary adenocarcinoma, *Cancer Res* 35(3):512–516, 1975.
148. Chambers AF, et al: Molecular biology of breast cancer metastasis. Clinical implications of experimental studies on metastatic inefficiency, *Breast Cancer Res* 2(6):400–407, 2000.
149. Paez D, et al: Cancer dormancy: a model of early dissemination and late cancer recurrence, *Clin Cancer Res* 2012.
150. Barkan D, et al: Inhibition of metastatic outgrowth from single dormant tumor cells by targeting the cytoskeleton, *Cancer Res* 68(15):6241–6250, 2008.
151. Barkan D, et al: Metastatic growth from dormant cells induced by a col-I-enriched fibrotic environment, *Cancer Res* 70(14):5706–5716, 2010.
152. Sica A, Allavena P, Mantovani A: Cancer related inflammation: The macrophage connection, *Cancer Lett* 267(2):204–215, 2008
153. Ben-Neriah Y, Karin M: Inflammation meets cancer, with NF-kappa B as the matchmaker, *Nat Immunol* 12(8):715–723, 2011.
154. Argyle DJ, Blacking T: From viruses to cancer stem cells: dissecting the pathways to malignancy, *Vet J* 177(3):311–323, 2008.
155. Blacking TM, Wilson H, Argyle DJ: Is cancer a stem cell disease? Theory, evidence and implications, *Vet Comp Oncol* 5(2):76–89, 2007.
156. Park CH, Bergsage DE, McCulloc EA: Mouse myeloma tumour stem cells: primary cell culture assay, *J Natl Cancer Inst* 46(2):411, 1971.
157. Huntly BJ, Gilliland DG: Leukaemia stem cells and the evolution of cancer-stem-cell research, *Nat Rev Cancer* 5(4):311–321, 2005.
158. Kamel-Reid S, et al: A model of human acute lymphoblastic leukemia in immune-deficient SCID mice, *Science* 246(4937):1597–1600, 1989.
159. Lapidot T, et al: A cell initiating human acute myeloid leukaemia after transplantation into SCID mice, *Nature* 367(6464): 645–648, 1994.
160. Sirard C, et al: Normal and leukemic SCID-repopulating cells (SRC) coexist in the bone marrow and peripheral blood from CML patients in chronic phase, whereas leukemic SRC are detected in blast crisis, *Blood* 87(4):1539–1548, 1996.
161. Bonnet D, Dick JE: Human acute myeloid leukemia is organized as a hierarchy that originates from a primitive hematopoietic cell, *Nat Med* 3(7):730–737, 1997.
162. Fidler IJ, Kripke ML: Metastasis results from preexisting variant cells within a malignant tumor, *Science* 197:893–895, 1977.
163. Heppner GH: Tumor heterogeneity. *Cancer Res* 44:2259–2265, 1984.
164. Nowell PC: Mechanisms of tumor progression, *Cancer Res* 46:2203–2207, 1986.
165. Southam CM, Brunschwig A: Quantitative studies of autotransplantation of human cancer, *Cancer* 14:971–978, 1961.
166. Pang LY, Argyle DJ: Using naturally occurring tumours in dogs and cats to study telomerase and cancer stem cell biology, *Biochim Biophys Acta* 1792(4):380–391, 2009.
167. Pang LY, Argyle D: Cancer stem cells and telomerase as potential biomarkers in veterinary oncology, *Vet J* 185(1):15–22, 2010.
168. Pang LY, Cervantes-Arias A, Else RW, et al: Canine mammary cancer stem cells are radio- and chemo-resistant and exhibit an epithelial-mesenchymal transition phenotype, *Cancer* 3(2):1744–1762, 2011.

The Pathology of Neoplasia

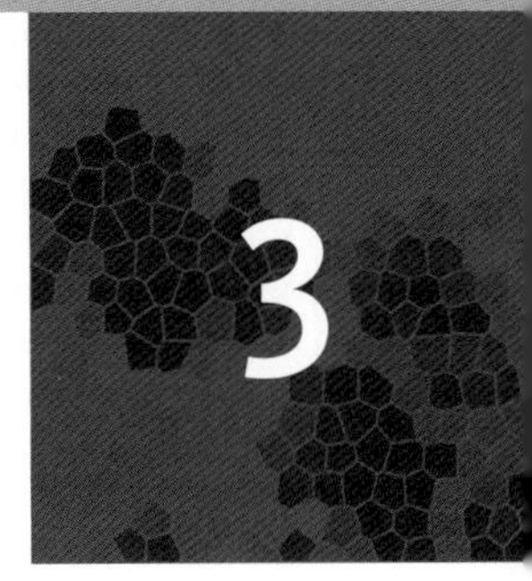

E.J. Ehrhart, Debra A. Kamstock, and Barbara E. Powers

Veterinary pathologists play a critical role in the management of neoplasia of companion animals by providing accurate diagnostic information to clinicians so that a prognosis can be determined and adequate treatment provided. The clinician needs to have knowledge of the pathology of neoplasia to understand neoplastic conditions and the limitations of histopathologic assessment in the diagnosis of neoplasia. Both the pathologist and the clinician must work together to determine optimal treatment for the patient because the diagnosis and treatment of neoplasia in veterinary medicine have become more complex. No longer is it adequate to simply determine if the tumor is benign or malignant. The tumor type needs to be identified as accurately as possible, and tumor subtypes should be identified if prognostically significant. Grading of tumors is increasingly important because the behavior of some tumors can be predicted by the grade of the tumor. In addition, the assessment of margins for completeness of surgical removal is very important. In some cases, the histologic assessment of tissue treated preoperatively is important in predicting treatment outcome. Special procedures such as immunohistochemistry (IHC), electron microscopy (EM), flow cytometry, or polymerase chain reaction (PCR) may be advantageous in some cases to correctly identify tumor type or subtype or to predict clinical behavior of certain tumors. Classification of neoplasia in veterinary medicine is becoming more commonly applied, and systems have become more advanced with application of molecular markers for more accurate classification and prognostic information. For example, a recently upgraded histopathologic classification and grading system for canine mammary tumors has been reported to better prognostically evaluate tumors and standardize studies for cross-comparison.[1] As more is learned about the diagnosis and treatment of neoplasia in veterinary medicine, newer predictive/prognostic classifications and grading schemes will continue to be developed.

Sample Handling

The biopsy sample should be visually inspected by the clinician to help determine that the appropriate tissue was obtained. If the biopsy was a needle core or incisional specimen, the sample should be of sufficient size and consistency so that it remains intact in formalin and does not become lost in processing. Samples less than 1 mm^3 are usually inadequate, although a needle core sample 1 mm wide but at least 5 mm long can be sufficient. If the biopsy samples are needle core samples, more than one core of tissue should be obtained, if possible.

Very small samples can easily be lost during shipping or in processing because sample shrinkage during fixation and processing is imminent. Given these precautions, some techniques can be utilized to maximize the chances that the sample will make it through the process. Samples less than 3 mm in size can be placed on paper (surgical glove paper is appropriate) before fixation. These samples will be tacky and adhere to the paper. Very small or pale samples can be circled with pencil to draw attention to the samples at the histology laboratory. The paper can then be folded around the sample, and the entire package can be placed in formalin for fixation and shipping. Alternatively, commercially available screened tissue cassettes can be used to house the sample during fixation and shipment. The sample is placed in the screened cassette at the time of surgery, and the cassette with the sample is placed directly into formalin for fixation. These techniques decrease the chance for small samples to be lost in larger formalin containers. Extremely small samples can also be dyed with India ink or other commercially available dyes to assist in the identification of the sample. Samples containing excessive blood, mucus, or necrotic material may not be diagnostic, and the biopsy procedure may need to be repeated. If the specimen was an excisional sample, the entire sample should be submitted if feasible, and margins of concern should be identified with suture or ink. For very large samples such as large splenic tumors, representative sections such as peripheral versus central or different-colored or textured areas can be submitted. Visualization by an experienced person is extremely important when selecting the sample so that viable tissue is selected. Usually it is best to submit at least three to five sections of large lesions in case some portions of the tumor have excessive distortion, necrosis, or inflammation. When taking representative samples, the tumor and normal tissue interface should be included so assessment of tumor invasiveness into normal tissue can be determined. Tissue samples should be handled gently because compression during biopsy sampling and excessive use of electrocautery, cryosurgery, or laser surgery can cause specimen artifact, which can prevent a definitive diagnosis from being made.[2]

The sample needs to be preserved in fixative. The most widely used fixative is 10% neutral buffered formalin, which is readily available and frequently supplied in individual specimen containers by most laboratories. During excessive cold conditions, samples can freeze during shipment and cause significant destructive tissue artifact. Addition of 20% ethylene glycol or ethanol to the formalin can prevent freezing and maintain tissue integrity. Prior to immersion in fixative, larger samples may need to be sliced, facilitating adequate fixation; however, one side such as the deep edge should be left intact rather than slicing all the way through the sample so that orientation and margin assessment are not lost. Slices less than 1 cm thick should be avoided because curling and distortion of the tissue during fixation can result. The volume of tissue to fixative should approximate 1 : 10. In cases in which this volume ratio is not feasible because of large tumor size, multiple representative sections can be obtained. It is advisable to save the remnants of the sample, if possible, in case these first sections are not adequate for a diagnosis. When mailing large samples, use of smaller volumes of fixative is acceptable if the specimen has been in the recommended initial volume for at least 12 hours.[3]

Sample containers must be properly labeled (on the container, not just the lid) prior to submission to the laboratory. During transportation by mail, courier, or unpacking at the laboratory, paperwork can be inadvertently separated from the sample container, and unless the container is properly labeled, samples could become mixed. Most important, adequate history, including signalment, pertinent clinical findings, radiographic findings, and pertinent treatment, should be provided to the pathologist. A drawing of the sample indicating the position of the tissue on the animal is helpful in some situations, especially when margin determination is needed. If margins or areas of special clinical interest are marked (labeled) on the sample, a clear description of these labels, margins, or areas should be present in the submission form. A proper history is crucial for accurate diagnosis; without this the pathologist can be severely handicapped. The end result might be an inaccurate diagnosis, culminating in an inaccurate prognosis and improper treatment.[2,4]

After arrival at the laboratory, the specimens are catalogued and assigned an identification number, visually examined, trimmed to fit into processing cassettes, processed into paraffin blocks, sectioned, and stained. These procedures are performed by trained technicians and automated laboratory equipment. In most laboratories, tissues are trimmed into cassettes on the day of arrival, processed overnight, and completed slides are ready for examination by the pathologist 24 hours after receipt. Hard tissue such as bone needs to be decalcified prior to sections and thus will take longer to process. Larger samples incompletely fixed, extremely bloody samples (e.g., spleen), or samples with abundant fatty tissue (e.g., mammary gland) may require additional time for fixation. This additional time is vital to assure fatty tissue at the margin of the surgically excised sample remains intact during trimming, processing, and sectioning. In the process of trimming in or sectioning on the microtome, margins could become distorted and orientation may be lost, in which case reexamination of the gross specimen by the pathologist may be necessary. Most laboratories will hold remnant wet tissues in formalin for 7 to 60 days in the event further examination or sectioning is needed. Most laboratories file paraffin blocks and glass slides indefinitely, permitting review of previously submitted tissue on a given patient or retrospective studies on a series of cases.

Although infrequent, frozen sections can be made during operative procedures to provide the surgeon with a more rapid diagnosis. Samples are quick-frozen, sectioned on a cryostat, fixed, stained, and examined within 20 to 35 minutes. This technique is often conducted during surgery to assist with intraoperative decisions and thus requires a diagnostic laboratory and facility on site. However, these tissue sections are inferior to those processed routinely into paraffin, and as a result diagnostic accuracy is not as high and is proportional to the experience of the pathologist interpreting frozen sections. Furthermore, only a few veterinary institutions provide this service. This procedure may be helpful in establishing the identity of the tissue, adequacy of surgical margins, or adequacy of the tissue for more routine processing. Sometimes a provisional diagnosis can be made or at least a distinction between benign and malignant processes can be determined. The frozen-section diagnosis is always confirmed by routine histopathologic assessment of a paraffin-embedded section, often using the same tissue sample.[4]

Molecular techniques are now routinely applied as diagnostic tests in veterinary medicine. Some of these such as PCR and IHC have been developed and characterized for use on formalin-fixed, paraffin-embedded samples. Once processed, these tissues are often viable indefinitely for these tests, although the time prior to fixation, the time in fixation, and the storage time can negatively affect test sensitivity. These factors need to be determined for individual tests, and their effect needs to be considered in interpretation of results. IHC on formalin-fixed tissues requires only unstained, routine sections on slides appropriate for IHC. Exposure to sunlight or extremes of temperature should be avoided. Requirements particular to individual testing laboratories should be determined prior to submitting samples for these tests. PCR requires thick sections (10 to 20 μm) to assure adequate DNA or RNA amounts. These are typically allowed to roll up during microtome sectioning and can be sent to the testing laboratory at room temperature in an air-tight container. Acquiring specifics of the test material needed and shipping requirements prior to collecting the sample or requesting the test is often beneficial and avoids frustration for the owner, submitter, and testing laboratory.

Terminology

Numerous terms associated with tumors or suspected tumors are encountered in the description of the features of a tissue sample. A clear understanding of this terminology is imperative to understand the implications of the histopathologic findings. A clinician's responsibility extends beyond collection of the tumor and treating the patient. A clinician has a responsibility to interpret the histopathology report, to identify details that might help subclassify a tumor beyond the base of tumor identification, and to assist in determining a tailored treatment protocol for individuals. A firm grasp on terminology is required for this interpretation and to discuss details of the tumor with the pathologist.

A *tumor* is any tissue mass or swelling and may be neoplastic or not, although this term today more typically is a generic term used to describe any neoplasm. *Neoplasia* is the abnormal growth of a tissue into a mass that is not responsive to normal control mechanisms and may be benign or malignant. Growth of this mass is not affected when the inciting stimulus is removed. *Cancer* refers to a malignant neoplasm.[5] All neoplasms arise in normal tissue and thus are composed of parenchymal and stromal cells—some can also incite secondary inflammation. Their differentiation state can be assessed with histopathology and is based on the appearance of the tumor cells, their organization, and their association with the supporting stroma. Differentiation is controlled at the molecular level by gene expression. Normal reversible processes of *hyperplasia* (a nonneoplastic increase in the number of cells present) and atrophy (a decrease in the number of cells present) are also composed of parenchymal cells and stroma. Their retention of near-normal architecture, just as well-differentiated neoplasms retain normal architecture, can make differentiation of the two processes difficult. At times, only removal of the inciting stimulus and time can distinguish between hyperplasia and well-differentiated cancer. One definition of cancer is a proliferation of a clonal population of cells that is no longer responsive to tissue homeostatic mechanisms. Molecular techniques to determine a clonal expansion of cells by their similar DNA sequence structure could help separate these conditions or identify occult cancer prior to tissue distortion at a microscopic level. These tests are few, but more are currently being developed, specifically for use in canine and feline lymphomas.[6] *Metaplasia* is the abnormal transformation of a differentiated tissue of one kind into a differentiated tissue of another kind and not a neoplastic condition. Metaplasia should reverse or not progress with cessation of the chronic inciting stimulus. An example is squamous metaplasia in the prostate gland, where normally columnar epithelium becomes squamous under the influence of estrogen. Metaplastic cells can be targets for carcinogenesis if continued carcinogenic promotional events occur (e.g., bronchial squamous metaplasia in human smokers). In such cases, metaplasia often progresses and acquires dysplastic changes. *Dysplasia* is abnormal tissue development and can be a feature of neoplasia, but it is not necessarily a neoplastic condition. Dysplasia such as epithelial dysplasia in the oral cavity can be a preneoplastic condition. *Anaplasia* is a loss of differentiation or atypical differentiation and is a feature of many, but not all, malignancies.

Terms associated with cellular or growth features are frequently encountered in descriptions of neoplasia. *Pleomorphism* is the occurrence of multiple forms, shapes, and sizes of cells and nuclei (cellular and nuclear pleomorphism respectively). *Anisocytosis* and *anisokaryosis* are greater than normal variations in cell and nuclear size, respectively. Round or polygonal cell shapes are usually associated with epithelial or hematologic tumors, whereas spindle cell shapes are usually associated with mesenchymal tumors. A *scirrhous* or *desmoplastic* response is an abundant fibroblastic proliferation with collagen formation that occurs in some malignant invasive cancers. *In situ* refers to a malignancy, usually limited to lesions of epithelial origin, that has not yet become invasive or invaded beyond the natural confines of its basement membrane.[2,4,5]

For each type of tumor, specific terminology is used to denote the origin of the tumor and whether the tumor is benign or malignant (Table 3-1). In basic terms, although benign tumors can cause tissue distortion, they typically do not have a high mortality. In contrast, malignant tumors (cancer) are more destructive of tissues and will often ultimately lead to death if the patient is left untreated. There are exceptions to these rules. Tumors can develop from any normal tissue type; therefore there are a considerable number of different tumor types. As more is learned about certain tumors, names and subclassifications may change, creating some confusion. More recent advances in molecular techniques applied to tumors have allowed additional subclassification of tumors beyond the histologic realm. More focused techniques such as IHC, targeted PCR for genetic alterations and mutations, and flow cytometry for cell surface markers can be applied once specific alterations in tumor types have been identified and determined to be markers in a specific tumor or tumor subtype. Broad encompassing techniques for large genomic, proteomic, and more recently metabolomic fingerprinting of tumors are used as discovery tools to scan for alterations that define subclasses of tumor types previously unidentified by more traditional methods. The identification of genetic mutations, varied cell surface receptor expression, altered signaling pathways, or altered cellular metabolic response to these genetic modifications may identify unique fingerprints for a tumor, which, combined with traditional histologic methods, might allow subclassification that is more accurate at identifying a tumor's behavior and its response to tailored cancer treatment (see Chapter 8).

Benign tumors of epithelial origin are termed *adenoma, papilloma,* or *epithelioma.* Benign tumors of mesenchymal origin are designated by the suffix *-oma* after the tissue type (e.g., fibroma, osteoma). Malignant tumors of epithelial origin are termed *carcinoma* or *adenocarcinoma* if forming glands and ducts, whereas malignant tumors of mesenchymal origin are termed *sarcoma.* In some cases, the *-oma* suffix is used when the tumor is malignant, as in malignant melanoma and lymphoma. *Leukemia,* a malignant neoplasia of blood cells (occasionally referred to as "liquid tumors") in hematopoietic tissues and usually in the blood, has no benign counterpart, although a leukemoid reaction is a nonmalignant condition that mimics leukemia.[2,4,7] Although nomenclature for human cancer can often be applied to animal cancer, all nomenclature cannot be directly applied across species due to differences in tumor types and tumor behavior. Similarities and differences must be taken into account when considering whether nomenclature can have cross-species application. For example, direct comparison of canine mammary gland tumors to those of the human mammary classification system have identified differences that require an independent classification system.[8]

Histologic Features of Neoplasia

Despite recent advances in a number of areas of pathology, including molecular techniques, evaluation of tissue by light microscopy remains the standard technique for tumor diagnosis.[3] Neoplasia has certain histologic features that distinguish it from hyperplasia or inflammation, and there are features that distinguish benign from malignant neoplasia. In some cases, these features can be difficult to observe. Definitive diagnosis of malignant versus benign versus inflammation or hyperplasia may not always be possible. In these cases, a repeat biopsy, either immediately or after a period of clinical observation, may facilitate a definitive diagnosis.

When inflammation is present, the cellular features of reactive fibroblasts and reactive endothelial cells can be misleading.[2,9] However, in reactive tissue with inflammation, the fibroblasts and endothelial cells usually are oriented perpendicular to one another (reactive granulation tissue) and usually a substantial amount of inflammation relative to reactive tissue is present. When granulomatous inflammation occurs, large reactive and epithelioid macrophages can be mistaken for tumor cells, but the pattern of tissue involvement and presence of other inflammatory cells helps rule out neoplasia. In some tumors, especially those with surface ulceration or necrosis (e.g., some synovial cell and soft tissue sarcomas), an extensive amount of inflammation can obscure neoplasia but is considered a secondary process.

Benign tumors may be most difficult to distinguish from hyperplasia (Table 3-2) because both have a proliferation of well-differentiated cells that are easy to identify. There is a distortion or loss of normal tissue architecture in benign neoplasia, and usually the tumor grows in an expansive manner, causing compression rather than invasion of adjacent tissue. These tumors are often defined by a fibrous tumor capsule. Hyperplasia tends to retain normal tissue orientation and does not compress adjacent tissue. It often lacks a fibrous capsule. In general, if allowed to grow, benign neoplasia will attain a larger size than a hyperplastic lesion. In some instances, such as thyroid gland adenoma versus adenomatous hyperplasia of the thyroid gland in cats or sebaceous gland adenoma versus sebaceous gland hyperplasia the distinction between benign tumor and hyperplasia is not clinically important.

Features that distinguish malignant from benign neoplasia include more dramatic loss of tissue organization, increased anisocytosis and anisokaryosis, increased nuclear and cellular pleomorphism, increased and variable nuclear : cytoplasmic ratio, abnormal nuclear chromatin, increased mitotic figures, increased and abnormal mitotic figures, abnormal large and/or multiple nucleoli, increased necrosis, amount and character of the supporting stroma, and invasiveness of malignant tumors (see Table 3-2). With invasion, individual cells or groups of tumor cells infiltrate extensively into surrounding tissue, may invade into vascular or lymphatic spaces, and may invoke a scirrhous or desmoplastic response characterized by an excessive fibrous reaction. A further feature of

TABLE 3-1 Nomenclature of Common Tumor Types in Veterinary Medicine

TISSUE OR CELL OF ORIGIN	BENIGN	MALIGNANT
Epithelial		
Squamous	Squamous papilloma	Squamous cell carcinoma
Transitional	Transitional papilloma	Transitional cell carcinoma
Glandular	Adenoma, cystadenoma	Adenocarcinoma
Nonglandular	Adenoma	Carcinoma
Mesenchymal		
Fibrous tissue	Fibroma	Fibrosarcoma
Fat	Lipoma, "infiltrative lipoma"	Liposarcoma
Cartilage	Chondroma	Chondrosarcoma
Bone	Osteoma	Osteosarcoma, multilobular osteochondrosarcoma
Muscle (smooth)	Leiomyoma	Leiomyosarcoma
Muscle (skeletal)	Rhabdomyoma	Rhabdomyosarcoma
Endothelial cells	Hemangioma	Hemangiosarcoma
Synovium	—	Synovial cell sarcoma
Mesothelium	—	Mesothelioma
Melanocytes	Benign melanoma, melanocytoma	Malignant melanoma, melanosarcoma
Peripheral nerve	—	Malignant schwannoma, neurofibrosarcoma, peripheral nerve sheath tumor
Uncertain origin*	—	Malignant fibrous histiocytoma, hemangiopericytoma
Hematopoietic and lymphoreticular		
Lymphocytes	—	Lymphoma with subclassifications and leukemic forms
Plasma cells	Cutaneous plasmacytoma	Multiple myeloma, plasmacytoid lymphoma
Granulocytes	—	Myeloid leukemia
Red blood cells	—	Erythroid leukemia
Macrophages	Histiocytoma	Histiocytic sarcoma (malignant histiocytosis)
Mast cells	—	Mast cell tumor†
Thymus	Thymoma, encapsulated	Invasive thymoma
Brain		
Glial cells	Astrocytoma, oligodendroglioma	Astrocytoma, glioblastoma multiforme, oligodendroglioma
Meninges	Meningioma	Malignant meningioma
Gonadal		
Germ cells‡	Seminoma, dysgerminoma	Seminoma, dysgerminoma
Supportive cells‡	Sertoli cell tumor, granulosa cell tumor	Sertoli cell tumor, granulosa cell tumor
Interstitial cells‡	Interstitial (Leydig) cell tumor, thecoma, luteoma	Interstitial (Leydig) cell tumor

*Pathologists disagree about the origin of these tumors; some feel they are a class of peripheral nerve sheath tumors or perivascular wall tumors.
†Theoretically, all mast cell tumors are potentially malignant, but grade 1 mast cell tumors are clinically benign.
‡Unfortunately, the terminology of these tumors does not distinguish between benign and malignant forms.

TABLE 3-2 Histologic Features of Hyperplasia and of Benign and Malignant Neoplasia

HISTOLOGIC FEATURE	HYPERPLASIA	BENIGN NEOPLASIA	MALIGNANT NEOPLASIA
Overall differentiation	Normal	Disorganized, but well differentiated	Disorganized, well to poorly differentiated
Cell and nuclear pleomorphism	None	Minimal	Moderate to marked
Mitotic index	Variable, usually low	Usually low	Often high
Nucleoli	Normal	Normal	Large and/or multiple
Amount of necrosis	None	Usually minimal	Minimal to abundant
Tissue demarcation	Blends with normal tissue	Expansive and/or compressive	Invasive

TABLE 3-3 Molecular Features Underlying Grading Criteria

GRADING CRITERIA	UNDERLYING MOLECULAR MECHANISMS
Mitotic index	Cyclins, cyclin-dependent kinases (CDKs), proliferating cell nuclear antigen (PCNA), Ki67, bromodeoxyuridine (BrdUrd), labeling index (LI)/growth fraction (GF)
Percent necrosis	Inflammatory mediators, including eicosanoids (prostaglandins), cytokines (interleukin [IL], tumor necrosis factor alpha [TNF-α]), microvessel density (MVD)
Invasiveness	Matrix metalloproteinases (MMPs), plasminogen activators (PA), integrin expression, CAM (cell adhesion molecules)
Stromal reaction	Transforming growth factor beta (TGF-β), platelet-derived growth factor (PDGF), basic fibroblast growth factor (bFGF), vascular endothelial growth factor (VEGF), MVD mediators
Nucleolar size	RNA transcriptional activity, silver staining nucleolar organizing regions (AgNORs)
Overall cellularity	Growth fraction, apoptosis factors (i.e., FasL, caspases), tumor doubling time
Inflammatory (lymphoid) response	TNF-α, interferon gamma (IFN-γ), IL-2, increased MHCII, intercellular adhesion molecule (ICAM)

malignancy is destruction of the normal tissue or obliteration of normal tissue architecture. Evidence of lymph node or more widespread metastasis obviously distinguishes malignant from benign tumors.[2,4,10] However, in certain tumors, histologic features do not correlate with behavior (e.g., canine histiocytoma and benign plasmacytoma). Both have histologic features of malignancy but are clinically benign. Histologically low-grade, yet biologically high-grade, fibrosarcomas of the canine head have histologic features of a benign condition but are clinically malignant.[11] Similarly, bronchial carcinomas in cats will retain organized epithelial structures composed of well-differentiated ciliated pseudostratified columnar epithelium even at distant metastatic sites, including the digit, eye, heart, and kidneys.[12] In these instances, knowledge of clinical history and tumor behavior is needed to distinguish benign from malignant neoplasia.

Generally, a pathologist makes the diagnosis of tumor versus reactive tissue and sometimes tumor type at relatively low magnification after evaluating the overall tissue pattern and behavior with respect to adjacent normal tissue. Higher magnification is then used to confirm the low magnification impression, to classify tumor type if not already done, and to assess nuclear features and mitotic index. Immediate use of high magnification is a mistake because very reactive tissue and inflammation, especially when macrophages are present, may be mistaken for neoplasia. For this reason, a definitive diagnosis may be difficult to establish with small samples or with samples that lack some normal tissue. There are numerous instances such as with osteosarcoma, mast cell tumor, transitional cell carcinoma, some soft tissue sarcomas, and squamous cell carcinoma in which histologic features are sufficiently distinct to make a definitive diagnosis on a small sample if the tumor was sampled correctly. In other cases such as with lymphoma or granulomatous inflammation, small samples may be inadequate to establish a final diagnosis because the overall cellular pattern and interaction with normal tissue is an important diagnostic feature.

Grading and Staging of Neoplasia

In certain tumors, grading the degree of malignancy is predictive of biologic behavior,[2,4,10] and, in the future, quite likely the behavior of more tumors will be shown to be related to histologic grade. Grading of tumors is somewhat subjective, and reproducibility between pathologists can be variable.[13] Despite this limitation, in one study of 440,000 cases of cancer in humans, interobserver variation did not have a sufficient impact to alter the relationship between grade and outcome.[14] A recent international study applying the World Health Organization (WHO) system of lymphoma classification to canine lymphomas demonstrated a reproducibility of 83% to 87% if the classification entities were well described and illustrated for reference by those applying the classification system. With preparative training of those using the system and careful application to well-described criteria, a high level of accuracy can be achieved in diagnosing canine lymphoma or any other disease entity.[15]

Another difficulty is that tumors are heterogeneous, and patterns as well as features of increased malignancy may vary from area to area. If heterogeneity is present, the most malignant areas are usually assessed for grading purposes. Sampling variation with small biopsy samples can dramatically affect the representation of different components in a heterogeneous tumor; therefore, if the sample is small, accurate grading is not possible and grades should be interpreted with caution.

Features of tumors that are often evaluated to assess grade include (1) degree of differentiation, (2) mitotic index (number of mitotic figures per 10 high-power 400× fields), (3) degree of cellular or nuclear pleomorphism, (4) amount of necrosis, (5) invasiveness, (6) stromal reaction, (7) nucleolar size and number, (8) overall cellularity, and (9) lymphoid response (Table 3-3). Of these features, mitotic index, amount of necrosis, and nucleolar features are the only objective, quantifiable features that can be quantified with manual counting, computerized morphometry, or chemical quantification.[2,4,10] Often, in determining a grade, individual features are scored, and then each score is added to obtain a total tumor score. The tumor scores are then separated into ranges that are associated with a tumor grade. Current grading scales are efficient, cost-effective, and involve no new technology. As the identification of molecular markers for tumor subtypes and prognostic or predictive parameters progresses and as the techniques become more time and cost efficient, yielding quicker turnaround times and easier application, they will become more routine and, likely, a valuable component of updated grading systems.

The quantifiable criteria previously mentioned for tumor grading have more recently been assessed with image analysis (computerized analytical morphometry). The use of image analysis allows for a more objective, repeatable measure decreasing interobserver variation and bias. Examples of this methodology demonstrate nuclear features such as nuclear area, mean diameter, and perimeter that correlate with mast cell tumor histologic grade, which is predictive of tumor biologic aggressiveness.[16,17] Currently, the routine application of computerized morphometry is not practical for routine use in diagnostic pathology due to time and effort restrictions, but it is only a matter of time before automation overcomes these limitations.

The rationale behind the effectiveness of tumor grade is the indirect assessment of molecular features. Many of the histologic criteria used in grading scales probably reflect the underlying molecular mechanisms (Table 3-4). One example would be the correlation between tumor necrosis evaluated in many tumor grades and the underlying mechanism of tumor microvessel density (MVD) and factors that affect the density of these vessels. Lack of adequate tumor vessel density will result in tumor hypoxia and thus tumor necrosis. An underlying mechanism of tumor vessel density includes the vascular endothelial growth factor (VEGF) signaling pathway. Studies have demonstrated the strong association of MVD and VEGF expression with tumor grade and biologic tumor aggressiveness.[52,53] Another example involves the induction of hypoxia-inducible factor-1α (HIF-1α) by hypoxic tumor cells. The HIF-1 gene product is the alpha subunit of transcription factor HIF-1 (http://www.ncbi.nlm.nih.gov/gene/3091). HIF-1α is a regulator of the cellular response to hypoxia by activating transcription of many genes involved in energy metabolism, angiogenesis, apoptosis, and other genes whose protein products increase oxygen delivery or facilitate metabolic adaptation to hypoxia. HIF-1α thus plays an essential role in angiogenesis and pathophysiology in the hypoxic environment present in many rapidly growing tumors. HIF-1α overexpression in brain, breast, cervical, esophageal, oropharyngeal, and ovarian cancers is correlated with treatment failure and mortality, as well as tumor progression.[54]

Tumor grade may correlate with survival, metastatic rate, disease-free interval, or with frequency and/or speed of local recurrence. Tumors in which grade or histologic features have been determined to be prognostic for biologic behavior in dogs include mast cell tumor[18-21]; lymphoma[24,25]; dermal, oral, and ocular melanoma[26,29,54,55]; mammary gland carcinoma[1,35]; synovial cell sarcoma[39,40]; multilobular osteochondrosarcoma[43,44]; hemangiosarcoma[47]; nonhematogenous sarcoma and fibrohistiocytic nodules of the spleen[48,49]; transitional cell carcinoma of the urinary bladder[50]; squamous cell carcinoma of the tongue[51]; lung carcinoma[33,34]; appendicular osteosarcoma[42,56]; mandibular osteosarcoma[45]; chondrosarcoma[46]; and soft tissue sarcoma[31,32,57] (see Table 3-3). In humans and dogs with soft tissue sarcoma, the histologic grade is more important than the tumor type.[2,32,58] Tumors whose grade or histologic features are predictive of biologic behavior in cats include lung carcinoma[34] and mammary gland carcinoma,[38] with conflicting reports regarding feline mast cell tumor and fibrosarcoma[22,23,59,60] (see Table 3-4).

Grading systems have not been well established for some malignant tumors, yet the pathologist can make an assessment of presumed biologic behavior based on the overall degree of tumor differentiation. In these cases, the terms *well differentiated, moderately differentiated* or *poorly differentiated* may be suggestive of a low-grade, medium-grade, and high-grade malignancy, respectively.[61] This type of assessment is most commonly done for squamous cell carcinomas, some sarcomas, and carcinomas of the mammary gland, salivary gland, gastrointestinal tract, liver, exocrine pancreas, and perianal gland. Tumor grading probably will become even more widespread and important in the future, especially as novel analytical techniques and molecular tumor markers are included. Not only can prognosis be determined based on tumor grade and differentiation, but also treatment may be modified to apply more aggressive therapies to tumors of higher grade.

The pathologist also may assist in staging of cancer by assessing tumor size, depth of tumor invasion, the presence of tumor in regional lymph nodes, and identification of tumor in distant sites. This information is needed to stage tumors into the *T* (tumor size and/or invasion), *N* (nodal involvement), and *M* (distant metastasis) system.[10] Cytologic assessment of draining lymph nodes has been shown as a sensitive alternative to histopathology for lymph node metastasis needed for staging.[62] For some tumors such as bladder cancer in humans, tumor staging is based largely on depth of tumor invasion into the bladder wall.[2,4] This may prove to be useful in cases of bladder cancer in pets and has been shown to correlate with tumor grade in dogs.[50] In both processes of tumor grading or tumor staging, these procedures are useful only if they have been shown to correlate with clinical behavior.

Assessment of Tumor Margins

Tumor margin assessment is an essential part of the pathology report whenever curative-intent surgical excision is attempted.[3] It may be the best determinant of adequate surgical treatment and may serve as a predictor of treatment outcome.[63] Grossly, the surgical margin can be defined as the margin beyond which tissue remains in the surgical bed or any region of the biopsy specimen adjacent to or contiguous with tissue that remains in vivo.[63] Microscopically, the surgical margin is the region between the neoplastic process and the surgical edge of the biopsy specimen. Margin assessment should be performed for both benign and malignant lesions, although detailed characterization of the margin (e.g., objective measurement, tissue constituents, viability) is typically more critical for malignancies. Obtaining accurate surgical margin information on the pathology report is critically dependent on (1) specimen handling and information submitted by the clinician, (2) method of tissue trimming at the diagnostic laboratory, and (3) observations reported by the pathologist.

Appropriate assessment of the surgical margin is at the onset critically dependent on information provided by the submitting clinician and moreover by appropriate tissue demarcation (e.g., inking) prior to submission. Inking is superior to other methods of denoting surgical margins (e.g., suture placement) because surgical ink is visible at both the gross and microscopic levels.[4,64] At the gross specimen level, the surgical ink impacts the regions of the specimen that are obtained by laboratory personnel during trimming for microscopic examination. At the microscopic level, assuming appropriate corresponding information was provided on the submission form by the clinician (e.g., yellow ink = deep margins, black ink = lateral margin), the ink allows the pathologist to appropriately assess and report the margins relative to a specific region. Surgical ink should only be placed on regions of the specimen that are *true* surgical margins or of specific concern to the clinician. The ink should also be allowed to dry (typically 5 to 10 minutes) prior to placement into a fixative (e.g., 10% neutral buffered formalin) to prevent the ink from washing off or unintentionally coating insignificant areas.[63]

Once at the laboratory, the specimen will be trimmed routinely with guidance from the information provided on the submission form and based on any tissue markings. If desired and if it enhances communication, annotated sketches or images of the specimen may also be submitted. The most common method of trimming for routine specimens is known as the *cross-sectioning method.* The mass is bisected along its short axis, after which each remaining half is bisected along its long axis, creating quarter sections. Ultimately, this method is perpendicular sectioning and allows for margin

TABLE 3-4 Neoplasia with Grades or Histologic Features Having Prognostic Significance

Tumor Type	Grades Given	Features of Importance	References
Mast cell tumor, cutaneous (dog)	I, II, III	Cellularity, nuclear:cytoplasmic ratio, cell morphology, mitotic index, depth, necrosis, granularity	18, 19
	2-tier: High, low	Mitotic index, karyomegaly, multinucleation, bizarre nuclei	20
	SQ: High, low	Mitotic index ≤4, >4; invasiveness; multinucleation	21
Mast cell tumor, cutaneous (cat)	Well and poorly differentiated, histiocytic	Cellular and nuclear pleomorphism, mitotic index	22, 23
Lymphoma	Low, intermediate, high	Architecture, mitotic index, nuclear size, morphology, T-cell/B-cell immunophenotype	24, 25
Dermal melanoma	Well and poorly differentiated	Mitotic index: ≥3/10 hpf	26, 27
Oral and lip melanomas	Well and poorly differentiated	Mitotic index: ≥3/10 hpf	28
Anterior uveal melanoma (cat, dog)	I-VI (or early, moderate, advanced); benign, malignant (dog)	Mitotic index, extent of invasion	29, 30
Soft tissue sarcoma (dog)	1, 2, 3 or mitotic index >9,* mitotic index <9*	Overall differentiation, mitotic index, necrosis	31, 32
Lung/pulmonary carcinoma (dog)	1, 2, 3	Overall differentiation, nuclear pleomorphism, mitotic index, necrosis, nucleolar size, fibrosis, invasion	33, 34
Lung/pulmonary carcinoma (cat)	Moderately and poorly differentiated	Organization, pleomorphism, pulmonary and vascular invasion	34
Mammary gland carcinoma (dog)	System 1: Well, moderately, and poorly differentiated grades	Invasion, nuclear differentiation, lymphoid response	35-37
	System 2: Grades I, II, III	Tubule formation, nuclear pleomorphism, mitotic index, simple carcinoma versus other, lymph node metastasis	
Mammary gland carcinoma (cat)	System 1: Well, moderately, and poorly differentiated grades	Differentiation, cellular pleomorphism, mitotic index	37, 38
	System 2: Grades I, II, III	Same as system 2 for dog	
Synovial cell sarcoma	1, 2, 3	Nuclear pleomorphism, mitotic index, necrosis	39-41
	Histiocytic or nonhistiocytic	CD18±	
	Myxoma or nonmyxoma	Abundant myxomatous matrix	
Primary and metastatic osteosarcoma (dog)	I-III	Tumor pleomorphism, mitoses, tumor matrix, cell density, necrosis, vascular invasion	42
Multilobular osteochondrosarcoma	1, 2, 3	Borders, lobule size, organization, mitotic index, nuclear pleomorphism, necrosis	43, 44
Mandibular osteosarcoma	1, 2, 3	Nuclear pleomorphism, mitotic index, necrosis	45
Appendicular chondrosarcoma	1, 2, 3	Tumor pleomorphism, mitoses, tumor matrix, cellularity, necrosis, architecture	46
Hemangiosarcoma	1, 2, 3	Overall differentiation, nuclear pleomorphism, mitotic index, necrosis	47
Nonlymphoid, nonangiomatous splenic sarcomas	Mitotic index 0-9,* mitotic index >9	Mitotic index	48
Fibrohistiocytic nodules of spleen	1, 2, 3	Proportion of lymphocytes and multinucleated cells, mitotic index	49
Transitional cell carcinoma	1, 2, 3	Cytoplasmic and nuclear variation, nuclear placement, nucleolar size/number, mitoses	50
Squamous cell carcinoma	1, 2, 3	Overall differentiation, mitotic index, nuclear pleomorphism, invasion, stromal reaction	51

SQ, Subcutaneous.

*Sum of mitoses in ten 400× fields.

evaluation at four lateral and four deep regions of the specimen.[65] Additional techniques exist that can increase the region of marginal tissue evaluated although increased costs may also be incurred. These techniques include "parallel" sectioning, "modified" sectioning (a combination of parallel and cross-sectioning), and "tangential" sectioning.[63] An additional method for evaluating excisional completeness is to evaluate the "tumor bed," which is the in vivo tissue that was adjacent to or contiguous with the excised specimen. Small regions/scrapings from the tumor bed may be submitted in addition to the excised mass but should be submitted in a separate container and clearly specified that it is "tumor bed" tissue. If neoplastic cells exist within the tumor bed tissue, this indicates presence of residual disease in the patient.

Specimens come in all shapes and sizes, thus no one blanket trimming method can be recommended. Additionally, each method has advantages and disadvantages. The most important fundamental aspects of trimming to recognize are that the regions selected for microscopic examination (1) adequately represent the mass lesion for diagnosis and (2) are the most appropriate for margin evaluation for that specific specimen. It is essential for clinicians to understand the various trimming methods that exist and the methods by which their own specimens are being trimmed, to have an understanding of the percentage of marginal tissue that is evaluated relative to the entire surgical margin, and to recognize that they can greatly influence the region of the tissue examined microscopically through inking and information provided on the submission form.

Assuming tissue demarcation, specimen submission, and tissue trimming have all been appropriately performed, microscopic reporting of the surgical margins should be clear, concise, and thorough, furnishing the clinician with essential information such that they can make informed decisions and recommendations regarding further management of the cancer patient. Thorough microscopic evaluation of the tissue margin should include (1) a description of the neoplastic cells closest to the margin (e.g., individual cells, nests of cells, cells at the periphery of the mass itself); (2) an objective measurement (via stage or ocular micrometer) from the tissue edge to the closest neoplastic cell (this parameter is precluded for tangentially trimmed sections); and (3) a description of the tissue constituents (e.g., adipose tissue, dense connective tissue, skeletal muscle) and quality of these constituents (e.g., normal, necrotic, inflamed) composing the margin because different tissue types provide variable barriers against invasion and infiltration of neoplastic cells.[63] Objective measurements may be provided in any appropriate metric (e.g., micrometers, millimeters), but the metric used should remain consistent for all margins reported for a given specimen. Vague and ambiguous terminology such as *clean, dirty, close,* or *narrow*, should be avoided, since these are subjective and introduce interpretative variability.

Microscopic evaluation of surgical margins to assess excisional completeness is not a perfect science but is approached to provide the best possible assessment. If surgical resection is determined to be complete by microscopic evaluation, the chance of local recurrence is reduced, but by no means is local tumor control guaranteed. Recurrence of soft tissue sarcomas in humans has been shown to occur in about 10% of cases in which margins were deemed complete[66]; a similar situation likely exists in veterinary medicine. Additionally, "complete excision" of local disease does not address the potential for systemic or metastatic disease and thus in no way can confirm a disease-free state.

Many tumor-specific (especially canine soft tissue sarcoma and mast cell tumor) studies have been performed with the goal of correlating surgical margins to clinical outcome.[32,67-73] To this end, it is important to note that tissue shrinkage subsequent to formalin fixation does occur and the degree of shrinkage varies relative to tissue type.[74-77] For cutaneous biopsies, shrinkage can occur up to 30%.[75,77] Additionally, tissue shrinkage is impacted by inherent postexcisional tissue retraction, as well as dehydration steps during processing. These changes may result in reported surgical margins that appear to be significantly less than the clinician believed were obtained at surgery.

Assessment of Treatment Response

Sometimes histologic assessment of preoperative treatment response may help predict outcome and could even alter subsequent therapeutic options. Assessment of preoperative therapy is most common with osteosarcoma and soft tissue sarcoma. Percent tumor necrosis is the most commonly used parameter to quantify the impact of presurgical chemotherapy or radiation therapy. In dogs with osteosarcoma, percent tumor necrosis is a good predictor for local recurrence following limb-sparing surgery subsequent to neoadjuvant radiation therapy and/or chemotherapy. Tumor necrosis rates of 90% or more, between 80% and 90%, and below 80% are associated with 91%, 78%, and 28% local control rates, respectively.[78,79] In humans, the percent of tumor necrosis in osteosarcoma following preoperative chemotherapy is also predictive for survival, and poor responders may be treated with more aggressive alternative chemotherapeutic regimes.[80] In soft tissue sarcomas, percent tumor necrosis has been used to assess presurgical therapy in humans[81] and could be done in companion animals.

The effect of previous treatment also may be evaluated histologically when there is progressive growth of tissue in an area treated previously with radiation, surgery, chemotherapy, or photodynamic therapy. In these cases, distinguishing between reactive tissue and neoplasia is important but also may be extremely difficult. Inflammation, fibrovascular proliferation (granulation tissue), or epithelial hyperplasia (if applicable) is usually present in the area. Furthermore, especially after radiation therapy, the area may contain some bizarre reactive cells, including fibroblasts (called *radiation atypical fibroblasts*) with many features of malignancy, although these cells are not neoplastic.[82] If tumor cells are identified, the clinician may wish to know if these cells are viable, dead, or rendered viable but sterilized (reproductively dead) by radiation or chemotherapy. Distinction between a viable and dead cell is often possible, but determining if a cell is viable but sterilized, or nonclonogenic, is not possible with routine microscopy. However, the presence of numerous mitotic figures in a viable-appearing tumor is suggestive of active regrowth.

Molecular techniques hold promise in identifying the adequacy of treatment and/or treatment response. Use of PCR to identify residual circulating lymphoma cells in dogs during clinical remission holds promise as an early indicator of tumor reoccurrence prior to clinical and histologic/cytologic identifiable disease. New techniques that identify large portions of the tumor's genomic expression (gene expression microarrays) and molecular phenotype (tissue microarrays, protein microarrays, and mass spectrometry) can identify tumor gene and phenotypic profiles that are predictive of a tumor's biologic behavior, a tumor's response to treatment, or early tumor recurrence.

Special Procedures

Approximately 90% of oncologic cases in humans can be diagnosed by light microscopy using hematoxylin and eosin (H&E) stains.[3] This likely approximates the situation in veterinary medicine as well. In the remaining 10% of cases, special stains or special procedures such as IHC or EM may help. IHC, flow cytometry, or other molecular techniques may also be useful in predicting tumor behavior or may help in distinguishing benign from malignant tumors (see Chapter 8).

Special Histochemical Stains

Histochemical stains consist of chemical substances that, when applied to tissue sections, result in a direct chemical reaction with tissue constituents. For all intents and purposes, routine H&E is a histochemical stain; however, many additional special histochemical stains exist. In veterinary oncologic pathology, these stains are most commonly used to assist in the diagnosis of certain poorly differentiated tumors.[10] Toluidine blue and Giemsa are two of the more common histochemical stains that aid in the identification of mast cell granules in poorly differentiated mast cell tumors. Periodic acid–Schiff (PAS), another histochemical stain, is often used in feline and ferret mast cell tumors because the granules in these species are often better visualized with PAS.

Silver stains such as Pascual's, Grimelius, or Sevier-Munger can aid in the identification of neuroendocrine tumors. Sudan black and Oil Red O stains are specific for lipid and thus may aid in the diagnosis of poorly differentiated liposarcomas or lipid-rich variants of some carcinomas and other tumor types.[83-86] It should be noted that these stains must be performed on nonprocessed tissue because exposure to xylene during processing will dissolve lipid components. A melanin bleach or iron stain (Prussian blue) may help distinguish between melanin and hemosiderin, respectively, in suspected cases of melanoma. Masson's trichrome or other trichrome stains may be used to identify collagen fibrils; this can help differentiate certain mesenchymal tumors, such as those derived from muscle (leiomyomas, leiomyosarcomas, rhabdomyoma, rhabdomyosarcomas), and those that produce collagen matrix (fibromas, fibrosarcomas). It is important to keep in mind, however, that muscle-derived tumors may have a small amount of collagen inherent in the surrounding microenvironment, and poorly differentiated fibrosarcomas may produce only minimal, if any, collagen. Phosphotungstic acid hematoxylin (PTAH) can aid in differentiating a rhabdomyosarcoma from leiomyosarcoma or other tumor as it enhances visibility of the cytoplasmic cross-striations present in skeletal muscle. Alcian blue stain may help identify ground substance glycosaminoglycans that may be seen in some neurofibrosarcomas or myxosarcomas. Mucicarmine stain or PAS is useful in mucosal tissues for identifying poorly differentiated carcinomas, whereas PAS is also helpful in the diagnosis of granular cell tumor as it reacts with the intracytoplasmic lysosomes.

With the advancement of IHC (discussed later), many histochemical stains have lost popularity but are still available and useful in the appropriate setting. Silver staining of nucleolar organizer regions (AgNOR) is an additional histochemical stain that has been shown to be prognostically relevant in canine malignant lymphoma[87] and mast cell tumors.[88]

Immunohistochemistry

Immunohistochemistry (IHC) can aid the classification of several tumors in veterinary medicine and is a widely used diagnostic technique. IHC is a staining procedure that employs commercial antibodies to identify specific cellular and extracellular molecules ex vivo, such as cytoplasmic intermediate filaments, secretory substances, and cell surface markers. IHC can be performed on frozen sections or specimens routinely fixed in formalin and processed into paraffin blocks. The tissue sections are incubated with primary antibodies to specific cell proteins (the antigens). These sections with bound primary antibody are then exposed to secondary antibodies directed against the primary antibody. The secondary antibodies are linked to peroxidase or avidin-biotin peroxidase complexes. The peroxidase catalyzes a reaction in the presence of dye that precipitates at the site of the complex and is visible with light microscopy.[3,89] As an alternative, alkaline phosphatase enzyme systems are also available. Commonly used immunohistochemical stains include those for intermediate filaments, such as vimentin for mesenchymal cells, cytokeratin for epithelial cells, and desmin or actin for muscle cells (myocytes).[3,90-92] A list of common diagnostic IHC markers used in veterinary oncology and the respective tumor types in which their use is indicated is provided in Table 3-5.

IHC can also be useful in determining cellular proliferation or the tumor growth fraction that may carry prognostic relevance.[116] This can be done using Ki-67 and PCNA staining, markers of multidrug resistance (e.g., P-glycoprotein),[136] or altered proto-oncogenes such as p53, CD117/c-Kit, p21, Rb, and PTEN.[137-139] Other markers that have been explored as potential prognostic markers via IHC in a variety of veterinary tumor types include VEGF, cyclooxygenase-2 (COX-2), epidermal growth factor receptor (EGFR), human epidermal growth factor receptor-2 (HER2), urokinase plasminogen activator (UPA), and heat shock proteins (HSPs), among others. As the realm of IHC in veterinary medicine continues to advance, so too will the discovery of tumor-specific diagnostic markers, as well as markers for prognostic (biologic aggressiveness) and predictive (response to therapy) utility.

Although IHC can be a valuable tool, some complicating factors exist. A negative stain does not exclude a certain cell type as technical difficulties or tumor cell dedifferentiation, causing loss of expression of expected proteins/markers, may result in a negative stain. One of the more common technical problems that can cause negative staining is prolonged formalin fixation that results in excessive cross-linking of the antigenic components or loss of soluble proteins into the fixative. Antibody-specific antigens (epitopes) that have been masked by protein cross-linking can often be "unmasked" by pretreating sections with trypsin or pepsin or by using heat-induced epitope retrieval (HIER) techniques.[89] Decalcification of tissue may also result in alteration of target proteins so that they are no longer recognized by the respective antibody; however, the type and duration of decalcifying solution may mitigate these deleterious effects.[89] Areas of tissue necrosis, autolysis, hemorrhage, section drying, and sometimes collagenous matrix components can cause excessive nonspecific background staining. A skilled pathologist who is familiar with the IHC stain should be asked to differentiate background stain from tumor-specific stain and to navigate technical difficulties. Additionally, IHC does not distinguish between neoplastic and nonneoplastic tissue, normal, or hyperplastic. For example, normal bladder mucosal epithelium (urothelium), urothelial hyperplasia, and urothelial carcinoma (transitional cell carcinoma) would all be immunopositive for cytokeratin. The differentiation between neoplastic and nonneoplastic is made via routine H&E light microscopy based on hallmark features of neoplasia (e.g., loss of organization, cellular atypica, invasion). IHC is an ancillary diagnostic tool that aids in determining histogenesis for poorly differentiated tumors. Considerable cross-reactivity of staining in different tumor types may occur because some markers lack specificity and can be found in a variety of cells or tumors (e.g., S-100 in melanomas, cartilage, and certain epithelial cells).[3,140] Because most tumor markers have limitations, the best and most reliable results may be obtained by using a panel of IHC stains wherein both marker-specific immunopositive and immunonegative results may be anticipated (e.g., rhabdomyosarcoma should be immunopositive for vimentin and desmin but

TABLE 3-5 Common Diagnostic Immunohistochemical Markers/Panels and Respective Tumor Types in Cats and Dogs

Tumor Type	Molecular Marker(s)	Localization/ Expression	Protein Family/Function	Comments	References
Carcinoma	Cytokeratin^{+}* Vimentin^{-}	Cyto	IFP		93-95
GIST	C-kit/CD117$^{+/-}$ SMA$^{+/-}$ Desmin^{-} S-100^{-} (Dog-1^{+})†	C-kit = PM & Cyto SMA, Desmin = Cyto S-100 = N & Cyto Dog-1 = PM & Cyto	C-kit = RTK SMA & Desmin = IFPs S-100 = Calcium flux regulator Dog-1 = Calcium-activated chloride channel protein	DOG1/TMEM16A	96-101
Hemangiosarcoma/ lymphangiosarcoma	Factor VIII-RAg/ vWF+ CD31/ PECAM-1^{+}	Factor VIII-RAg/vWF = Cyto CD31/PECAM-1 = PM & Cyto	Factor VIII-RAg = Polymeric protein synthesized by ECs and MKs; forms a circulating complex with factor VIII and plays a role in platelet aggregation. CD31/PECAM-1 = Adhesion molecule mediating leukocyte-endothelial, as well as endothelial-endothelial, cell interactions.	Factor VIII-RAg and CD31 do not differentiate between hematogenous and lymphatic endothelial origin; however, lymphatic endothelium-specific markers such as LYVE-1 and Prox-1 hold promise for future use. CD31/PECAM is also expressed, in lower levels, by monocytes, granulocytes, and subsets of T-cells.	102-107
Histiocytic sarcoma	CD18^{+}, CD3e^{-}, CD79a^{-}, Pax5^{-}, Lysozyme^{+}	CD18, CD3e, CD79a = PM Pax5 = N Lysozyme = Cyto	CD18 = Integrin β2 chain CD3e = Transmembrane protein (epsilon chain) of the T-cell receptor complex CD79a = Transmembrane protein (alpha chain) of the B-cell receptor complex Pax5 = Transcription factor Lysozyme = bacteriolytic enzyme	CD18 forms complexes with CD11a, b, c, & d, and is expressed on all leukocytes. Its expression is typically highest on yet not specific for histiocytic cells.	108-111
Leiomyoma, Leiomyosarcoma	C-kit/CD117^{-} SMA^{+} Desmin$^{+/-}$ S-100^{-} (Dog-1^{-})†	C-kit = PM & Cyto SMA, Desmin = Cyto S-100 = N & Cyto Dog-1 = PM & Cyto	C-kit = RTK SMA & Desmin = IFPs S-100 = Calcium flux regulator Dog-1= Chloride-channel protein		96-99
Lymphoma, B-cell	CD18^{-}, CD3^{-}, CD79a^{+}, Pax5^{+}‡	CD18, CD3e, CD79a = PM Pax5 = N	CD18 = Integrin β2 chain CD3e = Transmembrane protein (epsilon chain) of the T-cell receptor complex CD79a = Transmembrane protein (alpha chain) of the B-cell receptor complex Pax5 = Transcription factor involved in the	At the time of this writing, Pax5 immunopositivity in feline B-cell lymphoma is not reported in the literature but has been anecdotally observed by the authors.	112-115

Lymphoma, T cell	CD18^{-}, CD3^{+}, CD79a^{-}, Pax5^{-}	CD18, CD3e, CD79a = PM Pax5 = N	As above	Pax5 is also known as BSAP, a member of the highly conserved paired box (PAX)-domain family of transcription factors and is encoded for by the *Pax5* gene.	112-115
Lymphoma, null cell	CD18^{-}, CD3e^{-}, CD79a^{-}, Pax5^{-} (and exclusion of other round cell tumors)	CD18, CD3e, CD79a = PM Pax5 = N	As above		112
Mast cell tumor	Tryptase^{+} (C-kit/ CD117)§	Tryptase = Cyto	Tryptase = Mast cell–specific protease enzyme	*Histochemical* stains Toluidine blue and Giemsa are more commonly used to confirm mast cell origin. Tryptase IHC is fairly uncommon but is available if other diagnostic parameters are unrewarding.	116, 117
Melanocytic neoplasms (melanotic and amelanotic)	Melan-A$^{+/-}$‖ PNL2$^{+/-}$ Tyrosinase$^{+/-}$ TRP-1$^{+/-}$ TRP-2$^{+/-}$ Vim^{+} S-100$^{+/-}$	Melan-A = Cyto PNL2 = Cyto Tyrosinase = Cyto TRP-1&2 = Cyto Vim = Cyto S-100 = N & Cyto	Melan-A = Melanocyte antigen recognized by T-cells (melanocyte lineage–specific protein) PNL2 = Unknown Tyrosinase = Melanocyte differentiation protein involved in melanin synthesis TRP-1&2 = Glycoproteins involved in melanin synthesis Vimentin = IFPs S-100 = Calcium flux regulator	Melan-A/MART-1 PNL2 is melanocyte-specific save for myeloid cells, especially neutrophils	118-124
Neural astrocytic tumors (astrocytoma, glioblastoma, oligoastrocytoma)	GFAP^{+} S-100$^{+/-}$	GFAP = Cyto S-100 = N & Cyto	GFAP = IFP S-100 = Calcium flux regulator	Astrocytomas are glial tumors like oligodendrogliomas; however, oligodendrogliomas are negative for GFAP.	94, 125, 126
NE tumors	Chromogranin A^{+}¶ Synaptophysin^{+} NSE^{+}	Chromogranin = Cyto Synaptophysin = Cyto NSE = Cyto	Chromogranin = Soluble protein extract of neurosecretory granules in NE cells Synaptophysin = Gp and integral component of the NE secretory granule membrane NSE = Glycolytic isoenzyme involved in various reactions	NSE lacks NE specificity as it is found in a number of other normal and neoplastic cell types but is considered useful in combination with other NE markers.	93, 127, 128
Plasma cell tumor	MUM-1/IRF4^{+} CD18$^{+/-}$ CD3e^{-} CD79a$^{+/-}$ (Pax5^{-})	MUM-1 = N CD18, CD3e, CD79a = PM Pax5 = N	MUM-1 = Transcription factor involved in lymphoid differentiation. CD18, CD3e, CD79a Pax5 = As above	In humans, plasma cell neoplasms, multiple myeloma, and plasmablastic lymphomas typically are negative for Pax5; however, currently, similar tumors have not been evaluated in dogs.	129, 130

(continued)

TABLE 3-5 Common Diagnostic Immunohistochemical Markers/Panels and Respective Tumor Types in Cats and Dogs (continued)

Tumor Type	Molecular Marker(s)	Localization/Expression	Protein Family/Function	Comments	References
Rhabdomyosarcoma	Vim^{+} Desmin^{+} Myoglobin$^{+/-}$ SMA^{-}	Cyto	Vim, Desmin, & SMA = IFPs Myoglobin = Iron-binding protein exclusively in skeletal muscle	Myoglobin is typically a late-stage marker and thus may be negative in poorly differentiated rhabdomyosarcomas. Myo-D1 and myogenin are also skeletal muscle-specific markers but are not routinely used. PTAH is a histochemical stain that may assist in highlighting cyto cross-striations of skeletal muscle.	93, 131, 132
Sarcoma	Vimentin^{+}# Cytokeratin^{-}	Cyto	IFP		93-95
Thyroid tumor: Follicular epithelial origin (follicular carcinoma)	Thyroglobulin^{+} TTF-1^{+} Calcitonin^{-} Chromogranin A^{-} Synaptophysin^{-} NSE^{-}	Thyroglobulin = Cyto TTF-1 = N Calcitonin = Cyto	Thyroglobulin = Heavily glycosylated protein providing iodination sites for the production of thyroid hormones TTF-1 = Nuclear transcription factor specific to thyroid tissue save for pulmonary epithelium Calcitonin = Polypeptide hormone secreted by thyroid C-cells; counteracts effects of PTH by reducing blood Ca^{2+}		133-135
Thyroid tumor: C-cell/parafollicular cell origin (medullary C-cell carcinoma)	Thyroglobulin^{-} TTF-1^{+} Calcitonin^{+} Chromogranin A^{+} Synaptophysin^{+} NSE^{+}	As above	As above		133-135

This table provides common diagnostic immunohistochemical markers utilized in veterinary oncologic pathology. For a complete list of cell-specific markers available for use in veterinary samples, visit www.ihc.sdstate.org. Immunohistochemical stains should always be interpreted in conjunction with routine (hematoxylin & eosin [H&E]) histopathologic evaluation and in the presence of appropriately stained positive and negative control tissues.

BSAP, B-cell–specific activator protein; *Cyto,* cytoplasmic; *DOG1,* discovered on gastrointestinal tumor 1; *EC,* endothelial cell; *Factor VIII-RAg/vWF,* factor VIII–related antigen/von Willebrand factor; *GFAP,* glial fibrillary acidic protein; *GIST,* gastrointestinal stromal tumor; *Gp,* glycoprotein; *IFP,* intermediate filament protein; *IHC,* immunohistochemistry; *MKs,* megakaryocytes; *MUM-1/IRF4,* multiple myeloma 1/interferon regulatory factor 4; *N,* nuclear; *NE,* neuroendocrine; *NSE,* neuron-specific enolase; *PECAM,* platelet endothelial cell adhesion molecule; *PM,* plasma membrane; *PTH,* parathyroid hormone; *PTAH,* phosphotungstic acid hematoxylin; *RTK,* tyrosine kinase receptor; *SMA,* smooth muscle actin; *TRP,* tyrosinase-related protein; *TTF-1,* thyroid transcription factor-1; *Vim,* vimentin.

*Generic marker for tumors of epithelial origin.

†A well characterized diagnostic marker for GISTs in humans and, at the time of this writing, under investigation for veterinary application by one of the chapter authors (BEP).

‡At the time of this writing, reported only in the dog; however, anecdotally observed in feline lymphoma by the authors.

§c-kit/CD117 is *not* diagnostic for mast cell tumors because it is not mast-cell specific, but it has been shown to carry prognostic relevance in canine cutaneous mast cell tumor based on its cellular localization/expression pattern determined via immunohistochemistry.[116]

||Rare positivity in amelanotic melanomas.

¶Generic markers for tumors of neuroendocrine (NE) origin. A panel of all three markers is strongly recommended because NE tumors may be positive for only one of the three.

#Generic marker for tumors of mesenchymal cell origin.

immunonegative for smooth muscle actin) rather than relying on a single stain. Additionally, IHC stains can *only* be appropriately interpreted in the presence of appropriate species-specific controls. For example, if one seeks to support the diagnosis of or immunophenotype an intestinal lymphoma in a cat, the appropriate positive control tissue that must be run simultaneously would be a section of normal feline lymphoid tissue (e.g., lymph node, spleen, tonsil, or other). It must be of feline origin and contain normal lymphoid tissue in order for the pathologist to confirm that the IHC stain was successfully performed and to appropriately interpret the immunoreaction of the test tissue. Similarly, a negative control that consists of the test tissue treated either with nonspecific antibody or omission of the primary antibody must also be run to assist in ruling out background/nonspecific staining. Finally, IHC can be a powerful tool providing information that could not otherwise be determined on routine microscopy alone (e.g., confirmation of tumor histogenesis); however, an IHC stain should never be interpreted in and of itself but rather should always be evaluated in conjunction with routine light microscopic findings and knowledge of relevant clinical information.

Electron Microscopy

EM involves preserving very small representative tumor samples (1 × 1 mm) in special fixatives such as glutaraldehyde, processing tissue into epoxy-based plastic blocks, and sectioning at 1 μm for thick sections to determine the adequacy of the sample and inclusion of appropriate tumor cells. Subsequently, sectioning is done at about 600Å, stained with heavy-metal-based stains, and examined with the aid of the electron microscope. Samples fixed in formalin can be used, although the quality of the subsequent sections is less than ideal. EM may help identify certain specific features, such as intercellular junctions or basal lamina in epithelial cells, melanosomes in melanocytic cells, mast cell granules in mast cells, neurosecretory granules in neuroendocrine cells, or mucin droplets in certain epithelial cells. These features are useful in distinguishing carcinomas from lymphomas and identifying melanomas, mast cell tumors, and neuroendocrine tumors. Unless a specific feature is sought, however, EM will be no more useful than a higher magnification of a tumor that could not be diagnosed with the light microscope. Furthermore, EM is not useful for distinguishing benign from malignant cells in many cases because the magnification is too high and the tumor pattern in the tissue is not evident.[4,10] Not all veterinary diagnostic laboratories have the technical support and equipment needed for EM.

Flow Cytometry and Polymerase Chain Reaction

Flow cytometry is an analytic procedure that can be used to evaluate cell suspensions obtained from suspected neoplastic masses or fluids. In human medicine, this procedure is frequently used to diagnose and occasionally to monitor for the recurrence of various tumors, such as bladder carcinoma. Use of flow cytometry for humans is especially useful for detecting neoplastic cells in the urine of bladder cancer patients and in the evaluation of cell suspensions of suspected leukemia and lymphoma. In solid tumors, the cells must first be disassociated to create a single cell suspension. Cell suspensions are stained with specific fluorochromes, passed through the flow cytometer chamber, and analyzed and sorted by use of a focused laser beam. The most routine analysis is to determine DNA content or ploidy of the cells. Malignant cells may be diploid (normal DNA content) or aneuploid (nondiploid), but normal tissue, benign tumors, and reactive tissues are usually diploid. Occasionally, however, benign tumors and reactive tissue can be aneuploid. In some instances, aneuploidy may be prognostically significant and can be predictive of survival time. Flow cytometry also can be used to evaluate S-phase distribution or cell cycle time if the tumor is sampled at appropriate times after injecting the patient with bromodeoxyuridine (BrdUrd).[141]

Flow cytometry has been used to evaluate tumors in dogs and is becoming a more routine diagnostic procedure combined with other tests, including histopathology and cytopathology, immunocytochemistry, and PCR. In the earliest report, various canine tumors were characterized for DNA ploidy.[142] In subsequent studies, tumor cell heterogeneity, comparisons of primary and metastatic tumors, and the positive predictive value of kinetic parameters in canine osteosarcomas were evaluated.[143,144] Other studies have indicated the value of flow cytometry in predicting the behavior of various canine tumors, including lymphomas,[145,146] myeloproliferative disease,[147-149] mammary gland tumors,[150] melanomas,[151] osteosarcomas,[143] and plasmacytomas.[152] Flow cytometry can also be useful for analyzing abnormal populations of white blood cells in blood or fluid, helping to distinguish lymphoma from reactive processes. As samples to be evaluated by flow cytometry are often cell suspensions derived from tumor masses, a correlate sample from the same site or same specimen should always be taken for histopathologic assessment. Histologic correlation is necessary because flow cytometry cannot distinguish a benign from a malignant diploid tumor, nor can it always identify tumor type.[3] Currently the use of flow cytometry in diagnostic medicine to identify tumor subtypes, occult disease with a leukemic component, or cell surface prognostic markers is crossing over from investigational to practical diagnostic veterinary medicine.

PCR is a technique now commonly used to distinguish lymphoma from reactive processes by evaluating for the presence of antigen-receptor rearrangements (PARR) to determine clonality. The PCR is used to amplify DNA encoding the antigen-binding region of lymphocytes, and a clonal or single-size product indicates malignancy. In an early study, 91% of lymphomas were identified by this technique.[6] This technique also accurately identified B- or T-cell immunophenotype. Currently, air-dried aspirates, fresh, or formalin-fixed tissue can be used for this technique. Mutations resulting in internal tandem duplication in exon 11 of the *c-Kit* gene, CD117 or stem cell growth factor receptor, have been identified as a mutation constitutively activating this tyrosine kinase receptor, resulting in a more aggressive biologic behavior in canine mast cell tumors.[153,154] PCR is currently used to identify this mutation in a diagnostic setting as a biologic marker of prognosis.

Clinical-Pathologic Correlation and Second Opinions

Sometimes the pathologist cannot make an accurate diagnosis without clinical correlations.[2,4] This is especially true for some primary bone tumors or secondary tumors involving bone. Diagnosis of a surface or juxtacortical osteosarcoma is based on both radiographic and histologic features. An osteoma may be difficult to distinguish from reactive bone without a corroborative radiograph. A synovial cell sarcoma may be difficult to distinguish from other sarcomas or even inflammatory or immune-mediated joint disease unless there is radiographic or gross evidence of joint involvement and bone invasion. An acanthomatous epulis may be difficult to distinguish from a fibrous epulis unless there is bone invasion in the former that cannot be identified without appropriately deep biopsy samples that include underlying bone. The best example of the need for clinical and pathologic correlation is with histologically low-grade yet biologically high-grade fibrosarcomas of the canine head in which the histologic appearance is of benign fibrous tissue, but the clinical presentation is an aggressive invasive mass, often recurrent after conservative surgery, causing bone destruction.[11] These examples demonstrate the necessity for an accurate history with pertinent clinical results being provided to the pathologist along with the biopsy sample. In some cases, photographs of the tumor site or inclusion of radiographs or radiographic findings are most helpful.

Before any major treatment is undertaken or *if a pathology diagnosis is not consistent with clinical presentation,* a second opinion should be requested from the pathologist. In human medicine, a review of mandatory second-opinion surgical pathology at major hospitals revealed 1.4% to 5.8% major changes in diagnosis that resulted in change of therapy or prognoses. It was concluded that despite the extra cost, mandatory second opinions should be obtained whenever a major therapeutic endeavor is considered or if treatment decisions are based primarily on the pathologic diagnosis.[155-157]

The two major categories of errors that may occur at the pathology laboratory are technical errors and errors in interpretation of the tissue.[61] Technical errors may occur if the histotechnologist improperly labels specimens, tissue blocks, or slides or fails to process all the critical tissue submitted by the clinician. If tissue is improperly processed because of equipment malfunction or because it is poorly sectioned, artifacts can occur that make the tissue specimen impossible to interpret. Errors in interpretation by the pathologist may occur in difficult cases. If a pathology service staffed by physicians is used, certain tumors such as histiocytoma, mast cell tumor, transmissible venereal tumor, or perianal gland adenoma may be misdiagnosed, as these do not have a human counterpart. Many pathologists will obtain opinions from other pathologists when confronted with difficult cases, just as clinicians will seek second opinions on difficult radiographs or clinical problems. *The clinician should never hesitate to ask for a second opinion nor should the pathologist be offended by the request.* Each pathologist approaches a section differently and in some cases, one approach might prove more accurate than another. A second or even third pathologist can offer a different perspective on a difficult case, offer an alternative diagnosis, confirm the primary pathologist's diagnosis, or confirm that an accurate diagnosis is not possible. Since the patient's treatment options or decisions regarding euthanasia are often based on the final pathology diagnosis, it is not at all unreasonable for the clinician to request a second opinion. A misdiagnosis can result in costly, ineffective, and untimely treatments that can cause undo discomfort for patients. They can result in unnecessary surgery, unnecessary chemotherapy or radiation therapy, insufficient treatment resulting in cancer progression, and, worst of all, unwarranted euthanasia. Considering these possible scenarios, second opinions are not only prudent but highly recommended.

The clinician needs to have knowledge of the pathology of neoplasia to understand neoplastic conditions and understand the limitations of histopathologic assessment in the diagnosis of neoplasia. In the case of tumor diagnosis, histopathologic assessment of a thin slice of tissue may not always be an exact science. The pathologist and the clinician must work together to establish the most appropriate diagnosis so that proper treatment can be initiated.

REFERENCES

1. Goldschmidt M, et al: Classification and grading of canine mammary tumors, *Vet Pathol* 48(1):117–131, 2011.
2. Bonfiglio TA, Stoler MH: The pathology of cancer. In Rubin P, editor: *Clinical Oncology*, ed 7, Philadelphia, 1993, WB Saunders.
3. Pfeifer J, Wick M: The pathologic evaluation of neoplastic diseases, In Murphy G, Lawrence W, Lenhard R, editors: *Clinical oncology*, Washington, DC, 1991, Pan American Health Organization.
4. Pfeifer J, Wick M: The pathologic evaluation of neoplastic diseases, In Murphy G, Lawrence W, Lenhard R, editors: *Clinical oncology*, Washington, DC, 1995, Pan American Health Organization.
5. Stedman T: *Stedman's medical dictionary*, ed 23, Baltimore, 1976, Lippincott Williams & Wilkins.
6. Burnett RC, et al: Diagnosis of canine lymphoid neoplasia using clonal rearrangements of antigen receptor genes, *Vet Pathol* 40(1):32–41, 2003.
7. Jacobs R, Messick H, Valli V: Tumors of the hemolympatic system, In Meuten D, editor: *Tumors in domestic animals*, ed 4, Ames, Iowa, 2002, Iowa State Press.
8. Sorenmo KU, et al: Development, anatomy, histology, lymphatic drainage, clinical features, and cell differentiation markers of canine mammary gland neoplasms, *Vet Pathol* 48(1):85–97, 2011.
9. Misdorp W: General considerations. In Meuten J, editor: *Tumors of domestic animals*, ed 3, Berkeley, Calif, 1990, University of California Press.
10. Cullen J, Page R, Misdorp W: An overview of cancer pathogenesis, diagnosis and management. In Meuten D, editor: *Tumors in domestic animals*, ed 4, Ames, Iowa, 2002, Iowa State Press.
11. Ciekot PA, et al: Histologically low-grade, yet biologically high-grade, fibrosarcomas of the mandible and maxilla in dogs: 25 cases (1982-1991), *J Am Vet Med Assoc* 204(4):610–615, 1994.
12. Gottfried SD, et al: Metastatic digital carcinoma in the cat: a retrospective study of 36 cats (1992-1998), *J Am Anim Hosp Assoc* 36(6):501–509, 2000.
13. Northrup NC, et al: Variation among pathologists in histologic grading of canine cutaneous mast cell tumors, *J Vet Diagn Invest* 17(3):245–248, 2005.
14. Carriaga MT, Henson DE: The histologic grading of cancer, *Cancer* 75(1 Suppl):406–421, 1995.
15. Valli VE, et al: Classification of canine malignant lymphomas according to the World Health Organization criteria, *Vet Pathol* 48(1):198–211, 2011.
16. Maiolino P, et al: Nucleomorphometric analysis of canine cutaneous mast cell tumours, *J Comp Pathol* 133(2-3):209–211, 2005.
17. Strefezzi Rde F, Xavier JG, Catao-Dias JL: Morphometry of canine cutaneous mast cell tumors, *Vet Pathol* 40(3):268–275, 2003.
18. Patnaik AK, Ehler WJ, MacEwen EG: Canine cutaneous mast cell tumor: morphologic grading and survival time in 83 dogs, *Vet Pathol* 21(5):469–474, 1984.
19. Bostock DE: The prognosis following surgical removal of mastocytomas in dogs, *J Small Anim Pract* 14(1):27–41, 1973.
20. Kiupel M, et al: Proposal of a 2-tier histologic grading system for canine cutaneous mast cell tumors to more accurately predict biological behavior, *Vet Pathol* 48(1):147–155, 2011.
21. Thompson JJ, et al: Canine subcutaneous mast cell tumor: characterization and prognostic indices, *Vet Pathol* 48(1):156–168, 2011.
22. Wilcock BP, Yager JA, Zink MC: The morphology and behavior of feline cutaneous mastocytomas, *Vet Pathol* 23(3):320–324, 1986.
23. Molander-McCrary H, et al: Cutaneous mast cell tumors in cats: 32 cases (1991-1994), *J Am Anim Hosp Assoc* 34(4):281–284, 1998.
24. Carter RF, Valli VE, Lumsden JH: The cytology, histology and prevalence of cell types in canine lymphoma classified according to the National Cancer Institute Working Formulation, *Can J Vet Res* 50(2):154–164, 1986.
25. Teske E, et al: Prognostic factors for treatment of malignant lymphoma in dogs, *J Am Vet Med Assoc* 205(12):1722–1728, 1994.

26. Bostock DE: Prognosis after surgical excision of canine melanomas, *Vet Pathol* 16(1):32–40, 1979.
27. Laprie C, et al: MIB-1 immunoreactivity correlates with biologic behaviour in canine cutaneous melanoma, *Vet Dermatol* 12(3): 139–147, 2001.
28. Esplin DG: Survival of dogs following surgical excision of histologically well-differentiated melanocytic neoplasms of the mucous membranes of the lips and oral cavity, *Vet Pathol* 45(6): 889–896, 2008.
29. Wilcock BP, Peiffer RL Jr: Morphology and behavior of primary ocular melanomas in 91 dogs, *Vet Pathol* 23(4):418–424, 1986.
30. Kalishman JB, et al: A matched observational study of survival in cats with enucleation due to diffuse iris melanoma, *Vet Ophthalmol* 1(1):25–29, 1998.
31. Bostock DE, Dye MT: Prognosis after surgical excision of canine fibrous connective tissue sarcomas, *Vet Pathol* 17(5):581–588, 1980.
32. Kuntz CA, et al: Prognostic factors for surgical treatment of soft-tissue sarcomas in dogs: 75 cases (1986-1996), *J Am Vet Med Assoc* 211(9):1147–1151, 1997.
33. McNiel EA, et al: Evaluation of prognostic factors for dogs with primary lung tumors: 67 cases (1985-1992), *J Am Vet Med Assoc* 211(11):1422–1427, 1997.
34. Hahn KA, McEntee MF: Prognosis factors for survival in cats after removal of a primary lung tumor: 21 cases (1979-1994), *Vet Surg* 27(4):307–311, 1998.
35. Kurzman ID, Gilbertson SR: Prognostic factors in canine mammary tumors, *Semin Vet Med Surg (Small Anim)* 1(1):25–32, 1986.
36. Karayannopoulou M, et al: Histological grading and prognosis in dogs with mammary carcinomas: application of a human grading method, *J Comp Pathol* 133(4):246–252, 2005.
37. Misdorp W: Tumors of the mammary gland. In Meuten D, editor: *Tumors in Domestic Animals*, ed 4, Ames, Iowa, 2002, Iowa State Press, pp 575–606, 764.
38. Weijer K, et al: Feline malignant mammary tumors. I. Morphology and biology: some comparisons with human and canine mammary carcinomas, *J Natl Cancer Inst* 49(6):1697–1704, 1972.
39. Vail DM, et al: Evaluation of prognostic factors for dogs with synovial sarcoma: 36 cases (1986-1991), *J Am Vet Med Assoc* 205(9):1300–1307, 1994.
40. Craig LE, Julian ME, Ferracone JD: The diagnosis and prognosis of synovial tumors in dogs: 35 cases, *Vet Pathol* 39(1):66–73, 2002.
41. Craig LE, Krimer PM, Cooley AJ: Canine synovial myxoma: 39 cases, *Vet Pathol* 47(5):931–936, 2010.
42. Kirpensteijn J, et al: Prognostic significance of a new histologic grading system for canine osteosarcoma, *Vet Pathol* 39(2):240–246, 2002.
43. Straw RC, et al: Multilobular osteochondrosarcoma of the canine skull: 16 cases (1978-1988), *J Am Vet Med Assoc* 195(12):1764–1769, 1989.
44. Dernell WS, et al: Multilobular osteochondrosarcoma in 39 dogs: 1979-1993, *J Am Anim Hosp Assoc* 34(1):11–18, 1998.
45. Straw RC, et al: Canine mandibular osteosarcoma: 51 cases (1980-1992), *J Am Anim Hosp Assoc* 32(3):257–262, 1996.
46. Farese JP, et al: Biologic behavior and clinical outcome of 25 dogs with canine appendicular chondrosarcoma treated by amputation: a Veterinary Society of Surgical Oncology retrospective study, *Vet Surg* 38(8):914–919, 2009.
47. Ogilvie GK, et al: Surgery and doxorubicin in dogs with hemangiosarcoma, *J Vet Intern Med* 10(6):379–384, 1996.
48. Spangler WL, Culbertson MR, Kass PH: Primary mesenchymal (nonangiomatous/nonlymphomatous) neoplasms occurring in the canine spleen: anatomic classification, immunohistochemistry, and mitotic activity correlated with patient survival, *Vet Pathol* 31(1):37–47, 1994.
49. Spangler WL, Kass PH: Pathologic and prognostic characteristics of splenomegaly in dogs due to fibrohistiocytic nodules: 98 cases, *Vet Pathol* 35(6):488–498, 1998.
50. Valli VE, et al: Pathology of canine bladder and urethral cancer and correlation with tumour progression and survival, *J Comp Pathol* 113(2):113–130, 1995.
51. Carpenter L, Withrow S, Powers B: Squamous cell carcinoma of the tongue in 10 dogs, *J Am Anim Hosp Assoc* 29:17–24, 1993.
52. Pakos EE, et al: Expression of vascular endothelial growth factor and its receptor, KDR/Flk-1, in soft tissue sarcomas, *Anticancer Res* 25(5):3591–3596, 2005.
53. Yudoh K, et al: Concentration of vascular endothelial growth factor in the tumour tissue as a prognostic factor of soft tissue sarcomas, *Br J Cancer* 84(12):1610–1615, 2001.
54. Hansen AE, et al: Hypoxia-inducible factors–regulation, role and comparative aspects in tumourigenesis, *Vet Comp Oncol* 9(1):16–37, 2011.
55. Smedley RC, et al: Prognostic markers for canine melanocytic neoplasms: a comparative review of the literature and goals for future investigation, *Vet Pathol* 48(1):54–72, 2011.
56. Loukopoulos P, Robinson WF: Clinicopathological relevance of tumour grading in canine osteosarcoma, *J Comp Pathol* 136(1): 65–73, 2007.
57. Dennis MM, et al: Prognostic factors for cutaneous and subcutaneous soft tissue sarcomas in dogs, *Vet Pathol* 48(1):73–84, 2011.
58. Coindre JM, et al: Histopathologic grading in spindle cell soft tissue sarcomas, *Cancer* 61(11):2305–2309, 1988.
59. Bostock DE, Dye MT: Prognosis after surgical excision of fibrosarcomas in cats, *J Am Vet Med Assoc* 175(7):727–728, 1979.
60. Davidson EB, Gregory CR, Kass PH: Surgical excision of soft tissue fibrosarcomas in cats, *Vet Surg* 26(4):265–269, 1997.
61. Bonfiglio T, Terry R: The pathology of cancer. In Rubin P, editor: *Clinical oncology*, ed 6, 1983.
62. Langenbach A, et al: Sensitivity and specificity of methods of assessing the regional lymph nodes for evidence of metastasis in dogs and cats with solid tumors, *J Am Vet Med Assoc* 218(9):1424–1428, 2001.
63. Kamstock DA, et al: Recommended guidelines for submission, trimming, margin evaluation, and reporting of tumor biopsy specimens in veterinary surgical pathology, *Vet Pathol* 48(1):19–31, 2011.
64. Rochat MC, et al: Identification of surgical biopsy borders by use of india ink, *J Am Vet Med Assoc* 201(6):873–878, 1992.
65. Abide JM, Nahai F, Bennett RG: The meaning of surgical margins, *Plast Reconstr Surg* 73(3):492–497, 1984.
66. Rydholm A: Surgical margins for soft tissue sarcoma, *Acta Orthop Scand Suppl* 273:81–85, 1997.
67. Baker-Gabb M, Hunt GB, France MP: Soft tissue sarcomas and mast cell tumours in dogs; clinical behaviour and response to surgery, *Aust Vet J* 81(12):732–738, 2003.
68. Bacon NJ, et al: Evaluation of primary re-excision after recent inadequate resection of soft tissue sarcomas in dogs: 41 cases (1999-2004), *J Am Vet Med Assoc* 230(4):548–554, 2007.
69. Stefanello D, et al: Marginal excision of low-grade spindle cell sarcoma of canine extremities: 35 dogs (1996-2006), *Vet Surg* 37(5):461–465, 2008.
70. McSporran KD: Histologic grade predicts recurrence for marginally excised canine subcutaneous soft tissue sarcomas, *Vet Pathol* 46(5):928–933, 2009.
71. Simpson AM, et al: Evaluation of surgical margins required for complete excision of cutaneous mast cell tumors in dogs, *J Am Vet Med Assoc* 224(2):236–240, 2004.
72. Fulcher RP, et al: Evaluation of a two-centimeter lateral surgical margin for excision of grade I and grade II cutaneous mast cell tumors in dogs, *J Am Vet Med Assoc* 228(2):210–215, 2006.
73. Schultheiss PC, et al: Association of histologic tumor characteristics and size of surgical margins with clinical outcome after surgical removal of cutaneous mast cell tumors in dogs, *J Am Vet Med Assoc* 238(11):1464–1469, 2011.

74. Johnson RE, et al: Quantification of surgical margin shrinkage in the oral cavity, *Head Neck* 19(4):281–286, 1997.
75. Reimer SB, et al: Evaluation of the effect of routine histologic processing on the size of skin samples obtained from dogs, *Am J Vet Res* 66(3):500–505, 2005.
76. Wang L, et al: [The extensibility and retractility of surgical margins in digestive tract cancer], *Zhonghua Wai Ke Za Zhi* 40(4):271–273, 2002.
77. Kerns MJ, et al: Shrinkage of cutaneous specimens: formalin or other factors involved? *J Cutan Pathol* 35(12):1093–1096, 2008.
78. Powers BE, et al: Percent tumor necrosis as a predictor of treatment response in canine osteosarcoma, *Cancer* 67(1):126–134, 1991.
79. Withrow SJ, et al: Comparative aspects of osteosarcoma. Dog versus man, *Clin Orthop Relat Res* 270:159–168, 1991.
80. Rosen G, et al: Preoperative chemotherapy for osteogenic sarcoma: selection of postoperative adjuvant chemotherapy based on the response of the primary tumor to preoperative chemotherapy, *Cancer* 49(6):1221–1230, 1982.
81. Willett CG, et al: The histologic response of soft tissue sarcoma to radiation therapy, *Cancer* 60(7):1500–1504, 1987.
82. Fajardo LF, Berthrong M, Anderson RE: Differential diagnosis of atypical cells in irradiated tissues. In Berthrong M, Fajardo LF, Anderson RE, editor: *Radiation pathology*, New York, 2001, Oxford University Press.
83. Masserdotti C, et al: Use of Oil Red O stain in the cytologic diagnosis of canine liposarcoma, *Vet Clin Pathol* 35(1):37–41, 2006.
84. Kwon HJ, et al: Round cell variant of myxoid liposarcoma in a Japanese Macaque (Macaca fuscata), *Vet Pathol* 44(2):229–232, 2007.
85. Kamstock DA, Fredrickson R, Ehrhart EJ: Lipid-rich carcinoma of the mammary gland in a cat, *Vet Pathol* 42(3):360–362, 2005.
86. Avakian A, et al: Lipid-rich pleural mesothelioma in a dog, *J Vet Diagn Invest* 20(5):665–667, 2008.
87. Kiupel M, Teske E, Bostock D: Prognostic factors for treated canine malignant lymphoma, *Vet Pathol* 36(4):292–300, 1999.
88. Kravis LD, et al: Frequency of argyrophilic nucleolar organizer regions in fine-needle aspirates and biopsy specimens from mast cell tumors in dogs, *J Am Vet Med Assoc* 209(8):1418–1420, 1996.
89. Ramos-Vara JA: Technical aspects of immunohistochemistry, *Vet Pathol* 42(4):405–426, 2005.
90. Andreasen CB, Mahaffey EA, Duncan JR: Intermediate filament staining in the cytologic and histologic diagnosis of canine skin and soft tissue tumors, *Vet Pathol* 25(5):343–349, 1988.
91. Sandusky GE, Carlton WW, Wightman KA: Diagnostic immunohistochemistry of canine round cell tumors, *Vet Pathol* 24(6):495–499, 1987.
92. Espinosa de los Monteros A, et al: Coordinate expression of cytokeratins 7 and 20 in feline and canine carcinomas, *Vet Pathol* 36(3):179–190, 1999.
93. Dabbs D: *Diagnostic immunohistochemistry*, ed 2, Philadelphia, 2006, Churchill Livingstone Elsevier.
94. Moore AS, Madewell BR, Lund JK: Immunohistochemical evaluation of intermediate filament expression in canine and feline neoplasms, *Am J Vet Res* 50(1):88–92, 1989.
95. Desnoyers MM, Haines DM, Searcy GP: Immunohistochemical detection of intermediate filament proteins in formalin fixed normal and neoplastic canine tissues, *Can J Vet Res* 54(3):360–365, 1990.
96. Frost D, Lasota J, Miettinen M: Gastrointestinal stromal tumors and leiomyomas in the dog: a histopathologic, immunohistochemical, and molecular genetic study of 50 cases, *Vet Pathol* 40(1):42–54, 2003.
97. Russell KN, et al: Clinical and immunohistochemical differentiation of gastrointestinal stromal tumors from leiomyosarcomas in dogs: 42 cases (1990-2003), *J Am Vet Med Assoc* 230(9):1329–1333, 2007.
98. Fatima N, Cohen C, Siddiqui MT: DOG1 utility in diagnosing gastrointestinal stromal tumors on fine-needle aspiration, *Cancer Cytopathol* 119(3):202–208, 2011.
99. Espinosa I, et al: A novel monoclonal antibody against DOG1 is a sensitive and specific marker for gastrointestinal stromal tumors, *Am J Surg Pathol* 32(2):210–218, 2008.
100. West RB, et al: The novel marker, DOG1, is expressed ubiquitously in gastrointestinal stromal tumors irrespective of KIT or PDGFRA mutation status, *Am J Pathol* 165(1):107–113, 2004.
101. Morini M, et al: C-kit gene product (CD117) immunoreactivity in canine and feline paraffin sections, *J Histochem Cytochem* 52(5):705–708, 2004.
102. von Beust BR, Suter MM, Summers BA: Factor VIII-related antigen in canine endothelial neoplasms: an immunohistochemical study, *Vet Pathol* 25(4):251–255, 1988.
103. Ferrer L, et al: Immunohistochemical detection of CD31 antigen in normal and neoplastic canine endothelial cells, *J Comp Pathol* 112(4):319–326, 1995.
104. Wilting J, et al: The transcription factor Prox1 is a marker for lymphatic endothelial cells in normal and diseased human tissues, *FASEB J* 16(10):1271–1273, 2002.
105. Sagartz JE, et al: Lymphangiosarcoma in a young dog, *Vet Pathol* 33(3):353–356, 1996.
106. Galeotti F, et al: Feline lymphangiosarcoma–definitive identification using a lymphatic vascular marker, *Vet Dermatol* 15(1):13–18, 2004.
107. Sugiyama A, et al: Lymphangiosarcoma in a cat, *J Comp Pathol* 137(2-3):174–178, 2007.
108. Moore PF: Characterization of cytoplasmic lysozyme immunoreactivity as a histiocytic marker in normal canine tissues, *Vet Pathol* 23(6):763–769, 1986.
109. Affolter VK, Moore PF: Localized and disseminated histiocytic sarcoma of dendritic cell origin in dogs, *Vet Pathol* 39(1):74–83, 2002.
110. Thio T, et al: Malignant histiocytosis of the brain in three dogs, *J Comp Pathol* 134(2-3):241–244, 2006.
111. Fulmer AK, Mauldin GE: Canine histiocytic neoplasia: an overview, *Can Vet J* 48(10):1041–1043, 1046–1050, 2007.
112. Willmann M, et al: Pax5 immunostaining in paraffin-embedded sections of canine non-Hodgkin lymphoma: a novel canine pan pre-B- and B-cell marker, *Vet Immunol Immunopathol* 128(4): 359–365, 2009.
113. Ferrer L, et al: Immunohistochemical detection of CD3 antigen (pan T marker) in canine lymphomas, *J Vet Diagn Invest* 5(4):616–620, 1993.
114. Milner RJ, et al: Immunophenotypic classification of canine malignant lymphoma on formalin-mixed paraffin wax-embedded tissue by means of CD3 and CD79a cell markers, *Onderstepoort J Vet Res* 63(4):309–313, 1996.
115. Caniatti M, et al: Canine lymphoma: immunocytochemical analysis of fine-needle aspiration biopsy, *Vet Pathol* 33(2):204–212, 1996.
116. Webster JD, et al: The use of KIT and tryptase expression patterns as prognostic tools for canine cutaneous mast cell tumors, *Vet Pathol* 41(4):371–377, 2004.
117. Walls AF, et al: Immunohistochemical identification of mast cells in formaldehyde-fixed tissue using monoclonal antibodies specific for tryptase, *J Pathol* 162(2):119–126, 1990.
118. Smedley RC, et al: Immunohistochemical diagnosis of canine oral amelanotic melanocytic neoplasms, *Vet Pathol* 48(1):32–40, 2011.
119. Koenig A, et al: Expression of S100a, vimentin, NSE, and melan A/MART-1 in seven canine melanoma cells lines and twenty-nine retrospective cases of canine melanoma, *Vet Pathol* 38(4):427–435, 2001.
120. Giudice C, et al: Immunohistochemical investigation of PNL2 reactivity of canine melanocytic neoplasms and comparison with Melan A, *J Vet Diagn Invest* 22(3):389–394, 2010.
121. Ramos-Vara JA, Miller MA: Immunohistochemical identification of canine melanocytic neoplasms with antibodies to melanocytic antigen PNL2 and tyrosinase: comparison with Melan A, *Vet Pathol* 48(2):443–450, 2011.

122. Ramos-Vara JA, et al: Melan A and S100 protein immunohistochemistry in feline melanomas: 48 cases, *Vet Pathol* 39(1):127–132, 2002.
123. Kawakami Y, et al: Identification of the immunodominant peptides of the MART-1 human melanoma antigen recognized by the majority of HLA-A2-restricted tumor infiltrating lymphocytes, *J Exp Med* 180(1):347–352, 1994.
124. Schneider J, et al: Overlapping peptides of melanocyte differentiation antigen Melan-A/MART-1 recognized by autologous cytolytic T lymphocytes in association with HLA-B45.1 and HLA-A2.1, *Int J Cancer* 75(3):451–458, 1998.
125. Lipsitz D, et al: Glioblastoma multiforme: clinical findings, magnetic resonance imaging, and pathology in five dogs, *Vet Pathol* 40(6):659–669, 2003.
126. Stoica G, et al: Morphology, immunohistochemistry, and genetic alterations in dog astrocytomas, *Vet Pathol* 41(1):10–19, 2004.
127. Hawkins KL, et al: Immunocytochemistry of normal pancreatic islets and spontaneous islet cell tumors in dogs, *Vet Pathol* 24(2):170–179, 1987.
128. Leblanc B, et al: Immunocytochemistry of canine thyroid tumors, *Vet Pathol* 28(5):370–380, 1991.
129. Ramos-Vara JA, Miller MA, Valli VE: Immunohistochemical detection of multiple myeloma 1/interferon regulatory factor 4 (MUM1/IRF-4) in canine plasmacytoma: comparison with CD79a and CD20, *Vet Pathol* 44(6):875–884, 2007.
130. Feldman AL, Dogan A: Diagnostic uses of Pax5 immunohistochemistry, *Adv Anat Pathol* 14(5):323–334, 2007.
131. Andreasen CB, et al: Desmin as a marker for canine botryoid rhabdomyosarcomas, *J Comp Pathol* 98(1):23–29, 1988.
132. Murakami M, et al: Cytologic, histologic, and immunohistochemical features of maxillofacial alveolar rhabdomyosarcoma in a juvenile dog, *Vet Clin Pathol* 39(1):113–118, 2010.
133. Liptak JM, et al: Cranial mediastinal carcinomas in nine dogs, *Vet Comp Oncol* 6(1):19–30, 2008.
134. Ramos-Vara JA, Miller MA, Johnson GC: Usefulness of thyroid transcription factor-1 immunohistochemical staining in the differential diagnosis of primary pulmonary tumors of dogs, *Vet Pathol* 42(3):315–320, 2005.
135. Ramos-Vara JA., et al: Immunohistochemical detection of thyroid transcription factor-1, thyroglobulin, and calcitonin in canine normal, hyperplastic, and neoplastic thyroid gland, *Vet Pathol* 39(4):480–487, 2002.
136. Bergman PJ, Ogilvie GK, Powers BE: Monoclonal antibody C219 immunohistochemistry against P-glycoprotein: sequential analysis and predictive ability in dogs with lymphoma, *J Vet Intern Med* 10(6):354–359, 1996.
137. Sagartz JE, et al: p53 tumor suppressor protein overexpression in osteogenic tumors of dogs, *Vet Pathol* 33(2):213–221, 1996.
138. London CA, et al: Expression of stem cell factor receptor (c-kit) by the malignant mast cells from spontaneous canine mast cell tumours, *J Comp Pathol* 115(4):399–414, 1996.
139. Koenig A, et al: Expression and significance of p53, rb, p21/waf-1, p16/ink-4a, and PTEN tumor suppressors in canine melanoma, *Vet Pathol* 39(4):458–472, 2002.
140. Lewis RE, Johnson WW, Cruse JM: Pitfalls and caveats in the methodology for immunoperoxidase staining in surgical pathologic diagnosis, *Surv Synth Pathol Res* 1:134, 1983.
141. Nunez R: DNA measurement and cell cycle analysis by flow cytometry, *Curr Issues Mol Biol* 3(3):67–70, 2001.
142. Johnson TS, et al: Ploidy and DNA distribution analysis of spontaneous dog tumors by flow cytometry, *Cancer Res* 41(8):3005–3009, 1981.
143. LaRue SM, et al: Impact of heterogeneity in the predictive value of kinetic parameters in canine osteosarcoma, *Cancer Res* 54(14):3916–3921, 1994.
144. Fox MH, et al: Comparison of DNA aneuploidy of primary and metastatic spontaneous canine osteosarcomas, *Cancer Res* 50(19):6176–6178, 1990.
145. Gibson D, et al: Flow cytometric immunophenotype of canine lymph node aspirates, *J Vet Intern Med* 18(5):710–717, 2004.
146. Gelain ME, et al: Aberrant phenotypes and quantitative antigen expression in different subtypes of canine lymphoma by flow cytometry, *Vet Immunol Immunopathol* 121(3-4):179–188, 2008.
147. Weir EG, Borowitz MJ: Flow cytometry in the diagnosis of acute leukemia, *Semin Hematol* 38(2):124–138, 2001.
148. Wilkerson MJ, et al: Lineage differentiation of canine lymphoma/leukemias and aberrant expression of CD molecules, *Vet Immunol Immunopathol* 106(3-4):179–196, 2005.
149. Villiers E, et al: Identification of acute myeloid leukemia in dogs using flow cytometry with myeloperoxidase, MAC387, and a canine neutrophil-specific antibody, *Vet Clin Pathol* 35(1):55–71, 2006.
150. Hellmen E, et al: Prognostic factors in canine mammary tumors: a multivariate study of 202 consecutive cases, *Vet Pathol* 30(1):20–27, 1993.
151. Bolon B, Calderwood Mays MB, Hall BJ: Characteristics of canine melanomas and comparison of histology and DNA ploidy to their biologic behavior, *Vet Pathol* 27(2):96–102, 1990.
152. Frazier KS, et al: Analysis of DNA aneuploidy and c-myc oncoprotein content of canine plasma cell tumors using flow cytometry, *Vet Pathol* 30(6):505–511, 1993.
153. Letard S, et al: Gain-of-function mutations in the extracellular domain of KIT are common in canine mast cell tumors, *Mol Cancer Res* 6(7):1137–1145, 2008.
154. Webster JD, et al: The role of c-KIT in tumorigenesis: evaluation in canine cutaneous mast cell tumors, *Neoplasia* 8(2):104–111, 2006.
155. Abt AB, Abt LG, Olt GJ: The effect of interinstitution anatomic pathology consultation on patient care, *Arch Pathol Lab Med* 119(6):514–517, 1995.
156. Kronz JD, Westra WH, Epstein JI: Mandatory second opinion surgical pathology at a large referral hospital, *Cancer* 86(11):2426–2435, 1999.
157. Kronz JD, Westra WH: The role of second opinion pathology in the management of lesions of the head and neck, *Curr Opin Otolaryngol Head Neck Surg* 13(2):81–84, 2005.

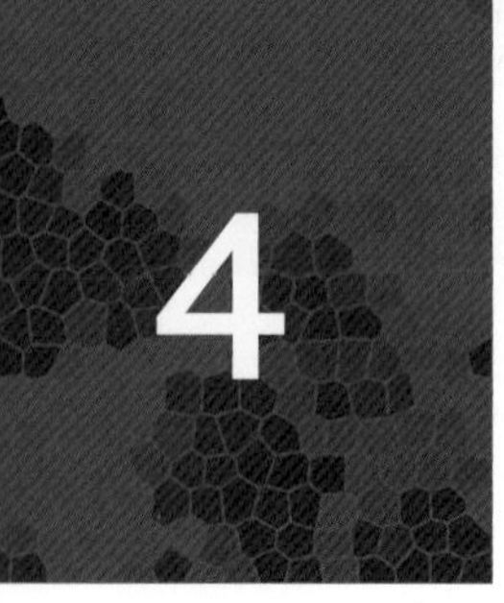

4 Epidemiology and the Evidence-Based Medicine Approach

Lesley M. Butler, Brenda N. Bonnett, and Rodney L. Page

Epidemiology has been traditionally defined as the study of the distribution and determinants of disease in populations. Although historically epidemiologic methods were primarily used for the investigation of outbreaks and/or epidemics of infectious disease, the philosophies, attitudes, methodologies, and application of epidemiology are in fact more broadly applicable to research and clinical practice, regardless of species, disease, or discipline. Evidence-based medicine (EBM) is an approach to the practice of health care that is now well-accepted in the human and veterinary fields. Using the EBM approach involves a commitment to base all decisions on the best available evidence and to be explicit about the level and quality of evidence on which decisions are based. Much of the underpinning of EBM, including study design and interpretation, are also facets of epidemiology. Extensive literature is available on EBM and evidence-based practice in the human field (e.g., The Cochrane Collaboration [http://www.cochrane.org/about-us/evidence-base-health-care/webliography/books/ebhc]).

The EBM approach can and should be applied to all interventions, including diagnosis and prognosis, and choice of preventive and clinical therapies applied to individuals, as well as decisions about health policy or control programs for populations. Pathophysiology forms the basis of our understanding of health and disease, but this knowledge, even combined with clinical acumen and experience, is not sufficient grounds for decision making across the spectrum of activities of health professionals. In order to have confidence that our interventions will be beneficial, we need to understand that personal and expert opinion are only anecdotal evidence, unless they are based on a valid appraisal of available evidence from the literature. In addition to embracing the philosophy of EBM, all clinicians must develop the knowledge and skills such as information management, critical appraisal, and causal reasoning that are needed to assess evidence in order to determine that their chosen interventions are both efficacious and effective (see glossary of terms in Table 4-1). Unfortunately, especially in veterinary medicine, there are many gaps in our evidence base, both in terms of validity and relevance of published studies.

In veterinary medicine, in general, and in certain specialties, including oncology, the trend has been toward a heightened sophistication of practice, including the use of advanced technologies in diagnostic testing (e.g., state-of-the-art imaging techniques and molecular characterization of tumors) and therapeutic interventions (e.g., interventional surgery and targeted, small molecule chemotherapy). This trend has been due in part to the presumption that most clients want care for their pets at more or less the level they themselves receive. Therefore many approaches and interventions have been adopted from human medicine and applied to animals despite considerable gaps in evidence as to their efficacy and/or effectiveness in the veterinary clinical situation. Additionally, even where a sufficient quantity of studies is present, the quality and consistency of reporting is frequently inadequate to allow systematic review or adequate comparison between studies.[1] This issue is not unique to oncology and has spawned efforts to improve the reporting of veterinary studies, with a longer term goal of improving the quality of work.[1-4] For example, the *Journal of Veterinary Internal Medicine* has initiated an effort to develop guidelines to improve the quality of reporting of therapeutic intervention studies in companion animals (e.g., the Companion Animal Reporting Expectations and Standards [CARES; Ken Hinchcliff, personal communication]) that are similar to the Consolidated Standards of Reporting Trials (CONSORT) guidelines used in the human field.[4] To approach a level of care in veterinary oncology truly similar to that in humans, there will need to be an increased focus on EBM, and the CARES reporting guidelines represent an initial step toward better clinical evidence. Further information and articles pertinent to challenges of applying EBM in practice can be found on the website of the Evidence-Based Veterinary Medicine Association (http://www.ebvma.org) and the Centre for Evidence-Based Veterinary Medicine (http://www.nottingham.ac.uk/cevm/index.aspx).

In this chapter, we will focus on quantifying the occurrence of cancer (incidence, prevalence) and risk factors for cancer (causal reasoning, associations). An evidence-based approach to diagnosis, prognosis, and selection of therapeutic interventions will be proposed, although other authors in this text will present specific details of diagnosis, prognosis, and therapy for specific cancers. Rather than presenting an exhaustive or systematic review of the literature in this chapter, we will highlight relevant literature. Our aim is to provide a guide for the application of epidemiologic principles to oncology, in general and for clinical practice.

Measures of Disease Occurrence

Complete and accurate cancer surveillance data are the foundation needed to make appropriate conclusions about the burden of disease, to make recommendations for cancer prevention and control, and for the design of analytic studies to identify causal associations between exposures and cancer risk. Here we cover the measures used to quantify cancer occurrence such as incidence, prevalence, and proportional measures and the types of data used to calculate them.

Incidence

Incidence, or the number of newly diagnosed cancer cases divided by the total population at risk over a specified period of time, is the most useful disease occurrence statistic for comparison between populations over time. Incidence data are especially valid when they are generated from a large population-based cancer registry with histologically confirmed cases and complete ascertainment of

TABLE 4-1 Glossary of Terms

TERM	DEFINITION	COMMENTS
Efficacy	How well a treatment works in those who receive it (e.g., correct formulation, dose).	May be proved in laboratory studies or clinical trials.
Effectiveness	How well a treatment works in those to whom it is offered.	Studies must occur in the environment and under conditions and with patients typical of those to whom it will be offered in practice.
Compliance	How closely a treatment protocol is followed.	Influenced by clinician, client, patient, formulation, duration, and so forth.
Coherence	How well findings reflect our understanding of biologic relationships/pathophysiology.	Limited by our current understanding.
Consistency	The extent to which new findings agree with previously published findings.	Limited by the current literature, traditional approaches, funding, and so forth.
Experimental studies	Traditional research approach done in a laboratory or highly controlled environment.	Potential for high validity, generally lower relevance to the clinical situation.
External validity	The extent to which a study's findings can be extrapolated to a wider population. Similar terms include relevance and generalizability.	A function of the study population, methods, data collection, treatments, and so forth.
Incidence rate	The rate at which new events occur in a population: (Number of new events in a specified period) ÷ (Number of individuals at risk during this period) $\times 10^n$	Cancer incidence rates are available from population-based data (e.g., cancer registry data) or prospective (cohort or longitudinal) studies.
Internal validity	The extent to which a study's findings are likely correct for that study population.	Likelihood that systematic bias is responsible for the study findings reduces its validity (e.g., due to bias in selecting study participants, measuring the exposure, and confounding).
Observational studies	Epidemiologic studies that use existing comparisons in the species of interest in its "natural" environment (often client-owned animals, perhaps in veterinary practice settings).	Examples: (1) Case-control study: Researcher observes/describes exposures in individuals selected based on presence/absence of the outcome; (2) Cohort study: Individuals with different exposures are followed and incidence of outcome(s) is observed.
Randomized controlled trial (RCT)	*Randomized* refers to the random allocation of exposure. *Controlled* refers to appropriate comparison groups (e.g., placebo or standard treatment). *Trial* is generally conducted in a clinical setting.	Researcher exerts control over which individuals receive which treatments or exposures and observes outcomes.
Prevalence	The number of events in a given population at a designated time: Number of events at a designated time ÷ Number of individuals at risk at the designated time	Taking the number of canine cancers that are observed in a clinic or several clinics during a designated period of time and dividing by the total number of patients seen during the same period is a proportional measure, *not* prevalence.
Proportional morbidity or mortality	The number of events (e.g., disease, death) in a limited population (e.g., animals presenting to the clinic, total deaths) at a designated time.	Proportional measures are used when the underlying population at risk is not known.

the population at risk within a defined geographic area or theoretically from large prospective, longitudinal or cohort studies.

Cancer incidence data has been provided from several population-based cancer registries (Table 4-2). Estimates of canine cancer incidence range from 99.3 to 272.1 per 100,000 dog-years.[5] Variation in estimates may be due in part to differences in actual cancer risks and/or variation in the base population. These registries included information from all cancer cases identified within a specified geographic region from a well-defined and enumerated population. One of the earliest, well-known cancer registries for companion animals was the California Animal Neoplasm Registry.[11,13] This comprehensive effort began in 1963 with the goal of identifying all neoplasms diagnosed over a 3-year period among animals living in the San Francisco Bay Area Counties of Alameda and Contra Costa. The denominator was estimated by conducting a survey in a probability sample of households in Alameda County to derive the age, sex, and breed distribution of pets and to determine whether the household had used veterinary services. Additional information on former and existing cancer registries for companion animals has been comprehensively reviewed.[14,15]

TABLE 4-2 Characteristics of Population-Based Companion Animal Cancer Registries and Cancer Incidence

Registry	Period	Cases/Population at Risk	Incidence/Prevalence
Genoa Registry of Animal Tumors[5] (Genoa, Italy)	1985-2002	3303/107,981; 1,943,725 dog-years	Males: 99.3/100,000 dog-years; females: 272.1/100,000 dog-years, for total tumors (malignant and benign).
Animal Tumor Registry[6] (Venice, Italy)	2005	2509 dogs; 494 cats/296,318 dogs; 214,683 cats	282, 143 and 140/100,000 dogs for total, malignant and benign tumors, respectively; 77, 63, 14/100,000 cats for total, malignant and benign tumors, respectively.
Danish Veterinary Cancer Registry (DVCR)[7]	2005-2008	1523 dogs/dogs registered in the Danish Dog Registry as of August 2006	Breeds with standardized morbidity ratios ≥2: Boxer, Bernese mountain dog, and West Highland white terrier. Measures for all dogs were not provided.
Norwegian Canine Cancer Registry[8,9] (Oslo, Norway)	1990-1998	14,401 tumors/census of dogs in Norway in 1992-93[10]	Boxers: 28 and 14/1000 dogs per year for total and malignant tumors, respectively. Bernese mountain dogs: 10 and 4/1000 dogs/year for total and malignant tumors, respectively.
California Animal Neoplasm Registry (CANR)[11,12]	1963-1966	1624/80,006 dogs 448/54,786 cats	381.2/100,000 dogs over 3-year period. 155.8/100,000 cats over the 3-year period.

Prevalence

Cancer prevalence information from population-based registries is also useful for surveillance and comparison between populations. Prevalence is the number of total cancer cases divided by the number of dogs in the population at risk at one point in time. For example, the prevalence of canine cancer in April 2005 was 143 per 100,000 dogs in an Italian population (see Table 4-2).[5,6]

Feline cancer prevalence has been reported from a population-based registry in Italy as 63 per 100,000 cats[6] (see Table 4-2). These data were based on a telephone survey conducted among 214,683 residents of two provinces in northern Italy over a 3-year period starting in 2005. Earlier prevalence data for feline cancers have ranged from 51.9/100,000 cat-years from the California Animal Neoplasm Registry[11,13] to 470.2/100,000 cat-years from the Tulsa Registry.[16]

In addition to population-based cancer registries, cancer occurrence data are abundantly available from veterinary teaching hospital databases as well as insurance databases. A caution to be noted when interpreting cancer occurrence information from hospital-based registries is that the size and characteristics of the underlying population at risk are not known[17]; thus neither true incidence nor prevalence measures can be calculated. Instead, the proportional morbidity ratio (PMR) is used to quantify cancer occurrence. For example, the PMR for a particular tumor type among a single breed is calculated as follows:

(# tumor type in breed ÷ # total tumors in breed) ÷
(# tumor type in all other breeds ÷ # total tumors in all other breeds)

Proportional measures are *not* to be interpreted as prevalence or incidence of cancer occurrence. As an example, Craig et al presents proportional statistics from a necropsy database and concludes that golden retrievers have an increased "risk" of tumors similar to that for Boxers.[18] However, only the proportion of dead dogs that had cancer are available in that study, and these data cannot be used to estimate risk. Although proportional measures, such as those presented in a recent article by Fleming et al,[19] have some usefulness for describing patterns within a breed, they are very risky to use for comparison across breeds in which population-based measures are unavailable and the degree of referral bias is unknown. In addition, in those data, 40% of deaths were unable to be classified pathologically and the unclassified proportion showed extreme variation across breed (e.g., from 16% to 60%). Using a subset of data from Bonnett et al, a study with information on the population at risk and data from the recent Veterinary Medical Database (VMDB) study, Figure 4-1 shows a comparison between proportional mortality ratios and true mortality rate.[19,20] For golden retrievers, 30% of deaths (before 10 years of age in the Swedish insurance population) were due to cancer. For Leonbergers and Boxers, the proportional mortality was 28% and 37%, respectively. Proportional values for these three breeds may be similar, but, in fact, Leonbergers and Boxers have a risk for death due to cancer (before 10 years of age) that is almost four times as high as that for golden retrievers (approximately 200 deaths per 10,000 years-at-risk versus 55 [$p > 0.05$]). Irish wolfhounds and Bernese mountain dogs have an equal risk (approximately 300 deaths due to tumors per 10,000 dog-years at risk [DYAR]), but tumors account for over 40% of deaths in Bernese mountain dogs and only 22% in Irish wolfhounds. Note that these are deaths before 10 years of age. Comparing the proportional mortality values between the two studies, values for Bernese mountain dogs are very similar (42%, 45%), perhaps because almost all dogs of this breed would die before 10 years of age, whereas the values for golden retrievers are somewhat different (30%, 50%). Of course, there may be true differences between the two study populations and/or the differences may be influenced by referral bias and the high proportion of unclassifiable deaths in the VMDB study.

To further illustrate this example, using just the breeds in Figure 4-1 and data from the Swedish insurance database, if one ranked the breeds based on actual numbers of dogs that died due to tumors (e.g., perhaps how an oncology clinician would perceive the "risk," based on dogs that present to a specialty clinic), golden retrievers would be number one because they are one of the more numerous breeds in this population. Likewise, if one ranked the breeds by the

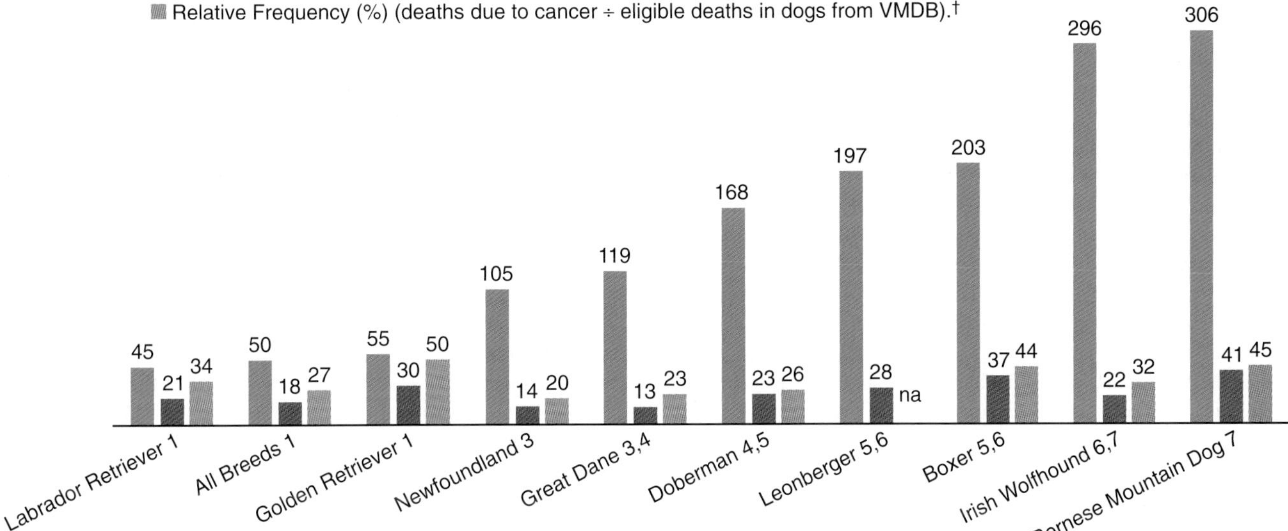

FIGURE 4-1 Comparison of true mortality rate and proportional mortality for selected breeds. The 95% confidence intervals for mortality rates overlap for breeds with the same number (e.g., mortality risk in Labrador retrievers and golden retrievers was not different from that for all breeds combined). *(Data from Bonnett BN, Egenvall A, Hedhammar A, et al: Mortality in over 350,000 insured Swedish dogs from 1995-2000: I. Breed-, gender-, age- and cause-specific rates,* Acta Vet Scand *46(3):105–120, 2005*; and Fleming JM, Creevy KE, Promislow DE: Mortality in North American dogs from 1984 to 2004: An investigation into age-, size-, and breed-related causes of death,* J Vet Intern Med *25(2):187–198, 2011.†)*

proportion of dead dogs that had tumors (e.g., similar to what would be reported in analysis of postmortem data), the top three would be Bernese mountain dogs, Boxers, and golden retrievers. So, in these examples, as has been frequently reported in the United States, based on proportional statistics, golden retrievers would be labeled as being one of the highest risk breeds. However, in looking at the true incidence based on these Swedish data, they do not have an increased risk compared to all breeds. There is likely considerable misunderstanding of the occurrence of cancer in dogs in the United States due to the lack of accurate incidence data and confusion about the interpretation of proportional statistics. Of course, where a breed is very common, like the golden retriever, and given that a considerable proportion of them die of cancer, that will represent an important population burden of disease, even if they are not truly the "highest risk" breed. Additionally, the Swedish data only include dogs up to 10 years of age; it is unknown how the statistics would look if dogs of all ages were included. As the authors (Bonnett et al) discuss, for cancer (or any cause of death) that occurs at older ages, a dog must live long enough to experience it (i.e., not die at a younger age due to any other cause) and deaths before 10 years of age are relevant to focus on for cancer prevention.[20]

Sources of Information on Cancer Occurrence

One of the largest clinic-based databases is the VMDB.[21] This database was started in 1964 by the National Cancer Institute, includes patient data from 26 university teaching hospitals in the United States and Canada, and contains over 7 million records from all species covering the full range of diagnoses, including cancer. This database is a widely used source of cancer surveillance information for companion animals; however, as was discussed previously (and presented in Figure 4-1), there is no information on the base population in these studies and only proportional measures can be calculated. Given that the data sources are teaching hospitals, patients, and diseases may not be typical of those seen in the general population. Therefore the results generated from passive surveillance such as the VMDB are likely to be influenced by referral bias. This type of selection bias affects estimates of disease frequency if the monitored clinics or hospitals have a predominance of patients that were referred for more specialized care. In fact, in a recent analysis using VMDB medical records from November 2006 to October 2007 for 9577 dogs and 4445 cats, it was concluded that substantial referral bias may exist.[22] The authors suggested that the accuracy of

*In total, there were over 350,000 insured Swedish dogs up to 10 years of age contributing to over one million dog-years at risk (DYAR) during 1995 to 2000 and a total of 43,172 deaths. Of these, 31,057 (72%) had a code for cause of death; however, of these, 6.8% were unclassified as to system or process.

†The authors use the term *relative frequency* but it is proportional mortality. There is no knowledge of total deaths in the referent population, but there were 80,306 deaths that met their inclusion criteria recorded in VMDB. Of these, 5750 were initially dropped because there was no cause of death recorded and 26,442 more were unclassifiable as to pathologic process, therefore, for approximately 40% of eligible deaths, cause was unknown. There was great between-breed variation (e.g., Bernese Mountain dogs had 16% and miniature dachshunds had 60% unclassified for pathologic process, not including those initially excluded). It is very likely that there is bias in types of disease, age, and other factors influencing whether a cause of death is recorded.

prevalence estimates measured from the VMDB could be improved by statistical adjustment on the basis of geographic proximity to the university teaching hospitals.[22]

Two well-established insurance databases are from the United Kingdom[23] and from Sweden.[20,24,25] A notable limitation of these databases is that not all cases are histologically confirmed. The benefits and limitations of these data have been discussed extensively in the literature.[26] From the U.K. database, using data from 1997 through 1998, cancer incidence among 130,684 dogs at risk was 747.9 per 100,000 dog-years.[23] From the Swedish data, the overall mortality rate for cancer was 50 per 10,000 dog-years-at-risk (which equates to 500 per 100,000).[20] The limitations with the Swedish data are that deaths are mainly in dogs 10 years of age or younger and it is unknown whether the diagnosis has been validated by histology.[17] Osteosarcoma incidence rates were 6.1 and 5.0 dogs per 10,000 dog-years for males and females, respectively,[27] and among females, breast cancer incidence was 111 dogs per 10,000 dog-years.[28] Comparison across breeds within the Swedish data is quite informative, given that the limitations occur equally across breeds. Crudely comparing overall mortality rates for cancer, Bernese mountain dogs were approximately 6 times more likely to die of cancer compared to all dogs, combined (306 versus 50 per 10,000 DYAR, respectively).[20] Where it was possible to do more sophisticated analyses, Bernese mountain dogs were shown to be 17 times more likely to die of cancer, compared to baseline, and adjusting for age, gender, and breed.[25] Even if specifics of the population may not be the same as other populations, data such as these are important for identifying high-risk breeds. Comparison across populations and over time is needed, with due consideration of data issues.

Studies on Swedish insurance data have presented statistics on morbidity and mortality in cats.[29,30] As with dogs, the diagnoses are made by veterinarians, but further details are unavailable. The overall age-standardized mortality rate for death due to cancer in insured Swedish cats (generally <12 years of age) was 37 per 10,000 cat-years at risk (95% confidence interval [CI]: 28, 46). The most common types of cancer in the Swedish data were mammary, stomach/intestinal, and lymphoma. Siamese breeds were at increased risk of death due to neoplasia; mammary cancer was the most common type,[31] in agreement with an earlier study.[32] Differences between populations and data are no doubt affected by differences in various factors (e.g., spay/neuter rates and age structure of the populations). Further study of neoplasia in cats is needed.

Notwithstanding the previous discussion on the relative paucity of population-based, histologically-confirmed data on the incidence of cancer, there is no doubt that certain breeds are at high risk for cancer (e.g., the Bernese mountain dog, flat-coated retrievers, Boxers, and Scottish terriers). In the section that follows, we will present an overview of known and suspected risk factors for specific cancers, including breed-specific risks, which is not strictly limited by the level of evidence or quality of studies or data but that reflects the current state of knowledge. An important concern for the future, however, is that without true incidence data we are limited in our ability to track changes in occurrence over time, as proportional measures are influenced both by changes in the numerator and denominator. In other words, an increase in the popularity of a breed may lead to its apparent overrepresentation in proportional cancer measures; a change in the distribution of breeds may affect cancer prevalence, without any actual change in breed risk. Without incidence measures, it would be impossible to accurately evaluate the effectiveness of programs aimed at preventing or controlling disease.

Factors Associated with Cancer Risk

Observational studies are the tools of epidemiology used to identify and characterize the determinants of cancer risk. Information from descriptive studies such as case series may help to generate hypotheses but is not adequate as a basis for evidence-based cancer prevention strategies. Results from case series are also no longer accepted for publication in at least one major veterinary medical journal.[4] Analytic observational studies such as case-control and cohort designs, on the other hand, are used to test research hypotheses, and when well-designed, can provide valuable information for cancer prevention strategies.

The case-control study design is the most commonly used observational study design in veterinary epidemiology research and in cancer epidemiology research in general. This is the most efficient study design, in terms of cost and time, when evaluating associations with relatively rare outcomes, such as specific cancers. Unfortunately, as data collection is often retrospective, many potential sources of bias must be considered. The features of an ideally conducted study (e.g., with the least opportunity for systematic bias) include the complete ascertainment of all newly diagnosed cases with histopathologic confirmation of primary tumors and a random (or matched) selection of controls from the same base population as the cases. In a population-based case-control study design,[33,34] we can assume that if a control subject had been diagnosed with the tumor of interest, that control would have been a case in the study (i.e., the controls are from the same base population as the cases). The goal of the control group is to represent the exposure experience of the base population. For this reason, we are not interested in selecting the "healthiest" subjects as our comparison group.

In a hospital-based case-control study, both cases and controls are selected from the same hospital(s). The limitation with this design is that we cannot generalize the study results to a clearly defined base population. This design, however, is valid and can still provide meaningful results. When using this design, it is preferable to randomly or systematically sample from the non-case population and to not include animals that have been diagnosed with other cancers.[35,36]

In a prospective cohort study, a group of animals is defined on the basis of exposure and followed over time to compare the incidence of disease (or other specified outcome) among the exposed and unexposed groups. The results obtained from a prospective cohort study are advantageous to results obtained from a case-control study for many reasons. One primary advantage is that we can assume temporality, or that the exposure came before the disease, when associations are observed from prospectively collected data. Systematic errors due to selection bias (e.g., referral bias) and differential recall bias (e.g., misclassification of exposure by disease status) are also not major concerns when interpreting results from a well-performed prospective cohort study. However, regardless of the observational study design, nondifferential exposure misclassification will be a major concern and the possibility and extent of misclassification should be considered when interpreting observational study results. Methods by which exposure misclassification can be reduced include using a precise and accurate questionnaire that has been properly validated or incorporating the use of biomarkers of exposure into the study design. There is a need for more longitudinal (as opposed to retrospective), preferably population-based studies in veterinary oncology.

To estimate the magnitude of an association between an exposure and a cancer type, the relative risk, or risk ratio (RR), and odds ratio (OR) are calculated from data collected from cohort studies or cross-sectional and case-control studies, respectively. The RR is calculated as follows:

RR = Incidence among exposed subjects ÷ Incidence among unexposed subjects

where incidence is the number of events divided by total animal-time of follow-up. The OR can be used to estimate the RR when incidence data are not available. The OR is calculated as follows:

OR = (Number exposed cases ÷ number unexposed cases) ÷ (number exposed controls ÷ number unexposed controls)

The RR and OR are similarly interpreted. A value greater than 1.0 indicates that the exposure is positively associated with disease (increases risk), whereas a value less than 1.0 indicates that the exposure is inversely associated with disease (decreases risk). A value of 1.0 indicates no association between exposure and disease. The 95% CI indicates the precision of the RR or OR, and if the 95% CI includes 1.0, we interpret the RR or OR to be statistically nonsignificant. It must be remembered, however, that statistical significance does not necessarily equate with clinical importance. For the latter, the magnitude of the effect is also important to consider. Table 4-3 shows suggested guidelines for interpretation of risk estimates. When considering whether to implement preventive measures or health interventions at the population level, the following, in addition to the risk estimate, are also relevant: Prevalence of the factor (i.e., likelihood of exposure) and the prevalence of the disease. These values are used to estimate the attributable risk or risk-reduction measures.

Findings from all observational studies are influenced by systematic error to some degree because there is inherent bias in the methods used to select the study population, measure exposures, and identify the outcome. The opportunity for any one study to report an association that is due in part to chance is a real concern, even with the use of valid study design methods and statistical analyses. Confidence in the evidence for a particular association is strengthened when it is observed repeatedly in multiple populations and with the use of more and more rigorous study design methods. Metaanalysis is a technique whereby results from multiple, similar studies can be combined to increase the power of findings. Several examples are available from the human literature relating to nutritional risk factors associated with pancreatic, breast, and colon cancer.[37-39] Unfortunately, in small animal oncology, studies have neither been performed nor reported consistently enough nor are there an adequate number of studies conducted to support metaanalyses at this time. Notwithstanding these limitations, Table 4-4 presents risk factors, including breed risks, for some of the more common cancers in dogs and cats for which there are at least reasonable estimations of association.

The identification of modifiable risk factors for canine cancers is the first step in eventually reducing incidence. Table 4-5 presents analytic studies used to test hypotheses that selected factors were

Text continued on page 78.

TABLE 4-3 Guidelines for Interpreting Clinical Relevance from Odds Ratios or Relative Risk Measures

Inverse Association ≈ Decreased Risk	Clinical Relevance	Positive Association ≈ Increased Risk
1.0	Not evident	1.0
0.7 to <1.0	Weak	>1.0 to 1.5
0.5 to <0.7	Moderate	>1.5 to 2.0
0.3 to <0.5	Strong	>2.0 to 3.5
<0.3	Very strong	>3.5

TABLE 4-4 Commonly Diagnosed Cancers and Suspected Risk Factors

Cancers	Suspected Risk Factors
Common Canine Cancers	
Mammary carcinoma	Obesity, high dietary fat intake, late age at spay, and some breeds (e.g., English Springer spaniel, Pointer, Poodle, Boston terrier, Dachshund, German shepherd, Chihuahua)
Osteosarcoma	High weight, high height, early castration/spay, some breeds (e.g., Irish wolfhound, Saint Bernard, Great Dane, Rottweiler, Irish setter, Doberman Pinscher, golden retriever, Labrador retriever, Leonberger)
Transitional cell carcinoma of the urinary bladder	Being neutered, exposure to phenoxy-acid containing herbicides, frequent flea dipping, some breeds (e.g., Scottish terrier, Beagle, Shetland sheepdog, Wirehaired fox terrier, West Highland white terrier)
Mast cell tumors	Some breeds (e.g., Boxer, Rhodesian ridgeback, Vizsla, Boston terrier, Weimaraner, Chinese Shar-Pei, Bullmastiff, Dutch pug, Labrador retriever, American Staffordshire terrier, golden retriever, English setter, English pointer)
Lymphoma	ETS, exposure to chemicals containing 2,4-dichlorophenoxyacetic acid, some breeds (e.g., Bullmastiff, Boxer, Scottish terrier, Gordon setter, Irish wolfhound, Basset hound, golden retriever)
Common Feline Cancers	
Lymphoma	FeLV, FIV, environmental tobacco smoke
Sarcoma	Vaccine injection
Cutaneous squamous cell carcinoma	Solar irradiation

ETS, Environmental tobacco smoke; *FeLV*, Feline leukemia virus; *FIV*, feline immunodeficiency virus.

TABLE 4-5 Selected Observational Studies of Canine and Feline Cancers by Type of Exposure

EXPOSURE	MAIN FINDINGS	STRENGTHS/LIMITATIONS
ETS		
Reif, 1998[40]	Positive trend for number of packs smoked by owner and increased risk of canine nasal cancer among long-nosed (dolichocephalic) dogs.	Strengths: Evaluation of nose size as an effect modifier with biologic plausibility; collected information on potential confounders. Limitations: Use of controls with cancer.
Reif, 1992[41]	Statistically nonsignificant positive association for living with ≥1 versus no smokers and canine lung cancer risk. Association was stronger among short-nosed dogs (brachycephalic or mesocephalic).	Strengths: High participation rates among cases and controls. Limitations: Use of controls with cancer; limited statistical power.
Marconato, 2009[34]	Any ETS exposure was positively associated with canine lymphoma, compared with no exposure.	Strengths: Population-based study design. Limitations: Use of controls with cancer; limited ETS exposure information was collected.
Bertone, 2002[42]	Strong, statistically significant association for any household ETS exposure and malignant lymphoma in cats. Statistically significant trend reported for a stronger association with increasing years of ETS exposure.	Strengths: Statistical power to evaluate trends; cases confirmed by biopsy; respectable response rate among the cases and controls (>65%); use of a detailed questionnaire to assess ETS and other environmental exposures. Limitations: No clear biologic mechanism for the observed association.
Bertone, 2003[43]	Clinic-based case-control study had ETS exposure positively associated with feline oral SCC. Overall, results do not support a causal relationship between ETS exposure and feline SCC.	Strengths: Cases confirmed by biopsy; good response rates; use of a detailed questionnaire (see previous entry). Limitations: Prevalence of ETS exposure was low; limiting the statistical power to evaluate more than two levels of exposure.
Pesticides		
Hayes, 1991[44]	Any use of chemicals containing 2,4-dichlorophenoxyacetic acid (2,4-D) positively associated with canine malignant lymphoma, compared with no use. Lymphoma risk increased with greater number of applications of 2,4-D–containing chemicals.	Strengths: Complete ascertainment of newly diagnosed cases; high participation rates among cases and controls; collected extensive information on chemical use on lawns/yards (self-applied and commercially applied). Limitations: One control group comprised of dogs with other cancers. NOTE: This and other limitations were addressed in subsequent analyses.
Glickman, 1989[45]	Residence location within one mile of a marsh (where chemicals were used for mosquito control) positively associated with canine TCC of the urinary bladder. Receiving flea dips more than two times/year versus no use was positively associated with TCC.	Strengths: Collected information on numerous sources of chemical exposure, including residential location to industries, pesticide use, flee/tick treatments. Limitations: 45% of control dogs had malignant neoplasia; information was not collected on individual dog exposure to the marsh or on specific chemicals used around the house/yard.
Glickman, 2004[35]	Access versus no access to phenoxy herbicide–treated lawns/yards positively associated with TCC of the urinary bladder among Scottish terriers. No association was observed for lawns/yards not treated with phenoxy herbicides.	Strengths: Collected information on brand name and active ingredients for household, lawn, and garden chemicals; results were specific for phenoxy herbicide exposure. Limitations: Limited statistical power to conduct subgroup analyses.
Raghavan, 2004[46]	Use of topical flea/tick products (e.g., shampoos, dips, powders, sprays, and collars) not associated with TCC of the urinary bladder among Scottish terriers.	Strengths: Collected detailed information on use of flea/tick products (e.g., type, brand, pattern of use) Limitation: 24% of control dogs had cancer; numbers for cases and controls were not presented by exposure level.
Environmental Pollutants		
Bettini, 2010[47]	Pulmonary anthracosis (high versus none) positively associated with canine lung cancer risk.	Strengths: Histologic confirmation of primary diagnosis of lung cancer; exposure assessment determined by histologic scoring of anthracosis; strong biologic mechanism supporting the a priori hypothesis. Limitations: Small number of cases limited the statistical analyses.

TABLE 4-5 Selected Observational Studies of Canine and Feline Cancers by Type of Exposure (continued)

EXPOSURE	MAIN FINDINGS	STRENGTHS/LIMITATIONS
Marconato, 2009[34]	Living in geographic areas exposed to toxic waste positively associated with canine cancer risk (all tumors and lymphoma), compared with living in an unexposed area. No associations observed for canine mast cell tumors, canine mammary cancer, or feline cancers.	Strengths: Population-based study design, histologic confirmation of cases; odds ratios were adjusted for age, sex, and breed. Limitations: Same eligibility criterion (i.e., living at same address for 2 years prior to enrollment) was not applied to controls.
Gavazza, 2001[48]	Living in an industrial neighborhood was positively associated with canine lymphoma risk, compared with living in any other neighborhood. Use or storage of paints and solvents was positively associated with lymphoma risk, compared with no use of chemicals.	Strengths: Histopathologic or cytologic confirmation of cases; information was collected on potential confounders. Limitations: Very low prevalence of exposed cases and controls; only univariate analyses were conducted.
Bukowski, 1998[49]	Cumulative kerosene or coal heat exposure was positively associated with sinonasal cancer risk.	Strengths: High participation rate; covariate information was compared between respondents and nonrespondents; histopathologic confirmation of cases. Limitations: Use of controls with cancer.
Endogenous/Exogenous Sex Hormones		
Sonnenschein, 1991[50]	Earlier age at spaying was inversely associated with canine mammary cancer. Trend of decreasing risk was observed for younger age at spaying.	Strengths: Cases were limited to mammary carcinoma or adenocarcinoma. Limitations: Controls may not be representative of the base population.
Ru, 1998[51]	Neutered dogs, regardless of gender, had a greater risk of osteosarcoma, compared to intact dogs.	Strengths: Histologic or radiologic confirmation; large study size; collected information on potential confounders. Limitations: Medical conditions of the controls were not clearly described.
Glickman, 2004[35]	Neutered status versus intact was a risk factor for TCC of the urinary bladder among Scottish terriers.	Strengths: Cases were histologically confirmed. Limitations: Small study size did not permit for analyses by age at neutering.
Dias Pereira, 2008[52]	No overall association was observed for COMT genotype and canine mammary cancer risk. Older age at mammary cancer diagnosis was observed by COMT genotype.	Strengths: Strong biologic rationale for research hypothesis; cases were histologically confirmed. Limitations: Very small numbers in subgroup analyses; selection methods were not provided; information was not collected on potential confounders (e.g., hormone-related exposures).
Cooley, 2002[53]	Neutering prior to 1 year of age increased risk of canine osteosarcoma among Rottweilers, regardless of gender. Incidence rates decreased with later age at neutering. Reproductive factors (number of litters, number of live births, age at first pregnancy) were not associated with osteosarcoma among female dogs.	Strengths: Radiographic or histologic confirmation of cases; retrospective cohort study design. Limitations: Low participation rate.
Stovring, 1997[33]	MPA use was positively associated with canine mammary cancer.	Strengths: Population-based study design; histologic confirmation of cases. Limitations: Information was not collected on details of MPA use (e.g., frequency, dose, age at first use).
Teske, 2002[54]	Castration was positively associated with canine prostate cancer risk, compared with intact status.	Strengths: Strong biologic plausibility. Limitations: Only cytology was used to make cancer diagnosis.
Bryan, 2007[55]	Neutered versus intact status was a risk factor for the following canine cancers: TCC of the urinary bladder, prostate carcinoma, prostate adenocarcinoma, and TCC of the prostate.	Strengths: Histopathologic confirmation of cases; included analyses by histologic subtype. Limitations: Statistically nonsignificant measures were not presented.

(continued)

TABLE 4-5 Selected Observational Studies of Canine and Feline Cancers by Type of Exposure (continued)

EXPOSURE	MAIN FINDINGS	STRENGTHS/LIMITATIONS
Misdorp, 1991[56]	Ovariectomy was inversely associated with feline mammary cancer risk. Regular administration of progestogens increased risk. No association was observed for irregular progestogen administration or for parity.	Strengths: Histologic confirmation of cases; collection of detailed exogenous progestogens (frequency, brand, type); large study size. Limitations: Cases and controls were selected over different time periods.
Overley, 2005[57]	Intact versus neutered status was a risk factor for feline mammary cancer. Cats spayed before 1 year of age were at lower risk of mammary cancer than those spayed after 6 months of age. There was no risk benefit in cats spayed after 2 years of age.	Strengths: Histologic confirmation of cases; large study size. Limitations: Univariate analyses were performed, although detailed information was collected on exogenous hormone use, parity, and number of litters; large amount of missing data due to veterinarian nonresponse.
Diet		
Perez Alenza, 1998[58]	Higher intake of red meat (as percentage of total calories) was positively associated with canine mammary carcinoma risk. No differences were observed for intake of fruits and vegetables, or biomarker levels of selenium, retinol, or individual fatty acids.	Strength: Used biomarkers of exposure; multivariable analyses included covariates for body conformation. Limitations: Use of a retrospective study design is not recommended for evaluating biomarkers of exposure and cancer risk because of possible disease and/or treatment effects on the biomarker measurement.
Sonnenschein, 1991[50]	Higher intake of fat and table food (as percentage of total calories) was inversely associated with canine mammary carcinoma. No associations were observed with protein or carbohydrates intake.	Strengths: Cases and controls were matched by age, spay status, and breed size, thus reducing the opportunity for confounding by these factors; the dietary assessment tool was validated using a 7-day food record, Limitations: Study size was too small to evaluate diet-cancer associations in subgroups.
Raghavan, 2005[59]	Vegetable intake (≥3 versus 0 times/week) was inversely associated with TCC of the urinary bladder in Scottish terriers. A trend was observed with greater servings of vegetables per week and decreased risk of TCC. No association was observed for weekly vitamin supplement intake, compared with no intake.	Strengths: Histopathology and/or cytology confirmation; use of a comprehensive dietary questionnaire; multivariable analyses. Limitations: Used a volunteer population; 61% of the cases were deceased at the start of the study; 24% of control dogs had neoplastic diseases.
Body Size		
Perez Alenza, 1998[58]	Obese body condition at 1 year of age and at 1 year before diagnosis was positively associated with canine mammary cancer, compared with normal or underweight body condition at the same time points.	Strengths: Objective measurements of weight and height were collected at presentation; body conformation was determined by a clinician at presentation. Limitations: Height, weight, and body conformation at 1 year of age and 1 year before diagnosis were based on owners' reports.
Sonnenschein, 1991[50]	Spayed dogs that were thin at 9 to 12 months of age had a lower risk of mammary cancer. Intact dogs that were not overweight in adulthood had a lower risk of mammary cancer.	Strengths: Cases were limited to mammary carcinoma or adenocarcinoma; designed to assess a timely hypothesis that early life factors are related to mammary cancer risk. Limitations: Controls may not be representative of the base population; subgroup analyses did not have ample statistical power to calculate precise measures.
Weeth, 2007[36]	BCSs ≥6 were inversely associated with canine cancer risk (all cancers, sarcomas, and carcinomas), compared with BCSs of 4 to 6. BCSs <3 were inversely associated with canine sarcoma risk, compared with scores of 4 to 6.	Strengths: Very large study size; 9-point BCS determined by physical examination; analyses were conducted by cancer type (sarcoma, carcinoma, round cell tumors) Limitations: Selection of cases and controls depended on availability of BCS in medical records; the inverse associations with higher BCS may be due to reverse causation.

TABLE 4-5 Selected Observational Studies of Canine and Feline Cancers by Type of Exposure (continued)

Exposure	Main Findings	Strengths/Limitations
Ru, 1998[51]	Height (>61 versus <35.5 cm) and weight (>45 versus <23 kg) were positively associated with canine osteosarcoma risk, after adjusting for age and standard weight and height, respectively. Longer length of hind limbs and front limbs was positively associated with canine osteosarcoma risk, compared with shortest length.	Strengths: Histologic or radiologic confirmation; large study size; collected information on potential confounders. Limitations: Medical conditions of the controls were not clearly described; a proxy measure for height was used; there was a large percentage (22.5%) with missing weight information.
Glickman, 2004[35]	Greater weight was positively associated with TCC urinary bladder risk in Scottish terriers, comparing third versus first tertile. Greater weight-to-height ratio was also a risk factor for TCC.	Strengths: Cases were histologically confirmed. Limitations: Weight and height information was based on owners' reports.
Vaccines/Injection Site		
Kass, 2003[60]	Cats with sarcomas at a vaccine injection site (n = 662) were compared with cats with basal cell tumors or noninjection site sarcomas (n = 473). Univariate analyses showed no difference in the vaccine type (FVRCP, rabies, FeLV) between cases and controls. There were no differences between time at vaccination and tumor diagnosis between the two groups.	Strengths: Histologic confirmation of cases and controls; collected extensive vaccine information (date of injection, manufacturer, type, brand, site of injection). Limitations: Cases were identified on a volunteer basis from participating clinics; heterogeneous sarcoma case group.
Kass, 1993[61]	In 345 cats diagnosed with fibrosarcoma, 53.6% had tumors at the vaccine injection site. The time from FeLV vaccination to tumor diagnosis was significantly shorter among cats that had tumors at the cervical/interscapular region than cats that had tumors at noninjection sites.	Strengths: Biopsy-confirmed diagnoses; vaccination history was validated by veterinarian; collected vaccination details allowing for analyses by type of vaccine, time since vaccination and location of injection site. Limitations: Differential missing data by exposure status.
FeLV/FIV		
Hutson, 1991[62]	Among 1160 cats identified from an oncology referral and a general practice clinic, 2.5% were FIV positive. Of the FIV-positive cats, 62% were diagnosed with neoplasia (myeloproliferative disease, lymphoma, and SCC).	Strengths: Descriptive information of neoplasia among FIV-positive cats. Limitations: No evident population base; only count data were presented.
Gabor, 2001[63]	Among 101 cats with lymphosarcoma, 50% were FIV positive. These cats were more likely to be male domestic crossbreeds.	Strengths: Histopathologic confirmation of cases; FIV antibodies were determined using Western blot. Limitations: Convenience study population was used.
Shelton, 1990[64]	Coinfection with FIV and FeLV was present in 14.4% of 353 cats collected in several US cities. FIV and FeLV infection were strongly associated with risk of leukemia or lymphoma. A very imprecise positive association was also reported for coinfection and leukemia/lymphoma risk.	Strengths: FIV antibodies were determined using ELISA and Western blot. Limitations: Base population and subject recruitment methods were not well defined; low prevalence of coinfection among controls limited statistical power.
Solar Irradiation		
Dorn, 1971[65]	Among white cats, the observed incidence of SCC of the skin was greater than the expected incidence ($p < 0.001$). For SCC of the mouth-pharynx, white cats had no difference between observed and expected incidence.	Strengths: Population-based study population. Limitations: Amount of sun exposure was not quantified; the number of cats with SCC of the mouth-pharynx was small (n = 29).

ETS, Environmental tobacco smoke; *SCC,* squamous cell carcinoma; *TCC,* transitional cell carcinoma; *COMT,* catechol-O-methyltransferase; *MPA,* medroxyprogesterone acetate; *BCS,* body condition score; *FeLV,* feline leukemia virus; *FIV,* feline immunodeficiency virus; *FVRCP,* feline viral rhinotracheitis-calicivirus-panleukopenia; *ELISA,* enzyme-linked immunosorbent assay.

either associated with an increased or decreased risk of canine and feline cancers. Characteristics of the study design and analytic methods are highlighted as strengths and weaknesses. Studies with the strongest level of evidence included several characteristics related to study design (e.g., hypothesis-driven, population-based, large study size, validated exposure assessment) and results (e.g., a precise measure of association, a modest-to-strong magnitude of association, statistically significant measure of association, statistically significant trend between exposure level and magnitude of association).

Highlighted Findings from Observational Studies

In this section, we discuss risk factors for which there is relatively strong evidence, those which relate to key issues in animal or human oncology, and those for which important controversies need to be addressed by further research. These categories coincide with those shown in Table 4-5.

Environmental Exposures

The identification of environmental exposures that are related to canine cancer risk have a broad public health interest, given the shared environments of companion animals and their owners, as well as similar etiology of some cancers.[66] In a recent review, a historic perspective is provided on how studies in pet populations have informed human health with respect to the specific exposures of air pollution, environmental tobacco smoke (ETS), and pesticides.[67] The shared etiologic characteristics of cancers such as lymphoma, osteosarcoma, and mammary cancer also support the utility of looking to both pet and human populations to investigate environmental-cancer associations.[68]

There is experimental evidence for an underlying biologic mechanism for the compounds of cigarette smoke to have a causal relationship with canine carcinogenesis.[69,70] There are few observational studies that were designed to specifically evaluate associations between ETS exposure and canine cancer risk.[40,41] There is support for a positive association (3.4-fold increased risk) between ETS and lymphoma[34] and sinonasal cancers[40] but not for lung cancer.[41] In a clinic-based case-control study, household ETS exposure was strongly associated with feline lymphoma.[42] The OR for any exposure, compared with no exposure was 2.4 (95% CI: 1.2, 4.5), and statistically significant trends were reported for more years of ETS exposure, more smokers in the household, and number of cigarettes smoked per day in the household. In contrast, there is only weak observational evidence for ETS as a risk factor for oral squamous cell carcinoma in cats.[43] In summary, avoiding ETS exposure may reduce the risk of lymphoma in cats and dogs and the risk of sinonasal cancers in dogs.

Pesticides are a heterogeneous group of chemicals, some of which are known human and canine carcinogens.[71-73] Dogs may be exposed to pesticides in the home, in the yard/garden, and upon application of flea and tick treatments. The most consistent observational evidence for pesticide exposure as a cancer risk factor is for phenoxy acid–containing herbicides and lymphoma risk, both in humans and dogs.[74] These data, however, have not been deemed strong enough to establish causality.[75] In a large case-control study ($n = 491$ cases and $n = 945$ controls) by Hayes et al, any use of pesticides that contained dichlorophenoxyacetic acid (2,4-D) was associated with a 30% increased risk of lymphoma, compared to no use.[44,76] Although modest, the positive association also demonstrated a dose-dependent effect, in which more frequent use of 2,4-D pesticides resulted in a stronger positive association with lymphoma risk (p for trend < 0.02). Additional support for 2,4-D and canine bladder cancer risk is from the result of a small case-control study in Scottish terriers.[33]

Residential proximity to environmental hazard–containing sites has been used to estimate chemical exposure and canine cancer risk in several observational studies.[34,45,48] A 2.4-fold increase in risk of lymphoma was observed among dogs living in the cities containing illegal waste sites, compared to dogs living in other cities.[34] No association was observed with mast cell tumors or breast cancer. Mortality due to cancer is also higher among human populations living near the same waste sites, compared with the general population.[77] Chemical mixtures that have been identified at hazard waste landfills include organic solvents, polychlorinated biphenyls, and heavy metals and can reach human and pet populations through contaminated air, water, and/or soil[78] and have been causally related to adverse human health effects, including childhood lymphoma.[79] The biologic plausibility and the observational findings from Marconato et al[34] both help strengthen the evidence that living near the waste sites increases risk of canine lymphoma.

Exposure misclassification is a primary limitation of using geographic proximity as a marker of exposure to an industrial or waste site because it may or may not be a good proxy for individual-level exposure. For example, a validation study would need to be conducted that provides information on whether dogs that live close to an industrial site are necessarily exposed at higher levels to environmental hazards, compared to dogs that live further from the site. Misclassification of exposure that does not differ by disease status (e.g., nondifferential misclassification) typically results in an underestimate of the exposure-cancer association, although there are situations when the observed association results in an overestimate of the true association.[80,81]

Hormones and Neuter Status

Hormones may act as either growth factors or inhibitors, depending on the sex of the dog and the tissue type.[53,82,83] For some cancers, such as breast, less exposure to sex hormones is protective, whereas for others, such as osteosarcoma and prostate cancer, less exposure increases risk. Neuter/spay status and age at neuter/spay are the most commonly used measures of endogenous hormone exposure. Given the widespread recommendation for early spay/neuter, especially in North America, this is a topic in need of further study.

In a mammary cancer case-control study by Sonnenschein et al, there was clear evidence that spayed dogs were at lower risk of mammary cancer.[50] In particular, the earlier age at which dogs were spayed the lower their mammary cancer risk, compared to dogs that were not spayed. This finding has been supported by other observational studies of spay status and mammary cancer risk.[84]

Contrary to human epidemiologic and experimental evidence,[85,86] exposure to sex hormones such as androgens may be protective for canine prostate cancer.[87] From two case-control studies using large veterinary teaching hospital databases, neutered dogs had a 2.8- and 3.4-fold increased risk of prostate cancer compared with intact dogs.[54,55] The apparent opposite associations between hormone exposure and prostate cancer risk in men and dogs are likely due to the higher rate of androgen-independent tumors in dogs than in men.[88,89]

Neuter status is also a risk factor for osteosarcoma and transitional cell carcinoma of the urinary bladder,[35,51,53,55] regardless of sex.[51,53] Cooley et al conducted a retrospective cohort study in 1999 among 683 Rottweilers and used a self-administered questionnaire to test the hypothesis that neuter/spay status was related to the development of osteosarcoma.[53] The owners were identified through eight national Rottweiler breed specialty clubs and had a purebred Rottweiler that was alive on January 1, 1995. The participation rate ([number of participants] ÷ [total number of invited owners] × 100) was 49%. This low participation rate suggests that selection bias may have influenced the results of this study. In other words, the participants of the study are likely to have systematic differences compared with those who did not participate. However, a strength of this study is the ability to calculate incidence because the total number of dog-months of observation were estimated retrospectively among dogs that were neutered/spayed and those that were not. During a total of 71,004 dog-months of observation, there were 86 cases of osteosarcoma. Collectively, the findings of a positive association between neuter/spay status and osteosarcoma from both case-control and cohort studies, as well as the biologic plausibility of the association, provide strong evidence that neutering/spaying dogs, regardless of sex, increases risk of osteosarcoma.

Risk Factors in Cats

In cats, the epidemiology of injection-site sarcomas has been well studied. A recent review provides information on the current epidemiology, etiology, and clinical knowledge of feline injection-site sarcomas (FISS).[90] Kass et al conducted one of the first epidemiologic studies investigating the hypothesis that vaccinations were related to feline fibrosarcoma risk in the early 1990s.[61] A main finding of this study was the shorter time interval from vaccination to FISS compared with the interval from vaccination to noninjection site fibrosarcomas. This finding was not supported by a second, larger case-control study conducted by Kass et al.[60] Although there is no doubt that the phenomenon of FISS exists, the administration of an injection itself is not sufficient to cause development of FISS. The component causes (e.g., the nature of vaccines and adjuvants in the injected material and the role of the resulting inflammatory reaction), in addition to the physical injection that leads to the development of FISS, are not well characterized. Further epidemiologic research designed with due consideration of the challenging methodologic issues is needed to identify the various factors associated with FISS.[91]

Cats infected with the feline immunodeficiency virus (FIV), the feline analog to the human immunodeficiency virus (HIV), are at increased risk of certain cancers.[92] FIV is a lentivirus typically transmitted by biting.[93] Lymphomas, particularly those of B-cell origin, are the most commonly diagnosed neoplasia among FIV-infected cats. Persistent feline leukemia virus (FeLV) infection is also known to have a strong role in feline neoplasia development,[94] and co-infection with FIV and FeLV may have synergistic effects on feline neoplasia risk.[64]

Diagnosis and Screening

As mentioned previously, numerous guidelines have been produced for the human medical literature (e.g., http://www.cochrane.org/about-us//evidence-base-health-care/webliography/books/reporting). One of these describes an approach to complete and accurate reporting of studies of diagnostic accuracy (Standards for Reporting of Diagnostic Accuracy [STARD]).[95,96] The application of this and another instrument in the veterinary field has been discussed.[97] Unfortunately, relatively few diagnostic interventions in veterinary medicine have been examined or evaluated as fully, in terms of reliability, accuracy, efficacy, and effectiveness, as is needed to support EBM practices. Guidelines for prognostic studies in veterinary oncology have also been reported.[98]

It may also be appropriate to use clinical trial methodology to evaluate the outcomes of diagnostic tests, for example, whether the animal is better off for having had the test performed.[99] In addition, recommendations about diagnostic tests and screening programs may have both positive and negative impacts beyond any individual, on populations of animals and owners. Although new, sophisticated diagnostic tests used in humans are being evaluated for use in companion animals, it is important to remember that beyond the benefit in a specific case, efficacy and effectiveness of tests should consider the broadest aspects of cost benefit. In human oncology, there has been much discussion about the problems inherent in certain widely applied screening processes and the consequences of false positives and negatives (e.g., prostate specific antigen test for prostate cancer[100]). Due to space constraints, we cannot expand on this crucially important area of cancer epidemiology.

Therapeutic Interventions

A recent review highlighted that the quality of reporting of oncology studies in dogs and cats published in the *Journal of Veterinary Internal Medicine* has not improved appreciably in the past 10 years and that quality of reporting is highly correlated with the rate of positive outcomes (i.e., well-described studies are more likely to report positive effects of a treatment).[101] This may also be exacerbated by the fact that the profession increasingly depends on corporate contracts for funding of research, and, in addition to this having a major impact on which treatments are investigated, there may also be underreporting of studies in which either beneficial effects were not seen or there were deleterious side effects. As mentioned previously, efforts are underway to produce reporting guidelines for companion animal intervention studies. However, guidelines for appropriate study design for clinical trials have been widely available for many decades, and the need for appropriate trials in oncology has been specifically advocated (see Chapter 17).[102] Longer-term analyses of survival following diagnosis and treatment, including both outcome and cost-benefit analysis, are needed to provide the information that owners and veterinarians need to choose the best options, with due consideration of quality-of-life issues.

Although there are good examples of randomized, controlled, blinded trials in veterinary oncology,[103,104] essentially all studies have some limitations in terms of either quality (validity) or relevance (extrapolation to other situations). For example, because many trials are performed on clients at specialty practices or veterinary teaching hospitals, animals have passed through numerous filters in order to be available for the study (e.g., referral, have a willing and capable owner, live long enough to have a confirmed diagnosis). Although this may improve the validity of the study (e.g., by increasing compliance and reducing loss to follow-up), it reduces the relevance to, for example, primary practice. Therefore clinicians must be able to apply the rules of evidence to determine both the quality and relevance of information for their specific situation and patients. Other authors in this text will present current information on treatments for cancer, and a further review of the literature is beyond the scope of this chapter. Hopefully, the quality of the veterinary literature will continue to improve over time, and the application of appropriate reporting guidelines and production of evidence-based reviews will assist clinicians to interpret and apply published information.

Knowledge Gaps and Future Directions

Even though systematic reviews and metaanalysis may not be currently possible, evidence-based reviews of the existing oncology literature in dogs and cats are needed to further elucidate what we know about breed risks, other risk factors, appropriate use of diagnostic and screening aids, therapies, prognoses, and so forth, and to identify the most crucial gaps in our knowledge. Appropriate assessment of existing oncology prevention and treatment strategies is also needed.

With increasingly available genomic information, our understanding of breeds and breed risk may change.[105,106] It is especially important to recognize the value of studying populations from different areas or countries. There are important differences and similarities in genetics (across and within breeds), environments, diets, and activities that will inform cancer etiology and management. Such complex relationships will only be fully understood by a multidisciplinary approach using various methodologies and study designs. These should include more population-based, longitudinal observational studies.[33,34,107] Although these may not yield results for many years, relying solely on traditional approaches (case-control studies and clinical trials of invasive or risky treatments) is not an effective strategy to reduce the population burden of cancer. In addition and beyond the scope of this chapter, there are important complex issues of human-animal interactions, in general and specifically related to the field of oncology. Thus there is a need for an increased understanding of the social and emotional factors underpinning many aspects of this diverse field.[108]

REFERENCES

1. Sargeant JM, O'Connor AM, Gardner IA, et al: The REFLECT statement: reporting guidelines for randomized controlled trials in livestock and food safety: explanation and elaboration, *J Food Prot* 73(3):579–603, 2010.
2. O'Connor AM, Sargeant JM, Gardner IA, et al: The REFLECT statement: methods and processes of creating reporting guidelines for randomized controlled trials for livestock and food safety, *J Food Prot* 73(1):132–139, 2010.
3. Rishniw M, Pion PD, Herndon WE, et al: Improving reporting of clinical trials in veterinary medicine, *J Vet Intern Med* 24(4): 799–800, 2010. Author reply 1-2.
4. Hinchcliff KW, DiBartola SP: Quality matters: publishing in the era of CONSORT, REFLECT, and EBM, *J Vet Intern Med* 24(1):8–9, 2010 Jan-Feb.
5. Merlo DF, Rossi L, Pellegrino C, et al: Cancer incidence in pet dogs: findings of the Animal Tumor Registry of Genoa, Italy, *J Vet Intern Med* 22(4):976–984, 2008.
6. Vascellari M, Baioni E, Ru G, et al: Animal tumour registry of two provinces in northern Italy: incidence of spontaneous tumours in dogs and cats, *BMC Vet Res* 5:39, 2009.
7. Bronden LB, Nielsen SS, Toft N, et al: Data from the Danish veterinary cancer registry on the occurrence and distribution of neoplasms in dogs in Denmark, *Vet Rec* 166(19):586–590, 2010.
8. Moe L, Gamlem H, Dahl K, et al: Canine neoplasia–population-based incidence of vascular tumours, *APMIS Suppl* (125):63–68, 2008.
9. Nodtvedt A, Gamlem H, Gunnes G, et al: Breed differences in the proportional morbidity of testicular tumours and distribution of histopathologic types in a population-based canine cancer registry, *Vet Comp Oncol* 9(1):45–54, 2011.
10. Moe L, Bredal WP, Glattre E: *Census of dogs in Norway*, Oslo, 2001, Norwegian School of Veterinary Science; (ISBN 82-7725-062-2).
11. Dorn CR, Taylor DO, Frye FL, et al: Survey of animal neoplasms in Alameda and Contra Costa Counties, California. I. Methodology and description of cases, *J Natl Cancer Inst* 40(2):295–305, 1968.
12. Dorn CR, Taylor DO, Schneider R, et al: Survey of animal neoplasms in Alameda and Contra Costa Counties, California. II. Cancer morbidity in dogs and cats from Alameda County, *J Natl Cancer Inst* 40(2):307–318, 1968.
13. Priester WA, McKay FW: The occurrence of tumors in domestic animals, *Natl Cancer Inst Monogr* (54):1–210, 1980.
14. Bronden LB, Flagstad A, Kristensen AT: Veterinary cancer registries in companion animal cancer: a review, *Vet Comp Oncol* 5(3):133–144, 2007.
15. Nødtvedt A, Berke O, Bonnett BN, et al: Current status of canine cancer registration: Report from an international workshop, *Vet Comp Oncol* 2011. doi: 10.1111/j.1476-5829.2011.00279.x.
16. MacVean DW, Monlux AW, Anderson PS Jr, et al: Frequency of canine and feline tumors in a defined population, *Vet Pathol* 15(6):700–715, 1978.
17. Nødtvedt A, Berke O, Bonnett BN, et al: Current status of canine cancer registration: Report from an international workshop, *Vet Comp Oncol* 2011: doi: 10.1111/j.1476-5829.2011.00279.x epub ahead of print.
18. Craig LE: Cause of death in dogs according to breed: a necropsy survey of five breeds, *J Am Anim Hosp Assoc* 37(5):438–443, 2001.
19. Fleming JM, Creevy KE, Promislow DE: Mortality in north american dogs from 1984 to 2004: an investigation into age-, size-, and breed-related causes of death, *J Vet Intern Med* 25(2):187–198, 2011.
20. Bonnett BN, Egenvall A, Hedhammar A, et al: Mortality in over 350,000 insured Swedish dogs from 1995-2000: I. Breed-, gender-, age- and cause-specific rates, *Acta Vet Scand* 46(3):105–120, 2005.
21. Veterinary Medical Database (VMDB) www.vmdb.org. accessed: 06/08/2011.
22. Bartlett PC, Van Buren JW, Neterer M, et al: Disease surveillance and referral bias in the veterinary medical database, *Prev Vet Med* 94(3-4):264–271, 2010.
23. Dobson JM, Samuel S, Milstein H, et al: Canine neoplasia in the UK: estimates of incidence rates from a population of insured dogs, *J Small Anim Pract* 43(6):240–246, 2002.
24. Egenvall A, Hedhammar A, Bonnett BN, et al: Survey of the Swedish dog population: age, gender, breed, location and enrollment in animal insurance, *Acta Vet Scand* 40(3):231–240, 1999.
25. Egenvall A, Bonnett BN, Hedhammar A, et al: Mortality in over 350,000 insured Swedish dogs from 1995-2000: II. Breed-specific age and survival patterns and relative risk for causes of death, *Acta Vet Scand* 46(3):121–136, 2005.
26. Egenvall A, Nodtvedt A, Penell J, et al: Insurance data for research in companion animals: benefits and limitations, *Acta Vet Scand* 51:42, 2009.
27. Egenvall A, Nodtvedt A, von Euler H. Bone tumors in a population of 400 000 insured Swedish dogs up to 10 y of age: incidence and survival, *Can J Vet Res* 71(4):292–299, 2007.
28. Egenvall A, Bonnett BN, Ohagen P, et al: Incidence of and survival after mammary tumors in a population of over 80,000 insured female dogs in Sweden from 1995 to 2002, *Prev Vet Med* 69 (1-2):109–127, 2005.
29. Egenvall A, Nodtvedt A, Haggstrom J, et al: Mortality of life-insured Swedish cats during 1999-2006: age, breed, sex, and diagnosis, *J Vet Intern Med* 23(6):1175–1183, 2009.
30. Egenvall A, Bonnett BN, Haggstrom J, et al: Morbidity of insured Swedish cats during 1999-2006 by age, breed, sex, and diagnosis, *J Feline Med Surg* 12(12):948–959, 2010.
31. Rissetto K, Villamil JA, Selting KA, et al: Recent trends in feline intestinal neoplasia: an epidemiologic study of 1,129 cases in the veterinary medical database from 1964 to 2004, *J Am Anim Hosp Assoc* 47(1):28–36, 2011.
32. Hayes HM Jr., Milne KL, Mandell CP: Epidemiological features of feline mammary carcinoma, *Vet Rec* 108(22):476–479, 1981.

33. Stovring M, Moe L, Glattre E: A population-based case-control study of canine mammary tumours and clinical use of medroxyprogesterone acetate, *APMIS* 105(8):590–596, 1997.
34. Marconato L, Leo C, Girelli R, et al: Association between waste management and cancer in companion animals, *J Vet Intern Med* 23(3):564–569, 2009.
35. Glickman LT, Raghavan M, Knapp DW, et al: Herbicide exposure and the risk of transitional cell carcinoma of the urinary bladder in Scottish Terriers, *J Am Vet Med Assoc* 224(8):1290–1297, 2004.
36. Weeth LP, Fascetti AJ, Kass PH, et al: Prevalence of obese dogs in a population of dogs with cancer, *Am J Vet Res* 68(4):389–398, 2007.
37. Paluszkiewicz P, Smolinska K, Debinska I, et al: Main dietary compounds and pancreatic cancer risk. The quantitative analysis of case-control and cohort studies, *Cancer Epidemiol* 2011 Oct 20.
38. Sun CL, Yuan JM, Koh WP, et al: Green tea, black tea and breast cancer risk: a meta-analysis of epidemiological studies, *Carcinogenesis* 27(7):1310–1315, 2006.
39. Aune D, Chan DS, Lau R, et al: Dietary fibre, whole grains, and risk of colorectal cancer: systematic review and dose-response meta-analysis of prospective studies, *BMJ* 343, 2011. d6617.
40. Reif JS, Bruns C, Lower KS: Cancer of the nasal cavity and paranasal sinuses and exposure to environmental tobacco smoke in pet dogs, *Am J Epidemiol* 147(5):488–492, 1998.
41. Reif JS, Dunn K, Ogilvie GK, et al: Passive smoking and canine lung cancer risk, *Am J Epidemiol* 135(3):234–239, 1992.
42. Bertone ER, Snyder LA, Moore AS: Environmental tobacco smoke and risk of malignant lymphoma in pet cats, *Am J Epidemiol* 156(3):268–273, 2002.
43. Bertone ER, Snyder LA, Moore AS: Environmental and lifestyle risk factors for oral squamous cell carcinoma in domestic cats, *J Vet Intern Med* 17(4):557–562, 2003.
44. Hayes HM, Tarone RE, Cantor KP, et al: Case-control study of canine malignant lymphoma: positive association with dog owner's use of 2,4-dichlorophenoxyacetic acid herbicides, *J Natl Cancer Inst* 83(17):1226–1231, 1991.
45. Glickman LT, Schofer FS, McKee LJ, et al: Epidemiologic study of insecticide exposures, obesity, and risk of bladder cancer in household dogs, *J Toxicol Environ Health* 28(4):407–414, 1989.
46. Raghavan M, Knapp DW, Dawson MH, et al: Topical flea and tick pesticides and the risk of transitional cell carcinoma of the urinary bladder in Scottish Terriers, *J Am Vet Med Assoc* 225(3):389–394, 2004.
47. Bettini G, Morini M, Marconato L, et al: Association between environmental dust exposure and lung cancer in dogs, *Vet J* 186(3):364–369, 2010.
48. Gavazza A, Presciuttini S, Barale R, et al: Association between canine malignant lymphoma, living in industrial areas, and use of chemicals by dog owners, *J Vet Intern Med* 15(3):190–195, 2001 May-Jun.
49. Bukowski JA, Wartenberg D, Goldschmidt M: Environmental causes for sinonasal cancers in pet dogs, and their usefulness as sentinels of indoor cancer risk, *J Toxicol Environ Health A* 54(7):579–591, 1998.
50. Sonnenschein EG, Glickman LT, Goldschmidt MH, et al: Body conformation, diet, and risk of breast cancer in pet dogs: a case-control study, *Am J Epidemiol* 133(7):694–703, 1991.
51. Ru G, Terracini B, Glickman LT: Host related risk factors for canine osteosarcoma, *Vet J* 156(1):31–39, 1998.
52. Dias Pereira P, Lopes CC, Matos AJ, et al: Influence of catechol-O-methyltransferase (COMT) genotypes on the prognosis of canine mammary tumors, *Vet Pathol* 46(6):1270–1274, 2009.
53. Cooley DM, Beranek BC, Schlittler DL, et al: Endogenous gonadal hormone exposure and bone sarcoma risk, *Cancer Epidemiol Biomarkers Prev* 11(11):1434–1440, 2002.
54. Teske E, Naan EC, van Dijk EM, et al: Canine prostate carcinoma: epidemiological evidence of an increased risk in castrated dogs, *Mol Cell Endocrinol* 197(1-2):251–255, 2002.
55. Bryan JN, Keeler MR, Henry CJ, et al: A population study of neutering status as a risk factor for canine prostate cancer, *Prostate* 67(11):1174–1181, 2007.
56. Misdorp W, Romijn A, Hart AA: Feline mammary tumors: a case-control study of hormonal factors, *Anticancer Res* 11(5):1793–1797, 1991.
57. Overley B, Shofer FS, Goldschmidt MH, et al: Association between ovarihysterectomy and feline mammary carcinoma, *J Vet Intern Med* 19(4):560–563, 2005.
58. Perez Alenza D, Rutteman GR, Pena L, et al: Relation between habitual diet and canine mammary tumors in a case-control study, *J Vet Intern Med* 12(3):132–139, 1998.
59. Raghavan M, Knapp DW, Bonney PL, et al: Evaluation of the effect of dietary vegetable consumption on reducing risk of transitional cell carcinoma of the urinary bladder in Scottish Terriers, *J Am Vet Med Assoc* 227(1):94–100, 2005.
60. Kass PH, Spangler WL, Hendrick MJ, et al: Multicenter case-control study of risk factors associated with development of vaccine-associated sarcomas in cats, *J Am Vet Med Assoc* 223(9):1283–1292, 2003.
61. Kass PH, Barnes WG Jr, Spangler WL, et al: Epidemiologic evidence for a causal relation between vaccination and fibrosarcoma tumorigenesis in cats, *J Am Vet Med Assoc* 203(3):396–405, 1993.
62. Hutson CA, Rideout BA, Pedersen NC: Neoplasia associated with feline immunodeficiency virus infection in cats of southern California, *J Am Vet Med Assoc* 199(10):1357–1362, 1991.
63. Gabor LJ, Love DN, Malik R, Canfield PJ: Feline immunodeficiency virus status of Australian cats with lymphosarcoma, *Aust Vet J* 79(8):540–545, 2001.
64. Shelton GH, Grant CK, Cotter SM, et al: Feline immunodeficiency virus and feline leukemia virus infections and their relationships to lymphoid malignancies in cats: a retrospective study (1968-1988), *J Acquir Immune Defic Syndr* 3(6):623–630, 1990.
65. Dorn CR, Taylor DO, Schneider R: Sunlight exposure and risk of developing cutaneous and oral squamous cell carcinomas in white cats, *J Natl Cancer Inst* 46(5):1073–1078, 1971.
66. Backer LC, Grindem CB, Corbett WT, et al: Pet dogs as sentinels for environmental contamination, *Sci Total Environ* 274(1-3):161–169, 2001.
67. Reif JS: Animal sentinels for environmental and public health, *Public Health Rep* 126(Suppl 1):50–57, 2011.
68. Kelsey JL, Moore AS, Glickman LT: Epidemiologic studies of risk factors for cancer in pet dogs, *Epidemiol Rev* 20(2):204–217, 1998.
69. Hernandez JA, Anderson AE Jr, Holmes WL, et al: Pulmonary parenchymal defects in dogs following prolonged cigarette smoke exposure, *Am Rev Respir Dis* 93(1):78–83, 1966.
70. Cross FT, Palmer RF, Filipy RE, et al: Carcinogenic effects of radon daughters, uranium ore dust and cigarette smoke in beagle dogs, *Health Phys* 42(1):33–52, 1982.
71. Dich J, Zahm SH, Hanberg A, et al: Pesticides and cancer, *Cancer Causes Control* 8(3):420–443, 1997.
72. Hardell L: Pesticides, soft-tissue sarcoma and non-Hodgkin lymphoma—historical aspects on the precautionary principle in cancer prevention, *Acta Oncol* 47(3):347–354, 2008.
73. Andrade FH, Figueiroa FC, Bersano PR, et al: Malignant mammary tumor in female dogs: environmental contaminants, *Diagn Pathol* 5:45, 2010.
74. Zahm SH, Blair A: Pesticides and non-Hodgkin's lymphoma, *Cancer Res* 52(19 Suppl):5485s–5488s, 1992.
75. Garabrant DH, Philbert MA: Review of 2,4-dichlorophenoxyacetic acid (2,4-D) epidemiology and toxicology, *Crit Rev Toxicol* 32(4):233–257, 2002.
76. Hayes HM, Tarone RE, Cantor KP: On the association between canine malignant lymphoma and opportunity for exposure to 2,4-dichlorophenoxyacetic acid, *Environ Res* 70(2):119–125, 1995.
77. Comba P, Bianchi F, Fazzo L, et al: Cancer mortality in an area of Campania (Italy) characterized by multiple toxic dumping sites, *Ann N Y Acad Sci* 1076:449–461, 2006.

78. Upton AC, Kneip T, Toniolo P: Public health aspects of toxic chemical disposal sites, *Annu Rev Public Health* 10:1–25, 1989.
79. Vrijheid M: Health effects of residence near hazardous waste landfill sites: a review of epidemiologic literature, *Environ Health Perspect* 108(Suppl 1):101–112, 2000.
80. Dosemeci M, Wacholder S, Lubin JH: Does nondifferential misclassification of exposure always bias a true effect toward the null value? *Am J Epidemiol* 132(4):746–748, 1990.
81. Wacholder S, Hartge P, Lubin JH, et al: Non-differential misclassification and bias towards the null: a clarification, *Occup Environ Med* 52(8):557–558, 1995.
82. Millanta F, Calandrella M, Bari G, et al: Comparison of steroid receptor expression in normal, dysplastic, and neoplastic canine and feline mammary tissues, *Res Vet Sci* 79(3):225–232, 2005.
83. Rhodes L, Ding VD, Kemp RK, et al: Estradiol causes a dose-dependent stimulation of prostate growth in castrated beagle dogs, *Prostate* 44(1):8–18, 2000.
84. Perez Alenza MD, Pena L, del Castillo N, et al: Factors influencing the incidence and prognosis of canine mammary tumours, *J Small Anim Pract* 41(7):287–291, 2000.
85. Heinlein CA, Chang C: Androgen receptor in prostate cancer, *Endocr Rev* 25(2):276–308, 2004.
86. Gann PH, Hennekens CH, Ma J, et al: Prospective study of sex hormone levels and risk of prostate cancer, *J Natl Cancer Inst* 88(16):1118–1126, 1996.
87. Johnston SD, Kamolpatana K, Root-Kustritz MV, et al: Prostatic disorders in the dog, *Anim Reprod Sci* 60-61:405–415, 2000.
88. Sorenmo KU, Goldschmidt M, Shofer F, et al: Immunohistochemical characterization of canine prostatic carcinoma and correlation with castration status and castration time, *Vet Comp Oncol* 1(1):48–56, 2003.
89. Navarro D, Luzardo OP, Fernandez L, et al: Transition to androgen-independence in prostate cancer, *J Steroid Biochem Mol Biol* 81(3):191–201, 2002.
90. Martano M, Morello E, Buracco P: Feline injection-site sarcoma: past, present and future perspectives, *Vet J* 188(2):136–141, 2011.
91. Kass PH: Methodological issues in the design and analysis of epidemiological studies of feline vaccine-associated sarcomas, *Anim Health Res Rev* 5(2):291–293, 2004.
92. Magden E, Quackenbush SL, Vandewoude S: FIV associated neoplasms-A mini-review, *Vet Immunol Immunopathol* 143(3-4):227–234, 2011.
93. Yamamoto JK, Hansen H, Ho EW, et al: Epidemiologic and clinical aspects of feline immunodeficiency virus infection in cats from the continental United States and Canada and possible mode of transmission, *J Am Vet Med Assoc* 194(2):213–220, 1989.
94. Rezanka LJ, Rojko JL, Neil JC: Feline leukemia virus: pathogenesis of neoplastic disease, *Cancer Invest* 10(5):371–389, 1992.
95. Bossuyt PM, Reitsma JB: The STARD initiative, *Lancet* 361(9351):71, 2003.
96. Bossuyt PM, Reitsma JB, Bruns DE, et al: Towards complete and accurate reporting of studies of diagnostic accuracy: The STARD initiative. Standards for Reporting of Diagnostic Accuracy, *Clin Chem* 49(1):1–6, 2003.
97. Gardner IA: Quality standards are needed for reporting of test accuracy studies for animal diseases, *Prev Vet Med* 97(3-4):136–143, 2010.
98. Webster JD, Dennis MM, Dervisis N, et al: Recommended guidelines for the conduct and evaluation of prognostic studies in veterinary oncology, *Vet Pathol* 48(1):7–18, 2011.
99. Lawrence J, Rohren E, Provenzale J: PET/CT today and tomorrow in veterinary cancer diagnosis and monitoring: fundamentals, early results and future perspectives, *Vet Comp Oncol* 8(3):163–187, 2010.
100. Chou R, Croswell JM, Dana T, et al: Screening for prostate cancer: a review of the evidence for the U.S. Preventive Services Task Force, *Ann Intern Med* 155(11):762–771, 2011.
101. Sargeant JM, Thompson A, Valcour J, et al: Quality of reporting of clinical trials of dogs and cats and associations with treatment effects, *J Vet Intern Med* 24(1):44–50, 2010.
102. Vail DM: Cancer clinical trials: development and implementation, *Vet Clin North Am Small Anim Pract* 37(6):1033–1057, 2007.
103. London CA, Malpas PB, Wood-Follis SL, et al: Multi-center, placebo-controlled, double-blind, randomized study of oral toceranib phosphate (SU11654), a receptor tyrosine kinase inhibitor, for the treatment of dogs with recurrent (either local or distant) mast cell tumor following surgical excision, *Clin Cancer Res* 15(11):3856–3865, 2009.
104. Rau SE, Barber LG, Burgess KE: Efficacy of maropitant in the prevention of delayed vomiting associated with administration of doxorubicin to dogs, *J Vet Intern Med* 24(6):1452–1457, 2010.
105. Scott MC, Sarver AL, Gavin KJ, et al: Molecular subtypes of osteosarcoma identified by reducing tumor heterogeneity through an interspecies comparative approach, *Bone* 49(3):356–367, 2011.
106. Modiano JF, Breen M, Burnett RC, et al: Distinct B-cell and T-cell lymphoproliferative disease prevalence among dog breeds indicates heritable risk, *Cancer Res* 65(13):5654–5661, 2005.
107. Akesson A, Julin B, Wolk A: Long-term dietary cadmium intake and postmenopausal endometrial cancer incidence: a population-based prospective cohort study, *Cancer Res* 68(15):6435–6441, 2008.
108. Shaw J: Chapter 15c: Relationship-Centered Approach to Cancer Communication. In Withrow SJ, MacEwen EG, Page RL, editors: *Small Animal Clinical Oncology*, St. Louis, 2012, Saunders Elsevier.

Paraneoplastic Syndromes

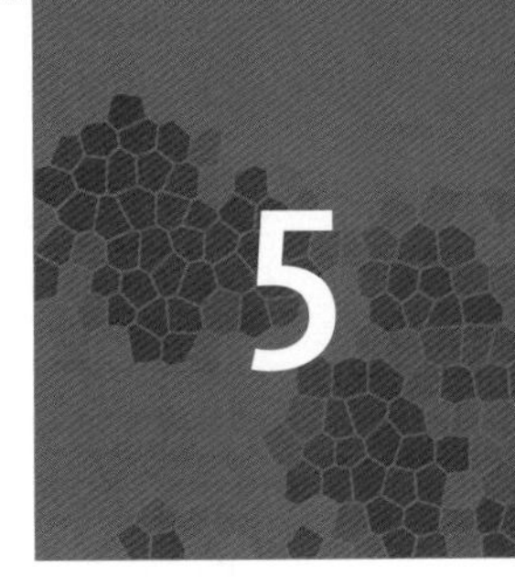

Philip J. Bergman

Paraneoplastic syndromes (PNSs) are neoplasm-associated alterations in bodily structure and/or function that occur distant to the tumor. They are a diverse group of clinical aberrations that are associated with the noninvasive actions of the tumor. In many situations, the PNS parallels the underlying malignancy; therefore successful treatment of the tumor leads to disappearance of the PNS. Alternatively, recurrence of the PNS after successful treatment signals tumor recurrence and often significantly precedes clinically detectable tumor.

PNSs are often the first sign of malignancy, and the PNS may be a hallmark of a certain tumor histology. Therefore an understanding and appreciation for the types and causes of these syndromes are paramount for early cancer detection and appropriate therapy. In addition, a PNS may result in greater morbidity than that associated with the actual tumor.

The causes of PNSs are quite variable; they are usually caused by the production of small molecules (e.g., hormones, cytokines, or peptides) that are released into the circulation to cause effects at distant sites or by immune cross-reactivity between malignant and normal tissues. Some PNSs are due to functional mutations that result in overexpression of the small molecule in question, whereas many nonendocrine PNSs have no known etiology. PNSs are recognized commonly in both human and companion animal cancer patients.[1] Box 5-1 summarizes the most common PNSs of dogs and cats and the tumors associated with them.

Gastrointestinal Manifestations of Cancer

Cancer Cachexia and Anorexia

An important systemic effect of cancer in animals is profound malnutrition and wasting. The weight loss and metabolic alterations observed in cancer patients despite adequate nutritional intake are termed *cancer cachexia,* whereas alterations observed as the result of poor nutritional intake are termed *cancer anorexia.* The clinical outcome of either cancer cachexia and/or anorexia is a progressive wasting (Figure 5-1). The weight loss endured by these patients is more than a simple cosmetic abnormality as human patients with cancer cachexia can have significantly reduced survival times, and many patients are unable to undergo appropriate therapy because of their poor clinical status.

Cancer cachexia occurs frequently in human oncology, with estimated incidences from 40% to approximately 90% of hospitalized patients.[2,3] Importantly, cancer cachexia accounts for approximately 20% of cancer deaths.[4,5] The incidence of cancer cachexia in veterinary oncology patients is presently unknown, although this author believes that an estimated incidence of cancer cachexia in dogs is realistically 10% or less. For example, only 4% of dogs presenting to an academic oncology center were found to have cachexia, although referral bias likely results in some reporting artifact.[6] The metabolic alterations associated with this PNS usually occur before weight loss is detected in both human and veterinary cancer patients.[3,7-11] These metabolic alterations may last for some time after the patient is tumor free making it difficult for the clinician to reverse the weight loss.[8,10] A plasmid-DNA–mediated approach utilizing growth hormone–releasing hormone (GHRH) in dogs appears to increase insulin-like growth factor-1 (IGF-1) levels (a measure of GHRH activity) and may represent a mechanism for attenuating cancer cachexia.[12-15]

In the clinical evaluation of a veterinary patient for the possibility of cancer cachexia/anorexia, a detailed history and physical examination are crucial. The prognostic importance of the presence of cancer cachexia in human cancer patients cannot be overstated because many studies show that this PNS is the only or one of very few independent multivariate negative prognostic factors for a variety of malignancies.[2,3] A more detailed discussion of this syndrome is found in Chapter 15, Section B.

Protein-Losing Enteropathy

Protein-losing enteropathy (PLE) is a syndrome whereby excessive serum proteins are lost into the gastrointestinal (GI) tract, leading to hypoproteinemia.[16] The hypoproteinemia seen in cancer patients can be due to impaired synthesis and/or increased loss into the GI tract or urine (see Renal Manifestations of Cancer later in this chapter). Once the loss of proteins becomes greater than the body's ability to synthesize them, serum protein levels begin to decrease. The half-life of many serum proteins is long, and patients with hypoproteinemia caused by PLE or some other cancer-related protein loss may represent long-standing protein loss.[2,16] PLE is thought to result from an increase in mucosal serum protein permeability because of mucosal erosion, ulceration, or lymphatic obstruction.

The diagnosis of PLE is made by noting hypoproteinemia on serum chemistry evaluation with subsequent exclusion of severe malnutrition and liver disease. Confirmation of the diagnosis is made in humans with PLE by alpha-1-antitrypsin detection,[17] but this methodology has not been validated in veterinary medicine.[18] In addition, nuclear scintigraphy appears to be a reliable methodology for the diagnosis of PLE.[19] The incidence of PLE as a PNS is unknown in veterinary medicine but is likely to be rare. The treatment for PLE consists of treating the primary malignancy; however, those patients with a lymphangiectasia-related PLE may also be treated with medium-chain triglycerides that do not undergo transport by intestinal lymphatics.

BOX 5-1 Paraneoplastic Syndromes and Associated Tumors

Gastrointestinal Manifestations of Cancer

Cancer Cachexia
Multiple tumor types

Gastroduodenal Ulceration
Mast cell tumor
Gastrinoma

Endocrinologic Manifestations of Cancer

Hypercalcemia of Malignancy
Lymphoma
Anal sac apocrine gland adenocarcinoma
Multiple myeloma
Parathyroid tumors
Mammary tumors
Thymoma
Others

Hypoglycemia
Insulinoma
Hepatic tumors
Salivary tumors
Leiomyoma/leiomyosarcoma
Plasma cell tumors
Lymphoma
Mammary tumors
Others

Ectopic ACTH
Primary lung tumors

Hematologic Manifestations of Cancer

Hypergammaglobulinemia
Multiple myeloma
Lymphoma

Anemia
Multiple tumors

Erythrocytosis
Renal tumors (increased erythropoietin)
Lymphoma
Nasal fibrosarcoma
TVT
Hepatic tumors

Neutrophilic Leukocytosis
Lymphoma
Multiple tumors

Thrombocytopenia/Coagulopathies/DIC
Lymphoma
Mast cell tumor
Hemangiosarcoma
Thyroid tumors
Mammary tumors
Nasal tumors
Inflammatory carcinomas
Others

Cutaneous Manifestations of Cancer

Alopecia
Pancreatic carcinoma (feline)
Others

Flushing
Mast cell tumor
Pheochromocytoma
Others

Nodular Dermatofibrosis
Renal cystadenoma/cystadenocarcinoma

Necrolytic Migratory Erythema/Superficial Necrolytic Dermatitis
Glucagonoma

Cutaneous Necrosis of the Hind Feet
Lymphoma (cat)

Pemphigus Vulgaris
Lymphoma (dog and horse)

Renal Manifestations of Cancer

Glomerulonephritis/Nephrotic Syndrome
Multiple myeloma
Polycythemia vera
Lymphocytic leukemia
Others

Neurologic Manifestations of Cancer

Myasthenia Gravis
Thymoma
Osteosarcoma
Biliary carcinoma
Others

Peripheral Neuropathy
Insulinoma
Others

Miscellaneous Manifestations of Cancer

Hypertrophic Osteopathy
Primary lung tumor
Urinary bladder rhabdomyosarcoma
Esophageal tumors
Metastatic tumors
Others

Fever
Multiple tumors

ACTH, Adrenocorticotropic hormone; *DIC*, disseminated intravascular coagulation; *TVT*, transmissible venereal tumor.

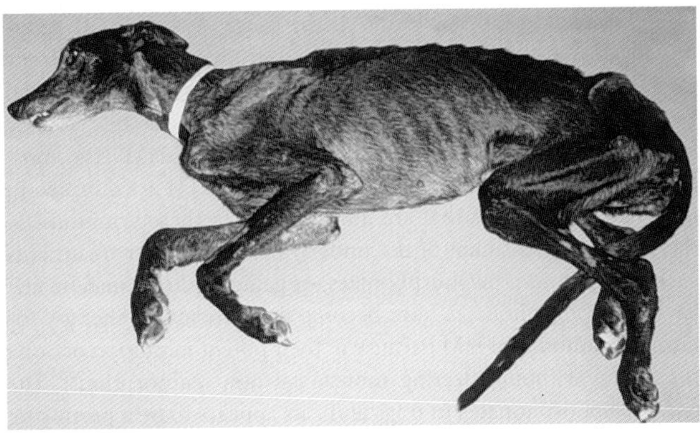

FIGURE 5-1 Dog with lymphoma and secondary severe cachexia. Cancer cachexia can be a common paraneoplastic syndrome (PNS) in dogs and cats. The weight loss noted in cases of paraneoplastic cancer cachexia occurs despite adequate nutritional intake. The metabolic alterations associated with cancer cachexia usually occur before clinical signs of the inciting malignancy appear and unfortunately may continue after the patient is successfully treated for the tumor.

Gastroduodenal Ulceration

The most common cause of PNS-associated gastroduodenal ulceration is mast cell tumor (MCT). The excess histamine seen in MCTs stimulates gastric H_2 receptors, leading to increased gastric acid secretion. Clinical manifestations of mucosal damage and/or ulceration with gastric vessel thrombosis occur in association with gastric hyperacidity. Plasma histamine concentrations are elevated in approximately 75% of dogs with macroscopic MCT, although only 30% have GI signs.[20,21] Abnormally elevated plasma histamine concentrations have also been found to be a negative prognostic factor in dogs with MCT.[21] Symptomatic therapies such as proton-pump inhibitors, H_2 blockers, misoprostol, sucralfate, and rehydration may be helpful in combating PNS-associated gastroduodenal ulceration. MCTs are covered in greater detail in Chapter 20.

An additional cause of PNS-associated gastroduodenal ulceration is gastrinoma (gastrin-secreting non–islet cell pancreatic tumor). Although these tumors are relatively rare, they have been reported in both dogs and cats.[22-26] Gastrinomas can be associated with vomiting, lethargy, anorexia, blood loss, and abdominal pain. Many of these features are also seen in humans with gastrinoma-related Zollinger-Ellison syndrome. Gastrinomas are covered in greater detail in Chapter 25.

Endocrinologic Manifestations of Cancer

Hypercalcemia

The most common cause of hypercalcemia in the dog is cancer. A variety of tumors have been associated with hypercalcemia of malignancy (HM), and neoplasia is diagnosed in approximately two-thirds of dogs[27,28] and one-third of cats with hypercalcemia.[29] Lymphoma is the most common cause of HM (10% to 35% occurrence). Other tumor types associated with HM in dogs and cats include anal sac apocrine gland adenocarcinoma (≥25%), thyroid carcinoma, multiple myeloma (20%), bone tumors, thymoma, squamous cell carcinoma, mammary gland carcinoma/adenocarcinoma, melanoma, primary lung tumors, chronic lymphocytic leukemia, renal angiomyxoma, and parathyroid gland tumors.[30-40] The causes of HM are varied and include ectopic production of parathormone (PTH) or PTH-related peptide (PTH-rp) by the tumor, extensive and usually multifocal lytic bone metastases, primary hyperparathyroidism, tumor-associated prostaglandins ($PGE_{1/2}$), interleukin-1-β (IL-1β, previously known as osteoclast-activating factor [OAF]), transforming growth factor-β (TGF-β), and receptor activator of nuclear factor kappa-B ligand (RANKL).[2,34,41-46] Interestingly, TGF-β1 regulates the mRNA stability of PTH-rp.[47] The HM seen in lymphoma and anal sac apocrine gland adenocarcinoma is commonly caused by tumor-associated PTH-rp.[48,49] PTH-rp is a 16-kDa protein with significant sequence identity to PTH, suggesting it may act and function like PTH. In addition to HM, other hypercalcemia differential diagnoses include "lab error" (lipemia and hemolysis), acute renal failure, hypervitaminosis D, hypoadrenocorticism, and granulomatous disease.

In addition to ensuring the hypercalcemia is not due to lipemia or hemolysis, it is important to interpret the calcium value in relation to the level of serum albumin if ionized calcium determination is not available. Two commonly utilized correction formulas that controversially attempt to account for the level of serum albumin follow:

$$\text{Adjusted calcium (mg/dL)} = [\text{Calcium (mg/dL)} - \text{albumin (g/dL)}] + 3.5$$

or

$$\text{Adjusted calcium (mg/dL)} = \text{Calcium (mg/dL)} - [\text{total serum protein (g/dL)} \times 0.4] + 3.3$$

Similarly, an increase in the free ionized fraction of calcium can occur with acidosis. Acidotic HM patients may have an increase in clinical signs of hypercalcemia when compared to nonacidotic HM patients.

The primary clinical manifestations of HM are due to renal function impairment. Severe HM (calcium > 18 mg/dL) should be considered a *medical emergency.* An inability to concentrate urine is the initial manifestation of hypercalcemia and is due to decreased responsiveness to antidiuretic hormone (ADH) at the distal tubule; the calcium then decreases renal blood flow and glomerular filtration rate (GFR) as the result of severe vasoconstriction. Calcium salt deposition in the renal parenchyma may also contribute to renal azotemia, although this is uncommon. The urinary epithelium may then undergo degeneration, and in severe cases, necrosis results in exposure of the basement membrane of the renal tubule. The situation worsens as the patient becomes polyuric and polydipsic, resulting in progressive dehydration. In addition to effects on the renal system, severe HM may cause constipation, hypertension, twitching, weakness, shaking, depression, vomiting, bradycardia, stupor, and possibly coma and/or death.

When HM is diagnosed, appropriate steps for identification of the underlying neoplasm cause are necessary, and if azotemia accompanies HM, appropriate therapy to support renal function should be instituted quickly. The diagnostic evaluation of HM should begin with procedures used in the staging of lymphoma (as outlined in Chapter 32, Sections A and B) in addition to a rectal palpation and examination for anal sac apocrine gland adenocarcinoma. If these diagnostics do not confirm the specific cause of the HM, then the aforementioned hypercalcemia differential diagnoses should be considered and appropriately pursued. Dogs and cats with HM will typically have low PTH and high PTH-rp concentrations; however, the cause of the HM can usually be delineated with appropriate diagnostics before the return of PTH/PTH-rp assay results and such tests may not be routinely needed. Since HM is a potential medical emergency, the primary goal is elucidation of the underlying cause in order to institute the appropriate therapy for the specific tumor. Symptomatic therapy must be judiciously utilized while searching for the underlying cause of the HM. The premature administration of symptomatic therapy that includes the use of corticosteroids prior to the confirmation of the cause of the HM can have serious consequences. If lymphoma is the underlying cause of the HM, the use of corticosteroids may interfere with the ability to confirm a diagnosis, necessitating either additional diagnostics and/or waiting to determine if the lymphoma reappears after glucocorticoid withdrawal. In addition, glucocorticoids may induce resistance to other chemotherapy agents with a decrease in the ability to induce a complete remission, as well as a decrease in the length of survival.[50] Therefore the use of corticosteroids in cases of undiagnosed hypercalcemia is strongly discouraged.

Symptomatic therapies that promote external loss of calcium, increase renal excretion of calcium, and inhibit bone reabsorption may be utilized in HM patients. The severity of clinical signs and associated hypercalcemia determine the preferred therapy (Box 5-2). The use of 0.9% NaCl intravenously (IV) is recommended for management of existing dehydration and to expand the extracellular fluid volume, increase GFR, increase calciuresis and natriuresis, and decrease calcium reabsorption by the kidneys. Once rehydrated, the loop diuretic furosemide with continued normosaline diuresis can be utilized to potentially inhibit calcium reabsorption in the ascending loop of Henle. If the cause of the HM is determined, corticosteroids can be extremely effective as adjunct therapy for HM by their inhibition of PGE, OAF (IL-1β), vitamin D, and intestinal calcium absorption. Corticosteroids can also be cytotoxic to lymphoma cells, the most common cause of HM. The most common therapies utilized in the treatment of HM are outlined in Box 5-2. In rare cases that are unresponsive to these symptomatic therapies and treatment of the underlying cause, other treatments such as calcitonin, bisphosphonates, or gallium nitrate may be utilized.[51] Bisphosphonates have become the standard of therapy for human nonhumoral HM because of their potent inhibition of bone resorption without affecting tubular calcium reabsorption.[52] The use of bisphosphonates in dogs and cats appears to be a promising treatment for hypercalcemia but requires additional study.[53,54] In the future, treatment options for refractory HM may include osteoprotegerins, more potent bisphosphonates, anti-PTH-rp antibodies, noncalcemic calcitriol analogs, distal tubule calcium reabsorption inhibitors, RANKL antagonists, and new bone resorption inhibitors.[52,55]

BOX 5-2 Treatment for Hypercalcemia of Malignancy

Elimination of the inciting tumor is the primary goal for all categories of hypercalcemia.

Mild Hypercalcemia and Minimal Clinical Signs

Rehydration with normosaline (0.9% NaCl)

Moderate Hypercalcemia and Clinical Signs

Rehydration with normosaline (0.9% NaCl)

Continue normosaline diuresis (urine output >2 mL/kg/hr)

Furosemide (1-4 mg/kg every 8-24 hours IV or PO)

NOTE: Only use after patient is fully rehydrated.

Prednisone (1 mg/kg daily to BID PO)

NOTE: Only use after diagnosis obtained (see text).

Severe Hypercalcemia and Severe Clinical Signs

ONCOLOGIC EMERGENCY

See moderate hypercalcemia treatments

For refractory cases:

- Bisphosphonates
- Pamidronate (1-1.5 mg/kg IV every 2-3 weeks)
- Salmon calcitonin (4-10 MRC units/kg SQ daily)
- Mithramycin (25 μg/kg IV 1-2 times/week)

NOTE: Sclerosing agent and hepatotoxin at higher doses—rarely used.

NaCl, Sodium chloride; *IV,* intravenous; *PO,* by mouth; *BID,* twice a day.

Hypoglycemia

The most common cause of cancer-induced hypoglycemia (<65 to 70 mg/dL serum glucose) in the dog is insulinoma (beta-islet cell tumor), and the reader is directed to Chapter 25 for a discussion of insulinomas.[56] Nonislet cell tumors can also serve as sources of ectopic hormone production with resultant hypoglycemia in dogs and humans. Nonislet cell tumors with PNS hypoglycemia have been most commonly associated with hepatocellular carcinomas; however, lymphoma, hemangiosarcoma, oral melanoma, hepatoma, plasma cell tumor, multiple myeloma, smooth muscle tumors (leiomyoma and leiomyosarcoma), mammary tumors, renal tumors, and salivary gland tumors have also been reported.[57-62] The hypoglycemia of extrapancreatic tumors has interestingly been associated with low insulin levels, whereas pancreatic beta-islet cell tumors (insulinomas) induce hypoglycemia by excessive circulating insulin levels. Nonislet cell tumors may induce hypoglycemia by increased tumor utilization of glucose, decreased hepatic glycogenolysis or gluconeogenesis, or the secretion of insulin or IGF-1 and IGF-2. Additional mechanisms include upregulation of insulin receptors, increased insulin binding by M proteins in myeloma, and increased production of somatomedins.[2,63] The differential diagnoses of hypoglycemia include insulinoma, nonislet cell tumor hyperinsulinism, nonislet cell tumor, hypoadrenocorticism, starvation, sepsis, liver dysfunction, and laboratory error (lack of timely serum separation). Tumors associated with extrapancreatic hypoglycemia are often extremely large and therefore radiographs/ultrasound of the abdomen and/or thorax may be helpful. Exploratory laparotomy may be necessary if a space-occupying mass is not identified. Provocative testing via glucagon or glucose tolerance testing may be useful in cases when the diagnosis is uncertain. The reader is directed to Chapter 25 for an extensive discussion of the clinical consequences, diagnosis, and therapy of tumor-induced hypoglycemia.

Syndrome of Inappropriate Secretion of Antidiuretic Hormone

Syndrome of inappropriate secretion of ADH (SIADH) is a PNS widely recognized in lung, head, neck, and many other tumors in humans[1,2]; however, it continues to be essentially unrecognized in veterinary oncology. SIADH has been reported in dogs associated with heartworm disease, congenital hydrocephalus, and granulomatous amebic meningoencephalitis.[64-66] In addition to

PNS-associated SIADH, chemotherapy agents and other drugs (vincristine, cyclophosphamide, cisplatin, thiazides, morphine, and chlorpropamide), pulmonary and/or central nervous system (CNS) infections, and a variety of other conditions can cause SIADH.[67,68] The initial finding in SIADH patients is hyponatremia. In addition to hyponatremia, serum hypo-osmolarity, hypernatriuresis, urine hyperosmolarity, and euvolemia with normal renal, thyroid, and adrenal function is noted.[2,67] Although most human SIADH patients are asymptomatic, clinical signs can develop due to hyponatremia that result in CNS signs such as fatigue, anorexia, confusion and potentially seizures. The treatment of choice for PNS-associated SIADH is removal of the underlying cause. In addition, water restriction, demeclocycline (ADH antagonist), and hypertonic sodium chloride may be useful in SIADH cases.[69]

Ectopic Adrenocorticotropic Hormone Syndrome

The ectopic production of adrenocorticotropic hormone (ACTH) or ACTH-like substances is the second most common PNS reported in humans.[2] This PNS is associated with small cell lung tumors, pancreatic tumors, and a wide variety of other human tumors.[2,67] In the dog, this PNS is reported to occur in primary lung tumors and a single case of an abdominal neuroendocrine tumor.[70,71] The predominant active molecules in this PNS are ACTH, ACTH precursors, endorphins, enkephalins, and melanocyte-stimulating hormone (MSH).[2,67] All result in excessive production of steroids from the adrenal glands resulting in clinical signs similar to those seen in hyperadrenocorticism (Cushing's disease). Invariably, tumors that cause this PNS are dexamethasone insuppressible. The diagnosis of this PNS is made by the concomitant presentation of Cushing's-like signs with an abnormal dexamethasone suppression test and a localizable tumor. The treatment of choice is removal of the underlying cause by surgical extirpation of the tumor. When necessary, the medical therapy for this PNS centers on inhibiting cortisol production by mitotane or ketoconazole. The use of selegiline (Anipryl) in the management of this PNS in dogs has not been evaluated to date in veterinary medicine.

Hypocalcemia/Hyperglycemia

Paraneoplastic hypocalcemia and hyperglycemia are extremely rare. Tumors associated with lytic bone metastases and tumors that secrete calcitonin (medullary carcinoma of the thyroid) are the most common causes of human PNS hypocalcemia.[2] A variety of nonthyroid cancers such as breast cancer, GI cancer, carcinoids, and lung cancer in humans have been reported to secrete calcitonin.[72] Most cases of PNS hypocalcemia are asymptomatic, although human patients may have neuromuscular irritability and/or tetany. A gingival vascular hamartoma in a 4-month-old kitten has been reported to be associated with PNS hyperglycemia, and the hyperglycemia resolved within 24 hours on removal of the tumor.[73] Treatment of choice for either PNS is eradication of the primary tumor whenever possible, calcium infusion in severe hypocalcemia cases, and diabetes-like support for severe hyperglycemia cases.

Hematologic Manifestations of Cancer

Hypergammaglobulinemia

Monoclonal gammopathies can be common in animals and people with cancer and they are termed *M-component disorders.*[1,2,74-76] The hypergammaglobulinemia seen as a PNS is due to the excessive production of proteins from a monoclonal line of immunoglobulin (Ig)-producing plasma cells or lymphocytes. When production of these Igs, partial Igs, heavy chains, and/or light chains becomes extreme, clinical signs of hyperviscosity (ataxia, depression, dementia, cardiac disease and/or failure, seizures, and coma), tissue hypoxia, bleeding (poor platelet aggregation, platelet coating with Igs, and release of platelet factor III), and/or ocular disorders (e.g., papilledema, retinal hemorrhage, detachment) may occur. These proteins may be identified by performing a protein electrophoresis on the serum and/or urine.[76] Similarly, light chain production may be detected in the urine as Bence-Jones proteins. In addition to the hypergammaglobulinemia PNS seen in plasma cell tumors (multiple myeloma and extramedullary plasmacytoma), lymphomas, lymphocytic leukemias, and primary macroglobulinemia can also cause this PNS.[75,76] Further discussion of plasma cell tumors, myeloma and lymphoma/leukemia can be found in Chapter 32.

Anemia

Anemia is one of the most common PNSs seen in veterinary and human oncology. Approximately 20% to 25% of human cancer patients have PNS anemia, and although the exact incidence of PNS anemia in veterinary oncology is unknown, it is thought to be a significant problem.[77] There are numerous possible causes for PNS anemia in veterinary oncology patients, and the vast majority are due to either anemia of chronic disease (ACD), immune-mediated hemolytic anemia (IMHA), blood loss anemia, or microangiopathic hemolytic anemia (MAHA).

ACD is extremely common in veterinary and human oncology patients with disseminated and/or metastatic tumors. This anemia is due to disordered iron storage and metabolism, shortened red blood cell (RBC) lifespan, and occasionally decreased bone marrow response.[77] The anemia seen in ACD is normocytic/normochromic, and evaluation of the bone marrow does not suggest significant problems with cellularity. Treatment of choice is removal of the tumor.

IMHA can be triggered by tumors in animals and humans. Immune mechanisms then result in the premature destruction of RBCs.[78] The diagnosis of PNS IMHA is typically established by a Coombs' slide agglutination test, and many patients will have concurrent spherocytosis and a regenerative anemia. The treatment of choice is removal of the tumor; however, if this is not immediately possible, the use of immunosuppressive dosages of prednisone (1 to 2 mg/kg daily to two times a day by mouth [BID PO]) may be indicated if a diagnosis has been established. Similar to non-PNS IMHA, the use of additional agents such as azathioprine (1 to 2 mg/kg daily for 4 to 7 days, then 0.5 to 1 mg/kg every 48 hrs PO), cyclosporine, cyclophosphamide, and others may be necessary for complicated IMHA cases.[78-81]

Blood loss anemia can be a sequela to many types of cancer. Due to decreased hemoglobin content, the RBCs in blood loss anemia are microcytic/hypochromic. In addition, decreased serum iron, increased total iron-binding capacity, and poikilocytosis may also be noted.[82,83] The blood loss may be readily apparent in some patients (e.g., bleeding splenic tumor or bleeding superficial tumor), whereas others may not have a readily identifiable source for the loss (e.g., GI tumors). The treatment of choice is removal of the tumor, although severe anemia may necessitate blood transfusions. The use of oral and/or injectable iron may be a useful adjunct therapy.

MAHA is a secondary phenomenon to hemolysis and is typically due to fibrin deposition and/or endothelial damage.[77] The most common causes of MAHA are PNS disseminated intravascular coagulation (DIC) and RBC shearing as the result of hemangiosarcoma.[77,80] Schistocytosis and hemolysis are common indicators of ongoing MAHA. While any tumor can cause DIC and subsequent MAHA, hemangiosarcoma is most common.[84] The treatment of choice is removal of the tumor; however, additional ancillary treatments such as aggressive supportive therapy and transfusions may be useful.

Chemotherapy-induced anemia can be quite common in people because of more aggressive chemotherapy protocols[2]; however, this is rarely seen in veterinary patients.[77,82,83] The degree of anemia seen in veterinary cancer patients undergoing chemotherapy is generally mild, with typical packed cell volumes hovering in the 28% to 32% range for dogs and 24% to 28% range for cats. This anemia rarely necessitates therapy and resolves on discontinuation of the chemotherapy protocol.

A relatively uncommon cause of PNS-associated anemia is myelophthisis (bone marrow invasion/crowding out), and it is most commonly caused by leukemias.[2] Another uncommon cause of PNS-associated anemia is bone marrow hypoplasia resulting from hyperestrogenism. Sertoli cell tumors in the male dog and granulosa cell tumors of the female dog are commonly associated with hyperestrogenism, and anemia is a common presenting feature.[85-87]

Erythrocytosis

Erythrocytosis is a relatively uncommon PNS. Tumors that have been associated with PNS erythrocytosis include renal tumors (primary and secondary), lymphoma (including renal origin), lung or liver tumors, cecal leiomyosarcoma, nasal fibrosarcoma, and transmissible venereal tumor (TVT).[62,88-93] The erythrocytosis seen in cancer patients can be due directly to overproduction of erythropoietin, indirect excess erythropoietin from renal hypoxia, or increased production of hypoxia-inducible factors such as HIF-1.[94] Interestingly, some tumor suppressor genes (TSG) are important proteosomal regulators of HIF-1, which may explain some of the vascular diseases seen in human patients with certain TSG mutations.[95] Other differential diagnoses for polycythemia include arteriovenous shunts, severe dehydration, hyperadrenocorticism, polycythemia vera (primary polycythemia), and a variety of cardiac and/or pulmonary diseases.

It is important to differentiate primary and secondary causes of erythrocytosis. Polycythemia vera is a myeloproliferative disorder resulting in clonal proliferation of RBCs with splenomegaly and possibly pancytosis most commonly associated with acquired recurrent mutation in JAK2.[1,2,96] Secondary polycythemia results from decreased arterial oxygen saturation. PNS erythrocytosis is best treated by removal of the erythropoietin-producing tumor whenever possible; phlebotomy can be a useful temporary adjunct therapy. Unfortunately, the volumes typically needed for a therapeutic phlebotomy in PNS erythrocytosis cases necessitates administration of fluids and potentially readministration of plasma. The use of hydroxyurea (40 to 50 mg/kg divided BID PO)[91] as a chemotherapeutic agent for polycythemia vera has been previously recommended; however, this author has noted limited benefit with use of this agent.

Neutrophilic Leukocytosis

Increases in the number of circulating neutrophils have occasionally been associated with a variety of tumors in humans and dogs. Unfortunately, a leukemoid reaction of this nature can be difficult to distinguish from a true leukemia without extensive diagnostics. Neutrophilic leukocytosis has been reported in dogs with lymphoma, renal carcinoma, primary lung tumor, rectal polyp, and metastatic fibrosarcoma.[97-100] The exact mechanism of PNS leukemoid reactions is unknown; however, the production of a colony-stimulating factor such as granulocyte colony-stimulating factor (G-CSF) or granulocyte-macrophage colony-stimulating factor (GM-CSF) is considered likely. Reports have documented tumor-produced G-CSF and GM-CSF in dogs with primary lung tumor and renal transitional cell carcinoma, whereas tumor-produced G-CSF has been documented in a cat with dermal adenocarcinoma and suspected in a cat with pulmonary squamous cell carcinoma.[101-103] This PNS is generally of minimal clinical significance, and normalization of the PNS is possible following removal of the inciting tumor.

Thrombocytopenia

Thrombocytopenia in human and veterinary cancer patients is typically secondary to chemotherapy administration; however, the incidence of thrombocytopenia in tumor-bearing dogs prior to chemotherapy administration has been reported to be as high as 36%.[80] Dogs with lymphoproliferative tumors have been reported to have thrombocytopenia in 58% of cases.[104] Dogs with Sertoli cell tumors (or occasionally seminomas) that excessively produce estrogen are also prone to thrombocytopenia.[85,87] Twenty percent of the cases of thrombocytopenia in cats have been reported to be due to cancer, most commonly associated with lymphoma.[105]

Numerous mechanisms for PNS thrombocytopenia are possible and include platelet destruction, sequestration, or consumption and/or decreased platelet production. The most common tumors associated with PNS thrombocytopenia are vascular tumors of the spleen and tumors infiltrating the marrow, such as lymphoma or leukemias.[106] Immune-mediated thrombocytopenia (ITP) is an additional significant cause of thrombocytopenia.[107] The treatment of PNS-associated thrombocytopenia is removal of the inciting tumor; however, adjunctive therapies such as intravenous fluids, plasma, and heparin may be beneficial. For those cases secondary to ITP, the use of immunosuppressive drugs such as corticosteroids (≥2 mg/kg PO daily) and azathioprine (2 mg/kg PO daily then 0.5 to 1 mg/kg PO every other day) may be necessary.

Coagulopathies and Disseminated Intravascular Coagulation

Alterations in hemostasis can be common in human and veterinary cancer patients. PNS coagulopathies are most commonly associated with tumors that cause thrombocytopenia, thrombocytosis, DIC, platelet dysfunction, changes in platelet aggregation, or hyperheparinemia (due to MCT).[108,109] Trousseau's syndrome is a carcinoma-associated human coagulopathy that appears to be related to excess production of hypoxia factors leading to angiogenesis and a procoagulant state.[110] PNS-associated DIC has been reported to be the cause of consumptive thrombocytopenia in almost 40% of DIC cases,[80] suggesting this PNS may be an important clinical syndrome based on the potentially devastating morbidity and mortality associated with DIC. The diagnosis of DIC is made when the patient has thrombocytopenia, prolongation of activated partial thromboplastin time (aPTT), elevated fibrin degradation products (FDP), and hypofibrinogenemia.[80,111,112] A reduction in serum antithrombin III levels appears to be one of the most reliable and prognostic measurements for the presence of DIC.[104,113,114]

The incidence of DIC in dogs with malignant tumors is approximately 10%.[115] A variety of tumors have been associated with DIC; hemangiosarcoma is the most common in dogs. Other associated tumors include inflammatory mammary gland tumors, thyroid carcinomas, primary lung tumors, and intraabdominal carcinomas.[113,115-117] DIC has not been evaluated as a prognostic factor in veterinary cancer patients to date; however, the presence and severity of DIC in human cancer patients is a significant negative prognostic factor. Although not specifically related to DIC, the hyperheparinemia associated with MCTs can be associated with prolonged bleeding times and poor hemostasis during and after biopsy or surgery.[20]

Miscellaneous

Thrombocytosis is a common PNS in humans with lymphomas and leukemias, although it is rarely noted in veterinary oncology. Myeloproliferative disorders appear to be the most common cause of PNS thrombocytosis in dogs and cats.[118-120] Important differential diagnoses include causes of primary thrombocytosis such as inflammatory processes, some hemolytic anemias, posthemorrhage, iron deficiency, and postsplenectomy.

PNS eosinophilia is rarely reported in veterinary medicine. Dogs with mammary tumors, leiomyosarcoma, T-cell lymphosarcoma (LSA), or fibrosarcoma and cats with a variety of tumors (lymphoma, sarcomas, MCT, and bladder tumors) have been reported to have tumor-associated eosinophilia.[121-125] In addition, eosinophilic effusions have been documented in dogs and cats with cancer and nonneoplastic conditions.[126] The cause of eosinophilia in these cases is poorly understood; however, the production of eosinophilic substances such as GM-CSF, various interleukins (e.g., IL-5, -13, and -17), and eotaxins are likely. PNS eosinophilia should be distinguished from eosinophilic leukemia and hypereosinophilia syndrome. The treatment for PNS eosinophilia is removal of the inciting tumor; PNS-associated eosinophilia is typically of little clinical significance.

Although lymphocytosis can be noted with various lymphocytic neoplasms and reactive nonneoplastic conditions, it is rarely noted as a PNS. T-cell lymphocytosis has been recently reported as a PNS in association with thymoma in a dog.[127]

Platelets may play a role in cancer progression and metastasis attributable to platelet aggregation–mediated augmentation of tumor cell extravasation, survival, and angiogenesis. Platelet aggregation was investigated in a study of 59 dogs with cancer.[109] When compared to control dogs, the platelets of dogs with cancer exhibited significantly higher maximum aggregation, higher adenosine triphosphate (ATP) secretion, and shorter delays in the aggregation response. In addition to aiding the metastatic process, platelet hyperaggregation may also lead to thromboembolism.[128]

Cutaneous Manifestations of Cancer

A wide variety of cutaneous syndromes are associated with malignancies in humans,[129] whereas relatively few are noted in veterinary medicine.[130] For example, Sweet syndrome is a human PNS associated with hematologic and solid tumors that causes acute febrile neutrophilic dermatosis but has not been reported to date in veterinary patients.[131] As with any PNS, cutaneous-associated PNS lesions may precede, coexist with, or follow the diagnosis of the underlying tumor.

Alopecia

Pancreatic carcinoma has been reported in cats as the cause of a progressive, nonscarring PNS alopecia.[132-135] The alopecia is acute, bilaterally symmetric (ventrum and limbs), and ventrally glistening. The hair easily epilates from nonalopecic areas and histologically exhibits severe follicular and adnexal atrophy with absence of stratum corneum in many areas, including the foot pads. Clinical signs include anorexia, weight loss, lethargy, and difficulty walking and/or standing, which is most likely due to the aforementioned foot pad histologic changes. In two reports, a similar presentation was noted in cats with bile duct carcinoma.[134,136] The cause of this PNS is presently unknown.

Cutaneous Flushing

When the skin episodically turns various shades of red because of changes in cutaneous blood vessel vasodilation, it is termed *cutaneous flushing*. Intermittent or paroxysmal cutaneous flushing can be associated with pheochromocytoma (see Chapter 25).[2,137,138] This PNS has also been reported in a dog with primary lung tumor and concomitant intrathoracic MCT.[139] Dogs that undergo MCT degranulation may also have cutaneous flushing. Important nonneoplastic diagnoses to rule out for this PNS include drug reactions, demodicosis, and systemic lupus erythematosus. In addition to pheochromocytoma, humans may experience cutaneous flushing caused by Zollinger-Ellison syndrome, carcinoids, leukemias, renal cell carcinoma, and many other conditions.[2,140]

Nodular Dermatofibrosis

Nodular dermatofibrosis (ND) is a well-recognized PNS of multiple, slowly growing cutaneous nodules in dogs with bilateral renal cysts or cystadenocarcinomas (Figure 5-2).[141-144] The nodules are

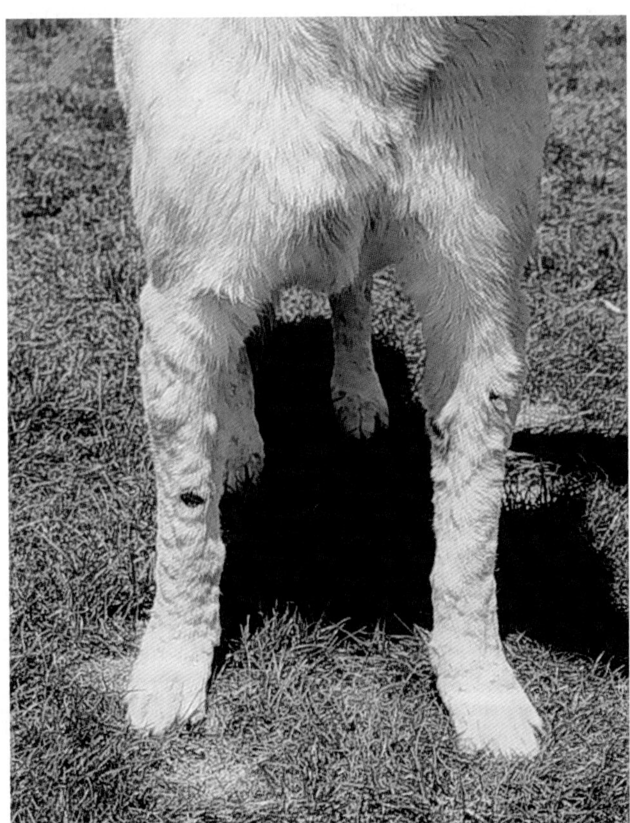

FIGURE 5-2 Diffuse nodular dermatofibrosis (ND) in a German shepherd dog. The nodules are composed of extremely dense but well-differentiated collagen tissue (collagenous nevi) and are found predominately on the limbs, although the head and trunk may be affected in advanced cases.

composed of dense but well-differentiated collagen tissue (collagenous nevi) and are found predominately on the limbs, although the head and trunk may be affected in advanced cases. ND appears to be inherited in an autosomal dominant fashion and is most commonly seen in middle-aged German shepherd dogs.[141-143,145] The ND-associated mutation was mapped to exon 7 of the Birt-Hogg-Dube (BHD) locus on canine chromosome 5, which is the same locus for a phenotypically similar human disease.[146] Intact females with ND are also at increased risk for the development of uterine leiomyomas, and the BHD mutation appears to be homozygous lethal.[143,146,147] The pathogenesis of ND is unknown; however, the BHD mutation in humans leads to a novel protein called *folliculin,* which may be related to the mTOR pathway.[148,149] Currently, there is no effective therapy for the underlying tumor; however, palliative therapy via surgical removal of nodules may be utilized in cases in which the nodules are ulcerated, cosmetically displeasing, or interfering with function.

Necrolytic Migratory Erythema/ Superficial Necrolytic Dermatitis

Superficial necrolytic dermatitis (SND) is a rare PNS in humans and dogs characterized by circinate and gyrate areas of erosive blistering and erythema as the result of glucagonomas (glucagon-secreting pancreatic alpha-cell tumors).[2,150-153] Marked fissuring, ulceration, and crusting of foot pads have also been noted in dogs. Nonneoplastic differential diagnoses for SND include hepatic disease and diabetes mellitus. Necrolytic migratory erythema, metabolic epidermal necrosis, diabetic dermatopathy, and hepatocutaneous syndrome are terms that have been previously used to describe SND. This PNS resolves in people after surgical extirpation of the glucagonoma, although the prognosis may be poor in dogs due to multiple postoperative complications.[154] Octreotide (2 to 3 µg/kg BID) has been reported to successfully treat paraneoplastic SND.[155] Although not specifically related to hepatocutaneous syndrome, a dog with sarcomatoid renal cell carcinoma and paraneoplastic hepatopathy with similarities to Stauffer's syndrome in humans has been reported.[152,156]

Miscellaneous Syndromes

The number of recognized cutaneous PNSs in humans easily reaches into the dozens; however, the specificity of which we are able to delineate similar PNS in veterinary oncology is limited.[130] Ischemic necrosis of the digits and/or feet is a common human PNS associated with lymphoma, adenocarcinoma, and occasionally other malignancies.[157] Symmetric cutaneous necrosis of the hind feet has been reported in a cat with multicentric follicular lymphoma.[158] Interestingly, the necrosis was not associated with a neoplastic infiltrate and thrombotic/vasculitic causes were not seen histologically, suggesting it was of paraneoplastic origin.

Malassezia-associated dermatitis was first reported in a cat with paraneoplastic alopecia from a metastatic exocrine pancreatic carcinoma.[159] A study of over 500 feline skin biopsies found fifteen (2.7%) of the submissions contained Malassezia organisms. Ten of the 15 cats also had neoplasia, suggesting that Malassezia yeast in feline skin biopsies should prompt a clinical workup for neoplasia.[160]

Pemphigus vulgaris (PV) is a dermatopathy characterized by intraepidermal bullae and erosions of the skin and oral mucosa.[161,162] In humans, paraneoplastic PV (PPV) can be associated with lymphoma, Kaposi's sarcoma, and various carcinomas.[2] PPV has been reported in association with mediastinal lymphoma and splenic sarcoma in dogs.[163,164] Canine paraneoplastic pemphigus may be an excellent comparative model to human pemphigus PNS.[165] Recent reports suggest that paraneoplastic pemphigus is due to circulating IgG autoantibodies against desmoglein 3 across species.[161,166,167]

Erythema multiforme has been associated with thymoma in a dog.[168] The erythema multiforme resolved after thymectomy, suggesting it was paraneoplastic in origin and may be similar to feline thymoma-associated exfoliative dermatitis.[169,170] The variety noted in miscellaneous reports should serve as a reminder that there are likely many other uncharacterized cutaneous PNSs in veterinary oncology.

Renal Manifestations of Cancer

Human and veterinary cancer patients alike can develop important renal complications. Most are iatrogenic in nature and include chemotherapy-related toxicity (e.g., cisplatin), antibiotic toxicity (e.g., aminoglycoside), and contrast-associated nephropathy. In addition, infiltrative diseases such as lymphoma can have renal consequences. Biochemical alterations that can lead to nephrotoxicity include tubular precipitations from hypercalcemia, protein casts, glomerulopathies due to amyloidosis and/or membranous glomerulopathy, and fluid and electrolyte disorders due to hypercalcemia, hyponatremia, and acute tumor lysis syndrome. Nephrogenic diabetes insipidus may be a renal PNS in dogs with intestinal leiomyosarcoma.[171]

Approximately 6% to 10% of human cancer patients have significant glomerulonephritis and protein loss in the urine.[172,173] Similarly, 11% of humans with nephrotic syndrome have a concurrent diagnosis of cancer.[174] The most common malignancies associated with PNS glomerulonephritis in humans are carcinomas of the lung and GI tract.[175] Immune complexes are thought to play a central role.[176,177] The prevalence of glomerulonephritis in veterinary cancer patients is unknown; however, immune complex glomerulonephritis has been reported in a dog with polycythemia vera and a dog with lymphocytic leukemia.[178,179]

Neurologic Manifestations of Cancer

Greater than 50% of human cancer patients have a mild degree of neuromuscular dysfunction (myopathy and/or peripheral neuropathy); however, the frequency of a specific neurologic PNS is low.[1,2,180-182] Human neurologic PNSs are separated into anatomic categories (brain, spinal cord, peripheral nerve, muscle, neuromuscular junction). The prevalence of neurologic PNSs in veterinary medicine is unknown, and presently there are examples of neurologic PNSs reported in the dog for the brain, peripheral nerves, and neuromuscular junction.[183-189] Many non-PNS causes of neurologic complications from cancer such as metabolic encephalopathy, brain metastasis, cerebrovascular incidents, neurotoxicity from radiation and/or chemotherapy, and neurologic infections due to altered immunity are possible.

Myasthenia Gravis

Myasthenia gravis (MG) is an acquired or congenital disorder of the neuromuscular junction that results from a failure of synaptic transmission. Antibodies to nicotinic acetylcholine receptors (nACHRs) can be documented in dogs with MG and are useful in the diagnosis and follow-up.[183,190] In a similar fashion, Lambert-Eaton syndrome in humans occurs as the result of calcium-channel autoantibody formation from predominately lung tumors, which then result in an MG-like syndrome caused by poor calcium influx from the presynaptic neuromuscular junction.[191,192]

The most common cause of acquired MG in the dog is thymoma, although it has also been reported in association with osteosarcoma, lymphoma, and bile duct carcinoma.[184,193-199] The clinical signs revolve around intermittent mild-to-severe muscular weakness, exercise intolerance, dysphagia, and megaesophagus (and possible secondary aspiration pneumonia). Rapid clinical improvement and decreases in nACHR antibodies have been noted after surgical extirpation of thymoma.[194,200] The use of immunosuppressive doses of prednisone (>2 mg/kg PO daily) may be a useful adjunct in the treatment of paraneoplastic MG.[195]

Peripheral Neuropathy

Peripheral nerve lesions that are the result of cancer are a relatively common event in humans and animals. When nerve fibers were analyzed from dogs with a wide variety of malignancies, a significant percentage of abnormal findings such as demyelination, myelin globulation, and axonal degeneration were noted in some specific malignancies.[185] Tumors associated with large numbers of peripheral nerve changes included primary lung tumors, insulinoma, MCT, thyroid adenocarcinoma, melanoma, and mammary tumors.[185] In contrast, clinically apparent PNS of the peripheral nerves in veterinary medicine is rare. Tumors associated with PNS peripheral neuropathy in dogs and cats include primary lung tumor, leiomyosarcoma, undifferentiated sarcoma, hemangiosarcoma, mammary tumor, multiple myeloma, lymphoma, and insulinoma.[185-187,201-203] A multisystemic PNS in humans caused by plasma cell dyscrasia or tumor is termed *POEMS syndrome* for *p*olyneuropathy, *o*rganomegaly, *e*ndocrinopathy, *M* protein, and *s*kin changes. The treatment for paraneoplastic peripheral neuropathy is removal of the inciting tumor.

Diencephalic Syndrome and Miscellaneous Neuromuscular Syndromes

Diencephalic syndrome is a PNS seen in infants with rostral hypothalamic tumors that undergo extreme emaciation despite normal to increased caloric intake.[2] All cases occur in association with a tumor in the diencephalic region that secretes excess growth hormone. Only one case has been reported in the veterinary literature to date (affecting a 3-year-old Doberman pinscher).[188] Similar to human cases of diencephalic syndrome, this dog had extreme emaciation despite increased caloric intake with a growth-hormone producing astrocytoma in the diencephalic region. The cause for the lack of acromegalic and accelerated growth signs in this case is unknown.

Miscellaneous Manifestations of Cancer

Hypertrophic Osteopathy

Hypertrophic osteopathy (HO) is a syndrome characterized by periosteal proliferation of new bone along the shafts of long bones in response to malignant and nonmalignant diseases (Figure 5-3). HO has been present in the medical literature for over 25 centuries—Hippocrates described "Hippocratic fingers" (digital clubbing seen in humans with HO). As a PNS, HO is reported most commonly with primary lung tumors[2,204]; however, in clinical veterinary practice, HO secondary to pulmonary metastatic disease (especially osteosarcoma) is common. It has also been reported with urinary bladder rhabdomyosarcoma, esophageal tumors, malignant Sertoli cell tumor, renal TCC, and nephroblastoma and in cats with renal adenoma, papillary carcinoma, and adrenocortical carcinoma.[102,205-213] Nonmalignant conditions such as heartworms, heart disease, focal lung atelectasis, pregnancy, abscesses, granulomas, foreign bodies, and pneumonia have also been associated with HO.

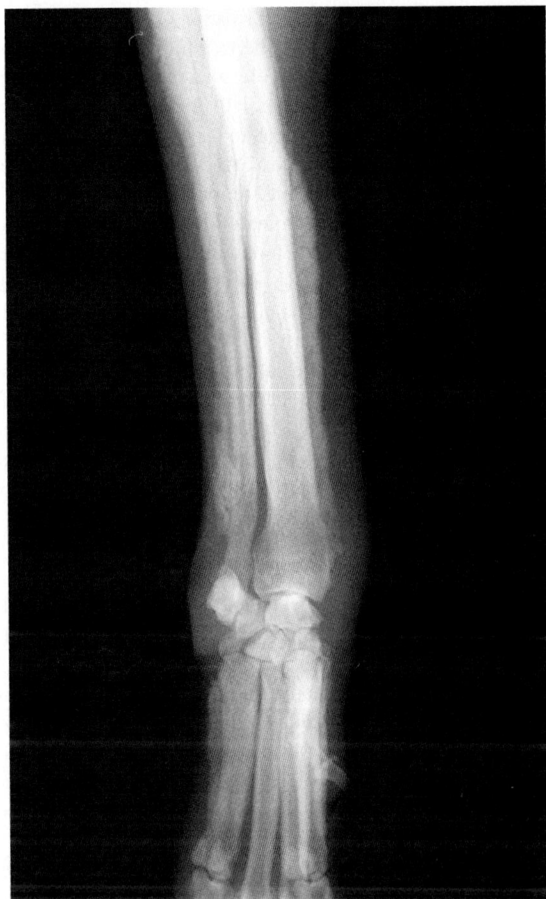

FIGURE 5-3 Hypertrophic osteopathy (HO) in the front limb of a dog with a primary lung tumor. This paraneoplastic syndrome (PNS) is a bony disease that results in periosteal proliferation and subsequent lameness. This syndrome is seen in a wide variety of malignant and nonmalignant diseases.

The clinical signs of dogs or cats afflicted with HO typically include a history of shifting-leg lameness and/or reluctance to move with all four limbs affected. The limbs are typically warm to the touch and swollen with occasional cases having involvement of the ribs and/or pelvis. The diagnosis of HO is made by radiography of the affected bones (starts distally and moves proximally) and finding the unique 90-degree periosteal reaction seen in Figure 5-3. The search for the inciting tumor begins with radiographs of the thorax, and if negative, radiographs and/or ultrasound of the abdomen with blood work and urinalysis should be pursued.

The etiology of HO is still unknown; however, based on measurable increase in blood flow to extremities and resultant connective tissue and periosteal proliferation, it has been well accepted that HO likely develops in part as a result of afferent neurologic stimulation.[214] This is further supported by the resolution of HO after vagotomy; however, this therapy is not routinely used in veterinary patients.[215] Recent work suggests that excess production of GHRH and/or vascular endothelial growth factor (VEGF) by the tumor may also contribute to HO.[12,216] The treatment for HO is removal of the inciting tumor when possible, and reports have been published documenting resolution of HO in dogs treated for their primary tumor.[217,218] Prednisone (1 to 2 mg/kg PO daily) or nonsteroidal antiinflammatory drugs (NSAIDs) may be a useful adjunct therapy for HO when the inciting tumor cannot be removed (i.e., diffuse metastasis). Other treatments for HO such as intercostal nerve resection, unilateral vagotomy, bilateral cervical vagotomy, analgesics, and subperiosteal rib resection have been suggested; however, these therapies have not been evaluated extensively in veterinary patients.[204,219] The use of bisphosphonates has become more common for human patients with HO[220] and likely represents an exciting new therapeutic modality in veterinary medicine for a variety of indications.[53,54] Furthermore, the use of agents such as toceranib phosphate (Palladia),[221] in light of its antiangiogenic mechanisms of action, may warrant investigation for patients with resistant HO.

Fever

Although the most common causes of fever are infection, inflammation, autoimmune disease, or drug/blood product reactions, cancer can cause fever as a PNS and should remain an important differential diagnosis. Paraneoplastic fever can accompany a wide variety of tumors in human and veterinary patients. The incidence of fever as a PNS in veterinary medicine is unknown; however, in human patients presenting with fever of unknown origin, cancer is the cause in over one-third of the cases, with the most commonly diagnosed cancers being lymphoma, hepatoma, and renal cell carcinoma.[2] Approximately 10% of human cancer patients develop noninfectious/inflammation-related fever at some point during the course of their disease.[222] The pathogenesis of PNS fever is predominately due to excess production of cytokines (IL-1, IL-6, TNF-α, and interferons) and febrile-promoting prostaglandins.[1,222,223]

The most important point in managing fever in veterinary patients with cancer is the evaluation for the presence of concurrent infection. Cancer patients with neutropenia and fever represent a medical emergency. Cancer patients with fever in the absence of neutropenia are not generally medical emergencies but should still be worked up to determine the presence or absence of an infectious and/or inflammatory nidus. If one is not found, then PNS fever is more likely the cause. If the fever is severe and threatens quality of life, the use of an NSAID such as indomethacin or naproxen is commonly utilized in humans with PNS fever. The best therapy for PNS fever is removal of the inciting tumor; however, if this cannot be accomplished, NSAIDs may be useful.

REFERENCES

1. Pelosof LC, Gerber DE: Paraneoplastic syndromes: an approach to diagnosis and treatment, *Mayo Clin Proc* 85(9):838–854, 2010.
2. John WJ, Patchell RA, Foon KA: Paraneoplastic syndromes. In DeVita VT, Hellman S, Rosenberg SA, editors: *Cancer: Principles & Practice of Oncology*, ed 5, Philadelphia, 1997, Lippincott-Raven Publishers, pp 2397–2422.
3. Coss CC, Bohl CE, Dalton JT: Cancer cachexia therapy: a key weapon in the fight against cancer, *Curr Opin Clin Nutr Metab Care* 14(3):268–273, 2011.
4. Muscaritoli M, Bossola M, Bellantone R, et al: Therapy of muscle wasting in cancer: what is the future? *Curr Opin Clin Nutr Metab Care* 7(4):459–466, 2004.
5. Crowe SE, Oliver J: Cancer cachexia, *Compend Contin Educ Pract Vet* 3:681–690, 1981.
6. Michel KE, Sorenmo K, Shofer FS: Evaluation of body condition and weight loss in dogs presented to a veterinary oncology service, *J Vet Intern Med* 18(5):692–695, 2004.
7. Ogilvie GK, Walters LM, Salman MD, et al: Resting energy expenditure in dogs with nonhematopoietic malignancies before and after excision of tumors, *Am J Vet Res* 57:1463–1467, 1996.
8. Chlebowski RT, Herber D: Metabolic abnormalities in cancer patients: carbohydrate metabolism, *Surg Clin North Am* 66:957–968, 1986.
9. Herber D, Byerly LO, Chi J, et al: Pathophysiology of malnutrition in the adult cancer patient, *Cancer* 58:1867–1873, 1986.
10. McAndrew PF: Fat metabolism and cancer, *Surg Clin North Am* 66:1003–1012, 1986.
11. Ogilvie GK, Vail DM, Wheeler SL, et al: Effects of Chemotherapy and Remission on Carbohydrate Metabolism in Dogs with Lymphoma, *Cancer* 69(1):233–238, 1992.
12. Mito K, Maruyama R, Uenishi Y, et al: Hypertrophic pulmonary osteoarthropathy associated with non-small cell lung cancer demonstrated growth hormone-releasing hormone by immunohistochemical analysis, *Intern Med* 40(6):532–535, 2001.
13. Draghia-Akli R, Hahn KA, King GK, et al: Effects of plasmid-mediated growth hormone-releasing hormone in severely debilitated dogs with cancer, *Mol Ther* 6(6):830–836, 2002.
14. Tone CM, Cardoza DM, Carpenter RH, et al: Long-term effects of plasmid-mediated growth hormone releasing hormone in dogs, *Cancer Gene Ther* 11(5):389–396, 2004.
15. Bodles-Brakhop AM, Brown PA, Pope MA, et al: Double-blinded, Placebo-controlled plasmid GHRH trial for cancer-associated anemia in dogs, *Mol Ther* 16(5):862–870, 2008.
16. Fossum TW: Protein-losing enteropathy, *Semin Vet Med Surg (Small Anim)* 4(3):219–225, 1989.
17. Strygler B, Nicor MJ, Santangelo WC, et al: Alpha1-anti-trypsin excretion in stool in normal subjects and in patients with gastrointestinal disorders, *Gastroenterology* 99:1380–1387, 1990.
18. Ruaux CG, Steiner JM, Williams DA: Protein-losing enteropathy in dogs is associated with decreased fecal proteolytic activity, *Vet Clin Pathol* 33(1):20–22, 2004.
19. Berry CR, Guilford WG, Koblik PD, et al: Scintigraphic evaluation of four dogs with protein-losing enteropathy using 111indium-labeled transferrin, *Vet Radiol Ultrasound* 38(3):221–225,1997.
20. Fox LE, Rosenthal RC, Twedt DC, et al: Plasma histamine and gastrin concentrations in 17 dogs with mast cell tumors, *J Vet Intern Med* 4(5):242–246, 1990.
21. Ishiguro T, Kadosawa T, Takagi S, et al: Relationship of disease progression and plasma histamine concentrations in 11 dogs with mast cell tumors, *J Vet Intern Med* 17(2):194–198, 2003.
22. English RV, Breitschwerdt EB, Grindem CB, et al: Zollinger-Ellison syndrome and myelofibrosis in a dog, *J Am Vet Med Assoc* 192:1430–1434, 1988.
23. Drazner FH: Canine gastrinoma: a condition analogous to the Zollinger-Ellison syndrome in man, *California Vet* 11:6–11, 1981.
24. Middleton DJ: Duodenal ulceration associated with gastrin-secreting pancreatic tumor in a cat, *J Am Vet Med Assoc* 183:461–462, 1983.
25. Straus E, Johnson GF, Yalow RS: Canine Zollinger-Ellison syndrome, *Gastroenterology* 72:380–381, 1977.
26. Hayden DW, Henson MS: Gastrin-secreting pancreatic endocrine tumor in a dog (putative Zollinger-Ellison syndrome), *J Vet Diagn Invest* 9:100–103, 1997.
27. Uehlinger P, Glaus T, Hauser B, et al: [Differential diagnosis of hypercalcemia–a retrospective study of 46 dogs], *Schweiz Arch Tierheilkd* 140(5):188–197, 1998.
28. Elliott J: Hypercalcemia in the dog: A study of 40 cases, *J Small Anim Pract* 32:564–567, 1991.
29. Savary KC, Price GS, Vaden SL: Hypercalcemia in cats: a retrospective study of 71 cases (1991-1997), *J Vet Intern Med* 14(2):184–189, 2000.
30. Sheafor SE, Gamblin RM, Couto CG: Hypercalcemia in two cats with multiple myeloma, *J Am Anim Hosp Assoc* 32:503–508, 1996.

31. Pressler BM, Rotstein DS, Law JM, et al: Hypercalcemia and high parathyroid hormone-related protein concentration associated with malignant melanoma in a dog, *J Am Vet Med Assoc* 221(2):263–265, 240, 2002.
32. Kleiter M, Hirt R, Kirtz G, Day MJ: Hypercalcaemia associated with chronic lymphocytic leukaemia in a Giant Schnauzer, *Aust Vet J* 79(5):335–338, 2001.
33. Anderson TE, Legendre AM, McEntee MM: Probable hypercalcemia of malignancy in a cat with bronchogenic adenocarcinoma, *J Am Anim Hosp Assoc* 36(1):52–55, 2000.
34. Weller RE, Hoffman WE: Renal function in dogs with lymphosarcoma and associated hypercalcemia, *J Small Anim Pract* 33:61–66, 1992.
35. Klausner JS, Bell FW, Hayden DW, et al: Hypercalcemia in two cats with squamous cell carcinoma, *J Am Vet Med Assoc* 196:103–105, 1990.
36. Elliott J, Dobson JM, Dunn JK, et al: Hypercalcemia in the dog: a study of 40 cases, *J Small Anim Pract* 32:564–571, 1991.
37. Messinger JS, Windham WR, Ward CR: Ionized hypercalcemia in dogs: a retrospective study of 109 cases (1998-2003), *J Vet Intern Med* 23(3):514–519, 2009.
38. Gajanayake I, Priestnall SL, Benigni L, et al: Paraneoplastic hypercalcemia in a dog with benign renal angiomyxoma, *J Vet Diagn Invest* 22(5):775–780, 2010.
39. Ross JT, Scavelli TD, Matthieson DT, et al: Adenocarcinoma of the apocrine glands of the anal sac in dogs: a review of 32 cases, *J Am Anim Hosp Assoc* 27:349–355,1991.
40. Meuten DJ, Cooper BJ, Capen CC, et al: Hypercalcemia associated with an adenocarcinoma derived from the apocrine glands of the anal sac, *Vet Pathol* 18:454–471, 1981.
41. Hofbauer LC, Neubauer A, Heufelder AE: Receptor activator of nuclear factor-kappaB ligand and osteoprotegerin: potential implications for the pathogenesis and treatment of malignant bone diseases, *Cancer* 92(3):460–470, 2001.
42. Rosol TJ, Nagode LA, Couto CG, et al: Parathyroid hormone (PTH)-related protein, PTH, and 1,25-dihydroxyvitamin D in dogs with cancer-associated hypercalcemia, *Endocrinology* 131:1157–1164, 1992.
43. Forrester SD, Fallin EA: Diagnosing and managing the hypercalcemia of malignancy, *Vet Med* 1(26):39, 1992.
44. Cryer PE, Kissane JM: Clinicopathologic conference: Malignant hypercalcemia, *Am J Med* 65:486–494, 1979.
45. Weir EC, Norrdin RW, Matus RE, et al: Humoral hypercalcemia of malignancy in canine lymphosarcoma, *Endocrinology* 122:602–608, 1988.
46. Barger AM, Fan TM, de Lorimier LP, et al: Expression of receptor activator of nuclear factor kappa-B ligand (RANKL) in neoplasms of dogs and cats, *J Vet Intern Med* 21(1):133–140, 2007.
47. Sellers RS, Capen CC, Rosol TJ: Messenger RNA stability of parathyroid hormone-related protein regulated by transforming growth factor-beta1, *Mol Cell Endocrinol* 188(1-2):37–46, 2002.
48. Bolliger AP, Graham PA, Richard V, et al: Detection of parathyroid hormone-related protein in cats with humoral hypercalcemia of malignancy, *Vet Clin Pathol* 31(1):3–8, 2002.
49. Weir EC, Burtis WJ, Morris CA, et al: Isolation of 16000-dalton parathyroid hormone-like proteins from two animal tumors causing humoral hypercalcemia of malignancy, *Endocrinology* 123(6):2744–2751, 1988.
50. Price GS, Page RL, Fischer B, et al: Efficacy and toxicity of doxorubicin/cyclophosphamide maintenance therapy in dogs with multicentric lymphosarcoma, *J Vet Intern Med* 5:259–262, 1991.
51. Nelson KA, Walsh D, Abdullah O, et al: Common complications of advanced cancer, *Semin Oncol* 27(1):34–44, 2000.
52. Hurtado J, Esbrit P: Treatment of malignant hypercalcaemia, *Expert Opin Pharmacother* 3(5):521–527, 2002.
53. Milner RJ, Farese J, Henry CJ, et al: Bisphosphonates and cancer, *J Vet Intern Med* 18(5):597–604, 2004.
54. Hostutler RA, Chew DJ, Jaeger JQ, et al: Uses and effectiveness of pamidronate disodium for treatment of dogs and cats with hypercalcemia, *J Vet Intern Med* 19(1):29–33, 2005 Jan.
55. Sato K, Onuma E, Yocum RC, et al: Treatment of malignancy-associated hypercalcemia and cachexia with humanized anti-parathyroid hormone-related protein antibody, *Semin Oncol* 30(5 Suppl 16):167–173, 2003.
56. Caywood DD, Klausner JS, O'Leary TP, et al: Pancreatic insulin-secreting neoplasms:clinical, diagnostic, and prognostic features in 73 dogs, *J Am Anim Hosp Assoc* 24:577–584, 1988.
57. Boari A, Venturoli M, Minuto F: Non-islet cell tumor hypoglycemia in a dog associated with high levels of insulin-like growth factor II. XVII World Small Animal Veterinary Association Proceedings 678–679, 1992.
58. Beaudry D, Knapp DW, Montgomery T, et al: Smooth muscle tumors associated with hypoglycemia in four dogs. Clinical presentation, treatment, and tumor immunohistochemical staining, *J Vet Intern Med* 9:415–418m, 1995.
59. Rossi G, Errico G, Perez P, Rossi G, et al: Paraneoplastic hypoglycemia in a diabetic dog with an insulin growth factor-2-producing mammary carcinoma, *Vet Clin Pathol* 39(4):480–484, 2010.
60. Zini E, Glaus TM, Minuto F, et al: Paraneoplastic hypoglycemia due to an insulin-like growth factor type-II secreting hepatocellular carcinoma in a dog, *J Vet Intern Med* 21(1):193–195, 2007.
61. Battaglia L, Petterino C, Zappulli V, et al: Hypoglycaemia as a paraneoplastic syndrome associated with renal adenocarcinoma in a dog, *Vet Res Commun* 29(8):671–675, 2005.
62. Snead EC: A case of bilateral renal lymphosarcoma with secondary polycythaemia and paraneoplastic syndromes of hypoglycaemia and uveitis in an English Springer Spaniel, *Vet Comp Oncol* 3(3):139–144, 2005.
63. Zapf J: Role of insulin-like growth factor (IGF) II and IGF binding proteins in extrapancreatic tumour hypoglycaemia, *J Intern Med* 234(6):543–552, 1993.
64. Breitschwerdt EB, Root CR: Inappropriate secretion of antidiuretic hormone in a dog, *J Am Vet Med Assoc* 175(2):181–186, 1979.
65. Brofman PJ, Knostman KA, DiBartola SP: Granulomatous amebic meningoencephalitis causing the syndrome of inappropriate secretion of antidiuretic hormone in a dog, *J Vet Intern Med* 17(2):230–234, 2003.
66. Shiel RE, Pinilla M, Mooney CT: Syndrome of inappropriate antidiuretic hormone secretion associated with congenital hydrocephalus in a dog, *J Am Anim Hosp Assoc* 45(5):249–252, 2009.
67. Pierce ST: Paraendocrine syndromes, *Curr Opin Oncol* 5(4):639–645, 1993.
68. Sorensen JB, Andersen MK, Hansen HH: Syndrome of inappropriate secretion of antidiuretic hormone (SIADH) in malignant disease, *J Intern Med* 238(2):97–110, 1995.
69. Kinzie BJ: Management of the syndrome of inappropriate secretion of antidiuretic hormone, *Clin Pharm* 6(8):625–633, 1987.
70. Ogilvie GK, Weigel RM, Haschek WM, et al: Prognostic factors for tumor remission and survival in dogs after surgery for primary lung tumor: 76 cases (1975-1985), *JAVMA* 195:109–112, 1989.
71. Galac S, Kooistra HS, Voorhout G, et al: Hyperadrenocorticism in a dog due to ectopic secretion of adrenocorticotropic hormone, *Domest Anim Endocrinol* 28(3):338–348, 2005.
72. Hillyard V, Coombes RC, Greenberg PB, et al: Calcitonin in breast and lung cancer, *Clin Endocrinol* 5:1–8, 1976.
73. Padgett SL, Tillson DM, Henry CJ, et al: Gingival vascular hamartoma with associated paraneoplastic hyperglycemia in a kitten, *J Am Vet Med Assoc* 210:914–915, 1997.
74. Forrester SD, Greco DS, Relford RL: Serum hyperviscosity syndrome associated with multiple myeloma in two cats, *JAVMA* 200(1):79–82, 1992.
75. Forrester SD, Reeford RL: Serum hyperviscosity syndrome: Its diagnosis and treatment, *Vet Med* 1:48–54, 1992.

76. MacEwen EG, Hurvitz AI: Diagnosis and management of monoclonal gammopathies, *Vet Clin North Am* 7:119–132, 1977.
77. Madewell BR, Feldman BF: Characterization of anemias associated with neoplasia in small animals, *J Am Vet Med Assoc* 176:419–425, 1980.
78. Dodds WJ: Autoimmune hemolytic disease and other causes of immune-mediated anemia: an overview, *J Am Anim Hosp Assoc* 13:437–441, 1977.
79. Ogilvie GK, Felsberg PJ, Harris SW: Short term effect of cyclophosphamide and azathioprine on the selected aspects of the canine immune system, *J Vet Immunol Immunopathol* 18:119–127, 1988.
80. Madewall BR, Feldman BF, O'Neil S: Coagulation abnormalities in dogs with neoplastic disease, *Thromb Haemost* 44:35–38, 1980.
81. Mason N, Duval D, Shofer FS, et al: Cyclophosphamide exerts no beneficial effect over prednisone alone in the initial treatment of acute immune-mediated hemolytic anemia in dogs: a randomized controlled clinical trial, *J Vet Intern Med* 17(2):206–212, 2003.
82. Feldman BF: Management of the anemic dog. In Kirk RW, editor: *Current Veterinary Therapy*, VIII ed, Philadelphia, 1983, Saunders, pp 395–400.
83. Comer KM: Anemia as a feature of prmary gastrointestinal neoplasia, *Compend Contin Educ Pract Vet* 12:13–19, 1990.
84. Hammer AS, Couto CG, Swardson C, et al: Hemostatic abnormalities in dogs with hemangiosarcoma, *J Vet Intern Med* 5:11–14, 1991.
85. Sherding RG, Wilson GP: Bone marrow hypoplasia in eight dogs with Sertoli cell tumor, *J Am Vet Med Assoc* 178:497–501, 1982.
86. Sanpera N, Masot N, Janer M, et al: Oestrogen-induced bone marrow aplasia in a dog with a Sertoli cell tumour, *J Small Anim Pract* 43(8):365–369, 2002.
87. Morgan RW: Blood dyscrasias associated with testicular tumors in the dog, *J Am Anim Hosp Assoc* 18:971–975, 1982.
88. Peterson ME: Inappropriate erythropoietin production from a renal carcinoma in a dog with polycythemia, *J Am Vet Med Assoc* 179:995–996, 1981.
89. Scott RC, Patnaik AK: Renal carcinoma with secondary polycythemia in the dog, *J Am Anim Hosp Assoc* 8:275–283, 1972.
90. Nelson RW, Hager D: Renal lymphosarcoma with inappropriate erythropoietin production in a dog, *J Am Vet Med Assoc* 182: 1396–1397, 1983.
91. Couto CG, Boudrieau RJ, Zanjani ED: Tumor-associated erthrocytosis in a dog with a nasal fibrosarcoma, *J Vet Intern Med* 3:183–185, 1989.
92. Gorse MJ: Polycythemia associated with renal fibrosarcoma in a dog, *J Am Vet Med Assoc* 192:793–794, 1988.
93. Durno AS, Webb JA, Gauthier MJ, et al: Polycythemia and inappropriate erythropoietin concentrations in two dogs with renal T-cell lymphoma, *J Am Anim Hosp Assoc* 47(2):122–128, 2011.
94. Yeo EJ, Chun YS, Park JW: New anticancer strategies targeting HIF-1, *Biochem Pharmacol* 68(6):1061–1069, 2004.
95. Czyzyk-Krzeska MF, Meller J: von Hippel-Lindau tumor suppressor: not only HIF's executioner, *Trends Mol Med* 10(4):146–149, 2004.
96. Beurlet S, Krief P, Sansonetti A, et al: Identification of JAK2 mutations in canine primary polycythemia, *Exp Hematol* 39(5): 542–545, 2011.
97. Lappin MR, Lattimer KS: Hematuria and extreme neutrophilic leukocytosis in a dog with renal tubular carcinoma, *J Am Vet Med Assoc* 192:1289–1292, 1988.
98. Thompson JP, Christopher MM, Ellison GW, et al: Paraneoplastic leukocytosis associated with a rectal adenomatous polyp in a dog, *J Am Vet Med Assoc* 201:737–738, 1992.
99. Chinn DR, Myers RK, Matthews JA: Neutrophilic leukocytosis associated with metastatic fibrosarcoma in a dog, *J Am Vet Med Assoc* 186:806–809, 1985.
100. Madewell BR, Wilson DW, Hornoff WJ, et al: Leukemoid blood response and bone infarcts in a dog with renal tubular adenocarcinoma, *J Am Vet Med Assoc* 197:1623–1625, 1990.
101. Sharkey LC, Rosol TJ, Grone A, et al: Production of granulocyte colony-stimulating factor and granulocyte-macrophage colony-stimulating factor by carcinomas in a dog and a cat with paraneoplastic leukocytosis, *J Vet Intern Med* 10:405–408, 1996.
102. Peeters D, Clercx C, Thiry A, et al: Resolution of paraneoplastic leukocytosis and hypertrophic osteopathy after resection of a renal transitional cell carcinoma producing granulocyte-macrophage colony-stimulating factor in a young Bull Terrier, *J Vet Intern Med* 15(4):407–411, 2001.
103. Dole RS, MacPhail CM, Lappin MR: Paraneoplastic leukocytosis with mature neutrophilia in a cat with pulmonary squamous cell carcinoma, *J Feline Med Surg* 6(6):391–395, 2004.
104. Ruslander D, Page RL: Perioperative management of paraneoplastic syndromes, *Vet Surg* 25:47–62, 1995.
105. Jordan HL, Grindem CB, Breitschwerdt EB: Thrombocytopenia in cats: a retrospective study of 41 cases, *J Vet Intern Med* 7:261–265, 1993.
106. Hatgis AM, Feldman BF: Evaluation of hemostatic defects secondary to vascular tumors in dogs: 11 cases (1983-1988), *J Am Vet Med Assoc* 198:891–894, 1991.
107. Helfand SC, Couto CG, Madewell BR: Immune-mediated thrombocytopenia associated with solid tumors in dogs, *J Am Anim Hosp Assoc* 21:787–794, 1985.
108. Rogers KS: Coagulation disorders associated with neoplasia in the dog, *Vet Med* 1:55–61, 1992.
109. McNiel EA, Ogilvie GK, Fettman MJ, et al: Platelet hyperfunction in dogs with malignancies, *J Vet Intern Med* 11:178–182, 1997.
110. Denko NC, Giaccia AJ: Tumor hypoxia, the physiological link between Trousseau's syndrome (carcinoma-induced coagulopathy) and metastasis, *Cancer Res* 61(3):795–798, 2001.
111. Ratnoff OD: Hemostatic emergencies in malignancy, *Semin Oncol* 16(6):561–571, 1989.
112. Sarris AH, Kempin S, Berman E, et al: High incidence of disseminated intravascular coagulation during remission induction of adult patients with acute lymphoblastic leukemia, *Blood* 79:1305–1310, 1992.
113. Feldman BF, Madewell BR, O'Neil S: Disseminated intravascular coagulation: anti-thrombin, plasminogen, and coagulation abnormalities in 41 dogs, *J Am Vet Med Assoc* 179:151–154, 1981.
114. Green RA: Clinical Implications of antithrombin III deficiency in animal diseases, *Comp Cont Ed* 6(6):537–546, 1984.
115. Maruyama H, Miura T, Sakai M, et al: The incidence of disseminated intravascular coagulation in dogs with malignant tumor, *J Vet Med Sci* 66(5):573–575, 2004.
116. Stockhaus C, Kohn B, Rudolph R, et al: Correlation of haemostatic abnormalities with tumour stage and characteristics in dogs with mammary carcinoma, *J Small Anim Pract* 40(7):326–331, 1999.
117. Susaneck SJ, Allen TA, Hoopes J, et al: Inflammatory mammary carcinoma in the dog, *J Am Anim Hosp Assoc* 19:971–976, 1983.
118. Hammer AS, Couto CG, Bailey MQ: Essential thrombocythemia in a cat, *Proc Vet Cancer Soc* 8:18, 1988.
119. Hogan DF, Dhaliwal RS, Sisson DD, et al: Paraneoplastic thrombocytosis-induced systemic thromboembolism in a cat, *J Am Anim Hosp Assoc* 35(6):483–486, 1999.
120. Degen MA, Feldman BF, Turrel JM, et al: Thrombocytosis associated with myeloproliferative disorder in a dog, *J Am Vet Med Assoc* 194:1457–1459, 1989.
121. Sellon RK, Rottman JB, Jordan HL, et al: Hypereosinophilia associated with transitional cell carcinoma in a cat, *J Am Vet Med Assoc* 201:591–593, 1992.
122. Barrs VR, Beatty JA, McCandlish IA, et al: Hypereosinophilic paraneoplastic syndrome in a cat with intestinal T cell lymphosarcoma, *J Small Anim Pract* 43(9):401–405, 2002.
123. Couto CG: Tumor associated eosinophilia in a dog, *J Am Vet Med Assoc* 184:837–838, 1984.
124. Fews D, Scase TJ, Battersby IA: Leiomyosarcoma of the pericardium, with epicardial metastases and peripheral eosinophilia in a dog, *J Comp Pathol* 138(4):224–228, 2008.

125. Marchetti V, Benetti C, Citi S, et al: Paraneoplastic hypereosinophilia in a dog with intestinal T-cell lymphoma, *Vet Clin Pathol* 34(3):259–263, 2005.
126. Fossum TW, Wellman M, Relford RL, et al: Eosinophilic pleural or peritoneal effusions in dogs and cats: 14 cases (1986-1992), *J Am Vet Med Assoc* 202:1873–1876, 1993.
127. Batlivala TP, Bacon NJ, Avery AC, et al: Paraneoplastic T cell lymphocytosis associated with a thymoma in a dog, *J Small Anim Pract* 51(9):491–494, 2010.
128. Honn KV, Tang DG, Crissman JD: Platelets and cancer metastasis: a causal relationship? *Cancer Metastasis Rev* 11(3-4):325–351, 1992.
129. Boyce S, Harper J: Paraneoplastic dermatoses, *Dermatol Clin* 20(3):523–532, 2002.
130. Turek MM: Cutaneous paraneoplastic syndromes in dogs and cats: a review of the literature, *Vet Dermatol* 14(6):279–296, 2003.
131. Cohen PR, Holder WR, Tucker SB, et al: Sweet syndrome in patients with solid tumors, *Cancer* 72:2723–2731, 1993.
132. Brooks DG, Campbell KL, Dennis JS, et al: Pancreatic paraneoplastic alopecia in three cats, *J Am Anim Hosp Assoc* 30:557–563, 1994.
133. Tasker S, Griffon DJ, Nuttall TJ, et al: Resolution of paraneoplastic alopecia following surgical removal of a pancreatic carcinoma in a cat, *J Small Anim Pract* 40(1):16–19, 1999.
134. Pascal-Tenorio A, Olivry T, Gross TL, et al: Paraneoplastic alopecia associated with internal malignancies in the cat, *Vet Dermatol* 8:47–51, 1997.
135. Godfrey DR: A case of feline paraneoplastic alopecia with secondary Malassezia-associated dermatitis, *J Small Anim Pract* 39:394–396, 1998.
136. Barrs VR, Martin P, France M, et al: What is your diagnosis? Feline paraneoplastic alopecia associated with pancreatic and bile duct carcinomas, *J Small Anim Pract* 40(12):559, 595, 596, 1999.
137. Barthez PY, Marks SL, Woo J, et al: Pheochromocytoma in dogs: 61 cases (1984-1995), *J Vet Intern Med* 11:272–278, 1997.
138. Herrera MF, Stone E, Deitel M, Asa SL: Pheochromocytoma producing multiple vasoactive peptides, *Arch Surg* 127:105–108, 1992.
139. Miller WH: Cutaneous flushing associated with intrathoracic neoplasia in a dog, *J Am Anim Hosp Assoc* 28:217–219, 1992.
140. Shepherd JJ, Challis DR, Davies PF, et al: Multiple endocrine neoplasm, type 1: Gastrinomas, pancreatic neoplasms, microcarcinoids, the Zollinger-Ellison syndrome, lymph nodes, and hepatic metastases, *Arch Surg* 128:1133–1142, 1993.
141. Gilbert PA, Griffin CE, Walder EJ: Nodular dermatofibrosis and renal cystadenoma in a German Shepherd dog, *J Am Anim Hosp Assoc* 26:253–256, 1990.
142. Lium G, Moe E: Hereditary multifocal renal cystadenocarcinomas and nodular dermatofibrosis in the German Shepherd dog: macroscopic and histopathologic changes, *Vet Pathol* 22:447–455, 1985.
143. Atlee BA, DeBoer DJ, Ihrke PJ, et al: Nodular dermatofibrosis in German Shepherd dogs as a marker for renal cystadenocarcinoma, *J Am Anim Hosp Assoc* 27:481–487, 1991.
144. Suter M, Lott-Stoltz G, Wild P: Generalized nodular dermatofibrosis in six Alsatians, *Vet Pathol* 20:632–634, 1983.
145. Jonasdottir TJ, Mellersh CS, Moe L, et al: Genetic mapping of a naturally occurring hereditary renal cancer syndrome in dogs, *Proc Natl Acad Sci U S A* 97(8):4132–4137, 2000.
146. Lingaas F, Comstock KE, Kirkness EF, et al: A mutation in the canine BHD gene is associated with hereditary multifocal renal cystadenocarcinoma and nodular dermatofibrosis in the German Shepherd dog, *Hum Mol Genet* 12(23):3043–3053, 2003.
147. Moe L, Lium B: Hereditary multifocal renal cystadenocarcinomas and nodular dermatofibrosis in 51 German shepherd dogs, *J Small Anim Pract* 38(11):498–505, 1997.
148. Warren MB, Torres-Cabala CA, Turner ML, et al: Expression of Birt-Hogg-Dube gene mRNA in normal and neoplastic human tissues, *Mod Pathol* 17(8):998–1011, 2004.
149. Menko FH, van Steensel MA, Giraud S, et al: Birt-Hogg-Dube syndrome: diagnosis and management, *Lancet Oncol* 10(12):1199–1206, 2009.
150. Allenspach K, Arnold P, Glaus T, et al: Glucagon-producing neuroendocrine tumour associated with hypoaminoacidaemia and skin lesions, *J Small Anim Pract* 41(9):402–406, 2000.
151. Byrne KP: Metabolic epidermal necrosis-hepatocutaneous syndrome, *Vet Clin North Am Small Anim Pract* 29(6):1337–1355, 1999.
152. Gross TL, Song MD, Havel PJ, et al: Superficial necrolytic dermatitis (necrolytic migratory erythema) in dogs, *Vet Pathol* 30:75–81, 1993.
153. Cave TA, Evans H, Hargreaves J, et al: Metabolic epidermal necrosis in a dog associated with pancreatic adenocarcinoma, hyperglucagonaemia, hyperinsulinaemia and hypoaminoacidaemia, *J Small Anim Pract* 48(9):522–526, 2007.
154. Torres SMF, Caywood DD, O'Brien TD, et al: Resolution of superficial necrolytic dermatitis following excision of a glucagon-secreting pancreatic neoplasm in a dog, *J Am Anim Hosp Assoc* 33:313–319, 1997.
155. Oberkirchner U, Linder KE, Zadrozny L, et al: Successful treatment of canine necrolytic migratory erythema (superficial necrolytic dermatitis) due to metastatic glucagonoma with octreotide, *Vet Dermatol* 21(5):510–516, 2010.
156. Zini E, Bovero A, Nigrisoli E, et al: Sarcomatoid renal cell carcinoma with osteogenic differentiation and paraneoplastic hepatopathy in a dog, possibly related to human Stauffer's syndrome, *J Comp Pathol* 129(4):303–307, 2003.
157. Poszepczynska-Guigne E, Viguier M, et al: Paraneoplastic acral vascular syndrome: epidemiologic features, clinical manifestations, and disease sequelae, *J Am Acad Dermatol* 47(1):47–52, 2002.
158. Ashley PA, Bowman LA: Symmetric cutaneous necrosis of the hind feet and multicentric follicular lymphoma in a cat, *J Am Vet Med Assoc* 214:211–214, 1999.
159. Godfrey DR: A case of feline paraneoplastic alopecia with secondary Malassezia-associated dermatitis, *J Small Anim Pract* 39(8):394–396, 1998.
160. Mauldin EA, Morris DO, Goldschmidt MH: Retrospective study: The presence of Malassezia in feline skin biopsies. A clinicopathological study, *Vet Dermatol* 13(1):7–13, 2002.
161. Schmidt E, Zillikens D: Modern diagnosis of autoimmune blistering skin diseases, *Autoimmun Rev* 10(2):84–89, 2010.
162. Olivry T, Linder KE: Dermatoses affecting desmosomes in animals: a mechanistic review of acantholytic blistering skin diseases, *Vet Dermatol* 20(5-6):313–326, 2009.
163. Lemmens P, De Bruin A, De Meulemeester J, et al: Paraneoplastic pemphigus in a dog, *Vet Dermatol* 9:127–134, 1998.
164. Elmore SA, Basseches J, Anhalt GJ, et al: Paraneoplastic pemphigus in a dog with splenic sarcoma, *Vet Pathol* 42(1):88–91, 2005.
165. De Bruin A, Muller E, Wyder M, et al: Periplakin and envoplakin are target antigens in canine and human paraneoplastic pemphigus, *J Am Acad Dermatol* 40(5 Pt 1):682–685, 1999.
166. Nishifuji K, Olivry T, Ishii K, et al: IgG autoantibodies directed against desmoglein 3 cause dissociation of keratinocytes in canine pemphigus vulgaris and paraneoplastic pemphigus, *Vet Immunol Immunopathol* 117(3-4):209–221, 2007.
167. Nishifuji K, Tamura K, Konno H, et al: Development of an enzyme-linked immunosorbent assay for detection of circulating IgG autoantibodies against canine desmoglein 3 in dogs with pemphigus, *Vet Dermatol* 20(5-6):331–337, 2009.
168. Tepper LC, Spiegel IB, Davis GJ: Diagnosis of erythema multiforme associated with thymoma in a dog and treated with thymectomy, *J Am Anim Hosp Assoc* 47(2):e19–e25, 2011.
169. Singh A, Boston SE, Poma R: Thymoma-associated exfoliative dermatitis with post-thymectomy myasthenia gravis in a cat, *Can Vet J* 51(7):757–760, 2010.
170. Rottenberg S, Von TC, Roosje PJ: Thymoma-associated exfoliative dermatitis in cats, *Vet Pathol* 41(4):429–433, 2004.

171. Cohen M, Post GS: Nephrogenic diabetes insipidus in a dog with intestinal leiomyosarcoma, *J Am Vet Med Assoc* 215(12):1818–1820, 1806, 1999.
172. Zimmerman SW, Vishnu-Moorthy A, Burkholder PM: Glomerulopathies associated with neoplastic disease. In Rieselbach RE, Garnick NB, editors: *Cancer in the kidney*, Philadelphia, 1982, Lea & Febiger.
173. Lien YH, Lai LW: Pathogenesis, diagnosis and management of paraneoplastic glomerulonephritis, *Nat Rev Nephrol* 7(2):85–95, 2011.
174. Lee JC, Yamauchi H, Hopper J: The association of cancer and nephrotic syndrome, *Ann Intern Med* 64:41–47, 1966.
175. Alpers CE, Cotran RS: Neoplasia and glomerular injury, *Kidney Int* 30(4):465–473, 1986.
176. Dinh BL, Brassard A: Renal lesion associated with the Walker 256 adenocarcinoma in the rat, *Br J Exp Pathol* 49:145–148, 1968.
177. Norris SH: Paraneoplastic glomerulopathies, *Semin Nephrol* 13(3):258–272, 1993.
178. Page RL, Stiff ME, McEntee MC, et al: Transient glomerulonephropathy associated with primary erythrocytosis in a dog, *J Am Vet Med Assoc* 196:620–622, 1990.
179. Willard MD, Krehbiel JD, Schmidt GM, et al: Serum and urine protein abnormalities associated with lymphocytic leukemia and glomerulonephritis in a dog, *J Am Anim Hosp Assoc* 17:381 386, 1981.
180. Waterhouse DM, Natale RB, Cody RL: Breast cancer and paraneoplastic cerebellar degeneration, *Cancer* 68:1835–1841, 1991.
181. Nishi Y, Yufu Y, Shinomiya S, et al: Polyneuropathy in acute megakaryoblastic leukemia, *Cancer* 68:2033–2036, 1991.
182. Braik T, Evans AT, Telfer M, et al: Paraneoplastic neurological syndromes: unusual presentations of cancer. A practical review, *Am J Med Sci* 340(4):301–308, 2010.
183. Shelton GD, Willard MD, Cardinet GH, et al: Acquired myasthenia gravis: selective involvement of esophageal, pharyngeal, and facial muscles, *J Vet Intern Med* 4:281–284, 1990.
184. Ridyard AE, Rhind SM, French AT, et al: Myasthenia gravis associated with cutaneous lymphoma in a dog, *J Small Anim Pract* 41(8):348–351, 2000.
185. Braund KG: Remote effects of cancer on the nervous system, *Semin Vet Med Surg (Sm Anim)* 5:262–270, 1990.
186. Bergman PJ, Bruyette DS, Coyne BE, et al: Canine clinical peripheral neuropathy associated with pancreatic islet cell carcinoma, *Prog Vet Neurol* 5:57–62, 1994.
187. Braund KG, Steiss JE, Amling KA, et al: Insulinoma and subclinical peripheral neuropathy in two dogs, *J Vet Intern Med* 1:86–90, 1987.
188. Nelson RW, Morrison WB, Lurus AG, et al: Diencephalic syndrome secondary to intracranial astrocytoma in a dog, *J Am Vet Med Assoc* 179:1004–1010, 1981.
189. Inzana KD: Paraneoplastic neuromuscular disorders, *Vet Clin North Am Small Anim Pract* 34(6):1453–1467, 2004.
190. Shelton GD: Routine and specialized laboratory testing for the diagnosis of neuromuscular diseases in dogs and cats, *Vet Clin Pathol* 39(3):278–295, 2010.
191. Leys K, Lang B, Johnston I, et al: Calcium channel autoantibodies in the Lambert-Eaton myasthenic syndrome, *Ann Neurol* 29:307–310, 1991.
192. Mareska M, Gutmann L: Lambert-Eaton myasthenic syndrome, *Semin Neurol* 24(2):149–153, 2004.
193. Krotje LJ, Fix AS, Potthoff AD: Acquired myasthenia gravis and cholangiocellular carcinoma in a dog, *J Am Vet Med Assoc* 197(4):488–490, 1990.
194. Lainesse MFC, Taylor SM, Myers SL, et al: Focal myasthenia gravis as a paraneoplastic syndrome of canine thymoma: Improvement following thymectomy, *J Am Anim Hosp Assoc* 32:111–117, 1996.
195. Moore AS, Madewell BR, Cardinet III GH, et al: Osteogenic sarcoma and myasthenia gravis in a dog, *J Am Vet Med Assoc* 197(2):226–227, 1990.
196. Joseph RJ, Carrillo JM, Lennon VA: Myasthenia gravis in the cat, *J Vet Intern Med* 2:75–79, 1988.
197. Klebanow ER: Thymoma and acquired myasthenia gravis in the dog: a case report and review of 13 additional cases, *J Am Anim Hosp Assoc* 28:63–69, 1992.
198. Atwater SW, Powers BE, Park RD, et al: Thymoma in dogs: 23 cases (1980-1991), *J Am Vet Med Assoc* 205(7):1007–1013, 1994.
199. Moffet AC: Metastatic thymoma and acquired generalized myasthenia gravis in a beagle, *Can Vet J* 48(1):91–93, 2007.
200. Zitz JC, Birchard SJ, Couto GC, et al: Results of excision of thymoma in cats and dogs: 20 cases (1984-2005), *J Am Vet Med Assoc* 232(8):1186–1192, 2008.
201. Villiers E, Dobson J: Multiple myeloma with associated polyneuropathy in a German shepherd dog, *J Small Anim Pract* 39(5):249–251, 1998.
202. Mariani CL, Shelton SB, Alsup JC: Paraneoplastic polyneuropathy and subsequent recovery following tumor removal in a dog, *J Am Anim Hosp Assoc* 35(4):302–305, 1999.
203. Cavana P, Sammartano F, Capucchio MT, et al: Peripheral neuropathy in a cat with renal lymphoma, *J Feline Med Surg* 11(10):869–872, 2009.
204. Ogilvie GK: Paraneoplastic syndromes. In Withrow SJ, MacEwen EG, editors: *Small animal clinical oncology*, ed 2, Philadelphia, 1996, Saunders, pp 32–42.
205. Gram WD, Wheaton LG, Snyder PW, et al: Feline hypertrophic osteopathy associated with pulmonary carcinoma, *J Am Anim Hosp Assoc* 26:425–428, 1990.
206. Seaman RL, Patton CS: Treatment of renal nephroblastoma in an adult dog, *J Am Anim Hosp Assoc* 39(1):76–79, 2003.
207. Barrand KR, Scudamore CL: Canine hypertrophic osteoarthropathy associated with a malignant Sertoli cell tumour, *J Small Anim Pract* 42(3):143–145, 2001.
208. Becker TJ, Perry RL, Watson GL: Regression of hypertrophic osteopathy in a cat after surgical excision of an adrenocortical carcinoma, *J Am Anim Hosp Assoc* 35(6):499–505, 1999.
209. Randolph JF, Center SA, Flanders JA, et al: Hypertrophic osteopathy associated with adenocarcinoma of the esophageal glands in a dog, *J Am Vet Med Assoc* 184:98–99, 1984.
210. Halliwell WH, Ackerman N: Botryoid rhabdomyosarcoma of the urinary bladder and hypertrophic osteoarthropathy in a young dog, *J Am Vet Med Assoc* 165:911–913, 1974.
211. Caywood DD, Osborne CA, Stevens JB, et al: Hypertrophic osteoarthropathy associated with an atypical nephroblastoma in a dog, *J Am Anim Hosp Assoc* 16:855–865, 1980.
212. Rendano VT, Slauson DO: Hypertrophic osteopathy in a dog with prostatic adenocarcinoma and without thoracic metastasis, *J Am Anim Hosp Assoc* 18:905–909, 1982.
213. Johnson RL, Lenz SD: Hypertrophic osteopathy associated with a renal adenoma in a cat, *J Vet Diagn Invest* 23(1):171–175, 2011.
214. Uchiyama G, Ishizuka M, Sugiura N: Hypertrophic pulmonary osteoarthropathy inactivated by antitumor chemotherapy, *Radiat Med* 3(1):25–28, 1985.
215. Hara Y, Tagawa M, Ejima H, et al: Regression of hypertrophic osteopathy following removal of intrathoracic neoplasia derived from vagus nerve in a dog, *J Vet Med Sci* 57(1):133–135, 1995.
216. Abe Y, Kurita S, Ohkubo Y, et al: A case of pulmonary adenocarcinoma associated with hypertrophic osteoarthropathy due to vascular endothelial growth factor, *Anticancer Res* 22(6B):3485–3488, 2002.
217. Madewell BR, Nyland TG, Weigel JE: Regression of hypertrophic osteopathy following pneumonectomy in a dog, *J Am Vet Med Assoc* 172:818–821, 1978.
218. Hahn KA, Richardson RC: Use of cisplatin for control of metastatic malignant mesenchymoma and hypertrophic osteopathy in a dog, *J Am Vet Med Assoc* 195:351–353, 1989.
219. Brodey RS: *Hypertrophic osteoarthropathy. Spontaneous animal models of human disease*, San Diego, 1980, Academic Press.

220. Amital H, Applbaum YH, Vasiliev L, et al: Hypertrophic pulmonary osteoarthropathy: control of pain and symptoms with pamidronate, *Clin Rheumatol* 23(4):330–332, 2004.
221. London CA, Malpas PB, Wood-Follis SL, et al: Multi-center, placebo-controlled, double-blind, randomized study of oral toceranib phosphate (SU11654), a receptor tyrosine kinase inhibitor, for the treatment of dogs with recurrent (either local or distant) mast cell tumor following surgical excision, *Clin Cancer Res* 15(11):3856–3865, 2009.
222. Greenberg SB, Taber L: Fever of unknown origin. In Mackowiak PA, editor: *Fever: Mechanisms and management*, New York, 1991, Raven Press, pp 183.
223. Saper CB, Breder CD: The neurologic basis of fever, *N Engl J Med* 330:1880–1886, 1994.

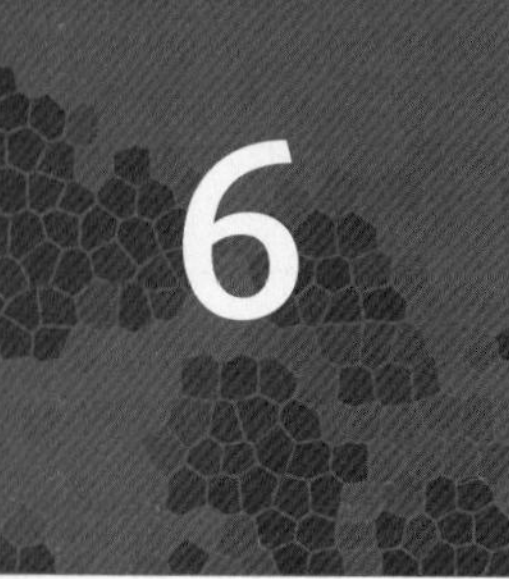

Imaging in Oncology

Lisa J. Forrest and Susan L. Kraft

Diagnostic imaging plays an essential role in the management of the cancer patient. The initial diagnosis, staging, surgical and radiation treatment planning and response to therapy all involve imaging to a varying extent. Routine radiographs, ultrasound, nuclear medicine, and cross-sectional imaging in the form of computed tomography (CT) and magnetic resonance imaging (MRI) are routinely used in veterinary oncology. The choice of imaging modality depends on many factors, including the desired outcome. The biologic behavior of the tumor directs the imaging choice in cancer staging, and imaging may play an important role in guiding serial tumor biopsy during the course of therapy. The sophistication of imaging modalities continues to increase exponentially. Each modality has advantages and disadvantages with regard to cost, availability, sensitivity, specificity, and qualities of anatomic versus functional imaging (Table 6-1). Advanced molecular imaging techniques, which measure biologic processes at the cellular level,[1-3] are quickly becoming commonplace in physician-based oncology and have the potential to play an important role in the tailoring of cancer therapy in veterinary patients.

Imaging Modalities

Radiography

Conventional radiography has been the mainstay of cancer imaging for many years because of its accessibility and low cost. However, it usually is relegated to a screening test and is often followed by other imaging modalities to better differentiate and define tumor extent (Figure 6-1).[4,5] Radiographic images are produced by the differential absorption of x-rays as the primary beam passes through the patient. Some x-ray photons are absorbed by the body and some pass through. Absorption depends on the thickness, physical density, and effective atomic number of the tissues of the patient's body. The x-rays that are not absorbed reach the radiographic film and determine the blackness and gray scale of the image.

Two of the strengths of radiography are the global information it provides and its excellent utility for bone imaging, especially the appendicular skeleton.[6] Thoracic and abdominal radiographs are excellent screening tools for feline and canine lymphoma patients to determine thoracic lymph node and pulmonary involvement, as well as liver, spleen, and abdominal lymph node neoplastic spread.[7,8] Radiography's greatest weaknesses are the superimposition of overlying structures and that only a few radiographic opacities are depicted. CT and MRI have replaced radiography for imaging of the head and, in some circumstances, the axial skeleton.[9-12]

Computed Tomography

As does radiography, CT relies on the physical density differences between tissues to form the image. Unlike radiography, CT portrays *slices* of the patient without superimposition of structures because the images are computer generated and the gray scale display is superior. Although thoracic radiographs are routinely used as a screening method for evaluation of primary and metastatic tumors of the lung, mediastinum, and ribs, CT provides superior information for characterizing and anatomically localizing thoracic lesions for their diagnosis and treatment (see Figure 6-1). Compared with radiography, CT is more sensitive for identifying pulmonary nodules (Figure 6-2), mediastinal lymphadenopathy, and pleural and other masses.[5,13-17] CT should be used to ascertain the full extent of pulmonary nodules from metastatic disease and when a primary lung tumor has been identified to evaluate for intrathoracic metastases and tracheobronchial lymphadenopathy.

CT is more sensitive than radiography to osteolysis and osteoproduction associated with neoplasia, and its three-dimensional (3D) information is especially useful for skeletal structures such as the sinonasal region, orbit (Figure 6-3), ear canals, and skeleton (Figure 6-4).[9] CT is also useful to determine the origin and extent of abdominal mass lesions, and compared to ultrasonography, CT can better document the relationship of a mass with surrounding anatomic structures (Figure 6-5).[18,19] Infiltrative muscular lesions such as infiltrative lipomas and soft tissue sarcomas are routinely imaged with CT for both surgical and radiotherapy planning.[12,20] A contrast-enhanced scan is essential during CT to improve visualization of tumor margins, especially for infiltrative tumors such as feline vaccine–associated sarcomas.[21]

CT is exceedingly useful for both surgical and radiotherapy planning. Although MRI has better tissue differentiation, CT is used most often for radiotherapy treatment planning because there is no image distortion and the physical tissue density is available for input into treatment planning computers.[22,23] It is extremely important to position the radiotherapy patient for the CT scan done for radiation treatment planning in a manner that can reliably be repeated during therapy. This will ensure the treatment is delivered as planned. CT is also amenable to obtaining image-guided biopsy of masses that are not readily obtained with ultrasound guidance, and is particularly helpful for thoracic, brain, spinal, and skeletal lesion biopsy (Figure 6-6).[24-28] Contrast-enhanced CT angiography (CTA) is now also becoming more routine due to the increasing availability of multidetector CT scanners in veterinary medicine. CTA allows detection of tumor vascular invasion and can also depict tumor vascular supply for interventional therapies (Figure 6-7). Dynamic multiphase CT can also improve detection of metastases and small tumors such as insulinomas and may distinguish benign from malignant hypervascular primary hepatic tumors.[29-32]

Tumor perfusion, vascular permeability, and tumor blood volume can predict tumor aggressiveness through the use of

TABLE 6-1 Comparison of Imaging Modalities Used in Veterinary Medicine

MODALITY	COST	SENSITIVITY	SPECIFICITY	AVAILABILITY
Radiography*	Low	Moderate-high for bone lesions only	High for bone lesions only	High
Ultrasound*†	Moderate	High	Low-moderate	Moderate-high
CT*†	High	Moderate-high	Moderate-high	Moderate-high
MRI*†	High	High	Moderate-high	Moderate-low
NM†	Moderate-high	Moderate-high	Low	Moderate-low
SPECT and PET†	High	High	Moderate	Low
PET/CT*†	High	High	High	Low

CT, Computed tomography; *MRI,* magnetic resonance imaging; *NM,* nuclear medicine; *SPECT,* single-photon emission computed tomography; *PET,* positron emission tomography.

*Anatomic imaging.

†Functional/physiologic imaging.

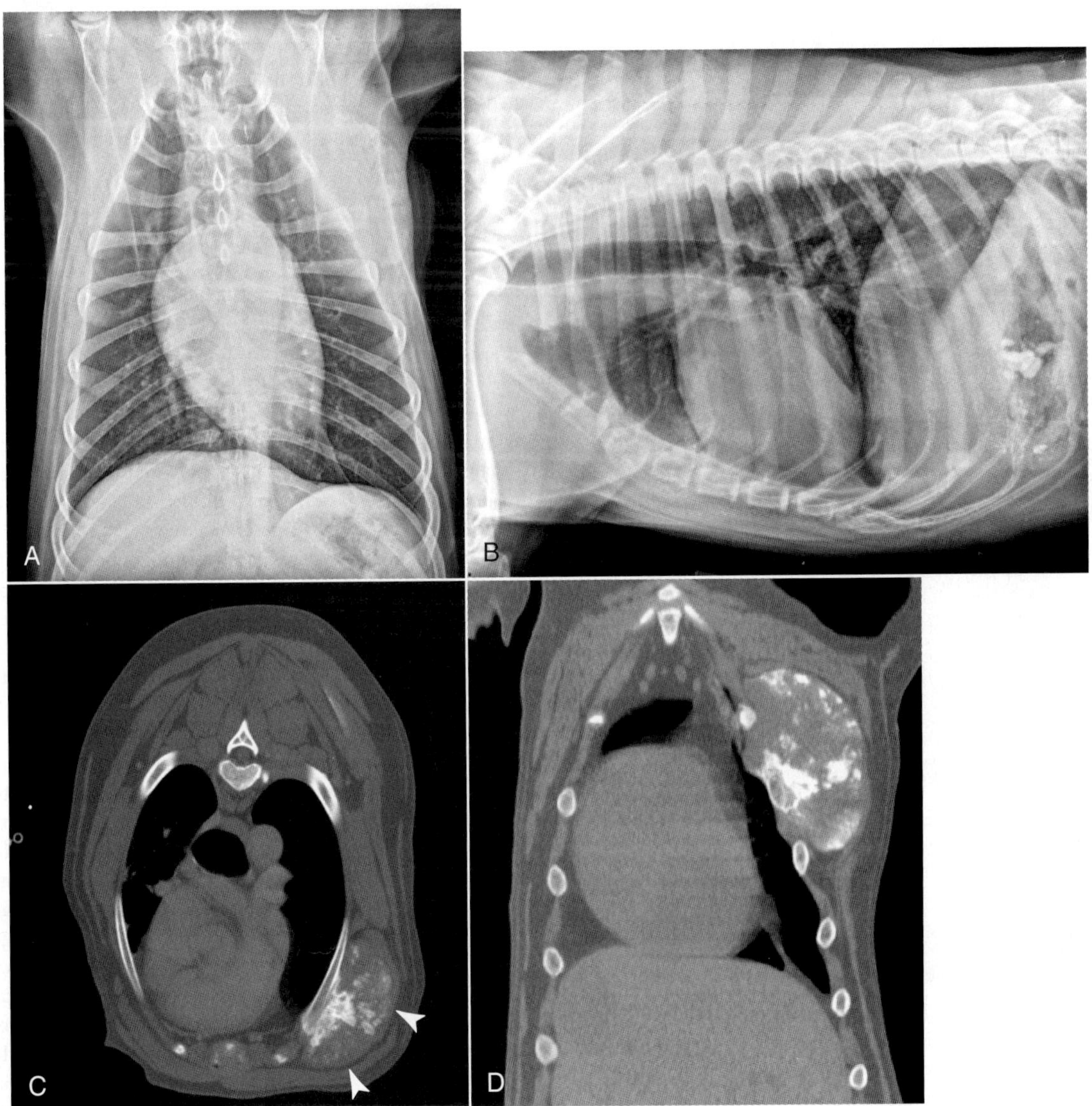

FIGURE 6-1 Lateral and ventral dorsal thoracic radiographs (**A** and **B**) and corresponding CT images (**C,** transverse image and, **D,** dorsal reconstruction) of a dog with a thoracic wall osteosarcoma. Note that the mass is only faintly visible on lateral and ventral dorsal radiographic images, whereas CT provides complete information about tumor margins and extent of rib involvement *(white arrows).*

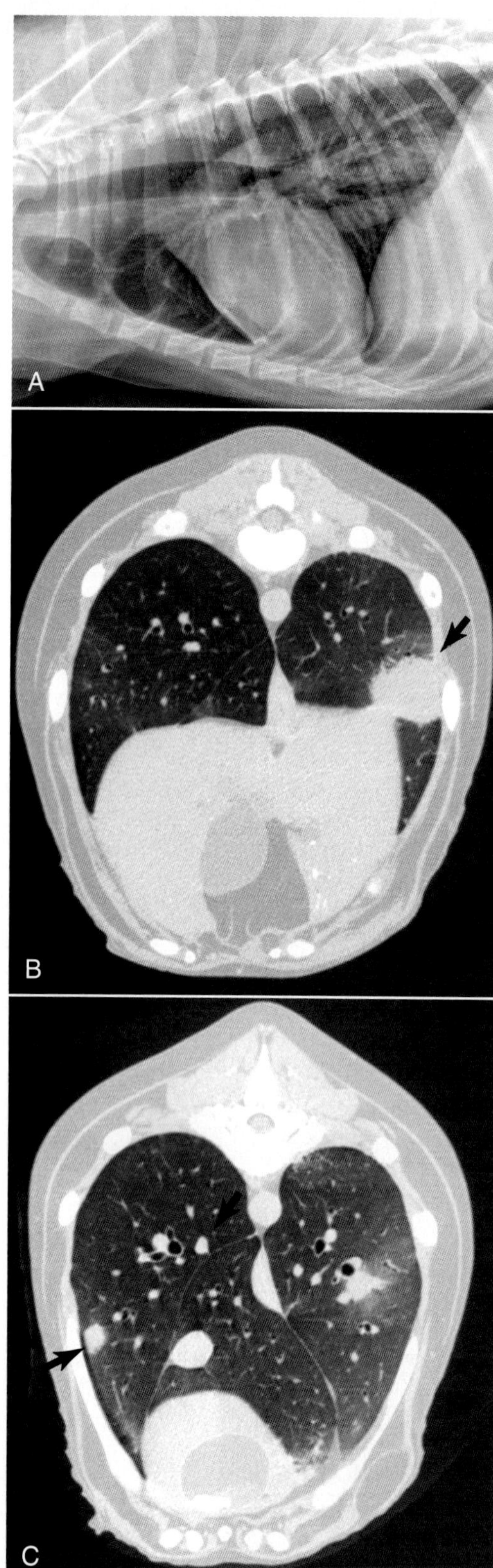

FIGURE 6-2 This large pulmonary mass is barely visible on the right lateral thoracic radiograph due to its superimposition over the esophagus **(A)** but is clearly visible on CT (*black arrow*, **B**) along with additional metastatic nodules that were too small to see on radiographs **(C)**.

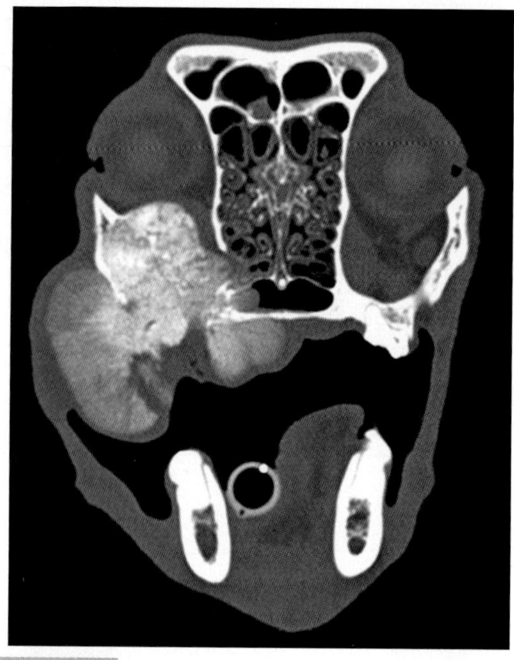

FIGURE 6-3 CT transverse image of a dog with a multilobular osteochondrosarcoma; note the nodular bone formations arising from the zygoma and palate that are encroaching on the orbit and displacing the eye.

dynamic contrast-enhanced CT, which estimates tumor wash-in and wash-out contrast kinetics.[33,34]

Ultrasonography

Ultrasound imaging's ability to evaluate the internal structure of organs and to image body cavities when effusion is present has made it an essential diagnostic tool that has replaced abdominal radiography as the first-line choice in evaluation of the abdomen. The information provided by ultrasound is based on differences in acoustic impedance. The acoustic impedance of a material is a product of its physical density and the velocity of sound in the material. As sound waves pass from tissue to tissue, the amount of sound reflected (echoes) is determined by the impedance difference between tissues. The reflected echoes are detected by the transducer and processed into an image.

Ultrasound is superior to radiographs in instances of pleural or peritoneal effusion due to the loss of visceral detail that occurs on radiographs as the fluid will efface the margins of organs.[35] Ultrasound is also useful in guidance for biopsy or fine-needle aspiration of an observed abnormality. It is more sensitive than survey radiographs for detecting abdominal lymphadenopathy[36-38] and size, shape, margins, heterogeneity, perinodal fat appearance, and vascular pattern of lymph nodes are useful in determining malignancy.[38-42] However, radiographs are superior for detection of bony invasion that may be associated with malignant medial iliac lymph node enlargement, often seen with tumors of the urinary bladder, prostate,[43] and anal glands. Ultrasound is sensitive in the detection of adrenal abnormalities, including vessel invasion, which is usually associated with malignancy (Figure 6-8).[19,44] Ultrasound is routinely used to stage and monitor cats and dogs with mast cell disease, which has a varied appearance.[45,46] It is used extensively in

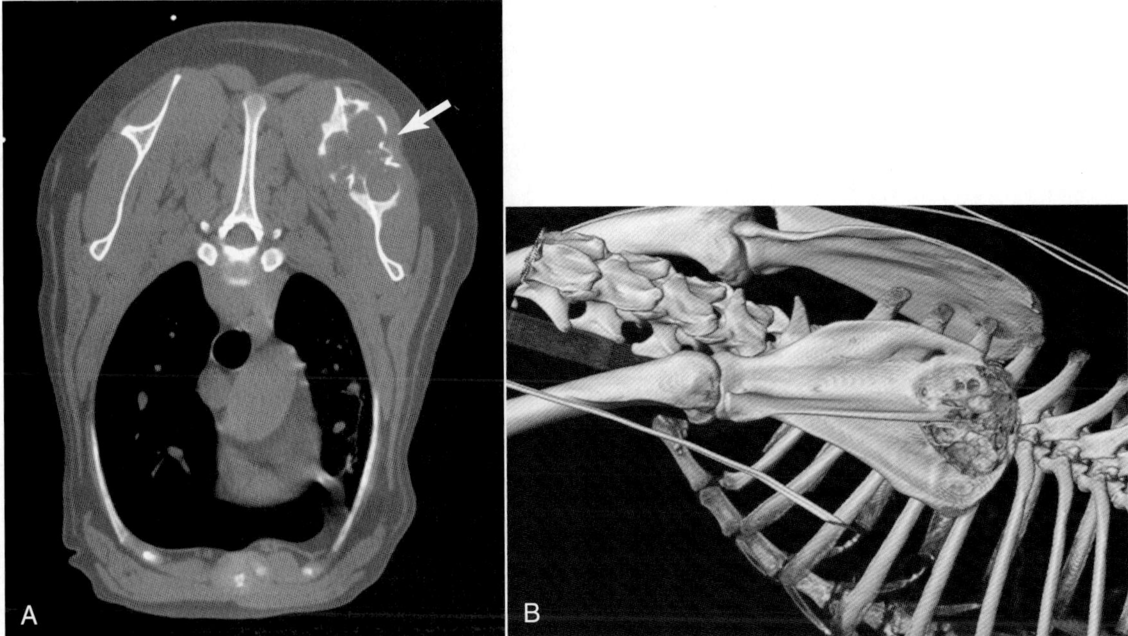

FIGURE 6-4 **A,** CT transverse image *(white arrow)*. **B,** Three-dimensional reconstructed image of a dog with scapular osteosarcoma, which provides an excellent visual assessment for surgical planning.

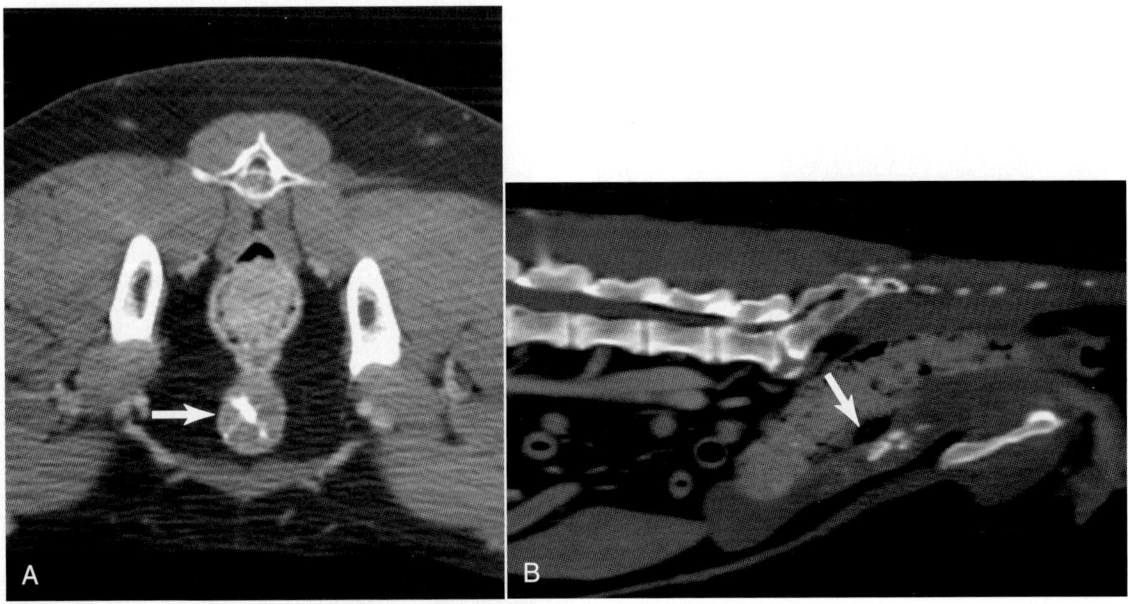

FIGURE 6-5 CT images of the urethra of a dog with transitional cell carcinoma (TCC). Note the thickened urethra with multifocal calcifications on the transverse image **(A)** and sagittal reconstructed image **(B).**

patients with gastrointestinal disease for initial diagnosis and monitoring of therapy.[47-52]

Ultrasonography is sensitive for lesion detection, but it is not specific for disease etiology. Many studies have attempted unsuccessfully to differentiate benign from malignant lesions based on sonographic appearance.[44,46,50,53-55] Therefore biopsy or fine-needle aspirates of lesions are necessary. Ultrasound-guided sampling of tissue can be performed quickly, accurately, and safely.[56-60] A caveat is the potential seeding of tumor cells from ultrasound-guided percutaneous sampling of transitional cell carcinoma.[61]

Advances in ultrasound equipment and the development of sonographic contrast agents are increasing the specificity of ultrasound.[62] Doppler techniques are used to assess tumor vasculature, which is found generally to be tortuous with high velocity as compared to normal tissues.[40,42,63,64] Tissue harmonic imaging transmits at one frequency and receives at twice that frequency. This technique has advantages over fundamental imaging.[62,65] Harmonic imaging and/or ultrasound contrast agents have been used to differentiate benign from malignant lesions[64-76] and continued exploration of this imaging modality is warranted.

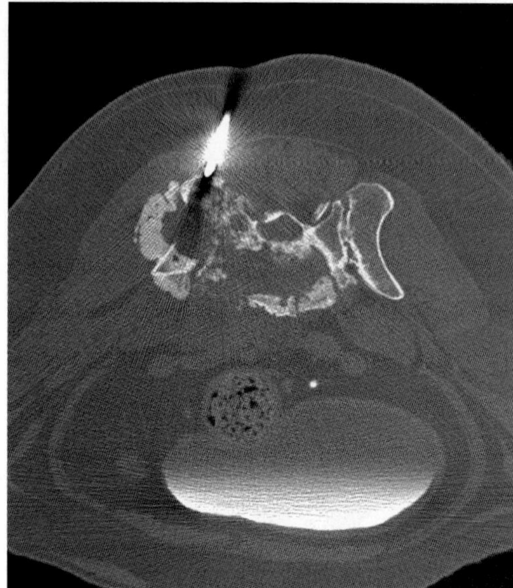

FIGURE 6-6 CT transverse image of a biopsy needle being directed into an aggressive osteolytic bone tumor within the ilial wing of the pelvis. The metallic biopsy needle creates a metal streak artifact *(black lines above and below the visible portion of the needle)* on this image.

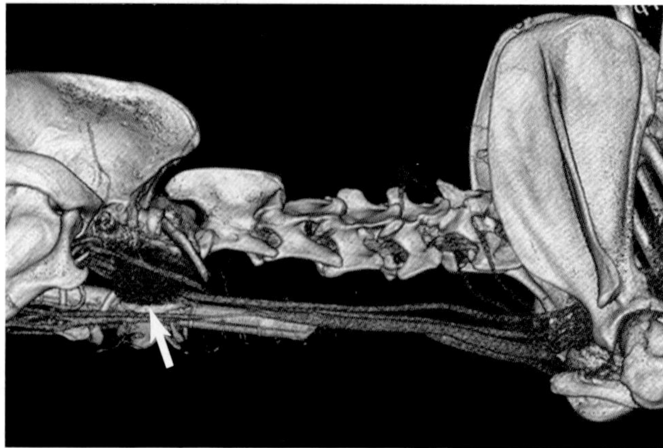

FIGURE 6-7 Lateral view of a 3D-reconstructed CT angiogram of a highly vascular thyroid carcinoma *(white arrow)*. This technique can be useful for identifying the larger vascular territory supplying a tumor.

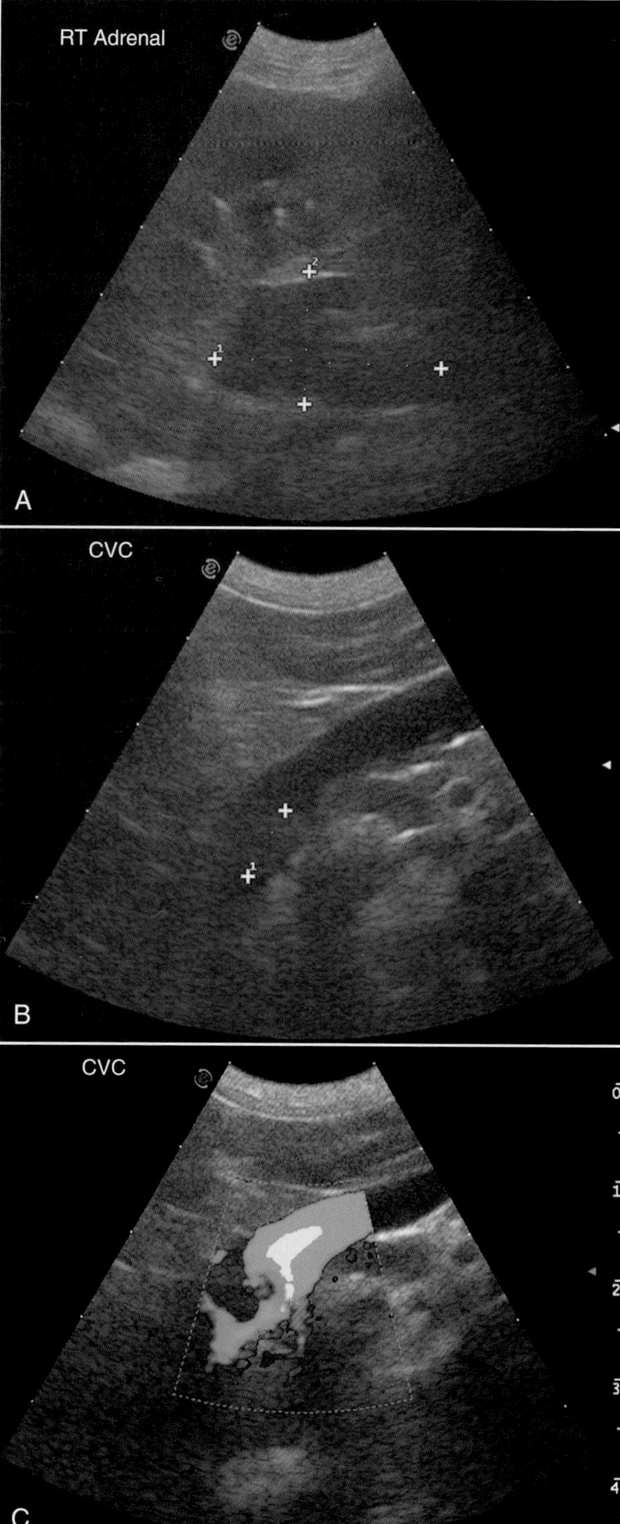

FIGURE 6-8 Ultrasound images of a right adrenal gland tumor with invasion into the caudal vena cava and probable tumor thrombus. **A,** Note the large heterogeneous mass (2.93 × 1.68 cm). **B,** A tumor thrombus or tumor extension is present. **C,** Note the turbulent Doppler flow in the caudal vena cava, indicating invasion of the right adrenal tumor into the vessel.

Magnetic Resonance Imaging

MRI is an advanced imaging technique that provides superb soft tissue images and sensitive detection of pathology based on properties of hydrogen atoms when placed in magnetic and radiofrequency fields. Images can be acquired directly in any plane with MRI, compared to CT in which sagittal and dorsal images are made by reconstructing transverse image data. MRI is the imaging modality of choice for the evaluation of the central nervous system, and the characteristics of the common canine and feline neurologic tumors are now well described (Figure 6-9).[77-82] MRI provides better anatomic detail and more sensitive detection of neuropathology than CT but is less useful for assessing cortical bone because of the number and characteristics of hydrogen protons in bone. Bone landmarks, areas of mineralization, and periosteal bone production are not as obvious with MRI as with CT. Nevertheless, MRI provides excellent anatomic detail and sensitive detection of infiltrative diseases affecting the musculoskeletal soft tissues, including joints, ligaments and tendons, and bone marrow, and is most accurate in determining the extent of canine appendicular osteosarcoma for limb-sparing procedures (Figure 6-10).[83]

As advanced MR equipment becomes more common in veterinary medicine, MRI's use in cancer diagnosis and staging will increase because of its value in determining tumor morphology, margins, characteristics, and composition.[32,84] MRI is excellent for tumors of the head, neck, and torso, although special measures are sometimes needed to minimize respiratory motion in certain anatomic sites.[85,86] Whole-body MR is under evaluation as a sensitive method for cancer staging that is superior to CT and scintigraphy, and in human clinical trials it can rival the results of positron-emission tomography-CT (PET-CT) without the use of ionizing radiation.[87] Whole-body MRI does require ultrafast imaging methods, so it would be limited to veterinary sites having newer and high-field MR instruments.[84,87] Although CT scans are most often used for radiation therapy planning, MRI provides advantages in select situations, including the ability to anatomically define small at-risk structures such as the optic chiasm and to contour margins of lesions where beam-hardening artifact is problematic with CT.[84] MRI is also quite useful for detecting residual or recurring tumors due to its sensitivity to early disease. New MRI techniques are being developed that allow the study of tumor physiology and metabolism and valuable information about treatment response. Dynamic contrast-enhanced MRI provides information about tumor vascularity, perfusion, and angiogenesis that has been shown to have predictive value for treatment response and outcome (Figure 6-11).[88,89] Diffusion MRI evaluates the mobility of tumor water molecules as a function of cell density and tissue architecture, with an increase in tumor diffusion indicating a positive treatment response and cell death.[32,88,90,91] In vivo MR spectroscopy for measuring malignant metabolic biomarkers such as choline relative to normal surrounding tissue is moving from the research realm into human clinical use for brain and prostatic cancer and also has future potential for veterinary diagnosis.[84,92]

Nuclear Medicine

Diagnostic nuclear medicine, or scintigraphy, involves the administration of radiopharmaceuticals that localize to an area of interest in the body by physiologic processes. Images obtained from nuclear medicine studies do not provide the anatomic detail attainable with other imaging techniques; however, the functional dependence on physiologic processes adds important information. Technetium-99m (^{99m}Tc) is the most commonly used radionuclide because it has excellent imaging qualities and a short half-life (6 hours) and is easily bound to localizing pharmaceuticals. Bone scintigraphy using ^{99m}Tc methylene diphosphonate (^{99m}Tc-MDP) is frequently used in veterinary medicine because it is a simple, sensitive, and noninvasive method of evaluating the entire skeleton.[93] Other commonly used nuclear imaging studies include renal, thyroid, lung,

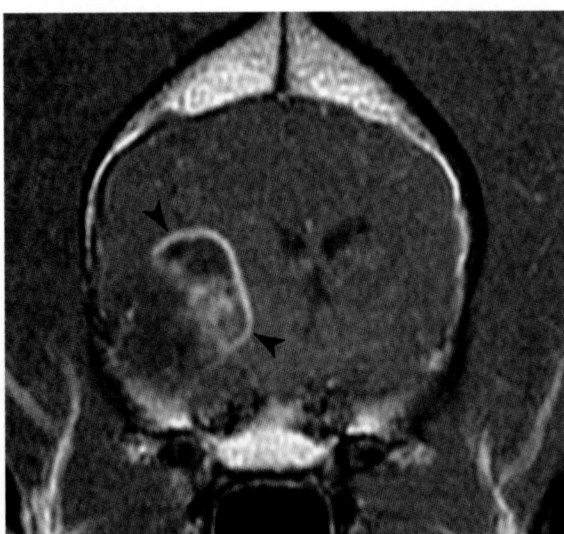

FIGURE 6-9 Postcontrast T1-weighted transverse MR image of a canine oligodendroglioma *(black arrowheads)*. Note its intraaxial location and ring enhancement around a hypointense less enhancing center.

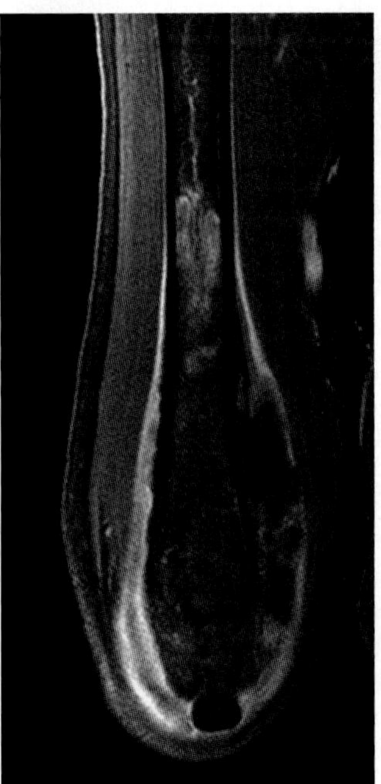

FIGURE 6-10 Fat-saturated postcontrast T1-weighted coronal MR image of a canine femur showing contrast-enhancing infiltrative tumor within the bone marrow and extramedullary extension from osteosarcoma.

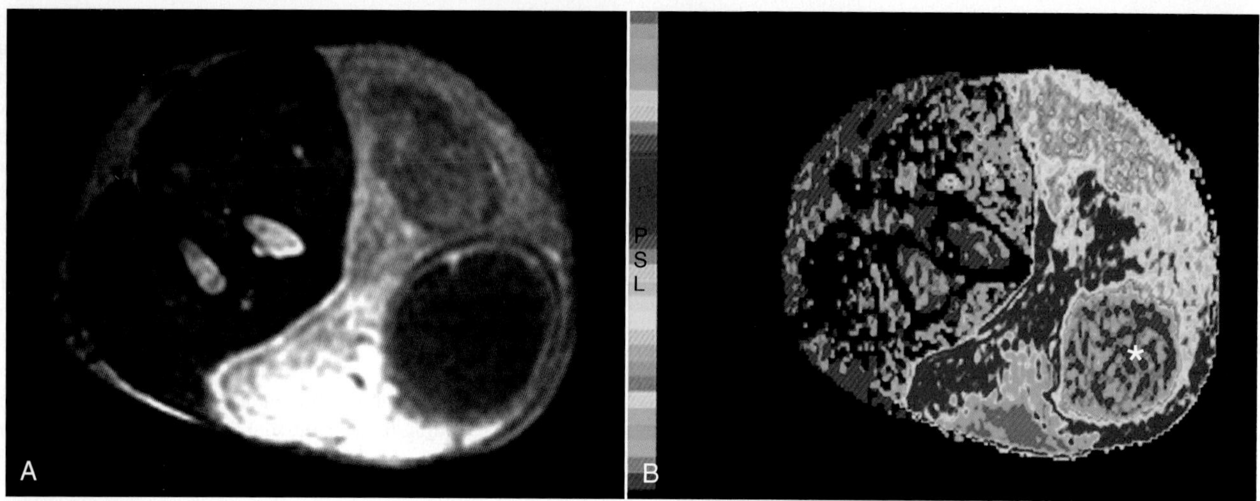

FIGURE 6-11 **A,** Transverse MR images of a soft tissue sarcoma of a canine forelimb. **B,** A color map of maximum slope of increase indicating the most rapidly contrast-enhancing tumor regions and also showing poor uptake in the necrotic core *(*)*. Compare to the normal musculature and cross-sectional views of the radius and ulna in the left of the image.

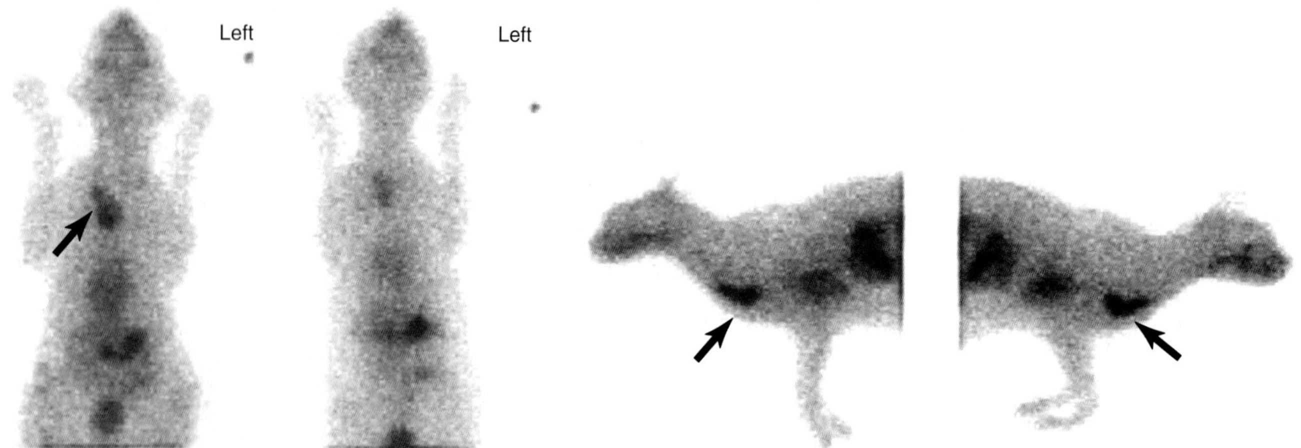

FIGURE 6-12 Ventral, dorsal, and left and right lateral scintigraphic images of a cat with ectopic thyroid carcinoma *(black arrows)*. Images were obtained 20 minutes after intravenous administration of technetium-99m (^{99m}Tc).

and liver scintigraphy (Figure 6-12). Parathyroid scintigraphy has been performed using dual-phase imaging[94] but due to lack of sensitivity was not recommended for identification of abnormal parathyroid glands in hypercalcemic dogs. At this author's (LJF) institution, ultrasound is used primarily to locate parathyroid masses in hypercalcemic dogs and cats.[95,96]

In general, nuclear medicine studies are sensitive for lesion detection but are nonspecific for disease etiology. Benign and malignant lesions can have similar scintigraphic appearances. Bone metastases can be detected earlier with scintigraphy, before clinical and radiographic recognition, and scintigraphy can aid in the selection of the best site for biopsy (Figure 6-13).[93,97] Once a lesion is identified, additional imaging (radiography, ultrasonography, CT, MRI) may be necessary.

Single-Photon Emission Computed Tomography and Positron Emission Tomography

Two advanced radionuclide imaging techniques used extensively in human medicine are single-photon emission computed tomography (SPECT) and positron emission tomography (PET). SPECT utilizes traditional gamma ray–emitting radionuclides, often with a rotating gamma camera or stationary ring, which reconstructs the images in cross-sections. SPECT provides better lesion localization as compared to planar scintigraphy, and hybrid instruments coupling functional SPECT information with CT for anatomy are now in use for oncology.[98] PET detectors also register gamma rays in a cross-section to reconstruct a 3D image, but these gamma rays are produced during annihilation of another emitted particle, the positron.[99] Positron-emitting radionuclides are closer in identity to physiologic atoms than gamma ray–emitting radionuclides, allowing synthesis of compounds of more biologic relevance. Dual-modality hybrid PET/CT and, most recently, PET/MRI scanners are now commercially available with widespread use in oncology. The systems are housed in the same instrument allowing for almost simultaneous acquisition of both images and their fusion, providing both anatomic and physiologic information. The complementary data provided by the two imaging procedures provide the most accurate cancer staging for oncology patients.[100]

Compared with normal cells, tumor cells have increased glucose utilization through glycolysis; this makes glucose an appropriate molecule for modification and labeling with a positron-emitting radionuclide. The increased energy demand of tumors is met through upregulation of the hexose monophosphate pathway, cell membrane glucose transporter proteins, and hexokinase. A glucose analog, ^{18}F-fluorodeoxyglucose (FDG) acts as a glucose molecule and is transported by membrane proteins and becomes phosphorylated by hexokinase in the cell. However, phosphorylated FDG is not used in the glycolytic pathway and remains trapped intracellularly, as tumor cells are deficient in glucose-6-phosphatase. The differential uptake of FDG by tumor cells forms the basis for contrast in images.

Whole-body FDG PET/CT imaging has been utilized extensively for human cancer imaging for cancer staging and detecting metastases and is also proving useful for target definition for radiation therapy.[3,99,101] Its use has been demonstrated not only for staging and follow-up of human lymphoma but also for prognostication and response evaluation.[102,103] FDG PET/CT is now also available and being actively studied for use in veterinary cancer patients (Figure 6-14).[104-107] Its utility for cancer staging of canine mast cell tumor and lymphoma has already been demonstrated.[108] However, there are limitations to the interpretation of FDG PET images. The uptake of FDG in normal tissues must be understood relative to veterinary species to avoid false-positive diagnoses because some normal tissues are also highly metabolic.[109-112] Normal gray matter of the brain can confound interpretation of intracranial tumor images because of its high glucose utilization normally. Inflammatory processes also have increased FDG uptake, and post-radiation tissue reaction can be difficult to distinguish from tumor recurrence during the early posttherapy time period.[113] Also, certain low-grade or poorly differentiated tumors do not show sufficient FDG uptake to be distinguished from background. Although FDG is still the most commonly used commercial PET agent for cancer imaging, limitations of FDG PET have led to exploration of other novel PET probes.[101]

Thymidine, the only nucleoside used solely in construction of DNA and not in RNA, provides an accurate measurement of increased cellular proliferation in a tumor both before and after treatment.[105,114,115] Two fluorinated compounds that have been proved stable to degradation and useful in tumor imaging are 2′-fluoro-5-methyldeoxyuracil (FMAU) and 3′-deoxy-3′-fluorothymidine (FLT). Both compounds are phosphorylated by thymidine kinase (TK) intracellularly and incorporated into DNA to variable degrees. Although FLT acts as a chain terminator in DNA synthesis and has limited incorporation into DNA, for imaging purposes it remains trapped intracellularly by TK and indirectly reflects cellular proliferation. Early studies show normal FLT distribution within the bone marrow, liver, and urinary system as a result of excretion. Research using dogs with spontaneous tumors continues to look at the utility of FLT as a marker of tumor proliferation.[114] Figure 6-15 is a sagittal reconstruction PET

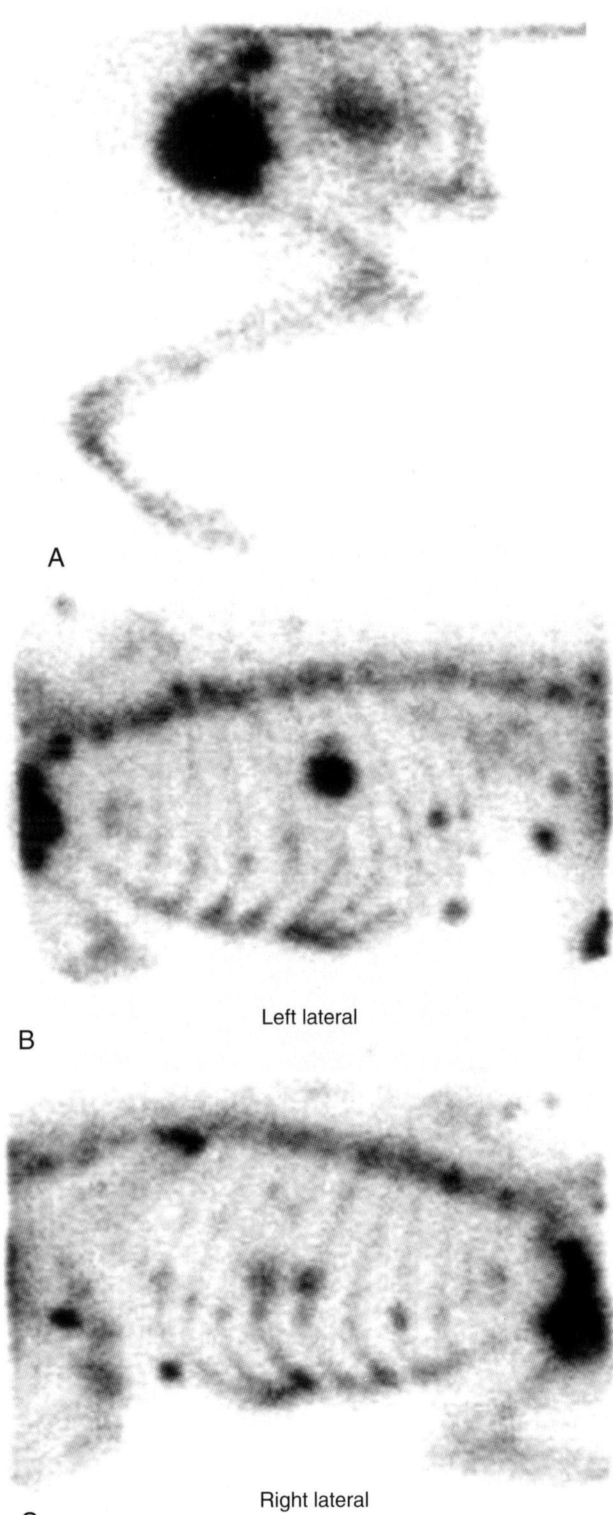

FIGURE 6-13 Bone scan images of a dog with primary osteosarcoma of the left proximal humerus **(A)** with subcutaneous and rib metastases (**B** and **C**). Images were obtained 2 hours after intravenous administration of technetium-99m methylene diphosphonate (^{99m}Tc MDP). Note the large mass with associated radiopharmaceutical uptake in the left proximal humerus **(A)** and the focal increased uptake in multiple ribs and in subcutaneous tissue overlying the thoracic spine and dorsal to the scapula (**B** and **C**).

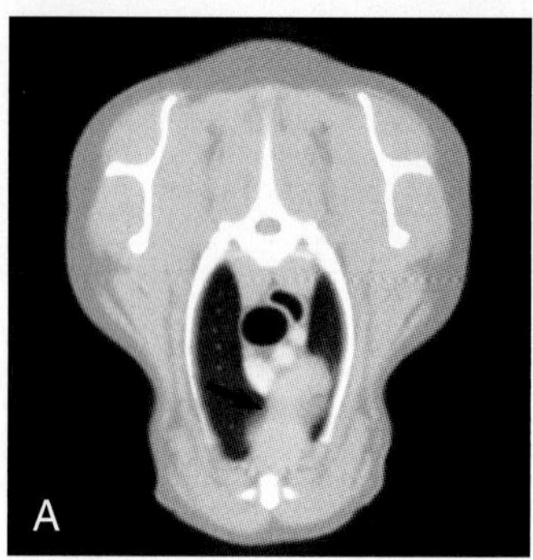

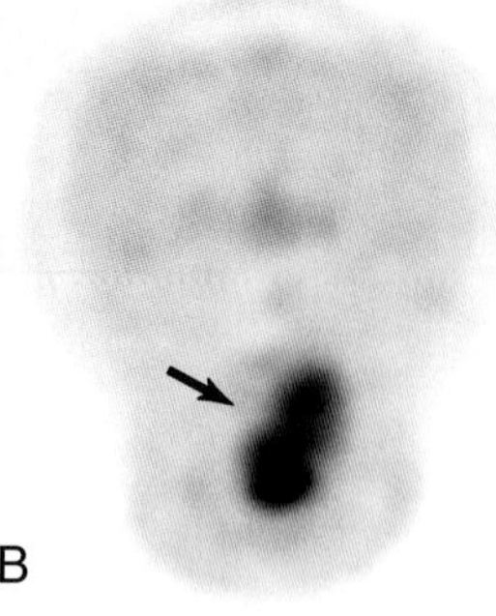

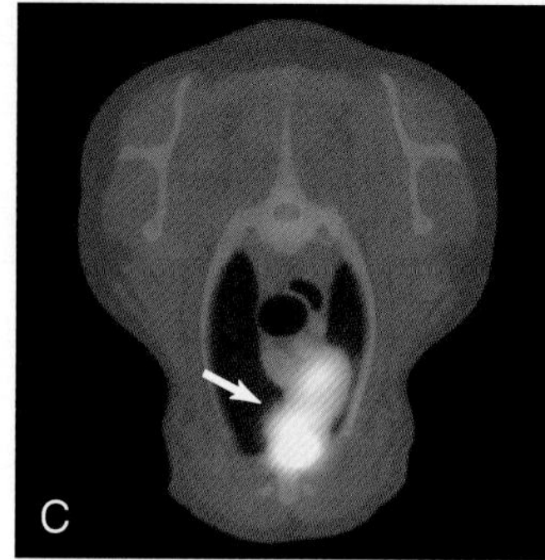

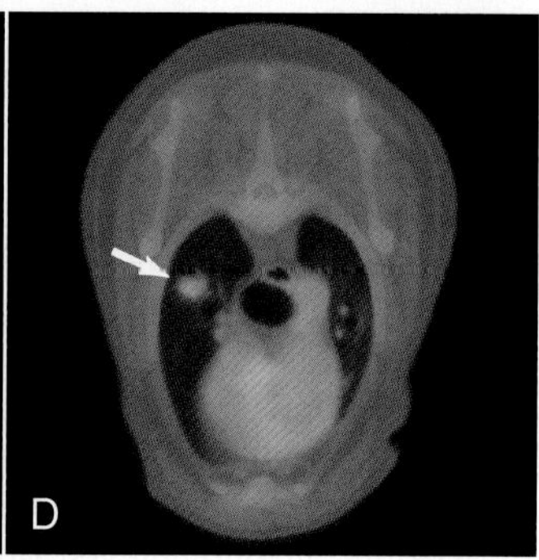

FIGURE 6-14 Transverse CT **(A)**, PET **(B)**, and fused PET/CT image **(C)** of a thymoma in the cranial mediastinum of a dog *(arrows)*. **D,** A small hypermetabolic pulmonary adenocarcinoma *(white arrow)*, which was not visible radiographically, was found incidentally on fused PET/CT image and also surgically removed.

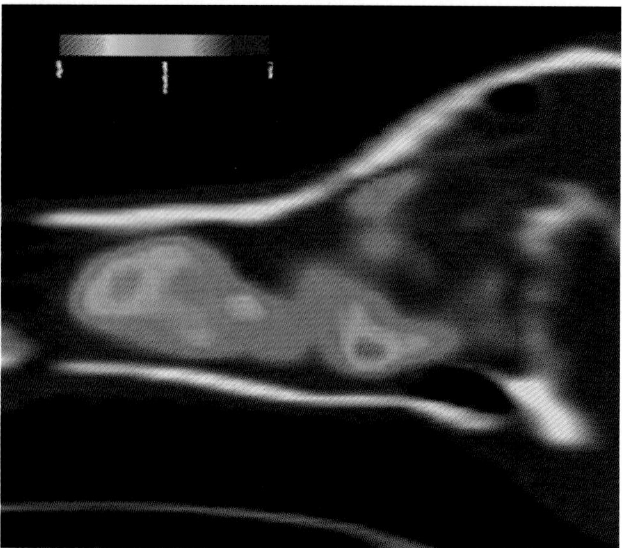

FIGURE 6-15 3′-Deoxy-3′-fluorothymidine (FLT) sagittal reconstruction of dog with nasal adenocarcinoma.

FLT scan of a dog with a nasal adenocarcinoma. PET radiotracers for noninvasive imaging of tumor hypoxia have been found in human cancer trials to have value in prognostication, predicting response, and better defining hypoxic tumor volumes for boost radiation therapy.[99,116] Hypoxic radiotracers include several in the nitroimidazole class, including ^{18}F-misonidazole, the more hydrophilic ^{18}F-fluoroazomycin (FAZA), and the more lipophilic version 2-(2-nitro-1H-imidazol-1-yl)-N-(2,2,3,3,3pentafluoropropyl)-acetamide (^{18}F-EF5). ^{60}Cu-labeled diacetyl-bis(N^4-methylthiosemicarbazone (^{60}Cu-ATSM) is a non-nitroimidazole tracer that is also being evaluated as a hypoxic tracer.

^{18}F-sodium fluoride (^{18}F-NaF) is a PET tracer that is now commercially available for bone scans. ^{18}F-NaF localizes to areas of high bone turnover similar to ^{99m}Tc-MDP that is used for bone scintigraphy. PET imaging with this tracer provides 3D, highly detailed whole-body skeletal images that are superior to bone scintigraphy and SPECT imaging for bone metastases.[117-119] Its use is being evaluated in veterinary patients for detection of skeletal metastases and other bone disease processes (Figure 6-16).

Advances

The state of the art in human radiotherapy is represented by conformal radiotherapy and intensity-modulated radiotherapy (IMRT). In the former technique, the treatment beam is conformed to the tumor volume. In the latter technique, in addition to shaping the treatment beam to the tumor, beam intensity is modulated to maximize the tumor dose and minimize the dose to normal tissue.[120,121] These advanced treatment modalities require imaging periodically through the radiation course.

In particular, IMRT requires precise and accurate tumor and normal tissue localization due to its high-dose gradients and maximal sparing of surrounding normal structures. This is accomplished through image-guided radiation therapy (IGRT) via a range of on-board imaging incorporated with IMRT linear accelerators.[122] In addition to traditional portal image options, IGRT also includes the ability to use kV x-ray and cone-beam CT (CBCT) systems to image the patient at the time of setup so that slight movements can be made with the therapy table to perfectly match bone and soft tissue landmarks on the digitally reconstructed radiographic images and 3D–planning CT scan. These advances in technology make it possible to perform adaptive radiotherapy by taking into consideration changes in size and shape of the target volumes during a treatment course. Tumor motion can be a problem for many sites, especially as oncologists attempt to balance increased tumor dose with reduced normal tissue complications while attempting to improve overall survival. To this end, 4-dimensional (4D) CT imaging, in which respiratory motion is taken into account in the treatment planning process and delivery, is being implemented in human radiation oncology centers.[120,123-125]

Another advance is helical tomotherapy, which integrates a linear accelerator with a helical CT scanner, allowing IGRT.[126] Each day before treatment, a CT scan is obtained with the linear accelerator; this scan is fused with the planning CT image, and the patient is moved accordingly to ensure precise treatment delivery.[127] CT imaging is an integral part of radiotherapy planning and delivery.

Advances are also being made in the area of molecular imaging.[1-3,101,104,106] These techniques can be used to characterize and measure biologic processes, assess molecular targets, and monitor treatment at the cellular level.[1,128] Molecular imaging can be used to assess gene delivery and identify marker proteins for apoptosis, angiogenesis, hypoxia, and other growth factors.[1,3,101,116,129] Moreover, treatment of cancer using molecular targets holds great promise for individualized cancer therapy.[116,130-132]

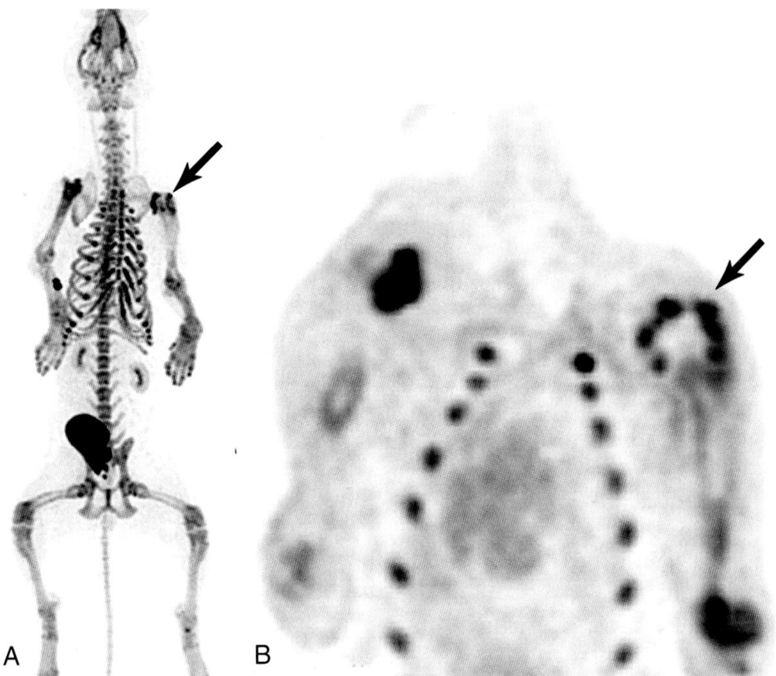

FIGURE 6-16 **A,** ^{18}F-sodium fluoride (^{18}F-NaF) PET bone scan 3D maximum intensity projection (MIP) image of a dog with a proximal humeral osteosarcoma *(black arrow)* 6-months poststereotactic radiation therapy. Note the excellent skeletal image with multifocal uptake at the costochondral junctions, the injection catheter, the opposite shoulder joint, and the urinary bladder due to excretion. **B,** The irradiated tumor *(black arrow)* on the dorsal plane PET image exhibits a photopenic center consistent with inactive bone remodeling and/or necrosis.

REFERENCES

1. Higgins LJ, Pomper MG: The evolution of imaging in cancer: current state and future challenges, *Semin Oncol* 38:3–15, 2011.
2. Smith RA, Guleryuz S, Manning HC: Molecular imaging metrics to evaluate response to preclinical therapeutic regimens, *Front Biosci* 16:393–410, 2011.
3. Zhu A, Lee D, Shim H: Metabolic positron emission tomography imaging in cancer detection and therapy response, *Semin Oncol* 38:55–69, 2011.
4. Prather AB, Berry CR, Thrall DE: Use of radiography in combination with computed tomography for the assessment of noncardiac thoracic disease in the dog and cat, *Vet Radiol Ultrasound* 46:114–121, 2005.
5. Nemanic S, London CA, Wisner ER: Comparison of thoracic radiographs and single breath-hold helical CT for detection of pulmonary nodules in dogs with metastatic neoplasia, *J Vet Intern Med* 20:508–515, 2006.
6. Schultz RM, Puchalski SM, Kent M, et al: Skeletal lesions of histiocytic sarcoma in nineteen dogs, *Vet Radiol Ultrasound* 48:539–543, 2007.
7. Blackwood L, Sullivan M, Lawson H: Radiographic abnormalities in canine multicentric lymphoma: a review of 84 cases, *J Small Anim Pract* 38:62–69, 1997.
8. Geyer NE, Reichle JK, Valdes-Martinez A, et al: Radiographic appearance of confirmed pulmonary lymphoma in cats and dogs, *Vet Radiol Ultrasound* 51:386–390, 2010.
9. Forrest LJ: The head: excluding the brain and orbit, *Clin Tech Small Anim Pract* 14:170–176, 1999.
10. Kraft SL, Gavin PR: Intracranial neoplasia, *Clin Tech Small Anim Pract* 14:112–123, 1999.
11. Thomas WB: Nonneoplastic disorders of the brain, *Clin Tech Small Anim Pract* 14:125–147, 1999.
12. Rudich SR, Feeney DA, Anderson KL, et al: Computed tomography of masses of the brachial plexus and contributing nerve roots in dogs, *Vet Radiol Ultrasound* 45:46–50, 2004.
13. Swensen SJ, Jett JR, Hartman TE, et al: CT Screening for lung cancer: Five-year prospective experience, *Radiology* 235(1):259–265, 2005.
14. Yoon J, Feeney DA, Cronk DE, et al: Computed tomographic evaluation of canine and feline mediastinal masses in 14 patients, *Vet Radiol Ultrasound* 45:542–546, 2004.
15. Li F, Sone S, Abe H, et al: Malignant versus benign nodules at CT screening for lung cancer: comparison of thin-section CT findings, *Radiology* 233:793–798, 2004.
16. Ballegeer EA, Adams WM, Dubielzig RR, et al: Computed tomography characteristics of canine tracheobronchial lymph node metastasis, *Vet Radiol Ultrasound* 51:397–403, 2010.
17. Eberle N, Fork M, von Babo V, et al: Comparison of examination of thoracic radiographs and thoracic computed tomography in dogs with appendicular osteosarcoma, *Vet Comp Oncol* 9:131–140, 2010.
18. Fife WD, Samii VF, Drost WT, et al: Comparison between malignant and nonmalignant splenic masses in dogs using contrast-enhanced computed tomography, *Vet Radiol Ultrasound* 45:289–297, 2004.
19. Rosenstein DS: Diagnostic imaging in canine pheochromocytoma, *Vet Radiol Ultrasound* 41:499–506, 2000.
20. McEntee MC, Thrall DE: Computed tomographic imaging of infiltrative lipoma in 22 dogs, *Vet Radiol Ultrasound* 42:221–225, 2001.
21. McEntee MC, Page RL: Feline vaccine-associated sarcomas, *J Vet Intern Med* 1:176–182, 2001.
22. Peters TM, Slomka PJ, Fenster A: Imaging for radiation therapy planning (MRI, nuclear medicine, ultrasound). In Van Dyk J, editor: *The modern technology of radiation oncology*, Madison, WI, 1999, Medical Physics Publishing.
23. Van Dyk J, Barnett RB, Battista JJ: Computerized radiation treatment planning systems. In Van Dyk J, editor: *The modern technology of radiation oncology*, Madison, Wisconsin, 1999, Medical Physics Publishing.
24. Giroux A, Jones JC, Bohn JH, et al: A new device for stereotactic CT-guided biopsy of the canine brain: design, construction, and needle placement accuracy, *Vet Radiol Ultrasound* 43:229–236, 2002.

25. Tidwell AS, Johnson KL: Computed tomography-guided percutaneous biopsy in the dog and cat: description of technique and preliminary evaluation in 14 patients, *Vet Radiol Ultrasound* 35:445–456, 1994.
26. Tidwell AS, Johnson KL: Computed tomography-guided percutaneous biopsy: criteria for accurate needle tip identification, *Vet Radiol Ultrasound* 35:440–444, 1994.
27. Troxel MT, Vite CH: CT-guided stereotactic brain biopsy using the Kopf stereotactic system, *Vet Radiol Ultrasound* 49:438–443, 2008.
28. Zekas LJ, Crawford JT, O'Brien RT: Computed tomography-guided fine-needle aspirate and tissue-core biopsy of intrathoracic lesions in thirty dogs and cats, *Vet Radiol Ultrasound* 46:200–204, 2005.
29. Robben JH, Pollak YWEA, Kirpensteijn J, et al: Comparison of ultrasonography, computed tomography, and single-photon emission computed tomography for the detection and localization of canine insulinoma, *J Vet Intern Med* 19:15–22, 2005.
30. Taniura T, Marukawa K, Yamada K, et al: Differential diagnosis of hepatic tumor-like lesions in dog by using dynamic CT scanning, *Hiroshima J Med Sci* 58:17–24, 2009.
31. Mai W, Caceres AV: Dual-phase computed tomographic angiography in three dogs with pancreatic insulinoma, *Vet Radiol Ultrasound* 49:141–148, 2008.
32. Kanematsu M, Kondo H, Goshima S, et al: Imaging liver metastases: Review and update, *Euro J Radiol* 58:217–228, 2006.
33. Pollard RE, Garcia TC, Stieger SS, et al: Quantitative evaluation of perfusion and permeability of peripheral tumors using contrast-enhanced computed tomography, *Invest Radiol* 39:340–349, 2004.
34. Van Camp S, Fisher P, Thrall DE: Dynamic CT measurement of contrast medium washin kinetics in canine nasal tumors, *Vet Radiol Ultrasound* 41:403–408, 2000.
35. Monteiro CB, O'Brien RT: A retrospective study on the sonographic findings of abdominal carcinomatosis in 14 cats, *Vet Radiol Ultrasound* 45:559–564, 2004.
36. Llabres-Diaz FJ: Ultrasonography of the medial iliac lymph nodes in the dog, *Vet Radiol Ultrasound* 45:156–165, 2004.
37. Nyman HT, Kristensen AT, Flagstad A, et al: A review of the sonographic assessment of tumor metastases in liver and superficial lymph nodes, *Vet Radiol Ultrasound* 45:438–448, 2004.
38. Nyman HT, O'Brien RT: The sonographic evaluation of lymph nodes, *Clin Tech Small Anim Pract* 22:128–137, 2007.
39. Kinns J, Mai W: Association between malignancy and sonographic heterogeneity in canine and feline abdominal lymph nodes, *Vet Radiol Ultrasound* 48:565–569, 2007.
40. Prieto S, Gomez-Ochoa P, De Blas I, et al: Pathologic correlation of resistive and pulsatility indices in canine abdominal lymph nodes, *Vet Radiol Ultrasound* 50:525–529, 2009.
41. de Swarte M, Alexander K, Rannou B, et al: Comparison of sonographic features of benign and neoplastic deep lymph nodes in dogs, *Vet Radiol Ultrasound*, 2011.
42. Della Santa D, Gaschen L, Doherr MG, et al: Spectral waveform analysis of intranodal arterial blood flow in abnormally large superficial lymph nodes in dogs, *Am J Vet Res* 69:478–485, 2008.
43. Bradbury CA, Westropp JL, Pollard RE: Relationship between prostatomegaly, prostatic mineralization, and cytologic diagnosis, *Vet Radiol Ultrasound* 50:167–171, 2009.
44. Besso JG, Penninck DG, Gliatto JM: Retrospective ultrasonographic evaluation of adrenal lesions in 26 dogs, *Vet Radiol Ultrasound* 38:448–455, 1997.
45. Sato AF, Solano M: Ultrasonographic findings in abdominal mast cell disease: a retrospective study of 19 patients, *Vet Radiol Ultrasound* 45:51–57, 2004.
46. Hanson JA, Papageorges M, Girard E, et al: Ultrasonographic appearance of splenic disease in 101 cats, *Vet Radiol Ultrasound* 42:441–445, 2001.
47. Beck C, Slocombe RF, O'Neill T, et al: The use of ultrasound in the investigation of gastric carcinoma in a dog, *Aust Vet J* 79:332–334, 2001.
48. Paoloni MC, Penninck DG, Moore AS: Ultrasonographic and clinicopathologic findings in 21 dogs with intestinal adenocarcinoma, *Vet Radiol Ultrasound* 43:562–567, 2002.
49. Penninck DG, Moore AS, Gliatto J: Ultrasonography of canine gastric epithelial neoplasia, *Vet Radiol Ultrasound* 39:342–348, 1998.
50. Penninck DG, Smyers B, Webster CR, et al: Diagnostic value of ultrasonography in differentiating enteritis from intestinal neoplasia in dogs, *Vet Radiol Ultrasound* 44:570–575, 2003.
51. Rivers BJ, Walter PA, Johnston GR, et al: Canine gastric neoplasia: utility of ultrasonography in diagnosis, *J Am Anim Hosp Assoc* 33:144–155, 1997.
52. Gaschen L: Ultrasonography of small intestinal inflammatory and neoplastic diseases in dogs and cats, *Vet Clin North Am Small Anim Pract* 41:329–344, 2011.
53. Cruz-Arambulo R, Wrigley R, Powers B: Sonographic features of histiocytic neoplasms in the canine abdomen, *Vet Radiol Ultrasound* 45:554–558, 2004.
54. Cuccovillo A, Lamb CR: Cellular features of sonographic target lesions of the liver and spleen in 21 dogs and a cat, *Vet Radiol Ultrasound* 43:275–278, 2002.
55. Ramirez S, Douglass JP, Robertson ID: Ultrasonographic features of canine abdominal malignant histiocytosis, *Vet Radiol Ultrasound* 43:167–170, 2002.
56. Crystal MA, Penninck DG, Matz ME, et al: Use of ultrasound-guided fine-needle aspiration biopsy and automated core biopsy for the diagnosis of gastrointestinal diseases in small animals, *Vet Radiol Ultrasound* 34:438–444, 1993.
57. Penninck DG, Crystal MA, Matz ME, et al: The technique of percutaneous ultrasound guided fine-needle aspiration biopsy and automated microcore biopsy in small animal gastrointestinal diseases, *Vet Radiol Ultrasound* 34:433–436, 1993.
58. Wang KY, Panciera DL, Al-Rukibat RK, et al: Accuracy of ultrasound-guided fine-needle aspiration of the liver and cytologic findings in dogs and cats: 97 cases (1990-2000), *J Am Vet Med Assoc* 224:75–78, 2004.
59. Wood EF, O'Brien RT, Young K: Ultrasound-guided fine-needle aspiration of focal parenchymal lesions of the lung in dogs and cats, *J Vet Intern Med* 12:338–342, 1998.
60. Samii VF, Nyland TG, Werner LL, et al: Ultrasound-guided fine-needle aspiration biopsy of bone lesions: a preliminary report, *Vet Radiol Ultrasound* 40:82–86, 1999.
61. Nyland TG, Wallack ST, Wisner ER: Needle-tract implantation following ultrasound-guided fine-needle aspiration biopsy of transitional cell carcinoma of the bladder, urethra, and prostate, *Vet Radiol Ultrasound* 43:50–53, 2002.
62. Wisner ER, Pollard RE: Trends in veterinary cancer imaging, *Vet Comparative Oncology* 2:49–74, 2004.
63. Nyman HT, Kristensen AT, Lee MH, et al: Characterization of canine superficial tumors using gray-scale B mode, color flow mapping, and spectral Doppler ultrasonography–a multivariate study, *Vet Radiol Ultrasound* 47:192–198, 2006.
64. Salwei RM, O'Brien RT, Matheson JS: Characterization of lymphomatous lymph nodes in dogs using contrast harmonic and power Doppler ultrasound, *Vet Radiol Ultrasound* 46:411–416, 2005.
65. Ziegler LE, O'Brien RT: Harmonic ultrasound: a review, *Vet Radiol Ultrasound* 43:501–509, 2002.
66. Bahr A, Wrigley R, Salman M: Quantitative evaluation of Imagent as an abdominal ultrasound contrast medium in dogs, *Vet Radiol Ultrasound* 41:50–55, 2000.
67. Haers H, Vignoli M, Paes G, et al: Contrast harmonic ultrasonographic appearance of focal space-occupying renal lesions, *Vet Radiol Ultrasound* 51:516–522, 2010.
68. Kanemoto H, Ohno K, Nakashima K, et al: Characterization of canine focal liver lesions with contrast-enhanced ultrasound using a novel contrast agent—Sonazoid, *Vet Radiol Ultrasound* 50:188–194, 2009.

69. Matheson JS, O'Brien RT, Delaney F: Tissue harmonic ultrasound for imaging normal abdominal organs in dogs and cats, *Vet Radiol Ultrasound* 44:205–208, 2003.
70. Nakamura K, Sasaki N, Murakami M, et al: Contrast-enhanced ultrasonography for characterization of focal splenic lesions in dogs, *J Vet Intern Med* 24:1290–1297, 2010.
71. Nakamura K, Takagi S, Sasaki N, et al: Contrast-enhanced ultrasonography for characterization of canine focal liver lesions, *Vet Radiol Ultrasound* 51:79–85, 2010.
72. O'Brien RT: Improved detection of metastatic hepatic hemangiosarcoma nodules with contrast ultrasound in three dogs, *Vet Radiol Ultrasound* 48:146–148, 2007.
73. O'Brien RT, Iani M, Matheson J, et al: Contrast harmonic ultrasound of spontaneous liver nodules in 32 dogs, *Vet Radiol Ultrasound* 45:547–553, 2004.
74. Szatmari V, Harkanyi Z, Voros K: A review of nonconventional ultrasound techniques and contrast-enhanced ultrasonography of noncardiac canine disorders, *Vet Radiol Ultrasound* 44:380–391, 2003.
75. Taeymans O, Penninck D: Contrast enhanced sonographic assessment of feeding vessels as a discriminator between malignant vs. benign focal splenic lesions, *Vet Radiol Ultrasound* 52(4):457–461, 2011.
76. Ziegler LE, O'Brien RT, Waller KR, et al: Quantitative contrast harmonic ultrasound imaging of normal canine liver, *Vet Radiol Ultrasound* 44:451–454, 2003.
77. Pollard RE, Reilly CM, Uerling MR, et al: Cross-sectional imaging characteristics of pituitary adenomas, invasive adenomas and adenocarcinomas in dogs: 33 cases (1988-2006), *J Vet Intern Med* 24:160–165, 2010.
78. Westworth DR, Dickinson PJ, Vernau W, et al: Choroid plexus tumors in 56 dogs (1985-2007), *J Vet Intern Med* 22:1157–1165, 2008.
79. Wisner ER, Dickinson PJ, Higgins RJ: Magnetic resonance imaging features of canine intracranial neoplasia, *Vet Radiol Ultrasound* 52:S52–S61, 2011.
80. Sturges BK, Dickinson PJ, Bollen AW, et al: Magnetic resonance imaging and histological classification of intracranial meningiomas in 112 dogs, *J Vet Intern Med* 22:586–595, 2008.
81. Kraft S, Ehrhart EJ, Gall D, et al: Magnetic resonance imaging characteristics of peripheral nerve sheath tumors of the canine brachial plexus in 18 dogs, *Vet Radiol Ultrasound* 48:1–7, 2007.
82. Petersen SA, Sturges BK, Dickinson PJ, et al: Canine intraspinal meningiomas: Imaging features, histopathologic classification, and long-term outcome in 34 dogs, *J Vet Intern Med* 22:946–953, 2008.
83. Wallack ST, Wisner ER, Werner JA, et al: Accuracy of magnetic resonance imaging for estimating intramedullary osteosarcoma extent in preoperative planning of canine limb-salvage procedures, *Vet Radiol Ultrasound* 43:432–441, 2002.
84. Kraft SL: Cancer imaging. In Gavin PR, Bagley RS, editors: *Practical small animal MRI*, Vol 1. Ames, 2009, Wiley-Blackwell, pp 333–358.
85. Clifford CA, Pretorius ES, Weisse C, et al: Magnetic resonance imaging of focal splenic and hepatic lesions in the dog, *J Vet Intern Med* 18:330–338, 2004.
86. Yasuda D, Fujita M, Yasuda S, et al: Usefulness of MRI compared with CT for diagnosis of mesenteric lymphoma in a dog, *J Vet Med Sci* 66:1447–1451, 2004.
87. Schmidt GP, Kramer H, Reiser MF, et al: Whole-body magnetic resonance imaging and positron emission tomography-computed tomography in oncology, *Top Magn Reson Imagining* 18:193–202, 2007.
88. Yankeelov TE, Arlinghaus LR, Li X, et al: The role of magnetic resonance imaging biomarkers in clinical trials of treatment response in cancer, *Semin Oncol* 38:16–25, 2011.
89. Zhao Q, Lee S, Kent M, et al: Dynamic contrast-enhanced magnetic resonance imaging of canine brain tumors, *Vet Radiol Ultrasound* 51:122–129, 2010.
90. Thamm DH, Kurzman ID, Clark MA, et al: Preclinical investigation of PEGylated tumor necrosis factor alpha in dogs with spontaneous tumors: Phase I evaluation, *Clin Cancer Res* 16:1498–1508, 2010.
91. Lin C, Luciani A, El-Gnaoui IE, et al: Whole-body diffusion-weighted magnetic resonance imaging with apparent diffusion coefficient mapping for staging patients with diffuse large B-cell lymphoma, *Eur Radiol* 20:2027–2038, 2010.
92. Glunde K, Bhujwalla ZM: Metabolic tumor imaging using magnetic resonance spectroscopy, *Semin Oncol* 38:26–41, 2011.
93. Forrest LJ, Thrall DE: Bone scintigraphy for metastasis detection in canine osteosarcoma, *Vet Radiol Ultrasound* 35:124–130, 1994.
94. Matwichuk CL, Taylor SM, Daniel GB, et al: Double-phase parathyroid scintigraphy in dogs using technetium-99M-sestamibi, *Vet Radiol Ultrasound* 41:461–469, 2000.
95. Sueda MT, Stephanacci JD: Ultrasound evaluation of the parathyroid glands in two hypercalcemic cats, *Vet Radiol Ultrasound* 41:448–451, 2000.
96. Wisner ER, Penninck DG, Biller DS, et al: High-resolution parathyroid sonography, *Vet Radiol Ultrasound* 38:462–466, 1997.
97. Head LL, Daniel GB: Scintigraphic diagnosis-an unusual presentation of metastatic pheochromocytoma in a dog, *Vet Radiol Ultrasound* 45:574–576, 2004.
98. Brandon D, Alazraki A, Halkar RK, et al: The role of single-photon emission computed tomography and SPECT/computed tomography in oncologic imaging, *Semin Oncol* 38:87–108, 2011.
99. Nestle U, Weber W, Hentschel M, et al: Biological imaging in radiation therapy: role of positron emission tomography, *Phys Med Biol* 54:R1–R25, 2009.
100. Bar-Shalom R, Valdiva AY, Blaufox MD: PET imaging in oncology, *Semin Nucl Med* 30:150–185, 2010.
101. Chen K, Chen X: Positron emission tomography imaging of cancer biology: current status and future prospects, *Semin Oncol* 38:70–86, 2011.
102. Terasawa T, Lau J, Bardet S, et al: Fluorine-18-fluorodeoxyglucose positron emission tomography for interim response assessment of advanced-stage Hodgkin's lymphoma and diffuse large B-cell lymphoma: a systematic review, *J Clin Oncol* 27:1906–1914, 2009.
103. Wahl RL, Jacene H, Kasamon Y, et al: From RECIST to PERCIST: evolving considerations for PET response criteria in solid tumors, *J Nucl Med* 50 Suppl 1:122S–150S, 2009.
104. Lawrence J, Rohren E, Provenzale J: PET/CT today and tomorrow in veterinary cancer diagnosis and monitoring: fundamentals, early results and future perspectives, *Vet Comp Oncol* 8:163–187, 2010.
105. Ballegeer EA, Forrest LJ, Jeraj R, et al: PET/CT for primary lung tumor in a dog, *Vet Radiol Ultrasound* 47:228–233, 2006.
106. Hansen AE, McEvoy F, Engelholm SA, et al: FDG PET/CT imaging in canine cancer patients, *Vet Radiol Ultrasound* 52:201–206, 2011.
107. Kang B-Y, Park C, Yoo J-H, et al: 18F-fluorodeoxyglucose positron emission tomography and magnetic resonance imaging findings of primary intracranial histiocytic sarcoma in a dog, *J Vet Med Sci* 71:1397–1401, 2009.
108. LeBlanc AK, Jakoby BW, Townsend DW, et al: 18FDG-PET imaging in canine lymphoma and cutaneous mast cell tumor, *Vet Radiol Ultrasound* 50:215–223, 2009.
109. LeBlanc AK, Wall JS, Morandi F, et al: Normal thoracic and abdominal distribution of 2-deoxy-2-[18F]fluoro-D-glucose (18FDG) in adult cats, *Vet Radiol Ultrasound* 50:436–441, 2009.
110. LeBlanc AK, Jakoby B, Townsend DW, et al: Thoracic and abdominal organ uptake of 2-deoxy-2-[18F]Fluoro-D-Glucose (18FDG) with positron emission tomography in the normal dog, *Vet Radiol Ultrasound* 49:182–188, 2008.
111. Lee AR, Lee MS, Jung IS, et al: Imaging diagnosis—FDG-PET/CT of a canine splenic plasma cell tumor, *Vet Radiol Ultrasound* 51:145–147, 2010.
112. Lee MS, Lee AR, Jung MA, et al: Characterization of physiologic 18F-FDG uptake with PET-CT in dogs, *Vet Radiol Ultrasound* 51:670–673, 2010.

113. Greven KM: Positron-emission tomography for head and neck cancer, *Semin Radiat Oncol* 14:121–129, 2004.
114. Lawrence J, Vanderhoek M, Barbee D, et al: Use of 3′-deoxy-3′-[18F] fluorothymidine PET/CT for evaluating response to cytotoxic chemotherapy in dogs with non-Hodgkin's lymphoma, *Vet Radiol Ultrasound* 50:660–668, 2009.
115. Barwick T, Bencherif B, Mountz JM, et al: Molecular PET and PET/CT imaging of tumour cell proliferation using F-18 fluoro-L-thymidine: a comprehensive evaluation, *Nucl Med Commun* 30:908–917, 2009.
116. Chitneni SK, Palmer GM, Zalutsky MR, et al: Molecular imaging of hypoxia, *J Nucl Med* 52:165–168, 2011.
117. Grant FD, Fahey FH, Packard AB, et al: Skeletal PET with 18F-fluoride: applying new technology to an old tracer, *J Nucl Med* 49:68–78, 2008.
118. Even-Sapir E: PET/CT in malignant bone disease, *Semin Musculoskelet Radiol* 11:312–321, 2007.
119. Bridges RL, Wiley CR, Christian JC, et al: An introduction to Na(18)F bone scintigraphy: basic principles, advanced imaging concepts, and case examples, *J Nucl Med Technol* 35:64–76; quiz 78–79, 2007.
120. Keall P: 4-Dimensional computed tomography imaging and treatment planning, *Semin Radiat Oncol* 14:81–90, 2004.
121. Staffurth J: A review of the clinical evidence for intensity-modulated radiotherapy, *Clin Oncol* 22:643–657, 2010.
122. Bhide SA, Nutting CM: Recent advances in radiotherapy, *BMC Med* 8:25, 2010.
123. Underberg RW, Lagerwaard FJ, Cuijpers JP, et al: Four-dimensional CT scans for treatment planning in stereotactic radiotherapy for stage I lung cancer, *Int J Radiat Oncol Biol Phys* 60:1283–1290, 2004.
124. Chang JY, Cox JD: Improving radiation conformality in the treatment of non-small-cell lung cancer, *Semin Radiat Oncol* 20:171–177, 2010.
125. Jiang SB: Radiotherapy of mobile tumors, *Semin Radiat Oncol* 16:239–248, 2008.
126. Mackie TR, Balog J, Ruchala K, et al: Tomotherapy, *Semin Radiat Oncol* 9:108–117, 1999.
127. Forrest LJ, Mackie TR, Ruchala K, et al: The utility of megavoltage computed tomography images from a helical tomotherapy system for setup verification purposes, *Int J Radiat Oncol Biol Phys* 60:1639–1644, 2004.
128. Zaidi H, Vees H, Wissmeyer M: Molecular PET/CT imaging-guided radiation therapy treatment planning, *Acad Radiol* 16:1108–1133, 2009.
129. Bogdanov A Jr, Mazzanti ML: Molecular magnetic resonance contrast agents for the detection of cancer: past and present, *Semin Oncol* 38:42–54, 2011.
130. Bentzen SM: Dose painting and theragnostic imaging: towards the prescription, planning and delivery of biologically targeted dose distributions in external beam radiation oncology, *Cancer Treat Res* 139:41–62, 2008.
131. Thorwarth D, Geets X, Paiusco M: Physical radiotherapy treatment planning based on functional PET/CT data, *Radiother Oncol* 96:317–324, 2010.
132. Thorwarth D, Alber M: Implementation of hypoxia imaging into treatment planning and delivery, *Radiother Oncol* 97:172–175, 2010.

Diagnostic Cytopathology in Clinical Oncology

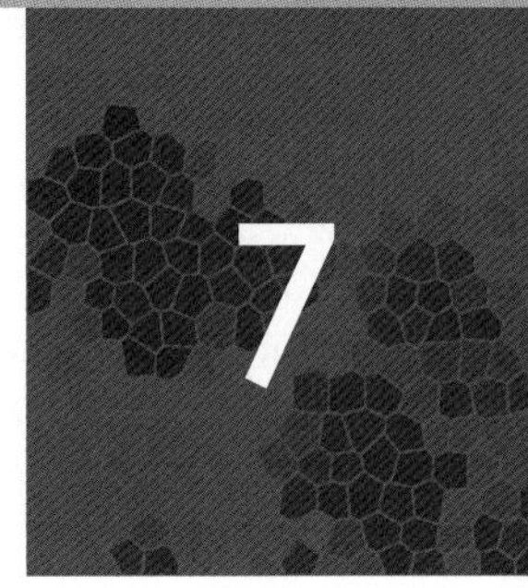

7

KRISTEN R. FRIEDRICHS AND KAREN M. YOUNG

Cytologic evaluation plays several important roles in veterinary oncology that aid in clinical decision making, including making a preliminary or definitive diagnosis, planning diagnostic and treatment strategies, determining prognosis through staging, detecting recurrence, and monitoring response to therapy. An understanding of the advantages and limitations of cytologic evaluation is necessary to utilize this diagnostic modality effectively in clinical oncology.

Advantages of cytologic evaluation include the ability to evaluate the morphologic appearance of individual cells, the relatively low risk of procedures to the animal patient, the lower cost compared with biopsy, and the speed with which results can be obtained. Cytologic evaluation also has several limitations. The amount of tissue sampled is small compared with that obtained from a biopsy; therefore cytologic specimens may not be fully representative of the lesion. Sample quality may be poor because of factors intrinsic to the lesion or poor collection technique. Importantly, the inability to evaluate architectural relationships among cells in cytologic specimens may prevent distinction between reactive and neoplastic processes. Examination of histologic samples, in which tissue architecture is preserved, may be required to make a definitive diagnosis of neoplasia, determine tumor type, and assess the extent of the lesion, including metastasis. Even then, ancillary tests like immunohistochemical staining or tests for clonality may be required. Often cytologic evaluation precedes a biopsy and provides information that assists in formulating subsequent diagnostic and treatment procedures.

Some tumors, such as lymphoma, may be diagnosed and staged using cytologic evaluation exclusively, and treatment can be initiated without the need to collect histologic specimens. For other tumors, such as well-differentiated hepatocellular carcinoma, cytologic examination permits formulation of a list of differential diagnoses, and histologic evaluation must be performed for definitive diagnosis. At a minimum, categorization of a tumor as an epithelial, mesenchymal, or discrete round cell tumor often can be determined cytologically; this may be sufficient for initial discussions with the owner about diagnosis and prognosis. Staging the malignancy, monitoring therapy, and detecting recurrence using cytologic evaluation is more easily accomplished once a definitive diagnosis has been made and cytomorphologic features of the tumor described.

Sample Collection

Proper collection and preparation techniques are prerequisites to obtaining diagnostic samples of high quality. Supplies necessary for collecting cytologic samples from a variety of tissues, body cavities, and mucosal surfaces are available in most clinics. These include hypodermic needles and syringes, scalpel blades and handles, propylene urinary catheters, bone marrow aspiration needles, cotton swabs, clean glass slides, marking pencils, and collection vials and tubes (tubes with ethylenediaminetetraacetic acid [EDTA] and plain sterile tubes). For aspiration of internal lesions, obtained by guidance with ultrasonography or computed tomography (CT), longer spinal needles and butterfly catheters (used to connect the spinal needle to the aspirating syringe) are useful. Cytologic specimens also can be made from tissues collected during biopsy (see Chapter 9). All supplies should be assembled in one location for ready access. Although life-threatening situations are rarely encountered when collecting cytologic specimens, supplies and medications should be available to control bleeding and to treat anaphylaxis. The latter occurs rarely when aspirating mast cell tumors because of release of histamine.

For external or easily accessible lesions, such as cutaneous and subcutaneous masses or enlarged lymph nodes, aspiration simply requires stabilization of the mass and consideration of underlying structures, such as large vessels and nerves. Some large abdominal masses can be aspirated blindly if they can be stabilized and if they are unlikely to be highly vascular or an abscess, aspiration of which may result in hemorrhage or dissemination of infection, respectively. Aspiration of intrathoracic and intraabdominal lesions is typically accomplished with guidance by imaging, either by ultrasonography or by CT, to aid in targeting the lesion and avoiding large vessels and other sensitive areas. Defects in cortical bone also can be identified with imaging, which can facilitate needle placement for aspiration of bone lesions. Cavity effusions are collected easily without imaging if fluid volume is significant; however, imaging can target smaller accumulations of fluid and provide a measure of safety. If there is particular concern for hemorrhage following aspiration, imaging can be repeated to look for evidence of bleeding at the aspiration site. Collection of cytologic specimens from the eye, brain, and lung requires special consideration and expertise.

Collection Techniques

Fine-needle aspiration (FNA) is by far the most common method for collecting cytologic specimens. Small-gauge needles (22 to 25 g) are sufficient for smaller lesions and result in less hemorrhage. Large-gauge needles (18 to 20 g) may be required to collect sufficient material from masses containing abundant matrix (i.e., firm masses and sarcomas), but specimens may contain more blood. Medium-sized syringes (12 to 15 cc) yield more vacuum for aspiration than smaller syringes (3 to 6 cc). The intent of aspiration is to draw cells into the needle shaft, not to fill the syringe with material unless the lesion is fluid-filled. After the needle is inserted into the lesion, vacuum is maintained in the syringe while the needle is redirected into the tissue several times to collect a broad representation of cells. This is especially important when aspirating lymph nodes to search for metastasis. Following aspiration, vacuum is released prior to removing the needle from the tissue, the needle is removed from the tissue and then from the syringe, the syringe is filled with air and reattached to the needle, and the cells are expelled onto a glass slide. An alternative technique is to obtain cells without aspiration by holding the needle by the hub between the thumb and middle finger while covering the hub opening with the forefinger (to prevent blood or other fluids from escaping) and rapidly and repeatedly inserting the needle into the lesion with redirection until cells are packed into the needle shaft.[1] This method often yields as much cellular material as the aspiration technique and produces less hemorrhage and patient discomfort. Similar to the aspiration technique, a syringe is used to expel the material in the needle onto a glass slide. A second clean slide is then placed on top of the sample and the two slides are pulled apart in parallel, taking care not to exert pressure on the sample. The aim is to obtain a monolayer of intact cells. Failure to spread the specimen immediately leads to a sample that is too thick to interpret; conversely, aggressive pressure on the sample may rupture many if not all cells, also leading to a nondiagnostic specimen.

Cytologic material may be collected from mucosal surfaces such as the respiratory, gastrointestinal, and genital tracts by saline washes or with a brush or biopsy forceps inserted through an endoscope. Cytologic materials collected using an endoscopic brush are gently rolled onto a glass slide and often result in highly cellular smears. In contrast, rolling a cotton swab over the surface of a lesion is only moderately successful at collecting sufficient material for cytologic evaluation of tumors. Traumatic catheterization is the best method for collecting material from bladder masses because of the risk of seeding tumor cells when transitional cell carcinomas (TCCs) are aspirated transabdominally. Traumatic catheterization is accomplished with an open-ended polypropylene urinary catheter attached to a large (50 to 60 cc) syringe. The catheter is inserted into the urethra and bounced off the bladder wall in the region of the lesion (typically using ultrasound guidance), taking care not to perforate the bladder wall. Saline can be flushed into the bladder to facilitate collection of cells and cellular particles, some of which may be large enough to process for histologic evaluation.

Imprinting and scraping are excellent means of preparing cytologic specimens from biopsied tissues. When making imprints, a fresh surface should be exposed on the piece of tissue using a scalpel blade and then gently blotted on absorbent paper until little blood or tissue fluid appears on the paper. The tissue is held with forceps, and the fresh surface is gently pressed repeatedly onto the glass slide, using slightly different pressure with each imprint. The final specimen will contain a row of imprints of varying thickness, one or more of which should be suitable for evaluation. Common mistakes when preparing imprints include insufficient blotting and application of too much pressure, resulting in excessive blood or cellular disruption, respectively. Sometimes mucosal or connective tissue is obtained instead of tumor cells if the incorrect surface is imprinted onto the slide. When tumors such as sarcomas contain abundant matrix, imprinting will often not yield sufficient numbers of cells for evaluation. The surface of these lesions should be crosshatched with a scalpel blade and imprinted without blotting; this may liberate cells embedded in matrix. Alternatively, the surface of firm lesions can be scraped several times in one direction with a scalpel blade held at 45 degrees to the tissue. The material on the edge of the blade is then gently spread on a glass slide. When using biopsy tissue to prepare cytologic specimens, care must be taken not to disrupt surfaces or margins important for histologic evaluation, especially for excisional biopsies in which assessment of tumor margins is fundamental to the evaluation.

Tissue particles or mucus collected by saline washes or by traumatic catheterization can be retrieved with a pipette and gently pressed between two glass slides. If washes or cavity fluids are cell-poor, the cells in the fluid must be concentrated to prepare slides of sufficient cellularity. Collection fluid can be centrifuged, the supernatant decanted, and the cell pellet or sediment resuspended in a small amount of remaining fluid and then spread on a glass slide. Similar to preparation of blood smears, the feathered edge of the fluid should be included on the slide because nucleated cells will accumulate there and may be best evaluated at the edge. Alternatively, when spreading the suspended cell pellet fluid on a glass slide, the spreader slide can be abruptly lifted off the slide, leaving a line of fluid—and concentrated cells—on the slide instead of a feathered edge. The best method to concentrate cells in cell-poor fluid samples is to use a cytocentrifuge, but most practices lack this equipment.

Cytologic Stains

A variety of quick stains are available for immediate examination of cytologic specimens and include quick Romanowsky stains, such as Diff-Quik. A specific set of staining jars should be kept exclusively for cytologic specimens and not used concurrently for dermatologic specimens. The jars containing the stain components should be capped between uses to prevent evaporation and contamination of the fixative and stains. Maintenance, including scheduled replacement of stain components, is important to avoid artifacts such as stain precipitate and contamination with organisms or debris that might be misinterpreted. Slides should be completely air-dried prior to fixation in the methanol fixative. Stains must thoroughly penetrate the smear, and in well-stained smears nuclei should be purple (Figure 7-1, *A*). A thick sample requires more contact time with the stains; understained slides (Figure 7-1, *B*) can be restained for a longer period of time, and overstained slides can be destained with methanol and restained for a shorter period of time. If the slides will be sent to an outside diagnostic laboratory, clinicians are encouraged to stain a slide to ensure that sufficient material was collected and that cells are intact prior to submitting additional unstained slides for evaluation. Additional specimens should be collected if only noncellular material is present or if all the cells are lysed. For some lesions, the first slide prepared may be the only slide that contains cellular material. It is best to send this slide unstained to the diagnostic laboratory, but, if it is stained, be sure to include it with the other slides.

Quick Romanowsky stains provide good nuclear detail and usually sufficient cytoplasmic detail for cytologic interpretation. Mast cell granules occasionally fail to stain with aqueous quick stains (Figure 7-2, *A*). Wright-Giemsa and modified Wright stains provide a broader palette of colors and excellent staining of cytoplasmic granules (Figure 7-2, *B*) but require more steps and longer staining times or use of an automated stainer. Fixation of wet smears is required for Papanicolaou staining, which is not frequently used in veterinary cytology. Heat fixation is not required or recommended for cytologic specimens.

Cytochemical and immunocytochemical staining may be necessary to determine the specific tumor type. A complete list of available special stains and antibodies is beyond the scope of this chapter; consultation with a veterinary cytopathologist is recommended when considering the necessity and use of these stains.

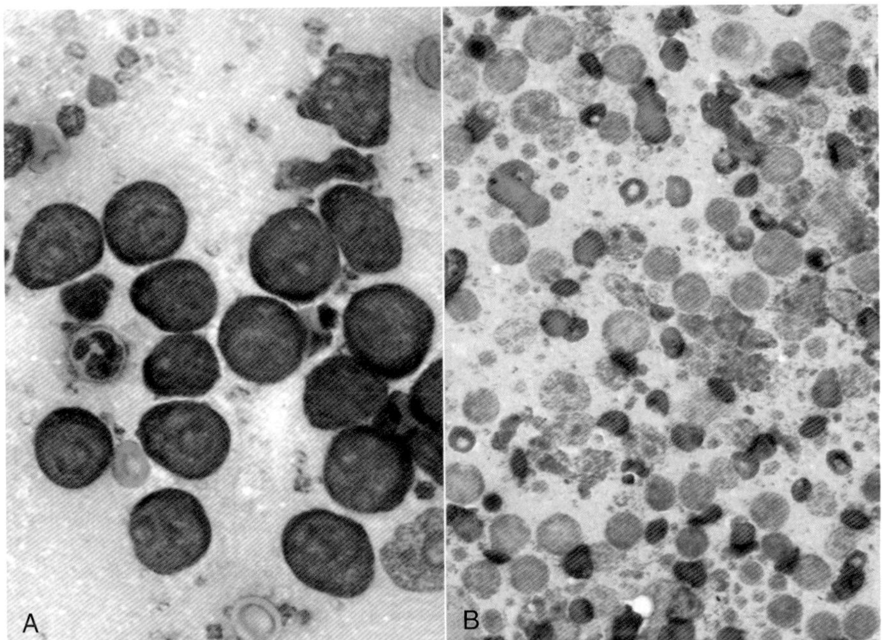

FIGURE 7-1 Fine-needle aspirate of a lymph node from a dog with lymphoma. **A,** Well-stained specimen. Lymphocytes are three times the diameter of an erythrocyte and larger than a neutrophil and have multiple prominent nucleoli. Cytoplasmic fragments are visible in the background. **B,** Poorly stained specimen. Cytoplasmic fragments are visible, but cellular detail is poor.

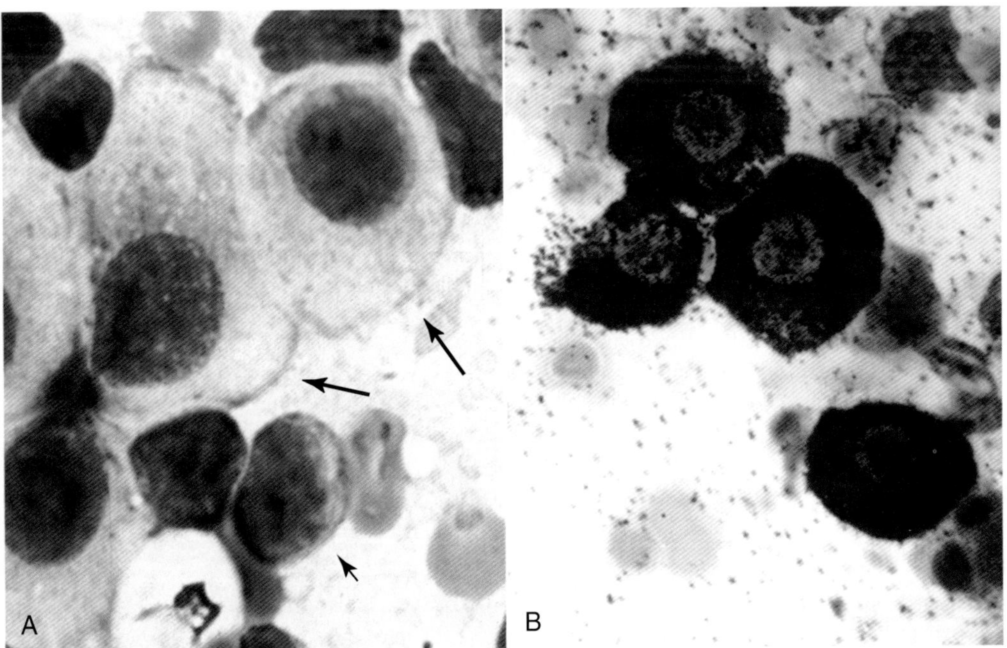

FIGURE 7-2 Fine-needle aspirate of a mast cell tumor. **A,** Granules in mast cells *(large arrows)* fail to stain when the specimen is stained with an aqueous quick stain. Small lymphocytes *(small arrow)* are also present. **B,** Granules are prominent in a Wright-stained specimen from the same tumor.

Cytochemical stains identify specific chemical compounds or structures within the cytoplasm or nucleus and include stains such as Prussian blue for iron, periodic acid-Schiff (PAS) for carbohydrates, alkaline phosphatase for identifying osteoblasts,[2] and a wide variety of leukocyte markers, including Sudan black B, peroxidase, chloracetate esterase, and nonspecific esterases. Immunocytochemical staining procedures utilize antibodies to identify specific proteins or peptides within or on the surface of the cells. Common antibodies used in veterinary oncology include those directed against CD3 (T-cells), CD79a and CD20 (B-cells), cytokeratin (epithelial cells), vimentin (mesenchymal cells), and Melan A (melanocytes). Use of a single stain or antibody is discouraged, as cell lineage is rarely identified and aberrant expression by neoplastic cells may lead to an erroneous diagnosis if a single marker is evaluated; a panel of stains or antibodies usually is necessary for complete identification.

Examination and Description of Cytologic Specimens

A good microscope, ideally equipped with a digital camera to document cytologic findings for the medical record or for consultation, should be used for examining cytologic specimens. The 4×, 10×, and 20× objectives are useful for scanning the slide and assessing cellular arrangements and general cell shape, whereas the 40× ("high dry") and 50× or 100× (oil-immersion) objectives are required for examining cellular detail. To improve clarity the 40× objective requires an additional optical interface, which can be provided by applying a drop of immersion oil or permanent mounting medium to the slide followed by a coverslip. As a note of warning, the 40× objective lens is easily coated with oil applied to the slide for viewing the specimen with oil-immersion objectives; if this occurs, the lens should be cleaned immediately with glass cleaner and lens paper to prevent accumulation of oil inside the objective lens. Proper use, including correct placement of the condenser for viewing stained and unstained specimens, and maintenance of the microscope are essential to adequate examination of cytologic specimens.

Consider the following when examining the slide preparation: (1) Is the specimen of sufficient quality to permit a clinically useful interpretation? Clinical decisions should not be made from specimens that are poorly cellular or have too many ruptured cells. (2) Based on the tissue sampled, do the cells represent the expected population, an abnormal population, or both? It is important to become familiar with the cytologic appearance of "normal" cells in frequently aspirated tissues, such as lymph node and liver. (3) Does the abnormal population represent inflammation or a neoplasm? Whenever inflammation is found in a lesion suspected to be a tumor, caution is advised in making a definitive diagnosis of neoplasia. Although some tumors are accompanied by neutrophilic inflammation, experienced cytopathologists recognize that primary inflammatory lesions can convincingly mimic neoplastic lesions. (4) If neoplasia is likely, what is the tissue of origin and is the tumor benign or malignant? These questions can sometimes be answered by cytologic evaluation of the tumor but often require confirmation with histologic examination.

Specimens of Diagnostic Quality

What constitutes adequate cellularity depends on the type of tumor. Aspirates of mesenchymal tumors, which often contain extracellular matrix, tend to be less cellular than those of epithelial and discrete round cell tumors. The degree of cellularity also has an impact on the level of confidence expressed in the interpretation, and diagnostic opinions are often qualified with "possible" or "probable" for poorly cellular specimens compared with "diagnostic for" or "consistent with" for highly cellular specimens. All cytologic specimens contain some ruptured cells, but to render a meaningful interpretation the majority of cells should be intact. Material from ruptured cells is recognized as stringy strands of chromatin or swollen magenta nuclei, often with obvious nucleoli, and free cytoplasmic fragments (see Figure 7-1, *A*). Large lymphocytes and cells from endocrine tumors are highly susceptible to lysis, and extra care should be taken not to exert pressure on the cells when preparing cytologic specimens from these lesions.

Nonneoplastic Cells and Noncellular Material Found in Cytologic Specimens

The submandibular salivary gland occasionally is aspirated instead of the mandibular lymph node and is recognized by clusters of foamy cells in a background of mucin and blood. When tissue containing a metastatic tumor is aspirated, the specimen may contain only neoplastic cells or may contain normal cells from the tissue (e.g., lymphoid populations in a lymph node), which helps confirm location of the tumor. Necrosis can be found in tumors that have outgrown their blood supply. Necrotic cells lack detail and consist of gray-pink, indistinct cytoplasm and amorphous nuclei (Figure 7-3); they should not be confused with apoptotic or pyknotic cells, which retain distinct cytoplasmic borders that surround condensed nuclear fragments.

Aspiration usually results in some degree of sampling hemorrhage leading to the presence of few or many erythrocytes admixed with nucleated cells. Aspiration of splenic lesions and thyroid and vascular tumors may result in pronounced hemorrhage and abundant blood in the cytologic specimen. Preexisting intralesional hemorrhage is indicated by the presence of macrophages containing erythrocytes or hemosiderin. Small numbers of peripheral leukocytes, primarily neutrophils, will accompany hemorrhage, but the presence of neutrophils in numbers greater than their proportion in blood is supportive of inflammation. Neutrophilic inflammation may accompany tumors, most notably squamous cell carcinoma and large tumors with necrotic centers; however, inflammation can induce criteria of malignancy in nonneoplastic populations, especially fibroblasts and squamous cells, and biopsy may be required to confirm suspected neoplasia when inflammation is prominent. Some tumors are associated with infiltration of specific inflammatory cells (e.g., eosinophils in mast cell tumors).

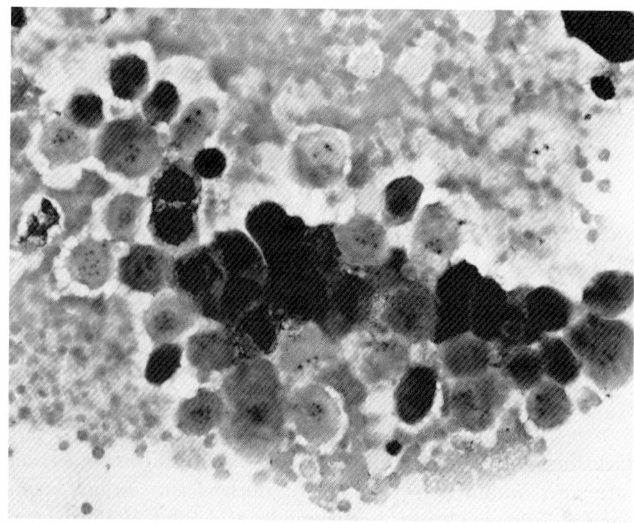

FIGURE 7-3 Cells from a mass in the bladder obtained by traumatic catheterization. The cells are gray and have indistinct morphologic features, typical of necrotic cells.

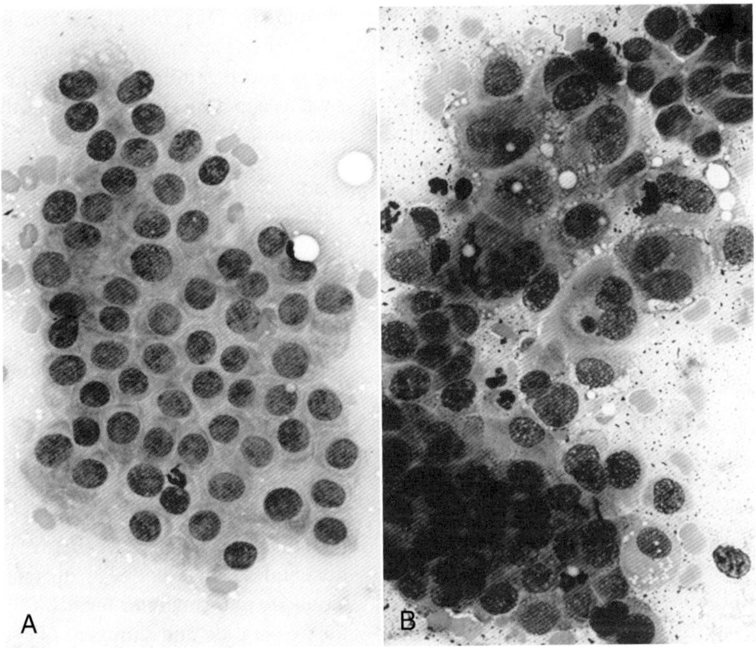

FIGURE 7-4 Cells from a pulmonary carcinoma **(A)** and a transitional cell carcinoma (TCC) **(B).** Note that in both specimens, cells comprise a homogeneous population of epithelial cells. However, cells from the pulmonary carcinoma are monomorphic, whereas those from the TCC are pleomorphic.

For tumors that produce ground substance(s), such as sarcomas, or that elicit a scirrhous response, such as some carcinomas, extracellular matrix may be observed in cytologic specimens. Collagen and osteoid consist of collections of smooth or fibrillar magenta material, whereas chondroid matrix typically forms larger lakes of bright pink-to-purple material. Mucin may be secreted by a variety of tumors, including salivary, biliary, and intestinal carcinomas and synovial and myxomatous sarcomas. Mucin is pale blue to pink, and cells surrounded by mucin are often aligned in rows. Ultrasound gel may be a contaminant of slides prepared from ultrasound-guided aspirates if the needle is not cleaned prior to expelling cells onto the slide. Ultrasound gel appears as granular, bright magenta material when stained with cytologic stains and, if abundant, may impair cytologic examination.

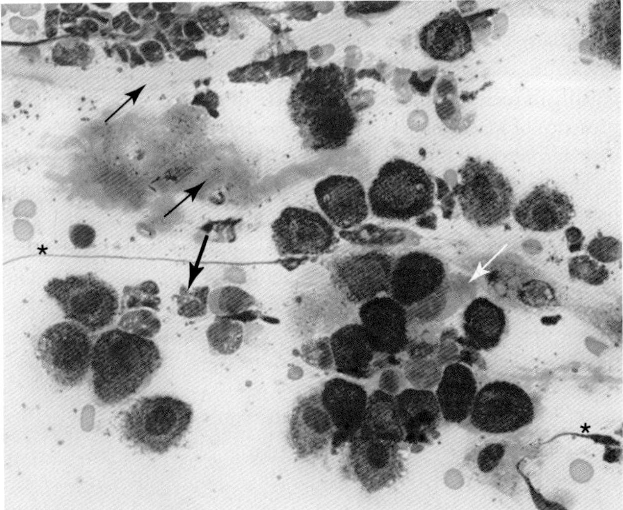

FIGURE 7-5 Fine-needle aspirate of a mast cell tumor. Note the heterogeneous populations of cells, including mast cells, eosinophils *(thick arrow)*, fibroblasts *(white arrow)*, and lymphocytes. Extracellular matrix *(thin arrows)*, likely collagen, is also present and stringy chromatin *(asterisks)* from broken nuclei is noted.

Description of Neoplastic Populations

Determination of the number of cells exfoliated and the shape and arrangement of cells early in the cytologic evaluation aids in formulating an initial list of differential diagnoses, permitting placement of tumors in three broad categories: epithelial, mesenchymal, and discrete round cell tumors. Briefly, cells from epithelial tumors exfoliate well and are round, cuboidal, columnar, or polygonal cells arranged in cohesive sheets or clusters; cells from mesenchymal tumors exfoliate poorly and are spindle-shaped, stellate, or oval cells arranged individually or in noncohesive aggregates; and cells from discrete round cell tumors exfoliate well and are individualized round cells that are arranged in a monolayer. Cellular arrangements observed in cytologic specimens and their associated histologic correlates and tissue types have been described.[3]

Proper terminology should be used to succinctly describe cell populations and convey important information. The terms *homogeneous* and *heterogeneous* describe cell populations (Figures 7-4 and 7-5). Homogeneous denotes a population of one cell type (excluding erythrocytes and associated leukocytes), which is typical of most tumors. Heterogeneous refers to mixed populations of cells, which are commonly found in aspirates of inflammatory lesions; however, some neoplasms will contain heterogeneous populations of cells (e.g., mast cell tumors accompanied by eosinophils and fibroblasts [see Figure 7-5] and squamous cell carcinomas with associated neutrophilic inflammation [see later]). The terms *monomorphic* and *pleomorphic* describe the morphologic appearance of cells within a single population. Monomorphic describes cells of a single lineage in which the cells have a uniform morphologic appearance (see Figure 7-4, *A*). Monomorphic features typically are associated with benign tumors, but a number of malignant tumors are cytologically monomorphic. In contrast, pleomorphic is used to describe cells of a single lineage that have variable morphologic features (see Figure 7-4, *B*). Pleomorphic features comprise a set of criteria of malignancy and suggest malignant behavior, but can be observed in nonneoplastic cells found in primary inflammatory lesions.

Criteria of malignancy are cellular features within a single population that suggest malignant behavior, with greater emphasis placed on nuclear criteria. The more criteria observed, the more likely the tumor is malignant. Cellular and cytoplasmic criteria of malignancy include variation in cell size *(anisocytosis),* abnormal cellular arrangement (3-dimensional [3D] clusters instead of a monolayer), cells that are smaller or larger than their normal counterpart, variable nuclear-to-cytoplasmic (N:C) ratios or N:C ratios that differ from what is expected for the cell type, intensely basophilic cytoplasm *(hyperchromasia),* abnormal vacuolation or granulation, and aberrant phagocytic activity. The nucleus is the most important component of the cell when determining the biologic behavior of a neoplasm. Nuclear criteria of malignancy include variation in nuclear size *(anisokaryosis),* unusual nuclear shape, multinuclearity, variation in nuclear size within the same multinucleated cell, nuclear fragments, multiple nucleoli that vary in size and shape within the same nucleus or among cells, increased mitoses, and nonsymmetric mitoses (Figure 7-6). When Papanicolaou stain is used, additional nuclear features such as irregular thickening of the nuclear membrane can be evaluated. Cellular gigantism (cell >10 times the diameter of an erythrocyte) and the presence of macronuclei (>5 times the diameter of an erythrocyte) or macronucleoli (larger than an erythrocyte) are particularly disturbing criteria of malignancy. In nonneoplastic cells the chromatin pattern is finely stippled in replicating or metabolically active cells and condensed in mature quiescent cells. Finely stippled chromatin is also common in rapidly proliferating neoplastic cells, and chromatin that is irregularly clumped or ropy is unusual and suggestive of a neoplastic process. Some nonneoplastic cells, including mesothelial cells, fibroblasts, and squamous epithelial cells, may have criteria of malignancy when they are highly proliferative in the presence of inflammation. Conversely, some malignant tumors such as apocrine gland tumors of the anal sac have few criteria of malignancy.

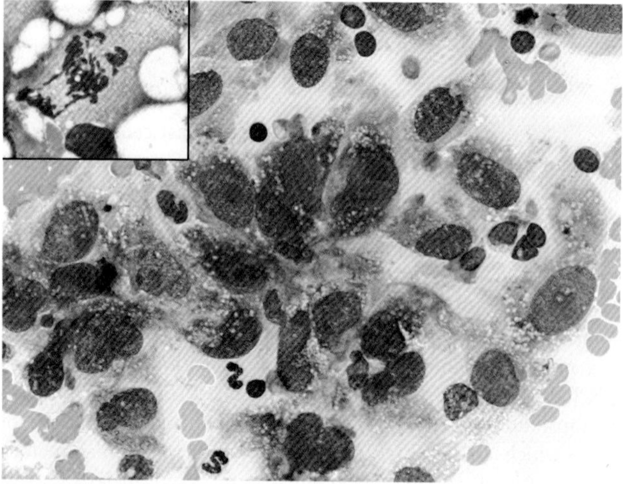

FIGURE 7-6 Fine-needle aspirate of hemangiosarcoma with multiple criteria of malignancy. *Inset*, An atypical mitotic figure from a liposarcoma.

Sending Cytologic Samples to a Diagnostic Laboratory

When using a referral diagnostic laboratory, two to four unstained smears should be sent. If a highly cellular smear has been stained and examined by the oncologist for confirmation of sample quality and the cellularity of the remaining unstained smears is in question, send the stained smear in addition to the unstained smears. Pack all slides in rigid slide containers to prevent breakage during shipment. For shipment by commercial mail services, place slide holders in a cardboard box with sufficient padding; padded envelopes are not recommended because these may not provide sufficient protection. Slides should not be refrigerated prior to or during shipment. Exposure to formalin or formalin fumes should be avoided during the preparation and shipment of cytologic specimens because this will permanently alter staining characteristics and render the sample nondiagnostic; biopsy specimens preserved in formalin should be sent separately from cytologic specimens, or each type of sample should be sealed in separate plastic bags. If cavity fluids or mucosal washes are submitted, include two freshly made unstained smears along with the fluid (in EDTA) or wash (sealed container). Plain tubes (red top) or sterile vials are required for specimens that may be cultured. For all submitted glass slides, indicate how the slides were prepared and whether a concentration method was used for cavity effusions.

Interpretation of Cytologic Specimens

The final interpretation of a cytologic specimen should be based not only on the cytologic findings but also on signalment, history, clinicopathologic findings, and imaging results. This information should be provided in a concise but complete summary to the individual evaluating the sample. When submitting samples to a cytopathologist, the exact location of the lesion should be clearly described because "thoracic mass" could indicate a mass located in the skin, subcutis, body wall, mediastinum, thoracic cavity, or pulmonary parenchyma; the differential diagnoses will be different for different locations. For clinicians who perform an initial evaluation of the cytologic specimen, observational and interpretative skills can be developed by comparing your findings with those described in the cytopathologist's complete report and by considering the information obtained from other diagnostic tests.

Confidence in cytologic interpretation is based on the quality of the specimen, the completeness of the clinical information provided, and the experience of the cytopathologist. Terms that express the degree of certainty, such as "consistent with," "diagnostic for," "cannot rule out," "probable," and "possible," may be used and interpreted differently by cytopathologists and clinicians, respectively.[4] If the certainty of an interpretation or diagnosis is unclear, the clinician should consult the cytopathologist. Correlations between cytologic and histologic interpretations or diagnoses are highly variable, depending on tissue types, disease processes, and methods of collection and preparation.

Epithelial, Mesenchymal, and Discrete Round Cell Tumors

The ability to identify specific tumor types by cytologic evaluation can aid in treatment planning and prognostication. Even if a specific diagnosis cannot be made, classification of the tumor as an epithelial, mesenchymal, or discrete round cell neoplasm can provide sufficient information to formulate a differential diagnosis and plan additional diagnostic procedures.

Tumors of Epithelial Tissues

Tumors derived from epithelial tissue comprise the largest category of neoplasms and include tumors of epithelial surfaces, such as the skin and respiratory, gastrointestinal, and urogenital tracts, as well as tumors of glands and organs. Given their diverse origin, the cytomorphologic appearance of these neoplasms can be highly variable; however, some features are shared by most epithelial tumors. Epithelial cells have intercellular junctions that connect the cells to each other and do not elaborate extracellular matrix. Therefore the cells exfoliate well, resulting in highly cellular specimens, and are arranged in cohesive sheets or clusters in cytologic smears (Figure 7-7). The cytoplasmic borders of individual cells typically are distinct, but this can vary in certain types of tumors. Poorly differentiated epithelial tumors have few or no identifying features and tend to be round cells with moderate-to-high N:C ratios and basophilic cytoplasm. In some cases, the cells no longer have intercellular junctions and appear as discrete round cells (Figure 7-8). Determining the tissue of origin in these cases is difficult, and histologic evaluation, with or without immunohistochemical analysis, is necessary to define the specific tumor type.

Tumors of Hair Follicles and Sebaceous Glands

Differentiating among adnexal tumors of skin by cytologic evaluation may be difficult when identifying features are absent or when multiple cell types are present. Many adnexal tumors have a large component of basilar cells that are small cuboidal or round cells with high N:C ratios and are arranged in tightly cohesive sheets or in palisading rows (see Figure 7-7). Nuclei are uniformly round with condensed to reticular chromatin, and nucleoli are indistinct or appear as a small single nucleolus. The cytoplasm is lightly basophilic and may contain black melanin granules (Figure 7-9). Tumors of hair follicle origin and matrical cysts often have a central cystic space filled with mature squamous cells, keratin flakes, or keratin debris, and this material may be aspirated when the mass is sampled. Tumors with sebaceous differentiation contain clusters of large round cells filled with oily-appearing vacuoles that partially obscure the small central nucleus (Figure 7-10). Tumors of basal cell origin (cutaneous basilar epithelial neoplasms) include trichoblastoma, pilomatricoma, basal cell epithelioma, sebaceous epithelioma, and others, and histologic examination is usually required to identify the specific type. Fortunately, the majority of adnexal tumors are benign; malignant types can occur and typically have pleomorphic features that predict their biologic behavior.

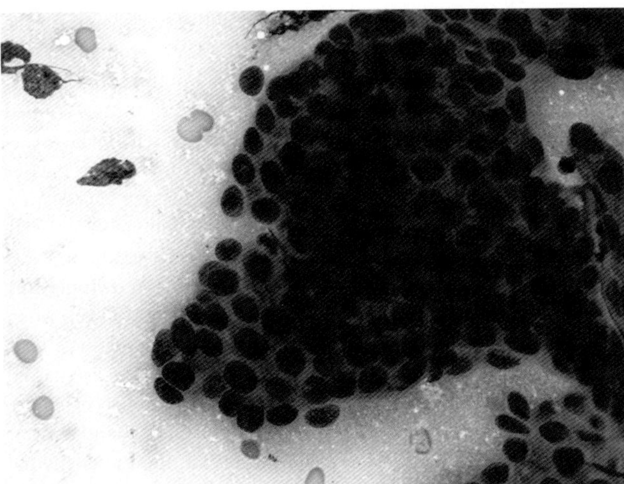

FIGURE 7-7 Fine-needle aspirate of a basal cell tumor (epithelioma). Note the monomorphic population of cohesive cells aligned in rows.

Tumors of the Epidermis

Squamous cell carcinoma (SCC) is the most common malignancy of the epidermis; the tumor has varying degrees of differentiation, even within a single tumor, and the cytologic specimen may consist primarily of basilar cells, more mature keratinized cells, or both

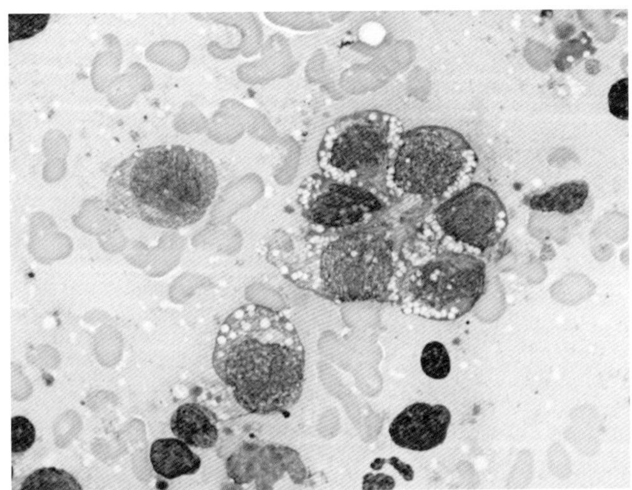

FIGURE 7-8 Fine-needle aspirate of an anaplastic colonic carcinoma. The tumor cells have high N:C ratios and are sometimes individualized.

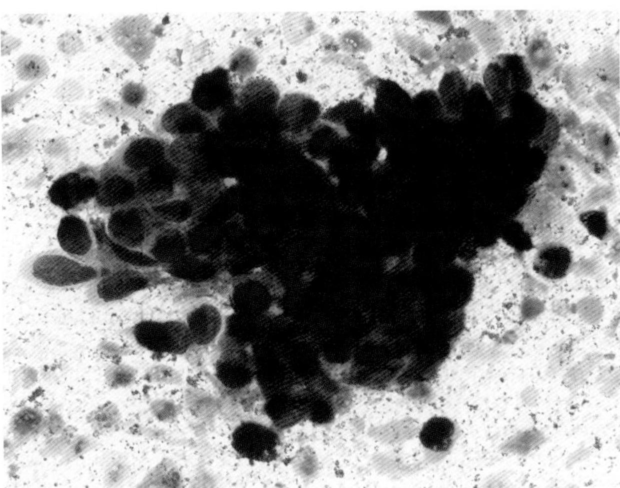

FIGURE 7-9 Fine-needle aspirate of a basal cell tumor in which the cells are heavily pigmented.

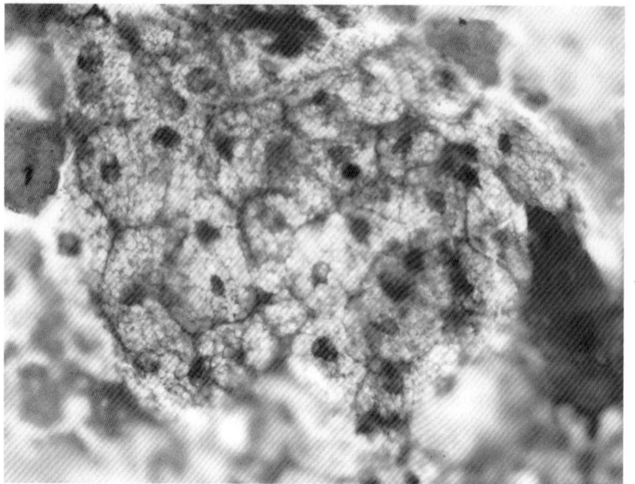

FIGURE 7-10 Fine-needle aspirate of a sebaceous adenoma.

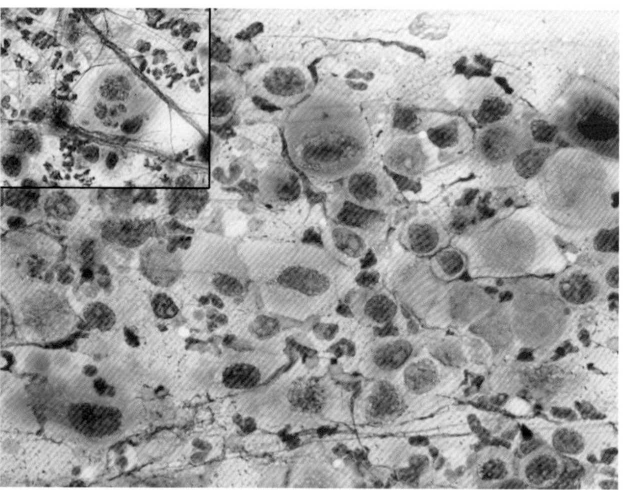

FIGURE 7-11 Fine-needle aspirate of a squamous cell carcinoma (SCC). Note the marked anisocytosis and anisokaryosis, variable N:C ratios, perinuclear vacuolation, and angular cytoplasmic borders in some cells. *Inset,* A neutrophilic infiltrate often accompanies SCC.

(Figure 7-11). Pleomorphism can be marked, including moderate-to-marked anisocytosis and anisokaryosis, hyperchromasia, and marked nuclear atypia. Keratin does not stain with Romanowsky stains, and cytologic features suggestive of keratinization include individualization of cells, sharp angular cytoplasmic margins, and smooth and glassy turquoise cytoplasm. Cells that appear keratinized may have small condensed nuclei or absent nuclei, representing a normal maturational process, but may have a large intact nucleus with fine-to-reticular chromatin and multiple visible nuclei. An immature nucleus concurrent with mature cytoplasm signifies "asynchronous maturation." Perinuclear vacuolation or magenta cytoplasmic inclusions (keratohyaline granules) may be observed in the more mature squamous cells. Keratinization within a tumor typically is accompanied by neutrophilic inflammation (Figure 7-11, *inset*). Differentiating between SCC and a primary inflammatory lesion with dysplastic squamous epithelium is a cytologic dilemma: in both cases the cells may have criteria of malignancy and asynchronous maturation. Location, appearance of the lesion,

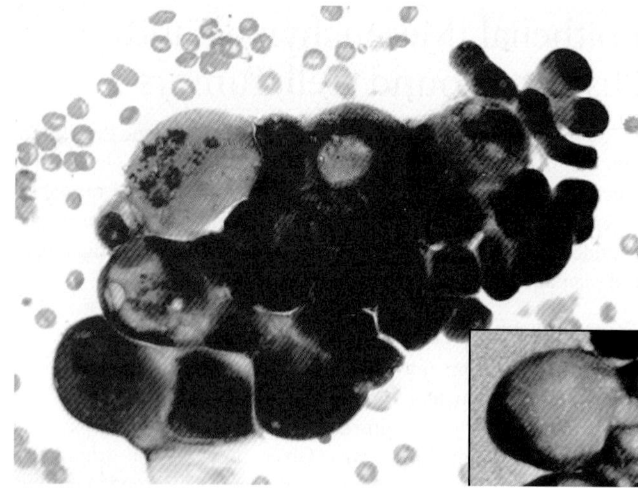

FIGURE 7-12 Fine-needle aspirate of a mammary adenocarcinoma. *Inset*, Signet-ring cell.

and ultimately histologic examination aid in differentiating inflammatory and neoplastic lesions.

Tumors of Glands

Salivary Gland Tumors Salivary gland tumors may be neoplasms of ductular cells, secretory cells, or both. In ductular tumors, the cells resemble basilar epithelial cells. Pleomorphism typically is minimal even when these tumors are malignant, although mild-to-moderate anisokaryosis may be present and nucleoli may be prominent. Tumors of secretory origin often are more pleomorphic. The neoplastic cells are arranged in 3D clusters, sometimes resembling acini seen histologically, and have moderate and variable N:C ratios. The cytoplasm contains few-to-many secretory vacuoles of varying sizes. Cells with a single large vacuole that displaces the nucleus to an eccentric location may be noted and are referred to as *signet-ring cells.* Anisokaryosis and the presence of visible nucleoli of varying number, shape, and size are typical. Tumors may produce mucin, which appears as pale pink or blue material that aligns surrounding erythrocytes into streaming rows.

Mammary Gland Tumors Mammary gland tumors are classified histologically into benign and malignant tumors based on the type, arrangement, and invasiveness of neoplastic epithelium and on the presence or absence of neoplastic and nonneoplastic mesenchymal components. This classification system cannot be applied to cytologic specimens, nor can biologic behavior reliably be ascertained by cytology. Cytologic specimens from mammary masses may contain ductular cells, secretory cells, mesenchymal cells, or a combination of these. Cells from ductular or tubular mammary tumors resemble basilar epithelial cells with low-to-moderate N:C ratios and occasionally contain basophilic granular cytoplasmic inclusions. Pleomorphic features are mild-to-moderate, even when these tumors are malignant. Tumors of secretory origin have few-to-many criteria of malignancy, including moderate-to-marked anisocytosis and anisokaryosis, variably sized secretory vacuoles within the cytoplasm with some signet-ring formation, and nuclear criteria of malignancy (Figure 7-12). If present, the mesenchymal component may consist of mildly to moderately pleomorphic spindle-shaped cells with or without fibrillar magenta extracellular matrix. The spindle cells represent myoepithelial cells or fibroblasts and may be neoplastic or nonneoplastic. The background of many mammary tumors contains lakes of blue secretory material, vacuolated macrophages containing a similar material, and low numbers of neutrophils. Although biologic behavior is difficult to determine cytologically, the greater the number of malignant criteria present within any of the cell types, the more likely the tumor is malignant. However, even tumors with mild pleomorphism may be malignant. Features that define inflammatory mammary carcinomas histologically, such as the presence of tumor emboli in lymphatic vessels, cannot be appreciated cytologically, and this diagnosis is suspected when epithelial cells have cytologic criteria of malignancy and when typical clinical signs such as erythema, swelling, and warmth are identified. Mammary hyperplasia cannot be differentiated cytologically from neoplastic proliferation of tubular cells in the absence of pleomorphic features, and knowing the stage of the reproductive cycle in intact females can be helpful.

Perianal Gland Tumors Perianal gland tumors, also called *circumanal* or *hepatoid tumors,* have a characteristic appearance and with experience can be differentiated from tumors of the apocrine gland of the anal sac. Cells are arranged in cohesive clusters and resemble hepatocytes, having uniformly low N:C ratios and abundant amphophilic granular cytoplasm with distinct margins (Figure 7-13). Nuclei are uniformly round and centrally located, with reticular chromatin and a single nucleolus. A population of reserve cells with high N:C ratios may be found at the periphery of the clusters. Occasionally, a perianal gland tumor may consist exclusively of reserve cells and is termed a *hepatoid gland epithelioma.* Although the majority of these tumors are benign, pleomorphic features are not prominent even in the malignant tumors.

Tumors of the Apocrine Gland of the Anal Sac Tumors of the apocrine gland of the anal sac and perianal gland tumors are the most common tumors in the perianal region and with experience can be reliably differentiated cytologically. Although not of neuroendocrine origin, apocrine adenocarcinomas resemble other tumors with a neuroendocrine appearance (see later). Even though pleomorphism is minimal, these tumors usually are malignant and frequently metastasize to the medial iliac lymph nodes.

Tumors of the Prostate Gland Tumors of the prostate gland have features similar to other glandular tumors. Sometimes the cells contain circular granular eosinophilic inclusions (see section on transitional cell carcinomas). Primary prostatic carcinomas cannot be easily differentiated cytologically from transitional cell carcinomas that arise within the prostate.

Tumors of the Urogenital System

Transitional Cell Carcinoma TCC may be located in the bladder, urethra, ureter, prostate, or vagina. Needle aspiration of tumor tissue is avoided to prevent seeding of tumor cells along the needle tract. Traumatic catheterization of the bladder and prostatic washes are the preferred means of obtaining cytologic specimens. Cells from a TCC are individualized round cells with some cells forming cohesive sheets and clusters. Criteria of malignancy typically are prominent and include marked anisocytosis and anisokaryosis, variation in N:C ratios, marked basophilia, coarse chromatin patterns, and variation in nucleolar size, shape, and number (see Figure 7-4, *B*). Multinuclearity is common. Large circular eosinophilic or magenta granular inclusions, representing accumulations of glycosaminoglycans, occasionally are found in the cytoplasm, but this feature is not pathognomonic for TCC (Figure 7-14). Moderately pleomorphic TCC must be differentiated from hyperplastic transitional epithelium that occurs secondary to inflammatory processes in the bladder; this can be challenging because inflammation sometimes is present in TCCs. Transitional cell polyps are sampled infrequently and typically consist of sheets of epithelial cells with a uniform or mildly pleomorphic appearance.

Tumors of Organs

Hepatocellular Tumors In the liver, primary tumors may arise from hepatocytes or from biliary epithelium. Hepatic carcinoids may be considered as primarily hepatic in origin (see neuroendocrine tumors below). Hepatocellular tumors include benign adenomas, or hepatomas, and carcinomas. Unfortunately, hepatic nodules and masses, whether areas of hyperplasia, benign tumors, or malignant tumors, may be indistinguishable cytologically because all of these entities may consist of well-differentiated hepatocytes with some atypia. Histologic examination is recommended for a definitive diagnosis. Features of hepatocellular atypia that should raise concern for a neoplastic process include anisocytosis and

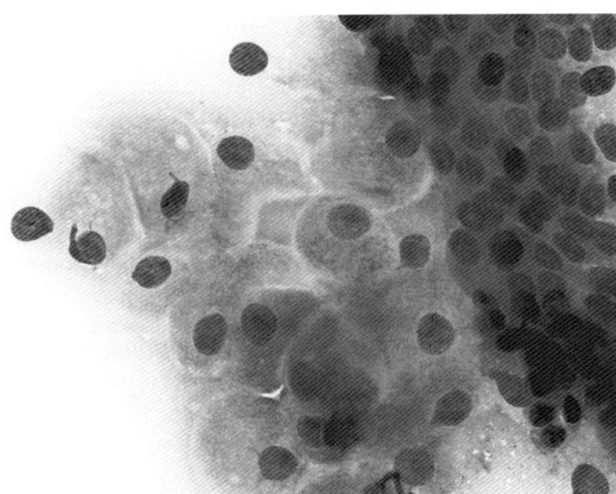

FIGURE 7-13 Fine-needle aspirate of a perianal adenoma with characteristic hepatoid cells *(left)* and reserve cells *(right).*

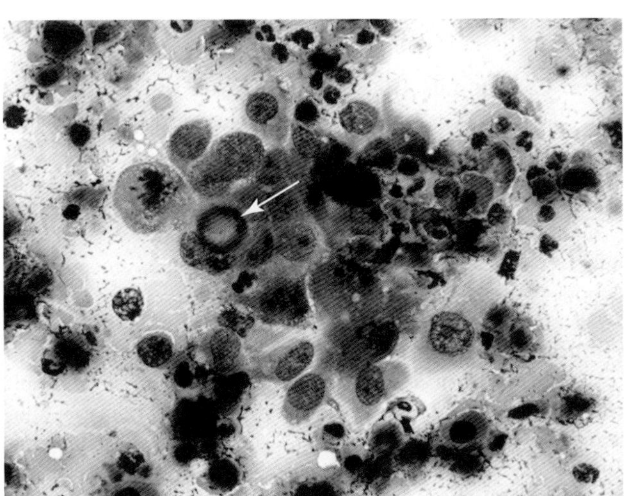

FIGURE 7-14 Cells from a transitional cell carcinoma (TCC) of the prostate. The arrow indicates a cytoplasmic eosinophilic inclusion that represents an accumulation of glycosaminoglycans.

anisokaryosis, variations in N:C ratios, decreased volume and increased basophilia of the cytoplasm, and the presence of more than two nuclei per cell and multiple visible nucleoli. In addition, the cells may appear disorganized and form 3D clusters rather than appearing in a uniform monolayer. The presence of capillaries coursing through the hepatocellular sheets is suggestive of hepatocellular carcinoma.[5] In our experience, the absence of cytoplasmic lipofuscin granules suggests formation of new cells and thus a benign or malignant neoplasm. However, all these features may be observed in hyperplastic or regenerative hepatic nodules. Undifferentiated hepatocellular carcinomas may have few cytologic features that identify them as hepatocellular in origin and may resemble other undifferentiated carcinomas that have metastasized to the liver.

Biliary Tumors Biliary tumors include both benign biliary cystadenomas and carcinomas. Biliary cystic tumors consist of cystic spaces lined by attenuated biliary epithelium that is indistinguishable from normal biliary epithelium. Cytologic specimens consist of small-to-large sheets of monomorphic cuboidal epithelial cells, arranged in a monolayer, with moderately high N:C ratios, basophilic cytoplasm, and uniform central round nuclei. The cytoplasm may contain secretory vacuoles. Biliary carcinomas also may have a monomorphic appearance or may be pleomorphic with polygonal cells arranged in sheets and 3D clusters; in this case, the cells may have variable N:C ratios, deeply basophilic cytoplasm, and central-to-eccentric oval nuclei. Secretory vacuoles may be numerous, single, or absent. Nuclear and nucleolar pleomorphism is prominent. A mucinous background that aligns erythrocytes in streaming rows may be associated with the tumor cells and is suggestive that the cells are of biliary origin.

Tumors of the Exocrine Pancreas Tumors of the exocrine pancreas may arise from ductular or acinar epithelium. Cells from ductular carcinomas resemble biliary carcinomas and consist of monomorphic sheets of cuboidal cells with high N:C ratios, basophilic cytoplasm, and central round nuclei. Nuclear pleomorphism is typically mild, but criteria of malignancy may be present. Exocrine pancreatic adenocarcinoma typically has markedly pleomorphic features. The distinctive cytoplasm of exocrine pancreas, consisting of intensely basophilic cytoplasm with numerous small eosinophilic globules, may be observed in a proportion of cells supporting pancreatic origin.

Renal Carcinomas Renal carcinomas have few defining cytologic characteristics. Variably pleomorphic cuboidal epithelial cells may be arranged in loose sheets, clusters, tubules, and acini. The cells have moderate-to-high N:C ratios and may contain a few discrete cytoplasmic vacuoles. Nuclei are generally round and centrally or basally located, with variably distinct nucleoli. Cytologically, renal carcinomas may be mistaken for neuroendocrine tumors.

Pulmonary Carcinomas or Adenocarcinomas Pulmonary carcinomas or adenocarcinomas may occur in animals with respiratory signs or may be found incidentally when thoracic radiographs are taken for another reason. Cats with primary pulmonary tumors may be presented for lameness resulting from metastasis to the digits. Primary lung tumors are often minimally pleomorphic (see Figure 7-4, *A*), although moderately to markedly pleomorphic features may be observed. Cells are cuboidal to polygonal, are arranged in cohesive sheets and clusters, and have moderate-to-high N:C ratios. Within a single tumor, some cells may contain many discrete vacuoles (Figure 7-15). Apical cilia typically are lacking. If the tumor is large and has outgrown its blood supply, there may be large amounts of necrotic cellular debris accompanied by neutrophilic inflammation. Aspirates from the center of necrotic lesions may not contain intact epithelial cells, and repeat aspiration from the periphery of the lesion is recommended. When numerous large sheets and clusters of epithelial cells are aspirated from a pulmonary mass, a diagnosis of neoplasia is straightforward. However, when only a few small sheets of deeply basophilic epithelium are found, it is difficult to differentiate a pulmonary neoplasm from consolidated hyperplastic respiratory epithelium resulting from a primary inflammatory process.

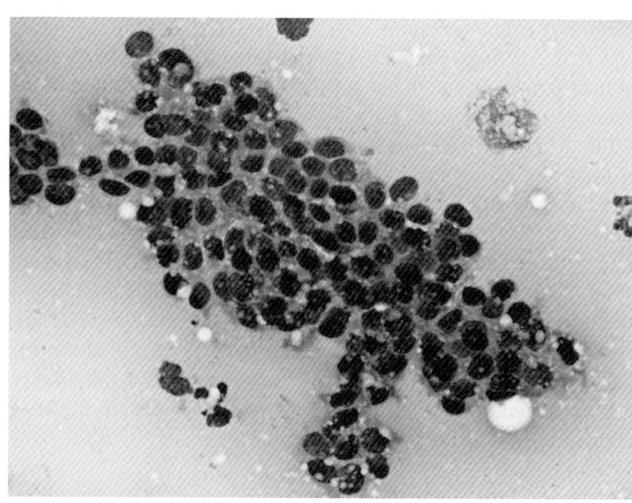

FIGURE 7-15 Fine-needle aspirate of a pulmonary carcinoma. Note the monomorphic population with numerous small cytoplasmic vacuoles.

Thymoma and Thymic Carcinoma Thymoma and thymic carcinoma result from neoplastic transformation of the supporting epithelium in the thymus. However, neoplastic epithelial cells often comprise only a small proportion of cells aspirated from a thymoma. The majority of cells are small lymphocytes, and in dogs, well-differentiated mast cells often are present (Figure 7-16). Epithelial cells, when observed, are polyhedral cells with abundant cytoplasm and central oval nuclei and are arranged individually or in small sheets. Criteria of malignancy among the epithelial cells are minimal in thymomas. In thymic carcinomas, the epithelial component is much more prominent as are criteria of malignancy.

Nasal Carcinomas and Adenocarcinomas Nasal carcinomas and adenocarcinomas, like primary lung tumors, typically are only mildly to moderately pleomorphic. Cytoplasmic vacuolation also may vary, with the majority of cells having few-to-no secretory vacuoles. Apical cilia are typically lacking. Small numbers of highly pleomorphic epithelial cells arranged in sheets or clusters accompanied by marked neutrophilic inflammation likely represent hyperplastic respiratory epithelium and not a tumor. Biopsy is often required to make a diagnosis of neoplasia, especially when cytoplasmic features are not definitive and when inflammation is concurrently present.

Gastrointestinal Tumors Gastrointestinal tumors include adenocarcinomas of the stomach, small intestine, and large

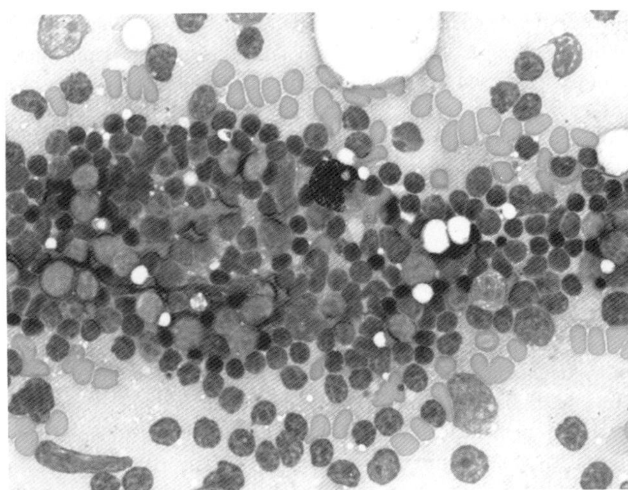

FIGURE 7-16 Fine-needle aspirate of a thymoma in a dog. The majority of cells are small lymphocytes. A mast cell and an eosinophil also are present.

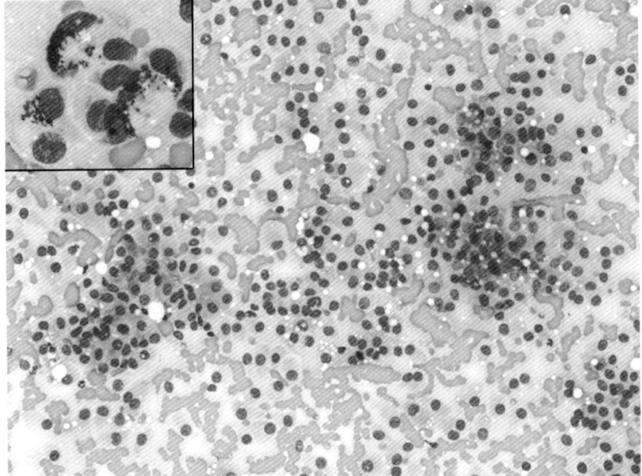

FIGURE 7-17 Fine-needle aspirate of a thyroid carcinoma in a dog. Note the loosely cohesive sheets of cells in a background of abundant blood. *Inset,* Some of the tumor cells contain blue-black granules thought to be tyrosine granules.

intestine, and these tumors have similar cytologic features. Aspirates of these tumors typically consist of highly pleomorphic epithelial cells arranged in sheets and clusters. The cells typically contain few-to-many secretory vacuoles. The background may contain abundant mucus produced by the tumor cells or pink fibrillar collagen representing a scirrhous response secondary to the tumor.

Endocrine and Neuroendocrine Tumors Endocrine and neuroendocrine tumors comprise a diverse collection of tumor types. If the primary location of the tumor is not known, specific tumor type may be impossible to determine owing to the cytologic similarity among these tumors. In general, aspirates of endocrine and neuroendocrine tumors are highly cellular and consist of loosely cohesive sheets and clusters of epithelial cells with ill-defined intercellular junctions and cytoplasmic margins (Figure 7-17). The cells are fragile, and numerous free nuclei from ruptured cells are scattered in the background. Nuclei of intact cells may be

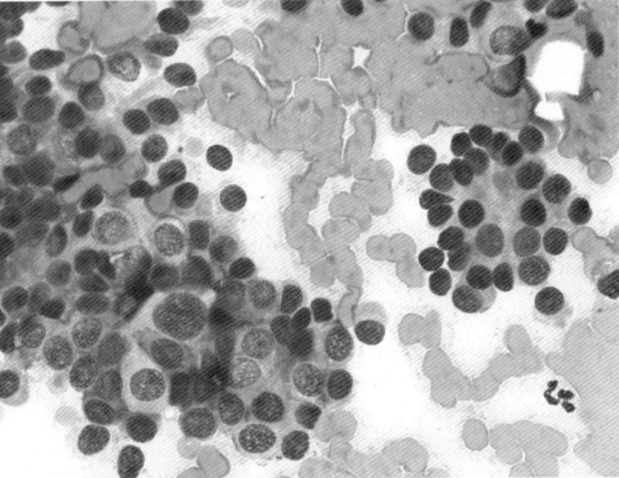

FIGURE 7-18 Fine-needle aspirate of an anal sac apocrine adenocarcinoma. Note the rosette of tumor cells *(right).*

arranged in a rosette (Figure 7-18), suggestive of acinar formation. Within intact cells, nuclei are round and centrally located with reticular chromatin. Nucleoli are often indistinct, but one to two nucleoli may be observed. The cytoplasm may contain a few clear, distinct vacuoles. There are usually few criteria of malignancy, even in carcinomas, and anisocytosis and anisokaryosis are mild to moderate with large nuclei observed occasionally. Mitotic figures may be present. Some tumors of endocrine origin are biologically active, and tumor type may be identified based on clinical presentation and laboratory findings.

Thyroid Carcinomas Thyroid carcinomas in dogs are highly vascularized, and aspirates may yield abundant blood as well as some hemosiderophages. In addition to displaying general features of endocrine tissue, cells from thyroid tumors may contain blue-black cytoplasmic granules (see Figure 7-17, *inset*), believed to represent tyrosine granules, and amorphous pink material that may represent colloid. In the absence of these features, thyroid tumors cannot be differentiated cytologically from C-cell tumors and parathyroid tumors that occur in the same location. Most thyroid tumors in dogs are nonfunctional carcinomas, whereas in cats thyroidal masses or nodules are functional adenomas or adenomatous hyperplasia. Ectopic thyroid tissue may undergo transformation and be found in unexpected locations, such as the thoracic inlet and mediastinum.

Parathyroid Tumors Parathyroid tumors are typically adenomas but are often functional and result in hypercalcemia through the systemic actions of parathyroid hormone. Parathyroid tumors have the typical features of endocrine tissue. Occasionally, eosinophilic spiculate inclusions are found in the cytoplasm.[6]

Chemodectomas Chemodectomas are neuroendocrine tumors of chemoreceptor cells found in the carotid or aortic bodies located in the submandibular region and at the base of the heart, respectively. They do not have cytologic features that distinguish them from other endocrine tumors, such as ectopic thyroid tumors.

Adrenal Cortical and Medullary Tumors Adrenal cortical and medullary tumors are cytologically similar and have a typical neuroendocrine appearance. Adrenal cortical tumors of the zona glomerulosa and fasciculata often contain few-to-many discrete clear vacuoles. Pleomorphism is minimal and differentiation between adrenal adenoma and adenocarcinoma is not always possible cytologically. Pheochromocytomas of the adrenal medulla lack distinct cytoplasmic vacuoles and will stain positively with silver stains and express synaptophysin and chromogranin A.[7]

Insulinomas Insulinomas or beta-cell tumors have typical neuroendocrine features without additional defining characteristics except for the clinical presentation of hypoglycemia. Insulinomas may metastasize to liver, regional lymph nodes, mesentery, and omentum.

Carcinoids of Lung, Liver, Intestine, and Colon Carcinoids of lung, liver, intestine, and colon are rare neuroendocrine tumors. They must be distinguished from other neuroendocrine tumors that have metastasized based on history, clinical presentation, presence of other primary tumors, and histologic examination.

Tumors of Mesenchymal Tissues

Tumors derived from mesenchymal or connective tissues can be diverse in their cytologic appearances, but they have some common features. Cells are often embedded in extracellular matrix produced by tumor cells and exfoliate poorly. Thus cytologic samples tend to have low cellularity, although exceptions occur. Cells do not have intercellular junctions and are individually arranged (Figure 7-19); however, in cases in which cellularity is high or when scraping and imprint methods are used to prepare slides, cells may be found in dense noncohesive aggregates that are disorganized. Cell shape is typically oval, spindle-shaped, or stellate, and the tumors are often grouped according to the most common shape. Cytoplasmic margins are characteristically indistinct, and nuclei are generally round, oval, or elongate. Some mesenchymal tumors lack further distinguishing features, and knowledge of the location and other clinical information is necessary to formulate a list of differential diagnoses in anticipation of the definitive diagnosis based on histologic and immunochemical staining.

Reactive or hyperplastic mesenchymal cells that accompany inflammatory and neoplastic lesions present a diagnostic dilemma because these cells may have criteria of malignancy (Figure 7-20). When a mass is composed of heterogeneous cell populations, caution is advised in making a definitive cytologic diagnosis of a mesenchymal tumor; this is especially true when concurrent neutrophilic inflammation is present. Additional diagnostic measures should be taken to confirm the presence of a neoplasm prior to making major treatment decisions.

Mesenchymal Tumors Composed of Spindle-Shaped and Stellate Cells

Tumors of Fibroblasts Tumors of fibroblasts may have morphologic features of well-differentiated fibroblasts, including monomorphic elongate spindle-shaped or fusiform cells with moderate N:C ratios, basophilic cytoplasm, and central oval nuclei with one to several small nucleoli. However, a population of well-differentiated fibroblasts may represent reactive fibroplasia, as is found in scars or granulation tissue (see Figure 7-20), a fibroma, or a well-differentiated fibrosarcoma. Unfortunately, there are no clear cytomorphologic characteristics that can reliably differentiate among these entities. The presence of accompanying inflammation warrants an interpretation of reactive fibroblasts even when pleomorphic features are present. Epithelioid macrophages found in pyogranulomatous lesions are frequently mistaken for neoplastic fibroblasts by inexperienced clinicians. High cellularity, marked pleomorphism, especially with respect to the nucleus, and absence of inflammation along with a supportive clinical picture lend credible evidence for a cytologic diagnosis of fibrosarcoma. Malignant fibroblasts may vary in shape and N:C ratio and may have numerous nuclear criteria of malignancy. Anisocytosis and anisokaryosis may be moderate to marked (Figure 7-21). Neoplastic fibroblasts may contain pink cytoplasmic granules. Accompanying collagen, consisting of fibrillar bands of pink extracellular material, may support the origin of the cells as fibroblasts; however, similar matrix can be seen with a variety of other mesenchymal neoplasms. Cells from myxosarcoma resemble cells of fibrosarcoma, but are embedded in a lightly eosinophilic matrix that aligns the cells in streaming rows (Figure 7-22; see Figure 7-19). Feline vaccine-associated sarcomas (VAS) are highly pleomorphic mesenchymal tumors, primarily of fibroblastic origin, that occur at sites of previous injections, most often of vaccines containing adjuvant. In

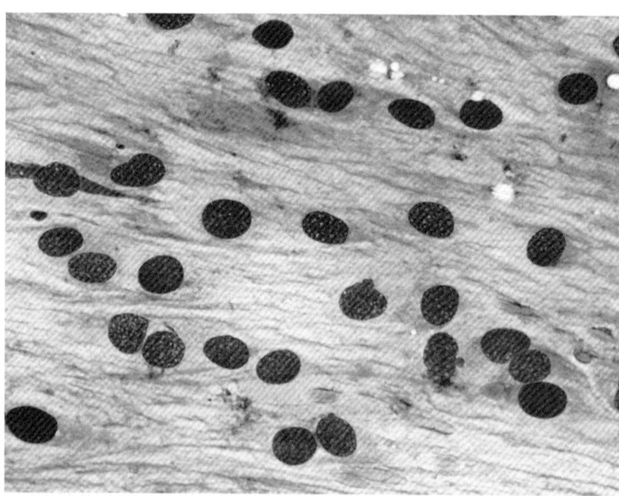

FIGURE 7-19 Fine-needle aspirate of a myxosarcoma in a dog. Note the individualized spindle-shaped cells.

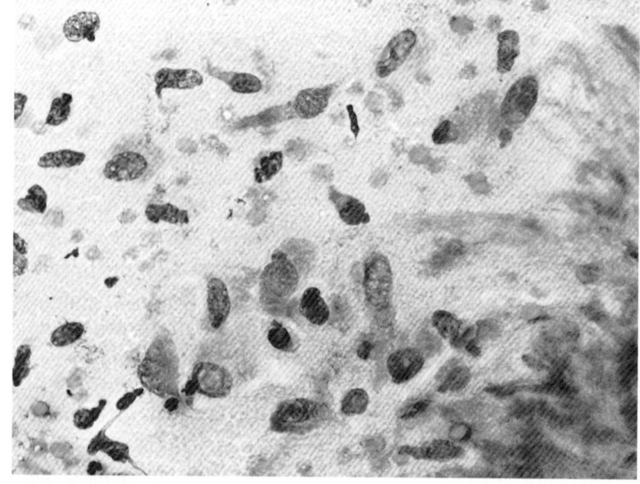

FIGURE 7-20 Imprint of granulation tissue composed of pleomorphic fibroblasts.

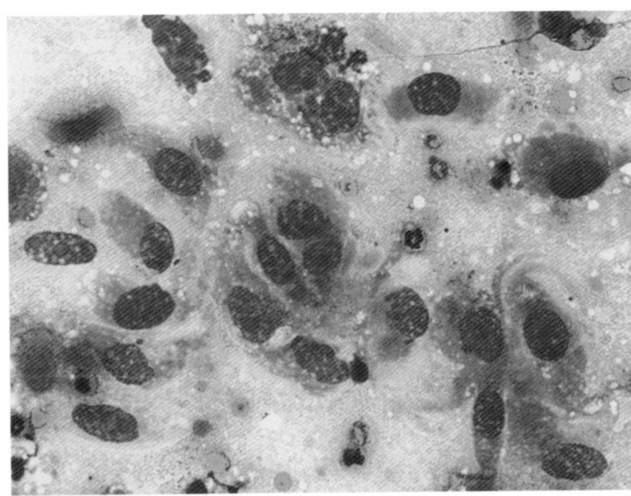

FIGURE 7-21 Fine-needle aspirate of a fibrosarcoma in a dog. Note the cellular pleomorphism and pink background, possibly glycosaminoglycans.

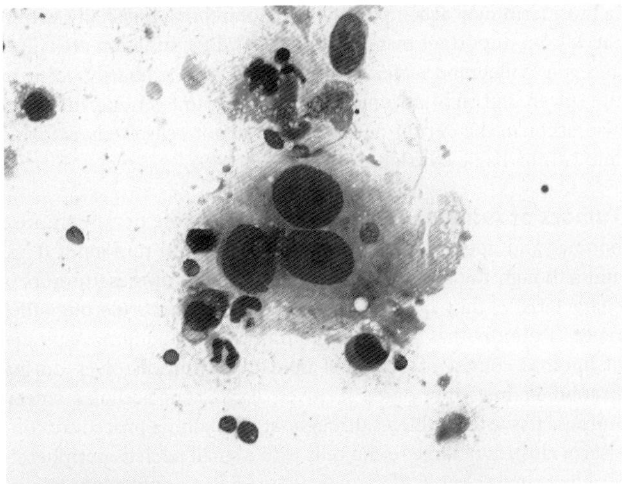

FIGURE 7-23 Fine-needle aspirate of a vaccine-associated fibrosarcoma in a cat. Note the extreme atypia in the multinucleated tumor cell.

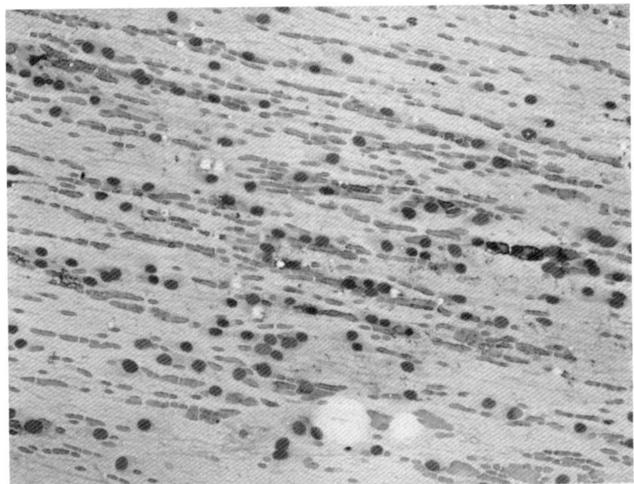

FIGURE 7-22 Fine-needle aspirate of a myxosarcoma (same tumor as Figure 7-19). Note the myxomatous background in which tumor cells and erythrocytes are streaming.

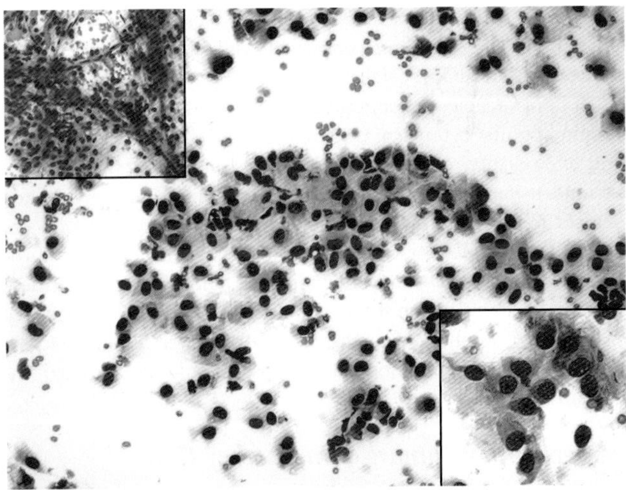

FIGURE 7-24 Fine-needle aspirate of a perivascular wall tumor (hemangiopericytoma). Note how well the cells exfoliated. *Upper left inset,* Vessels are often associated with the tumor cells. *Lower right inset,* Cells are spindle-shaped, stellate, or oval.

addition to containing pleomorphic mesenchymal cells, aspirates of feline VAS may contain large multinucleated tumor cells (Figure 7-23) and moderate numbers of small lymphocytes.

Tumors of the Perivascular Wall or Nerve Sheath Tumors of the perivascular wall or nerve sheath, such as hemangiopericytoma, peripheral nerve sheath tumor (PNST), and schwannoma, often exfoliate well; samples are highly cellular with cells arranged both individually and in dense aggregates (Figure 7-24). Cells are usually spindle-shaped and plump with wispy cytoplasmic extensions; oval-to-stellate forms also are found. The lightly basophilic cytoplasm frequently contains a few small clear round vacuoles. Nuclei are oval and centrally located with finely stippled chromatin and often one to three small nucleoli. Binuclearity is observed in a small proportion of cells. Anisocytosis and anisokaryosis are mild to moderate. Linear capillaries may be embedded within aggregates of tumor cells in aspirates of hemangiopericytomas.

Tumors of Vascular Endothelium Tumors of vascular endothelium include hemangioma and hemangiosarcoma. Aspirates of hemangioma may contain a uniform population of long thin spindle-shaped cells in a background of abundant blood; however, cellularity is rarely sufficient for a definitive diagnosis of this benign vascular tumor. Aspiration of suspected hemangiosarcoma is approached cautiously because of the potential consequence of hemorrhage, but cellular yields may be sufficient to reach a tentative diagnosis. The neoplastic cells are often markedly pleomorphic and consist of spindle-shaped, stellate, and oval cells that have deeply basophilic cytoplasm containing punctate vacuoles (see Figure 7-6).[8] Large, irregular, or indented oval nuclei typically have coarse chromatin and multiple prominent nucleoli that vary in shape and size. Multinucleated cells are found occasionally. Anisocytosis and anisokaryosis are often marked. A small amount of pink extracellular matrix may be associated with the neoplastic cells. Erythroid precursors and macrophages containing erythrocytes or hemosiderin may accompany hemangiosarcoma, especially within the spleen. Important markers of vascular differentiation are CD31 and von Willebrand factor. Hemangiosarcomas primarily occur in the spleen and right atrium with metastasis to liver and lung, but also occur in the dermis and subcutis. Tumor cells rarely exfoliate into hemorrhagic effusions.

Tumors of Adipose Tissue Tumors of adipose tissue comprise lipomas and liposarcomas. Lipomas are common tumors of dogs, and although the gross appearance and texture of these tumors is characteristic, they often are aspirated in order to rule out other types of tumors that require more immediate attention. Aspirates of lipomas consist of abundant lipid that often dissolves during fixation in methanol-based fixatives, leaving an acellular smear. Adipose tissue that adheres throughout the staining procedure consists of clusters of large round cells with a small nucleus peripheralized by a single clear lipid vacuole (Figure 7-25). Supporting stromal strands and capillary vessels are sometimes visible within the cluster of adipocytes, and free fat may be present. Normal subcutaneous adipose tissue cannot be differentiated from a lipoma or infiltrating lipoma cytologically; therefore caution is recommended when making a conclusive cytologic diagnosis of lipoma if the gross appearance or texture of the mass is not typical. Liposarcomas are uncommon and can adopt a variety of cytologic appearances. Cells may be spindle-shaped, stellate, or round with variable N:C ratios. Clear lipid vacuoles of varying sizes are present within a basophilic or amphophilic cytoplasm (Figure 7-26). Nuclei are round to oval and often display criteria of malignancy. Confirming the presence of lipid using Oil Red O stain is best accomplished on unfixed smears. With inflammation of adipose tissue (panniculitis or steatitis), the sample often contains moderately pleomorphic fibroblasts and histiocytes that contain lipid or lipid-like vacuoles; these cells are easily mistaken for a neoplastic population. The presence of even low numbers of neutrophils within these lesions favors a conservative interpretation, and biopsy should be pursued for definitive diagnosis.

Mesenchymal Tumors Composed of Thin Elongate Cells

Tumors of Smooth Muscle and Stroma Tumors of smooth muscle and stroma, such as leiomyoma, leiomyosarcoma, and gastrointestinal stromal tumor (GIST), have a similar cytologic appearance. Aspirates of these tumors, whether benign or malignant, often are highly cellular and consist of long thin mesenchymal cells arranged in aggregates and linear bundles. Nuclei are often elongate or "cigar-shaped" (Figure 7-27). Pleomorphism is typically mild. The most common sites for these tumors are the gastrointestinal tract and female reproductive tract, especially the uterus and vagina. Immunohistochemical detection of smooth muscle actin or c-kit expression in smooth muscle tumors and GIST, respectively, is required to distinguish these tumors.

Tumors of Striated Muscle Tumors of striated muscle, rhabdomyoma and rhabdomyosarcoma, are uncommon and can have a variety of cytomorphologic appearances. Rhabdomyomas occurring in the tongue and pharynx may present cytologically as a "granular cell tumor" composed of individual round or polygonal cells containing numerous fine pink cytoplasmic granules and a central round nucleus. Electron microscopic examination reveals the pink granules to be numerous mitochondria. Rhabdomyosarcomas typically comprise individualized pleomorphic

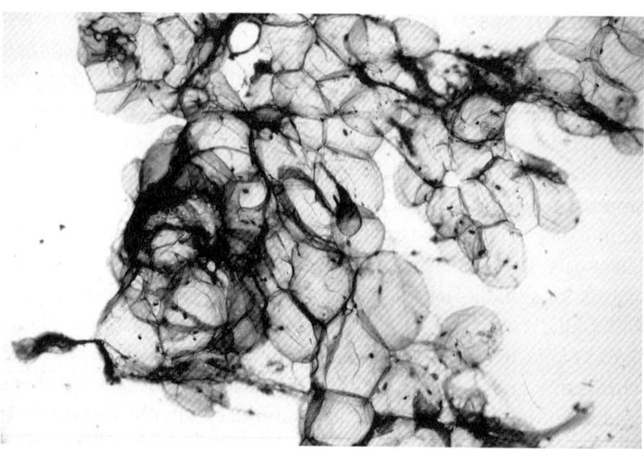

FIGURE 7-25 Fine-needle aspirate of well-differentiated adipocytes from a lipoma.

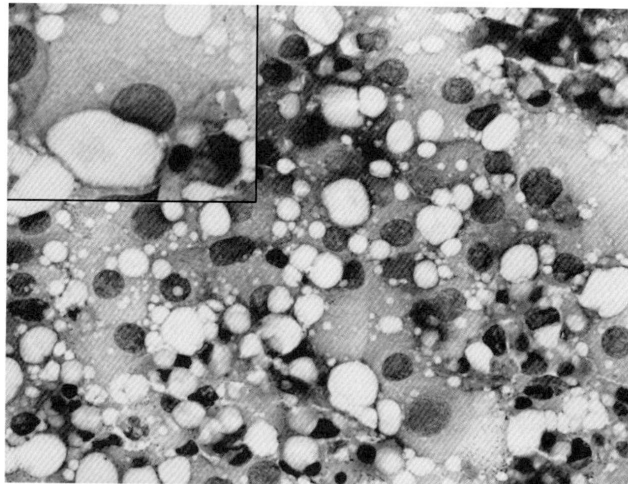

FIGURE 7-26 Fine-needle aspirate of a liposarcoma in a dog. Note that the polygonal cells contain lipid vacuoles. *Inset*, A large lipid vacuole in a tumor cell.

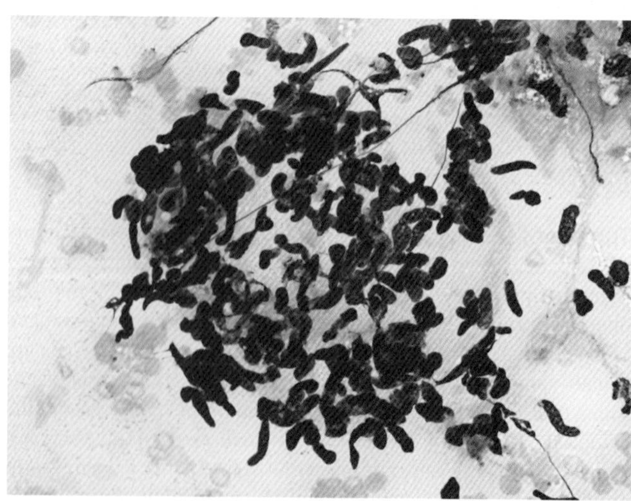

FIGURE 7-27 Fine-needle aspirate of a gastrointestinal stromal tumor (GIST). Many cells are disrupted, but elongated (cigar-shaped) nuclei are visible.

spindle-shaped cells with low numbers of elongate strap cells that may or may not demonstrate cross-striations within the cytoplasm. Strap cells characteristically have several round-to-oval nuclei arranged in a linear row. Normal muscle fibers are bright blue, with prominent cross-striations when viewed at high magnification, and have randomly distributed pale oval nuclei.

Mesenchymal Tumors Composed of Round or Oval Cells

Tumors of Bone Origin Tumors of bone origin include osteosarcoma, osteoma, multilobular tumor of bone, and giant cell tumor of bone. Osteosarcoma is the most common tumor of bone in dogs and results in a mixed osteolytic and osteoproliferative lesion radiographically. Aspirates of osteosarcoma may be highly or poorly cellular, depending on the collection technique and the nature of the lesion. Cytologic features that support osteoblasts as the cells of origin include oval cells with indistinct margins, basophilic cytoplasm containing a distinct paranuclear clearing, and eccentric nuclei with criteria of malignancy (Figure 7-28). The cytoplasm occasionally contains fine-to-coarse magenta granules. N:C ratios are moderate to high, and anisocytosis is moderate to occasionally marked. Often, bright magenta extracellular matrix or osteoid is found. Large multinucleated osteoclasts are typically scattered among the neoplastic osteoblasts. Multilobular tumor of bone and giant cell tumor of bone are tumors of osteoblasts and osteoclasts, respectively, that have characteristic locations or radiographic appearances. The cytologic appearance of plasma cell tumor and osteosarcoma may overlap because both contain cells with eccentric nuclei and paranuclear clearing; for inexperienced clinicians, this may constitute a diagnostic dilemma in dogs, and less frequently in cats, that have osteolytic lesions. Clinical presentation and laboratory abnormalities may be useful in distinguishing these malignancies. Caution is recommended when making a cytologic diagnosis of osteosarcoma at the site of a pathologic fracture as hyperplastic and reactive osteoblasts may have a degree of pleomorphism that can be mistaken for a well-differentiated neoplasm.

Tumors of Chondrocytes Tumors of chondrocytes are less common than osteosarcoma and may arise in any location where cartilage occurs, including epiphyseal bone, nasal cavity, and trachea. Although the amount of matrix present in any given tumor can vary, the most characteristic cytologic finding in aspirates of chondrosarcoma is the large amount of purple extracellular matrix that envelops and often obscures the neoplastic chondroblasts (Figure 7-29). Neoplastic chondroblasts are round with moderate-to-high N:C ratios but may be spindle-shaped or stellate. A few cytoplasmic vacuoles or magenta granules are common, and nuclei are round with finely stippled chromatin and variably prominent nucleoli.

Tumors of Synovial Cells Tumors of synovial cells or synovial cell sarcomas are periarticular tumors. The cells are arranged individually or in noncohesive aggregates and are round to spindle-shaped with moderate N:C ratios. Pleomorphism can vary from mild to marked, including marked anisocytosis and anisokaryosis and nuclear criteria of malignancy. For highly pleomorphic synovial cell sarcomas, immunohistochemical staining may be necessary to distinguish them from periarticular histiocytic sarcomas.

Tumors of Melanocytes

In malignant melanoma, the cells can adopt the appearance of epithelial (sheets of cohesive cells), mesenchymal (individualized oval or spindle-shaped cells), or discrete round cell tumors. Individual melanoblasts are round, oval, or spindle-shaped cells with moderately high N:C ratios, lightly basophilic cytoplasm, and round or oval nuclei with fine chromatin and distinct nucleoli. Criteria of malignancy consist primarily of anisokaryosis and nucleolar pleomorphism. Melanized tumors do not present a diagnostic challenge, and fine black melanin granules may be so numerous that they obscure all cellular detail. Cells with varying degrees of melanization are typically found within the same tumor, and melanin granules may be sparse in some cells (Figure 7-30). Amelanotic tumors present a greater diagnostic challenge. Usually, a faint scattering of fine gray-black melanin granules are found in a few cells to support a diagnosis, but cells may be completely devoid of pigmentation (Figure 7-31). In these circumstances, moderately

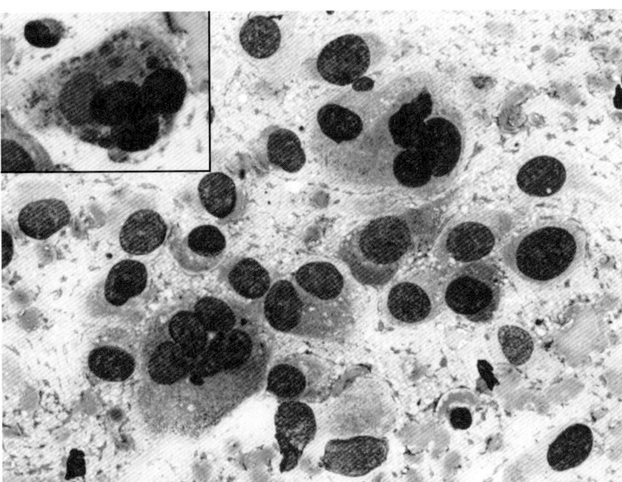

FIGURE 7-28 Fine-needle aspirate of a proliferative and lytic lesion in bone. The diagnosis was osteosarcoma. The pleomorphic cells tend to be round or oval with eccentric nuclei and sometimes paranuclear clear zones. *Inset*, A multinucleated tumor cell contains prominent pink granules.

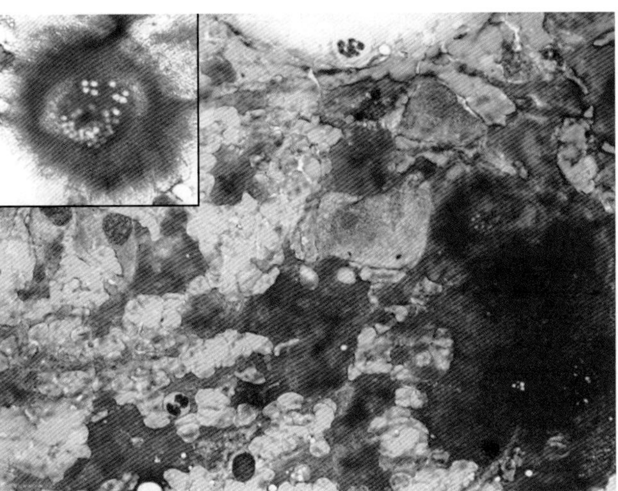

FIGURE 7-29 Fine-needle aspirate of a chondrosarcoma with pleomorphic tumor cells and abundant magenta matrix that sometimes surrounds the tumor cells *(inset)*.

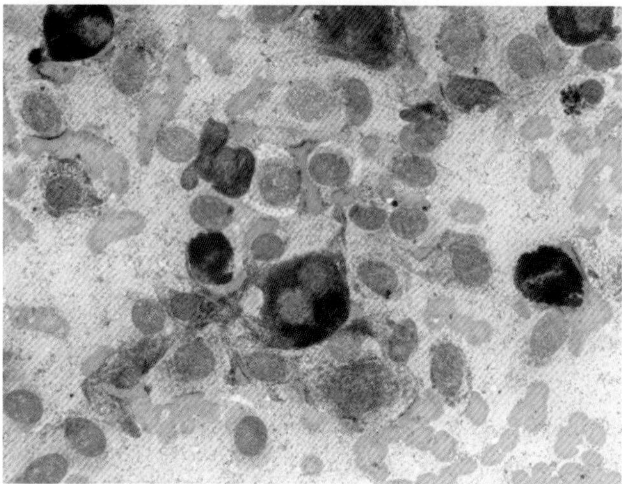

FIGURE 7-30 Fine-needle aspirate of a melanoma in a dog. Note the fine melanin granules in the tumor cells and in the background.

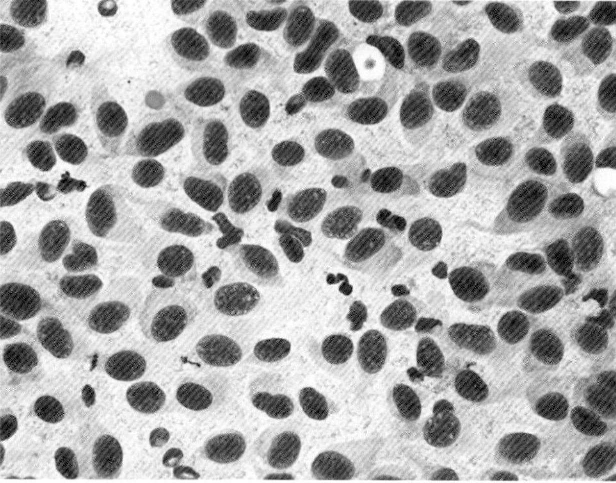

FIGURE 7-31 Fine-needle aspirate of a melanoma in which melanin granules are not visible (amelanotic melanoma).

pleomorphic tumor cells aspirated from masses on the digits or in the oral cavity should alert the clinician to the possibility of this highly malignant tumor. Because melanocytes are of neuroectodermal origin, the cells may express certain neural markers, such as S-100 and neuron-specific enolase, in addition to vimentin and often Melan A.

An additional cytologic challenge is the identification of metastatic lesions within lymph nodes. Most lymph nodes draining pigmented melanomas contain melanophages, which are macrophages containing abundant melanin; in the authors' experience, this is especially true following surgical removal or biopsy of the primary mass. These melanophages may be mistaken for metastatic cells, but they differ from neoplastic melanoblasts as melanophages typically contain coarse collections of melanin within phagolysosomes rather than the fine granulation typically found within melanoblasts.

Most dermal tumors of melanocytic origin are benign and are termed *melanocytomas.* They consist of polygonal or spindle-shaped cells containing black cytoplasmic granules. Other dermal tumors containing melanin pigment, such as basal cell tumor (epithelioma), must be differentiated from melanocytomas. These typically are of epithelial origin and should be distinguished by their cellular arrangement in cohesive sheets (see Figure 7-9).

Mesenchymal Tumors Composed of Cells Arranged in Dense Aggregates

Cells aspirated from some mesenchymal tumors, including rhabdomyosarcoma, perivascular wall tumor, PNST, amelanotic melanoma, and the epithelioid form of hemangiosarcoma, form dense aggregates and clusters that are more characteristic of epithelial cells. Careful examination typically reveals some spindle-shaped cells with indistinct margins and spaces between the closely packed cells indicating the lack of intercellular junctions. Slide preparation by imprinting and scraping also may yield clusters and sheets of mesenchymal cells that mimic epithelial populations.

Mesenchymal Tumors with Frequent Multinucleated Cells

Although any neoplasm can have a few multinucleated cells, multinuclearity is especially common in certain sarcomas. These include histiocytic sarcoma, feline VAS, malignant fibrous histiocytosis, and rhabdomyosarcoma, in which the multinucleated cells are part of the tumor population. In osteosarcoma, multinucleated osteoclasts are often present and are not part of the neoplastic population of cells.

Discrete Round Cell Tumors

The majority of discrete round cell tumors are of hematopoietic (and mesenchymal) origin, including neoplasms of mast cells, plasma cells, lymphocytes, and histiocytes. Transmissible venereal tumors (TVTs) are also included in this category, and there are a variety of epithelial and mesenchymal tumors that sometimes appear as round cell tumors. These tumors share certain cytomorphologic features. Cells exfoliate easily leading to highly cellular specimens in which the cells are individualized in noncohesive monolayers. As the moniker indicates, the cells are round and have distinct cytoplasmic margins and round nuclei, although nuclear shape may vary in pleomorphic forms of these tumors.

Mast Cell Tumors

Mast cell tumors consist of cells with numerous purple cytoplasmic granules that fill the cytoplasm and often obscure the nucleus (see Figures 7-2 and 7-5). In cats, granules are finer than they are in canine mast cells. Even in poorly granulated mast cell tumors, there often are enough granules in some cells to suggest that they are mast cells. One notable exception is when the granules fail to take up stain when one of the aqueous quick stains is used, so clinicians using these stains should be alert to this artifact (see Figure 7-2). The nucleus is generally centrally located, but may be eccentric. Criteria of malignancy are observed infrequently and may include anisocytosis, anisokaryosis, binuclearity, multinuclearity, multiple visible nucleoli, and frequent mitotic figures. Marked pleomorphism is uncommon and when present suggests a higher grade tumor; however, at present grading is based on histologic findings. Markedly pleomorphic mast cells may have sparse or absent granulation, marked variation in cell and nuclear size, and lobulated or ameboid nuclei. In dogs, aspirates of mast cell tumors often contain numerous eosinophils along with a small proportion of reactive fibroblasts and thick bands of collagen (see Figure 7-5).

Determining the presence of metastasis in tissues, including lymph node, liver, and spleen, that have resident mast cells may be difficult. Additional features that support metastatic disease include the presence of large numbers of mast cells suggestive of tissue effacement, mast cells with pleomorphic features, and mast cells arranged in groups instead of singly. If cytologic evaluation cannot distinguish between resident mast cells and metastasis, a biopsy should be evaluated.

Other neoplasms in which the cells contain cytoplasmic granules may be mistaken for mast cell tumors and include granulated T-cell lymphoma, natural killer (NK) cell lymphoma, and granular cell tumors. When cells from mast cell tumors are agranular or when the granules fail to stain with aqueous stains, the tumor may be mistaken for plasmacytoma, histiocytoma, or atypical lymphoma. Reactive nonneoplastic mast cells may be found in increased numbers at sites of fibrosis because of the role mast cells play in wound healing.

Plasma Cell Tumors

Plasma cell tumors composed of well-differentiated plasma cells are easily recognized owing to the characteristic features of plasma cells—abundant royal blue cytoplasm, paranuclear clear zone (Golgi apparatus), eccentric round nucleus, and clumped chromatin. Multinuclearity is common in plasmacytomas, and in more pleomorphic forms of this tumor the nuclei may be multilobulated (Figure 7-32). Neoplastic plasma cells may appear immature and resemble large lymphocytes with higher N:C ratios and finer chromatin. Sometimes the cells contain Russell bodies, collections of immunoglobulin within the endoplasmic reticulum, and are termed *Mott cells*. Plasma cell tumors may occur in the skin, oral mucosa, bone marrow, liver, and spleen, and the specific diagnostic criteria for plasma cell myeloma, extramedullary plasma cell myeloma, and plasmacytoma are presented in Chapter 32, Section D. Reactive plasma cell proliferations consist of a mixture of inflammatory cells and are rarely mistaken for a neoplastic process in a cutaneous mass; however, when plasmacytosis is identified in bone marrow, reactive and neoplastic conditions must be distinguished.

Lymphoma

Lymphoma comprises many variants, and entire chapters are written on their cytologic features. Definitive diagnosis of lymphoma based on examination of cytologic specimens is often possible; however, some types of lymphoma or lymphoma in certain tissues may be difficult to diagnose cytologically. As with many discrete round cell neoplasms, it is the homogeneity of the population, rather than the morphologic features, that suggest a neoplastic process. In lymphoid organs or other tissues in which there is a reactive or polyclonal infiltrate of lymphocytes, small lymphocytes should predominate and comprise more than 50% of the lymphoid cells, even as the proportion of large and intermediate lymphocytes increases. Plasma cells and other inflammatory cells also may be found in these reactive lesions. As the proportion of intermediate and large lymphocytes approaches or exceeds 50%, it becomes more difficult to differentiate between a reactive and neoplastic process; this is especially true for the spleen and certain lymph nodes, such as mandibular and mesenteric nodes, that are continuously exposed to antigen. Because of this, sampling of other nodes or tissues is preferred. In addition, cats can mount strong lymphocytic responses that can cytologically resemble lymphoma. In contrast, there are certain types of lymphoma, such as T-cell rich B-cell lymphoma and Hodgkin's-like lymphoma, that contain a mixture of clonal (neoplastic) and polyclonal (nonneoplastic) populations of lymphocytes. When a diagnosis of lymphoma is not obvious from the cytologic specimen, additional procedures should be performed, including biopsy with histologic evaluation, immunophenotyping, assessment of clonality, or a combination of these (see Chapter 32, Sections A and B).

Lymphoma can be diagnosed cytologically when large or intermediate lymphocytes comprise the majority of the nodal population. Large and intermediate lymphocytes are defined as those larger than or the same size as a neutrophil, respectively, or that are greater than two times or one-and-a-half to two times the diameter of an erythrocyte, respectively. Cytologic types include immunoblastic or centroblastic types, composed of large cells with visible nucleoli and deeply basophilic cytoplasm (see Figure 7-1, *A*), and types composed of medium-sized cells often having indistinct nucleoli (Figure 7-33). Mitotic figures and tingible-body macrophages, which are macrophages containing nuclear debris from tumor cells, may be increased, but this is not a defining characteristic. Cytologic diagnosis of small cell lymphoma is more challenging, especially in tissues such as lymph node and spleen with a resident population of small lymphocytes or in tissues such as

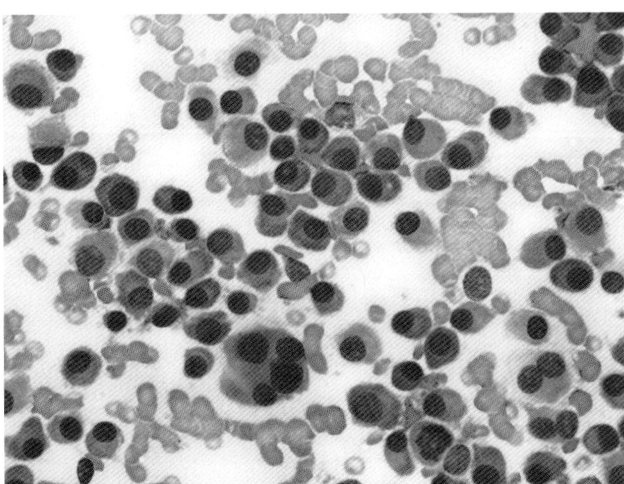

FIGURE 7-32 Fine-needle aspirate of a plasmacytoma. Many cells have the characteristic appearance of plasma cells. Multinuclearity is a common feature of this tumor.

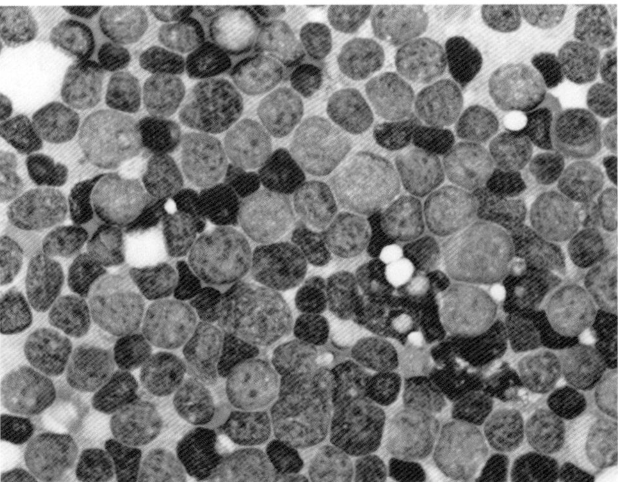

FIGURE 7-33 Fine-needle aspirate of a lymph node from a dog with T-cell lymphoma. Note that most of the cells are about two times the diameter of an erythrocyte and that nucleoli are indistinct in many cells.

liver and small intestine in which lymphocytic inflammation is common. In these cases, additional diagnostic testing is required for confirmation and may include one or more of the following: histologic examination, preferably of a whole node or full-thickness piece of intestine; immunophenotyping by immunocytochemical/histochemical staining or flow cytometry; and polymerase chain reaction (PCR) for antigen receptor rearrangement to detect clonality. Because lymphocytes are fragile, free nuclei and cytoplasmic fragments frequently are observed in aspirates of lymphoma (see Figure 7-1, *A*); however, these features can be found in samples from reactive lymphocytic populations and are not criteria for neoplasia.

Infrequently, neoplastic lymphocytes are highly pleomorphic and exhibit moderate to marked anisocytosis, indented or deeply clefted nuclei, ameboid nuclei, multinuclearity, cytoplasmic vacuoles, and aberrant phagocytic behavior. When present, a few, some, or most of the neoplastic lymphocytes in a given tumor may have these features and may be mistaken for neoplastic histiocytes.[9] Sometimes neoplastic lymphocytes contain fine or coarse pink cytoplasmic granules, suggestive of a T- or NK-cell phenotype. In large granular lymphoma, the lymphocytes contain large, coarse, pink granules and are thought to be cytotoxic T- or NK-cells (Figure 7-34).

Tumors of Histiocytic Origin

Cutaneous Histiocytoma Cutaneous histiocytoma originates from epidermal dendritic or Langerhans cells and is typically found on the head or limbs of young dogs. The cells are round and have pale blue to colorless cytoplasm and a round, sometimes indented, central nucleus with fine to reticular chromatin and indistinct nucleoli (Figure 7-35). Occasionally, the cytoplasm is more basophilic, and the nucleus more eccentrically located; in these cases, the cells may be mistaken for immature plasma cells and the mass called a plasmacytoma. Finding a few mitotic figures is common, but binuclearity is infrequent. Often the tumor cells are highlighted by a pale purple proteinaceous background. In mature lesions, there may be an infiltrate of small lymphocytes representing the T-cell–mediated immune response that leads to the spontaneous resolution of these tumors. Presumed histiocytomas that do not resolve or that increase in size should be biopsied to rule out cutaneous lymphoma.

Histiocytic Sarcomas of Dendritic and Macrophage Lineage Histiocytic sarcomas of dendritic and macrophage lineage are malignant tumors and are variably called *histiocytic sarcoma* (HS), *malignant histiocytosis* (MH), and *hemophagocytic histiocytic sarcoma* (HHS), depending on clinical presentation, cytomorphologic appearance, and specific cell lineage (see Chapter 33, Section F). These tumors have at least three cytologic appearances. First, the tumor may be composed of a highly pleomorphic population of discrete round cells with extreme variations in N:C ratios, cell size, and nuclear size (Figure 7-36).[10] The cytoplasm is basophilic and may contain numerous vacuoles, thought to be lysosomes, or phagocytosed erythrocytes, leukocytes, other tumor cells,

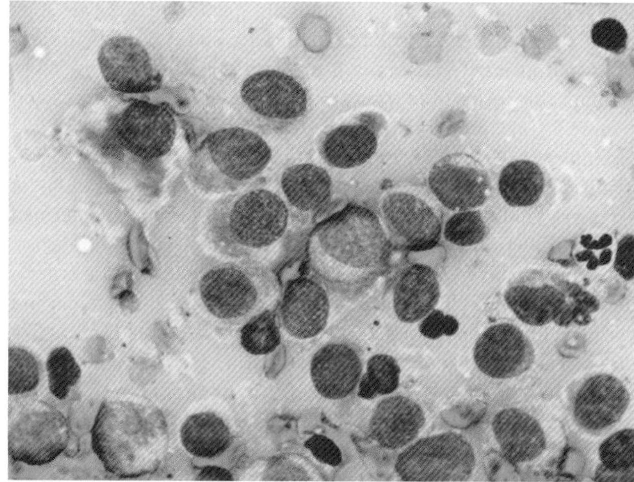

FIGURE 7-35 Fine-needle aspirate of a histiocytoma. Note the discrete round cells with a variable appearance. A few small lymphocytes are also present.

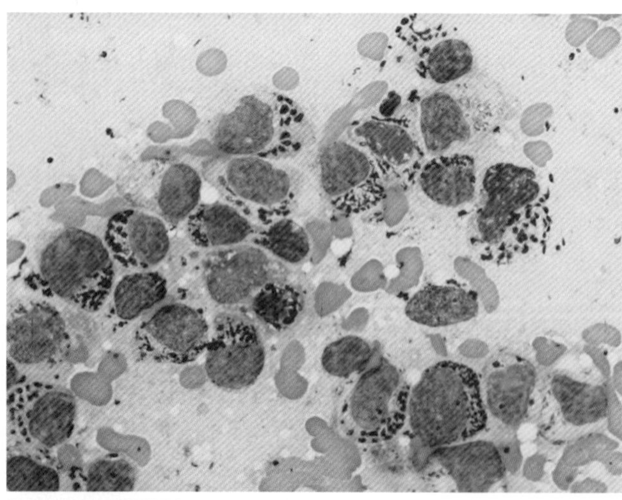

FIGURE 7-34 Fine-needle aspirate of a mesenteric lymph node from a cat with large granular lymphoma. Note the prominent coarse eosinophilic granules in the tumor cells.

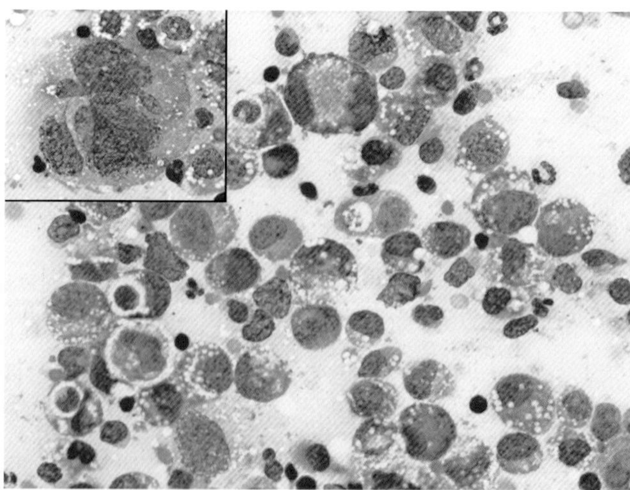

FIGURE 7-36 Fine-needle aspirate of a histiocytic sarcoma. Note extreme pleomorphism, phagocytosis, and bizarre multinucleated cell *(inset)*.

or cellular debris. Nuclei are typically round but may vary in shape and have indented or irregular margins. Chromatin is coarse to clumped, and nucleoli are prominent and vary in number, size, and shape. Multinuclearity and bizarre mitotic figures are common. Many of these tumors are infiltrated by small lymphocytes, plasma cells, and neutrophils. The second form comprises round, oval, and spindle-shaped cells with a more sarcoma-like appearance. Pleomorphism is less striking, but criteria of malignancy are present and warrant a cytologic interpretation of malignancy. Cytoplasmic vacuolation and phagocytic behavior also are less frequent. Nuclear shape is typically round to oval or elongate. These two forms are consistent with a tumor of dendritic cell origin.

The third form is hemophagocytic histiocytic sarcoma in which neoplastic macrophages constitute a "wolf in sheep's clothing" because the cells resemble phagocytic macrophages found in inflammatory lesions and seldom exhibit criteria of malignancy.[11] The cells have moderate N:C ratios; vacuolated cytoplasm that frequently contains hemosiderin or phagocytosed erythrocytes, neutrophils, or platelets; and round central nuclei with reticular chromatin and one to two variably prominent nucleoli. More prominent pleomorphic features may be seen in a few cells. The neoplastic macrophages may form dense sheets in spleen, liver, or bone marrow, which may be the sole warning of their malignant nature. Rarely is a definitive diagnosis of HHS made cytologically and biopsy is required; a clinical presentation of hemolytic anemia nonresponsive to immunosuppressive therapy, with or without other peripheral blood cytopenias, warrants consideration of HHS. In the absence of defined masses, a histologic diagnosis may also be difficult.

Differential diagnoses for these tumors depend on cytologic appearance. Few tumors are as pleomorphic as the round cell variant of HS; however, differential diagnoses may include anaplastic carcinoma and synovial cell sarcoma, depending on location. Differential diagnoses for the spindle-cell variant include a variety of other sarcomas. Differentials for HHS are not tumors at all, but include reactive macrophage proliferations secondary to other tumors or other inflammatory processes (hemophagocytic syndrome).

Transmissible Venereal Tumor TVT is a unique transmissible tumor thought to be of histiocytic origin. Its morphologic appearance is distinctive, and cytologic evaluation can provide a definitive diagnosis, especially when the tumor is located in typical locations, such as mucous membranes of external genitalia and nasal cavity. The N:C ratio is moderate to high. The nucleus is centrally or eccentrically located and has coarse chromatin and one or more prominent nucleoli (Figure 7-37). The cytoplasm is lightly basophilic and contains characteristic clear vacuoles. Mitotic figures are frequent. Mature lesions may contain infiltrating small lymphocytes. When found in atypical locations, such as the torso, limbs, and lymph nodes, TVT may be mistaken for lymphoma, histiocytic sarcoma, or amelanotic melanoma.

Mesenchymal and Epithelial Tumors That May Appear as Discrete Round Cell Tumors

Mesenchymal and epithelial tumors that may appear as discrete round cell tumors include amelanotic melanoma, granular cell tumor, anaplastic carcinoma, osteosarcoma, chondrosarcoma, rhabdomyosarcoma, and liposarcoma. Histologic examination of the tumor and immunohistochemical evaluation may be required to ascertain the lineage of these round cell imposters.

Tumor Metastases and Tumors Exfoliating into Cavity Effusions

Specific tumor types preferentially metastasize to certain organs or sites, depending on location of the primary tumor, vascular or lymphatic dissemination, and many other factors. Regional lymph nodes, lung, liver, and spleen are common metastatic sites, but any tissue or organ can be involved, including skin, bone, bone marrow, and the central nervous system. Cytologic identification of tumor metastases begins with recognizing an abnormal population of cells in the metastatic site followed by determining the tissue of origin, if possible, based on cytomorphologic features.

Both primary and metastatic tumors may exfoliate into cavities, including the thoracic, abdominal, and pericardial cavities, or into cerebrospinal or synovial fluid. Although neoplastic cells in these abnormal locations may be categorized as epithelial, mesenchymal,

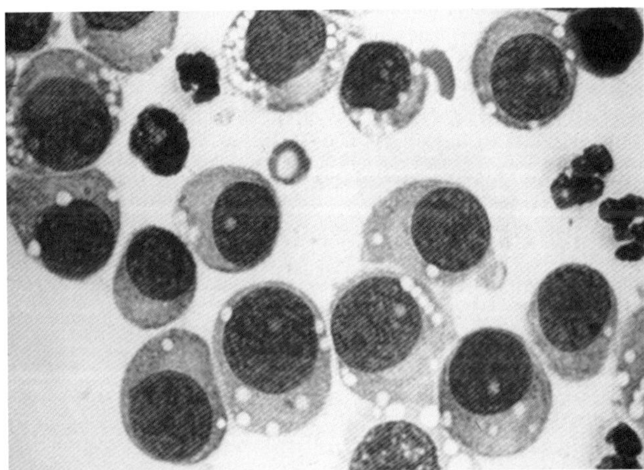

FIGURE 7-37 Fine-needle aspirate of a transmissible venereal tumor (TVT). Note the coarse chromatin and small discrete vacuoles in the cytoplasm that are often referred to as a "string of pearls." *(Courtesy Dr. Robert Hall.)*

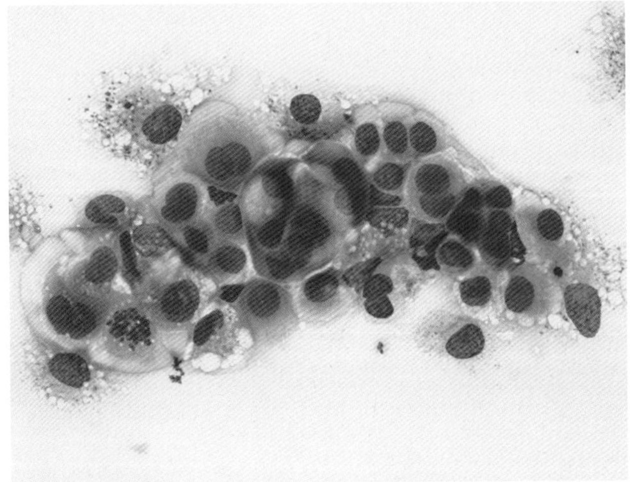

FIGURE 7-38 Reactive mesothelial cells in pleural fluid from a cat with chylothorax. These cells may be highly pleomorphic and have criteria of malignancy, but represented hyperplastic mesothelium in this cat.

or discrete round cell tumors, the specific origin of the primary tumor is only rarely determined by examining cells in the effusion. A major cytologic challenge when examining cells in cavity effusions is distinguishing reactive mesothelium, mesothelioma, and carcinoma. Mesothelium undergoes hyperplasia and exfoliation whenever an effusion forms in the thoracic, abdominal, or pericardial cavities, and reactive mesothelial cells can adopt all the criteria of malignancy described for tumor cells, including marked anisocytosis and anisokaryosis, macrocytosis and macrokaryosis, multinuclearity, variation of nuclear size within the same cell, nucleolar pleomorphism, and abnormal mitotic figures (Figure 7-38). Identification of a mass and histologic examination often are required for a definitive diagnosis.

REFERENCES

1. Akhtar M, Ali MA, Huq M, et al: Fine-needle biopsy: comparison of cellular yield with and without aspiration, *Diagn Cytopathol* 5:162–165, 1989.
2. Barger A, Graca R, Bailey K, et al: Use of alkaline phosphatase staining to differentiate canine osteosarcoma from other vimentin-positive tumors, *Vet Pathol* 42:161–165, 2005.
3. Masserdotti C: Architectural patterns in cytology: correlation with histology, *Vet Clin Pathol* 35:388–396, 2006.
4. Christopher MM, Hotz CS, Shelly SM, et al: Interpretation by clinicians of probability expressions in cytology reports and effect on clinical decision-making, *J Vet Intern Med* 24:496–503, 2010.
5. Masserdotti C, Drigo M: Retrospective study of cytologic features of canine well-differentiated hepatocellular carcinoma, *Vet Clin Pathol* (In press).
6. Alleman AR, Choi US: Endocrine system. In Raskin RE, Meyer DJ, editors: *Canine and feline cytology: A color atlas and interpretation guide*, ed 2, St Louis, 2010, Saunders.
7. Barthez PY, Marks SL, Woo J, et al: Pheochromocytoma in dogs: 61 cases (1984-1995), *J Vet Intern Med* 11:272–278, 1997.
8. Bertazzolo W, Dell'Orco M, Bonfanti U, et al: Canine angiosarcoma: cytologic, histologic, and immunohistochemical correlations, *Vet Clin Pathol* 34:28–34, 2005.
9. Flatland B, Fry MM, Newman SJ, et al: Large anaplastic spinal B-cell lymphoma in a cat, *Vet Clin Pathol* 37:389–396, 2008.
10. Affolter VK, Moore PF: Localized and disseminated histiocytic sarcoma of dendritic cell origin in dogs, *Vet Pathol* 39:74–83, 2002.
11. Moore PF, Affolter VK, Vernau W: Canine hemophagocytic histiocytic sarcoma: a proliferative disorder of CD11d^{+} macrophages, *Vet Pathol* 43:632–645, 2006.

Molecular Diagnostics

8

Anne C. Avery, Christine Olver, Chand Khanna, and Melissa C. Paoloni

Goals of Molecular Diagnostic Testing in Oncology

Since the mid-1980s, advances in the fields of molecular biology and genetics have changed our understanding of the biology of cancer. Technologic advances now provide the opportunity for applying this advanced understanding to the clinical arena in the form of novel diagnostic tests and management strategies. Molecular approaches for cancer diagnosis are now part of the standard of care for most human patients.[1] Technologic advances have reduced the unit cost for many of these approaches, and their use and commercialization is increasingly taking hold within the veterinary field. It is now feasible to assess proteins, RNA, DNA, or their metabolites in tumors, effusions, blood, saliva, and urine to more accurately classify and detect various forms of neoplasia.

Recently, the National Comprehensive Cancer Network (NCCN) defined molecular testing in oncology as "procedures designed to detect somatic or germline mutations in DNA and changes in gene or protein expression that could impact the diagnosis, prognosis, prediction and evaluation of therapy for patients with cancer."[1] Molecular assays are used for a variety of reasons in the diagnostic evaluation of malignancy. For example, the presence or absence of individual oncogene mutations or chromosomal abnormalities has significant prognostic implications in many types of malignancies. In people, finding a mutation in the nucleophosmin gene in cases of acute myelogenous leukemia (AML) predicts a significantly better prognosis, independent of other factors.[2] In canine mast cell disease, the presence of a mutation in the *c-kit* gene suggests a worse prognosis than for patients without such a mutation.[3] In lymphoma, the phenotype (B- versus T-cell) plays a large role in determining prognosis in both veterinary and human patients. A variety of molecular diagnostic tests, including DNA-based and various methods of protein detection, can establish the phenotype of lymphoma.

The presence of a particular mutation or chromosomal abnormality can help to subclassify a tumor. For example, chronic lymphocytic leukemia/small cell lymphoma (CLL/SCL) and mantle cell lymphoma in humans are both neoplasms of mature B-cells, with a similar (but not identical) immunophenotype. Mantle cell lymphoma, however, almost always has a rearrangement between the immunoglobulin heavy chain locus (IgH) and the *CCND1* (encoding cyclinD1) gene, whereas this rearrangement is very rare in CLL/SCL.[4] The prognosis and treatment of these two diseases is quite different, so the distinction is important to make.

Molecular diagnostic testing also helps guide therapy. This may be best illustrated by the development of tyrosine kinase inhibitors (TKIs). These drugs inhibit signaling through tyrosine kinase receptors, such as *c-kit,* platelet-derived growth factor (PDGF) receptor, and epidermal growth factor (EGF) receptor. Tumors with mutations in these receptors that result in their constitutive activation respond well to TKIs, whereas those without may require different kinds of chemotherapy. Thus testing for mutations in these genes has become commonplace in human medicine—EGF receptor in small cell lung carcinoma and stem cell factor (SCF) receptor *(c-kit)* in gastrointestinal stromal cell tumors. Similarly, mast cell tumors in dogs that harbor a *c-kit* mutation respond better to TKIs than those without the mutation.[3]

Finally, oncogenes and chromosomal translocations uniquely distinguish neoplastic from normal tissue. As such, sensitive detection of mutations can be used to quantify residual disease in patients that have been treated. The best example of this is detection of the *bcr-abl* fusion gene, which can allow oncologists to detect as few as $1:10^6$ neoplastic cells in peripheral blood.[5] Tumor-specific primers that recognize the unique immunoglobulin genes found in both canine and human B-cell lymphomas have been used to quantify tumor burden and monitor disease in both dogs and people with lymphoma.

The goal of this chapter is to review several molecular techniques useful in the diagnosis and classification of cancer. It is likely that advanced molecular methodologies and diagnostics will continue to improve, become increasingly inexpensive and simpler to use, and be more broadly available to veterinarians over the next few years.

Methods for Analyzing Genes

DNA represents the genetic code of all species. This code consists of a series of continuous nucleic acid sugar strands linked through hydrogen bonds. This series of nucleic acids takes on a tertiary folded structure through modification by binding proteins called *histones.* The folded and wrapped DNA strand is packaged within the chromosomes of the cell. The earliest techniques used to assess the genetic changes of cancer were those that defined gains, losses, or structural changes in chromosomes, referred to as *cytogenetics.* Subsequently, polymerase chain reaction (PCR)–based methods and high-throughput sequencing have allowed us to detect smaller discrete mutations in DNA that do not involve changes in large portions of the chromosome. Small deletions and insertions in genes, as well as single nucleotide changes, are now routinely detected.

Detection of Chromosomal Abnormalities

Historically, these techniques involved the examination of metaphase preparations made from chromosomes. Metaphase preparations were then stained (banded) to help in the identification of distinct chromosome morphologies. Using these techniques, detection of gross abnormalities in chromosome number (ploidy) and of the presence of chromosomal translocations was possible and led to the identification of genes associated with tumor development and progression. Cytogenetic analysis has been most useful in the clinical assessment of leukemias, in which metaphase preparations are relatively easy to develop from whole blood samples.[6] For most human leukemias, cytogenetic descriptors are used to define distinct subgroups into prognostic groups and to guide treatment decisions. The use of cytogenetic approaches in the management of companion animals has been limited due to the difficulty in using conventional chromosomal banding to identify canine chromosomes. The development of chromosome-specific "paints" that allow the identification of specific canine chromosomes has improved the opportunity to apply cytogenetic descriptors to canine cancers. Using these techniques, Breen and colleagues have identified a chromosomal translocation in canine chronic myelogenous leukemia (CML) and chronic monocytic leukemia that is the equivalent of the *bcr-abl* Philadelphia chromosome found in human CML.[7,8]

For the most part, traditional cytogenetic techniques, including the use of chromosome-specific paints, are labor intensive and have been replaced by alternative modalities. Comparative genomic hybridization (CGH) arrays can define gains and losses in chromosome number within tumor specimens rapidly and with highly reproducible results. In CGH analysis, the investigator labels genomic DNA from a normal individual and from tumor cells of the patient with two different color fluorescent probes. The labeled DNA is then hybridized to an array of DNA probes that span the majority of the genome. These probes are printed onto a chip or slide, such that the location of each individual probe is identified. The degree of hybridization to each probe is then determined by the level of fluorescence detected by laser excitation. Equal hybridization of the DNA from both sources to an individual probe indicates normal copy number, whereas increased binding by the tumor DNA indicates the presence of chromosomal duplication in the area of the genome covered by that probe (Figure 8-1). Similarly, higher binding by the DNA from the normal individual indicates chromosomal loss in the area.

CGH arrays are useful for localizing chromosomal regions where investigators should focus their search for genes important to that cancer. A canine CGH array with 2 megabase resolution has been reported.[9] Using this array, Breen and colleagues have shown that a subset of T-cell lymphomas (histologically defined as peripheral T-cell lymphoma, unspecified) exhibits copy number gain in regions common to most examples of this histologic type but not present in other T-cell lymphoma subtypes.[10] This finding will help to identify genes within the duplicated areas that might be useful for diagnostics and therapy and for understanding the genesis of the neoplasm. A similar study in canine malignant histiocytosis (MH) demonstrated that MH frequently exhibits loss of chromosomal regions that contain tumor suppressor genes.[11] Such genetic characterization of a diverse group of cancers, with distinct biologic behaviors but similar histologic descriptions, will significantly improve opportunities to target specific therapies and management strategies to distinct biologic subgroups of these diseases.

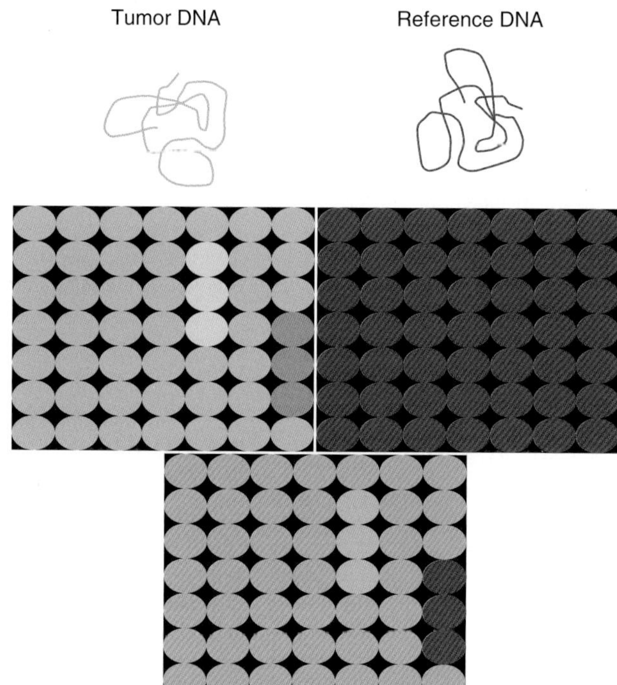

FIGURE 8-1 The principle of array analysis. A chip or slide is printed so that each position on the chip (there are thousands) has a single probe, which can range in size, depending on the type of array. DNA from a tumor tested is labeled with one dye *(green)* and DNA from the reference sample with another *(red)*. Both samples are hybridized to the same chip. The separate red and green panels indicate that the tumor DNA exhibits both chromosomal gain (increased green fluorescence) and loss (decreased green fluorescence). When the two DNA preparations are co-hybridized, a yellow signal indicates equal degrees of red and green fluorescence. When there is a gain in copy number in a region of DNA, the signal will be green. When there is a loss in copy number, the signal will be red.

Polymerase Chain Reaction–Based Techniques: Detection of Mutations, Novel Genes, and Assessment of Clonality

PCR is the process of amplifying a small specific segment of DNA for the purpose of further analysis. Two small segments of DNA (commonly about 20 bases long), which are complementary to the DNA sequence surrounding the area to be amplified, are synthesized. These primers are then used to amplify the DNA, which lies between them (typically less than 1000 bases). This amplified DNA product can then be analyzed in a number of ways for mutations to quantify the product for measurement of gene expression, or in the case of lymphoid malignancy the DNA can be separated by size in order to look for clonal populations of B- and T-cells. The same methods can be applied to the analysis of RNA, once the RNA has been transcribed into DNA.

Primer synthesis typically requires that the sequence of the target gene is known. The publication of the canine genome in 2005[12] has been invaluable in this regard, since it is now possible to simply use the known canine sequences rather than hope for sequence similarities with mice and humans.

Detection of Genetic Insertions and Deletions

PCR-based assays are commonly used in human oncology to detect insertions or deletions in genes relevant to the prognosis or treatment of a neoplasm. In veterinary medicine, detection of internal tandem duplications (ITD) in the *c-kit* gene in canine mast cell tumors is now a routine part of the diagnosis for the purpose of determining the most effective treatment. *C-kit* is a TK receptor for the growth factor SCF and is mutated in some cases of canine mast cell tumors.[13] The primary mutations described are internal ITD in two different exons, exon 8 and 11.[14] The mutations involve the duplication of a small segment of DNA so that it is repeated, resulting in a larger gene (Figure 8-2). Approximately 14% to 20% of canine mast cell tumors have a duplication in either exon 8 or 11.[14] Since mast cell tumors containing the ITD respond better to TK inhibitors than tumors with wild-type *c-kit*,[15] testing for *c-kit* mutations has become a routine part of the diagnostic work-up for mast cell tumors.

Detection of this type is fairly simple, since the presence of a larger (or smaller, in the case of deletions) PCR product is determined by size separation. It is likely that as more genes are identified as being targets of therapy, such assays will become more frequent. Recently, Suter et al identified an internal duplication in the *FLT3* gene[16] in acute lymphocytic leukemia (ALL) using the same methods and provided preliminary evidence that response to a small molecule inhibitor is predicted by the presence of the mutation in lymphoid cell lines. We are likely to see routine use of mutation detection grow in the near future and continue to guide treatment decisions.

Detection of Single-Base Mutations

Single-base mutations are more difficult to detect, since the base-pair change does not confer a size difference to the PCR product. Several strategies are used in human medicine for detecting these kinds of mutations. First, mutations can be detected by synthesizing primers that are complementary to the mutation, rather than to the wild-type version of the gene. In theory, a PCR product would only be seen if the mutation is present. This approach has to be tested empirically for each individual mutation, since such primers may also anneal to the wild-type gene, although with less affinity. There are a variety of ways to produce primers that are more discriminating, and different methods will be more or less effective for individual mutations.

Another approach employs direct sequencing of the PCR product. Sequencing is now inexpensive and widely available. The limitation of direct sequencing is that the sample must contain a significant percentage of tumor cells for the mutation to be detected—most estimates suggest 10% or more. This is because at best only one-half of the DNA sequenced will have the individual mutation (assuming the tumor also has a wild-type copy of the gene), and the presence of nonneoplastic tissue in most clinically derived samples will serve to further dilute the amount of mutated DNA. Thus, unless the PCR products are cloned and sequenced individually, a significant portion of the DNA must be tumor derived.

Detection of Fusion Gene Products by PCR

One mechanism by which chromosomal translocation causes malignant transformation of cells is to create novel proteins with altered function. The best studied of these fusion genes, the Philadelphia chromosome, is the breakpoint cluster region-Abelson (*bcr-abl*) fusion gene found in greater than 90% of all human CMLs and occasionally ALL and AML.[17] *abl* is a tyrosine kinase that has myriad activities involved in cell growth and differentiation. It is encoded on human chromosome 9, and in CML, it is translocated to chromosome 22. The site of the translocation varies within the *bcr* gene, so that a new fusion gene, *bcr-abl*, is formed. The new fusion protein allows for the constitutive activation of the *abl* tyrosine kinase, which in turn promotes the development of CML (Figure 8-3).

This fusion protein is the product of a novel RNA transcript, which can be readily detected by PCR. To accomplish this, RNA is extracted from blood containing potentially neoplastic cells and reverse transcribed to cDNA. The cDNA is then amplified with two primers, one which anneals to the *bcr* gene, and the other to the *abl* gene. Since these two genes are normally on different chromosomes, no product will be seen in the absence of a translocation, but will be detected if the genes have been brought together to form a single messenger RNA (mRNA). This assay can detect as few as $1:10^6$ tumor cells[5] and can therefore be used for both diagnosis of CML and quantifying residual disease after treatment.

Assays for a large number of translocations have been developed over the past 10 years.[18] These assays are now routinely available for characterization of human tumors, particularly leukemia. The finding that canine leukemia and lymphoma can exhibit the same translocations as their human counterparts[8] suggests that detection of this novel fusion gene would aid in the diagnosis of canine chronic myelogenous leukemia.

Assessment of Clonality in Lymphoma and Leukemia

A clonality assay demonstrates that a group of cells is derived from a single clone. The term is usually used to refer to detection of the unique genes found in each individual B- or T-cell—immunoglobulin genes in B-cells and T-cell receptor (TCR) genes in T-cells. The portion of these genes that encodes the antigen-binding region is the portion that varies between cells, both in size and sequence. When B- or T-cells divide, the immunoglobulin and TCR genes are passed on to the daughter cells.[19,20]

In the course of a normal immune response to a pathogen, B- and T-cells are activated, expand, and eventually die, leaving behind a small number of residual memory cells. On the other hand, when a cell becomes neoplastic, it no longer responds to growth controls and undergoes unlimited expansion. Therefore, if one can establish that the majority of cells in a particular collection of lymphocytes have the same immunoglobulin or TCR gene, it is most likely that these cells are neoplastic rather than reactive.[21]

When immunoglobulin and TCR genes rearrange during the course of B-cell and T-cell development, respectively, the length and sequence of the resultant gene differs from cell to cell. There are many reasons for this, including the fact that nucleotides are added between V, D, and J segments as they rearrange into a contiguous formation. The clonality assay takes advantage of this fact. In a sample consisting of many different lymphocytes, as in a reactive process (the lymph nodes of a dog with chronic pyoderma or poor dental hygiene, for example), there will be multiple different-sized TCR and immunoglobulin genes. On the other hand, in a sample consisting of neoplastic lymphocytes, the immunoglobulin gene or the TCR gene (depending on whether it is a B-cell or a T-cell lymphoma) will be a single size (Figure 8-4).

Clonality assays are accomplished by isolating DNA from cells suspected to be neoplastic and then using PCR primers directed at the conserved regions of TCR or immunoglobulin genes. The primers amplifying the variable regions and the PCR products are separated by size using a variety of possible methods. The presence of a single-sized PCR product is indicative of clonality, whereas the presence of multiple PCR products supports a reactive process. This assay has now been reported by a number of laboratories[22-25] and used to answer a variety of clinical questions.[26-28] This assay is termed the *PCR for antigen receptor rearrangement* (PARR) assay in order to distinguish it from other types of clonality assays.[23] It should be noted, however, that the term *PARR* is not used in the human literature, where the assay instead is referred to as a *clonality assay.*

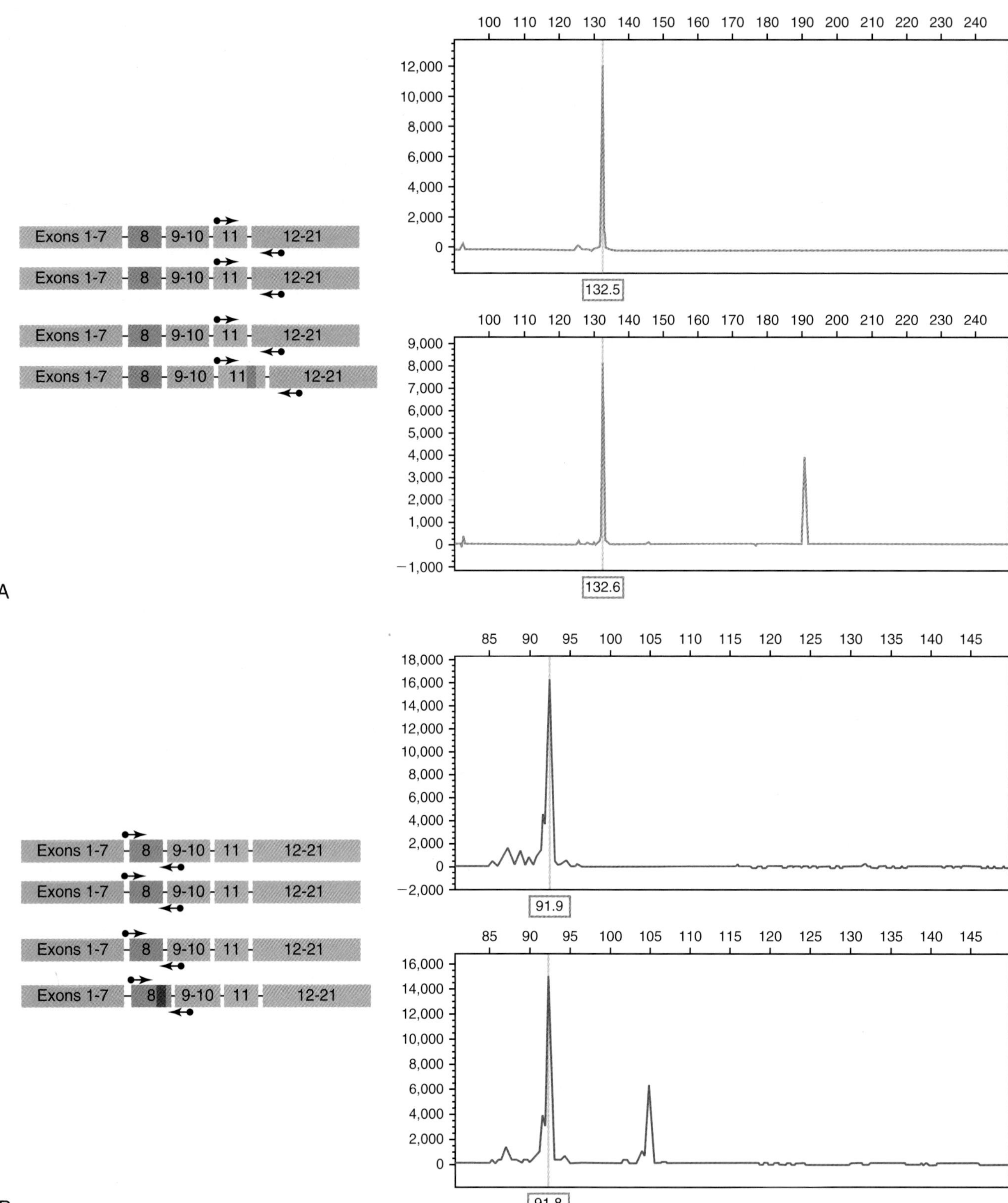

FIGURE 8-2 Detection of *c-kit* mutations by PCR. **A,** Two different tumor types are depicted—one has two copies of a wild type *c-kit* gene, and the second has one copy of a *c-kit* gene containing an internal tandem mutation in exon 11. The PCR products detected after amplification with primers surrounding the duplication *(arrows)* for each tumor are shown on the right. **B,** Same as in **A,** but in this case, the second tumor has an internal duplication in exon 8, and the PCR products are amplified with primers flanking the region of the duplication.

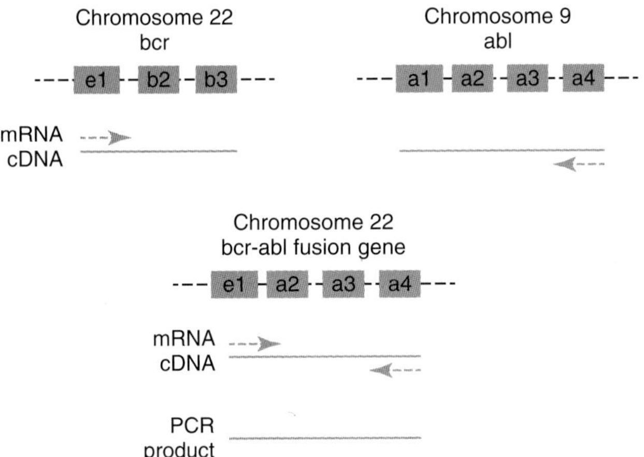

FIGURE 8-3 Translocation of the *abl* gene to the *bcr* gene creates a fusion gene that can be detected by PCR. In nonleukemic cells, primers located as indicated *(arrows)* will not amplify any product, because they anneal to two distinct cDNAs. When *bcr* and *abl* are brought together, the primers are both annealing to the same cDNA and will amplify this product. e1, b2, and so forth refer to exon numbers.

The PARR assay is able to detect approximately 1 : 100 neoplastic cells. The sensitivity and specificity of the assay will differ between laboratories because the results are highly sensitive to the conditions under which the assay is run and to the technique used to separate the PCR products. Capillary gel electrophoresis has the highest resolution, but high percentage polyacrylamide gels may also be used. Agarose gels, even high-resolution agarose gels, provide insufficient resolution for this assay and should not be used.

The main application of the PARR assay is to establish clonality in a sample that is cytologically or histologically ambiguous—cases in which there are rare cytologically suspicious cells within the context of a reactive node, for example, or a lymph node that was interpreted as "atypical lymphoid hyperplasia" on histology. Clonality assays can sometimes be useful for establishing the lineage (B- versus T-cell) in cytologically unambiguous lymphomas if additional case material is not obtainable from the patient, but in general flow cytometry, immunohistochemistry, or immunocytochemistry are preferable for this purpose. This is because aberrant rearrangements can occasionally be seen in nonlymphoid tumors such as myelogenous leukemias and also in a neoplasm of the opposite phenotype (TCR rearrangement in a B-cell lymphoma, for example). The rate at which this occurs also probably differs from laboratory to laboratory and depends on the subtype of lymphoma being examined.

The principle of the clonality assay can also be used to quantify tumor cells in blood or node and to monitor minimum residual disease. For this type of analysis, PCR primers specific for the immunoglobulin or TCR gene that is carried by the tumor are used, instead of the broadly reactive primers used to screen samples. In this way the investigator is certain that only tumor DNA is being amplified and not nonneoplastic lymphocytes. The specificity of this reaction permits determination of the number of tumor cells in a sample of blood, even when those cells are as rare as 1 : 10,000 cells. Yamazaki et al[28] demonstrated that with current chemotherapy protocols, all seven dogs they examined had at least 1 : 10,000 cells in their peripheral blood, even though the dogs achieved clinical remission. Although this kind of analysis may not be practical for routine diagnostics, it is a powerful research tool to compare the efficacy of novel chemotherapy regimens.

Single Nucleotide Polymorphism Analysis

A great deal of interpatient variability in the biology of cancers is based on the presence or absence of mutations in a cancer. However, small differences in host genes—referred to as single nucleotide polymorphisms (SNPs)—have been shown to be important in defining these interindividual differences in disease progression and response to treatment. SNPs can result in a change in the structure or function of a gene. SNPs are considered to be distinct from mutations since they are present in a subset of the population and do not cause disease themselves. A number of SNPs in genes that function in hepatic metabolism in the human population have been identified and can predict increased risk for toxicity to some drugs. Similarly, SNPs in other genes have been shown to predict an increased risk for a more aggressive course of metastatic progression once a patient develops a cancer.[29] The release of the canine genome sequence has made possible the high-throughput detection of SNPs—using an array platform[30]—within a population of dogs. It is likely that SNP-based diagnostics will emerge from these discovery efforts and will contribute to the individualization of therapy of dogs and cats with otherwise similar diseases. SNP-based diagnostics are also helpful in providing an opportunity to attempt to predict or define individual differences seen between patients treated in the same way for the same disease. These differences may include toxicities experienced after receiving a treatment, beneficial response to a therapy, or progression rates for patients with a similar disease stage. These forms of individualized therapy are on the horizon for both human and veterinary cancer patients.

Quantifying Genes and Gene Expression

The complete genetic code, or DNA sequence, is present within every cell in the body. The effective genetic information that uniquely defines each cell type within the body is defined by the genes expressed (transcribed) as mRNA. The expression of mRNA is more responsible for the phenotype of a cancer than the individual genes and mutations harbored by the tumor. When assessing the level of expression of one or a few genes, real time PCR is most commonly used. Assessment of the global level of gene expression is carried out with microarrays and is called *gene expression profiling*. Both methods measure relative expression of message when compared to a control gene whose expression is thought to be more or less constant in all cells and universal. These methods are both likely to be replaced over the next 10 years with new technologies, which allow investigators to count the absolute number of genes or transcripts in a sample.

Real-Time Polymerase Chain Reaction

Real-time PCR (also called *Q-PCR*) refers to the quantitative measurement of DNA—either genes, or more commonly, RNA that has been reverse transcribed to cDNA. The principle of real-time PCR is that DNA is amplified using primers, just as in a routine PCR reaction, but at each round of amplification, fluorescence relative to the amount of PCR product is quantified. Unlike endpoint PCR, in which the reaction runs to completion and the product is separated by size, real-time PCR is highly quantitative.

The two main methods for quantifying DNA in real-time PCR have different advantages and disadvantages. The simplest and least expensive method is the use of the DNA-binding dyes, such as *SYBR green* (pronounced cyber). This dye fluoresces when it

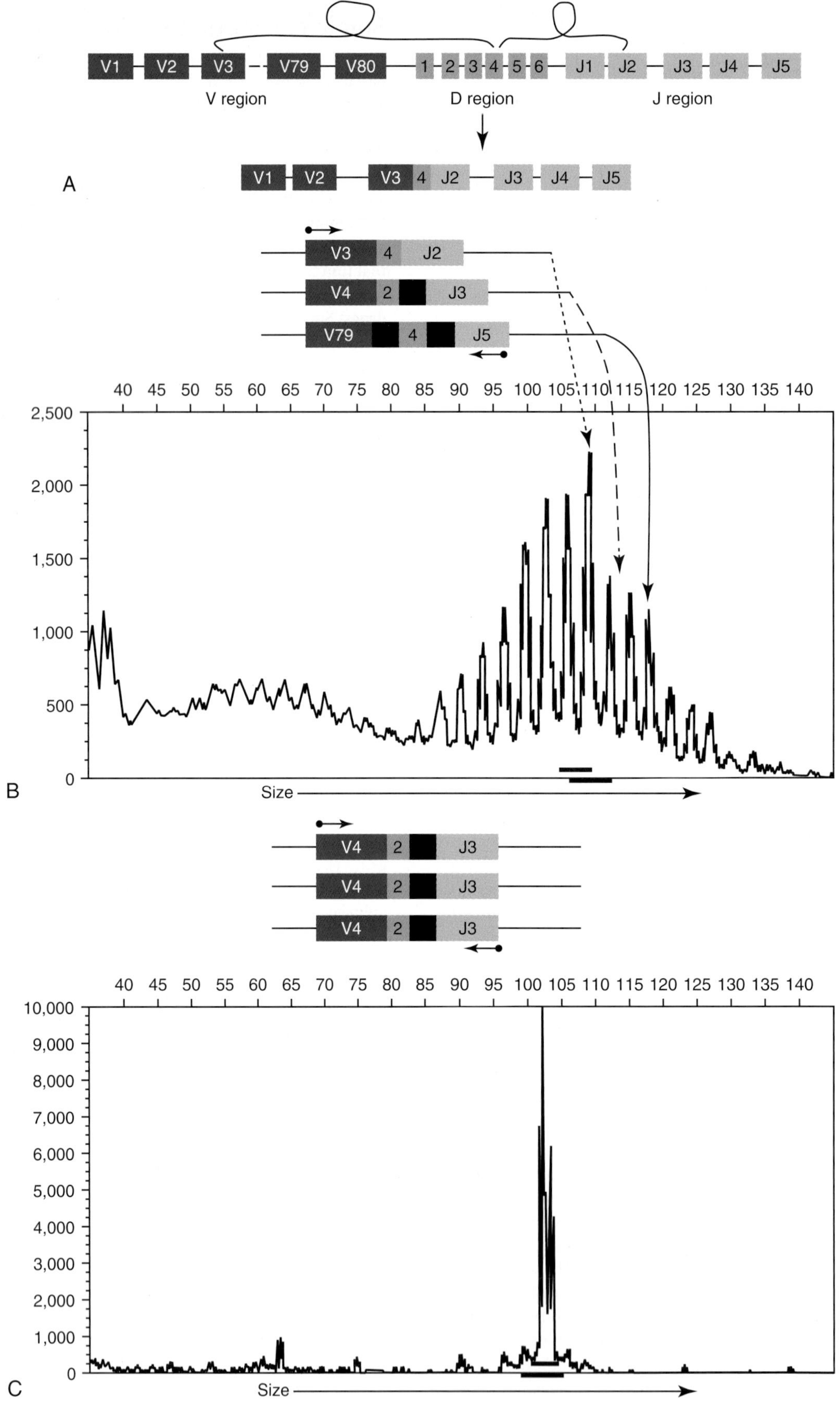

V1
V2
V3
V79
V80
1
2
3
4
5
6
J1
J2
J3
J4
J5
V region
D region
J region
A
B
C
Size

intercollates into DNA. Therefore, at each round of amplification, more dye is intercollated and the degree of fluorescence increases. Eventually, the fluorescence reaches saturation, but the endpoint is less important than the log phase of DNA increase. The amount of starting material is compared between samples by determining at which amplification cycle the degree of fluorescence crosses a given threshold. SYBR green will intercollate into any DNA product, so this method is only accurate when the primers are highly specific and amplify only one gene product.

An alternative method uses fluorescently labeled DNA probes. These are short segments of DNA complementary to the target sequence between the two primer sites. A fluorescent molecule attached to the probe is quenched until the 5′ to 3′ exonuclease activity of the Taq polymerase releases the fluorescent molecule. As the amount of PCR product increases proportional to the starting material, the amount of fluorescence increases. The advantage of the probe method is that instead of two primers providing specificity to the reaction, there are three. In order to detect a product, these three different segments of DNA need to bind to the target sequence in three separate places. The assay may be less robust at low target numbers and is slightly more expensive but also significantly more specific. This assay with its increased specificity was used by Yamazaki et al[28] to quantify individual neoplastic lymphocytes in a background of heterogenous lymphocytes and thus quantify minimal residual disease.

Real-time PCR can quickly allow for precise quantification of mRNA levels within samples and has a number of defined clinical applications. It is commonly used in the quantification of aberrant oncogenic fusion products. Promyelocytic leukemia gene–retinoic acid receptor (PML-RAR) fusion transcripts in acute promyelocytic leukemia (APL) are identified by this method[31] and can be used to define molecular remission in patients with APL. Molecular remissions are defined by the absence of not only clinically detectable disease but by the absence of any tumor-associated transcript in blood, bone marrow, or lymph node. Achieving a molecular remission in patients with leukemias and lymphoma is a superior measure of prognosis over clinical assessments of remission that are based on clinical examination, imaging techniques, or histologic or cytologic assessments of at-risk tissues.

Gene Expression Profiling

Gene expression profiling refers to the quantification of thousands of mRNAs simultaneously to create a picture of global gene expression in the cell population. The pattern of gene expression is called a *gene expression profile.* A variety of different software tools are available for identifying patterns of expression involved in a common pathway or function. The companies that produce these tools mine the literature for information about the function(s) of different genes, and then place these genes into pathways. A collection of genes involved in a particular pathway are frequently referred to as *signatures.* For example, if the gene expression profile shows a proliferation signature, then the genes involved in the regulation of cell division are upregulated. If the cells show a nuclear factor kappa B (NFκB) signature, expression of genes regulated by the transcription factor NFκB are increased.

Gene expression profiling is performed using similar tools as CGH arrays. Oligonucleotides complementary to thousands of different genes are printed on a slide or chip, usually more than one oligo for each gene. mRNA from the sample in question is isolated, reverse transcribed to DNA, and labeled with a fluorescent probe. This fluorescent cDNA is then hybridized to the chip, and the degree of fluorescence is proportional to the amount of mRNA present in the original sample. A variety of controls are built into the chip and are used during the analysis to look at gene expression relative to standard housekeeping genes, such as *GAPDH.*

Gene expression profiling is comparative. Investigators can compare expression profiles of tumor cells to the normal cellular counterpart, to similar tumors with different clinical outcomes, and to tumor cells from the same patient before chemotherapy; can compare primary lesions to metastatic lesions; and can make other comparisons to ask how different pathways have changed. Such information has proved invaluable in a variety of settings. For example, in a study of cervical cancer in humans, investigators analyzed gene expression profiles of tumors that responded to chemotherapy and radiation and compared those with tumors that did not respond. Their study revealed that activation of the PI3K/Akt signaling pathway was associated with a poor response, suggesting one potential therapeutic target.[32] Another example of how gene expression profiling has advanced oncology are the studies of B-cell lymphoma by Staudt and colleagues. Noting that diffuse large B-cell lymphoma (DLBCL) has a heterogeneous outcome in people, this group compared the gene expression profiles of 96 DLBCL with B-cells derived from different stages of normal B-cell development.[33] They found that the gene expression profile of DLBCL could either be categorized as similar to germinal center B-cells or similar to activated B-cells. Importantly, these two categories had prognostic significance: germinal center-like DLBCL cases had a better prognosis. The distinction between germinal center DLBCL and activated B-cell DLBCL is now well established as a prognostic indicator.

This same group made another important discovery about B-cell lymphoma using gene expression profiling, which provided insights into immunity to cancer. Expression profiles of lymph nodes from patients with follicular B-cell lymphoma demonstrated that the type of immune response signature was prognostic in this disease. Patients whose lymph node gene expression patterns exhibited evidence of T-cell activation had a better overall survival than patients whose gene expression patterns resembled activated

FIGURE 8-4 Rearrangement of immunoglobulin genes. **A,** There are approximately 80 V-region genes, 6 D-region genes, and 5 J-region genes. A single V, D, and J are brought together at random to create a single VDJ gene segment that encodes the antigen-binding portion of an antibody, and the intervening sequence is removed. **B,** In the process of bringing together V, D, and J genes, a variable number of nucleotides *(black)* are added between V and D and D and J. As a result, each individual B-cell will have a VDJ gene segment with a unique length. When DNA from a heterogeneous population of B-cells is isolated and amplified with primers bracketing the VDJ gene segment *(small arrows),* the PCR products will be different lengths. The lower panel shows the PCR products separated by size using capillary gel electrophoresis and illustrates multiple different-sized PCR products. **C,** When a population of B-cells is comprised of cells derived from a single clone, all the VDJ gene segments will be identically sized. PCR amplification of the VDJ gene segment will yield a single-sized product as shown in the lower panel. All the principles illustrated here also apply to T-cell receptor (TCR) genes. For the clonality assay, the TCR γ-chain is amplified, although in theory TCR β-chain could also be used.

macrophages.[34] The expression profile of the tumor cells themselves was not predictive. This finding suggests that the immune response contributes to survival in patients with follicular B-cell lymphoma, a result which was corroborated in other types of B-cell lymphoma.[35,36]

Gene expression profiling is now a readily accessible tool in canine oncology because of the availability of the Affymetrix Canine Genome 2.0 and Agilent (V2) Gene Expression microarrays, and investigators have begun to examine gene expression profiles in a variety of canine neoplasms, including hemangiosarcoma,[37-39] lymphoma, and osteosarcoma.[40,41]

On the Horizon—Counting Genes

The next generation of genetic analysis uses a new paradigm for evaluating individual genes, gene expression (cDNA analysis), and whole genomes. The old paradigm has been to use fluorescent or other types of DNA labels to quantify copies of DNA—more fluorescence means more copies. For example, if we want to quantify *bcr-abl* fusion messenger RNA for determining the number of circulating cells present before and after treatment, a fluorescent based real time PCR method would be used. Fluorescently labeled probes, corresponding to a portion of the *bcr-abl* fusion gene, would be added to a PCR reaction where that gene is specifically amplified. The amount of fluorescence is directly proportional to the amount of product, which is proportional to the amount of starting cDNA. This is usually compared with the amount of message from a housekeeping gene to give a relative quantity of *bcr-abl* message.

In the new paradigm, the number of cDNAs corresponding to *bcr-abl* in a blood sample would be counted in absolute numbers. One name given to this idea is "digital PCR." There are many methods to accomplish this kind of quantification, but they all share the idea that millions of isolated PCR reactions are being carried out on single DNA molecules. In the *bcr-abl* example, millions of individual cDNAs from a blood sample, together with *bcr-abl* primers and polymerase, would be isolated on a solid matrix or in individual droplets in an emulsion; the result of that amplification would be positive (if the *bcr-abl* cDNA is present) or negative (if the *bcr-abl* DNA is absent). Presence or absence of a product can still be a fluorescent readout, but the message is quantified by the percentage of individual reactions that are positive. The advantage of this method is the elimination of the need for standard curves and reference samples. In addition, these methods are likely to be significantly more sensitive since thousands to millions of DNA molecules are analyzed at one time. Thus one has the possibility of measuring as few as 1 in 10^6 copies of a gene or message. The first generation of instruments that can carry out this kind of analysis are now commercially available, and it is likely that these will eventually become commonplace.

Next generation whole genome sequencing works on a similar principle. A variety of instruments are now available with the capability of sequencing an entire mammalian genome within days (including setup and DNA isolation) at a cost of about $10,000 to $20,000. This is accomplished by carrying out millions of sequencing PCR reactions simultaneously. Whole genomic DNA is sheared into small fragments, and individual sequencing PCR reactions are carried out on each fragment. The result is that the investigator obtains millions of short sequences, which must then be interpreted by extensive software analysis. It is certain that the cost of this type of analysis and its complexity will both decrease in the near future. Current efforts are underway to sequence both whole genome and exons of a number of canine cancers that will continue to identify and characterize important targets and pathways in their pathogenesis. The day when a patient's entire tumor genome is sequenced as a routine part of diagnostics is imaginable and not that far in the future.

Methods for Protein Analysis

Protein expression represents the accumulation or end product of genetic information. DNA is transcribed into RNA, which is then translated into proteins. Therefore the detection of proteins and their active forms (most often phosphorylated) represents an important step in the global understanding of cancer biology. Protein measurements can be both qualitative and quantitative and can include a variety of candidate approaches, including Western blotting, immunohistochemistry, and various novel noncandidate proteomic platforms, collectively referred to as *proteomic approaches.*

Western Blots

Western blots allow for the detection of a protein within a sample through the use of an antibody that is specific to that protein. Western blots are used widely as a diagnostic modality that has recently seen expanded clinical use in the field of oncology through the availability of antibodies that are specific for phosphorylated forms of proteins and for mutated proteins. As treatment modalities for cancer have become more target-dependent, the need has increased to define the presence of the target protein in a clinical sample. Documentation of HER2/neu oncogene expression in human breast cancer patients has the dual utility of contributing to prognosis (expression of this protein carries a negative prognostic value) and guiding the rational use of trastuzumab (Herceptin), a therapeutic monoclonal antibody that has been shown to improve time to progression and overall survival in metastatic breast cancer patients when combined with chemotherapy.[42]

In the veterinary field, Western blots have been part of the diagnosis and management of animals with tick-borne infectious disease and feline immunodeficiency virus. The use of in-house "snap" test technology is based on a similar technique of antibody-based detection, including enzyme-linked immunosorbent assay (ELISA) and radioimmunoassay (RIA). In these assays, rather than using gel electrophoresis, the probing antibody is affixed to a substrate for detection of antigen in material passed over or through this substrate. As such, the specificity and sensitivity of antigen-antibody interactions needed for these tests are greater than what are needed for a Western blot. In the field of oncology, these snap tests have been limited by a lack of tumor-specific antibodies (with high sensitivity and specificity) that could aid in the diagnosis of cancer.

Immunohistochemistry and Flow Cytometry

As in the case of Western blots, advances in antibody development have similarly improved the opportunity to define patient groups and direct therapy through the use of immunohistochemistry (IHC; the assessment of protein expression in fixed tissue sections) or by flow cytometry.

Immunohistochemical staining is carried out on formalin-fixed, paraffin-embedded tissue or, less commonly, on frozen sections. Immunocytochemistry (ICC) uses the same methods and reagents but on fine-needle aspirates. Antibodies to specific proteins are applied to the tissue, generally followed by a secondary antibody of a different species than the patient or the primary antibody. The secondary antibodies are conjugated to enzymes that catalyze a color change when substrate is added. This method allows pathologists to identify individual cells that do or do not express the protein of interest and to put these cells in the context of tissue architecture.

In veterinary oncology, IHC is most commonly used to distinguish sarcomas from carcinomas and to phenotype lymphomas. The first application involves staining tumor sections with antibodies to the cytoskeletal proteins vimentin and cytokeratin. Vimentin is found in mesenchymal origin tumors (e.g., osteosarcomas, fibrosarcomas). Cytokeratin is expressed by epithelial origin cancers (carcinomas). Although the distinction between these two types of tumors is generally straightforward, when there is doubt, it is common to request vimentin/cytokeratin staining (see Chapter 3).

IHC is particularly important in subclassifying lymphoma. The 2008 World Health Organization (WHO) classification of lymphomas describes greater than 40 lymphoproliferative disorders (lymphoma and leukemia) in humans.[43] All subclassifications begin with phenotype (B- versus T-cell). The origin and biologic behavior of different subclassifications of lymphoma are different enough that it is not scientifically justified to consider lymphoma a single disease. Therefore, when conducting therapeutic trials, epidemiologic studies, and any other types of analyses on canine lymphoma, it will be necessary to examine individual subtypes separately (Figure 8-5).

The antibodies used to determine the B- or T-cell origin of lymphoma in formalin-fixed sections are anti-CD3 (which identifies T-cells) and one of several anti–B-cell antibodies, including CD79a, Pax5, and CD20. All of these antibodies recognize the cytoplasmic portions of the target antigen—the process of fixation permeabilizes cells to allow antibodies access to these epitopes. The antibodies also recognize conserved regions of the proteins and are therefore useful in a variety of different species. Further subclassification of lymphoma is possible based on the distribution of neoplastic cells within the lymph node. For example, there are a number of neoplasms of mature B-cells with very different outcomes: SCL, mantle cell lymphoma, and follicular lymphoma (FL). These can be differentiated by examining architecture of a lymph node stained with B-cell antibodies. In human patients, they can also be differentiated by flow cytometry (see later) or cytogenetic studies. The human classification has been applied to canine lymphoma by a consortium of pathologists who reached broad but not perfect agreement about histologic subtypes.[44] There is still a paucity of data, however, on the biologic behavior of these subtypes in dogs.

An alternative method of immunophenotyping lymphomas is flow cytometry. Flow cytometry analyzes cells in single-cell suspension. The flow cytometer uses lasers to identify characteristics of the cells, including their size, their complexity, and the proteins they express on their cell surface. The latter requires that the cells are stained with antibodies, which are conjugated to various fluorescent proteins. Flow cytometry is an extremely powerful tool because for each individual cell in the suspension, the expression of up to 10 different proteins can be analyzed routinely, and even higher numbers are possible. The value of this kind of analysis is highlighted in human medicine by the approach to a patient with circulating neoplastic mature B-cells. The differential diagnosis includes CLL, leukemic mantle cell lymphoma, marginal zone lymphoma, and FL. In all four entities, the cells will express the B-cell antigen CD20, but only mantle cell lymphoma and CLL express CD5. The latter two can then be distinguished from one another by expression of a series of additional surface proteins, which can be examined simultaneously by flow cytometry.[45]

Flow cytometric phenotyping has advantages and disadvantages compared with IHC. As noted above, the advantages are that multiple parameters can be analyzed at once and objective data obtained about each parameter. Information about cell size and granularity and the levels of expression of different antigens have prognostic significance.[46-48] Because formalin fixation damages proteins, most of the cell surface proteins examined by flow cytometry cannot be identified in tissue sections, so less information about protein expression is available by IHC. Flow cytometry can be carried out on lymph node aspirates, precluding the requirement of sedation and a biopsy.

IHC, however, allows the pathologist to view the architecture of the node. Veterinary pathologists recognize many of the WHO categories of lymphoma, including diffuse large B-cell lymphoma, FL, and mantle cell lymphoma. One study systematically evaluated outcome using contemporary classifications and found that small cell T-zone lymphoma had the most favorable outcome, whereas Burkitt-like B-cell lymphoma had the worst.[49] This study was small but revealed the value of classifying and subclassifying lymphomas using contemporary standards. More recently, an investigation of canine indolent T-cell lymphoma, which is a diagnosis that can only be made by histology coupled with IHC, revealed that treatment of this form of lymphoma with a CHOP-based protocol resulted in the same outcome as treatment with chlorambucil and prednisone. This is the first study clearly demonstrating the utility of histology and IHC in guiding treatment decisions.[50] When additional outcome-based investigations are performed and veterinary pathologists are more widely knowledgeable about the WHO classification scheme, the added expense and invasiveness of a biopsy over flow cytometry will be justified.

Proteomics

Proteomics is the large-scale and high-throughput study of proteins, including their identification, structure (e.g., posttranslational modifications), and function.[51] Proteomics, like gene expression profiling, is often comparative, and differences in protein expression in cell lysates or tissues in various conditions (e.g., neoplastic versus normal) are measured. The proteome is a dynamic entity that is much less stable and more complicated than the genome. Protein expression is influenced by translation, protein activation (most often by phosphorylation) or other posttranslational modifications, and also protein turnover and degradation. Thus the protein complement in a disease state is not solely defined by its genetic expression pattern and can change quickly over time. Because proteins are the molecules that execute cell or tissue processes, their identification globally is thought to be a more accurate "snapshot" of cell status than either the genomic sequence or gene expression at the RNA level. Thus far, proteomics has led to better understanding of cancer and identification of potential markers for diagnosis and prognosis. However, routine clinical application of proteomics is still developing.

A recent review describes proteomics and proteomics techniques in detail.[52] A typical proteomics experiment, the aim of which is to identify a large number of proteins in a complex mixture, requires multiple steps. These steps can include protein solubilization, separation into less complex fractions, mass spectrometric measurement of peptide masses, and finally protein identification via database searching. Separation of a mixture of proteins can be performed using one-dimensional polyacrylamide gel electrophoresis (1D-PAGE) (separation by size), two-dimensional PAGE (separation by isoelectric point, then size), liquid chromatography (separation of soluble proteins or peptides based on their physical

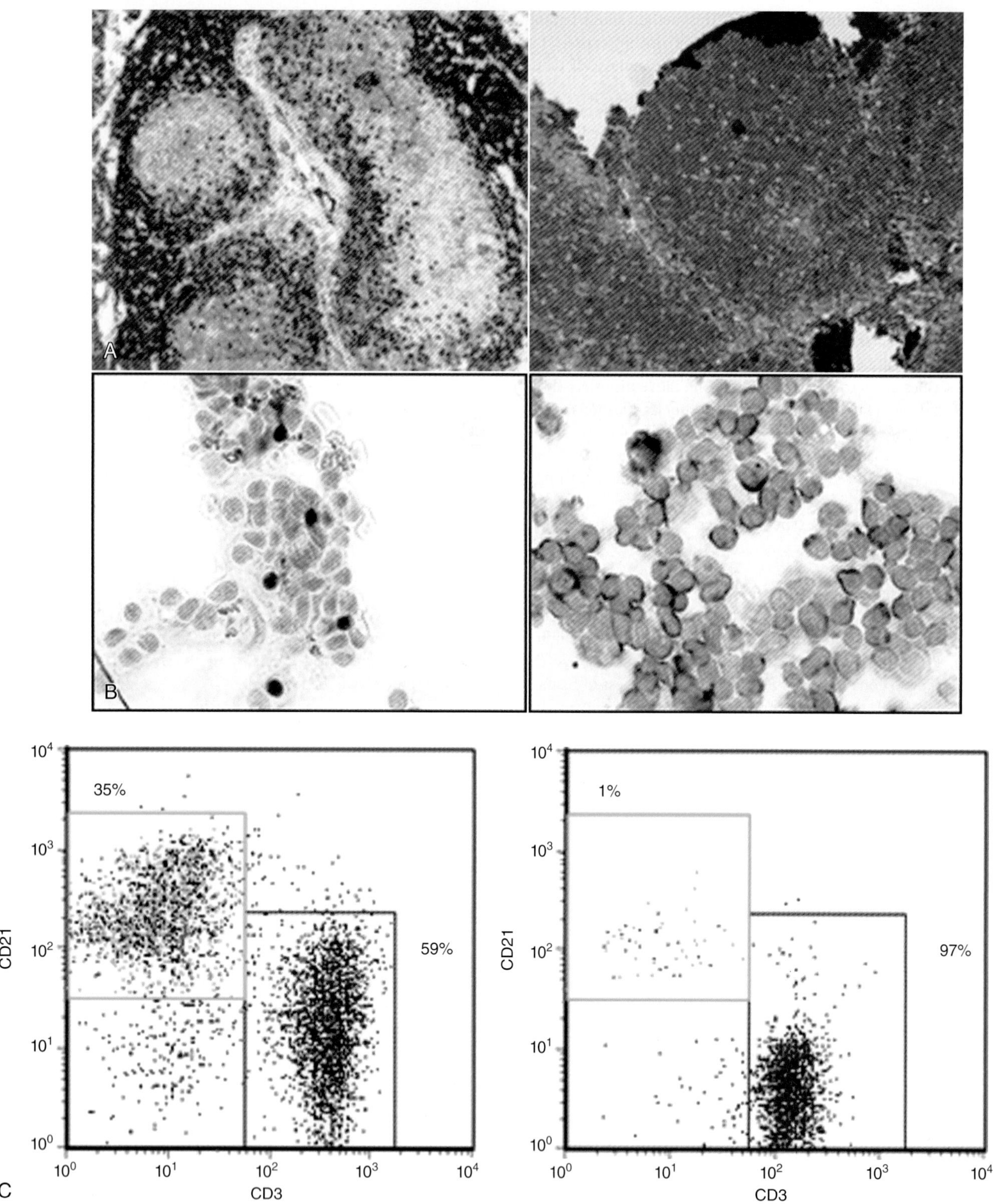

FIGURE 8-5 Two methods for determining immunophenotype in a T-cell lymphoma. **A,** Immunohistochemical staining of a normal lymph node *(left)* and a T-cell lymphoma *(right)*. The brown stain in the left panel is the result of binding by anti-CD79a, and indicates the B-cell regions of the lymph node. The red staining indicates binding by anti-CD3 and highlights the T-cell regions of the lymph node. The panel on the right reveals a node effaced by T-cells (T-cell lymphoma). **B,** Immunocytochemical staining of a T-cell lymphoma, showing staining with anti-Pax5 on the left (a B-cell specific antibody) and anti-CD3 on the right. **C,** Flow cytometry staining of a T-cell lymphoma *(right panel)* and a normal lymph node *(left panel)*. Each dot represents a cell, which is plotted on the histogram based on the amount of CD3 staining *(x axis, red box)* and CD21 staining *(y axis, green box)* for identifying T-cells and B-cells, respectively. The percentage of total cells in the node is indicated in each box. The lymph node from the dog with T-cell lymphoma contains T-cells almost exclusively, which, in a separate staining reaction, were shown to be CD4+.

properties), or a combination. Once proteins are separated, they are digested with an enzyme into a mixture of peptides. These peptides are applied to a mass spectrometer and their mass-to-charge ratio is measured. A list of measured masses is searched against theoretical peptide masses generated from "in silico" digestion of proteins translated from genomic databases.

There are several types of spectrometers, which vary by their ionization technique and method of mass-to-charge measurement. Briefly, electrospray ionization introduction and ionization of the sample occur in the liquid phase. For matrix-assisted laser desorption ionization (MALDI), the sample is mixed with a matrix (organic acid) and allowed to co-crystallize on a target (metal plate). Biomarker discovery has been performed using a specific application of MALDI-mass spectrometry called *surface-enhanced laser desorption/ionization* (SELDI) mass spectrometry. The separation of proteins for SELDI is performed directly on the plate, which contains specific materials designed to retain certain proteins. SELDI produces a profile of mass spectrometric masses (protein profiling), rather than actual protein identification. This technique was originally described as being highly sensitive and specific for identifying individuals with ovarian cancer,[53] although the interpretation of the spectral data has been difficult to reproduce.[54] This underscores the fact that, regardless of the initial promise of a diagnostic method, it is still necessary to use appropriate study design and statistical analysis (as with any other test).

A recent study demonstrates the utility of proteomic analysis in the study of cancer. Klose et al[55] asked if progression from hyperplastic mammary tissue to neoplastic and then metastatic disease was associated with changes in protein expression in humans. They compared normal mammary tissue, mammary adenomas, mammary carcinomas (nonmetastatic), and carcinomas that had metastasized. Among their most significant findings was that, while the histologic appearance of nonmetastatic and metastatic tumors was not different, the proteins they express were significantly different. This kind of study can lead directly to the development of prognostic markers, which can be used in routine IHC, and also serves to identify good and poor prognosis patients.

Summary

Molecular diagnostics is becoming more integrated into veterinary medicine and at the same time becoming more affordable. One important feature of such advanced diagnostics is that many of them save money for owners and preclude invasive procedures for their pets. Sensitive methods for detecting lymphoma through a combination of cytology, flow cytometry, and PARR assays, for example, can mean that a diagnosis of splenic lymphoma can be made without splenectomy. Detection of the *c-kit* mutation can guide therapy so that the most efficacious (and therefore cost-effective) drugs are used. More expensive exploratory techniques such as whole genome sequencing and proteomic analysis of tumors will almost certainly lead to discovery of new testing that can further simplify diagnoses. Veterinarians are encouraged to participate in these developmental studies when they can, by providing biologic materials and clinical data to researchers, because ultimately patients and their owners will derive great benefit from current research.

REFERENCES

1. Engstrom PF, Bloom MG, Demetri GD, et al: NCCN Molecular Testing White Paper: Effectiveness, efficiency, and reimbursement, *J Natl Compr Canc Netw* 9(suppl 6):S1–S16, 2011.
2. Grimwade D, Hills RK, Moorman AV, et al: Refinement of cytogenetic classification in acute myeloid leukemia: determination of prognostic significance of rare recurring chromosomal abnormalities among 5876 younger adult patients treated in the United Kingdom Medical Research Council trials, *Blood* 116:354–365, 2010.
3. London CA, Malpas PB, Wood-Follis SL, et al: Multi-center, placebo-controlled, double-blind, randomized study of oral toceranib phosphate (SU11654), a receptor tyrosine kinase inhibitor, for the treatment of dogs with recurrent (either local or distant) mast cell tumor following surgical excision, *Clin Canc Res* 15:3856–3865, 2009.
4. Jevremovic D, Viswanatha DS: Molecular diagnosis of hematopoietic and lymphoid neoplasms, *Hematol Oncol Clin North Am* 23:903–933, 2009.
5. Morley A: Quantifying leukemia, *N Engl J Med* 339:627–629, 1998.
6. Knuutila S: Cytogenetics and molecular pathology in cancer diagnostics, *Ann Med* 36:162–171, 2004.
7. Cruz Cardona JA, Milner R, Alleman AR, et al: BCR-ABL translocation in a dog with chronic monocytic leukemia, *Vet Clin Path* 40:40–47, 2011.
8. Breen M, Modiano JF: Evolutionarily conserved cytogenetic changes in hematological malignancies of dogs and humans—man and his best friend share more than companionship, *Chromosome Res* 16:145–154, 2008.
9. Thomas R, Scott A, Langford CF, et al: Construction of a 2-Mb resolution BAC microarray for CGH analysis of canine tumors, *Genome Res* 15:1831–1837, 2005.
10. Thomas R, Seiser EL, Motsinger-Reif A, et al: Refining tumor-associated aneuploidy through 'genomic recoding' of recurrent DNA copy number aberrations in 150 canine non-Hodgkin lymphomas, *Leuk Lymphoma* 52:1321–1335, 2011.
11. Hedan B, Thomas R, Motsinger-Reif A, et al: Molecular cytogenetic characterization of canine histiocytic sarcoma: A spontaneous model for human histiocytic cancer identifies deletion of tumor suppressor genes and highlights influence of genetic background on tumor behavior, *BMC Cancer* 11:201–215, 2011.
12. Lindblad-Toh K, Wade CM, Mikkelsen TS, et al: Genome sequence, comparative analysis and haplotype structure of the domestic dog, *Nature* 438:803–819, 2005.
13. London CA, Galli SJ, Yuuki T, et al: Spontaneous canine mast cell tumors express tandem duplications in the proto-oncogene c-kit, *Exp Hematol* 27:689–697, 1999.
14. Letard S, Yang Y, Hanssens K, et al: Gain-of-function mutations in the extracellular domain of KIT are common in canine mast cell tumors, *Mol Cancer Res* 6:1137–1345, 2008.
15. Hahn KA, Ogilvie G, Rusk T, et al: Masitinib is safe and effective for the treatment of canine mast cell tumors, *J Vet Int Med* 22:1301–1309, 2008.
16. Suter SE, Small GW, Seiser EL, et al: FLT3 mutations in canine acute lymphocytic leukemia, *BMC Cancer* 11:38–46, 2011.
17. Wong S, Witte ON: The BCR-ABL story: bench to bedside and back, *Annu Rev Immunol* 22:247–306, 2004.
18. Osumi K, Fukui T, Kiyoi H, et al: Rapid screening of leukemia fusion transcripts in acute leukemia by real-time PCR, *Leuk Lymphoma* 43:2291–2299, 2002.
19. Delves PJ, Roitt IM: The immune system. First of two parts, *N Engl J Med* 343:37–49, 2000.
20. Blom B, Spits H: Development of human lymphoid cells, *Annu Rev Immunol* 24:287–320, 2006.
21. Swerdlow SH: Genetic and molecular genetic studies in the diagnosis of atypical lymphoid hyperplasias versus lymphoma, *Hum Pathol* 34:346–351, 2003.
22. Vernau W, Moore PF: An immunophenotypic study of canine leukemias and preliminary assessment of clonality by polymerase chain reaction, *Vet Immunol Immunopath* 69:145–164, 1999.

23. Burnett RC, Vernau W, Modiano JF, et al: Diagnosis of canine lymphoid neoplasia using clonal rearrangements of antigen receptor genes, *Vet Path* 40:32–41, 2003.
24. Tamura K, Yagihara H, Isotani M, et al: Development of the polymerase chain reaction assay based on the canine genome database for detection of monoclonality in B cell lymphoma, *Vet Immunol Immunopath* 115:163–167, 2006.
25. Yagihara H, Tamura K, Isotania M, et al: Genomic organization of the T-cell receptor γ gene and PCR detection of its clonal rearrangement in canine T-cell lymphoma/leukemia, *Vet Immunol Immunopath* 115:375–382, 2007.
26. Burnett RC, Blake MK, Thompson LJ, et al: Evolution of a B-Cell lymphoma to multiple myeloma after chemotherapy, *J Vet Int Med* 18:768–771, 2004.
27. Keller RL, Avery AC, Burnett RC, et al: Detection of neoplastic lymphocytes in peripheral blood of dogs with lymphoma by polymerase chain reaction for antigen receptor gene rearrangement, *Vet Clin Path* 33:145–149, 2004.
28. Yamazaki J, Baba K, Goto-Koshino Y, et al: Quantitative assessment of minimal residual disease (MRD) in canine lymphoma by using real-time polymerase chain reaction, *Vet Immunol Immunopath* 126:321–331, 2008.
29. Hoque MO, Lee CC, Cairns P, et al: Genome-wide genetic characterization of bladder cancer: A comparison of high-density single-nucleotide polymorphism arrays and PCR-based microsatellite analysis, *Cancer Res* 63:2216–2222, 2003.
30. Heller MJ: DNA microarray technology: devices, systems, and applications, *Annu Rev Biomed Eng* 4:129–153, 2002.
31. Gallagher RE, Yeap BY, Bi W, et al: Quantitative real-time RT-PCR analysis of PML-RAR alpha mRNA in acute promyelocytic leukemia: Assessment of prognostic significance in adult patients from intergroup protocol 0129, *Blood* 101:2521–2528, 2003.
32. Schwarz JK, Payton JE, Rashmi R, et al: Pathway-specific analysis of gene expression data identifies the PI3K/Akt pathway as a novel therapeutic target in cervical cancer, *Clin Canc Res* 18(5):1464–1471 2012.
33. Alizadeh AA, Eisen MB, Davis RE, et al: Distinct types of diffuse large B-cell lymphoma identified by gene expression profiling, *Nature* 403:503–511, 2000.
34. Dave SS, Wright G, Tan B, et al: Prediction of survival in follicular lymphoma based on molecular features of tumor-infiltrating immune cells, *N Engl J Med* 351:2159–2169, 2004.
35. Rimsza LM, Roberts RA, Miller TP, et al: Loss of MHC class II gene and protein expression in diffuse large B-cell lymphoma is related to decreased tumor immunosurveillance and poor patient survival regardless of other prognostic factors: A follow-up study from the Leukemia and Lymphoma Molecular Profiling Project, *Blood* 103:4251–4258, 2004.
36. Lenz G, Wright G, Dave SS, et al: Stromal gene signatures in large-B-cell lymphomas, *N Engl J Med* 359:2313–2323, 2008.
37. Tamburini BA, Phang TL, Fosmire SP, et al: Gene expression profiling identifies inflammation and angiogenesis as distinguishing features of canine hemangiosarcoma, *BMC Cancer* 10:619, 2010.
38. Tamburini BA, Trapp S, Phang TL, et al: Gene expression profiles of sporadic canine hemangiosarcoma are uniquely associated with breed, *PLoS One* 4:e5549, 2009.
39. Starkey MP, Murphy S: Using lymph node fine needle aspirates for gene expression profiling of canine lymphoma, *Vet Comp Oncol* 8:56–71, 2010.
40. Scott MC, Sarver AL, Gavin KJ, et al: Molecular subtypes of osteosarcoma identified by reducing tumor heterogeneity through an interspecies comparative approach, *Bone* 49:356, 2011.
41. Paoloni M, Davis S, Lana S, et al: Canine tumor cross-species genomics uncovers targets linked to osteosarcoma progression, *BMC Genomics* 10:625, 2009.
42. Masood S, Bui MM: Prognostic and predictive value of HER2/neu oncogene in breast cancer, *Microsc Res Tech* 59:102–108, 2002.
43. Jaffe ES: The 2008 WHO classification of lymphomas: implications for clinical practice and translational research, *Hematology Am Soc Hematol Educ Program* 523–531, 2009.
44. Valli VE, San Myint M, Barthel A, et al: Classification of canine malignant lymphomas according to the World Health Organization criteria, *Vet Path* 48:198–211, 2011.
45. Hsi ED: The leukemias of mature lymphocytes, *Hematol Oncol Clin North Am* 23:843–871, 2009.
46. Rao S, Lana S, Eickhoff J, et al: Class II major histocompatibility complex expression and cell size independently predict survival in canine b-cell lymphoma, *J Vet Int Med* 25:1097–1105, 2011.
47. Williams MJ, Avery AC, Lana SE, et al: Canine lymphoproliferative disease characterized by lymphocytosis: Immunophenotypic markers of prognosis, *J Vet Int Med* 22:596–601, 2008.
48. Comazzi S, Gelain ME, Martini V, et al: Immunophenotype predicts survival time in dogs with chronic lymphocytic leukemia, *J Vet Int Med* 25:100–106, 2011.
49. Ponce F, Magnol JP, Ledieu D, et al: Prognostic significance of morphological subtypes in canine malignant lymphomas during chemotherapy, *Vet J* 167:158–166, 2004.
50. Flood-Knapik KE, Durham AC, Gregor TP, et al: Clinical, histopathological and immunohistochemical characterization of canine indolent lymphoma, *Vet Comp Onc* epub 2-2-12, 2012.
51. Cristea IM, Gaskell SJ, Whetton AD: Proteomics techniques and their application to hematology, *Blood* 103:3624–3634, 2004.
52. Prenni JE, Avery AC, Olver CS: Proteomics: a review and an example using the reticulocyte membrane proteome, *Vet Clin Path* 36:13–24, 2007.
53. Petricoin EF, Ardekani A, Hitt B, et al: Use of proteomic patterns in serum to identify ovarian cancer, *Lancet* 359:572–577, 2002.
54. Baggerly KA, Morris JS, Coombes KR: Reproducibility of SELDI-TOF protein patterns in serum: comparing datasets from different experiments, *Bioinformatics* 20:777–785, 2004.
55. Klose P, Weise C, Bondzio A, et al: Is there a malignant progression associated with a linear change in protein expression levels from normal canine mammary gland to metastatic mammary tumors? *J Proteome Res* 10:4405–4415, 2011.

Biopsy Principles

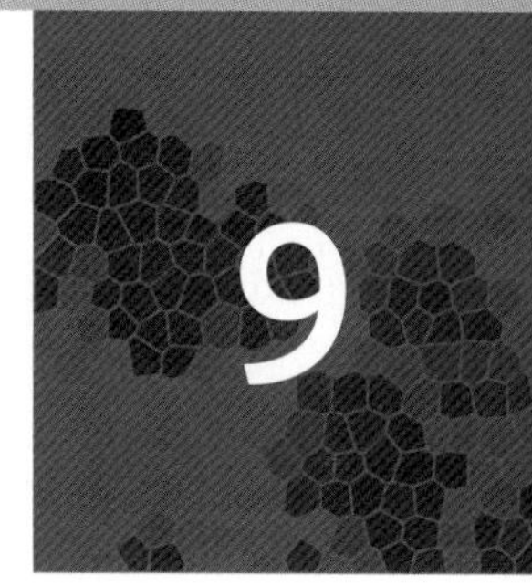

Nicole P. Ehrhart and Stephen J. Withrow

A biopsy refers to a procedure that obtains a tissue specimen for microscopic (i.e., histopathologic) analysis to establish a precise diagnosis. Histopathologic interpretation of tissue removed from a tumor is not infallible and is highly dependent on the quality of the biopsy sample submitted. Therefore it is important to understand basic principles of biopsy procurement and submission in order to obtain an accurate diagnosis. If the tissue diagnosis is incorrect, all subsequent steps in the treatment of the patient will also be incorrect.

Fine-needle aspiration cytology (FNAC) is a simple and rapid way to obtain information about a tumor and is often the first step in the diagnostic work-up (see Chapter 7). Results of FNAC help guide the diagnostic tests for staging. Studies have shown that FNAC is a reliable and useful method to guide further work-up when neoplasia is suspected or, in many cases, to help rule out neoplasia altogether.[1,2] Nonetheless, FNAC gives only limited information and may be nondiagnostic or equivocal. Inflammation, necrosis, and hemorrhage may result in cytopathologic changes that do not accurately represent the underlying disease process. Histologic confirmation is therefore required for definitive diagnosis of neoplasia.

Many techniques are available for obtaining tissue specimens—ranging from needle-core techniques to complete excision. The choice of technique depends on the anatomic location of the tumor, the patient's overall health, the suspected tumor type, and the clinician's preference. Biopsy techniques can be grouped under one of two major categories: pretreatment biopsy (e.g., needle core biopsy, punch biopsy, wedge biopsy) or excisional biopsy. Pretreatment biopsy is performed in order to obtain additional information about the tumor prior to definitive treatment. Posttreatment (i.e., excisional) biopsy refers to the process of obtaining histopathologic information following surgical removal of the tumor. Excisional biopsy is best used to obtain a more complete picture of the disease process (e.g., histologic subtype, tumor grade, degree of invasion into regional vasculature and lymphatics) and provides an opportunity to evaluate completeness of excision. It is rarely the best first step in obtaining a tissue diagnosis. Although excisional biopsy is attractive to many clinicians because it allows for definitive treatment and diagnosis in one step, it is often used inappropriately in the management of a cancer patient, resulting in incomplete surgical margins. Incomplete surgical margins may result in local recurrence, the need for radiation therapy, or a wider, more extensive surgery. All of these sequelae represent compromise of the optimum treatment pathway for the patient and will involve more morbidity and expense than a properly performed first excision. The issue to be determined before surgery is: how aggressive should the surgery to remove the tumor be? It is intuitive that wide, ablative surgery (e.g., body wall resection) would be inappropriate for a simple lipoma. It also follows that marginal excision ("shell out") is inappropriate for definitive treatment of an aggressive tumor, such as a soft tissue sarcoma. Thus thorough knowledge of the tumor type is imperative prior to attempting surgical excision. The best way to obtain this information is often via pretreatment biopsy.

Specific indications for pretreatment biopsy are as follows:

1. When fine-needle aspirate cytology is nondiagnostic or equivocal.
2. When the *type* of recommended treatment (radiation versus chemotherapy versus surgery) would be altered by knowledge of the tumor type or grade.
3. When the *extent* of recommended treatment (ablative surgery versus wide excision versus marginal excision) would be altered by knowledge of the tumor type or grade.
4. When the tumor is in a *difficult area to reconstruct* (maxillectomy, locations requiring extensive flaps, head and neck) and planning is needed to prepare the patient and client appropriately.
5. When knowledge of the tumor type or grade would *change the owner's willingness to go forward* with curative-intent treatment.

If any one of the listed criteria is met, a pretreatment biopsy should be pursued.

There are occasions when pretreatment biopsy would be contraindicated. These include cases when the type of treatment or extent of surgery would not be changed by knowing the tumor type (e.g., testicular mass, solitary splenic mass) or when the surgical procedure to obtain the biopsy is as risky as definitive removal (e.g., spinal cord biopsy). In these cases, the patient would best be served by excisional biopsy of the tumor if staging results support this choice.

Biopsy Methods

The more commonly used methods of tissue procurement are needle core biopsy, punch biopsy, incisional (wedge) biopsy, and excisional biopsy.

Needle Core Biopsy

Needle core biopsy utilizes various types of needle core instruments (e.g., Tru-Cut [Baxter General Healthcare, Deerfield, IL] or ABC needle [Kendall Sherwood-Davis & Geck, St. Louis, MO]) to obtain soft tissue (Figure 9-1). Most of these needles are manually operated, although spring and pneumatically powered needles are available as well. Specialized core instruments are used for bone biopsies and will be covered in Chapter 24. These instruments are generally 14-g in diameter and procure a piece of tissue that is about 1 mm wide and 1.0 to 1.5 cm long. In spite of this small sample size, the

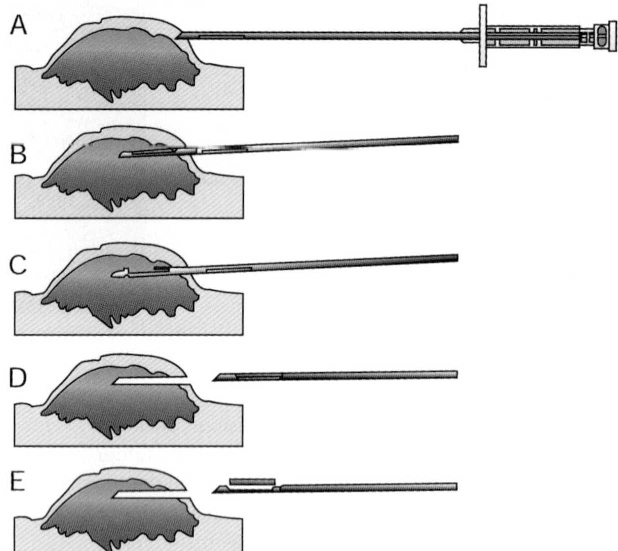

FIGURE 9-1 Mechanism of action of needle core biopsy needle for typical nodular tumor. **A,** A small skin incision is made with a Number 11 blade to allow insertion of the instrument. With the instrument closed, the outer capsule is penetrated. **B,** The outer cannula is fixed in place, and the inner cannula with the specimen notch is thrust into the tumor. The tissue then protrudes into the notch. **C,** The inner cannula is now held steady while the outer cannula is moved forward to cut off the biopsy specimen. **D,** The entire instrument is removed closed with the tissue contained within it. **E,** The inner cannula is pushed ahead to expose the tissue in the specimen notch.

structural relationship of the tissue and tumor cells can usually be visualized by the pathologist. Virtually any accessible mass can be sampled by this method. It may be used for externally located lesions or for deeply seated lesions (e.g., in the kidney, liver, or prostate) with image-guidance via closed methods or at the time of open surgery.

The most common usage of the needle core biopsy is for externally palpable masses. Except for highly inflamed and necrotic cancers (especially in the oral cavity), in which incisional biopsy is preferred, most biopsies can be done on an outpatient basis with local anesthesia and sedation. The area to be biopsied should be clipped of hair and sterilely prepared. The skin or overlying tissue is prepared as for minor surgery. If the overlying tissue (usually skin and muscle) is intact, it is anesthetized using local anesthetic in the region that the biopsy needle will penetrate. Tumor tissue itself is very poorly innervated and generally does not require local anesthesia. The mass is then fixed in place with one hand or by an assistant. A small 1- to 2-mm stab incision is made in the overlying skin with a scalpel blade to allow insertion of the biopsy instrument. The stab incision is necessary to prevent dulling of the needle tip and allow better penetration into the underlying tissue. Through the same skin hole, several needle cores are removed from different sites to get a "cross-section" of tissue types within the mass. The stab incision can be sutured with a single interrupted suture. The tissue is gently removed from the instrument with a scalpel blade or hypodermic needle and placed in formalin. For smaller-gauge biopsy needle instruments, the tissue may be flushed off the needle with saline. Samples may be gently rolled on a glass slide for cytologic preparations before fixation. With experience, the operator can generally tell from the appearance of the core sample whether diagnostic material has been attained. Small, discontinuous bits of tissue and fluid within the trough will only rarely be diagnostic and usually imply the need for incisional biopsy. Soft tissue sarcomas in particular may not yield good tissue cores because of necrosis and fibrous septa that often permeate the mass. Cystic masses are also problematic.

Needle biopsy tracts are of minimal risk for local tumor seeding but should be removed en bloc with the tumor at subsequent resection. Therefore it is important to plan where the stab incision and needle biopsy tract are placed in order to make the subsequent excision simpler. Avoid excessive tunneling through uninvolved tissues by choosing the most direct path from the skin to the tumor to obtain a representative sample.

Many of these needles are "disposable" with plastic casings and therefore cannot be steam sterilized. It is not uncommon, however, for veterinary practices to resterilize these instruments (using ethylene oxide or hydrogen peroxide gas) and use them repeatedly until they become dull.

Needle core biopsy instruments are inexpensive and easy to use, and needle core biopsy procedures can be performed as outpatient procedures. They are generally more accurate than cytology but likely have lower accuracy than larger incisional or excisional biopsy, especially when a tumor is heterogeneous, inflamed, or cystic or contains a large amount of necrosis. It is important to understand that for a 5-cm diameter mass, one needle core biopsy sample represents less than 1% of the tumor tissue. The smaller the biopsy specimen obtained, the less representative it may be for the entire tumor.

Needle core biopsy can be performed with the aid of image-guidance (discussed in greater detail later). Utilization of image-guidance for needle core biopsy is helpful for obtaining tissue from deeply seated lesions. Ultrasound-, fluoroscopic-, and computed tomographic-assistance may be used to obtain samples from tumors located in areas where percutaneous biopsy would be risky or unlikely to yield a representative sample. In situations in which the lesion is located within a body cavity, the risk of tumor seeding from uncontrolled hemorrhage or fluid leakage as a result of image-guided biopsy must be taken into account when determining if image-guided needle core biopsy techniques hold an advantage over more direct access in a given circumstance.

Punch Biopsy

Punch biopsy tools were originally designed for biopsy of the skin (Figure 9-2). They deliver a shorter and wider (2 to 8 mm) biopsy than does the needle core technique. They can be used on any external tumor (skin, oral, perianal) or tumors where there is direct access (e.g., liver biopsy during laparotomy). Preparation of the site is the same as for needle core biopsy. If the lesion is cutaneous, the punch biopsy instrument is placed on the surface of the area of interest and rotated back and forth using pressure to penetrate the involved tissue. If the skin is intact over the tumor, the skin is first incised using a scalpel. The punch is then introduced through the skin incision to the surface of the tumor. Once the punch has cut into the tumor, the core is gently lifted and the base of the core is cut off with scissors. One or two sutures may be placed to close the skin incision.

Incisional Biopsy

Incisional biopsy is utilized when fine-needle cytology or needle core biopsy has not yielded or is unlikely to yield diagnostic material (Figure 9-3). Additionally, it is preferred for ulcerated and

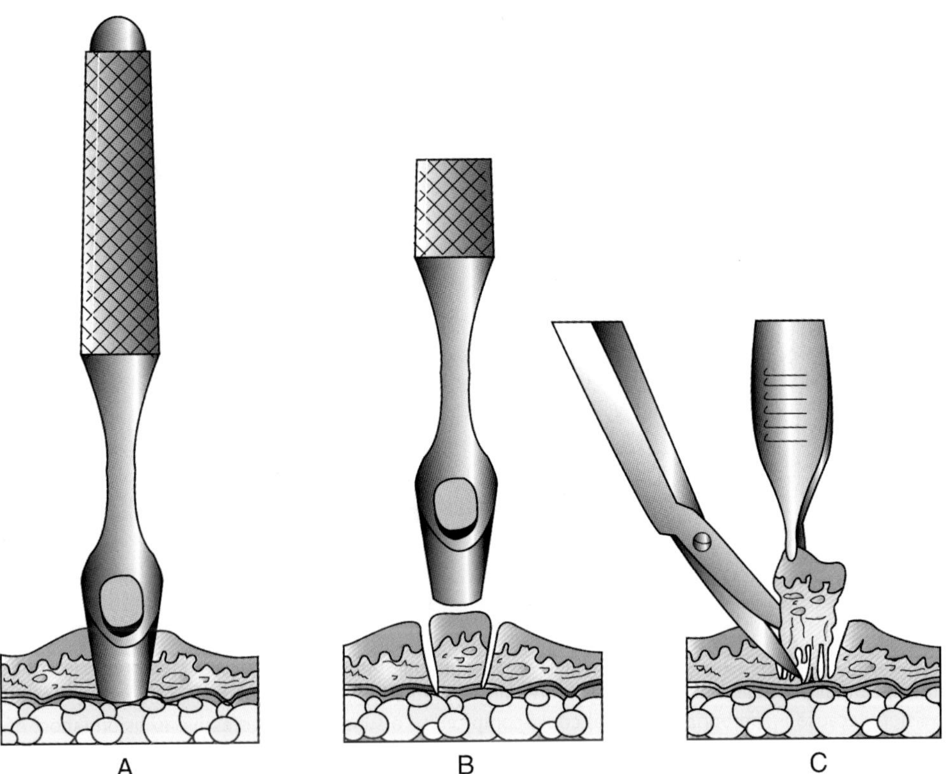

FIGURE 9-2 Mechanism of punch biopsy. **A,** Punch is rotated back and forth over suspect lesion until sufficient depth has been attained. **B,** Punch is removed or angled across base to sever deep attachments. **C,** Specimen may be "gently" grasped with thumb forceps and cut off deeply.

necrotic lesions because larger samples can be obtained, making it more likely to sample representative areas. Most tumors are poorly innervated and may be biopsied without the need for local anesthesia or sedation as long as the overlying normal skin and tissue has been anesthetized. Preparation involves clipping the hair over the incision site. After performing a sterile surgical preparation, surgical drapes are used to protect the field from the surrounding environment. Under sterile conditions, the skin over the tumor, if intact, is incised and a wedge of tumor tissue is removed from the mass. It is not necessary to remove a wedge of intact skin overlying the tumor if it appears to be normal and not fixed to the underlying tumor. The surgeon should confirm at the time of the biopsy that they have not simply removed a small section of the reactive tissue surrounding the tumor. This can be difficult in some cases, however, because most tumors have coloration and texture that is distinct from the surrounding normal and reactive tissue. If needed, "touch-prep" cytology slides can be made using the resected tissue prior to fixation to confirm that neoplastic cells are present in the removed tissue.

Many authors have recommended that the surgeon acquire a composite biopsy of normal and abnormal tissue to ensure accuracy in diagnosis on histopathologic examination. Although this may be helpful to the pathologist in benign skin disease and subtle lesions, it is not recommended in cases where neoplasia is suspected because this may compromise the surgical margin needed to remove the mass entirely at the time of definitive surgery and exposes previously uninvolved tissues to freshly incised tumor. Instead, a representative sample of the tumor itself should be submitted. This may require obtaining multiple samples via the same incision to ensure that a representative sample has been achieved. Care must be taken to ensure that any biopsy tract (incisional or other) will not compromise subsequent curative resection or contaminate uninvolved tissue needed for reconstruction. The surgeon should avoid wide exposure of uninvolved tissue planes that could become contaminated with released tumor cells. Small incisions, even through expendable muscle bellies, are preferred to contaminating the entire intramuscular compartment. The incisional biopsy tract is always removed in continuity with the tumor at the time of curative-intent resection.

Specialized Biopsy Techniques

Specialized biopsy techniques will generally be covered under the specific individual tumors. However, some general comments follow.

Endoscopic Biopsies

Endoscopic biopsy techniques use flexible or occasionally rigid scopes that allow visualized or blind biopsy of hollow lumens, especially gastrointestinal, respiratory, and urogenital systems. Although these techniques are convenient, cost effective, and generally safe, they may suffer from inadequate visualization and limited biopsy sample size when compared with other techniques. For example, an endoscopic biopsy result of ulcerative gastritis in a dog with a firm, infiltrative mass of the lesser curvature of the stomach does not rule out gastric adenocarcinoma.

Laparoscopy and Thoracoscopy

Evaluation of the abdomen and thorax via minimally invasive techniques, when performed by an experienced operator, can procure tissue for biopsy and yield important information regarding the

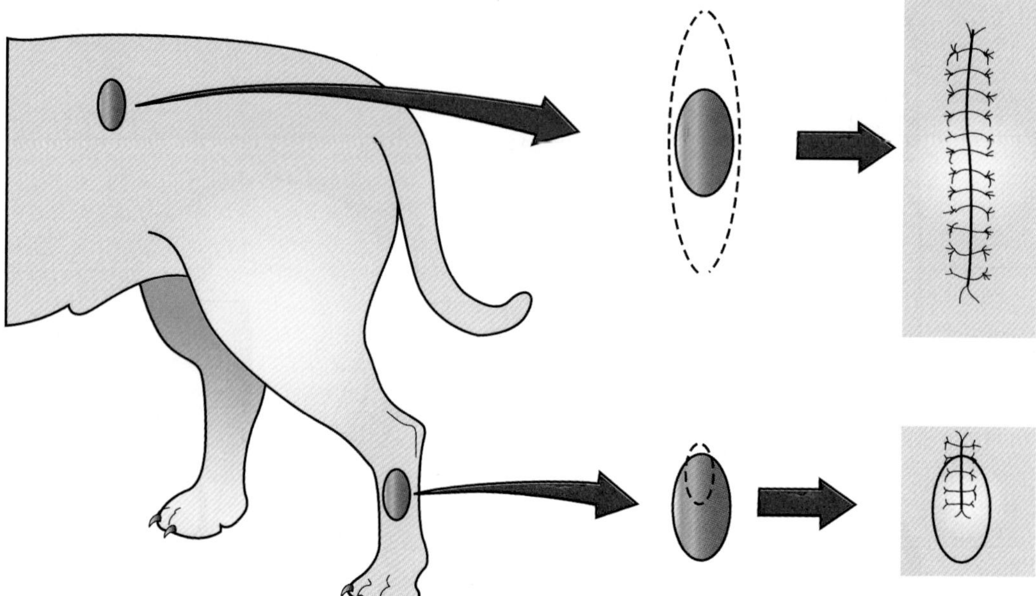

FIGURE 9-3 Excisional *(top)* contrasted with incisional *(bottom)* biopsy. The top tumor may be as easy to remove as to biopsy, and removal may not negatively influence other possible treatments (e.g., more surgery, radiation). The bottom tumor, however, requires knowledge of the tumor type prior to excision because inappropriate removal could compromise a subsequent aggressive excision (short of amputation). Note that the biopsy incision is in a plane that would be included in a subsequent resection.

locoregional stage of disease. Additionally, laparoscopic- and thoracoscopic-assisted removal results in smaller incisions and rapid recovery times when compared with open procedures. The option to convert to an open procedure is available if problems are encountered that cannot be adequately addressed using minimally invasive methods. As operators become more proficient at these techniques, more options become available for tumor removal.

Image-Guided Biopsy

Diagnostic imaging has greatly expanded the ability to stage various neoplasias. The use of positron emission tomography-computed tomography (PET-CT) in veterinary medicine has also led to significant advances in sentinel node mapping, novel staging methods, and the ability to assess response to treatment. In addition, the use of radiographic, fluoroscopic, ultrasonographic, computed tomographic, and magnetic resonance image–guided needle aspirates or core biopsies can obviate the need for more invasive diagnostic procedures. Common sites for image-guided biopsy include lung, kidney, liver, spleen, prostate, and, more recently, brain.

Excisional Biopsy

Excisional biopsy is utilized when definitive treatment would not be altered by knowledge of tumor type (e.g., "benign" skin tumor, solitary splenic mass, testicular tumor). It is more frequently performed than indicated, but, when used on properly selected cases, it can be both diagnostic and therapeutic, as well as cost effective.

General Guidelines for Tissue Procurement and Fixation

- When properly performed, a pretreatment biopsy will *not* negatively influence survival.[3] The metastatic cascade involves a series of complex events that are not altered by the number of neoplastic cells in circulation. On the other hand, neoplastic cells can contaminate the *local* tissues surrounding the mass and in some cases, successfully attach and grow within these normal tissues. Careful hemostasis, obliteration of dead space, and avoidance of seromas or hematomas will minimize local contamination of the incisional biopsy site. Definitive surgery to remove the tumor along with the associated biopsy tract should take place as soon as possible following the biopsy procedure. If possible, surgical drains should not be placed in biopsy sites because the drain tract can become contaminated with tumor cells and seed them through uninvolved tissue planes. In particular, care should be taken not to "spill" cancer cells within the thoracic or abdominal cavities during biopsy where they may seed pleural or peritoneal surfaces.
- When biopsies are performed on the legs or the tail, the incision should be longitudinal and not transverse. Transverse incisions are much harder to completely resect. If a biopsy is near midline, the incision should be oriented parallel to midline.
- Avoid taking the junction of normal and abnormal tissue for pretreatment biopsy unless a margin is likely necessary for differentiating benign or malignant tumors (e.g., perianal adenoma or adenocarcinoma often can only be differentiated histologically by observing local tissue infiltration). Care should be taken not to incise normal tissue that cannot be resected or would be used in reconstructing the surgical defect. Avoid biopsies that contain only ulcerated or inflamed tissues.
- The larger the sample, the more likely it is to be diagnostic. Tumors are not homogeneous and usually contain areas of necrosis, inflammation, and reactive tissue. Several samples from one mass are more likely to yield an accurate diagnosis than a single sample.
- Biopsies should not be obtained with electrocautery because it tends to deform (autolysis or polarization) the cellular

architecture. Electrocautery is better utilized for hemostasis after blade removal of a diagnostic specimen.

- Care should be taken not to unduly deform the specimen with forceps, suction, or other handling methods prior to fixation.
- Intraoperative diagnosis of disease by frozen sections, although not routinely available in veterinary medicine, has enjoyed widespread use in human oncology. Special equipment and training are required for this technique to be fully utilized. One study in veterinary medicine revealed an accurate and specific diagnosis rate of 83%.[4]
- If evaluation of excisional margins is desired, the surgeon should indicate the surgical margin on the specimen using tissue ink. Several commercial inking systems are available for this use. The resected tissue should be blotted with a paper towel because dyes will adhere better to the tissue when it is slightly tacky. The tissue ink is "painted" on the surgical margins using a cotton swab. The dye is allowed to dry for up to 20 minutes before the tissue is placed in formalin. Tissue already fixed in formalin can be marked; however, dye adherence is lessened and drying time is extended. When the pathologist sees tumor cells at the inked edge, it is a certainty that tumor cells have been left in the patient. Different-colored inks can also be used to denote different sites on the tumor, such as proximal margin or deep margin near nerve. Even with inking, proper fixation, and processing, the clinician must realize the entire margin will not be examined by the pathologist. Rather, representative sections will be obtained from the inked margin. Therefore any guidance that the clinician can give to the pathologist as to the most important sections to look for tumor cells will help the pathologist pay closer attention to such areas. It is vital that the pathologist and the clinician communicate if the pathology report is confusing or does not match the clinical picture. Of course, margin evaluation is only necessary for excisional biopsy or curative-intent surgery and does not apply to needle core biopsies or incisional biopsies, which by definition will have inadequate margins. Incomplete surgical resection of malignant disease is best detected early so that further surgery or other adjuvant therapies can be instituted immediately, as opposed to waiting for local recurrence or metastasis.
- Stainless steel vascular clips in the resected specimen will damage the microtomes used by the pathology laboratory. Remove them before the tissue is submitted.
- Proper fixation is vital. Tissue is generally fixed in 10% buffered neutral formalin with 1 part tissue to 10 parts fixative. If more than one lesion has been biopsied, they should each be placed in a separate container. Certain tissues such as eye, nerve, and muscle may require special fixation techniques. The clinician may want to consult with the pathologist on how to submit tissue for special circumstances.
- Tissue should not be thicker than 1 cm or it will not fix properly. Masses greater than 1 cm in diameter can be sliced like a loaf of bread, leaving the deep-inked margin intact, to allow fixation. Extremely large masses can be incompletely sliced as described above, fixed in a large bucket of formalin for 2 to 3 days and then shipped in a container with 1 part tissue to 1 part formalin. A less ideal but alternative approach is to have the surgeon take representative smaller samples from the mass (e.g., soft and hard pieces, red and pale pieces, deep and superficial pieces) in the hope that one of them is diagnostic. The rest of the mass can be saved in the clinic in formalin in case more tissue needs to be evaluated. This extra tissue should never be frozen. Freezing causes severe tissue artifact.
- A *detailed* history should accompany all biopsy requests. Interpretation of surgical biopsies is a combination of art and science. Without vital diagnostic information (e.g., signalment, history of recurrences, invasion into bone, rate of growth), the pathologist will be significantly compromised in his or her ability to deliver accurate and clinically useful information.
- A veterinary-trained pathologist is preferred over a pathologist trained in human diseases. Although many cancers are histologically similar across species lines, enough differences exist to result in interpretive errors.

In 2011, the American College of Veterinary Pathologists, along with several medical and surgical oncologists, published a comprehensive set of recommendations and guidelines for submission, trimming, margin evaluation, and reporting of tumor biopsy specimens.[5] This seminal paper was the first collaborative attempt to standardize pathology reporting in veterinary oncology and has been endorsed by a large international group of veterinary pathologists and oncology specialists. It is recommended that clinicians utilize diagnostic laboratories that adhere to these guidelines so that results are standardized and easier to interpret.

Interpretation of Results

The pathologist's task is to determine (1) tumor versus no tumor, (2) benign versus malignant, (3) histologic type, (4) grade (if applicable), and (5) margins (if excisional). Making an accurate diagnosis is not as simple as putting a piece of tissue in formalin and waiting for results. Many pitfalls can occur that render the end result inaccurate. Potential errors can take place at any level of the process, and it is up to the clinician to interpret the full meaning of the biopsy result. In cases in which the biopsy result does not correlate with the clinical scenario, a second opinion should be pursued. A study published in 2009 reviewed first and second opinion histopathology reports.[6] In 70% of cases, there was diagnostic agreement between first and second opinion results. In 20% of cases, there was partial agreement where the diagnosis did not change, but information such as grade or presence of lymphatic or vascular invasion was disparate. In 10% of cases reviewed, there was complete diagnostic disagreement. Of these, 7% were a disagreement between malignant versus nonmalignant and 3% were disagreements about cell origin. If the biopsy result does not correlate with the clinical scenario, the following several options are possible:

1. Call the pathologist and express your concern over the biopsy result. This exchange of information should be helpful for both parties and not looked on as an affront to the pathologist's authority or expertise. It may lead to the following:
   a. Resectioning of available tissue or paraffin blocks.
   b. Special stains for further discrimination of tumor types (e.g., toluidine blue for mast cells).
   c. A second opinion by another pathologist.
2. If the tumor is still present in the patient and particularly if widely varied options exist for therapy, a second (or third) biopsy should be performed.

A carefully performed, submitted, and interpreted biopsy is the most important step in management and subsequent prognosis of the patient with cancer. The biopsy report is key in decisions regarding prognosis, therapeutic options, and overall case management. All too often tumors are not submitted for histologic evaluation after removal because "the owner didn't want to pay for it." Histopathologic interpretation should not be an elective owner decision. Instead, it should be as automatic as closing the skin after surgery. The charge for submission and interpretation of the biopsy should be included in the surgery fee if need be, but histopathology interpretation is not optional. Because of increasing medicolegal concerns, it is not medical curiosity alone that mandates knowledge of tumor type. Understanding how and when to perform a biopsy, how to submit a biopsy specimen, and how to interpret the report is of paramount importance in the treatment of veterinary cancer patients.

REFERENCES

1. Ghisleni G, Roccabianca P, Ceruti R, et al: Correlation between fine-needle aspiration cytology and histopathology in the evaluation of cutaneous and subcutaneous masses from dogs and cats, *Vet Clin Path* 35(1):24–30, 2006.
2. Sharkey LC, Wellman ML: Diagnostic cytology in veterinary medicine: A comparative and evidence-based approach, *Clin Lab Med* 31(1):1–19, 2011.
3. Klopfleisch R, Sperling C, Kershaw O, et al: Does the taking of biopsies affect the metastatic potential of tumors? A systematic review of reports on veterinary and human cases and animal models, *Vet J* 190(2):e31–e42, 2011.
4. Whitehair JG, Griffey SM, Olander HJ, et al: The accuracy of intraoperative diagnoses based on examination of frozen sections. A prospective comparison with paraffin-embedded sections, *Vet Surg* 22(4):255–259, 1993.
5. Kamstock DA, Ehrhart EJ, Getzy DM, et al: Recommended guidelines for submission, trimming, margin evaluation, and reporting of tumor biopsy specimens in veterinary surgical pathology, *Vet Pathol* 48(1):19–31, 2011.
6. Regan RC, Rassnick KM, Balkman CE, et al: Comparison of first-opinion and second-opinion histopathology from dogs and cats with cancer: 430 cases (2001-2008), *Vet Comp Oncol* 8(1):1–10, 2010.

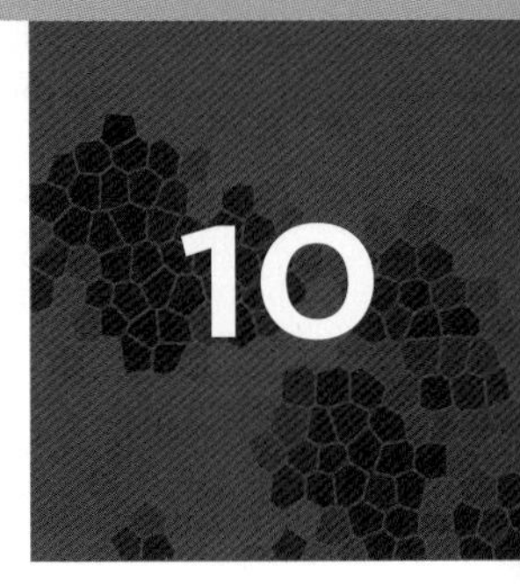

Surgical Oncology

James P. Farese and Stephen J. Withrow

Complete surgical removal of localized cancer cures more cancer patients than any other form of treatment,[1] in part because this modality is generally applied as sole treatment for local disease, early stage disease, or tumors with limited potential to metastasize. In humans, 60% of patients who are cured of cancer are cured by surgery alone.[2] Before this hope for cure can be realized in veterinary medicine, surgeons must have a thorough understanding of anatomy, physiology, resection, and reconstruction options for all organs; expected tumor behavior; and the various alternatives or adjuvants to surgery. Surgical oncologists should not only be good technical surgeons, but also dedicated tumor biologists. Surgery will likely play a role at one point or another in the management of most cancer patients. Surgical procedures may include any of the following: diagnosis (biopsy), resection for cure, palliation of symptoms, debulking (tumor cell cytoreduction), and a wide variety of ancillary procedures to enhance and complement other forms of treatment.

Surgical resection of cancer was introduced in the sixteenth century BCE and remained relatively underutilized until general anesthesia (1840s), antisepsis (1860s), and pain management made aggressive resection safe and tolerable for the patient. Dr. William Halstead developed the basic principles of surgical oncology in the 1890s. The radical resection of the twentieth century has increasingly been customized to meet the needs of the patient and has frequently been reduced in magnitude. Further refinements in surgery have been made possible with newer equipment (e.g., staples, endoscopy), advanced imaging, pain management, use of blood products, and critical care services.

Most patients with cancer are "old." However, "old" is a relative term, and a geriatric dog or cat with normal organ function should not be denied treatment simply on the basis of age. Age has not been shown to impact tumor-related prognosis. In fact, dogs with osteosarcoma that are less than 2 years of age do worse than dogs that are more than 2 years of age after amputation alone.[3] "Old" animals, in most instances, will tolerate aggressive surgical intervention as well or as poorly as "young" patients.

Surgery for Diagnosis

Although biopsy principles are covered in Chapter 9, it bears emphasizing that properly timed, performed, and interpreted biopsies are one of the most crucial steps in the management of the cancer patient. Not only does the surgeon need to procure adequate and representative tissue to establish a diagnosis, but also the biopsy must not compromise subsequent curative surgical resection or radiation field planning.

Surgery for Cure

Before a surgeon can be in a position to provide the optimal operation for the patient with cancer, the following questions need to be considered:

1. What is the histologic type, stage, and grade of cancer to be treated?
2. What are the expected local and systemic effects of this tumor type, grade, and stage?
3. Is a cure possible and at what price in terms of cosmetics and function?
4. Is an operation indicated at all?
5. What are the options for alternative or planned combination treatment?

A recurring theme in surgical management of cancer is that the first surgery has the best chance of cure. Several mechanisms for this improvement in survival have been advanced. Untreated tumors have had less chronologic time to metastasize than recurrent primary cancer. Untreated tumors and proximate normal tissues have near normal anatomy, which will facilitate operative orientation and maneuvers. Recurrent tumors may have had seeding of previously noninvolved tissue planes, requiring wider resection than would have been required on the initial tumor. If one thinks about a given cancer as resembling a crab, incomplete surgery removes the body of the crab and leaves the legs behind. The "body" of most tumors is often quiescent and hypoxic, whereas the leading edge of the tumor (legs) is the most invasive and well vascularized. Subtotal removal may actually selectively leave behind the most aggressive components of the tumor. Patients with recurrent cancer will often have less normal tissue for closure. An ill-defined negative aspect of recurrent cancer is reported to be related to changes in vascularity and local immune responses. Regardless of the mechanism, curative-intent surgery is best performed at the first operation and the surgeon should have all the necessary diagnostic information in hand when constructing a treatment plan. Radiography and ultrasonography have been routine for many years, and the increased availability of computed tomography (CT) has added greatly to our ability to determine the extent of a solid tumor and optimize the surgical approach. CT allows good visualization of muscle bellies/fascial planes, intraabdominal/intrathoracic organs, lymph nodes, and bone detail. Three-dimensional (3D) CT reconstructions are particularly useful for planning procedures for skull-based tumors.

Advanced imaging has greatly enhanced the surgeon's ability to assess the anatomic location and extent of various cancers; however, we must remember that imaging of any kind needs to be paired with clinical palpation, assessment of mobility, and expected biologic behavior. Some cancers deemed inoperable by imaging are in fact mobile and operable. Leading edges of some cancers are compressed against adjacent tissue and appear more invasive. Surgeons should always take the opportunity to palpate the local tumor before or after imaging, explore the history of the tumor's growth pattern, and in many cases obtain a tissue sample (i.e., histopathology or cytology when appropriate) before declaring a mass inoperable. Positive prognostic factors typically include slow growth rate, mobility within proximate tissues, first attempt at surgery, discrete tumor borders, small tumor size, and low grade nature. Conversely, surgery may be less effective for the same tumor type and grade if the mass is ill-defined, is recurrent, or has a recent history of rapid growth. Palpation under heavy sedation or anesthesia may suggest that resection is possible in spite of imaging findings (e.g., unilateral thyroid masses, some soft tissue sarcomas). Deeper masses from locations such as ribs and liver may appear inoperable due to inflammation or compression of adjacent organs and structures; however, there actually may be no invasion present.

The surgical oncologist must be able to assimilate all of the information and make an informed decision. We must also remind ourselves and our clients that there is much we do not know (e.g., incomplete margins do not necessarily ensure later local recurrence[4]) and that surgical judgment regarding expected local behavior and likely resection is often qualitative and is an imperfect "science."

The actual surgical technique will vary with the site, size, and stage of the tumor, as well as the skill and experience of the surgeon. The same tumor type in dogs and cats may vary in surgical approach, technique, and prognosis. Some general statements that need to be emphasized with surgical oncology are as follows:

1. All incisional biopsy tracts should be excised in continuity with the primary tumor because tumor cells are capable of growth in these wounds. Fine-needle aspiration (FNA) cytology tracts are of minor, but not zero, concern, whereas punch biopsy tracts are of intermediate concern.[5] With this in mind, all biopsies should be positioned in such a manner that they can be removed at surgery.
2. Early vascular ligation (especially venous) should be attempted to diminish release of large tumor emboli into the systemic circulation. This is probably only clinically meaningful for those tumors with a well-defined venous supply, such as splenic tumors, retained testicles, and lung tumors. Small numbers of cancer cells are constantly being released into the venous (and lymphatic) circulation by most tumors. Larger, macroscopic cell aggregates may be more dangerous, however, and these may be prevented from vascular escape with early venous ligation.
3. Local control of malignant cancer requires that a margin of normal tissue be removed around the tumor. Resection of the "bad from the good" can and should be classified in more detail than radical versus conservative (Table 10-1).[6] Tumors with high probability of local recurrence (e.g., high-grade soft tissue sarcoma, high-grade mast cell tumors, feline mammary adenocarcinoma) should have 2- to 3-cm margins removed in three dimensions. Tumors are not flat, and wide removal in one plane does not ensure complete excision. Fixation of cancer to adjacent structures mandates removal of the adherent area in continuity with the tumor. This is commonly seen with oral cancer that is firmly adherent to the underlying mandible or maxilla. Invasive cancer should not be peeled out, shelled out, enucleated, or curetted if a cure is expected. Many cancers are surrounded by a pseudocapsule. This capsule is almost invariably composed of compressed and viable tumor cells, not healthy reactive host cells. If a malignant tumor is entered at the time of resection, or if the margins are incomplete, that procedure is often no better therapeutically than a large incisional biopsy. When possible, resection of the previous scar and the entire wound bed with "new" margins (never entering the old wound cavity) is indicated. One should strive for a level of dissection that is one tissue plane away from the mass (Figure 10-1). For example, invasion of cancer into the medullary cavity of a bone requires subtotal or total bone resection and not curettage.

   The width of surgical margins necessary for a complete excision for a given tumor type is an ongoing debate, and our current practices are based on little objective data. As a community, we have answered most of the questions about how much tissue we can safely remove, but it will serve our patients well to determine how little extra tissue is necessary to excise and consistently achieve the same success. We must challenge recommendations that are reported in the literature if based solely on a surgeon's personal experience or opinion in the absence of objective findings.
4. Tumors should be handled gently to avoid risk of breaking off tumor cells into the operative wound, where they may thrive.[7] Copious lavage of all cancer wound beds will help mechanically remove small numbers of exfoliated tumor cells but should not replace gentle tissue handling and avoidance of entering the tumor bed.
5. If more than one malignant mass is being removed, separate surgical packs should be used for each site to avoid iatrogenic tumor cell implantation from site to site.

The aggressiveness of resection should only rarely be tempered by fears of wound closure. It is better to leave a wound partially or even in some cases completely open with no cancer than closed with residual cancer. Numerous innovative reconstructive techniques are available for closure of cancer wounds, and the surgeon is only limited by his or her ingenuity.[8] Reliable microvascular-free composite transfers of muscle and skin are somewhat hampered due to unique canine skin/muscle anatomy but are being developed.[9]

TABLE 10-1 Classification and Resection of Wound Margins

TYPE	PLANE OF DISSECTION	RESULT
Intracapsular	Tumor removed in pieces or curetted, "debulking"	Macroscopic disease left behind
Marginal	Removal just outside or on pseudocapsule or reactive capsule, "shelled out"	Usually leaves microscopic disease
Wide	Tumor and capsule never entered, normal tissue surrounds specimen	Possible skip lesions
Radical	Entire compartment or structure removed (e.g., amputation)	No local residual cancer

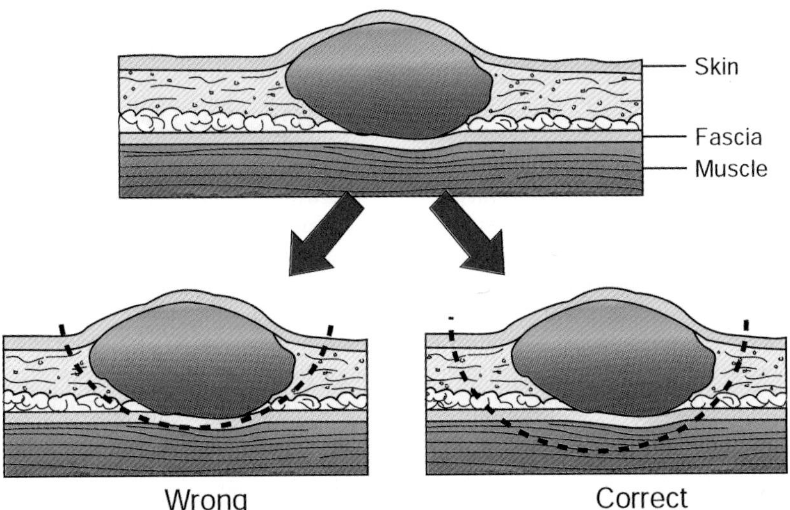

FIGURE 10-1 Typical soft tissue cancer is in proximity to skin and underlying fascia. Inappropriate removal is to "peel it off" the deeper fascia, where microscopic extension is probable. Correct removal entails wide three-dimensional (3D) margins, including underlying skin and underlying fascia.

Lymph Node Removal

Controversy surrounds the surgical management of regional lymph nodes draining the primary tumor site.[10,11] As a general rule, epithelial cancers are more likely to metastasize to lymph nodes than are mesenchymal cancers. However, any enlarged regional lymph node requires investigation for complete staging. Lymphadenopathy may be from metastasis of cancer (firm, irregular, and sometimes fixed to surrounding tissue) or from hyperplasia and reactivity to various tumor factors, infection, or inflammation.[12] The former cause is a poor prognostic sign, and the latter may be a beneficial host response. Enlarged lymph nodes as a result of cancer metastasis and invasion are generally effaced by tumor cells and can often be diagnosed by FNA. Histologically, positive lymph nodes at diagnosis usually are a sign of impending emergence of systemic metastasis. Removal of lymph nodes should be considered under the following circumstances:

1. If the lymph node is positive for cancer and not fixed to surrounding normal tissues, it may be possible to remove the node with some therapeutic intent. Frequently, however, many lymph nodes drain a primary tumor site (e.g., oral cavity) and lymphadenectomy is incomplete. Lymph node metastasis at the time of initial diagnosis is a poor prognostic sign. However, patients that develop metastasis in a delayed fashion (1 to 2 years) after local tumor control may benefit from lymphadenectomy. Although it is usually not practical, removal of the primary tumor, intervening lymphatic ducts, and draining lymph node has been recommended (en bloc resection). En bloc resection may be possible for a malignant toe tumor with metastasis to the popliteal lymph node but is usually only accomplished with amputation. A mastectomy that includes the regional lymph node (e.g., glands four and five with the inguinal lymph node) is another example of en bloc resection. Few other anatomic sites are routinely amenable to this therapy. A specific instance where local lymphadenectomy may be beneficial is in removal of iliac/sublumbar lymph nodes in patients with metastatic apocrine or sebaceous gland adenocarcinomas of the perineum. Although removal of these lymph nodes is rarely curative, it may help increase the benefit of adjuvant radiation or chemotherapy and should help alleviate, at least in the short term, the paraneoplastic syndrome of hypercalcemia by reducing levels of parathormone-like substances. Regional lymphadenectomy may also prevent or improve obstruction of the large bowel and urinary tract and can be repeated as necessary in the absence of overt systemic metastasis (e.g., metastasis to lungs, liver).
2. It is well estabished that normal-sized lymph nodes may contain micrometastasis, and this point should always be explained clearly to a client. Normal-appearing lymph nodes that are known to drain a primary tumor site may be randomly sampled (biopsy or cytology) to gain further staging information. This is particularly important if adjuvant therapy decisions (irradiation or chemotherapy) would be predicated on confirmation of residual or metastatic cancer. Intrathoracic or intraabdominal lymph nodes are perhaps most crucial because they are not readily accessible to histologic or cytologic follow-up examination. However, in some instances, lymph nodes that are not enlarged cannot be sampled safely due to proximity to vital structures (e.g., sublumbar lymph nodes at the aortic bifurcation), even under ultrasound guidance. In such cases, the surgeon must educate the client about the situation and either remove the primary tumor without further knowledge of regional lymph node involvement or recommend removal of the normal-sized nodes concurrently for staging (and possibly therapeutic) purposes. For dogs with malignant anal sac tumors, this approach involves an exploratory surgery of the sublumbar nodal bed and dissection/removal of all nodal tissue encountered.

In human medicine, the concept of the sentinel lymph node (first node to receive lymphatic flow from a primary tumor) has become important in the management of select malignancies, most notably breast cancer.[12] Basically, the area of the primary tumor is injected with blue dye or a low dose of a radionuclide or both. The first draining node is detected visually or with a handheld gamma camera probe and removed for frozen section analysis. If the first node is negative for metastasis, subsequent nodal dissection often is avoided. If the sentinel node is positive, further nodal dissection is performed. Targeting the sentinel node is most valuable in an anatomic location in which there is an extensive nodal bed[12] and hence numerous potential paths for regional metastasis. The benefits of such an approach in humans are readily apparent because many patients have been spared extensive nodal resections if the sentinel lymph node has been determined to be free of cancer cells. The topic of the sentinel lymph node has only recently emerged in veterinary medicine but is gathering some momentum.[13] Several techniques have been described, including microbubble detection via ultrasound,[14] fluorescein, and blue dye.[15] Although sentinel lymph node staging may not yet have the relevance and importance that have been demonstrated in humans due to less complex nodal networks, there are several potential indications (e.g., tumors of the head and neck) that should be investigated in clinical studies. Histologically positive lymph nodes will alter prognosis and stage and will also be informative for decisions related to postoperative chemotherapy and radiation.

Lymph node removal is generally *not* performed under the following circumstances:

1. Lymph nodes in critical areas (retropharyngeal, hilar, mesenteric) that have eroded through the capsule and become adherent (fixed) to surrounding tissues. In this scenario, lymph nodes may not be removeable without leaving residual disease in the wound bed (necessitating adjuvant therapy to achieve local control) or an attempt at removal may cause serious harm to the patient by injuring important adjacent structures. In such instances, it is usually prudent to aspirate or biopsy the node to confirm involvement in the disease process and leave the node in situ or treat with other modalities. One example of an exception to this scenario is metastasis of limb and paw tumors to prescapular and popliteal lymph nodes that can be removed with amputation (radical en bloc resection).
2. Prophylactic removal of "normal" draining lymph nodes or chains of lymph nodes (as opposed to sampling for stage) is not beneficial and may be harmful.[9] Regional lymph nodes may in fact be the initiator of favorable local and systemic immune responses, and elective removal has been associated with poor survival in certain human cancers.[10,16,17]

Surgery for Distant Disease

Metastasectomy for pulmonary metastasis of sarcoma *in some instances* has been accepted therapy in humans and dogs. Resection of liver metastasis for carcinomas (especially gastrointestinal cancers) is increasing in human oncology. As more effective adjuvant therapies evolve and minimally invasive techniques are further developed, the need for cytoreductive metastasectomy will increase.

Palliative Surgery

Palliative surgery is an attempt to improve the quality of the patient's life (pain relief or improved function) but not necessarily the length of the patient's life.[18] This type of surgery requires careful consideration of the expected morbidity of the procedure versus the expected gain to the patient and the client. In essence, it comes down to a decision of when to discontinue therapy. One of the most difficult decisions in surgical oncology is the decision not to operate. Treatment of any kind should never be worse than no treatment.

Certain situations do exist, however, in which palliative surgery may be beneficial. If an infected and draining mammary tumor in a patient with asymptomatic lung metastasis is the limiting factor in the patient's life, mastectomy may still be a logical procedure. Splenectomy for ruptured hemangiosarcoma is commonly performed but probably has little impact on long-term survival and can be considered palliative because it will stop the immediate threat of hemorrhage.

Cytoreductive Surgery

Incomplete removal of a tumor (planned or unplanned) is referred to as debulking or cytoreductive surgery. It is commonly performed but rarely indicated.[19] Its theoretical indication is to enhance the efficacy of other treatment modalities. Debulking is a practical consideration prior to cryosurgery to decrease the amount of tissue to freeze and the time it will take. It may also help the treatment planning and dosimetry with certain forms of irradiation, but the improved cancer control achieved is more a result of geometric and dosimetry considerations than intentional and incomplete removal of tumor cells. Removing 99.9% of a 1-cm tumor (1×10^9 cells, one billion) still leaves a million cancer cells behind. Immunotherapy and chemotherapy could theoretically be helped by tumor volume reduction (such as lymph node removal for oral melanoma with the use of a melanoma vaccine),[20,21] but few well-controlled clinical trials have shown a benefit to date in veterinary medicine. A variety of soft tissue sarcomas in dogs and cats will have better local control when radiation is given adjuvantly rather than for bulky measurable disease. Amputation or limb sparing of dogs with osteosarcoma is essentially an extreme cytoreductive procedure and clearly requires postoperative chemotherapy for prolongation of life. If tumors are debulked with the anticipation of postoperative radiation therapy, the margins of known tumor or the operative field should be marked with radiopaque metal clips to allow proper treatment planning from radiographs or CT. The orientation of the incision should be considered carefully if radiation therapy is possible postoperatively.

Nonsurgical Locally Ablative Procedures

Ablative techniques to eradicate local (or metastatic) disease have a place in oncology but often suffer from "sales before science" and are only rarely based on evidence of outcomes.[22] Several of these techniques will be mentioned later, and the reader is referred to accompanying references for details. Indications for the use of local ablative therapy vary but are generally limited to "small" (less than 2 cm diameter) discrete lesions. A limitation of all of the techniques is that completeness of cell kill and margin analysis cannot be determined after treatment. If the operator picked the correct tumor, site, and "dose" delivery, then local control may be achieved; however, monitoring for regrowth is the only way to ensure this. As a general rule, recurrent disease tends to be more invasive and difficult to control than the primary intervention, so the first ablative maneuver is hopefully well planned and executed. All of the local ablative treatments require special equipment and training to properly perform. Selective tumor cell kill while sparing all normal tissue is often claimed for these techniques but is unlikely to be true.

Radiofrequency Ablation

The most common nonsurgical locally ablative procedures in human medicine include radiofrequency (RF), microwave, and cryoablation. RF ablation involves delivery of a high frequency (300 to 500 KHz) alternating current via a needle-like probe. The procedure is typically performed via image guidance (e.g., ultrasound or CT) and is commonly used to treat both primary and secondary hepatic tumors. The minimally invasive nature of the technique makes it ideal for the latter application. With hepatic metastatic colorectal cancer, RF rivals surgery for increasing 5-year survival. Microwave ablation is similar to RF, but higher frequency current (900 to 2459 MHz) is delivered through the probe. It is a newer technology with less evidence supporting its use but is often used for the same indications as RF ablation. Neither the RF nor microwave procedures have been evaluated for clinical applications in veterinary patients[23,24]; however, some of the work done to evaluate the safety of these procedures in humans was performed experimentally in dogs.

Cryoablation

Cryosurgery, or cryoablation, is a much older form of local therapy that impacts tumors via direct cell kill and vascular collapse. It has been used extensively in veterinary medicine, most commonly for skin, nasal planum, eyelid, perianal, and oral cavity neoplasms.[25-27] It continues to be an attractive treatment option for clients not interested in invasive procedures and for palliation of advanced (i.e., nonresectable or metastatic) oral disease and can be used as an adjunct to debulking surgery. There is a recent report of image-guided cryoablation of a nasal mass in a dog that recurred following intensity-modulated radiation therapy (IMRT).[28] In humans, laparoscopic and percutaneous cryoablation of select neoplasms (e.g., breast and renal tumors) has become an attractive, minimally invasive treatment option.[29,30]

Hyperthermia

Hyperthermia is the elevation of tissue temperature above normal physiologic levels. Thus the term *hyperthermia* encompasses a wide range of temperatures and modalities. A variety of methods and devices are used clinically to induce hyperthermia in tissues. Noninvasive methods using RF currents, microwaves, or ultrasound are the most common. Heating of solid tumors is typically nonuniform, due in part to the heating devices available and in part to nonuniform distribution of blood flow in the tumor and heat-dissipating activity of surrounding normal tissue. A number of studies demonstrate improved outcome when hyperthermia is added to radiation therapy of solid tumors in dogs.[31-34] The ideal strategy for clinical hyperthermia treatment, including thermal dose, fractionation, and time and temperature goals, has yet to be identified.

Photodynamic Therapy

The practice of using sunlight to treat disease is ancient, but modern refinements have allowed the interactions between light and drugs to evolve into a highly effective cancer treatment called *photodynamic therapy* (PDT). PDT relies on light of an appropriate activating wavelength, oxygen, and a photosensitizer (PS) that accumulates within a tumor. The excited PS interacts with molecular oxygen, creating reactive oxygen species that are responsible for causing vascular stasis and necrosis, membrane damage, and apoptosis and for initiating a signaling cascade resulting in an influx of inflammatory cells. Although initially studied as a single modality, PDT may also be useful when combined with other cancer treatments. Early studies show that a combination of PDT and low-dose cisplatin increases efficacy in both in vitro and murine models, and similar synergy has been observed when doxorubicin is combined with PDT.[35,36] In veterinary medicine, PDT has been most commonly used in the treatment of squamous cell carcinoma (SCC). Most SCCs are superficial, localized, and do not metastasize until late in the course of the disease, making them well suited for treatment with PDT. An early description of chloro-aluminum sulfonated phthalocyanine–based PDT in 10 cats with superficial SCC or carcinoma in situ reported a 70% complete response rate, demonstrating the potential for PDT as a skin cancer treatment.[37] With a number of recent technologic improvements, PDT has the potential to become integrated into the mainstream of cancer treatment.[38]

Surgery and Chemotherapy

The combined use of chemotherapy and surgery is becoming more commonplace in veterinary oncology, and the knowledge an oncologic surgeon must possess to master the use of combination therapy is ever expanding.[39,40] Many chemotherapy agents will impede wound healing to some extent. In spite of this risk, few clinically relevant problems occur when surgery is performed on a patient receiving chemotherapy.[41,42] General recommendations are to wait 7 to 10 days after surgery to begin chemotherapy, especially for high-risk procedures such as intestinal anastomosis.[43] The use of intraoperative[44]or perioperative chemotherapy is receiving increased attention[45,46] and could have greater implications for wound healing. Neoadjuvant chemotherapy is also becoming more popular and in some instances may greatly facilitate excision of a solid tumor. Such an approach is commonly used with some canine mast cell tumors, but there remain unanswered questions, such as what characteristics identify the indications for such an approach? Also, if a tumor reduction occurs, should the location of the original tumor border be used to make measurements for margins or the new outer edge?

Surgery and Radiation

Theoretical advantages can be advanced for both preoperative and postoperative radiation.[40,47] Either way, some impairment of wound-healing potential will exist and need to be considered.[48] Radiation damage to normal tissues (stem cells, blood vessels, lymphatics) may be progressive and potentially permanent as total radiation dose, dose per fraction, and field size increase. Therefore close collaboration between the radiation oncologist and surgeon is critical when designing the most effective regimen. If radiation therapy is given preoperatively, surgery can be performed after acute radiation reactions have resolved (generally 3 to 4 weeks). Postoperative radiation is recommended after a 7- to 14-day delay to allow for adequate wound healing. In spite of the theoretical problems, surgery can often be safely performed on irradiated tissues and complications are not prohibitive.

The benefit of surgery and radiation is clear for some tumor types; however, in some instances the improvement in outcome over single modality therapy is controversial. One such debate is that of canine nasal tumors.[49,50] Early reports did not show benefit of postoperative radiation over radiation alone. A recent report demonstrated preoperative radiation as beneficial when followed by exenteration of the nasal cavity 6 to 10 weeks later.[50] With the advent of stereotactic radiation therapy (SRT) and IMRT (see Chapter 12), such approaches are even more attractive because the overlying skin or underlying mucosa in the case of nasal tumors can be spared from the full effects of the radiation, thereby diminishing concerns about incisional healing. In the past, surgeons would be reluctant to operate in a radiation field; thus these more focused forms of radiation therapy will hopefully allow the surgeon to operate with fewer wound healing complications and create novel treatment plans that combine radiation and surgery for select tumors. Radiation side effects are greatly diminished with a more conformal approach, and this in turn makes clients more willing to have their pets undergo radiotherapy.

Access to more sophisticated radiation techniques such as SRT and IMRT is rapidly increasing throughout the world, and with this development, a new paradigm is emerging in veterinary radiation oncology. For example, bone sarcomas in locations not amenable to limb-sparing surgery can now be treated with curative intent therapy[51] and treatment protocols for large solid tumors previously deemed nonresectable are currently being investigated. Combinations of SRT and surgery are also being explored. However, while these new treatment options represent great advances, familiar challenges remain. In the case of dogs with appendicular osteosarcoma, fracture may occur after SRT and while some of these cases are amenable to surgical stabilization, healing of the fracture does not occur normally due to the effects of radiation on bone healing. Thus the role of the surgeon continues to evolve in the management of cases treated with radiation.

Prevention of Cancer

Certain common cancers in dogs and cats can be prevented. The recent elucidation of the canine genome as it relates to genetic susceptibility will likely increase the surgical indications for prevention. It is well known that early (<1 year) oophorectomy will reduce the risk of mammary cancer in the dog by 200-fold compared to intact bitches (and to a lesser degree the cat). Castration of the male dog will help prevent perianal adenomas and obviously testicular cancer. Removal of in situ SCC (precancerous) from the skin of white cats or removal of in situ adenomatous polyps from the rectum of dogs may also prevent subsequent development of cancer. Elective removal of cryptorchid testes, which are at high risk for tumor development, is another example of preventive surgery.

Miscellaneous Oncologic Surgery

Veterinary surgeons are being called on increasingly to facilitate the medical management of cancer patients. The placement of long-term vascular access catheters for delivery of fluids, chemotherapy, or anesthesia and pain relief agents has become commonplace, and ports are routinely placed to aid in the evacuation of malignant thoracic effusions (e.g., mesothelioma). Operative placement of various enteral and parenteral feeding tubes is also commonly performed.

Surgeons and radiotherapists may work together for the operative exposure of nonresectable cancer so that large doses of irradiation may be delivered to the tumor or tumor bed after exclusion of radiosensitive tissues. Surgical intervention for oncologic emergencies such as intractable pain, bleeding, pathologic fracture, infection, and bowel perforation or obstruction may also arise.

The comprehensive veterinary oncology team also now includes the discipline of interventional radiology to help manage/palliate certain malignancies. Examples include the use of self-expanding nitinol stents to treat dogs with malignant urethral obstruction[52] and double pigtail stents for the treatment of malignant ureteral obstructions resulting from trigonal transitional cell carcinoma (TCC) of the urinary bladder.[53]

Equipment advances are facilitating tumor excisions (e.g., harmonic scalpel[54] and LigaSure for splenectomy and liver masses), and laparoscopic and thoracoscopic evaluation of body cavities for staging is increasingly being performed on animals. Cancer resections with this technique are also on the rise and given the potential for decreased morbidity, veterinary surgeons may feel more comfortable performing surgery in the face of advanced disease for certain solid cancers (e.g., thoracoscopic removal of a solitary metastatic lung nodule at the time of amputation for an appendicular osteosarcoma). A few other examples of minimally invasive surgery performed in companion animals for cancerous diseases include prostatic biopsy,[55] thoracoscopic pericardiectomy for heart-based tumors, laparoscopy-assisted intestinal biopsy, liver biopsy, pancreatic biopsy, splenectomy,[56] and adrenalectomy.[57] Further definition of appropriate case selection and increased access to equipment and training will ultimately expand these techniques because the rising popularity of minimally invasive surgery in the pet-owning public is driving this technology.

Discussion

It is clear that surgery will be the mainstay of local or regionally confined cancer treatment in veterinary medicine for many years to come. It is also clear that just because a surgical procedure is possible, this is not the best reason to do it. It was not long ago that surgical resection of the external genitalia was routine treatment for dogs with transmissible venereal tumors. It is now recognized that chemotherapy alone is curative in over 90% of dogs, and surgery is needed for biopsy only. Simple versus radical mastectomy in the dog and humans does not influence survival for most mammary gland tumors, but more aggressive surgery may indeed be beneficial in the cat.[58-60] More surgery is not always better surgery. Long-term follow-up of well-staged and graded tumors with defined surgical technique and margins is necessary to demonstrate the true value of any operation. A great deal of progress in surgical technique and surgical thinking needs to take place before the use of surgery can be optimized.

It is hoped that a better understanding of expected tumor biology and more precise staging methods (e.g., molecular diagnostics, angiograms, ultrasound, CT scans, magnetic resonance imaging [MRI], positron emission tomography [PET]/CT) will facilitate more precise surgical operations to be performed. Surgical techniques will continue to improve and undergo refinements,[54,61-63] but until surgeons become biologists, the big breakthroughs will be slow in coming. Surgeons should be investigating the influence of anesthesia, infection, immune function, blood transfusions, growth factors, oncogenes, and cytokines, to name a few, on the outcome of our patients.[64-70] In spite of these anticipated advances in technology and biology, the most difficult aspect to learn is surgical judgment. "Biology is king; selection of cases is queen, and the technical details of surgical procedures are the princes and princesses of the realm who frequently try to overthrow the powerful forces of the king or queen, usually to no long-term avail, although with some temporary apparent victories."[71]

REFERENCES

1. Chabner BA, Curt GA, Hubbard SM: Surgical oncology research development: the perspective of the National Cancer Institute, *Cancer Treat Rep* 68:825–829, 1984.
2. Poston GJ: Is there a surgical oncology? In *Textbook of surgical oncology*, London, 2007, Informa Healthcare.
3. Spodnick GJ, Berg J, Rand WM, et al: Prognosis for dogs with appendicular osteosarcoma treated by amputation alone: 162 cases (1978–1988), *J Am Vet Med Assoc* 200:995–999, 1992.
4. Bacon NJ, Dernell WS, Ehrhart N, et al: Evaluation of primary re-excision after recent inadequate resection of soft tissue sarcomas in dogs: 41 cases (1999–2004), *J Am Vet Med Assoc* 230(4):548–554, 2007.

5. Withrow SJ: Risk associated with biopsies for cancer. Kirk's current veterinary therapy, XII. In Bonagura J, editor: *Small animal practice*, Philadelphia, 1995, Saunders.
6. Enneking WF: *Musculoskeletal tumor surgery*, New York, 1983, Churchill-Livingstone.
7. Gilson SK, Stone EA: Surgically induced tumor seeding in eight dogs and two cats, *J Am Vet Med Assoc* 196:1811–1815, 1990.
8. Pavletic M: *Atlas of small animal reconstructive surgery*, Philadelphia, 1993, JB Lippincott.
9. Dundas JM, Fowler JD, Schmon CL: Modification of the superficial cervical axial pattern skin flap for oral reconstruction, *Vet Surg* 34:206–213, 2005.
10. Cady B: Lymph node metastases: Indicators, but not governors of survival, *Arch Surg* 119:1067–1072, 1984.
11. Gilson SD: Clinical management of the regional lymph node, *Vet Clin North Am Small Anim Pract* 25:149–167, 1995.
12. Nyman HT, Kristensen AT, Skovgaard IM, et al: Characterization of normal and abnormal canine superficial lymph nodes using gray-scale B-mode, color flow mapping, power, and spectral Doppler ultrasonography: a multivariate study, *Vet Radiol Ultrasound* 46:404–410, 2005.
13. Tuohy JL, J Milgram J, Worley DR, et al: A review of sentinel lymph node evaluation and the need for its incorporation into veterinary oncology, *Vet Comp Oncol* 7(2):81–91, 2009.
14. Lurie DM, Seguin B, Schneider PD, et al: Contrast-assisted ultrasound for sentinel lymph node detection in spontaneously arising canine head and neck tumors, *Invest Radiol* 41(4):415–421, 2006.
15. Wells S, Bennett A, Walsh P, et al: Clinical usefulness of intradermal fluorescein and patent blue violet dyes for sentinel lymph node identification in dogs, *Vet Comp Oncol* 4(2):114–122, 2006.
16. Olson RM, Woods JE, Soule EH: Regional lymph node management and outcome in 100 patients with head and neck melanoma, *Am J Surg* 142:470–473, 1981.
17. Veronesi U, Adamus J, Bandiera DC, et al: Delayed regional lymph node dissection in stage I melanoma of the skin of the lower extremities, *Cancer* 49:2420–2430, 1982.
18. Milch RA: Surgical palliative care, *Semin Oncol* 32:165–168, 2005.
19. Moore GE: Debunking debulking, *Surg Gyn Obstet* 150:395–396, 1980.
20. Morton DL: Changing concepts of cancer surgery: surgery as immunotherapy, *Am J Surg* 135:367–371, 1978.
21. Broomfield S, Currie A, van der Most RG, et al: Partial, but not complete, tumor-debulking surgery promotes protective antitumor memory when combined with chemotherapy and adjuvant immunotherapy, *Cancer Res* 65:7580–7584, 2005.
22. Withrow SJ, Poulson JM, Lucroy MD: *Miscellaneous treatments for solid tumors in Withrow and MacEwen's small animal clinical oncology*, ed 4, St Louis, 2007, Saunders.
23. Huang J, Li T, Liu N, et al: Safety and reliability of hepatic radiofrequency ablation near the inferior vena cava: an experimental study, *Int J Hyperthermia* 27(2):116–123, 2011.
24. Qiu-Jie S, Zhi-Yu H, Xiao-Xia N: Feasible temperature of percutaneous microwave ablation of dog liver abutting the bowel, *Int J Hyperthermia* 27(2):124–131, 2011.
25. Harvey HJ: Cryosurgery of oral tumors in dogs and cats, *Vet Clin North Am Small Anim Pract* 10(4):821–830, 1980.
26. Holmberg DL: Cryosurgical treatment of canine eyelid tumors, *Vet Clin North Am Small Anim Pract* 10(4):831–836, 1980.
27. Fernandez De Queiroz G, Matera JM, Dagli M: Clinical study of cryosurgery efficacy in the treatment of skin and subcutaneous tumors in dogs and cats, *Vet Surg* 37:438–443, 2008.
28. Murphy SM, Lawrence JA, Schmiedt CW, et al: Image-guided transnasal cryoablation of a recurrent nasal adenocarcinoma in a dog, *J Small Anim Pract* 52(6):329–333, 2011.
29. Manenti G, Perretta T, Gaspari E, et al: Percutaneous local ablation of unifocal subclinical breast cancer: clinical experience and preliminary results of cryotherapy, *Eur Radiol* 21(11):2344–2353, 2011.
30. Klatte T, Grubmüller B, Waldert M, et al: Laparoscopic cryoablation versus partial nephrectomy for the treatment of small renal masses: Systematic review and cumulative analysis of observational studies, *Eur Urol* 60(3):435–443, 2011.
31. Dewhirst MW, Sim DA, Sapareto S, et al: Importance of mini- mum tumor temperature in determining early and long-term responses of spontaneous canine and feline tumors to heat and radiation, *Cancer Res* 44:43–50, 1984.
32. Thrall DE, LaRue SM, Yu D, et al: Thermal dose is related to duration of local control in canine sarcomas treated with thermoradiotherapy, *Clin Cancer Res* 11(14):5206–5214, 2005.
33. Gillette EL, McChesney SL, Dewhirst MW, et al: Response of canine oral carcinomas to heat and radiation, *Int J Radiat Oncol Biol Phys* 13:1861–1867, 1987.
34. Gillette SM, Dewhirst MW, Gillette EL, et al: Response of canine soft tissue sarcomas to radiation or radiation plus hyperthermia: a randomized phase II study, *Int J Hyperthermia* 8:309–320, 1992.
35. Casas A, Fukuda H, Riley P, et al: Enhancement of aminolevulinic acid based photodynamic by Adriamycin, *Cancer Lett* 121:105, 1997.
36. Lanks KW, Gao JP, Sharma T: Photodynamic enhancement of doxorubicin cytotoxicity, *Cancer Chemother Pharmacol* 35:17, 1994.
37. Roberts WG, Klein MK, Loomis M, et al: Photodynamic therapy of spontaneous cancers in felines, canines, and snakes with chloro-aluminum sulfonated phthalocyanine, *J Natl Cancer Inst* 83:18, 1991.
38. Agostinis P, Berg K, Cengel KA, et al: Photodynamic therapy of cancer: an update, *CA Cancer J Clin* 61(4):250–281, 2011.
39. Cornell K, Waters DJ: Impaired wound healing in the cancer patient: effects of cytotoxic therapy and pharmacologic modulation by growth factors, *Vet Clin North Am Small Anim Pract* 25:111–131, 1995.
40. McEntee MC: Principles of adjunct radiotherapy and chemotherapy, *Vet Clin North Am Small Anim Pract* 25:133–148, 1995.
41. Ferguson MK: The effect of antineoplastic agents on wound healing, *Surg Gyn Obstet* 154:421–429, 1982.
42. Graves G, Cunningham P, Raaf JH: Effect of chemotherapy on the healing of surgical wounds, *Clin Bull* 10:144–149, 1980.
43. Laing EJ: The effects of antineoplastic agents on wound healing: guidelines for combined use of surgery and chemotherapy, *Compend Contin Educ Pract Vet* 11:136–143, 1989.
44. Dernell WS, Withrow SJ, Straw RC, et al: Intracavitary treatment of soft tissue sarcomas in dogs using cisplatin in a biodegradable polymer, *Anticancer Res* 17:4499–4506, 1997.
45. Fisher B, Gunduz N, Saffer EA: Influence of the interval between primary tumor removal and chemotherapy on kinetics and growth of metastases, *Cancer Res* 43:1488–1492, 1983.
46. Fisher B: Cancer surgery: A commentary, *Cancer Treat Rep* 68:31–41, 1984.
47. Tepper J, Million RR: Radiation therapy and surgery, *Cancer Treat Symposia* 1:111–117, 1984.
48. Sequin B, McDonald DE, Kent MS, et al: Tolerance of cutaneous or mucosal flaps placed into a radiation therapy field of dogs, *Vet Surg* 34:214–222, 2005.
49. MacEwen EG, Withrow SJ, Patnaik AK: Nasal tumors in the dog: retrospective evaluation of diagnosis, prognosis, and treatment, *J Am Vet Med Assoc* 170:45–48, 1977.
50. Adams WM, Bjorling DE, McAnulty JF, et al: Outcome of accelerated radiotherapy alone or accelerated radiotherapy followed by exenteration of the nasal cavity in dogs with intranasal neoplasia: 53 cases (1990–2002), *J Am Vet Med Assoc* 227:936–941, 2005.
51. Farese JP, Milner R, Thompson MS, et al: Stereotactic radiosurgery for the treatment of lower extremity osteosarcoma in dogs, *J Am Vet Med Assoc* 225(10):1567–1572, 2004.
52. Weisse C, Berent A, Todd K, et al: Evaluation of palliative stenting for management of malignant urethral obstructions in dogs, *J Am Vet Med Assoc* 229(2):226–234, 2006.
53. Berent AC, Weisse C, Beal MW, et al: Use of indwelling, double-pigtail stents for treatment of malignant ureteral obstruction in dogs: 12 cases (2006–2009), *J Am Vet Med Assoc* 238(8):1017–1025, 2011.

54. Royals SR, Ellison GW, Adin CA: Use of an ultrasonically activated scalpel for splenectomy in 10 dogs with naturally occurring splenic disease, *Vet Surg* 34:174–178, 2005.
55. Holak P, Adamiak Z, Jałyński M, et al: Laparoscopy-guided prostate biopsy in dogs–a study of 13 cases, *Pol J Vet Sci* 13(4):765–766, 2010.
56. Collard F, Nadeau ME, Carmel EN: Laparoscopic splenectomy for treatment of splenic hemangiosarcoma in a dog, *Vet Surg* 39:870–872, 2010.
57. Mayhew PD: Advanced laparoscopic procedures (hepatobiliary, endocrine) in dogs and cats, *Vet Clin North Am Small Anim Pract* 39(5):925–939, 2009.
58. MacEwen EG, Hayes AA, Harvey HJ, et al: Prognostic factors for feline mammary tumors, *J Am Vet Med Assoc* 185:201–204, 1984.
59. Golinger RC: Breast cancer controversies: surgical decisions, *Semin Oncol* 7:444–459, 1980.
60. Kurzman ID, Gilbertson SR: Prognostic factors in canine mammary tumors, *Semin Vet Med Surg* 1:25–32, 1988.
61. Bartels KE: Lasers in veterinary medicine: where have we been, and where are we going? *Vet Clin North Am Small Anim Pract* 32:495–515, 2002.
62. Gillams AR: Mini-review: The use of radiofrequency in cancer, *Br J Cancer* 92:1825–1829, 2005.
63. Kennedy JE: High-intensity focused ultrasound in the treatment of solid tumours, *Nature Rev* 5:321–327, 2005.
64. Kodama M, Kodama T, Nishi Y, et al: Does surgical stress cause tumor metastasis? *Anticancer Res* 12:1603–1616, 1992.
65. Blumberg N, Heal JM: Perioperative blood transfusion and solid tumor recurrence: a review, *Cancer Invest* 5:615–625, 1987.
66. Pollock RE, Lotzová E, Stanford SD: Surgical stress impairs natural killer cell programming of tumor for lysis in patients with sarcomas and other solid tumors, *Cancer* 70:2192–2202, 1992.
67. Medleau L, Crowe DT, Dawe DL: Effect of surgery on the in vitro response of canine peripheral blood lymphocytes to phytohemagglutinin, *Am J Vet Res* 44:859–860, 1983.
68. Murthy SM, Goldschmidt RA, Rao LN, et al: The influence of surgical trauma on experimental metastasis, *Cancer* 64:2035–2044, 1989.
69. Navarro M, Lozano R, Román A, et al: Anesthesia and immunosuppression in an experimental model, *Eur Surg Res* 22:317–322, 1990.
70. Meakins JL: Surgeons, surgery, and immunomodulation, *Arch Surg* 126:494–498, 1991.
71. Cady B: Basic principles in surgical oncology, *Arch Surg* 132:338–346, 1997.

Cancer Chemotherapy

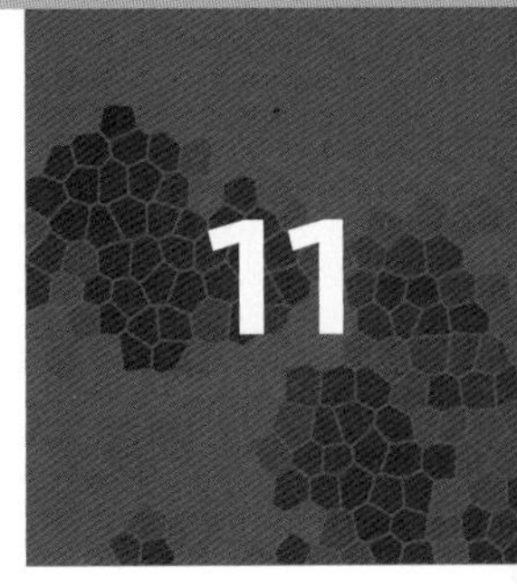

Daniel L. Gustafson and Rodney L. Page

General Principles of Cancer Chemotherapy

Mechanism of Cancer Therapy

The use of chemical elixirs for the treatment of cancer can be traced through the medicinal customs and practices of a number of cultures.[1] The modern use of pharmacologic agents to treat cancer began in the mid-1940s when Alfred Gilman and Louis Goodman showed the efficacy of nitrogen mustard in tumor-bearing mice, and these results were quickly translated and verified in human patients. These results and the efforts of others such as Sydney Farber with antifolates and George Hitchings and Gertrude Elion with purine analogs rapidly advanced the growing interest of treating cancer with drugs. The beginning of a systematic screening program for anticancer drugs at the National Cancer Institute (NCI) in 1955 set the framework for cancer chemotherapy development in both the public and private sectors and led to the characterization of many of the agents still in clinical use today.[2,3]

The basis of anticancer drug activity is the targeting of dividing cells through interference with processes involved in progression through the cell cycle. As shown in Figure 11-1, the major classes of drugs used to treat cancer work at various steps in the processes of DNA replication (S phase) and subsequent cell division (M phase). Another set of therapeutic agents, the signal transduction inhibitors, work by interfering with the signaling processes that trigger entry into the cell cycle and continuing cellular proliferation. This newer class of agents is discussed in Chapter 14, Section B, of this text. DNA synthesis is a complicated process involving anabolic processes to create the purine and pyrimidine nucleotide triphosphates required for replication, unwinding of the template DNA to provide access to the replication machinery, and the high fidelity process of creating complementary strands. Anticancer drugs work at all of these levels of DNA synthesis, including the antimetabolites that inhibit anabolic processes required for providing the nucleotide building blocks, topoisomerase inhibitors that interfere with the enzymatic process of DNA unwinding, cross-linking agents that through either interstrand or intrastrand interactions block the processes of strand separation and template processing, and the alkylating agents that interfere with the replication machinery through multiple mechanisms of altered binding and base recognition. The resulting effects of interacting at these levels of DNA replication can include the generation of DNA strand breaks, incomplete replication, and triggering of apoptotic signaling such that cell death is the ultimate result.

Processes in cell division not involving DNA replication are also targets for anticancer agents. The most prominent of these targets is tubulin with several classes of drugs having antitubulin activity. The mechanism of action of these agents involves either inhibiting the polymerization of tubulin or stabilizing the polymerized form so that depolymerization is blocked. The result of blocking either of these processes is the inhibition of microtubule function in the dividing cell. Microtubule function is critical to progression through mitosis via the spindle fiber formation and the separation of chromosome pairs into daughter cells. Blockade of this process by antitubulin agents has proved to be a very effective strategy of antiproliferation because cells blocked in this part of the cell cycle (M phase) can trigger apoptosis or undergo other mechanisms of cell death and loss of viability.

Terminology and Concepts

Terms that are related to the efficacy and toxicity of cancer chemotherapy are important concepts for understanding their pharmacologic activity. The *therapeutic index* for a given chemotherapeutic agent is the ratio between the toxic dose and the therapeutic dose for that drug. For most cytotoxic chemotherapy used to treat cancer, the therapeutic index is an abstract parameter because the administered dose is based on the *maximum tolerated dose* (MTD) rather than dose response. The MTD is an empirically derived value that represents the highest dose of a given drug that can be administered in the absence of unacceptable or irreversible side effects to a limited population sample. This is an important concept in cancer drug administration in that drug doses are generally based on this value rather than assessments of efficacy. A newer concept for drugs used to treat cancer is the *biologically effective dose* (BED), based on a measured response at a putative target or surrogate that is related to the mechanism of action of the agent. Determination of the BED is currently more related to the use of signal transduction inhibitors and molecularly targeted agents; however, the concept is not exclusive to these agents and this approach may be useful when applied to cytotoxic chemotherapy using dosing protocols not based on the MTD. *Dose intensity* (DI) is a measure of dose per unit of time and thus allows comparisons between protracted and compacted dosing schedules. Comparisons of DI between, for example, every 3 weeks and every week dosing allows for determining whether the total dose of the drug or the DI relates to toxicity or therapeutic outcome and the impact that altering dosing schedules can have on outcome. *Therapeutic gain* is often evaluated when combining two drugs or drug-radiation therapy combinations and quantitatively describes any improved tumor response relative to increased normal tissue toxicity when agents are used in a planned schedule. The basis for a positive therapeutic gain is the additive or synergistic tumor effects that exceed any summative toxicity patterns in normal tissues accomplished with combination therapy.

Indications and Goals of Therapy

The therapeutic intent and goals of a given chemotherapeutic regimen are important contributors to how a given drug is selected

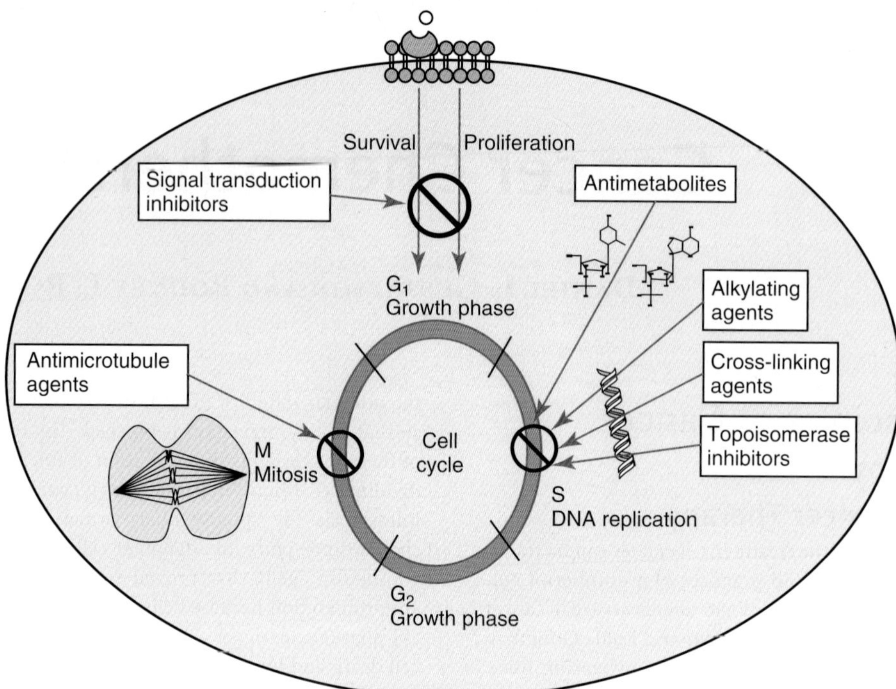

FIGURE 11-1 Cell cycle specificity of the major classes of drugs used in cancer chemotherapy. Although agents may have effects throughout the cell cycle, the phase where the major impact is realized is highlighted.

or assessed. *Adjuvant therapy* is the treatment with chemotherapeutic drugs following the surgical removal or radiation control of the primary tumor. The purpose is to treat occult disease and usually involves systemic drug exposure. *Primary* or *neoadjuvant therapy* is the utilization of chemotherapeutic drugs prior to treatment with other modalities, primarily surgical removal of the primary tumor, with the intent of decreasing tumor size for increased control and preventing possible postoperative growth of micrometastasis. *Induction therapy* is a similar concept to neoadjuvant therapy; however, this refers to the initial drug treatment phase with the intent of inducing remission in lymphoid or hematopoietic cancers. *Maintenance therapy* involves the use of chemotherapy in an ongoing basis to maintain remission. *Consolidation therapy* is intended to sustain an achieved remission. *Rescue* or *salvage therapy* is the use of chemotherapy after a tumor fails to respond to a previous therapy or after tumor recurrence. *Palliative chemotherapy* is delivered to decrease clinical signs in the case of unresectable or disseminated disease that is associated with functional disturbances or pain. The outcome of this therapy is based more on quality of life issues as opposed to other metrics of tumor response. The more subjective nature of assessing the effect of palliative chemotherapy, especially in terms of pain control, makes systematic testing of protocols difficult and treatment recommendations more at the discretion of the clinician and client. In the cases where organ function is impacted by tumor growth, more objective endpoints may exist in terms of functional improvements following treatment. Doses and scheduling of palliative intent therapies may also differ as strict adherence to schedules originating from trials where objective responses were measured may not be relevant and more patient-based endpoints employed. *Radiosensitization* is the enhancement of cytotoxicity when irradiation and chemotherapeutic agents are combined such that a therapeutic gain is obtained. The basis for chemotherapeutic exposure leading to enhanced radiosensitivity can be multifaceted and involve: (1) the enrichment of the tumor cell population in a more sensitive phase of the cell cycle, (2) increased tumor oxygenation through cytoreduction or alterations in tumor vascularization, and (3) selective killing of inherently radioresistant hypoxic cell fractions.

As a preliminary metric, the clinical measurements of the tumor response to cancer chemotherapy are useful for predicting the impact of treatment on the extent of disease or time interval of tumor control. Table 11-1 describes conventional measures of treatment response.

Tumor Susceptibility and Resistance

Tumor Cell Sensitivity

Individual cell sensitivity to anticancer agents has been addressed empirically through the screening of tumor cell panels associated with a given histotype. The NCI60 human tumor cell line panel is the most well characterized and studied compilation with more than 100,000 compounds and 50,000 extracts from natural products screened to date.[4] Further, rich gene expression and other characterizations of these cell lines exist in public databases so that drug sensitivity and genotypic characteristics can be considered.[5] The use of canine tumor cell line panels to screen drug sensitivity is becoming established[6] as a viable way to identify potential drug combinations for further testing as well.

Chemosensitivity depends on a number of factors, including drug uptake into the cell, interaction with a cellular target, generation of lethal damage to important cellular macromolecules, repair of potentially lethal damage, and the cell's response to generated damage as depicted in Figure 11-2. Uptake of some cancer chemotherapeutic agents occurs via passive diffusion due to their lipid-soluble properties; other compounds are actively transported into tumor cells. Melphalan is actively transported into cells by two amino acid transporters,[7] and blocking transport with amino acid substrates or analogs can significantly reduce cytotoxicity.[8] Other examples include nucleoside transporters used by Ara-C[9]

TABLE 11-1 Measures of Response in Cancer Therapy and Treatment

Response Term	Abbreviation	Description
Complete remission/response	CR	Complete disappearance of tumor(s) and symptoms of disease.
Partial remission/response	PR	Decrease in tumor volume of ≥50% or decrease in tumor maximum diameter of >30%.
Stable disease	SD	Neither an increase nor a decrease in tumor size or disease symptoms (e.g., ±20% diameter changes).
Progressive disease	PD	Increase in tumor volume of >25% or increase of tumor maximum diameter of >20%; appearance of new lesions.
Median duration of response/ median duration of survival	MDR/MDS	The median value for a group of individuals treated with a given therapy in terms of the length of time they achieved a complete or partial remission (MDR) or length of survival following implementation of therapy (MDS).
Progression-free interval/ progression-free survival	PFI/PFS	The amount of time elapsed without evidence of progressive tumor growth (PFI) or survival without progressive growth of the tumor from treatment start (PFS).
Disease-free interval/disease-free survival	DFI/DFS	The amount of time that elapses without disease recurrence (DFI) or survival (DFS) of the patient following therapy.

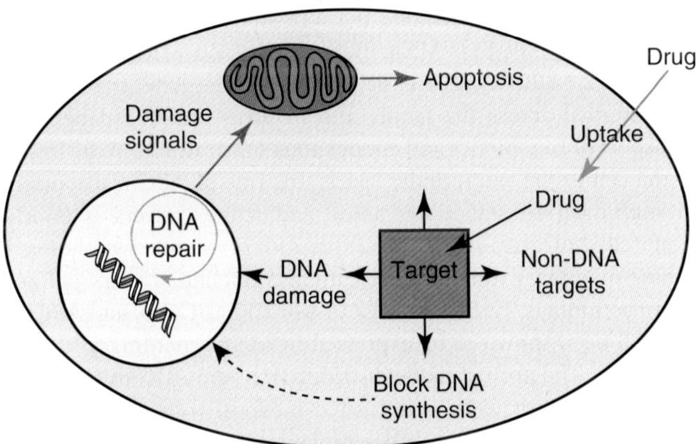

FIGURE 11-2 Processes involved in the pharmacologic activity and associated chemosensitivity of chemotherapeutic agents in tumor cells. Associated processes include drug uptake, interaction with drug target, impact on DNA and associated DNA repair, and the cellular response to these effects.

and gemcitabine[10] and the reduced folate carrier system involved in methotrexate uptake.[11] The intracellular target(s) for specific chemotherapeutic agents can play a role in determining sensitivity based on their levels and the nature of the interaction. For example, topoisomerase IIα levels can play a role in the sensitivity of tumor cells to doxorubicin[12,13] as altered levels via decreased gene copy or transcriptional downregulation leads to a decrease in sensitivity (resistance). The opposite is true for thymidylate synthetase levels and 5-fluorouracil (5-FU) toxicity where increased levels of enzyme correlate to a decrease in sensitivity to 5-FU.[14] Although the nature of the interaction with the target is different for doxorubicin and 5-FU, the fact that altered target levels can modulate response shows how quantitative interactions with the target can alter drug sensitivity.

The extent of cellular damage, potential repair of that damage, and the cellular response occur in a tightly knit continuum that determines cellular fate. The generation of cellular damage is a consequence of interaction with a cellular target and can be either a primary or secondary event. In general for DNA-damaging agents, the resulting DNA lesions are caused by the interplay of DNA binding and DNA repair. For example, DNA strand breaks that result from O-6-methyl guanine lesions are due to aberrant mismatch repair processes and subsequent replication.[15] DNA damage also triggers response pathways that can result in cell cycle arrest to allow for repair and subsequent survival or the triggering of apoptotic machinery that ultimately results in cell death. The definition of cellular response, whether mitotic catastrophe, apoptosis, necrosis, autophagy, or cellular stasis, depends on an intricate interplay of survival and death signaling and is often specific to the agent, dose at the critical target, and the cell lineage.[16] Alterations in proapoptotic and antiapoptotic signaling clearly play a role in tumorigenesis and response to therapy,[17] and the impact of antiapoptotic signaling in lymphoma by the mediators, bcl-2 and survivin, seem the most clear in regards to both chemosensitivity[18-20] and response to therapy in humans and dogs.[21-23] However, a clear understanding of the role of damage response and active cell death pathways in chemotherapeutic sensitivity and response in solid tumors is still lacking.

Tumor Cell Resistance

Acquired resistance, or selection of resistant cells, during the treatment process is thought to be one of the major mechanisms of therapeutic failure during cancer drug therapy. Resistance of tumor cells to chemotherapeutic agents can depend on the drug and its mechanism or be through a multidrug mechanism. In general, the development of acquired resistance to a specific agent can come via a variety of mechanisms associated with drug uptake, drug metabolism/detoxification, target modification, damage repair, or damage recognition and response. Changes in cellular drug levels can come about due to either a decrease in drug uptake or through increased efflux. Decreased expression of transporters known to play a role in drug uptake have been observed in response to treatment with melphalan in human breast cancer cells[24] and acquired resistance to methotrexate in KB cells,[25] with the resulting cells showing drug resistance that correlated with the lower intracellular drug levels. The induction of drug efflux pumps in response to drug treatment is a primary mechanism for multidrug resistance and will be discussed later in this section.

Alterations in metabolic or detoxification pathways within tumor cells are another mechanism by which acquired resistance occurs. Due to the fact that many chemotherapeutic agents are electrophilic based on their DNA-binding properties, enhancement of conjugation reactions with nucleophiles such as glutathione is a plausible mechanism of resistance.[26] Induction of glutathione S-transferases has been shown to be a mechanism by which tumor cells can acquire resistance to nitrogen mustards.[27,28] Although tumor cells themselves generally have limited drug metabolism capabilities, some metabolic pathways can play a role in the resistance phenotype. For example, the sensitivity of tumor cells to 5-FU is inversely correlated with the expression of dihydropyrimidine dehydrogenase,[29-31] the enzyme predominantly responsible for the metabolism of 5-FU to the inactive 5-FUH$_2$ metabolite.[32] For prodrugs such as gemcitabine, which must be phosphorylated to the di- and tri-phosphate forms prior to eliciting an inhibitory effect on DNA synthesis,[33,34] the enzyme responsible for this metabolic activation, deoxycytidine kinase,[35,36] has been shown to be decreased in pancreatic tumor cells made resistant to this drug.[37,38] This interplay between metabolic detoxification and activation, predominantly with drugs that are nucleotide analogs, leads to complex scenarios involving the upregulation of catabolic processes and the downregulation of anabolic processes regarding the cellular pharmacology of these cytotoxic agents.

Modifications in the cellular target of a given drug usually pertain to mutations in the target protein leading to a decrease in affinity or absence of drug interaction. These modifications can include a decrease in the levels of a specific target responsible for the generation of a toxic product, increases in target levels to ameliorate the effect of target inhibition, or target mutations such that the drug can no longer interact in a manner detrimental to the tumor cell. Decreased topoisomerase II gene expression and activity has been observed in human lung and colon cells with acquired resistance to the epipodophyllotoxins,[39] etoposide, and teniposide, whose antitumor activity involves topoisomerase II–dependent DNA strand break formation.[40,41] Target amplification as a mechanism of acquired resistance has been observed in methotrexate resistance where gene amplification and increased dihydrofolate reductase (DHFR) levels allow for cells to overcome DHFR inhibition by this agent.[42] Mutations in targets such as β-tubulin in the case of paclitaxel[43] and topoisomerase I for camptothecin[44] affect binding of drug and interaction with the target, thus generating tumor cells resistant to the toxic mechanism of these agents. These examples of altered target levels and structures show that drug resistance can come about via either quantitative or qualitative change in the nature of the interaction of drug and target and will depend on the impact of these changes on tumor cell growth both in the absence and presence of the selective agent.

Damage repair in cancer cells treated with chemotherapy commonly refers to DNA repair processes since a majority of chemotherapy agents work at the level of the DNA. Resistance conferred through alteration in DNA repair include not only the induction of specific processes to repair discrete lesions but also more global DNA repair processes, such as postreplication and mismatch repair.[45] Multiple studies have shown that enhanced removal of platinum adducts from tumor cell DNA correlate with acquired resistance[46-48] to cisplatin, although the exact mechanism(s) and protein(s) responsible for repair of these lesions are unknown. The bulky DNA adducts generated by many cancer chemotherapeutic agents can cause replicative gaps in DNA that require postreplication surveillance and repair. The ability of cells to bypass these bulky lesions and interstrand cross-links during DNA replication has been found to be an important process in tolerance to agents causing these types of DNA damage (cisplatin, mitomycin C, melphalan); multiple DNA repair pathways can account for this release from DNA replication block.[49] The fact that DNA repair pathways and processes are redundant and nondiscrete and that both lesion specific and global processes seem to play a role in determining drug resistance highlights the problems associated with attributing specific proteins or pathways to specific resistance phenotypes.

Some mechanisms of acquired resistance result in a phenotype in which the tumor is resistant to multiple chemotherapeutic agents or multidrug resistant (MDR). Some of the mechanisms discussed previously, including DNA repair, enhanced metabolism, or detoxification, and resistance to apoptosis can result in resistance to multiple agents; however, the MDR phenotype generally refers to tumor cells expressing individual or multiple members of the adenosine triphosphate (ATP)-binding cassette (ABC) transporter family who play a primary role in active efflux of drugs from cells. Forty-eight ABC genes have been identified in the human genome,[50] and currently, fifteen members of the ABC transporter family have been recognized that include a cancer chemotherapeutic as a substrate for transport.[51] These include the well-studied and characterized PGP/MDR1 *(ABCB1)*, MXR/BCRP *(ABCG2)*, MRP1 *(ABCC1)*, and MRP2 *(ABCC2)*. The basic function of the ABC transporters is conserved across the family and involves the ATP-dependent transport of xenobiotics and endogenous substrates from the inside of the cell to the extracellular space. The role of ABC transporters in multidrug resistance of canine and feline cancers is poorly explored; however, *ABCB1* is expressed in canine lymphoma,[52] canine mammary tumors,[53] and canine and feline primary pulmonary carcinomas.[54] *ABCC1, ABCC2, ABCC5, ABCC10,* and *ABCG2* have all been shown to be expressed in canine mammary tumors as well.[53,55] The normal tissue distribution of the ABC transporters is also beginning to be investigated in dogs, with initial studies showing similar tissue distributions and presumed function, although there appears to be some partial differences in relative expression in various tissues.[56,57] A recent study has shown that feline *ABCG2* has specific amino acid changes that lead to transporter dysfunction with regard to a number of substrates, suggesting that cats may have altered pharmacokinetic disposition for drugs that are *ABCG2* substrates.[58]

Combination Therapies

The success of combination chemotherapy as compared to single-agent treatment is attributed to the overcoming of both natural and acquired resistance of tumor cells, as well as use of agents that differ in dose-limiting side effects. A premise of cancer chemotherapy is to kill the largest fraction of tumor cells possible with each dose, with the dose and timing of each therapy based on the normal tissue tolerance. Therefore a strategy that allows for more intensive cycles of fractional cell killing without exacerbating the recovery of normal tissue damage is preferred. Combination chemotherapy has been shown to be curative in humans with acute lymphocytic leukemia (ALL), Hodgkin's disease, histiocytic lymphoma, and testicular carcinoma, whereas single-agent therapy was not.[59] The success of combination therapies as opposed to single-agent therapy is best illustrated in veterinary oncology by treatment protocols for canine lymphoma. Doxorubicin is the most active single-agent therapy tested against canine lymphoma; other combination protocols that generally consist of cyclophosphamide, vincristine, and prednisone

TABLE 11-2 Response of Canine Lymphoma to Single-Agent Doxorubicin, Combination Protocols, and Combination Protocols Including Doxorubicin*

TREATMENT	DOGS†	REMISSION RATE (%)	MEDIAN REMISSION (MO)	MEDIAN SURVIVAL (MO)
Doxorubicin alone‡	243 (5)	74.2 ± 9.5	5.3 ± 1.1	7.3 ± 1.3
Combination§	324 (5)	76.6 ± 8.0	4.7 ± 1.0	8.0 ± 1.1
Combination + doxorubicin‖	618 (9)	80.0 ± 9.5	8.8 ± 2.3	11.9 ± 3.9

*Values represent the mean ± standard deviation (SD) from the cited studies. The combination protocols used included cyclophosphamide, vincristine, and prednisone, with methotrexate and actinomycin D included in some.

†Number represents the total number of dogs, with the number of individual studies in parentheses.

‡Data for doxorubicin alone studies were from references 60-64.

§Data for combination studies were from references 61, 65-68.

‖Data for combination studies, including doxorubicin, were from references 68-76.

result in similar outcomes (Table 11-2). However, these same combination protocols with doxorubicin included empirically seem to increase both the median remission and median survival times over either doxorubicin alone or a combination protocol that excludes doxorubicin. It should be noted that the populations represented in Table 11-2 may not be homogeneous, and this data does not represent a formal reanalysis of these data sets.

Toxicities Associated with Drug Therapy of Cancer

Chemotherapy may fail to produce a positive clinical benefit for the reasons described previously but may also fail due to unacceptable toxicity. Anticipating and managing adverse events requires a thorough understanding of drug activity profiles and clinical experience modifying chemotherapeutic administration. The first step in the process of successfully managing cancer in companion animals is always a clear and frank discussion with the owner regarding the potential for benefit, toxicity, cost, and time commitment. A common understanding of the goals of therapy and committing to a continuing dialog as needs may change throughout treatment cannot be underestimated.

Dosing conventions have been developed from formal phase I studies for an increasing number of agents investigated specifically in companion animals. Nonetheless, suggested starting doses represent an estimate of the MTD from a small population of animals and safe individual patient dosing may vary substantially. There are numerous reasons for pharmacokinetic variability in cancer chemotherapy among a population of patients.[77] Concurrent illness or organ dysfunction, extreme tumor burden, specific breed sensitivities (e.g., Collie with *ABCB1 mut/mut*) or idiosyncratic considerations (anticipated drug-drug interactions or drug allergies) will mandate modification of the protocol and dosing. Concurrent illness and organ dysfunction can also have profound effects on selection of anticancer agents and dosing. In general, predictable dose adjustments for pets with renal or hepatic disease have not been developed and treatment should be approached conservatively. Interestingly, in cats, the glomerular filtration rate (GFR) can be used to define an individual dose for carboplatin that will permit some patients with renal disease to be safely dosed that would not have been safe if dosed by conventional methods.[78] Dose adjustments of 30% to 40% have been recommended for drugs that are *ABCB1* substrates in Collie-type breeds in which an *ABCB1 (mut/mut)* phenotype is confirmed, and even in dogs with an *ABCB1 (wt/mut)* phenotype, dose adjustments may need to be made.[79] Chemotherapeutic dosing in obese patients often raises questions about drug partitioning in lipid storage sites around the body. Distribution of many pharmaceutical agents may be affected in obese patients; however, there is no accepted scale for empiric dose adjustments in humans. Individual factors such as the specific drug, degree of obesity, and other comorbidities may convince a clinician to dose reduce or cap the dose of a chemotherapeutic agent.[80] Some reviews suggest that dose reductions based on body mass may ultimately be detrimental to outcomes in obese patients.[81] It is the initial chemotherapeutic intervention that is expected to result in the greatest opportunity to benefit the patient; therefore taking the time to assess the patient's specific medical limitations and then proceeding with thoughtfully designing, administering, and completing a therapeutically robust protocol are highly desirable.

As individual patient tolerance and response to each compound in a multiagent protocol is observed, future modifications may be anticipated more accurately. The greatest benefit achievable with anticancer cytotoxic therapy requires a commitment to dose intensity. Optimal dose intensity demands therapeutic monitoring in order to either reduce *or* increase the dose based on the patient's capacity to maintain a high quality lifestyle during effective therapy. The decision to increase the dose of an agent is conceptually challenging but important. In order to make a recommendation to increase dosing of a cytotoxic compound, owner understanding and monitoring of the patient's white blood cell values and clinical events during the first treatment cycle are critical. A dose of a cytotoxic agent that does not result in any change in the target normal tissue (e.g., blood neutrophil count) is likely ineffective and could be increased 10% at the next infusion with continued follow-up to determine adequacy of dose adjustments (Figure 11-3). Dose reductions are deleterious to the optimum delivery of chemotherapy but are to be anticipated. Specific guidelines for dose adjustments of antineoplastic agents are not standardized. In general, a 20% to 25% reduction is recommended for the subsequent dose for patients experiencing a moderate or severe dose-limiting toxicity, such as neutropenia or emesis. Close monitoring and preemptive handling of signs may permit successful management of some potential future clinical signs, and clinical decisions are based on the extent and severity of the resulting signs as described in Table 11-3.

The toxicity profile for anticancer agents may be categorized into immediately evident toxicities (at the time or within 24 to 48 hours after treatment), acute delayed effects (2 to 14 days), or cumulative/chronic toxicity (weeks, months, or years). Immediate toxicity may include infusion hypersensitivities due to histamine release associated with allergic reactions (L-asparaginase) or vehicle-induced mast cell degranulation (e.g., paclitaxel, etoposide). Routine

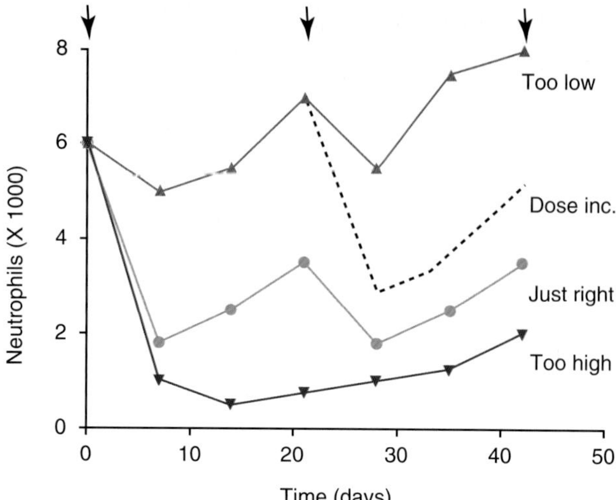

FIGURE 11-3 Blood neutrophil patterns following chemotherapy treatments *(arrows)*. The appropriate dose *(circles)* results in noticeable nadirs with return to normal prior to the next dose. Doses that are too high or too low should prompt dose adjustments, including potential dose increases *(dashed line)*.

management of these events with antihistamines and steroids may significantly reduce or eliminate this problem. Acute nausea and vomiting may occur with specific agents (e.g., cisplatin) or when the infusion is too rapid (e.g., doxorubicin). Preemptive antiemetic management is able to manage these situations well. Chemotherapeutics with vesicant properties can cause moderate-severe tissue necrosis if not administered safely through a suitable catheter. Vinca alkaloid and doxorubicin extravasations can be a very severe situation that should be avoided even if sedation is required or rescheduling must be recommended for safe catheter placement. Owners may need to be informed about this possibility prior to treatment and a management plan for this situation should be developed. Management recommendations for extravasations are included in the individual drug descriptions later.

Delayed acute effects from chemotherapy often include bone marrow suppression and nausea, vomiting, and diarrhea. In the majority of instances, these effects are self limiting and the incidence of hospitalization for such problems is low. Table 11-3 reviews the general therapeutic strategies for management of the most common types of adverse events experienced in companion animals following chemotherapy.[82]

Examples of potential cumulative and/or chronic toxicity include hepatic dysfunction after multiple doses of

TABLE 11-3 Guidelines for Common Chemotherapy-Induced Toxicity

	PROPHYLAXIS	GRADE 2/MILD TOXICITY	GRADE 3/MODERATE TOXICITY	GRADE 4/SEVERE TOXICITY
Neutropenia		1000/μL	500-999/μL	<500/μL, with or without fever
Broad-spectrum aerobic antibiotics*	Not recommended	No	Oral. Repeat CBC in 2-3 days. Do not hospitalize.	Oral. IV if fever. CBC in 24 hours.
Broad-spectrum anaerobic antibiotics†	No	No	No	Not routine unless refractory to aerobic antibiotics.
Parenteral fluids (SQ or IV) and supportive care	No	No	Not routine unless febrile.	Hospitalize if febrile.
Nausea/vomiting		<3 vomiting episodes	3-5 episodes/day for 2-4 days.	>5 episodes/24 hrs or >4 days.
Antiemetics‡	Oral, if prior experience warrants.	Oral or IV as indicated.	IV	IV
H_2 blocker,§ proton pump inhibitor‖	Oral, if prior experience warrants.	Oral or IV as indicated.	IV	IV
Parenteral fluids (SQ or IV) and supportive care	No	As indicated.	Yes	Yes, hospitalize.
Diarrhea		2 stools/day over baseline.	3-6 stools/day over baseline.	>6 stools/day.
Diet adjustment	Yes	Yes	Yes	Yes
Antidiarrheals¶	Yes	Yes	Yes	Yes
Parenteral fluids (SQ or IV) and supportive care	No	No	Yes	Yes, hospitalize.

SQ, Subcutaneous; *IV,* intravenous; *CBC,* complete blood count.
*Fluoroquinolone (enrofloxacin 5-10 mg/kg once daily).
†Ampicillin 20 mg/kg oral (PO) or IV three times/day (TID) ± cephalosporin 20 mg/kg oral or IV TID.
‡Maropitant 2 mg/kg PO or SQ once daily × 3-5 days—dogs; 1 mg/kg PO or SQ once daily × 3-5 days—cats (not labeled for cats).
§Famotidine 0.5-1.0 mg/kg PO, SQ, or IV.
‖Pantoprazole 1 mg/kg IV or SQ as needed.
¶Loperamide 0.08 mg/kg PO TID; tylosin 10 mg/kg PO TID; metronidazole 15-25 mg/kg PO BID.

cyclohexylchloroethylnitrosourea (CCNU), cardiac abnormalities after exceeding a safe cumulative dose of doxorubicin, and renal disease after cisplatin use in dogs or doxorubicin use in cats. Screening recommendations and strategies to reduce the risks of such chronic effects have been developed and are incorporated into standard protocol procedures. It is critical to the success of treatment that owners be thoroughly informed about monitoring guidelines for the general signs and symptoms of chemotherapy-induced toxicity. Online educational resources for owners are readily available at www.csuanimalcancercenter.org. It is advisable to instruct the owner regarding monitoring and early responses when their pet experiences nausea and vomiting, diarrhea, or hematuria and it is important to inform the owner about how to obtain an accurate body temperature. These "at home" aids will allow the clinician to assess the management options should a concern arise.

Safety Concerns of Cancer Drug Therapy

In general, safety concerns for cancer therapy are only applied to the patient with regard to the impact of drug treatment. An issue with cytotoxic chemotherapy, however, is the preparation and distribution of the drugs, as well as active drug eliminated in the urine and feces of the patient and the potential exposure of health professionals, caregivers, and others in the home. The preparation of these drugs should be done under strict regulations and involves the use of protective clothing, gloves, masks, and chemical hoods. Studies have characterized the potential impact of secondary exposure to these agents on oncology health workers in human medicine with regard to cancer prevalence, reproductive risks, and acute toxicities, and the results show little risk.[83] However, these results are a reflection of exposure in trained cohorts of individuals working in human medicine where fecal and urinary exposures are more limited. Clients with animals undergoing cancer therapy need to be informed of potential risks and safety precautions that need to be adhered to when dealing with oral medications and pet excrement. Simple precautions such as wearing gloves when handling oral medications and not opening capsules or splitting tablets are essential. Oral suspensions of these agents should be avoided. Urinary levels of some active drugs may remain high for days after treatment[84] and fecal excretion may also be expected. Therefore careful avoidance, collection, and disposal of urine and feces must be recommended, as well as having pregnant women, small children, and immunosuppressed individuals in particular avoid any contact with pet wastes for a defined time period following treatments. Preparation of guidelines for minimizing exposure to individuals and the environment should be prepared and distributed to clients for general, as well as drug-specific, instructions.

Pharmacologic Principles in Cancer Therapy

Pharmacokinetics

Pharmacokinetic (PK) considerations in cancer drug therapy are important due to the relationship between drug exposure and pharmacodynamic (PD) response, whether efficacy or toxicity, that is more exact than the relationship between drug dose and PD response.[85] PK considerations are also important with regard to interactions with other drugs,[86] herbal products,[87,88] and genetic differences among breeds and individuals[89] that can cause changes in drug exposure at a given dose. Cytotoxic chemotherapy is usually dosed on an MTD-based schedule reflecting only acceptable toxicity and thus limits any informative role of drug half-life and

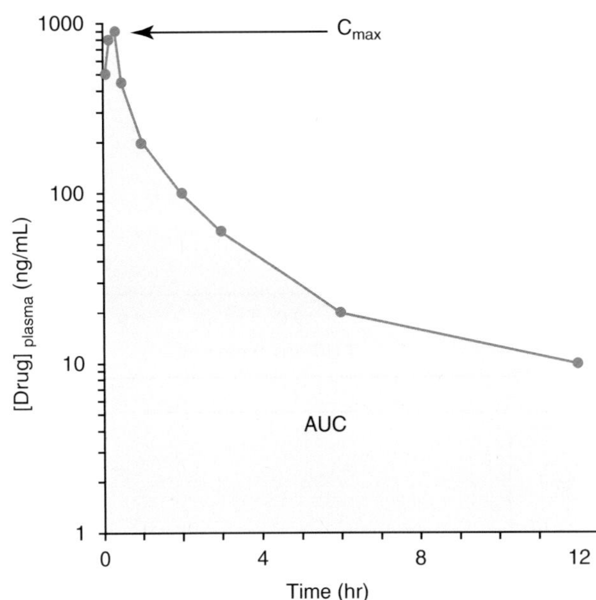

FIGURE 11-4 Illustration of pharmacokinetic parameters C_{max} and AUC in a theoretical drug plasma concentration versus time plot.

effective therapeutic concentrations from initial dosing considerations. The most important PK parameters are those that have a relationship with either a response to therapy (efficacy) or toxicity, which is most often either the area under the plasma/serum concentration versus time curve (AUC) or the maximum drug concentration (C_{max}) achieved, illustrated in Figure 11-4. The relationships of AUC and C_{max} in the clinical pharmacology of doxorubicin illustrate the complex associations with PK considerations. The C_{max} during doxorubicin infusion in humans is related to the incidence of cardiotoxicity both in adult[90] and pediatric[91] patients but is also associated with longer remissions in leukemia patients.[92] A relationship between AUC values and decreased white blood cells has also been established with doxorubicin.[93] However, no clear relationships between AUC and efficacy exist.[94] These data have allowed for adjustments in doxorubicin dosing protocols so that intermediate infusion times (10 to 30 minutes) are utilized to decrease the C_{max} and thus cardiotoxicity while still maintaining peak levels associated with effective therapy.

PK studies that relate drug exposure to responses are an important first step in establishing relationships that may be exploited for dose modification based on patient characteristics or therapeutic drug monitoring. These data are generally lacking for drugs used to treat cancer in companion animals with a few exceptions. Studies on the PK and myelotoxicity of carboplatin in cats have shown a clear relationship between drug exposure and the neutrophil nadir as well as drug clearance and GFR (Figure 11-5). The fact that PK parameters can be correlated both with a toxic endpoint and a physiologic function allows for the calculation of a dosing metric relating the GFR of an individual cat to a dose that produces a drug exposure (AUC) that results in acceptable toxicity.[78] It remains to be determined whether such individualized dosing results in improved outcome in a heterogeneous population. Current drug-dosing convention for cancer chemotherapeutic agents is the use of body surface area (BSA) for dose normalization (mg/m^2). Exceptions to this paradigm are the use of body weight (mg/kg) for dogs that weigh less than 15 kg and for cats with doxorubicin dosing based on empiric evidence showing a better toxicity

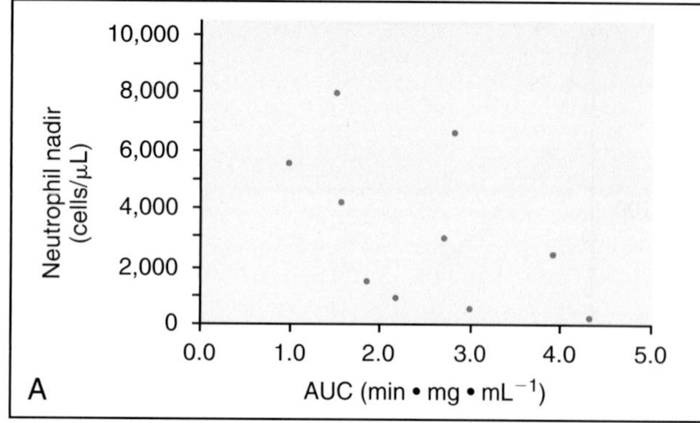

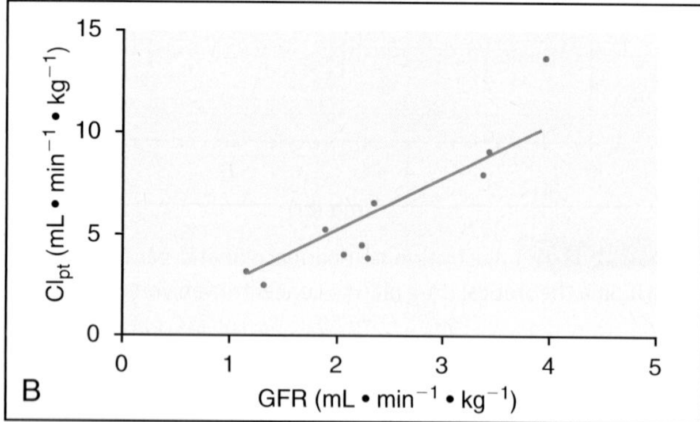

FIGURE 11-5 Relationship between **(A)** neutrophil nadir and carboplatin exposure and **(B)** platinum clearance and glomerular filtration rate (GFR) in cats being treated for cancer. *(From Bailey DB, Rassnick KM, Erb HN, et al: Effect of glomerular filtration rate on clearance and myelotoxicity of carboplatin in cats with tumors,* Am J Vet Res *65:1502, 2004.)*

profile for smaller dogs when mg/kg dosing is used.[95] The approximate calculation for BSA in dogs and cats based on weight is as follows:

$$m^2 = \frac{A \times (\text{weight in grams})^{2/3}}{10{,}000}$$

where *A* is equal to 10.1 for dogs and 10.0 for cats. The implementation of this equation relating body weight in kilograms to BSA in meters squared is shown for dogs and cats in Table 11-4.

TABLE 11-4 Relationship of Body Surface Area (BSA) to Weight in Dogs and Cats

Weight to Body Surface Area—Dogs					
kg	m^2	kg	m^2	kg	m^2
3.0	0.210	20.0	0.744	48.0	1.334
4.0	0.255	21.0	0.769	50.0	1.371
5.0	0.295	22.0	0.785	52.0	1.412
6.0	0.333	23.0	0.817	54.0	1.448
7.0	0.370	24.0	0.840	56.0	1.484
8.0	0.404	25.0	0.864	58.0	1.519
9.0	0.437	26.0	0.886	60.0	1.554
10.0	0.469	28.0	0.931	62.0	1.588
11.0	0.500	30.0	0.975	64.0	1.622
12.0	0.529	32.0	1.018	66.0	1.656
13.0	0.553	34.0	1.060	68.0	1.689
14.0	0.581	36.0	1.101	70.0	1.722
15.0	0.608	38.0	1.142	72.0	1.755
16.0	0.641	40.0	1.181	74.0	1.787
17.0	0.668	42.0	1.220	76.0	1.819
18.0	0.694	44.0	1.259	78.0	1.851
19.0	0.719	46.0	1.297	80.0	1.882
Weight to Body Surface Area—Cats					
kg	m^2	kg	m^2	kg	m^2
1.0	0.100	4.8	0.285	8.6	0.420
1.2	0.113	5.0	0.292	8.8	0.426
1.4	0.125	5.2	0.300	9.0	0.433
1.6	0.137	5.4	0.307	9.2	0.439
1.8	0.148	5.6	0.315	9.4	0.445
2.0	0.159	5.8	0.323	9.6	0.452
2.2	0.169	6.0	0.330	9.8	0.458
2.4	0.179	6.2	0.337	10.0	0.464
2.6	0.189	6.4	0.345	10.2	0.472
2.8	0.199	6.6	0.352	10.4	0.478
3.0	0.208	6.8	0.360	10.6	0.484
3.2	0.217	7.0	0.366	10.8	0.490
3.4	0.226	7.2	0.373	11.0	0.496
3.6	0.235	7.4	0.380	11.2	0.502
3.8	0.244	7.6	0.387	11.4	0.508
4.0	0.252	7.8	0.393	11.6	0.514
4.2	0.260	8.0	0.400	11.8	0.520
4.4	0.269	8.2	0.407	12.0	0.526
4.6	0.277	8.4	0.413	12.2	0.532

Pharmacodynamics

PD considerations for cytotoxic chemotherapy are generally related to standard measures of response (i.e., complete remission [CR], partial remission [PR], stable disease [SD]) and toxicity.[96] A majority of the literature in veterinary oncology relates PD responses to specific drugs or combinations, doses, or schedules. Figure 11-6 shows the relationships between vinblastine doses and the incidence of grade III or IV neutropenia observed in a phase I cohort of dogs.[97] These results relate a dose to a PD response with the absence of exposure PK data. PD endpoints can also be used as indicators of efficacy and potentially as targets of therapy. The proportion of dogs in remission following treatment for lymphoma is increased in the subgroup experiencing grade III or IV neutropenia compared to the group that did not show that level of observed toxicity (Figure 11-7).[98] In this example, the therapeutic response was related to overall drug effects on normal tissues as indicated by the degree of neutropenia (PD response), whereas DI did not show a significant difference. Again, these data did not include exposure PK assessment and in this case only relate the therapeutic outcome to an observed drug response. A lack of complete PK/PD data relationships in veterinary medicine reduces the opportunities for therapeutic drug monitoring and the potential for optimizing efficacy.

Pharmaceutics

Pharmaceutics is the science associated with dosage form design with regard to formulation and optimizing drug delivery via a

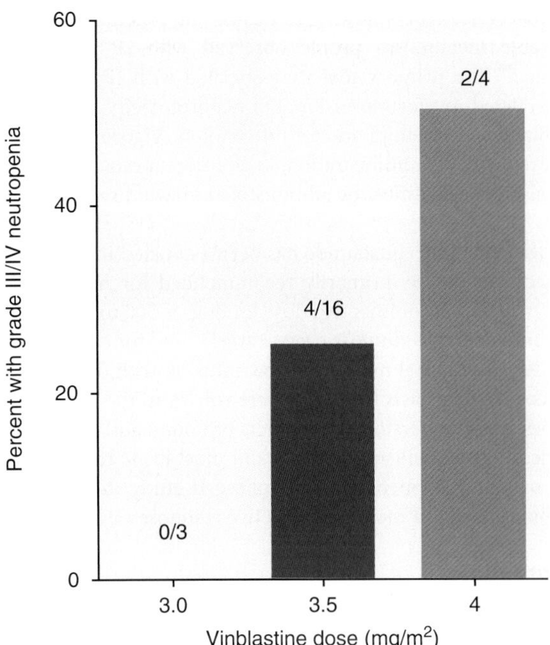

FIGURE 11-6 Relationship of prevalence of grade III/IV neutropenia with vinblastine dose in dogs being treated for cancer. *(Data from Bailey DB, Rassnick KM, Kristal O, et al: Phase I dose escalation of single-agent vinblastine in dogs,* J Vet Intern Med *22:1397, 2008.)*

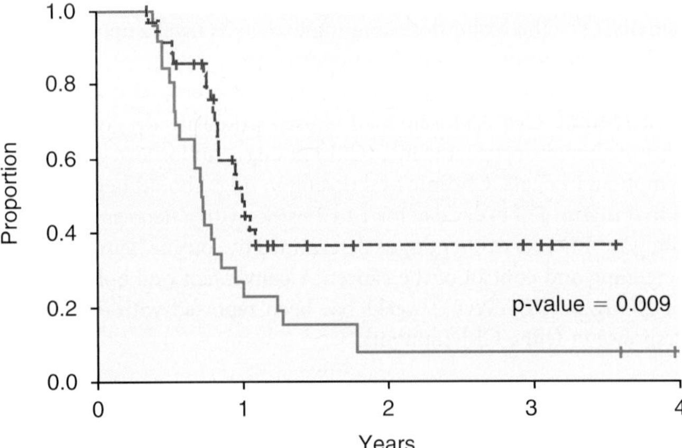

FIGURE 11-7 Proportion of dogs in remission following chemotherapy treatment for lymphoma. The dashed line represents those animals experiencing grade III/IV neutropenia, whereas the solid line represents those animals that did not show that level of toxicity. *(From Ghan A, Johnson JL, Williams LE: Impact of chemotherapeutic dose intensity and hematologic toxicity on first remission duration in dogs with lymphoma treated with a chemoradiotherapy protocol,* J Vet Intern Med *21:1332, 2007.)*

specific route. For example, improved formulations of clinical agents such as paclitaxel have made these compounds available for use in veterinary patients. The excipient (drug carrier) used in the original clinical formulation of paclitaxel (Taxol) was Cremophor EL, which causes histamine release and unacceptable toxicity when used in dogs and cats.[99,100] A new water-soluble formulation of paclitaxel (Paccal Vet) has been tested and shown to be effective without associated hypersensitivity reactions in dogs with mast cell tumors. The ability of new formulations and delivery methods to alter the efficacy and toxicity profile of agents is a rapidly expanding field. It is expected that new technologies in drug formulation and targeting will be incorporated into veterinary medicine to alter drug delivery and distribution in a more favorable manner.

Specific Chemotherapeutic Agents

Alkylating Agents

The alkylating agents are comprised of antitumor drugs whose mechanism of action involves the covalent binding of alkyl groups to cellular macromolecules. The cellular target of these agents is DNA in which they form monofunctional or bifunctional adducts that generate interstrand or intrastrand cross-links.

Nitrogen Mustards

Mechlorethamine

Basic Pharmacology Mechlorethamine is frequently referred to as "nitrogen mustard" and was the first cytotoxic agent to show antineoplastic activity.[101-103] Mechlorethamine undergoes spontaneous hydrolysis to 2-hydroxyethyl-2-chloroethylmethylamine and bis-2-hydroxyethylmethylamine, yielding nucleophilic reactive centers capable of forming DNA cross-links.[104]

Clinical Pharmacology Mechlorethamine rapidly disappears from the plasma following intravenous (IV) administration primarily through spontaneous degradation, although some percentage of the drug is enzymatically metabolized.[105] Mechlorethamine uptake into cells seems to be carrier mediated with decreased uptake as a mechanism for resistance.[106]

Clinical Use Mechlorethamine is used predominantly in multiagent protocols for lymphoma in dogs.[107-109] Experience with mechlorethamine as a single agent is not reported, although gastrointestinal (GI) and bone marrow toxicity are dose-limiting toxicities of conventional mustargen, vincristine, prednisone, and procarbazine (MOPP) protocols. Dosing of mechlorethamine in these protocols is reported as 3 mg/m^2 IV on days 0 and 7 of a 21-day cycle.

Melphalan

Basic Pharmacology Melphalan (L-phenylalanine mustard) is a nitrogen mustard containing DNA cross-linking agent with a similar structure and pharmacology to chlorambucil. The major difference is that melphalan is actively transported into tumor cells by amino acid transporters[7] and its uptake can be blocked by the amino acid leucine. Melphalan has direct alkylating activity and does not require metabolic activation.

Clinical Pharmacology Melphalan can be given orally with an oral bioavailability of approximately 30%. A relatively high percentage of melphalan (20% to 35%) is excreted unchanged in the urine with a majority of the remainder of the dose undergoing spontaneous chemical decomposition to inert products.[110] The primary toxicity is myelosuppression.

Clinical Use The primary indication for melphalan in companion animals is for management of myeloma. The initial dose of 0.1 mg/kg PO daily for 10 to 14 days should be reduced to 0.05 mg/kg PO daily based on control of the paraproteinemia and hematologic screening for both dogs and cats. Alternate dosing regimens have also been used for dogs: 7 mg/m^2 PO daily for 5 days every 3 weeks or 2 mg/m^2 PO daily for 10 days with a 10-days-off cycle and repeated as needed.

Cyclophosphamide

Basic Pharmacology Cyclophosphamide (CP) is a nitrogen mustard–containing prodrug that is inactive in the absence of metabolic activation that occurs via microsomal mixed function oxidases predominantly in the liver.[111] The activation of CP involves ring oxidation to 4-hydroxycyclophosphamide (4-OHCP), spontaneous and reversible ring opening to the amino aldehyde aldophosphamide, and the subsequent irreversible breakdown of aldophosphamide to phosphoramide mustard and acrolein. Phosphoramide mustard is considered the most active CP metabolite and is capable of bifunctional alkylation and cross-link production.[112]

Clinical Pharmacology Recent studies have characterized the PK of CP and the 4-OHCP metabolite following both IV and oral dosing in dogs.[113] The results of this study show that although exposure to CP is decreased following oral dosing, the overall exposure of 4-OHCP is similar when CP is dosed either intravenously or orally. The major dose-limiting side effects of CP are neutropenia and thrombocytopenia. GI toxicity (nausea and vomiting) is not common in dogs but has been observed in cats.[114] Other common toxicities include alopecia in dog breeds with continually growing hair and hemorrhagic cystitis. Although hemorrhagic cystitis is uncommon at conventional doses, furosemide is often administered (1 mg/kg subcutaneous [SQ] or IV) prior to IV injection and precautions are taken at home to encourage vigorous hydration and frequent urination. CP should be discontinued permanently if hemorrhagic cystitis occurs and chlorambucil may be substituted in a multiagent protocol. Urine culture, antiinflammatory drugs, and antispasmodics should be initiated at the onset of clinical signs of cystitis. Aggressive intravesical therapy or even surgery may be necessary in severe instances.

Clinical Use CP is commonly included in multiagent protocols for lymphoma in both dogs and cats. It is effectively administered as a bolus dose (250 mg/m^2) by either an oral (PO) or IV route in the dog.[113] A fractionated dosing schedule is also used in some protocols (50 mg/m^2 for 3 to 4 consecutive days after doxorubicin).[115] Metronomic therapy, the use of very low dosing for prolonged periods, has also been developed for CP. The rationale and application of metronomic therapy is covered extensively in Chapter 14, Section C, of this text. CP is administered IV (200 to 250 mg/m^2) in many multiagent protocols for lymphoma in cats. The efficacy of oral dosing of CP has not been as carefully investigated in cats compared to dogs although it may be safely administered at doses of 300 mg/m^2 PO every 3 weeks in multiagent protocols.[116]

Ifosfamide

Basic Pharmacology Ifosfamide (IP) is a nitrogen mustard–containing prodrug that like CP requires metabolic activation by microsomal mixed function oxidases prior to generating the isofosforamide mustard metabolite capable of bifunctional alkylation.[117]

Clinical Pharmacology The major difference between the clinical use of IP and CP is due to differences in the relative metabolism of the parent drugs, with dechloroethylation accounting for up to 25% of the metabolism of IP,[118] whereas this number is much smaller for CP. This difference in metabolism accounts for an increase in the formation of the neurotoxic metabolite chloroacetaldehyde following IP dosing and potentially for the less favorable metabolism profile observed with IP following oral dosing.[119] The primary toxicity associated with IP treatment is a dose-related myelosuppression, but nephrotoxicity and damage to the bladder epithelium are not uncommon. Vigorous hydration is required with IP administration; in addition, mesna, a urinary epithelial protectant, must be administered to avoid severe cystitis.

Clinical Use Ifosfamide has been evaluated in dogs and cats with cancer and is primarily recommended for management of sarcomas. The recommended dose for dogs is 300 to 350 mg/m^2 IV slow infusion with diuresis every 3 weeks, and for cats, the recommended dose is 900 mg/m^2 IV slow infusion with diuresis every 3 weeks.[120,121] The basis for such discrepancies in the MTD between species is not understood but reflects profound and interesting differences in metabolism pathways and most likely reduced generation of bioactive metabolites. A phase II study in feline vaccine sarcomas reported moderate objective response rates.[122]

Chlorambucil

Basic Pharmacology Chlorambucil (*p*-bis[chloro-2-ethyl] amino-phenyl-4-butanoic acid) is a nitrogen mustard derivative that enters cells via passive diffusion[123] and has direct bifunctional alkylating ability[124] that is responsible for the cytotoxic activity.

Clinical Pharmacology Chlorambucil is orally bioavailable with rapid absorption. Hepatic metabolism is extensive with the pharmacologically active phenylacetic acid being the primary metabolite and is presumably responsible for much of the clinical activity.[125,126] The major dose-limiting toxicity is myelosuppression, including neutropenia and thrombocytopenia.

Clinical Use Chlorambucil is used primarily for control of chronic lymphocytic leukemia (CLL) in dogs and for low-grade GI lymphoma in cats. Chronic oral dosing in dogs should begin with 3 to 6 mg/m^2 PO every day for 1 to 2 weeks with a decrease to 3 to 6 mg/m^2 PO every other day as determined by routine hematologic screening and control of the cancer. A convenient oral bolus dose of 20 mg/m^2 PO every 2 weeks has been reported with excellent response in feline GI lymphoma.[127]

Nitrosoureas

Lomustine (Cyclohexylchloroethylnitrosourea)

Basic Pharmacology Lomustine (CCNU, CeeNU) is a nitrosourea-based agent that is highly lipid soluble and enters cells by passive diffusion.[128] Under aqueous conditions and at physiologic pH, lomustine will spontaneously decompose to a reactive center capable of DNA alkylation[129,130] and DNA-DNA and DNA-protein cross-links.[131]

Clinical Pharmacology The highly lipophilic properties of lomustine allows for rapid crossing of biologic membranes, including the blood-brain barrier. Lomustine undergoes extensive hepatic metabolism,[132] predominantly by hydroxylation of the cyclohexyl ring, to metabolites with at least equivalent alkylating activity[133] that presumably play an important role in the cytotoxic activity. This extensive hepatic metabolism is presumably responsible for the lack of oral bioavailability of the parent compound but rapid appearance of metabolites following oral dosing.[134] The major dose-limiting toxicity is myelosuppression with acute neutropenia followed by a thrombocytopenia.[135] Chronic administration may result in hepatic dysfunction requiring discontinuation of the drug temporarily or permanently.[136] A recent report investigating coadministration of Denamarin, a product that increases glutathione levels and provides antioxidant properties, with CCNU reported reduced frequency of grade 4 hepatic toxicity.[137] Further evaluation of whether this strategy should be routinely employed to reduce chronic hepatic toxicity is needed.

Clinical Use CCNU (70 to 80 mg/m^2 PO every 3 weeks) is most often used alone or in multiagent protocols for canine multicentric lymphoma, epitheliotropic lymphoma, mast cell tumors, and histiocytic sarcoma. In cats, CCNU (50 to 60 mg/m^2 PO every 4 to 6 weeks) is used primarily for mast cell tumors and lymphoproliferative disorders.

Streptozotocin

Basic Pharmacology Streptozotocin is a naturally occurring nitrosourea capable of DNA alkylation and inhibition of DNA synthesis in both bacteria and mammalian cells.[138,139] Cellular uptake of streptozotocin depends on the glucose transporter 2 (GLUT2) transporter and expression of this transporter determines sensitivity of both insulinoma[140] and pancreatic beta cells.[141]

Clinical Pharmacology Streptozotocin is rapidly cleared from the blood following IV administration with reported half-life of 15 to 40 minutes in humans.[142] Streptozotocin has unique activities for nitrosoureas, including inducing diabetes in animals[143,144] and a lack of any significant bone marrow toxicity.[145,146]

Clinical Use Streptozotocin is used to manage malignant insulinoma. Limited reports of efficacy have appeared in the literature, although transient normoglycemia occurred in the experience of these authors.[147] The drug is dosed at 500 mg/m^2 as an IV infusion with diuresis to avoid renal toxicity, similar to the protocol for cisplatin.

Other Alkylating Agents

Dacarbazine

Basic Pharmacology Dacarbazine, or DTIC, is a prodrug that requires metabolic activation by the hepatic cytochrome P450 system[148,149] to the resulting 5-aminoimidazole carboxamide and the active methylating intermediate methyldiazonium ion.[150] Resulting DNA methylation products are 3-methyl adenine, 7-methyl guanine, and O-6-methyl guanine,[151] which are presumably responsible for the cytotoxic activity.

Clinical Pharmacology Dacarbazine has poor oral bioavailability and is administered intravenously. Use in cats is not recommended due to a lack of information regarding their ability to convert the parent drug to the active form. Dacarbazine is extensively metabolized in the liver and excreted in the urine. The major dose-limiting toxicity is GI toxicity, although occasional severe myelosuppression can be observed.

Clinical Use In dogs, dacarbazine is used as a component of protocols for lymphoproliferative diseases in a relapse setting and historically for melanoma. As a single agent, an IV infusion dose of 800 to 1000 mg/m^2 every 3 weeks has been used.[152] When combined with other cytotoxics, the dose of 600 mg/m^2 IV has been reported.[153]

Procarbazine

Basic Pharmacology Procarbazine (PCB), like dacarbazine, is a prodrug requiring chemical or metabolic alteration for the generation of active, toxic metabolites.[154,155] The mechanism of action of PCB could involve multiple interactions, including inhibition of DNA and RNA synthesis, but a predominant role for DNA methylation to form O-6-methyl guanine seems likely.[156]

Clinical Pharmacology PCB is rapidly and completely absorbed after oral administration followed by rapid disappearance of the parent compound and subsequent appearance of metabolites.[157] PCB and/or metabolites equilibrate rapidly between the blood and cerebrospinal fluid.[158] IV delivery has been tested in humans with the appearance of neurotoxicity not seen with oral delivery, suggesting that first-pass metabolism associated with oral dosing significantly alters the spectrum of exposure to parent drug versus metabolites.[159]

Clinical Use PCB is used in multiagent protocols for lymphoma.[107-109] It is dosed at 50 mg/m^2 PO for 14 days of a 28-day cycle. Every-other-day dosing is required for some dogs due to the limitations of available tablet sizes, and reformulation of the available product is required for small dogs.

Antitumor Antibiotics

The antitumor antibiotics consist of natural products from microbial fermentation including the anthracyclines, mitomycins, and actinomycins that have yielded clinically useful compounds with diverse mechanisms of action. Included in the discussion here are the anthracycline doxorubicin and a synthetic analog of the anthracenediones (mitoxantrone) and actinomycin D.

Doxorubicin

Basic Pharmacology The cellular pharmacology of doxorubicin (DOX) is dominated by its ability to react with a number of cellular components and a multimodal mechanism of cellular toxicity. Its activities include DNA intercalation and inhibition of RNA and DNA polymerases[160] and topoisomerase II,[161] alkylation of DNA,[162] reactive oxygen generation,[163,164] perturbation of cellular Ca^{2+} homeostasis,[165,166] inhibition of thioredoxin reductase,[167] and interaction with plasma membrane components.[168] These processes are involved in both the antitumor and dose-limiting side effects of DOX, with their relative contributions still open to some debate.

Clinical Pharmacology Following intravenous dosing, DOX is extensively distributed to tissues, with binding to cellular DNA[169] and anionic lipids[170,171] determining the magnitude of tissue uptake.[172] The elimination of DOX occurs through renal and biliary elimination of parent drug, as well as metabolism to doxorubicinol and the 7-hydroxy aglycone. Metabolism to doxorubicinol is via side chain reduction mediated by aldo-keto reductases[173] and 7-hydroxy aglycone by reductive cleavage of the sugar moiety both by the liver and extrahepatic tissues.[174] The dose-limiting toxicities associated with DOX treatment are infusion-rate–dependent hypersensitivity, myelosuppression, GI toxicity, and a well-established cumulative dose-related cardiotoxicity.[175] In addition, cats may develop renal tubular damage following repeated dosing.[176]

Clinical Use DOX is the most active single agent available for a wide variety of cancers in companion animals. The drug may be used alone or in combination protocols for lymphoma, osteosarcoma (OSA), and most mesenchymal and epithelial neoplasms. Conventional dosing regimens are 30 mg/m^2 slow IV bolus or infusion (10 to 30 minutes) every 3 weeks in dogs larger than 15 kg, 1 mg/kg for dogs smaller than 15 kg, and for all cats. This nonuniform dosing formula reflects the cumulative experience of specialists realizing that small dogs and cats are often overdosed with DOX using the BSA prescription base. Unfortunately, a uniform prescription model has not been developed, and thus dose adjustments should be anticipated following the initial DOX administration. The drug is diluted in saline and administered as a slow bolus or infusion over 10 to 30 minutes. Vigilant observation during the infusion is required to ensure proper IV delivery. Any concern about catheter placement should result in replacement using an alternate vein before beginning the infusion. Sedation may be required. If it is suspected that the drug has been delivered external to the vein, stop the infusion, aspirate remaining product out of the catheter, and remove it. Dexrazoxane (Zinecard) is used to reduce cardiac toxicity in humans, and infusion within a 3-hour period at 10 times the prescribed DOX dose may be useful for DOX extravasation.[177] Additional infusions at 24 and 48 hours may be useful as well. If DOX is being administered, a source for dexrazoxane should be identified through a local hospital pharmacy because it is expensive and sometimes difficult to obtain rapidly. Despite active management, DOX extravasations may progress to extensive tissue necrosis requiring surgical intervention, including potential amputation.

Cardiac performance should be carefully evaluated prior to each DOX infusion to detect any new murmurs, arrhythmias, or pulse deficits. Routine electrocardiography or echocardiography is not necessary due to limited sensitivity and specificity of these monitoring procedures for DOX cardiotoxicity in dogs and cats. However, any abnormalities that develop during treatment should be pursued with full diagnostic evaluation. Most protocols ostensibly limit the DOX cumulative dose to 120 to 150 mg/m^2 (4 to 5 doses) in order to limit potential toxicity in the general population and particularly in certain at-risk breeds, such as the Boxer and Doberman Pinscher. The cumulative dose of DOX may be increased as dictated by the need for additional treatment, such as in relapsed lymphoma following a formal cardiac evaluation. A complete blood count (CBC) is recommended prior to each DOX infusion, and in cats, a serum creatinine and urine specific gravity are recommended to identify any changes in renal function.[176]

Mitoxantrone

Basic Pharmacology Mitoxantrone is a synthetic DOX analog and maintains similar activity as DOX in terms of DNA intercalation and the inhibition of RNA and DNA polymerases and topoisomerase II.[178,179] However, mitoxantrone does not cause oxidative damage to cells[180] and has a reduced potential to undergo one-electron reduction and generate reactive oxygen species.[181]

Clinical Pharmacology Following IV administration, mitoxantrone is extensively distributed to tissues with residual levels being long lasting. Mitoxantrone is not extensively metabolized and a fraction of the drug (<30%) is excreted unchanged in the urine and feces.[182-184] Dose-limiting toxicities include GI disturbances and myelosuppression. Cardiotoxicity has not been reported in dogs and only rarely in humans.

Clinical Use Mitoxantrone (5 to 6 mg/m^2 IV slow bolus every 3 weeks) is used as a cardiac-sparing anthracycline in dogs that have reached the cumulative level of DOX or with evidence of cardiomyopathy and is at risk of further damage with doxorubicin administration. The clinical indications for mitoxantrone include lymphoproliferative disorders and, most recently, transitional cell carcinoma (TCC) of the bladder and urethra.[185]

Actinomycin D (Dactinomycin)

Basic Pharmacology Actinomycin D, or dactinomycin (DACT), consists of two symmetric polypeptide chains attached to a central phenoxazone ring. DACT has been shown to interact with double-stranded DNA in multiple ways in a sequence-dependent manner,[186-188] and also bind to single-stranded DNA.[189] The resulting interactions of DACT with both double- and single-stranded DNA results in a potent inhibition of transcription, thus inhibiting RNA and protein synthesis.[190,191] DACT is taken up into cells by passive diffusion,[192] and the sensitivity of cells may depend on uptake and retention[193] with *ABCB1* playing a role in DACT efflux.[194]

Clinical Pharmacology Following IV administration, DACT is rapidly distributed to tissues and then slowly eliminated from tissues. Metabolism is minimal with 20% of DACT excreted unchanged in the urine and 14% in the feces.[195] The major dose-limiting toxicities of DACT are myelosuppression and GI toxicity.[195]

Clinical Use Actinomycin D is used in multi-agent protocols for dogs with lymphoproliferative diseases in the relapse setting or as a doxorubicin substitute in dogs with cardiac abnormalities. It is administered IV at 0.5 to 0.75 mg/m^2 every 3 weeks. There is risk of perivascular damage following extravasation.

Antimetabolites

The antimetabolites are comprised of agents that inhibit the use of cellular metabolites in the course of cell growth and division. Therefore these agents are generally analogs of compounds used in the normal course of metabolism and in the case of cancer chemotherapeutics, specifically anabolic processes associated with DNA replication.

Cytosine Arabinoside (Cytarabine)

Basic Pharmacology Cytosine arabinoside (Ara-C), or cytarabine, acts as an analog to deoxycytidine and is phosphorylated in cells to generate arabinosylcytosine triphosphate (ara-CTP), which acts as a competitive inhibitor of DNA polymerase α.[196] Ara-CTP is also incorporated into DNA, which correlates with cytotoxicity[197] and thus presumably is the primary mechanism of action. Once incorporated into DNA, it cannot be excised[198] and inhibits both the function of the DNA template and subsequent synthesis.[199] Ara-C has also been reported to have a differentiating function in leukemic cells through decreased *c-myc* expression.[200] Ara-C is actively transported into tumor cells via nucleoside transporters[201] and is phosphorylated sequentially by deoxycytidine kinase, deoxycytidine monophosphate (dCMP) kinase, and nucleoside diphosphate kinase.[202]

Clinical Pharmacology Ara-C is water-soluble and dosed by IV infusion or SQ bolus injection. It distributes rapidly in total body water and crosses into the central nervous system (CNS), reaching levels 20% to 40% of those observed in the plasma.[203] The primary mode of metabolism is deamination by the liver and extrahepatic tissues. Observed dose-limiting toxicities are myelosuppression and occasionally GI disturbances.

Clinical Use Ara-C is an infrequent component of combination protocols for leukemias and lymphomas in dogs and cats. It is more often incorporated into treatment protocols for patients with a potential for CNS involvement. Ara-C is ideally administered as a constant rate infusion over a 4 to 5 day period. However, a more convenient method of administration in dogs and cats is SQ injection twice daily for 2 consecutive days at 150 mg/m^2 (total dose = 600 mg/m^2). Low-dose SQ Ara-C (50 mg/m^2 twice daily for 2 days or 100 mg/m^2 as a constant rate infusion for 1 day) has been reported to improve clinical signs in dogs with meningoencephalitis of undetermined origin when combined with prednisone.[204,205] The collective reported data regarding efficacy of Ara-C for this condition are not sufficient to make a treatment recommendation at this time to use Ara-C in addition to prednisone. Results of a recent small study suggest improved responses in dogs with naïve stage V multicentric lymphoma when Ara-C (150 mg/m^2/day as a continuous rate infusion) was infused over 5 days following the first and second cycle of a conventional cyclophosphamide, hydroxydaunorubicin (DOX), vincristine (Oncovin), prednisone (CHOP)-based protocol compared to the CHOP protocol alone.[206] Bone marrow support with human granulocyte colony-stimulating factor (G-CSF) and erythropoietin were co-administered with Ara-C, and patients in this treatment group did not experience increased adverse events. Further investigation of this protocol is certainly of interest.

Methotrexate

Basic Pharmacology Methotrexate (MTX) is a folate analog that inhibits the enzyme dihydrofolate reductase, thus depleting reduced folate pools required for purine and thymidylate biosynthesis.[207] MTX is also converted to polyglutamates that act as direct inhibitors of folate-dependent enzymes that play a role in de novo purine and thymidylate synthesis.[208,209] MTX enters cells via active transport through the reduced folate carrier.[11]

Clinical Pharmacology The oral bioavailability of MTX is high at lower doses but becomes variable as doses increase[210]; thus it is usually dosed orally at lower doses and intravenously at higher doses. The PK of MTX is well understood across species[211] and is dominated by enterohepatic recycling that accounts for the observed GI side effects at doses that do not cause hematopoietic toxicities. At higher doses, both GI toxicity and myelosuppression are observed. MTX does not undergo substantial hepatic metabolism except when administered at high doses and is primarily excreted unchanged in the urine.[211]

Clinical Use MTX was used in original multiagent protocols for treatment of lymphoproliferative disorders in dogs and cats. With the development of other less toxic and more potent agents, MTX has been eliminated from conventional treatment regimens and is rarely used in veterinary oncology.

Gemcitabine

Basic Pharmacology Gemcitabine, or 2,2-difluorodeoxycytidine (dFdC), is actively transported into cells by nucleoside transporters[212] and metabolized by phosphorylation to dFdC monophosphorylated (dFdCMP), dFdC diphosphorylated (dFdCDP), and dFdC triphosphorylated (dFdCTP) species.[202] The effect of dFdC treatment on cells is the inhibition of DNA synthesis through dFdCTP inhibition of DNA polymerase,[213] dFdCDP inhibition of ribonucleotide reductase and subsequent depletion of deoxyribonucleotide pools,[33] and dFdCTP incorporation into DNA leading to strand termination.[34] The dFdCTP incorporated into newly synthesized DNA appears resistant to normal DNA repair,[214] and its presence is critical for triggering apoptosis by this agent.[215] Recent studies suggest that the primary deamination metabolite of dFdC, difluorodeoxyuridine (dFdU), may also play a role in cytotoxicity.[216]

Clinical Pharmacology Gemcitabine is dosed intravenously because oral dosing leads to low systemic exposure[217] presumably due to extensive first-pass metabolism in the liver through deamination to the dFdU metabolite.[218] The length of the infusion also seems to be a potentially important variable as longer, constant rate infusions have been shown to lead to increased intracellular dFdCTP levels and enhanced response as opposed to shorter infusions.[219] The dose-limiting toxicity of dFdC is hematologic in both humans and dogs.[202,220]

Clinical Use Gemcitabine use has been reported infrequently in clinical studies in dogs and cats. Recent reports have used gemcitabine as a single agent or in combination with other antineoplastic agents or combined with radiation therapy. Dosing regimens employed in dogs involve either high dose (800 mg/m^2 IV over 20 to 30 minutes every week for 4 weeks) or low dose (25 to 50 mg/m^2 IV once or twice a week per protocol) options, depending on the use of other cytotoxics in the protocol. Cats have been treated with low-dose regimens (20 to 25 mg/m^2 or 2 mg/kg weekly to biweekly) in combination with full-dose carboplatin or radiation therapy.[221-223] All reports indicate that bone marrow and GI toxicity is moderate to significant with high-dose gemcitabine but manageable with routine prophylaxis. Results to date with current administration schedules support only limited, if any, gemcitabine-specific antitumor activity.[220,221,224-227]

5-Fluorouracil

Basic Pharmacology 5-Fluororacil (5-FU) is a halogenated analog of uracil that enters cells using a facilitated-transport system shared by adenine, uracil, and hypoxanthine.[228] 5-FU is converted to active nucleotide forms intracellularly by a series of phosphorylase and kinase reactions to yield monophosphate, diphosphate, and triphosphate forms of both fluorouridine and fluorodeoxyuridine,[229,230] which are incorporated into RNA and DNA interfering[231] with synthesis and function.[232-234] The 5-FU metabolite, FdUMP, is an inhibitor of thymidylate synthetase leading to depletion of thymidine 5′ monophosphate and thymidine 5′ triphosphate.[235] The alterations in thymidine and deoxyuridine phosphate pools caused by thymidylate synthetase inhibition, effects on DNA synthesis and integrity, as well as effects on RNA synthesis and processing, are all thought to play a role in cytotoxicity induced by 5-FU.

Clinical Pharmacology 5-FU is dosed intravenously and is extensively metabolized in many tissues by dihydropyrimidine dehydrogenase to dihydrofluorouracil, which is further catabolized to α-fluoro-β-alanine, ammonia, and carbon dioxide (CO_2).[236,237] Approximately 90% of an administered dose is metabolized, and both 5-FU and its catabolites undergo biliary excretion with less than 5% of the parent drug renally excreted. 5-FU causes a dose-dependent myelosuppression, GI toxicity, and neurotoxicity in dogs. Inadvertent ingestion of a topical 5-FU cream is toxic and/or fatal.[231] 5-FU is *contraindicated* in cats due to severe CNS toxicity.

Clinical Use 5-FU is infrequently used for management of epithelial tumors (e.g., hepatic, pancreatic, renal, mammary). The reported dose is 150 mg/m^2 IV weekly. It also may be administered topically and intralesionally to dogs, although convincing reports of efficacy are not available.

Antimicrotubule Agents

The antimicrotubule agents currently used in veterinary medicine are structurally complex agents belonging to the taxane or vinca alkaloid classes of compounds. These agents have a mechanism of action involving interference with the polymerization or depolymerization of the microtubules that play critical roles in cell function and division.

Taxanes (Paclitaxel and Docetaxel)

Basic Pharmacology The clinically used taxanes (paclitaxel and docetaxel) both act by stabilizing microtubules against depolymerization and thus inhibit reorganization dynamics required for carrying out cellular functions.[238-240] This alteration in microtubule function causes an abnormal organization of spindle microtubules involved in chromosome segregation during mitosis, leading to mitotic arrest.[241] Paclitaxel and docetaxel share identical mechanisms of action, with the increased potency of docetaxel[242] attributable to an approximately twofold higher affinity for tubulin binding as compared to paclitaxel.[243]

Clinical Pharmacology The clinical use of the taxanes is complicated by their poor solubility and the use of excipients, including Cremophor EL (paclitaxel) and polysorbate 80 (docetaxel) to allow for IV administration. Both paclitaxel and docetaxel are rapidly distributed throughout the body and eliminated slowly primarily by hepatic metabolism and biliary excretion. Renal elimination is 10% or less for both compounds. Toxicities associated with taxanes include hypersensitivity reactions that are attributable to the Cremophor EL and polysorbate 80 utilized in formulation. Diarrhea and neutropenia are the major dose-limiting, taxane-specific toxicities observed.

Clinical Use The use of paclitaxel has not been frequently described in either dogs or cats. This is likely due to the requirement for significant pretreatment with antihistamines and steroids followed by a prolonged infusion with continued monitoring for acute hypersensitivity. One report documented several responses in dogs treated with paclitaxel at a dose of 165 mg/m^2 slow IV infusion every 3 weeks.[100] Hypersensitivity was frequent despite pretreatment, and significant bone marrow toxicity was observed, leading to the conclusion that the recommended dose for further evaluation is 132 mg/m^2 as a slow IV infusion every 3 weeks in dogs. Paclitaxel in cats has been anecdotally used at 80 mg/m^2 slow IV infusion every 3 weeks in anecdotal reports with similar need for pretreatment. As discussed earlier in the section on pharmaceutics, a water-soluble formulation of paclitaxel (Paccal Vet) is currently under development for veterinary use, with dose regimens and safety profiles still to be determined.

Docetaxel has been investigated in dogs and cats. In order to overcome hypersensitivity reactions, a strategy was developed to administer oral docetaxel with cyclosporine as an absorption aid. Docetaxel and cyclosporine compete with *ABCB1*-mediated excretion mechanisms on the enterocytes, and both are substrates for CYP3A—the phase I enzymes found in enterocytes and the liver. This was initially studied in normal beagle dogs, confirming acceptable docetaxel bioavailability.[244] This strategy was subsequently investigated in phase I studies in dogs and cats with cancer in which the MTD of docetaxel is 1.63 mg/kg and 1.75 mg/kg PO (by gavage) every 2 to 3 weeks, respectively, when combined with cyclosporine (5 mg/kg PO).[245,246] Although no hypersensitivities were reported, diarrhea was the dose-limiting adverse event. A recent report of IV docetaxel in cats indicates that hypersensitivity in cats is less difficult to manage compared to hypersensitivity in dogs.[247] The MTD for docetaxel in cats is 2.25 mg/kg IV infused over 1 hour with routine pretreatment (antihistamine, steroids, famotidine). Tumor response data following oral or IV docetaxel have not been reported to date.

Vinca Alkaloids (Vinblastine and Vincristine)

The vinca alkaloids as a class of antitumor agents consist of the naturally occurring vincristine (VCR) and vinblastine (VBL), as well as a semisynthetic derivative and metabolite of VBL, vindesine (VDS), and the semisynthetic derivative of VBL, vinorelbine (VRL). These agents all share a similar mechanism of action; however, focus will be on VCR and VBL in this section due to their use in veterinary medicine.

Basic Pharmacology The vinca alkaloids bind to a distinct site on tubulin[248] and inhibit microtubule assembly.[249] This inhibition of microtubule function leads to a disruption in the mitotic spindle apparatus resulting in metaphase arrest and cytotoxicity.[250,251] The vinca alkaloids enter cells by a simple diffusion process. Exposure time and concentration seem to be important variables in determining cytotoxicity.

Clinical Pharmacology The vinca alkaloids are administered by IV infusion, rapidly distribute to tissues, and are slowly eliminated primarily by hepatic metabolism and biliary excretion of parent drug and metabolites. Urinary excretion of parent drug and metabolites is relatively low: 10% to 20%. One of the metabolites of VBL is desacetylvinblastine (vindesine), which is active and has been identified in dogs.[252] VBL and VCR differ in their respective toxicities with VCR being less myelosuppressive than VBL but causing more peripheral neurotoxic and GI effects, including significant ileus.

Clinical Use Vincristine is used predominantly as a component in multiagent protocols for dogs and cats with lymphoma. It is also used as a single agent for dogs with transmissible venereal tumor. The dose for vincristine is 0.5 to 0.75 mg/m^2 IV bolus weekly in both dogs and cats or as defined in the protocol. All vinca alkaloids are tissue vesicants if delivered extravascularly, although not as serious as doxorubicin. Extreme care should be taken with the injection.

Vinblastine is most often used to manage canine mast cell tumors, either as a single agent or in combination with other agents. Several dose-schedule variations have been developed in the last 5 years. Vinblastine as a single agent or when appropriately combined with other cytotoxic agents may be administered at 2.5 mg/m^2 IV every 1 to 2 weeks[253] or 3.0 to 3.5 mg/m^2 IV every 2 to 3 weeks.[97]

Vinorelbine is a synthetic vinca alkaloid and has been used in dogs with a variety of tumors at a starting dose of 15 mg/m^2 IV over 5 minutes once weekly. There are insufficient numbers of dogs evaluated to accurately quantify tumor response at this time.[254,255]

Topoisomerase Inhibitors

The topoisomerase inhibitors represent classes of drugs that inhibit either the type I or type II topoisomerase enzymes that are involved in the unlinking and unwinding of the DNA strand for replication and transcription. The major classes of topoisomerase II inhibitors used in veterinary oncology are the anthracyclines, which have already been discussed, and the epipodophyllotoxins, of which etoposide and teniposide are the clinically relevant members. The major class of topoisomerase I inhibitors used in human oncology are the camptothecins, which have found little use so far in veterinary medicine and will not be discussed here.

Epipodophyllotoxins (Etoposide and Teniposide)

Basic Pharmacology Etoposide (VP-16) and teniposide (VM-26) both inhibit the catalytic activity of topoisomerase II[256] by stabilizing a protein-DNA cleavage complex[257] that ultimately results in the generation of single- and double-strand DNA breaks.[258] These compounds enter tumor cells by simple diffusion across the cell membrane, and increased levels of topoisomerase II in proliferating tumor cells increases selectivity.[259]

Clinical Pharmacology Etoposide has been evaluated in dogs both intravenously and orally. Etoposide administered IV is associated with severe histamine release in dogs associated with the polysorbate 80 vehicle as described previously with the use of IV docetaxel. Oral dosing has shown low and highly variable bioavailability in dogs, making this route of delivery difficult to use.[260] Etoposide is eliminated following dosing by hepatic metabolism and renal elimination of both parent drugs (30% to 40% of the dose) and glucuronide metabolites. The major dose-limiting toxicity of IV etoposide in the dog is hypersensitivity.[261]

Clinical Use Based on the hypersensitivity reactions experienced in dogs following IV etoposide and the low bioavailability of orally administered etoposide, it is not recommended for use. Strategies to overcome the vehicle-induced hypersensitivity by reformulation or to improve bioavailability are required to continue evaluating etoposide. No studies have been reported in cats.

Steroids

Prednisone

Basic Pharmacology Prednisone, or prednisolone, is a corticosteroid that presumably induces killing of hematopoietic cancer cells through interaction with the glucocorticoid receptor[262] and the induction of apoptosis.[263] Mechanisms of apoptosis induction by corticosteroids in hematologic cancers is still not completely understood, and multiple mechanisms exist whereby tumor cells of hematopoietic origin resist steroid-induced killing.[264]

Clinical Pharmacology Prednisone is generally well tolerated in dogs over short time periods (weeks) when administered on a tapering schedule to a tolerable baseline dose dependent on the response of the patient and the cancer. The adrenal-pituitary axis can become suppressed, with signs of iatrogenic hyperadrenocorticism occurring if prednisone is continued at immunosuppressive doses.

Clinical Use Prednisone is widely used for management of lymphoid malignancies, mast cell tumors, and brain tumors in dogs and cats. Dogs are often dosed at 2 mg/kg (or 40 mg/m^2) PO daily at the beginning of multiagent protocols for lymphoma and are weaned off the drug over 3 to 4 weeks. Cats are tolerant of prednisone or prednisolone and are maintained at 5 mg PO every 24 hours or twice a day as needed. Prednisone is also used to manage signs and side effects of chemotherapy-induced toxicity, such as hypersensitivities or hemorrhagic cystitis. Antiinflammatory doses are used in dogs (0.5 to 1.0 mg/kg PO once daily and reduced as indicated by signs).

Others

Platinum (Carboplatin and Cisplatin)

Basic Pharmacology The activity of platinum-containing antitumor agents is through covalent binding to DNA through displacement reactions resulting in bifunctional lesions and interstrand or intrastrand cross-links.[265] The formation of interstrand cross-links has been shown to correlate to cytotoxicity,[266] presumably by blocking strand separation required for replication and transcription. Reactions with water are an important component of the pharmacology of cisplatin due to some of the aquatic species potentially crossing cell membranes more rapidly.[267]

Clinical Pharmacology Both cisplatin and carboplatin are administered intravenously. Metabolism of both cisplatin and carboplatin occurs primarily through reactions with water and elimination by binding to plasma and tissue proteins. Urinary elimination of unbound and bound forms accounts for nearly 50% of the cisplatin dose 5 days after administration. Carboplatin is predominantly excreted in the urine with approximately 65% of the dose recovered in the urine 24 hours after administration.[267] Strong correlations exist between carboplatin exposure and renal function such that simple formulas have been derived in both humans[268] and cats[269] for dosing calculations based on renal function. The most common toxicities associated with platinum therapies are vomiting and myelosuppression. Nephrotoxicity can occur with cisplatin therapy, and vigorous diuresis is required to avoid or decrease renal toxicity.

Clinical Use Cisplatin (50 to 70 mg/m^2 IV infusion administered with diuresis and antiemetics every 3 weeks) is indicated primarily for canine OSA. A variety of other tumor types have been reported to be marginally sensitive to cisplatin. Cisplatin is *contraindicated* in cats.

Carboplatin (300 mg/m^2 IV over 10 to 15 minutes every 3 weeks) is preferred to cisplatin because of the reduced incidence of nausea/vomiting, the absence of nephrotoxicity, and ease of administration. Myelosuppression is the dose-limiting toxicity. It is used for management of OSA in dogs, as well as a variety of sarcomas and carcinomas. The traditional dose of carboplatin in cats is 240 mg/m^2 IV over 10 minutes every 3 weeks.[270] It has a reported indication for sarcomas and carcinomas. As in humans, an individualized dose of carboplatin may be calculated based on GFR.[78] This provides a uniform systemic dose exposure in cats that may have impaired but subclinical renal disease, as well as makes treatment potentially feasible in cats with overt renal disease. Measurement of GFR requires some extra time and expense but increases the dose intensity and may thus improve response, although no response data using this dosing strategy have been reported to date.

Hydroxyurea

Basic Pharmacology Hydroxyurea enters cells via passive diffusion[271] and is an inhibitor of ribonucleotide reductase[272] resulting in depletion of deoxyribonucleotide pools.[273] This interaction with ribonucleotide reductase can also lead to the allosteric inhibition of other enzymes in the DNA precursor synthesis pathway that make up the replitase complex.[274] The magnitude of decrease in cellular deoxyribonucleotide pools induced by hydroxyurea treatment correlates with inhibition of DNA synthesis observed.[275]

Clinical Pharmacology Hydroxyurea is dosed orally and distributes rapidly to all tissues. Elimination is through hepatic metabolism, as well as urinary elimination of the parent compound. Toxicities associated with hydroxyurea treatment include GI effects, myelosuppression, onycholysis, and pulmonary fibrosis; cats are more susceptible to myelosuppressive effects and potentially methemoglobinemia at higher doses.

Clinical Use Hydroxyurea is used primarily for management of bone marrow disorders such as polycythemia vera and granulocytic leukemias. Hydroxyurea is safe to use at 50 to 60 mg/kg orally once daily initially for several weeks followed by a decreasing dose adjustment as needed to maintain a low red blood cell count in the case of polycythemia vera. It has been recently evaluated as an alternative agent for advanced mast cell tumors in dogs.[276]

L-Asparaginase

Basic Pharmacology The enzymatic function of L-asparaginase is the hydrolysis of L-asparagine to L-aspartic acid. This depletion of circulating L-asparagine leads to inhibition of protein synthesis in tumor cells lacking L-asparagine synthetase, causing induction of apoptosis.[277]

Clinical Pharmacology L-Asparaginase can be dosed subcutaneously, intramuscularly, or intraperitoneally, and blood levels of the protein remain for weeks. Hypersensitivity reactions can lead to a shorter half-life through enhanced clearance. The toxicities associated with L-asparaginase treatment are due to either hypersensitivity reactions, which may be accentuated following repeated exposures, or to decreased protein synthesis from depleted L-asparagine pools.[278] Hypersensitivity may be managed through pretreatment with antihistamines and dexamethasone, although owners should be advised to observe the dog for 1 to 4 hours after treatment for signs of hypersensitivity.

Clinical Use L-Asparaginase (400 IU/kg IM or SQ or 10,000 IU/m^2 IM or SQ) is used exclusively for lymphoproliferative disorders. In order to avoid development of resistance to L-asparaginase it is often used only for patients with relapsed lymphoma.

Future Directions in Drug Therapies for Cancer

Individualized Dosing

Population Pharmacokinetics

The convention for drug dosing is to normalize the dose to the weight or surface area of the patient. This is done even though there is often no data to support a relationship between a given drug's exposure in the patient and either of these parameters. These conventions are based on the idea that body weight or BSA is related to drug distribution and/or elimination in a manner that allows for consistent drug exposure in treated individuals. Dosing in mg/kg or mg/m^2 is a crude attempt at individualized dosing, and for some drugs, substantial variability is expected. Studies specifically aimed at determining what demographic characteristics in the patient population determine variability in drug exposure are termed *population pharmacokinetic studies.*

Molecular Profiling

Tumor Sensitivity

Tumors have traditionally been classified by descriptive characteristics, such as tissue or organ of origin, histology, aggressiveness, and extent of spread. That empiric rubric is being challenged, as molecular classifications made possible by microarrays and other profiling technologies become increasingly common and persuasive.[279,280] The reductionist program would suggest that eventually all differences among traditional tumor types will be reduced to statements about molecules in the tumors and about the interactions among those molecules. Hence it might then be possible to study physiologic processes in one type of cancer and extrapolate the results in a predictive manner to another type through commonalities in their molecular constitutions. But what if we want to do the same thing at the pharmacologic level—to extrapolate and predict drug sensitivity based on molecular characteristics of the tumor? These types of decisions are already being used in human medicine at a discrete level for the use of antiestrogens in estrogen receptor–positive breast cancers,[281] and the use of select molecularly targeted agents based on the mutation status of target molecules.[282,283] However, responses to traditional chemotherapy agents, which still make up the backbone of available therapies both in human and veterinary medicine, are more complex and do not generally sort as responders and nonresponders based on single, or even a few, molecular characteristics. Examples do exist in which this is the case such as overexpression of *ABCB1* and the multidrug resistance phenotype,[284] but generally, a multitude of genes involved in drug activation, detoxification, DNA repair, stress responses, and a myriad of other known and unknown pathways play a role in determining tumor cell chemosensitivity. Therefore a mechanism that can evaluate multiple factors in a tumor indiscriminately and determine whether it is sensitive or insensitive to a given chemotherapeutic agent would be an invaluable adjunct in determining which drugs to utilize for which individual tumor.

Prognostic Evaluation

Current clinical practice in both human and veterinary oncology bases the choice of cytotoxic chemotherapy on descriptive histopathology characteristics. For example, a diagnosis of OSA in a veterinary patient would lead to the use of adjuvant DOX and/or a platinum-based drug (carboplatin or cisplatin) following surgical resection of the tumor. Why are these drugs used? The easy answer is that studies have shown that dogs receiving either of these drugs following surgery live significantly longer than dogs receiving surgery alone.[285] Studies in human patients have shown in a variety of tumor types that in vitro chemosensitivity testing of tumor biopsies and tailoring therapy can lead to increases in antitumor response.[286-289] Therefore basing therapy on an empiric assessment of drug sensitivity rather than on tumor type alone is a strategy that can lead to preferred outcomes. Issues with the use of chemosensitivity assessment in clinical practice are the technical difficulties associated with tissue procurement and culturing and measures of drug response. Another approach to predicting the chemosensitivity of tumors has evolved around gene expression profiling and informatics.[290,291] Although much attention has been focused on recent evidence of research impropriety and improper validation of predictors used for clinical trials in human lung and breast cancers[292,293] and this has dampened some enthusiasm for using genomic predictors in chemosensitivity profiling, it should be noted that extensive review of these data by statisticians[294] and NCI review panels has found that the errors made were in data handling and consistency in analysis. Thus these unfortunate events should not be an indictment of "omics" approaches in making clinical decisions but rather a stark reminder that correct and careful research approaches and data analysis must be adhered to.

Novel Combinations

The approval of the first targeted agent for veterinary applications in the United States (Palladia) has provided access to a multitargeted tyrosine kinase inhibitor. Biologic agents, including species-specific cytokines, peptides, monoclonal antibodies, chimeric molecules, and targeted toxins will also invariably become more prevalent as experimental therapies in veterinary medicine. The use of these novel agents in combination with traditional cytotoxic chemotherapy will likely follow the development pathway seen in human oncology, which includes adding these agents to standard protocols in a disease-specific manner. Thus changes to current standards of practice and care should be expected as these newer agents are incorporated and tested.

REFERENCES

1. Morrison WB: Cancer chemotherapy: an annotated history, *J Vet Intern Med* 24:1249, 2010.
2. Chabner BA, Roberts TG Jr: Timeline: Chemotherapy and the war on cancer, *Nat Rev Cancer* 5:65, 2005.
3. DeVita VT Jr, Chu E: A history of cancer chemotherapy, *Cancer Res* 68:8643, 2008.
4. Shoemaker RH: The NCI60 human tumour cell line anticancer drug screen, *Nat Rev Cancer* 6:813, 2006.
5. Sharma SV, Haber DA, Settleman J: Cell line-based platforms to evaluate the therapeutic efficacy of candidate anticancer agents, *Nat Rev Cancer* 10:241, 2010.
6. Thamm DH, Rose B, Kow K, et al: Masitinib as a chemosensitizer of canine tumor cell lines: A proof of concept study, *Vet J* 191(1):131–134, 2011.
7. Begleiter A, Lam H-YP, Grover J, et al: Evidence for active transport of melphalan by two amino acid carriers in L5178Y lymphoblasts in vitro, *Cancer Res* 39:353, 1979.
8. Vistica D: Cytotoxicity as an indicator for transport mechanism: evidence that murine bone marrow progenitor cells lack a high-affinity leucine carrier that transports melphalan in murine L1210 leukemia cells, *Blood* 56:427, 1980.
9. Wiley JS, Jones SP, Sawyer WH, et al: Cytosine arabinoside influx and nucleoside transport sites in acute leukemia, *J Clin Invest* 69:479, 1982.
10. Mackey JR, Mani RS, Selner M, et al: Functional nucleoside transporters are required for gemcitabine influx and manifestation of toxicity in cancer cell lines, *Cancer Res* 58:4349, 1998.
11. Goldman ID, Lichtenstein NS, Oliverio VT: Carrier-mediated transport of the folic acid analogue, methotrexate, in the L1210 leukemia cell, *J Biol Chem* 243:5007, 1968.
12. Withoff S, Keith WN, Knol AJ, et al: Selection of a subpopulation with fewer DNA topoisomerase II alpha gene copies in a doxorubicin-resistant cell line panel, *Br J Cancer* 74:502, 1996.
13. Wang H, Jiang Z, Wong YW, et al: Decreased CP-1 (NF-Y) activity results in transcriptional down-regulation of topoisomerase IIalpha in a doxorubicin-resistant variant of human multiple myeloma RPMI 8226, *Biochem Biophys Res Commun* 237:217, 1997.
14. Moran RG, Spears CP, Heidelberger C: Biochemical determinants of tumor sensitivity to 5-fluorouracil: ultrasensitive methods for the determination of 5-fluoro-2′-deoxyuridylate, 2′-deoxyuridylate, and thymidylate synthetase, *Proc Natl Acad Sci U S A* 76:1456, 1979.
15. Karran P, Bignami M: DNA damage tolerance, mismatch repair and genome instability, *BioEssays* 16:833, 1994.
16. Brown JM, Attardi LD: The role of apoptosis in cancer development and treatment response, *Nat Rev Cancer* 5:231, 2005.
17. Igney FH, Krammer PH: Death and anti-death: tumour resistance to apoptosis, *Nat Rev Cancer* 2:277, 2002.
18. Reed JC, Kitada S, Takayama S, et al: Regulation of chemoresistance by the bcl-2 oncoprotein in non-Hodgkin's lymphoma and lymphocytic leukemia cell lines, *Ann Oncol* 5(Suppl 1):61, 1994.
19. Schmitt CA, Rosenthal CT, Lowe SW: Genetic analysis of chemoresistance in primary murine lymphomas, *Nat Med* 6:1029, 2000.
20. Ambrosini G, Adida C, Altieri DC: A novel anti-apoptosis gene, survivin, expressed in cancer and lymphoma, *Nat Med* 3:917, 1997.
21. Kramer M, Hermans J, Parker J, et al: Clinical significance of bcl2 and p53 protein expression in diffuse large B-cell lymphoma: a population-based study, *J Clin Oncol* 14:2131, 1996.
22. Sohn SK, Jung JT, Kim DH, et al: Prognostic significance of bcl-2, bax, and p53 expression in diffuse large B-cell lymphoma, *Am J Hematol* 73:101, 2003.
23. Rebhun RB, Lana SE, Ehrhart EJ, et al: Comparative analysis of survivin expression in untreated and relapsed canine lymphoma, *J Vet Intern Med* 22:989, 2008.
24. Moscow JA, Swanson CA, Cowan KH: Decreased melphalan accumulation in a human breast cancer cell line selected for resistance to melphalan, *Br J Cancer* 68:732, 1993.
25. Saikawa Y, Knight CB, Saikawa T, et al: Decreased expression of the human folate receptor mediates transport-defective methotrexate resistance in KB cells, *J Biol Chem* 268:5293, 1993.
26. Tew KD: Glutathione-associated enzymes in anticancer drug resistance, *Cancer Res* 54:4313, 1994.
27. Wang AL, Tew KD: Increased glutathione-S-transferase activity in a cell line with acquired resistance to nitrogen mustards, *Cancer Treat Rep* 69:677, 1985.
28. Lewis AD, Hickson ID, Robson CN, et al: Amplification and increased expression of alpha class glutathione S-transferase-encoding genes associated with resistance to nitrogen mustards, *Proc Natl Acad Sci U S A* 85:8511, 1988.
29. Beck A, Etienne MC, Cheradame S, et al: A role for dihydropyrimidine dehydrogenase and thymidylate synthase in tumour sensitivity to fluorouracil, *Eur J Cancer* 30A:1517, 1994.
30. Ishikawa Y, Kubota T, Otani Y, et al: Dihydropyrimidine dehydrogenase activity and messenger RNA level may be related to the antitumor effect of 5-fluorouracil on human tumor xenografts in nude mice, *Clin Cancer Res* 5:883, 1999.
31. Scherf U, Ross DT, Waltham M, et al: A gene expression database for the molecular pharmacology of cancer, *Nat Genet* 24:236, 2000.
32. Heggie GD, Sommadossi JP, Cross DS, et al: Clinical pharmacokinetics of 5-fluorouracil and its metabolites in plasma, urine, and bile, *Cancer Res* 47:2203, 1987.
33. Heinemann V, Xu YZ, Chubb S, et al: Inhibition of ribonucleotide reduction in CCRF-CEM cells by 2′,2′-difluorodeoxycytidine, *Mol Pharmacol* 38:567, 1990.
34. Huang P, Chubb S, Hertel LW, et al: Action of 2′,2′-difluorodeoxycytidine on DNA synthesis, *Cancer Res* 51:6110, 1991.
35. Heinemann V, Hertel LW, Grindey GB, et al: Comparison of the cellular pharmacokinetics and toxicity of 2′,2′-difluorodeoxycytidine and 1-beta-D-arabinofuranosylcytosine, *Cancer Res* 48:4024, 1988.
36. Bouffard DY, Laliberte J, Momparler RL: Kinetic studies on 2′,2′-difluorodeoxycytidine (Gemcitabine) with purified human deoxycytidine kinase and cytidine deaminase, *Biochem Pharmacol* 45:1857, 1993.
37. Ohhashi S, Ohuchida K, Mizumoto K, et al: Down-regulation of deoxycytidine kinase enhances acquired resistance to gemcitabine in pancreatic cancer, *Anticancer Res* 28:2205, 2008.
38. Nakano Y, Tanno S, Koizumi K, et al: Gemcitabine chemoresistance and molecular markers associated with gemcitabine transport and metabolism in human pancreatic cancer cells, *Br J Cancer* 96:457, 2007.
39. Long BH, Wang L, Lorico A, et al: Mechanisms of resistance to etoposide and teniposide in acquired resistant human colon and lung carcinoma cell lines, *Cancer Res* 51:5275, 1991.
40. Minocha A, Long BH: Inhibition of the DNA catenation activity of type II topoisomerase by VP16–213 and VM26, *Biochem Biophys Res Commun* 122:165, 1984.

41. Chen GL, Yang L, Rowe TC, et al: Nonintercalative antitumor drugs interfere with the breakage-reunion reaction of mammalian DNA topoisomerase II, *J Biol Chem* 259:13560, 1984.
42. Alt FW, Kellems RE, Bertino JR, et al: Selective multiplication of dihydrofolate reductase genes in methotrexate-resistant variants of cultured murine cells, *J Biol Chem* 253:1357, 1978.
43. Giannakakou P, Sackett DL, Kang Y-K, et al: Paclitaxel-resistant human ovarian cancer cells have mutant β-tubulins that exhibit impaired paclitaxel-driven polymerization, *J Biol Chem* 272:17118, 1997.
44. Andoh T, Ishii K, Suzuki Y, et al: Characterization of a mammalian mutant with a camptothecin-resistant DNA topoisomerase I, *Proc Natl Acad Sci U S A* 84:5565, 1987.
45. Chaney SG, Sancar A: DNA repair: Enzymatic mechanisms and relevance to drug response, *J Natl Cancer Inst* 88:1346, 1996.
46. Behrens BC, Hamilton TC, Masuda H, et al: Characterization of a cis-diamminedichloroplatinum(II)-resistant human ovarian cancer cell line and its use in evaluation of platinum analogues, *Cancer Res* 47:414, 1987.
47. Masuda H, Tanaka T, Matsuda H, et al: Increased removal of DNA-bound platinum in a human ovarian cancer cell line resistant to cis-diamminedichloroplatinum(II), *Cancer Res* 50:1863, 1990.
48. Parker RJ, Eastman A, Bostick-Bruton F, et al: Acquired cisplatin resistance in human ovarian cancer cells is associated with enhanced repair of cisplatin-DNA lesions and reduced drug accumulation, *J Clin Invest* 87:772, 1991.
49. Nojima K, Hochegger H, Saberi A, et al: Multiple repair pathways mediate tolerance to chemotherapeutic cross-linking agents in vertebrate cells, *Cancer Res* 65:11704, 2005.
50. Borst P, Elferink RO: Mammalian ABC transporters in health and disease, *Annu Rev Biochem* 71:537, 2002.
51. Fletcher JI, Haber M, Henderson MJ, et al: ABC transporters in cancer: more than just drug efflux pumps, *Nat Rev Cancer* 10:147, 2010.
52. Lee JJ, Hughes CS, Fine RL, et al: P-glycoprotein expression in canine lymphoma: a relevant, intermediate model of multidrug resistance, *Cancer* 77:1892, 1996.
53. Honscha KU, Schirmer A, Reischauer A, et al: Expression of ABC-transport proteins in canine mammary cancer: Consequences for chemotherapy, *Reprod Domest Anim* 44(Suppl 2):218, 2009.
54. Hifumi T, Miyoshi N, Kawaguchi H, et al: Immunohistochemical detection of proteins associated with multidrug resistance to anti-cancer drugs in canine and feline primary pulmonary carcinoma, *J Vet Med Sci* 72:665, 2010.
55. Nowak M, Madej JA, Dziegiel P: Expression of breast cancer resistance protein (BCRP-1) in canine mammary adenocarcinomas and adenomas, *In Vivo* 23:705, 2009.
56. Conrad S, Viertelhaus A, Orzechowski A, et al: Sequencing and tissue distribution of the canine MRP2 gene compared with MRP1 and MDR1, *Toxicology* 156:81, 2001.
57. Yabuuchi H, Tanaka K, Maeda M, et al: Cloning of the dog bile salt export pump (BSEP; ABCB11) and functional comparison with the human and rat proteins, *Biopharm Drug Dispos* 29:441, 2008.
58. Ramirez CJ, Minch JD, Gay JM, et al: Molecular genetic basis for fluoroquinolone-induced retinal degeneration in cats, *Pharmacogenet Genomics* 21:66, 2011.
59. Chabner BA: Clinical strategies for cancer treatment: the role of drugs. In Chabner BA, Collins JM, editors: *Cancer chemotherapy: Principles and practice*, Philadelphia, 1990, JB Lippincott.
60. Page RL, Macy DW, Ogilvie GK, et al: Phase III evaluation of doxorubicin and whole-body hyperthermia in dogs with lymphoma, *Int J Hyperthermia* 8:187, 1992.
61. Carter RF, Harris CK, Withrow SJ, et al: Chemotherapy of canine lymphoma with histopathological correlation- doxorubicin alone compared to COP as 1st treatment regimen, *J Am Anim Hosp Assoc* 23:587, 1987.
62. Postorino NC, Susaneck SJ, Withrow SJ, et al: Single agent therapy with adriamycin for canine lymphosarcoma, *J Am Anim Hosp Assoc* 25:221, 1989.
63. Valerius KD, Ogilvie GK, Mallinckrodt CH, et al: Doxorubicin alone or in combination with asparaginase, followed by cyclophosphamide, vincristine, and prednisone for treatment of multicentric lymphoma in dogs: 121 cases (1987–1995), *J Am Vet Med Assoc* 210:512, 1997.
64. Mutsaers AJ, Glickman NW, DeNicola DB, et al: Evaluation of treatment with doxorubicin and piroxicam or doxorubicin alone for multicentric lymphoma in dogs, *J Am Vet Med Assoc* 220:1813, 2002.
65. Cotter SM: Treatment of lymphoma and leukemia with cyclophosphamide, vincristine, and prednisone. 1. Treatment of Dogs, *J Am Anim Hosp Assoc* 19:159, 1983.
66. MacEwen EG, Brown NO, Patnaik AK, et al: Cyclic combination chemotherapy of canine lymphosarcoma, *J Am Vet Med Assoc* 178:1178, 1981.
67. MacEwen EG, Hayes AA, Matus RE, et al: Evaluation of some prognostic factors for advanced multicentric lymphosarcoma in the dog—147 Cases (1978–1981), *J Am Vet Med Assoc* 190:564, 1987.
68. Khanna C, Lund EM, Redic KA, et al: Randomized controlled trial of doxorubicin versus dactinomycin in a multiagent protocol for treatment of dogs with malignant lymphoma, *J Am Vet Med Assoc* 213:985, 1998.
69. Greenlee PG, Filippa DA, Quimby FW, et al: Lymphomas in dogs. A morphologic, immunologic, and clinical study, *Cancer* 66:480, 1990.
70. Stone MS, Goldstein MA, Cotter SM: Comparison of 2 protocols for induction of remission in dogs with lymphoma, *J Am Anim Hosp Assoc* 27:315, 1991.
71. Myers NC 3rd, Moore AS, Rand WM, et al: Evaluation of a multidrug chemotherapy protocol (ACOPA II) in dogs with lymphoma, *J Vet Intern Med* 11:333, 1997.
72. Boyce KL, Kitchell BE: Treatment of canine lymphoma with COPLA/LVP, *J Am Anim Hosp Assoc* 36:395, 2000.
73. Morrison-Collister KE, Rassnick KM, Northrup NC, et al: A combination chemotherapy protocol with MOPP and CCNU consolidation (Tufts VELCAP-SC) for the treatment of canine lymphoma, *Vet Comp Oncol* 1:180, 2003.
74. Zemann BI, Moore AS, Rand WM, et al: A combination chemotherapy protocol (VELCAP-L) for dogs with lymphoma, *J Vet Intern Med* 12:465, 1998.
75. Keller ET, MacEwen EG, Rosenthal RC, et al: Evaluation of prognostic factors and sequential combination chemotherapy with doxorubicin for canine lymphoma, *J Vet Intern Med* 7:289, 1993.
76. Garrett LD, Thamm DH, Chun R, et al: Evaluation of a 6-month chemotherapy protocol with no maintenance therapy for dogs with lymphoma, *J Vet Intern Med* 16:704, 2002.
77. Undevia SD, Gomez-Abuin G, Ratain MJ: Pharmacokinetic variability of anticancer agents, *Nat Rev Cancer* 5:447, 2005.
78. Bailey DB, Rassnick KM, Erb HN, et al: Effect of glomerular filtration rate on clearance and myelotoxicity of carboplatin in cats with tumors, *Am J Vet Res* 65:1502, 2004.
79. Mealey KL, Fidel J, Gay JM, et al: ABCB1-1Delta polymorphism can predict hematologic toxicity in dogs treated with vincristine, *J Vet Intern Med* 22:996, 2008.
80. Thompson LA, Lawson AP, Sutphin SD, et al: Description of current practices of empiric chemotherapy dose adjustment in obese adult patients, *J Oncol Pract* 6:141, 2010.
81. Hunter RJ, Navo MA, Thaker PH, et al: Dosing chemotherapy in obese patients: actual versus assigned body surface area (BSA), *Cancer Treat Rev* 35:69, 2009.
82. Vail DM: Supporting the veterinary cancer patient on chemotherapy: neutropenia and gastrointestinal toxicity, *Top Companion Anim Med* 24:122, 2009.
83. Dranitsaris G, Johnston M, Poirier S, et al: Are health care providers who work with cancer drugs at an increased risk for toxic events? A systematic review and meta-analysis of the literature, *J Oncol Pharm Pract* 11:69, 2005.

84. Hamscher G, Mohring SA, Knobloch A, et al: Determination of drug residues in urine of dogs receiving anti-cancer chemotherapy by liquid chromatography-electrospray ionization- tandem mass spectrometry: is there an environmental or occupational risk? *J Anal Toxicol* 34:142, 2010.
85. Evans WE, Relling MV: Clinical pharmacokinetics-pharmacodynamics of anticancer drugs, *Clin Pharmacokinet* 16:327, 1989.
86. Eckhoff GA: Mechanisms of adverse drug-reactions and interactions in veterinary-medicine, *J Am Vet Med Assoc* 176:1131, 1980.
87. He SM, Yang AK, Li XT, et al: Effects of herbal products on the metabolism and transport of anticancer agents, *Expert Opin Drug Metab Toxicol* 6:1195, 2010.
88. Tarirai C, Viljoen AM, Hamman JH: Herb-drug pharmacokinetic interactions reviewed, *Expert Opin Drug Metab Toxicol* 6:1515, 2010.
89. Mealey KL: Therapeutic implications of the MDR-1 gene, *J Vet Pharmacol Ther* 27:257, 2004.
90. Legha SS, Benjamin RS, Mackay B, et al: Reduction of doxorubicin cardiotoxicity by prolonged continuous intravenous infusion, *Ann Intern Med* 96:133, 1982.
91. Berrak SG, Ewer MS, Jaffe N, et al: Doxorubicin cardiotoxicity in children: reduced incidence of cardiac dysfunction associated with continuous-infusion schedules, *Oncol Rep* 8:611, 2001.
92. Preisler HD, Gessner T, Azarnia N, et al: Relationship between plasma adriamycin levels and the outcome of remission induction therapy for acute nonlymphocytic leukemia, *Cancer Chemother Pharmacol* 12:125, 1984.
93. Piscitelli SC, Rodvold KA, Rushing DA, et al: Pharmacokinetics and pharmacodynamics of doxorubicin in patients with small cell lung cancer, *Clin Pharmacol Ther* 53:555, 1993.
94. Danesi R, Fogli S, Gennari A, et al: Pharmacokinetic-pharmacodynamic relationships of the anthracycline anticancer drugs, *Clin Pharmacokinet* 41:431, 2002.
95. Arrington KA, Legendre AM, Tabeling GS, et al: Comparison of body surface area-based and weight-based dosage protocols for doxorubicin administration in dogs, *Am J Vet Res* 55:1587, 1994.
96. Veterinary co-operative oncology group—common terminology criteria for adverse events (VCOG-CTCAE) following chemotherapy or biological antineoplastic therapy in dogs and cats v1.0, *Vet Comp Oncol* 2:195, 2004.
97. Bailey DB, Rassnick KM, Kristal O, et al: Phase I dose escalation of single-agent vinblastine in dogs, *J Vet Intern Med* 22:1397, 2008.
98. Vaughan A, Johnson JL, Williams LE: Impact of chemotherapeutic dose intensity and hematologic toxicity on first remission duration in dogs with lymphoma treated with a chemoradiotherapy protocol, *J Vet Intern Med* 21:1332, 2007.
99. Eschalier A, Lavarenne J, Burtin C, et al: Study of histamine release induced by acute administration of antitumor agents in dogs, *Cancer Chemother Pharmacol* 21:246, 1988.
100. Poirier VJ, Hershey AE, Burgess KE, et al: Efficacy and toxicity of paclitaxel (Taxol) for the treatment of canine malignant tumors, *J Vet Intern Med* 18:219, 2004.
101. Goodman LS, Wintrobe MM, et al: Nitrogen mustard therapy; use of methyl-bis (beta-chloroethyl) amine hydrochloride and tris (beta-chloroethyl) amine hydrochloride for Hodgkin's disease, lymphosarcoma, leukemia and certain allied and miscellaneous disorders, *J Am Med Assoc* 132:126, 1946.
102. Jacobson LO, Spurr CL, et al: Studies on the effect of methyl bis (beta-chloroethyl) amine hydrochloride on diseases of the hemopoietic system, *J Clin Invest* 25:909, 1946.
103. Rhoads CP: Nitrogen mustards in the treatment of neoplastic disease; official statement, *J Am Med Assoc* 131:656, 1946.
104. Kohn KW, Spears CL, Doty P: Inter-strand crosslinking of DNA by nitrogen mustard, *J Mol Biol* 19:266, 1966.
105. Skipper HE, Bennett LL Jr, Langham WH: Over-all tracer studies with C14 labeled nitrogen mustard in normal and leukemic mice, *Cancer* 4:1025, 1951.
106. Goldenberg GJ, Vanstone CL, Israels LG, et al: Evidence for a transport carrier of nitrogen mustard in nitrogen mustard-sensitive and -resistant L5178Y lymphoblasts, *Cancer Res* 30:2285, 1970.
107. Rassnick KM, Mauldin GE, Al-Sarraf R, et al: MOPP chemotherapy for treatment of resistant lymphoma in dogs: a retrospective study of 117 cases (1989–2000), *J Vet Intern Med* 16:576, 2002.
108. Rassnick KM, Bailey DB, Malone EK, et al: Comparison between L-CHOP and an L-CHOP protocol with interposed treatments of CCNU and MOPP (L-CHOP-CCNU-MOPP) for lymphoma in dogs, *Vet Comp Oncol* 8:243, 2010.
109. Brodsky EM, Maudlin GN, Lachowicz JL, et al: Asparaginase and MOPP treatment of dogs with lymphoma, *J Vet Intern Med* 23:578, 2009.
110. Tew KD, Colvin OM, Chabner BA: Alkylating agents. In Chabner BA, Longo DL, editors: *Cancer chemotherapy & biotherapy: principles and practice*, Philadelphia, 2001, Lippincott Williams & Wilkins.
111. Cohen JL, Jao JY: Enzymatic basis of cyclophosphamide activation by hepatic microsomes of the rat, *J Pharmacol Exp Ther* 174:206, 1970.
112. Colvin M, Brundrett RB, Kan MN, et al: Alkylating properties of phosphoramide mustard, *Cancer Res* 36:1121, 1976.
113. Warry E, Hansen RJ, Gustafson DL, et al: Pharmacokinetics of cyclophosphamide after oral and intravenous administration to dogs with lymphoma, *J Vet Intern Med* 25:903, 2011.
114. Fetting JH, McCarthy LE, Borison HL, et al: Vomiting induced by cyclophosphamide and phosphoramide mustard in cats, *Cancer Treat Rep* 66:1625, 1982.
115. Lori JC, Stein TJ, Thamm DH: Doxorubicin and cyclophosphamide for the treatment of canine lymphoma: a randomized, placebo-controlled study, *Vet Comp Oncol* 8:188, 2010.
116. Hadden AG, Cotter SM, Rand W, et al: Efficacy and toxicosis of VELCAP-C treatment of lymphoma in cats, *J Vet Intern Med* 22:153, 2008.
117. Creaven PJ, Allen LM, Alford DA, et al: Clinical pharmacology of isophosphamide, *Clin Pharmacol Ther* 16:77, 1974.
118. Norpoth K: Studies on the metabolism of isopnosphamide (NSC-109724) in man, *Cancer Treat Rep* 60:437, 1976.
119. Lind MJ, Roberts HL, Thatcher N, et al: The effect of route of administration and fractionation of dose on the metabolism of ifosfamide, *Cancer Chemother Pharmacol* 26:105, 1990.
120. Rassnick KM, Frimberger AE, Wood CA, et al: Evaluation of ifosfamide for treatment of various canine neoplasms, *J Vet Intern Med* 14:271, 2000.
121. Rassnick KM, Moore AS, Northrup NC, et al: Phase I trial and pharmacokinetic analysis of ifosfamide in cats with sarcomas, *Am J Vet Res* 67:510, 2006.
122. Rassnick KM, Rodriguez CO, Khanna C, et al: Results of a phase II clinical trial on the use of ifosfamide for treatment of cats with vaccine-associated sarcomas, *Am J Vet Res* 67:517, 2006.
123. Begleiter A, Goldenberg GJ: Uptake and decomposition of chlorambucil by L5178Y lymphoblasts in vitro, *Biochem Pharmacol* 32:535, 1983.
124. Jiang BZ, Bank BB, Hsiang YH, et al: Lack of drug-induced DNA cross-links in chlorambucil-resistant Chinese hamster ovary cells, *Cancer Res* 49:5514, 1989.
125. Mitoma C, Onodera T, Takegoshi T, et al: Metabolic disposition of chlorambucil in rats, *Xenobiotica* 7:205, 1977.
126. Goodman GE, McLean A, Alberts DS, et al: Inhibition of human tumour clonogenicity by chlorambucil and its metabolites, *Br J Cancer* 45:621, 1982.
127. Stein TJ, Pellin M, Steinberg H, et al: Treatment of feline gastrointestinal small-cell lymphoma with chlorambucil and glucocorticoids, *J Am Anim Hosp Assoc* 46:413, 2010.
128. Begleiter A, Lam HP, Goldenberg GJ: Mechanism of uptake of nitrosoureas by L5178Y lymphoblasts in vitro, *Cancer Res* 37:1022, 1977.

129. Montgomery JA, James R, McCaleb GS, et al: The modes of decomposition of 1,3-bis(2-chloroethyl)-1-nitrosourea and related compounds, *J Med Chem* 10:668, 1967.
130. Colvin M, Brundrett RB, Cowens W, et al: A chemical basis for the antitumor activity of chloroethylnitrosoureas, *Biochem Pharmacol* 25:695, 1976.
131. Kohn KW: Interstrand cross-linking of DNA by 1,3-bis(2-chloroethyl)-1-nitrosourea and other 1-(2-haloethyl)-1-nitrosoureas, *Cancer Res* 37:1450, 1977.
132. Hill DL, Kirk MC, Struck RF: Microsomal metabolism of nitrosoureas, *Cancer Res* 35:296, 1975.
133. Wheeler GP, Johnston TP, Bowdon BJ, et al: Comparison of the properties of metabolites of CCNU, *Biochem Pharmacol* 26:2331, 1977.
134. Lee FY, Workman P, Roberts JT, et al: Clinical pharmacokinetics of oral CCNU (lomustine), *Cancer Chemother Pharmacol* 14:125, 1985.
135. Heading KL, Brockley LK, Bennett PF: CCNU (lomustine) toxicity in dogs: a retrospective study (2002–07), *Aust Vet J* 89:109, 2011.
136. Hosoya K, Lord LK, Lara-Garcia A, et al: Prevalence of elevated alanine transaminase activity in dogs treated with CCNU (Lomustine), *Vet Comp Oncol* 7:244, 2009.
137. Skorupski KA, Hammond GM, Irish AM, et al: Prospective randomized clinical trial assessing the efficacy of denamarin for prevention of CCNU-induced hepatopathy in tumor-bearing dogs, *J Vet Intern Med* 25:838, 2011.
138. Reusser F: Mode of action of streptozotocin, *J Bacteriol* 105:580, 1971.
139. Bhuyan BK: The action of streptozotocin on mammalian cells, *Cancer Res* 30:2017, 1970.
140. Schnedl WJ, Ferber S, Johnson JH, et al: STZ transport and cytotoxicity. Specific enhancement in GLUT2-expressing cells, *Diabetes* 43:1326, 1994.
141. Hosokawa M, Dolci W, Thorens B: Differential sensitivity of GLUT1- and GLUT2-expressing beta cells to streptozotocin, *Biochem Biophys Res Commun* 289:1114, 2001.
142. Adolphe AB, Glasofer ED, Troetel WM, et al: Preliminary pharmacokinetics of streptozotocin, an antineoplastic antibiotic, *J Clin Pharmacol* 17:379, 1977.
143. Schein PS, Cooney DA, Vernon ML: The use of nicotinamide to modify the toxicity of streptozotocin diabetes without loss of antitumor activity, *Cancer Res* 27:2324, 1967.
144. Schein PS, Rakieten N, Cooney DA, et al: Streptozotocin diabetes in monkeys and dogs, and its prevention by nicotinamide, *Proc Soc Exp Biol Med* 143:514, 1973.
145. Schein PS: 1-methyl-1-nitrosourea and dialkylnitrosamine depression of nicotinamide adenine dinucleotide, *Cancer Res* 29:1226, 1969.
146. Panasci LC, Fox PA, Schein PS: Structure-activity studies of methylnitrosourea antitumor agents with reduced murine bone marrow toxicity, *Cancer Res* 37:3321, 1977.
147. Moore AS, Nelson RW, Henry CJ, et al: Streptozocin for treatment of pancreatic islet cell tumors in dogs: 17 cases (1989–1999), *J Am Vet Med Assoc* 221:811, 2002.
148. Audette RC, Connors TA, Mandel HG, et al: Studies on the mechanism of action of the tumour inhibitory triazenes, *Biochem Pharmacol* 22:1855, 1973.
149. Reid JM, Kuffel MJ, Miller JK, et al: Metabolic activation of dacarbazine by human cytochromes P450: the role of CYP1A1, CYP1A2, and CYP2E1, *Clin Cancer Res* 5:2192, 1999.
150. Nagasawa HT, Shirota FN, Mizuno NS: The mechanism of alkylation of DNA by 5-(3-methyl-1-triazeno)imidazole-4-carboxamide (MIC), a metabolite of DIC (NSC-45388). Non-involvement of diazomethane, *Chem Biol Interact* 8:403, 1974.
151. Kleihues P, Kolar GF, Margison GP: Interaction of the carcinogen 3,3-dimethyl-1-phenyltriazene with nucleic acids of various rat tissues and the effect of a protein-free diet, *Cancer Res* 36:2189, 1976.
152. Griessmayr PC, Payne SE, Winter JE, et al: Dacarbazine as single-agent therapy for relapsed lymphoma in dogs, *J Vet Intern Med* 23:1227, 2009.
153. Flory AB, Rassnick KM, Al-Sarraf R, et al: Combination of CCNU and DTIC chemotherapy for treatment of resistant lymphoma in dogs, *J Vet Intern Med* 22:164, 2008.
154. Gale GR, Simpson JG, Smith AB: Studies of the mode of action of N-isopropyl-alpha-(2-methylhydrazino)-p-toluamide, *Cancer Res* 27:1186, 1967.
155. Moloney SJ, Wiebkin P, Cummings SW, et al: Metabolic activation of the terminal N-methyl group of N-isopropyl-alpha-(2-methylhydrazino)-p-toluamide hydrochloride (procarbazine), *Carcinogenesis* 6:397, 1985.
156. Schold SC Jr, Brent TP, von Hofe E, et al: O6-alkylguanine-DNA alkyltransferase and sensitivity to procarbazine in human brain-tumor xenografts, *J Neurosurg* 70:573, 1989.
157. Shiba DA, Weinkam RJ: Quantitative analysis of procarbazine, procarbazine metabolites and chemical degradation products with application to pharmacokinetic studies, *J Chromatogr* 229:397, 1982.
158. Oliverio VT, Denham C, Devita VT, et al: Some pharmacologic properties of a new antitumor agent, N-isopropyl-alpha-(2-methylhydrazino)-p-toluamide, hydrochloride (Nsc-77213), *Cancer Chemother Rep* 42:1, 1964.
159. Chabner BA, Sponzo R, Hubbard S, et al: High-dose intermittent intravenous infusion of procarbazine (NSC-77213), *Cancer Chemother Rep* 57:361, 1973.
160. Zunino F, Gambetta R, Di Marco A: The inhibition in vitro of DNA polymerase and RNA polymerase by daunomycin and Adriamycin, *Biochem Pharmacol* 24:309, 1975.
161. Tewey KM, Chen GI, Nelson EM, et al: Intercalative anti-tumor drugs interfere with the breakage-reunion reaction of mammalian DNA topoisomerase, *J Biol Chem* 259:9182, 1984.
162. Taatjes DJ, Gaudiano G, Resing K, et al: Alkylation of DNA by the anthracycline, antitumor drugs adriamycin and daunomycin, *J Med Chem* 39:4135, 1996.
163. Doroshow JH: Role of hydrogen peroxide and hydroxyl radical in the killing of ehrlich tumor cells by anticancer quinones, *Proc Natl Acad Sci U S A* 83:4514, 1985.
164. Bachur NR, Gordon SL, Gee MV: A general mechanism for microsomal activation of quinone anticancer agents to free radicals, *Cancer Res* 38:1745, 1978.
165. Pessah IN, Durie EL, Schiedt MJ, et al: Anthraquinone-sensitized Ca + release channel from rat cardiac sarcoplasmic reticulum: possible receptor-mediated mechanism of doxorubicin cardiomyopathy, *Mol Pharmacol* 37:503, 1990.
166. Oakes SG, Schlager JJ, Santone KS, et al: Doxorubicin blocks the increase in intracellular Ca ++, part of a second messenger system in N1E-115 murine neuroblastoma cells, *J Pharmacol Exp Ther* 252:979, 1990.
167. Mau BL, Powis G: Inhibition of cellular thioredoxin reductase by diaziquone and doxorubicin: relationship to the inhibition of cell proliferation and decreased ribonucleotide reductase activity, *Biochem Pharmacol* 43:1621, 1992.
168. Morre DJ, Kim C, Paulik M, et al: Is the drug-responsive NADH oxidase of the cancer cell plasma membrane a molecular target for adriamycin? *J Bioenerg Biomembr* 29:269, 1997.
169. Terasaki T, Iga T, Sugiyama Y, et al: Experimental evidence of characteristic tissue distribution of Adriamycin: tissue DNA concentration as a determinant, *J Pharm Pharmacol* 34:597, 1982.
170. Nicolay K, Timmers RJM, Spoelstra E, et al: The interaction of adriamycin with cardiolipin in model and rat liver mitochondrial membranes, *Biochim Biophys Acta* 778:359, 1984.
171. Goormaghtigh E, Chatelain P, Caspers J, et al: Evidence of a specific complex between adriamycin and negatively-charged phospholipids, *Biochim Biophys Acta* 597:1, 1980.
172. Gustafson DL, Rastatter JC, Colombo T, et al: Doxorubicin pharmacokinetics: macromolecule binding, metabolism and

elimination in the context of a physiological model, *J Pharm Sci* 91:1488, 2002.

173. Ahmed NK, Felsted RL, Bachur NR: Daunorubicin reduction mediated by aldehyde and ketone reductases, *Xenobiotica* 11:131, 1981.
174. Pan SS, Bachur NR: Xanthine oxidase catalyzed reductive cleavage of anthracycline antibiotics and free radical formation, *Mol Pharmacol* 17:95, 1980.
175. Young RC, Ozols RF, Myers CE: The anthracycline neoplastic drugs, *N Engl J Med* 305:139, 1981.
176. O'Keefe DA, Sisson DD, Gelberg HB, et al: Systemic toxicity associated with doxorubicin administration in cats, *J Vet Intern Med* 7:309, 1993.
177. Thamm DH, Vail DM: Aftershocks of cancer chemotherapy: managing adverse effects, *J Am Anim Hosp Assoc* 43:1, 2007.
178. Foye WO, Vajragupta O, Sengupta SK: DNA-binding specificity and RNA polymerase inhibitory activity of bis(aminoalkyl) anthraquinones and bis(methylthio)vinylquinolinium iodides, *J Pharm Sci* 71:253, 1982.
179. Crespi MD, Ivanier SE, Genovese J, et al: Mitoxantrone affects topoisomerase activities in human breast cancer cells, *Biochem Biophys Res Commun* 136:521, 1986.
180. Patterson LH, Gandecha BM, Brown JR: 1,4-Bis(2-[(2-hydroxyethyl) amino]ethylamino)-9,10-anthracenedione, an anthraquinone antitumour agent that does not cause lipid peroxidation in vivo; comparison with daunorubicin, *Biochem Biophys Res Commun* 110:399, 1983.
181. Nguyen B, Gutierrez PL: Mechanism(s) for the metabolism of mitoxantrone: electron spin resonance and electrochemical studies, *Chem Biol Interact* 74:139, 1990.
182. Alberts DS, Peng YM, Leigh S, et al: Disposition of mitoxantrone in cancer patients, *Cancer Res* 45:1879, 1985.
183. Lu K, Savaraj N, Loo TL: Pharmacological disposition of 1,4-dihydroxy-5-8-bis[[2 [(2-hydroxyethyl)amino]ethyl]amino]-9,10-anthracenedione dihydrochloride in the dog, *Cancer Chemother Pharmacol* 13:63, 1984.
184. Chiccarelli FS, Morrison JA, Cosulich DB, et al: Identification of human urinary mitoxantrone metabolites, *Cancer Res* 46:4858, 1986.
185. Henry CJ, McCaw DL, Turnquist SE, et al: Clinical evaluation of mitoxantrone and piroxicam in a canine model of human invasive urinary bladder carcinoma, *Clin Cancer Res* 9:906, 2003.
186. Takusagawa F, Dabrow M, Neidle S, et al: The structure of a pseudo intercalated complex between actinomycin and the DNA binding sequence d(GpC), *Nature* 296:466, 1982.
187. Takusagawa F, Goldstein BM, Youngster S, et al: Crystallization and preliminary X-ray study of a complex between d(ATGCAT) and actinomycin D, *J Biol Chem* 259:4714, 1984.
188. Brown SC, Mullis K, Levenson C, et al: Aqueous solution structure of an intercalated actinomycin D-dATGCAT complex by two-dimensional and one-dimensional proton NMR, *Biochemistry* 23:403, 1984.
189. Wadkins RM, Jovin TM: Actinomycin D and 7-aminoactinomycin D binding to single-stranded DNA, *Biochemistry* 30:9469, 1991.
190. Goldberg IH, Rabinowitz M, Reich E: Basis of actinomycin action. I. DNA binding and inhibition of RNA-polymerase synthetic reactions by actinomycin, *Proc Natl Acad Sci U S A* 48:2094, 1962.
191. Reich E, Franklin RM, Shatkin AJ, et al: Action of actinomycin D on animal cells and viruses, *Proc Natl Acad Sci U S A* 48:1238, 1962.
192. Kessel D, Wodinsky I: Uptake in vivo and in vitro of actinomycin D by mouse leukemias as factors in survival, *Biochem Pharmacol* 17:161, 1968.
193. Inaba M, Johnson RK: Decreased retention of actinomycin D as the basis for cross-resistance in anthracycline-resistant sublines of P388 leukemia, *Cancer Res* 37:4629, 1977.
194. Diddens H, Gekeler V, Neumann M, et al: Characterization of actinomycin-D-resistant CHO cell lines exhibiting a multidrug-resistance phenotype and amplified DNA sequences, *Int J Cancer* 40:635, 1987.
195. Galbraith WM, Mellett LB: Tissue disposition of 3H-actinomycin D (NSC-3053) in the rat, monkey, and dog, *Cancer Chemother Rep* 59:1601, 1975.
196. Furth JJ, Cohen SS: Inhibition of mammalian DNA polymerase by the 5′-triphosphate of 1-beta-d-arabinofuranosylcytosine and the 5′-triphosphate of 9-beta-d-arabinofuranoxyladenine, *Cancer Res* 28:2061, 1968.
197. Kufe DW, Major PP, Egan EM, et al: Correlation of cytotoxicity with incorporation of ara-C into DNA, *J Biol Chem* 255:8997, 1980.
198. Major PP, Egan EM, Herrick DJ, et al: Effect of ARA-C incorporation on deoxyribonucleic acid synthesis in cells, *Biochem Pharmacol* 31:2937, 1982.
199. Mikita T, Beardsley GP: Functional consequences of the arabinosylcytosine structural lesion in DNA, *Biochemistry* 27:4698, 1988.
200. Bianchi Scarra GL, Romani M, Coviello DA, et al: Terminal erythroid differentiation in the K-562 cell line by 1-beta-D-arabinofuranosylcytosine: accompaniment by c-myc messenger RNA decrease, *Cancer Res* 46:6327, 1986.
201. Plagemann PG, Marz R, Wohlhueter RM: Transport and metabolism of deoxycytidine and 1-beta-D-arabinofuranosylcytosine into cultured Novikoff rat hepatoma cells, relationship to phosphorylation, and regulation of triphosphate synthesis, *Cancer Res* 38:978, 1978.
202. Garcia-Carbonero R, Ryan DP, Chabner BA: Cytidine analogs. In Chabner BA, Longo DL, editors: *Cancer chemotherapy & biotherapy: Principles and practice*, Philadelphia, 2001, Lippincott Williams & Wilkins.
203. Ho DH, Frei E 3rd: Clinical pharmacology of 1-beta-d-arabinofuranosyl cytosine, *Clin Pharmacol Ther* 12:944, 1971.
204. Menaut P, Landart J, Behr S, et al: Treatment of 11 dogs with meningoencephalomyelitis of unknown origin with a combination of prednisolone and cytosine arabinoside, *Vet Rec* 162:241, 2008.
205. Smith PM, Stalin CE, Shaw D, et al: Comparison of two regimens for the treatment of meningoencephalomyelitis of unknown etiology, *J Vet Intern Med* 23:520, 2009.
206. Marconato L, Bonfanti U, Stefanello D, et al: Cytosine arabinoside in addition to VCAA-based protocols for the treatment of canine lymphoma with bone marrow involvement: does it make the difference? *Vet Comp Oncol* 6:80, 2008.
207. Allegra CJ, Fine RL, Drake JC, et al: The effect of methotrexate on intracellular folate pools in human MCF-7 breast cancer cells. Evidence for direct inhibition of purine synthesis, *J Biol Chem* 261:6478, 1986.
208. Allegra CJ, Chabner BA, Drake JC, et al: Enhanced inhibition of thymidylate synthase by methotrexate polyglutamates, *J Biol Chem* 260:9720, 1985.
209. Fabre I, Fabre G, Goldman ID: Polyglutamylation, an important element in methotrexate cytotoxicity and selectivity in tumor versus murine granulocytic progenitor cells in vitro *Cancer Res* 44:3190, 1984.
210. Wan SH, Huffman DH, Azarnoff DL, et al: Effect of route of administration and effusions on methotrexate pharmacokinetics, *Cancer Res* 34:3487, 1974.
211. Bischoff KB, Dedrick RL, Zaharko DS, et al: Methotrexate pharmacokinetics, *J Pharm Sci* 60:1128, 1971.
212. Mackey JR, Mani RS, Selner M, et al: Functional nucleoside transporters are required for gemcitabine influx and manifestation of toxicity in cancer cell lines, *Cancer Res* 58:4349, 1998.
213. Gandhi V, Plunkett W: Modulatory activity of 2′,2′-difluorodeoxycytidine on the phosphorylation and cytotoxicity of arabinosyl nucleosides, *Cancer Res* 50:3675, 1990.
214. Gandhi V, Legha J, Chen F, et al: Excision of 2′,2′-difluorodeoxycytidine (gemcitabine) monophosphate residues from DNA, *Cancer Res* 56:4453, 1996.
215. Huang P, Plunkett W: Fludarabine- and gemcitabine-induced apoptosis: incorporation of analogs into DNA is a critical event, *Cancer Chemother Pharmacol* 36:181, 1995.

216. Veltkamp SA, Pluim D, van Eijndhoven MA, et al: New insights into the pharmacology and cytotoxicity of gemcitabine and 2′,2′-difluorodeoxyuridine, *Mol Cancer Ther* 7:2415, 2008.
217. Veltkamp SA, Jansen RS, Callies S, et al: Oral administration of gemcitabine in patients with refractory tumors: a clinical and pharmacologic study, *Clin Cancer Res* 14:3477, 2008.
218. Veltkamp SA, Pluim D, van Tellingen O, et al: Extensive metabolism and hepatic accumulation of gemcitabine after multiple oral and intravenous administration in mice, *Drug Metab Dispos* 36:1606, 2008.
219. Tempero M, Plunkett W, Ruiz Van Haperen V, et al: Randomized phase II comparison of dose-intense gemcitabine: thirty-minute infusion and fixed dose rate infusion in patients with pancreatic adenocarcinoma, *J Clin Oncol* 21:3402, 2003.
220. Turner AI, Hahn KA, Rusk A, et al: Single agent gemcitabine chemotherapy in dogs with spontaneously occurring lymphoma, *J Vet Intern Med* 20:1384, 2006.
221. LeBlanc AK, LaDue TA, Turrel JM, et al: Unexpected toxicity following use of gemcitabine as a radiosensitizer in head and neck carcinomas: a veterinary radiation therapy oncology group pilot study, *Vet Radiol Ultrasound* 45:466, 2004.
222. Martinez-Ruzafa I, Dominguez PA, Dervisis NG, et al: Tolerability of gemcitabine and carboplatin doublet therapy in cats with carcinomas, *J Vet Intern Med* 23:570, 2009.
223. Jones PD, de Lorimier LP, Kitchell BE, et al: Gemcitabine as a radiosensitizer for nonresectable feline oral squamous cell carcinoma, *J Am Anim Hosp Assoc* 39:463, 2003.
224. Dominguez PA, Dervisis NG, Cadile CD, et al: Combined gemcitabine and carboplatin therapy for carcinomas in dogs, *J Vet Intern Med* 23:130, 2009.
225. Marconato L, Lorenzo RM, Abramo F, et al: Adjuvant gemcitabine after surgical removal of aggressive malignant mammary tumours in dogs, *Vet Comp Oncol* 6:90, 2008.
226. Marconato L, Zini E, Lindner D, et al: Toxic effects and antitumor response of gemcitabine in combination with piroxicam treatment in dogs with transitional cell carcinoma of the urinary bladder, *J Am Vet Med Assoc* 238:1004, 2011.
227. McMahon M, Mathie T, Stingle N, et al: Adjuvant carboplatin and gemcitabine combination chemotherapy postamputation in canine appendicular osteosarcoma, *J Vet Intern Med* 25:511, 2011.
228. Wohlhueter RM, McIvor RS, Plagemann PG: Facilitated transport of uracil and 5-fluorouracil, and permeation of orotic acid into cultured mammalian cells, *J Cell Physiol* 104:309, 1980.
229. Reyes P: The synthesis of 5-fluorouridine 5′-phosphate by a pyrimidine phosphoribosyltransferase of mammalian origin. I. Some properties of the enzyme from P1534J mouse leukemic cells, *Biochemistry* 8:2057, 1969.
230. Houghton JA, Houghton PJ: Elucidation of pathways of 5-fluorouracil metabolism in xenografts of human colorectal adenocarcinoma, *Eur J Cancer Clin Oncol* 19:807, 1983.
231. Snavely NR, Snavely DA, Wilson BB: Toxic effects of fluorouracil cream ingestion on dogs and cats, *Arch Dermatol* 146:1195, 2010.
232. Kufe DW, Major PP: 5-Fluorouracil incorporation into human breast carcinoma RNA correlates with cytotoxicity, *J Biol Chem* 256:9802, 1981.
233. Kufe DW, Major PP, Egan EM, et al: 5-Fluoro-2′-deoxyuridine incorporation in L1210 DNA, *J Biol Chem* 256:8885, 1981.
234. Tanaka M, Yoshida S, Saneyoshi M, et al: Utilization of 5-fluoro-2′-deoxyuridine triphosphate and 5-fluoro-2′-deoxycytidine triphosphate in DNA synthesis by DNA polymerases alpha and beta from calf thymus, *Cancer Res* 41:4132, 1981.
235. Santi DV, McHenry CS, Sommer H: Mechanism of interaction of thymidylate synthetase with 5-fluorodeoxyuridylate, *Biochemistry* 13:471, 1974.
236. Naguib FN, el Kouni MH, Cha S: Enzymes of uracil catabolism in normal and neoplastic human tissues, *Cancer Res* 45:5405, 1985.
237. Grem JL: 5-fluoropyrimidines. In Chabner BA, Longo DL, editors: *Cancer chemotherapy & biotherapy: principles and practice*, Philadelphia, 2001, Lippincott Williams & Wilkins.
238. Schiff PB, Fant J, Horwitz SB: Promotion of microtubule assembly in vitro by taxol, *Nature* 277:665, 1979.
239. Schiff PB, Horwitz SB: Taxol stabilizes microtubules in mouse fibroblast cells, *Proc Natl Acad Sci U S A* 77:1561, 1980.
240. Ringel I, Horwitz SB: Studies with RP 56976 (taxotere): a semisynthetic analogue of taxol, *J Natl Cancer Inst* 83:288, 1991.
241. Jordan MA, Toso RJ, Thrower D, et al: Mechanism of mitotic block and inhibition of cell proliferation by taxol at low concentrations, *Proc Natl Acad Sci U S A* 90:9552, 1993.
242. Bissery MC, Guenard D, Gueritte-Voegelein F, et al: Experimental antitumor activity of taxotere (RP 56976, NSC 628503), a taxol analogue, *Cancer Res* 51:4845, 1991.
243. Diaz JF, Andreu JM: Assembly of purified GDP-tubulin into microtubules induced by taxol and taxotere: reversibility, ligand stoichiometry, and competition, *Biochemistry* 32:2747, 1993.
244. McEntee M, Silverman JA, Rassnick K, et al: Enhanced bioavailability of oral docetaxel by co-administration of cyclosporin A in dogs and rats, *Vet Comp Oncol* 1:105, 2003.
245. McEntee MC, Rassnick KM, Bailey DB, et al: Phase I and pharmacokinetic evaluation of the combination of orally administered docetaxel and cyclosporin A in tumor-bearing cats, *J Vet Intern Med* 20:1370, 2006.
246. McEntee MC, Rassnick KM, Lewis LD, et al: Phase I and pharmacokinetic evaluation of the combination of orally administered docetaxel and cyclosporin A in tumor-bearing dogs, *Am J Vet Res* 67:1057, 2006.
247. Shiu KB, McCartan L, Kubicek L, et al: Intravenous administration of docetaxel to cats with cancer, *J Vet Intern Med* 25:916, 2011.
248. Correia JJ: Effects of antimitotic agents on tubulin-nucleotide interactions, *Pharmacol Ther* 52:127, 1991.
249. Wilson L, Jordan MA, Morse A, et al: Interaction of vinblastine with steady-state microtubules in vitro, *J Mol Biol* 159:125, 1982.
250. Bruchovsky N, Owen AA, Becker AJ, et al: Effects of vinblastine on the proliferative capacity of L cells and their progress through the division cycle, *Cancer Res* 25:1232, 1965.
251. Tucker RW, Owellen RJ, Harris SB: Correlation of cytotoxicity and mitotic spindle dissolution by vinblastine in mammalian cells, *Cancer Res* 37:4346, 1977.
252. Creasey WA, Marsh JC: Metabolism of vinblastine (VBL) in the dog, *Proceedings of the American Association for Cancer Research* 14:57 (abstract), 1973.
253. Vickery KR, Wilson H, Vail DM, et al: Dose-escalating vinblastine for the treatment of canine mast cell tumour, *Vet Comp Oncol* 6:111, 2008.
254. Grant IA, Rodriguez CO, Kent MS, et al: A phase II clinical trial of vinorelbine in dogs with cutaneous mast cell tumors, *J Vet Intern Med* 22:388, 2008.
255. Poirier VJ, Burgess KE, Adams WM, et al: Toxicity, dosage, and efficacy of vinorelbine (Navelbine) in dogs with spontaneous neoplasia, *J Vet Intern Med* 18:536, 2004.
256. Minocha A, Long BH: Inhibition of the DNA catenation activity of type II topoisomerase by VP16–213 and VM26, *Biochem Biophys Res Commun* 122:165, 1984.
257. Chen GL, Yang L, Rowe TC, et al: Nonintercalative antitumor drugs interfere with the breakage-reunion reaction of mammalian DNA topoisomerase II, *J Biol Chem* 259:13560, 1984.
258. Long BH, Musial ST, Brattain MG: Single- and double-strand DNA breakage and repair in human lung adenocarcinoma cells exposed to etoposide and teniposide, *Cancer Res* 45:3106, 1985.
259. Sullivan DM, Latham MD, Ross WE: Proliferation-dependent topoisomerase II content as a determinant of antineoplastic drug action in human, mouse, and Chinese hamster ovary cells, *Cancer Res* 47:3973, 1987.

260. Flory AB, Rassnick KM, Balkman CE, et al: Oral bioavailability of etoposide after administration of a single dose to tumor-bearing dogs, *Am J Vet Res* 69:1316, 2008.
261. Pommier YG, Goldwasser F, Strumberg D: Topoisomerase II inhibitors: epipodophyllotoxins, acridines, ellipticines, and bisdioxopiperazines. In Chabner BA, Longo DL, editors: *Cancer chemotherapy & biotherapy: principles and practice*, Philadelphia, 2001, Lippincott Williams & Wilkins.
262. Baxter JD, Harris AW, Tomkins GM, et al: Glucocorticoid receptors in lymphoma cells in culture: relationship to glucocorticoid killing activity, *Science* 171:189, 1971.
263. Greenstein S, Ghias K, Krett NL, et al: Mechanisms of glucocorticoid-mediated apoptosis in hematological malignancies, *Clin Cancer Res* 8:1681, 2002.
264. Moalli PA, Rosen ST: Glucocorticoid receptors and resistance to glucocorticoids in hematologic malignancies, *Leuk Lymphoma* 15:363, 1994.
265. Fichtinger-Schepman AM, van der Veer JL, den Hartog JH, et al: Adducts of the antitumor drug cis-diamminedichloroplatinum(II) with DNA: formation, identification, and quantitation, *Biochemistry* 24:707, 1985.
266. Zwelling LA, Anderson T, Kohn KW: DNA-protein and DNA interstrand cross-linking by cis- and trans-platinum(II) diamminedichloride in L1210 mouse leukemia cells and relation to cytotoxicity, *Cancer Res* 39:365, 1979.
267. Reed E, Kohn KW, Chabner BA, et al: Platinum analogues. In *Cancer chemotherapy: principles and practice*, Philadelphia, 1990, JB Lippincott.
268. Calvert AH, Newell DR, Gumbrell LA, et al: Carboplatin dosage: prospective evaluation of a simple formula based on renal function, *J Clin Oncol* 7:1748, 1989.
269. Bailey DB, Rassnick KM, Erb HN, et al: Effect of glomerular filtration rate on clearance and myelotoxicity of carboplatin in cats with tumors, *Am J Vet Res* 65:1502, 2004.
270. Kisseberth WC, Vail DM, Yaissle J, et al: Phase I clinical evaluation of carboplatin in tumor-bearing cats: a Veterinary Cooperative Oncology Group study, *J Vet Intern Med* 22:83, 2008.
271. Morgan JS, Creasey DC, Wright JA: Evidence that the antitumor agent hydroxyurea enters mammalian cells by a diffusion mechanism, *Biochem Biophys Res Commun* 134:1254, 1986.
272. Turner MK, Abrams R, Lieberman I: Meso-alpha, beta-diphenylsuccinate and hydroxyurea as inhibitors of deoxycytidylate synthesis in extracts of Ehrlich ascites and L cells, *J Biol Chem* 241:5777, 1966.
273. Skoog L, Nordenskjold B: Effects of hydroxyurea and 1-beta-D-arabinofuranosyl-cytosine on deoxyribonucleotide pools in mouse embryo cells, *Eur J Biochem* 19:81, 1971.
274. veer Reddy GP, Pardee AB: Inhibitor evidence for allosteric interaction in the replitase multienzyme complex, *Nature* 304:86, 1983.
275. Bianchi V, Pontis E, Reichard P: Changes of deoxyribonucleoside triphosphate pools induced by hydroxyurea and their relation to DNA synthesis, *J Biol Chem* 261:16037, 1986.
276. Rassnick KM, Al-Sarraf R, Bailey DB, et al: Phase II open-label study of single-agent hydroxyurea for treatment of mast cell tumours in dogs, *Vet Comp Oncol* 8:103, 2010.
277. Story MD, Voehringer DW, Stephens LC, et al: L-asparaginase kills lymphoma cells by apoptosis, *Cancer Chemother Pharmacol* 32:129, 1993.
278. Chabner BA, Sallan SE: Enzyme therapy: L-asparaginase. In Chabner BA, Longo DL, editors: *Cancer chemotherapy & biotherapy: principles and practice*, Philadelphia, 2001, Lippincott Williams & Wilkins.
279. Su AI, Welsh JB, Sapinoso LM, et al: Molecular classification of human carcinomas by use of gene expression signatures, *Cancer Res* 61:7388, 2001.
280. Golub TR, Slonim DK, Tamayo P, et al: Molecular classification of cancer: class discovery and class prediction by gene expression monitoring, *Science* 286:531, 1999.
281. Moseson DL, Sasaki GH, Kraybill WG, et al: The use of antiestrogens tamoxifen and nafoxidine in the treatment of human breast cancer in correlation with estrogen receptor values. A phase II study, *Cancer* 41:797, 1978.
282. Flaherty KT, Puzanov I, Kim KB, et al: Inhibition of mutated, activated BRAF in metastatic melanoma, *N Engl J Med* 363:809, 2010.
283. Paez JG, Janne PA, Lee JC, et al: EGFR mutations in lung cancer: correlation with clinical response to gefitinib therapy, *Science* 304:1497, 2004.
284. Ueda K, Cornwell MM, Gottesman MM, et al: The mdr1 gene, responsible for multidrug-resistance, codes for P-glycoprotein, *Biochem Biophys Res Commun* 141:956, 1986.
285. Mauldin G, Matus R, Patnaik A, et al: Efficacy and toxicity of doxorubicin and cyclophosphamide used in the treatment of selected malignant tumors in 23 cats, *J Vet Intern Med* 2:60, 1988.
286. Herzog TJ, Krivak TC, Fader AN, et al: Chemosensitivity testing with ChemoFx and overall survival in primary ovarian cancer, *Am J Obstet Gynecol* 203:68 e1, 2010.
287. Wakatsuki T, Irisawa A, Imamura H, et al: Complete response of anaplastic pancreatic carcinoma to paclitaxel treatment selected by chemosensitivity testing, *Int J Clin Oncol* 15:310, 2010.
288. Ugurel S, Schadendorf D, Pfohler C, et al: In vitro drug sensitivity predicts response and survival after individualized sensitivity-directed chemotherapy in metastatic melanoma: a multicenter phase II trial of the Dermatologic Cooperative Oncology Group, *Clin Cancer Res* 12:5454, 2006.
289. Staib P, Staltmeier E, Neurohr K, et al: Prediction of individual response to chemotherapy in patients with acute myeloid leukaemia using the chemosensitivity index Ci, *Br J Haematol* 128:783, 2005.
290. Lee JK, Havaleshko DM, Cho H, et al: A strategy for predicting the chemosensitivity of human cancers and its application to drug discovery, *Proc Natl Acad Sci U S A* 104:13086, 2007.
291. Staunton JE, Slonim DK, Coller HA, et al: Chemosensitivity prediction by transcriptional profiling, *Proc Natl Acad Sci U S A* 98:10787, 2001.
292. Potti A, Dressman HK, Bild A, et al: Retraction: Genomic signatures to guide the use of chemotherapeutics, *Nat Med* 17: 135, 2011.
293. Bonnefoi H, Potti A, Delorenzi M, et al: Retraction–Validation of gene signatures that predict the response of breast cancer to neoadjuvant chemotherapy: a substudy of the EORTC 10994/BIG 00-01 clinical trial, *Lancet Oncol* 12:116, 2011.
294. Baggerly KA, Coombes KR: Deriving chemosensitivity from cell lines: Forensic bioinformatics and reproducible research in high-throughput biology, *Ann Appl Stat* 3:1309, 2009.

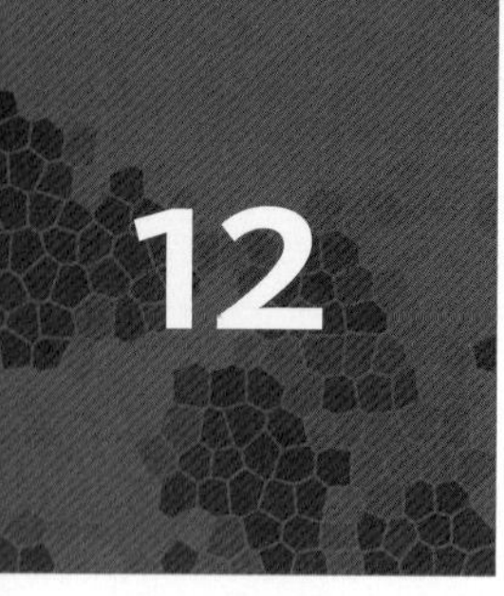

12 Radiation Therapy

Susan M. LaRue and Ira K. Gordon

Radiation therapy has been used in veterinary medicine since shortly after the discovery of x-rays by Roentgen in 1895. Alois Pommer, an Austrian veterinarian, published extensively on the irradiation of benign and malignant diseases and established a radiation therapy protocol widely used for many years.[1] Technologic advances improving our understanding of the radiation biology of normal and tumor tissues have enabled development of contemporary radiation therapy techniques and protocols.

Over half of human patients with serious cancers undergo radiation therapy at some point during treatment.[2] Radiation therapy is an effective treatment modality for animal cancer patients with solid tumors; however, early use of the modality was limited due to the sparse availability of veterinary treatment centers. The last decade has been marked by the opening of numerous veterinary radiation therapy centers and the commissioning of more advanced radiation therapy technologies. More than 60 facilities in North America are actively treating animals with radiation therapy and the American College of Veterinary Radiology (Specialty in Radiation Oncology) has residency training programs at 17 treatment centers.[3]

The management of cancer patients is complex, and determining the best treatment modality or combination of modalities can be challenging. In most instances, when local control of a solid tumor cannot be obtained surgically without excessively compromising an animal's function, appearance, or quality of life, a consultation with a radiation oncologist should be considered. In many such instances, combining surgery with radiation therapy will allow a more conservative surgery and yield comparable or better tumor control and/or functional outcome than either surgery or radiation alone. In other cases, radiation alone may be a preferred alternative to surgery (i.e., intranasal tumors).

In addition to treating serious cancers with what is referred to as "curative intent," radiation therapy also plays an important role in the palliative treatment of advanced cancers, the treatment of endocrinopathies associated with endocrine adenomas, and as an adjuvant treatment for lymphoma patients.

New modalities such as stereotactic radiation therapy (SRT), image-guided radiation therapy (IGRT), and intensity-modulated radiation therapy (IMRT) are also changing the treatment paradigm by providing improved radiation options for tumors in a variety of locations. Keeping abreast of ongoing clinical evaluation of these modalities is important for optimal patient management.

Biologic Principles of Radiation Oncology

Radiation dose is described by the amount of energy absorbed by the tissue. The unit of absorbed dose is the Gray (Gy); one Gy equals one joule absorbed per kilogram of tissue. Ionizing radiation kills cells by damaging critical molecules in the cell, primarily DNA, which eventually leads to cell death. Megavoltage photons, the predominant form of radiation used in veterinary medicine, interact with tissue primarily by the Compton effect, producing high energy electrons that cause ionization events either to critical molecules (direct effect) or from water molecules located within nanometers of critical molecules (indirect effect). These events produce highly reactive free radicals that result in biologic damage that may kill the cell or render it incapable of reproducing. In most cells, death from exposure to ionizing radiation results from chromosomal aberrations.

Repair of Radiation Damage

A critical determinant of a cell population's sensitivity to radiation is the ability of cells to repair DNA damage caused by radiation. One Gy of radiation from photons causes approximately 2500 base damages, 1000 single-strand breaks, and 40 double-strand breaks in DNA in each cell.[4] Most of this damage is repaired by cells within 6 to 24 hours; the double-strand breaks are the most lethal because they may lead to severe chromosomal aberrations. A given dose of radiation is preferentially cytotoxic to proliferating cells, including tumor cells and renewing cell populations (e.g., epithelial stem cells), although slowly dividing and nondividing cells (e.g., bone and cells of the nervous system) are also affected by radiation.

Cell Cycle Effects

The period of the cell cycle in which DNA undergoes synthesis is known as *S-phase*. Before and after S-phase are periods without overt activity by the DNA; these periods are called *G_1 phase* and *G_2 phase*. G_2 phase is followed by mitosis. Cells are distributed throughout the cell cycle in a tumor or tissue at a given time. The individual cell sensitivity to irradiation varies, depending on the phase of the cell cycle at the time of irradiation. Cells in late S-phase are most resistant to irradiation, and cells in late G_2 or mitosis are most sensitive.

Oxygen Effects

Because of their rapid growth and abnormal vasculature, tumors often become partially hypoxic. This results in upregulation of hypoxia-inducible proteins that may prepare the tumor cells to handle stresses. Oxygen is also a critical factor in the response to irradiation because reactive oxygen species (ROS) generate much of the damage from radiation. As a result, normoxic cells are up to threefold more sensitive to radiation than hypoxic cells.

Relative Biologic Effectiveness

Although this chapter primarily discusses the effects of photons (x-rays and gamma rays) and electrons, there are many other forms of radiation that can be used in oncology, including protons and neutrons. The biologic effects of 1 Gy of electrons are the same as 1 Gy of photons, but 1 Gy of protons or neutrons may cause substantially more damage than 1 Gy of photons or electrons. This difference is known as the relative biologic effectiveness (RBE) of the type of radiation.

Time, Dose, and Fractionation

Early radiation oncologists found that higher total doses could be given if the doses were divided into smaller fractions. They observed that tumor response was improved, and less injury of normal tissue occurred. In veterinary medicine, standard fractionation denotes a regimen delivering 2.7 to 4 Gy per fraction, 3 to 5 times per week to a total dose of 42 to 57 Gy, although several other regimens are currently being used or investigated. Hyperfractionation refers to schedules in which the dose per fraction is reduced and the total dose is increased. Accelerated fractionation describes a treatment regimen in which the overall time of treatment is reduced, but the dose per fraction and total dose are unchanged. Hypofractionation describes the administration of high doses per fraction given in a small number of fractions to a lower total dose. The response of tumor and normal tissues between fractions throughout the course of radiation therapy has been described by Withers[5] as the "four Rs" of radiation therapy: repair of DNA damage, redistribution of cells in the cell cycle, reoxygenation of tumor cells, and repopulation of tumor and normal tissues.

Division of the total radiation dose into fractions is important for a number of reasons. The first reason is to exploit potential differences in repair capabilities between tumors and normal tissues. Slowly dividing cells are somewhat less sensitive to small doses of radiation than more rapidly dividing cells; however, they appear to become relatively more sensitive if radiation is delivered in larger doses per fraction. If smaller doses per fraction are used, normal tissues with slowly dividing cells can be spared relative to tumor tissues with rapidly dividing cells.

Other events that occur between radiation fractions are cell cycle redistribution and reoxygenation. When a fraction of radiation therapy is administered, many of the cells in the sensitive portions of the cell cycle are killed. During the interval between fractions, cells from the late S-phase, which are more likely to be alive than other cells, progress to more sensitive parts of the cell cycle. This is known as *redistribution.* Reoxygenation also occurs during the interval between radiation fractions when many of the hypoxic tumor cells become aerobic and thus more sensitive to irradiation.

The length of time over which radiation therapy is administered is important, primarily because of tumor repopulation but also because of rapidly proliferating normal tissues, such as mucosa and skin. Tumor cells that have not been destroyed by irradiation continue to replicate during the course of therapy. This process is exacerbated by a phenomenon known as *accelerated repopulation.* Some have suggested that after approximately 4 weeks of therapy, tumors repopulate more rapidly than initially.[6] The reason for this is not clear, but the phenomenon could be related to (1) a reduction in the cell cycle time, (2) an increase in the number of tumor cells that are actively dividing, or (3) a reduction in the number of tumor cells that normally die (cell loss factor). Regardless of the cause, when treatment lasts longer than 4 weeks, repopulation may affect the outcome unless total dose is increased to account for this phenomenon. Repopulation may have a greater impact on rapidly dividing tumors than on slowly dividing tumors.

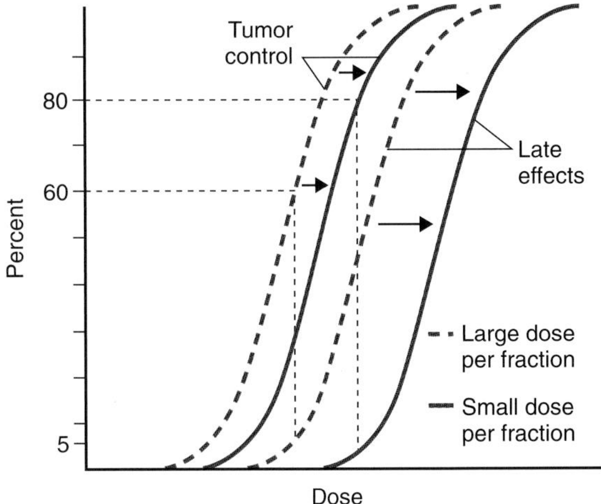

FIGURE 12-1 Radiotherapy delivered in small fractions *(solid lines)* can produce a higher probability of tumor control with the same level of late effects as radiotherapy delivered in large fractions *(broken lines).*

Repopulation of proliferating (also known as acutely responding) normal tissues is also affected by time. The same total dose of radiation administered over a short period results in somewhat more severe acute effects than if administered over a longer course. Nonproliferating (late-responding) normal tissues are not significantly affected by the length of time over which therapy is administered. Fraction size and the interval between treatment fractions are more important in late-responding tissues. Fractions should be separated by at least 6 hours to allow repair of DNA damage to normal tissues. Cells of the brain and spinal cord may require additional time for complete repair, and the impact of multiple fractions per day on these late-responding tissues is not clearly understood.

The total dose administered to a patient should have a low probability for causing significant late normal tissue reactions in the region of therapy. However, the response of tissues also depends on the fraction size. For example, 48 Gy administered in 4 Gy fractions has a higher probability of causing late effects than 48 Gy administered in 3 Gy fractions (Figure 12-1). The probability of tumor control is not as affected because rapidly proliferating tissues, including tumors, are not as sensitive to the change in dose per fraction. The benefits of protocols that use small doses per fraction are clear: they allow a higher total dose to be administered without increasing the probability of damage to late-responding normal tissues.

The total dose tolerated depends on the specific normal tissues present in the irradiated field. For example, brain and spinal cord are less tolerant to the effects of irradiation than muscle or bone. Another factor that must be considered when selecting the appropriate dose is the volume of tissue in the field. Large volumes of normal tissues are more susceptible to damage from irradiation than smaller volumes.

Although time, dose and fractionation are still the underpinnings of SRT, the paradigm is different than for fractionated radiation therapy. SRT involves the use of high doses per fraction but overcomes the radiobiologic limitations with stereotactically verified positioning and treatment delivery techniques that leave a minimal volume of normal tissue in the high dose area. Stereotactic radiation therapy, by definition, requires (1) a tumor for targeting (not microscopic disease), (2) treatment planning and administration that will provide a dramatic dose drop-off between the tumor and the surrounding normal tissue structures, and (3) a method of stereotactically verifying patient positioning. The result is that normal late-responding tissue structures are spared through dose avoidance rather than by administering small doses per fraction. The normal tissue structures still receive dose, and the dose per fraction is higher than for traditional radiation therapy. However, the total dose to the normal structures is lower than what is typical for fractionated radiation therapy. Normal tissue tolerance data are just evolving for SRT, as is long-term follow-up. Estimates of tolerance have been based on limited clinical data, toxicity observation, and educated guessing.[7] It is inappropriate to extrapolate dose constraints from fractionated protocols. An additional difference between SRT and fractionated radiation therapy is that with SRT, acutely responding normal tissues in the surrounding region such as skin, esophagus, and colon may be susceptible to consequential late effects. A consequential late effect is a late effect that develops from severe acute effects that may be associated with stem cell depletion. Dose constraints therefore must also be applied to these tissues. SRT treatment is generally delivered in 1 to 5 fractions over a period of 1 week or less for most tumors; therefore accelerated repopulation is unlikely to impact tumor control. Although historically stereotactic treatment was delivered in a single fraction (referred to as stereotactic radiosurgery), current technology allowing precise repositioning makes limited fractionation feasible. Even this minimal fractionation should allow higher total doses to be administered safely to late-responding tissues in the region and presumably take advantage of tumor reoxygenation and redistribution. However, biologic response following SRT has not been comprehensively evaluated. From a practical standpoint, SRT minimizes the number of anesthesia episodes to these older and sometimes debilitated patients and is also generally more convenient for the owner. Acute effects are minimal and tumor-associated signs such as discomfort or dysfunction often improve rapidly. Long-term tumor control and late effects need to be quantitated.

No perfect radiation therapy protocol exists, and all protocols commonly used in veterinary and human medicine have advantages and disadvantages. It is not within the scope of this chapter to prescribe specific radiation doses or fractionation schedules because many factors must be considered. Rather, referring veterinarians must know what to expect when sending patients to a radiation oncology center, and they should be able to explain some of the fundamental principles to clients. The radiation oncologist should inform the referring veterinarian and owner of the probabilities of late effects and tumor control and estimate the degree of acute effects expected with a specific protocol. The goal of radiation therapy is to destroy the reproductive capacity of the tumor without excessive damage to surrounding normal tissues. This goal is best achieved by dividing the total dose into a number of smaller fractions (fractionation) that are administered over a period of time or by applying stereotactic technology. Regardless of the approach, the relationship of these three parameters (time-dose-fractionation) must be carefully considered in the development of radiation treatment plans for successful therapy.

Acute and Late Effects

Reactions from radiation therapy are classified as acute (also called early) or late. Acute effects occur during or shortly after radiation therapy. Acute effects involve rapidly proliferating tissues, such as the oral mucosa, intestinal epithelium, and epithelial structures of the eyes and skin. Concurrent chemotherapy can exacerbate acute effects from radiation. These effects generally are self-limiting, and recovery is rapid. However, acute effects can be unpleasant for the patient and distressing to the owner, and in rare instances they can be life-threatening if the proper care is not given. The referring veterinarian often is called on to treat recently irradiated patients. Acute effects will heal without medical intervention in the vast majority of cases over the course of weeks or occasionally months. In veterinary patients, the most important provision to allow healing during this time is prevention of self-trauma of the radiation site by the patient. Therefore pain management plays an important role and should be addressed. Pain management for cancer patients is discussed in Chapter 15, Section A, of this text, and specific protocols have been published.[8] Additional treatment is based on common sense, supportive care, and the knowledge that the signs will resolve with time.

Late effects involve more slowly proliferating tissues, such as bone, lung, heart, kidneys, and nervous system. The dose of radiation administered is limited by the tolerance of these normal tissue structures in the field. Late reactions can be difficult to treat; it is the radiation oncologist's obligation to minimize the incidence of late effects with appropriate dose prescriptions and careful radiation planning and treatment. When late effects occur, they may be quite severe, resulting in fibrosis, necrosis, loss of function, or even death.[9] Late effects occur from thc loss of normal tissue stem cells with concurrent radiation-induced vascular changes and inflammation. These changes are multifactorial, but the cytokine transforming growth factor-β (TGF-β) is believed to play a critical role in radiation fibrosis. Strategies attempted in human radiation oncology to mitigate late radiation effects include the use of antioxidants and free radical scavengers (superoxide dismutase, vitamin E, thiol radioprotectors), vascular-directed therapies (clopidogrel, statins, pentoxifylline), antiinflammatory agents (corticosteroids), inhibitors of the renin-angiotensin system (angiotensin-converting enzyme [ACE] inhibitors), and stem cell therapies.[9] In veterinary patients, severe late reactions such as fibrosis and tissue necrosis should be managed under the guidance of or referred to a surgeon and/or radiation oncologist experienced in dealing with radiation injury.

Radiation-Induced Neoplasia

Ionizing radiation is a complete carcinogen, capable of initiating, promoting, and progressing cellular changes that lead to cancer. Therefore it is possible to see radiation-induced neoplasia develop in a radiation treatment field. It appears that orthovoltage radiation and radiation with high linear energy transfer (high-LET) such as neutrons result in carcinogenesis at a higher frequency than the megavoltage photons typically used in veterinary radiation therapy.[10] Other factors that influence the risk of radiation carcinogenesis include the age of the patient (young patients are more likely to develop subsequent tumors) and the tissues irradiated. Certain tissues are also more prone to development of radiation-induced tumors, such as the thyroid gland. For a tumor to be considered radiation induced, the following criteria must be met[10,11]:

1. The malignancy must arise within the irradiated field.
2. Sufficient latency must have elapsed between the time of irradiation and development of the tumor (typically at least 1 year).
3. The original tumor and the new tumor must have different histologic diagnoses.
4. The tissue in which the new tumor forms must have been normal prior to radiation exposure.

The overall incidence of radiation-induced tumors in patients treated with radiotherapy is thought to be extremely low (<1% to 2% of patients treated).[11]

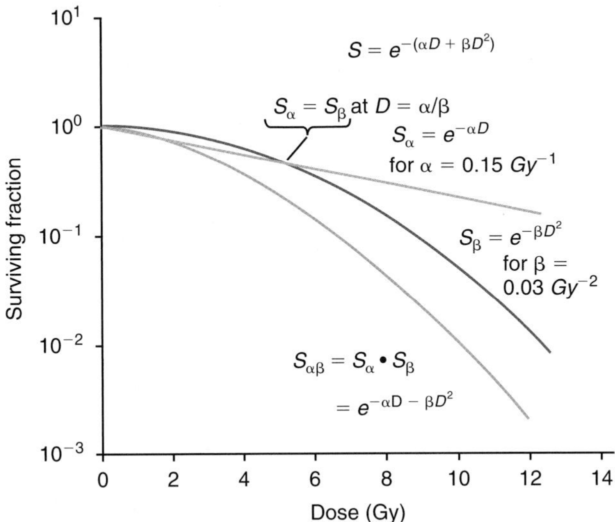

FIGURE 12-2 Illustration of the alpha/beta (α/β) model in which cell killing occurs by either a single-even process or a double-even process so that the overall killing by either process is the product of the two, and the (α/β) ratio is the dose at which both processes contribute equally to the total killing. Note that the upper curve is survival for the α component only, the middle curve is for the β component only, and the lower curve is for both components. *(Redrawn from Wilson PF, Bedford JS. In Hoppe RT, Phillips TL, Roach M III, editors:* Leibel and Phillips textbook of radiation oncology, *ed 3, St. Louis, 2010, Elsevier.)*

Cell Survival After Irradiation

After a tissue or population of cells is exposed to any dose of radiation, a fraction of the cells will be killed. The proportion of remaining cells is known as the *surviving fraction* (S). The sensitivity of a tumor or tissue to radiation can be shown as a graph of the radiation dose (D) versus the surviving fraction (Figure 12-2).[12] The relationship between a dose of radiation and the surviving fraction of cells is commonly described by the linear quadratic equation:

$$S(D) = e^{-(\alpha D + \beta D^2)}$$

where *S* is the surviving fraction at a dose *(D)*.[13] Alpha (α) and beta (β) are constants that vary according to the tissue with α corresponding to the cell death that increases linearly with dose and β corresponding to cell death that increases in proportion to the square of the dose (also known as the *quadratic component*). The α/β ratio is a useful number that is the dose in Gy when cell kill from the linear and quadratic components of the cell survival curve is equal. Cells with a higher α/β ratio have a more linear appearance when plotted on a log scale, and cells with a low α/β ratio have a parabolic shape. The α/β ratio is also an important description of the radiosensitivity of a cell. At low-dose fractions, tissues or cells with low α/β ratio are relatively radiation resistant compared to tissues or cells with high α/β ratio. It has been suggested that tissues and cells with low α/β ratios have a greater capacity for repair of sublethal radiation damage. Sublethal radiation damage is defined as damage that can become lethal if it interacts with additional damage. Sublethal damage repair is the reason that cell survival increases when a radiation dose is split into two fractions separated by a time interval.

Most early responding tissues and tumors have a high α/β ratio, whereas late-responding tissues have a low α/β ratio.[13] There are some tumors that may have a low α/β ratio, which can influence the optimal radiation prescription in terms of total dose, time, and fractionation. Tumors that may have lower α/β ratios include melanoma, prostatic tumors, soft tissue sarcomas, transitional cell carcinoma, and osteosarcomas.[14-16]

The concept of biologic effective dose (BED) is used to predict how changes in dose prescription may preferentially affect different cells or tissues based on their α/β ratio in the linear quadratic model of survival. The formula for BED is as follows:

$$BED = nd\,[1 + d/(\alpha/\beta)]$$

where *n* is the number of fractions and *d* is the dose per fraction. If the α/β ratio of a tissue is known or can be estimated, one can calculate the BED for any dose prescription. It is possible to use this formula to assess how dosimetry changes or errors alter the effective dose of a protocol. It is important to note that there are several limitations to the use of this equation, including that it does not account for differences in the overall length of time of the radiation protocol or accelerated repopulation. There are other formulas that can be used to account for time. Also, the true α/β ratio of any cell or tissue is rarely known; therefore calculations made with this model involve making assumptions or predictions that may be incorrect. Nevertheless, this formula is a useful tool when considering hyperfractionating or hypofractionating a standard radiation protocol in order to create a new protocol that will have expected outcomes related to either tumor control or tissue complications. However, the validity of BED for SRT is unclear.

Alternative Mechanisms of Radiation Injury

In addition to direct radiation cytotoxicity, the extracellular matrix and local microenvironment also appear to play an important role in radiation response. Some evidence suggests that apoptosis of endothelial cells may precede damage to proliferating cells and cause some of the effects observed after radiation. Apoptosis of endothelium primarily occurs when high-dose fractions are administered and may play a more important role when hypofractionated and radiosurgical doses of radiation are delivered.

Chemical Modifiers of Radiation

Although rarely used clinically in veterinary medicine, many drugs can modify the cellular and tissue response to radiation. Radioprotectors (e.g., amifostine/WR-2721) are compounds that decrease the amount of radiation damage to targeted normal cells without providing similar protection to tumor cells. Radiosensitizers are chemicals that achieve greater tumor inactivation than would be expected from the additive effect of treatment with either radiation or the chemical alone. Mechanisms of action of radiation sensitizers include hypoxic cell sensitizers or cytotoxins and agents that damage or incorporate into DNA.

Palliative Radiation Therapy

Palliative radiation therapy is commonly used in human medicine, and its use in veterinary medicine has increased in recent years. Palliative radiation is generally hypofractionated compared to curative intent protocols, often administered in larger doses per fraction (6 to 10 Gy per fraction) in 1 to 4 total fractions once or twice weekly. Conversely, palliative therapy can be delivered in conventional doses or modestly hypofractionated daily or twice daily for a short but intense treatment regimen. The goal of palliative radiation therapy is not to provide long-term or definitive tumor control; rather, it is intended to relieve pain or improve function or quality of life in patients in which other factors (e.g., advanced metastatic disease) are likely to lead to early demise. Palliative radiation therapy has been used most often for metastatic or primary bone tumors, principally canine osteosarcoma (see Chapter 24). Palliative therapy is more convenient for the owner, and the cost is modest compared with curative radiation therapy because fewer fractions are administered. It is, however, important to remember that palliative radiation is not a substitute for curative-intent protocols despite the convenience. Some palliative therapy protocols may have an increased probability of causing late radiation effects but because they are prescribed to patients that have a poor long-term prognosis, these late effects may not have time to manifest. Curative-intent radiation protocols require strict adherence to radiation biologic principles; palliative radiation protocols, on the other hand, are far more flexible. As in human hospital settings, the protocols may vary dramatically from radiation center to radiation center.

Radiation Therapy Equipment

Ionizing radiation can be administered by an external source (teletherapy), through placement of radioactive isotopes interstitially (brachytherapy), or by systemic or cavitary injection of radioisotopes, such as iodine-131 (^{131}I). Teletherapy, also referred to as *external-beam radiation therapy,* is the most commonly used method of radiation therapy in veterinary medicine. External-beam radiation therapy usually is classified as orthovoltage or megavoltage radiotherapy, based on the energy of the photon. Orthovoltage machines produce x-rays with an energy of 150 to 500 kVp; megavoltage radiation emits photons with an average energy greater than 1 million electron volts (1 MeV). Although some veterinary radiation oncology centers continue to treat with orthovoltage machines, megavoltage radiation is primarily used. Megavoltage radiation for therapy can be obtained from cobalt machines or linear accelerators. Because megavoltage radiation has excellent tissue-penetrating capabilities, radiation therapy can be performed on deeply seated tumors for which orthovoltage therapy would not be an option.

Orthovoltage x-rays, which have low energy, distribute maximum doses to the skin surface. Acute effects to the skin can be quite severe, causing discomfort to the patient, and late effects to the skin and subcutaneous tissues can be dose limiting. Megavoltage radiation has a higher energy than orthovoltage, and the photons must interact with tissues, allowing the dose to build up, before the maximum dose can be achieved. The skin therefore can receive a significantly weaker dose than the underlying tumor. This skin-sparing effect of megavoltage radiation allows the optimal dose to be administered to a more deeply seated tumor without causing severe reactions to the skin. When the tumor involves the skin or is in proximity of skin, megavoltage radiation can be used successfully by placing a sheet of tissue-equivalent material, called a *bolus,* over the tumor. This allows the dose build up to occur before reaching the skin, so that the skin and associated tumor can receive the maximum dose of radiation.

The absorption of megavoltage radiation, unlike that of orthovoltage radiation, is minimally dependent on the composition of the tissue. This characteristic permits even distribution of the dose throughout the tissues in the field. Orthovoltage radiation is preferentially absorbed by bone. If a tumor adjacent to or overlying bone is administered a meaningful dose of orthovoltage radiation, the probability that late effects to the bone (bone necrosis) will develop is quite high. Treatment with orthovoltage should be limited to small, superficial tumors such as nasal planum tumors or to superficial tumor beds after surgical excision. The interaction of megavoltage radiation with tissues is quite predictable, which has allowed the development of computerized treatment planning systems. These planning systems allow treatment of the tumor with multiple beams administered from different angles. Beam modifiers, such as wedges and blocks, can be incorporated into the treatment plan. Wedges are triangular-shaped pieces of lead that can be placed between the beam and the patient. Less radiation penetrates the thick side of the wedge, which modifies the dose distribution. The goal of computerized treatment planning is to ensure a desired minimum tumor dose to a region specified by the radiation oncologist and to spare normal tissue structures when possible. Conventional radiation therapy uses a limited number of computed tomography (CT) or magnetic resonance imaging (MRI) images, which are imported or contoured using a tablet. The summation of multiple beams coming from different directions provides a higher dose to the tumor than surrounding tissues.

Advances in treatment planning and imaging over the past decade have led to the development of image-based, three-dimensional (3D) conformal radiation therapy (3DCRT), which permits better conformity between the irradiated high-dose volume and the geometric shape of the tumor (Figure 12-3). 3DCRT requires importation of CT, MRI, or positron emission tomography (PET) imaging into the treatment planning system. The animal must be positioned for the imaging in a fashion that can be replicated precisely on a day-to-day basis for treatment. Alpha cradles, acrylic face masks, bite plates, and/or Vac-Lok Cushions (Figure 12-4) often are used as positional aids. The radiation oncologist identifies important normal tissue structures, as well as the gross tumor volume (GTV), clinical target volume (CTV), and planning target volume (PTV) on these images. By definition, the GTV only includes gross tumor, and the CTV includes the GTV plus an expansion based on the known clinical behavior of the specific tumor to account for regional microscopic disease. For example, the CTV expansion for a sarcoma is generally larger than for a carcinoma. If the patient has had cytoreductive surgery and only microscopic tumor remains, there is no GTV, and the CTV is based on the scar, regions of surgical disruption, and an expansion for microscopic disease beyond the surgical site. In addition to the GTV and CTV, the PTV includes expansion for an internal margin (IM) that accounts for variations in size and shape relative to anatomic landmarks (filling of bladder, respiratory movements) and set-up margin (SM). The SM accounts for uncertainties in patient positioning and alignment during planning imaging and subsequent treatments. The better the immobilization device, the smaller the SM expansion can be. SM expansions will vary based on the location of the tumor because some sites such as the head are more amenable to rigid immobilization devices such as bite blocks, which provide better replicability. The IM expansion is impacted more by the radiation therapy device. Machines with on-board-imaging devices such as kV x-ray or cone-beam CT (CBCT) can have more confidence in smaller IM expansions. Decreasing the PTV expansion by using good immobilization and available imaging impacts the volume of normal tissue treated and is a key component to successful 3DCRT and is critical to other advanced treatment modalities. More sophisticated beam shaping is performed by taking advantage of fixed multileaf collimators or custom-made blocks. A major advantage of 3DCRT is that dose-volume

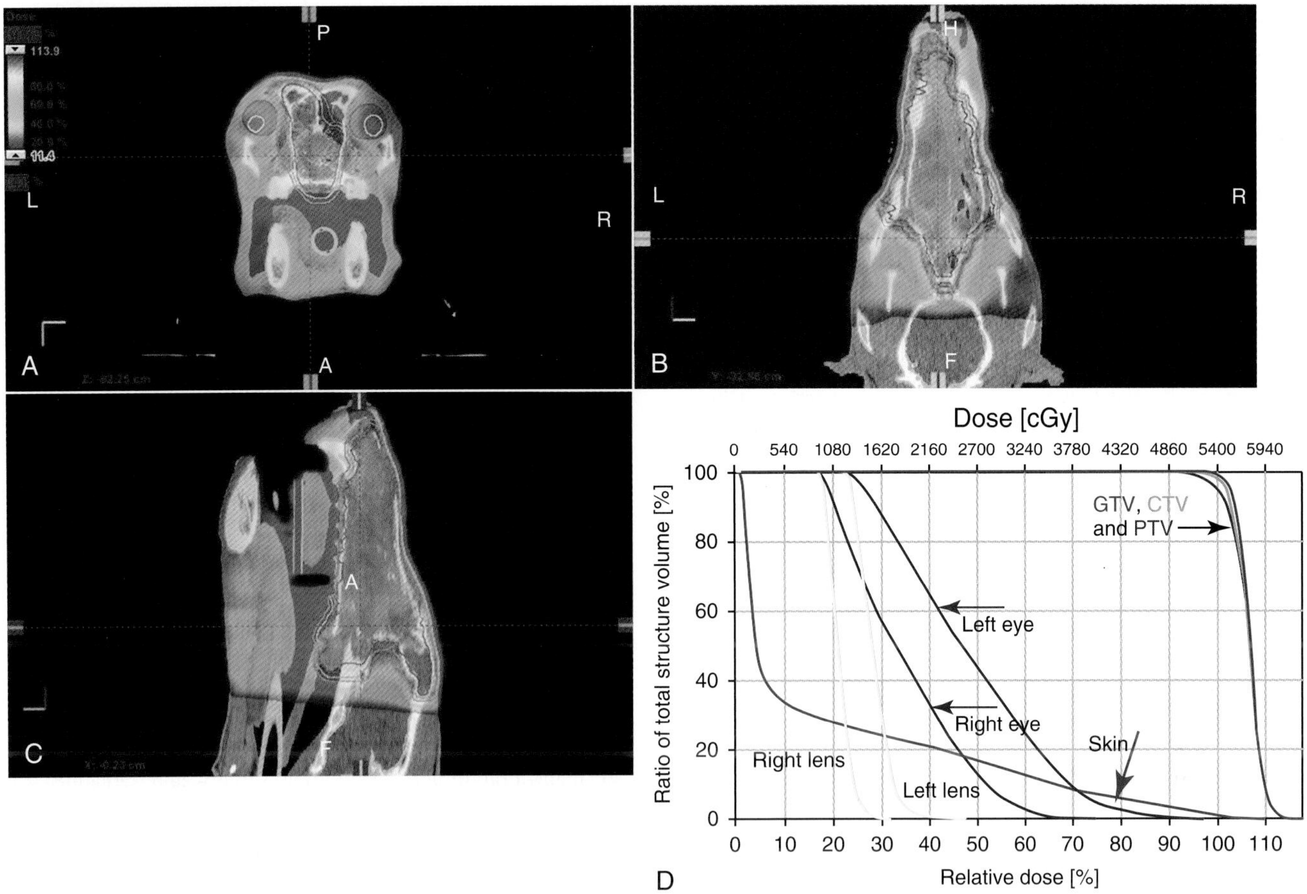

FIGURE 12-3 **A** to **C,** The axial, dorsal, and sagittal sections through a canine nasal tumor. Dose is in color wash, with the prescribed dose in orange. **D,** The dose-volume histogram. Note the high dose to the tumor compared to regional normal tissue structures.

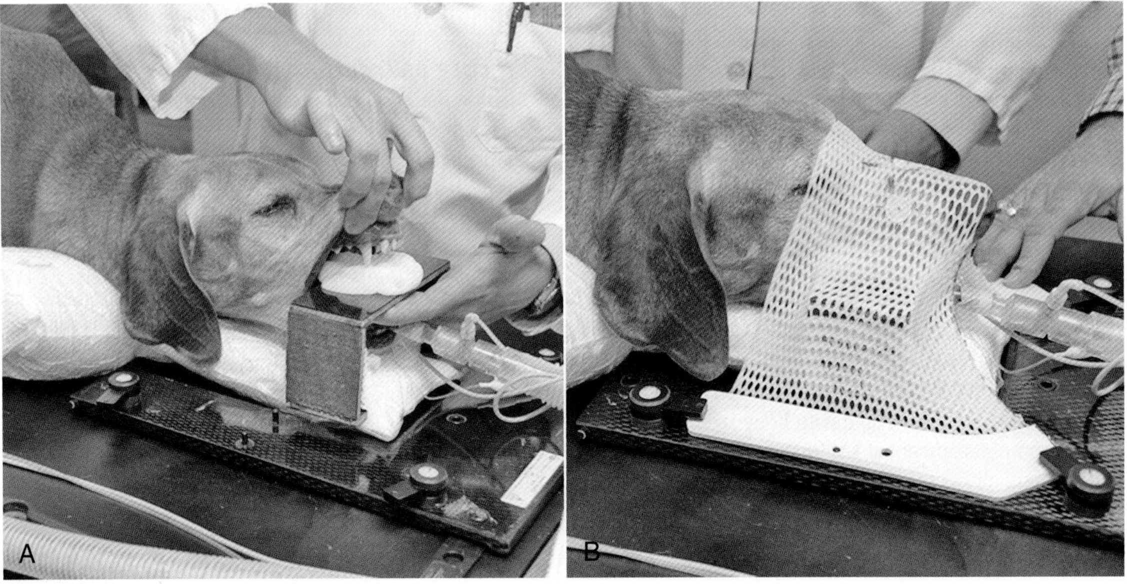

FIGURE 12-4 **A,** Teeth being placed in preformed acrylic bite block that is inserted into a carbon fiber–indexed frame. Neck is resting on a vacuum lock bag. **B,** Acrylic face mask being placed.

histograms can be obtained for the tumor and normal tissue structures. This provides a quantitative method of evaluating treatment plans and enhances quality assurance. Defined dosimetric parameters may be useful predictors of outcome.

IMRT and related modalities such as tomotherapy allow even greater sculpting of the radiation dose. These modalities require strategies for patient positioning and immobilization. IMRT requires a specific treatment planning system that uses *inverse planning*. Inverse planning requires that the various tumor structures (GTV, CTV, and PTV), as well as critical normal tissue structures, be identified and contoured into the planning system. Optimization objectives for each structure are entered, and a sophisticated algorithm attempts to meet all objectives. This is the standard of care for treatment of prostate tumors, head and neck cancers, vertebral cancers, some brain cancers, and pelvic cancers in humans. A major benefit associated with IMRT is that the dose to adjacent normal tissue structures can be minimized, dramatically reducing acute effects. Patients are more comfortable and require less pain medication.[17] In addition, the tumor dose can be increased without exceeding normal tissue tolerance, presumably leading to improved tumor control. Fractionation schedules similar to those for conventional radiation therapy are used. Tomotherapy, a form of IMRT that uses a helical delivery system to sculpt the beam, is also being used in veterinary medicine.[18,19] IMRT is proving useful for the treatment of tumors or tumor beds with complex geometry located near important normal tissues, such as nasal tumors, oral tumors, urogenital tumors, and in cats, vaccine-associated sarcomas.[17]

SRT describes an emerging field in radiation oncology that uses advanced technology to achieve a different biologic approach. It was originally coined *stereotactic radiosurgery* (SRS) when the gamma knife was first developed for treatment of inoperable brain tumors in the 1950s by Lars Leksell.[20] The gamma knife uses hundreds of small cobalt sources that can converge in 3 dimensions to focus precisely on a small volume of tumor. The gamma knife initially required a rigid frame-based positioning device that was bolted into the patient's skull prior to imaging and treatment planning. Therefore it was primarily used as a single fraction treatment. CyberKnife is a robotic radiosurgery system incorporating a small linear accelerator on a movable robotic arm, integrating advances in robotic technology and real-time computer-tracking technology.[21] The small linear accelerator is moved around the patient and tumor by the robotic device, while the tracking system verifies position by tracking fiducial markers placed in the tumor prior to treatment planning. This frameless tracking system makes repeat fractions feasible, allowing the benefits of modest fractionation. It also makes treating tumors in other parts of the body possible. SRT can also be delivered by specially designed linear accelerators that have designated beams with attributes conducive to small fields and on-board imaging (OBI) capability. Patients are placed in positioning devices such as bite blocks, face masks, and Vac-Lok cushions prior to imaging. For tumors associated with bony structures such as nasal or brain tumors, orthogonal kV images are obtained and the operating software allows the patient's treatment position to be "matched" to the original imaging positioning. The couch will then make an automatic adjustment. For tumors that may move relative to adjacent bone, CBCT is used and a 3D match is used to verify tumor position.[22] The benefits of accelerator-based SRT are that treatment times are generally short, almost any tumor location is accessible, and tumors with larger volumes can be treated.

A number of acronyms are used to describe hypofractionated stereotactic radiation treatment. SRS refers primarily to treatment of brain tumors and generally, but not always, refers to a single fraction treatment. *Stereotactic body radiation therapy* (SBRT), SRT, and *stereotactic ablative radiation therapy* (SAbR) are interchangeable terms used to describe 1 to 5 fraction treatment regimens, regardless of method of administration. Of key importance is the recognition that these stereotactic procedures require gross tumor as a target, must have dramatic dose drop-off between tumor and normal tissues, and must have a method of stereotactic verification.

Radiosurgery has been used on a limited basis in veterinary medicine for brain and bone tumors[23-25] and more recently for nasal tumors, multilobular osteochondromas, pituitary tumors, thyroid tumors, heart-based tumors, sarcomas, and tumors in the pelvic canal (personal communications, James Custis, Susan LaRue).[26] Technologic advances such as those described previously are likely to become available on a limited basis over the next decade. An important consideration is identifying which tumor types will benefit most from such approaches.

Tumors Commonly Treated with Radiation Therapy

Oral Tumors

Many oral tumors (see Chapter 22, Section A) are responsive to radiation therapy. The region is anatomically complex, and aggressive surgery often can leave functional and cosmetic abnormalities. For many oral tumors, combining surgery and radiation will provide the best outcomes; however, the optimal time to begin irradiation after surgery (or surgery after irradiation) has not been determined. If difficulty in obtaining primary wound healing appears likely, radiation can be delayed. However, the therapeutic gain from combining modalities will be lost if the tumor recurs in the interim. Initiating radiation therapy immediately after surgery does not appear to be a problem if the suture line is tension free and well vascularized. Mucosal flaps can be used successfully to close surgical defects in the oral cavity of patients that will receive postoperative radiotherapy, but complications are common.[27]

Efficacy of Treatment

Acanthomatous ameloblastomas, previously called adamantinomas or acanthomatous epulides, are very radiation responsive. Tumor control with radiation therapy can be close to 90%.[28] A relationship has been demonstrated between tumor (T) stage and local control.[29] The reported 3-year, progression-free survival (PFS) for T1 tumors (less than 2 cm) and T2 tumors (2 to 4 cm) is 86%; it is only about 30% for T3 tumors (over 4 cm).[29] In 2004 a retrospective study of 57 dogs with epulides that were treated with irradiation reported that the overall median time to first event and overall survival were 1210 and 1441 days, respectively.[30] Dogs younger than 8.3 years old (the median age in the study) had a significantly longer median survival time (2322 days) than dogs older than 8.3 years (1106 days). Dogs that received doses higher than 40 Gy had significantly longer survival times than dogs that received 40 Gy or less (2994 days versus 143 days).

Canine oral squamous cell carcinomas (SCCs) are responsive to radiation, although the prognosis is site dependent with tumors located more rostrally having better probability of control.[31] Tumors of the base of the tongue and tonsil are highly metastatic and are likely to recur locally or regionally. In these locations, radiation therapy has an advantage over surgery because it includes associated lymphatic structures in the treatment field. A 1987 study of oral SCC treated with a coarse fractionation protocol of 10 4.5-Gy fractions resulted in tumor control at 1 year of about 75%.[32] Another study of oral tumors reported a PFS at 1 and 3 years of 72% and 40% for SCC of all T stages.[33] A 1996 study of fractionated radiotherapy (48 to 57 Gy in 3 to 4 Gy fractions) in 14 dogs with SCC reported a median disease-free interval and survival of 365 and 450 days, respectively.[34]

In cats, oral SCC has a very poor prognosis.[35] Although many cats show an initial response and may even show dramatic reductions in tumor size, rapid tumor recurrence is common. Combining curative-intent radiation with etanidazole or mitoxantrone therapy has resulted in median survival times of 116 to 170 days.[36,37] In one study, seven cats with mandibular SCCs that were treated with hemimandibulectomy and mandibular node excision followed by radiation therapy had a median survival time of 420 days.[38] Although the numbers are limited, mandibular SCCs may have a better prognosis than sublingual SCC. Recent studies have indicated that palliative (coarsely fractioned) radiation therapy, with or without chemotherapy, for cats with oral SCC is of dubious value.[39,40] Another approach investigated in nine cats with oral SCC was accelerated radiotherapy (14 fractions of 3.5 Gy in 9 days), which resulted in a median survival of 86 days although three cats had a complete response with a median survival of 298 days.[41] Although radiation is likely to play a role in the treatment of this disease, new approaches are indicated.

Oral fibrosarcomas are unlikely to metastasize but can be difficult to control locally. The histologic appearance can be deceptive; tumors diagnosed as fibromas or low-grade fibrosarcomas can be extremely aggressive locally.[42] If clinical evidence of rapid growth, invasion into bone, or tumor recurrence exists, the tumor should be treated aggressively in spite of more benign pathologic features. En bloc surgical resection often is curative but difficult to accomplish because of the invasive nature of the tumor. Oral fibrosarcomas are less radiosensitive than epulides and SCC, although tumor control probabilities ranging from 33% to 67% at 1 year have been reported.[43,44] One study of oral fibrosarcomas reported a PFS at 1 year and 3 years of 76% and 55%, respectively.[33] Surgical cytoreduction improves the probability of tumor control by radiation therapy, and this should be taken into consideration during surgical planning with a focus on removing clinical disease (avoiding extensive local dissection, which increases the radiation field size) and obtaining a tension-free closure provided that all macroscopic tumor is removed. Forrest and colleagues[45] reported a median survival time of 540 days in eight dogs with oral sarcomas treated with surgery followed by irradiation. In tumors too large to be surgically resected to a subclinical level, radiation therapy alone is indicated; the probability of long-term tumor control is low with conventional radiation therapy, but new strategies using IMRT or SRT are currently being evaluated.

Malignant melanoma is the most common oral tumor in dogs and is associated with a high rate of regional and distant metastasis.[46] Higher doses of radiation per fraction (4 Gy and above) are believed to improve response rates for melanoma. In one study, 38 dogs with oral melanoma without evidence of metastasis were treated with 48 Gy delivered in 4 Gy fractions on a Monday-Wednesday-Friday schedule.[33] The median PFS was 17.8 months for all dogs and was stage dependent; for T1 tumors, it was 38 months; for T2 tumors, 11.7 months, and for T3 tumors, 12 months. A retrospective study of 140 dogs evaluated a population of dogs, most of which had regional or distant metastasis at presentation.[47] Coarsely fractionated (9 to 10 Gy weekly fractions to a total dose of 30 to 36 Gy) and conventionally fractionated (2 to 4 Gy fractions to as high as 45 Gy or more) protocols were used with or without surgery or chemotherapy. The median times to first event and survival were 5 and 7 months, respectively. Tumor recurrence was the first event in only 27% of the dogs, with new metastases or death accounting for the other 63%. In a retrospective study of 39 dogs with incompletely resected oral melanoma treated with coarsely fractionated radiation therapy plus platinum-based chemotherapy, the median survival time was 363 days.[48] The dogs received 6 weekly fractions of 6 Gy, with cisplatin (10 to 30 mg/m^2) or carboplatin (90 mg/m^2) administered 1 hour before irradiation. Fifteen percent of the dogs failed locally, and the median time to metastasis was 311 days.

Melanoma is frequently treated with immunotherapy to potentially prevent or delay the onset of metastasis. Immunotherapy is unlikely to be successful if the primary tumor is not controlled locally with radiation therapy and/or surgery. It is not currently known whether concurrent administration of a melanoma vaccine with radiation therapy may enhance or diminish the effectiveness or toxicities associated with each treatment.

Five cats with oral malignant melanoma were treated with 8 Gy delivered on days 0, 7, and 21. All died from progressive disease, and median survival was 146 days.[49]

Radiation Considerations

Reproducibility of treatment fields for oral tumors can be aided by positioning and immobilization devices. Depending on the size and location of the target, IMRT allows better sparing of surrounding normal structures, such as the eyes and salivary glands. Melanoma may have a low α/β ratio, making them more responsive to coarsely fractionation protocols.[50]

Treatment-Related Toxicities

Treatment toxicity depends on the time-dose-fractionation of the protocol and the specific normal structures in the treatment field. For oral tumors, this can include the skin, nasal cavity, and eyes, which are discussed in subsequent sections. The major acute complication associated with radiation treatment of the oral cavity is mucositis. Mucositis always occurs to some degree in patients that have received irradiation to the oral cavity, pharynx, and/or esophagus. Mucositis typically begins during the second week of therapy and reaches a maximum severity during or shortly after the last week of therapy. Clinical signs include thickened saliva and tenderness of the mouth. These patients occasionally become reluctant to eat or drink and require supportive care. Low-salt foods are more palatable and less irritating to the oral mucosa than regular commercial diets. Rarely, placement of a gastrostomy or esophagostomy tube may be necessary to facilitate feeding. Oral mucositis should subside 1 to 2 weeks after therapy. Rarely, animals treated with chemotherapy subsequent to a course of radiotherapy can develop a return of radiation side effects such as mucositis, which is a phenomenon known as *radiation recall.*

Late complications of radiation specific to the oral cavity include osteoradionecrosis, xerostomia, and oronasal fistula development. Xerostomia (dryness of the mouth due to salivary dysfunction) is a common complication in human patients undergoing radiation therapy of the head and neck region; however, clinically significant xerostomia is not commonly recognized in animals. IMRT technology should provide improved sparing of salivary glands and may decrease the volume of tissue with mucositis. Osteoradionecrosis or development of nonvital bone susceptible to pathologic fracture after radiotherapy is an uncommon complication that can occur in any bone in a radiation field, typically years after treatment. The mandible is the most susceptible bone to osteoradionecrosis but as with most late effects, the risk can be minimized by administering radiation in lower dose per fraction. Oronasal fistula development after radiation is rare unless the hard or soft palate has been disrupted by an aggressive tumor or oral surgery. At one time, it was suggested that radiation therapy could result in transformation of epulides into malignant epithelial tumors, but this possibility has since been refuted.[28,30]

Nasal Tumors

Nasal tumors (see Chapter 23, Section B) in dogs are difficult to control. Surgery, chemotherapy, cryosurgery, or immunotherapy alone does not appear to improve survival over no treatment.[51-56] Radiation therapy provides the best reported tumor control for canine nasal tumors and likely needs to be part of any curative-intent treatment regimen.

Efficacy of Treatment

Radiation therapy has long been the standard of care for nasal and sinonasal tumors. The location is not generally amenable to complete surgical resection, and most reports combining radiation therapy and surgery have not demonstrated therapeutic gain compared to radiation alone. Interestingly, over the last 20 years, advancement in treatment planning technology from point calculations to 2-dimensional (2D), 2.5-dimensional, and 3DCRT technologies has not been associated with improved tumor control or survival. Megavoltage radiation therapy alone has been reported to provide a median survival of about 1 year.[57-59] Histologic subpopulations may be prognostically significant; however, most publications are hampered by inadequate patient numbers. Nasal SCCs, undifferentiated carcinomas, and anaplastic carcinomas have been reported to have survival times of 4 to 6 months, and chondrosarcomas have been reported to have survival times up to 15 months. Cribriform erosion has been associated with a poor prognosis.[60] Adams and colleagues[61] reported a median survival time of 47.7 months in a small group of dogs that underwent surgery in cases in which a nasal tumor did not regress at least 80% 6 weeks after radiation. Late effects were significant; 9 of 13 dogs developed rhinitis, and 4 progressed to osteonecrosis. Surgery and coarse fractionation reduce normal tissue tolerance to radiation, which likely contributed to the high percentage of patients with late effects in this study. The role of chemotherapy combined with radiation therapy for nasal tumors is still unclear. Studies using conventional or low-dose chemotherapy have not improved the outcome over radiation alone.[52,58] Radiation therapy combined with slow-release cisplatin implanted intramuscularly in a small group of dogs significantly improved survival compared with a group of historic controls with sarcomas and carcinomas treated with radiation therapy alone.[62] The median survival time for 14 dogs in the combined radiation-cisplatin protocol was 580 days, compared to 325 days for the 13 dogs in the radiation-only group. In a follow-up study of 51 dogs treated with the same radiation-cisplatin regimen, the median survival time was 474 days.[63]

Two recent publications evaluated outcome in dogs with nasal tumors treated with IMRT.[17,64] Thirty-one dogs treated with IMRT were compared to 36 historic controls treated with the same prescription using 2D treatment planning. Duration of survival was 420 days and 410 days, respectively.[64] In another report, twelve dogs treated with IMRT to a dose commonly used for 2D or 3DCRT planning had a median survival of 446 days.[17] Patient numbers in both studies were low, and there was no stratification for prognostic factors. Although conclusions cannot be made regarding tumor control, the decrease in acute effects to the region in both studies was profound. Although it seems intuitively obvious that improved tumor control would require dose escalation, reducing acute effects and keeping patients more comfortable during treatment may allow more patients to complete treatment as prescribed.

SRT, delivered in 3 daily fractions of 9 to 10 Gy, has been used to treat over 40 dogs with nasal tumors. Treatment was well tolerated with few acute effects, and early improvement in clinical signs was noted. Median survival time was 411 days.[65] Lymphoproliferative nasal tumors in cats respond well and durably to radiation therapy (these are addressed later in the chapter in the section on lymphoma; also see Chapter 32).[66] Carcinomas and sarcomas in cats respond comparably to nasal tumors in dogs: 48 Gy administered in 4 Gy fractions over 4 weeks had a 1-year survival rate of 44.3% and a 2-year survival rate of 16.6%.[67] The histologic type and clinical stage of the tumor did not affect the prognosis.

Nine dogs with recurrent nasal tumors previously treated with 3DCRT (median 50 Gy), were reirradiated.[68] Overall median survival from initial treatment was 31 months with an increased incidence of late effects. Retreatment becomes a more viable option with new modalities that spare local normal tissues.

The response to planum nasale SCC is affected by the tumor type and stage.[69] Cats with T1 tumors had a 1-year survival rate of 85% and a 5-year survival rate of 56%, and the mean was 53 months (the median was not calculable). However, larger, more invasive tumors showed a less favorable response when treated with 40 Gy in 4 Gy fractions over 3.5 weeks. Tumor control should be improved by reducing the dose per fraction and increasing the total dose. For small, superficial SCC lesions of the planum nasale in cats, strontium (Sr)-90 plesiotherapy is a viable option. Because Sr-90 emits a low-energy β particle, very high doses can be administered to the surface of a lesion without unacceptable complications or damage to underlying tissue. In one study, 49 cats with SCC of the planum nasale were administered a median of 128 Gy in a single fraction, with a complete response rate of 88% and median progression-free interval of 1710 days. Larger, invasive SCC lesions are usually not amenable to treatment with Sr-90.[70]

Radiation Considerations

Canine and feline sinonasal tumors are challenging to treat with radiation because they are anatomically complex; they frequently involve the nasal sinuses, the cribriform plate, and the nasal pharynx. The geometry of the nasal cavity is problematic because the target is larger caudally than rostrally, making it difficult to achieve even dose distribution. The dose-sculpting benefits of IMRT and SRT decrease acute effects. Optimizing protocols, including modest dose escalation, may lead to improved tumor control. Evidence-based studies need to thoroughly evaluate the impact of IMRT and SRT on acute responding tissues, tumor control, and late effects.

Treatment-Related Toxicities

Because nasal tumors are immediately adjacent to the oral cavity, radiation toxicities of nasal treatment are similar to those described previously for the oral cavity. Radiation side effects in the nasal cavity may mimic signs of the tumor, such as nasal discharge, sneezing, and epistaxis. In most dogs, these clinical signs actually improve rather than worsen during treatment despite acute radiation effects because of the response of the tumor. Recurrence of clinical signs of an intranasal tumor (nasal discharge, sneezing, epistaxis) may indicate chronic radiation effects or tumor recurrence. Ocular radiation complications are extremely common because of the proximity of the nasal cavity and frontal sinus to the orbit. Effects to the eyes are dose related and vary in severity.[71] Acute effects include blepharitis, blepharospasm, conjunctivitis, and the development of keratoconjunctivitis sicca (KCS). KCS is treated with artificial tears and steroids to prevent corneal ulceration. If corneal ulceration is present, healing may be delayed as a result of radiation damage to the corneal stem cells. KCS may be temporary or permanent, depending on the dose administered and the sensitivity of the patient. Late effects include vascular changes, which may have subtle effects on vision but in most cases do not result in blindness. Radiation-induced cataracts may occur, and the latent period is related to dose. These cataracts can be removed with phacoemulsification. Eyes that are in the field of irradiation may receive the full treatment dose. At doses above 40 Gy, degenerative angiopathy of retinal vessels can progress over 2 years and result in retinal degeneration. Optic nerve axonal degeneration has occurred secondary to the retinal changes.[72] IMRT decreases dose to the ocular region, resulting in limited acute and late toxicities.[64]

Brain Tumors and Pituitary Tumors

Brain tumors can be treated successfully with radiation therapy (see Chapter 30). In the treatment of brain tumors, surgery may be indicated to relieve life-threatening clinical signs. Although appropriate studies are still needed, for animals with less severe clinical signs, reported survival times after radiation for brain tumors in dogs are frequently comparable to surgery alone. Adjuvant radiation is indicated in patients with incomplete surgical resection; combined surgery and radiation may provide the best long-term control. Radiation therapy alone should be performed in dogs with cancer at surgically inaccessible sites or in locations in which surgical morbidity is high. SRT is being evaluated for treatment of a wide variety of brain tumors in dogs and cats.

Efficacy of Treatment

Published survival times of canine brain tumors treated with radiotherapy compare favorably to surgery, although directly comparable data is lacking, and combined surgical and radiation treatment may be superior. In one study, 46 dogs with brain tumors that initially had shown neurologic signs were treated with radiation alone.[69] The median overall survival time was 23.3 months; 69% of the dogs survived 1 year, and 47% survived 2 years. The outcome in this study was superior to those from previous reports, in which the median survival time was about 1 year. No prognostic clinical factors (e.g., tumor size or location or clinical signs) were identified.[73-75] Differences may be due to improved treatment planning capabilities. In another study by Axlund et al of 31 dogs with meningioma, postoperative radiation improved the median survival time from 7 months with surgery alone to 16.5 months with surgery followed by radiation therapy. Stereotactic radiation therapy has been used to treat brain tumors.[23] In a recent preliminary summary of 20 dogs with presumed meningiomas treated with 3 fractions of SRT, median survival was 594 days, and treatment was well tolerated (personal communication, Lynn Griffin, CSU).

Radiation therapy should be used in dogs and cats with pituitary macroadenomas because pituitary tumors generally are responsive to radiation, and surgical access is limited. Dogs with pituitary tumors have been reported to have median survival times varying between 1 and 2 years.[76,77] A study comparing 19 dogs with pituitary tumors receiving radiation therapy (48 Gy in 16 daily fractions of 3 Gy) to untreated dogs found 1-, 2-, and 3-year survival rates of 93%, 87%, and 55% in the irradiated group and 45%, 32%, and 25% in the unirradiated group. Tumor size as assessed by relative tumor area to brain area was prognostic in the irradiated patients. Fractionated pituitary irradiation in dogs is more effective at delaying tumor growth than in controlling adrenocorticotropic hormone (ACTH) secretion. Eucortisolism is seen in some patients after irradiation; however, pre-ACTH and post-ACTH cortisol levels should be monitored at regular intervals so that medications can be modified, if indicated.

Cats seem to have marked clinical improvement of associated endocrinopathies. In one study, eight cats with pituitary tumors were treated with radiation therapy, and neurologic signs improved within 2 months in all cats.[78] Endocrinopathies, including hyperadrenocorticism, acromegaly, and insulin-resistant diabetes, were dramatically improved. The median survival time, regardless of cause of death, was 17.4 months. A study evaluating conformal radiation–focused treatment of 11 cats (single dose of 15 to 20 Gy) found improved regulation of diabetes mellitus in 5/9 cats and improved neurologic function in 2/2 cats, with a median survival time of 25 months. SRT was administered in 3 to 4 fractions to 19 acromegalic cats with macroscopic or microscopic pituitary tumors. Median survival has not been reached, with 90% of cats alive at 1 and 2 years. Insulin-resistant diabetes and other associated endocrinopathies improved. The treatment was well tolerated acutely[26] (see Chapter 25).

Radiation Considerations

The integration of 3D imaging, patient-positioning devices, and advanced treatment planning techniques have the potential to improve tumor targeting and sparing of normal brain tissue. For many brain tumors, IMRT will not provide an improved dose distribution compared to 3DCRT; however, dose sculpting may be beneficial for cranial nerve tumors. An additional consideration in patients undergoing radiation therapy for a brain tumor is anesthetic risk related to increased intracranial pressure or brainstem disease; an appropriate anesthetic regimen should be selected to minimize the risk of complications. Specifically, patients should be ventilated while under anesthesia to decrease partial pressure of carbon dioxide (P_{CO_2}) in the blood, and anesthetic agents that decrease (or at least do not increase) intracranial pressure should be selected. SRT limits the number of anesthetic episodes, which may be beneficial in unstable patients. SRT can be used with curative intent or in a single fraction for palliative purposes.

Treatment-Related Toxicities

For most brain tumors, acute effects to the skin can be avoided with megavoltage treatments. Occasionally, ocular and auricular side effects or mucositis to the caudal oral cavity may be seen if in or adjacent to the treatment field. The radiation tolerance is lower when the entire brain is treated; this limits prescription of a dose that is adequate for tumor control but still has an acceptable probability of late effects. The radiation tolerance of brain and spinal tissues is generally considered to be less than that of other commonly treated tissues, and volume may be an important factor for brain and spinal lesions. Early delayed effects can occur 1 to 3 months after treatment and may be due to transient demyelination. Animals with early delayed effects may have signs similar to those of the initial presentation, or they may be generally stuporous. Early delayed effects occur in up to 40% of humans undergoing brain irradiation; symptoms include headache, lethargy, and exacerbation of focal neurologic signs.[79] In animals, clinical signs often are transient, but response time can be slow. Sometimes administration of systemic cortisone and aggressive supportive care are required. CT and MRI may show an apparent increase in tumor size and tumor enhancement during this time. Focal enhancement in normal brain associated with edema and demyelination may also be present.[80]

Late effects probably occur in veterinary patients more often than identified and should be considered as a differential diagnosis for signs that occur during that interval. Late delayed effects (more commonly referred to simply as late effects) generally occur at least 6 months after treatment but can also occur years later. Late effects are associated with brain necrosis. The probability of late brain effects depends on the total dose, the fraction size, and the volume of brain irradiated. In a study of 83 dogs with brain masses treated with a hypofractionated protocol (38 Gy administered in 5 weekly fractions), brain necrosis was confirmed or suspected in 14% of dogs (32.7 months).[81] The signs are similar to those associated with early delayed effects, although the response to steroids is limited. Clinically, distinguishing between late effects and tumor recurrence can often be difficult. CT or MRI evaluation can be misleading. Not all brain tumors completely recede after treatment; therefore the presence of a mass does not always indicate a recurring tumor. A prudent course is to obtain a CT or MRI evaluation 6 months after treatment to serve as a reference if clinical signs develop in the future.

Superficial Tumors of the Trunk and Extremities

Many tumors involving the trunk or extremities are amenable to treatment by radiation therapy. Combining radiation therapy with surgery enhances tumor control and improves the functional outcome better than surgery or radiation alone. For tumors in nonresectable locations, radiation alone may provide a good outcome depending on tumor type and volume. The surgeon and radiation oncologist should consult before therapeutic intervention is started to develop an overall treatment approach.

Hemangiopericytomas, fibrosarcomas, neurofibrosarcomas, myxosarcomas, and nerve sheath tumors are classified together as soft tissue sarcomas because of their similar biologic behavior (see Chapter 21). Metastases are uncommon with grade 1 and grade 2 sarcomas; therefore local tumor control is the primary concern. Soft tissue sarcomas are locally invasive, and tumor cells may extend far beyond the bulk of the tumor. Surgery alone is curative if the tumor can be removed completely.[82] If surgical resection is attempted, the margins should be closely examined by a pathologist for evidence of tumor infiltration. If tumor cells extend out to the margin, radiation therapy should be recommended if further resection is not possible. If it is apparent that a tumor cannot be excised completely, treatment combining radiation and surgery can be beneficial. Radiation therapy can be administered first with the hope of converting an inoperable tumor into an operable one. This approach has the benefit of reducing the volume of normal tissues irradiated. As an alternative, surgical excision can be performed first as a cytoreductive procedure and then followed by radiation therapy to kill the residual subclinical disease. In one study, 48 dogs with soft tissue sarcomas were treated with surgical cytoreduction followed by radiation therapy; only 8 dogs (16%) developed tumor recurrence, and the 5-year survival rate was 78%.[83] In a different study, which involved 38 dogs with soft tissue sarcomas of the body and extremities, treatment with surgery followed by irradiation provided a median survival time of 2270 days.[45] In comparison, soft tissue sarcomas treated by narrow surgical excision alone have recurrence rates of 17% to 40%.[84-89]

Soft tissue sarcomas can be treated with radiation therapy alone; however, tumor control is not as durable as with a combination of radiation therapy and surgery.[43] Radiation therapy alone is useful for tumors near the pads, where surgical options are limited. Pads in the irradiation field initially may slough; however, if appropriate fractionation schemes are used, the pads regrow and can function normally. Local hyperthermia has been used effectively with radiation therapy to improve local tumor control in canine soft tissue sarcomas.[90] Currently, no facilities are able to administer hyperthermia. Adjuvant chemotherapy has been considered for grade 3 soft tissue sarcomas because of the higher metastatic potential of these tumors; however, definitive evidence of improvement in local tumor control or survival is lacking.

Cutaneous mast cell tumors (grades 1 and 2) can be treated successfully with radiation therapy (see Chapter 20). The obvious advantage is that greater margins can be obtained with radiation than with surgery. The probability of control may be improved if surgical cytoreduction is performed first. In a study involving 37 dogs with grade 2 tumors treated with cytoreduction and radiation therapy, tumor control at 1 and 2 years exceeded 90%.[91] In 56 dogs with incompletely resected mast cell tumors, the medium disease-free interval was 32.7 months.[92] Radiotherapy also is indicated for cutaneous mast cell tumors with regional lymph node metastasis. In one study, 19 dogs with mast cell tumors and regional node involvement were treated with surgical cytoreduction of the primary site, radiation to the primary tumor and regional node, and prednisone.[93] The median disease-free survival time was 1240 days. Palliative radiation therapy is commonly used to treat locoregional mast cell tumors in dogs when systemic spread has occurred.

Vaccine-associated soft tissue sarcomas are a significant problem in cats (see Chapter 21). These tumors are challenging to control locally and seem unresponsive to aggressive radiation therapy or conservative surgery alone. In one study, 33 cats with histologically confirmed fibrosarcomas were treated with radiation therapy followed by surgery.[94] The median disease-free interval and the overall survival time were 398 and 600 days, respectively. In another study, 25 cats with subclinical disease after surgery were treated with radiation therapy alone (57 Gy delivered in 3 Gy fractions) and in some cases with adjuvant chemotherapy.[95] The overall median survival time was 701 days. Recurrence was seen in 7 cases (5 of 18 [27.8%] in the group treated with doxorubicin and 2 of 7 [28.6%] in the group not treated with doxorubicin). In the recurrence cases, one tumor developed outside the treatment field and the others arose in the area treated with radiation. Metastases to the lung or other sites were not seen in this group of cats. Similar findings were evident in 78 cats treated with surgical cytoreduction followed by radiation.[96] In this study, cats that underwent only one surgery before radiation had a lower recurrence rate than cats that had more than one surgery. The survival time and the disease-free interval shortened as the time between surgery and the start of radiation therapy lengthened. In a study of 79 cats treated with either preoperative or postoperative radiation therapy, packed cell volume (PCV) higher than 25 was associated with better outcome (median survival 760 days) than cats with PCV lower than 25 (306 days).[97]

Cats with surgically nonresectable disease present a greater challenge. Escalation of the radiation dose by delivering the dose in smaller fractions probably is necessary for these patients. IMRT or SRT may be beneficial for obtaining adequate dose to the tumor because appropriate sparing of the lungs, viscera, and spinal cord is critical in these patients.

Radiation Considerations

Many tumors of the limbs and trunk extend very close to the skin surface. Application of an appropriate thickness of a bolus material over the skin is frequently needed when treating with megavoltage photons in order to avoid underdosing the superficial region. When treating a sloped surface such as around a limb, side-scatter equilibrium is lost, resulting in heterogeneous dose distribution that can lead to significant underdosing of tumor and/or overdosing of the skin. The use of tapered bolus can reduce such dose inhomogeneity. Whenever possible, when an extremity is in a radiation field, a 1 to 2 cm strip of tissue should be shielded to avoid the risk of lymphedema, which can present as painful swelling of the distal limb.

Treatment-Related Toxicities

When treating superficial tumors, early effects to the skin are expected and are restricted to the radiation field. The severity of effect is dose related, and the patient may have a variety of lesions. Epilation is common and in some cases may be permanent. The hair may not return for several months, and the amount of regrowth varies in relation to the dose administered to the skin and the individual patient's sensitivity. Damage to the melanocytes may result in hypopigmentation or hyperpigmentation of the skin and/or alteration of the coat color when regrowth occurs, often resulting in whitish-gray fur (leukotrichia). Dry desquamation may accompany epilation; this generally does not cause any problem or discomfort for the patient and usually is not treated. Moist desquamation, which usually appears 3 to 5 weeks after the start of therapy, is associated with pruritus, which can vary in severity. Self-inflicted mutilation exacerbates the problem and may lead to ulceration or necrosis. Severe late effects to the skin are rare in fractionated therapy but include fibrosis and necrosis.

Bone Tumors

Although osteosarcomas are not considered highly radiation-responsive tumors, radiation may be considered as part of a multimodality therapy when surgical excision is not an option. (Radiation therapy for osteosarcoma is discussed at length in Chapter 24.) Radiation therapy can be combined with chemotherapy and surgery for limb-sparing protocols.[98,99] In a retrospective study of multimodality therapy for axial skeletal osteosarcoma, dogs that underwent curative-intent radiation protocols had a longer duration of tumor control (265 days) than those treated with a palliative regimen (79 days).[100] SRT is currently being evaluated as a limb-sparing alternative. In one study, stereotactic radiosurgery was performed on 11 dogs with appendicular osteosarcomas,[24] and although radiation dose varied and not all dogs received adjuvant chemotherapy, good limb function and tumor control were observed in some of the patients. Fifty dogs with appendicular osteosarcoma underwent treatment with SRT followed by chemotherapy. Sites included distal radius and proximal and distal humerus, femur, and tibia. All dogs had improved limb function with no clinical recurrences.[25] Fracture was observed in dogs with severely lytic lesions at or before 90 days.[101] Criteria were established for patient selection, including evaluation of radiographs and CT scans, reducing fracture rate to less than 20% (personal communication, James Custis). Prophylactic stabilization is indicated in dogs with severely lytic lesions. The mechanism of the amelioration of pain caused by bony neoplasia is not completely understood. Relief of pain may occur almost immediately or may be delayed, sometimes as long as 2 weeks. Human studies have indicated that single, coarsely fractionated radiation may be comparable or superior to multifraction protocols using more conventional doses per fraction.[102] In a recent study of 58 dogs, 8 Gy was administered on 2 consecutive days, providing onset of pain relief within 2 days in 91% of patients.[103] Commonly in veterinary medicine, 7 to 10 Gy fractions have been administered on days 0, 7, and 21.[104,105] In one study, 12 of 15 dogs with appendicular bone tumors treated with palliative radiation therapy had improved limb function, and the median survival time was 130 days.[105] In another study, dogs with appendicular osteosarcoma were given either 3 fractions of 10 Gy or 2 fractions of 8 Gy.[106] Seventy of the 95 dogs experienced pain relief, with a median duration of 73 days. No difference in response was found between the two treatment groups. Sometimes, localized pain recurs before metastatic disease becomes life limiting. Palliative radiation can be readministered as long as the owners understand that continued administration of large doses per fraction eventually leads to late effects.

Radiation Considerations

Radiation is unlikely to have a substantial palliative effect if a pathologic fracture from a bone tumor is already present. Additional padding and support during anesthetic recovery is important to prevent a recovering patient from trying to stand prematurely and injuring the affected limb.

Treatment-Related Toxicities

The most common and concerning bone tumor treatment–related toxicity is pathologic fracture. Most likely, the bone tumor itself rather than any effects of radiation makes the bone susceptible to fracture; however, the pain-relieving effects of radiation and/or other treatments may make animals more likely to put significant weight on the affected limb, resulting in fracture.

Other Tumors

Radiation therapy is used for a variety of tumors in the thoracic and abdominal cavities (Table 12-1). The principles of patient selection for radiation therapy with tumors in these regions are the same as for any other region. Radiation therapy should be considered for any tumor that cannot be excised completely. In one study, dogs with thyroid carcinomas treated with 48 Gy delivered in 4 Gy fractions had PFS rates of 80% at 1 year and 72% at 3 years.[119] Thymomas are radiation responsive in human patients.[120] In a study of seven cats with thymoma that were treated with radiation therapy, the median survival time was close to 2 years (see Chapter 33, Section B).

Palliative radiation therapy can be useful for tumors that may be causing airway, bowel, or urinary tract obstruction or neurologic dysfunction. Mediastinal lymphoma often responds rapidly to irradiation. Relief from respiratory distress can be achieved within hours of a single dose of radiation.

Eighteen dogs with primary disease of the urinary bladder (7), urethra (1), or prostate (10) were treated with IMRT assisted by image guidance to verify tumor position (personal communication, Michael Nolan). The majority of patients were treated with adjuvant chemotherapy and nonsteroidal antiinflammatory drugs (NSAIDs). In all dogs, the radiation dose ranged from 54 to 58 Gy, delivered in 20 daily fractions. Acute and late tissue toxicity was limited, and treatment was well tolerated. Overall median survival time was 654 days. Location of primary tumor had no demonstrable effect on either local tumor control or survival.

Perianal adenocarcinomas and anal sac adenocarcinomas (see Chapter 22, Section H) can be difficult to control locally with surgery alone and are likely to spread to regional lymph nodes. One hundred and thirteen dogs with carcinomas of the apocrine gland were treated with surgery, radiation therapy, chemotherapy, or multimodal treatment. Overall median survival was 544 days. Dogs treated with chemotherapy alone had significantly shorter survival

Table 12-1 Tumors Commonly Treated with Radiation Therapy

Tumor Location/Type	Treatment Modality	Control or Survival Data	Comments	References
Brain Tumors				
Brain tumors, various types and locations—dogs	Radiation	Median survival: 23.3 months.		69
Pituitary macroadenomas and carcinomas—dogs	Radiation only	1 year: 93%, 2 years: 87%, and 3 years: 55% survival.		107
Pituitary macroadenomas and carcinomas—cats	Radiation only	Overall median survival: 17.4 months, but tumor-related median not reached.	May produce profound improvement in endocrinopathies.	78
	Conformal single fraction	Median survival: 25 months.	55% improved insulin response.	108
	SRT	1 and 2 year: 85% survival.	Decreased insulin requirements in all patients.	26
Tumors of the Extremities and Body—Dogs				
Soft tissue sarcomas	Radiation only	1-year control: 67%. 2-year control: 33%.		43
	Surgery plus radiation	Median control: 86%. Median survival: 5-6 years.	Conservative surgery followed by radiation.	45, 83
Mast cell tumors	Radiation only	1-year control: 44%-78%.		109, 110
	Surgery plus radiation	1-year control: About 90%. Median disease-free interval: 33 months.	For grade 2 tumors.	91
	Surgery plus radiation	Disease-free survival: 3.4 years.	Primary tumor with regional node involvement.	93
Ceruminous gland tumors—dogs and cats	Surgery plus radiation	1-year control: 56%. Mean control: 39.5 months.		111
Tumors of the Extremities and Body—Cats				
Vaccine-associated sarcomas	Radiation followed by surgery	Median disease-free interval: 13-20 months. Median survival: 20 months.	PCV >25, good prognostic indicator.	92, 94, 97, 112
	Surgery followed by radiation	Median survival: 23-43 months.		95, 113
Lymphoma (localized)	Radiation ± chemotherapy	Median survival: 28 months.	Nonnodal, localized forms.	114
Nasal Tumors—Dogs				
Carcinomas (all)	Megavoltage radiation therapy	Median control: 8-12.8 months.	The role of adjuvant chemotherapy has not been determined. Preoperative surgery does not appear to improve tumor control.	52, 57, 58, 60
	IMRT	Median control: 14-15 months.	Dramatically reduced acute effects.	17, 64
Adenocarcinomas	Megavoltage radiation therapy	Median control: 10-12.8 months.		52, 57, 58, 60
Squamous cell tumors	Megavoltage radiotherapy	Median control: 5-8 months.		
Sarcomas (all)	Megavoltage radiotherapy	Median control: 8-12.8 months.		
Chondrosarcomas	Megavoltage radiotherapy	Median control: 12-15 months.		
Carcinomas and sarcomas (all)	Megavoltage radiotherapy	Median control: 16-19 months.	Slow-release cisplatin–impregnated polymer used for sensitization.	62, 63

TABLE 12-1 Tumors Commonly Treated with Radiation Therapy continued

TUMOR LOCATION/TYPE	TREATMENT MODALITY	CONTROL OR SURVIVAL DATA	COMMENTS	REFERENCES
Nasal Tumors—Cats				
Lymphoma	Orthovoltage or megavoltage radiotherapy	Median survival: 20.8 months.		115
Sarcomas and carcinomas	Megavoltage radiotherapy	Median survival: 11.5 months.		66
Oral Tumors—Dogs				
Acanthomatous ameloblastoma	Radiation only	1-year survival: 85% Median: 48 months.	No evidence of malignant transformation.	29, 30
Squamous cell carcinoma	Radiation only	1-year survival: 65%.		31, 33, 116
Fibrosarcoma	Radiation only	Median control: 4 months.	Surgical cytoreduction followed by radiation therapy improves tumor control.	43, 44
Melanoma	Radiation ± surgery and chemotherapy	Median survival: 8-10 months.	A variety of fractionation schedules. Metastatic disease is a major obstacle to survival.	33, 47, 117, 118
Osteosarcoma—Dogs				
Extremities	SRT limb sparing Radiation (palliative)	10-12 months. Median survival: 4 months.	Multiple sites feasible. Provides pain relief.	24, 106
Axial skeleton	Radiation ± surgery and chemotherapy	Median survival: 4.5 months.	Surgery is performed for cytoreduction if paralysis and/or severe pain are present; cisplatin is used as a radiosensitizer.	100, 104

SRT, Stereotactic radiation therapy; *IMRT,* intensity-modulated radiation therapy; *PCV,* packed cell volume.

than those receiving other treatments, whereas the addition of surgery was beneficial.[121] Late effects from radiation therapy to the pelvic region can occur and be clinically significant.[122] This can be addressed by administering the radiation in smaller doses per fraction. Perianal gland tumors are generally slow to disseminate systemically, so full-course treatment of involved regional nodes may be warranted. Intraoperative therapy as a boost to external-beam radiation therapy may also be useful in the treatment of the regional nodes or associated tumor bed following excision.

Mucositis also can occur whenever any portion of the alimentary system receives radiation therapy. Colitis is a common acute effect during radiation therapy for bladder or colorectal tumors. Severe large bowel diarrhea may be seen. Anusitis from irradiation is worsened by the diarrhea, making the patient quite uncomfortable. High-bulk diets are recommended, along with good hygiene in the region. Steroid enemas seem beneficial in some patients with colitis.[123]

Lymphoma

Radiation therapy can be important in the treatment of localized lymphoma, and it has an emerging role as an adjuvant therapy in the treatment of systemic lymphoma. Lymphocytes are exquisitely radiation sensitive[124] and may undergo apoptosis in addition to classic mitotic death after exposure to radiation.[125] Human patients with non-Hodgkin's lymphoma commonly receive combined modality treatment with radiation therapy and chemotherapy, primarily for stage I or stage II disease,[126] although this treatment may have a role in more advanced stages as well.[127] Combined modality treatment or radiotherapy alone also is beneficial in humans for primary lymphomas of bone, cutaneous B-cell lymphoma, and mycosis fungoides.[128-131]

In one study, a series of feline extranodal lymphomas (nasal cavity, retrobulbar area, mediastinum, subcutaneous tissue, maxilla, and mandible) were treated with megavoltage radiotherapy with or without concurrent chemotherapy.[114] Eight of 10 cats attained a complete local remission; one cat with retrobulbar involvement and one with mandibular involvement attained a partial remission. The median remission time for the cats that attained complete remission was 114 weeks, and three cats were alive and disease free at 131 weeks. Three cats developed disease outside the radiation field, which suggests that adjuvant chemotherapy or extending the field for part of the treatment to include additional nodes may improve locoregional control.

Radiation has also been used to treat cutaneous lymphoma in dogs. Radiotherapy of localized lymphoma has been reported to result in prolonged remission times.[132] Humans with cutaneous B-cell lymphoma commonly undergo radiation therapy, which generally results in long-term control of disease. The extent of skin involvement and the presence of extracutaneous disease are prognostic.[131]

Mycosis fungoides is sometimes treated with total skin electron irradiation in humans. As with cutaneous B-cell lymphoma, the stage of disease is prognostic, but human patients with disease confined to the skin may have prolonged remission times.

Interest has developed in the use of half-body radiotherapy to treat canine lymphoma. A dosage of 8 Gy to lymphoma cells reduces the surviving fraction to 0.005, which is much greater than the estimated cell kill from one cycle of chemotherapy.[124] The rationale for adding radiation to a chemotherapy protocol is that the projected improvement in cell kill would improve the duration of remission and perhaps result in a cure. However, because of the impact of radiation on normal bone marrow cells, the radiation can be administered only to one-half of the body at a time. (8 Gy delivered to the entire body is lethal.) In one study, induction chemotherapy (11 weeks) was administered to 94 dogs, 52 of which received subsequent half-body irradiation.[133] Half-body irradiation was administered in 2 daily fractions of 4 Gy to the cranial half of the body; 1 month later, the same protocol was used for the caudal half of the body. No additional chemotherapy was administered because the main purpose of the study was to see whether the half-body irradiation could serve as a substitute for long-term chemotherapy. The median survival of 311 days was comparable to but no better than many chemotherapy-only protocols.

In another study, half-body irradiation was interposed within a 25-week protocol based on cyclophosphamide, doxorubicin, Oncovin, and prednisone (CHOP). The radiation was well tolerated, and the median remission and survival times were 455 and 560 days, respectively. Although these results are very encouraging, the study involved only eight dogs, and the role of radiation in the treatment of systemic lymphoma requires further evaluation. Nevertheless, the addition of irradiation represents a new approach to a disease for which the duration of remission with chemotherapy alone has not improved over the past 10 years. Interestingly, the two half-body studies described previously differed from earlier reports in which each half-body treatment was delivered in a single 7 to 8 Gy fraction (personal communication, A. Abrams-Ogg). Dividing the dose into 4 Gy fractions delivered on consecutive days reduced the number and severity of acute effects. Diarrhea, the most common effect, was seen in about two-thirds of the dogs after the caudal half of the body was treated.[134]

An emerging approach in the management of dogs with lymphoma is total body irradiation (TBI) with autologous transplantation of hematopoietic peripheral blood progenitor cells. In one protocol, following treatment with a standard chemotherapy regimen, dogs are given 500 to 650 mg/m^2 of cyclophosphamide intravenously. They are then treated with recombinant human granulocyte colony-stimulating factor (rhG-CSF) and undergo apheresis to separate CD34+ progenitor cells followed by two 5 Gy fractions of TBI, 3 hours apart. Immediately after TBI, the cell harvest from apheresis is infused intravenously. In a toxicity study of 10 dogs, all dogs experienced grade 4 neutropenia, lymphopenia, and thrombocytopenia. Neutrophils recovered to at least 500 neutrophils/μL by day 12, but thrombocytopenia often persisted for weeks. Collection of long-term outcome data is still ongoing, as are attempts to escalate TBI dose.[135]

REFERENCES

1. Pommer A: X-ray therapy in veterinary medicine. In Brandly CA, Jungher EL, editors: *Advances in veterinary science*, New York, 1958, Academic Press.
2. DeVita VT Jr: Progress in cancer management. Keynote address, *Cancer* 51:2401–2409, 1983.
3. Farrelly J, McEntee MC: *A survey of veterinary radiation facilities in the United States during 2010.* In 2011 Annual Meeting of the American College of Veterinary Radiology, 2011, Albuquerque, New Mexico.
4. Ward JF: DNA damage produced by ionizing radiation in mammalian cells: identities, mechanisms of formation, and reparability, *Prog Nucleic Acid Res Mol Biol* 35:95 125, 1988.
5. Withers HR: The four R's of radiotherapy. In Lett J, Adler H, editors: *Advances in radiation biology*, New York, 1975, Academic Press.
6. Schmidt-Ullrich RK, Contessa JN, Dent P, et al: Molecular mechanisms of radiation-induced accelerated repopulation, *Radiat Oncol Investig* 7:321–330, 1999.
7. Benedict SH, Yenice KM, Followill D, et al: Stereotactic body radiation therapy: the report of AAPM Task Group 101, *Med Phys* 37:4078–4101, 2010.
8. Carsten RE, Hellyer PW, Bachand AM, et al: Correlations between acute radiation scores and pain scores in canine radiation patients with cancer of the forelimb, *Vet Anaesth Analg* 35:355–362, 2008.
9. Stewart FA, Dorr W: Milestones in normal tissue radiation biology over the past 50 years: from clonogenic cell survival to cytokine networks and back to stem cell recovery, *Int J Radiat Biol* 85:574–586, 2009.
10. Halperin EC, Perez CA, Brady LW: The discipline of radiation oncology. In Halperin EC, Perez CA, Brady LW, editors: *Perez and Brady's principles and practice of radiation oncology*, ed 5, Philadelphia, PA, 2008, Lippincott Willams & Wilkins.
11. Hall EJ, Wuu CS: Radiation-induced second cancers: the impact of 3D-CRT and IMRT, *Int J Radiat Oncol Biol Phys* 56:83–88, 2003.
12. Wilson PF, Bedford JS: Radiobiological principles. In Hoppe RT, Phillips TL, Roach M III, editors: *Leibel and Phillips textbook of radiation oncology*, ed 3, St. Louis, 2010, Elsevier.
13. Fowler JF: The linear-quadratic formula and progress in fractionated radiotherapy, *Br J Radiol* 62:679–694, 1989.
14. van den Aardweg GJMJ, Kilic E, de Klein N, et al: Dose fractionation effects in primary and metastatic human uveal melanoma cell lines, *Invest Ophthalmol Vis Sci* 44:4660–4664, 2003.
15. Fitzpatrick CL, Farese JP, Milner RJ, et al: Intrinsic radiosensitivity and repair of sublethal radiation-induced damage in canine osteosarcoma cell lines, *Am J Vet Res* 69:1197–1202, 2008.
16. Parfitt SL, Milner RJ, Salute ME, et al: Radiosensitivity and capacity for radiation-induced sublethal damage repair of canine transitional cell carcinoma (TCC) cell lines, *Vet Comp Oncol* 9:232–240, 2011.
17. Hunley DW, Mauldin GN, Shiomitsu K, et al: Clinical outcome in dogs with nasal tumors treated with intensity-modulated radiation therapy, *Can Vet J* 51:293–300, 2010.
18. Yang JN, Mackie TR, Reckwerdt P, et al: An investigation of tomotherapy beam delivery, *Med Phys* 24:425–436, 1997.
19. Forrest LJ, Mackie TR, Ruchala K, et al: The utility of megavoltage computed tomography images from a helical tomotherapy system for setup verification purposes, *Int J Radiat Oncol Biol Phys* 60:1639–1644, 2004.
20. Leksell L: The stereotaxic method and radiosurgery of the brain, *Acta Chir Scand* 102:316–319, 1951.
21. Adler JR Jr, Chang SD, Murphy MJ, et al: The Cyberknife: a frameless robotic system for radiosurgery, *Stereotact Funct Neurosurg* 69:124–128, 1997.
22. Nieset JR, Harmon JF, LaRue SM: Characterization of canine bladder variations to optimize fractionated radiation therapy protocols using cone-beam computed tomography, *Vet Radiol Ultrasound* 51(2):235, 2009.
23. Lester NV, Hopkins AL, Bova FJ, et al: Radiosurgery using a stereotactic headframe system for irradiation of brain tumors in dogs, *J Am Vet Med Assoc* 219:1562–1567, 2001.
24. Farese JP, Milner R, Thompson MS, et al: Stereotactic radiosurgery for treatment of osteosarcomas involving the distal portions of the limbs in dogs, *J Am Vet Med Assoc* 225:1567–1572, 2004.

25. Ryan SD, Ehrhart NE, Worley D, et al: Stereotactic radiation therapy for appendicular bone tumors, *Vet Radiol Ultrasound* 51(2):234, 2010
26. Lunn KF, LaRue SM: Endocrine function in cats after stereotactic radiosurgery treatment for acromegally, *J Vet Intern Med* 23:698, 2009.
27. Seguin B, McDonald DE, Kent MS, et al: Tolerance of cutaneous or mucosal flaps placed into a radiation therapy field in dogs, *Vet Surg* 34:214–222, 2005.
28. Thrall DE: Orthovoltage radiotherapy of acanthomatous epulides in 39 dogs, *J Am Vet Med Assoc* 184:7:826–829, 1984.
29. Theon AP, Rodriguez C, Griffey S, et al: Analysis of prognostic factors and patterns of failure in dogs with periodontal tumors treated with megavoltage irradiation, *J Am Vet Med Assoc* 210:785–788, 1997.
30. McEntee MC, Page RL, Theon A, et al: Malignant tumor formation in dogs previously irradiated for acanthomatous epulis, *Vet Radiol Ultrasound* 45:357–361, 2004.
31. Evans SM, Shofer F: Canine oral nontonsillar squamous cell carcinomas: Prognostic factors for recurrence and survival following orthovoltage radiation therapy, *Vet Radiol* 29:133–137, 1988.
32. Gillette EL, McChesney SL, Dewhirst MW, et al: Response of canine oral carcinomas to heat and radiation, *Int J Radiat Oncol Biol Phys* 13:1861–1867, 1987.
33. Theon AP, Rodriquez C, Madewell BR: Analysis of prognostic factors and patterns of failure in dogs with malignant oral tumors treated with megavoltage irradiation, *J Am Vet Med Assoc* 210:778–784, 1997.
34. LaDueMiller T, Price GS, Page RL, et al: Radiotherapy of canine non-tonsillar squamous cell carcinoma, *Vet Radiol Ultrasound* 37:74–77, 1996.
35. Postorino-Reeves NC, Turrel JM, Withrow SJ: Oral squamous cell carcinoma in the cat, *J Am Anim Hosp Assoc* 29:1–4, 1993.
36. Evans SM, LaCreta F, Helfand S, et al: Technique, pharmacokinetics, toxicity, and efficacy of intratumoral etanidazole and radiotherapy for treatment of spontaneous feline oral squamous cell carcinoma, *Int J Radiat Oncol Biol Phys* 20:703–708, 1991.
37. Ogilvie GK, Moore AS, Obradovich JE: Toxicoses and efficacy associated with administration of mitoxantrone to cats with malignant tumors, *J Am Vet Med Assoc* 202:1839–1844, 1993.
38. Hutson CA, Willauer CC, Walder EJ, et al: Treatment of mandibular squamous cell carcinoma in cats by use of mandibulectomy and radiotherapy: seven cases (1987–1989), *J Am Vet Med Assoc* 201:777–781, 1992.
39. Bregazzi VS, LaRue SM, Powers BE, et al: Response of feline oral squamous cell carcinoma to palliative radiation therapy, *Vet Radiol Ultrasound* 42:77–79, 2001.
40. Jones PD, de Lorimier LP, Kitchell BE, et al: Gemcitabine as a radiosensitizer for nonresectable feline oral squamous cell carcinoma, *J Am Anim Hosp Assoc* 39:463–467, 2003.
41. Fidel JL, Sellon RK, Houston RK, et al: A nine-day accelerated radiation protocol for feline squamous cell carcinoma, *Vet Radiol Ultrasound* 48:482–485, 2007.
42. Ciekot PA, Powers BE, Withrow SJ, et al: Histologically low-grade, yet biologically high-grade, fibrosarcomas of the mandible and maxilla in dogs: 25 cases (1982–1991), *J Am Vet Med Assoc* 204:4:610–615, 1994.
43. McChesney SL, Withrow SJ, Gillette EL, et al: Radiotherapy of soft tissue sarcomas in dogs, *J Am Vet Med Assoc* 194:1:60–63, 1989.
44. Gillette SM, Dewhirst MW, Gillette EL, et al: Response of canine soft tissue sarcomas to radiation or radiation plus hyperthermia: a randomized phase II study, *Int J Hyperthermia* 8:309–320, 1992.
45. Forrest LJ, Chun R, Adams WM, et al: Postoperative radiotherapy for canine soft tissue sarcoma, *J Vet Intern Med* 14:578–582, 2000.
46. Todoroff RJ, Brodey RS: Oral and pharyngeal neoplasia in the dog: a retrospective survey of 361 cases, *J Am Vet Med Assoc* 175:567–571, 1979.
47. Proulx DR, Ruslander DM, Dodge RK, et al: A retrospective analysis of 140 dogs with oral melanoma treated with external beam radiation, *Vet Radiol Ultrasound* 44:352–359, 2003.
48. Freeman KP, Hahn KA, Harris FD, et al: Treatment of dogs with oral melanoma by hypofractionated radiation therapy and platinum-based chemotherapy (1987–1997), *J Vet Intern Med* 17:96–101, 2003.
49. Farrelly J, Denman DL, Hohenhaus AE, et al: Hypofractionated radiation therapy of oral melanoma in five cats, *Vet Radiol Ultrasound* 45:91–93, 2004.
50. Bentzen SM, Overgaard J, Thames HD, et al: Clinical radiobiology of malignant melanoma, *Radiother Oncol* 16:169–182, 1989.
51. Hahn KA, Knapp DW, Richardson RC, et al: Clinical response of nasal adenocarcinoma to cisplatin chemotherapy in 11 dogs, *J Am Vet Med Assoc* 200:355–357, 1992.
52. Henry CJ, Brewer WG Jr, Tyler JW, et al: Survival in dogs with nasal adenocarcinoma: 64 cases (1981–1995), *J Vet Intern Med* 12:436–439, 1998.
53. Holmberg DL, Fries C, Cockshutt J, et al: Ventral rhinotomy in the dog and cat, *Vet Surg* 18:446–449, 1989.
54. Langova V, Mutsaers AJ, Phillips B, et al: Treatment of eight dogs with nasal tumours with alternating doses of doxorubicin and carboplatin in conjunction with oral piroxicam, *Aust Vet J* 82:676–680, 2004.
55. MacEwen G, Withrow SJ, Patnaik AK: Nasal tumors in the dog: retrospective evaluation of diagnosis, prognosis and treatment, *J Am Vet Med Assoc* 170:45–48, 1977.
56. MacMillan R, Withrow SJ, Gillette EL: Surgery and regional irradiation for treatment of canine tonsillar squamous cell carcinoma: retrospective review of eight cases, *J Am Anim Hosp Assoc* 18:311–314, 1982.
57. McEntee MC, Page RL, Heidner GL, et al: A retrospective study of 27 dogs with intranasal neoplasms treated with cobalt radiation, *Vet Radiol* 32:3:135–139, 1991.
58. Nadeau M, Kitchell BE, Rooks RL, et al: Cobalt radiation with or without low-dose cisplatin for treatment of canine naso-sinus carcinomas, *Vet Radiol Ultrasound* 45:362–367, 2004.
59. Theon AP, Madewell BR, Harb MF, et al: Megavoltage irradiation of neoplasms of the nasal and paranasal cavities in 77 dogs, *J Am Vet Med Assoc* 202:1469–1475, 1993.
60. Adams WM, Withrow SJ, Walshaw R, et al: Radiotherapy of malignant nasal tumors in 67 dogs, *J Am Vet Med Assoc* 191:3:311–315, 1987.
61. Adams WM, Bjorling DE, McAnulty JE, et al: Outcome of accelerated radiotherapy alone or accelerated radiotherapy followed by exenteration of the nasal cavity in dogs with intranasal neoplasia: 53 cases (1990–2002), *J Am Vet Med Assoc* 227:936–941, 2005.
62. Lana SE, Dernell WS, LaRue SM, et al: Slow release cisplatin combined with radiation for the treatment of canine nasal tumors, *Vet Radiol Ultrasound* 38:474–478, 1997.
63. Lana SE, Dernell WS, Lafferty MH, et al: Use of radiation and a slow-release cisplatin formulation for treatment of canine nasal tumors, *Vet Radiol Ultrasound* 45:577–581, 2004.
64. Lawrence JA, Forrest LJ, Turek MM, et al: Proof of principle of ocular sparing in dogs with sinonasal tumors treated with intensity-modulated radiation therapy, *Vet Radiol Ultrasound* 51:561–570, 2010.
65. Custis JT, Harmon JF, Ryan SD, et al: *Canine nasal tumors: A stereotactic radiation therapy approach.* Presented at the ACVIM, Denver, June 16, 2011.
66. Straw RC, Withrow SJ, Gillette EL, et al: Use of radiotherapy for the treatment of intranasal tumors in cats: six cases (1980–1985), *J Am Vet Med Assoc* 189:8:927–929, 1986.
67. Theon AP, Peaston AE, Madewell BR, et al: Irradiation of nonlymphoproliferative neoplasms of the nasal cavity and paranasal sinuses in 16 cats, *J Am Vet Med Assoc* 204:78–83, 1994.
68. Bommarito DA, Kent MS, Selting KA, et al: Reirradiation of recurrent canine nasal tumors, *Vet Radiol Ultrasound* 52:207–212, 2011.

69. Bley CR, Sumova A, Roos M, et al: Irradiation of brain tumors in dogs with neurologic disease, *J Vet Intern Med* 6:849–854, 2005.
70. Hammond GM, Gordon IK, Theon AP, et al: Evaluation of strontium Sr 90 for the treatment of superficial squamous cell carcinoma of the nasal planum in cats: 49 cases (1990–2006), *J Am Vet Med Assoc* 231:736–741, 2007.
71. Roberts SM, Lavach JD, Severin GA, et al: Ophthalmic complications following megavoltage irradiation of the nasal and paranasal cavities in dogs, *J Am Vet Med Assoc* 190:1:43–47, 1987.
72. Ching SV, Gillette SM, Powers BE, et al: Radiation-induced ocular injury in the dog: a histological study, *Int J Radiat Oncol Biol Phys* 19:321–328, 1990.
73. Evans SM, Dayrell-Hart B, Powlis W, et al: Radiation therapy of canine brain masses, *J Vet Intern Med* 7:216–219, 1993.
74. Theon AP, LeCouteur RA, Carr EA, et al: Influence of tumor cell proliferation and sex-hormone receptors on effectiveness of radiation therapy for dogs with incompletely resected meningiomas, *J Am Vet Med Assoc* 216:701–707, 684–685, 2000.
75. Turrel JM, Fike JR, LeCouteur RA, et al: Radiotherapy of brain tumors in dogs, *J Am Vet Med Assoc* 184:82–86, 1984.
76. Dow SW, LeCouteur RA, Rosychuk RAW, et al: Response of dogs with functional pituitary macroadenomas and macrocarcinomas to radiation, *J Small Anim Pract* 31:287–294, 1990.
77. Theon AP, Feldman EC: Megavoltage irradiation of pituitary macrotumors in dogs with neurologic signs, *J Am Vet Med Assoc* 213:225–231, 1998.
78. Mayer MN, Greco DS, LaRue SM: Outcomes of pituitary tumor irradiation in eight cats, *J Vet Intern Med* 20:1151–1154, 2006.
79. Leibel SA, Sheline GE: Tolerance of the central and peripheral nervous system in therapeutic irradiation. In Lett JT, Altman KI, editors: *Advances in Radiation Biology*, New York, 1987, Academic Press.
80. Graeb DA, Steinbok P, Robertson WD: Transient early computed tomographic changes mimicking tumor progression after brain tumor irradiation, *Radiology* 144:813–817, 1982.
81. Brearley MJ: Hypofractionated radiation therapy of brain masses in dogs: a retrospective analysis of survival in 83 cases (1991–1996), *J Vet Intern Med* 13(5), 408–412, 1999.
82. Kuntz CA, Dernell WS, Powers BE, et al: Prognostic factors for surgical treatment of soft-tissue sarcomas in dogs: 75 cases (1986–1996), *J Am Vet Med Assoc* 211:1147–1151, 1997.
83. McKnight JA, Mauldin GN, McEntee MC, et al: Radiation treatment for incompletely resected soft-tissue sarcomas in dogs, *J Am Vet Med Assoc* 217:205–210, 2000.
84. Bostock DE, Dye MT: Prognosis after surgical excision of canine fibrous connective tissue sarcomas, *Vet Pathol* 17:581–588, 1980.
85. Graves GM, Bjorling DE, Mahaffey E: Canine hemangiopericytoma: 23 cases (1967–1984), *J Am Vet Med Assoc* 192:99–102, 1988.
86. Ettinger SN, Scase TJ, Oberthaler KT, et al: Association of argyrophilic nucleolar organizing regions, Ki-67, and proliferating cell nuclear antigen scores with histologic grade and survival in dogs with soft tissue sarcomas: 60 cases (1996–2002), *J Am Vet Med Assoc* 228:1053–1062, 2006.
87. Stefanello D, Morello E, Roccabianca P, et al: Marginal excision of low-grade spindle cell sarcoma of canine extremities: 35 dogs (1996–2006), *Vet Surg* 37:461–465, 2008.
88. McSporran KD: Histologic grade predicts recurrence for marginally excised canine subcutaneous soft tissue sarcomas, *Vet Pathol* 46:928–933, 2009.
89. Chase D, Bray J, Ide A, et al: Outcome following removal of canine spindle cell tumours in first opinion practice: 104 cases, *J Small Anim Pract* 50:568–574, 2009.
90. Thrall DE, LaRue SM, Yu D, et al: Thermal dose is related to duration of local control in canine sarcomas treated with thermoradiotherapy, *Clin Cancer Res* 11:5206–5214, 2005.
91. Frimberger AE, Moore AS, LaRue SM, et al: Radiotherapy of incompletely resected, moderately differentiated mast cell tumors in the dog: 37 cases (1989–1993), *J Am Anim Hosp Assoc* 33:320–324, 1997.
92. Ladue T, Price GS, Dodge R, et al: Radiation therapy for incompletely resected canine mast cell tumors, *Vet Radiol Ultrasound* 39:57–62, 1998.
93. Chaffin K, Thrall DE: Results of radiation therapy in 19 dogs with cutaneous mast cell tumor and regional lymph node metastasis, *Vet Radiol Ultrasound* 43:392–395, 2002.
94. Cronin K, Page RL, Spodnick G, et al: Radiation therapy and surgery for fibrosarcoma in 33 cats, *Vet Radiol Ultrasound* 39:51–56, 1998.
95. Bregazzi VS, LaRue SM, McNiel E, et al: Treatment with a combination of doxorubicin, surgery, and radiation versus surgery and radiation alone for cats with vaccine-associated sarcomas: 25 cases (1995–2000), *J Am Vet Med Assoc* 218:547–550, 2001.
96. Cohen M, Wright JC, Brawner WR, et al: Use of surgery and electron beam irradiation, with or without chemotherapy, for treatment of vaccine-associated sarcomas in cats: 78 cases (1996–2000), *J Am Vet Med Assoc* 219:1582–1589, 2001.
97. Mayer MN, Treuil PL, LaRue SM: Radiotherapy and surgery for feline soft tissue sarcoma, *Vet Radiol Ultrasound* 50:669–672, 2009.
98. LaRue SM, Withrow SJ, Powers BE, et al: Limb-sparing treatment for osteosarcoma in dogs, *J Am Vet Med Assoc* 195:1734–1744, 1989.
99. Thrall DE, Dewhirst MW, Page RL, et al: A comparison of temperatures in canine solid tumours during local and whole-body hyperthermia administered alone and simultaneously, *Int J Hyperthermia* 6:305–317, 1990.
100. Dickerson ME, Page RL, LaDue TA, et al: Retrospective analysis of axial skeleton osteosarcoma in 22 large-breed dogs, *J Vet Intern Med* 15:120–124, 2001.
101. Custis JT, Ryan SD, Valdes-Martinez A, et al: Identifying factors predictive of osteosarcoma related pathologic fracture following stereotactic radiation therapy, *Vet Radiol Ultrasound* 51(2):234. 2009.
102. Steenland E, Leer JW, van Houwelingen H, et al: The effect of a single fraction compared to multiple fractions on painful bone metastases: a global analysis of the Dutch Bone Metastasis Study, *Radiother Oncol* 52:101–109, 1999.
103. Knapp-Hoch HM, Fidel JL, Sellon RK, et al: An expedited palliative radiation protocol for lytic or proliferative lesions of appendicular bone in dogs, *J Am Anim Hosp Assoc* 45:24–32, 2009.
104. Dernell WS, Van Vechten BJ, Straw RC, et al: Outcome following treatment of vertebral tumors in 20 dogs (1986–1995), *J Am Anim Hosp Assoc* 36:245–251, 2000.
105. McEntee MC, Page RL, Novotney CA, et al: Palliative radiotherapy for canine appendicular osteosarcoma, *Vet Radiol Ultrasound* 34:367–370, 1993.
106. Ramirez O III, Dodge RK, Page RL, et al: Palliative radiotherapy of appendicular osteosarcoma in 95 dogs, *Vet Radiol Ultrasound* 40:517–522, 1999.
107. Kent MS, Bommarito D, Feldman E, et al: Survival, neurologic response, and prognostic factors in dogs with pituitary masses treated with radiation therapy and untreated dogs, *J Vet Intern Med* 21:1027–1033, 2007.
108. Sellon RK, Fidel J, Houston R, et al: Linear-accelerator-based modified radiosurgical treatment of pituitary tumors in cats: 11 cases (1997–2008), *J Vet Intern Med* 23:1038–1044, 2009.
109. Allan GS, Gillette EL: Response of canine mast cell tumors to radiaton, *J Natl Cancer Inst* 63(3):691–694, 1979.
110. Turrel JM: Prognostic factors for radiation treatment of mast cell tumor in 85 dogs, *J Am Vet Med Assoc* 193:936–940, 1988.
111. Theon AP, Barthez PY, Madewell BR, et al: Radiation therapy of ceruminous gland carcinomas in dogs and cats, *J Am Vet Med Assoc* 205:566–569, 1994.
112. Kobayashi T, Hauck ML, Dodge R, et al: Preoperative radiotherapy for vaccine associated sarcoma in 92 cats, *Vet Radiol Ultrasound* 43:473–479, 2002.

113. Eckstein C, Guscetti F, Roos M, et al: A retrospective analysis of radiation therapy for the treatment of feline vaccine-associated sarcoma, *Vet Comp Oncol* 7:54–68, 2009.
114. Elmslie RE, Ogilvie GK, Gillette EL, et al: Radiotherapy with and without chemotherapy for localized lymphoma in 10 cats, *Vet Radiol* 32:277–280, 1991.
115. North SM, Meleo KA, Mooney S, et al: *Radiation therapy in the treatment of nasal lymphoma in cats*. Proceedings of the Veterinary Cancer Society 14th Annual Conference Townsend, Tennessee, 21. 1994.
116. Gillette EL, McChesney SL, Dewhirst MW, et al: Response of canine oral carcinomas to heat and radiation, *Int J Radiat Oncol Biol Phys* 13:1861–1867, 1987.
117. Bateman KE, Catton PA, Pennock PW, et al: 0-7-21 Radiation therapy for the treatment of canine oral melanoma, *J Vet Intern Med* 8:267–272, 1994.
118. Blackwood L, Dobson JM: Radiotherapy of oral malignant melanomas in dogs, *J Am Vet Med Assoc* 209:98–102, 1996.
119. Theon AP, Marks SL, Feldman ES, et al: Prognostic factors and patterns of treatment failure in dogs with unresectable differentiated thyroid carcinomas treated with megavoltage irradiation.[see comment], *J Am Vet Med Assoc* 216:1775–1779, 2000.
120. Ohara K, Tatsuzaki H, Fuji H, et al: Radioresponse of thymomas verified with histologic response, *Acta Oncologica* 37:471–474, 1998.
121. Williams LE, Gliatto JM, Dodge RK, et al: Carcinoma of the apocrine glands of the anal sac in dogs: 113 cases (1985–1995), *J Am Vet Med Assoc* 223:825–831, 2003.
122. Anderson CR, McNiel EA, Gillette EL, et al: Late complications of pelvic irradiation in 16 dogs, *Vet Radiol Ultrasound* 43:187–192, 2002.
123. Fuccio L, Guido A, Laterza L, et al: Randomised clinical trial: preventive treatment with topical rectal beclomethasone dipropionate reduces post-radiation risk of bleeding in patients irradiated for prostate cancer, *Aliment Pharmacol Ther* 34:628–637, 2011.
124. Fertil B, Malaise E: Intrinsic radiosensitivity of human cell lines is correlated with radioresponsiveness of human tumors: Analysis of 101 published survival curves. *Int J Rad Onc Biol Phys* 11(9):1699–1707, 1985.
125. Bump EA, Braunhut SJ, Palayoor ST, et al: Novel concepts in modification of radiation sensitivity, *Int J Radiat Oncol Biol Phys* 29:249–253, 1994.
126. Vose JM: Current approaches to the management of non-Hodgkin's lymphoma, *Semin Oncol* 25:483–491, 1998.
127. Yahalom J: Radiation therapy in the treatment of lymphoma, *Curr Opin Oncol* 11:370–374, 1999.
128. Fidias P, Spiro I, Sobczak ML, et al: Long-term results of combined modality therapy in primary bone lymphomas, *Int J Radiat Oncol Biol Phys* 45:1213–1218, 1999.
129. Giger U, Evans SM, Hendrick MJ, et al: Orthovoltage radiotherapy of primary lymphoma of bone in a dog, *J Am Vet Med Assoc* 195:627–630, 1989.
130. Kirova YM, Piedbois Y, Haddad E, et al: Radiotherapy in the management of mycosis fungoides: indications, results, prognosis. Twenty years experience, *Radiother Oncol* 51:147–151, 1999.
131. Kirova YM, Piedbois Y, Le Bourgeois JP: Radiotherapy in the management of cutaneous B-cell lymphoma. Our experience in 25 cases, *Radiother Oncol* 52:15–18, 1999.
132. Meleo KA: The role of radiotherapy in the treatment of lymphoma and thymoma, *Vet Clin North Am Small Anim Pract* 27(1):115–129, 1997.
133. Williams LE, Johnson JL, Hauck ML, et al: Chemotherapy followed by half-body radiation therapy for canine lymphoma, *J Vet Intern Med* 18:703–709, 2004.
134. Gustafson NR, Lana SE, Mayer MN, et al: A preliminary assessment of whole-body radiotherapy interposed within a chemotherapy protocol for canine lymphoma, *Vet Comp Oncol* 2:125–131, 2005.
135. Escobar C, Grindem C, Neel JA, et al: Hematologic changes after total body irradiation and autologous transplantation of hematopoietic peripheral blood progenitor cells in dogs with lymphoma, *Vet Pathol* 49(2):341–343, 2012.

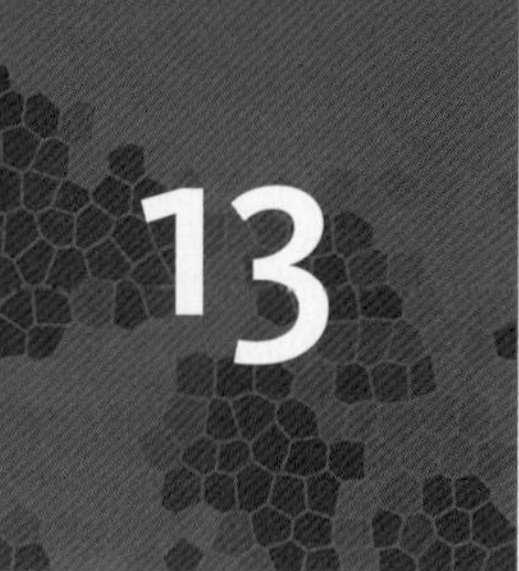

13 Cancer Immunotherapy

AMANDA M. GUTH AND STEVEN DOW

The main role of the immune system is recognition of "foreign" proteins, including mutated or altered forms of self-proteins that arise during tumorigenesis, which are commonly referred to as *tumor antigens* (TAs). However, it is now apparent that powerful regulatory cells whose main function is to prevent rampant, uncontrolled immune responses also serve to block natural development of potent antitumor immune response. Therefore the role of immunotherapy in treatment of various cancers must take into account the ability to overcome these regulators in order to be successful.

It has long been known that the immune system is capable of controlling cancer. For example, it is well established that cancer incidence is increased in immunosuppressed individuals. Moreover, in some cases, spontaneous remission of tumors is observed without any therapeutic intervention, most likely attributed to a successful immune response. Biologically, tumor-specific T-cells are observed in the tumor tissue and tumor-draining lymph nodes, providing evidence that these cells have encountered and recognized the tumor cells as foreign. Finally, in some cases, there is the development of paraneoplastic autoimmunity, suggesting that the antitumor immune response has somehow gone unchecked by the regulator cells.

With the advancement and sophistication of techniques used to study the immune system comes the increased ability to precisely target the malignant cells while leaving normal tissues intact. One of the major goals of immunotherapy is to develop a potent, long-lasting antitumor immune response without producing untoward side effects. However, it is difficult to develop an immunotherapy that is not affected by tumor-induced immune tolerance or even the immune system itself. For example, therapy with the T-cell growth factor cytokine, interleukin-2 (IL-2), leads to expansion of regulatory T-cells, known for their powerful immunosuppressive abilities.[1] In addition, when considering monoclonal antibody (MAb) immunotherapy in companion animals, one must account for the fact that the Fc region of the MAb, the part not involved in antigen recognition, is typically derived from mice or human protein sequences and thus is considered foreign by the immune system. Hence, repeated treatment with a non–canine-based antibody leads to a robust inactivation of the MAb, as well as systemic toxicity, thus eliminating its effectiveness over time.

Knowing more about the immune system and the way it is regulated will increase our ability to design better immunotherapies. In addition, immunotherapy has the potential to work in conjunction with and perhaps enhance the effectiveness of chemotherapies, radiation therapy, surgery, and other adjunct therapies. In this chapter, we will first discuss the role of the immune system in tumor development, then the various classes of immunotherapies both currently in use and those under investigation as part of clinical trials. We will discuss the biologic basis for the therapies, their use in human and companion animals, and their limitations.

Immune System Control of Tumor Development and Growth

Immune Surveillance of Cancer

Forty years ago, Thomas and Burnet, while studying how lymphocytes could respond to newly formed antigens on transformed cells, put forth the concept that the immune system could actively respond to and eliminate cancerous cells, an idea known as *immune surveillance*.[2] In contrast, later studies[3,4] showed that genetically manipulated immunodeficient (athymic) mice did not demonstrate an increased incidence of cancer—either spontaneously or carcinogen induced. Such observations were proposed to be due to residual immunity, leading to the immune surveillance concept falling out of favor.

Since the development of more sensitive and sophisticated technologies, many of the ideas behind the concept of the immune surveillance hypothesis are now more accepted, and currently, this modification of the original hypothesis is referred to as the *immunoediting hypothesis*.[5] Pivotal studies by Robert Schreiber's group showed that lymphocytes (T-cells) could directly or indirectly through production of a cytokine, interferon γ (IFN-γ), protect mice against the development of methylcholanthrene (MCA)-induced sarcomas.[6,7] Moreover, they demonstrated that tumors from immunodeficient mice were more immunogenic than tumors from immunocompetent mice, thus leading to the immunoediting hypothesis.[7,8] This hypothesis consists of three phases: (1) *elimination:* removal of the immunogenic tumor cells by the immune system; however, weakly immunogenic cells can survive; (2) *equilibrium:* tumor growth and immune destruction are equal; and (3) *escape:* tumor growth ensues as the result of decreased immunogenicity, immune suppression, and rapid tumor cell growth.[5] However, despite recent data, there is still a controversy that remains around the immune surveillance hypothesis, discussed in a review by Schreiber et al.[5]

Mechanisms of Immune Evasion by Tumors

Given the fact that cancer can develop in immunocompetent individuals, some tumor cells are able to avoid recognition by the immune system.[9] This is accomplished by various mechanisms (discussed later) that involve both changes in the tumor cells themselves and ways in which the tumor and the tumor stromal environment can manipulate the immune system and prevent antitumor immunity. These mechanisms of immune evasion pose a significant challenge to the development of effective immunotherapies. Figure 13-1 demonstrates some of these key mechanisms.

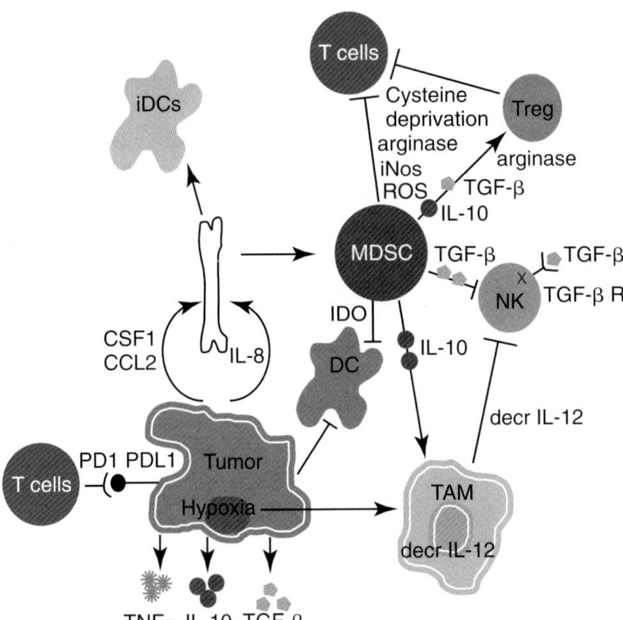

FIGURE 13-1 Mechanisms of tumor cell evasion via hijacking the immune system. *DC,* Dendritic cell; *iDC,* immature dendritic cell; *MDSC,* myeloid-derived suppressor cell; *TAM,* tumor-associated macrophage; *Treg,* regulatory T-cell.

Active Immune Suppression by Myeloid-Derived Suppressor Cells

One population of immune cells that play a major role in tumor immunosuppression are myeloid-derived suppressor cells (MDSCs). These cells consist of immature monocytes and granulocytes released from the bone marrow into the blood during pathologic conditions, including cancer. Sometimes included in the functional description of this group of cells are tumor-associated macrophages (TAMs), which have the same ability and use similar mechanisms as MDSCs to induce potent tumor immunosuppression.[10,11] Numerous studies demonstrate increased numbers of MDSCs in humans with cancer[12-14] and in mouse models of cancer.[15,16] Furthermore, it has been shown that the presence of these cells correlates with clinical disease stage and metastatic tumor burden in humans with solid tumors.[13] MDSCs are recruited to the tumor microenvironment through various chemoattractants,[10] many of which are induced by the tumor during times of hypoxia and are directly released by the effects of hypoxia-inducible factor-1α (HIF-1α) production.[17-20] Once at the tumor, MDSCs intercalate into the microenvironment and actively suppress the local antitumor immune response and promote tumor invasion and metastasis via the production of matrix metalloproteinases (MMPs) and various chemoattractants.[21,22] Moreover, these cells, including the TAMs, contribute to increased tumor vessel growth, a process referred to as *angiogenesis.*[10] Of note, although cell surface markers are used to identify these cells in mice and humans, similar markers have yet to be discovered for dogs, thus the role that MDSCs play in canine cancer is currently unknown.

The ability of MDSCs to suppress the antitumor response is the subject of many recent studies.[23-25] Numerous mechanisms of suppression have been reported, and MDSCs have the ability to suppress not only T-cells, but also natural killer (NK) cells and dendritic cells (DCs) and they also are able to potentiate T-regulatory cells (Tregs), which are discussed later, and TAMs in the tumor (see Figure 13-1). Currently known mechanisms of immune suppression by MDSCs include suppression of T-cells through production of inducible nitric oxide (NO) species (iNOS), reactive oxygen species (ROS) and arginase, as well as cysteine deprivation.[23] MDSCs can produce transforming growth factor-β (TGF-β) and IL-10, which stimulate Tregs and TAMs, and MDSCs can cause downregulation of the IL-12 production by TAMs, a cytokine involved in T-cell activation.[24] MDSCs cause NK cell anergy (lack of function) also by this decreased IL-12 production and through membrane-bound TGF-β.[24,25] Thus, given the ability of these cells to use multiple pathways to induce tumor immunosuppression, the development of effective immunotherapies that can target these cells and either eliminate them or lead to their maturation, rather than ones that target specific pathways of suppression, is critical for that therapy's success.

Induction of Regulatory T-Cells by Tumors

Another population of cells that are significantly increased in tumor-bearing humans and animals are Tregs. These cells are phenotypically defined by surface expression of CD4 and CD25 but are most specifically identified by the intracellular transcription factor, forkhead box P3 (foxp3).[26,27] Other surface markers used to characterize these cells have been described, including cytotoxic T-lymphocyte antigen-4 (CTLA-4), glucocorticoid-induced tumor necrosis factor (TNF) receptor family-regulated gene (GITR), lymphocyte-activation gene 3 (Lag3), and folate receptor-4 (FR-4).[28-31] This distinct subset of CD4+ T-cells is capable of directly suppressing tumor-specific CD4+ and CD8+ T-cells and NK cells and are enriched in the tumor microenvironment by conversion of CD4 T-cells to Tregs by DCs or TGF-β,[32-35] proliferation of tumor-specific Tregs following antigen recognition, or recruitment of these cells via chemokine signaling (i.e., CCR5).[36] Recent work has also suggested a role for the chemokine CCL-1 in specifically converting T-cells to Tregs and inducing their suppressive nature.[37]

Many studies demonstrate that increased numbers of Treg cells are correlated with a poor prognosis.[38-41] Additionally, Tregs present in metastatic lymph nodes inhibit the ability of tumor-infiltrating lymphocytes to mount an effective antitumor response.[42] Work in our laboratory demonstrated that canine Treg cells can also be identified via the expression of CD4 and foxp3.[43] Moreover, we saw that cancer-bearing dogs had increased numbers of Tregs compared to healthy dogs and that this difference was greater in certain types of canine cancers.[43,44] Therefore current therapies aimed at depleting Treg cells in humans could be applied to veterinary medicine. In particular, many studies have shown that the use of cyclophosphamide or anti–Treg-specific antibodies decreases the numbers of Tregs present in tumors and in circulation of tumor-bearing patients.[45-49]

Impaired Dendritic Cell Activation and Function

Another important mechanism of tumor suppression is through impairment of the potent antigen-presenting cells, dendritic cells (DCs). Numerous studies have denoted that overall numbers of DCs are decreased in various human cancers studied, including head and neck squamous cell carcinomas (HNSCCs),[50] breast and prostate cancers, and malignant gliomas.[51] A recent study showed that indoleamine 2,3-dioxygenase 1 (IDO1) expression in the tumor microenvironment led to increased DC apoptosis.[52] Some tumor studies also demonstrated fewer circulating myeloid DCs and a concurrent increase in immature DCs (iDCs) that reduce presentation of antigens and stimulation of T-cells; thus they induce T-cell tolerance rather than activate T-cells.[51,53,54] Thus the

DCs present in the tumor tend to be immature and dysfunctional. Studies of DCs in numerous human cancers demonstrate minimal activation, decreased ability to stimulate in an alloreactive fashion, and decreased expression of co-stimulatory molecules.[50,51,55-60] A similar study done in dogs with canine transmissible venereal tumors (CTVT) showed that the tumor environment caused downregulation of DC surface markers of activation and major histocompatibility (MHC), as well as decreased endocytic capabilities and decreased allogenic mixed lymphocyte reaction (MLR) responses.[61] Possible mechanisms causing the DC dysfunction include the overexpression of the protein S100A9,[62] accumulation of triglycerides in the DCs that leads to decreased capacity to present antigen,[63] and downregulation of toll-like receptor 9 (TLR9).[64] Moreover, factors such as IL-10 and vascular endothelial growth factor (VEGF) can negatively affect DC function and maturation.[65,66] Finally, some DCs in the tumor are considered to be regulatory based on low expression of surface markers MHC II, CD86, and CD11c with high expression of co-stimulatory molecules CD80, CD40, CD106, and CD11b. These cells secrete regulatory factors such as IL-10 and NO and inhibit proliferation of naïve CD4+ T cells to antigen presented by mature, functional DCs.[67] Overall, the microenvironment of the tumor leads to attraction of immature and regulatory DCs that due to their decreased activation and function can potently inhibit the development of antitumor T-cell responses even when copious amounts of antigen are present.

Production of Immunosuppressive Cytokines

In addition to the suppressive milieu established by tumor-infiltrating cells, the tumor cells themselves are capable of producing immunosuppressive cytokines.[68] A few key cytokines produced by tumor cells are IL-10, TGF-β, and tumor necrosis factor-α (TNF-α).[68,69] These cytokines act to suppress antitumor T-cell responses and inhibit DC function. IL-10 promotes Treg production and function[70] and, in an autocrine and/or paracrine fashion, may potentially affect tumor cell proliferation and survival.[71] In human cancer patients, increased levels of serum IL-10 is observed in patients with pancreatic carcinoma and non-Hodgkin's lymphoma (NHL).[72,73] In addition, elevated levels of IL-10 in diffuse large B-cell lymphoma in humans correlate with a poor prognosis.[74] TGF-β acts similarly to IL-10 in that it is a potent immunosuppressive cytokine that can potentiate Treg proliferation and function.[33,75-77] It can also enhance tumor progression; carcinomas can produce excess TGF-β, which in turn increases epithelial-to-mesenchymal transition, tumor invasion, and metastasis, and inhibit tumor-specific CD8+ T-cells.[77] Moreover, tumor-produced TNF-α leads to promotion of tumor cell survival via induction of antiapoptotic proteins.[78] Finally, TNF-α has been shown to promote tumor angiogenesis and metastasis and hamper cytotoxic T-cell and macrophage responses.[79]

One study in veterinary medicine examined a lymph node of a dog with metastatic melanoma. This study revealed an overexpression of IL-10 and TGF-β concurrent with a lack of expression of IL-2, IL-4, or IFN-γ—cytokines typically associated with antitumor immunity—thus demonstrating that tumor immunosuppression occurs in veterinary patients as well.[80] For a review of cytokines relevant to tumor immunotherapy, see Table 13-1.

Failure of Tumor Cells to Activate Immune System

Tumor cells are also capable of avoiding immune elimination by failing to be recognized by the immune system in the first place. For example, some tumor cells can downmodulate MHC surface expression to escape recognition by T-cells. MHC class I expression can be lost on tumor cells due to changes in protein synthesis, structure, or allelic loss.[81,82] Moreover, defects in antigen processing and presentation can occur that can also lead to decreased MHC expression.[81,82] A decrease in class II expression is also observed in certain human hematopoietic cancers, although it should be noted that most tumors are normally MHC class II negative.[83,84] Reduced expression of MHC class II has been recently correlated with poor outcome in dogs with B-cell lymphoma.[85]

In addition, tumor cells can express co-inhibitory surface molecules, such as CD73 and/or PD-L1. CD73 is an ecto-5′-nucleotidase that catalyzes the breakdown of adenosine monophosphate (AMP) to adenosine. When expressed on tumors, this creates a local microenvironment rich in adenosine, which is immunosuppressive.[52] The programmed death-1/programmed death ligand-1 (PD-1/PD-L1) axis also plays an immunosuppressive role in cancer. PD-L1 expression on tumors downmodulates antitumor T-cell function[86-88] and NK cell[89] activity via interaction through the PD-L1 expressed on these immune cells. Thus tumor cells themselves can actively and directly suppress antitumor T-cell responses

TABLE 13-1 Biologic Activities of Key Cytokines Relevant to Tumor Immunotherapy

CYTOKINE	MAJOR ACTIVITY
IL-2	▪ Growth factor for T-cells, including regulatory T-cells. ▪ Induces proliferation and differentiation of T-cells to effector T-cells. ▪ Enhances CTL and NK cell cytotoxicity, production of LAK cells. ▪ Induces B-cell proliferation. ▪ Approved for use clinically by the FDA.
IL-3	▪ Multicolony-stimulating factor. ▪ Promotes production/differentiation and proliferation of macrophages, monocytes, granulocytes, and DCs. ▪ Secreted by activated T-cells and supports growth and differentiation of T-cells.
IL-4	▪ Key Th2 cytokine. ▪ Induces differentiation of naïve CD4 T-cells toward Th2 phenotype. ▪ Inhibits macrophage activation. ▪ Induces B-cell growth and differentiation. ▪ Stimulates isotype switching and IgG and IgE production. ▪ Upregulates MHC class II production.

TABLE 13-1 Biologic Activities of Key Cytokines Relevant to Tumor Immunotherapy continued

CYTOKINE	MAJOR ACTIVITY
IL-6	▪ Supports B-cell proliferation and differentiation to plasma cells. ▪ Proinflammatory, antiapoptotic cytokine that may contribute to tumor development associated with chronic inflammation. ▪ Causes upregulation of PD-1 on monocytes that are triggered to produce IL-10 following ligation of this receptor.
IL-8	▪ Chemotactic/activation factor for neutrophils and T-cells. ▪ Induces MMP2 activity; plays a role in inflammation and tumor metastasis.
IL-10	▪ Immunosuppressive cytokine produced by activated DCs, macrophages, and T-cells. ▪ Induces regulatory T-cell function. ▪ Also overexpressed by some tumors and tumor-associated leukocytes.
IL-11	▪ Stimulates proliferation of hematopoietic stem cells. ▪ Induces megakaryocyte maturation, resulting in increased platelet production.
IL-12	▪ Key Th1 cytokine produced by DCs, macrophages. ▪ Stimulates synthesis of IFN-γ and TNF-α by T-cells and NKs, thus decreasing angiogenesis. ▪ Enhances cytotoxicity of CTLs and NK cells. ▪ Stimulates differentiation of naïve CD4+ T-cells to T-cells with the Th1 phenotype.
IL-13	▪ Th2-promoting cytokine, produced by NKT cells. ▪ Inhibits inflammatory cytokine production by macrophages. ▪ Possible inhibitory role in tumor immunosurveillance.
IL-15	▪ T-cell growth factor. ▪ Supports survival of memory CD8+ T-cells. ▪ Promotes NK cell activation and survival and triggers cytotoxic activity.
IL-17	▪ Induces proinflammatory response. ▪ Role in cancer is currently controversial, depending on context, may either promote or inhibit tumor growth.
IL-19	▪ Promotes T-cell differentiation toward the Th2 phenotype.
IL-21	▪ Member of IL-2 cytokine family. ▪ Enhances cytotoxicity and proliferation of CTLs and NK cells.
IL-23	▪ Member of IL-12 cytokine family. ▪ Upregulates the production of MMP9 in tumors. ▪ Increases angiogenesis, while reducing CD8 TILs. ▪ Stimulates CD4+ T-cells to become Th17 cells.
GM-CSF	▪ Promotes growth and differentiation of pluripotent progenitor cells. ▪ Stimulates growth of cells of the granulocyte, macrophage, and eosinophil lineage.
CSF-1	▪ Promotes differentiation of stem cells into monocytes and macrophages.
G-CSF	▪ Stimulates bone marrow to produce granulocytes and stem cells. ▪ Stimulates neutrophil survival, function, and maturation.
IFN-α, IFN-β	▪ Induces apoptosis of tumor cells. ▪ Enhances CTL effector function. ▪ Activates NK cells. ▪ Modulates MHC class I/II expression. ▪ Inhibits tumor angiogenesis.
IFN-γ	▪ Key Th1 cytokine produced by activated T-cells and NK cells. ▪ Promotes the differentiation of naïve CD4+ T cells to Th1 phenotype. ▪ Activates macrophages. ▪ Increases MHC class I/II expression.
TNF-α	▪ Produced by Th1 cells, CTLs, activated DCs, and macrophages. ▪ Induces NO production by macrophages. ▪ Induces tumor apoptosis. ▪ Important proinflammatory cytokine.
TGF-β	▪ Immunosuppressive cytokine. ▪ Inhibits macrophage activation and B-cell growth. ▪ Overexpressed by some tumors.

CTL, Cytotoxic T-lymphocyte; *CSF-1*, colony-stimulating factor-1; *DCs*, dendritic cells; *FDA*, Food and Drug Administration; *G-CSF*, granulocyte colony-stimulating factor; *GM-CSF*, granulocyte-macrophage colony-stimulating factor; *IFN*, interferon; *IgE*, immunoglobulin E; *IgG*, immunoglobulin G; *IL*, interleukin; *LAK*, lymphokine-activated killer; *MHC*, major histocompatibility; *MMP*, matrix metalloproteinase; *NK*, natural killer; *NKT*, natural killer T-cell; *NO*, nitric oxide; *PD-1*, programmed death-1; *Th1*, T-helper 1; *Th2*, T-helper 2; *TGF*, transforming growth factor; *TILs*, tumor-infiltrating lymphocytes; *TNF*, tumor necrosis factor.

through such mechanisms as decreased expression of MHC molecules and increased expression of inhibitory molecules.

Strategies to Control Tumor Growth through Immune Activation

Depletion of Immunosuppressive Myeloid-Derived Suppressor Cells to Allow for Effective Immunotherapy

In light of many recent studies, it has become clear that in order to develop an effective immunotherapy, it must be able to overcome, or be combined with other treatments that can overcome, the immunosuppression present in the tumor microenvironment. As mentioned previously, MDSCs are a key component of such immunosuppression. Box 13-1 lists the various potential ways in which MDSCs can be manipulated in order to enhance the effectiveness of immunotherapy.

Nonspecific Immune Activation to Generate Antitumor Activity Using Biologic-Response Modifiers

In the 1900s, William Coley observed that cancer patients who developed bacterial infections survived longer than those that did not (reviewed in Richardson and colleagues[110]). Building on these observations, Coley developed "Coley's toxins," which consisted of killed cultures of *Streptococcus pyogenes* and *Serratia marcescens* that he gave to patients with inoperable sarcomas. Although with this "vaccine," Coley saw cure rates of approximately 15%, his therapy was discontinued because of its significant failure rate and intolerable side effects. However, this seminal work laid the foundation for further studies aimed at nonspecific, pan-immune activation to treat cancer through the use of biologic-response modifiers (BRMs).

Bacillus Calmette-Guérin and Corynebacterium parvum

One of the most well-known and clinically utilized BRMs is bacillus Calmette-Guérin (BCG), a live, attenuated strain of *Mycobacterium bovis.* Currently, in human medicine, BCG is intravesically instilled into the bladder where it is considered to be effective as a means to treat and prevent relapse of noninvasive transitional cell carcinoma (TCC).[111,112] One proposed mechanism for its antitumor effects relates to the recruitment of neutrophils and their ability to promote urothelial cell turnover.[113] This recruitment most likely relates to the ability of BCG to elicit T-helper 1 (Th1) inflammatory cytokines.[114,115]

The use of BCG in veterinary medicine is rather limited. Although its efficacy has been tested on numerous forms of canine cancer,[116] its use as an immunotherapy in dogs is limited. BCG can be safely instilled into canine bladders,[117] but the rate of true superficial bladder cancers is extremely low in dogs as compared to humans.[118] Recent uses of BCG in canines include treatment of CTVT in conjunction with vincristine[119] or, in combination with human chorionic gonadotropin (hCG; LDI-100), treatment of mast cell tumors (MCTs).[120] In this study, response rates for grade I and II MCTs were comparable to single-agent vinblastine but without the myelosuppression.

Another BRM that has been studied in human and veterinary medicine is *Corynebacterium parvum.* In human and dog melanoma studies, *C. parvum* displayed antitumor activity as an adjunct to surgery.[121,122] However, efficacy of *C. parvum* as an immunotherapy in other canine cancers has been disappointing.[123]

Salmonella

As a tumor grows, the core may become necrotic as the initial tumor cells are deprived of nutrients. Layered on this necrotic core are tumor cells that exist in an area of hypoxia, which puts them out of reach of blood vessels that can supply them with oxygen. These cells are able to remain viable and pose a challenge to most immunotherapies, chemotherapies, and even small molecule drugs due to their restricted location. Recently, researchers have begun to

Box 13-1 Ways to Manipulate Myeloid-Derived Suppressor Cells to Decrease Immunosuppression

Depletion/Inhibit Proliferation
Liposomal clodronate (unpublished data)
Gemcitabine[90]
5-Fluorouracil (5-FU)[91]
Sunitinib[92]
Docetaxel[93]
Cyclooxygenase 2 (COX2) inhibitor (SC58236)[94]
KIT-specific Ab[95]
25-hydroxyvitamin D3[96]
CXCR2 antagonist (S-265610)[20]
CXCR4 antagonist (AMD3100)[20]
PROK2-specific Ab[97]

Promote Maturation
Zoledronate[98]
All-*trans* retinoic acid (ATRA)[99]
Docetaxel[93]
Sunitinib[92]
Decitabine[100]
Activated natural killer T-cells[101]
Very small size proteoliposome (VSSP) vaccine[102]

Inhibit Recruitment
cFMS kinase inhibitor (GW2580)[103]
Nonsteroidal antiinflammatories (NSAIDs)[94]

Block Interactions
Anti-CD40 Ab[104]
Anti-programmed death-1/programmed death ligand-1 (PD-1/PD-L1) Ab[105]

Block Function
Nitroaspirin[106]
Arginase 1 inhibitor: N hydroxyl arginine (NOHA)[107]
Triterpenoid[108]
Sildenafil[109]

genetically modify facultative anaerobic bacteria that can penetrate and survive in these regions. In fact, it has been shown that several strains of Salmonella, including *S. typhimurium* and *S. choleraesuis*, target tumors following systemic administration. These bacteria penetrate the necrotic core and feed on the dead cells while also emitting natural toxins that will destroy surrounding, viable cells. Using a mouse melanoma model, treatment with VNP20009, an attenuated *S. typhimurium*, was able to slow tumor growth and specifically target primary tumor and metastatic lesions.[124] Although this study showed that the effects were independent of B- and T-cells, possible indirect effects of the Salmonella include production of inflammatory cytokines, such as TNF-α.[125] Recently, another proposed mechanism involves the ability of Salmonella to induce melanoma cells to express gap junctions that can interact with DCs and cause bits of tumor cell proteins to be loaded and expressed on the surface of these DCs for presentation to T cells.[126] Unfortunately, in human trials, the bacteria failed to colonize some patients and did not provide any antitumor activity.[127]

Administration of VNP20009 in dogs resulted in a more positive outcome than in humans. In a phase I clinical trial, VNP20009 was administered to dogs with a variety of malignant tumors.[128] In this study, 41 dogs received intravenous infusions of VNP20009 either weekly or biweekly at escalating doses. Fever and vomiting were reported as dose-limiting toxicities. Bacterial colonization was seen in approximately 40% of dogs, and significant clinical responses were observed in 15% of patients, with an overall rate of 37% of dogs experiencing either a transient response or stable disease. Thus the use of VNP20009 in specific dog tumors should be further investigated, perhaps in combination with modified Salmonella engineered to deliver tumor cytotoxic agents.

Superantigens

Bacteria, such as *Staphylococcus aureus*, produce enterotoxins known as *superantigens* (SAgs). Two of these *S. aureus* enterotoxins, referred to as *SEA* or *SEB*, stimulate T-cell proliferation and Th1 cytokine production (IL-2, TNF-α, and IFN-γ) via their ability to cross-link the T-cell receptor and MHC class II molecules. These activated T-cells are highly cytolytic and antitumorigenic in mouse models of cancer.[129,130] Moreover, the potency of SAgs is increased when delivered with stimulatory cytokines.[131,132] However, when these SAgs were injected into humans, toxic shock syndrome was elicited.[133] Therefore genetically modified versions of the SAgs that maintain their immune potency have been evaluated in humans. In a study of patients with non–small-cell lung carcinoma using a modified SAg, stable disease occurred in 42% of patients with decreased tumor burdens of up to 50%. The dose-limiting side effect noted in this study was hypotension.[134] SAgs and modified versions are still currently being evaluated for potential use as a human cancer therapeutic.[135,136]

In veterinary medicine, SAgs were evaluated for efficacy and safety in dogs with oral melanoma and soft tissue sarcoma (STS). Dow et al assessed the efficacy of intratumoral injection of lipid-complexed plasmid DNA that encoded for SEB and either granulocyte-macrophage colony-stimulating factor (GM-CSF) or IL-2.[131] Complete or partial remission was seen in 46% of dogs and increased survival time for stage III diseased dogs was observed. There were no toxicities noted, and analysis of tissue sections revealed increased infiltration of tumors with T-cells and macrophages. Thamm et al assessed the efficacy of a lipid-DNA-SEA/IL-2 therapy in dogs with STS.[137] In this study, dogs received once weekly intratumoral injections and surgery was done after the 12-week treatment. In the 25% of dogs that responded to the therapy (3 complete responders, 1 partial), a diffuse lymphoplasmacytic infiltrate was observed on histologic evaluation of the tumors. Thus SAgs show some promise for use in veterinary medicine.

Liposome-Encapsulated Muramyl Tripeptide

Similar to SAgs, bacterial cell components such as peptides derived from mycobacterial cell walls were evaluated for potential immunogenicity. One such product is muramyl tripeptide (MTP), which, when encapsulated in a phosphatidylethanolamine-based liposome (L-MTP-PE), can efficiently activate monocytes and macrophages to produce proinflammatory cytokines, such as IL-1α and β, IL-6, IL-7, IL-8, IL-12, and TNF-α.[138] The use of L-MTP-PE as a therapeutic was assessed in phase I and II trials of people with osteosarcoma (OSA), renal carcinoma, and metastatic melanoma.[138-140] Moreover, this drug has been approved for use in treating pediatric osteosarcoma in Europe under the name Mifamurtide.[141]

L-MTP-PE has been evaluated in veterinary medicine in a variety of studies.[142-146] The survival benefit of L-MTP-PE therapy has been most clearly demonstrated in dogs with appendicular OSA.[147] In this study, dogs receiving L-MTP-PE following limb amputation had a median survival time (MST) of 222 days, whereas dogs that received placebo had an MST of 77 days. However, since most of the dogs in both groups developed metastatic disease, further studies evaluated the efficacy of L-MTP-PE in conjunction with chemotherapy.[142] In one study, dogs receiving L-MTP-PE after treatment with cisplatin had an MST of 14.4 months versus 9.8 months in dogs that received cisplatin only. Interestingly, only 73% of dogs receiving L-MTP-PE developed metastatic disease compared to 93% in the cisplatin only group. However, in a second trial, these investigators saw no significant survival advantage in dogs with OSA that received L-MTP-PE concurrently with cisplatin. The authors postulated that cisplatin obviated antimetastatic potential of L-MTP-PE due to impaired immune effectors. L-MTP-PE was also evaluated for efficacy in canine hemangiosarcoma (HSA).[144] Dogs that received L-MTP-PE with chemotherapy following splenectomy had an MST of 9 months versus the 5.7 months seen with dogs receiving chemotherapy alone. In another study, only dogs with stage I oral melanoma that received L-MTP-PE had an increased survival over placebo-treated dogs.[145] No differences were seen within the dogs with more advanced disease.

Liposome-DNA Complexes

Bacterial DNA can also stimulate the innate immune system via its CpG-oligonucleotides (CpG-ODNs), particularly when complexed with cationic liposomes, in a form known as cationic lipid-DNA complexes (CLDC).[148] Complexing bacterial plasmid DNA to liposomes allows for more efficient delivery of the CpG DNA to the endosomal compartment of antigen-presenting cells such as DCs, in which it is released from the liposomes and binds to its receptor, TLR9.[149,150] In mouse studies, CLDC stimulates the immune system largely through induction of NK cell activity and release of IFN-γ.[148] Moreover, CLDC was also shown to stimulate the production of type I IFN[151] and thus is a potent nonspecific immunostimulant.

The use of CLDC in dogs has been evaluated in metastatic OSA and in dogs with STS.[152,153] Intravenous administration of a modified CLDC that encodes for IL-2 was performed in dogs with stage IV OSA.[152] Dogs that received CLDC developed fevers and showed changes in their leukogram profile indicative of immune stimulation. Moreover, NK cell activity was observed, as assessed by target cell lysis, and monocytes showed increased expression of B7.2 on their surface, indicating activation. Treatment was associated with a significant increase in survival times compared to historic controls. Another study examined the use of CLDC in canine STS. Administration of CLDC intravenously once weekly for 6 weeks resulted in an objective response in 15% of the dogs and a decrease in tumor mean vessel density in half of the dogs receiving treatment.[153] Thus CLDC has potential to be used as a stand-alone immunotherapeutic in veterinary medicine for a variety of cancer types.

Oncolytic Viruses

Oncolytic viruses are defined as viruses capable of replicating in and lysing tumor cells, thus making them a likely candidate for drug or gene delivery to tumors. A beneficial side effect of these viruses is that they can kill the tumor cell, thus providing release of TAs for processing by the immune system. Adenoviruses that have undergone genetic modification of their early genes, 1A (E1A) and 1B (E1B), preferentially target rapidly dividing tumor cells and have been used to target canine OSA cells.[154-156] Canine distemper virus (CDV) has also been investigated as a treatment for B- and T-cell lymphoma in dogs.[157] In vitro studies using fluorescently labeled, attenuated CDV and canine lymphoma cells demonstrated that CDV infected lymphoid cells via binding of the cell membrane protein CD150, which is overexpressed on malignant B cells, and induced cellular apoptosis.[157]

Nonspecific Tumor Immunotherapy Using Recombinant Cytokine Therapy

Interleukin-2

IL-2 is a cytokine that is released by T-cells following their activation via interactions of antigen-loaded MHC and co-stimulatory molecules expressed on the surface of antigen-presenting cells. Its function is to induce clonal expansion of T-cells in an antigen-specific fashion and activate DCs, macrophages, and B-cells, which in turn release proinflammatory cytokines. Moreover, IL-2 stimulates NK cells, thus playing an important role in inducing both the innate and adaptive arms of the immune system.

The therapeutic use of IL-2 in humans is fraught with toxicity.[158-160] However, the use of IL-2 therapy in veterinary medicine holds some promise as a therapeutic. First, Helfand et al demonstrated that intravenously injected recombinant human IL-2 (rhIL-2) activates canine lymphocytes, causing only mild gastrointestinal toxicity, even at high doses for 4 consecutive days.[161] Another study demonstrated the ability of rhIL-2 to induce canine lymphokine-activated killer (LAK) cells and incidentally showed that LAK cells from tumor-bearing dogs did not kill tumor cells as efficiently as compared to normal dogs.[162] Further evaluation of toxicity and efficacy of rhIL-2 was done using dogs with primary lung cancer and with lung metastases in an aerosol formulation.[163] In this study, complete regression was seen in two of the four dogs with pulmonary metastases, and these dogs remained disease free for at least 12 months after treatment. One of the two dogs with a primary lung tumor had disease stabilization for more than 8 months, whereas the other dog had progressive disease. Assessment of the lymphocytes obtained from bronchoalveolar lavage showed increased cytolytic activity following 15 days of IL-2 treatment. In addition, minimal toxicity was noted in this study. Finally, IL-2 gene therapy using viral vectors has been examined for treatment of feline fibrosarcomas and canine melanoma and was shown to be safe and effective.[164-166] Therefore, given its low toxicity and promising effectiveness, rhIL-2 therapy is a plausible treatment for canine cancer.

Interleukin-12

IL-12, produced by antigen-stimulated DCs, macrophages, and B-cells, plays a role in stimulating the growth and function of T-cells and enhances the cytolytic activity of both T-cells and NK cells. Similar to IL-2, IL-12 therapy in humans leads to serious side effects; currently, it is not used clinically. Current investigation into the use of IL-12 in veterinary medicine revolves around recombinant gene therapy for treatment of canine head and neck tumors,[167] with some in vitro work looking at its use in feline hyperthermia-induced gene therapy.[168]

Interleukin-15

IL-15 is structurally similar to and uses similar signaling molecules as IL-2. IL-15 plays a role in stimulation of NK cells and promoting proliferation of T-cells. However, from an immunotherapy standpoint, IL-15 holds more promise than IL-2 in that (1) it does not cause activation-induced cell death of CD4+ T-cells following prolonged periods of exposure; rather it sustains T cell proliferation,[169] (2) IL-15 plays a critical role in CD8+ T-cell memory formation and maintenance,[170] and (3) unlike IL-2, IL-15 does not appear to play a role in the development of Tregs.[1]

Clinical investigation of IL-15 will begin soon. An initial safety study in nonhuman primates was recently conducted.[171] Twelve daily doses of clinical grade rhIL-15 revealed that neutropenia was the dose-limiting toxicity and documented an increase in circulating NK cells and memory CD8+ T-cells.

In veterinary medicine, one study used plasmid IL-15 in combination with plasmid IL-6 in beagles with CTVT.[172] A threefold increase in the proportion of CD8+ T-cells that infiltrated the tumors and an enhancement of IFN-γ–producing cells and increased cytolytic activity against the tumor were observed. Thus IL-15 therapy shows promise as an effective immunotherapy in both human and veterinary medicine.

Interferons

IFNs are proteins produced by lymphocytes that play an important role in immune responses to pathogens and cancer. Broadly, they can influence cell proliferation, play a role in the induction of apoptosis, upregulate antigen presentation to T-cells, and enhance the ability of the adaptive immune system to mount a cytolytic immune response. Moreover, IFNs have antiangiogenic properties. The IFNs are typically classified as either type I (IFN-α, -β, and -ω) or type II (IFN-γ).

Interferon-α, Interferon-β, and Interferon-ω Type I IFNs can affect cellular proliferation through various mechanisms, including interactions with cell cycle proteins (i.e., c-myc and retinoblastoma) and induction of apoptosis via Bcl-2/Bax and TNF/Fas interactions. Their antiangiogenic properties of downregulating VEGF and basic fibroblast growth factor (bFGF)[173] make them attractive as immunotherapies, and they have been used successfully to treat pediatric hemangiomas.[174]

Clinical trials using type I IFNs have met limited success due to the high occurrence of severe toxicity in light of overall limited response rates. Nonetheless, their effectiveness was assessed in melanoma, multiple myeloma, renal cell carcinoma, leukemia, and other cancers, as well as in conjunction with chemotherapies. The best response, in terms of disease-free survival, was seen in renal cell carcinoma and melanoma when used as single agents.[175,176]

The use of type I IFNs in veterinary medicine is limited and mostly used for feline viral therapies.[177] One study showed that recombinant feline IFN-ω was safe and easy to use for treating feline fibrosarcomas. As this was a safety study, the therapeutic effects of this treatment were not evaluated. Another recently published study also used recombinant feline IFN-ω with or without chemotherapy to study its effects in treating mammary tumors in vitro.[178] This study reported that the antitumor cell effects of recombinant IFN and chemotherapy were additive and suggested further investigation into its clinical use as an adjuvant therapy.

Interferon-γ IFN-γ plays an important role in stimulating the immune system. It is secreted mostly by NK cells, DCs, and antigen-activated T-cells and counteracts the effects of many of the immunosuppressive cytokines. It is a physiologic activator of macrophages, leading to increased antigen presentation and increased lysosomal function and NO production by macrophages. NO production by macrophages is an efficient mechanism of tumor cytolysis. IFN-γ can also cause increased MHC class I and II expression on a variety of cells, including tumors. Increased MHC expression has been confirmed to occur on in vitro IFN-γ–treated canine tumor cells lines[179] and in vivo following treatment with INF-γ.[180] Thus its role in antitumor immunity is characterized by increased tumor cell lysis and increased tumor antigen presentation to the adaptive immune response.

The use of IFN-γ in veterinary medicine is currently being investigated. A recently published study examined the use of IFN-γ in combination with a single injection of autologous, ex vivo activated DCs in dogs with various malignant or benign tumors.[181] In the seven dogs enrolled in the study, the investigators noted four complete responses and two partial responses against malignant tumors and saw moderate partial responses against fast-growing benign tumors. Another study looked at the use of adenoviral IFN-γ gene transfer as an adjuvant therapy to treat a dog with astrocytoma.[182] Following therapy and surgery, the dog was tumor free for greater than 450 days. Finally, a safety study was done in cats with fibrosarcomas using a triple-gene therapy that included IFN-γ along with IL-2 and GM-CSF.[166] In this study, cats tolerated the therapy, although six of the eight cats developed local recurrence of disease within 1 year of treatment.

Specific Immunotherapy for Cancer: Tumor Vaccines

The development of a tumor vaccine that is safe, effective, and long-lasting is an ultimate goal of immunotherapy. Whereas the effects of traditional cancer treatments such as chemotherapy, surgery, and radiation therapy typically result in noticeable clinical responses within hours to days following treatment, cancer vaccine therapeutic responses typically take weeks to months to lead to an appreciable clinical response. This difference in response time, coupled with the lack of congruent and objective ways to measure efficacy, make it difficult to develop tumor vaccines.

In an attempt to alleviate the lack of objectivity in assessing responses to cancer therapy, the National Cancer Institute (NCI) created an objective way to measure clinical responses, termed *response evaluation criteria in solid tumors* (RECIST). Under RECIST criteria, a clinical response is defined as a 30% reduction in the total sum of the maximum diameter of all lesions concurrent with the lack of appearance of new lesions or progression of current lesions.[183] The RECIST criteria were modified in 2009 to include changes to the number of lesions assessed, evaluation of pathologic lymph nodes, confirmation of response to treatments, clarification of disease progression, and incorporation of imaging modalities into the RECIST criteria.[184]

Nonetheless, despite the challenges to tumor vaccine development, there are many different varieties of tumor vaccines currently in use either clinically or as part of phase I, II, and III clinical trials. In fact, in April of 2010, the first therapeutic cancer vaccine for human prostate cancer was approved by the Food and Drug Administration (FDA). In this section, we will discuss only those vaccines showing success in human trials and those relevant to veterinary medicine.

Tumor Antigen Targets for Immunization

Mutations or differential expression of tumor-derived proteins are referred to as *tumor antigens* (TAs). These proteins include the broad categories of oncogenes, oncofetal proteins, and cancer testes antigens. Although TAs offer potential targets for vaccine development, their downside is that some of them tend to be individual or tumor type specific. Nonetheless, much work has been accomplished characterizing TAs for various forms of cancer, and a table of currently studied TAs can be found in a 2009 publication by a panel of experts organized by the NCI.[185] Whereas numerous TAs exist, the use of these TAs in tumor vaccines is not trivial. As mentioned previously, the tumor is highly capable of inducing a potent, immunosuppressive microenvironment by various mechanisms, thus standard vaccine procedures using TAs can be rendered useless in this powerful environment. In fact, there are little data available showing a clear correlation between in vitro TA responses and prognosis. Success of most tumor vaccines has been limited to animal models of induced disease.[186,187] However, through the use of better vaccine strategies and by combining therapies that can ultimately overcome tumor immunosuppression, more promising specific immunotherapies are being developed. Next, we will discuss the various platforms used to develop tumor vaccines.

Tumor Vaccine Approaches

Whole Tumor Cell and Tumor Cell Lysate Vaccines

One of the more simple approaches to tumor vaccine development is through the use of whole tumor cell or tumor cell lysate vaccines. These can either be made directly from the patient in the form of an autologous vaccine or from cell lines of similar tumor types from the same species as an allogeneic vaccine. Whole cell preparations are made by rendering tumor cells and/or tissues nonfunctional, typically via gamma irradiation. Tumor lysate vaccines, including membrane protein fraction vaccines, are made by mechanically disrupting the tumor cells and/or tissues. Both whole cell and tumor lysate vaccines are typically administered with some form of adjuvant to enhance the immune response. These polyvalent vaccines are superior to specific peptide or protein (subunit) vaccines in that they contain a heterogeneous population of TAs.

One study out of our laboratory assessed the use of an allogeneic HSA tumor lysate vaccine in combination with chemotherapy.[188] In this phase I/II study, 28 dogs were evaluated and received eight immunizations of tumor lysate plus liposome-DNA adjuvant (see Liposome-DNA Complexes) over a 22-week period while concurrently receiving doxorubicin. The vaccine was well tolerated; side effects were limited to moderate diarrhea and anorexia. Tumor-specific antibody responses were detected in four to five of the six dogs tested, depending on which HSA cell-line they were screened against. Moreover, overall survival times of dogs receiving the combination treatment were significantly better than historic controls treated with only chemotherapy.

Whole cell and tumor lysate vaccines can also be modified to enhance their immunogenicity. Aside from different adjuvant strategies, combination of these vaccines with modifiers such as immunostimulatory cytokines has been examined. One clinical trial of 16 dogs with STS or melanoma assessed the use of an autologous, whole cell vaccine transfected with human GM-CSF.[189] Three dogs in the study demonstrated objective tumor responses that included regression of primary and metastatic lesions. On histologic examination of tumor tissue in the dogs that received the vaccine, an impressive inflammatory response was noted. Another recent study using a similar human GM-CSF vaccine looked at its efficacy in treating dogs with B-cell lymphoma.[190] Dogs in remission following a 19-week standard CHOP protocol (cyclophosphamide, hydroxydaunorubicin [doxorubicin], vincristine [Oncovin], prednisone) were randomized into placebo or vaccine treatment groups. Although no changes in median length of remission were seen, dogs receiving the vaccine demonstrated a significant increase in overall survival. Lastly, a recent study investigated the use of an allogeneic melanoma vaccine in combination with a xenogenic melanoma protein, human glycoprotein 100 (hgp100).[191] In this phase II trial, the vaccine was well tolerated, and the researchers observed an overall response rate of 17% and a tumor control rate (including complete and partial responses as well as stable disease greater than 6 weeks duration) of 35%.

Immunization Against Defined Tumor Antigens Using Plasmid DNA

Vaccines that use specific gene sequences of TAs encoded in plasmid DNA have shown some clinical promise with their ability to invoke both cellular and humoral immunity. The ease of working with bacterial DNA and the ability to quickly produce large quantities of plasmid DNA make this an attractive vaccine platform. Moreover, the DNA sequences of a majority of TAs are known and can be easily inserted into the plasmid DNA and expressed under the control of a constitutively active bacterial promoter. Typically given intradermally or intramuscularly, the proteins expressed by transcription and translation of the plasmid are readily picked up by DCs, processed, and presented in the context of MHC class I and II, thus providing a more "natural" stimulation of the immune system. Moreover, the unmethylated dinucleotide-CpG residues, or CpG motifs, present in high frequency in the bacterial DNA, provide additional stimulation of DCs, triggering them to induce a Th1-type immune response.[192]

No DNA vaccines have been licensed for human use yet. However, many DNA vaccines have been tested in clinical trials, and results have thus far been disappointing for various reasons (see review in Liu[193]). Nonetheless, the first conditionally licensed (by the U.S. Department of Agriculture [USDA]) veterinary cancer vaccine is based off of the DNA plasmid technology.[194] The ONCEPT vaccine (Merial, Duluth, GA) for canine malignant melanoma (CMM) uses xenogeneic DNA plasmids that contain the gene-encoding human tyrosinase (huTyr). Initial studies showed the development of an antibody-mediated immune response against the huTyr protein that cross-reacted to canine tyrosinase.[195] Improved survival of dogs treated with this vaccine compared to historical control animals has been reported with no severe side effects noted.[194,196] Further studies of this plasmid DNA technology demonstrated that the vaccine could induce antigen-specific IFN-γ+ T-cells in normal beagle dogs.[197] Finally, the same group that developed the CMM vaccine has reportedly completed phase I trials of murine CD20 for treatment of canine B-cell lymphoma and is initiating a phase II trial soon.[198]

Tumor Vaccination Using Viral Vector Vaccines

As discussed previously, viruses have been used to target tumor cells, particularly those with innate oncolytic properties. However, viruses can also be used as vectors for expression of particular TAs. Typically, attenuated or replication-defective forms of the virus are used to allow for effective stimulation of the innate and adaptive immune responses without the risk of spreading and rapidly dividing within the host. The most commonly used viral platform for both human and veterinary studies is the Poxviridae family. The poxviruses are easy to work with, amenable to large amounts of foreign DNA, and highly immunogenic, allowing for strong immune responses against weak TAs, such as carcinoembryonic antigen (CEA).[199] In humans, one of the most commonly used viral vaccine platforms is the canarypox virus ALVAC. Recent published human clinical trials using ALVAC include combining CEA-expressing ALVAC with chemotherapy for metastatic colorectal cancer,[200] ALVAC-expressing human GM-CSF or IL-2 for treatment of melanoma or leiomyosarcoma,[201] and intranodal injection of ALVAC-expressing gp100 in high-risk melanoma patients.[202] Interestingly, although all of these studies reported that the vaccine was safe to use and that immunologic responses were observed, efficacy of these therapies is limited.[203]

Vaccination Against Tumor Antigens Using Dendritic Cells

Dendritic cells (DCs) possess very potent antigen-presenting abilities and are an attractive target for cancer vaccine strategies. Besides their role in vivo in processing and presenting TAs derived either naturally or from tumor vaccines, there are many clinical trials published that examine the use of ex vivo activated and expanded DCs injected back into the donor as a way of activating tumor-specific T-cells in vivo. The drawback to this method is that the ex vivo processing of DCs typically takes about 7 to 10 days, requires growth in a combination of cytokines, and can only be used autologously. Nonetheless, ex vivo prepared DCs have shown clinical efficacy, particularly in human patients with metastatic disease.[204,205] Recently, it has been determined that the potency of the DCs produced ex vivo depends on the combination of cytokines used.[206] DCs generated with GM-CSF and IFN-α or GM-CSF and IL-15 display potent priming of T-cell–mediated and CD8+ T-cell–mediated immune responses in vitro. Moreover, the use of mature DCs is better then immature DCs, since immature DCs actually induce immune tolerance via expansion of IL-10–secreting T-cells.[207] However, the methods of maturation matter as well, with studies showing DCs activated with a mixture of IFN-α, polyinosinic-polycytidylic acid, IL-1β, TNF, and IFN-γ elicit many more anti-melanoma cytotoxic T-lymphocytes (CTLs) in vitro than the standard IL-1β, TNF, IL-6, and prostaglandin E_2 (PGE_2) cocktail.[208] Finally, new methods of targeting antigens to DCs through anti-DC receptor (i.e., lectin receptors such as DEC-205, DC-SIGN, or DNGR-1) antibody-TA fusions, appropriate selection of adjuvants to deliver antigens to DCs, and combination therapies using chemotherapy and DC activation are being investigated.[204,206]

Of note, the first FDA-approved therapeutic cancer vaccine, Provenge (sipuleucel-T, Dendreon, Seattle) is derived from peripheral blood mononuclear cells (PBMCs) removed from patients with castration-refractory prostate cancer that are cultured and activated ex vivo with a fusion protein of human recombinant prostatic acid phosphatase (PAP) and human GM-CSF prior to transfusion back into the donor.[209] This vaccine has demonstrated an increase in survival time that was a little over 4 months compared to the placebo group in a multicenter clinical trial of over 500 patients. Besides consisting of activated DCs, this vaccine also contains autologous lymphocytes that may be playing a role in its efficacy.[210]

DC vaccination in veterinary medicine has been and is still currently being explored. An initial study of three dogs with oral melanoma showed that bone marrow–derived DCs transduced with an adenovirus expressing human gp100 could safely be used. In this study, dogs received three subcutaneous vaccines over 4 months.[211] One of the dogs that had a complete response with no evidence of disease 4 years later developed a robust CTL response against the gp100. Another dog that relapsed after 22 months had no evidence of anti-gp100 CTLs. A similar study performed in normal dogs was done to assess the immune response of DCs pulsed with canine melanoma cell (CMM2) lysates, in which a good delayed-type hypersensitivity response was seen against CMM2 following vaccination.[212]

Another study described previously saw success using ex vivo activated DCs and IFN-γ for treating canine solid tumors. Finally, a very recent study looked at the safety of using a DC-mammary tumor cell fusion hybrid vaccine.[213] In this case, normal dog PBMCs were used to generate DCs that were subsequently fused to canine mammary tumor cells. Injection of normal Beagle dogs with this fusion plus CpG adjuvant resulted in a robust antibody response against the fusion partner tumor cell line, as well as three unrelated canine mammary tumor cells. However, no CTL responses were noted. Hence development of DC vaccines for use in veterinary medicine is currently being explored in various tumor models and by using various strategies to optimize the induced antitumor immune response.

Antibody Therapy for Cancer

Monoclonal Antibodies

The use of monoclonal antibody (MAb) therapy for cancer has been studied for over a quarter century, following the development of hybridoma technology by Kohler and Milstein in 1975.[214] This technique consisted of antibody-producing cells fused with mouse myeloma cells, thus becoming immortalized and capable of continuously producing antibody that can be purified out of the culture media. Initially, the use of MAbs clinically was limited due to the responses mounted by the host against the foreign mouse proteins. However, recent technology allowed for "humanizing" these antibodies by genetically grafting the mouse hypervariable region of interest onto the human immunoglobulin, thus resulting in an antibody that is 95% human. Moreover, mice genetically rendered to express human immunoglobulins can successfully generate 100% human antibodies in response to various antigens.[215] Using humanized antibodies improves antibody-dependent cell-mediated cytotoxicity (ADCC), improves antibody stability, and decreases immunogenicity of the antibody itself. The use of MAbs in human medicine has increased over the years. Several MAbs are approved by the FDA for use as human cancer treatments, and many are in active development and currently undergoing testing in human clinical trials.[216] As a general guide, MAb names ending in -omab are murine based, -ximab and -zumab are chimeric, and -umab are humanized versions of the antibodies.

Unfortunately, the generation of canine versions of antibodies for use in veterinary medicine has yet to occur. Nonetheless, one recent study looked at the use of a murine (L243) and humanized form (IMMU-114) of an anti-HLA-DR MAb in normal dogs and dogs with B-cell lymphoma.[217] In vitro studies demonstrated that both of these antibodies bound normal and malignant canine lymphocytes, inducing apoptosis in some. In vivo administration to normal dogs provided safety and pharmacokinetic data. A pilot study was then performed on seven dogs with either lymphoma or plasmacytomas; these dogs received 1 to 4 treatments with L243 MAb every 2 weeks. Myelosuppression was a cumulative-dose adverse effect, but some dogs displayed a transient response to the treatments. Thus future investigation of the use of this MAb in canine lymphoma is warranted.

Conjugated Monoclonal Antibodies

Another use of MAbs is linking them to potential toxins or radioisotopes. Initial studies involved linking chemical toxins to immunoglobulins to generate molecules called *immunotoxins.* Such chemicals tested were ricin and diphtheria toxins, but these conjugates were immunogenically and chemically unstable. Development of recombinant immunotoxins helped address this issue, although the current concern with immunotoxins is their ability to nonspecifically kill any cell expressing the antibody-specific receptor.

MAbs can also be linked to radionuclides. The concept behind these antibodies is that the antibody targets tumor tissue and the energy released by the radioisotope attached to the antibody can penetrate bulky solid tumors and may also kill surrounding tumor and stromal cells. Examples of radiolabeled MAbs in clinical therapeutic use in humans currently exist. The current use of radiolabeled MAbs in dogs is limited to imaging modalities rather than treatment of cancer.

Cancer Immunotherapy Using Adoptive Transfer of T-Cells

Adoptive T-cell transfer (ACT) is a technique in which cells are collected from a cancer patient, expanded and activated in culture, and then transferred back into the patient. Although this technique allows for the enhancement of tumor-specific T-cells, it is labor intensive and time consuming, thus its use is limited in both human and veterinary patients. Below, we will discuss a couple of historic methods used to generate these cells, as well as new techniques currently being investigated to improve this form of immunotherapy.

Transfer of Lymphokine-Activated Killer Cells

Initial T-cell transfer studies involved the generation of LAK cells. This was done by culturing PBMCs in high concentrations of IL-2, thus selecting for a population of cells with potent tumor cell-lysis ability. Clinical trials using this technique in humans were disappointing and unfeasible, despite promising mouse studies.[218] Use of LAK cells in veterinary medicine is limited to studies of cats with feline leukemia virus (FeLV) or feline immunodeficiency virus (FIV).[219]

Transfer of Tumor-Infiltrating Lymphocytes

One source of potent antitumor T-cells is in the tumor itself. These cells, called *tumor-infiltrating lymphocytes* (TILs), when expanded using IL-2, exhibit potent cytolytic activity that is many times higher than LAK cells against tumors in both a specific and nonspecific way.[220] Although they are considered the best source of T-cells for ACT,[221,222] their use in human medicine is limited because of a few variables such as time of isolation, the tumor they were isolated from, and the functional state of the cells when isolated.[218] Nonetheless, limited success has been observed in cases of treating human melanoma with TILs, particularly when combined with nonmyeloablative chemotherapy such as fludarabine and cyclophosphamide, which deplete lymphocytes but spare bone marrow stem cells.[223] In one study, six of thirteen melanoma patients had significant tumor regression and four had a mixed response including regression of some lesions and growth of others.[223] In a follow-up study involving a larger number of patients (34 in total), tumor regression was seen in 51% of the patients that received chemotherapy prior to the TIL transfer and IL-2 treatment.[224] In addition to the use of nonmyeloablative treatments, recent studies have investigated the use of other forms of Th1 stimulation along with ACT. One group has investigated the use of adding CpG-ODNs to their TILs to increase their efficacy.[225] In a study using ex vivo isolated human TILs, instillation of the activated TILs with CpG-ODN into athymic nude, tumor-bearing mice resulted in decreased tumor burden and prolonged survival. Regardless of the human clinical trials' results, TILs have not been used in veterinary medicine, perhaps due to the lack of reliable efficacy across multiple tumor types.

New Approaches to Adoptive T-Cell Transfers

As mentioned at the beginning of this chapter, one limitation to most immunotherapies is the fact that tumors can orchestrate an immunosuppressive environment. Thus, even if one instilled thousands of activated, tumor-specific T-cells into a cancer patient, the majority of these cells will become inactivated on reaching the tumor, particularly when dealing with solid tumors.[226] It is currently being recognized that strategies to overcome immunosuppression must be implemented in order to enhance the efficiency of tumor-specific T-cells in ACT studies. One technique to address this suppression is performing lymphodepletion prior to ACT.[227-229] Recent studies have also suggested the isolation of CD4+ T-cells for ACT, rather than cytotoxic CD8+ T-cells because CD4+ T-cells are capable of activating both innate immune cells and CD8+ T-cells.[230,231] However, CD4+ T-cells contain Treg cells, thus strategies to block the development of Treg cells during CD4+ T-cell ACT have also been investigated.[230] In addition, the availability of TAs also appears to play a role in the strength of CD4+ ACT therapy.[232] Similarly, the addition of cytokines and/or blocking antibodies against suppressor cells, along with ACTs, has been shown to enhance the effectiveness of this therapy.[230,233-235]

The Future of Cancer Immunotherapy

The use of immunotherapy for the treatment of cancer is an exciting and ever-evolving field of research and application. With the advancement of techniques used to assess immune responses to tumors; better ways of predicting responses, including development of RECIST; and an understanding that tumor responses to immunotherapies may be delayed as compared to conventional chemotherapy, radiation therapy, and surgery, one can more reliably assess the clinical efficacy and safety of novel immunotherapies. Moreover, a better understanding of the disease pathology in our veterinary patients has led to a movement toward using spontaneous canine and feline cancers as models for human disease, thus allowing for testing of novel immunotherapies in our small animal patients that will not only benefit them, but benefit human cancer patients as well.[236,237]

However, the development of a successful immunotherapy protocol is not without limitations. One of the main reasons for failure of many immunotherapies is due to the immunosuppressive microenvironment established by the tumor. Thus immunotherapies that are best able to overcome this suppression will prove the most successful.[238] In addition, certain drugs and/or proteins that can deplete or inactivate the key players in immune suppression (i.e., MDSCs and Tregs) may be best used in concert with novel vaccines or other immunotherapies in order to optimize their effectiveness. Along those lines, the use of newer and more potent adjuvants such as various preparations of CpG motifs to stimulate the immune system will be a critical component of newer vaccines. It has now become clear that the most successful adjuvants are those that not only stimulate a strong primary response against the tumor, but also lead to the development of a robust central memory response.

One of the more successful categories of immunotherapies currently used in human medicine is MAbs. Advances in technology led to the development of humanized, nonimmunogenic forms of antibodies against key cellular receptors, either to activate key antitumor immune cells or lead to cytolytic activity against tumor cells. However, similar advances in treating dogs with MAbs are lacking, although some promising preliminary results have been seen using human or mouse antibodies to treat canine lymphoma.[217]

It should be understood that many, if not all, immunotherapies developed should work in concert and synergize with current cancer treatment modalities. Given the ability of tumor cells to become resistant to chemotherapy and radiation therapy and their ability to suppress the immune system, one would be naïve to think that a single-modality treatment is the most effective means of tumor control. While the immune system can be manipulated to mount an effective antitumor immune response, it is best utilized in cases of minimal residual and metastatic disease, in which radiation therapy, chemotherapy, and/or surgery are used to cytoreduce large tumors. Moreover, it is becoming very clear that the immune system is a key player involved in the tumor response to radiation and chemotherapy; thus finding ways to incorporate immunotherapy into current standards of care may actually enhance the effectiveness of these modalities. For example, we have observed that the use of liposomal clodronate therapy to eliminate MDSCs can enhance the tumor response to lomustine (CCNU) in dogs with malignant histiocytosis (unpublished observation). We hypothesize that the immunosuppressive cells present in the tumor microenvironment are capable of protecting tumor cells from the effects of chemotherapy, thus by removing these tumor cells we can enhance the effectiveness of the chemotherapy. We predict that the use of immunotherapy as part of a protocol to treat canine and feline diseases should soon become routine. By understanding the role of the immune system in cancer in our small animal patients, we can develop not only better immunotherapies that will benefit these patients, but also therapies that will be applicable to human medicine.

REFERENCES

1. Antony PA, Restifo NP: CD4+CD25+ T regulatory cells, immunotherapy of cancer, and interleukin-2, *J Immunother* 28:120–128, 2005.

2. Burnet M: Cancer; a biological approach. I. The processes of control, *Br Med J* 1:779–786, 1957.
3. Stutman O: Tumor development after 3-methylcholanthrene in immunologically deficient athymic-nude mice, *Science* 183:534–536, 1974.
4. Rygaard J, Povlsen CO: The mouse mutant nude does not develop spontaneous tumours. An argument against immunological surveillance, *Acta Pathol Microbiol Scand B Microbiol Immunol* 82:99–106, 1974.
5. Schreiber TH, Podack ER: A critical analysis of the tumour immunosurveillance controversy for 3-MCA-induced sarcomas, *Br J Cancer* 101:381–386, 2009.
6. Kaplan DH, Shankaran V, Dighe AS, et al: Demonstration of an interferon gamma-dependent tumor surveillance system in immunocompetent mice, *Proc Natl Acad Sci U S A* 95:7556–7561, 1998.
7. Shankaran V, Ikeda H, Bruce AT, et al: IFNgamma and lymphocytes prevent primary tumour development and shape tumour immunogenicity, *Nature* 410:1107–1111, 2001.
8. Dunn GP, Bruce AT, Ikeda H, et al: Cancer immunoediting: from immunosurveillance to tumor escape, *Nat Immunol* 3:991–998, 2002.
9. Rabinovich GA, Gabrilovich D, Sotomayor EM: Immunosuppressive strategies that are mediated by tumor cells, *Annu Rev Immunol* 25:267–296, 2007.
10. Murdoch C, Muthana M, Coffelt SB, et al: The role of myeloid cells in the promotion of tumour angiogenesis, *Nat Rev Cancer* 8:618–631, 2008.
11. Qian BZ, Pollard JW: Macrophage diversity enhances tumor progression and metastasis, *Cell* 141:39–51, 2010.
12. Almand B, Clark JI, Nikitina E, et al: Increased production of immature myeloid cells in cancer patients: a mechanism of immunosuppression in cancer, *J Immunol* 166:678–689, 2001.
13. Diaz-Montero CM, Salem ML, Nishimura MI, et al: Increased circulating myeloid-derived suppressor cells correlate with clinical cancer stage, metastatic tumor burden, and doxorubicin-cyclophosphamide chemotherapy, *Cancer Immunol Immunother* 58:49–59, 2009.
14. Mandruzzato S, Solito S, Falisi E, et al: IL4Ralpha+ myeloid-derived suppressor cell expansion in cancer patients, *J Immunol* 182:6562–6568, 2009.
15. Bunt SK, Yang L, Sinha P, et al: Reduced inflammation in the tumor microenvironment delays the accumulation of myeloid-derived suppressor cells and limits tumor progression, *Cancer Res* 67:10019–10026, 2007.
16. Melani C, Chiodoni C, Forni G, et al: Myeloid cell expansion elicited by the progression of spontaneous mammary carcinomas in c-erbB-2 transgenic BALB/c mice suppresses immune reactivity, *Blood* 102:2138–2145, 2003.
17. Bosco MC, Puppo M, Blengio F, et al: Monocytes and dendritic cells in a hypoxic environment: Spotlights on chemotaxis and migration, *Immunobiology* 213:733–749, 2008.
18. Du R, Lu KV, Petritsch C, et al: HIF1alpha induces the recruitment of bone marrow-derived vascular modulatory cells to regulate tumor angiogenesis and invasion, *Cancer Cell* 13:206–220, 2008.
19. Sawanobori Y, Ueha S, Kurachi M, et al: Chemokine-mediated rapid turnover of myeloid-derived suppressor cells in tumor-bearing mice, *Blood* 111:5457–5466, 2008.
20. Yang L, Huang J, Ren X, et al: Abrogation of TGF beta signaling in mammary carcinomas recruits Gr-1+CD11b+ myeloid cells that promote metastasis, *Cancer Cell* 13:23–35, 2008.
21. Ye XZ, Yu SC, Bian XW: Contribution of myeloid-derived suppressor cells to tumor-induced immune suppression, angiogenesis, invasion and metastasis, *J Genet Genomics* 37:423–430, 2010.
22. Joyce JA, Pollard JW: Microenvironmental regulation of metastasis, *Nat Rev Cancer* 9:239–252, 2009.
23. Ostrand-Rosenberg S, Sinha P: Myeloid-derived suppressor cells: linking inflammation and cancer, *J Immunol* 182:4499–4506, 2009.
24. Sinha P, Clements VK, Bunt SK, et al: Cross-talk between myeloid-derived suppressor cells and macrophages subverts tumor immunity toward a type 2 response, *J Immunol* 179:977–983, 2007.
25. Li H, Han Y, Guo Q, et al: Cancer-expanded myeloid-derived suppressor cells induce anergy of NK cells through membrane-bound TGF-beta1, *J Immunol* 182:240–249, 2009.
26. Nomura T, Sakaguchi S: Naturally arising CD25+CD4+ regulatory T cells in tumor immunity, *Curr Top Microbiol Immunol* 293:287–302, 2005.
27. Fontenot JD, Rudensky AY: A well adapted regulatory contrivance: regulatory T cell development and the forkhead family transcription factor Foxp3, *Nat Immunol* 6:331–337, 2005.
28. Camisaschi C, Casati C, Rini F, et al: LAG-3 expression defines a subset of CD4(+)CD25(high)Foxp3(+) regulatory T cells that are expanded at tumor sites, *J Immunol* 184:6545–6551, 2010.
29. Shimizu J, Yamazaki S, Takahashi T, et al: Stimulation of CD25(+) CD4(+) regulatory T cells through GITR breaks immunological self-tolerance, *Nat Immunol* 3:135–142, 2002.
30. Wing K, Onishi Y, Prieto-Martin P, et al: CTLA-4 control over Foxp3+ regulatory T cell function, *Science* 322:271–275, 2008.
31. Yamaguchi T, Hirota K, Nagahama K, et al: Control of immune responses by antigen-specific regulatory T cells expressing the folate receptor, *Immunity* 27:145–159, 2007.
32. Qin FX: Dynamic behavior and function of Foxp3+ regulatory T cells in tumor bearing host, *Cell Mol Immunol* 6:3–13, 2009.
33. Chen W, Jin W, Hardegen N, et al: Conversion of peripheral CD4+CD25- naive T cells to CD4+CD25+ regulatory T cells by TGF-beta induction of transcription factor Foxp3, *J Exp Med* 198:1875–1886, 2003.
34. Chen W, Wahl SM: TGF-beta: the missing link in CD4+CD25+ regulatory T cell-mediated immunosuppression, *Cytokine Growth Factor Rev* 14:85–89, 2003.
35. Hawiger D, Wan YY, Eynon EE, et al: The transcription cofactor Hopx is required for regulatory T cell function in dendritic cell-mediated peripheral T cell unresponsiveness, *Nat Immunol* 11:962–968, 2010.
36. Huehn J, Hamann A: Homing to suppress: address codes for Treg migration, *Trends Immunol* 26:632–636, 2005.
37. Hoelzinger DB, Smith SE, Mirza N, et al: Blockade of CCL1 inhibits T regulatory cell suppressive function enhancing tumor immunity without affecting T effector responses, *J Immunol* 184:6833–6842, 2010.
38. Curiel TJ, Coukos G, Zou L, et al: Specific recruitment of regulatory T cells in ovarian carcinoma fosters immune privilege and predicts reduced survival, *Nat Med* 10:942–949, 2004.
39. Miller AM, Lundberg K, Ozenci V, et al: CD4+CD25high T cells are enriched in the tumor and peripheral blood of prostate cancer patients, *J Immunol* 177:7398–7405, 2006.
40. Sasada T, Kimura M, Yoshida Y, et al: CD4+CD25+ regulatory T cells in patients with gastrointestinal malignancies: possible involvement of regulatory T cells in disease progression, *Cancer* 98:1089–1099, 2003.
41. Turk MJ, Guevara-Patino JA, Rizzuto GA, et al: Concomitant tumor immunity to a poorly immunogenic melanoma is prevented by regulatory T cells, *J Exp Med* 200:771–782, 2004.
42. Viguier M, Lemaitre F, Verola O, et al: Foxp3 expressing CD4+CD25(high) regulatory T cells are overrepresented in human metastatic melanoma lymph nodes and inhibit the function of infiltrating T cells, *J Immunol* 173:1444–1453, 2004.
43. Biller BJ, Elmslie RE, Burnett RC, et al: Use of FoxP3 expression to identify regulatory T cells in healthy dogs and dogs with cancer, *Vet Immunol Immunopathol* 116:69–78, 2007.
44. O'Neill K, Guth A, Biller B, et al: Changes in regulatory T cells in dogs with cancer and associations with tumor type, *J Vet Intern Med* 23:875–881, 2009.

45. Teng MW, Swann JB, von Scheidt B, et al: Multiple antitumor mechanisms downstream of prophylactic regulatory T-cell depletion, *Cancer Res* 70:2665–2674, 2010.
46. Piconese S, Valzasina B, Colombo MP: OX40 triggering blocks suppression by regulatory T cells and facilitates tumor rejection, *J Exp Med* 205:825–839, 2008.
47. Berraondo P, Nouze C, Preville X, et al: Eradication of large tumors in mice by a tritherapy targeting the innate, adaptive, and regulatory components of the immune system, *Cancer Res* 67:8847–8855, 2007.
48. Matar P, Rozados VR, Gonzalez AD, et al: Mechanism of antimetastatic immunopotentiation by low-dose cyclophosphamide, *Eur J Cancer* 36:1060–1066, 2000.
49. Ghiringhelli F, Menard C, Puig PE, et al: Metronomic cyclophosphamide regimen selectively depletes CD4+CD25+ regulatory T cells and restores T and NK effector functions in end stage cancer patients, *Cancer Immunol Immunother* 56:641–648, 2007.
50. Hoffmann TK, Muller-Berghaus J, Ferris RL, et al: Alterations in the frequency of dendritic cell subsets in the peripheral circulation of patients with squamous cell carcinomas of the head and neck, *Clin Cancer Res* 8:1787–1793, 2002.
51. Pinzon-Charry A, Ho CS, Laherty R, et al: A population of HLA-DR+ immature cells accumulates in the blood dendritic cell compartment of patients with different types of cancer, *Neoplasia* 7:1112–1122, 2005.
52. Jin D, Fan J, Wang L, et al: CD73 on tumor cells impairs antitumor T-cell responses: a novel mechanism of tumor-induced immune suppression, *Cancer Res* 70:2245–2255, 2010.
53. Steinman RM, Hawiger D, Nussenzweig MC: Tolerogenic dendritic cells, *Annu Rev Immunol* 21:685–711, 2003.
54. Fuchs EJ, Matzinger P: Is cancer dangerous to the immune system? *Semin Immunol* 8:271–280, 1996.
55. Enk AH, Jonuleit H, Saloga J, et al: Dendritic cells as mediators of tumor-induced tolerance in metastatic melanoma, *Int J Cancer* 73:309–316, 1997.
56. Nestle FO, Burg G, Fah J, et al: Human sunlight-induced basal-cell-carcinoma-associated dendritic cells are deficient in T cell co-stimulatory molecules and are impaired as antigen-presenting cells, *Am J Pathol* 150:641–651, 1997.
57. Chaux P, Favre N, Martin M, et al: Tumor-infiltrating dendritic cells are defective in their antigen-presenting function and inducible B7 expression in rats, *Int J Cancer* 72:619–624, 1997.
58. Ishida T, Oyama T, Carbone DP, et al: Defective function of Langerhans cells in tumor-bearing animals is the result of defective maturation from hemopoietic progenitors, *J Immunol* 161:4842–4851, 1998.
59. Almand B, Resser JR, Lindman B, et al: Clinical significance of defective dendritic cell differentiation in cancer, *Clin Cancer Res* 6:1755–1766, 2000.
60. Troy AJ, Summers KL, Davidson PJ, et al: Minimal recruitment and activation of dendritic cells within renal cell carcinoma, *Clin Cancer Res* 4:585–593, 1998.
61. Liu CC, Wang YS, Lin CY, et al: Transient downregulation of monocyte-derived dendritic-cell differentiation, function, and survival during tumoral progression and regression in an in vivo canine model of transmissible venereal tumor, *Cancer Immunol Immunother* 57:479–491, 2008.
62. Cheng P, Corzo CA, Luetteke N, et al: Inhibition of dendritic cell differentiation and accumulation of myeloid-derived suppressor cells in cancer is regulated by S100A9 protein, *J Exp Med* 205:2235–2249, 2008.
63. Herber DL, Cao W, Nefedova Y, et al: Lipid accumulation and dendritic cell dysfunction in cancer, *Nat Med* 16:880–886, 2010.
64. Hartmann E, Wollenberg B, Rothenfusser S, et al: Identification and functional analysis of tumor-infiltrating plasmacytoid dendritic cells in head and neck cancer, *Cancer Res* 63:6478–6487, 2003.
65. Gerlini G, Tun-Kyi A, Dudli C, et al: Metastatic melanoma secreted IL-10 down-regulates CD1 molecules on dendritic cells in metastatic tumor lesions, *Am J Pathol* 165:1853–1863, 2004.
66. Gabrilovich DI, Chen HL, Girgis KR, et al: Production of vascular endothelial growth factor by human tumors inhibits the functional maturation of dendritic cells, *Nat Med* 2:1096–1103, 1996.
67. Zhang M, Tang H, Guo Z, et al: Splenic stroma drives mature dendritic cells to differentiate into regulatory dendritic cells, *Nat Immunol* 5:1124–1133, 2004.
68. Lin WW, Karin M: A cytokine-mediated link between innate immunity, inflammation, and cancer, *J Clin Invest* 117:1175–1183, 2007.
69. Ridge J, Terle DA, Dragunsky E, et al: Effects of gamma-IFN and NGF on subpopulations in a human neuroblastoma cell line: flow cytometric and morphological analysis, *In Vitro Cell Dev Biol Anim* 32:238–248, 1996.
70. Maloy KJ, Salaun L, Cahill R, et al: CD4+CD25+ T(R) cells suppress innate immune pathology through cytokine-dependent mechanisms, *J Exp Med* 197:111–119, 2003.
71. Sredni B, Weil M, Khomenok G, et al: Ammonium trichloro(dioxoethylene-o,o')tellurate (AS101) sensitizes tumors to chemotherapy by inhibiting the tumor interleukin 10 autocrine loop, *Cancer Res* 64:1843–1852, 2004.
72. Ebrahimi B, Tucker SL, Li D, et al: Cytokines in pancreatic carcinoma: correlation with phenotypic characteristics and prognosis, *Cancer* 101:2727–2736, 2004.
73. Ozdemir F, Aydin F, Yilmaz M, et al: The effects of IL-2, IL-6 and IL-10 levels on prognosis in patients with aggressive non-Hodgkin's lymphoma (NHL), *J Exp Clin Cancer Res* 23:485–488, 2004.
74. Lech-Maranda E, Bienvenu J, Michallet AS, et al: Elevated IL-10 plasma levels correlate with poor prognosis in diffuse large B-cell lymphoma, *Eur Cytokine Netw* 17:60–66, 2006.
75. Becker C, Fantini MC, Neurath MF: TGF-beta as a T cell regulator in colitis and colon cancer, *Cytokine Growth Factor Rev* 17:97–106, 2006.
76. Ghiringhelli F, Puig PE, Roux S, et al: Tumor cells convert immature myeloid dendritic cells into TGF-beta-secreting cells inducing CD4+CD25+ regulatory T cell proliferation, *J Exp Med* 202:919–929, 2005.
77. Derynck R, Akhurst RJ, Balmain A: TGF-beta signaling in tumor suppression and cancer progression, *Nat Genet* 29:117–129, 2001.
78. Luo JL, Maeda S, Hsu LC, et al: Inhibition of NF-kappaB in cancer cells converts inflammation- induced tumor growth mediated by TNFalpha to TRAIL-mediated tumor regression, *Cancer Cell* 6:297–305, 2004.
79. Elgert KD, Alleva DG, Mullins DW: Tumor-induced immune dysfunction: the macrophage connection, *J Leukoc Biol* 64:275–290, 1998.
80. Catchpole B, Gould SM, Kellett-Gregory LM, et al: Immunosuppressive cytokines in the regional lymph node of a dog suffering from oral malignant melanoma, *J Small Anim Pract* 43:464–467, 2002.
81. Reinis M: Immunotherapy of MHC class I-deficient tumors, *Future Oncology* 6:1577–1589, 2010.
82. Garrido F, Algarra I, Garcia-Lora AM: The escape of cancer from T lymphocytes: immunoselection of MHC class I loss variants harboring structural-irreversible "hard" lesions, *Cancer Immunol Immunother* 59:1601–1606, 2010.
83. Rimsza LM, Farinha P, Fuchs DA, et al: HLA-DR protein status predicts survival in patients with diffuse large B-cell lymphoma treated on the MACOP-B chemotherapy regimen, *Leuk Lymphoma* 48:542–546, 2007.
84. Rimsza LM, Roberts RA, Miller TP, et al: Loss of MHC class II gene and protein expression in diffuse large B-cell lymphoma is related to decreased tumor immunosurveillance and poor patient survival regardless of other prognostic factors: a follow-up study from the Leukemia and Lymphoma Molecular Profiling Project, *Blood* 103:4251–4258, 2004.

85. Rao S, Lana S, Eickhoff J, et al: Class II major histocompatibility complex expression and cell size independently predict survival in canine B-cell lymphoma, *J Vet Intern Med* 25(5):1097–1105, 2011.
86. Shi F, Shi M, Zeng Z, et al: PD-1 and PD-L1 upregulation promotes CD8(+) T-cell apoptosis and postoperative recurrence in hepatocellular carcinoma patients, *Int J Cancer* 128:887–896, 2011.
87. Mu CY, Huang JA, Chen Y, et al: High expression of PD-L1 in lung cancer may contribute to poor prognosis and tumor cells immune escape through suppressing tumor infiltrating dendritic cells maturation, *Med Oncol* 28(3):682–688, 2010.
88. Nomi T, Sho M, Akahori T, et al: Clinical significance and therapeutic potential of the programmed death-1 ligand/ programmed death-1 pathway in human pancreatic cancer, *Clin Cancer Res* 13:2151–2157, 2007.
89. Benson DM, Jr., Bakan CE, Mishra A, et al: The PD-1/PD-L1 axis modulates the natural killer cell versus multiple myeloma effect: a therapeutic target for CT-011, a novel monoclonal anti-PD-1 antibody, *Blood* 116:2286–2294, 2010.
90. Suzuki E, Kapoor V, Jassar AS, et al: Gemcitabine selectively eliminates splenic Gr-1+/CD11b+ myeloid suppressor cells in tumor-bearing animals and enhances antitumor immune activity, *Clin Cancer Res* 11:6713–6721, 2005.
91. Vincent J, Mignot G, Chalmin F, et al: 5-Fluorouracil selectively kills tumor-associated myeloid-derived suppressor cells resulting in enhanced T cell-dependent antitumor immunity, *Cancer Res* 70:3052–3061, 2010.
92. Ko JS, Zea AH, Rini BI, et al: Sunitinib mediates reversal of myeloid-derived suppressor cell accumulation in renal cell carcinoma patients, *Clin Cancer Res* 15:2148–2157, 2009.
93. Kodumudi KN, Woan K, Gilvary DL, et al: A novel chemoimmunomodulating property of docetaxel: suppression of myeloid-derived suppressor cells in tumor bearers, *Clin Cancer Res* 16:4583–4594, 2010.
94. Sinha P, Clements VK, Fulton AM, et al: Prostaglandin E2 promotes tumor progression by inducing myeloid-derived suppressor cells, *Cancer Res* 67:4507–4513, 2007.
95. Pan PY, Wang GX, Yin B, et al: Reversion of immune tolerance in advanced malignancy: modulation of myeloid-derived suppressor cell development by blockade of stem-cell factor function, *Blood* 111:219–228, 2008.
96. Lathers DM, Clark JI, Achille NJ, et al: Phase 1B study to improve immune responses in head and neck cancer patients using escalating doses of 25-hydroxyvitamin D3, *Cancer Immunol Immunother* 53:422–430, 2004.
97. Shojaei F, Singh M, Thompson JD, et al: Role of Bv8 in neutrophil-dependent angiogenesis in a transgenic model of cancer progression, *Proc Natl Acad Sci U S A* 105:2640–2645, 2008.
98. Melani C, Sangaletti S, Barazzetta FM, et al: Amino-biphosphonate-mediated MMP-9 inhibition breaks the tumor-bone marrow axis responsible for myeloid-derived suppressor cell expansion and macrophage infiltration in tumor stroma, *Cancer Res* 67:11438–11446, 2007.
99. Mirza N, Fishman M, Fricke I, et al: All-trans-retinoic acid improves differentiation of myeloid cells and immune response in cancer patients, *Cancer Res* 66:9299–9307, 2006.
100. Daurkin I, Eruslanov E, Vieweg J, et al: Generation of antigen-presenting cells from tumor-infiltrated CD11b myeloid cells with DNA demethylating agent 5-aza-2′-deoxycytidine, *Cancer Immunol Immunother* 59:697–706, 2010.
101. Ko HJ, Lee JM, Kim YJ, et al: Immunosuppressive myeloid-derived suppressor cells can be converted into immunogenic APCs with the help of activated NKT cells: an alternative cell-based antitumor vaccine, *J Immunol* 182:1818–1828, 2009.
102. Fernandez A, Mesa C, Marigo I, et al: Inhibition of tumor-induced myeloid-derived suppressor cell function by a nanoparticulated adjuvant, *J Immunol* 186:264–274, 2011.
103. Priceman SJ, Sung JL, Shaposhnik Z, et al: Targeting distinct tumor-infiltrating myeloid cells by inhibiting CSF-1 receptor: combating tumor evasion of antiangiogenic therapy, *Blood* 115:1461–1471, 2010.
104. Pan PY, Ma G, Weber KJ, et al: Immune stimulatory receptor CD40 is required for T-cell suppression and T regulatory cell activation mediated by myeloid-derived suppressor cells in cancer, *Cancer Res* 70:99–108, 2010.
105. Curran MA, Montalvo W, Yagita H, et al: PD-1 and CTLA-4 combination blockade expands infiltrating T cells and reduces regulatory T and myeloid cells within B16 melanoma tumors, *Proc Natl Acad Sci U S A* 107:4275–4280, 2010.
106. De Santo C, Serafini P, Marigo I, et al: Nitroaspirin corrects immune dysfunction in tumor-bearing hosts and promotes tumor eradication by cancer vaccination, *Proc Natl Acad Sci U S A* 102:4185–4190, 2005.
107. Serafini P, Mgebroff S, Noonan K, et al: Myeloid-derived suppressor cells promote cross-tolerance in B-cell lymphoma by expanding regulatory T cells, *Cancer Res* 68:5439–5449, 2008.
108. Nagaraj S, Youn JI, Weber H, et al: Anti-inflammatory triterpenoid blocks immune suppressive function of MDSCs and improves immune response in cancer, *Clin Cancer Res* 16:1812–1823, 2010.
109. Serafini P, Meckel K, Kelso M, et al: Phosphodiesterase-5 inhibition augments endogenous antitumor immunity by reducing myeloid-derived suppressor cell function, *J Exp Med* 203:2691–2702, 2006.
110. Richardson MA, Ramirez T, Russell NC, et al: Coley toxins immunotherapy: a retrospective review, *Altern Ther Health Med* 5:42–47, 1999.
111. Alexandroff AB, Jackson AM, O'Donnell MA, et al: BCG immunotherapy of bladder cancer: 20 years on, *Lancet* 353:1689–1694, 1999.
112. van der Meijden AP: Non-specific immunotherapy with bacille Calmette-Guerin (BCG), *Clin Exp Immunol* 123:179–180, 2001.
113. Vita F, Siracusano S, Abbate R, et al: BCG prophylaxis in bladder cancer produces activation of recruited neutrophils, *Can J Urol* 18:5517–5523, 2011.
114. Ludwig AT, Moore JM, Luo Y, et al: Tumor necrosis factor-related apoptosis-inducing ligand: a novel mechanism for Bacillus Calmette-Guerin-induced antitumor activity, *Cancer Res* 64:3386–3390, 2004.
115. Herr HW, Morales A: History of bacillus Calmette-Guerin and bladder cancer: an immunotherapy success story, *J Urol* 179:53–56, 2008.
116. Klein WR, Rutten VP, Steerenberg PA, et al: The present status of BCG treatment in the veterinary practice, *In Vivo* 5:605–608, 1991.
117. Debruyne FM, van der Meijden AP, Schreinemachers LM, et al: Intravesical and intradermal BCG-RIVM application: a toxicity study, *Prog Clin Biol Res* 185B:151–159,1985.
118. Knapp DW, Glickman NW, Denicola DB, et al: Naturally-occurring canine transitional cell carcinoma of the urinary bladder: a relevant model of human invasive bladder cancer, *Urol Oncol* 5:47–59, 2000.
119. Mukaratirwa S, Chitanga S, Chimatira T, et al: Combination therapy using intratumoral bacillus Calmette-Guerin (BCG) and vincristine in dogs with transmissible venereal tumours: therapeutic efficacy and histological changes, *J S Afr Vet Assoc* 80:92–96, 2009.
120. Henry CJ, Downing S, Rosenthal RC, et al: Evaluation of a novel immunomodulator composed of human chorionic gonadotropin and bacillus Calmette-Guerin for treatment of canine mast cell tumors in clinically affected dogs, *Am J Vet Res* 68:1246–1251, 2007.
121. Lipton A, Harvey HA, Balch CM, et al: Corynebacterium parvum versus bacille Calmette-Guerin adjuvant immunotherapy of stage II malignant melanoma, *J Clin Oncol* 9:1151–1156, 1991.
122. MacEwen EG, Patnaik AK, Harvey HJ, et al: Canine oral melanoma: comparison of surgery versus surgery plus Corynebacterium parvum, *Cancer Invest* 4:397–402, 1986.
123. Misdorp W: Incomplete surgery, local immunostimulation, and recurrence of some tumour types in dogs and cats, *Vet Q* 9:279–286, 1987.

124. Luo X, Li Z, Lin S, et al: Antitumor effect of VNP20009, an attenuated Salmonella, in murine tumor models, *Oncol Res* 12:501–508, 2001.
125. Leschner S, Westphal K, Dietrich N, et al: Tumor invasion of Salmonella enterica serovar Typhimurium is accompanied by strong hemorrhage promoted by TNF-alpha, *PLoS One* 4:e6692, 2009.
126. Saccheri F, Pozzi C, Avogadri F, et al: Bacteria-induced gap junctions in tumors favor antigen cross-presentation and antitumor immunity, *Sci Transl Med* 2:44–57, 2010.
127. Toso JF, Gill VJ, Hwu P, et al: Phase I study of the intravenous administration of attenuated Salmonella typhimurium to patients with metastatic melanoma, *J Clin Oncol* 20:142–152, 2002.
128. Thamm DH, Kurzman ID, King I, et al: Systemic administration of an attenuated, tumor-targeting Salmonella typhimurium to dogs with spontaneous neoplasia: phase I evaluation, *Clin Cancer Res* 11:4827–4834, 2005.
129. Ochi A, Migita K, Xu J, et al: In vivo tumor immunotherapy by a bacterial superantigen, *J Immunol* 151:3180–3186, 1993.
130. Newell KA, Ellenhorn JD, Bruce DS, et al: In vivo T-cell activation by staphylococcal enterotoxin B prevents outgrowth of a malignant tumor, *Proc Natl Acad Sci U S A* 88:1074–1078, 1991.
131. Dow SW, Elmslie RE, Willson AP, et al: In vivo tumor transfection with superantigen plus cytokine genes induces tumor regression and prolongs survival in dogs with malignant melanoma, *J Clin Invest* 101:2406–2414, 1998.
132. Sun D, Woodland DL, Coleclough C, et al: An MHC class II-expressing T cell clone presenting conventional antigen lacks the ability to present bacterial superantigen, *Int Immunol* 7:1079–1085, 1995.
133. Kotzin BL, Leung DY, Kappler J, et al: Superantigens and their potential role in human disease, *Adv Immunol* 54:99–166, 1993.
134. Forsberg G, Ohlsson L, Brodin T, et al: Therapy of human non-small-cell lung carcinoma using antibody targeting of a modified superantigen, *Br J Cancer* 85:129–136, 2001.
135. Xu Q, Zhang X, Yue J, et al: Human TGFalpha-derived peptide TGFalphaL3 fused with superantigen for immunotherapy of EGFR-expressing tumours, *BMC Biotechnol* 10:91, 2010.
136. Imani Fooladi AA, Sattari M, Reza Nourani M: Synergistic effects between staphylococcal enterotoxin type B and monophosphoryl lipid A against mouse fibrosarcoma, *J BUON* 15:340–347, 2010.
137. Thamm DH, Kurzman ID, Macewen EG, et al: Intralesional lipid-complexed cytokine/superantigen immunogene therapy for spontaneous canine tumors, *Cancer Immunol Immunother* 52:473–480, 2003.
138. Kleinerman ES, Jia SF, Griffin J, et al: Phase II study of liposomal muramyl tripeptide in osteosarcoma: the cytokine cascade and monocyte activation following administration, *J Clin Oncol* 10:1310–1316, 1992.
139. Asano T, Kleinerman ES: Liposome-encapsulated MTP-PE: a novel biologic agent for cancer therapy, *J Immunother Emphasis Tumor Immunol* 14:286–292, 1993.
140. Gianan MA, Kleinerman ES: Liposomal muramyl tripeptide (CGP 19835A lipid) therapy for resectable melanoma in patients who were at high risk for relapse: an update, *Cancer Biother Radiopharm* 13:363–368, 1998.
141. Anderson PM, Tomaras M, McConnell K: Mifamurtide in osteosarcoma—a practical review, *Drugs Today (Barc)* 46:327–337, 2010.
142. Kurzman ID, MacEwen EG, Rosenthal RC, et al: Adjuvant therapy for osteosarcoma in dogs: results of randomized clinical trials using combined liposome-encapsulated muramyl tripeptide and cisplatin, *Clin Cancer Res* 1:1595–1601, 1995.
143. Fox LE, King RR, Shi F, et al: Induction of serum tumor necrosis factor-alpha and interleukin-6 activity by liposome-encapsulated muramyl tripeptide-phosphatidylethanolamine (L-MTP-PE) in normal cats, *Cancer Biother* 9:329–340, 1994.
144. Vail DM, MacEwen EG, Kurzman ID, et al: Liposome-encapsulated muramyl tripeptide phosphatidylethanolamine adjuvant immunotherapy for splenic hemangiosarcoma in the dog: a randomized multi-institutional clinical trial, *Clin Cancer Res* 1:1165–1170, 1995.
145. MacEwen EG, Kurzman ID, Vail DM, et al: Adjuvant therapy for melanoma in dogs: results of randomized clinical trials using surgery, liposome-encapsulated muramyl tripeptide, and granulocyte macrophage colony-stimulating factor, *Clin Cancer Res* 5:4249–4258, 1999.
146. Teske E, Rutteman GR, vd Ingh TS, et al: Liposome-encapsulated muramyl tripeptide phosphatidylethanolamine (L-MTP-PE): a randomized clinical trial in dogs with mammary carcinoma, *Anticancer Res* 18:1015–1019, 1998.
147. MacEwen EG, Kurzman ID, Rosenthal RC, et al: Therapy for osteosarcoma in dogs with intravenous injection of liposome-encapsulated muramyl tripeptide, *J Natl Cancer Inst* 81:935–938, 1989.
148. Dow SW, Fradkin LG, Liggitt DH, et al: Lipid-DNA complexes induce potent activation of innate immune responses and antitumor activity when administered intravenously, *J Immunol* 163:1552–1561, 1999.
149. Zaks K, Jordan M, Guth A, et al: Efficient immunization and cross-priming by vaccine adjuvants containing TLR3 or TLR9 agonists complexed to cationic liposomes, *J Immunol* 176:7335–7345, 2006.
150. Hemmi H, Takeuchi O, Kawai T, et al: A toll-like receptor recognizes bacterial DNA, *Nature* 408:740–745, 2000.
151. Sellins K, Fradkin L, Liggitt D, et al: Type I interferons potently suppress gene expression following gene delivery using liposome(-) DNA complexes, *Mol Ther* 12:451–459, 2005.
152. Dow S, Elmslie R, Kurzman I, et al: Phase I study of liposome-DNA complexes encoding the interleukin-2 gene in dogs with osteosarcoma lung metastases, *Hum Gene Ther* 16:937–946, 2005.
153. Kamstock D, Guth A, Elmslie R, et al: Liposome-DNA complexes infused intravenously inhibit tumor angiogenesis and elicit antitumor activity in dogs with soft tissue sarcoma, *Cancer Gene Ther* 13:306–317, 2006.
154. Smith BF, Curiel DT, Ternovoi VV, et al: Administration of a conditionally replicative oncolytic canine adenovirus in normal dogs, *Cancer Biother Radiopharm* 21:601–606, 2006.
155. Le LP, Rivera AA, Glasgow JN, et al: Infectivity enhancement for adenoviral transduction of canine osteosarcoma cells, *Gene Ther* 13:389–399, 2006.
156. Hemminki A, Kanerva A, Kremer EJ, et al: A canine conditionally replicating adenovirus for evaluating oncolytic virotherapy in a syngeneic animal model, *Mol Ther* 7:163–173, 2003.
157. Suter SE, Chein MB, von Messling V, et al: In vitro canine distemper virus infection of canine lymphoid cells: a prelude to oncolytic therapy for lymphoma, *Clin Cancer Res* 11:1579–1587, 2005.
158. Siegel JP, Puri RK: Interleukin-2 toxicity, *J Clin Oncol* 9:694–704, 1991.
159. Vial T, Descotes J: Clinical toxicity of interleukin-2, *Drug Saf* 7:417–433, 1992.
160. Margolin KA, Rayner AA, Hawkins MJ, et al: Interleukin-2 and lymphokine-activated killer cell therapy of solid tumors: analysis of toxicity and management guidelines, *J Clin Oncol* 7:486–498, 1989.
161. Helfand SC, Soergel SA, MacWilliams PS, et al: Clinical and immunological effects of human recombinant interleukin-2 given by repetitive weekly infusion to normal dogs, *Cancer Immunol Immunother* 39:84–92, 1994.
162. Funk J, Schmitz G, Failing K, et al: Natural killer (NK) and lymphokine-activated killer (LAK) cell functions from healthy dogs and 29 dogs with a variety of spontaneous neoplasms, *Cancer Immunol Immunother* 54:87–92, 2005.
163. Khanna C, Anderson PM, Hasz DE, et al: Interleukin-2 liposome inhalation therapy is safe and effective for dogs with spontaneous pulmonary metastases, *Cancer* 79:1409–1421, 1997.

164. Jourdier TM, Moste C, Bonnet MC, et al: Local immunotherapy of spontaneous feline fibrosarcomas using recombinant poxviruses expressing interleukin 2 (IL2), *Gene Ther* 10:2126–2132, 2003.
165. Quintin-Colonna F, Devauchelle P, Fradelizi D, et al: Gene therapy of spontaneous canine melanoma and feline fibrosarcoma by intratumoral administration of histoincompatible cells expressing human interleukin-2, *Gene Ther* 3:1104–1112, 1996.
166. Jahnke A, Hirschberger J, Fischer C, et al: Intra-tumoral gene delivery of feIL-2, feIFN-gamma and feGM-CSF using magnetofection as a neoadjuvant treatment option for feline fibrosarcomas: a phase-I study, *J Vet Med A Physiol Pathol Clin Med* 54:599–606, 2007.
167. Cutrera J, Torrero M, Shiomitsu K, et al: Intratumoral bleomycin and IL-12 electrochemogenetherapy for treating head and neck tumors in dogs, *Methods Mol Biol* 423:319–325, 2008.
168. Siddiqui F, Li CY, Zhang X, et al: Characterization of a recombinant adenovirus vector encoding heat-inducible feline interleukin-12 for use in hyperthermia-induced gene-therapy, *Int J Hyperthermia* 22:117–134, 2006.
169. Marks-Konczalik J, Dubois S, Losi JM, et al: IL-2-induced activation-induced cell death is inhibited in IL-15 transgenic mice, *Proc Natl Acad Sci U S A* 97:11445–11450, 2000.
170. Zhang X, Sun S, Hwang I, et al: Potent and selective stimulation of memory-phenotype CD8+ T cells in vivo by IL-15, *Immunity* 8:591–599, 1998.
171. Waldmann TA, Lugli E, Roederer M, et al: Safety (toxicity), pharmacokinetics, immunogenicity, and impact on elements of the normal immune system of recombinant human IL-15 in rhesus macaques, *Blood* 117(18):4787–4795, 2011.
172. Chou PC, Chuang TF, Jan TR, et al: Effects of immunotherapy of IL-6 and IL-15 plasmids on transmissible venereal tumor in beagles, *Vet Immunol Immunopathol* 130:25–34, 2009.
173. Streck CJ, Zhang Y, Miyamoto R, et al: Restriction of neuroblastoma angiogenesis and growth by interferon-alpha/beta, *Surgery* 136:183–189, 2004.
174. Folkman J: Successful treatment of an angiogenic disease, *N Engl J Med* 320:1211–1212, 1989.
175. Coates A, Rallings M, Hersey P, et al: Phase-II study of recombinant alpha 2-interferon in advanced malignant melanoma, *J Interferon Res* 6:1–4, 1986.
176. Rosenthal MA, Cox K, Raghavan D, et al: Phase II clinical trial of recombinant alpha-2 interferon for biopsy-proven metastatic or recurrent renal carcinoma, *Br J Urol* 69:491–494, 1992.
177. Zeidner NS, Mathiason-DuBard CK, Hoover EA: Reversal of feline leukemia virus infection by adoptive transfer of activated T lymphocytes, interferon alpha, and zidovudine, *Semin Vet Med Surg (Small Anim)* 10:256–266, 1995.
178. Penzo C, Ross M, Muirhead R, et al: Effect of recombinant feline interferon-omega alone and in combination with chemotherapeutic agents on putative tumour-initiating cells and daughter cells derived from canine and feline mammary tumours, *Vet Comp Oncol* 7:222–229, 2009.
179. Whitley EM, Bird AC, Zucker KE, et al: Modulation by canine interferon-gamma of major histocompatibility complex and tumor-associated antigen expression in canine mammary tumor and melanoma cell lines, *Anticancer Res* 15:923–929, 1995.
180. Hsiao YW, Liao KW, Chung TF, et al: Interactions of host IL-6 and IFN-gamma and cancer-derived TGF-beta1 on MHC molecule expression during tumor spontaneous regression, *Cancer Immunol Immunother* 57:1091–1104, 2008.
181. Mito K, Sugiura K, Ueda K, et al: IFNγ markedly cooperates with intratumoral dendritic cell vaccine in dog tumor models, *Cancer Res* 70:7093–7101, 2010.
182. Pluhar GE, Grogan PT, Seiler C, et al: Anti-tumor immune response correlates with neurological symptoms in a dog with spontaneous astrocytoma treated by gene and vaccine therapy, *Vaccine* 28:3371–3378, 2010.
183. Duffaud F, Therasse P: [New guidelines to evaluate the response to treatment in solid tumors], *Bull Cancer* 87:881–886, 2000.
184. Eisenhauer EA, Therasse P, Bogaerts J, et al: New response evaluation criteria in solid tumours: revised RECIST guideline (version 1.1), *Eur J Cancer* 45:228–247, 2009.
185. Cheever MA, Allison JP, Ferris AS, et al: The prioritization of cancer antigens: a National Cancer Institute pilot project for the acceleration of translational research, *Clin Cancer Res* 15:5323–5337, 2009.
186. Smyth MJ, Dunn GP, Schreiber RD: Cancer immunosurveillance and immunoediting: the roles of immunity in suppressing tumor development and shaping tumor immunogenicity, *Adv Immunol* 90:1–50, 2006.
187. Whiteside TL: Immune responses to malignancies, *J Allergy Clin Immunol* 125:S272–S283, 2010.
188. U'Ren LW, Biller BJ, Elmslie RE, et al: Evaluation of a novel tumor vaccine in dogs with hemangiosarcoma, *J Vet Intern Med* 21:113–120, 2007.
189. Hogge GS, Burkholder JK, Culp J, et al: Preclinical development of human granulocyte-macrophage colony-stimulating factor-transfected melanoma cell vaccine using established canine cell lines and normal dogs, *Cancer Gene Ther* 6:26–36, 1999.
190. Turek MM, Thamm DH, Mitzey A, et al: Human granulocyte-macrophage colony-stimulating factor DNA cationic-lipid complexed autologous tumour cell vaccination in the treatment of canine B-cell multicentric lymphoma, *Vet Comp Oncol* 5:219–231, 2007.
191. Alexander AN, Huelsmeyer MK, Mitzey A, et al: Development of an allogeneic whole-cell tumor vaccine expressing xenogeneic gp100 and its implementation in a phase II clinical trial in canine patients with malignant melanoma, *Cancer Immunol Immunother* 55:433–442, 2006.
192. Mutwiri G, Pontarollo R, Babiuk S, et al: Biological activity of immunostimulatory CpG DNA motifs in domestic animals, *Vet Immunol Immunopathol* 91:89–103, 2003.
193. Liu MA: DNA vaccines: an historical perspective and view to the future, *Immunol Rev* 239:62–84, 2011.
194. Bergman PJ, Camps-Palau MA, McKnight JA, et al: Development of a xenogeneic DNA vaccine program for canine malignant melanoma at the Animal Medical Center, *Vaccine* 24:4582–4585, 2006.
195. Liao JC, Gregor P, Wolchok JD, et al: Vaccination with human tyrosinase DNA induces antibody responses in dogs with advanced melanoma, *Cancer Immun* 6:8, 2006.
196. Bergman PJ, McKnight J, Novosad A, et al: Long-term survival of dogs with advanced malignant melanoma after DNA vaccination with xenogeneic human tyrosinase: a phase I trial, *Clin Cancer Res* 9:1284–1290, 2003.
197. Goubier A, Fuhrmann L, Forest L, et al: Superiority of needle-free transdermal plasmid delivery for the induction of antigen-specific IFNgamma T cell responses in the dog, *Vaccine* 26:2186–2190, 2008.
198. Bergman PJ: Cancer immunotherapy, *Vet Clin North Am Small Anim Pract* 40:507–518, 2010.
199. von Mehren M, Arlen P, Tsang KY, et al: Pilot study of a dual gene recombinant avipox vaccine containing both carcinoembryonic antigen (CEA) and B7.1 transgenes in patients with recurrent CEA-expressing adenocarcinomas, *Clin Cancer Res* 6:2219–2228, 2000.
200. Kaufman HL, Lenz HJ, Marshall J, et al: Combination chemotherapy and ALVAC-CEA/B7.1 vaccine in patients with metastatic colorectal cancer, *Clin Cancer Res* 14:4843–4849, 2008.
201. Hofbauer GF, Baur T, Bonnet MC, et al: Clinical phase I intratumoral administration of two recombinant ALVAC canarypox viruses expressing human granulocyte-macrophage colony-stimulating factor or interleukin-2: the transgene determines the composition of the inflammatory infiltrate, *Melanoma Res* 18:104–111, 2008.
202. Spaner DE, Astsaturov I, Vogel T, et al: Enhanced viral and tumor immunity with intranodal injection of canary pox viruses expressing the melanoma antigen, gp100, *Cancer* 106:890–899, 2006.

203. Lech PJ, Russell SJ: Use of attenuated paramyxoviruses for cancer therapy, *Expert Rev Vaccines* 9:1275–1302, 2010.
204. Melief CJ: Cancer immunotherapy by dendritic cells, *Immunity* 29:372–383, 2008.
205. Palucka K, Ueno H, Roberts L, et al: Dendritic cells: are they clinically relevant? *Cancer J* 16:318–324, 2010.
206. Palucka K, Ueno H, Banchereau J: Recent developments in cancer vaccines, *J Immunol* 186:1325–1331, 2011.
207. Slingluff CL Jr, Petroni GR, Yamshchikov GV, et al: Clinical and immunologic results of a randomized phase II trial of vaccination using four melanoma peptides either administered in granulocyte-macrophage colony-stimulating factor in adjuvant or pulsed on dendritic cells, *J Clin Oncol* 21:4016–4026, 2003.
208. Giermasz AS, Urban JA, Nakamura Y, et al: Type-1 polarized dendritic cells primed for high IL-12 production show enhanced activity as cancer vaccines, *Cancer Immunol Immunother* 58:1329–1336, 2009.
209. Kantoff PW, Higano CS, Shore ND, et al: Sipuleucel-T immunotherapy for castration-resistant prostate cancer, *N Engl J Med* 363:411–422, 2010.
210. Carballido E, Fishman M: Sipuleucel-T: Prototype for development of anti-tumor vaccines, *Curr Oncol Rep* 13:112–119, 2011.
211. Gyorffy S, Rodriguez-Lecompte JC, Woods JP, et al: Bone marrow-derived dendritic cell vaccination of dogs with naturally occurring melanoma by using human gp100 antigen, *J Vet Intern Med* 19:56–63, 2005.
212. Tamura K, Yamada M, Isotani M, et al: Induction of dendritic cell-mediated immune responses against canine malignant melanoma cells, *Vet J* 175:126–129, 2008.
213. Bird RC, Deinnocentes P, Church Bird AE, et al: An autologous dendritic cell canine mammary tumor hybrid-cell fusion vaccine, *Cancer Immunol Immunother* 60:87–97, 2011.
214. Kohler G, Milstein C: Continuous cultures of fused cells secreting antibody of predefined specificity, *Nature* 256:495–497, 1975.
215. Osbourn J, Jermutus L, Duncan A: Current methods for the generation of human antibodies for the treatment of autoimmune diseases, *Drug Discov Today* 8:845–851, 2003.
216. Abes R, Teillaud JL: Modulation of tumor immunity by therapeutic monoclonal antibodies, *Cancer Metastasis Rev* 30:111–124, 2011.
217. Stein R, Balkman C, Chen S, et al: Evaluation of anti-human leukocyte antigen-DR monoclonal antibody therapy in spontaneous canine lymphoma, *Leuk Lymphoma* 52:273–284, 2011.
218. Yannelli JR, Wroblewski JM: On the road to a tumor cell vaccine: 20 years of cellular immunotherapy, *Vaccine* 23:97–113, 2004.
219. Blakeslee J, Noll G, Olsen R, et al: Adoptive immunotherapy of feline leukemia virus infection using autologous lymph node lymphocytes, *J Acquir Immune Defic Syndr Hum Retrovirol* 18:1–6, 1998.
220. Yron I, Wood TA, Jr., Spiess PJ, et al: In vitro growth of murine T cells. V. The isolation and growth of lymphoid cells infiltrating syngeneic solid tumors, *J Immunol* 125:238–245, 1980.
221. Rosenberg SA, Restifo NP, Yang JC, et al: Adoptive cell transfer: a clinical path to effective cancer immunotherapy, *Nat Rev Cancer* 8:299–308, 2008.
222. Dudley ME, Rosenberg SA: Adoptive-cell-transfer therapy for the treatment of patients with cancer, *Nat Rev Cancer* 3:666–675, 2003.
223. Dudley ME, Wunderlich JR, Yang JC, et al: A phase I study of nonmyeloablative chemotherapy and adoptive transfer of autologous tumor antigen-specific T lymphocytes in patients with metastatic melanoma, *J Immunother* 25:243–251, 2002.
224. Rosenberg SA, Dudley ME: Cancer regression in patients with metastatic melanoma after the transfer of autologous antitumor lymphocytes, *Proc Natl Acad Sci U S A* 101(Suppl 2):14639–14645, 2004.
225. Xu L, Wang C, Wen Z, et al: CpG oligodeoxynucleotides enhance the efficacy of adoptive cell transfer using tumor infiltrating lymphocytes by modifying the Th1 polarization and local infiltration of Th17 cells, *Clin Dev Immunol* 2010:410893, 2010.
226. Rosenberg SA, Yang JC, Restifo NP: Cancer immunotherapy: moving beyond current vaccines, *Nat Med* 10:909–915, 2004.
227. Gattinoni L, Finkelstein SE, Klebanoff CA, et al: Removal of homeostatic cytokine sinks by lymphodepletion enhances the efficacy of adoptively transferred tumor-specific CD8+ T cells, *J Exp Med* 202:907–912, 2005.
228. Paulos CM, Wrzesinski C, Kaiser A, et al: Microbial translocation augments the function of adoptively transferred self/tumor-specific CD8+ T cells via TLR4 signaling, *J Clin Invest* 117:2197–2204, 2007.
229. Dudley ME, Yang JC, Sherry R, et al: Adoptive cell therapy for patients with metastatic melanoma: evaluation of intensive myeloablative chemoradiation preparative regimens, *J Clin Oncol* 26:5233–5239, 2008.
230. Quezada SA, Simpson TR, Peggs KS, et al: Tumor-reactive CD4(+) T cells develop cytotoxic activity and eradicate large established melanoma after transfer into lymphopenic hosts, *J Exp Med* 207:637–650, 2010.
231. Xie Y, Akpinarli A, Maris C, et al: Naive tumor-specific CD4(+) T cells differentiated in vivo eradicate established melanoma, *J Exp Med* 207:651–667, 2010.
232. Corthay A, Lorvik KB, Bogen B: Is secretion of tumour-specific antigen important for cancer eradication by CD4(+) T cells?—Implications for cancer immunotherapy by adoptive T cell transfer, *Scand J Immunol* 73(6):527–530, 2011.
233. Hanson HL, Donermeyer DL, Ikeda H, et al: Eradication of established tumors by CD8+ T cell adoptive immunotherapy, *Immunity* 13:265–276, 2000.
234. Klebanoff CA, Finkelstein SE, Surman DR, et al: IL-15 enhances the in vivo antitumor activity of tumor-reactive CD8+ T cells, *Proc Natl Acad Sci U S A* 101:1969–1974, 2004.
235. May KF, Jr., Chen L, Zheng P, et al: Anti-4–1BB monoclonal antibody enhances rejection of large tumor burden by promoting survival but not clonal expansion of tumor-specific CD8+ T cells, *Cancer Res* 62:3459–3465, 2002.
236. Khanna C, London C, Vail D, et al: Guiding the optimal translation of new cancer treatments from canine to human cancer patients, *Clin Can Res* 15:5671–5677, 2009.
237. Withrow SJ, Khanna C: Bridging the gap between experimental animals and humans in osteosarcoma, *Cancer Treat Res* 152:439–446, 2009.
238. Stewart TJ, Smyth MJ: Improving cancer immunotherapy by targeting tumor-induced immune suppression, *Cancer Metastasis Rev* 30:125–140, 2011.

Molecular/Targeted Therapy of Cancer

14

SECTION A

Gene Therapy for Cancer

DAVID J. ARGYLE

Since its development, recombinant DNA technology has been vigorously applied to the advancement of medicine. New molecular techniques have been used to study the role of specific genes and their products in disease, to improve diagnosis, and to produce novel therapeutics. Gene therapy, in its simplest definition, is the introduction of genes into cells in vivo to treat a disease.[1] Although one may recognize this as one of the newest areas of medicine, the actual concept of gene therapy is not a new idea. In the late 1960s, the idea of gene therapy was hypothesized by many working in the field of molecular biology, in particular the use of gene therapy to deliver a normal copy of a gene into a patient with a single gene defect, such as hemophilia. However, the technology to manipulate genes and be able to deliver them safely to patients was not available until very recently. Even now and despite improvements in technologies involving gene manipulation and delivery, there are still many technical hurdles to overcome before gene therapy can become accepted clinical practice.[1,2]

Efficient Gene Delivery: The Major Hurdle to Clinical Benefits

In simple terms, gene therapy is the introduction of nucleic acid into a cell to ameliorate a disease process. For this to be effective, the gene has to be delivered to sufficient numbers of target cells in the body, and this requires a vehicle or vector for delivery. In addition, the gene has to be expressed at a sufficient level and for a length of time appropriate for the disease.[2]

Early studies on how viruses were able to cause tumors by delivery of their own DNA to foreign cells made them ideal candidates for vectors for gene therapy (i.e., the vehicles by which we could transfer therapeutic genes to patients). However, it was not until the 1980s when work on the retroviral life cycle started to revolutionize the development of gene therapy. In these early studies, it was demonstrated that retroviruses could transfer DNA to cells and this DNA could be stably integrated into the host cell's genome. Since these early experiments, a number of viruses have been manipulated to act as vehicles for gene delivery. In addition, because of concerns over safety of viral vectors for gene delivery, a number of workers have also explored the possibility of using naked DNA (a therapeutic gene delivered in a bacterial plasmid or lipid/DNA complexes) with some success. The vehicles used for gene delivery and their associated problems are shown in Table 14-1.

The ideal vector would efficiently deliver the gene of interest (transgene) specifically to the cancer cell. It would be easy and cheap to manufacture and would be nonimmunogenic. Obviously the ideal vector does not exist, but there have been great advances in both viral and nonviral delivery systems.[2]

Viral Vectors

The great advantage to viral vectors for gene delivery is their ability to infect cells and our ability to exploit their replicative machinery. The majority of systems utilize replicative-defective viruses to overcome concerns that recombination within the host may lead to the production of wild-type virus with pathogenic potential. The common systems rely on oncogenic retroviruses (e.g., murine leukemia virus [MuLV]) or adenoviruses (e.g., human adenovirus type 5 [AD5]), but great strides are also being made with lentiviral vectors (particularly human immunodeficiency virus-1 [HIV-1]).[3-8] Most of the systems described involve the local delivery of virus to tumor deposits (e.g., by intratumoral injection). Systemic delivery is hindered by rapid clearance of viruses from the body by the immune and complement systems. To overcome this, work is in progress to explore cellular delivery of viruses by the systemic route. In this delivery system, viral producer cells are delivered to the patient, and virus production is triggered when the cells reach the tumor. Endothelial cell cultures lend themselves well to this technology because they specifically home in to areas of neoangiogenesis. However, T-cells, macrophages, and dendritic cells are also being explored as potential cell delivery systems. The advantage of this system is that virus could potentially be delivered to metastatic disease, as well as primary tumors.[9-13] Recent evidence suggests that mesenchymal stem cells also have homing ability to tumors and could be used to deliver "suicide" genes (see later).

Nonviral Gene Delivery

Concerns relating to virus safety and an inability to produce high enough viral titers have led to the development of nonviral delivery systems for gene therapy.[14] Liposomes have been used to safely and efficiently deliver genes to tumor cells through direct injection.[15,16] Further, naked DNA delivery (the delivery of plasmid DNA alone containing the gene of interest) has been shown to be taken up by tumor cells and antigen-presenting cells after simple direct injection. A modification of this is particle-mediated gene delivery using a "gene gun." In this approach, DNA is adsorbed on to gold particles and fired into tissues under high pressure (using helium as the

TABLE 14-1 Gene Therapy Vector Systems

VECTORS	COMMENTS
Viral Vectors	
Retroviruses (oncoviruses)	Originally the gold-standard vector, the gene is packaged into replication-defective viral particles using a packaging cell line. The therapeutic gene is integrated into the host cell genome when the virus is delivered to the target cell. Limited by their inability to infect postmitotic cells.
Retroviruses (lentivirus)	Many based on HIV-1. These vectors have become significantly safer in recent years and have many of the benefits of the oncoviruses and also will infect postmitotic cells. Construction of the vector takes place in a packaging cell line, and the therapeutic gene is integrated into the host cell genome.
Adenoviruses	Have become the most popular viral delivery mechanism. Gene is packaged into a replication-incompetent adenovirus (usually E1 deleted). Gene expression remains episomal when delivered to the host cell. Concerns have been raised about the safety of adenoviral vectors, particularly potential toxic side effects at high doses. Adenoviruses can infect a wide range of premitotic and postmitotic cells. Conditionally replicating adenoviruses are being explored as oncolytic vectors.
Adeno-associated viruses (AAV)	Gaining popularity as a vector because they are potentially safer than adenoviruses. They infect a wide variety of mammalian cell types but are limited by the amount of DNA they can deliver. Gene expression in the host cell is episomal. However, in the natural host, integration is possible.
Nonviral Vectors	
Naked DNA	Simple form of gene delivery in which "naked" plasmid DNA is directly injected into the tumor. Vectors are derived from bacterial plasmids and are engineered to express the therapeutic gene under the control of a strong promoter. Naked DNA can be taken up by many tissues, but typically the efficiency for delivery is lower than that for viral gene delivery.
Particle bombardment (gene gun)	A more sophisticated approach to the delivery of naked DNA. In this system, plasmid DNA is typically adsorbed onto gold particles. Helium is then used as a motive force to fire the gold particles into cells or tissues via a handheld "gene gun."
Liposome/DNA conjugates	In this system, naked DNA is coated with liposome to improve uptake by endocytosis. This enhances the efficiency of gene delivery.
Ligand/DNA conjugates	Ligands are used to specifically target DNA to tumor tissue.

HIV-1, Human immunodeficiency virus-1.

motive force).[17,18] However, the majority of these techniques are still inefficient vehicles for delivery and are not able to be given systemically (Figure 14-1; see Table 14-1).

Targeted Gene Delivery

One of the major barriers to gene therapy becoming accepted in clinical practice is the ability to give vectors systemically and to ensure that therapeutic transgenes are not expressed in normal cells. Numerous strategies have been attempted to provide levels of targeting to spare normal tissue. In a later section, we describe the use of conditionally replicating viruses, which is one method of targeting. Surface modification of viruses (transductional targeting) is also being explored. An example of this is the use of modified fibers on the surface of adenoviruses that only allow the virus to enter cells with specific receptors (Figure 14-2).

A further targeting strategy is transcriptional targeting once the vector has entered the cell.[19-26] Although every gene is represented in every cell of the body, expression of any one gene requires specific transcription factors that may be unique to a particular cell or tissue type. Certain genes have been identified that are expressed in cancer cells but are not expressed in normal cells (e.g., telomerase) or are only expressed in a specific tissue type (e.g. prostate-specific antigen [PSA]). By using the promoter sequences for these genes to drive transgene expression, targeted expression in cancer cells only (e.g., using the promoter for telomerase) or to a specific tissue type (e.g., to the prostate using the promoter for PSA) can be achieved (see Figure 14-2).

Gene Therapy Strategies for Cancer

Despite advances in surgical techniques and the use of radiotherapy and chemotherapy, cancer still remains a disease of high mortality in both human and veterinary medicine, warranting the investigation of alternative treatments. Gene therapy has the potential to play a major role in the development of new cancer therapeutic agents, and there are four broad approaches that can be applied, as follows.

Rescue of the Cancer Cell Through Gene Replacement Technologies

The increased understanding of the molecular events in cancer has made possible the identification of defective genes involved in the cancer phenotype. One of the most studied genes in cancer development has been the tumor suppressor gene *p53. p53* acts as a genomic guardian for the cell; it is switched on when a cell's DNA is damaged. The product of this gene causes the cell to either stop

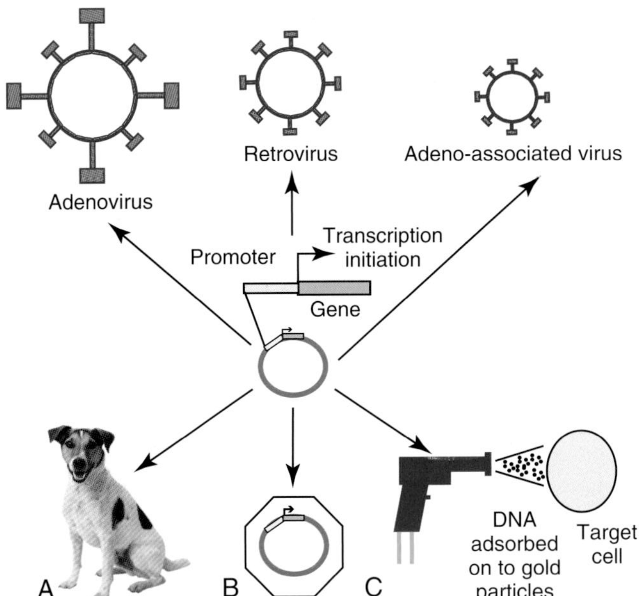

FIGURE 14-1 Viral and nonviral gene delivery. Adenoviral vectors are produced in "producer cell lines." They enter the cell by transduction, and their genetic material is transported to the nucleus. In contrast to retroviruses, the DNA is not integrated into the host genome—gene expression is achieved episomally. Retroviral vectors are also produced in specialized producer cell lines. They enter the cell by transduction, but their RNA genome is reverse transcribed into proviral DNA. This integrates into the host genome in which expression of the transgene takes place. DNA plasmid vectors contain a gene cassette that incorporates the therapeutic transgene under the control of a promoter. The plasmid can be delivered by direct injection as naked or liposome-encapsulated DNA **(A),** by direct injection or systemically wrapped in nanomedicine particles **(B),** or by direct injection utilizing a helium-driven "biolistic" gene gun **(C).**

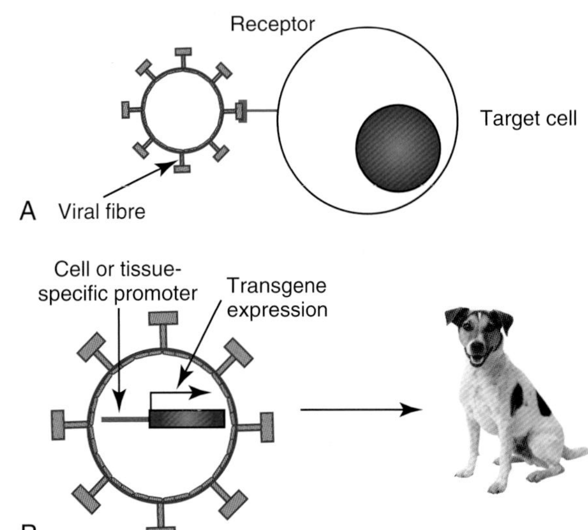

FIGURE 14-2 Vector targeting. The specificity of viral vectors can be improved utilizing either transductional targeting **(A)** where the viral surface proteins are modified so they will only enter the cell of interest or transcriptional targeting **(B)** where the expression of the therapeutic transgene is under the control of a tissue or cell-specific promoter. Transcriptional targeting can also be employed in nonviral vectors and directly delivered to the patient.

dividing or become apoptotic (programmed cell death), depending on the degree of damage. In many cancers, this gene is defective; thus damaged cells fail to stop dividing and can accumulate further damaging events, which can allow selection for a malignant phenotype. A number of studies have addressed this by attempting to replace the defective *p53* gene with its normal counterpart.[27] However, problems associated with this approach include the following:

- The inability of our current technology to be able to efficiently deliver a normal *p53* gene to every cancer cell in a tumor mass.
- Cancer is a multigenetic abnormality, and the delivery of one correct gene to a tumor cell may still not have the desired phenotypic effect.

A more promising approach has been to use the lack of a normal functioning *p53* gene to target viruses to kill cells. The use of E1b-deleted adenoviruses to specifically cause oncolysis in p53 null cells is described later and has proved successful in some human clinical models.[28] p53 mutations in domestic species such as the dog and cat have also been well characterized, and these may provide targets for therapy, particularly for diseases such as canine osteosarcoma (OSA) and feline vaccine-associated sarcomas (FVAS).

Destruction of Cancer Cells Through Delivery of "Suicide Genes"

Typically, the "suicide gene" approach involves the delivery of a gene (usually an enzyme) to cancer cells that has the ability to convert a relatively nontoxic prodrug to an active compound within the cancer cell (gene-directed enzyme prodrug therapy [GDEPT]) (Figure 14-3). At the clinical level, the gene would be delivered to the patient's tumor and the enzyme activity would be confined to the cancer cells.[29] The patient would then be given a prodrug systemically. In the cancer cells, this novel enzyme can convert the prodrug to a more active compound that has the ability to kill the cancer cell (see Figure 14-3). A number of successful approaches have been developed based on this system. For example, the *Escherichia coli* nitroreductase gene has been used in preclinical models to cause reduction of an inactive prodrug (CB1954, a weak alkylating agent) to promote cell killing in cancer cells.[29] However, due to the low efficiency of existing vectors, the success of this therapy will largely depend on the extent of the bystander effect. In this, the activation of the prodrug in the cell causes cell death and also leakage of toxic metabolites to neighboring cells. Consequently, it is estimated that only a small fraction of the cells need receive the gene for there to be a dramatic effect on tumor volume. Further, in mouse models, a distant bystander effect on tumor metastases has been demonstrated that is mediated through the patient's immune system.[22] The in-situ destruction of tumor cells is mediated through necrosis rather than apoptosis, creating an ideal inflammatory environment for the exposure and presentation of tumor antigens to the immune system. This allows the patient's immune system to recognize tumor metastases and has caused regression in a number of preclinical model systems. These systems have been combined with

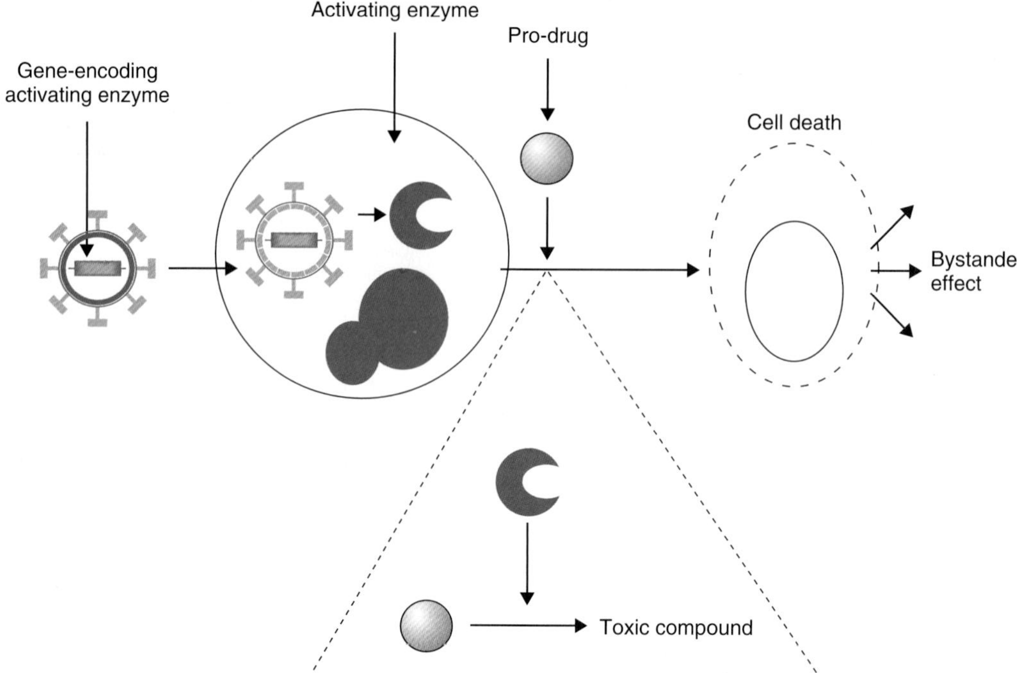

FIGURE 14-3 In gene-directed enzyme prodrug therapy (GDEPT), an activating gene is delivered to the cancer cells. A relatively inactive prodrug is then given to the patient systemically. In cells processing the activating gene, the prodrug is converted to a highly toxic drug, which can kill the cancer cell. The advantage of this system is evidence of the bystander effect. In this, only a small proportion of cancer cells need to receive the activating gene, as toxic metabolites leak across gap junctions and kill surrounding cancer cells.

transcriptionally targeted vectors (described previously) to improve the eventual therapeutic index.

Utilizing Stem Cells to Deliver "Suicide Genes"

The attractiveness of prodrug cancer gene therapy has been described earlier, but it does rely on the ability to specifically target prodrugs to tumors. This can be achieved using transcriptional targeting of vectors (i.e., the use of cell-specific promoters to drive prodrug gene expression). However, this targeting needs an effective and efficient delivery vehicle, and viruses demonstrate some severe deficiencies in this role. The use of stem cells to target tumors can avoid systemic toxicity. Tumor stroma is composed of a variety of cells, including proliferating tumor cells, cancer stem cells (CSCs), tumor fibroblasts, endothelial cells, lymphocytes, and other cells. Many therapeutic strategies are now geared toward killing both tumor cells and CSCs. Prodrug cancer gene therapy driven by mesenchymal stem cells (MSCs) has been suggested as a treatment modality that could achieve this.[30] It represents an attractive tool for activating the prodrug directly within the tumor mass, thus avoiding systemic toxicity. In addition, MSCs lack major histocompatibility complex (MHC)-II and show only minimal MHC-I expression.[31-33] Thanks to their immunosuppressive properties, allogeneic MSCs can substitute for autologous stem cells in delivering the therapeutic agent in targeted tumor therapy. Stem cell–driven cancer gene therapy is based on the tumor-trophic property of MSCs. Tumor-homing ability of MSCs holds therapeutic advantages compared to vehicles such as proteins, antibodies, nanoparticles, and to some extent viruses. The success of an enzyme-prodrug gene therapy depends on several factors. The catalytic activity of the enzyme encoded by a suicide gene, a suitable prodrug-enzyme combination, ability of the vector to target tumor cells, sufficient transgene expression, and, importantly, the extent of the bystander effect are the main indicators of effective and successful suicide gene therapy. Various combinations of suicide genes, prodrugs, and gene transfer technologies have been investigated in order to find the most suitable and effective system in combating the otherwise incurable tumors. The failures of the present suicide gene therapies were mainly caused by the inability of vectors carrying the suicide gene to reach invasive tumor cells distant from the tumor bulk, as well as inefficient spread of the vectors within the tumor. Therefore the stem cell–based suicide gene therapy based on the inherent and privileged tumor-trophic nature of MSCs holds great potential for moving suicide gene therapy closer to translation (Figure 14-4).

Gene-Directed Immunotherapy

The search for an effective cancer vaccine over the past 150 years has led to extensive studies of the immune response of cancer patients. These studies have suggested that cell-mediated immune responses are important components of the antitumor immune response. Cytokines are small glycoprotein molecules that orchestrate the immune response, tissue repair, and hemopoiesis, and it has been demonstrated that the relative amounts of individual cytokines can direct the immune system toward either a mainly humoral or a mainly cell-mediated response. In particular, cytokines such as interleukin-2 (IL-2), interferon-γ (IFN-γ), IL-12, and IL-18 have the ability to promote cell-mediated responses. Further, evidence derived from animal models suggested that local production of cytokines around a tumor mass can lead to production of an antitumor immune response and a reversal of T-cell anergy (nonresponsiveness).[34,35] Thus there appears a rationale for using cytokine molecules in cancer patients to improve the antitumor immune response to tumors that present weakly antigenic epitopes or

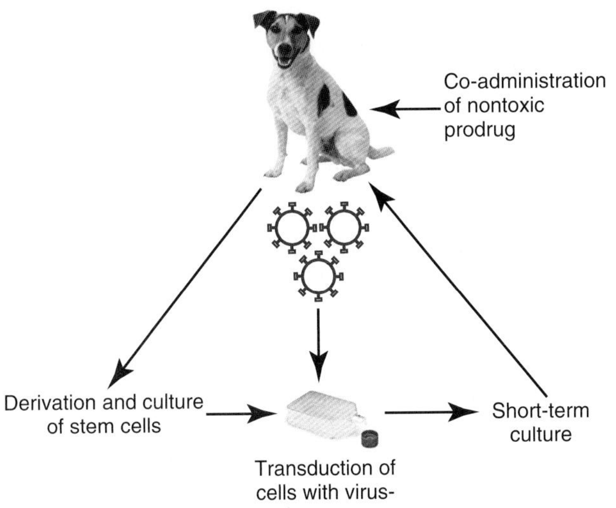

FIGURE 14-4 Mesenchymal stem cell (MSC)–targeted cancer gene therapy. MSCs are isolated from patients. Bone marrow-MSCs (BM-MSCs) are isolated from mononuclear fraction of bone marrow obtained by Percoll density gradient centrifugation. Obtained cells are plated in a plastic dish and expanded. Stem cells are transduced with virus containing a suicide gene and gene encoding resistance to antibiotic G418. Transduced cells are exposed to selective medium containing antibiotic G418. The population of selected therapeutic stem cells is expanded and used for systemic or intratumoral injections. Therapeutic cells migrate to the tumor site. Subsequently, nontoxic prodrug is administered and converted at the tumor site to toxic drug killing tumor cells and therapeutic cells as well. No adverse systemic toxicities have been observed.

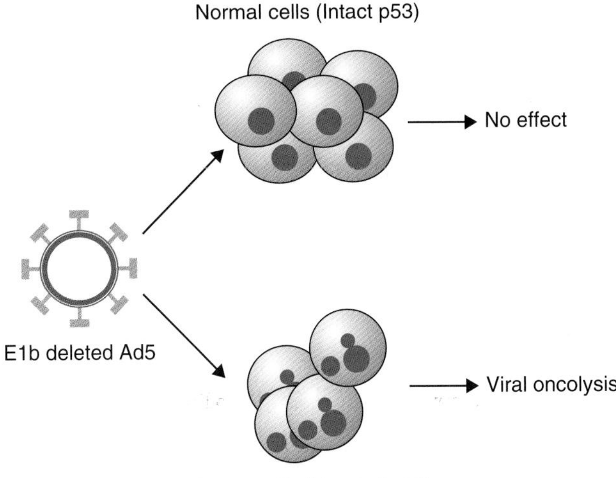

FIGURE 14-5 Conditionally replicating adenovirus. The Onyx 015 vector is an E1b-deleted adenovirus that conditionally replicates in cells with a nonfunctional *p53* gene. p53 protein has the potential to shut down cell cycling when infected with wild-type adenovirus but is prevented from doing so through the actions of the product of viral E1b. E1b-deficient viruses cannot replicate in normal cells with p53 intact. However, in cells that have no functional p53 protein, viral replication can proceed and cause cell lysis.

epitopes that evade immune recognition. In the 1980s and 1990s, a number of clinical studies were undertaken using recombinant cytokine proteins to improve the survival of human cancer patients. However, cytokines tend to be autocrine or paracrine in nature and the levels of protein required to demonstrate a biologic effect were often too toxic for the patient to withstand. However, a more promising approach has been to deliver the actual cytokine genes to cancer cells rather than delivery of the protein to the whole patient.[36-38] This approach has also been adopted in a number of small-scale veterinary studies, including one on canine malignant melanoma, which used cells to deliver IL-2 to tumors.[39] These studies have had encouraging results and warrant further larger scale trials.

In the preceding section, we described how the in-situ destruction of tumor cells by enzymes can lead to a distant bystander effect mediated by the immune system. Many trials have now combined this approach with gene-directed immunotherapy. In this approach, cytokine genes, as well as the prodrug-activating gene, are delivered to cancer cells. The conversion of an inactive prodrug by the activating gene leads to destruction of the cancer cells by necrosis. The co-delivery of cytokines that enhance cell-mediated immune responses such as IL-2, IFN-γ, IL-12, and IL-18 enhances the antitumor response and may potentially improve the distant bystander effect against micrometastatic disease.[1,2]

Delivery of Chemoprotective Genes

An alternative approach to gene therapy for cancer involves the delivery of genes to normal cells of the bone marrow to protect them against the cytotoxic effects of conventional chemotherapeutic drugs. In particular, the multidrug resistance (MDR) gene has been cloned and delivered to normal bone marrow cells. When patients are given high doses of chemotherapy, the normal cells with the MDR gene are able to export the toxic drugs across their membranes and reduce potential side effects.[40-42] However, this approach does not protect gastrointestinal cells, which limit this approach. Further, there is also a danger that the MDR gene could transfer to malignant cells, rendering them insensitive to the effects of standard drugs.

The Use of Replication-Competent Viral Vectors

Progress has been made in the development of replication-competent viruses that conditionally replicate in cancer cells.[43-48] As an example, the Onyx 015 vector is an E1b-deleted adenovirus that conditionally replicates in cells with a nonfunctional *p53* gene. p53 protein has the potential to shut down cell cycling when infected with wild-type adenovirus but is prevented from doing so through the actions of the product of viral E1b. E1b-deficient viruses cannot replicate in normal cells with p53 intact. However, in cells that have no functional p53 protein, viral replication can proceed and cause cell lysis (Figure 14-5). Many other conditionally replicating viruses are being developed that rely on specific cancer cell defects (e.g., Reo viruses that conditionally replicate in cells with intact Ras signalling pathways) or are transcriptionally targeted. p53 mutations in domestic species such as the dog and cat have also been well characterized, and this may provide targets for therapy, particularly for diseases such as canine OSA and feline vaccine-associated sarcomas. In one study, researchers have utilized the osteocalcin promoter for restricting the replication of a canine adenovirus to dog OSA cells.[47] This has shown promise in preclinical evaluations and has been shown to yield a therapeutic benefit in vivo. A cautionary note, however, is that the majority of dogs in the United States and Europe are vaccinated against canine adenovirus, and these vectors may not be able to overcome host immunity.

Miscellaneous Approaches to Cancer Gene Therapy

The multigenetic abnormalities of cancer lend themselves to multiple gene therapy approaches. In addition to those approaches described previously, there is vigorous exploration of the following:

- Gene delivery of sodium iodide symporter genes to tumors to allow them to concentrate radioactive iodine.[1]
- Delivering proapoptotic genes to cancer cells.[1]
- Delivering antiangiogenesis genes to cancers to inhibit growth of their blood supply.[1]

It is highly likely that one individual approach to cancer will be insufficient to cure or control particular cancers. However, it is possible that a combination of treatments, with or without conventional therapies, will prove to provide the best therapeutic solution.

Safety Considerations in Gene Therapy

One of the major considerations in gene therapy revolves around issues of safety, in particular the safety of the vectors used for gene delivery. In 1999, gene therapy suffered a major setback with the death of a patient as a direct result of adenovirus gene therapy. Problems associated with vector delivery include inappropriate inflammatory responses caused by vector delivery (e.g., adenoviruses), the generation of replication-competent viruses (although this is unlikely with new generation vectors), and insertional mutagenesis caused by integrating viruses (e.g., retroviruses).

Until recently, many gene therapy trials had utilized retroviral vectors for gene delivery. There are many advantages to using retroviruses as outlined in Table 14-1. However, retroviruses are also associated with serious diseases of domestic animals and the use of these in gene therapy poses a risk of insertional mutagenesis or the production of replication-competent viruses during the manufacturing process. Realistically, insertional mutagenesis leading to a malignant transformation is an unlikely event because cancer is a multistep process. In fact, there may be a greater risk of malignant transformation from external beam radiation than from the use of retroviruses to treat cancer. The production of replication-competent retroviruses during the production process would also be unlikely because of the rigorous testing that is required prior to clinical application. Many of these issues are resolving with the development of new generation vectors.[1] As an example, in the use of retroviruses and to prevent insertional mutagenesis in normal tissues, one group recently described the use of zinc finger nucleases (engineered DNA-editing enzymes) that allows the insertion of DNA to a site of choice within the genome.[49] This adds a further level of safety in a high-risk procedure.

In recent years, there has been a shift from using retroviruses in gene therapy to using viruses such as adenovirus and the human adeno-associated viruses (AAV). Adenoviruses may also pose some risks, including inappropriate inflammatory responses leading to serious clinical complications. However, a great deal of work is currently underway to improve viral vectors by removing most of their genetic material to produce "ghost vectors." These would be potentially less toxic and offer a brighter future for virally mediated gene transfer.

One might imagine that the delivery of naked DNA may offer a safer alternative. However, all of the potential safety issues using this technology are still not fully answered. These include potential risks of autoimmunity and also the actual fate of the DNA when it has been delivered to the patient; in the case of the former, however, there would appear to be no evidence of autoimmunity being a problem in preclinical models.

One of the most exciting developments in cancer gene therapy is the use of conditionally replicating viruses. However, the safety of these vector systems needs special consideration as many of them in their native form could pose a risk to both human and animal health.

New Horizons

Gene therapy promises a completely new approach to the treatment of cancer and represents the newest area of pharmacology. It has suffered over the past 10 years as clinical trials in human medicine have not delivered what they had originally promised. However, one has to put this into context in that many of these studies were conducted in patients with high-grade or end-stage disease and many studies were conducted prematurely without refining the delivery technologies. Clearly, there are a number of technical issues such as safety issues surrounding the delivery and efficiency of the vectors that need to be resolved before gene therapy becomes established clinical practice. Despite gene therapy being very much in its infancy, the field is advancing at a rapid rate. A number of clinical trials have begun in companion animals, and products are in development for clinical application. However, although these treatments would appear to be powerful in preclinical models, it is likely that their greatest benefit will be in the management of patients with minimal disease states. Thus gene therapy will probably have its greatest advantage not as a stand-alone treatment but as an adjunct to more conventional therapies such as surgery, radiation, or chemotherapy.

REFERENCES

1. Argyle DJ: Gene therapy in veterinary medicine, *Vet Rec* 144:369–376, 1999.
2. Harris J, Sikora, K. (1993): Gene therapy in the clinic, *Aspects Med* 14:251–546, 1993.
3. Bartosch B, Cosset FL: Strategies for retargeted gene delivery using vectors derived from lentiviruses, *Curr Gene Ther* 4(4):427–443, 2004.
4. Tomanin R, Scarpa M: Why do we need new gene therapy viral vectors? Characteristics, limitations and future perspectives of viral vector transduction, *Curr Gene Ther* 4(4):357–372, 2004.
5. Lachmann RH: Herpes simplex virus-based vectors, *Int J Exp Path* 85(4):177–190, 2004.
6. Buning H, Braun-Falco M, Hallek M: Progress in the use of adeno-associated viral vectors for gene therapy, *Cells Tissues Organs* 177(3):139–150, 2004.
7. Mah C, Byrne BJ, Flotte TR: Virus-based gene delivery systems, *Clin Pharmacokinet* 41(12):901–911, 2002.
8. Dornburg R: The history and principles of retroviral vectors, *Front Biosci* 8:D818–D835, 2003.
9. Culver KW, Ram Z, Wallbridge S, et al: In vivo gene transfer with retroviral vector-producer cells for treatment of experimental brain tumors, *Science* 256:1550–1552, 1992.
10. Gomez Navarro J, Contreras JL, Arafat W, et al: Genetically modified CD34+ cells as cellular vehicles for gene delivery into areas of angiogenesis in a rhesus model, *Gene Ther* 7:1 43–52, 2000.

11. Harrington K, Alvarez-Vallina L, Crittenden M, et al: Cells as vehicles for cancer gene therapy: the missing link between targeted vectors and systemic delivery? *Hum Gene Ther* 13(11):1263–1280, 2002.
12. Muta M, Matsumoto G, Hiruma K, et al: Study of cancer gene therapy using IL-12-secreting endothelial progenitor cells in a rat solid tumor model, *Oncol Rep* 10(6):1765–1769, 2003.
13. Pereboeva L, Komarova S, Mikheeva G, et al: Approaches to utilize mesenchymal progenitor cells as cellular vehicles, *Stem Cells* 21:4 389–404, 2003.
14. Annier AK, Shea LD: Controlled release systems for DNA delivery, *Mol Ther* 10(1):19–26, 2004.
15. Tranchant I, Thompson B, Nicolazzi C, et al: Physicochemical optimisation of plasmid delivery by cationic lipids, *J Gene Med* 6:S24–S35, 2004.
16. Hirko A, Tang FX, Hughes JA: Cationic lipid vectors for plasmid DNA delivery, *Curr Med Chem* 10(14):1185–1193, 2003.
17. Yang N, Sun WH: Gene and non-viral approaches to cancer gene therapy, *Nat Med* 1:481–483, 1995.
18. Keller ET, Burkholder JK, Shi Pugh TD, et al: In-vivo particle mediated cytokine gene transfer into canine oral mucosa and epidermis, *Cancer Gene Therapy* 3:186–191, 1996
19. Dachs GU, Dougherty GJ, Stratford IJ, et al: Targeting gene therapy to cancer, *Oncol Res* 9:313–325, 1997.
20. Scanlon KJ: Cancer gene therapy: Challenges and opportunities, *Anticancer Res* 24(2A):501–504, 2004.
21. Blackwood L, Onions DE, Argyle DJ: The feline thyroglobulin promoter: towards targeted gene therapy of hyperthyroidism, *Domest Anim Endocrinol* 20(3):185–201, 2001.
22. Vile RG, Hart IR: In-vitro and in-vivo targeting of gene expression to melanoma cells, *Cancer Res* 53(5):962–967, 1993.
23. Gu R, Fang BL: Telomerase promoter-driven cancer gene therapy, *Cancer Biol Ther* 2(4):S64–S70, 2003.
24. Song JS: Adenovirus-mediated suicide SCLC gene therapy using the increased activity of the hTERT promoter by the MMRE and SV40 enhancer, *Biosci Biotechnol Biochem* 69(1):56–62, 2005.
25. Helder MN, Wiseman GBA, van der Zee AGJ: Telomerase and telomeres: From basic biology to cancer treatment, *Cancer Invest* 20(1):82–101, 2002.
26. Fullerton NE, Boyd M, Mairs RJ, et al: Combining a targeted radiotherapy and gene therapy approach for adenocarcinoma of prostate, *Prostate Cancer Prostatic Dis* 7(4):355–363, 2004.
27. Edelman J, Edelman J, Nemunaitis J: Adenoviral p53 gene therapy in squamous cell cancer of the head and neck region, *Curr Opin Mol Ther* 5(6):611–617, 2003.
28. Bortolanza S, Hernandez-Alcoceba R, Kramer G, et al: Evaluation of the tumor specificity of a conditionally replicative adenovirus controlled by a modified human core telomerase promoter, *Mol Ther* 9:S375, 2004.
29. Blackwood L, O'Shaughnessy PJ, Reid SJ, et al: *E. coli* Nitroreductase/CB1954: In vitro studies into a potential system for feline cancer gene therapy? *Vet J* 161:269–279, 2001.
30. Cihova M, Altanerova V, Altaner C: Stem cell based cancer gene therapy, *Mol Pharma* 8(5):1480–1487, 2011.
31. Le Blanc K: Immunomodulatory effects of fetal and adult mesenchymal stem cells, *Cytotherapy* 5:485–489, 2003.
32. Koppula PR, Chelluri LK, Polisetti N, et al: Histocompatibility testing of cultivated human bone marrow stromal cells—a promising step towards pre-clinical screening for allogeneic stem cell therapy, *Cell Immunol* 259:61–66, 2009.
33. Griffin MD, Ritter T, Mahon BP: Immunological aspects of allogeneic mesenchymal stem cell therapies, *Hum Gene Ther* 21:1641–1655, 2010.
34. Lasek W, Basak G, Switaj T, et al: Complete tumour regressions induced by vaccination with IL-12 gene-transduced tumour cells in combination with IL-15 in a melanoma model in mice, *Cancer Immunol Immunother* 53(4):363–372, 2004.
35. Yamazaki M, Straus FH, Messina M, et al: Adenovirus-mediated tumor-specific combined gene therapy using Herpes simplex virus thymidine/ganciclovir system and murine interleukin-12 induces effective antitumor activity against medullary thyroid carcinoma, *Cancer Gene Ther* 11(1):8–15, 2004.
36. Nagayama Y, Nakao K, Mizuguchi H, et al: Enhanced antitumor effect of combined replicative adenovirus and nonreplicative adenovirus expressing interleukin-12 in an immunocompetent mouse model, *Gene Ther* 10(16):1400–1403, 2003.
37. Liu YQ, Huang H, Saxena A, et al: Intratumoral co-injection of two adenoviral vectors expressing functional interleukin-18 and inducible protein-10, respectively, synergizes to facilitate regression of established tumors, *Cancer Gene Therapy* 9(6):533–542, 2002.
38. Goto H, Osaki T, Nishino K, et al: Construction and analysis of new vector systems with improved interleukin-18 secretion in a xenogeneic human tumor model, *J Immunother* 25:S35–S41, 2002.
39. Quintin-Colonna F, Devauchelle P, Fradelizi D, et al: Gene therapy of spontaneous canine melanoma and feline fibrosarcoma by intratumoral administration of histoincompatible cells expressing human interleukin-2, *Gene Ther* 3(12):1104–1112, 1996.
40. Carpinteiro A, Peinert S, Ostertag W, et al: Genetic protection of repopulating hematopoietic cells with an improved MDR1-retrovirus allows administration of intensified chemotherapy following stem cell transplantation in mice, *Int J Cancer* 98(5):785–792, 2002.
41. Schiedlmeier B, Schilz AJ, Kuhlcke K, et al: Multidrug resistance 1 gene transfer can confer chemoprotection to human peripheral blood progenitor cells engrafted in immunodeficient mice, *Hum Gene Ther* 13(2):233–242, 2002.
42. Fairbairn LJ, Rafferty JA, Lashford LS: Engineering drug resistance in human cells, *Bone Marrow Transplant* 25:S110–S113, 2000.
43. Chiocca EA, Abbed KM, Tatter S, et al: A phase I open-label, dose-escalation, multi-institutional trial of injection with an E1B-attenuated adenovirus, ONYX-015, into the peritumoral region of recurrent malignant gliomas, in the adjuvant setting, *Mol Ther* 10(5):958–966, 2004.
44. Post DE, Fulci G, Chiocca EA, et al: Replicative oncolytic herpes simplex viruses in combination cancer therapies, *Curr Gene Ther* 4(1):41–51, 2004.
45. Shah AC, Benos D, Gillespie GY, et al: Oncolytic viruses: clinical applications as vectors for the treatment of malignant gliomas, *J Neuroncol* 65(3):203–226, 2003.
46. Dirven CMF, van Beusechem VW, Lamfers MLM, et al: Oncolytic adenoviruses for treatment of brain tumours, *Exp Opin Biol Ther* 2(8):943–952, 2002.
47. Hemminki A, Kanerva A, Kremer EJ, et al: A canine conditionally replicating adenovirus for evaluating oncolytic virotherapy in a syngeneic animal model, *Mol Ther* 7(2):163–173, 2003.
48. Zhan JH, Gao Y, Wang WS, et al: Tumor-specific intravenous gene delivery using oncolytic adenoviruses, *Cancer Gene Therapy* 12(1):19–25, 2005.
49. Lombardo A, Genovese P, Beausejour CM, et al: Gene editing in human stem cells using zinc finger nucleases and integrase-defective lentiviral vector delivery, *Nat Biotechnol* 25:1298–1306, 2007.

SECTION B

Signal Transduction and Cancer

Cheryl A. London

In normal cells, signals are generated that begin at the outside of the cell and transmit through the cytoplasm to the nucleus, regulating cell growth, differentiation, survival, and death. Over the past few years, researchers have recognized that many of the components of the signal transduction pathways are dysregulated in cancer cells, leading to uncontrolled cell growth and thereby contributing to tumorigenesis. Because many tumors have similar alterations in signal transduction components, these have become promising targets for therapeutic intervention. This section primarily focuses on the role of a particular group of signal transducers called *protein kinases,* their role in normal cells, the mechanisms by which they contribute to tumorigenesis, and the use of agents designed to inhibit them when they become dysfunctional.

Protein Kinases and Normal Cells

Protein kinases play critical roles in normal cell signal transduction, acting to tightly regulate critical cellular processes such as growth and differentiation. These proteins work through phosphorylation; that is, they bind adenosine triphosphate (ATP) and use it to add phosphate groups to key residues on themselves (a process called *autophosphorylation*) and on other molecules, thereby stimulating a downstream signal inside the cell. This process typically occurs in response to external signals generated by growth factors (GFs) or other stimuli that initiate the cascade. Protein kinases are classified as tyrosine kinases (TKs) if they phosphorylate proteins on tyrosine residues or serine/threonine kinases if they phosphorylate proteins on serine and threonine residues. In some cases the kinases perform both functions (i.e., dual function kinases). These kinases can be expressed on the cell surface, in the cytoplasm, and in the nucleus. The human genome encodes approximately 518 kinases, of which 90 are classified as TKs.[1]

TKs on the cell surface that are activated through binding of GFs are called receptor TKs (RTKs). Of the 90 identified TKs, 58 are known to be RTKs. Each RTK contains an extracellular domain that binds the GF, a transmembrane domain, and a cytoplasmic kinase domain that positively and negatively regulates phosphorylation of the RTK (Figure 14-6).[2-4] Most RTKs are monomers on the cell surface and are dimerized through the act of GF binding; this changes the three-dimensional structure of the receptor, permitting ATP to bind and autophosphorylation to occur, resulting in generation of a downstream signal through subsequent binding of adaptor proteins and nonreceptor kinases.[2] Dysregulation of RTKs resulting in pathway activation/uncontrolled signaling is known to contribute to several human cancers, and work is ongoing to characterize such abnormalities in canine and feline cancers. Examples of RTKs known to play prominent roles in specific cancers include KIT, MET, epidermal growth factor receptor (EGFR), and anaplastic lymphoma kinase (ALK), which can be activated by overexpression, mutation, and chromosomal translocation.[5-9]

RKT signaling is critical for regulating typical cell functions and is also an important regulator of angiogenesis, a process known to be essential for continued tumor cell growth. The RTKs involved in angiogenesis include vascular endothelial growth factor receptor (VEGFR), platelet-derived growth factor receptor (PDGFR), fibroblast growth factor receptor (FGFR), and Tie-1 and Tie-2 (receptors for angiopoietin).[10-13] VEGFRs are expressed on vascular endothelium, and VEGFR signaling drives endothelial migration and proliferation.[10] PDGFR is expressed on stroma and pericytes that are critical for the maintenance of newly formed blood vessels. It also supports angiogenesis by inducing VEGF transcription and secretion.[12,13] FGFR is expressed on vascular endothelium and works with VEGFR to promote increased expression of VEGF.[12] Tie-1 and Tie-2 are expressed on blood vessels in tumors and are important in the recruitment of pericytes and smooth muscle cells to the newly forming vascular channels.[14]

Kinases in the cytoplasm act as a bridge, conducting signals generated by RTKs to the nucleus through a series of intermediates that become phosphorylated.[15] The cytoplasmic kinases may be directly on the inside of the cell membrane or free in the cytoplasm. With respect to tumor cell biology, two particular cytoplasmic pathways are often dysregulated in a number of cancers. The first includes members of the RAS-RAF-MEK-ERK/p38/JNK families (Figure 14-7).[16,17] Most of these are serine/threonine kinases, and their activation leads to ERK phosphorylation, translocation into the nucleus, and subsequent alteration of transcription factors and nuclear kinase activity important for controlling the cell cycle. Examples of dysregulation in human cancers include RAS mutations in lung cancer, colon cancer, and several hematologic

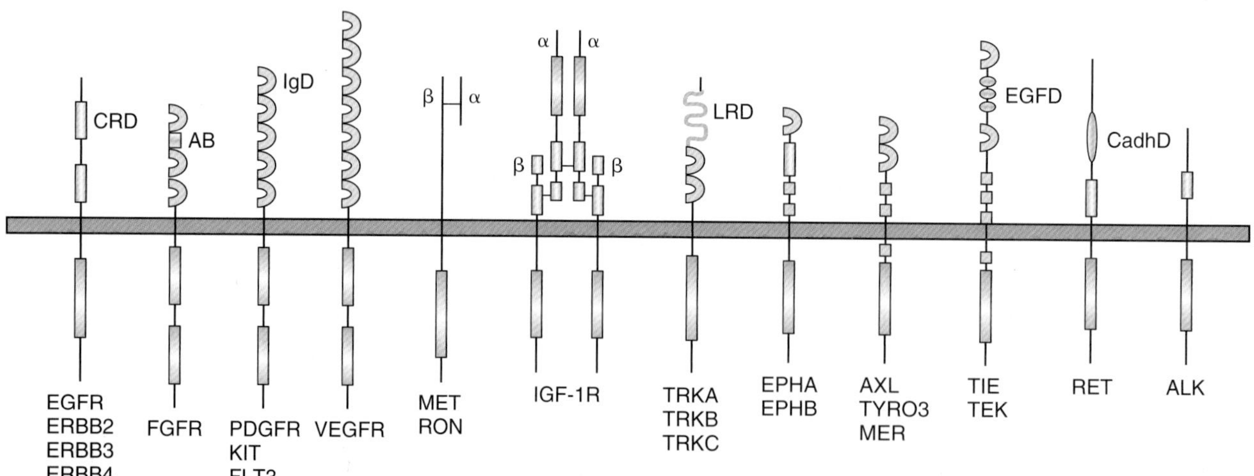

FIGURE 14-6 The structures of receptor tyrosine kinase (RTK) families implicated in a variety of malignancies are shown. The symbols α and β indicate specific RTK subunits. *AB,* Acid box; *ALK,* anaplastic lymphoma kinase; *CadhD,* cadherin-like domain; *CRD,* cysteine-rich domain; *EGFD,* epidermal growth factor-like domain; *EGFR,* epidermal growth factor receptor; *EPH,* member of ephrin receptor family; *FGFR,* fibroblast growth factor receptor; *IgD,* immunoglobulin-like domain; *IGF-1R,* insulin-like growth factor receptor 1; *LRD,* leucine-rich domain; *PDGFR,* platelet-derived growth factor receptor; *Tie,* tyrosine kinase receptor on endothelial cells; *TRK,* member of nerve growth factor receptor family; *VEGFR,* vascular endothelial growth factor receptor. *(From London CA: Kinase inhibitors in cancer therapy,* Vet Comp Oncol *2:177–193, 2004. Reprinted with permission from Blackwell Publishing.)*

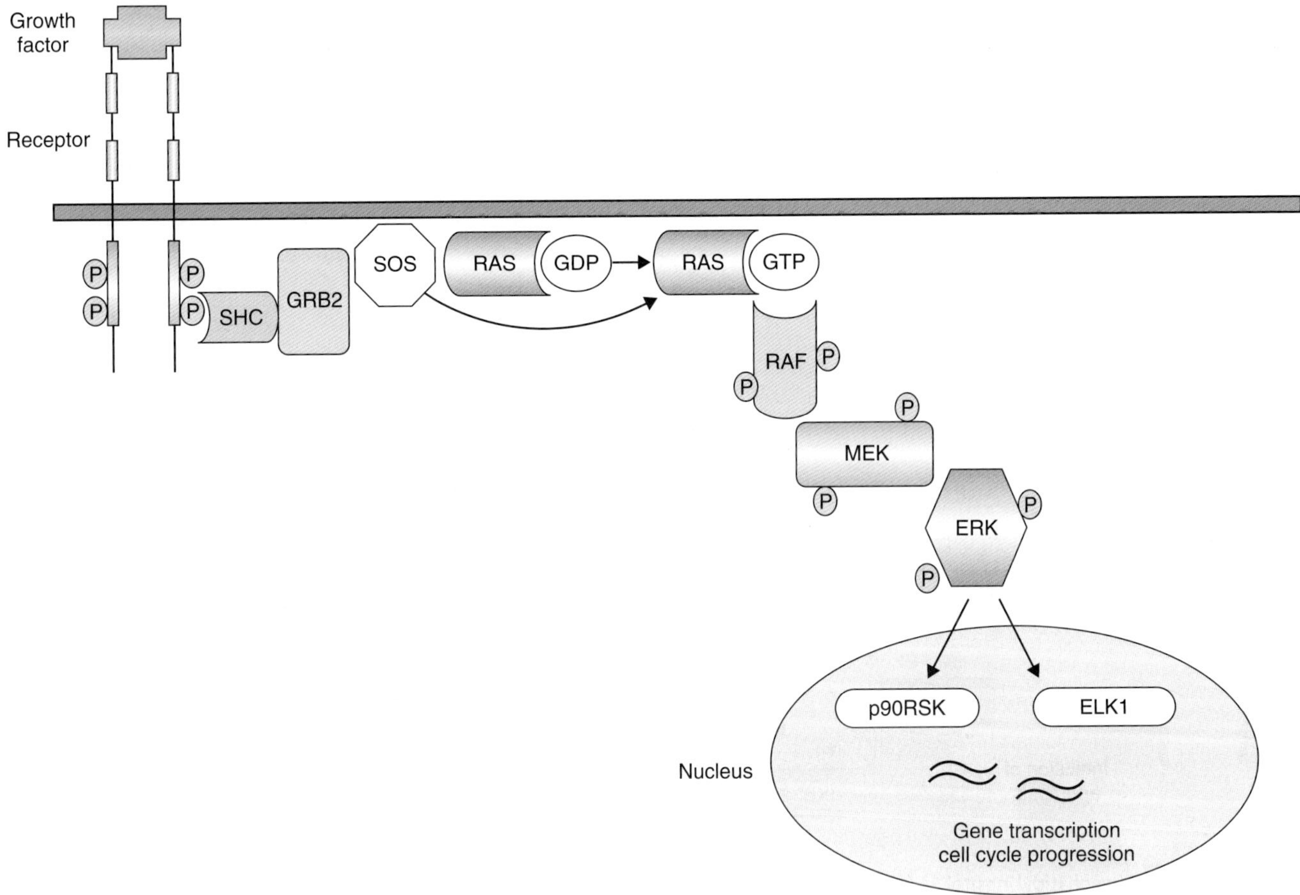

FIGURE 14-7 RAS signal transduction. Activated receptor tyrosine kinases recruit SOS to the plasma membrane through binding of SHC and GRB2. SOS replaces bound GDP with GTP, thereby activating RAS. The downstream target RAF is then phosphorylated by RAS, leading to subsequent activation of MEK, then ERK. ERK has several substrates both in the nucleus and in the cytoplasm, including ETS transcription factors such as ELK1 and RSK, which regulate cell cycle progression. *(From London CA: Kinase inhibitors in cancer therapy,* Vet Comp Oncol *2:177–193, 2004. Reprinted with permission from Blackwell Publishing.)*

malignancies and BRAF mutations in cutaneous melanomas and papillary thyroid carcinomas.[18-20]

The second cytoplasmic pathway includes phosphatidyl inositol-3 kinase (PI3K) and its associated downstream signal transducers AKT, nuclear factor κB (NFκB), and mTOR, among others (Figure 14-8).[21,22] PI3K is activated by RTKs and in turn activates AKT, which alters several additional proteins involved in the regulation of cell survival, cycling, and growth.[23] AKT phosphorylates targets that promote apoptosis (BAD, procaspase-9, and Forkhead transcription factors) and activates NFκB, a transcription factor that has antiapoptotic activity.[21-23] AKT also phosphorylates other proteins such as mTOR, p21, p27, and glycogen synthase kinase 3 (GSK3). This leads to redistribution of these proteins either in or out of the nucleus, ultimately inhibiting apoptosis while promoting cell cycling.[21-23] Abnormalities of PI3K resulting in pathway activation are commonly found in human cancers, including mutations (breast and colorectal cancers and glioblastoma) and gene amplification (gastric, lung, ovarian cancers).[24] This pathway may also become dysregulated through loss of activity of PTEN, a phosphatase that normally acts to dephosphorylate AKT and terminate signaling.[21,25,26] PTEN mutations and/or decreased PTEN expression are found in several human cancers (e.g., glioblastoma and prostate cancer)[24,25] and have been documented in canine cancers (OSA, melanoma).[27-29]

RTK-induced signaling ultimately influences cellular events by affecting transcription and the proteins that control cell cycling. The cyclins and their kinase partners (cyclin-dependent kinases [CDKs]) act to regulate the progression of cells through various phases of the cell cycle (Figure 14-9).[30-32] The cyclins comprise several families. Cyclins D and E control restriction point passage by activating their respective CDKs (CDK4 and CDK6 for cyclin D and CDK2 for cyclin E). Coordinated function of cyclins D and E is required for cells to progress from G_1 into S phase (see Figure 14-9). In many cases, RTK-generated signals induce expression of cyclin D, which complexes with CDK4 and CDK6, resulting in phosphorylation of the tumor suppressor Rb, partially repressing its function.[31,32] Functional cyclin D/CDK complexes induce transcription of cyclin E, and active cyclin E/CDK complexes further reduce Rb activity through phosphorylation. This in turn initiates the process of DNA replication important for cell cycling. Dysregulation of the cyclins and CDKs is common in human cancers; for example, overexpression of cyclins D and E is often present in breast, pancreas, and head and neck carcinomas.[32]

Protein Kinases and Cancer Cells

Dysfunction of protein kinases is now recognized to be a common event in tumors. Although this has been best characterized in

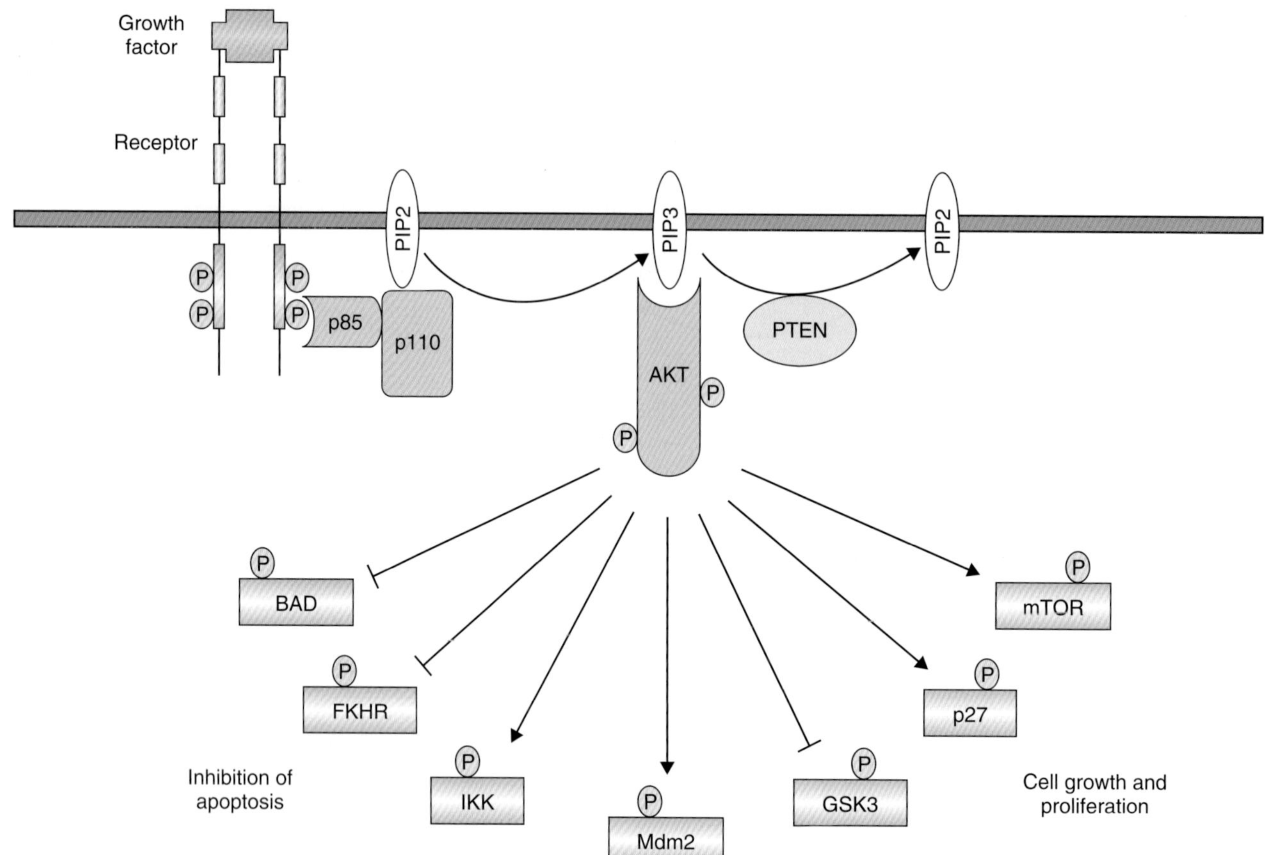

FIGURE 14-8 Phosphatidyl inositol-3 kinase (PI3K) signal transduction. Following receptor tyrosine kinase (RTK) activation, PI3K is recruited to the phosphorylated receptor through binding of the p85 adaptor subunit, leading to activation of the catalytic subunit (p110). This activation results in the generation of the second messenger phosphatidyl inositol-3,4,5-triphosphate (PIP3). PIP3 recruits AKT to the membrane and following its phosphorylation, several downstream targets are subsequently phosphorylated, leading to either their activation or inhibition. The cumulative effect results in cell survival, growth, and proliferation. *(From London CA: Kinase inhibitors in cancer therapy,* Vet Comp Oncol *2:177–193, 2004. Reprinted with permission from Blackwell Publishing.)*

humans, recent data indicate that dog and cat cancers experience similar dysregulation (Table 14-2). Kinases may be dysregulated through a variety of mechanisms, including mutation, overexpression, fusion proteins, or autocrine loops. In the case of mutations, these may result in phosphorylation of the kinase in the absence of an appropriate signal. Such mutations can consist of a single amino acid change through a point mutation, deletion of amino acids, or insertion of amino acids, usually in the form of an internal tandem duplication (ITD). For example, a point mutation occurs in the BRAF gene (V600E, exon 15) in approximately 60% of human cutaneous melanomas.[18,33,34] This amino acid change causes a conformation change in BRAF that mimics its activated form, thereby inducing constitutive downstream ERK signaling and abnormal promotion of cell growth and survival.[35,36] RAS is another kinase that is dysregulated through point mutation in several hematopoietic neoplasms (multiple myeloma, juvenile chronic myelogenous leukemia [CML], acute myelogenous leukemia [AML], and chronic myelomonocytic leukemia [CMML]) and in lung cancer, colon cancer, and many others.[17,37,38]

Another example of a mutation involves KIT, an RTK that normally is expressed on hematopoietic stem cells, on melanocytes, in the central nervous system, and on mast cells.[39] In approximately 25% to 30% of canine grade 2 and grade 3 mast cell tumors (MCTs), mutations consisting of ITDs are found in the juxtamembrane domain of KIT, resulting in constitutive activation in the absence of ligand binding. These mutations are associated with a higher risk of local recurrence and metastasis.[40-42] KIT mutations consisting of deletions in the juxtamembrane domain are also found in approximately 50% of human patients with gastrointestinal stromal tumors (GISTs) and are also found in GISTs in dogs.[43-45] There are now several well-characterized mutations involving RTKs in human cancers, including FLT3 ITDs in AML,[46-49] EGFR point mutations in lung carcinomas,[50,51] and PI3K mutations in several types of carcinomas.[24]

Overexpression of kinases usually involves the RTKs and may result in enhanced response of the cancer cells to normal levels of growth factor; or, if the levels are high enough, the kinase may become activated through spontaneous dimerization in the absence of signal/growth factor. In humans, the RTK human epidermal growth factor receptor 2 (HER2; also known as ErbB2, a member of the EGFR family) is overexpressed in both breast and ovarian carcinomas and often correlates with a more aggressive phenotype.[4,52,53] EGFR is also overexpressed in human lung, bladder, cervical, ovarian, renal, and pancreatic cancers, and some tumors have as many as 60 copies of the gene per cell.[7,54,55] As with HER2, such overexpression is linked to a worse outcome in affected patients.[7]

Fusion proteins are generated when a portion of the kinase becomes attached to another gene through chromosomal

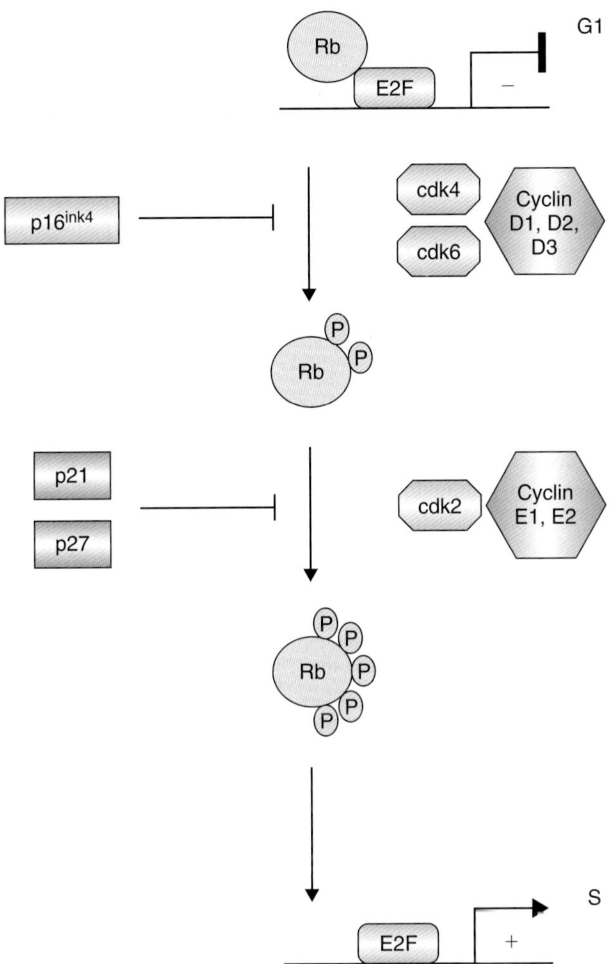

FIGURE 14-9 Cyclin and cyclin-dependent kinase (CDK) regulation of G1-S transition. CDK inhibitors such as p16ink4 and p21 restrict the activity of cyclin D- and cyclin E-dependent kinases. Progressive Rb phosphorylation by the cyclins results in liberation of E2F and the resultant transcription of S-phase genes. *(From London CA: Kinase inhibitors in cancer therapy,* Vet Comp Oncol *2:177–193, 2004. Reprinted with permission from Blackwell Publishing.)*

rearrangement and the normal mechanisms that control protein function are disrupted. One of the best characterized fusion proteins is BCR-ABL, which is found in 90% of patients with CML.[56-59] ABL is a cytoplasmic tyrosine kinase that, when fused to BCR, results in dysregulation of ABL, inappropriate activity of the protein, and resultant malignant transformation. Other examples include TEL-PDGFRβ in CMML, FIP1-PDGFRα in hypereosinophilic syndrome with mastocytosis, and (EML4)-ALK in non–small-cell lung cancer (NSCLC).[60]

Autocrine loops of activation primarily occur when the tumor cell expresses both the RTK and the growth factor; in most cases, one or the other usually is also overexpressed, resulting in constitutive activation of the RTK. Examples include coexpression of transforming growth factor α (TGFα) and EGFR in glioblastoma and squamous cell carcinoma, insulin-like growth factor (IGF) and its ligand, IGF-1R, in breast and colorectal cancer, and VEGF and VEGFR in melanoma.[4,61-63] In canine cancers, possible autocrine loops have been documented in OSA (co-expression of MET and its ligand, HGF) and hemangiosarcoma (HSA; co-expression of KIT and its ligand, SCF).[64-66]

TABLE 14-2 Receptor Tyrosine Kinases Associated with Cancer

TYROSINE KINASE	CANCER ASSOCIATION
EGFR family	Breast, ovary, lung, stomach, colon, glioblastoma
Insulin receptor family	Sarcomas, cervix, kidney
PDGFR family	Glioblastoma, ovary, CMML, GIST
KIT	AML, GIST, seminoma, MCT, melanoma
Flt3	AML
VEGFR family	Angiogenesis, Kaposi's sarcoma, hemangiosarcoma, melanoma
FGFR family	AML, lymphoma, breast, prostate, multiple myeloma, TCC
NGFR family	Thyroid cancer, neuroblastoma, fibrosarcoma, AML
Met/Ron	Thyroid cancer, osteosarcoma, rhabdomyosarcoma, liver, kidney, colon
EPHR family	Melanoma, stomach, colon, breast, esophagus
AXL	AML
Tie family	Angiogenesis, stomach, hemangioblastoma
RET family	Thyroid cancer, multiple endocrine neoplasia
ALK	Non-Hodgkin's lymphoma, lung

ALK, Anaplastic lymphoma kinase; *AML,* acute myelogenous leukemia; *CMML,* chronic myelomonocytic leukemia; *EGFR,* epidermal growth factor receptor; *EPHR,* ephrin receptor; *FGFR,* fibroblast growth factor receptor; *GIST,* gastrointestinal stromal tumors; *MCT,* mast cell tumors; *NGFR,* nerve growth factor receptor; *PDGFR,* platelet-derived growth factor receptor; *TCC,* transitional cell carcinoma; *Tie,* tyrosine kinase receptor on endothelial cells; *VEGFR,* vascular endothelial growth factor receptor.

Inhibition of Kinases

Given the detailed molecular characterization of signal transducer dysregulation in cancer cells, significant efforts have been directed at developing strategies to inhibit those transducers that participate in tumorigenesis through direct effects on the cancer cell or through modulation of tumor microenvironment (stroma and neovasculature). The two most successful approaches to date have been monoclonal antibodies (MAbs) and small molecule inhibitors.

Several antibodies have been developed to target the extracellular domain of RTKs known to be important in a variety of tumors. These antibodies may prevent the growth factor from binding, may promote internalization of the RTK and subsequent degradation, or may induce an immune response against the cancer cell. One of the most successful examples is a humanized MAb called *trastuzumab* (Herceptin). This antibody targets HER2, which as previously discussed is overexpressed in approximately 30% of breast cancers, as well as other cancers, including prostate cancer, ovarian cancer, and NSCLC.[67] In initial clinical trials, trastuzumab treatment of HER2-positive breast cancer resulted in a response rate of approximately 25% in patients with metastatic disease.[68] The response rate approached 50% when trastuzumab was combined with chemotherapy.[69] When used in the adjuvant setting, multiple studies have demonstrated that trastuzumab markedly improves survival rates of women with HER2-positive disease; trastuzumab is now part of the routine standard of care for this disease.[70,71] Other examples of MAbs that have demonstrated significant activity in human cancers include rituximab (Rituxan) that targets CD20 expressed in a number of B-cell lymphomas[72,73] and cetuximab (Erbitux) that targets ERBB1/HER1 EGFR known to be overexpressed in several carcinomas.[7,67,74]

Small molecule inhibitors work primarily by blocking the ATP-binding site of kinases, essentially acting as competitive inhibitors; a smaller number of these inhibitors work by preventing necessary protein-protein interactions (allosteric inhibition).[75] In the absence of ATP, the kinase is unable to phosphorylate itself or downstream signaling elements, thereby interrupting a survival/growth signal essential to the tumor cell, ultimately resulting in cell death. As the molecular characterization of tumors has improved, the development and application of small molecule inhibitors have rapidly expanded in human oncology and their use is markedly altering how cancers are managed. Such inhibitors often are easy to synthesize in large quantities, frequently orally bioavailable, and can readily enter cells to bind the intended target.

The first small molecule inhibitor to be approved for human use was imatinib (Gleevec), an orally administered drug that binds the ATP pocket of ABL, as well as the RTKs KIT and PDGFRα.[76] As previously discussed, BCR-ABL fusion proteins are present in 90% of human patients with CML, making ABL a good target for therapeutic intervention. The application of imatinib to CML has been transformative, with significant biologic activity demonstrated in several clinical trials, resulting in the approval of imatinib for up-front care of affected individuals.[77-82] In the chronic phase of CML, imatinib induces a remission rate of close to 95%, and most patients remain in remission for longer than 1 year. Unfortunately, the remission rate is much lower for patients in blast crisis (20% to 50%), often lasting less than 10 months. Resistance to imatinib has been well characterized and is primarily due to the development of mutations in ABL that preclude drug binding, although gene amplification has also been documented.[83,84] Imatinib also has clinical activity against human GIST in which 60% to 80% of the tumors have point mutations or deletions in the juxtamembrane domain of KIT, resulting in constitutive activation.[85,86] Response rates of 50% to 70% have been reported with imatinib, far better than the 5% response rate seen with standard chemotherapy.[87,88] A small number of GISTs have activating mutations in PDGFRα instead of KIT mutations; these patients also respond to imatinib.[89]

There are now several small molecule inhibitors approved for the treatment of human cancers that possess specific mutations in kinases known to drive tumor growth and survival. A subset of patients with NSCLC have tumors with activating mutations in EGFR that respond to erlotinib (Tarceva) or gefitinib (Iressa), small molecule inhibitors of EGFR.[90] Response rates in patients with EGFR mutations can be as high as 80% compared to less than 10% to 20% for those without, demonstrating that efficacy of targeted therapies often depends on the presence of a known activated signaling element. A small number of patients with NSCLC also exhibit activation of the RTK ALK through its fusion to EML4.[91] A small molecule inhibitor of ALK, crizotinib (Xalkori), has demonstrated significant activity against lung cancer patients whose tumors express the EML4-ALK translocation. In a recent phase II study, an objective response rate of 56% was achieved in this subset of patients, with another 31% of patients experiencing stable disease.[91,92] As expected with a targeted therapeutic that disrupts key cell-signaling events, responses were rapid with most occurring by 8 weeks of treatment.

Vemurafenib (Zelboraf) is a small molecule inhibitor of BRAF that has shown significant activity against cutaneous malignant melanomas that possess activating mutations in BRAF. Most patients treated with vemurafenib experienced tumor shrinkage, with close to 50% meeting the criteria for objective response.[93] This compares to an objective response rate of only 5% in patients treated with dacarbazine. Inhibition of mTOR has become of interest in several cancers given the activation of the PI3K pathway and the critical role of mTOR in mediating its effects. Rapamycin, a drug used for many years as an immunosuppressive agent, is the prototypical mTOR inhibitor.[94,95] Temsirolimus and everolimus, two rapamycin analogs, have already been approved for use in patients with metastatic renal carcinoma and other mTOR inhibitors are currently under investigation for their potential utility in treating soft tissue sarcomas and bone sarcomas.[94,95]

Flavopiridol, a partly synthetic flavonoid derived from an indigenous plant (rohitukine) found in India, sits in the ATP-binding pocket of CDK2, acting as a competitive inhibitor.[89,90] This compound has been shown to inhibit most of the CDKs evaluated, although some less potently than others.[91,92] Although flavopiridol initially failed to demonstrate significant efficacy when used as a single agent,[89] recent pharmacokinetic data demonstrated activity in some patients, particularly those with chronic lymphocytic leukemia (CLL), when an alternative dosing schedule that enhanced the area under the curve was employed.[96]

The inhibitors discussed previously tend to affect a restricted set of kinases, although other drugs exhibit much more broadly targeted inhibition. Sunitinib (Sutent) is a small molecule inhibitor of several RTKs, including VEGFR1, VEGFR2, PDGFRα/β, KIT, FLT3, receptor of colony-stimulating factor 1 (CSFR1), and rearranged during transfection receptor (RET).[97] The multitargeted nature of this inhibitor may be responsible for its observed activity in several types of cancer, including GIST, renal cell carcinoma, thyroid carcinoma, and insulinoma, among others.[97] Although such agents often have significant clinical activity, they are typically associated with a broader range of toxicities that may limit their use.

Kinase Inhibitors in Veterinary Medicine

There are now two small molecule inhibitors approved for use in dogs in veterinary medicine. Toceranib (Palladia) is a multitargeted inhibitor closely related to sunitinib that exhibits a similar target profile, including VEGFR, PDGFR, KIT, FLT3, and CSF1R. Toceranib has demonstrated activity against MCT, as well as sarcomas and carcinomas. In the original phase I study, 28% of dogs experienced objective responses to treatment, with an additional 26% experiencing stable disease for an overall biologic activity of 54%.[98] A pivotal study of toceranib was subsequently conducted in dogs with recurrent or metastatic intermediate or high grade MCT resulting in an objective response rate of 42.8% (21 complete responses, 42 partial responses), with an additional 16 dogs experiencing stable disease for an overall biologic activity of 60%.[99] Dogs whose MCT harbored activating mutations in KIT were roughly twice as likely to respond to toceranib than those without mutation (69% versus 37%). Following approval of toceranib in 2009, it has been used to treat a number of different solid tumors.[100] Preliminary observations of biologic activity were reported in dogs with anal sac adenocarcinoma, thyroid carcinoma, head and neck carcinoma, nasal carcinoma, and OSA. Several studies are ongoing to more clearly define the role of toceranib in the treatment of canine and feline cancer.

Masitinib (Kinavet) is a small molecule inhibitor of KIT, PDGFRα/β, and Lyn. In dogs with MCTs, masitinib significantly improved time to progression compared to placebo, and outcome was improved in dogs with MCT harboring KIT mutations.[101] Subsequent follow-up of patients treated with long-term masitinib identified an increased number of patients with long-term disease control compared to those treated with placebo (40% versus 15% alive at 2 years).[102] Finally, small studies have evaluated the efficacy of imatinib for the treatment of canine and feline MCT.[103-105] Imatinib was well tolerated, and objective antitumor responses were observed in dogs with both mutant and wild-type KIT. Responses have also been observed in cats with MCT.[106,107]

Conclusion

With the advent of molecular techniques, the characterization of signal transduction pathways that are dysfunctional in cancer cells has become commonplace. Advances in computer modeling and small molecule engineering have led to the rapid development of inhibitors capable of blocking specific pathways critical for cancer cell survival. The success of inhibitors such as imatinib and crizotinib indicate that the application of this therapeutic strategy can markedly improve clinical outcome. Perhaps the greatest challenges will be determining how these novel therapeutics can be effectively combined with standard treatment regimens such as chemotherapy and radiation therapy to provide optimal anticancer efficacy without enhancing toxicity and identifying strategies to use these therapeutics in ways that are less likely to result in drug resistance.

REFERENCES

1. Manning G, Whyte DB, Martinez R, et al: The protein kinase complement of the human genome, *Science* 298:1912–1934, 2002.
2. Lemmon MA, Schlessinger J: Cell signaling by receptor tyrosine kinases, *Cell* 141:1117–1134, 2010.
3. Madhusudan S, Ganesan TS: Tyrosine kinase inhibitors in cancer therapy, *Clin Biochem* 37:618–635, 2004.
4. Zwick E, Bange J, Ullrich A: Receptor tyrosine kinases as targets for anticancer drugs, *Trends Mol Med* 8:17–23, 2002.
5. Barreca A, Lasorsa E, Riera L, et al: Anaplastic lymphoma kinase in human cancer, *J Mol Endocrinol* 47:R11–R23, 2011.
6. Fletcher JA: Role of KIT and platelet-derived growth factor receptors as oncoproteins, *Semin Oncol* 31:4–11, 2004.
7. Laskin JJ, Sandler AB: Epidermal growth factor receptor: a promising target in solid tumours, *Cancer Treat Rev* 30:1–17, 2004.
8. Ma PC, Jagadeeswaran R, Jagadeesh S, et al: Functional expression and mutations of c-Met and its therapeutic inhibition with SU11274 and small interfering RNA in non-small cell lung cancer, *Cancer Res* 65:1479–1488, 2005.
9. Ma PC, Maulik G, Christensen J, et al: c-Met: structure, functions and potential for therapeutic inhibition, *Cancer Metastasis Rev* 22:309–325, 2003.
10. Thurston G, Gale NW: Vascular endothelial growth factor and other signaling pathways in developmental and pathologic angiogenesis, *Int J Hematol* 80:7–20, 2004.
11. Eskens FA: Angiogenesis inhibitors in clinical development; where are we now and where are we going? *Br J Cancer* 90:1–7, 2004.
12. Cherrington JM, Strawn LM, Shawver LK: New paradigms for the treatment of cancer: the role of anti-angiogenesis agents, *Adv Cancer Res* 79:1–38, 2000.
13. McCarty MF, Liu W, Fan F, et al: Promises and pitfalls of anti-angiogenic therapy in clinical trials, *Trends Mol Med* 9:53–58, 2003.
14. Thurston G: Role of Angiopoietins and Tie receptor tyrosine kinases in angiogenesis and lymphangiogenesis, *Cell Tissue Res* 314:61–68, 2003.
15. Blume-Jensen P, Hunter T: Oncogenic kinase signalling, *Nature* 411:355–365, 2001.
16. Johnson GL, Lapadat R: Mitogen-activated protein kinase pathways mediated by ERK, JNK, and p38 protein kinases, *Science* 298:1911–1912, 2002.
17. Downward J: Targeting RAS signalling pathways in cancer therapy, *Nat Rev Cancer* 3:11–22, 2003.
18. Davies H, Bignell GR, Cox C, et al: Mutations of the BRAF gene in human cancer, *Nature* 417:949–954, 2002.
19. Kumar R, Angelini S, Snellman E, et al: BRAF mutations are common somatic events in melanocytic nevi, *J Invest Dermatol* 122:342–348, 2004.
20. Mercer KE, Pritchard CA: Raf proteins and cancer: B-Raf is identified as a mutational target, *Biochim Biophys Acta* 1653:25–40, 2003.
21. Fresno Vara JA, Casado E, de Castro J, et al: PI3K/Akt signalling pathway and cancer, *Cancer Treat Rev* 30:193–204, 2004.
22. Franke TF, Hornik CP, Segev L, et al: PI3K/Akt and apoptosis: size matters, *Oncogene* 22:8983–8998, 2003.
23. Mitsiades CS, Mitsiades N, Koutsilieris M: The Akt pathway: molecular targets for anti-cancer drug development, *Curr Cancer Drug Targets* 4:235–256, 2004.
24. Markman B, Atzori F, Perez-Garcia J, et al: Status of PI3K inhibition and biomarker development in cancer therapeutics, *Ann Oncol* 21:683–691, 2010.
25. Simpson L, Parsons R: PTEN: Life as a tumor suppressor, *Exp Cell Res* 264:29–41, 2001.
26. Weng LP, Smith WM, Dahia PL, et al: PTEN suppresses breast cancer cell growth by phosphatase activity-dependent G1 arrest followed by cell death, *Cancer Res* 59:5808–5814, 1999.
27. Kanae Y, Endoh D, Yokota H, et al: Expression of the PTEN tumor suppressor gene in malignant mammary gland tumors of dogs, *Am J Vet Res* 67:127–133, 2006.
28. Koenig A, Bianco SR, Fosmire S, et al: Expression and significance of p53, rb, p21/waf 1, p16/ink-4a, and PTEN tumor suppressors in canine melanoma, *Vet Pathol* 39:458–472, 2002.
29. Levine RA, Forest T, Smith C: Tumor suppressor PTEN is mutated in canine osteosarcoma cell lines and tumors, *Vet Pathol* 39:372–378, 2002.
30. Swanton C: Cell-cycle targeted therapies, *Lancet Oncol* 5:27–36, 2004.
31. Ortega S, Malumbres M, Barbacid M: Cyclin D-dependent kinases, INK4 inhibitors and cancer, *Biochim Biophys Acta* 1602:73–87, 2002.
32. Malumbres M, Barbacid M: To cycle or not to cycle: a critical decision in cancer, *Nat Rev Cancer* 1:222–231, 2001.
33. Wellbrock C, Ogilvie L, Hedley D, et al: V599EB-RAF is an oncogene in melanocytes, *Cancer Res* 64:2338–2342, 2004.
34. Pollock PM, Meltzer PS: A genome-based strategy uncovers frequent BRAF mutations in melanoma, *Cancer Cell* 2:5–7, 2002.
35. Wan PT, Garnett MJ, Roe SM, et al: Mechanism of activation of the RAF-ERK signaling pathway by oncogenic mutations of B-RAF, *Cell* 116:855–867, 2004.
36. Dhillon AS, Kolch W: Oncogenic B-Raf mutations: crystal clear at last, *Cancer Cell* 5:303–304, 2004.
37. Brose MS, Volpe P, Feldman M, et al: BRAF and RAS mutations in human lung cancer and melanoma, *Cancer Res* 62:6997–7000, 2002.
38. Malumbres M, Barbacid M: RAS oncogenes: the first 30 years, *Nat Rev Cancer* 3:459–465, 2003.
39. Galli SJ, Zsebo KM, Geissler EN: The kit ligand, stem cell factor, *Adv Immunol* 55:1–95, 1994.
40. Downing S, Chien MB, Kass PH, et al: Prevalence and importance of internal tandem duplications in exons 11 and 12 of c-kit in mast cell tumors of dogs, *Am J Vet Res* 63:1718–1723, 2002.
41. London CA, Galli SJ, Yuuki T, et al: Spontaneous canine mast cell tumors express tandem duplications in the proto-oncogene c-kit, *Exp Hematol* 27:689–697, 1999.

42. Zemke D, Yamini B, Yuzbasiyan-Gurkan V: Mutations in the juxtamembrane domain of c-KIT are associated with higher grade mast cell tumors in dogs, *Vet Pathol* 39:529–535, 2002.
43. Demetri GD: Targeting the molecular pathophysiology of gastrointestinal stromal tumors with imatinib. Mechanisms, successes, and challenges to rational drug development, *Hematol Oncol Clin North Am* 16:1115–1124, 2002.
44. Demetri GD: Differential properties of current tyrosine kinase inhibitors in gastrointestinal stromal tumors, *Semin Oncol* 38(Suppl 1):S10–S19, 2011.
45. Frost D, Lasota J, Miettinen M: Gastrointestinal stromal tumors and leiomyomas in the dog: a histopathologic, immunohistochemical, and molecular genetic study of 50 cases, *Vet Pathol* 40:42–54, 2003.
46. Kondo M, Horibe K, Takahashi Y, et al: Prognostic value of internal tandem duplication of the FLT3 gene in childhood acute myelogenous leukemia, *Med Pediatr Oncol* 33:525–529, 1999.
47. Nakoa M, Yokota S, Iwai T, et al: Internal tandem duplication of the flt3 gene found in acute myeloid leukemia, *Leukemia* 10:1911–1918, 1996.
48. Yokota S, Kiyoi H, Nakao M, et al: Internal tandem duplication of the FLT3 gene is preferentially seen in acute myeloid leukemia and myelodysplastic syndrome among various hematological malignancies. A study on a large series of patients and cell lines, *Leukemia* 11:1605–1609, 1997.
49. Iwai T, Yokota S, Nakao M, et al: Internal tandem duplication of the FLT3 gene and clinical evaluation in childhood acute myeloid leukemia. The Children's Cancer and Leukemia Study Group, Japan, *Leukemia* 13:38–43, 1999.
50. Pao W, Chmielecki J: Rational, biologically based treatment of EGFR-mutant non-small-cell lung cancer, *Nat Rev Cancer* 10:760–774, 2010.
51. Wen J, Fu J, Zhang W, et al: Genetic and epigenetic changes in lung carcinoma and their clinical implications, *Mod Pathol* 24:932–943, 2011.
52. Paik S, Hazan R, Fisher ER, et al: Pathologic findings from the National Surgical Adjuvant Breast and Bowel Project: prognostic significance of erbB-2 protein overexpression in primary breast cancer, *J Clin Oncol* 8:103–112, 1990.
53. Slamon DJ, Clark GM, Wong SG, et al: Human breast cancer: correlation of relapse and survival with amplification of the HER-2/neu oncogene, *Science* 235:177–182, 1987.
54. Libermann TA, Nusbaum HR, Razon N, et al: Amplification, enhanced expression and possible rearrangement of EGF receptor gene in primary human brain tumours of glial origin, *Nature* 313:144–147, 1985.
55. Libermann TA, Nusbaum HR, Razon N, et al: Amplification and overexpression of the EGF receptor gene in primary human glioblastomas, *J Cell Sci Suppl* 3:161–172, 1985.
56. Golub TR, Barker GF, Lovett M, et al: Fusion of PDGF receptor beta to a novel ets-like gene, tel, in chronic myelomonocytic leukemia with t(5;12) chromosomal translocation, *Cell* 77:307–316, 1994.
57. Gotlib J, Cools J, Malone JM, 3rd, et al: The FIP1L1-PDGFRalpha fusion tyrosine kinase in hypereosinophilic syndrome and chronic eosinophilic leukemia: implications for diagnosis, classification, and management, *Blood* 103:2879–2891, 2004.
58. Melo JV, Hughes TP, Apperley JF: Chronic myeloid leukemia, *Hematology (Am Soc Hematol Educ Program)* 2003:132–152, 2003.
59. Van Etten RA: Mechanisms of transformation by the BCR-ABL oncogene: new perspectives in the post-imatinib era, *Leuk Res* 2004;28(Suppl 1):S21–S28, 2004.
60. Medves S, Demoulin JB: Tyrosine kinase gene fusions in cancer: Translating mechanisms into targeted therapies, *J Cell Mol Med* 16(2):237–248, 2012.
61. Sciacca L, Costantino A, Pandini G, et al: Insulin receptor activation by IGF-II in breast cancers: evidence for a new autocrine/paracrine mechanism, *Oncogene* 18:2471–2479, 1999.
62. Ekstrand AJ, James CD, Cavenee WK, et al: Genes for epidermal growth factor receptor, transforming growth factor alpha, and epidermal growth factor and their expression in human gliomas in vivo, *Cancer Res* 51:2164–2172, 1991.
63. Graeven U, Fiedler W, Karpinski S, et al: Melanoma-associated expression of vascular endothelial growth factor and its receptors FLT-1 and KDR, *J Cancer Res Clin Oncol* 125:621–629, 1999.
64. Fosmire SP, Dickerson EB, Scott AM, et al: Canine malignant hemangiosarcoma as a model of primitive angiogenic endothelium, *Lab Invest* 84:562–572, 2004.
65. MacEwen EG, Kutzke J, Carew J, et al: c-Met tyrosine kinase receptor expression and function in human and canine osteosarcoma cells, *Clin Exp Metastasis* 20:421–430, 2003.
66. Ferracini R, Angelini P, Cagliero E, et al: MET oncogene aberrant expression in canine osteosarcoma, *J Orthop Res* 18:253–256, 2000.
67. Harris M: Monoclonal antibodies as therapeutic agents for cancer, *Lancet Oncol* 5:292–302, 2004.
68. Vogel CL, Cobleigh MA, Tripathy D, et al: First-line Herceptin monotherapy in metastatic breast cancer, *Oncology* 61(Suppl 2):37–42, 2001.
69. Slamon DJ, Leyland-Jones B, Shak S, et al: Use of chemotherapy plus a monoclonal antibody against HER2 for metastatic breast cancer that overexpresses HER2, *N Engl J Med* 2001;344:783–792, 2001.
70. Arteaga CL, Sliwkowski MX, Osborne CK, et al: Treatment of HER2-positive breast cancer: current status and future perspectives, *Nat Rev Clin Oncol* 9(1):16–32, 2011.
71. Mukai H: Treatment strategy for HER2-positive breast cancer, *Int J Clin Oncol* 15:335–340, 2010.
72. Cabanillas F: Front-line management of diffuse large B cell lymphoma, *Curr Opin Oncol* 22:642–645, 2010.
73. Vidal L, Gafter-Gvili A, Salles G, et al: Rituximab maintenance for the treatment of patients with follicular lymphoma: an updated systematic review and meta-analysis of randomized trials, *J Natl Cancer Inst* 103:1799–1806, 2001.
74. Brand TM, Iida M, Wheeler DL: Molecular mechanisms of resistance to the EGFR monoclonal antibody cetuximab, *Cancer Biol Ther* 11:777–792, 2011.
75. Zhang J, Yang PL, Gray NS: Targeting cancer with small molecule kinase inhibitors, *Nat Rev Cancer* 9:28–39, 2009.
76. de Kogel CE, Schellens JH: Imatinib, *Oncologist* 12:1390–1394, 2007.
77. Mauro MJ, Druker BJ: STI571: targeting BCR-ABL as therapy for CML, *Oncologist* 6:233–238, 2001.
78. Kantarjian H, Sawyers C, Hochhaus A, et al: Hematologic and cytogenetic responses to imatinib mesylate in chronic myelogenous leukemia, *N Engl J Med* 346:645–652, 2002.
79. Beham-Schmid C, Apfelbeck U, Sill H, et al: Treatment of chronic myelogenous leukemia with the tyrosine kinase inhibitor STI571 results in marked regression of bone marrow fibrosis, *Blood* 99:381–383, 2002.
80. Druker BJ, Talpaz M, Resta DJ, et al: Efficacy and safety of a specific inhibitor of the BCR-ABL tyrosine kinase in chronic myeloid leukemia, *N Engl J Med* 344:1031–1037, 2001.
81. Druker BJ, Sawyers CL, Kantarjian H, et al: Activity of a specific inhibitor of the BCR-ABL tyrosine kinase in the blast crisis of chronic myeloid leukemia and acute lymphoblastic leukemia with the Philadelphia chromosome, *N Engl J Med* 344:1038–1042, 2001.
82. Sawyers CL: Rational therapeutic intervention in cancer: Kinases as drug targets, *Curr Opin Genet Dev* 12:111–115, 2002.
83. Weisberg E, Griffin JD: Resistance to imatinib (Glivec): update on clinical mechanisms, *Drug Resist Updat* 6:231–238, 2003.
84. Nardi V, Azam M, Daley GQ: Mechanisms and implications of imatinib resistance mutations in BCR-ABL, *Curr Opin Hematol* 11:35–43, 2004.
85. Duffaud F, Blay JY: Gastrointestinal stromal tumors: Biology and treatment, *Oncology* 65:187–197, 2003.
86. Heinrich MC, Rubin BP, Longley BJ, et al: Biology and genetic aspects of gastrointestinal stromal tumors: KIT activation and cytogenetic alterations, *Hum Pathol* 33:484–495, 2002.

87. Miettinen M, Sarlomo-Rikala M, Lasota J: Gastrointestinal stromal tumors: recent advances in understanding of their biology, *Hum Pathol* 30:1213–1220, 1999.
88. Miettinen M, Sarlomo-Rikala M, Lasota J: Gastrointestinal stromal tumours, *Ann Chir Gynaecol* 87:278–281, 1998.
89. Heinrich MC, Corless CL, Duensing A, et al: PDGFRA activating mutations in gastrointestinal stromal tumors, *Science* 299:708–710, 2003.
90. Peled N, Yoshida K, Wynes MW, et al: Predictive and prognostic markers for epidermal growth factor receptor inhibitor therapy in non-small cell lung cancer, *Ther Adv Med Oncol* 1:137–144, 2009.
91. Bang YJ: The potential for crizotinib in non-small cell lung cancer: A perspective review, *Ther Adv Med Oncol* 3:279–291, 2011.
92. Shaw AT, Yeap BY, Solomon BJ, et al: Effect of crizotinib on overall survival in patients with advanced non-small-cell lung cancer harbouring ALK gene rearrangement: a retrospective analysis, *Lancet Oncol* 12:1004–1012, 2011.
93. Chapman PB, Hauschild A, Robert C, et al: Improved survival with vemurafenib in melanoma with BRAF V600E mutation, *N Engl J Med* 364:2507–2516, 2011.
94. Markman B, Dienstmann R, Tabernero J: Targeting the PI3K/Akt/mTOR pathway–beyond rapalogs, *Oncotarget* 1:530–543, 2010.
95. Vilar E, Perez-Garcia J, Tabernero J: Pushing the envelope in the mTOR pathway: the second generation of inhibitors, *Mol Cancer Ther* 10:395–403, 2011.
96. Christian BA, Grever MR, Byrd JC, et al: Flavopiridol in the treatment of chronic lymphocytic leukemia, *Curr Opin Oncol* 19:573–578, 2007.
97. Papaetis GS, Syrigos KN: Sunitinib: a multitargeted receptor tyrosine kinase inhibitor in the era of molecular cancer therapies, *BioDrugs* 23:377–389, 2009.
98. London CA, Hannah AL, Zadovoskaya R, et al: Phase I dose-escalating study of SU11654, a small molecule receptor tyrosine kinase inhibitor, in dogs with spontaneous malignancies, *Clin Cancer Res* 9:2755–2768, 2003.
99. London CA, Malpas PB, Wood-Follis SL, et al: Multi-center, placebo-controlled, double-blind, randomized study of oral toceranib phosphate (SU11654), a receptor tyrosine kinase inhibitor, for the treatment of dogs with recurrent (either local or distant) mast cell tumor following surgical excision, *Clin Cancer Res* 15:3856–3865, 2009.
100. London C, Mathie T, Stingle N, et al: Preliminary evidence for biologic activity of toceranib phosphate (Palladia) in solid tumours, *Vet Comp Oncol* June 1, 2011. Epub ahead of print.
101. Hahn KA, Ogilvie G, Rusk T, et al: Masitinib is safe and effective for the treatment of canine mast cell tumors, *J Vet Intern Med* 22:1301–1309, 2008.
102. Hahn KA, Legendre AM, Shaw NG, et al: Evaluation of 12- and 24-month survival rates after treatment with masitinib in dogs with nonresectable mast cell tumors, *Am J Vet Res* 71:1354–1361, 2010.
103. Isotani M, Ishida N, Tominaga M, et al: Effect of tyrosine kinase inhibition by imatinib mesylate on mast cell tumors in dogs, *J Vet Intern Med* 22(4):985–988, 2008.
104. Marconato L, Bettini G, Giacoboni C, et al: Clinicopathological features and outcome for dogs with mast cell tumors and bone marrow involvement, *J Vet Intern Med* 22(4):1001–1007, 2008.
105. Yamada O, Kobayashi M, Sugisaki O, et al: Imatinib elicited a favorable response in a dog with a mast cell tumor carrying a c-kit c.1523A>T mutation via suppression of constitutive KIT activation, *Vet Immunol Immunopathol* 142:101–106, 2011.
106. Isotani M, Tamura K, Yagihara H, et al: Identification of a c-kit exon 8 internal tandem duplication in a feline mast cell tumor case and its favorable response to the tyrosine kinase inhibitor imatinib mesylate, *Vet Immunol Immunopathol* 114:168–172, 2006.
107. Isotani M, Yamada O, Lachowicz JL, et al: Mutations in the fifth immunoglobulin-like domain of kit are common and potentially sensitive to imatinib mesylate in feline mast cell tumours, *Br J Haematol* 148:144–153, 2009.

SECTION C
Antiangiogenic and Metronomic Therapy

ANTHONY J. MUTSAERS

Tumor Angiogenesis

Angiogenesis has emerged as a validated therapeutic target in oncology over the last several years, particularly with the widespread approval of drugs that target the proangiogenic vascular endothelial growth factor (VEGF) signaling pathway.[1-5] Drugs such as bevacizumab (Avastin), the humanized anti-VEGF monoclonal antibody, and small molecule RTK inhibitors (RTKIs) such as sunitinib (Sutent) and sorafenib (Nexavar) in human oncology and toceranib (Palladia) in veterinary medicine are all considered to be efficacious, at least in part, because of an antiangiogenic mechanism of action.[6,7] The guiding principle of tumor angiogenesis states that in order for a solid tumor to grow beyond a few millimeters in size, it must recruit its own blood supply to provide adequate nutrients and oxygen to the dividing cell mass, as well as the removal of waste products.[8,9] Inducing angiogenesis is considered a hallmark of cancer progression,[10] yet angiogenesis is a prominent aspect of normal physiology and transient pathology (e.g., in wound healing) and is tightly regulated. A large number of proangiogenic growth factors and signaling pathways promote the process of blood vessel growth.[8] Similarly, endogenous inhibitors of angiogenesis are temporally expressed to suppress vessel expansion and maintain angiogenic balance.[11] The net effect depends on this relative balance, which is tipped toward promoting angiogenesis during tumor growth. Therapeutic interventions aim to tip the scales back toward inhibition of tumor angiogenesis.[12]

Angiogenesis occurs through the sprouting of new vessels from existing vasculature, whereas the term *vasculogenesis* is generally used to describe the de novo formation of new blood vessels from bone marrow–derived progenitor cell populations that respond to locally produced proangiogenic signals.[13,14] In addition, although controversial, circulating endothelial progenitor cells (CEPs) from the bone marrow may contribute to tumor angiogenesis by travelling to tumor sites and incorporating into existing vessel walls.[15-18] Finally, mature endothelial cells originating from the growing vasculature itself may be shed into the bloodstream, and are referred to as circulating endothelial cells (CECs).[19] These CECs may represent a byproduct of local angiogenesis rather than an indicator of bone marrow involvement. At the present time, there is still much to learn regarding the morphology, surface marker expression, and relative contribution circulating cell populations make to tumor blood vessel growth and maintenance.[20,21]

Despite the principles of angiogenesis finding extensive application in the field of solid tumor growth, blood vessels are also a normal component of the bone marrow microenvironment, and angiogenesis is a prominent feature of malignant bone marrow disorders. Many of the same growth factor and inhibitory pathway components described in solid tumor angiogenesis contribute to the biology of myelodysplasia, leukemias, myeloma, and lymphoma, among other "liquid" tumors.[22] As a result, targeting angiogenesis is being investigated for the treatment of blood and bone marrow neoplasia and, indeed, one such agent with demonstrated antiangiogenic effects, thalidomide, has been approved for treatment of human multiple myeloma.[23]

In addition to blood vessels, lymphatics are an important component of the tumor microenvironment and a prominent feature of tissue homeostasis, immunosurveillance, and a gateway to metastatic spread.[24] The regulation of lymphatic vessel growth is physiologically similar in principle to that of blood vessels, although the contribution of cells from the bone marrow to the formation and maintenance of lymphatic channels may be equally controversial.[25] Similar to angiogenesis, targeting lymphangiogenesis is an attractive prospect in clinical oncology that is receiving an increased research focus.[26]

Antiangiogenic Therapy

There are multiple theories to explain the potential antitumor effects that result from antiangiogenic therapies.[3] The first and most intuitive is vascular collapse resulting in impaired oxygen delivery to the tumor, leading to nutrient starvation, hypoxia, and death of cancer cells that cannot survive in this oxygen-deprived environment. Conversely, a second mechanism actually involves more efficient delivery of oxygen, nutrients, and indeed other drugs (such as chemotherapeutics) to tumor cells by a process termed *vessel normalization*.[27,28] Normalization occurs when smaller, tortuous, inefficient, and leaky tumor vessels are selectively destroyed, resulting in improved blood flow through the tumor as a whole.[29] Vascular normalization has been demonstrated clinically using functional magnetic resonance imaging (fMRI) methods in patients undergoing treatment with VEGF pathway inhibitors.[30,31] The most common clinical approach to targeting tumor angiogenesis has been either inhibition of overexpressed proangiogenic stimuli or supplementation of factors that inhibit angiogenesis. Targeting vasculogenesis through neutralization of CEPs is also a potential treatment strategy.[32]

Inhibition of Proangiogenic Factors—Receptor Tyrosine Kinase Inhibitors

Currently, most RTKIs target numerous receptors to a varying degree.[7,33] Toceranib is an example of an RTKI approved for veterinary use that complements its direct effects on tumor cells (e.g., via mutated *c-kit* inhibition) with angiogenesis inhibition because it directly targets VEGF receptors (VEGFR).[34] Binding to VEGFR results in blockade of the most powerful endothelial growth and survival factor. Additionally, through inhibition of platelet-derived growth factor receptors (PDGFR), toceranib and another veterinary approved RTKI, masitinib (Masivet, Kinavet), disrupt signaling pathways for blood vessel support structures, such as the stromal pericyte component of larger vessels.[35,36] The relative antiangiogenic and direct antitumor effect of these RTKIs is made more complicated by the fact that some angiogenesis receptors such as VEGFR and PDGFR may also be concomitantly expressed by certain cancer cell types, resulting in an autocrine growth factor loop.[37,38] The end result is that in certain cases targeting angiogenic pathways may have concurrent antitumor cell and antiangiogenic effects.

Significant cross-talk exists between growth signaling pathways, and as a result there is strong interaction between tumor cell–based oncogene or tumor suppressor gene expression and regulation of blood vessel growth *via* factors such as VEGF. Therefore many drugs designed to target oncogenes have demonstrated antiangiogenic "off-target" effects as a byproduct of VEGF inhibition.[39-41] For example, the anti-HER2 *(ErbB-2)* human MAb trastuzumab (Herceptin) and anti-EGFR antibodies such as cetuximab (Erbitux) are examples of drugs that indirectly suppress angiogenesis because neutralization of their oncogenic targets leads to a dramatic reduction in tumor cell VEGF production, which increases again at the time of targeted drug resistance.[42,43] Through reduction in VEGF or other growth factor levels, there is an antiangiogenic component inherent in many forms of cancer treatment, including not only targeted inhibitors but also cytotoxic chemotherapy and radiation therapy. As a result, antiangiogenic mechanisms are not necessarily restricted to treatment modalities that target known angiogenesis pathways directly.

Angiogenic Inhibitor Supplementation

Since the discovery of endogenous proteins and protein fragments that inhibit blood vessel growth such as angiostatin, endostatin, and thrombospondins, there has been clinical interest in using angiogenesis inhibitors as cancer therapeutics.[11,44] In veterinary medicine, thrombospondin-1 mimetic peptides have been evaluated as an antiangiogenic strategy in dogs with multiple tumor types. Treatment with the mimetic peptides ABT-526 and ABT-510 in a prospective clinical trial of 242 dogs with multiple tumor types showed an objective response or substantially stabilized disease in 42 dogs and a lack of dose-limiting toxicity.[45] Interestingly, most objective responses were recorded after 60 days of continuous drug treatment. A prospective randomized placebo-controlled clinical trial has also been reported in dogs with multicentric lymphoma treated at first relapse.[46] Results revealed a significant improvement in time to tumor progression and remission duration, but not remission rate, when ABT-526 was used in combination with lomustine, compared to dogs treated with lomustine alone, with no ABT-526–specific toxicities noted. In addition to thrombospondin-1, preliminary studies documenting detection of the endogenous inhibitors angiostatin and endostatin in normal and tumor-bearing dogs have been reported.[47,48] In a preliminary study of endostatin as a therapeutic agent, 13 dogs with soft tissue sarcomas were treated with the canine endostatin gene delivered via liposome-DNA complexes.[49] Although endostatin gene expression was not detected in the tumors following treatment, objective responses were documented in 2 dogs, and 8 dogs experienced stable disease, suggesting potential nonspecific antitumor activity.

Direct Targeting of Tumor Endothelial Cell Surface Markers

Tumor endothelial cells differ from normal endothelia in their genetic and protein composition.[50] These differences may represent an opportunity for a favorable therapeutic index when drugs are designed to bind differentially expressed targets on tumor-specific endothelium. If not naturally destructive to these cells, drugs can be designed to carry a payload to induce local cytotoxicity, resulting in an antiangiogenic effect. A phage vector delivering tumor necrosis factor (RGD-A-TNF) to αV integrins on tumor endothelium is one example of such a strategy that has undergone evaluation in dogs.[51] Through serial biopsy, this dose escalation trial was able to demonstrate selective targeting of tumor endothelium via αV integrin-targeted expression of TNF, and treatment of a cohort of tumor-bearing dogs with the maximum tolerated dose (MTD) resulting in partial remission in 2/14 and stable disease in 6/14 dogs.

Other Antiangiogenic Agents

A vast array of drugs not necessarily designed as anticancer therapeutics may derive at least a portion of their activity through inhibition of angiogenesis. Two examples investigated in a veterinary setting include inhibitors of matrix metalloproteinase (MMP) and cyclooxygenase (COX). The MMPs are a family of enzymes that degrade the extracellular matrix and basement membrane, thereby mediating tumor invasion, angiogenesis, and metastasis.[52] Unfortunately, clinical evaluation of compounds that inhibit these enzymes has to date been largely unrewarding,[53,54] including results from a large randomized trial of 303 dogs with OSA, in which treatment with the MMP inhibitor Bay12-9566 or placebo after doxorubicin chemotherapy did not improve overall survival.[55] Inhibition of the proinflammatory COX enzymes has been commonly studied in numerous tumor types in veterinary oncology.[56-58] The effects of COX inhibition on reducing angiogenesis specifically have been evaluated with piroxicam treatment of canine transitional cell carcinoma (TCC). In a study of 18 dogs, piroxicam treatment was associated with reduced urinary concentrations of the proangiogenic growth factor basic fibroblast growth factor (bFGF) and induction of apoptosis.[59] In a subsequent study evaluating these parameters in 12 dogs treated with piroxicam in combination with cisplatin, reductions in urinary bFGF and VEGF were associated with response to the combination regimen.[60]

Metronomic Chemotherapy

Conventional cytotoxic chemotherapy agents that have been in clinical use for many decades also achieve at least a portion of their therapeutic efficacy by inhibition of tumor angiogenesis.[61,62] The basis for this notion likely originated with the observation that tumor endothelial cell populations are much more proliferative than the quiescent endothelium found elsewhere in the body. These rapidly dividing endothelial cells would be targets of chemotherapy in the same way that other proliferative cells such as intestinal epithelia and bone marrow precursors are damaged. The key to maximizing the antiangiogenic potential of chemotherapeutic drugs was considered to be through reduction or elimination of the break period between doses. It is during this break period that repair and repopulation of endothelial cells were likely to occur, as they do for other cell populations.[61] However, conventional chemotherapeutic protocols are largely based on the principle of MTD, which originated through models of optimized tumor cell kill that require a break period to allow recovery of normal cell populations.[63,64] Despite the success of MTD chemotherapy protocols for the treatment and outright cure of certain cancers, critics of such models point out that the preclinical experiments were performed in exponential growth phase cell culture models, and the exposure time of the cells to chemotherapy was not an included variable.[65] More continuous exposure to chemotherapy, with reduction or elimination of the break period between each dose, has come to be known as "metronomic" delivery.[66] Not surprisingly, dose reduction is required to provide a more continuous treatment schedule. Generally speaking, metronomic chemotherapy protocols are well tolerated. The low toxicity profile, combined with ease of administration when oral drugs are used, and often lower cost make metronomic chemotherapy protocols appealing in veterinary oncology. However, mechanistic and clinical evaluation in veterinary patients is still at an early stage.

Mechanisms of Treatment

When different types of dividing cells in culture are exposed to continuous ultra-low doses of chemotherapy, endothelial cell populations display an exquisite sensitivity compared to other cell types, including tumor cells in many instances.[67,68] Although the reasons for this selectivity are not entirely clear, the explanation likely goes beyond mere targeting of rapidly dividing cells. Experimental evidence has suggested that upregulation of the endogenous angiogenesis inhibitor thrombospondin-1 occurs during treatment with metronomic cyclophosphamide and possibly other agents.[69,70] The resulting angiogenic suppression is likely reinforced by a decrease in tumor cell production of proangiogenic growth factors such as VEGF. Decreased VEGF production may be accomplished through reduced tumor cell mass as a result of direct cancer cell killing by chemotherapy. This explains why the antiangiogenic actions of metronomic chemotherapy may be enhanced when there is concomitant tumor cell kill; however, in theory, antiangiogenic targeting of chemotherapy drugs does not require drug sensitivity from the tumor cell population. Targeting the genetically stable endothelial component of the tumor microenvironment instead of the genetically unstable tumor cell population was promoted early on as a potential advantage of antiangiogenic treatment strategies.[71]

Other components of the tumor microenvironment may also be targeted by metronomic delivery of certain cytotoxic chemotherapy drugs. As mentioned earlier, tumor angiogenesis may involve recruitment of CEPs.[17] These cells, if they play a significant role in the growth of tumor blood vessels, may be most influential after the acute damage that would occur in the early break period of MTD chemotherapy schedules.[72] Preclinical models have demonstrated that CEPs acutely decrease with MTD treatment, only to rapidly rebound during the break period, when they may contribute to endothelial cell repopulation.[73] In contrast, metronomic chemotherapy delivery does not appear to be associated with this CEP surge, leading instead to a sustained antiangiogenic effect.[73-75]

Other cells also compose a significant component of the tumor microenvironment. Immune effector cells such as lymphocytes and macrophages influence tumor biology and may be affected by chemotherapy treatment. As such, the potential immunomodulatory antitumor mechanisms of metronomic chemotherapy, particularly with the alkylating agent cyclophosphamide, are receiving significant investigation. Low doses of cyclophosphamide influence the T-lymphocyte subset population by decreasing levels of CD4+CD25+ regulatory T-cells.[76] Regulatory T-cells (Tregs) inhibit the immune response, thereby suppressing tumor immunosurveillance. In dogs with various malignancies, regulatory T-cells have been quantified by flow cytometry[77,78] and have been shown to decrease in blood samples taken from dogs with soft tissue sarcoma treated with low-dose cyclophosphamide chemotherapy.[79] Further effects of metronomic cyclophosphamide on tumor immunology remain to be determined, and the nature of potential immunomodulatory mechanisms for other chemotherapeutics delivered metronomically is currently largely unexplored.

Clinical Trial Evaluation

Recent small retrospective and phase II clinical trials have been reported in human and veterinary oncology with a variety of chemotherapy drugs and combinations.[80-86] Most clinical trial evaluations to date have paired conventional chemotherapy drugs with noncytotoxic drugs that target angiogenesis directly or indirectly. Preclinical results demonstrated over a decade ago that such combinations resulted in superior outcomes, likely due to more robust neutralization of the prosurvival functions of VEGF in the tumor endothelium.[87,88] As a result, most clinical trials have evaluated combination approaches without necessarily any clear prior documentation of single-agent clinical activity for each drug. Bevacizumab has been a popular choice to pair with human metronomic chemotherapy schedules and is FDA-approved for multiple indications.[83,89-92] Other, more readily available "targeted" drugs, shown

Table 14-3 Reported Veterinary Metronomic Chemotherapy Protocols with Alkylating Agents

Tumor	Chemotherapy Drug	Dose	Other Drugs	Setting
Hemangiosarcoma[100]	Cyclophosphamide	12.5-25 mg/m^2 daily for 3 weeks, alternating with etoposide	Etoposide 50 mg/m^2 daily for 3 weeks Piroxicam daily 0.3 mg/kg	Adjuvant
Soft tissue sarcoma[101]	Cyclophosphamide	10 mg/m^2 daily or every other day	Piroxicam daily 0.3 mg/kg	Adjuvant
Soft tissue sarcoma[78]	Cyclophosphamide	12.5 mg/m^2 or 15 mg/m^2 daily	None	Gross disease
Multiple tumor types[102]	Cyclophosphamide	25 mg/m^2 daily	Celecoxib daily 2 mg/kg	First-line metastatic
Multiple tumor types[103]	Chlorambucil	4 mg/m^2 daily	None	Any
Multiple tumor types[104]	Lomustine	2.84 mg/m^2 daily	None	Any

to have at least indirect antiangiogenic effects, are also commonly utilized. Examples include COX inhibitors,[81,93-97] tetracyclines, thalidomide,[23,98] and others.[99] Generally speaking, in contrast to MTD chemotherapy protocols, targeted drugs are often given for longer periods of time at their optimal biologic dose (OBD). As a result, targeted drug combinations with metronomic chemotherapy may be an effective treatment strategy, as each follows a similar dose and scheduling principle. In addition, it is possible that there may be a role for targeted antiangiogenic treatment or metronomic chemotherapy in combination with MTD chemotherapy schedules to neutralize rebound angiogenic responses that occur during the break period. This approach has been demonstrated successfully in preclinical studies.[72,100] Ultimately, rigorous clinical trials are necessary to identify and optimize successful drug combinations and schedules of antiangiogenic drugs and chemotherapy.

Veterinary Trials with Cyclophosphamide

Cyclophosphamide has been the most common drug by far to be studied in low-dose metronomic treatment protocols in both human and veterinary oncology. At this time, metronomic chemotherapy protocols have only been evaluated in small retrospective studies and phase I and II veterinary clinical trials (Table 14-3).[78,100-104] A protocol of low-dose cyclophosphamide (12.5 to 25 mg/m^2 orally daily) alternating with etoposide (50 mg/m^2 orally daily) and paired with continuous piroxicam treatment has been evaluated for adjuvant treatment of splenic HSA in dogs.[105] The survival time of 9 dogs treated with this regimen was not different from a historic control group of 24 dogs treated with doxorubicin alone. The metronomic protocol was well tolerated over a 6-month period. Pharmacokinetic analysis of etoposide in 3 dogs revealed detectable drug levels. Another report of etoposide administration in dogs demonstrated a low and variable oral bioavailability with this drug.[101]

Low-dose continuous cyclophosphamide and piroxicam were also studied for the adjuvant treatment of canine incompletely resected soft tissue sarcoma.[102] Unlike the HSA study, in this trial the dose of cyclophosphamide was 10 mg/m^2 daily or every other day. The disease-free interval was significantly prolonged in the treated group of 30 dogs compared to an age, site, and grade-matched contemporary control group of 55 dogs treated with surgery alone. Again, the protocol was well tolerated, although 40% of dogs experienced mild toxicity at some point of the treatment, and 1 dog experienced grade 4 sterile hemorrhagic cystitis. The every-other-day dosing regimen was better tolerated than daily cyclophosphamide dosing.

Metronomic cyclophosphamide treatment was also recently reported for first-line therapy of metastatic canine tumors of varying histologies.[106] Fifteen dogs were treated with daily oral cyclophosphamide at 25 mg/m^2 combined with the COX-2 inhibitor celecoxib at 2 mg/kg. One dog had a complete response, and five dogs had stable disease with a treatment protocol that was devoid of toxicity. All dogs were reported to have improved quality of life scores. Most of the tumors treated were carcinomas, and as with many other trials it is not apparent what the relative contribution of each drug may have been to the overall response rate, as single-agent responses to COX inhibitors have been documented in cancer-bearing dogs.[58] Interestingly, the authors measured circulating VEGF and IL-6 and observed that pretreatment plasma VEGF levels were significantly lower in responders than nonresponders,[106] as has been observed in other clinical trials of metronomic cyclophosphamide.[103]

Other Alkylating Agents

Chlorambucil has been used in many veterinary treatment protocols, such as first-line treatment of canine chronic lymphocytic leukemia (CLL), low-grade lymphoma, MCTs, and as a cyclophosphamide replacement for cases that develop sterile hemorrhagic cystitis.[107] A recent prospective clinical trial of daily single-agent metronomic chlorambucil therapy at a dose of 4 mg/m^2 in 36 dogs with tumors of varying histologies and prior therapies revealed a complete response over 35 weeks duration in 3 dogs, a partial response in 1 dog, and stable disease in 17 dogs.[104] The median progression-free interval was 61 days, and there were no grade 3 or 4 toxicities noted.

Lomustine (CCNU) has also been evaluated in a metronomic protocol at a dose of 2.84 mg/m^2 by mouth, which corresponds to the conversion of a 60 mg/m^2 every 3 week dose into a daily schedule.[108] A total of 81 dogs with various primary and metastatic tumors were treated with this single-agent regimen for a median of 98 days. Twenty-two dogs had treatment discontinued for adverse events of gastrointestinal, bone marrow, hepatic, or renal origin, although the authors concluded that the treatment was generally well tolerated.

Platinum Compounds

While not designed to be administered in a metronomic fashion per se, the various slow-release and oral formulations of platinum compounds that have been evaluated in veterinary oncology may represent metronomic application of these drugs. Slow-release cisplatin using delivery systems such as the open-cell polylactic acid polymer impregnated with drug (OPLA-Pt) has been studied in a variety of scenarios, including treatment of canine OSA, soft tissue sarcoma, and nasal tumors with desirable efficacy and manageable toxicity.[109-111] A dose escalation and pharmacokinetic study of satraplatin, the first orally bioavailable platinum agent, has recently been reported.[112] The aim of this study was to determine the MTD; however, the fact that this drug is administered orally makes possible the future investigation of satraplatin in a metronomic-dosing schedule. These studies with platinum compounds raise the general question of whether forms of slow-release chemotherapeutic delivery such as liposome encapsulation represent a form of metronomic drug delivery.

Biomarkers for Antiangiogenic and Metronomic Therapy

The identification and application of biomarkers is becoming increasingly important as the field of oncology moves further into clinical application of targeted therapeutics.[113] The aims of validated biomarkers are to (1) predict patient populations that will or will not respond to treatment, (2) monitor response to therapy on a cellular or molecular level, or (3) determine the proper therapeutic dose for targeted agents that often possess optimal biologic activity at doses well below the traditionally defined MTD. The use of biomarkers for antiangiogenic agents is valid in all three categories.

Tumor tissue expression and/or blood-based circulating growth factor levels have been the most popular approaches to predicting response to angiogenesis inhibitors, with VEGF being the most studied molecule.[114-116] For example, in the study of metronomic cyclophosphamide and celecoxib by Marchetti and colleagues, low baseline plasma VEGF was predictive of response.[106] In many cases it may be through comparison of pretreatment to posttreatment levels that insight will be gained from this surrogate marker, as was demonstrated with urinary bFGF and VEGF with piroxicam treatment of canine TCC.[59,60] The most important biomarker in angiogenesis may be one that defines tumor response because inhibition of angiogenesis does not necessarily correspond to a reduction in tumor volume. This static response sits in sharp contrast to MTD chemotherapy approaches that result in measureable tumor shrinkage. Systems for clinical evaluation of tumor response to therapy are often formally based on World Health Organization (WHO) criteria or response evaluation criteria in solid tumors (RECIST), which equate tumor shrinkage with positive outcome. Therefore there may be a need for both recognition of sustained stable disease as a desirable clinical trial endpoint and biomarkers to evaluate angiogenic function during treatment. Imaging modalities that can provide information about vascular function are a potentially valuable tool for monitoring tumor angiogenesis and the effects of antiangiogenic therapy.[114] Dynamic contrast-enhanced MRI (DCE-MRI) has been studied for its ability to quantitatively assess vascular parameters.[117] A study by MacLeod and colleagues demonstrated blood volume and permeability measurements in canine intracranial masses using this modality.[118]

The area of dose optimization also represents an unmet need for biomarkers in antiangiogenic and metronomic chemotherapy. Tregs are providing insight in this regard. Recent results from Burton and coworkers demonstrated a dose-dependent reduction in Tregs with metronomic cyclophosphamide treatment, observed at 15 mg/m^2 but not 12.5 mg/m^2 doses, leading the investigators to conclude that 15 mg/m^2 may be a more appropriate dose for future clinical trials.[79] In addition to Treg levels, temporal evaluation of other markers has been studied. Assessment of CECs and/or CEPs has been applied for biomarker analysis of dosing antiangiogenic and metronomic therapy.[75,97,119] For example, in the study by Rusk and colleagues, decreasing CEC levels in dogs treated with the thrombospondin-1 mimetic peptide ABT-526 may have indicated adequate exposure to the antiangiogenic drug, which in this study was utilized at a single dose.[45]

Side Effects (Adverse Events)

Despite the therapeutic index achieved by treating activated versus dormant vasculature, there is still potential risk that drug effects on vessels have unwanted consequences. For bevacizumab, potential side effects of a vascular etiology include hypertension, edema, hemorrhage, thromboembolism, proteinuria, intestinal perforation, and impaired wound healing.[120] Through further clinical evaluation, we will learn the relative risks for different antiangiogenic drugs applied to a number of tumor settings. Resistance to antiangiogenic therapy has also become evident from early clinical data. Given the genetically stable nature of the blood vessel/endothelial cell target compared to the mutationally prone cancer cell population, antiangiogenic treatment was originally postulated to be less likely to demonstrate drug resistance.[71] Proposed mechanisms of resistance to antiangiogenic therapies involve both tumor and host-mediated pathways that can be intrinsic or induced by treatment.[121] One alarming consequence of antiangiogenic treatment that has emerged from recent preclinical studies is the potential that certain drugs may alter the host microenvironment, leading to metastatic conditioning.[122,123] This phenomenon of increased invasion and metastasis as a result of antiangiogenic drug treatment, despite successful suppression of primary tumor growth, has been demonstrated in preclinical models with certain antiangiogenic RTKIs. The drugs studied include sunitinib, an RTKI with a similar target spectrum to toceranib.[123] Further validation and investigation into potential explanations for these provocative results are ongoing.

Finally, it is worth noting that similar to most other drugs, antiangiogenic agents are not innocuous and may have a unique side-effect profile that is independent of their effects on blood vessels or the tumor microenvironment. Side effects for toceranib include dose-dependent gastrointestinal upset, including bleeding, myelosuppression, azotemia, anemia, lethargy, or lameness.[124-126] Masitinib's side effects include gastrointestinal upset, regenerative or nonregenerative anemia, and protein-losing nephropathy.[35,124] Cyclophosphamide has become a popular drug for metronomic scheduling but is associated with the potential for sterile hemorrhagic cystitis.[127] It is currently unknown whether cystitis is more frequent in metronomic protocols; however, close urinary monitoring is strongly recommended for these patients. Similarly, chlorambucil has been clinically evaluated for metronomic use[104] and can be used as an alternative to cyclophosphamide, although it is still not known whether drug efficacy will be similar for different drugs applied across multiple tumor types.

REFERENCES

1. Potente M, Gerhardt H, Carmeliet P: Basic and therapeutic aspects of angiogenesis, *Cell* 146:873–887, 2011.
2. Kerbel RS: Tumor angiogenesis, *N Engl J Med* 358:2039–2049, 2008.
3. Kerbel RS: Antiangiogenic therapy: A universal chemosensitization strategy for cancer? *Science* 312:1171–1175, 2006.
4. Khosravi SP, Fernandez PI: Tumoral angiogenesis: review of the literature, *Cancer Invest* 26:104–108, 2008.
5. Carmeliet P, Jain RK: Molecular mechanisms and clinical applications of angiogenesis, *Nature* 473:298–307, 2011.
6. Motzer RJ, Hoosen S, Bello CL, et al: Sunitinib malate for the treatment of solid tumours: a review of current clinical data, *Expert Opin Investig Drugs* 15:553–561, 2006.

7. Ivy SP, Wick JY, Kaufman BM: An overview of small-molecule inhibitors of VEGFR signaling, *Nat Rev Clin Oncol* 6:569–579, 2009.
8. Folkman J: Angiogenesis in cancer, vascular, rheumatoid and other disease, *Nat Med* 1:27–31, 1995.
9. Folkman J: Tumor angiogenesis: therapeutic implications, *N Engl J Med* 285:1182–1186, 1971.
10. Hanahan D, Weinberg RA: Hallmarks of cancer: the next generation, *Cell* 144:646–674, 2011.
11. Folkman J: Endogenous angiogenesis inhibitors, *APMIS* 112:496–507, 2004.
12. Ferrara N, Kerbel RS: Angiogenesis as a therapeutic target, *Nature* 438:967–974, 2005.
13. Patel-Hett S, D'Amore PA: Signal transduction in vasculogenesis and developmental angiogenesis, *Int J Dev Biol* 55:353–363, 2011.
14. Stewart KS, Kleinerman ES: Tumor Vessel Development and Expansion in Ewing's Sarcoma: A Review of the Vasculogenesis Process and Clinical Trials with Vascular-Targeting Agents, *Sarcoma* 2011:165837, 2011.
15. Asahara T, Murohara T, Sullivan A, et al: Isolation of putative progenitor endothelial cells for angiogenesis, *Science* 275:964–967, 1997.
16. Purhonen S, Palm J, Rossi D, et al: Bone marrow-derived circulating endothelial precursors do not contribute to vascular endothelium and are not needed for tumor growth, *Proc Natl Acad Sci U S A* 105:6620–6625, 2008.
17. Shaked Y, Ciarrocchi A, Franco M, et al: Therapy-induced acute recruitment of circulating endothelial progenitor cells to tumors, *Science* 313:1785–1787, 2006.
18. Kerbel RS, Benezra R, Lyden DC, et al: Endothelial progenitor cells are cellular hubs essential for neoangiogenesis of certain aggressive adenocarcinomas and metastatic transition but not adenomas, *Proc Natl Acad Sci USA* 105:E54, 2008.
19. Bertolini F, Mancuso P, Braidotti P, et al: The multiple personality disorder phenotype(s) of circulating endothelial cells in cancer, *Biochim Biophys Acta* 1796:27–32, 2009.
20. Bertolini F, Shaked Y, Mancuso P, et al: The multifaceted circulating endothelial cell in cancer: towards marker and target identification, *Nat Rev Cancer* 6:835–845, 2006.
21. Yoder MC, Ingram DA: Endothelial progenitor cell: Ongoing controversy for defining these cells and their role in neoangiogenesis in the murine system, *Curr Opin Hematol* 16:269–273, 2009.
22. Vacca A, Ribatti D: Angiogenesis and vasculogenesis in multiple myeloma: role of inflammatory cells, *Recent Results Cancer Res* 183:87–95, 2011.
23. Suvannasankha A, Fausel C, Juliar BE, et al: Final report of toxicity and efficacy of a phase II study of oral cyclophosphamide, thalidomide, and prednisone for patients with relapsed or refractory multiple myeloma: A Hoosier Oncology Group Trial, HEM01-21, *Oncologist* 12:99–106, 2007.
24. Tammela T, Alitalo K: Lymphangiogenesis: Molecular mechanisms and future promise, *Cell* 140:460–476, 2010.
25. Adams RH, Alitalo K: Molecular regulation of angiogenesis and lymphangiogenesis, *Nat Rev Mol Cell Biol* 8:464–478, 2007.
26. Holopainen T, Bry M, Alitalo K, et al: Perspectives on lymphangiogenesis and angiogenesis in cancer, *J Surg Oncol* 103:484–488, 2011.
27. Jain RK: Normalization of tumor vasculature: An emerging concept in antiangiogenic therapy, *Science* 307:58–62, 2005.
28. Carmeliet P, Jain RK: Principles and mechanisms of vessel normalization for cancer and other angiogenic diseases, *Nat Rev Drug Discov* 10:417–427, 2011.
29. Goel S, Duda DG, Xu L, et al: Normalization of the vasculature for treatment of cancer and other diseases, *Physiol Rev* 91:1071–1121, 2011.
30. Sorensen AG, Emblem KE, Polaskova P, et al: Increased survival of glioblastoma patients who respond to antiangiogenic therapy with elevated blood perfusion, *Cancer Res* 72(2):402–407, 2012.
31. Batchelor TT, Sorensen AG, di TE, et al: AZD2171, a pan-VEGF receptor tyrosine kinase inhibitor, normalizes tumor vasculature and alleviates edema in glioblastoma patients, *Cancer Cell* 11:83–95, 2007.
32. Shaked Y, Henke E, Roodhart JM, et al: Rapid chemotherapy-induced acute endothelial progenitor cell mobilization: implications for antiangiogenic drugs as chemosensitizing agents, *Cancer Cell* 14:263–273, 2008.
33. Fabian MA, Biggs WH, III, Treiber DK, et al: A small molecule-kinase interaction map for clinical kinase inhibitors, *Nat Biotechnol* 23:329–336, 2005.
34. London CA, Malpas PB, Wood-Follis SL, et al: Multi-center, placebo-controlled, double-blind, randomized study of oral toceranib phosphate (SU11654), a receptor tyrosine kinase inhibitor, for the treatment of dogs with recurrent (either local or distant) mast cell tumor following surgical excision, *Clin Cancer Res* 15:3856–3865, 2009.
35. Hahn KA, Ogilvie G, Rusk T, Devauchelle P, Leblanc A, Legendre A, et al: Masitinib is safe and effective for the treatment of canine mast cell tumors, *J Vet Intern Med* 22:1301–1309, 2008.
36. Pietras K, Hanahan D: A multitargeted, metronomic, and maximum-tolerated dose "chemo-switch" regimen is antiangiogenic, producing objective responses and survival benefit in a mouse model of cancer, *J Clin Oncol* 23:939–952, 2005.
37. Mentlein R, Forstreuter F, Mehdorn HM, et al: Functional significance of vascular endothelial growth factor receptor expression on human glioma cells, *J Neurooncol* 67:9–18, 2004.
38. Jackson MW, Roberts JS, Heckford SE, et al: A potential autocrine role for vascular endothelial growth factor in prostate cancer, *Cancer Res* 62:854–859, 2002.
39. Kerbel RS, Viloria-Petit A, Klement G, et al: "'Accidental" anti-angiogenic drugs: anti-oncogene directed signal transduction inhibitors and conventional chemotherapeutic agents as examples, *Eur J Cancer* 36:1248–1257, 2000.
40. Lopez-Ocejo O, Viloria-Petit A, Bequet-Romero M, et al: Oncogenes and tumor angiogenesis: the HPV-16 E6 oncoprotein activates the vascular endothelial growth factor (VEGF) gene promoter in a p53 independent manner, *Oncogene* 19:4611–4620, 2000.
41. Ebos JM, Tran J, Master Z, et al: Imatinib mesylate (STI-571) reduces Bcr-Abl-mediated vascular endothelial growth factor secretion in chronic myelogenous leukemia, *Mol Cancer Res* 1:89–95, 2002.
42. du Manoir JM, Francia G, Man S, et al: Strategies for delaying or treating in vivo acquired resistance to trastuzumab in human breast cancer xenografts, *Clin Cancer Res* 12:904–916, 2006.
43. Viloria-Petit A, Crombet T, Jothy S, et al: Acquired resistance to the antitumor effect of epidermal growth factor receptor-blocking antibodies in vivo: a role for altered tumor angiogenesis, *Cancer Res* 61:5090–5101, 2001.
44. O'Reilly MS, Boehm T, Shing Y, et al: Endostatin: an endogenous inhibitor of angiogenesis and tumor growth, *Cell* 88:277–285, 1997.
45. Rusk A, McKeegan E, Haviv F, et al: Preclinical evaluation of antiangiogenic thrombospondin-1 peptide mimetics, ABT-526 and ABT-510, in companion dogs with naturally occurring cancers, *Clin Cancer Res* 12:7444–7455, 2006.
46. Rusk A, Cozzi E, Stebbins M, et al: Cooperative activity of cytotoxic chemotherapy with antiangiogenic thrombospondin-I peptides, ABT-526 in pet dogs with relapsed lymphoma, *Clin Cancer Res* 12:7456–7464, 2006.
47. Pirie-Shepherd SR, Coffman KT, Resnick D, et al: The role of angiostatin in the spontaneous bone and prostate cancers of pet dogs, *Biochem Biophys Res Commun* 292:886–891, 2002.
48. Troy GC, Huckle WR, Rossmeisl JH, et al: Endostatin and vascular endothelial growth factor concentrations in healthy dogs, dogs with selected neoplasia, and dogs with nonneoplastic diseases, *J Vet Intern Med* 20:144–150, 2006.
49. Kamstock D, Guth A, Elmslie R, et al: Liposome-DNA complexes infused intravenously inhibit tumor angiogenesis and elicit

antitumor activity in dogs with soft tissue sarcoma, *Cancer Gene Ther* 13:306–317, 2006.
50. St CB, Rago C, Velculescu V, Traverso G, Romans KE, Montgomery E, et al: Genes expressed in human tumor endothelium, *Science* 289:1197–1202, 2000.
51. Paoloni MC, Tandle A, Mazcko C, et al: Launching a novel preclinical infrastructure: comparative oncology trials consortium directed therapeutic targeting of TNFalpha to cancer vasculature, *PLoS One* 4:e4972, 2009.
52. Hua H, Li M, Luo T, et al: Matrix metalloproteinases in tumorigenesis: an evolving paradigm, *Cell Mol Life Sci* 68:3853–3868, 2011.
53. Hirte H, Vergote IB, Jeffrey JR, et al: A phase III randomized trial of BAY 12-9566 (tanomastat) as maintenance therapy in patients with advanced ovarian cancer responsive to primary surgery and paclitaxel/platinum containing chemotherapy: A National Cancer Institute of Canada Clinical Trials Group Study, *Gynecol Oncol* 102:300–308, 2006.
54. Moore MJ, Hamm J, Dancey J, et al: Comparison of gemcitabine versus the matrix metalloproteinase inhibitor BAY 12-9566 in patients with advanced or metastatic adenocarcinoma of the pancreas: a phase III trial of the National Cancer Institute of Canada Clinical Trials Group, *J Clin Oncol* 21:3296–3302, 2003.
55. Moore AS, Dernell WS, Ogilvie GK, et al: Doxorubicin and BAY 12-9566 for the treatment of osteosarcoma in dogs: a randomized, double-blind, placebo-controlled study, *J Vet Intern Med* 21:783–790, 2007.
56. Mohammed SI, Khan KN, Sellers RS, et al: Expression of cyclooxygenase-1 and 2 in naturally-occurring canine cancer, *Prostaglandins Leukot Essent Fatty Acids* 70:479–483, 2004.
57. Knapp DW, Richardson RC, Chan TC, et al: Piroxicam therapy in 34 dogs with transitional cell carcinoma of the urinary bladder, *J Vet Intern Med* 8:273–278, 1994.
58. Knapp DW, Richardson RC, Bottoms GD, et al: Phase I trial of piroxicam in 62 dogs bearing naturally occurring tumors, *Cancer Chemother Pharmacol* 29:214–218, 1992.
59. Mohammed SI, Bennett PF, Craig BA, et al: Effects of the cyclooxygenase inhibitor, piroxicam, on tumor response, apoptosis, and angiogenesis in a canine model of human invasive urinary bladder cancer, *Cancer Res* 62:356–358, 2002.
60. Mohammed SI, Craig BA, Mutsaers AJ, et al: Effects of the cyclooxygenase inhibitor, piroxicam, in combination with chemotherapy on tumor response, apoptosis, and angiogenesis in a canine model of human invasive urinary bladder cancer, *Mol Cancer Ther* 2:183–188, 2003.
61. Kerbel RS, Kamen BA: The anti-angiogenic basis of metronomic chemotherapy, *Nat Rev Cancer* 4:423–436, 2004.
62. Pasquier E, Kavallaris M, Andre N: Metronomic chemotherapy: new rationale for new directions, *Nat Rev Clin Oncol* 7:455–465, 2010.
63. Skipper HE, Schabel FM Jr, Mellett LB, et al: Implications of biochemical, cytokinetic, pharmacologic, and toxicologic relationships in the design of optimal therapeutic schedules, *Cancer Chemother Rep* 54:431–450, 1970.
64. Skipper HE, Perry S: Kinetics of normal and leukemic leukocyte populations and relevance to chemotherapy, *Cancer Res* 30:1883–1897, 1970.
65. Kamen BA, Glod J, Cole PD: Metronomic therapy from a pharmacologist's view, *J Pediatr Hematol Oncol* 28:325–327, 2006.
66. Hanahan D, Bergers G, Bergsland E: Less is more, regularly: metronomic dosing of cytotoxic drugs can target tumor angiogenesis in mice, *J Clin Invest* 105:1045–1047, 2000.
67. Drevs J, Fakler J, Eisele S, et al: Antiangiogenic potency of various chemotherapeutic drugs for metronomic chemotherapy, *Anticancer Res* 24:1759–1763, 2004.
68. Bocci G, Nicolaou KC, Kerbel RS: Protracted low-dose effects on human endothelial cell proliferation and survival in vitro reveal a selective antiangiogenic window for various chemotherapeutic drugs, *Cancer Res* 62:6938–6943, 2002.
69. Bocci G, Francia G, Man S, et al: Thrombospondin 1, a mediator of the antiangiogenic effects of low-dose metronomic chemotherapy, *Proc Natl Acad Sci U S A* 100:12917–12922, 2003.
70. Hamano Y, Sugimoto H, Soubasakos MA, et al: Thrombospondin-1 associated with tumor microenvironment contributes to low-dose cyclophosphamide-mediated endothelial cell apoptosis and tumor growth suppression, *Cancer Res* 64:1570–1574, 2004.
71. Kerbel RS: A cancer therapy resistant to resistance, *Nature* 390:335–336, 1997.
72. Shaked Y, Kerbel RS: Antiangiogenic strategies on defense: on the possibility of blocking rebounds by the tumor vasculature after chemotherapy, *Cancer Res* 67:7055–7058, 2007.
73. Bertolini F, Paul S, Mancuso P, et al: Maximum tolerable dose and low-dose metronomic chemotherapy have opposite effects on the mobilization and viability of circulating endothelial progenitor cells, *Cancer Res* 63:4342–4346, 2003.
74. Daenen LG, Shaked Y, Man S, et al: Low-dose metronomic cyclophosphamide combined with vascular disrupting therapy induces potent antitumor activity in preclinical human tumor xenograft models, *Mol Cancer Ther* 8:2872–2881, 2009.
75. Shaked Y, Emmenegger U, Man S, et al: Optimal biologic dose of metronomic chemotherapy regimens is associated with maximum antiangiogenic activity, *Blood* 106:3058–3061, 2005.
76. Ghiringhelli F, Menard C, Puig PE, et al: Metronomic cyclophosphamide regimen selectively depletes CD4+CD25+ regulatory T cells and restores T and NK effector functions in end stage cancer patients, *Cancer Immunol Immunother* 56:641–648, 2007.
77. Biller BJ, Elmslie RE, Burnett RC, et al: Use of FoxP3 expression to identify regulatory T cells in healthy dogs and dogs with cancer, *Vet Immunol Immunopathol* 116:69–78, 2007.
78. O'Neill K, Guth A, Biller B, et al: Changes in regulatory T cells in dogs with cancer and associations with tumor type, *J Vet Intern Med* 23:875–881, 2009.
79. Burton JH, Mitchell L, Thamm DH, et al: Low-dose cyclophosphamide selectively decreases regulatory T cells and inhibits angiogenesis in dogs with soft tissue sarcoma, *J Vet Intern Med* 25:920–926, 2011.
80. Sanborn SL, Cooney MM, Dowlati A, et al: Phase I trial of docetaxel and thalidomide: a regimen based on metronomic therapeutic principles, *Invest New Drugs* 26:355–362, 2008.
81. Bhatt RS, Merchan J, Parker R, et al: A phase 2 pilot trial of low-dose, continuous infusion, or "metronomic" paclitaxel and oral celecoxib in patients with metastatic melanoma, *Cancer* 116:1751–1756, 2010.
82. Wong NS, Buckman RA, Clemons M, et al: Phase I/II trial of metronomic chemotherapy with daily dalteparin and cyclophosphamide, twice-weekly methotrexate, and daily prednisone as therapy for metastatic breast cancer using vascular endothelial growth factor and soluble vascular endothelial growth factor receptor levels as markers of response, *J Clin Oncol* 28:723–730, 2010.
83. Garcia AA, Hirte H, Fleming G, et al: Phase II clinical trial of bevacizumab and low-dose metronomic oral cyclophosphamide in recurrent ovarian cancer: a trial of the California, Chicago, and Princess Margaret Hospital phase II consortia, *J Clin Oncol* 26:76–82, 2008.
84. Gorn M, Habermann CR, Anige M, et al: A pilot study of docetaxel and trofosfamide as second-line 'metronomic' chemotherapy in the treatment of metastatic non-small cell lung cancer (NSCLC), *Onkologie* 31:185–189, 2008.
85. Bottini A, Generali D, Brizzi MP, et al: Randomized phase II trial of letrozole and letrozole plus low-dose metronomic oral cyclophosphamide as primary systemic treatment in elderly breast cancer patients, *J Clin Oncol* 24:3623–3628, 2006.
86. Kieran MW, Turner CD, Rubin JB, et al: A feasibility trial of antiangiogenic (metronomic) chemotherapy in pediatric patients

with recurrent or progressive cancer, *J Pediatr Hematol Oncol* 27:573–581, 2005.

87. Klement G, Huang P, Mayer B, et al: Differences in therapeutic indexes of combination metronomic chemotherapy and an anti-VEGFR-2 antibody in multidrug-resistant human breast cancer xenografts, *Clin Cancer Res* 8:221–232, 2002.
88. Browder T, Butterfield CE, Kraling BM, et al: Antiangiogenic scheduling of chemotherapy improves efficacy against experimental drug-resistant cancer, *Cancer Res* 60:1878–1886, 2000.
89. Reardon DA, Desjardins A, Vredenburgh JJ, et al: Metronomic chemotherapy with daily, oral etoposide plus bevacizumab for recurrent malignant glioma: a phase II study, *Br J Cancer* 101(12):1986–1994, 2009.
90. Dellapasqua S, Bertolini F, Bagnardi V, et al: Metronomic cyclophosphamide and capecitabine combined with bevacizumab in advanced breast cancer, *J Clin Oncol* 26:4899–4905, 2008.
91. Garcia-Saenz JA, Martin M, Calles A, et al: Bevacizumab in combination with metronomic chemotherapy in patients with anthracycline- and taxane-refractory breast cancer, *J Chemother* 20:632–639, 2008.
92. Jurado JM, Sanchez A, Pajares B, et al: Combined oral cyclophosphamide and bevacizumab in heavily pre-treated ovarian cancer, *Clin Transl Oncol* 10:583–586, 2008.
93. Buckstein R, Kerbel RS, Shaked Y, et al: High-Dose celecoxib and metronomic "low-dose" cyclophosphamide is an effective and safe therapy in patients with relapsed and refractory aggressive histology non-Hodgkin's lymphoma, *Clin Cancer Res* 12:5190–5198, 2006.
94. Andre N, Rome A, Coze C, et al: Metronomic etoposide/cyclophosphamide/celecoxib regimen given to children and adolescents with refractory cancer: a preliminary monocentric study, *Clin Ther* 30:1336–1340, 2008.
95. Krzyzanowska MK, Tannock IF, Lockwood G, et al: A phase II trial of continuous low-dose oral cyclophosphamide and celecoxib in patients with renal cell carcinoma, *Cancer Chemother Pharmacol* 60:135–141, 2007.
96. Stempak D, Gammon J, Halton J, et al: A pilot pharmacokinetic and antiangiogenic biomarker study of celecoxib and low-dose metronomic vinblastine or cyclophosphamide in pediatric recurrent solid tumors, *J Pediatr Hematol Oncol* 28:720–728, 2006.
97. Twardowski PW, Smith-Powell L, Carroll M, et al: Biologic markers of angiogenesis: circulating endothelial cells in patients with advanced malignancies treated on phase I protocol with metronomic chemotherapy and celecoxib, *Cancer Invest* 26:53–59, 2008.
98. D'Amato RJ, Loughnan MS, Flynn E, et al: Thalidomide is an inhibitor of angiogenesis, *Proc Natl Acad Sci U S A* 91:4082–4085, 1994.
99. Hafner C, Reichle A, Vogt T: New indications for established drugs: combined tumor-stroma-targeted cancer therapy with PPARgamma agonists, COX-2 inhibitors, mTOR antagonists and metronomic chemotherapy, *Curr Cancer Drug Targets* 5:393–419, 2005.
100. Shaked Y, Emmenegger U, Francia G, et al: Low-dose metronomic combined with intermittent bolus-dose cyclophosphamide is an effective long-term chemotherapy treatment strategy, *Cancer Res* 65:7045–7051, 2005.
101. Flory AB, Rassnick KM, Balkman CE, et al: Oral bioavailability of etoposide after administration of a single dose to tumor-bearing dogs, *Am J Vet Res* 69:1316–1322, 2008.
102. Elmslie RE, Glawe P, Dow SW: Metronomic therapy with cyclophosphamide and piroxicam effectively delays tumor recurrence in dogs with incompletely resected soft tissue sarcomas, *J Vet Intern Med* 22:1373–1379, 2008.
103. Calleri A, Bono A, Bagnardi V, et al: Predictive potential of angiogenic growth factors and circulating endothelial cells in breast cancer patients receiving metronomic chemotherapy plus bevacizumab, *Clin Cancer Res* 15:7652–7657, 2009.
104. Leach TN, Childress MO, Greene SN, et al: Prospective trial of metronomic chlorambucil chemotherapy in dogs with naturally occurring cancer, *Vet Comp Oncol* 10(2):102–112, 2011.
105. Lana S, U'ren L, Plaza S, et al: Continuous low-dose oral chemotherapy for adjuvant therapy of splenic hemangiosarcoma in dogs, *J Vet Intern Med* 21:764–769, 2007.
106. Marchetti V, Giorgi M, Fioravanti A, et al: First-line metronomic chemotherapy in a metastatic model of spontaneous canine tumours: a pilot study, *Invest New Drugs* 2011.
107. Taylor F, Gear R, Hoather T, et al: Chlorambucil and prednisolone chemotherapy for dogs with inoperable mast cell tumours: 21 cases, *J Small Anim Pract* 50:284–289, 2009.
108. Tripp CD, Fidel J, Anderson CL, et al: Tolerability of metronomic administration of lomustine in dogs with cancer, *J Vet Intern Med* 25:278–284, 2011.
109. Withrow SJ, Liptak JM, Straw RC, et al: Biodegradable cisplatin polymer in limb-sparing surgery for canine osteosarcoma, *Ann Surg Oncol* 11:705–713, 2004.
110. Lana SE, Dernell WS, Lafferty MH, et al: Use of radiation and a slow-release cisplatin formulation for treatment of canine nasal tumors, *Vet Radiol Ultrasound* 45:577–581, 2004.
111. Havlicek M, Straw RS, Langova V, et al: Intra-operative cisplatin for the treatment of canine extremity soft tissue sarcomas, *Vet Comp Oncol* 7(2):122–129, 2009.
112. Selting KA, Wang X, Gustafson DL, et al: Evaluation of satraplatin in dogs with spontaneously occurring malignant tumors, *J Vet Intern Med* 25:909–915, 2011.
113. Park JW, Kerbel RS, Kelloff GJ, et al: Rationale for biomarkers and surrogate end points in mechanism-driven oncology drug development, *Clin Cancer Res* 10:3885–3896, 2004.
114. Drevs J, Schneider V: The use of vascular biomarkers and imaging studies in the early clinical development of anti-tumour agents targeting angiogenesis, *J Intern Med* 260:517–529, 2006.
115. Sandri MT, Johansson HA, Zorzino L, et al: Serum EGFR and serum HER-2/neu are useful predictive and prognostic markers in metastatic breast cancer patients treated with metronomic chemotherapy, *Cancer* 110:509–517, 2007.
116. Lindauer A, Di GP, Kanefendt F, et al: Pharmacokinetic/Pharmacodynamic modeling of biomarker response to sunitinib in healthy volunteers, *Clin Pharmacol Ther* 87:601–608, 2010.
117. Morgan B, Thomas AL, Drevs J, et al: Dynamic contrast-enhanced magnetic resonance imaging as a biomarker for the pharmacological response of PTK787/ZK 222584, an inhibitor of the vascular endothelial growth factor receptor tyrosine kinases, in patients with advanced colorectal cancer and liver metastases: results from two phase I studies, *J Clin Oncol* 21:3955–3964, 2003.
118. MacLeod AG, Dickinson PJ, LeCouteur RA, et al: Quantitative assessment of blood volume and permeability in cerebral mass lesions using dynamic contrast-enhanced computed tomography in the dog, *Acad Radiol* 16:1187–1195, 2009.
119. Bertolini F, Mancuso P, Shaked Y, et al: Molecular and cellular biomarkers for angiogenesis in clinical oncology, *Drug Discov Today* 12:806–812, 2007.
120. Shih T, Lindley C: Bevacizumab: an angiogenesis inhibitor for the treatment of solid malignancies, *Clin Ther* 28:1779–1802, 2006.
121. Ebos JM, Lee CR, Kerbel RS: Tumor and host-mediated pathways of resistance and disease progression in response to antiangiogenic therapy, *Clin Cancer Res* 15:5020–5025, 2009.
122. Paez-Ribes M, Allen E, Hudock J, et al: Antiangiogenic therapy elicits malignant progression of tumors to increased local invasion and distant metastasis, *Cancer Cell* 15:220–231, 2009.
123. Ebos JM, Lee CR, Cruz-Munoz W, et al: Accelerated metastasis after short-term treatment with a potent inhibitor of tumor angiogenesis, *Cancer Cell* 15:232–239, 2009.
124. London CA: Tyrosine kinase inhibitors in veterinary medicine, *Top Companion Anim Med* 24:106–112, 2009.
125. London CA, Hannah AL, Zadovoskaya R, et al: Phase I dose-escalating study of SU11654, a small molecule receptor tyrosine kinase inhibitor, in dogs with spontaneous malignancies, *Clin Cancer Res* 9:2755–2768, 2003.

126. London CA, Malpas PB, Wood-Follis SL, et al: Multi-center, placebo-controlled, double-blind, randomized study of oral toceranib phosphate (SU11654), a receptor tyrosine kinase inhibitor, for the treatment of dogs with recurrent (either local or distant) mast cell tumor following surgical excision, *Clin Cancer Res* 15:3856–3865, 2009.
127. Charney SC, Bergman PJ, Hohenhaus AE, et al: Risk factors for sterile hemorrhagic cystitis in dogs with lymphoma receiving cyclophosphamide with or without concurrent administration of furosemide: 216 cases (1990-1996), *J Am Vet Med Assoc* 222:1388–1393, 2003.

SECTION D
Novel and Emerging Therapeutic Targets

DOUGLAS H. THAMM AND DAVID J. ARGYLE

The recent explosion in available cancer bioinformatics, rational and combinatorial drug design, and high-throughput drug screening has resulted in a massive increase in potential therapeutic targets and anticancer treatment strategies. An exhaustive survey of all potential novel targets for cancer therapy would be impossible; thus this review is designed to present a brief overview of some of the more promising and well-developed "druggable" targets that have been discovered recently and, when applicable, their potential application to veterinary oncology.

DNA Methylation

In addition to the information encoded within the genome sequence, it has been shown that epigenetic changes are of great importance in the modification and maintenance of gene expression. These changes take place through a number of mechanisms, including polymerase enzyme modulation, chromatin condensation, and DNA methylation. Mammalian DNA is methylated at cytosines within cytosine-guanine (CpG) dinucleotide sequences. During tissue differentiation, the methylation pattern is one governor of tissue-specific gene expression and thus phenotype.[1-3]

Two different methylation-related phenomena have been identified in cancer. First, tumor cell DNA has been shown in both dogs and other mammals to be globally hypomethylated,[4,5] specifically in pericentromeric satellite sequences. This may lead to decreased genome stability and an increase in the incidence of oncogenic chromosome defects. Indeed, the purposeful induction of genomic hypomethylation by reduction in germline DNA methyltransferase-1 (DNMT1) levels in genetically engineered mice is associated with a high incidence of T-cell lymphomas displaying trisomy 15.[6] Second, cancer cells also acquire sequence-specific promoter hypermethylation and transcriptional repression in normally unmethylated regions, several of which have been shown to be associated with known tumor suppressor genes, including *Rb, p16, p73,* and the von Hippel-Lindau protein *(VHL),*[1,2,7-9] or other important tumor-associated genes such as *E-cadherin* and estrogen and retinoic acid receptors.[10]

The methylation of DNA is controlled by four known DNMTs, of which DNMT1 may be the most important in cancer.[1-3] A variety of agents can inhibit DNMT function. The two best studied are 5-azacytidine (Vidaza) and 5-aza-deoxycitidine (decitabine, Dacogen), which are nucleoside analogs that incorporate into DNA and inhibit DNMT activity but allow replication to proceed. A large number of single-agent clinical trials with these agents have been reported, and significant activity has been demonstrated in hematopoietic neoplasia, leading to the Food and Drug Administration (FDA) approval of 5-azacytidine and decitabine for the treatment of myelodysplastic syndrome.[11,12] Encouraging response rates to the nucleoside analog decitabine have also been seen in human patients with imatinib-refractory CML.[13,14] Results in advanced solid tumors have been generally disappointing[15,16]; however, studies in combination with standard antineoplastic therapy and other targeted agents (e.g., histone deacetylase inhibitors) are ongoing.[17] One drawback of these drugs is the requirement of DNA replication for activity. There are various other drugs that have DNMT inhibitory activity in nonreplicating cells, including green tea polyphenols[1] and marine products of the psammaplin class,[18] a synthetic derivative of which concurrently inhibits histone deacetylase (see later) and is in human clinical trials.[19] Interestingly, the commonly used cardiac medications procainamide and hydralazine also possess demethylating activity,[10,20] and clinical trials have demonstrated alterations in promoter methylation and reactivation of silenced genes following administration of well-tolerated doses of hydralazine to human cervical cancer patients.[21] Hydralazine-valproic acid combinations have demonstrated activity in myelodysplastic syndrome in early human trials.[22] Procainamide and hydralazine have a long track record of use in veterinary medicine and as such could serve as interesting and readily available drugs for the initial evaluation of methylation inhibition in veterinary cancer patients.

Two potential problems exist regarding the wide clinical implementation of DNMT inhibitors for cancer treatment. As discussed previously, induction of long-term genome-wide hypomethylation could decrease chromosome stability leading to potentially tumorigenic chromosome rearrangements.[3] Demethylation could also trigger the reactivation of genes promoting a more aggressive or metastatic phenotype.[3] In support of this theory, treatment of non-metastatic breast cancer cells with 5-azacytidine was shown to upregulate expression of urokinase-like plasminogen activator, an enzyme important in tumor invasion and metastasis, leading to enhanced metastatic potential.[23]

Histone Deacetylase

Another critical determinant of gene expression is the condensation of chromatin in the form of heterochromatin, which results in transcriptional silencing and enhanced genome stability. This is accomplished by a number of pathways, one of which is the acetylation and deacetylation of histones, controlled by histone acetyltransferases and histone deacetylases (HDACs).[24] The HDACs specifically maintain chromatin in a condensed form, and can associate with specific transcription factors resulting in transcription repression. The acetylation of histones may be key in regulating the expression of genes associated with cellular proliferation, differentiation, and survival, both in development and carcinogenesis.[25,26] Studies suggest that histone acetylation reduces electrostatic charge interactions between histones, leading to chromatin decondensation, and more recent work has suggested that HDAC enzymes' effects may also be indirect through modulation of other proteins important in chromatin condensation, including DNMT1.[27] Induction of HDAC expression, leading to transcriptional repression, is a common feature in human cancers such as colon cancer[28] and negatively regulates the expression of several tumor suppressor genes, including *p53* and *VHL.*[29] Differential expression of certain HDAC isoforms has been associated with outcome in a variety of human tumors, with HDAC2 and 6 studied most completely.[30]

Pharmacologic inhibition of HDAC can affect multiple facets of the malignant phenotype. HDAC inhibition inhibits colon carcinogenesis in the adenomatosis polyposis coli (APC) mouse model.[28] Angiogenesis can be inhibited through upregulation of VHL and subsequent inhibition of hypoxia-inducible factor-1α (HIF-1α) function and VEGF production[29,31,32]; decreased expression of other proangiogenic factors such as bFGF, angiopoietin-2, and Tie2[31,32]; inhibition of endothelial nitric oxide (NO) synthase and endothelial cell proliferation and tube formation[33,34]; and inhibition of the commitment of endothelial progenitor cells to the endothelial lineage.[35] Inhibition of HDAC can enhance apoptosis in tumor and endothelial cells[32,36-38] and directly inhibit tumor cell proliferation.[37,39-41] Consistent with its role as a transcription repressor, inhibition of HDAC has been shown to induce differentiation in thyroid and prostate cancers, neuroblastoma, and the leukemias.[42-46] HDAC inhibition dramatically enhances the in vitro and in vivo efficacy of multiple standard cytotoxic therapies, as well as novel antibodies and small molecules.[27,32,38,47-54]

Two HDAC inhibitors, vorinostat (suberoylanilide hydroxamic acid [SAHA], Zolinza) and romidepsin (FK228, Istodax), have recently been approved by the FDA for the treatment of cutaneous T-cell lymphoma (CTCL),[55-57] and a large number of additional agents are in intermediate to late-stage clinical trials. A number of studies are being conducted evaluating HDAC inhibitors for various other hematologic and solid tumors, and early studies combining these drugs with other targeted and cytotoxic therapies have been reported.[58-61]

A recent in vitro study demonstrated potent induction of histone acetylation, growth inhibition, and induction of apoptosis in a variety of canine tumor cell lines treated with either vorinostat or the novel HDAC inhibitor OSU-HDAC42 (AR42).[62] The commercially available anticonvulsant drug valproic acid (VPA) can function as an HDAC inhibitor and is capable of inhibiting tumor cell invasion, P-glycoprotein expression, proliferation, and angiogenesis and enhancing chemosensitivity.[24,27,43] VPA was recently shown to enhance the antiproliferative and proapoptotic effects of doxorubicin in canine OSA cell lines in vitro and to synergize with doxorubicin in a canine OSA xenograft.[53]

There is a single case report describing administration of vorinostat to a dog with microscopic HSA.[63] Although apparently well tolerated, the dose was empirically chosen, there was no pharmacokinetic analysis or demonstration of target inhibition, and the drug's impact on the course of the disease could not be unequivocally determined. A recent study demonstrated that VPA could be administered prior to a standard dose of doxorubicin in tumor-bearing dogs, at dosages sufficient to enhance histone acetylation in tumor and peripheral blood mononuclear cells, but was not associated with toxicity or apparent potentiation of doxorubicin's adverse effects.[54]

The Proteasome

The abundance of cellular proteins is tightly controlled at the levels of both production and destruction. Protein production can be modified at the transcriptional and posttranscriptional level, and therapies based on these approaches are relatively abundant. Until recently, relatively little attention has been paid to the manipulation of protein degradation as a therapeutic modality. The ubiquitin-proteasome pathway (UPP) is responsible for the degradation of the majority of intracellular proteins and for the regulation of many proteins with key roles in cancer.

The 26S proteasome is a large multiprotein complex containing ubiquitin recognition domains, which bind ubiquitinated proteins tagged for degradation, and proteolytic domains with trypsin-like, chymotrypsin-like, and caspase-like activity, which degrade proteins into short polypeptide sequences.[64] It is responsible for the degradation of a variety of proteins responsible for cell-cycle regulation, angiogenesis, apoptosis, and chemotherapy and radiation sensitivity (Table 14-4).[64-66]

Tumor cells are generally more sensitive to the effects of proteasome inhibition than are normal cells. Various studies have demonstrated a threefold to fortyfold increase in susceptibility to proteasome inhibitor–associated apoptosis when comparing tumor cells to corresponding normal tissues.[66-70] The mechanisms for this differential sensitivity are unclear, but proliferating cells generally appear more sensitive than do quiescent cells.[64,66] Additionally, dysregulation of UPP function appears to occur in many cancer cells, thus potentially rendering them more sensitive to inhibition.[66,71] Recent studies implicate profound upregulation of the proapoptotic factor Noxa as being a key mediator of proteasome inhibitor–induced tumor cell apoptosis.[72,73]

Although a number of chemicals appear capable of proteasome inhibition in vitro, only the boronic acid derivatives appear suitable for clinical use and only one drug, bortezomib (Velcade, PS-341), has received FDA approval for the treatment of multiple myeloma.[74-77] Several additional proteasome inhibitors are in clinical development. Meaningful antitumor activity has been observed in patients with other hematopoietic neoplasms,[78-80] but less activity has been seen in solid tumors to date.[81-84] Although toxicology studies with bortezomib have been performed in dogs,[85] there is no information available to date regarding the safety or biologic effect of proteasome inhibitors in veterinary patients or tumor cells.

Heat Shock Protein 90

Given the complex nature of cancer and the multiple pathways that can be subjugated to contribute to the malignant phenotype, an optimal cancer drug might target a variety of oncogenic pathways simultaneously. One molecular target that has the potential to interrupt a wide variety of pathways important in cancer is heat shock protein 90 (HSP90), a molecular chaperone responsible for the conformational maturation of many proteins involved in diverse oncogenic activities such as cell adhesion/migration/invasion, signal transduction, cell cycle progression, angiogenesis, and survival (Table 14-5).[86-111] HSP90 and other chaperones are responsible for ensuring the correct folding and prevention of aggregation of their client proteins.[112] Misfolding and aggregation of proteins lead to ubiquitination and proteasomal destruction, resulting in proteins with diminished function and greatly shortened half-lives.[113] Although several classes of compound are capable of inhibiting HSP90 chaperone function,[97,98,103] the best studied are ansamycin antibiotics of the geldanamycin class.

Many HSP90 inhibitors appear to demonstrate significant preferential activity against malignant versus normal somatic cells. The HSP90 derived from most tumor cells has a binding affinity for 17-allylaminogeldanamycin (17-AAG) approximately 100-fold higher than HSP90 derived from normal cells. This may occur as a result of the overaccumulation of mutated, misfolded, and overexpressed signaling proteins in tumor cells, leading to increased HSP90 chaperone activity and a greater proportion of the molecule in the bound, active, and 17-AAG–sensitive state.[114]

Tumor cells display considerable variation in sensitivities to HSP90 inhibition. Although the mechanisms underlying this

TABLE 14-4 Molecular Targets and Consequences of Proteasome Inhibition

PROCESS	PROTEINS DEGRADED BY PROTEASOME	CELLULAR CONSEQUENCES
Nuclear factor-κB (NF-κB) activation	IκB	Accumulation of IκB inhibits nuclear translocation and activity of NF-κB, leading to decreased proliferation, survival, invasion, angiogenesis
Apoptosis	p53, Bax, tBid, Smac, JNK, Noxa	Accumulation of these proteins directly or indirectly promotes apoptosis through various pathways.
Cell cycle regulation	p21, p27, other cyclin-dependent kinase (CDK) inhibitors, cyclins, p53	Accumulation of CDK inhibitors can cause cell-cycle arrest and apoptosis. The dysregulated elevation of multiple cyclins can send contradictory signals to the cell resulting in apoptosis.
Signal transduction	Mitogen-activated protein (MAP) kinase (MKP-1) phosphatase	Accumulation dephosphorylates p44/42 MAP kinase, leading to decreased MAP kinase pathway signaling, proliferation, survival, ± angiogenesis.
Oncogenic transformation	c-Fos, c-jun, c-myc, N-myc	Unclear how overabundance of these proteins exerts an antitumor effect.
Unfolded protein response	Various damaged/misfolded proteins	Accumulation of damaged proteins leads to endoplasmic reticulum stress and apoptosis.
Chemo/radiation sensitivity	IκB, P-glycoprotein, topoisomerase IIα, DNA damage repair enzyme downregulation	NF-κB is induced in response to DNA damage; normal proteasome function is required for correct folding of P-glycoprotein; downregulation of topoisomerase IIα may reduce sensitivity to doxorubicin.

Adapted from Adams J: The development of proteasome inhibitors as anticancer drugs, *Cancer Cell* 5:417–421, 2004; Rajkumar SV, Richardson PG, Hideshima T, et al: Proteasome inhibition as a novel therapeutic target in human cancer, *J Clin Oncol* 23:630–639, 2005; and Voorhees PM, Dees EC, O'Neil B, et al: The proteasome as a target for cancer therapy, *Clin Cancer Res* 9:6316–6325, 2003.

TABLE 14-5 Molecules Targeted by Heat Shock Protein 90 (HSP90) Inhibition

PROCESS	TARGETS	REFERENCES
Invasion and migration	Urokinase-like plasminogen activator,* focal adhesion kinase (FAK) phosphorylation	86-88
Cell cycle progression	Cyclin D3, cyclin-dependent kinase 4 (CDK4)	89
Signal transduction	AKT, KIT, RAF-1, EGFR, *HER2,* Jun, Lyn, Src, IGF-1R, PDGFR, Met, *Bcr-Abl,* ILK, androgen receptor, progesterone receptor, glucocorticoid receptor	89-96
Hypoxic response/angiogenesis	HIF-1, VEGF, Glut-1, nitric oxide synthase	90, 97-102
Antiapoptosis	Wild-type and mutant p53, survivin	103-109
Cell senescence	Telomerase	110, 111

EGFR, Epidermal growth factor receptor; *HIF-1,* hypoxia-inducible factor-1; *IGF-1R,* insulin-like growth factor receptor 1; *ILK,* integrin-linked kinase; *PDGFR,* platelet-derived growth factor receptor; *VEGF,* vascular endothelial growth factor.

*Urokinase-like plasminogen activator activity appears to be inhibited by geldanamycin class drugs through a mechanism other than heat shock protein 90 (HSP90) inhibition.

differential sensitivity are incompletely characterized, some important characteristics include reliance on certain kinase cascades, expression of apoptotic and cell-cycle regulators, and p-glycoprotein expression.[90]

Many RTKs targeted by the geldanamycins may have an important role in canine and feline tumors. For example, they are capable of inhibiting the function of mutant and wild-type KIT,[91] important in canine mast cell neoplasia[115]; Met,[92] expressed in multiple canine tumor types[116,117]; PDGFR,[118] expressed in FVAS and OSA[119,120]; and IGF-1R,[91] which is expressed and functional in canine OSA and melanoma.[121-123] The geldanamycins are likewise able to attenuate the function of the HIF-1α protein, a key transcription factor responsible for sensing and responding to hypoxia and activating the angiogenic switch.[97,99,100] They are additionally able to deplete key antiapoptotic proteins such as mutant *p53* and survivin,[104-107] contributing to enhanced in vitro sensitivity to standard cytotoxic therapies such as radiation and chemotherapy when used in combination.[93,94,101,124-126]

Under certain circumstances, HSP90 inhibitors may have undesirable effects from the standpoint of cancer therapy. For example, 17-AAG has been shown to protect colon carcinoma cells from cisplatin-mediated toxicity,[95] whereas it has additive or synergistic activity when combined with cisplatin against human neuroblastoma and OSA cells.[124] Additionally, 17-AAG inhibited primary tumor formation, although it potentiated bone-specific mammary carcinoma metastasis by enhancing osteoclastogenesis in one murine model.[127]

The impressive preclinical data generated with compounds such as HSP90 inhibitors have led to phase I human clinical trials of multiple agents,[128-132] including some early combinatorial studies.[130-132] Evidence of biologic effect in the form of upregulation of HSP70 chaperone expression in peripheral blood cells has been observed. There is in vitro evidence of antitumor activity of HSP90 inhibitors in canine OSA and mast cell tumor cell lines[133,134]; however, no clinical evaluation of these agents has been reported to date.

Poly Adenosine Diphosphate Ribose Polymerase and Poly Adenosine Diphosphate Ribose Glycohydrolase

Poly adenosine diphosphate (ADP)-ribose polymerase (PARP) is a "nick-sensor" that signals the presence of DNA damage and facilitates DNA repair.[135] The first PARP enzyme was discovered by Chambon et al and is now recognized as a superfamily of 18 members,[136] although only PARP-1 and PARP-2 are known to act in DNA damage.[137] The PARP family is also involved in the regulation of several transcription factors such as NFκB in modulating the expression of chemokines, adhesion molecules, inflammatory cytokines, and mediators.[135] Poly ADP-ribose glycohydrolase (PARG) is the main enzyme in catabolizing poly ADP-ribose to ADP-ribose. To date, only one single PARG gene has been detected in mammals, encoding for three complementary DNAs (cDNA), which generate three isoforms.[135]

PARP has multiple intracellular functions, including signaling DNA damage, and recognizing and binding to DNA strand breaks generated by DNA-damaging agents (cytotoxic drugs and ionizing radiation).[138] Activation of PARP is one of the earliest DNA damage responses. PARP is also a modulator of DNA base excision repair (BER), which constitutes a major mechanism for genomic stability. There is increasing evidence demonstrating that both PARP and PARG repair DNA.[136] When PARP binds to DNA strand breaks, it activates an enzyme causing shuttling of PARP and, subsequently, opening of the chromatin. PARG enters the nucleus, it moves to the PARP substrate, and DNA strand breaks are repaired. Due to excessive PARG, poly ADP-ribose decreases and thus chromatin reverts back to its original structure.

PARP inhibition has been suggested as an important approach in sensitizing cancer cells to conventional cancer therapy, leading to early clinical trials with PARP inhibitors.[138] PARP inhibitors have been shown to be lethal in *BRCA*-deficient cells due to persistence of DNA lesions that would normally be repaired in a *BRCA*-dependent fashion,[139] suggesting that PARP inhibitors might be an effective monotherapy in these cancers. However, one might expect that their major benefit would be to enhance conventional cytotoxic drug treatment or radiation therapy, and studies have demonstrated that PARP inhibition potentiates the cytotoxicity of anticancer drugs and ionizing radiation through inhibition of DNA repair in cancer cells. PARG inhibition could also be one of the pathways selected for cancer management due to its effects on increased sensitivity to both radiation and chemotherapy.

Although PARG inhibitors have lagged behind PARP inhibitors, a number of molecules have been developed that target these pathways, with varying degrees of specificity. In experimental mouse models, these have shown promise in breast, colon, lung, and brain tumors and in melanoma, either as monotherapy or combined with conventional drugs or radiation.[140-144] Only PARP inhibitors have been used in early human clinical trials (phase I). It is too early to pass judgment on these early trials, and the next 5 years will demonstrate whether PARP inhibitors will have a place in the drug arsenal for cancer treatment.

Carbonic Anhydrase

Hypoxia in cancer tissues is emerging as a key negative prognostic marker in cancer survival. Carbonic anhydrase functions to interconvert carbon dioxide and bicarbonate to maintain acid-base balance in tissues and may play important roles in hypoxic states. In humans, there are 13 active isoenzymes of carbonic anhydrase (CA), and the transmembrane isoform CA IX has been linked with carcinogenesis.[145] High levels of CA IX expression have been demonstrated in human epithelial tumors such as carcinomas of the cervix, uterus, kidney, lung, esophagus, breast, and colon. Normally, this isoenzyme has restricted expression to the epithelia of the gastrointestinal tract, which is in contrast to studies in cancer where ectopic expression has been demonstrated in hypoxic tumors, participating in tumor cell environment acidosis and contributing to malignant progression and poor treatment outcome.[145] Modulation of extracellular tumor pH via inhibition of CA IX activity has been suggested as a promising approach to novel anticancer therapies. Much attention has recently been paid to the CA IX inhibitors' drug design, and efforts have been made to obtain isozyme IX inhibitors, with putative applications as antitumor drugs or diagnostic agents. A large number of selective CA IX inhibitors have been developed in the past 5 years in the sulfonamide, sulfamide, and sulfamate series.[146] Some of these compounds can constitute interesting leads for further development. Furthermore, new classes of prodrug have emerged in the design of new anticancer compounds, which can be activated under hypoxia. As yet, there is little clinical information regarding the efficacy of any of these compounds, but one may anticipate that these drugs could be beneficial in large hypoxic tumors that have failed conventional treatments or as possible sensitizers to radiation damage.[145,147]

REFERENCES

1. Brueckner B, Lyko F: DNA methyltransferase inhibitors: old and new drugs for an epigenetic cancer therapy, *Trends Pharmacol Sci* 25:551–554, 2004.
2. Herman JG, Baylin SB: Gene silencing in cancer in association with promoter hypermethylation, *N Engl J Med* 349:2042–2054, 2003.
3. Szyf M: DNA methylation and cancer therapy, *Drug Resist Update* 6:341–353, 2003.
4. Pelham JT, Irwin PJ, Kay PH: Genomic hypomethylation in neoplastic cells from dogs with malignant lymphoproliferative disorders, *Res Vet Sci* 74:101–104, 2003.
5. Ehrlich M: DNA methylation in cancer: too much, but also too little, *Oncogene* 21:5400–5413, 2002.
6. Gaudet F, Hodgson JG, Eden A, et al: Induction of tumors in mice by genomic hypomethylation, *Science* 300:489–492, 2003.
7. Catto JW, Azzouzi AR, Rehman I, et al: Promoter hypermethylation is associated with tumor location, stage, and subsequent progression in transitional cell carcinoma, *J Clin Oncol* 23:2903–2910, 2005.
8. Baylin SB, Herman JG: DNA hypermethylation in tumorigenesis: epigenetics joins genetics, *Trends Genet* 16:168–174, 2000.
9. van Doorn R, Zoutman WH, Dijkman R, et al: Epigenetic profiling of cutaneous T-cell lymphoma: promoter hypermethylation of multiple tumor suppressor genes including BCL7a, PTPRG, and p73, *J Clin Oncol* 23:3886–3896, 2005.

10. Segura-Pacheco B, Trejo-Becerril C, Perez-Cardenas E, et al: Reactivation of tumor suppressor genes by the cardiovascular drugs hydralazine and procainamide and their potential use in cancer therapy, *Clin Cancer Res* 9:1596–1603, 2003.
11. Silverman LR, Demakos EP, Peterson BL, et al: Randomized controlled trial of azacitidine in patients with the myelodysplastic syndrome: a study of the cancer and leukemia group B, *J Clin Oncol* 20:2429–2440, 2002.
12. Kantarjian H, Issa JP, Rosenfeld CS, et al: Decitabine improves patient outcomes in myelodysplastic syndromes: results of a phase III randomized study, *Cancer* 106:1794–1803, 2006.
13. Issa JP, Gharibyan V, Cortes J, et al: Phase II study of low-dose decitabine in patients with chronic myelogenous leukemia resistant to imatinib mesylate, *J Clin Oncol* 23:3948–3956, 2005.
14. Cashen AF, Schiller GJ, O'Donnell MR, et al: Multicenter, phase II study of decitabine for the first-line treatment of older patients with acute myeloid leukemia, *J Clin Oncol* 28:556–561, 2010.
15. Aparicio A, Eads CA, Leong LA, et al: Phase I trial of continuous infusion 5-aza-2'-deoxycytidine, *Cancer Chemother Pharmacol* 51:231–239, 2003.
16. Momparler RL, Bouffard DY, Momparler LF, et al: Pilot phase I-II study on 5-aza-2'-deoxycytidine (Decitabine) in patients with metastatic lung cancer, *Anticancer Drugs* 8:358–368, 1997.
17. Pohlmann P, DiLeone LP, Cancella AI, et al: Phase II trial of cisplatin plus decitabine, a new DNA hypomethylating agent, in patients with advanced squamous cell carcinoma of the cervix, *Am J Clin Oncol* 25:496–501, 2002.
18. Pina IC, Gautschi JT, Wang GY, et al: Psammaplins from the sponge *Pseudoceratina purpurea:* inhibition of both histone deacetylase and DNA methyltransferase, *J Org Chem* 68:3866–3873, 2003.
19. Remiszewski SW: The discovery of NVP-LAQ824: from concept to clinic, *Curr Med Chem* 10:2393–2402, 2003.
20. Villar Garea A, Fraga MF, Espada J, et al: Procaine is a DNA-demethylating agent with growth-inhibitory effects in human cancer cells, *Cancer Res* 63:4984–4989, 2003.
21. Zambrano P, Segura-Pacheco B, Perez-Cardenas E, et al: A phase I study of hydralazine to demethylate and reactivate the expression of tumor suppressor genes, *BMC Cancer* 5:44, 2005.
22. Candelaria M, Herrera A, Labardini J, et al: Hydralazine and magnesium valproate as epigenetic treatment for myelodysplastic syndrome. Preliminary results of a phase-II trial, *Ann Hematol* 90:379–387, 2011.
23. Guo Y, Pakneshan P, Gladu J, et al: Regulation of DNA methylation in human breast cancer. Effect on the urokinase-type plasminogen activator gene production and tumor invasion, *J Biol Chem* 277:41571–41579, 2002.
24. Blaheta RA, Michaelis M, Driever PH, et al: Evolving anticancer drug valproic acid: insights into the mechanism and clinical studies, *Med Res Rev* 25:383–397, 2005.
25. Berger SL: Histone modifications in transcriptional regulation, *Curr Opin Genet Dev* 12:142–148, 2002.
26. Jenuwein T, Allis CD: Translating the histone code, *Science* 293:1074–1080, 2001.
27. Marchion DC, Bicaku E, Daud AI, et al: Valproic acid alters chromatin structure by regulation of chromatin modulation proteins, *Cancer Res* 65:3815–3822, 2005.
28. Zhu P, Martin E, Mengwasser J, et al: Induction of HDAC2 expression upon loss of APC in colorectal tumorigenesis, *Cancer Cell* 5:455–463, 2004.
29. Kim MS, Kwon HJ, Lee YM, et al: Histone deacetylases induce angiogenesis by negative regulation of tumor suppressor genes, *Nat Med* 7:437–443, 2001.
30. Weichert W: HDAC expression and clinical prognosis in human malignancies, *Cancer Lett* 280:168–176, 2009.
31. Zgouras D, Becker U, Loitsch S, et al: Modulation of angiogenesis-related protein synthesis by valproic acid, *Biochem Biophys Res Commun* 316:693–697, 2004.
32. Qian DZ, Wang X, Kachhap SK, et al: The histone deacetylase inhibitor NVP-LAQ824 inhibits angiogenesis and has a greater antitumor effect in combination with the vascular endothelial growth factor receptor tyrosine kinase inhibitor PTK787/ZK222584, *Cancer Res* 64:6626–6634, 2004.
33. Michaelis M, Michaelis UR, Fleming I, et al: Valproic acid inhibits angiogenesis in vitro and in vivo, *Mol Pharmacol* 65:520–527, 2004.
34. Rossig L, Li H, Fisslthaler B, et al: Inhibitors of histone deacetylation downregulate the expression of endothelial nitric oxide synthase and compromise endothelial cell function in vasorelaxation and angiogenesis, *Circ Res* 91:837–844, 2002.
35. Rossig L, Urbich C, Bruhl T, et al: Histone deacetylase activity is essential for the expression of HoxA9 and for endothelial commitment of progenitor cells, *J Exp Med* 201(11):1825–1835, 2005.
36. Phillips A, Bullock T, Plant N: Sodium valproate induces apoptosis in the rat hepatoma cell line, FaO, *Toxicology* 192:219–227, 2003.
37. Tang R, Faussat AM, Majdak P, et al: Valproic acid inhibits proliferation and induces apoptosis in acute myeloid leukemia cells expressing P-gp and MRP1, *Leukemia* 18:1246–1251, 2004.
38. Roh MS, Kim CW, Park BS, et al: Mechanism of histone deacetylase inhibitor Trichostatin A induced apoptosis in human osteosarcoma cells, *Apoptosis* 9:583–589, 2004.
39. Maeda T, Nagaoka Y, Kawai Y, et al: Inhibitory effects of cancer cell proliferation by novel histone deacetylase inhibitors involve p21/WAF1 induction and G2/M arrest, *Biol Pharm Bull* 28:849–853, 2005.
40. Takai N, Desmond JC, Kumagai T, et al: Histone deacetylase inhibitors have a profound antigrowth activity in endometrial cancer cells, *Clin Cancer Res* 10:1141–1149, 2004.
41. Olsen CM, Meussen-Elholm ET, Roste LS, et al: Antiepileptic drugs inhibit cell growth in the human breast cancer cell line MCF7, *Mol Cell Endocrinol* 213:173–179, 2004.
42. Fortunati N, Catalano MG, Arena K, et al: Valproic acid induces the expression of the Na+/I- symporter and iodine uptake in poorly differentiated thyroid cancer cells, *J Clin Endocrinol Metab* 89:1006–1009, 2004.
43. Gottlicher M: Valproic acid: an old drug newly discovered as inhibitor of histone deacetylases, *Ann Hematol* 83(suppl 1):S91–S92, 2004.
44. Gottlicher M, Minucci S, Zhu P, et al: Valproic acid defines a novel class of HDAC inhibitors inducing differentiation of transformed cells, *EMBO J* 20:6969–6978, 2001.
45. Stockhausen MT, Sjolund J, Manetopoulos C, et al: Effects of the histone deacetylase inhibitor valproic acid on Notch signalling in human neuroblastoma cells, *Br J Cancer* 92:751–759, 2005.
46. Thelen P, Schweyer S, Hemmerlein B, et al: Expressional changes after histone deacetylase inhibition by valproic acid in LNCaP human prostate cancer cells, *Int J Oncol* 24:25–31, 2004.
47. Chobanian NH, Greenberg VL, Gass JM, et al: Histone deacetylase inhibitors enhance paclitaxel-induced cell death in ovarian cancer cell lines independent of p53 status, *Anticancer Res* 24:539–545, 2004.
48. Fuino L, Bali P, Wittmann S, et al: Histone deacetylase inhibitor LAQ824 down-regulates Her-2 and sensitizes human breast cancer cells to trastuzumab, Taxotere, gemcitabine, and epothilone B, *Mol Cancer Ther* 2:971–984, 2003.
49. Kim MS, Blake M, Baek JH, et al: Inhibition of histone deacetylase increases cytotoxicity to anticancer drugs targeting DNA, *Cancer Res* 63:7291–7300, 2003.
50. Maggio SC, Rosato RR, Kramer LB, et al: The histone deacetylase inhibitor MS-275 interacts synergistically with fludarabine to induce apoptosis in human leukemia cells, *Cancer Res* 64:2590–2600, 2004.
51. Watanabe K, Okamoto K, Yonehara S: Sensitization of osteosarcoma cells to death receptor-mediated apoptosis by HDAC inhibitors through downregulation of cellular FLIP, *Cell Death Differ* 12:10–18, 2005.

52. Chinnaiyan P, Vallabhaneni G, Armstrong E, et al: Modulation of radiation response by histone deacetylase inhibition, *Int J Radiat Oncol Biol Phys* 62:223–229, 2005.
53. Wittenburg LA, Bisson L, Rose BJ, et al: The histone deacetylase inhibitor valproic acid sensitizes human and canine osteosarcoma to doxorubicin, *Cancer Chemother Pharmacol* 67:83–92, 2011.
54. Wittenburg LA, Gustafson DL, Thamm DH: Phase I pharmacokinetic and pharmacodynamic evaluation of combined valproic acid/doxorubicin treatment in dogs with spontaneous cancer, *Clin Cancer Res* 16:4832–4842, 2010.
55. Whittaker SJ, Demierre MF, Kim EJ, et al: Final results from a multicenter, international, pivotal study of romidepsin in refractory cutaneous T-cell lymphoma, *J Clin Oncol* 28:4485–4491, 2010.
56. Duvic M, Talpur R, Ni X, et al: Phase 2 trial of oral vorinostat (suberoylanilide hydroxamic acid, SAHA) for refractory cutaneous T-cell lymphoma (CTCL), *Blood* 109:31–39, 2007.
57. Olsen EA, Kim YH, Kuzel TM, et al: Phase IIb multicenter trial of vorinostat in patients with persistent, progressive, or treatment refractory cutaneous T-cell lymphoma, *J Clin Oncol* 25:3109–3115, 2007.
58. Munster PN, Thurn KT, Thomas S, et al: A phase II study of the histone deacetylase inhibitor vorinostat combined with tamoxifen for the treatment of patients with hormone therapy-resistant breast cancer, *Br J Cancer* 104:1828–1835, 2011.
59. Kirschbaum M, Frankel P, Popplewell L, et al: Phase II study of vorinostat for treatment of relapsed or refractory indolent non-Hodgkin's lymphoma and mantle cell lymphoma, *J Clin Oncol* 29:1198–1203, 2011.
60. Otterson GA, Hodgson L, Pang H, et al: Phase II study of the histone deacetylase inhibitor Romidepsin in relapsed small cell lung cancer (Cancer and Leukemia Group B 30304), *J Thor Oncol* 5:1644–1648, 2010.
61. Stathis A, Hotte SJ, Chen EX, et al: Phase I study of decitabine in combination with vorinostat in patients with advanced solid tumors and non-Hodgkin's lymphomas, *Clin Cancer Res* 17:1582–1590, 2011.
62. Kisseberth WC, Murahari S, London CA, et al: Evaluation of the effects of histone deacetylase inhibitors on cells from canine cancer cell lines, *Am J Vet Res* 69:938–945, 2008.
63. Cohen LA, Powers B, Amin S, et al: Treatment of canine haemangiosarcoma with suberoylanilide hydroxamic acid, a histone deacetylase inhibitor, *Vet Compar Oncol* 2:243–248, 2004.
64. Adams J: The development of proteasome inhibitors as anticancer drugs, *Cancer Cell* 5:417–421, 2004.
65. Rajkumar SV, Richardson PG, Hideshima T, et al: Proteasome inhibition as a novel therapeutic target in human cancer, *J Clin Oncol* 23:630–639, 2005.
66. Voorhees PM, Dees EC, O'Neil B, et al: The proteasome as a target for cancer therapy, *Clin Cancer Res* 9:6316–6325, 2003.
67. Hideshima T, Richardson P, Chauhan D, et al: The proteasome inhibitor PS-341 inhibits growth, induces apoptosis, and overcomes drug resistance in human multiple myeloma cells, *Cancer Res* 61:3071–3076, 2001.
68. Masdehors P, Omura S, Merle-Beral H, et al: Increased sensitivity of CLL-derived lymphocytes to apoptotic death activation by the proteasome-specific inhibitor lactacystin, *Br J Haematol* 105:752–757, 1999.
69. Orlowski RZ, Eswara JR, Lafond-Walker A, et al: Tumor growth inhibition induced in a murine model of human Burkitt's lymphoma by a proteasome inhibitor, *Cancer Res* 58:4342–4348,1998.
70. Soligo D, Servida F, Delia D, et al: The apoptogenic response of human myeloid leukaemia cell lines and of normal and malignant haematopoietic progenitor cells to the proteasome inhibitor PSI, *Br J Haematol* 113:126–135, 2001.
71. Masdehors P, Merle-Beral H, Maloum K, et al: Deregulation of the ubiquitin system and p53 proteolysis modify the apoptotic response in B-CLL lymphocytes, *Blood* 96:269–274, 2000.
72. Fernandez Y, Verhaegen M, Miller TP, et al: Differential regulation of noxa in normal melanocytes and melanoma cells by proteasome inhibition: therapeutic implications, *Cancer Res* 65:6294–6304, 2005.
73. Qin JZ, Ziffra J, Stennett L, et al: Proteasome inhibitors trigger NOXA-mediated apoptosis in melanoma and myeloma cells, *Cancer Res* 65:6282–6293, 2005.
74. Jagannath S, Barlogie B, Berenson J, et al: A phase 2 study of two doses of bortezomib in relapsed or refractory myeloma, *Br J Haematol* 127:165–172, 2004.
75. Jagannath S, Durie BG, Wolf J, et al: Bortezomib therapy alone and in combination with dexamethasone for previously untreated symptomatic multiple myeloma, *Br J Haematol* 129:776–783, 2005.
76. Richardson PG, Sonneveld P, Schuster MW, et al: Bortezomib or high-dose dexamethasone for relapsed multiple myeloma, *N Engl J Med* 352:2487–2498, 2005.
77. Richardson PG, Barlogie B, Berenson J, et al: A phase 2 study of bortezomib in relapsed, refractory myeloma, *N Engl J Med* 348:2609–2617, 2003.
78. O'Connor OA, Wright J, Moskowitz C, et al: Phase II clinical experience with the novel proteasome inhibitor bortezomib in patients with indolent non-Hodgkin's lymphoma and mantle cell lymphoma, *J Clin Oncol* 23:676–684, 2005.
79. Goy A, Younes A, McLaughlin P, et al: Phase II study of proteasome inhibitor bortezomib in relapsed or refractory B-cell non-Hodgkin's lymphoma, *J Clin Oncol* 23:667–675, 2005.
80. Cortes J, Thomas D, Koller C, et al: Phase I study of bortezomib in refractory or relapsed acute leukemias, *Clin Cancer Res* 10:3371–3376, 2004.
81. Davis NB, Taber DA, Ansari RH, et al: Phase II trial of PS-341 in patients with renal cell cancer: a University of Chicago phase II consortium study, *J Clin Oncol* 22:115–119, 2004.
82. Maki RG, Kraft AS, Scheu K, et al: A multicenter Phase II study of bortezomib in recurrent or metastatic sarcomas, *Cancer* 103:1431–1438, 2005.
83. Markovic SN, Geyer SM, Dawkins F, et al: A phase II study of bortezomib in the treatment of metastatic malignant melanoma, *Cancer* 103:2584–2589, 2005.
84. Shah MH, Young D, Kindler HL, et al: Phase II study of the proteasome inhibitor bortezomib (PS-341) in patients with metastatic neuroendocrine tumors, *Clin Cancer Res* 10:6111–6118, 2004.
85. Bouchard PR, Juedes MJ, Nix D, et al: *Nonclinical discovery and development of Bortezomib (PS-341, VELCADE), a proteasome inhibitor for the treatment of cancer*. In Proceedings of the 55th Annual Meeting of the American College of Veterinary Pathology, Orlando, FL, 2004.
86. Xie Q, Gao CF, Shinomiya N, et al: Geldanamycins exquisitely inhibit HGF/SF-mediated tumor cell invasion, *Oncogene* 24:3697–3707, 2005.
87. Zagzag D, Nomura M, Friedlander DR, et al: Geldanamycin inhibits migration of glioma cells in vitro: a potential role for hypoxia-inducible factor (HIF-1alpha) in glioma cell invasion, *J Cell Physiol* 196:394–402, 2003.
88. Masson-Gadais B, Houle F, Laferriere J, et al: Integrin alphavbeta3, requirement for VEGFR2-mediated activation of SAPK2/p38 and for Hsp90-dependent phosphorylation of focal adhesion kinase in endothelial cells activated by VEGF, *Cell Stress Chaperones* 8:37–52, 2003.
89. Smith V, Sausville EA, Camalier RF, et al: Comparison of 17-dimethylaminoethylamino-17-demethoxy-geldanamycin (17DMAG) and 17-allylamino-17-demethoxygeldanamycin (17AAG) in vitro: effects on Hsp90 and client proteins in melanoma models, *Cancer Chemother Pharmacol* 56:126–137, 2005.
90. Maloney A, Clarke PA, Workman P: Genes and proteins governing the cellular sensitivity to HSP90 inhibitors: a mechanistic perspective, *Curr Cancer Drug Targets* 3:331–341, 2003.
91. Fumo G, Akin C, Metcalfe DD, et al: 17-Allylamino-17-demethoxygeldanamycin (17-AAG) is effective in down-regulating

mutated, constitutively activated KIT protein in human mast cells, *Blood* 103:1078–1084, 2004.
92. Maulik G, Kijima T, Ma PC, et al: Modulation of the c-Met/hepatocyte growth factor pathway in small cell lung cancer, *Clin Cancer Res* 8:620–627, 2002.
93. Machida H, Matsumoto Y, Shirai M, et al: Geldanamycin, an inhibitor of Hsp90, sensitizes human tumour cells to radiation, *Int J Radiat Biol* 79:973–980, 2003.
94. Solit DB, Basso AD, Olshen AB, et al: Inhibition of heat shock protein 90 function down-regulates Akt kinase and sensitizes tumors to Taxol, *Cancer Res* 63:2139–2144, 2003.
95. Vasilevskaya IA, Rakitina TV, O'Dwyer PJ: Geldanamycin and its 17-allylamino-17-demethoxy analogue antagonize the action of cisplatin in human colon adenocarcinoma cells: differential caspase activation as a basis for interaction, *Cancer Res* 63:3241–3246, 2003.
96. Aoyagi Y, Fujita N, Tsuruo T: Stabilization of integrin-linked kinase by binding to Hsp90, *Biochem Biophys Res Commun* 331:1061–1068, 2005.
97. Kurebayashi J, Otsuki T, Kurosumi M, et al: A radicicol derivative, KF58333, inhibits expression of hypoxia-inducible factor-1alpha and vascular endothelial growth factor, angiogenesis and growth of human breast cancer xenografts, *Jpn J Cancer Res* 92:1342–1351, 2001.
98. Osada M, Imaoka S, Funae Y: Apigenin suppresses the expression of VEGF, an important factor for angiogenesis, in endothelial cells via degradation of HIF-1alpha protein, *FEBS Lett* 575:59–63, 2004.
99. Mabjeesh NJ, Post DE, Willard MT, et al: Geldanamycin induces degradation of hypoxia-inducible factor 1alpha protein via the proteosome pathway in prostate cancer cells, *Cancer Res* 62:2478–2482, 2002.
100. Isaacs JS, Jung YJ, Mimnaugh EG, et al: Hsp90 regulates a von Hippel Lindau-independent hypoxia-inducible factor-1 alpha-degradative pathway, *J Biol Chem* 277:29936–29944, 2002.
101. Bisht KS, Bradbury CM, Mattson D, et al: Geldanamycin and 17-allylamino-17-demethoxygeldanamycin potentiate the in vitro and in vivo radiation response of cervical tumor cells via the heat shock protein 90-mediated intracellular signaling and cytotoxicity, *Cancer Res* 63:8984–8995, 2003.
102. Kaur G, Belotti D, Burger AM, et al: Antiangiogenic properties of 17-(dimethylaminoethyl amino)-17-demethoxygeldanamycin: An orally bioavailable heat shock protein 90 modulator, *Clin Cancer Res* 10:4813–4821, 2004.
103. Plescia J, Salz W, Xia F, et al: Rational design of shepherdin, a novel anticancer agent, *Cancer Cell* 7:457–468, 2005.
104. Muller L, Schaupp A, Walerych D, et al: Hsp90 regulates the activity of wild type p53 under physiological and elevated temperatures, *J Biol Chem* 279:48846–48854, 2004.
105. Muller P, Ceskova P, Vojtesek B: Hsp90 is essential for restoring cellular functions of temperature-sensitive p53 mutant protein but not for stabilization and activation of wild-type p53: implications for cancer therapy, *J Biol Chem* 280:6682–6691, 2005.
106. Walerych D, Kudla G, Gutkowska M, et al: Hsp90 chaperones wild-type p53 tumor suppressor protein, *J Biol Chem* 279:48836–48845, 2004.
107. Fortugno P, Beltrami E, Plescia J, et al: Regulation of survivin function by Hsp90, *Proc Natl Acad Sci U S A* 100:13791–13796, 2003.
108. Park JW, Yeh MW, Wong MG, et al: The heat shock protein 90-binding geldanamycin inhibits cancer cell proliferation, down-regulates oncoproteins, and inhibits epidermal growth factor-induced invasion in thyroid cancer cell lines, *J Clin Endocrinol Metab* 88:3346–3353, 2003.
109. Hawkins LM, Jayanthan AA, Narendran A: Effects of 17-allylamino-17-demethoxygeldanamycin (17-AAG) on pediatric acute lymphoblastic leukemia (ALL) with respect to Bcr-Abl status and imatinib mesylate sensitivity, *Pediatr Res* 57:430–437, 2005.
110. Villa R, Folini M, Porta CD, et al: Inhibition of telomerase activity by geldanamycin and 17-allylamino, 17-demethoxygeldanamycin in human melanoma cells, *Carcinogenesis* 24:851–859, 2003.
111. Haendeler J, Hoffmann J, Rahman S, et al: Regulation of telomerase activity and anti-apoptotic function by protein-protein interaction and phosphorylation, *FEBS Lett* 536:180–186, 2003.
112. Neckers L: Hsp90 inhibitors as novel cancer chemotherapeutic agents, *Trends Mol Med* 8:S55–S61, 2002.
113. Isaacs JS, Xu W, Neckers L: Heat shock protein 90 as a molecular target for cancer therapeutics, *Cancer Cell* 3:213–217, 2003.
114. Kamal A, Thao L, Sensintaffar J, et al: A high-affinity conformation of Hsp90 confers tumour selectivity on Hsp90 inhibitors, *Nature* 425:407–410, 2003.
115. Downing S, Chien MB, Kass PH, et al: Prevalence and importance of internal tandem duplications in exons 11 and 12 of c-kit in mast cell tumors of dogs, *Am J Vet Res* 63:1718–1723, 2002.
116. Liao AT, McMahon M, London CA: Characterization, expression and function of c-Met in canine spontaneous cancers, *Vet Compar Oncol* 3:61–72, 2005.
117. MacEwen EG, Kutzke J, Carew J, et al: c-Met tyrosine kinase receptor expression and function in human and canine osteosarcoma cells, *Clin Exp Metastasis* 20:421–430, 2003.
118. Sakagami M, Morrison P, Welch WJ: Benzoquinoid ansamycins (herbimycin A and geldanamycin) interfere with the maturation of growth factor receptor tyrosine kinases, *Cell Stress Chaperones* 4:19–28, 1999.
119. Katayama R, Huelsmeyer MK, Marr AK, et al: Imatinib mesylate inhibits platelet-derived growth factor activity and increases chemosensitivity in feline vaccine-associated sarcoma, *Cancer Chemother Pharmacol* 54:25–33, 2004.
120. Levine RA: Overexpression of the sis oncogene in a canine osteosarcoma cell line, *Vet Pathol* 39:411–412, 2002.
121. MacEwen EG, Pastor J, Kutzke J, et al: IGF-1 receptor contributes to the malignant phenotype in human and canine osteosarcoma, *J Cell Biochem* 92:77–91, 2004.
122. Serra M, Pastor J, Domenzain C, et al: Effect of transforming growth factor-beta1, insulin-like growth factor-I, and hepatocyte growth factor on proteoglycan production and regulation in canine melanoma cell lines, *Am J Vet Res* 63:1151–1158, 2002.
123. Thamm DH, Huelsmeyer MK, Mitzey AM, et al: RT-PCR-based tyrosine kinase display profiling of canine melanoma: IGF-1 receptor as a potential therapeutic target, *Melanoma Res* 20:35–42, 2010.
124. Bagatell R, Beliakoff J, David CL, et al: Hsp90 inhibitors deplete key anti-apoptotic proteins in pediatric solid tumor cells and demonstrate synergistic anticancer activity with cisplatin, *Int J Cancer* 113:179–188, 2005.
125. Jones DT, Addison E, North JM, et al: Geldanamycin and herbimycin A induce apoptotic killing of B chronic lymphocytic leukemia cells and augment the cells' sensitivity to cytotoxic drugs, *Blood* 103:1855–1861, 2004.
126. Munster PN, Basso A, Solit D, et al: Modulation of Hsp90 function by ansamycins sensitizes breast cancer cells to chemotherapy-induced apoptosis in an RB- and schedule-dependent manner, *Clin Cancer Res* 7:2228–2236, 2001.
127. Price JT, Quinn JMW, Sims NA, et al: The heat shock protein 90 inhibitor, 17-allylamino-17-demethoxygeldanamycin, enhances osteoclast formation and potentiates bone metastasis of a human breast cancer cell line, *Cancer Res* 65:4929–4938, 2005.
128. Goetz MP, Toft D, Reid J, et al: Phase I trial of 17-allylamino-17-demethoxygeldanamycin in patients with advanced cancer, *J Clin Oncol* 23:1078–1087, 2005.
129. Grem JL, Morrison G, Guo XD, et al: Phase I and pharmacologic study of 17-(allylamino)-17-demethoxygeldanamycin in adult patients with solid tumors, *J Clin Oncol* 23:1885–1893, 2005.
130. Pacey S, Wilson RH, Walton M, et al: A phase I study of the heat shock protein 90 inhibitor alvespimycin (17-DMAG) given intravenously to patients with advanced solid tumors, *Clin Cancer Res* 17:1561–1570, 2011.

131. Richardson PG, Chanan-Khan AA, Alsina M, et al: Tanespimycin monotherapy in relapsed multiple myeloma: results of a phase 1 dose-escalation study, *Br J Haematol* 150:438–445, 2010.
132. Ramanathan RK, Egorin MJ, Erlichman C, et al: Phase I pharmacokinetic and pharmacodynamic study of 17-dimethylaminoethylamino-17-demethoxygeldanamycin, an inhibitor of heat-shock protein 90, in patients with advanced solid tumors, *J Clin Oncol* 28:1520–1526, 2010.
133. Lin TY, Bear M, Du Z, et al: The novel HSP90 inhibitor STA-9090 exhibits activity against Kit-dependent and -independent malignant mast cell tumors, *Exper Hematol* 36:1266–1277, 2008.
134. McCleese JK, Bear MD, Fossey SL, et al: The novel HSP90 inhibitor STA-1474 exhibits biologic activity against osteosarcoma cell lines, *Int J Cancer* 125:2792–2801, 2009.
135. Fauzee NJ, Pan J, Wang YL: PARP and PARG inhibitors—new therapeutic targets in cancer treatment, *Pathol Oncol Res* 16:469–478, 2010.
136. D'Amours D, Desnoyers S, D'Silva I, et al: Poly (ADP-ribosyl) ation reactions in the regulation of nuclear functions, *Biochem J* 342(Pt 2):249–268,1999.
137. Hochegger H, Dejsuphong D, Fukushima T, et al: Parp-1 protects homologous recombination from interference by Ku and Ligase IV in vertebrate cells, *EMBO J* 25:1305–1314, 2006.
138. Plummer R, Jones C, Middleton M, et al: Phase I study of the poly (ADP-ribose) polymerase inhibitor, AG014699, in combination with temozolomide in patients with advanced solid tumors, *Clin Cancer Res* 14:7917–7923, 2008.
139. De Soto JA, Wang X, Tominaga Y, et al: The inhibition and treatment of breast cancer with poly (ADP-ribose) polymerase (PARP-1) inhibitors, *Int J Biol Sci* 2:179–185, 2006.
140. Albert JM, Cao C, Kim KW, et al: Inhibition of poly (ADP-ribose) polymerase enhances cell death and improves tumor growth delay in irradiated lung cancer models, *Clin Cancer Res* 13:3033–3042, 2007.
141. Donawho CK, Luo Y, Penning TD, et al: ABT-888, an orally active poly (ADP-ribose) polymerase inhibitor that potentiates DNA-damaging agents in preclinical tumor models, *Clin Cancer Res* 13:2728–2737, 2007.
142. Li M, Threadgill MD, Wang Y, et al: Poly(ADP-ribose) polymerase inhibition down-regulates expression of metastasis-related genes in CT26 colon carcinoma cells, *Pathobiology* 76:108–116, 2009.
143. Tentori L, Leonetti C, Scarsella M, et al: Systemic administration of GPI 15427, a novel poly(ADP-ribose) polymerase-1 inhibitor, increases the antitumor activity of temozolomide against intracranial melanoma, glioma, lymphoma, *Clin Cancer Res* 9:5370–5379, 2003.
144. Dungey FA, Caldecott KW, Chalmers AJ: Enhanced radiosensitization of human glioma cells by combining inhibition of poly(ADP-ribose) polymerase with inhibition of heat shock protein 90, *Mol Cancer Ther* 8:2243–2254, 2009.
145. Winum JY, Scozzafava A, Montero JL, et al: Inhibition of carbonic anhydrase IX: a new strategy against cancer, *Anticancer Agents Med Chem* 9:693–702, 2009.
146. El-Sayed NS, El-Bendary ER, El-Ashry SM, et al: Synthesis and antitumor activity of new sulfonamide derivatives of thiadiazolo [3, 2-a]pyrimidines, *Eur J Med Chem* 46:3714–3720, 2011.
147. Muller V, Riethdorf S, Rack B, et al: Prospective evaluation of serum tissue inhibitor of metalloproteinase 1 and carbonic anhydrase IX in correlation to circulating tumor cells in patients with metastatic breast cancer, *Breast Can Res* 13:R71, 2011.

Supportive Care for the Cancer Patient

15

SECTION A
Management of Chronic Cancer Pain

B. Duncan X. Lascelles

In 1978 Yoxall[1] stated: "It is surprising, for instance, how much a dog's quality of life, observed by the owner, may be improved by the administration of a simple analgesic if the dog is suffering from a tumor, which although painless on palpation, may be causing considerable chronic pain." Despite this statement and the fact that obvious pain associated with specific tumors such as osteosarcoma (OSA) has been emphasized for a long time as a diagnostic criterion, there is little literature specifically investigating cancer pain in companion animals.[2-14] However, it is very encouraging that since the previous edition of this book, there has been an approximately fourfold increase in published studies (from 4 to 17 using a PubMed search). Encouragingly, we have seen the first studies looking at mechanisms in companion animal cancer pain.[15,16]

This chapter will deal with the treatment of chronic cancer pain in dogs and cats. Given the relative lack of clinical work in dogs and cats, the information in this chapter cannot be based on peer-reviewed investigations. Rather, it is a combination of the authors' experience and the experience of others who are heavily involved in the treatment of cancer patients. It is also based on considered extrapolations from human medicine and from veterinary research in other chronically painful conditions, such as osteoarthritis. The control of acute perioperative pain in cancer patients is also very important (see section on relationship between cancer and pain), and readers are referred to appropriate texts for information on perioperative pain control.[17]

How Painful Is Cancer in Animals?

Not all tumors are painful, and the amount of pain is likely to vary considerably from one animal to another, even with similar tumor types. The author's experience and the experience of others would suggest that, using a conservative estimate, 30% of tumors in dogs and cats are associated with significant pain at the time of diagnosis. Tumors most likely to be associated with pain include those at the following sites: oral cavity, bone, urogenital tract, eyes, nose, nerve roots, gastrointestinal tract, and skin (Table 15-1). The 30% estimate is likely conservative since pain is experienced by 20% to 50% of human patients when the lesion is diagnosed, by nearly half undergoing active treatment, and by up to 90% with far advanced or terminal cancer. An overall average of about 70% of human patients with advanced cancer suffer pain.[18]

In addition to pain caused by the tumor itself, pain in cancer patients can also be caused by chemotherapy, radiation therapy, or surgery (perioperative pain, postoperative pain, and conditions such as "phantom limb" associated with some amputations) and by concurrent noncancerous disease, most notably osteoarthritis, gingivitis, and dermatologic conditions.

General Approach to Cancer Pain Management

The incidence of pain in animals caused by cancer is very difficult to estimate, as is the effectiveness of analgesic therapy. Recent surveys have found that significant numbers of animals in the perioperative setting were not receiving analgesic drugs,[19-26] although an overview of these studies seems to suggest the situation is improving. Analgesics are even less likely to be used for cancer pain. Glucocorticoids do provide some analgesia, and their use may be more widespread,[22] but the specific treatment of cancer pain in animals is still likely to be suboptimal.

Suboptimal treatment of cancer pain in animals probably results from a number of factors such as the following:

- Lack of appreciation that many cancers are associated with significant pain.
- Overly focusing on the cancer treatment, rather than patient comfort.
- Inability to assess pain in cancer patients.
- Lack of knowledge of drugs, drug therapy, and other pain-relieving techniques
- Lack of communication with clients and lack of involvement of clients in the assessment and treatment phases.
- Under-use of nursing staff for assessment and reevaluation of pain in cancer patients.

In large part, these factors associated with suboptimal treatment of cancer pain in animals result from a lack of published, scientifically sound information on the subject. Such information also stimulates presentation and discussion of the topic in continuing education forums. In many respects, continuing education in a topic is facilitated by having Food and Drug Administration (FDA)-approved drugs or proven treatments because industry then has a vested interest in improving knowledge of the subject. Unfortunately, there are no analgesics with FDA approval for cancer pain in animals.

Although drug treatment is the mainstay of cancer pain treatment, effective cancer pain treatment often involves a combination of drug therapy, nondrug therapies, and good communication between all parties involved. A basic approach to cancer pain management is summarized in Table 15-2.

TABLE 15-1 List of Tumors Most Likely to Be Associated with Pain

TUMOR CATEGORY	NOTES
Tumors involving bone	Primary bone tumors (both of the appendicular and axial skeleton) and metastasis to bone are painful. Just as in humans, sometimes metastasis to bone can be relatively nonpainful; however, this should be considered the exception.
Central nervous system tumors	Extradural tumors that expand and put pressure on neural tissue are often associated with pain. Tumors originating from within the neural tissue are often not associated with pain until later on in the course of the disease. In humans with primary brain tumors or metastases to brain, 60%-90% of them suffer from headaches; it should be presumed that animals also suffer such headaches.
Gastrointestinal	Especially esophagus, stomach, colon, and rectum. Such pain may be very difficult to localize, and it may manifest as vague signs and behavioral changes. Colonic and rectal pain is often manifested as perineal discomfort.
Inflammatory mammary carcinoma	This form of mammary cancer is very painful in humans, and dogs with this form of mammary cancer appear to exhibit obvious signs of pain.
Genitourinary tract tumors	Stretching of the renal capsule appears to produce significant pain. Bladder tumors appear to be predictably associated with pain. Tumors of the distal genitourinary tract are often manifested as perineal pain or pain apparently associated with the lower back.
Prostate	Prostatic tumors appear to be particularly painful, especially if local metastasis to bone is present, and the pain may be manifested as lower back or abdominal pain.
Oral and pharyngeal tumors	Soft tissue tumors that are growing by projecting from the surface (e.g., projecting from the gingival surface) appear to be relatively nonpainful. Tumors involving bone or those growing within the tissues of the maxilla or mandible appear to be significantly more painful. Soft tissue tumors of the pharynx and caudal oral cavity are particularly painful.
Intranasal tumors	Pain probably results both from the destruction of turbinates and from the destruction of bone of the nasal cavity.
Invasive soft tissue sarcomas	The aggressive vaccine-associated sarcomas in cats are particularly painful—the apparent size of the lesion does not correlate with the degree of pain. Other invasive sarcomas in both species are painful. Also, in both cats and dogs, noninvasive soft tissue sarcomas that are pressing on nerves and other sensitive structures will be painful. One form of soft tissue sarcomas, the peripheral nerve sheath tumor (PNST), is sometimes reported to be painful to the touch.
Invasive cutaneous tumors	Especially those that are ulcerative.
Liver and biliary tumors	Especially those that are expansile, stretching the liver capsule. Expansile liver tumors are reported to be painful in humans.
Disseminated intrathoracic and intraabdominal tumors (e.g., mesothelioma, malignant histiocytosis)	The signs associated with such tumors are particularly vague; however, often, intracavitary analgesia (such as intraabdominal local anesthetic) can markedly improve the animal's demeanor, and thus, just as in humans, it appears disseminated neoplasia of these cavities is associated with significant pain.
Lung tumors	Although significant pain is reported in humans with lung cancer, often animals appear to show few signs of pain. However, even in those animals, the provision of an analgesic can often improve demeanor.
Pain following surgical removal of a tumor	Pain well beyond the postoperative period occurs in animals that have undergone surgery and is probably neuropathic in nature. Phantom pain (such as phantom limb pain), a form of neuropathic pain, does appear to exist in animals. If tumor recurrence occurs, significant pain is usually associated with this.

The Importance of Alleviating Pain in the Cancer Patient

The alleviation of pain is important not only from a physiologic and biologic standpoint, but also from an ethical point of view.[27] To help in an evaluation of welfare, "five freedoms," initially proposed by the Brambell Committee in reference to farmed animals,[28] have been suggested. They may be applied equally in the context of companion animals[27] and are as follows:

- Freedom from hunger and thirst
- Freedom from physical and thermal discomfort
- Freedom from pain, injury, and disease
- Freedom to express normal behavior
- Freedom from fear and distress

For each freedom, there should be a consideration of the severity, incidence, and duration. As an example, consider a dog undergoing a maxillectomy. With such a surgery, it is possible that thirst and hunger may result from interference with the dog's ability to eat and drink. However, the dog could be hand-fed and gradually

TABLE 15-2 A Basic Approach to Cancer Pain Management

A	Assess the patient	Ask for the owner's perceptions of the pain present or of any compromise of the animal's quality of life. Assess the patient thoroughly, using palpation and observation.
B	Believe the owner	The owner sees the pet every day in its own environment and knows when alterations in behavior occur. They can rarely suggest diagnoses, but they do know when something is wrong and when their pet is in pain, just as a mother knows when something is wrong with her child.
C	Choose appropriate therapy	Anything other than mild pain should be treated with more than one class of analgesic, or an analgesic drug combined with nondrug adjunctive therapy. **Be aware of potential drug interactions.**
D	Deliver therapy	Deliver the therapy in a logical coordinated manner and explain carefully to the owner about any possible side effects.
E	Empower the client	Empower the clients to participate actively in their pet's treatment; ask for feedback and updates on how the therapy is working.

taught to eat and drink despite the facial alteration. If the dog was never able to eat or drink again on its own, the owners could hand-feed him for the rest of his life or the dog could be fed via a feeding tube. Although this may represent a compromise to his freedom to express normal eating behavior, he would not be hungry or thirsty. Such a surgery may result in a cure for the disease and eliminate pain. However, the surgery may also result in pain and distress. Fear and distress would result because of the unfamiliar surroundings and people during the hospital stay. With appropriate nursing care, the dog should not suffer any physical or thermal discomfort. It can be seen from this example how many factors are interrelated, and all need consideration in the cancer patient, including pain and consideration of the length and severity of pain.

Pain relief may affect survival in cancer patients. Immunosuppression has been shown to depend on the severity of surgery in clinical[29-31] and experimental animal studies.[32,33] Additionally, the severity of surgery has been shown to influence tumor metastasis.[34-37] In 2002, a human clinical study suggested that laparoscopic colectomy was associated with increased survival,[38] and although subsequent studies found no difference in long-term survival,[39] there is interest in the immunologic and oncologic implications of less-invasive surgery.[40] In 2001, Page and coworkers found that the provision of analgesics significantly reduced the tumor-promoting effects of undergoing and recovering from surgery in a rodent model.[41] The reduction of the tumor-promoting effects of surgery by analgesics may result from maintenance of natural killer (NK) cell function, but it is likely that other unrecognized factors also play a role.[41,42] More recently, it was found that spinal analgesia attenuated the laparotomy-induced suppression of tumoricidal function of liver mononuclear cells and decreased metastasis compared to rodents undergoing laparotomy without spinal analgesia.[43] This was considered to be due to preservation of T helper 1/T helper 2 (Th1/Th2) cytokine balance. Thus the provision of adequate perioperative pain management in oncologic surgery may be protective against metastatic sequelae in clinical patients. It is quite possible that chronic pain experienced by animals with cancer may also affect metastasis.

Assessment of Cancer Pain

Assessment of pain in animals, while often difficult, is extremely important. It is likely that the tolerance of pain by an individual animal varies greatly and is further complicated by the innate ability of dogs and cats to mask significant disease and pain. Physiologic variables such as heart rate, respiratory rate, temperature, and pupil size are not reliable measures of acute perioperative pain in dogs[44] and are unlikely to be useful in chronic pain states. The mainstay of pain assessment in cats and dogs suffering from cancer is likely to be changes in behavior. Table 15-3 outlines behaviors that are probably indicative in certain situations of pain. In general, if a tumor is considered to be painful in humans, it is appropriate to give an animal with a similar condition the benefit of the doubt and treat it for pain.

One of the most useful ways of determining if a tumor is painful is to palpate the area and evaluate the animal's response. This may not correlate precisely with the amount of pain the animal spontaneously experiences, but if a tumor is painful on manipulation or palpation, it is highly likely there is spontaneous pain associated with it. As veterinarians, we struggle to measure spontaneous pain. It is perhaps reassuring that there is tremendous debate in the research community on how to measure spontaneous pain in rodent models.

Veterinarians should involve technicians and other staff members in the assessment process because they are usually the ones spending the most time with the patients in the hospital and may have more time to converse in a relaxed and informal way with owners.

The most important people in the assessment process are the owners. The veterinarian must work closely with the owner to capture this information. Often, owners need to be educated as to what signs to look for and that certain behaviors may be indicative of pain. Once very specific changes in behavior can be identified and recorded, these behaviors can be used to monitor the effectiveness of analgesic therapy. Furthermore, these specific activities can be used to create goals and therapy tailored to try to meet these goals. The importance of patient-reported outcomes (PROs) in human medicine is widely recognized.[45] These PROs may refer to a large variety of different health data reported by patients, such as symptoms, functional status, quality of life (QOL), and health-related quality of life (HRQOL).[45] In humans, QOL is a complex, abstract, multidimensional concept defining an individual's satisfaction with life in domains he or she considers important. The term *HRQOL* reflects an attempt to restrict this complex concept to those aspects of life specifically related to the individual's health and potentially modifiable by healthcare.[46] Both QOL and HRQOL have been used in veterinary medicine. Questionnaires have been developed to assess HRQOL in dogs[47,48] and cats[49] with cancer. Although pain certainly appears to be assessed in these HRQOL tools, it is not known how specific or sensitive these tools are to changing pain status.

The author's approach to the evaluation of pain at each visit is to evaluate each of the following three aspects:

1. Palpation-induced pain
2. Activity parameters
3. Behavioral parameters

TABLE 15-3 Outline of Behaviors that May Be Seen with Cancer-Associated or Cancer Therapy–Associated Pain in Cats and Dogs

BEHAVIOR	NOTES
Activity	Less activity than normal; may be very specific activities that are changed; decreased jumping; less playing; less venturing outside; less willing to go on walks (dogs); stiff gait, altered gait, or lameness can be associated with generalized pain but is more often associated with limb or joint pain; slow to rise and get moving after rest (osteoarthritis is often concurrently present).
Appetite	Often decreased with chronic pain.
Attitude	Any change in behavior can be associated with cancer pain—aggressiveness, dullness, shyness, "clinginess," increased dependence
Facial expression	Head hung low, squinted eyes in cats. Sad expression in dogs, head carried low.
Grooming	Failure to groom can be due to either a painful oral lesion or generalized pain.
Response to palpation	This is one of the best ways to diagnose and monitor pain. Pain can be elicited by palpation of the affected area, or manipulation of the affected area, which exacerbates the pain present. This is manifested as an aversion response from the animal (i.e., the animal attempts to escape the procedure, or yowls, cries, hisses, or bites). Pain is inferred when this occurs.
Respiration	May be elevated with severe cancer pain.
Self-trauma	Licking at an area (e.g., joint with osteoarthritis, bone with primary bone cancer, the abdomen with intraabdominal cancer) can indicate pain; scratching can indicate pain (e.g., scratching at cutaneous tumors, scratching and biting at the flank with prostatic or colonic neoplasia).
Urinary and bowel elimination	Failure to use litter box (cats); urinating and defecating inside (dogs).
Vocalization	Vocalization is rare in response to chronic pain in dogs and cats; however, owners of dogs will often report frequent odd noises (whining, grunting) associated with cancer pain. Occasionally, cats will hiss, utter spontaneous plaintive meows, or purr in association with cancer pain

Follow-up is important, and the assessment of activity and behavioral parameters can be evaluated over the telephone.

Principles of Alleviation of Cancer Pain

Pharmacologic Therapy

Drugs are the mainstay of cancer pain management, although nondrug adjunctive therapies are becoming recognized as increasingly important. The World Health Organization (WHO) has outlined a general approach to the management of cancer pain based on the use of the following groups of analgesics:

- Nonopioid analgesics (e.g., nonsteroidal antiinflammatory drugs [NSAIDs], acetaminophen)
- Weak opioid drugs (e.g., codeine)
- Strong opioid drugs (e.g., morphine)
- Adjuvant drugs (e.g., corticosteroids, tricyclic antidepressants, anticonvulsants, *N*-methyl D-aspartate [NMDA] antagonists).

The general approach of the WHO ladder is a three-step hierarchy. Initially, pain is treated with a nonopioid (usually an NSAID), ± an adjuvant drug. The next two stages add on a "weak" opioid, then a "strong" opioid. There are several problems with this approach. First, it is naïve because our current understanding of pain indicates that drugs are not "strong" and "weak" but rather "appropriate" and "less appropriate." Furthermore, there is little information from human medicine and virtually none from veterinary medicine on which drugs are most effective for particular types of cancer pain. It may well be that "third-tier" drugs might be most effective for a particular condition and therefore used upfront.

The second problem is that the approach is not well suited to patients that present initially with significant-to-severe pain. Many veterinary cancer patients present at an advanced stage of disease and thus are already in moderate-to-severe pain. Once pain has been present for a period of time, changes take place in the central nervous system (CNS) that alter the way pain signals are processed. A better understanding of this is helped by understanding the classification of cancer pain.

Classification of Cancer Pain

Pain is a multifactorial experience with sensory (the sensation), affective/emotional (how it makes the subject feel), and functional (can the subject still perform particular functions) components. It can result from obvious causes (e.g., ulcerated skin tumor) and last an expected time. However, in many cases (e.g., postamputation pain) the pain persists after the original painful cancer has been removed or the surgical wound appears to be healed. In the past, pain has often been categorized as acute or chronic based solely on duration—the latter arbitrarily being pain that lasts more than 3 to 6 months. However, it is now accepted that this may not be a helpful classification. It has been suggested that the terms *adaptive* and *maladaptive* be adopted; adaptive infers a normal response to tissue damage and involves an inflammatory component (e.g., a surgical incision) and is reversible over an expected, relatively short time. Maladaptive pain results from changes in the spinal cord and brain that result in abnormal sensory processing and is usually persistent. Maladaptive pain can result from poorly treated adaptive pain, and maladaptive pain can occur quickly in some circumstances. A key feature of maladaptive pain is central sensitization—changes in the CNS (anywhere from the dorsal root ganglion rostrally) that are likely initiated by cellular wind-up and result in amplification and facilitation of nociceptive signal generation and transmission. *Until proved otherwise, cancer pain should be considered maladaptive, with both peripheral and central changes in the pain processing system contributing to the pain, in addition to noxious input from the cancer or pathologic area.*

Ideally, pain would be classified by the underlying mechanism, for example, inflammatory or neuropathic. However, many diseases are associated with overlapping "forms" of pain. Taken one step further, pain occurring in different diseases or conditions would be further classified by the underlying mechanisms in that particular disease and even patient. This could be referred to as the *neurobiologic signature* of pain in a particular disease or patient. Knowing this would better guide the practitioner in the choice of treatment. For example, a diagnosis of "cancer" pain is not very helpful since the cause could be mechanical compression of a nerve, inflammation from tissue necrosis, mechanical distension of an organ, neuropathic pain, or a combination of these. However, a diagnosis of "transitional cell carcinoma pain of the bladder," with the associated knowledge of the upregulation of peripheral sodium channel (e.g., NaV1.7) and acid-sensing ion channel (ASIC) receptors and nerve growth factor and central glial cell activity and cyclooxygenase-2 (COX-2) enzyme, is far more informative in terms of guiding clinical treatment. Without this information, treatment is empiric and it may be better termed "hit or miss."

Early intervention is recommended to limit cellular wind-up and prevent central sensitization. In patients experiencing long-lasting, persistent pain, as is the case with many types of cancer, changes within the peripheral and CNS may occur. These changes (peripheral or central sensitization) may contribute to the further development of pain, separate from the initial inciting cause and should be considered in patients with pain that is unresponsive to first-line or conventional analgesics. Pain syndromes commonly associated with sensitization include prolonged pain or pain experienced outside of the immediate area that is affected, hyperalgesia (increased sensitivity to noxious stimuli), and allodynia (pain after nonnoxious stimuli). The author has found altered sensory processing states to be associated with long-standing osteoarthritis-associated pain, and it is likely many cancers are associated with the same changes.

At the current time, with limited information as to what the "ideal" therapies are for individual cancer pains, the most important aspect to remember in the treatment of cancer pain is that for the majority of situations, *multimodal therapy* (i.e., concurrent use of more than one class of drug) *is required for successful alleviation of the pain.*

A general outline to approaching cancer pain is given in Figure 15-1. This figure can be used in combination with Tables 15-4 and 15-5. There are many different scenarios that the clinician may face when dealing with cancer pain, and this figure and these tables are only guides. The term *wind-down therapy* refers to admitting refractory pain patients into the hospital and treating them with multiple intravenous (IV) analgesic medications in the hope that the pain can be controlled, making it easier to subsequently manage the pain at home.

Drugs and Strategies Used for Management of Pain in Cancer Patients

The drugs that can be used for chronic cancer pain management are outlined in Tables 15-4 and 15-5. The following notes are not a comprehensive appraisal of each class of drug but are suggestions for their use for cancer pain.

Nonsteroidal Antiinflammatory Drugs

NSAIDs have been the mainstay of therapy for chronic pain, especially in osteoarthritis, and they are an excellent first line of treatment in cancer pain. There are several excellent reviews on NSAID use in small animals, and the reader is referred to these.[50-54] The choice of NSAIDs available can be bewildering, but a few key points are as follows:

- On a population basis, all NSAIDs are probably equally efficacious in relieving pain, but for a given patient, one drug is often more effective than another.
- Gastrointestinal side effects associated with NSAID use appear to be more common with drugs that preferentially block COX-1 over COX-2.
- There is no difference in renal toxicity between COX-1 selective drugs and COX-2 selective drugs.
- Liver toxicity can occur with any NSAID.
- There are no completely safe NSAIDs, but the approved NSAIDs are significantly safer than the older nonapproved NSAIDs.
- Longer term or continuous NSAID use appears to be more effective than short-term or reactive use,[52] but in relatively stable disease states, gradual dose reduction may be possible while maintaining efficacy.[55]

There are no licensed NSAIDs for long-term administration in cats other than meloxicam, which is approved in the European Union for long-term treatment of musculoskeletal pain. However, a number of these compounds can probably be used safely (see Table 15-5). The key to safe chronic NSAID administration in cats is the use of the smallest effective dose and avoiding use or using decreased doses in cats with renal disease. Choosing drugs with short half-lives is also considered important by the author.

The patient on NSAIDs should be monitored for toxicity by informing the owner of potential toxicity and what signs to watch for (lethargy, depression, vomiting, melena, increased water ingestion), as well as through the regular evaluation of blood work (and urinalysis) to evaluate renal and liver function. A baseline should be obtained when therapy is initiated and parameters monitored on a regular basis thereafter. The author repeats evaluations after 2 to 4 weeks and then at 1- to 4-month intervals as dictated by the individual patient and client.

If pain relief with NSAIDs is inadequate, oral opioid medications such as morphine or tramadol can be administered (see later). Acetaminophen or acetaminophen/codeine combinations can often be used in conjunction with NSAIDs. Transdermal fentanyl can also be used. Fentanyl, morphine, or tramadol can be used for dogs that cannot be given NSAIDs. Other agents that are used to treat chronic pain include: amantadine, an NMDA antagonist; anticonvulsants such as gabapentin; and tricyclic antidepressants such as amitriptyline. These can all be combined with NSAIDs, although we do not know the full extent of side effects. Readers are cautioned that they should not assume that combinations of different adjunctive drugs are without side effects—quite the contrary, there is much to be learned about potential adverse interactions, especially in cancer patients that may be on other therapies.

Acetaminophen

Acetaminophen is a nonacidic NSAID; many authorities do not consider it an NSAID as it probably acts by somewhat different mechanisms.[56] With any chronic pain, there are always CNS changes, so for what seems a "peripheral" problem such as many cancers, centrally acting analgesics can be very effective. *Although highly toxic in the cat, even in small quantities, it can be effectively used in dogs for pain control in the acute setting.*[57,58] No studies of

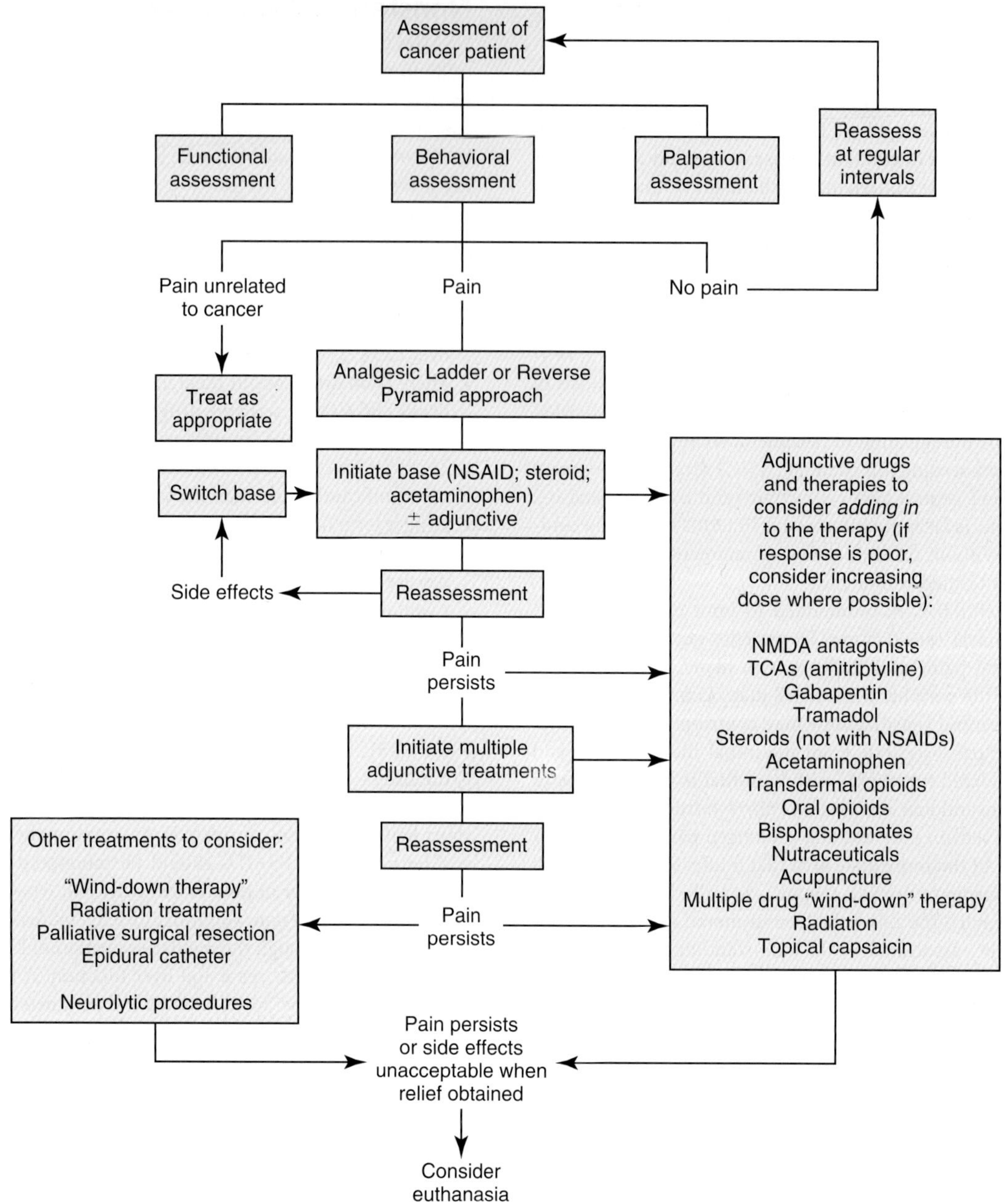

FIGURE 15-1 Outline to approaching cancer pain.

toxicity in dogs have been done, but if toxicity is seen, it will probably affect the liver; thus the drug, in common with all NSAIDs and opioids, should be used cautiously in dogs with liver dysfunction. It can be used on its own or in a preparation combined with codeine and is initially dosed at about 10 to 15 mg/kg twice a day (bid). The author often uses it as the first-line analgesic therapy in dogs with renal compromise in which NSAIDs cannot be used or in dogs that appear to be otherwise intolerant to NSAIDs (e.g., vomiting or gastrointestinal ulceration).

Opioids

Opioids can be an effective part of the management of cancer pain, particularly when used as part of a multimodal approach (i.e., including NSAIDs or adjunctive analgesics). Side effects of opioids include diarrhea, vomiting, sedation, and constipation with long-term use. It is often constipation and occasionally the sedation that owners object to most as a side effect in their pet. Oral morphine, transdermal fentanyl, oral butorphanol, sublingual buprenorphine (cats only), and oral codeine are used most often for the alleviation of chronic cancer pain. None of these drugs has been fully evaluated for clinical toxicity when administered long term nor for efficacy against chronic cancer pain. Dosing must be done on an individual basis, and adjustment of the dose to produce effective analgesia without undesirable side effects requires interaction and communication with clients. However, despite these suggestions, recent evidence has indicated that oral opioids may not reach effective plasma concentrations in dogs when dosed at the currently recommended levels.[59-62]

There is currently no information on the long-term use of oral opioids for chronic pain in the cat. There appears to be individual

TABLE 15-4 Suggested Doses of Analgesics that May Be Used for the Alleviation of Chronic Cancer Pain in the Dog

DRUG	DOSE FOR DOGS	COMMENTS
Paracetamol (acetaminophen)	10-15 mg/kg PO q12 hrs	Associated with fewer GI side effects than regular NSAIDs and has not been noted to be associated with renal toxicity. Toxicity has, however, not been evaluated clinically in dogs. Can be combined with regular NSAIDs in severe cancer pain, but this combination has not been evaluated for toxicity.
Paracetamol (acetaminophen) + codeine (30 or 60 mg)	10-15 mg/kg of acetaminophen	Sedation can be seen as a side effect with doses at or above 2 mg/kg codeine.
Amantadine	4.0-5.0 mg/kg PO q24 hrs	Loose stools and excess GI gas can be seen at higher doses for a few days. Should not be combined with drugs such as selegiline or sertraline until more is known about drug interactions. Should not be used in seizure patients or patients in heart failure.
Amitriptyline	0.5-2.0 mg/kg PO q24 hrs	Has not been evaluated for clinical toxicity in the dog. Should be used cautiously in combination with tramadol.
Butorphanol	0.2-0.5 mg/kg PO up to q8 hrs	May produce sedation at higher doses. Not a very predictable analgesic, especially in the dog, and best when used in combination with other analgesics (e.g., NSAIDs).
Codeine	0.5-2.0 mg/kg PO q8-12 hrs	Sedation can be seen at higher doses. Like all oral opioids, it is subject to significant first-pass effect at the liver, likely limiting its analgesic effect.
Fentanyl, transdermal	2-5 mcg/kg/hr	Can be very useful in the short-term control of cancer pain. For long-term therapy, usefulness is limited due to need to change the patch every 4 to 7 days.
Gabapentin	3-10 mg/kg PO q6-12 hrs	Has not been evaluated in dogs as an analgesic. The most likely side effect is sedation.
Glucosamine and chondroitin sulfate	13-15 mg/kg chondroitin sulfate PO q24 hrs	Can be used in a variety of cancer pains due to its mild antiinflammatory and analgesic effects.
Morphine, liquid	0.2-0.5 mg/kg PO q 6-8 hrs	Can be useful for dosing smaller dogs where the morphine tablets are not suitable. Sedation and particularly constipation are side effects that are seen as the dose is increased. Like all oral opioids, it is subject to significant first-pass effect at the liver, likely limiting its analgesic effect.
Morphine, sustained release	0.5-3.0 mg/kg PO q 8-12 hrs	Doses higher than 0.5-1.0 mg/kg are often associated with unacceptable constipation according to owners, so suggest using 0.5 mg/kg several times a day. Like all oral opioids, it is subject to significant first-pass effect at the liver, likely limiting its analgesic effect.
Pamidronate	1-1.5 mg/kg slowly IV diluted in 4 mL/kg normal saline, administered over 2 hrs; repeat every 4-6 weeks	Inhibits osteoclast activity and thus only provides analgesia in cases suffering from a primary or metastatic bone tumor that is causing osteolysis. Effect may be delayed days-weeks.
Prednisolone	0.25-1 mg/kg PO q12-24 hrs; taper to q48 hrs if possible after 14 days	Do NOT use concurrently with NSAIDs. Can be particularly useful in providing analgesia when there is a significant inflammatory component associated with the tumor and for CNS or nerve tumors.
Tramadol	4-5 mg/kg PO q6-12 hrs	This drug has not been evaluated for efficacy or toxicity in dogs.

PO, By mouth; *GI,* gastrointestinal; *NSAIDs,* nonsteroidal antiinflammatories; *IV,* intravenous.

None of these drugs have been evaluated for efficacy in the treatment of cancer pain.

None of these drugs are approved or licensed for use in chronic cancer pain. The NSAIDs have not been included in this table. NSAIDs should be used as a first line of pain relief if it is clinically appropriate to use them and should be used at their approved dose.

The doses given come from the author's experience and the experience of others working in the area of clinical cancer pain control.

TABLE 15-5 Suggested Doses of Analgesics that May Be Used for the Alleviation of Chronic Cancer Pain in the Cat

DRUG	CAT DOSE (MG/KG)	NOTES
Acetaminophen (Paracetamol)	**Contraindicated**	Small doses rapidly cause death in cats.
Amantadine	3.0-5.0 mg/kg PO q24 hrs	This drug has not been evaluated for toxicity but is well tolerated in dogs and humans, with occasional side effects of agitation and GI irritation. May be a useful addition to NSAIDs in the treatment of chronic cancer pain conditions. Amantadine powder can be purchased and formulated into appropriately sized capsules. The kinetics have recently been evaluated in cats.
Amitriptyline	0.5-2.0 mg/kg PO q24 hrs	This drug appears to be well tolerated for up to 12 months of daily administration. May be a useful addition to NSAIDs for treatment of chronic pain conditions.
Aspirin	10 mg/kg PO q48 hrs	Can cause significant GI ulceration.
Buprenorphine	0.01-0.02 mg/kg SL q8-12 hrs	SL route is not resented by cats and may be a good way to provide postoperative analgesia at home. Feedback from owners indicates that after 2-3 days dosing at this dose, anorexia develops. Smaller doses (5-10 μg/kg) may be more appropriate for "long-term" administration, especially in combination with other drugs.
Butorphanol	0.2-1.0 mg/kg PO q6 hrs	One study suggests using oral form after surgery may be beneficial. Generally considered to be a poor analgesic in cats except for visceral pain; however, the author has found it to be useful as part of a multimodal approach to cancer pain therapy.
Carprofen	Not enough data to enable recommendations for long-term administration.	—
Etodolac	Not recommended.	—
Firocoxib	—	Has not been reported in clinical cases, but it has a half-life of 8-12 hours in the cat, and at 3 mg/kg provided antipyretic effects in a pyrexia model.
Flunixin meglumine	1 mg/kg PO daily for 7 days	Daily dosing for 7 days results in increased rate of metabolism of the drug but a rise in liver enzymes, suggesting liver toxicity *may* be a problem with prolonged dosing.
Gabapentin	10 mg/kg q12 hrs	Appears to be particularly effective in chronic pain in cats where an increase in sensitivity has occurred, or where the pain appears to be excessive in comparison to the lesion present.
Glucosamine/chondroitin sulphate combinations	Approximately 15 mg/kg chondroitin sulphate PO q12-24 hrs	May be associated with mild analgesic effects.
Glucosamine/chondroitin sulphate combination with avocado/soya extracts	Labelled dose	May be associated with mild analgesic effects.
Ketoprofen	1 mg/kg PO q24 hrs	Probably well tolerated as pulse therapy for chronic pain, with a few days "rest" between treatments of approximately 5 days. Has also been used by some at 1 mg/kg every 3 days long term. Another approach has been to use 0.5 mg/kg daily for 5 days (weekdays) followed by no drug over the weekend and repeated.

TABLE 15-5 Suggested Doses of Analgesics that May Be Used for the Alleviation of Chronic Cancer Pain in the Cat (continued)

DRUG	CAT DOSE (MG/KG)	NOTES
Meloxicam	0.01 mg/kg PO on day 1, followed by 0.05 mg/kg PO daily for 4 days, then 0.05 mg/kg every other day thereafter. (Approval in the European Union at 0.05mg/kg daily indefinitely for musculoskeletal pain.)	Well received by cats due to its formulation as a honey syrup. Also, the drop formulation makes it very easy to gradually and accurately decrease the dose. A decreasing regimen has not been evaluated for efficacy in cats but has been found to be successful in dogs. Meloxicam should be dosed accurately using syringes.
Morphine (oral liquid)	0.2-0.5 mg/kg PO tid-qid	Best compounded into a palatable, flavored syrup; however, cats usually resent this medication. Morphine may not be as effective in cats as it is in dogs.
Morphine (oral sustained release)	Tablets too large for dosing cats.	—
Piroxicam	1 mg/cat PO daily for a maximum of 7 days. If longer term medication is considered, suggest every other day dosing.	Daily dosing for 7 days results in a slight increase in the half-life.
Prednisolone	0.5-1.0 mg/kg PO q24 hrs	Can be very effective. **NOT to be combined with concurrent NSAID administration.**
Polysulfated glycosaminoglycans (PSGAGs; Adequan)	5 mg/kg SQ twice weekly for 4 weeks; then once weekly for 4 weeks; then once monthly (other suggested regimens call for once weekly injections for 4 weeks, then once monthly).	There is no evidence-based medicine that it provides any analgesic effect, but anecdotal information suggests improvement can be seen after a few injections.
Robenacoxib	1-2 mg/kg q24 hrs	Has varying approvals in different parts of the world (approved for up to 11 days administration in Switzerland). First NSAID that is a COX-2 inhibitor, has a short half-life, and demonstrates tissue selectivity.
Tepoxalin	5-10 mg/kg q24 hrs	The author has used this successfully long-term in cats, likely due to its short half-life (5 hours) and true dual inhibition characteristics.
Tolfenamic acid	4 mg/kg PO q24 hrs for 3 days maximum	Has not been evaluated for chronic pain, but recent objective measurements demonstrate analgesia in the cat when administered perioperatively.
Tramadol	1-2 mg/kg once to twice daily	Main problem is dosing cats—the tablets are very bitter and aversive to cats.
Transdermal fentanyl patch	2-5 μg/kg/hrs	The patches may provide 5-7 days of analgesia in some cases and should be left on for longer than 3 days. Following removal, the decay in plasma levels following patch removal is slow.
Vedaprofen	0.5 mg/kg q 24 hrs for 3 days	Has not been evaluated for chronic pain but was evaluated for controlling pyrexia in upper respiratory infection, and for controlling postoperative pain following ovariohysterectomy.

PO, By mouth; *GI,* gastrointestinal; *NSAIDs,* nonsteroidal antiinflammatories; *SL,* sublingual; *SQ,* subcutaneous; *tid,* three times a day; *qid,* four times a day; *COX-2,* cyclooxygenase-2.

None of the drugs have been evaluated for efficacy in the treatment of cancer pain.

None of these drugs are approved or licensed for use in chronic cancer pain. Some drugs are approved for inflammatory or painful conditions in the cat in certain countries, and doses for the control of cancer pain are extrapolated from these. The doses given come from the author's experience and the experience of others working in the area of clinical cancer pain control.

variation in the level of analgesia obtained with certain opioids, especially morphine and butorphanol, in the acute setting.[63,64] Buprenorphine appears to produce predictable analgesia when given sublingually[65] and is well accepted by most cats. The small volume required (max 0.066 mL/kg [20 μg/kg]) makes administration simple. Based on clinical feedback from owners, this is an acceptable technique for home use. Inappetence can occur after several days of treatment and sometimes lower doses (5 to 10 μg/kg) can overcome this problem. When administered concurrently with other drugs, less frequent dosing is often required.[65]

N-Methyl D-Aspartate Antagonists

The NMDA receptor appears to be central to the induction and maintenance of central sensitization,[66-68] and the use of NMDA receptor antagonists would appear to offer benefit where central sensitization has become established (i.e., especially chronic pain). Ketamine, tiletamine, dextromethorphan, and amantadine possess NMDA antagonist properties, among other actions.

Ketamine is not obviously useful for the management of chronic pain due to the formulation available and the tendency for dysphoric side effects even at low doses. However, oral ketamine has not been evaluated in dogs or cats for long-term administration. Intraoperative microdose IV ketamine appears to provide beneficial effects for a variety of oncology surgical procedures, including limb amputations,[69] and this may decrease the incidence of chronic pain later. Other reports suggest a benefit of using ketamine perioperatively in low doses.[70] When used in this manner, ketamine should be administered as a bolus (0.5 mg/kg IV) followed by an infusion (10 μg/kg/min) prior to and during surgical stimulation. A lower infusion rate (2 μg/kg/min) may be beneficial for the first 24 hours postoperatively and an even lower rate (1 μg/kg/min) for the next 24 hours. In the absence of an infusion pump, ketamine can be mixed in a bag of crystalloid solutions for administration during anesthesia. Using anesthesia fluid administration rates of 10 mL/kg/hr, 60 mg (0.6 mL) of ketamine should be added to a 1-liter bag of crystalloid fluids to deliver ketamine at 10 μg/kg/min.

The active metabolite of dextromethorphan may not be produced in dogs, probably negating its use in the species for chronic pain.[61]

Amantadine has been used for the treatment of neuropathic pain in humans,[71] and one report suggests a benefit of adding amantadine to an NSAID in dogs that do not get complete relief from the NSAID alone.[72] Suggested dosages are given in Tables 15-4 and 15-5. The toxic side effects have been evaluated in the dog (but not the cat), and the dosages suggested are considered safe.[73] Amantadine should be avoided in patients with congestive heart failure, history of seizure, or those on selegiline, sertraline, or tricyclic antidepressants.

Combination Analgesics

Tramadol is a synthetic derivative of codeine and is classified as an opioidergic/monoaminergic drug.[74,75] It has been found to be effective in the alleviation of pain associated with osteoarthritis in humans. Tramadol's analgesic efficacy is a result of complex interactions between opiate, adrenergic, and serotonin receptor systems. Hepatic demethylation of tramadol produces the active metabolite, *O*-desmethyltramadol (M1). The different metabolites interact with different receptors; thus efficacy in different species is likely to depend on the metabolic characteristics in the particular species. Initial work in dogs suggested that tramadol was absorbed sufficiently, producing levels that would theoretically provide analgesia.[76] However, recently there has been some discussion about the actual amounts of the M1 metabolite that are formed in dogs, and the pharmacokinetics of tramadol does not favor an analgesic effect.[77-81] There is no published evidence of efficacy for canine pain.

Little is known about the side effects of tramadol in dogs, and almost nothing is known about the side effects seen when tramadol is combined with other drugs in human or canine medicine. In human medicine, a recent study found that for patients hospitalized for peptic ulcer treatment, tramadol use prior to admission was associated with just as high a risk of mortality as was NSAID use prior to admission. Additionally, mortality was 2.02- and 1.41-fold higher in these groups of patients, respectively, than in patients who used neither tramadol nor NSAIDs.[82] A recent study evaluating the analgesic effects of various doses of rofecoxib and tramadol alone and in combination found that the most analgesic combination of tramadol and rofecoxib produced gastric injury in rats that was more severe than with rofecoxib or tramadol alone.[83] Tramadol is metabolized differently in the cat[84,85] and appears to have clinical efficacy when administered intravenously perioperatively[86] and has shown antinociceptive activity when administered orally in an experimental setting.[87]

The dosages given in Tables 15-4 and 15-5 are for the regular (not prolonged release) form of the drug. It has not been thoroughly evaluated for toxicity in the dog or cat.

Anticonvulsant Drugs

Many anticonvulsants such as carbamazepine, phenytoin, baclofen, and more recently gabapentin have been used to treat chronic pain, including neuropathic pain in humans, as well as chemotherapy-induced peripheral neuropathies. Gabapentin and the more recently introduced pregabalin appear to be among the most effective drugs available for neuropathic pain in humans. While the exact mechanism of action of these drugs is unclear, one potential mode by which they exert their analgesic effect is by binding to the α_2-δ protein subunit of voltage-gated calcium channels, thereby reducing excitatory neurotransmitter release through channel modulation or channel trafficking. Although there is considerable information on gabapentin disposition in dogs[88,89] and some information on its use as an anticonvulsant in dogs,[90] there is as yet no information on its use for the control of chronic or long-term pain. However, a recent small study suggested no beneficial effect of perioperative gabapentin.[91] Information on the kinetics of gabapentin in cats has become available,[92] and one study found a lack of thermal antinociception.[93] There are no scientific publications demonstrating its efficacy for long-term pain in this species. While the indications for gabapentin (and pregabalin) are presently unclear in veterinary patients, they do appear to be useful for cancer pain in some patients and are probably particularly effective in cancers that have some neurogenic or nerve destruction component. Suggested dosages are in Tables 15-4 and 15-5.

Tricyclic Antidepressants

Tricyclic antidepressants have been used for many years for the treatment of chronic pain syndromes in people and are becoming widely used for the modulation of behavioral disorders in animals. Within the CNS, there are descending inhibitory serotonergic and noradrenergic pathways that reduce pain transmission in the spinal cord. Tricyclic antidepressants such as amitriptyline, clomipramine, fluoxetine, imipramine, maprotiline, and paroxetine primarily inhibit the reuptake of various monoamines (serotonin for clomipramine, fluoxetine, and paroxetine; noradrenaline for imipramine, amitriptyline, and maprotiline). Tricyclic antidepressants can also interact directly with 5-hydroxytryptamine (5-HT) and peripheral noradrenergic receptors and may also contribute other actions such as voltage-gated sodium channel blockade and reduction in peripheral prostaglandin E_2 (PGE_2)-like activity or tumor necrosis factor (TNF) production. However, in human medicine, there is a relative lack of controlled, clinical trials specifically evaluating the efficacy of antidepressants in treating cancer pain,[94] with the exception of two studies demonstrating a lack of efficacy in the treatment of chemotherapy-induced peripheral neuropathy.[95,96] If there are beneficial effects, it could be from modulation of pain or improvement in mood or feeling.

The tricyclic antidepressant amitriptyline appears to be effective in the cat for pain alleviation in interstitial cystitis,[97] and many practitioners are reporting efficacy in other chronically painful conditions in the cat, including osteoarthritis. Amitriptyline has been used daily for periods up to 1 year for interstitial cystitis, and few side effects are reported. The author has also used amitriptyline in the cat for cancer pain with some encouraging results. It should probably not be used concurrently with other drugs that modify the serotonergic system such as amantadine or tramadol until more is known about drug interactions.

Sodium Channel Blockade

Alterations in the level of expression, cellular localization, and distribution of sodium channels are seen in many pain states. These aberrantly expressed sodium channels result in hyperexcitability and ectopic activity in peripheral and central nerves that encode nociceptive information. Low doses of lidocaine and other sodium-channel blockers readily block these aberrantly expressed sodium channels, producing pain relief. Low-dose IV lidocaine has proven as effective as other commonly used medications for treatment of neuropathic pain in humans,[98] and the author uses such an approach to "downregulate" central sensitization in veterinary cancer patients. There is increasing interest in the use of transdermal lidocaine patches for treatment of cancer pain.[99] Much of this interest revolves around using the patch to administer a low systemic level of lidocaine that blocks the aberrantly expressed sodium channels. Studies have been performed evaluating the kinetics of lidocaine absorbed from patches applied to dogs and cats.[100-102] Peak plasma concentrations of lidocaine were obtained between 10 and 24 hours postapplication in dogs and at 65 hours postapplication in cats. The results of these studies indicate that, similar to humans, systemic absorption of lidocaine from the patch is minimal. Peak plasma concentrations were over 100 times below the level reported to induce neurologic signs and 10 times below the level reported to result in myocardial depression in dogs and 25 times lower than that observed following an IV injection of lidocaine (2 mg/kg) in cats. Potential systemic toxicity associated with lidocaine administration, including bradycardia, hypotension, cardiac arrest, muscle or facial twitching, tremors, seizures, nausea, and vomiting, were not noted in any study. Dosing guidelines have been suggested,[103] although to date there have been no published reports evaluating the analgesic efficacy of lidocaine patches in veterinary cancer patients, but the technique holds promise.

Steroids

Steroids have a mild analgesic action, can produce a state of euphoria, and are often used for these reasons to palliate cancer and cancer pain in cats and dogs. They should not be used concurrently with NSAIDs because the risk of side effects (especially gastrointestinal) is increased dramatically.

Bisphosphonates

Malignant bone disease creates a unique pain state, with a neurobiologic signature distinct from that of inflammatory and neuropathic pain.[104-106] Bone cancer–related pain is thought to be initiated and perpetuated by dysregulated osteoclast activity and activation of nociceptors by prostaglandins, cytokines, and H^+ ions. Therapies that block osteoclast activity not only have the potential to markedly reduce bone pain but may also mitigate other skeletal complications associated with neoplastic conditions, including pathologic fractures and hypercalcemia of malignancy. Bisphosphonates are synthetic analogs of pyrophosphate whose primary effect is to inhibit osteoclast activity. Bisphosphonates accumulate in bone, and following osteoclast-mediated bone resorption, bisphosphonates are released and disrupt cellular functions, resulting in osteoclast death. Oral absorption of bisphosphonates tends to be poor, and IV dosing is the preferred route of administration. Adverse effects include nephrotoxicity, electrolyte abnormalities, and acute-phase reactions.[107,108] In addition to the inhibitory effects of bisphosphonates on osteoclasts, reports suggest that they may also exert direct effects on cancer cells, including canine OSA and fibrosarcoma lines.[109,110] Studies have found beneficial effects of IV pamidronate for the treatment of malignant osteolysis associated with primary and secondary bone neoplasms.[10,11,108,111] These studies have also suggested analgesic effects; however, the positive assessments have been based on subjective evaluations. In a placebo-controlled study, there was no difference in the pain relief between placebo and bisphosphonates using either subjective or objective (force plate) evaluations.[9] Despite these results, it is believed that some patients attain pain relief from bisphosphonate administration, and a better and validated means of assessing cancer pain may help elucidate the degree of pain relief that can be achieved. Pamidronate may be administered at a dose of 1 to 2 mg/kg as a 2 to 4 hour infusion (diluted in saline) and repeated at 3 to 5 week intervals. Other examples of a bisphosphonate that can be used in dogs are clodronate, alendronate, and zoledronate.[111-113]

Neuronal Ablation or Exhaustion Therapy

Several new approaches to pain treatment revolve around the use of mechanisms to destroy or exhaust neurons involved in pain transmission. One approach is to use targeted neurotoxins to cause neuronal death.[114] An example of this is the combination of a neurotoxin (saponin) to substance P. Substance P, when administered, binds to the neurokinin receptor (NKR), and the conjugate is internalized (a normal phenomenon of the receptor-ligand interaction), resulting in cell death due to the neurotoxin.[115,116] Because sensory neurons are rich in NKRs, if the conjugate is targeted appropriately (e.g., given intrathecally), sensory neurons are killed. Basic science studies suggest that in models of chronic pain, general sensory function is left intact, whereas hyperalgesia associated with chronic pain is decreased. Some toxicity work has been performed in dogs,[117] and clinical trials in dogs with naturally occurring bone OSA are underway, with these being used as a model of human OSA pain. Another approach uses the transient receptor potential channel, vanilloid subfamily member 1 (TRPV1) to target neurons involved in pain. When drugs such as capsaicin and resiniferatoxin bind to TRPV1, the resulting calcium influx that is initiated results in an inability of the neuron to function. If the activation of TRPV1 occurs for long enough or is intense enough, the resulting calcium influx can cause the neurons to degenerate and undergo apoptosis.

Capsaicin is used in humans for neuropathic pain, and resiniferatoxin has been evaluated in dogs with naturally occurring bone cancer pain in which it provided prolonged pain relief, despite significant hemodynamic effects.[5]

Radiation Therapy

Radiation therapy is considered to palliate pain in canine OSA, although the evidence is largely anecdotal. A 0-7-21 palliative regimen, using 8 or 10 Gy fractions, has been reported to result in pain relief lasting about 70 days.[4,118] Additionally, two 8 Gy fractions over 2 consecutive days was reported to result in pain relief for a duration of 67 days.[13] The difficulty in interpreting the value of radiation therapy for pain relief in these studies is the lack of controls or objective measures. Indeed, the natural course of pain and lameness in dogs with appendicular OSA has not been determined. One study evaluating objective measure of limb use in dogs with OSA undergoing radiation therapy found no significant changes in kinetic parameters after one 8-Gy dose of radiation.[2]

Samarium is a radioisotope that has been evaluated for use in dogs.[119] Although the use of samarium Sm153 lexidronam in veterinary medicine is still limited, results of a noncontrolled clinical study with subjective assessments suggested improvement in lameness scores in 63% of dogs, suggesting that this therapy may be useful in the palliation of pain in dogs with bone tumors in which curative-intent treatment is not pursued.[3]

Acupuncture

Acupuncture can be provided through simple needle placement or by needle placement combined with electrical stimulation (of high or low frequency, although most types of pain respond to low-frequency stimulation). Results of a study in normal experimental dogs demonstrated a weak analgesic effect of electroacupuncture in anesthetized patients as evaluated by a reduction in the minimum alveolar concentration (MAC) of inhaled anesthetic agent.[120] Recent data utilizing a rodent model suggest that electroacupuncture may have beneficial effects in treatment of pain associated with bone cancer.[121,122] As yet, there is no evidence that acupuncture provides pain relief in veterinary patients.

The Future: Toward a Mechanistic Understanding of Cancer Pain

Over the last few years, it has become evident that the pain transmission system is plastic (i.e., it alters in response to inputs). This plasticity results in a unique neurobiologic signature within the CNS and peripheral nervous system for each painful disease. Understanding the individual neurobiologic signatures for different disease processes should allow novel, targeted, and more effective treatments to be established.[123] This approach should also allow for a more informed choice to be made regarding which of the currently available drugs might be most effective.

The *first relevant model* of cancer pain has been established in rats—an OSA model.[124] Prior to this model, evaluation of mechanisms and treatments were undertaken in chronic pain models such as sciatic nerve ligation or injection of chronic irritants—models that did not involve cancer. The introduction of clinically relevant cancer pain models is allowing tremendous progress to be made in the translation to effective human cancer pain treatment.[104] It is likely that spontaneous cancer in veterinary species will play a significant role in the future in the development of new analgesic approaches for humans, with an obvious benefit to canine and feline patients. Indeed, we are starting to see this with an exciting example being the evaluation of resiniferatoxin in dogs with bone cancer.[5]

REFERENCES

1. Yoxall AT: Pain in small animals—its recognition and control, *J Small Anim Pract* 19:423–438, 1978.
2. Weinstein JI, Payne S, Poulson JM, et al: Use of force plate analysis to evaluate the efficacy of external beam radiation to alleviate osteosarcoma pain, *Vet Radiol Ultrasound* 50:673–678, 2009.
3. Barnard SM, Zuber RM, Moore AS: Samarium Sm 153 lexidronam for the palliative treatment of dogs with primary bone tumors: 35 cases (1999-2005), *J Am Vet Med Assoc* 230:1877–1881, 2007.
4. Bateman KE, Catton PA, Pennock PW, et al: 0-7-21 radiation therapy for the palliation of advanced cancer in dogs, *J Vet Intern Med* 8:394–399, 1994.
5. Brown DC, Iadarola MJ, Perkowski SZ, et al: Physiologic and antinociceptive effects of intrathecal resiniferatoxin in a canine bone cancer model, *Anesthesiology* 103:1052–1059, 2005.
6. Carsten RE, Hellyer PW, Bachand AM, et al: Correlations between acute radiation scores and pain scores in canine radiation patients with cancer of the forelimb, *Vet Anaesth Analg* 35:355–362, 2008.
7. Coomer A, Farese J, Milner R, et al: Radiation therapy for canine appendicular osteosarcoma, *Vet Comp Oncol* 7:15–27, 2009.
8. Davis KM, Hardie EM, Lascelles BD, et al: Feline fibrosarcoma: perioperative management, *Compend Contin Educ Vet* 29:712–714, 716–720, 722–729 passim, 2007.
9. Fan TM, Charney SC, de Lorimier LP, et al: Double-blind placebo-controlled trial of adjuvant pamidronate with palliative radiotherapy and intravenous doxorubicin for canine appendicular osteosarcoma bone pain, *J Vet Intern Med* 23:152–160, 2009.
10. Fan TM, de Lorimier LP, Charney SC, et al: Evaluation of intravenous pamidronate administration in 33 cancer-bearing dogs with primary or secondary bone involvement, *J Vet Intern Med* 19:74–80, 2005.
11. Fan TM, de Lorimier LP, O'Dell-Anderson K, et al: Single-agent pamidronate for palliative therapy of canine appendicular osteosarcoma bone pain, *J Vet Intern Med* 21:431–439, 2007.
12. Karai L, Brown DC, Mannes AJ, et al: Deletion of vanilloid receptor 1-expressing primary afferent neurons for pain control, *J Clin Invest* 113:1344–1352, 2004.
13. Knapp-Hoch HM, Fidel JL, Sellon RK, et al: An expedited palliative radiation protocol for lytic or proliferative lesions of appendicular bone in dogs, *J Am Anim Hosp Assoc* 45:24–32, 2009.
14. Mueller F, Poirier V, Melzer K, et al: Palliative radiotherapy with electrons of appendicular osteosarcoma in 54 dogs, *IN VIVO* 19:713–716, 2005.
15. Fan TM, Barger AM, Fredrickson RL, et al: Investigating CXCR4 expression in canine appendicular osteosarcoma, *J Vet Intern Med* 22:602–608, 2008.
16. Fan TM, Barger AM, Sprandel IT, et al: Investigating TrkA expression in canine appendicular osteosarcoma, *J Vet Intern Med* 22:1181–1188, 2008.
17. Lascelles BDX: Surgical pain: Pathophysiology, assessment and treatment strategies. In Tobias KM, Johnston SA, editors: *Veterinary surgery small animal*, St. Louis, 2012, Elsevier Saunders.
18. Marcus DA: Epidemiology of cancer pain, *Curr Pain Headache Rep* 15:231–234, 2011.
19. Dohoo SE, Dohoo IR: Factors influencing the postoperative use of analgesics in dogs and cats by Canadian veterinarians, *Can Vet J* 37:552–556, 1996.
20. Dohoo SE, Dohoo IR: Postoperative use of analgesics in dogs and cats by Canadian veterinarians, *Can Vet J* 37:546–551, 1996.

21. Dohoo SE, Dohoo IR: Attitudes and concerns of Canadian animal health technologists toward postoperative pain management in dogs and cats, *Can Vet J* 39:491–496, 1998.
22. Watson AD, Nicholson A, Church DB, et al: Use of anti-inflammatory and analgesic drugs in dogs and cats, *Aust Vet J* 74:203–210, 1996.
23. Williams VM, Lascelles BD, Robson MC: Current attitudes to, and use of, peri-operative analgesia in dogs and cats by veterinarians in New Zealand, *N Z Vet J* 53:193–202, 2005.
24. Hugonnard M, Leblond A, Keroack S, et al: Attitudes and concerns of French veterinarians towards pain and analgesia in dogs and cats, *Vet Anaesth Analg* 31:154–163, 2004.
25. Raekallio M, Heinonen KM, Kuussaari J, et al: Pain alleviation in animals: attitudes and practices of Finnish veterinarians, *Vet J* 165:131–135, 2003.
26. Capner CA, Lascelles BD, Waterman-Pearson AE: Current British veterinary attitudes to perioperative analgesia for dogs, *Vet Rec* 145:95–99, 1999.
27. Lascelles BD, Main DC: Surgical trauma and chronically painful conditions–within our comfort level but beyond theirs? *J Am Vet Med Assoc* 221:215–222, 2002.
28. Brambell FWR: Report of technical committee to enquire into the welfare of animals kept under intensive husbandry systems (Cmnd 2836). In Vol. London, HM Stationery Office, 1965.
29. Baxevanis CN, Papilas K, Dedoussis GV, et al: Abnormal cytokine serum levels correlate with impaired cellular immune responses after surgery, *Clin Immunol Immunopathol* 71:82–88, 1994.
30. Lennard TW, Shenton BK, Borzotta A, et al: The influence of surgical operations on components of the human immune system, *Br J Surg* 72:771–776, 1985.
31. Kutza J, Gratz I, Afshar M, et al: The effects of general anesthesia and surgery on basal and interferon stimulated natural killer cell activity of humans, *Anesth Analg* 85:918–923, 1997.
32. Oka M, Hazama S, Suzuki M, et al: Depression of cytotoxicity of nonparenchymal cells in the liver after surgery, *Surgery* 116:877–882, 1994.
33. Sandoval BA, Robinson AV, Sulaiman TT, et al: Open versus laparoscopic surgery: a comparison of natural antitumoral cellular immunity in a small animal model, *Am Surg* 62:625–630; discussion 630–631, 1996.
34. Eggermont AM, Steller EP, Sugarbaker PH: Laparotomy enhances intraperitoneal tumor growth and abrogates the antitumor effects of interleukin-2 and lymphokine-activated killer cells, *Surgery* 102:71–78, 1987.
35. Allendorf JD, Bessler M, Horvath KD, et al: Increased tumor establishment and growth after open vs laparoscopic bowel resection in mice, *Surg Endosc* 12:1035–1038, 1998.
36. Allendorf JD, Bessler M, Horvath KD, et al: Increased tumor establishment and growth after open vs laparoscopic surgery in mice may be related to differences in postoperative T-cell function, *Surg Endosc* 13:233–235, 1999.
37. Allendorf JD, Bessler M, Kayton ML, et al: Increased tumor establishment and growth after laparotomy vs laparoscopy in a murine model, *Arch Surg* 130:649–653, 1995.
38. Lacy AM, Garcia-Valdecasas JC, Delgado S, et al: Laparoscopy-assisted colectomy versus open colectomy for treatment of non-metastatic colon cancer: a randomised trial, *Lancet* 359: 2224–2229, 2002.
39. A comparison of laparoscopically assisted and open colectomy for colon cancer, *N Engl J Med* 350:2050–2059, 2004.
40. Lee SW, Whelan RL: Immunologic and oncologic implications of laparoscopic surgery: what is the latest? *Clin Colon Rectal Surg* 19:5–12, 2006.
41. Page GG, Blakely WP, Ben-Eliyahu S: Evidence that postoperative pain is a mediator of the tumor-promoting effects of surgery in rats, *Pain* 90:191–199, 2001.
42. Lee SW, Gleason NR, Southall JC, et al: A serum-soluble factor(s) stimulates tumor growth following laparotomy in a murine model, *Surg Endosc* 14:490–494, 2000.
43. Wada H, Seki S, Takahashi T, et al: Combined spinal and general anesthesia attenuates liver metastasis by preserving TH1/TH2 cytokine balance, *Anesthesiology* 106:499–506, 2007.
44. Conzemius MG, Hill CM, Sammarco JL, et al: Correlation between subjective and objective measures used to determine severity of postoperative pain in dogs, *J Am Vet Med Assoc* 210:1619–1622, 1997.
45. Arpinelli F, Bamfi F: The FDA guidance for industry on PROs: the point of view of a pharmaceutical company, *Health Qual Life Outcomes* 4:85, 2006.
46. Apolone G, De Carli G, Brunetti M, et al: Health-related quality of life (HR-QOL) and regulatory issues. An assessment of the European Agency for the Evaluation of Medicinal Products (EMEA) recommendations on the use of HR-QOL measures in drug approval, *Pharmacoeconomics* 19:187–195, 2001.
47. Yazbek KV, Fantoni DT: Validity of a health-related quality-of-life scale for dogs with signs of pain secondary to cancer, *J Am Vet Med Assoc* 226:1354–1358, 2005.
48. Lynch S, Savary-Bataille K, Leeuw B, et al: Development of a questionnaire assessing health-related quality-of-life in dogs and cats with cancer, *Vet Comp Oncol* 9:172–182, 2011.
49. Tzannes S, Hammond MF, Murphy S, et al: Owners "perception of their cats" quality of life during COP chemotherapy for lymphoma, *J Feline Med Surg* 10:73–81, 2008.
50. Bergh MS, Budsberg SC: The coxib NSAIDs: potential clinical and pharmacologic importance in veterinary medicine, *J Vet Intern Med* 19:633–643, 2005.
51. Papich MG: An update on nonsteroidal anti-inflammatory drugs (NSAIDs) in small animals, *Vet Clin North Am Small Anim Pract* 38:1243–1266, 2008.
52. Innes JF, Clayton J, Lascelles BD: Review of the safety and efficacy of long-term NSAID use in the treatment of canine osteoarthritis, *Vet Rec* 166:226–230, 2010.
53. Lascelles BD, Court MH, Hardie EM, et al: Nonsteroidal anti-inflammatory drugs in cats: a review, *Vet Anaesth Analg* 34:228–250, 2007.
54. Kukanich B, Bidgood T, Knesl O: Clinical pharmacology of nonsteroidal anti-inflammatory drugs in dogs, *Vet Anaesth Analg* 39:69–90, 2012.
55. Wernham BG, Trumpatori B, Hash J, et al: Dose reduction of meloxicam in dogs with osteoarthritis-associated pain and impaired mobility, *J Vet Intern Med* 25:1298–1305, 2011.
56. Smith HS: Potential analgesic mechanisms of acetaminophen, *Pain Physician* 12:269–280, 2009.
57. Mburu DN: Evaluation of the anti-inflammatory effects of a low dose of acetaminophen following surgery in dogs, *J Vet Pharmacol Ther* 14:109–111, 1991.
58. Mburu DN, Mbugua SW, Skoglund LA, et al: Effects of paracetamol and acetylsalicylic acid on the post-operative course after experimental orthopaedic surgery in dogs, *J Vet Pharmacol Ther* 11:163–170, 1988.
59. Kukanich B, Lascelles BD, Aman AM, et al: The effects of inhibiting cytochrome P450 3A, p-glycoprotein, and gastric acid secretion on the oral bioavailability of methadone in dogs, *J Vet Pharmacol Ther* 28:461–466, 2005.
60. Kukanich B, Lascelles BD, Papich MG: Pharmacokinetics of morphine and plasma concentrations of morphine-6-glucuronide following morphine administration to dogs, *J Vet Pharmacol Ther* 28:371–376, 2005.
61. Kukanich B, Papich MG: Plasma profile and pharmacokinetics of dextromethorphan after intravenous and oral administration in healthy dogs, *J Vet Pharmacol Ther* 27:337–341, 2004.
62. KuKanich B: Pharmacokinetics of acetaminophen, codeine, and the codeine metabolites morphine and codeine-6-glucuronide in healthy Greyhound dogs, *J Vet Pharmacol Ther* 33:15–21, 2010.
63. Lascelles BD, Robertson SA: Use of thermal threshold response to evaluate the antinociceptive effects of butorphanol in cats, *Am J Vet Res* 65:1085–1089, 2004.

64. Robertson SA, Taylor PM, Lascelles BD, et al: Changes in thermal threshold response in eight cats after administration of buprenorphine, butorphanol and morphine, *Vet Rec* 153:462–465, 2003.
65. Lascelles BD, Robertson SA, Taylor PM, et al: Comparison of the pharmacokinetics and thermal antinociceptive pharmacodynamics of 20mcg/kg buprenorphine administered sublingually or intravenously in cats, *Vet Anaesth Analg* 30:109 (Abstr), 2003.
66. Woolf CJ, Thompson SWN: The induction and maintenance of central sensitization is dependent on N-methyl-D-aspartic acid receptor activation: implication for the treatment of post-injury pain hypersensitivity states, *Pain* 44:293–299, 1991.
67. Julius D, Basbaum AI: Molecular mechanisms of nociception, *Nature* 413:203–210, 2001.
68. Graven-Nielsen T, Arendt-Nielsen L: Peripheral and central sensitization in musculoskeletal pain disorders: an experimental approach, *Curr Rheumatol Rep* 4:313–321, 2002.
69. Wagner AE, Walton JA, Hellyer PW, et al: Use of low doses of ketamine administered by constant rate infusion as an adjunct for postoperative analgesia in dogs, *J Am Vet Med Assoc* 221:72–75, 2002.
70. Slingsby LS, Waterman-Pearson AE: The post-operative analgesic effects of ketamine after canine ovariohysterectomy–a comparison between pre- or post-operative administration, *Res Vet Sci* 69:147–152, 2000.
71. Eisenberg E, Pud D: Can patients with chronic neuropathic pain be cured by acute administration of the NMDA receptor antagonist amantadine? *Pain* 74:337–339, 1998.
72. Lascelles BD, Gaynor JS, Smith ES, et al: Amantadine in a multimodal analgesic regimen for alleviation of refractory osteoarthritis pain in dogs, *J Vet Intern Med* 22:53–59, 2008.
73. Vernier VG, Harmon JB, Stump JM, et al: The toxicologic and pharmacologic properties of amantadine hydrochloride, *Toxicol Appl Pharmacol* 15:642–665, 1969.
74. Dayer P, Desmeules J, Collart L: Pharmacology of tramadol, *Drugs* 53:18–24, 1997.
75. Oliva P, Aurilio C, Massimo F, et al: The antinociceptive effect of tramadol in the formalin test is mediated by the serotonergic component, *Eur J Pharmacol* 445:179–185, 2002.
76. KuKanich B, Papich MG: Pharmacokinetics of tramadol and the metabolite O-desmethyltramadol in dogs, *J Vet Pharmacol Ther* 27:239–246, 2004.
77. Giorgi M, Del Carlo S, Saccomanni G, et al: Pharmacokinetic and urine profile of tramadol and its major metabolites following oral immediate release capsules administration in dogs, *Vet Res Commun* 2009.
78. Giorgi M, Del Carlo S, Saccomanni G, et al: Pharmacokinetics of tramadol and its major metabolites following rectal and intravenous administration in dogs, *N Z Vet J* 57:146–152, 2009.
79. Giorgi M, Del Carlo S, Saccomanni G, et al: Biopharmaceutical profile of tramadol in the dog, *Vet Res Commun* 33(Suppl 1):189–192, 2009.
80. Giorgi M, Saccomanni G, Lebkowska-Wieruszewska B, et al: Pharmacokinetic evaluation of tramadol and its major metabolites after single oral sustained tablet administration in the dog: a pilot study, *Vet J* 180:253–255, 2009.
81. McMillan CJ, Livingston A, Clark CR, et al: Pharmacokinetics of intravenous tramadol in dogs, *Can J Vet Res* 72:325–331, 2008.
82. Torring ML, Riis A, Christensen S, et al: Perforated peptic ulcer and short-term mortality among tramadol users, *Br J Clin Pharmacol* 65:565–572, 2008.
83. Garcia-Hernandez L, Deciga-Campos M, Guevara-Lopez U, et al: Co-administration of rofecoxib and tramadol results in additive or sub-additive interaction during arthritic nociception in rat, *Pharmacol Biochem Behav* 87:331–340, 2007.
84. Papich MG, Bledsoe DL: Tramadol pharmacokinetics in cats after oral administration of an immediate release tablet, *J Vet Intern Med* 21:616 (abstr.), 2007.
85. Pypendop BH, Ilkiw JE: Pharmacokinetics of tramadol, and its metabolite O-desmethyl-tramadol, in cats, *J Vet Pharmacol Ther* 31:52–59, 2008.
86. Brondani JT, Luna SP, Marcello GC, et al: Perioperative administration of vedaprofen, tramadol or their combination does not interfere with platelet aggregation, bleeding time and biochemical variables in cats, *J Feline Med Surg* 11:503–509, 2009.
87. Pypendop BH, Siao KT, Ilkiw JE: Effects of tramadol hydrochloride on the thermal threshold in cats, *Am J Vet Res* 70:1465–1470, 2009.
88. Radulovic LL, Turck D, von Hodenberg A, et al: Disposition of gabapentin (neurontin) in mice, rats, dogs, and monkeys, *Drug Metab Dispos* 23:441–448, 1995.
89. Vollmer KO, von Hodenberg A, Kolle EU: Pharmacokinetics and metabolism of gabapentin in rat, dog and man, *Arzneimittelforschung* 36:830–839, 1986.
90. Platt SR, Adams V, Garosi LS, et al: Treatment with gabapentin of 11 dogs with refractory idiopathic epilepsy, *Vet Rec* 159:881–884, 2006.
91. Wagner AE, Mich PM, Uhrig SR, et al: Clinical evaluation of perioperative administration of gabapentin as an adjunct for postoperative analgesia in dogs undergoing amputation of a forelimb, *J Am Vet Med Assoc* 236:751–756, 2010.
92. Siao KT, Pypendop BH, Ilkiw JE: Pharmacokinetics of gabapentin in cats, *Am J Vet Res* 71:817–821, 2010.
93. Pypendop BH, Siao KT, Ilkiw JE: Thermal antinociceptive effect of orally administered gabapentin in healthy cats, *Am J Vet Res* 71:1027–1032, 2010.
94. Verdu B, Decosterd I, Buclin T, et al: Antidepressants for the treatment of chronic pain, *Drugs* 68:2611–2632, 2008.
95. Kautio AL, Haanpaa M, Leminen A, et al: Amitriptyline in the prevention of chemotherapy-induced neuropathic symptoms, *Anticancer Res* 29:2601–2606, 2009.
96. Kautio AL, Haanpaa M, Saarto T, et al: Amitriptyline in the treatment of chemotherapy-induced neuropathic symptoms, *J Pain Symptom Manage* 35:31–39, 2008.
97. Chew DJ, Buffington CA, Kendall MS, et al: Amitriptyline treatment for severe recurrent idiopathic cystitis in cats, *J Am Vet Med Assoc* 213:1282–1286, 1998.
98. Challapalli V, Tremont-Lukats IW, McNicol ED, et al: Systemic administration of local anesthetic agents to relieve neuropathic pain, *Cochrane Database Syst Rev* (4):CD003345, 2005.
99. Fleming JA, O'Connor BD: Use of lidocaine patches for neuropathic pain in a comprehensive cancer centre, *Pain Res Manag* 14:381–388, 2009.
100. Ko J, Weil A, Maxwell L, et al: Plasma concentrations of lidocaine in dogs following lidocaine patch application, *J Am Anim Hosp Assoc* 43:280–283, 2007.
101. Ko JC, Maxwell LK, Abbo LA, et al: Pharmacokinetics of lidocaine following the application of 5% lidocaine patches to cats, *J Vet Pharmacol Ther* 31:359–367, 2008.
102. Weiland L, Croubels S, Baert K, et al: Pharmacokinetics of a lidocaine patch 5% in dogs, *J Vet Med A Physiol Pathol Clin Med* 53:34–39, 2006.
103. Weil AB, Ko J, Inoue T: The use of lidocaine patches, *Compend Contin Educ Vet* 29:208–210, 212, 214–206, 2007.
104. Jimenez Andrade JM, Mantyh P: Cancer pain: From the development of mouse models to human clinical trials. In Kruger L, Light AR, editors: *Translational pain research: from mouse to man,* Boca Raton, FL, 2010, CRC Press.
105. Jimenez-Andrade JM, Mantyh WG, Bloom AP, et al: Bone cancer pain, *Ann N Y Acad Sci* 1198:173–181, 2010.
106. Sabino MA, Mantyh PW: Pathophysiology of bone cancer pain, *J Support Oncol* 3:15–24, 2005.
107. Milner RJ, Farese J, Henry CJ, et al: Bisphosphonates and cancer, *J Vet Intern Med* 18:597–604, 2004.
108. Fan TM: Intravenous aminobisphosphonates for managing complications of malignant osteolysis in companion animals, *Top Companion Anim Med* 24:151–156, 2009.

109. Ashton JA, Farese JP, Milner RJ, et al: Investigation of the effect of pamidronate disodium on the in vitro viability of osteosarcoma cells from dogs, *Am J Vet Res* 66:885–891, 2005.
110. Farese JP, Ashton J, Milner R, et al: The effect of the bisphosphonate alendronate on viability of canine osteosarcoma cells in vitro, *In Vitro Cell Dev Biol Anim* 40:113–117, 2004.
111. Fan TM, de Lorimier LP, Garrett LD, et al: The bone biologic effects of zoledronate in healthy dogs and dogs with malignant osteolysis, *J Vet Intern Med* 22:380–387, 2008.
112. de Lorimier LP, Fan TM: Bone metabolic effects of single-dose zoledronate in healthy dogs, *J Vet Intern Med* 19:924–927, 2005.
113. Tomlin JL, Sturgeon C, Pead MJ, et al: Use of the bisphosphonate drug alendronate for palliative management of osteosarcoma in two dogs, *Vet Rec* 147:129–132, 2000.
114. Wiley RG, Lappi DA: Targeted toxins in pain, *Adv Drug Deliv Rev* 55:1043–1054, 2003.
115. Wiley RG: Substance P receptor-expressing dorsal horn neurons: lessons from the targeted cytotoxin, substance P-saporin, *Pain* 136:7–10, 2008.
116. Wiley RG, Kline RH, Vierck CJ, Jr.: Anti-nociceptive effects of selectively destroying substance P receptor-expressing dorsal horn neurons using [Sar9,Met(O2)11]-substance P-saporin: behavioral and anatomical analyses, *Neuroscience* 146:1333–1345, 2007.
117. Allen JW, Horais KA, Tozier NA, et al: Intrathecal substance P-Saporin selectively lesions NK-1 receptor bearing neurons in dogs, *J Pain* 3(suppl 1):51, 2002.
118. Ramirez O, 3rd, Dodge RK, Page RL, et al: Palliative radiotherapy of appendicular osteosarcoma in 95 dogs, *Vet Radiol Ultrasound* 40:517–522, 1999.
119. Milner RJ, Dormehl I, Louw WK, et al: Targeted radiotherapy with Sm-153-EDTMP in nine cases of canine primary bone tumours, *J S Afr Vet Assoc* 69:12–17, 1998.
120. Culp LB, Skarda RT, Muir WW, 3rd: Comparisons of the effects of acupuncture, electroacupuncture, and transcutaneous cranial electrical stimulation on the minimum alveolar concentration of isoflurane in dogs, *Am J Vet Res* 66:1364–1370, 2005.
121. Zhang RX, Li A, Liu B, et al: Electroacupuncture attenuates bone-cancer-induced hyperalgesia and inhibits spinal preprodynorphin expression in a rat model, *Eur J Pain* 12:870–878, 2008.
122. Zhang RX, Li A, Liu B, et al: Electroacupuncture attenuates bone cancer pain and inhibits spinal interleukin-1 beta expression in a rat model, *Anesth Analg* 105:1482–1488, table of contents, 2007.
123. Mantyh PW: Neurobiology of substance P and the NK1 receptor, *J Clin Psychiatry* 63(Suppl 11):6–10, 2002.
124. Honore P, Menning PM, Rogers SD, et al: Neurochemical plasticity in persistent inflammatory pain, *Prog Brain Res* 129:357–363, 2000.

SECTION B

Nutritional Management of the Cancer Patient

JOSEPH J. WAKSHLAG

Over the past 75 years the examination of nutrients and their relationship to cancer control and cancer prevention has led to a better understanding of how nutrition may play a role in the management of neoplastic disease. The paucity of well-controlled studies in companion animals and the extrapolation of data derived from studies conducted in humans investigating tumor types uncommon to companion animals (colon, prostate, pancreas) are frustrating and make general recommendations for nutritional intervention challenging. However, owners often wish to alter their pet's feeding regimen regardless of proven efficacy. In this context, three areas of nutrition are often discussed with clients, including modification in tumor metabolism, adjustment of nutritional risk factors that may impact outcomes, and nutritional intervention during therapy, all of which will be addressed in this section.

Metabolism of Cancer: Substrate Utilization

Numerous neoplastic cell lines have been successfully propagated in culture allowing examination of cell biology. A fundamental observation is that the majority of neoplastic cells propagate better in a high glucose media, which is likely the result of limited fatty acid metabolism coupled with increases in metabolic pathways that utilize glucose. This has traditionally been termed the *Warburg effect* after Otto Warburg's seminal work suggesting that glycolysis is the primary pathway for energy production in neoplastic cells.[1,2] Studies in humans have shown that certain cancer patients liberate excessive lactate from solid tumors,[3,4] providing evidence that glycolysis and pyruvate production are critical to neoplastic cell metabolism. This has led to the Cori cycle hypothesis of neoplasia, whereby neoplastic tissues, much like skeletal muscle tissue, appear to undergo regeneration of glucose from lactate through hepatic resynthesis of glucose.[5] Unfortunately, this regeneration of glucose is an energy costly cycle and is thought to contribute to increases in resting energy requirements.

In veterinary medicine, there is a significant body of work examining metabolism and cancer, often through the application of indirect calorimetry assessments to study whole body metabolism. These studies have interrogated oxygen consumption and carbon dioxide liberation and such data provide an estimate of energy consumption (resting energy expenditure [REE]) and substrate utilization (respiratory quotient [RQ]). Healthy dogs display higher REE than dogs with stage III and IV lymphoma.[6] RQ values between the groups were not different, suggesting that all dogs were using similar substrate, and dogs with lymphoma were not preferentially consuming more glucose than their control counterparts.[6] In a separate study, dogs with lymphoma fed either a high-fat or high-carbohydrate diet during doxorubicin chemotherapy did not differ in remission times, survival times, or tumor burden, suggesting that dogs with lymphoma under treatment were not sensitive to this basic dietary alteration.[7] During this study the REE and RQ assessed during treatment did not change significantly when the tumor burden was eliminated with chemotherapy suggesting no significant changes in energy expenditure or metabolism. These data collectively indicate that there is no fundamental difference observed between normal healthy dogs and dogs with lymphoma and that removal of the tumor burden does not alter the resting energy requirement.

Canine nonhematopoietic malignancies were also examined before and 4 to 6 weeks after excision of their primary tumors, including mammary carcinoma, OSA, high-grade mast cell tumors, and lung carcinoma. As in dogs with lymphoma, REE was not different from control dogs nor was there any difference in REE between preexcision and postexcision of the primary tumor, suggesting no futile cycling of energy in these patients.[8] Interestingly, in this study the RQ values were above 0.8 for all control and tumor-bearing dogs, suggesting that the resting energy was not from lipolysis, which was contradictory to a follow-up study performed in dogs with OSA. In that follow-up study, there was an increase observed in the REE in dogs with OSA compared to control dogs but a RQ of 0.7 in both affected and control dogs.[9] This increased

REE persisted after excision of the primary lesion, suggesting that the modest increase in REE was due to factors other than the primary neoplasia and may be associated with micrometastasis, inflammation associated with neoplastic disease, or heightened pain response associated with the primary tumor and surgical procedure.[9] These findings were surprising in light of the previous studies mentioned but were likely more valid considering that the REE calculations in the OSA study were based on lean mass rather than total kilograms of body weight.[9] It is well known that fat mass is relatively metabolically inert; therefore REE based on lean body mass is more appropriate. The previous studies in nonhematopoietic malignancies and lymphoma did not adjust for body condition or lean body mass in tumor-bearing or normal populations under study,[7,8] and the inability to document differences in REE noted in these two studies may have been confounded by a lack of body condition assessment.

Specific metabolic changes have been reported in dogs with several types of cancer. Alterations in glucose metabolism (potentially higher glucose turnover), increased protein turnover, and urinary protein losses in dogs with OSA have been observed.[9] In addition, studies in dogs with lymphoma identified alterations in carbohydrate metabolism such as increased serum lactate and insulin concentrations during glucose tolerance testing that suggest insulin resistance.[6,10,11] This may be partially explained by aberrant interleukin-6 (IL-6) and other cytokine influences on glucose metabolism resulting in insulin resistance in dogs with lymphoma.[12] Insulin insensitivity and serum lactate did not change once remission was achieved in one of these studies.[6] Mild alterations in lipid metabolism in dogs with lymphoma were suggested by higher basal triglyceride and cholesterol concentrations compared to control dogs,[13] and treatment with doxorubicin lowered serum cholesterol, perhaps due to hepatic effects of chemotherapy.[13] However, the dyslipidemia present was not ameliorated once the primary tumor burden was eliminated, which is logical in light of the insulin resistance observed.

Cancer Anorexia and Cachexia

Anorexia or hyporexia (inadequate food intake) in cancer patients is a common occurrence and can be one of the presenting clinical signs of cancer. Inadequate appetite is often due to an enhanced inflammatory cytokine response (i.e., IL-6 and IL-1) associated with the tumor, resulting in hypothalamic arcuate nucleus suppression of appetite. In the case of gastrointestinal cancer, pain associated with eating, obstruction, or dysfunctional transit mechanisms can lead to anorexia. In patients undergoing treatment, anorexia may be partially explained by adverse events associated with the use of chemotherapy. Chemotherapeutics can cause a variety of alterations in olfactory and taste sensorium. Since dogs and cats rely heavily on olfactory cues, the loss of olfactory bulb stimulus diminishes palatability of foods.[13,14] Additionally, the loss or alteration of taste (ageusia or dysgeusia) can further complicate anorexia and may last for several months before neuronal regeneration can take place at the olfactory bulb and tongue.[13,14]

Cachexia, on the other hand, although identified in many human cancer patients, does not appear to be common in dogs with nonhematopoietic malignancies other than a predisposition toward insulin resistance.[6,10,15,16] Evidence in humans and mouse models suggests that the most prominent influence inciting the cachectic phenomenon may be excessive cytokine stimulation, which leads to insulin resistance, extensive lipolysis, and proteolysis of tissue stores.[17,18] The three primary cytokines thought to be involved in promoting enhanced proteolysis are TNF-α, IL-1β, and IL-6.[17,18] TNF-α and IL-1β have both been directly associated with anorexia and upregulation of mitochondrial uncoupling protein, whereas IL-6 and TNF-α have been observed to increase myofibrillar degradation machinery, all of which may play a role in the anorexia/cachexia syndrome associated with neoplasia.[19,20] IL-6 and c-reactive protein, both markers of inflammation, have been observed to increase in canine lymphoma patients.[12,21,22] Yet, it does not appear that cachexia is a common occurrence in dogs diagnosed with neoplasia since dogs examined 6 months prior to diagnosis of cancer showed no difference in body weight or body condition than at presentation for various neoplasms.[15] This may be partially explained by differences in common tumor types between species. Cachexia in humans is often associated with epithelial cancers such as pancreatic, colon, mammary, and prostate cancer. Additionally, human patients undergo dramatically different and more aggressive treatment protocols over lengthy time periods, which we typically do not encounter in veterinary medicine due to owner financial constraints and QOL considerations.

Cats on the other hand may show a more typical cachectic response involving excessive lean body mass wasting. Recent evidence suggests that approximately 56% of cats with lymphoma and other solid tumors have body condition scores of less than 5 out of 9.[23] More intriguing is that the survival time for cats with lymphoma with a body condition score of 5 or greater was 16.9 months, compared to those with lower scores (3.3 months).[23] This warrants monitoring of caloric intake and aggressive implementation of nutritional interventions in feline cancer patients.

Epidemiology, Prevention, and Risk Factors

In humans, the two major nutritional factors associated with risk of developing cancer are excess body weight (obesity) and low fruit and vegetable consumption.[24-27] Although these parameters may be interrelated, both appear to play a direct role in the risk of cancer development. Convincing data suggest that the westernized diet and lack of fruit and vegetable matter are linked to increased relative risk of nearly all types of neoplasia, including prostate, colon, breast, lymphoma, and leukemia.[28-30] Although the evidence is compelling, the data do not support a causal association, and it may be a combination of factors associated with diet, as well as confounding lifestyle differences in humans consuming higher amounts of fruits and vegetables, that may be important in deterring cancer.

In veterinary medicine, there are few studies examining the effects of dietary substrate (protein, fat, carbohydrate) and plant-based dietary intake and cancer incidence. Two epidemiologic studies using validated food frequency questionnaires examined the effect on survival of calories coming from fat, protein, and carbohydrate for 1 year prior to and after diagnosis of mammary carcinoma.[31,32] These data were contradictory to human findings, showing that dogs with increased protein intake had increased survival times and that fat and carbohydrate intake did not play a role in progression of disease.[31,32] Another study suggested that risk of neoplasia was increased in dogs receiving nontraditional, poorly balanced diets (i.e., table foods as primary consumption).[33] Further examination of this group showed no association between blood selenium concentration and mammary carcinoma when compared to healthy age-matched and hospitalized control dogs. Serum retinol (vitamin A) values were also decreased in dogs with mammary carcinoma in this study.[33] Whether the lower serum retinol was a reflection of poor retinol intake or a reflection of the disease manifestation was not determined. A diet high in red meat was also identified as a risk factor in this study. In many cases, a high-protein food may be evaluated as higher quality because protein is an expensive ingredient; however, many variables in addition to ingredients are important. Ingredient quality, digestibility, and socioeconomic factors such as veterinary care should be considered. It does suggest that feeding an incomplete diet is associated with increased cancer risk and provides justification for a complete and balanced diet (Association of American Feed Control Officials [AAFCO]-approved commercial dog food) throughout the life of a dog.

Nutritional risk factors examined in Scottish terriers, who have a genetic predisposition to develop transitional cell carcinoma (TCC), showed that the addition of vegetables to a dog's diet resulted in a lower incidence of the disease.[34] However, there are confounding lifestyle factors that cannot be accounted for in this epidemiologic investigation, including better health care, variation in nutrition supplied as commercial food, and other associated environmental exposures. Yet, this study is provocative and suggests further study is warranted.

Specific vitamins and their relationship to cancer development have received significant attention in humans, including retinol, ascorbic acid, vitamin E, selenium, and vitamin D. In veterinary medicine, these nutrients have not been thoroughly studied in relation to cancer risk. Human metaanalyses examining oral supplementation for single nutrients such as ascorbate, selenium, and vitamin E have been inconclusive or negative when examining protective, anticarcinogenic effects.[35-37] Other nutrients like β-carotene, the precursor to retinol, is currently thought to be ineffective as a chemopreventive agent and in some instances has proved to be harmful in certain populations (i.e., smoking populations).[38-40] Currently, vitamin D (25-hydroxyvitamin [OH] D_3) status and supplementation has been an area of vigorous epidemiologic investigation due to an increased relative risk of various neoplastic diseases associated with low serum vitamin D status.[41-43] In dogs and cats, unlike humans, vitamin D status is directly dependent on dietary intake since they cannot convert 7-OH-dehydrocholesterol to pre-vitamin D. One would expect that serum vitamin D concentrations would not fluctuate tremendously in dogs being fed commercial dog food.[44] A recent investigation suggests that Labrador retrievers with mast cell disease have lower serum vitamin D status than healthy Labrador retrievers, making vitamin D status an interesting area of future investigation.[45] Whether this is a direct reflection of dietary intake or a reflection of the biochemical disposition in affected dogs with cancer remains to be determined.

In humans, obesity has been associated with an increased risk of many cancers, including breast, prostate, colon, leukemia, lymphoma, and pancreatic neoplasia.[24-27] In companion species, studies examining this association are limited. The largest retrospective study in dogs showed no association between body condition and neoplastic disease,[15] whereas other epidemiologic studies suggested that obese cats and dogs may have a slightly higher rate of neoplastic disease.[46,47] Two other investigations revealed a more definitive link between obesity in female dogs and the onset of mammary carcinoma.[31,33] The risk of mammary carcinoma was greater in obese spayed dogs in one study, although obesity was an increased risk factor but independent of spay status in another.[31,33] Both studies suggest an increased risk when obesity is present at 1 year of age, and one suggested that obesity at 1 year before diagnosis also increased risk.[47] The question of whether early onset obesity, much like early spaying, epigenetically predisposes mammary glands to an altered risk of cancer remains to be addressed.

Implementing a Nutritional Plan for the Oncology Patient: Nutritional Assessment

To fully assess the cancer patient, information regarding body weight, body condition score, and diet history are crucial. Dietary history, before and during treatment, should be obtained to appropriately assess the kilocalorie intake. This information will allow the practitioner to feed the patient appropriately during hospitalization and, more importantly, to recognize hypophagic behaviors, allowing for proactive interventions. A typical diet history should include the forms of food (wet or dry), amounts fed daily, as well as treats, human table foods, and additional supplements provided. A food diary has been helpful for humans attempting to understand energy and nutrient intake and is likely to also be helpful for dogs in particular as a wide variety of food stuffs are offered to dogs.

Serial assessment of body weight is important, particularly where malnutrition is a consideration. Malnutrition is often associated with cachexia and/or anorexia. Anorexic behavior can be deduced from the diet history and can be treated aggressively with nutritional and/or pharmacologic intervention; however, if cachexia is suspected, then alternative treatments can be sought. The difficulty in clinically differentiating cachexia from anorexia is our inability to measure loss of lean versus fat mass. The loss of fat mass is typical during anorexia, and equal loss of lean and fat mass suggests cachexia. Although this cannot be deciphered efficiently in veterinary practice, overall weight loss guidelines have been offered in the human literature whereby body weight loss of 5% in 1 month or 10% in 3 months without conscientious dieting suggests cancer cachexia.[48] Two body condition scoring (BCS) systems have been adopted as a means of nutritional assessment in companion species; however, the 1 to 9 BCS system (Figure 15-2) has been more thoroughly validated in the literature.[49,50] Modest differences in BCS between dogs and cats exist due to preferential deposition of body fat along the inguinal and abdominal areas in cats, whereas dogs tend to have no preferential deposition. These differences may justify a muscle condition scoring system in cats (Table 15-6).[23]

The final component of nutritional assessment consists of a routine physical examination, complete blood cell count, and serum chemistry evaluation. Physical examination findings consistent with malnutrition include poor hair coat, chronic gastrointestinal disturbance, seborrhea, lethargy, and pallor. The first signs of chronic nutrient deficiency are often manifested in areas of rapid cellular turnover leading to skin, gastrointestinal, and hematologic

TABLE 15-6 Description of the Muscle Mass Scoring System (MMS)

SCORE	MUSCLE MASS
0	On palpation over the spine, muscle mass is severely wasted.
1	On palpation over the spine, mass is moderately wasted.
2	On palpation over the spine, muscle mass is mildly wasted.
3	On palpation over the spine, muscle mass is normal.

Nestlé PURINA

BODY CONDITION SYSTEM

TOO THIN

1 Ribs visible on shorthaired cats; no palpable fat; severe abdominal tuck; lumbar vertebrae and wings of ilia easily palpated.

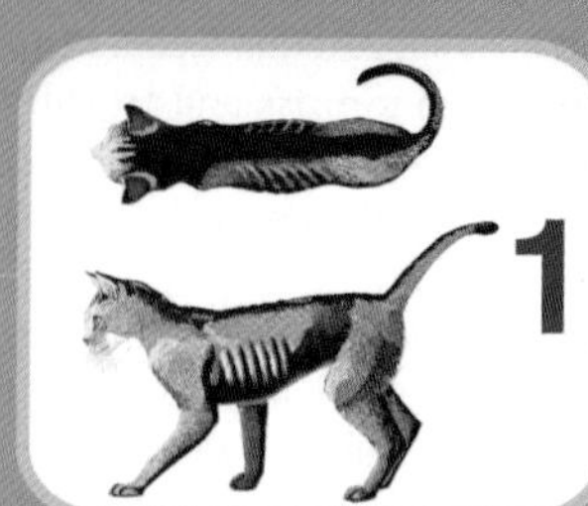

2 Ribs easily visible on shorthaired cats; lumbar vertebrae obvious with minimal muscle mass; pronounced abdominal tuck; no palpable fat.

3 Ribs easily palpable with minimal fat covering; lumbar vertebrae obvious; obvious waist behind ribs; minimal abdominal fat.

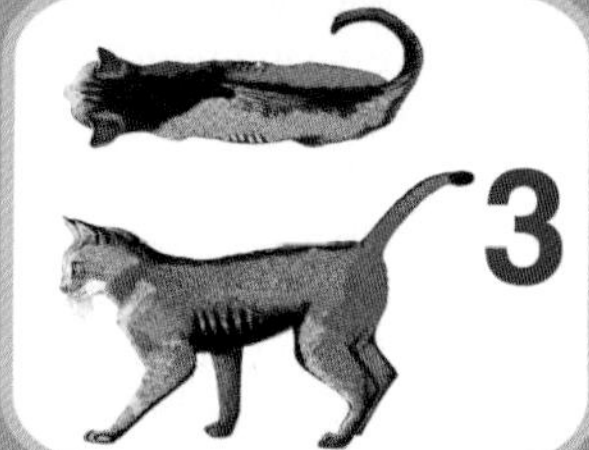

4 Ribs palpable with minimal fat covering; noticeable waist behind ribs; slight abdominal tuck; abdominal fat pad absent.

IDEAL

5 **Well-proportioned; observe waist behind ribs; ribs palpable with slight fat covering; abdominal fat pad minimal.**

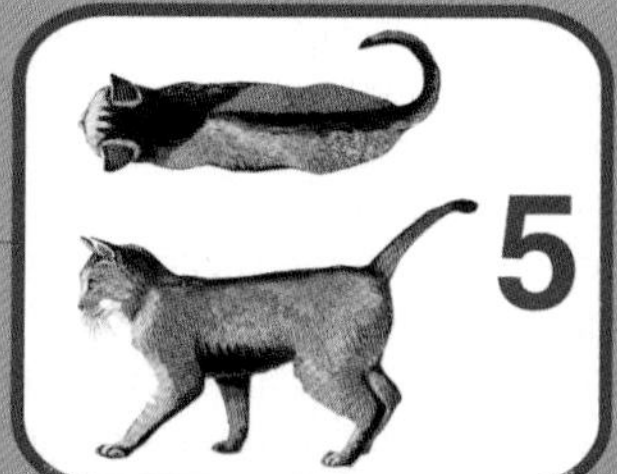

TOO HEAVY

6 Ribs palpable with slight excess fat covering; waist and abdominal fat pad distinguishable but not obvious; abdominal tuck absent.

7 Ribs not easily palpated with moderate fat covering; waist poorly discernible; obvious rounding of abdomen; moderate abdominal fat pad.

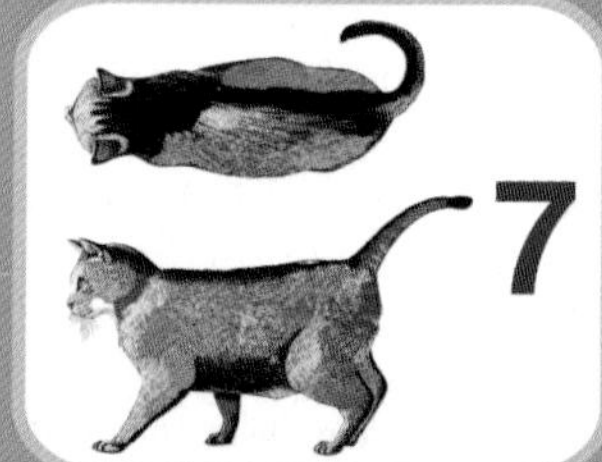

8 Ribs not palpable with excess fat covering; waist absent; obvious rounding of abdomen with prominent abdominal fat pad; fat deposits present over lumbar area.

9 Ribs not palpable under heavy fat cover; heavy fat deposits over lumbar area, face and limbs; distention of abdomen with no waist; extensive abdominal fat deposits.

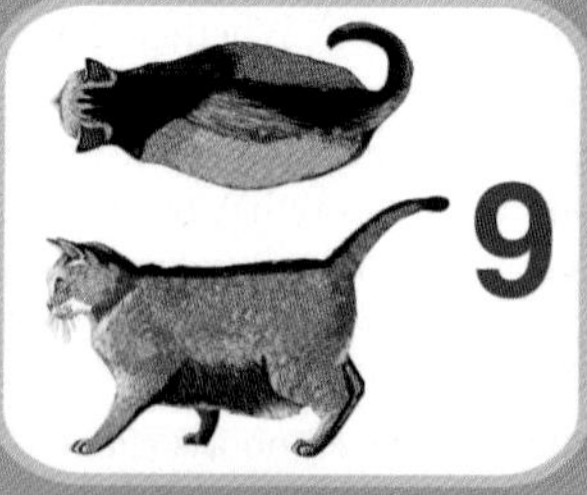

Call 1-800-222-VETS (8387), weekdays, 8:00 a.m. to 4:30 p.m. CT

Nestlé PURINA

FIGURE 15-2 Body condition scoring (BCS) scale (1-9) for a cat. A similar BCS scale exists for dogs. *(Reprinted with permission of Nestle Purina PetCare, St. Louis.)*

signs and should be considered in cases of prolonged anorexia. Chronic malnutrition can result in low hemoglobin and red blood cell counts, as well as hypoproteinemia and hypoalbuminemia. Additionally, with the trend toward nontraditional feeding practices, there is the potential for diets that lack sufficient mineral content (e.g., calcium, iron, and copper) resulting in bone and hematologic manifestations. Many homemade diets lacking supplementation with bone meal can lead to secondary hyperparathyroidism and clinical osteopenia.[51,52] Clients using nontraditional diets should be educated through consultation with a veterinary nutritionist.

In dogs, excess body condition (i.e., obesity) may be more of a concern than malnutrition or deficiency. Treatment of obesity is not a priority in many cancer patients, considering metabolic changes that may occur during chemotherapy and the potential for treatment-related eating pattern changes. One study suggests that body condition does not change from 6 months prior to diagnosis to the day of diagnosis,[15] whereas another study suggests that over 68% of dogs lose weight during treatment[53]; however, loss was less than 5% of body weight and nearly 30% of dogs were scored as obese prior to treatment. The occurrence of obesity in dogs with neoplasia appears to follow the national trends in canine obesity.

Feeding the Hospitalized Oncology Patient

Hospitalization of debilitated cancer patients undergoing evaluation or therapy has unique nutritional opportunities and challenges. Hospitalization during some fractionated radiation therapy is common, and the provision of more than the resting energy requirement (RER) during this period is often unnecessary unless extreme circumstances exist where extensive tissue repair is ongoing (e.g., postoperatively, epithelial mucositis). This increased energy requirement is known as the illness energy requirement (IER) and is often considered to be between 1.1 to 2 times the RER, particularly when transudates or exudates are involved with the repair process and protein losses are excessive. Energy requirements post-discharge may also be increased above hospitalization RER due to increased activity and neuter status, which is represented as the maintenance energy requirement (MER). Table 15-7 presents starting calculations for MER based on the linear equation used in veterinary patients taking into account the activity status. Exponential equations are preferred in dogs and cats under 2 kg or over 30 kg to derive a more accurate estimate of the RER:

$$\text{RER} = 70(\text{BW in kg})^{0.75}$$

TABLE 15-7 Maintenance Energy Requirement Equations for Adult Cats and Dogs

ANIMAL	MER EQUATION
Neutered adult dog	$(70 + 30\ [\text{BW}_{\text{kg}}]) \times 1.6$
Intact adult dog	$(70 + 30\ [\text{BW}_{\text{kg}}]) \times 1.8$
Obesity-prone adult dog	$(70 + 30\ [\text{BW}_{\text{kg}}]) \times 1.2$ to 1.4
Neutered adult cat	$(70 + 30\ [\text{BW}_{\text{kg}}]) \times 1.2$ to 1.4
Intact adult cat	$(70 + 30\ [\text{BW}_{\text{kg}}]) \times 1.4$ to 1.6
Inactive obesity-prone adult cat	$(70 + 30\ [\text{BW}_{\text{kg}}]) \times 1.0$

BW, Body weight; *MER*, maintenance energy requirement.

Evidence suggests that the exponent of the equation may be different for cats (e.g., 0.67).[54] Once a patient returns home, its RER typically increases slightly due to increased activity. Therefore clinicians should adjust the energy intake on discharge.

Coax Feeding and Pharmacologic Appetite Stimulation

Ensuring full energy requirement intake enterally may be difficult due to a diminished appetite in canine and feline cancer patients. There are many considerations when trying to promote adequate intake, and these may be different in dogs and cats. Hand-feeding in dogs and cats that enjoy this approach should be considered rather than putting a bowl in the cage and leaving it there. Hand-feeding may be best achieved during owner visits when the animal is most comfortable and often away from the busy atmosphere of most intensive care units or oncology wards.[55] For cats, having a quiet place away from distractions that create a fearful environment may be helpful to achieve adequate intake. Making one cage an eating cage that is covered and away from the litter box is ideal as some cats will not eat near the litter box during hospitalization.[55]

Addition of flavorings may also be helpful. Dogs have salt and sweet receptors, and the addition of sugar, syrups, or other sweeteners can sometimes improve appetite.[55] Cats do not have the lingual receptors to appreciate sweet flavors. Therefore salt can be used to entice cats to eat; however, they tend to be more averse to oversalted foods.[55] Additional protein added to the diet of both dogs and cats can improve appetite and enhance intake since dogs appear to prefer higher protein diets and cats have increased density of lingual amino acid receptors, making high protein choices logical.[55] The supplementation of animal-based or vegetable-based fat may increase palatability but must be monitored as additional fat can dilute the nutrient content of the feed. In the presence of nausea, introducing multiple foods can create long-term aversions limiting choices of form and texture once the nausea has resolved.[55] Using one or two foods to coax feed is ideal, rather than an entire array of products from the kitchen.

Pharmacologic approaches to improve enteral support may be attempted; however, many of the purported effects are anecdotal with little evidence of their true utility in veterinary medicine. Human studies suggest several approaches, including pharmacologic alterations in serotonergic stimulation in the brain, decreased cytokine stimulation, and the promotion of hypothalamic satiety center signaling.[56,57] Approaches in veterinary medicine have focused on the use of the antiserotonergics (e.g., cyproheptadine and mirtazapine). Unfortunately, no definitive clinical studies documenting the efficacy of these drugs in dogs and cats with cancer exist.[55] Of some interest is the use of valium to stimulate appetite in cats and the recommended dosing of 1 mg by mouth (PO) daily has proved useful.[58] However, the use of valium does not come without the potential for severe side effects (e.g., hepatic necrosis), making long-term use of valium ill advised.[59] In dogs, low-dose propofol is used to briefly stimulate eating behavior to test the integrity of the bowel (i.e., vomiting) when unsure about enteral functional status, although more prolonged use of propofol is not attempted.[60]

Assisted Enteral Support

In many instances, the use of assisted enteral nutrition should be considered, particularly if the animal is not consuming appropriate kilocalorie requirements. In the hypophagic cancer patient, it may be essential to provide assisted feeding through various techniques, including syringe, nasogastric, esophagostomy, or gastrostomy feeding. Syringe feeding is the easiest and requires the least attention to detail by owners and clinicians. In the nauseous and anosmic patient, this can be difficult to implement due to patient resistance. Nasogastric tubes can be easily placed without anesthesia and can be useful in hospitalized animals but are often problematic to manage at home and are limited to the use of liquid enteral products due to tube diameter. The two most widely accepted means of implementing long-term enteral support is the placement of an esophagostomy or gastrostomy tube. The esophagostomy tube is typically placed under anesthesia; techniques for placement have been described elsewhere.[61] Once secured, the tube site is typically wrapped, and the insertion site should be examined every 24 to 48 hours for signs of cellulitis and discharge. These tubes are typically recommended for intermediate to long-term feeding for a period of 2 to 3 weeks up to 2 to 3 months.

Gastrostomy tube placement should be considered when tube placement is required for longer than 6 to 8 weeks.[61,62] Advantages include direct gastric delivery of nutrients and prevention of tube eversion if emesis is encountered. Anesthesia is required for either surgical or percutaneous endoscopic placement approaches. The endoscopic approach is generally safe and effective, although associated with a higher risk of complications.[62] The author prefers surgical placement in large breed dogs because they may be predisposed to separation of the stomach from the body wall after endoscopic placement. Peritonitis is the most serious complication following tube placement since the peritoneum is disturbed with this approach and leads to a permanent stoma from the stomach to the outside of the body.[61,62] After successful gastrostomy tube placement, the tube can be used within 24 hours of placement but should not be removed before 2 weeks, allowing for adhesion and fibrosis of the gastric wall to the abdominal wall. Once a stoma has formed, the original surgically placed tube may be replaced with a low profile or "button" feeding device. Owners should be aware that these low profile devices need replacing every 6 to 8 months and will require mild sedation for replacement.[63]

Esophagostomy and gastrostomy tubes allow for a diverse number of products to be used for feeding beyond the liquid veterinary diets. Many over-the-counter and veterinary therapeutic diets can be blended for feeding; however, when some products are blended with water, they result in less than 1 kcal/mL. Diets that provide higher caloric density that can be passed through a 7 French or greater diameter catheter are listed in Table 15-8. These products tend to be higher in protein and fat and can be fed at reduced volumes and rates when nausea or food volume is an issue. A typical dog or cat receiving a slurry of food at 1 kcal/mL will also be meeting their fluid requirements.[64] Similarly, providing 1 kcal/mL for dogs and cats that are not actively consuming water at home is also advised.

Parenteral Support

If enteral support is not an option, then parenteral nutrition (PN) should be considered. Parenteral support can be either partial PN (PPN) or total PN (TPN). PPN has also been termed *peripheral parenteral nutrition* considering it is typically delivered through peripheral veins. Prospective studies examining outcome following parenteral support have not been performed in clinical veterinary medicine and only a handful of retrospective investigations characterize complication rates.[65-70] In veterinary patients, particularly cats, the metabolic complication most often encountered is hyperglycemia. Mechanical complications are also prevalent (i.e., feeding line problems, inadvertent patient removal). A common misconception is that sepsis is a common complication, but in fact it is quite rare.[65-70] Parenteral support should only be considered when enteral support is not an option due to medical complications; enteral support is considered superior as it prevents transmigration of bacteria to the portal blood and improves the immunologic status of patients.[71]

Parenteral support is not well studied in veterinary medicine, and the relative use and utility of the three main substrates (glucose, amino acid, and lipid) differ, depending on the source of information.[72-74] Some advocate using glucose and lipid to meet the energy requirements and then add in amino acids to the formulation based on the protein needs per kilogram of body weight. Others advocate adding just above the minimal protein requirement as amino acids making up part of the REE. The protein requirements for ill cats and dogs are currently unknown, and we can only assume the requirements are similar to those of healthy normal animals. Extrapolation from human data suggests that protein turnover may be higher during catabolic illness, and we often add slightly more protein than required. In an elegantly designed study, it was found that approximately 2.3 g protein/kg body weight is sufficient for IV amino acid solution in normal dogs.[75] This suggests that adding 2.5 to 3 g/kg amino acid solution for a dog appears sufficient and 4 g/kg is often used as a starting point for cats. Amino acids come in several different formulations and strengths (e.g., 5.5%, 8.5%, and 10%). Additionally, amino acid

TABLE 15-8 Selected High Protein/High Calorie Products for Tube Feeding Cancer Patients and the Amount of Water Needed to Make a 1 kcal/mL Mixture to Meet Daily Fluid Requirements

PRODUCT	CALORIES (KCAL/ML)	PROTEIN (G/100 KCAL)	FAT (G/100 KCAL)	WATER NEEDED FOR 1 KCAL/ML
Abbott Clinicare	1.0	9.1	5.3	—
Royal Canin Recovery RS (5.8 oz)	1.1	9.9	6.4	18
Hill's a/d (5.5 oz)	1.2	9.2	6.3	30
Eukanuba Max Cal (6 oz)	2.0	7.2	6.4	165
Impact (2 oz scoop; 56 gr)*	2.6	9.6	6.0	220
Carnivore Care (2 oz.; 56 gr)*	2.6	9.0	6.2	220

*Dry powdered products—50 cc of water is required for preparation with thorough mixing before administering.

RER = 30(kg BW) + 70 or 70(kg BW)$^{0.75}$ RER = ________.

A. Protein requirement:
DOGS: 3 grams/kg BW CATS: 4 grams/kg/BW

Protein requirement (gm/day) = ______ gm/kg × W kg = ______ gm/day

Protein calories (gm/day) × 4 kcal/gm = ________________ kcal/day

Total kcal − protein calories = ______________________ nonprotein calories

B. Nonprotein calories (NPC)

Glucose (40-60%) NPC = ________ × ________ NPC = ________ kcal glucose

Lipid (40-60%) NPC = ________ × ________ NPC = ________ kcal lipid.

C. Volumes of substrates

10% amino acid solution = 0.10 gm/mL

Protein gm req ________ / 0.10 gm = ________ mL of AA solution. ($\frac{1}{2}$ volume day 1 ________)

50% dextrose (kcals) ________ / 1.7 kcal/mL = ________ mL of 50% dextrose. ($\frac{1}{2}$ volume day 1 ________)

20% Lipid (kcals) ________ / 2.0 kcal/mL = ________ mL of 20% lipid. ($\frac{1}{2}$ volume day 1 ________)

Total volume of TPN solution = ________ mL/24 hrs / 24 hrs = ________ mL/hr. ($\frac{1}{2}$ rate day 1 ________)

Fluid req ________ mL − TPN volume ________ mL = Remaining fluid req ________ mL.

Remaining fluid requirement/24 hours = ________ mL/hr of fluids.

FIGURE 15-3 Small animal total parenteral nutrition (TPN) formulation sheet.

solutions come with and without electrolytes. Amino acids with electrolytes typically provide basal sodium, chloride, magnesium, phosphorus, and potassium when used at 1.5 to 2.5 g/kg body weight of protein; however, these are used less often in veterinary species, particularly in cats whose protein requirements are higher. When using amino acids with electrolytes, the electrolytes provided should be considered before supplementing additional electrolytes in fluids. Figure 15-3 describes a typical TPN feeding program for a cat or dog using a 10% amino acid solution without electrolytes. During the first day of TPN, it is recommended to provide only half of the calorie requirement, particularly if there has been a history of anorexia. This recommendation is due to the potential for refeeding syndrome, whereby rapid glucose metabolism can lead to hypophosphatemia, hypokalemia, and hypomagnesemia. This also illustrates the need to assess electrolyte status every 12 to 24 hours for the first 48 to 72 hours when implementing TPN.

PN formulation should be done in a laminar flow hood with appropriate aseptic procedures to prevent contamination of solutions. A sterile catheter should be used, and PN should be administered through its own port in a multilumen catheter with the most distal port reserved for PN. Avoid the addition of other medications or treatments because some medications are not compatible with PN. The typical osmolality and pH of a TPN solution will be far different than plasma osmolality (around 1000 to 1300 mOsmol and pH less than 7). This may be irritating to the vascular endothelium and requires a large vessel for administration.[74] Such high osmolar solutions cannot be used in a peripheral vein as they may induce thrombophlebitis, and this is the reason that 5% glucose is used to dilute PPN rather than the 50% glucose solution used in TPN solutions.[66,72] Using 5% dextrose creates an osmolality of less than 700 mOsmol, which is a guideline from human medicine that has been adopted by many veterinary nutritionists and internists.[76] Figure 15-4 describes guidelines for PPN formulation for dogs and cats.[66,72] Addition of B-complex vitamins should also be considered when using TPN and PPN. Most preparations do not include folate, and cobalamin may be insufficient or absent and should be considered separately if long-term support is required Furthermore, if chronic use of TPN is required, the addition of calcium to separate fluids and the use of amino acids with electrolytes and trace mineral additions to the TPN should be considered.

The proportions of glucose and lipids in parenteral solutions is a subject of much debate, particularly in the cancer patient, because of suggestions that neoplastic tissues utilize glucose more readily and the possibility of mild insulin resistance.[10,11] However, increasing lipid content to meet energy requirements has also been met with some trepidation due to lipid's potential to mildly suppress the immune system.[77] Lipid has also been incriminated as the cause of microemboli,[78] and some suggest placing a 1.5 to 2 μm filter in the line to remove lipid particles and microbes; however, recent evidence suggests that in a typical veterinary-formulated TPN solution the lipid particles remain well emulsified—no bacterial growth was evident for 3 days following formulation when kept refrigerated.[79] PPN, with its lower osmolality, is at an increased risk of sequestering microbial growth.

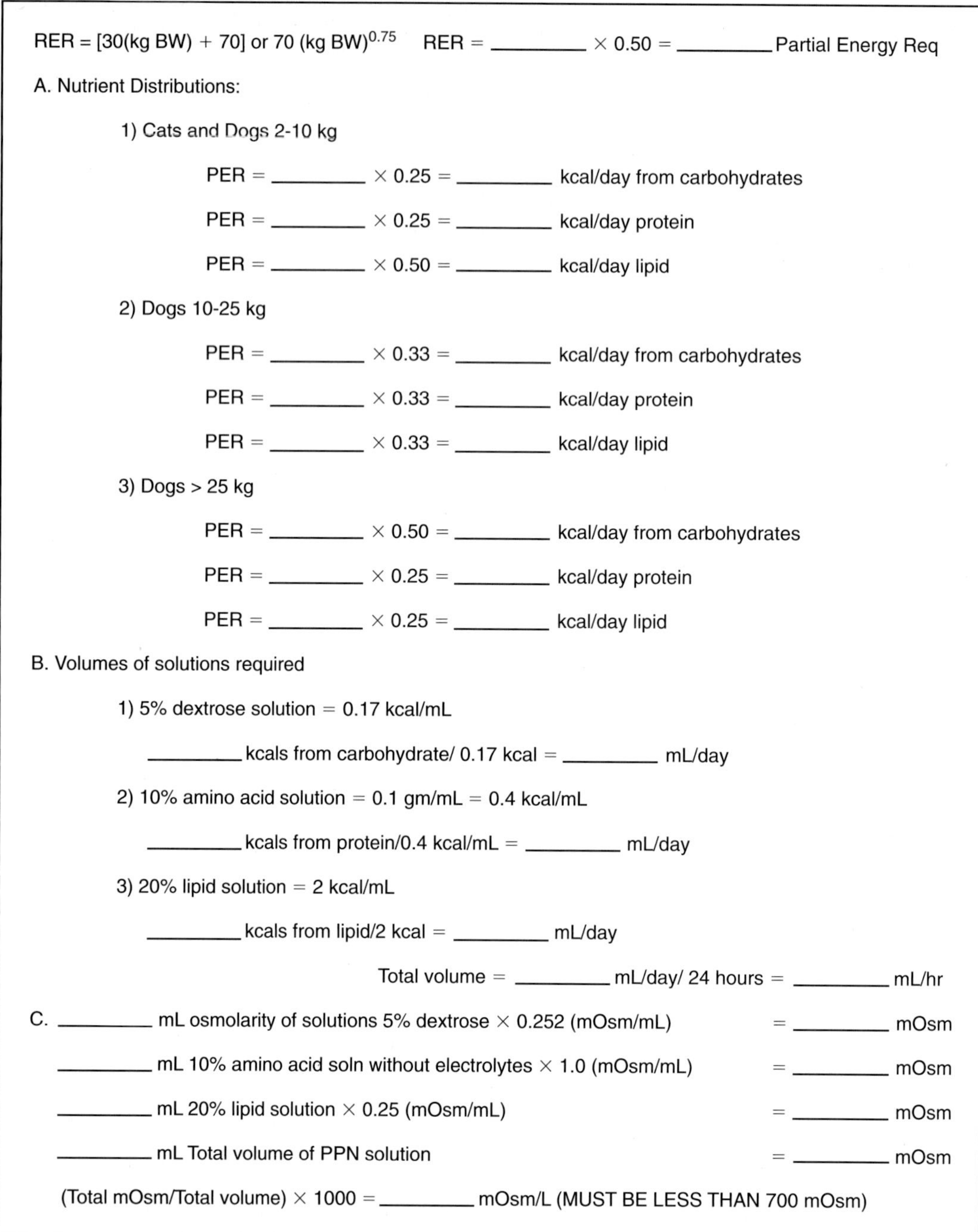

RER = [30(kg BW) + 70] or 70 (kg BW)$^{0.75}$ RER = _______ × 0.50 = _______ Partial Energy Req

A. Nutrient Distributions:

1) Cats and Dogs 2-10 kg

PER = _______ × 0.25 = _______ kcal/day from carbohydrates

PER = _______ × 0.25 = _______ kcal/day protein

PER = _______ × 0.50 = _______ kcal/day lipid

2) Dogs 10-25 kg

PER = _______ × 0.33 = _______ kcal/day from carbohydrates

PER = _______ × 0.33 = _______ kcal/day protein

PER = _______ × 0.33 = _______ kcal/day lipid

3) Dogs > 25 kg

PER = _______ × 0.50 = _______ kcal/day from carbohydrates

PER = _______ × 0.25 = _______ kcal/day protein

PER = _______ × 0.25 = _______ kcal/day lipid

B. Volumes of solutions required

1) 5% dextrose solution = 0.17 kcal/mL

_______ kcals from carbohydrate/ 0.17 kcal = _______ mL/day

2) 10% amino acid solution = 0.1 gm/mL = 0.4 kcal/mL

_______ kcals from protein/0.4 kcal/mL = _______ mL/day

3) 20% lipid solution = 2 kcal/mL

_______ kcals from lipid/2 kcal = _______ mL/day

Total volume = _______ mL/day/ 24 hours = _______ mL/hr

C. _______ mL osmolarity of solutions 5% dextrose × 0.252 (mOsm/mL) = _______ mOsm

_______ mL 10% amino acid soln without electrolytes × 1.0 (mOsm/mL) = _______ mOsm

_______ mL 20% lipid solution × 0.25 (mOsm/mL) = _______ mOsm

_______ mL Total volume of PPN solution = _______ mOsm

(Total mOsm/Total volume) × 1000 = _______ mOsm/L (MUST BE LESS THAN 700 mOsm)

FIGURE 15-4 Small animal partial parenteral nutrition (PPN) formulation sheet.

Nutritional Support in the Cancer-Bearing Patient

Substrate

Based on our present understanding, the use of specific dietary regimens in cancer patients is premature. It has been hypothesized that due to the glycolytic nature of neoplastic cell growth, altering the substrates to hypothetically "starve the tumor" by eliminating some carbohydrates may be indicated.[1,2,10,11] This argument falls short for a number of reasons. If carbohydrates are limited, energy sources are replaced with additional fat and/or protein. Added protein will lead to increased transaminase and deaminase activity causing conversion of the protein to glucose and carbon precursors for glucose or fatty acid synthesis, and serum glucose and delivery of glucose to the tumor tissue may still remain constant. If appetite is diminished, choosing a higher protein and higher fat food may enhance palatability and caloric density, making these foods appropriate for long-term management during treatment.[55] Previous sections have discussed the discordance of results of studies investigating low-carbohydrate, high-fat, and modified-fat diets.[7] One study documented slight increases in remission and survival times when a high polyunsaturated fat diet (high ω-3 fatty acids) and arginine diet was used, suggesting that the type of fats and amino acids may influence remission and survival (see subsequent discussion).[12]

Cats appear more prone to weight loss during hospitalization. Many cats receive inadequate caloric intake, particularly during radiation treatment when food availability is limited each day due to repeated anesthesia. Many cats will eat 12 to 20 small meals throughout the day and night based on observed feeding patterns.[80] The use of higher protein may be worthwhile because recent rodent data show that a high-protein and low-carbohydrate diet decreases tumor growth in a variety of different xenografted tumors.[81] In this diet study, calories were met with approximately 50% protein, implying that high protein may be the benefit, rather than low carbohydrate.[81] The use of high-protein diets may also have benefits in cats with lean body mass wasting issues.[82,83] Although these were small studies, it suggests that in cats, skeletal muscle may respond to higher protein by increasing lean mass to a small extent. With this in mind we often recommend feeding cats higher protein (>35% dry matter) and fat (>20% dry matter). Dogs can be fed similarly, even though many commercial dog foods will have lower protein (typically >30% dry matter is achievable) than cat food.

Amino Acids

The benefits of additional protein to the diet of cancer patients may result from increased circulating amino acids as inhibitory molecules in neoplastic cell proliferation.[81] Arginine has received considerable attention since low-millimolar concentrations of arginine can inhibit various neoplastic cell lines by altering cell cycle progression.[84-87] Additional xenograft data using human and mouse cell lines show diminished tumor growth when mice are provided foods with high dietary arginine, and a single study in dogs with lymphoma, using an arginine-enhanced diet in combination with enhanced ω-3 fatty acids, documented improved remission and survival times.[12] However, the practicality of using an amino acid supplement like arginine leaves much to be desired since the required dose is in excess of 100 mg/kg body weight. Additionally, the bitter taste of arginine and potential for creating amino acid imbalance also prevents its use in long-term feeding regimens. The benefits of glutamine have also been touted due to lean body mass preservation properties and its ability to enhance mucosal barrier function.[88,89] However, enterocytes' ability to utilize glutamine and first-pass hepatic metabolism do not allow glutamine to have any pronounced effects on lean mass. The use of high-protein mixed meals to support enterocyte health and mucosal barrier function is often recommended for general health.

Polyunsaturated Fats

Using fat in diets is helpful in increasing palatability and energy density, but in many instances the fatty acid constituents can influence neoplastic cell growth. Human and rodent studies suggest that consumption of high concentrations of ω-3 fatty acids, namely eicosapentaenoic acid (EPA) and docosahexaenoic acid (DHA), in the form of marine oils may perturb loss of lean body mass and possibly decrease tumor growth rate.[90-97] These fatty acids may transform into inert eicosanoids (PGE_3, leukotriene B_5 [LTB_5], 12-hydroxyeicosapentaenoic acid [12-HEPE], 5-HEPE) rather than proinflammatory eicosanoids (PGE_2, LTB_4, 12-hydroxyeicosatetraenoic acid [12-HETE], and 5-HETE). The pathways and eicosanoids liberated are highly dependent on the enzymatic machinery present in the cells. Although the addition of fatty acids into the cell membrane may affect intracellular signaling events, the intracellular enzymatic machinery that modifies the primary fatty acid into promitogenic or inert eicosanoids may be more important.[96-99] Cell signaling events that lead to liberation of arachidonic acid from the cell membrane can be converted to eicosanoids, which when released from the cell can have local or paracrine effects on cell growth through interactions with eicosanoid receptors (Figure 15-5). The two enzymes that have received the most attention are COX and 5-lipoxygenase (5-LOX) due to the promitogenic mechanisms of action observed by their respective eicosanoids, PGE_2 (COX) and 5-oxo-ETE/LTB_4 (5-LOX).[96-99]

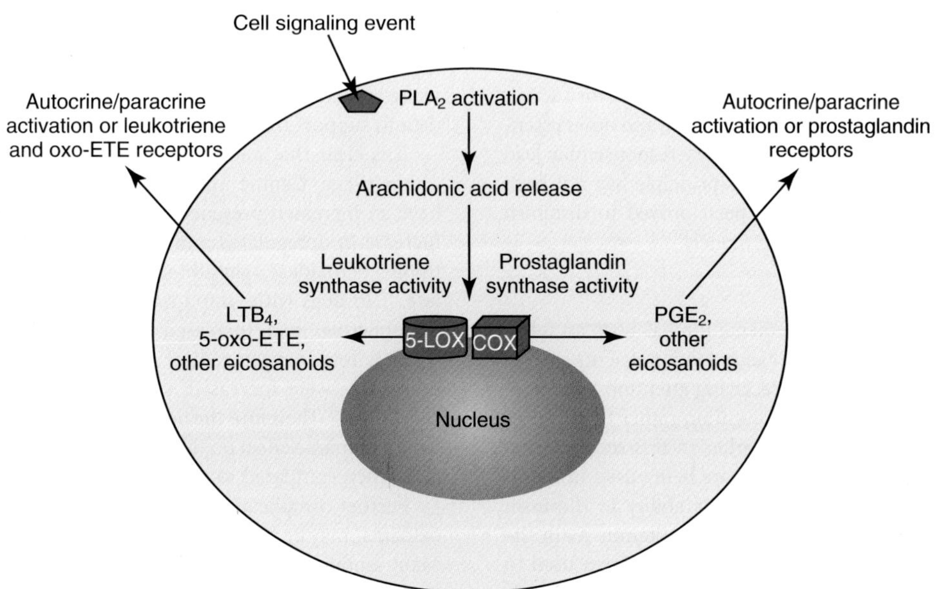

FIGURE 15-5 The liberation of arachidonic acid (AA) from the cell membrane due to cell signaling events leading to nuclear translocation of AA. Cyclooxygenase and lipoxygenase activity coupled with leukotriene synthase or prostaglandin synthase will allow for formation of bioactive eicosanoids that when released can have autocrine or paracrine cell proliferation signaling activities depending on receptor presence. *PLA2,* Phospholipase A_2; *LTB_4,* leukotriene B_4; *PGE_2,* prostaglandin E_2; *5-LOX,* 5-lipoxygenase; *COX,* cyclooxygenase.

Although possibly relevant to many types of human cancers, there is a paucity of data in companion animals, with the most intriguing studies documenting the use of COX inhibition in TCC.[100,101]

A single study in cancer-bearing dogs using a fish-based ω-3 fatty acid–enhanced diet showed a small improvement in survival times; however, there were multiple changes in the dietary trial, including arginine and energy substrate differences that may have played a role.[12] Although the biochemical principle that increased EPA in cells will inhibit promitogenic eicosanoid formation as an autocrine/paracrine signaling molecule is valid,[99] it is unclear what tumor types this may apply to. Some neoplastic tissues will utilize the proinflammatory cytokine milieu to promote proliferation or upregulate pathways that may promote metastasis.[102] The benefits of fish oils may go beyond mild suppression of tumor cell proliferation because the antiinflammatory effects of fish oil may also quench the inflammatory reactions associated with certain cancers.[103-105] Thus there is little downside to increasing ω-3 fatty acid consumption in the diet of cancer patients. The lack of clinical studies in this area precludes an optimal dosing regimen, and recent metaanalysis of human trials using fish oils for QOL issues were inconclusive.[106] Additionally, cats seem to be more sensitive to fish oil supplementation than dogs as the result of greater effects on platelet reactivity resulting in alterations of clotting times.[107] A safe and tolerable dose for fatty acids in dogs can be extrapolated from studies in cardiac cachexia in dogs,[108,109] in which EPA 45 mg and DHA 25 mg/kg body weight (e.g., 1 tsp/20 kg body weight) was used, but higher doses may be needed in dogs with cancer. Furthermore, the type of fish oil can significantly affect the ratio of EPA to DHA. Salmon oils tend to have higher DHA than EPA, and whitefish oils (e.g., herring, menhaden, cod) tend to have higher EPA than DHA; therefore whitefish oils are the preferred source. A safe and potentially effective dose in cats cannot be recommended.

During radiation therapy, the paradigm may be altered because radiation therapy causes irreparable damage to tumor cellular microstructure, resulting in apoptosis of cells and negative effects on surrounding tissues. The use of polyunsaturated fats (the longest, the ω-3 fatty acid DHA, has more double bonds) may be oxidized to a greater extent during radiation treatment, potentially leading to increased membrane compromise and cellular death.[110] Surrounding tissues may not exhibit an aggressive inflammatory action due to the hastened eicosanoid response with EPA, and other essential fatty acids quenching this proinflammatory response may lead to less surrounding tissue damage.[111] This principle has not been studied in veterinary patients but has been proved to diminish radiation-induced tissue damage in pig models.[111]

Vitamins and Minerals

Essential vitamin and mineral supplementation has been an interesting area of investigation in human cancer, with nutrients such as vitamin A, vitamin D, and selenium receiving attention.* Much of the research has centered on cancer prevention rather than cancer treatment, which has been addressed earlier in this section. That being said, certain vitamins and minerals are being used in therapeutic clinical trials in humans due to their ability to diminish tumor cell proliferation in preclinical models. Vitamin A, in the form of retinoic acid and synthetic derivatives, has been used to treat certain cancers; however, discordant effects on nuclear signaling occur with different heterodimers.[113,114] Some heterodimers drive the proliferative response, whereas others diminish cell proliferation.[115] Their use cannot be globally recommended at this time.

Regarding vitamin D, low concentrations of the precursor to active vitamin D (25, OH D3 calcidiol) in people may promote tumorigenesis and treatment with active vitamin D (1,25, OH D3 calcitriol) may cause tumor regression in some cases.[41-43,116] Although antiproliferative at high doses, calcitriol can lead to hypercalcemia and its sequelae, including calcification of soft tissues. This is illustrated in a recent trial characterizing dosing in dogs with mast cell tumors in which many patients developed clinical signs of hypercalcemia, inappetence, and vomiting.[116,117]

Selenium has generated considerable interest in certain human neoplastic diseases, such as lung, squamous cell, and prostatic carcinoma.[118-121] Low serum concentrations have been associated with an increased risk of prostatic cancer in humans.[118,120] Interestingly, the selenium requirement in most dog food based on the AAFCO is considerably lower than what the National Research Council deems adequate intake in dogs and cats.[122] Thus many pet foods may not have optimal concentrations of selenium, and modest supplementation may be considered.[118-121] However, recent metaanalysis of human intervention studies suggests no definitive benefits from selenium supplementation in treatment or prevention of neoplastic disease.[37]

B vitamins of interest include folate and vitamin B_{12} (cobalamin). The interest once again derives from human literature in which their effects on epigenetic alterations may affect tumor suppressor and oncogene expression over time.[122-124] Considering the consistent intake of folate and cobalamin in the pet population caused by commercial dog food consumption, there is a large gap in applying these paradigms of subclinical deficiency to pet populations. Furthermore, the lack of clinical or even canine or feline in-vitro investigation prevents any postulation as to their effects on cancer cells.

Antioxidants/Supplements

Utilization of supplements, most commonly substances termed *antioxidants,* has grown tremendously in the past 15 years. Studies suggest that approximately 65% of pet owners are using some sort of alternative treatments—over 30% are oral supplements and over 50% say their veterinarian approves of this use.[125] In oncology referral centers, the general recommendation to clients is to refrain from using antioxidants or herbal supplements due to the lack of clinical data to support their use.[126]

It is clear that antioxidant and oxidative balance is altered in tumor tissue. Canine mammary cancer tissue has been shown to have an increased presence of lipid peroxidation coupled with an increase in upregulated antioxidant mechanisms, including glutathione peroxidase, glutathione, superoxide dismutase, and catalase.[127] In dogs with lymphoma, reductions in serum antioxidants (tocopherols) and increased lipid peroxidation were observed, whereas total oxygen radical absorption capacity and glutathione peroxidase were increased, suggesting an increase in antioxidant capability.[128] Therefore the addition of an antioxidant is unlikely to have a dramatic effect on the overall antioxidant capability of tumor cells when compared to normal tissue.

Further complicating this issue, many substances given as "antioxidants" may be considered pro-oxidants in some environments.[129] Many isothiocyanates, flavonoids, and carotenoids that clients use may actually cause alteration of cell signaling or depletion of specific antioxidant systems.[129,130] Furthermore, there is increasing evidence that many of these compounds upregulate or downregulate specific or sometimes global cell signaling systems to alter the proliferative cycle from activities such as cell cycle disruption (cyclin-dependent

*References 35, 36, 41-43, 112-114.

kinase [CDKs], p16, p21), prosurvival signals (nuclear factor-κB [NF-κB], AKT), mitochondrial-induced apoptosis (bcl and bax family proteins), and proliferative signaling pathways (i.e., mitogen-activated protein [MAP] kinase, tyrosine kinase [TK] activity).[131-133] Recent primary cancer cell culture data in lymphoma and OSA support these principles. Astaxanthin and lycopene, two carotenoids, showed limited antioxidant capability in canine OSA cell lines, and when coupled with the chemotherapeutic agent doxorubicin or irradiation, there were no protective effects on cell proliferation indices or cell death,[134,135] whereas isoflavones appear to induce mitochondrial apoptosis in canine lymphoma cells.[136]

Even if some of these compounds have little to no detrimental effect on current chemotherapy or radiation protocols, the limiting factor to their effective use is absorption, hepatic metabolism, and the attainment of tissue concentrations that recapitulate what has been used *in vitro*.[131] Pharmacokinetic data have been collected on three nutraceuticals: genistein (an isoflavone) in cats, epigallocatechin gallate (EGCG, a flavone from green tea) in dogs, and lycopene in dogs (carotenoids). All of these nutraceuticals required dosing at very high concentrations, which may preclude their use. There is a tremendous disconnect from what is available and what may be required, as well as a lack of clinical investigation to assess efficacy and safety except for the few examples listed above. Furthermore, metabolism of these compounds may be different in cats and dogs; therefore caution is advised. Doses of over 150 mg/kg of EGCG in dogs caused hepatic necrosis, and the use of lipoic acid (an antioxidant thought to help salvage glutathione) has potential for toxicity and hepatic damage in cats, when used at doses thought safe in dogs and humans.[137,138]

In conclusion, set nutritional requirements for cancer-bearing companion species do not exist. In part, this is due to the variety of neoplastic diseases involved and the danger in trying to extrapolate data generated in human trials. There remain many aspects to address, including nutritional interventions (during treatment and remission) for anorexia/cachexia and nutrition recommendations based on specific disease processes. Therefore there is no one dietary recommendation for cancer patients; rather each case should be evaluated based on the body condition of the patient, the specific neoplastic process, and the treatment protocol initiated by the oncologist. The topics discussed are merely guidelines for interested clients and clinicians, and the most important factor in nutritional intervention is to supply a complete and balanced ration that meets the energy requirements of the patient to prevent weight loss.

REFERENCES

1. Koppenol WH, Bounds PL, Dang CV: Otto Warburg's contributions to current concepts of cancer metabolism, *Nat Rev Cancer* 11:325–337, 2011.
2. Cairns RA, Harris IS, Mak TW: Regulation of cancer cell metabolism, *Nat Rev Cancer* 11:85–95, 2011.
3. Walenta S, Schroeder T, Mueller-Klieser W: Lactate in solid malignant tumors: potential basis of a metabolic classification in clinical oncology, *Curr Med Chem* 11:2195–2204, 2004.
4. Vaupel P: Metabolic microenvironment of tumor cells: a key factor in malignant progression, *Exp Oncol* 32:125–127, 2010.
5. Ogilvie GK, Vail DM: Nutrition and cancer—recent developments, *Vet Clin North Am Small Anim Pract* 20:969–985, 1990.
6. Ogilvie GK, Vail DM, Wheeler SL, et al: Effects of chemotherapy and remission on carbohydrate metabolism in dogs with lymphoma, *Cancer* 69:233–238, 1992.
7. Ogilvie GK, Walters LM, Fettman MJ, et al: Energy expenditure in dogs with lymphoma fed two specialized diets, *Cancer* 71:3146–3152, 1993.
8. Ogilvie GK, Walters LM, Salman MD, et al: Resting energy expenditure in dogs with nonhematopoietic malignancies before and after excision of tumors, *Am J Vet Res* 57:1463–1467, 1996.
9. Mazzaferro EM, Hackett TB, Stein TP, et al: Metabolic alterations in dogs with osteosarcoma, *Am J Vet Res* 62:1234–1239, 2001.
10. Ogilvie GK, Walters L, Salman MD, et al: Alterations in carbohydrate metabolism in dogs with non hematopoietic malignancies, *Am J Vet Res* 58:277–281, 1997.
11. Vail DM, Ogilvie GK, Wheeler SL et al: Alterations in carbohydrate metabolism in canine lymphoma, *J Vet Int Med*, 4:8–11, 1990.
12. Ogilvie GK, Fettman MJ, Mallinckrodt CH et al: Effect of fish oil, arginine, and doxorubicin chemotherapy on remission and survival time for dogs with lymphoma: a double-blind, randomized placebo-controlled study, *Cancer* 88:1916–1928, 2000.
13. Ogilvie GK, Ford RB, Vail DM, et al: Alterations in lipoprotein profiles in dogs with lymphoma, *J Vet Intern Med* 8:62–66, 1994.
14. Ackerman BH, Kasbekar N: Disturbances of taste and smell induced by drugs, *Pharmacotherapy* 17:482–496, 1997.
15. Weeth LP, Fascetti AJ, Kass PH, et al: Prevalence of obese dogs in a population of dogs with cancer, *Am J Vet Res* 68:389–398, 2007.
16. Tisdale MJ: Are tumoral factors responsible for host tissue wasting in cancer cachexia? *Future Oncol* 6:503–513, 2010.
17. Penna F, Minero VG, Costamagna D, et al: Anti-cytokine strategies for the treatment of cancer-related anorexia and cachexia, *Expert Opin Biol Ther* 10:1241–1250, 2010.
18. Seruga B, Zhang H, Bernstein LJ, et al: Cytokines and their relationship to the symptoms and outcome of cancer, *Nat Rev Cancer* 8:887–899, 2008.
19. Pajak B, Orzechowska S, Pijet B, et al: Crossroads of cytokine signaling–the chase to stop muscle cachexia, *J Physiol Pharmacol* 59(Suppl 9):251–264, 2008.
20. Fearon KC: Cancer cachexia and fat-muscle physiology, *N Engl J Med* 365:565–567, 2011.
21. Merlo A, Rezende BC, Franchini ML, et al: Serum C-reactive protein concentrations in dogs with multicentric lymphoma undergoing chemotherapy, *J Am Vet Med Assoc* 230:522–526, 2007.
22. Tecles F, Caldín M, Zanella A, et al: Serum acute phase protein concentrations in female dogs with mammary tumors, *J Vet Diagn Invest* 21:214–219, 2009.
23. Baez JL, Michel KE, Sorenmo K, et al: A prospective investigation of the prevalence and prognostic significance of weight loss and changes in body condition in feline cancer patients, *J Feline Med Surg* 9:411–417, 2007.
24. Wolin KY, Carson K, Colditz GA: Obesity and cancer, *Oncologist* 15:556–565, 2010.
25. Roberts DL, Dive C, Renehan AG: Biological mechanisms linking obesity and cancer risk: new perspectives, *Ann Rev Med* 61:301–316, 2010.
26. Calle EE, Rodriguez C, Walker-Thurmond K, et al: Overweight, obesity, and mortality from cancer in a prospectively studied cohort of U.S. adults, *N Engl J Med* 348:1625–1638, 2003.
27. Lichtman MA: Obesity and the risk for a hematological malignancy: leukemia, lymphoma, or myeloma, *Oncologist* 15:1083–1101, 2010.
28. de Boer EJ, Slimani N, van 't Veer P, et al: The European Food Consumption Validation Project: conclusions and recommendations, *Eur J Clin Nutr* 65(Suppl 1):S102–S107, 2011.
29. Jansen RJ, Robinson DP, Stolzenberg-Solomon RZ, et al: Fruit and vegetable consumption is inversely associated with having pancreatic cancer, *Cancer Causes Control* [Epub ahead of print September 14, 2011].
30. Magalhães B, Peleteiro B, Lunet N: Dietary patterns and colorectal cancer: systematic review and meta-analysis, *Eur J Cancer Prev* [Epub ahead of print September 22, 2011].
31. Sonnenschein EG, Glickman LT, Goldschmidt MH, et al: Body conformation, diet, and risk of breast cancer in pet dogs: a case-control study, *Am J Epidemiol* 133:694–703, 1991.

32. Shofer FS, Sonnenschein EG, Goldschmidt MH, et al: Histopathologic and dietary prognostic factors for canine mammary carcinoma, *Breast Cancer Res Treat* 13:49–60, 1989.
33. Pérez Alenza D, Rutteman GR, Peña L, et al: Relation between habitual diet and canine mammary tumors in a case-control study, *J Vet Intern Med* 12:132 139, 1998.
34. Raghavan M, Knapp DW, Bonney PL, et al: Evaluation of the effect of dietary vegetable consumption on reducing risk of transitional cell carcinoma of the urinary bladder in Scottish Terriers, *J Am Vet Med Assoc* 227:94–100, 2005.
35. Fulan H, Changxing J, Baina WY, et al: Retinol, vitamins A, C, and E and breast cancer risk: a meta-analysis and meta-regression, *Cancer Causes Control* 22:1383–1396, 2011.
36. Arain MA, Abdul Qadeer A: Systematic review on "vitamin E and prevention of colorectal cancer," *Pak J Pharm Sci* 23:125–130, 2010.
37. Dennart G, Zwahlen M, Vinceti M, et al: Selenium for preventing cancer, *Cochrane Database Syst Rev* 11(5):CD005195, 2011.
38. Wu K, Erdman JW Jr, Schwartz SJ: Plasma and dietary carotenoids, and the risk of prostate cancer: a nested case-control study, *Cancer Epidemiol Biomarkers Prev* 13:260–269, 2004.
39. Bendich A: From 1989 to 2001: what have we learned about the "biological actions of beta-carotene"? *J Nutr* 134:225S–230S, 2004.
40. Cooper DA: Carotenoids in health and disease: recent scientific evaluations, research recommendations and the consumer, *J Nutr* 134:221S–224S, 2004.
41. Deeb KK, Trump DL, Johnson CS: Vitamin D signaling pathways in cancer: potential for anticancer therapeutics, *Nature Rev Canc* 7:684–700, 2007.
42. Abbas S, Linseisen J, Slanger T, et al: Serum 25-hydroxyvitamin D and risk of post-menopausal breast cancer—results of a large case-control study, *Carcinogenesis* 29:93–99, 2007.
43. Yin L, Grandi N, Raum E, et al: Meta-analysis: longitudinal studies of serum vitamin D and colorectal cancer risk, *Aliment Pharmacol Ther* 30:113–125, 2009.
44. How KL, Hazewinkel HA, Mol JA: Dietary vitamin D dependence of cat and dog due to inadequate cutaneous synthesis of vitamin D, *Gen Comp Endocrinol* 96:12–18, 1994.
45. Wakshlag JJ, Rassnick KM, Malone EK, et al: Cross sectional study to investigate the association between serum vitamin D and cutaneous mast cell tumours in Labrador retrievers, *Br J Nutr* 106:S60–S63, 2011.
46. Lund EM, Armstrong PJ, Kirk CA, et al: Prevalence and risk factors for obesity in adult cats from private US veterinary practices, *Int J Appl Res Vet Med* 3:88–96, 2005.
47. Lund EM, Armstrong PJ, Kirk CA, et al: Prevalence and risk factors for obesity in adult dogs from private US veterinary practices, *Int J Appl Res Vet Med* 4:177–186, 2006.
48. Inui A: Cancer anorexia-cachexia syndrome: current issues in research and management, *Cancer J Clin* 52:72–91, 2002.
49. Laflamme DP: Development and validation of a body condition score system for cats: a clinical tool, *Feline Pract* 25:5–6, 1997.
50. Mawby DI, Bartges JW, d'Avignon A, et al: Comparison of various methods for estimating body fat in dogs, *J Am Anim Hosp Assoc* 40:109–111, 2004.
51. de Fornel-Thibaud P, Blanchard G, et al: Unusual case of osteopenia associated with nutritional calcium and vitamin D deficiency in an adult dog, *J Am Anim Hosp Assoc* 43:52–60, 2007.
52. Taylor MB, Geiger DA, Saker KE, et al: Diffuse osteopenia and myelopathy in a puppy fed a diet composed of an organic premix and raw ground beef, *J Am Vet Med Assoc* 234:1041–1048, 2009.
53. Michel KE, Sorenmo K, Shofer FS: Evaluation of body condition and weight loss in dogs presented to a veterinary oncology service, *J Vet Intern Med* 18:692–695, 2004.
54. Kienzle E: Energy. In Beitz DC, editor: *National Research Council nutrient requirements of dogs and cats*, Washington DC, 2006, National Academies Press.
55. Delaney SJ: Management of anorexia in dogs and cats, *Vet Clin North Am Small Anim Pract* 36:1243–1249, 2006.
56. Fox CB, Treadway AK, Blaszczyk AT, et al: Megestrol acetate and mirtazapine for the treatment of unplanned weight loss in the elderly, *Pharmacotherapy* 29:383–397, 2009.
57. Braun TP, Marks DL: Pathophysiology and treatment of inflammatory anorexia in chronic disease, *J Cachex Sarcopenia Muscle* 1:135–145, 2010.
58. Bedford SW, Godsall SA: Diazepam for inappetence, *Vet Rec* 122:590–591, 1988.
59. Center SA, Elston TH, Rowland PH, et al: Fulminant hepatic failure associated with oral administration of diazepam in 11 cats, *J Am Vet Med Assoc* 209:618–625, 1996.
60. Long JP, Greco SC: The effect of propofol administered intravenously on appetite stimulation in dogs, *Contemp Top Lab Anim Sci* 39:43–46, 2000.
61. Remillard RL, Saker KE: Critical care nutrition and enteral-assisted feeding. In Hand MS, Thatcher CD, Remillard RL, et al, editors: *Small animal clinical nutrition*, ed 5, Topeka, 2010, Mark Morris Institute.
62. Salinardi BJ, Harkin KR, Bulmer BJ, et al: Comparison of complications of percutaneous endoscopic versus surgically placed gastrostomy tubes in 42 dogs and 52 cats, *J Am Anim Hosp Assoc* 42:51–56, 2006.
63. Yoshimoto SK, Marks SL, Struble AL, et al: Owner experiences and complications with home use of a replacement low profile gastrostomy device for long-term enteral feeding in dogs, *Can Vet J* 47:144–150, 2006.
64. Hill RC: Physical activity and environment. In Beitz DC, editor: *National Research Council nutrient requirements of dogs and cats*, Washington DC, 2006, National Academy Press.
65. Chandler ML, Payne-James JJ: Prospective evaluation of a peripherally administered three-in-one parenteral nutrition product in dogs, *J Am Anim Hosp Assoc* 47:518–523, 2006.
66. Chan DL, Freeman LM, Labata MA, et al: Retrospective evaluation of partial parenteral nutrition in dogs and cats, *J Vet Int Med* 16:440–445, 2002.
67. Pyle SC, Marks SL, Kass PH: Evaluation of complications and prognostic factors associated with administration of total parenteral nutrition in cats: 75 cases (1994-2001), *J Am Vet Med Assoc* 225:242–250, 2004.
68. Crabb SE, Freeman LM, Chan DL, et al: Retrospective evaluation of total parenteral nutrition in cats: 40 cases (1991-2003), *J Vet Emerg Crit Care* 16:S1–S26, 2006.
69. Lippert AC, Fulton RB, Parr, RB: A retrospective study of the use of total parenteral nutrition in dogs and cats, *J Vet Int Med* 7:52–64, 1993.
70. Queau Y, Larsen JA, Kass PH, et al: Factors associated with adverse outcomes during parenteral nutrition administration in dogs and cats, *J Vet Intern Med* 25:446–452, 2011.
71. Qin HL, Su ZD, Hu LG, et al: Effect of early intrajejunal nutrition on pancreatic pathological features and gut barrier function in dogs with acute pancreatitis, *Clin Nutr* 21:469–472, 2002.
72. Chan DL: Parenteral nutritional support. In Ettinger SL, Feldman EC, editor: *Textbook of veterinary internal medicine*, ed 6, St. Louis, 2005, Elsevier Saunders.
73. Remillard RL, Saker KE: Critical care nutrition and enteral-assisted feeding. In Hand MS, Thatcher CD, Remillard RL, et al, editors: *Small animal clinical nutrition*, ed 5, Topeka, 2010, Mark Morris Institute.
74. Wakshlag J, Schoeffler GL, Russell DS, et al: Extravasation injury associated with parenteral nutrition in a cat with presumptive gastrinomas, *J Vet Emerg Crit Care* 21:375–381, 2011.
75. Mauldin GE, Reynolds AJ, Mauldin GN, et al: Nitrogen balance in clinically normal dogs receiving parenteral nutrition solutions, *Am J Vet Res* 62:912–920, 2011.
76. ASPEN Board of Directors and the Clinical Guidelines Task Force: Guidelines for the use of parenteral and enteral nutrition in adult and pediatric patients, *J Parenter Enteral Nutr* 26(1 Suppl):1SA–138SA, 2002.

77. Gogos CA, Kalfarentzos F: Total parenteral nutrition and immune system activity: a review, *Nutrition* 11:339–344, 1995.
78. Kitchell CC, Balogh K: Pulmonary lipid emboli in association with long-term hyperalimentation, *Hum Pathol* 17:83–85, 1986.
79. Thomovsky EJ, Backus RC, Mann FA, et al: Effects of temperature and handling conditions on lipid emulsion stability in veterinary parenteral nutrition admixtured during simulated intravenous administration, *Am J Vet Res* 69:652–658, 2008.
80. Martin GJ, Rand JS: Food intake and blood glucose in normal and diabetic cats fed ad libitum, *J Feline Med Surg* 1:241–251, 1999.
81. Ho VW, Leung K, Hsu A, et al: A low carbohydrate, high protein diet slows tumor growth and prevents cancer initiation, *Cancer Res* 71:4484–4493, 2011.
82. Nguyen P, Lerray V, Dumon H, et al: High protein intake affects lean body mass but not energy expenditure in nonobese neutered cats, *J Nutr* 134:2084S–2086S, 2004.
83. Hannah SS, LaFlamme DP: Effect of dietary protein on nitrogen balance and lean body mass in cats, *Vet Clin Nutr* 3:30, 1996.
84. Burns RA, Milner JA: Effects of arginine on the carcinogenicity of 7,12-dimethylbenz(a)-anthracene and N-methyl-N-nitrosourea, *Carcinogenesis* 5:1539–1542, 1984.
85. Brittenden J, Heys SD, Ross J, et al: Natural cytotoxicity in breast cancer patients receiving neoadjuvant chemotherapy: effects of L-arginine supplementation, *Eur J Surg Oncol* 20:467–472, 1994.
86. Reynolds JV, Daly JM, Shou J, et al: Immunologic effects of arginine supplementation in tumor-bearing and non-tumor-bearing hosts, *Ann Surg* 211:202–210, 1990.
87. Wakshlag JJ, Kallfelz FA, Wakshlag RR, et al: The effects of branched-chain amino acids on canine neoplastic cell proliferation and death, *J Nutr* 136:2007S–2010S, 2006.
88. Kaufmann Y, Kornbluth J, Feng Z, et al: Effect of glutamine on the initiation and promotion phases of DMBA-induced mammary tumor development, *J Parenter Enteral Nutr* 27:411–418, 2003.
89. Yoshida S, Kaibara A, Ishibashi N, et al: Glutamine supplementation in cancer patients, *J Nutr* 17:766–768, 2001.
90. Wigmore SJ, Barber MD, Ross JA, et al: Effect of oral eicosapentaenoic acid on weight loss in patients with pancreatic cancer, *Nutr Cancer* 36:177–184, 2000.
91. Togni V, Ota CC, Folador A, et al: Cancer cachexia and tumor growth reduction in Walker 256 tumor-bearing rats supplemented with N-3 polyunsaturated fatty acids for one generation, *Nutr Cancer* 46:52–58, 2003.
92. Fearon KC, Von Meyenfeldt MF, Moses AG, et al: Effect of a protein and energy dense N-3 fatty acid enriched oral supplement on loss of weight and lean tissue in cancer cachexia: a randomized double blind trial, *Gut* 52:1479–1486, 2003.
93. Colas S, Paon L, Denis F, et al: Enhanced radiosensitivity of rat autochthonous mammary tumors by dietary docosahexaenoic acid, *Int J Cancer* 109:449–454, 2004.
94. Senzaki H, Iwamoto S, Ogura E, et al: Dietary effects of fatty acids on growth and metastasis of KPL-1 human breast cancer cells in vivo and in vitro, *Anticancer Res* 18:1621–1627, 1998.
95. Noguchi M, Earashi M, Minami M, et al: Effects of eicosapentaenoic and docosahexaenoic acid on cell growth and prostaglandin E and leukotriene B production by a human breast cancer cell line (MDA-MB-231), *Oncology* 52:458–464, 1995.
96. Hawcroft G, Loadman PM, Belluzzi A, et al: Effect of eicosapentaenoic acid on E-type prostaglandin synthesis and EP4 receptor signaling in human colorectal cancer cells, *Neoplasia* 12:618–627, 2010.
97. Hayashi T, Nishiyama K, Shirahama T: Inhibition of 5-lipoxygenase pathway suppresses the growth of bladder cancer cells, *Int J Urol* 13:1086–1091, 2006.
98. Schley PD, Brindley DN, Field CJ: (n-3) PUFA alter raft lipid composition and decrease epidermal growth factor receptor levels in lipid rafts of human breast cancer cells, *J Nutr* 137:548–553, 2007.
99. Furstenberger G, Krieg P, Muller-Decker K, et al: What are cyclooxygenases and lipoxygenases doing in the driver's seat of carcinogenesis? *Int J Cancer* 119:2247–2254, 2006.
100. Mohammed SI, Bennett PF, Craig BA, et al: Effects of the cyclooxygenase inhibitor, piroxicam, on tumor response, apoptosis and angiogenesis in a canine model of human invasive urinary bladder cancer, *Cancer Res* 62:356–358, 2002.
101. McMillan SK, Boria P, Moore GE, et al: Antitumor effects of deracoxib treatment in 26 dogs with transitional cell carcinoma of the urinary bladder, *J Am Vet Med Assoc* 239:1084–1089, 2011.
102. Hanahan D, Weinberg RA: Hallmarks of cancer: the next generation, *Cell* 144:646–674, 2011.
103. Weylandt KH, Krause LF, Gomolka B, et al: Suppressed liver tumorigenesis in fat-1 mice with elevated omega-3 fatty acids is associated with increased omega-3 derived lipid mediators and reduced TNF-α, *Carcinogenesis* 32:897–903, 2011.
104. Endres S, Ghorbani R, Kelley VE, et al: The effect of dietary supplementation with n-3 polyunsaturated fatty acids on the synthesis of interleukin-1 and tumor necrosis factor by mononuclear cells, *N Engl J Med* 320:265–271, 1989.
105. Purasiri P, Murray A, Richardson S, et al: Modulation of cytokine production in vivo by dietary essential fatty acids in patients with colorectal cancer, *Clin Sci (Lond)* 87:711–717, 1994.
106. Dewey A, Baughan C, Dean T, et al: Eicosapentaenoic acid (EPA, an omega-3 fatty acid from fish oils) for the treatment of cancer cachexia, *Cochrane Database Syst Rev* 24 (1):CD004597, 2007.
107. Saker KE, Eddy AL, Thatcher CD, et al: Manipulation of dietary (n-6) and (n-3) fatty acids alters platelet function in cats, *J Nutr* 128:2645s–2647s, 1998.
108. Freeman LM, Rush JE, Kehayias JJ, et al: Nutritional alterations and the effect of fish oil supplementation in dogs with heart failure, *J Vet Intern Med* 12:440–448, 1998.
109. Freeman LM, Rush JE: Cardiovascular diseases: nutritional modulation. In Pibot P, Elliot D, Biourge V, editors: *Encyclopedia of canine clinical nutrition*, Paris, 2006, Aniwa SAS.
110. Kikawa KD, Herrick JS, Tateo RE, et al: Induced oxidative stress and cell death in the A549 lung adenocarcinoma cell line by ionizing radiation is enhanced by supplementation with docosahexaenoic acid, *Nutr Cancer* 62:1017–1024, 2010.
111. Hopewell JW, van den Aardweg GJ, et al: Amelioration of both early and late radiation-induced damage to pig skin by essential fatty acids, *Int J Radiat Oncol Biol Phys* 30:1119–1125, 1994.
112. Paik J, Blaner WS, Sommer KM, et al: Retinoids, retinoic acid receptors, and breast cancer, *Cancer Invest* 21:304–312, 2003.
113. Tang XH, Gudas LJ: Retinoids, retinoic acid receptors, and cancer, *Annu Rev Pathol* 6:345–364, 2011.
114. Bushue N, Wan YJ: Retinoid pathway and cancer therapeutics, *Adv Drug Deliv Rev* 62:1285–1298, 2010.
115. Hayes KC: Nutritional problems in cats: taurine deficiency and vitamin A excess, *Can Vet J* 23:2–5, 1982.
116. Rassnick KM, Muindi JR, Johnson CS, et al: Oral bioavailability of DN101, a concentrated formulation of calcitriol, in tumor-bearing dogs, *Cancer Chemother Pharmacol* 67:165–171, 2011.
117. Malone EK, Rassnick KM, Wakshlag JJ, et al: Calcitriol enhances mast cell tumour chemotherapy and receptor tyrosine kinase inhibitor activity in-vitro and has single agent activity against spontaneously occurring canine mast cell tumours, *Vet Comp Oncol* 8:209–220, 2010.
118. Nelson MA, Porterfield BW, Jacobs ET, et al: Selenium and prostate cancer prevention, *Semin Urol Oncol* 17:91–96, 1999.
119. Reid ME, Duffield-Lillico AJ, Garland L, et al: Selenium supplementation and lung cancer incidence: an update of the nutritional prevention of cancer trial, *Cancer Epidemiol Biomarkers Prev* 11:1285–1291, 2002.
120. Duffield-Lillico AJ, Dalkin BL, Reid ME, et al: Selenium supplementation, baseline plasma selenium status and incidence of prostate cancer: an analysis of the complete treatment period of the Nutritional Prevention of Cancer Trial, *BJU Int* 91:608–612, 2003.

121. Clark LC, Comb GF Jr, Turnbull BW, et al: Effects of selenium supplementation for cancer prevention in patients with carcinoma of the skin. A randomized controlled trial. Nutritional Prevention of Cancer Study Group, *JAMA* 276:1957–1963, 1996.
122. Xiao SD, Meng XJ, Shi Y, et al: Interventional study of high dose folic acid in gastric carcinogenesis in beagles, *Gut* 50:61–64, 2002.
123. Jhaveri MS, Wagner C, Trepel JB: Impacts of extracellular folate levels on global gene expression, *Mol Pharmacol* 60:1288–1295, 2001.
124. Friso S, Choi SW: The potential cocarcinogenic effect of vitamin B12 deficiency, *Clin Chem Lab Med* 43:1158–1163, 2005.
125. Lana SE, Kogan LR, Crump KA, et al: The use of complementary and alternative therapies in dogs and cats with cancer, *J Am Anim Hosp Assoc* 42:361–365, 2006.
126. Seifried HE, McDonald SS, Anderson DE, et al: The antioxidant conundrum in cancer, *Cancer Res* 63:4295–4298, 2003.
127. Szczubial M, Kankofer M, Lopuszynski W, et al: Oxidative stress parameters in bitches with mammary gland tumors, *J Vet Med* 51:336–340, 2004.
128. Winter JL, Barber LG, Freeman TM, et al: Antioxidant status and biomarkers of oxidative stress in dogs with lymphoma, *J Vet Int Med* 23:311–316, 2009.
129. Chandhok D, Saha T: Redox regulation in cancer: a double-edged sword with therapeutic potential, *Oxid Med Cell Longev* 3:23–34, 2010.
130. Zhao CR, Gao ZH, Qu XJ: Nrf2-ARE signaling pathway and natural products for cancer chemoprevention, *Cancer Epidemiol* 34:523–533, 2010.
131. Crozier A, Jaganath IB, Clifford MN: Dietary phenolics: chemistry, bioavailability and the effects on health, *Nat Prod Rep* 26:1001–1043, 2009.
132. Khan N, Afaq F, Mukhtar H: Cancer chemoprevention through dietary antioxidants: progress and promise, *Antioxidants Redox Signal* 10:1–36, 2008.
133. Shanmugam MK, Kannaiyan R, Sethi G: Targeting cell signaling and apoptotic pathways by dietary agents: role in the prevention and treatment of cancer, *Nutr Cancer* 63:161–173, 2011.
134. Wakshlag JJ, Balkman CA, Morgan SK, et al: Evaluation of the protective effects of all-trans-astaxanthin on canine osteosarcoma cell lines, *Am J Vet Res* 71:89–96, 2010.
135. Wakshlag JJ, Balkman CE: Effects of lycopene on proliferation and death of canine osteosarcoma cells, *Am J Vet Res* 71:1362–1370, 2010.
136. Jamadar-Shroff V, Papich MG, Suter SE: Soy-derived isoflavones inhibit the growth of canine lymphoid cell lines, *Clin Cancer Res* 15:1269–1276, 2009.
137. Serisier S, Leray V, Poudroux W, et al: Effects of green tea on insulin sensitivity, lipid profile and expression of PPAR alpha and PPAR gamma and their target genes in dogs, *Br J Nutr* 99:1208–1216, 2008.
138. Kapetanovic IM, Crowell JA, Krishnaraj R, et al: Exposure and toxicity of green tea polyphenols in fasted and non-fasted dogs, *Toxicology* 260:28–36, 2009.

SECTION C

Relationship-Centered Approach to Cancer Communication

JANE R. SHAW

The increasing recognition of the relationships that people develop with their companion animals[1,2] brings an awareness of the impact of animal illness on pet caregivers and the veterinary team.[3] Rising acknowledgment of pets as family members has also been associated with increasing expectations of pet owners for the highest quality medical care for their companion animals, as well as compassionate care and respectful communication for themselves.[1,4,5] The human-animal bond is particularly stressed and fragile when an animal is sick and even more so with a cancer diagnosis. Appreciating the impact of animal companionship on the health and well-being of humans creates a new dimension in public health. The responsibilities of veterinary professionals have expanded to include the mental health and well being of their clients, as well as their clients' pets.[4]

Cancer communication presents challenges for both oncologists and clients. From the veterinarian's perspective, a number of factors[6,7] may contribute to discomfort, including lack of training, being short of time, practice culture, feeling responsible for the patient's illness, perceptions of failure, unease with death and dying, lack of comfort with uncertainty, impact on the veterinarian-client-patient relationship, worry about the patient's QOL, concerns about the client's emotional response, and their own emotional response to the circumstances. Some of these same reasons may account for client anxiety during difficult conversations. These include self-blame, unease with death and dying, anticipatory grief, effect on the human-animal bond, impact on the veterinarian-client-patient relationship, pet's QOL, and concerns about their emotional response to the situation. Research[6-9] in human medicine indicates that end-of-life discussions are often suboptimal due to many of these barriers and a lack of specific training in communication.

The content, duration, and methods of communication training in veterinary curricula are highly diverse and variable. Many practitioners have not received formal communication training and may feel unprepared to engage in difficult conversations.[10,11] The veterinary profession has identified a skills gap between the content of the veterinary school curriculum and the actual skills required to be a successful veterinarian.[12] Using experiential techniques, defining key skills, and creating opportunities to practice them enhance effective communication.[13-15] In accreditation standards, the American Veterinary Medical Association Council on Education recognizes communication as a core clinical competency for success.

Several aspects of cancer care make it a unique communication context.[16] The diagnosis is frequently made by the primary care veterinarian who may refer the client and patient to an oncologist. Therefore the first visit with the oncologist often occurs after the patient has been diagnosed and the focus of the conversation is on confirming the diagnosis, treatment information, and decision making. In this setting, tough conversations occur on the back of a newly formed veterinarian-client-patient relationship. Cancer is an emotionally laden diagnosis, and clients often present with high levels of uncertainty, anxiety, fear, frustration, and guilt, which heightens the stakes for both parties. Fortunately, today we can offer clients a menu of sophisticated diagnostic and therapeutic options to treat their companion animal's cancer. The challenge is navigating the complexity of the information and the decision-making process of making the "right choice" for their pet without overwhelming the client. It may require as much listening as talking to hear what is most important to your clients to address these challenges.

There are six functions of relationship-centered communication in cancer care: exchanging information, making decisions, fostering healing relationships, enabling clients to provide patient care, managing uncertainty, and responding to emotions.[17] Cancer communication is a process that occurs over time, starting with delivering the diagnosis (i.e., often delivering bad news), discussing prognosis, making decisions about treatment options, assessing QOL, transitioning to palliative or supportive care, and ending with preparing families for euthanasia, dying, and death.[18] These difficult conversations are spread throughout multiple visits, as the relationship grows and a partnership develops with the client in caring for the patient.

The purpose of this section is to present best practices for cancer communication. There are limited empiric studies in the veterinary literature concerning veterinarian-client-patient communication, and information pertaining specifically to oncology is based largely on clinical experience. In contrast, the literature on human medical communication contains a large number of empiric studies; however, in relation to cancer communication, what is available is based on expert opinion, case studies, reviews, and predominantly descriptive studies.[16,18] The objectives of this section are to describe relationship-centered care, define core cancer communication skills, and highlight communication approaches to difficult discussions. The medical cancer communication literature[7,9,18-20] and clinical experience provide the foundation for communication techniques presented here.

A Paradigm Shift: Paternalism to Partnership

Recent societal changes have caused a paradigm shift in the veterinarian-client-patient relationship. Growing client expectations, the strong attachment between people and their pets, and increasing consumer knowledge demand a shift in communication style from the traditional paternalistic approach to a collaborative partnership.[5,21,22] Many clients are no longer content with taking a passive role in their animal's healthcare, preferring to take an active role in the decision-making process.[5]

Paternalism is characterized as a relationship in which the oncologist sets the agenda for the appointment, assumes that the client's values are the same as the veterinarian's, and takes on the role of a guardian for the patient.[23,24] Traditionally, paternalism is the most common approach to medical and veterinary visits. In general practice, the veterinarian used a paternalistic approach in 31% of wellness visits and 85% of problem visits.[21] The topic of conversation is primarily biomedical in nature, focusing on the medical condition, diagnosis, treatment, and prognosis.[21]

In a paternalistic relationship, the oncologist does most of the talking and the client plays a passive role. This approach is often referred to as the *data dump* and symbolized by a shot-put.[25] Throwing a shot-put is unidirectional, the intent is on the delivery, the information to be delivered is large in mass and scale, and it is challenging to receive the message. Intuitively, it seems like this directive approach enhances efficiency and promotes time management. The challenge is that the agenda and subsequent diagnostic or treatment plan may not be shared between the oncologist and client, compromising the ability to reach agreement, move forward, and achieve full compliance. This could result in a roadblock and the need to take steps backward to recover and regain client understanding, commitment, and trust.

In contrast, partnership or relationship-centered care represents a balance of power between veterinarian and client and is based on mutuality.[23,24,26] In the relationship-centered model, the relationship between oncologist and client is characterized by negotiation between partners, resulting in creation of a joint venture, with the veterinarian taking on the role of advisor for the client. Respect for the client's perspective and values and recognition of the role the animal plays in the life of the client are incorporated into all aspects of care. In general practice, 69% of wellness visits and 15% of problem visits were characterized as relationship-centered.[21]

The conversation content of relationship-centered visits is broad, including biomedical topics, lifestyle discussion of the pet's daily activities (e.g., exercise regimen, environment, travel, diet, and sleeping habits) and social interactions (e.g., personality or temperament, behavior, human-animal interaction, and animal-animal interactions) that are key indicators of patient quality of life.[21] In addition, a relationship-centered approach encompasses building rapport, establishing a partnership, and encouraging client participation in the animal's care, all of which have the potential to enhance clinical outcomes.

This collaborative relationship is symbolized by a Frisbee.[25] In playing Frisbee, the interaction is reciprocal; the intent is on dialog; the delivery is airy, light, and free; small pieces of information are delivered at a time; and the deliverer and receiver adjust their message to stay on target. The emphasis of the Frisbee analogy is on eliciting client feedback to assess how the client perceives, processes, and understands the information presented.

Relationship-Centered Care

Combining several frameworks, Mead and Bower[27] identified the following five distinct dimensions of relationship or patient-centered care in the human medical setting:

1. The biopsychosocial perspective—a perspective on illness that includes the social and psychologic, as well as biomedical factors.
2. The "patient as a person"—understand the personal meaning of the illness for each individual patient.
3. Sharing power and responsibility—sensitivity to patients' preferences for information and shared decision making.
4. The therapeutic alliance—developing common therapeutic goals and enhancing the physician-patient relationship.
5. The "doctor as person"—awareness of the influence of the subjectivity of the doctor on the practice of medicine.

These principles translate readily to the veterinary context.[21,22] Expanding data gathering to explore the broader lifestyle of the client and pet enhances the understanding of the animal's illness. Discussing unique details such as financial resources, the role of the primary caregiver, feasibility of implementing the plan, and recent life events (i.e., new birth, death, new job, or moving) promotes compliance. With increased recognition of the human-animal bond, it is important to assess the level of attachment and the impact of the animal's illness on the family. Eliciting information on the client's expectations, thoughts, feelings, and fears about the pet's illness fosters client participation and satisfaction and promotes shared decision making.

Based on medical communication studies, the following principles of relationship-centered care are associated with significant clinical outcomes:

1. Broadening the explanatory perspective of disease beyond the biomedical to include lifestyle and social factors is related to expanding the field of inquiry and improved diagnostic reasoning and accuracy.[25]
2. Building a strong relationship is associated with increased accuracy of data gathering,[25] patient satisfaction,[28-30] and physician satisfaction.[31,32]
3. Encouraging participation, negotiation, and shared decision making promotes patient satisfaction,[28-30] adherence,[33] and improved health.[34]

In veterinary medicine, a study investigating the use of patient-centered communication in euthanasia discussions with undisclosed standardized clients identified that veterinarians did not fully explore client feelings, ideas, and expectations.[22] In these visits, veterinarians did not involve clients in defining the problem and identifying treatment goals. Shared decision making is a key component of relationship-centered care, in which there is two-way exchange between the veterinarian and client, identifying preferences and working toward consensus to achieve significant clinical outcomes for the veterinarian, client, and patient.

Core Communication Skills for Cancer Communication

The Calgary-Cambridge Guide[25] is an evidence-based communication model that provides structure to the clinical interview, describing the tasks and identifying key communication skills to help veterinarians achieve clinical outcomes. Defining and demonstrating specific skills and behaviors are instrumental first steps to enhancing communication approaches.[14,15] The communication tools described next were identified as core communication skills[15] in human cancer communication literature[7,13,18,20] and are highly applicable to veterinary oncologist-client-patient interactions.

Gathering Information

Identify the Client's Full Agenda

Eliciting the client's full agenda through open-ended inquiry promotes early detection of the problem(s) and sets a plan for the rest of the visit.[35] An open-ended question is designed to draw out a full response from the client rather than a brief one and usually begins with "how," "what," or "tell me or describe for me."[36]

"*What brings you and Mandy in today?*" [open-ended question]

"*What other questions do you have about Mandy's cancer?*" [open-ended question]

"*Anything else you would like to discuss?*" [open-ended question]

This process of questioning may seem redundant, but clients often bring a laundry list of concerns, questions, or topics that they would like to discuss with their oncologist. Given the overwhelming nature of cancer conversations, these steps help identify the key questions and information sought by the client. Helping to generate the client's list of concerns and melding it with your agenda will set the structure for the remainder of the appointment and optimizes use of the visit time.

Elicit the Client's Perspective

Invite the clients to share their thoughts, ideas, feelings, and perceptions.[22] How the client perceives the patient's illness can have a major impact on the decision-making process and compliance. Many clients have had previous experiences with cancer, and it is helpful to hear these stories to address client concerns, provide reassurance, and identify misconceptions or barriers to patient care. Pick up on client verbal cues (*"I am not sure how she will do with chemotherapy."* or *"I am really concerned about her loss of appetite."* or *"My big fear is that we won't get quality time"*). Knowing the client's expectations enables you to get on the same page and customize the message to the client's concerns and meet their needs.

"What are your goals for treating Mandy's cancer?"

"I am wondering about what experiences you have had with cancer in your life, as it may impact decisions we make for Mandy."

"How are you doing with all of this?"

"What are your greatest hopes in caring for Mandy?"

"What are your greatest fears in treating her cancer?"

Explaining and Planning

Assess the Client's Knowledge Level

Assessing the client's prior knowledge and experiences allows you to evaluate the client's understanding and determine what level to pitch the information.[25] An equally important goal is to ascertain the type and kind of information the client desires because not all clients may want the same degree of information. Client preferences for information may change over time; initially, overwhelmed clients may want just the big picture and as they absorb and process the information, they may produce a list of detailed questions for follow-up discussions.

"What have you heard or read about osteosarcoma?"

"I am wondering what your veterinarian told you about Mandy's cancer."

"What other questions would you like me to address today?"

"What additional information will be helpful to you?"

"Some clients prefer the big picture and for others it is important to get into the details. What is your preference?"

Give Information in Manageable Chunks and Checks

Chunks and checks (chunk-n-check) consists of giving information in small pieces (i.e., chunks), followed by checking for understanding before proceeding further (i.e., check)—the Frisbee approach in action.[25] Sharing small pieces of information, one to three sentences at a time, allows your client time to absorb the news, and checking-in encourages client participation in the discussion and ensures that the client stays with you to achieve shared understanding. This approach to information giving avoids lecturing to the client and aims to increase recall, understanding, and commitment to plans. In this manner, the information-giving process is responsive to the client's needs and provides an opportunity for the client to participate in the conversation, provide feedback, or ask for clarification. The check can take on various forms such as taking a pause, encouraging the client to contribute to the conversation (*"What questions do you have at this point?"*), picking up on client cues (*"You seem a little hesitant about surgery."*), asking for client suggestions (*"What options have you and your husband discussed?"*), and checking for the client's understanding (*"What part of the plan will be most difficult for you and Mandy?"*).

Building Relationships

Offer Partnership

Partnership is inclusive language (i.e., let's, we, together, our, or us), which reflects that you and the client are working as a team toward mutual goals. Offering partnership informs the client that they are not alone and that they have a working partner in their oncologist, who will guide and advise them at each stage. Often, clients may arrive at their oncology appointment on their own and it may be helpful to assess their support system and offer to include other key decision makers in the conversations.

"What else can I do for you and Mandy today?"

"We'll work together to determine the best treatment plan for Mandy."

"I'm here for you. Take your time. We have a few days to decide how to proceed."

"Who else will take part in making decisions in Mandy's care?"

Ask Permission

Asking permission is a gentle approach to assess the client's readiness to take the next step. This act of respect allows the client to ready their minds, be receptive to what you have to say, and pace the conversation with you. Asking permission is a method of structuring the conversation by proposing a transition to the client and to determine whether they would like to move on.

"Would it be all right if we sit down and I asked you some questions about Mandy?"

"I am wondering if we could talk more about pain management."

"Are you OK with talking about how we might debulk the tumor?"

"Maybe you could write down your specific questions before our next visit."

Express Empathy

The stress of cancer can result in intense emotions: sadness, fear, anxiety, uncertainty, and guilt, and acknowledging these emotions reduces client distress. Empathy is an affective response resulting from perceiving the situation of another, vicariously experiencing what it might be like, and paying deep attention to another person's emotions. As a result, there are three tasks to expressing empathy.[37] The first is to appreciate the client's situation, perspective, and feelings and their attached meanings. The second is to communicate that understanding back to the client and check its accuracy. The third is to move forward in the clinical interview and act on that understanding with the client and patient in a helpful way. Simply, empathy is putting yourself in the client's shoes and communicating that you understand where they are coming from. Expressing empathy acknowledges, validates, and normalizes the client's emotional response and is essential to establishing a trusting veterinarian-client-patient relationship.[36]

"I'm so sorry to tell you this. I know it was not what you were expecting."

"I can only imagine how hard this is to hear. Mandy has been your companion for so long."

"I can see that you are agonizing over the right decision for Mandy."

Demonstrate Appropriate Nonverbal Behavior

Expression of all of the verbal core communication skills is strengthened when accompanied by complementary nonverbal communication.[36] As much as 80% of communication is nonverbal in nature, whereas 20% is based on verbal content.[25] When verbal and nonverbal communication are incongruent with each other, the nonverbal behaviors reveal the truth. There are two areas of focus for nonverbal communication: the first is to increase your sensitivity to picking up on client cues and the second is enhanced awareness of the nonverbal messages you are sending out. Tune in closely to client nonverbal behaviors such as breaking eye contact, nervous body movements, or tone of voice because client nonverbal behaviors often reflect their true underlying feelings and responses. Out of respect for their relationship with their oncologist, clients often express hesitation indirectly through their nonverbal behaviors and may not feel comfortable with directly verbalizing their concerns. It is important to pick up on these client clues and follow-up on them with the client to explore the concerns (*"I sensed some hesitation when I mentioned chemotherapy as a treatment option."* or *"You seem worried about taking Mandy to surgery, what are you most scared about?"*).

Veterinarian nonverbal cues include attentive body posture, appropriate distance from the client, turning your body toward the client, sitting at the same level, maintaining good eye contact, and complementary gestures. Display your compassion through nonverbal cues such as sitting close to your client; using a gentle, calm tone and soft volume; slowing your pace of speech; and leaning forward and reaching out through touch. Use silence to create time for the client to examine his/her thoughts and feelings. It can be difficult at times to find the right words to say and simply being a caring presence can provide just as much comfort to the client as any spoken words. Being mindful of the messages sent is important because when veterinarians are triggered or feeling judgmental, these sentiments can be leaked to the client through nonverbal behaviors.

Providing Structure

Summarize

Summarizing is an explicit review of the information that has been discovered and discussed with the client. Therefore there are multiple opportunities to present a summary: reflect back what you heard and learned at several stages during information gathering, then take time to repeat the key aspects of the diagnostic and treatment plan, and finally provide a full and complete summary at the end of the clinical interview. Summarizing helps structure the conversation by reviewing what has been discussed, identifying data that needs further clarification, providing an opportunity for reflection on where the interview should go next, and managing effective use of time during the visit.[25] The skill of summary creates a window to inform the client that they have been heard and time for the clinician to gather their thoughts, synthesize and integrate the data, and work through the diagnostic reasoning process.

"So, if I understand it correctly, your referring veterinarian felt the large lymph nodes, took a sample, and diagnosed lymphoma. You were sent here for further testing to determine if the lymphoma has spread to other organs. Is that correct?"

"What we talked about doing today, is requesting a second opinion from our pathologist on the tumor sample and conducting an ultrasound exam to look at the abdominal lymph nodes, liver, and spleen for spread of the tumor."

"I Don't Have Time for This..."

Before moving on to how to use these skills in crucial cancer conversations, one of the most common concerns expressed in communication training is that there is not enough time in the clinical interview. It seems like the facilitative approach (i.e., Frisbee) of relationship-centered care takes more time; however, it was found in veterinary general practice visits that relationship-centered care appointments were shorter in length because the veterinarian and the client achieved common ground.[21] In human medicine, when patients are left to tell their story uninterrupted, their average talking time was 92 seconds, sharing key clues to the diagnosis.[25] Empathy can be expressed as well without prolonging the appointment time; in one study, as little as 40 seconds of empathy decreased the patient's anxiety level.[38,39] Although counterintuitive, evidence suggests that using the core communication skills actually saves time and allows for a more efficient veterinarian-client-patient interaction. In addition, spending time to build a relationship at the beginning of the evaluation process creates trust, which will pay dividends as the management process progresses through the diagnostic and treatment phases.

Approaches to Cancer Conversations

As presented in the introduction, cancer communication is a series of conversations over time, starting with delivering the diagnosis (i.e., delivering bad news), discussing prognosis, making decisions about treatment options, assessing QOL, transitioning to palliative or supportive care, and ending with preparing families for euthanasia, dying, and death.[18] These difficult conversations are spread throughout multiple visits. This step-by-step approach is guided by the veterinarian's expertise, the client's agenda and perspective, and the patient's condition, response to treatment, and QOL.

Delivering Bad News

Bad news is defined as any news that drastically and negatively alters the person's views of her or his future with their pet such as a cancer diagnosis.[7] Clients interpret bad news on an individual basis and their response is related to their relationship with their companion animal, severity of the diagnosis, past experiences, other stressors in their lives, and their support system. Grief often accompanies change, and clients may express a wide range of emotions that are largely unpredictable. One useful model for delivering bad news is the SPIKES six-step model developed by Buckman[7] and employed in many medical school curricula. The SPIKES model[7] (setting, perception, invitation, knowledge, empathize, and summarize) provides guidelines on how to present information, structure the conversation, and create a supportive environment. Communication techniques for delivering bad news in the veterinary setting were previously published.[40,41]

Discussing Prognosis

Three different approaches have been described in the medical communication literature for presenting prognostic information—realism, optimism, and avoidance.[9] The challenge with realism in human medicine is that approximately 20% of patients do not want full information about their prognosis,[42-45] and unfortunately such studies of client perceptions are lacking in veterinary medicine. The drawback of optimism is that clients may lose opportunities to fulfill last wishes, prepare themselves and their family, and spend quality time with their pet. Finally, the shortcoming of avoidance is appearing evasive or dishonest, risking the trust that has been built between veterinarian and client potentially compromising the care of the pet.

Based on recommendations in human medicine,[9,18,19] be mindful of making assumptions about what the client wants to know and instead explicitly ask if and how the client wants to talk about prognosis (*"How much would you like to know about the course of Mandy's cancer?"* or *"Some clients would like all the details and others would like the big picture. What works best for you?"*). It is effective to break the information into small pieces (i.e., chunk) and then to check for client understanding and for how the prognostic information is impacting the client (*"This is hard to talk about."* or *"I am wondering if this is the kind of information you need."*). Asking permission is a key skill in this conversation to assess the client's readiness to hear more information (*"What questions do you have at this point?"* or *"Would you like me to continue?"*), along with reading the client's nonverbal cues to assess how they are processing the information (*"I notice that you seem hesitant when I was talking about survival time with chemotherapy. Could you tell me more about this?"*). To balance sustaining *hope* and maintaining *reality*, it may be helpful to frame the prognosis, using both positive and negative language (*"Median survival time means that half of the patients live longer than 2 years and half the patients live less than 2 years."*).

Given the overwhelming nature of this discussion, take time to acknowledge the client's emotional reactions (*"This is a lot of information to take in. How are you doing?"* or *"This is really difficult to talk about and we can take it one step at a time."* or *"I can see how sad this is for you."*). Allowing for silence or offering to take a break creates space for clients to work through their emotions and process the information shared with them. It can be difficult for clients to recall and understand all of the data presented, so you may want them to invite friends or family to take part (*"Who else plays a role in caring for Mandy? I am wondering if they might want to be part of this discussion."*). As this is an emotionally laden conversation loaded with complex information and associated with decision-making, it is helpful to compose and center yourself beforehand, pace yourself with your client, and offer some time for reflection.

Assessing Quality of Life

In human medicine, a spectrum of hopes has been described from the initial cancer diagnosis to preparing for death.[46] With a cancer diagnosis, a client's initial hopes may center around curing the cancer and the pet living longer and then move toward spending special time with loved ones, finding meaning, and then seeking a peaceful death. This reflects the transition that many veterinary clients go through in caring for their companion animal with cancer. This breakpoint discussion is a crucial conversation that signals the transition from fighting for quantity of time to fighting for QOL.[47] It can be challenging for clients who have been working so hard to fight the cancer to shift their energy to living the fullest life with their pet right now and preparing to let go (*"It can be difficult to switch gears from fighting the cancer to preserving Mandy's quality of life."* or *"It seems like it may be helpful to focus on what time Mandy has left with you."* or *"Just because we can do something does not mean that we should."*).

Eliciting the client and patient goals may help in moving the conversation forward (*"Can we create a plan together to ensure Mandy's quality of life?"* or *"Let's focus on what we can do to help Mandy now."* or *"What is most important to you in caring for Mandy at the end of life?"*). A supportive way to acknowledge the client's desire to do more is through expressions of "I hope" or "I wish" statements (*"I wish there were something we could do to cure Mandy's cancer."* or *"I hope that Mandy has many good weeks ahead."*).[48] At this stage, it is equally important to reflect on the oncologist's conversational emphasis and what influence the presentation of information may have on client decision making[49] such as how much time is spent talking about anticancer therapy compared to QOL, supportive care, or euthanasia. Inadvertently, the veterinarian can influence the client's decisions because of the prioritization placed on the options for care.[49]

As a source of validation and support, clients may also need to hear from their oncologist that they did everything they could for their pet (*"You have given Mandy every chance possible."*).[50] Words of reassurance and partnership can be highly supportive such as *"All along you have made your decisions with Mandy's best interests in mind."* or *"We will do this together, just as we have done everything that got us to this point."*).[50] Clients are often overwhelmed and feel alone in the enormity of the decision to euthanize their pet, and it is comforting to know that their veterinarian will guide, advise, and inform them through the process.

Transitioning to Palliative Care

Fortunately, there is much that can be done for patient comfort, despite the inability to effect a cure, including symptom management, supportive care, and pain management to ease suffering. Depending on the resources in your region, it may be appropriate to refer the client and patient to a veterinary hospice service.[51,52] Veterinary hospice is the patient care provided after a terminal diagnosis of weeks to months has been given and includes providing palliative treatment for the animal and emotional support for the family to prepare for the imminent death of the animal and focus on spending quality time together. At-home patient care entails administering medications, assessing and monitoring pain management, evaluating proper hydration and nutrition, and educating families about euthanasia, the grief process, and death and dying.[51] Today, statements such as "there is nothing more we can do" can be replaced with words of encouragement and offers of partnership to comfort clients (*"There is still much that we can do to make sure that Mandy is content and comfortable."*).[49]

Client and patient abandonment may be a concern that arises during this stage of care. The value placed on the client's relationship with the oncologist may increase as the patient's cancer progresses, as the desire for information lessens and the need for support grows.[53] With the change in focus on the care provided from cancer treatment to palliative care, the client may perceive that the oncologist's relationship with the client and patient has ended. Offering partnership helps create a sense of support for the client (*"We will work through these decisions together."* or *"I will be here to help you and Mandy whatever your decisions may be."*) Clients may want to hear explicitly that the oncologist will still be taking care of their pet, even if they decide to discontinue treatment. Depending on the client's relationship with the oncologist and the primary care clinician, it may be critical to determine the client's expectations and offer to maintain the relationship to provide end-of-life care. Caring for clients and patients at the end of life can be a source of meaning and fulfillment for the oncologist as well and an opportunity to recognize the special relationships formed during this difficult time.

Preparing Families for Euthanasia

Clients may be waiting for the oncologist to raise the option of euthanasia to give them permission to consider euthanasia as a valid and supported option (*"One of the options that is important to discuss is hospice care and euthanasia"*). Clients may be worried that the oncologist may perceive them as "giving up" if they bring up the option of euthanasia and therefore clients may need your validation (*"It is a valid and caring decision to consider euthanasia at this time"* or *"Euthanasia is a humane option for Mandy given how the cancer has spread."*). Client anxiety results from the uncertainty that lies ahead, and a large part of these conversations is helping clients cope.[47] Previously, clients had a clear plan for how to treat the cancer, and it may be helpful to have a designated path for how to care for their animal at the end of life. Discussing end-of-life wishes for the patient is crucial to preparing the client for euthanasia decision making, and creating a euthanasia plan often eases the client's discomfort.[41] Once completed, it can be put on the shelf until it is needed and the client can focus their energies on being present with their pet during these final precious days, weeks, or months. Being prepared ensures that the client's needs are met and minimizes regrets during this difficult time of grief. Communication techniques for euthanasia decision making were previously published and provide guidelines on how to walk a client through making a euthanasia decision, discussing the procedure, and presenting options for location, body care, memorializing, and family presence.[41,54]

Providing Support for Grief and Loss

Research indicates that 70% of clients are affected emotionally by the death of their pet and that as many as 30% of clients experience severe grief in anticipation of or following the death of their pet.[3] In addition, approximately 50% of clients studied reported feeling guilty about their decision to euthanize their pet. One of the factors contributing to client grief was the perception of the professional support provided by the veterinarian. The manner in which the veterinarian provides care for a client whose pet has died has the potential to alleviate or aggravate grief. A thorough description of client grief responses and techniques for providing emotional support were outlined in the previous edition of this textbook.[54]

Caring for Yourself

Compassion fatigue is deep physical, emotional, and spiritual exhaustion that can result from working day to day in an intense caregiving environment.[55,56] The natural response to this downward spiral is to work harder until there is nothing left to give, which is counter to the adaptive response of taking a break. The symptoms are the same as those of chronic stress and are a consequence of caring for the needs of others before caring for your own needs.[54] Compassion fatigue results from a lack of daily self-care practices that create opportunities to reflect, refuel, and rejuvenate. The good news is that feeling compassion fatigue results from being a deeply caring person. When oncologists care for themselves, they can care for others from a place of abundance not scarcity. With development of healthy self-care routines, practitioners can continue to successfully provide compassionate care to others. Recognizing the signs of compassion fatigue is the first step toward positive change, and the second step is making a daily firm commitment to choices that lead to resiliency. A thorough description of caregiver stress and stress management strategies was provided in the previous edition of this textbook.[54]

Conclusion

Given the growing expectations of clients, the strength of the human-animal relationship, and the resultant emotional impact of cancer communication on pet caregivers and the oncology team, relationship-centered care is integral to providing quality cancer care.[5,21,22] Extrapolating from evidence in human medicine, compassionate cancer communication is related to significant clinical outcomes for the oncologist, client, and the patient, including enhancing client[28-30] and veterinarian satisfaction,[31,32] improving adherence to recommendations,[33] working through emotions,[38,39] and promoting patient health.[34] Effective techniques for cancer communication can be taught and are a series of learned skills.[15,25] Through supportive approaches, cancer communication can be made less distressing to the client, fostering client relationships and optimizing patient care while promoting professional fulfillment for the veterinarian.

REFERENCES

1. Brown JP, Silverman JD: The current and future market for veterinarians and veterinary medical services in the United States, *J Am Vet Med Assoc* 225:161–183, 2004.
2. Lue TW, Patenburg DB, Crawford PM: Impact of the owner-pet and client-veterinarian bond on the care that pets receive, *J Vet Med Assoc* 232:531–540, 2008.

3. Adams CL, Bonnett BN, Meek AH: Predictors of owner response to companion animal death in 177 clients from 14 practices in Ontario, *J Vet Med Assoc* 217:1303–1309, 2000.
4. Blackwell MJ: The 2001 Iverson Bell Symposium keynote address: beyond philosophical differences: the future training of veterinarians, *J Vet Med Educ* 28:148–152, 2001.
5. Coe JB, Adams CL, Bonnett BN: A focus group study of veterinarians' and pet owners' perceptions of veterinarian-client communication in companion animal practice, *J Vet Med Assoc* 233:1072–1080, 2008.
6. Gorman TE, Ahern SP, Wiseman J, et al: Residents' end-of-life decision making with adult hospitalized patients: a review of the literature, *Acad Med* 80:622–633, 2005.
7. Buckman R: *Practical plans for difficult conversations in medicine: Strategies that work in breaking bad news*, Baltimore, 2010, Johns Hopkins University Press.
8. Girgis A, Sanson-Fisher RW: Breaking bad news: current best advice for clinicians, *Behav Med* 24:53–60, 1998.
9. Back AL, Arnold RM: Discussing prognosis: "How much do you want to know?" Talking to patients who are prepared for explicit information, *J Clin Oncol* 24:4209–4213, 2006a.
10. Tinga, CE, Adams CL, Bonnett BN, et al: Survey of veterinary technical and professional skills in students and recent graduates of a veterinary college, *J Am Vet Med Assoc* 219:924–931, 2001.
11. Butler C, William S, Koll S: Perceptions of fourth-year veterinary students regarding emotional support of clients in veterinary practice and in veterinary college curriculum, *J Am Vet Med Assoc* 221:360–363, 2002.
12. North American Veterinary Medical Education Consortium: *Roadmap for veterinary medical education in the 21st century: responsive, collaborative, flexible*. American Association of Veterinary Medical Colleges, 2010, Draft Report.
13. Bylund CL, Brown R, Gueguen JA, et al: The implementation and assessment of a comprehensive communication skills training curriculum for oncologists, *Psycho-Onc* 19:583–593, 2010.
14. Shaw JR, Barley GE, Hill AE, et al: Communication skills education onsite in a veterinary practice, *Patient Educ Couns* 80:337–344, 2010.
15. Kurtz SM, Silverman J, Draper J: *Teaching and learning communication skills in medicine*, Abingdon UK, 2005, Radcliffe Medical Press
16. Venetis MK, Robinson JD, LaPlant Turkiewics K, et al: An evidence base for patient-centered cancer care: a meta-analysis of studies of observed communication between cancer specialists and their patients, *Patient Educ Couns* 77:379–383, 2009.
17. Epstein RM, Street RL: *Patient-centered communication in cancer care: Promoting healing and reducing suffering. Publication No. 07-6225*, Bethesda, MD, 2007, National Institutes of Health.
18. Back AL, Anderson WG, Bunch L, et al: Communication about cancer near the end of life, *Cancer* 113:1897–1910, 2008.
19. Back AL, Arnold RM: Discussing prognosis: "How much do you want to know?" Talking to patients who do not want information or who are ambivalent, *J Clin Oncol* 24:4214–4217, 2006b.
20. Roter DL, Larson S, Rischer GS, et al: Experts practice what they preach: A descriptive study of best and normative practices in end-of-life discussions, *Arch Intern Med* 160:3477–3485, 2000.
21. Shaw JR, Bonnett BN, Adams CL, et al: Veterinarian-client-patient communication patterns used during clinical appointments in companion animal practice, *J Am Vet Med Assoc* 228:714, 2006.
22. Nogueira Borden LJ, Adams CL, Bonnett BN, et al: Use of the measure of patient-centered communication to analyze euthanasia discussions in companion animal practice, *J Am Vet Med Assoc* 237:1275–1286, 2010.
23. Emanual EJ, Emanual LG: Four models of the physician-patient relationship, *JAMA* 267:2221–2226, 1992.
24. Roter DL: The enduring and evolving nature of the patient-physician relationship, *Patient Educ Couns* 39:5–15, 2000.
25. Silverman J, Kurtz SM, Draper J: *Skills for communicating with patients*, Abingdon UK, 2005, Radcliffe Medical Press.
26. Tresolini C: Pew-Fetzer Task Force. *Health professional education and relationship-centered care*. San Francisco: The Pew-Fetzer Task Force on Advancing Psychosocial Health Education, 1994, Pew Health Professions Commission on the Fetzer Institute.
27. Mead N, Bower P: Patient-centredness: a conceptual framework and review of the empirical literature, *Soc Sci Med* 51:1087–1110, 2000.
28. Bertakis KD, Roter DL, Putnam SM: The relationship of physician medical interview style to patient satisfaction, *J Fam Pract* 32:175–181, 1991.
29. Buller MK, Buller DB: Physicians' communication style and patient satisfaction, *J Health Soc Behav* 28:375–388, 1987.
30. Hall JA, Dornan MC: Meta-analyses of satisfaction with medical care: description of research domain and analysis of overall satisfaction levels, *Soc Sci Med* 27:637–644, 1988.
31. Levinson W, Stiles WB, Inui TS, et al: Physician frustration in communicating with patients, *Med Care* 31:285–295, 1993.
32. Roter DL, Stewart M, Putnam SM, et al: Communication patterns of primary care physicians, *JAMA* 277:350–356, 1997.
33. DiMatteo MR, Sherbourne CD, Hays RD: Physicians' characteristics influence patient's adherence to medical treatments: results from the medical outcomes study, *Health Psychology* 12:93–102, 1993.
34. Stewart MA: Effective physician-patient communication and health outcomes: a review, *Can Med Assoc J* 152:1423–1433, 1995.
35. Dysart LM, Coe JB, Adams CL: Analysis of solicitation of client concerns in companion animal practice, *J Am Vet Med Assoc* 238:1609–1615, 2011.
36. Shaw JR: Four core communication skills of highly effective practitioners, *Vet Clinic Small Anim* 36:385–396, 2006.
37. Neumann M, Bensing J, Mercer S, et al: Analyzing the "nature" and "specific effectiveness" of clinical empathy: A theoretical overview and contribution towards a theory-based research agenda, *Patient Educ Couns* 74:339–346, 2009.
38. Fogarty LA, Curbow BA, Wingard JR, et al: Can 40 seconds of compassion reduce patient anxiety? *J Clin Oncol* 17:371, 1999.
39. Roter DL, Hall JA, Kern DE, et al: Improving physicians' interviewing skills and reducing patients' emotional distress. A randomized clinical trial, *Arch Intern Med* 155:1877, 1995.
40. Allen E, Shaw JS: Delivering bad news: a crucial conversation, *Except Vet Team* 2:17–19, 2010.
41. Shaw JR, Lagoni L: End-of- life communication in veterinary medicine: delivering bad news and euthanasia decision making, *Vet Clin Small Anim Pract* 37:95, 2007.
42. Fried TR, Bradley EH, O'Leary J: Prognosis communication in serious illness: Perceptions of older patients, caregivers and clinicians, *J Am Geriatr Soc* 51:1398–1403, 2003.
43. Leydon GM, Boulton M, Moynihan C, et al: Faith, hope and charity: An in-depth interview study of cancer patients' information needs and information-seeking behavior, *West J Med* 173:26–31, 2000.
44. Jenkins V, Fallowfield L, Poole K: Information needs of patients with cancer: Results from a large study in UK Cancer Centres, *Br J Cancer* 84:322–331, 2001.
45. Cassileth BR, Zupkis RV, Sutton-Smith K, et al: Information and participation preferences among cancer patients, *Ann Intern Med* 92:832–836, 1980.
46. Clayton JM, Butow PN, Arnold RM, et al: Fostering coping and nurturing hope when discussing the future with terminally ill cancer patients and their caregivers, *Cancer* 103:164, 2005.
47. Gawande A: Letting go: What should medicine do when it can't save your life? *The New Yorker* August 2, 2010.
48. Pantilat SZ: Communication with seriously ill patients: Better words to say, *JAMA* 301:1279–1281, 2009.
49. Yeates JW, Main DC: The ethics of influencing clients, *J Vet Med Assoc* 237:263–267, 2010.
50. Harpham WS: View from the other side of the stethoscope: "It's okay", *Oncology Times* 40, February 25, 2011.
51. Bishop GA, Long CC, Carlsten KS, et al: The Colorado State University pet hospice program: end-of-life care for pets and their families, *J Vet Med Educ* 35:525–531, 2008.

52. Johnson CL, Patterson-Kane E, Lamison A, et al: Elements of and factors important in veterinary hospice, *J Vet Med Assoc* 238:148–150, 2011.
53. Graugaard PK, Holgersen K, Eide H, et al: Changes in physician-patient communication from initial to return visits: a prospective study in a haematology outpatient clinic, *Patient Educ Couns* 57:22, 2005.
54. Lagoni L: Bond-centered cancer care: an applied approach to euthanasia and grief support for your clients, your staff, and yourself. In Withrow SJ, Vail DM, editors: *Withrow and McEwen's small animal clinical oncology*, ed 4, St. Louis, 2007, Saunders Elsevier.
55. Pfifferling JH, Gilley K: Overcoming compassion fatigue, *Fam Prac Mngmt* April:39–44, 2000.
56. Figley CR, Roop RG: *Compassion fatigue in the animal-care community*, Washington, DC, 2006, Humane Society Press.

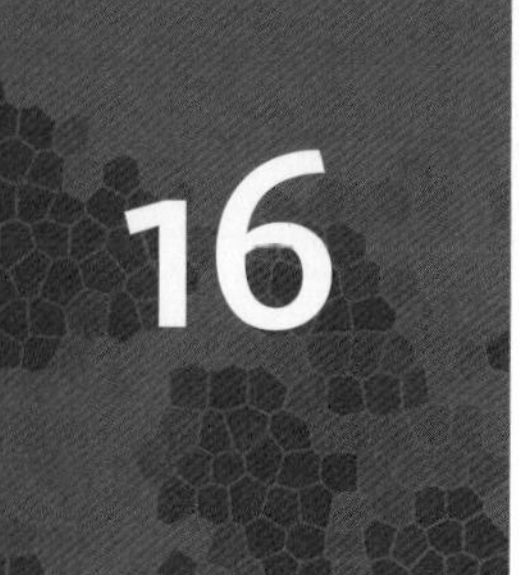

Complementary and Alternative Medicine for Cancer: The Good, the Bad, and the Dangerous

NARDA G. ROBINSON

Complementary and alternative medicine (CAM) constitutes a diverse and often controversial group of treatments that exist outside of mainstream medicine. Although CAM has yet to produce a single, proven cancer cure,[1] this does not stop some veterinarians and lay healers from continuing to claim that these products can "stop cancer in its tracks" or eliminate neoplasia. Other claims for CAM cancer treatments are not as extreme, and scientific evidence shows that some methods or products actually do benefit oncology patients.

Clients need their veterinarians' help in navigating both factual and fictitious CAM options for their animal companions with cancer. As one human oncologist wrote,

> It is no longer acceptable to patients for physicians to label all of these alleged treatments as ludicrous and unfounded. Medical professionals must be able to converse intelligently about them with patience and learn not to denigrate out of hand those who utilize alternative and complementary techniques, as long as they are safe. Physicians must also warn patients of danger and hoaxes when that is appropriate.[2]

One way to assist clients is by indicating which CAM treatments have evidence of both efficacy and safety and which ones are deemed ineffective or unsafe.[3,4]

The popularity of CAM is undeniable. For human patients with cancer, the usage rate is well over 50%.[5] A 2006 survey of clients who brought their pet to the Colorado State University Animal Cancer Center found that 76% of surveyed owners used CAM to improve well being. Other reasons they provided included attempting to reduce pain and treatment toxicity, as well as to improve appetite.[6] However, a majority of those surveyed had not yet spoken to their veterinarian about CAM. If clients seek input and treatment from nonveterinarian practitioners in lieu of science-based veterinary professionals, patient health and safety could be jeopardized. Lay healers' lack of formal veterinary medical training hinders their capacity to coordinate medically sound recommendations for animals. Nonveterinarians are, for the most part, unable to rapidly identify health problems and intervene effectively in disease progression. For cancer patients, delays in prompt and appropriate medical attention may make an otherwise treatable condition resistant to therapy.[7]

The veterinary medical profession and educational institutions owe their students and graduates scientific, evidence-informed CAM instruction in both undergraduate curricula and continuing education courses. As Memon et al found in their 2011 survey of veterinary college academic deans,

> ... CAVM [Complementary and alternative veterinary medicine] is an important topic that should be addressed in veterinary medical education.... The most common comment reflected strong opinions that inclusion of CAVM ... must be evidence-based.... [S]tudents should be aware of CAVM modalities because of strong public interest in CAVM and because practitioners should be able to address client questions from a position of knowledge.[8]

Still, a client's desperate search for nontoxic alternative or adjunctive therapy can lead some to consider unproven remedies. The penchant of some practitioners to promote products designed to treat cancer is too often based on belief systems rather than strong science and evidence. Even within the veterinary profession, holistic "healers" continue to claim to have found a "powerful" mixture of Chinese herbs, homeopathic remedies, or invisible energy manipulations that will cure, treat, or prevent cancer. This belief-system basis of CAM practice has prevailed entirely too long. It perpetuates learning CAM methods in the absence of critical thinking and sidesteps concerns about best practices and evidence-informed options. This puts clients in the difficult position of all too often opting for CAM approaches based on their faith in a charismatic practitioner rather than evidence-driven outcomes.

Thankfully, research on integrative approaches for humans with cancer is building steadily. As such, elevating CAM cancer care by replacing folklore with facts and metaphors with meaningful mechanisms is becoming a real possibility. The information in this chapter is designed to help veterinary professionals sort between a range of CAM modalities according to their scientific basis (or lack thereof) and evidenced-based insights concerning their potential to impart real benefits to patients with cancer. For each treatment type included here, the discussion will address the good, bad, or dangerous aspects about the therapy.

Acupuncture

What Is Acupuncture?

Acupuncture involves the insertion of thin, sterile needles into certain sites on the body corresponding to influential neurovascular or myofascial zones that, when stimulated, promote analgesia, recovery of normal circulation and immune function, overall physiologic restoration, and homeostasis. In addition to needling, other forms of somatic afferent stimulation include acupressure, laser acupuncture, and electroacupuncture, wherein one clips electrode wires to the needles in order to augment the stimulation and neurologic response.

How Does Acupuncture Work?

Acupuncture counteracts pain and other adverse sequelae of cancer treatment through neuromodulation. It may reduce the levels of medication required.[9] Nerve fiber stimulation begins at the needle-tissue interface, where local alterations in cytokines and inflammatory mediators lead to modulation (i.e., normalization) of circulation and immune function in the immediate area surrounding the site around the needle. From there, agitation of the connective tissue and subsequent tugging of the collagen fibers, fibroblasts, and myofascia in the region produce activation of sensory somatic and autonomic nerve fibers. When excited, afferent pathways ferry action potentials along large nerve axons that underlie and often define the trajectory of acupuncture channels. A cascade of simultaneous central nervous system (CNS) and autonomic nervous system (ANS) changes follow soon thereafter, producing somatosomatic, somatoautonomic, and somatovisceral reflexes in spinal cord segments related to the excited nerve(s). In addition to propriospinal signaling, acupuncture incites a barrage of brain stimulation in the limbic system, the cerebellum, the cortex, and the brainstem. Functional brain imaging research illustrates, through changes in neuronal metabolism, which centers process pain, regulate autonomic function, and affect moods in response to acupuncture. This aids in the ever deepening understanding of the neurophysiologic premise underlying acupuncture.

How Might Acupuncture Benefit a Veterinary Patient with Cancer?

Human integrative oncology clinics have found acupuncture to be a safe, inexpensive, and valuable intervention for several problems that cancer patients often encounter, including leukopenia, gastrointestinal upset, and systemic reactions.[9-12] Acupuncture is often effective in reducing emetic effects of chemotherapy and opioids.[13-18] For pain, acupuncture provides benefits along several routes, including normalizing muscle tone, deactivating myofascial trigger points, upregulating analgesic gene expression in the spinal cord, promoting segmental analgesia, reducing neuropathic pain, elevating endogenous opioid release, and promoting a sense of well being through pathways that influence the limbic system.[19-28] Acupuncture also activates natural killer (NK) cells that aid in anticancer immune mechanisms at least in part through its effects on neural circuitry connected to somatosympathetic reflexes.[29-32]

Through neurologic and circulatory modulation, acupuncture affects the diameter of arterial, venous, and lymphatic vessels, working to assist in the alleviation of chronic lymphedema, and accelerates wound healing.[33,34] Patients with head and neck cancer also appear to benefit from acupuncture's effects on glandular function by helping to minimize xerostomia following radiation.[35-38] Even for human patients with advanced, incurable cancer, acupuncture has been shown to alleviate a wide range of symptoms with no significant or unexpected adverse effects.[39] Any acupuncturist treating animals should have a thorough understanding of animal health and disease, as well as acupuncture anatomy and physiology, in order to minimize risk of injury.[40]

Although acupuncture provides repeatable and measurable benefits for patients with advanced cancer, the treatment is underutilized.[41] Whether due to lack of knowledge about the evidential support for acupuncture in cancer, its scientifically based mechanisms of action, or unsubstantiated bias against the technique, oncologists may forget to recommend it or resist requests for it.

The Importance of Approaching Acupuncture Scientifically

Despite accruing facts regarding the mechanisms and clinical benefits of acupuncture, a notable subset of practitioners continue to believe that acupuncture point stimulation moves invisible energy (qi) through invisible pathways on the body (meridians). Although this misconception may not directly harm a patient, metaphysical misimpressions about how needling works may mislead veterinarians and clients in a number of ways. For example, certain energy-based acupuncture courses teach that veterinarians could successfully and easily treat cancer by selecting and stimulating a single acupuncture point chosen according to abstract ideas and psychic powers. The inventor of this technique alludes to "total disappearance or significant regression" of cancer in 80% of patients.[42-44] This claim has no rational scientific mechanism nor has it been submitted to experimental scrutiny. It risks delaying proper treatment through conventional means and allowing the cancer to progress to an untreatable stage.

Conversely, myths have circulated within the veterinary acupuncture community for decades that acupuncture could raise the risk of metastasis by increasing blood flow to a tumor. This has led to unnecessary underutilization in patients who stood to benefit from this palliative, pain-reducing, and quality-of-life–supporting modality.[45]

Herbs

Herbs for oncology clients typically offer anticancer, antiinflammatory, antioxidant, and/or analgesic benefits. Herbs to support quality of life include those that support wound healing (for example, during or after radiation therapy), anxiolytics to reduce the burden of cancer and conventional treatment on the psyche, and antiemetics. The pros and cons of representatives from each herbal category follow.

Do Herbs Have Anticancer Benefits?

Several phytomedicinals influence the activity of cancer (whether in vitro cell cultures or in vivo). Perhaps the most common products include Asian mushrooms for their immune-enhancing benefits, curcumin (a component of the spice turmeric) and *Boswellia* (an oleoresin gum from the frankincense tree) for their antitumor and antiinflammatory activities, and topical bloodroot (sanguinarine) for its tumor-dissolving value. Most plant-based substances confer an antioxidant benefit; some phytotherapeutics such as green tea are strong enough that clinicians should consider the risk of antagonizing the benefits of chemotherapy if the two are co-administered.

How Do Herbs Work to Fight Cancer?

Natural products from both Asian and Western herbs have the capacity to inhibit proliferation, induce apoptosis, reduce angiogenesis, retard metastasis, and even enhance the effects of chemotherapy.[46-48] The challenge, however, is to know which herbs to prescribe for each specific cancer type. Another mystery entails how the herbs' biochemistries interact and possibly interfere with conventional medication or chemotherapy.

The pharmacokinetics and pharmacodynamics of herbs are mostly a mystery for nonhuman animals, leading to questions about how the various veterinary species that receive these products metabolize and clear the xenobiotics (herbs). What is more concerning is the multiplicity and undisclosed quantities of herbs, animal residues, and toxic substances such as strychnine and aconite included in traditional Chinese veterinary medicine (TCVM) products.[49] Many TCVM practitioners have little to no understanding of the biochemical actions of a plant product, instead relying on metaphoric descriptions of the remedies' properties. In addition, TCVM practitioners may utilize unvalidated, primitive, folkloric diagnostic methods in order to arrive at a quasi-diagnosis. They assemble subjective impressions derived from various physical observations and pulse palpation into a "pattern," which is then matched to a TCVM compound that is supposed to address that pattern. This method is fraught with problems and pitfalls but is important to note because a large segment of veterinary herbalists adhere to this approach.

Veterinarians treating cancer patients should be conversant with not only the potential value of unconventional cancer approaches[50-52] but also their dangers. The likelihood of TCVM herbal toxicity and interactions is in part due to the sheer number of herbal (and animal) ingredients in each mixture. Most have never been tested in typical veterinary species, worsening confusion.

Recommending TCVM herbs based on rigorously derived discoveries in botanical research allows practitioners to discard untestable, abstract mechanisms of action such as claiming that they "resolve stagnation, invigorate Qi, and remove phlegm/damp accumulation."[53] Medical professionals should, in contrast, insist on instruction that describes Chinese herb effects in simple, biologic language, especially when scientific investigations have already shown how they work. For example, astragalus upregulates host immune response and reduces chemotherapy toxicity, and *Oldenlandia diffusa* directly attacks tumor cells through apoptosis. One could then conceive of incorporating these two herbs into a combination with others that work through additive or synergistic means, rather than guessing at their metaphoric effects. An oncologist might choose a third herb that inhibits abnormal gene transcription activity *(Coix lachrymal)* and a fourth that promotes tumor necrosis *(Glycyrrhiza glabra)*.[54]

Until more becomes known about how Chinese herbs affect chemotherapy in veterinary cancer patients,

> Caution should be taken when anticancer drugs are used in combination with herbal medicines, particularly for cytotoxic anticancer drugs with narrow therapeutic indices. Monitoring plasma concentrations of concurrently administered anticancer drugs and observing for possible signs of clinical toxicity are necessary when herbal remedies are used concurrently.[55]

Computerized databases are further assisting oncologists by enabling determination of relevant, potential interactions between anticancer drugs and Chinese herbs.[56] Even oncologists in China are encouraging their colleagues to maintain a watchful eye for surprise sequelae. For example, one paper warned:

> [P]rofessional complacency about TCM [Traditional Chinese Medicine] use is becoming less acceptable as the knowledge base of TCM-induced toxicities and interactions expands. Being rich sources of bioactive xenobiotics, TCMs are frequent causes of puzzling complications, including hepatotoxicity, nephrotoxicity, and hematologic disorders.[57]

Some traditional Chinese herbal medicines (TCHMs) are chemosensitizing or radiosensitizing and thus may cause conventional treatment to work more robustly, whereas others directly antagonize medication through one or more mechanisms. Toxicity from Chinese herbs co-administered with chemotherapy may lead to diagnostic dilemmas when clinicians misattribute problems to the drug rather than the TCHM product, thereby delaying discontinuation of the appropriate compound.[57] In fact, Chinese herbalists in Taiwan who work directly with herbs in the raw form are finding themselves at increased risk of liver and bladder cancer, possibly due to the heavy metal contamination of TCHMs and/or the intrinsic toxicity of some ingredients.[58] This heightened risk for urologic cancers, chronic and unspecified nephritis, renal failure, and renal sclerosis "highlights the urgent need for safety assessments of Chinese herbs."[59]

Public perception holds that TCHMs protect cancer patients' health and well being during chemotherapy.[57] A double-blind, randomized, placebo-controlled study questioned this assumption, showing that TCHMs did not significantly reduce any of the hematologic toxicities (leukopenia, neutropenia, and thrombocytopenia) associated with adjuvant chemotherapy for breast and colon cancer.[60] Three licensed, experienced TCHM practitioners from China prescribed herbal formulas to patients on an individualized basis, since many believe this approach yields superior benefits. Even the myth that individualizing TCHMs produces better outcomes could be more folklore than fact.[61] According to some critics, "[A]lmost all individualized herbal medicine is practiced without the support of any rigorous evidence about effectiveness whatsoever."[62] They continue,

> The lack of standardisation and use of multiple herbs in a single prescription also greatly multiply the safety risks. There are additional risks associated with variability in the diagnostics skills of the practitioner, their awareness or lack of awareness of potential interactions, and their ability or inability to identify red flag symptoms indicating serious diseases requiring immediate mainstream medical treatment. Given the risks and lack of supporting evidence, the use of individualised herbal medicine cannot be recommended in any indication.

Despite these limitations, the potential for Chinese herbs to one day participate legitimately within a methodic, evidence-informed herb and chemotherapy regimen seems imminent. To this end, one group, the nonprofit Consortium for Globalization of Chinese Medicine (http://www.tcmedicine.org) has assembled a broad collective of scientists from academia and industry. Researchers are conducting national and international collaborative clinical trials along with experimental animal and in vitro studies. They aim to fulfill four basic regulatory requirements: batch-to-batch consistency in Chinese herbal preparations; evidence-based clinical effectiveness; safety; and rational understanding of mechanisms of actions, sites of biochemical impact, active ingredients, and drug-herb interactions.[63]

For the most up-to-date information on the mechanisms, safety, and effectiveness of a given herb, veterinarians should consult the scientific medical databases. Literature searches through PubMed and CAB abstracts provide rational, up-to-date information and impartial reviews that are unavailable through herbal practitioners who base their recommendations on centuries-old folkloric practices and metaphoric mechanisms.

Additional Issues with Herbs for Cancer Patients

Herbs may interfere with blood coagulation, upregulate or downregulate drug metabolism systems, or otherwise interact unpredictably with conventional treatments.

Many common herbal products modulate intestinal P-glycoprotein and/or cytochrome P450 (CYP450) enzymes, producing clinically important herb-drug interactions.[64] Because of this, owners should disclose all dietary supplements and/or herbs they are giving the patient. The veterinarian should then weigh the potential for interactions between the conventional treatment and the supplement against the proven benefits of the product and determine prior to treatment whether or not the patient should stop the product.

Whether an herb will interact with chemotherapy and/or radiation therapy is often unknown, although research is gradually illuminating when and how this can happen.[65-67] Garlic, often recommended by holistic practitioners for cancer, induces the P-glycoprotein drug efflux transport system to aid the body in ridding itself of perceived toxins, such as chemotherapeutics.[68]

Clinicians unaware of herbal antiplatelet effects may find themselves surprised by bleeding during biopsies or surgeries. Because of this, the American Society of Anesthesiologists recommends that human patients discontinue dietary supplements at least 2 weeks prior to surgery.[69] Botanicals such as angelica root (dong quai), German chamomile, red clover, and ginseng increase the risk of bleeding. Garlic, ginkgo, and saw palmetto also may have significant anticoagulant actions. Cancer patients may already have thrombocytopenia from chemotherapy or myelosuppression from bone marrow invasion that compromises their capacity to clot.

Herbs that have anticancer effects but contain phytoestrogens such as *Angelica sinensis* may adversely affect patients with hormone-sensitive cancer.[70]

The task of assessing complex herb-drug interactions even in one species, the human, reveals the daunting number of considerations involved when designing research strategies. For example, the herb astragalus is a plant commonly employed for cancer treatment that potentiates host immune function. A 2006 metaanalysis of randomized trials concluded that, when combined with platinum-based chemotherapy, Chinese herbal formulations with astragalus improved survival, increased tumor response, and reduced toxicity from the chemotherapy in human patients with non–small-cell lung cancer.[71] Critics of this metaanalysis questioned the findings, citing unevenness in treatment methods.[72] Only two of the 30 studies utilized astragalus as a single agent; the rest involved combinations of plants. In addition, the species of astragalus studied in each case was unclear; was it *Astragalus membranaceus* (huang qi), whose major constituents include triterpene saponins and polysaccharides in the roots, or was another plant in the astragalus genus substituted in some cases? How did the amount of astragalus in each mixture compare, given that single herb preparations putatively contained 100% astragalus, whereas in others it was only one of up to 17 herbs. Finally, which part of the plant was used and how was it prepared? Decoctions, fluid extracts, and dry matter vary considerably in their concentration of active constituents; thus their biochemical make-up and resultant pharmacologic activity may differ dramatically.

Examples of Herbs for Patients with Cancer

Some of the most common herbs sought for their anticancer properties are presented next in order to illustrate the breadth of their mechanisms of action, as well as clinical considerations regarding toxicity and possible interactions with chemotherapy.

Asian Mushrooms

Mushroom mixtures and mushroom-derived polysaccharide preparations modify tumor response and improve immune function in patients with solid tumors.[73] The active agents in Asian mushrooms, polysaccharides, also possess antitumor effects through inhibition of cellular proliferation and tumor growth, invasion, and angiogenesis.[74]

A proprietary, protein-bound polysaccharide extract of *Coriolis versicolor* reduced serum levels of immunosuppressive acidic protein in stage II and III colorectal cancer patients, increased 5-year disease-free survival, and decreased relative risk of regional metastases.[75] A metaanalysis of three trials involving over a thousand subjects with colorectal cancer confirmed these results.[76] A variety of other medicinal mushrooms and extracts have proved beneficial, improving immune parameters such as NK cell activity and cytokines, without significant toxicity.

The still-unanswered question regarding medicinal mushrooms pertains to their risk or value in lymphoma, given their immunostimulatory effects. A study of a standardized extract of Maitake mushroom in dogs with lymphoma reported no objective value, although two dogs did develop hyphema and one developed petechiae.[77] These agents can inhibit platelet function; whether the bleeding noted in this study related to the Maitake mushroom or the lymphoma remained unknown.

Curcumin

Cancer cells employ various pathways to evade host defenses. This means that a drug or herb works best against cancer when it takes more than one route of action to attack the disease. In its interaction with several cellular proteins, curcumin[78,79] constituents induce phase II detoxification enzymes, suppress tumor cell proliferation in several cancer cell lines, and downregulate transcription factors (nuclear factor-κB [NF-κB], activator protein 1 [AP-1], early growth response 1 [EGR-1]). Curcumin downregulates enzymes such as cyclooxygenase-2 (COX-2), lipoxygenase (LOX), nitric oxide synthase (NOS), matrix metalloproteinase 9 (MMP9), urokinase-type plasminogen activator, and more. Curcumin also downregulates other factors and receptors such as tumor necrosis factor, chemokines, cell surface adhesion molecules, and growth factor receptors (e.g., epidermal growth factor receptor [EGFR], human EGFR 2 [HER2]). Curcumin acts antiangiogenically and enhances the cytotoxicity of certain chemotherapy drugs.

Curcumin causes cell death in several human cancer cell lines, including breast, lung, prostate, colon, melanoma, kidney, hepatocellular, ovarian, and leukemia. The effect curcumin has on cell death involves both the usual apoptotic mechanisms such as oligonucleosomal DNA degradation and alternative means. When resistance develops to apoptosis-inducing factors, curcumin can overcome this impediment through alternative cell-signaling pathways, such as mitotic catastrophe.[80] Mitotic catastrophe involves a morphologically distinct and aberrant mitotic process that distinguishes it from apoptosis, characterized by the formation of giant, multinucleated cells carrying uncondensed chromosomes. Curcumin may also counteract the induction of prosurvival factors in cells generated by radiation therapy and chemotherapy.

Human clinical trials demonstrate no dose-limiting toxicity when given up to 10 g of curcumin in 1 day.[81] The amount of curcumin contained in turmeric averages only about 3% by weight[82]; concentrated curcumin supplements therefore supposedly provide higher levels of the active constituent, provided that the label and actual contents agree. The hurdles of maintaining adequate blood levels of curcumin pertain to its low bioavailability, although absorption varies between species. One way to overcome delivery challenges could include coupling it with compounds that focus curcumin's activity toward specific target cells.

Curcumin could hypothetically negate some of the effects of chemotherapy because it affects so many pathways. Research suggests that curcumin can inhibit chemotherapy-induced apoptosis in breast cancer cells, specifically in combination with camptothecin, mechlorethamine, or doxorubicin. The potential benefits of certain herbs should be considered and compared against the risks. For example, a synthetic analog of curcumin helped reduce doxorubicin-induced cardiotoxicity through an anticancer-antioxidant dual function in vitro.[83] Additionally, curcumin and catechin (from green tea) may work synergistically against cancer through cytotoxicity, nuclear fragmentation, and antiproliferative and proapoptotic effects.[84]

Boswellia

Boswellic acids exhibit potent antiinflammatory properties in vitro and in vivo. Triterpenes in boswellic acid reduce the synthesis of leukotrienes in intact neutrophils by inhibiting 5-LOX, the key enzyme involved in the biosynthesis of leukotrienes, which mediate inflammation.[85,86] *Boswellia* extracts exert immunomodulatory benefits by simultaneously inhibiting T-helper 1 (Th1) and promoting Th2 cytokine production.[87] They regulate vascular responses to inflammation[86] and stabilize mast cells.[89] In cases of intestinal inflammation, boswellic acids may modulate the adhesive interactions between leukocytes and endothelial cells by countering the activation of leukocytes and/or downregulating the expression of endothelial cell-adhesion molecules.[90,91]

Specific to their anticancer properties, boswellic acids induce antiproliferation, differentiation, and apoptosis in leukemia cell lines.[92-95] They exert cytotoxic effects on established human glioblastoma and leukemia cell lines, as well as on primary human meningioma cells.[96] Boswellic acids may help reduce cerebral edema in patients with brain tumors.[97]

Side effects of boswellic acids include abdominal discomfort, nausea, epigastric pain, hyperacidity,[98] and diarrhea.[99]

The presence of food in the stomach, as well as the type of food eaten, dramatically alters the bioavailability of boswellic acids, and bile acids significantly affect their absorption.[100] When human subjects ingested boswellic acids along with a high-fat meal, the areas under the plasma concentration-time curves and peak concentrations totaled several times higher than when the herbal preparations are taken in the fasting condition. A human study showed that the elimination half-life for *Boswellia* was approximately 6 hours, suggesting that oral administration would require dosing every 6 to 8 hours.[101]

Frankincense extracts, as well as boswellic acids themselves, display moderate-to-potent inhibition of human drug-metabolizing CYP450 enzymes,[102] but the clinical significance and comparative effects on nonhuman P450 enzyme systems remain largely unexplored.

Milk Thistle

Most veterinarians are familiar with milk thistle as a liver support supplement, but its value as an adjunct for cancer patients should not be overlooked. The most salient new applications for milk thistle arise in its role as an adjunct for cancer chemoprevention and treatment and to reduce side effects of treatment.[103,104] Specifically, silymarin has led to reductions in tumor incidence and a number of chemically induced tumors in rat models for colon, tongue, and bladder cancer. It inhibits the growth of human prostate cancer and lung cancer xenografts in mice.[105] Milk thistle derivatives protect the kidneys from radiation injury and cisplatin nephrotoxicity.[104,106] They may also protect the heart from doxorubicin-induced lipid peroxidation, as well as the liver from CCNU (lomustine) toxicity (see Chapter 11). When combined with ω-3 fatty acids, milk thistle has reduced the number of radionecrosis sites in cancer patients and prolonged survival.[104] Milk thistle potentiated antitumor effects of drugs like cisplatin in both in vivo and in vitro studies.[104]

The risk of herb-drug interactions from milk thistle appears to be low but not nonexistent. Milk thistle may inhibit certain isoforms of the CYP450 family, namely CYP3A4 and CYP2C9. This becomes significant when combined with agents that depend on CYP3A4 for metabolism, raising concerns about adding milk thistle for "liver protection" during chemotherapy, especially at high doses.[107] Silymarin has potentiated chemotherapy toxicity in at least one study.[104] However, a recent investigation testing its effects on the disposition of irinotecan as a model drug indicated that milk thistle poses little risk of interfering with agents of similar metabolic profile.[108] Still, evaluating clinically significant interactions for each target species will likely prove necessary, given the large interspecies differences in CYP450-mediated metabolic activities between humans, horses, dogs, and cats.[109]

Milk thistle's ability to promote liver regeneration could conceivably stimulate tumor growth in cases of hepatocellular carcinoma.[104] An in vitro study showed that milk thistle demonstrated strong anticancer (i.e., proapoptotic and growth-inhibiting) activity against human hepatocellular carcinoma cells.[110] However, silymarin/silibinin promoted mammary tumor growth in two rodent models. This likely occurred through stimulation of estrogen-receptor signaling by silymarin,[105] which raises caution about its safety in cases of breast cancer. Overall, the majority of patients tolerate even high doses of milk thistle. As with most herbs, adverse effects typically involve gastrointestinal upset, diarrhea, or inappetence, although practitioners should monitor blood chemistries and platelet function on a regular basis (at least every 6 months), if animals are taking herbs for months or years.

Bloodroot

Bloodroot extract is an escharotic that may be topically applied in a salve or injected directly into tumors.[111,112] The "black salve" version of bloodroot *(Sanguinaria canadensis)* may come admixed with mineral agents such as zinc chloride, chromium chloride, or arsenic trisulfide and possibly other herbs. Bloodroot pastes became popular in the mid-twentieth century and have persisted despite risks of serious injury. It causes strong and rapid apoptotic responses through several modes of cell death, including an early and severe glutathione-depleting effect.

Sanguinarine, the active ingredient in bloodroot, supposedly targets only cancer cells, according to its enthusiastic supporters. Sanguinarine does appear to selectively target cancer cells over normal ones in vitro, and it may sensitize these cells to chemotherapy-mediated growth inhibition and apoptosis.[113] Sanguinarine has also been reported to provide dose-dependent differential antiproliferative and apoptotic effects on cancer and normal cells.[114] How tissue levels in vivo would compare to those tested in vitro is unknown, although high concentrations of sanguinarine can cause normal keratinocytes to necrose.[112]

Websites selling black salves for veterinary cancer patients generate undeniable excitement. One website lists pages of testimonials claiming quick and complete resolution of tumors deemed untreatable by conventional practitioners. Pictures of these tumors disappearing in a wide variety of animals make the message even more convincing. Even Dr. Andrew Weil, the author of the bestseller *Spontaneous Healing* and director of the Program in Integrative Medicine (PIM) at the University of Arizona in Tucson, claims that black salve cured a tumor on his dog. Further, he advocates the use of black salve for skin growths on his website.[115]

However, the toxicity of bloodroot in dogs with cancer was recently reported.[112] Childress et al describe the case of two dogs from the same household who were submitted to intratumoral injection of a preparation commonly employed by holistic veterinarians who treat tumors with bloodroot. Both underwent surgical excision of the tumors following bloodroot extract injection. In one dog, histologic evaluation revealed severe necrosis and inflammation; this dog developed postsurgical wound complications and required rehabilitation to treat wound contracture. The other dog had a less severe response and an uncomplicated recovery. The authors

> believe that bloodroot and other escharotics constitute potentially harmful herbal products, and that their use in the treatment of cutaneous neoplasia in domestic animals should be discouraged.… [E]scharotics may be manufactured without regard to accepted standards and therefore may contain unknown quantities of pharmacologically active compounds or toxic adulterants. Second, in the absence of biopsy prior to escharotic administration, escharotic treatment precludes accurate histologic identification of tumor type. Third, escharotic treatment prevents accurate in vivo or histologic assessment of tumor margins.… Fourth, escharotic treatment is painful and cosmetically unappealing. Fifth, escharotic treatment has no documented history of success in the human or veterinary medical literature. Sixth, escharotic treatment may be unnecessary [given the percentage of benign tumors that appear in veterinary patients that do not require aggressive treatment]. Finally, and most importantly, escharotic administration may delay or prevent definitive treatment by a more effective means, notably surgical excision, which is curative for many cutaneous tumors.[112]

They conclude

> Veterinarians should be aware of the potential deleterious consequences of escharotic administration and should likewise discourage clients from using escharotics on their animals until indications for their use, appropriate dosages, and incidences and types of adverse effects are established in well-designed clinical trials.[112]

Yunnan Baiyao

Yunnan Baiyao (also known as Yunnan Paiyao) is a Chinese herbal mixture consisting primarily of notoginseng that has become a popular product among veterinary clients, particularly those caring for animals with hemangiosarcoma. This popularity is the result of the claim that Yunnan Baiyao regulates bleeding. Therefore patients with a high risk of hemorrhage might be less likely to bleed if Yunnan Baiyao was indeed effective.

Westerners first learned of the Chinese herbal mixture "Yunnan Baiyao," meaning "the white medicine of Yunnan," during the Vietnam War. Members of the U.S. military discovered that prisoners from North Vietnam often carried with them a tiny bottle of this product to take in the event that they were injured and bleeding, either internally or externally.[116] Over the ensuing decades, Yunnan Baiyao has grown in popularity among complementary medical practitioners and even in some conventional medicine practices for its hemostatic and thrombolytic properties.

At first glance, the foil packet of Yunnan Baiyao capsules may seem puzzling because an unidentified little red pill lies at one end. Folklore has it that the North Vietnamese soldiers would take this red "hit pill" when seriously wounded, as in receiving a gunshot wound, and this would check the bleeding. The *Chinese Herbal Patent Formulas* contain an equally curious recommendation for the hit pill: "In cases of serious wounds or bleeding, take the single red pill that comes with each bottle first, with wine."[117] The contents of this "hit pill" remain a mystery.

The Chinese doctor Qu Huangzhang developed Yunnan Baiyao in the Yunnan province of China in the early 1900s. The Yunnan province is known as "the Kingdom of Fauna and Flora" for its vast supply of plants and animals used in Chinese medicinals. Although the capsule's contents remained a manufacturing secret until fairly recently, suspicion grew that its main active ingredient consisted of pseudoginseng root, now called *Panax notoginseng*, notoginseng, "tien chi," or "san qi."[117] Notoginseng is a type of ginseng that offers the highest concentration of hemostatic constituents among all seven major ginseng types.[118] Its origin in Yunnan makes sense because the notoginseng grown there outperforms that grown elsewhere in terms of crop yield and quality.[119] Other substances in Yunnan Baiyao formulations vary between manufacturers and may include myrrh, ox bile, Chinese yam, sweet geranium, lesser galangal root, and possibly other antiseptics or astringent substances in a starch base. No contents of the hit pill specifically appear on the Yunnan Baiyao label, although it may contain a concentrated dose of notoginseng.

Studies done decades ago showed that Yunnan Baiyao activates platelets and decreases bleeding and clotting times. However, much more remains to be known about the effects of this Chinese herb on various species and for those patients with cancer. Limited information is available documenting the value of this product in both human and nonhuman patients. A prospective, randomized, double-blind, placebo-controlled study on Yunnan Baiyao for human patients undergoing bimaxillary orthognathic surgery found significant reduction in intraoperative blood loss when Yunnan Baiyao was administered presurgically for 3 days.[120] No thrombolic events or other side effects were noted during this short-term administration.

Additional indications in the future may arise for cancer treatment due to the cytotoxic effects of notoginseng,[121] as well as its capacity to specifically sensitize tumor cells to ionizing radiation.[122]

High doses of notoginseng could be toxic to bone marrow stem cells.[122] In addition, the usual drawbacks to Chinese herbal products apply—lack of quality control, manufacturing regulations, and standardization.

In summary, as is so often the case for Chinese herbs, although Yunnan Baiyao appears to offer possible value, at this time its anecdotal acclaim outweighs the evidence, and unknowns regarding dosage, purity, and long-term benefits or risks persist.

Massage

What Is Massage and How Can It Help Cancer Patients?

Massage incorporates several methods of hands-on, low-force techniques that target restrictions and pain, mostly in the soft tissues of the body. The benefits that massage may hold for cancer patients encompass quality of life, control of postoperative or postprocedural pain and stress, and support of improved mobility and functional recovery following amputation. Cancer and its treatments can make people and animals physically uncomfortable. A 2011 study of patients with metastatic bone cancer, reported in the journal *Pain*, found that "[T]he reduction in pain with massage was both statistically and clinically significant, and the massage-related effects on relaxation were sustained for at least 16-18 hours postintervention."[123] Massage was also shown to benefit subjects in terms of mood, muscle relaxation, and sleep quality. Research on massage supports its value for treating pain and stress[124-131]; immune dysfunction[132]; lymphedema[133-137]; relief of anxiety, nausea, depression, and fatigue[138]; and chemotherapy-induced peripheral neuropathy.[139]

How Does Massage Work?

Thanks to the rapidly expanding paradigm of autonomic neuromodulation and the desire by medical massage therapists to explain how their treatments work, a unifying theory is beginning to emerge: neurophysiology explains how and why soft tissue therapy improves many bodily processes, including—but not limited to—digestion, emotional states, sleep, weight regulation, pain control, and immune function.[140,141]

The recognition that moderate pressure massage gave patients slower heart rates, lower blood pressure, and reduced cortisol levels pointed to changes within the ANS.[140] Eventually, investigations led to the vagal nerve network as the final common pathway. This tenth cranial nerve and associated brainstem nuclei affect nearly every bodily function, serving as a neural expressway mediating the tightly orchestrated, restorative parasympathetic nervous system. Some of the most compelling research on massage and the vagus nerve involves term and preterm infants. For example, massage allows preterm infants to better autoregulate their body temperature.[142] Properly massaged infants show less physiologic stress and reactivity,[143] higher vagal tone, and significantly less fussing, crying, and stress behavior such as hiccups.

Vagal afferent fibers on the body wall innervate pressure-sensitive mechanoreceptors; massage applied to the skin, subcutaneous tissue, and underlying myofascia activates these nerve endings. Signals then travel to brainstem nuclei and cerebral centers that coordinate ANS homeostasis by means of moment-to-moment alterations in parasympathetic and sympathetic output.

Ordinarily, animals suffering from acute and chronic illness exhibit heightened sympathetic tone that can cause maladaptive changes. The complementary, dualistic reciprocity encoded within the ANS dictates that as parasympathetic tone increases, sympathetic (fight-or-flight) activity calms down.[144] Consequently, reducing sympathetic hyperactivity by means of massage can benefit patients by countering peripheral vasoconstriction, inflammation, muscle tension, spinal cord wind-up, and pain.[145,146] For older veterinary patients suffering from cancer, as well as those recovering from surgery and experiencing postoperative ileus, regulation of digestive function through massage may provide much-needed parasympathetic support.[147,148]

The relaxing benefits of medical massage would assist veterinary oncology patients in counteracting stress during minimally invasive procedures, although it should never be relied on to replace conventional anesthesia and analgesia for more painful events. Facial massage calms patients at least in part by activating trigeminal-vagal reflexes.[149] Veterinary technicians can include certain techniques while assisting with gentle restraint; slow, up-and-down moderate pressure massage along the midline between the nose and forehead can sometimes induce a quasi-hypnotic state in patients.[150]

How Does Massage Benefit Cancer Patients?

Massage offers additional attributes such as improved immune, circulatory, and visceral functions. Veterinary massage, although lacking in research, is growing in popularity.[151,152] The benefits of massage may include relief of pain, anxiety, and nausea, as well as alleviation of lymphedema and chemotherapy-related neuropathy. Home-care providers can be instructed in several of these procedures to assist in patient recovery and providing comfort.

What Are the Risks of Massage for Cancer Patients?

Patients with osteosarcoma, skeletal metastasis, spinal instability, low platelet count, or osteopenia should avoid deep massage. Light or moderate pressure, delivered through skilled hands after informed palpation, would not be contraindicated, except over areas of recent surgery, instability, or infection. Massage should be avoided over implantations to deliver chemotherapy or other drugs. Massage to sites containing stents or prostheses may cause displacement. Tissues subjected to prior surgery or radiation therapy may be fragile, and massage to these areas should either be avoided or be done gently. Hypercoagulable patients may experience emboli subsequent to deep pressure over a thrombus; patients who are prone to bleeding may develop hematomas secondary to pressures that in normal patients would not cause problems. Deep abdominal massage has caused internal bleeding even in the absence of bleeding disorders. Although no evidence exists to indicate that massage promotes the likelihood of tumor metastasis, one should avoid massage directly over known tumors or predictable metastasis sites.

Laser Therapy

What Is Laser Therapy?

The acronym "laser" stands for *Light Amplification by Stimulated Emission of Radiation.* Low-level laser therapy (LLLT) and laser therapy (LT) refer to similar applications, but in LLLT, the instrument utilized does not produce heat (i.e., in the Class IIIb category, delivering <500 mW per laser), whereas Class IV units can in fact warm tissue (>500 mW, up to 12 W or higher).

Evidence is accruing that LT can provide safe and cost-effective treatment for wound healing, neurologic recovery, and pain reduction. Investigations into the benefits of LT are taking place in a number of areas, including oncology. Lasers are usually considered contraindicated in cancer patients, although a body of evidence suggests that LT may help to alleviate oral mucositis.[153,154]

How Does Laser Therapy Work?

In contrast to acupuncture, in which input begins with the microtraumatic mechanical effects of the needle on local tissue, LT relies on the absorption and scattering of light within tissue. LT imparts a monochromatic, narrow-band, coherent light source. Photons from the laser create a stimulating, biomodulatory effect, which is probably the main reason why LT has typically been avoided for cancer patients.

Physiologic responses from LT's photobiomodulation include increased phagocytosis, vasodilation, increased rate of regeneration of lymphatic and blood vessels, stimulation of enzyme activity at the wound edges, fibroblast stimulation, keratinocyte and fibroblast proliferation, scar and keloid reduction, increased adenosine triphosphate (ATP) and DNA synthesis, and stimulation of muscle, tendon, and nerve regeneration.[155]

How Might Laser Therapy Benefit Cancer Patients?

A 2007 phase III, randomized, double-blind, placebo-controlled clinical trial that evaluated the efficacy of LLLT for the prevention of oral mucositis (OM) indicated that laser with a 650-nm wavelength reduced the severity of OM as well as pain scores.[156] No adverse effects were noted in this study.

In 2011, a systematic review of studies on this topic concluded that

> [T]here is moderate to strong evidence in favour of LLLT applied with doses of 1-6 J per point in the oropharyngeal area in cancer patients receiving chemotherapy or radiation therapy. There are limitations to the material in terms of small sample size in the included trials. However, the material was consistently in favour of LLLT in both the prevention of OM occurrences and reductions of severity, pain, and duration of OM ulcers.[157]

How Might Laser Therapy Harm Cancer Patients?

Little in vivo research is currently available pertaining to the risk of LT stimulating cancer growth. However, prudent practice warrants avoiding LT in cancer patients or at least, tumor sites. Furthermore, LT's immunostimulatory effects make this therapy contraindicated for lymphoma patients.

Homeopathy

What Is Homeopathy?

Homeopathy is conceptually difficult for scientifically oriented practitioners to grasp due to its irrational philosophic basis that the more dilute a remedy is, the more potent it is. Homeopathic remedies exist in moderate-to-extremely dilute concentrations, wherein the homeopathic solution is nearly pure water.

Homeopathic practitioners claim that they prescribe minute dilutions of natural substances (from plants, minerals, or animals) in order to stimulate that individual's natural healing response. According to homeopathic principles, a natural substance that causes symptoms of illness in a healthy person can cure that same sickness in an unhealthy person suffering from those same symptoms, when it is administered in a highly dilute form. When selecting a remedy for a patient, a homeopath first determines which substance most closely resembles the symptoms of that patient's disease and then selects a specific remedy to match the clinical picture.

Contrary to conventional medical pharmacotherapeutic principles, homeopathic doctrine states that remedies are more powerful as they become more dilute. A matter of confusion among those accustomed to conventional medical approaches is the fact that highly diluted remedies may not even contain one molecule of the original substance.[158] The mechanism of purported action of homeopathy, other than its placebo effects, remains unknown. Proponents speculate that homeopathic remedies may have properties distinct from those of water, although skeptics would argue that there is little, if any, difference between homeopathic remedies and water.

As difficult as homeopathic theory is to understand, the remedies are as easy to administer as sugar pills because for many remedies the pills are just that: lactose tablets impregnated on the outer surface with the diluted homeopathic mixture. Most remedies are available over the counter. Although most states consider the practice of homeopathy on animals as part of veterinary medicine, clients can and do self-prescribe and self-administer the medication to their animals. Several do-it-yourself books on veterinary homeopathy are available.

How Does Homeopathy Work?

First, there is the question of whether homeopathy does, in fact, work. Most systematic reviews and metaanalyses find that the effects of homeopathy resemble the strength of placebos. The benefits seen in humans receiving homeopathy may be due to the lengthy interviewing process itself rather than the homeopathic remedies per se.[159] Currently, there is no repeatable, rigorous evidence that homeopathy works for veterinary patients. Similarly, there is no rational mechanism of action.

Despite this lack of scientific substantiation, veterinary homeopaths claim that homeopathy is "powerful medicine." In one popular instructor's words, "In my experience, the potential of homeopathy is to cure at the deepest level, with all symptoms resolving and the animal living a long and healthy life."[160] She continues, "[F]rom day one homeopathy can improve the overall well being and health of the animal in spite of the continuing presence of the original, uncured pathology such as renal disease, Cushing's, cancer, diabetes and more." These are big claims for a small or nonexistent dose of plant, mineral, or animal matter.

How Might Homeopathy Benefit Patients with Cancer?

Evidence for the incorporation of homeopathy for symptom control in cancer patients is weak and burdened with methodologic flaws, uncontrolled trials, and/or small subject numbers. Reports from these types of studies suggest a benefit from homeopathy for symptoms of pain, fatigue, hot flushes, and mood disturbances[161,162]; control of skin reactions during radiotherapy for breast cancer[163,164]; chemotherapy-induced stomatitis in children[165]; and hot flushes for women receiving Tamoxifen.[166] One study investigating the effects of a homeopathic drug, Chelidonium, reported antitumor and nongenotoxic activity, as well as favorable modulation of certain marker enzymes.[167,168] Nevertheless, studies such as these are usually unreplicated and positive benefits disappear when the study is repeated with larger numbers and controls.

Thus the most reliable benefit from homeopathy may be its placebo effects on the client (i.e., bolstering a feeling that they are doing something safe and supportive for their animal with cancer). This false sense of assurance could work against the animal's best interests if it delays meaningful diagnosis and effective care, as illustrated in a human study on the effect of antecedent use of CAM in delaying medical advice sought for breast cancer.[7]

One of the strongest studies for what has been called "homeopathy" involves assessment of a mouth rinse containing Traumeel S. The product tested, however, is not homeopathic in the classic sense. Classic homeopathy usually relies on remedies of higher dilutions with only a single substance. It also entails tailoring that substance to the individual's constitution and symptom picture; the highly diluted homeopathic remedies are given one time. In contrast, this small, randomized, double-blind, placebo-controlled clinical trial looked at the effects of a "homotoxicologic" remedy (often confused with homeopathy) containing Traumeel S that was given to children with either lymphoma or acute myelogenous leukemia.[169] These patients received stem cell transplantation and subsequently developed chemotherapy-induced stomatitis. All children underwent standard oral care for the stomatitis along with a 5-times-a-day mouth rinse of either placebo or Traumeel S. Of the 15 patients in the treatment group, 5 (33%) did not develop stomatitis, whereas only 1 (7%) out of the 15 children receiving placebo avoided it. Stomatitis worsened in 47% of the individuals receiving Traumeel S, as compared to 93% worsening in the placebo group. The benefits of Traumeel S were statistically significant.

Traumeel S differs from many homeopathic remedies in terms of the concentration of its ingredients in which it more resembles a weak extract of agents (in this case plants and minerals), rather than a solution of infinitesimal dilution. It also contains 14 components rather than only one. Instead of working through "vibrational frequencies" as many ascribe to homeopathic remedies, homotoxicologic agents likely confer benefits through pharmacologic activities because they are actually weak solutions of plant, mineral, or animal matter.

Thus far, this study has not been replicated.[170]

Can Homeopathy Harm Cancer Patients?

Although homeopaths may administer remedies to serve as a complementary treatment to minimize side effects of conventional treatment methods, they have not as often attempted to treat the cancer itself.[171] Homeopathy in general is unlikely to harm patients unless it is used as a substitute for proper conventional care.[172]

Edzard Ernst, a well-respected and prolific author from the University of Exeter in the United Kingdom, critic of CAM, and former homeopath summarized the "intangible risks of complementary and alternative medicine" for patients with cancer.[173] Ernst noted,

> [C]omplementary therapies, particularly those popular in palliative and supportive cancer care (e.g., acupressure, homeopathy, reflexology, and spiritual healing), might be judged as entirely free of direct risks; nevertheless they are associated with indirect risks. The most obvious of such risks is the use of complementary therapies as true alternatives to conventional cancer treatments.[173]

Ernst continues, referencing a "nonmedically qualified CAM practitioner" acquaintance who self-medicated with homeopathic remedies for a brown lesion on her arm. When she finally consulted an allopathic physician, she discovered it was advanced malignant melanoma; she died shortly thereafter. Ernst continues, "Complementary therapists assure us that such disasters almost never happen, but I find this hard to believe. Underreporting is probably close to 100%, and very little systematic research exists in this area…"[173]

Words of Caution

Oncology clients today have access to an information overload on CAM for cancer. The Internet provides, literally at clients' fingertips, abundant opportunities to purchase remedies from companies and even holistic veterinarians who have neither taken a history nor examined the animal with cancer. The lay literature on alternative treatments for cancer recommends well over a hundred approaches for cancer, with little consensus among authors and even less scientific or evidential support.[174]

One author provided the following alerts regarding "signs of a hoax" to help human patients and their healthcare providers with detection of fraudulent treatments[175]:

- "The treatment is a 'secret' that only specific individuals can provide."
- "Patients are told not to use conventional medical treatment."
- "The treatment promises a cure for almost all cancers or medical conditions."
- "The treatment is promoted only in the mass media such as the Internet, television, or radio 'talk shows,' and books instead of reputable scientific journals."
- "The promoters claim that they are persecuted by the medical establishment."
- "Advertisements for the treatment claim to 'cleanse the body of poisons and toxins.'"
- "The treatment will help the patient by 'strengthening the immune system.'"
- "Testimonials and case reports are used to promote a specific treatment or product."
- "Catch phrases such as 'nontoxic,' 'no side effects,' and 'painless' are used."
- "The promoters attack the medical community."

General Considerations When Recommending Integrative Care for Oncology Patients

CAM practitioners are not subject to litigation as often as physicians, but referrals to CAM practitioners are not without risk.[176] A referral to a CAM practitioner that delays, prevents, or minimizes the opportunity for the patient to receive necessary care via conventional means and which subsequently causes the patient suffering may be considered negligent, as can referrals made to incompetent practitioners.

According to the January 1999 issue of the *Journal of the American Veterinary Medical Association*, "More inquiries and complaints are directed to the AVMA (American Veterinary Medical Association) about alternative and complementary therapies than any other issue."[177] Referring animals for unconventional care can raise issues of CAM provider credibility, especially if the practitioner is not a licensed doctor of veterinary medicine. To quote the AVMA committee studying this matter:

> the veterinary profession wants to assure the public that, when alternative and complementary modalities are being used, they are being used by persons rendered capable and responsible through education and regulation, and that, as a result, these practitioners will "do no harm." Licensed professionals who have not received adequate education or who do not submit themselves to a required standard of practice in these modalities, and unlicensed nonprofessionals who possess minimal acquired or practical experience, both pose a danger to clients and patients. Furthermore, the committee encourages the use of these modalities within the context of a valid veterinarian/client/patient relationship.[178]

As more academic institutions provide courses and training programs in CAM techniques, a greater emphasis on scientific exploration will arise, along with substantially more opportunities for methodical and in-depth study. For the treatment of cancer in particular, evidence-based clinical research on the safety and efficacy of CAM modalities in veterinary cancer patients must take place in order to determine where these approaches best partner and synergize with conventional veterinary cancer care. Indeed, as concluded by the American Veterinary Medical Law Association in 2004, veterinarians offering complementary or alternative therapies: "[S]hould remain vigilant to use only what has been demonstrated to be scientifically reliable treatments or therapies. In other words, treatments and therapies that have been subjected to the same critical analysis and assessment as conventional treatments and therapies."[179]

REFERENCES

1. Ernst E: Complementary therapies in palliative cancer care, *Cancer* 91:2181–2185, 2001.
2. Metz JM: "Alternative medicine" and the cancer patient: an overview, *Med Pediatr Oncol* 34:20–26, 2000.
3. Weiger WA, et al: Advising patients who seek complementary and alternative medical therapies for cancer, *Ann Intern Med* 137: 889-903, 2002.
4. Kehr RW: DMSO – Colloidal Silver Protocol for Cancer. Independent Cancer Research Foundations, Inc. Accessed at http://www.new-cancer-treatments.org/Cancer/DMSO_CS.html on 11–18–11.
5. Zappa SB, Cassileth BR: Complementary approaches to palliative oncological care, *J Nurs Care Qual* 18:22–26, 2003.
6. Lana SE, Kogan LR, Crump KA, et al: The use of complementary and alternative therapies in dogs and cats with cancer, *J Am Anim Hosp Assoc* 42:361–365, 2006.
7. Malik IA, Gopalan S: Use of CAM results in delay in seeking medical advice for breast cancer, *Eur J Epidemiol* 18:817–822, 2003.
8. Memon MA, Sprunger LK: Survey of colleges and schools of veterinary medicine regarding education in complementary and alternative veterinary medicine, *J Am Vet Med Assoc* 239:619–623, 2011.
9. Cassileth BR, Deng GE, Gomez JE, et al: Complementary therapies and integrative oncology in lung cancer: ACCP evidence-based clinical practice guidelines (2nd edition), *Chest* 132(3 Suppl): 340S-354S, 2007.
10. Junqin Z, Zhihua L, Pule Jin: A clinical study on acupuncture for prevention and treatment of toxic side-effects during radiotherapy and chemotherapy, *J Trad Chin Med* 19(1):16–21, 1999.
11. Johnstone PAS, Polston GR, Niemtzow RC, et al: Integration of acupuncture into the oncology clinic, *Palliat Med* 16:235–239, 2002.
12. Wong R, Sagar CM, Sagar SM: Integration of Chinese medicine into supportive cancer care: a modern role for an ancient tradition, *Cancer Treat Rev* 27:235–246, 2001.
13. Dundee JW, Ghaly RG, Fitzpatrick KT, et al: Acupuncture prophylaxis of cancer chemotherapy-induced sickness, *J R Soc Med* 82(5):268–271, 1989.
14. Al-sadi M, Newman B, Julious SA, et al: Acupuncture in the prevention of postoperative nausea and vomiting, *Anesthesia* 52:658–661, 1997.
15. Reference deleted in pages.
16. Parfitt A: Acupuncture as an antiemetic treatment, *J Alt Compl Med* 2(1):167–173, 1996.
17. Vickers AJ: Can acupuncture have specific effects on health? A systematic review of acupuncture antiemesis trials, *J R Soc Med* 89:303–311, 1996.
18. McMillan C, Dundee JW, Abram WP: Enhancement of the antiemetic action of ondansetron by transcutaneous electrical stimulation of the P6 antiemetic point, in patients having highly emetic cytotoxic drugs, *Br J Cancer* 64:971–972, 1991.
19. Paley CA, Bennett MI, Johnson MI: Acupuncture for cancer-induced bone pain? *Evid Based Complement Alternat Med* 2011:671043, 2011.
20. Dillon M, Lucas C: Auricular stud acupuncture in palliative care patients, *Palliative Medicine* 13:253–254, 1999.
21. Alimi D, Rubino C, Leandri EP, et al: Analgesic effects of auricular acupuncture for cancer, *J Pain Symptom Manage* 19(2):81–82, 2000.
22. Alimi D, Rubino C, Pichard-Léandri E, et al: Analgesic effect of auricular acupuncture for cancer pain: A randomized, blinded, controlled trial, *J Clin Oncol* 21:4120–4126, 2003.
23. Omura Y, Losco BM, Omura AK, et al: Common factors contributing to intractable pain and medical problems with insufficient drug uptake in areas to be treated, and their pathogenesis and treatment: Part I. Combined use of medication with acupuncture, (+) Qi Gong energy-stored material, soft laser or electrical stimulation, *Acupunc Electrother Res* 17:107–148, 1992.
24. Nordenström BEW: An electrophysiologic view of acupuncture: role of capacitive and closed circuit currents and their clinical effects in the treatment of cancer and chronic pain, *Am J Acupuncture* 17(2):105–117, 1989.
25. Filshie J: The non-drug treatment of neuralgic and neuropathic pain of malignancy, *Cancer Surv* 7(1):161–193, 1988.
26. Filshie J, Redman D: Acupuncture and malignant pain problems, *Eur J Surg Onc* 11:389–394, 1985.
27. Filshie J: Acupuncture for malignant pain. Presented to the BMAS Spring Meeting at Warwick, 1990.
28. Liaw M, Wong AM, Cheng P: Therapeutic trial of acupuncture in phantom limb pain of amputees, *Am J Acupuncture* 22:205–213, 1994.
29. Johnston MF, Sanchez EO, Vujanovic NL, et al: Acupuncture may stimulate anticancer immunity via activation of natural killer cells, *Evid Based Complement Alternat Med* 2011:481625, 2011.
30. Sato T, Yu Y, Guo SY, et al: Acupuncture stimulation enhances splenic natural killer cell cytotoxicity in rats, *Japan J Physiol* 46(2):131–136, 1996.
31. Chin TF, Lin JG, Wang SY: Induction of circulating interferon in humans by acupuncture, *Am J Acupuncture* 16(4):319–322, 1988.
32. Yu Y, Kasahara T, Sato T, et al: Enhancement of splenic interferon-γ, interleukin-2, and NK cytotoxicity by S36 acupoint acupuncture in F344 rats, *Japan J Physiol* 47:173–178, 1997.
33. Cassileth BR, Van Zee KJ, Chan Y, et al: A safety and efficacy pilot study of acupuncture for the treatment of chronic lymphedema, *Acupunct Med* 29(3):170–172, 2011.
34. Muxeneder R: Die konservative Behandlung chronischer Hautver nderungen des Pferdes durch Laserpunktur, *Der Praktische Tierarzt* 69:12–21, 1988.
35. Braga Fdo P, Lemos Junior CA, Alves FA, et al: Acupuncture for the prevention of radiation-induced xerostomia in patients with head and neck cancer, *Braz Oral Res* 25(2):180–185, 2011.
36. Blom M, Dawidson I, Fernberg JO, et al: Acupuncture treatment of patients with radiation-induced xerostomia, *Oral Oncol* 32B(3): 182–190, 1996.
37. Dawidson I, et al: The influence of sensory stimulation (acupuncture) on the release of neuropeptides in the saliva of healthy subjects, *Life Sci* 63(8):659–674, 1998.
38. Wong RKW, Jones GW, Sagar SM, et al: A Phase I-II study in the use of acupuncture-like transcutaneous nerve stimulation in the treatment of radiation-induced xerostomia in head-and-neck cancer patients treated with radial radiotherapy, *Int J Radiat Oncol Biol Phys* 57(2):472–480, 2003.
39. Lim JT, Wong ET, Aung SK: Is there a role for acupuncture in the symptom management of patients receiving palliative care for cancer? A pilot study of 20 patients comparing acupuncture with nurse-led supportive care, *Acupunct Med* 29(3):173–179, 2011.
40. Shen J, Glaspy J: Acupuncture: evidence and implications for cancer supportive care, *Cancer Practice* 9:147–150, 2001.
41. Dean-Clower E, Doherty-Gilman AM, Keshaviah A, et al: Acupuncture as palliative therapy for physical symptoms and quality of life for advanced cancer patients, *Integr Cancer Ther* 9(2):158–167, 2010.
42. Thoresen A: Acupuncture and cancer therapy, Obtained at http://home.online.no/~arethore/engelsk/foredrag/kreft.html on 05–26–08.
43. Thoresen A: Small animal cancer, Obtained at http://med-vetacupuncture.org/english/articles/an-canc.html on 05–26–08.
44. Kaphle K, Wu YL, Lin JH: Thirtieth Annual Congress on Veterinary Acupuncture: IVAS Report, *eCAM* 2(2):239–242, 2005.
45. Personal communication with clients who sought acupuncture for their animal with cancer, most commonly for palliative care, pain control, and other quality of life issues but were refused care by energy-based veterinary acupuncturists.
46. Tan W, Lu J, Huang M, et al: Anti-cancer natural products isolated from Chinese medicinal herbs, *Chin Med* 6:27, 2011.
47. Li-Weber M: Targeting apoptosis pathways in cancer by Chinese medicine, *Cancer Lett* 2010 [Epub ahead of print].

48. Wang S, Penchala S, Prabhu S, et al: Molecular basis of traditional Chinese medicine in cancer chemoprevention, *Curr Drug Discov Technol* 7(1):67–75, 2010.
49. Robinson NG: TCVM's Silk Road may lead to detour. *Veterinary Practice News* April 7, 2010. Accessed on 08–08–11 at http://www.veterinarypracticenews.com/vet-practice-news columns/complementary-medicine/tcvm-silk-road-may-lead-to-detour.aspx.
50. McCulloch M, See C, Shu XJ, et al: Astragalus-based Chinese herbs and platinum-based chemotherapy for advanced non-small-cell lung cancer: meta-analysis of randomized trials, *J Clin Oncol* 24:419–430, 2006.
51. Senthilnathan P, Padmavathi R, Banu SM, et al: Enhancement of antitumor effect of paclitaxel in combination with immunomodulatory *Withania somnifera* on benzo(*a*)pyrene induced experimental lung cancer, *Chem Biol Interact* 159:180–185, 2006.
52. Shu X, McCulloch M, Xiao H, et al: Chinese herbal medicine and chemotherapy in the treatment of hepatocellular carcinoma: a meta-analysis of randomized controlled trials, *Integr Cancer Ther* 4:219–229, 2005.
53. DiNatale C: Clinical application of Chinese herbal medicine for companion animals. In Xie H, Preast V, editors: *Xie's Chinese veterinary herbology*, Ames, Iowa, 2010, Blackwell Publishing.
54. McCulloch MF, See C, Shu XJ, et al: Important bias in the *Astragalus* meta-analysis [Reply], *J Clin Oncol* 24(19):3216–3217, 2006.
55. Yang AK, He SM, Liu L, et al: Herbal interactions with anticancer drugs: mechanistic and clinical considerations, *Curr Med Chem* 17:1635–1678, 2010.
56. Yap KY, Kuo EY, Lee JJ, et al: An onco-informatics database for anticancer drug interactions with complementary and alternative medicines used in cancer treatment and supportive care: An overview of the OncoRx project, *Support Care Cancer* 18:883–891, 2010.
57. Chiu J, Yau T, Epstein RJ: Complications of traditional Chinese/herbal medicines (TCM)—a guide for perplexed oncologists and other cancer caregivers, *Support Care Cancer* 17:231–240, 2009.
58. Liu SH, Liu YF, Liou SH, et al: Mortality and cancer incidence among physicians of traditional Chinese medicine: A 20 year national follow-up study, *Occup Environ Med* 67:166–169, 2010.
59. Yang HY, Wang JD, Lo TC, et al: Increased mortality risk for cancers of the kidney and other urinary organs among Chinese herbalists, *J Epidemiol* 19(1):17–23, 2009.
60. Mok TSK, Yeo W, Johnson PJ, et al: A double-blind placebo-controlled randomized study of Chinese herbal medicine as complementary therapy for reduction of chemotherapy-induced toxicity, *Ann Oncol* 18:768–774, 2007.
61. DiNatale C: Clinical application of Chinese herbal medicine for companion animals. In Xie H, Preast V, editors: *Xie's Chinese veterinary herbology*, Ames, Iowa, 2010, Blackwell Publishing.
62. Guo R, Canter PH, Ernst E: A systematic review of randomized clinical trials of individualized herbal medicine in any indication, *Postgrad Med J* 83:633–637, 2007.
63. Sze DM, Chan GC: Supplements for immune enhancement in hematologic malignancies, *Hematology* 2009:313–319, 2009.
64. Zhou S, Lim LY, Chowbay B: Herbal modulation of p-glycoprotein, *Drug Metab Rev* 36(1):57–104, 2004.
65. Shord SS, Shah K, Lukose A: Drug-botanical interactions: a review of the laboratory, animal, and human data for 8 common botanicals, *Integr Cancer Ther* 8(3):208–227, 2009.
66. Davis VL, Jayo MJ, Ho A, et al: Black cohosh increases metastatic mammary cancer in transgenic mice expressing c-*erb*B2, *Cancer Res* 68(20):8377–8383, 2008.
67. Hwang SW, Han HS, Lim KY: Drug interaction between complementary herbal medicines and gefitinib, *J Thorac Oncol* 3(8):942, 2008.
68. Engdal S, Klepp O, Nilsen OG: Identification and exploration of herb-drug combinations used by cancer patients, *Integr Cancer Ther* 8(1):29–36, 2009.
69. Michaud LB, Karpinski JP, Jones KL, et al: Dietary supplements in patients with cancer: risks and key concepts, part 1, *Am J Health Syst Pharm* 64:369–381, 2007.
70. Piersen CE: Phytoestrogens in botanical dietary supplements: Implications for cancer, *Integr Cancer Ther* 2(2):120–136, 2003.
71. McCulloch M, See C, Shu X-J, et al: Astragalus-based Chinese herbs and platinum-based chemotherapy for advanced non-small-cell lung cancer: meta-analysis of randomized trials, *J Clin Oncol* 24:419–430, 2006.
72. Firenzuoli F, Gori L, Di Simone L, et al: Important bias in the *Astragalus* meta-analysis, *J Clin Oncol* 24(19):3215–3216, 2006.
73. Hardy ML: Dietary supplement use in cancer care: help or harm, *Hematol Oncol Clin North Am* 22(4):581–617, 2008.
74. Song KS, Kim JS, Jing K, et al: Protein-bound polysaccharide from *Phellinus linteus* inhibits tumor growth, invasion, and angiogenesis and alters Wnt/beta-catenin in SW480 human colon cancer cells, *BMC Cancer* 11:307, 2011.
75. Ohwada S, Ikeya T, Yokomori T: Adjuvant immunochemotherapy with oral Tegafur/Uracil plus PSK in patients with stage II or III colorectal cancer: a randomised controlled study, *Br J Cancer* 90:1003–1010, 2004.
76. Sakamoto J, Morita S, Oba K, et al: Efficacy of adjuvant immunochemotherapy with polysaccharide K for patients with curatively resected colorectal cancer: a meta-analysis of centrally randomized controlled clinical trials, *Cancer Immunol Immunother* 55(4):404–411, 2006.
77. Griessmayr PC, Gautheir M, Barber LG, et al: Mushroom-derived maitake PET fraction as a single agent for the treatment of lymphoma in dogs, *J Vet Intern Med* 21(6):1409–1412, 2007.
78. Zhu HL, Ji JL, Huang XF: Curcumin and its formulations: Potential anti-cancer agents, *Anticancer Agents Med Chem* 12(3):210–218, 2011.
79. Schaffer M, Schaffer PM, Zidan J, et al: Curcuma as a functional food in the control of cancer and inflammation, *Curr Opin Clin Nutr Metab Care* 14(6):588–597, 2011.
80. Salvioli S, Sikora E, Cooper EL, et al: Curcumin in cell death processes: a challenge for CAM of age-related pathologies, *eCAM* 4(2):181–190, 2007.
81. Aggarwal BB, Kumar A, Bharti AC: Review. Anticancer potential of curcumin: preclinical and clinical studies, *Anticancer Res* 23:363–398, 2003.
82. Tayyem RF, Heath DD, Al-Delaimy WK, et al: Curcumin content of turmeric and curry powders, *Nutr Cancer* 55(2):126–131, 2006.
83. Dayton A, Selvendiran K, Meduru S, et al: Amelioration of doxorubicin-induced cardiotoxicity by an anticancer-antioxidant dual-function compound, HO-3867, *J Pharmacol Exp Ther* 339(2):350–357, 2011.
84. Manikandan R, Beulaja M, Arulvasu C, et al: Synergistic anticancer activity of curcumin and catechin: An in vitro study using human cancer cell lines, *Microsc Res Tech* 75(2):112–116, 2012.
85. Hostanska K, Daum G, Saller R: Cytostatic and apoptosis-inducing activity of boswellic acids toward malignant cell lines in vitro, *Anticancer Res* 22(5):2853–2862, 2002.
86. Roy S, Khanna S, Krishnaraju AV, et al: Regulation of vascular responses to inflammation: inducible matrix metalloproteinase-3 expression in human microvascular endothelial cells is sensitive to anti-inflammatory *Boswellia*, *Antioxid Redox Signal* 8(3&4):653–660, 2006.
87. Chevrier MR, Ryan AE, Lee DYW, et al: *Boswellia carterii* extract inhibits TH1 cytokines and promotes TH2 cytokines in vitro, *Clin Diagn Lab Immunol* 12(5):575–580, 2005.
88. Reference deleted in pages.
89. Pungle P, Banayalikar M, Suthar A, et al: Immunomodulatory activity of boswellic acids of *Boswellia serrata* Roxb, *Indian J Exp Biol* 41:1460–1462, 2003.
90. Krieglstein CE, Anthoni C, Rijcken EJM, et al: Acetyl-11-keto-beta-boswellic acid, a constituent of a herbal medicine from *Boswellia*

serrata resin, attenuates experimental ileitis, *Int J Colorectal Dis* 16:88–95, 2001.

91. Anthoni C, Laukoetter MG, Rijcken E, et al: Mechanisms underlying the anti-inflammatory actions of boswellic acid derivatives in experimental colitis, *Am J Physiol Gastro Liver Physiol* 290: G1131-G1137, 2006.
92. Jing Y, Nakajo S, Xia L, et al: Boswellic acid acetate induces differentiation and apoptosis in leukemia cell lines, *Leukemia Res* 23:43–50, 1999.
93. Hostanska K, Daum G, Saller R: Cytostatic and apoptosis-inducing activity of boswellic acids toward malignant cell lines in vitro, *Anticancer Res* 22(5):2853–2862, 2002.
94. Zhao W, Entschladen F, Liu H, et al: Boswellic acid acetate induces differentiation and apoptosis in highly metastatic melanoma and fibrosarcoma cells, *Cancer Detect Prev* 27:67–75, 2003.
95. Shao Y, Ho CT, Chin CK, et al: Inhibitory activity of boswellic acids from *Boswellia serrata* against human leukemia HL-60 cells in culture, *Planta Med* 64:328–331, 1998.
96. Park YS, Lee JH, Bondar J, et al: Cytotoxic action of acetyl-11-keto-beta-boswellic acid (AKBA) on meningioma cells, *Planta Med* 68:397–401, 2002.
97. Reising K, Meins J, Bastian B, et al: Determination of boswellic acids in brain and plasma by high-performance liquid chromatography/tandem mass spectrometry, *Anal Chem* 77:6640–6645, 2005.
98. Gupta I, Gupta V, Parihar A, et al: Effects of *Boswellia serrata* gum resin in patients with bronchial asthma: results of a double-blind, placebo-controlled, 6-week clinical study, *Eur J Med Res* 3:511–514, 1998.
99. Kimmatkar N, Thawani V, Hingorani L, et al: Efficacy and tolerability of *Boswellia serrata* extract in treatment of osteoarthritis of knee—a randomized double-blind placebo controlled trial, *Phytomedicine* 10:3–7, 2003.
100. Sterk V, Buchele B, Simmet T: Effect of food intake on the bioavailability of boswellic acids from a herbal preparation in healthy volunteers, *Planta Med* 70:1155–1160, 2004.
101. Sharma S, Thawani V, Hingorani L, et al: Pharmacokinetic study of 11-keto beta-boswellic acid, *Phytomedicine* 11:255–260, 2004.
102. Frank A, Unger M: Analysis of frankincense from various *Boswellia* species with inhibitory activity on human drug metabolizing cytochrome P450 enzymes using liquid chromatography mass spectrometry after automated on-line extraction, *J Chromatogr A* 1112:255–262, 2006.
103. Kroll DJ, Shaw KS, Oberlies NH: Milk thistle nomenclature: why it matters in cancer research and pharmacokinetic studies, *Integr Cancer Ther* 6(2):110–119, 2007.
104. Greenlee H, Abascal K, Yarnell E, et al: Clinical applications of Silybum marianum in oncology, *Integr Cancer Ther* 2007 6(2): 158–166, 2007.
105. Malewicz B, Wang Z, Jiang C, et al: Enhancement of mammary carcinogenesis in two rodent models by silymarin dietary supplements, *Carcinogenesis* 27:1739–1747, 2006.
106. Gaedeke J, Fels LM, Bokemeyer C, et al: Cisplatin nephrotoxicity and protection by silibinin, *Nephrol Dial Transplant* 11(1):55–62, 1996.
107. Kroll DJ, Shaw KS, Oberlies NH: Milk thistle nomenclature: why it matters in cancer research and pharmacokinetic studies, *Integr Cancer Ther* 6(2):110–119, 2007.
108. Van Erp NPH, Baker SD, Zhao M, et al: Effect of milk thistle (Silybum marianum) on the pharmacokinetics of irinotecan, *Clin Cancer Res* 11(21):7800–7805, 2005.
109. Chauret N, Gauthier A, Martin J, et al: In vitro comparison of cytochrome P450-mediated metabolic activities in human, dog, cat, and horse, *Drug Metab Disp* 25(10):1130–1136, 1997.
110. Varghese L, Agarwal C, Tyagi A, et al: Silibinin efficacy against human hepatocellular carcinoma, *Clin Cancer Res* 11(23):8441–8448, 2005.
111. Cienki JJ, Zaret L: An internet misadventure: bloodroot salve toxicity, *J Alt Comp Med* 16(10):1125–1127, 2010.
112. Childress MO, Burgess RC, Holland CH, et al: Consequences of intratumoral injection of a herbal preparation containing blood root (Sanguinaria canadensis) extract in two dogs, *J Am Vet Med Assoc* 239(3):374–379, 2011.
113. Sun M, Lou W, Chun JY, et al: Sanguinarine suppresses prostate tumor growth and inhibits survivin expression, *Genes Cancer* 1(3):283–292, 2010.
114. Ahmad N, Gupta S, Husain MM, et al: Differential antiproliferative and apoptotic response of sanguinarine for cancer cells versus normal cells, *Clin Cancer Res* 6(4):1524–1528, 2000.
115. Weil A: Q&A Library: Accessed at http://www.drweil.com/drw/u/id/QAA269352 on November 18, 2011.
116. Bergner P: *Panax notoginseng (Yunnan bai yao)*: A must for the first aid kit, *Medical Herbalism* October 31:12, 1994.
117. Fratkin J: *Chinese herbal patent formulas: A practical guide*, Santa Fe, 1986, Shya Publications.
118. Zheng YN: Comparative analysis of the anti-haemorrhagic principle in ginseng plants, *Acta Agri Univ Jilin* 11(1):24–27, 102, 1989. [Article in Chinese.]
119. Jin H, Cui XM, Zhu Y, et al: Effects of meteorological conditions on the quality of radix Notoginseng, *Southwest China J Agri Sci* 18(6):825–828, 2005.
120. Tang ZL, Wang X, Yi B, et al: Effects of the preoperative administration of Yunnan Baiyao capsules on intraoperative blood loss in bimaxillary orthognathic surgery: a prospective, randomized, double-blind, placebo-controlled study, *Int J Oral Maxillofac Surg* 38:261–266, 2009.
121. Chung VQ, Tattersall M, Cheung HTA: Interactions of a herbal combination that inhibits growth of prostate cancer cells, *Cancer Chemo Pharmcol* 53:384–390, 2004.
122. Chen FD, Wu MC, Wang HE, et al: Sensitization of a tumor, but not normal tissue, to the cytotoxic effect of ionizing radiation using Panax notoginseng extract, *Am J Chin Med* 29(3/4):517–524, 2001.
123. Jane SW, Chen SL, Wilkie DJ, et al: Effects of massage on pain, mood status, relaxation, and sleep in Taiwanese patients with metastatic bone pain: a randomized clinical trial, *Pain* 152(10):2432–2442, 2011.
124. Martin LA, Hagen NA: Neuropathic pain in cancer patients: mechanisms, syndromes, and clinical controversies, *J Pain Symptom Manage* 14(2):99–117, 1997.
125. Ferrell-Torry AT, Glick OJ: The use of therapeutic massage as a nursing intervention to modify anxiety and the perception of cancer pain, *Cancer Nurs* 16(2):93–101, 1993.
126. Burke C, Macnish S, Saunders J, et al: The development of a massage service for cancer patients, *Clin Oncol (R Coll Radiol)* 6(6):381–384, 1994.
127. Field T: Massage therapy for infants and children, *Dev Behav Pediatr* 16(2):105–111, 1995.
128. Francke AL, Luiken JB, Garssen B, et al: Effects of a pain programme on nurses' psychosocial, physical, and relaxation interventions, *Patient Educ Couns* 28:221–230, 1996.
129. Smith M, Stallings MA, Mariner S, et al: Benefits of massage therapy for hospitalized patients: a descriptive and qualitative evaluation, *Altern Ther* 5(4):64–71, 1999.
130. Smith MC, Reeder F, Daniel L, et al: Outcomes of touch therapies during bone marrow transplant, *Altern Ther* 9(1):40–49, 2003.
131. Post-White J, Kinney ME, Savik K, et al: Therapeutic massage and healing touch improve symptoms in cancer, *Integr Cancer Ther* 2(4):332–344, 2003.
132. Ironson G: Massage therapy is associated with enhancement of the immune system's cytotoxic capacity, *Int J Neurosci* 84(1–4):205–217, 1996.
133. Cornish BH, Bunce IH, Ward LC, et al: Bioelectrical impedance for monitoring the efficacy of lymphoedema treatment programmes, *Breast Cancer Res Treat* 38(2):169–176, 1996.
134. Mortimer PS: Therapy approaches for lymphedema, *Angiology* 48(1):87–91, 1997.

135. Woods M: The experience of manual lymph drainage as an aspect of treatment for lymphoedema, *Int J Palliat Nurs* 9(8):337–342, 2003.
136. Kirschbaum M: Using massage in the relief of lymphoedema, *Professional Nurse* 11(4):230–232, 1996.
137. McNeely ML, Peddle CJ, Yurick JL, et al: Conservative and dietary interventions for cancer-related lymphedema: a systematic review and meta-analysis, *Cancer* 117(6):1136–1148, 2011.
138. Cassileth BR, Vickers AJ: Massage therapy for symptom control: outcome study at a major cancer center, *J Pain Symptom Manage* 28:244–249, 2004.
139. Cunningham JE, Kelechi T, Sterba K, et al: Case report of a patient with chemotherapy-induced peripheral neuropathy treated with manual therapy (massage), *Support Care Cancer* 19(9):1473–1476, 2011.
140. Diego MA, Field T: Moderate pressure massage elicits a parasympathetic nervous system response, *Int J Neurosci* 119: 630–638, 2009.
141. Touch Research Institute: Massage therapy research, *Touchpoints* 17(3):1, 2010. Accessed at http://www6.miami.edu/touch-research/Touchpoints%20Summer%202010.pdf on 07–20–10.
142. Diego MA, Field T, Hernandez-Reif M: Temperature increases in preterm infants during massage therapy, *Infant Behav Dev* 31(1):149–152, 2008.
143. Feldman R, Singer M, Zagoory O: Touch attenuates infants' physiological reactivity to stress, *Dev Sci* 13(2):271–278, 2010.
144. Gellhorn E: *Principles of autonomic-somatic integrations: Physiologic basis and psychological and clinical implications*, Minneapolis, 1967, University of Minnesota Press.
145. Huang SY, Di Santo M, Wadden KP, et al: Short-duration massage at the hamstrings musculotendinous junction induces greater range of motion, *J Strength Cond Res* 24(7):1917–1924, 2010.
146. Huang J, Wang Y, Jiang D, et al: The sympathetic-vagal balance against endotoxemia, *J Neural Transm* 117:729–735, 2010.
147. Gao Z, Muller MH, Karpitschka M, et al: Role of the vagus nerve on the development of postoperative ileus, *Langenbecks Arch Surg* 395:407–411, 2010.
148. Lubbers T, Buurman W, Luyer M: Controlling postoperative ileus by vagal activation, *World J Gastroenterol* 16(14):1683–1687, 2010.
149. Hatayama T, Kitamura S, Tamura C, et al: The facial massage reduced anxiety and negative mood status, and increased sympathetic nervous activity, *Biomed Res* 29(6):317–320, 2008.
150. Personal experience of the author.
151. Mowen K: For the love of Fido, *Massage and Bodywork* Feb/Mar:36–42, 1999.
152. Bane R: Promoting better health through massage, *Cats* May/June:38–40, 1993.
153. Jaguar GC, Prado JD, Nishimoto IN, et al: Low-energy laser therapy for prevention of oral mucositis in hematopoietic stem cell transplantation, *Oral Dis* 13(6):538–543, 2007.
154. Alterio D, Jereczek-Fossa BA, Fiore MR, et al: Cancer treatment-induced oral mucositis, *Anticancer Res* 27(2):1105–1125, 2007.
155. Chung H, Dai T, Sharma SK, et al: The nuts and bolts of low-level laser (light) therapy, *Ann Biomed Eng* 40(2):516–533, 2012.
156. Schubert MM, Eduardo FP, Guthrie KA, et al: A phase III randomized double-blind placebo-controlled clinical trial to determine the efficacy of low level laser therapy for the prevention of oral mucositis in patients undergoing hematopoietic cell transplantation, *Support Care Cancer* 15(10):1145–1154, 2007.
157. Bjordal JM, Bensadoun RJ, Tuner J, et al: A systematic review with meta-analysis of the effect of low-level laser therapy (LLLT) in cancer therapy-induced oral mucositis, *Support Care Cancer* 19:1069–1077, 2011.
158. Benjamin SD: Homeopathy: can like cure like? *Patient Care* 16–27, 1999. http://business.highbeam.com/436950/article-1G1-58546345/homeopathy-can-like-cure-like.
159. Rostock M, Naumann J, Guethlin C, et al: Classical homeopathy in the treatment of cancer patients—a prospective observational study of two independent cohorts, *BMC Cancer* 11:19, 2011.
160. Chambreau C: A1—Controversies in alternative medicine. Practical use of homeopathy in your practice. 2006 World Congress Proceedings. 31st World Small Animal Association Congress, 12th European Congress FECAVA, & 14th Czech Small Animal Veterinary Association Congress, Prague, Czech Republic, 11–14 October, 2006.
161. Rajendran ES: Homeopathy as a supportive therapy in cancer, *Homeopathy* 93:99–102, 2004.
162. Thompson EA: The homeopathic approach to symptom control in the cancer patient: a prospective observational study, *Palliat Med* 16:227–233, 2002.
163. Balzarini A, Felisi E, Martini A, et al: Efficacy of homeopathic treatment of skin reactions during radiotherapy for breast cancer: a randomized, double-blind clinical trial, *Br Homeopath J* 89(1):8–12, 2000.
164. Schlappack O: Homeopathic treatment of radiation-induced itching in breast cancer patients. A prospective observational study, *Homeopathy* 93:210–215, 2004.
165. Oberbaum M, Yaniv I, Ben-Gal Y, et al: A randomized, controlled clinical trial of the homeopathic medication TRAUMEEL S in the treatment of chemotherapy-induced stomatitis in children undergoing stem cell transplantation, *Cancer* 92(3):684–690, 2001.
166. Clover A, Ratsey D: Homeopathic treatment of hot flushes: a pilot study, *Homeopathy* 91(2):75–79, 2002.
167. Biswas SJ, Khuda-Bukhsh AR: Effect of a homeopathic drug, Chelidonium, in amelioration of p-DAB induced hepatocarcinogenesis in mice, *BMC Complement Altern Med* 2:4, 2002.
168. Seligmann IC, et al: The anticancer homeopathic composite "Canova Method" is not genotoxic for human lymphocytes *in vitro*, *Genet Mole Res* 2(2):223–228, 2003.
169. Oberbaum M, Yaniv I, Ben-Gal Y, et al: A randomized, controlled clinical trial of the homeopathic medication TRAUMEEL S(r) in the treatment of chemotherapy-induced stomatitis in children undergoing stem cell transplantation, *Cancer* 92:684–690, 2001.
170. Kassab S, Cummings M, Berkovitz S, et al: Homeopathic medicines for adverse effects of cancer treatments, *Cochrane Database Syst Rev* Apr 15(2):CD004845, 2009.
171. Montfort H: Education and debate: a new homeopathic approach to neoplastic diseases: from cell destruction to carcinogen-induced apoptosis, *Br Homeopath J* 89:78–83, 2000.
172. Larkin M: Homeopathy & cancer: What to tell your patients, *Oncology Times* 19:68, 73, 1997.
173. Ernst E: Intangible risks of complementary and alternative medicine, *J Clin Oncol* 19(8):2365–2366, 2001.
174. Ernst E, Armstrong NC: Lay books on complementary/alternative medicine: a risk factor for good health? *Int J Risk Safety Med* 11:209–215, 1998.
175. Metz J: Watch out for a hoax when considering unconventional medical treatments. *OncoLink* Accessed at http://oncolink.org/oncotips/article.cfm?c=2&s=8&ss=16&id=53 on November 18, 2011.
176. Grandinetti D: Will alternative-medicine referrals get you sued? *Med Econ* 76(10):38–51, 1999.
177. Anonymous: Alternative and complementary therapies task force, convention program coordinator position created, *J Am Vet Med Assoc* 214(2):173, 1999.
178. Anonymous: House approves guidelines on alternative, complementary medicine, *J Am Vet Med Assoc* 209(6):1026–1028, 1996.
179. American Veterinary Medical Law Association: *The law and complementary & alternative veterinary medicine.* 2004, Prepared for the American Holistic Veterinary Medical Association, October 7.

Clinical Trials and Developmental Therapeutics

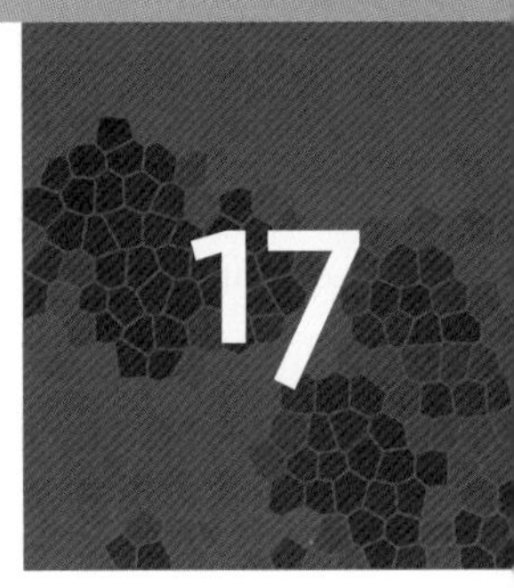

MELISSA C. PAOLONI AND DAVID M. VAIL

Clinical research is essential to improving patient outcome and quality of life (QOL). This is never more important than in the field of oncology in which scientific and technologic advances must translate to novel therapies or approaches that benefit patients. Clinical trials in veterinary oncology have gained interest and focus over the last decade, with both veterinary and comparative oncology drug development leading the effort. There have also been a growing number of consortia and cooperative groups that have functioned successfully by uniting multiinstitutional efforts, advocating for veterinary clinical trials, and emphasizing the synergy between basic science and clinical progress. With support from clients who are motivated to seek advanced care for their pets and to enroll them in investigational trials that offer new therapies, clinical research in veterinary oncology is growing in scope and importance.

Oncology clinical trials attempt to answer questions and find better ways to prevent, diagnose, or treat cancer. Their model is different from trials involving infectious or even chronic diseases because the risks involved have greater morbidity and mortality. Traditional drug development follows a strict, step-wise paradigm that begins with a phase I dose-finding trial, followed by a phase II efficacy/activity trial, and concludes with a phase III "pivotal" trial that pits a novel agent against or with the current standard of care (Table 17-1).[1,2] Although veterinary oncology trials sometimes combine these concepts, their individual descriptions serve as the framework for new drug development. Clinical designs, pertinent endpoints and analyses, the process for drug approval, and clinical trial ethics will be explored in the following sections.

Phase I Trials (Dose Finding)

Phase I trials are the first step in the evaluation of a new agent or biologic. The primary goal is to determine a tolerable dose to be used in future studies by evaluating safety, tolerance, and dose-limiting toxicity (DLT).[2-4] Typically, safety is determined in increasing dosing cohorts that escalate toward the goal of a maximum tolerated dose (MTD) or, for targeted therapies, biologically optimal dose (BOD). Activity/efficacy is not a primary goal. In fact, response rates in phase I trials are seldom more than 10%.[2-4] Secondary goals of phase I trials may include scheduling issues, response rate, pharmacokinetic (PK) information (absorption, distribution, metabolism, and elimination [ADME]), and effects on molecular targets or pathways (pharmacodynamics [PD]). These later biologic endpoints are increasingly important components of phase I trials as dose determinants are inherently linked to drug exposure and effect, especially as we move away from more indiscriminant cytotoxic agents and toward the study of molecular-focused therapeutics. These biologic questions are also the basis of comparative oncology modeling of drug development and are emphasized in their design.[5,6]

Human oncology phase I trials are typically small, single-arm trials that include patients who have failed standard therapies. As such, subjects are generally heavily pretreated with advanced disease. In veterinary medicine, the phase I patient may have failed standard of care or have a condition for which no effective standard of care exists, the standard of care is beyond the client's financial wherewithal, or the client is interested in investigational therapy. Additionally, since standard of care is not necessarily requisite, phase I veterinary trials can proceed in patients with naïve disease. Many veterinary oncology trials provide financial support for enrolled patients and/or include the provision of funds for traditional therapies if novel ones fail. Incentivization enhances accrual. Phase I trial designs must take into account patient selection, starting dose, dose escalation method, definition of MTD or BOD, and target toxicity criteria.

Phase I starting dose selection is a critical design question.[7] Dose is based on data in normal research on Beagle dogs, extrapolation from rodent data, and even human patient data if such exist.[1,3,4] Different options include starting with one-third of the "no observable adverse event level" (NOAEL), or one-tenth of the severe toxicity dose in the most sensitive species, or if normal dog data are available, one-half of the MTD in Beagles as they seem to be less sensitive to adverse events (i.e., toxicity) than are more age-advanced, tumor-bearing patient dogs. Phase I design is integral to the long-term success or failure of an agent's development. Therefore, if the starting dose is too low, the length of the trials is longer, there is poor use of resources, and the number of patients exposed to suboptimal doses is increased. For targeted therapies, it also makes defining the BOD or therapeutic index more difficult.[8,9]

As with starting dose, escalation strategies greatly affect the number of patients treated at a potentially ineffective dose, the length of the trial, the use of resources, and the risk of adverse events.[7] The traditional method of escalation, outlined in Table 17-2, uses a "3 × 3" cohort design, wherein dose escalations are made with three dogs per dose level and the MTD is set based on the number of patients experiencing a DLT. A DLT is defined as grade III or greater toxicity in any category (except hematologic) according to predefined adverse event categories, such as those in the Veterinary Cooperative Oncology Group—Common Terminology Criteria for Adverse Events (VCOG-CTCAE version 1.1).[2,7,10] Grade IV is the cutoff most preferred for myelosuppression DLTs because these events are usually considered manageable with supportive care, generally transient, and often clinically silent.[1-4] Additional DLTs are defined on an agent-by-agent basis due to expected toxicities. These can include or exclude some grade III events from being DLTs, again if transient and clinically silent in nature and are prospectively defined in the study protocol. The MTD is defined as the highest dose level in which no more than one of six dogs develops a DLT. Traditionally, a fixed-dose modified

TABLE 17-1 Goals of Phase I–III Clinical Trials

	Phase of Clinical Trial		
Characteristic	**Phase I (Dose Finding)**	**Phase II (Activity/Efficacy)**	**Phase III (Pivotal)**
Primary goals	▪ Determine MTD ▪ Define DLT ▪ Characterize type and severity of adverse events	▪ Determine activity/efficacy in defined populations ▪ Inform the decision to move to a Phase III trial	▪ Compare a new drug or combination to therapy currently regarded as standard of care
Secondary goals	▪ PK/PD issues ▪ Scheduling issues ▪ Target modulation effects ▪ Preliminary efficacy data ▪ Investigate surrogate biomarkers of response	▪ Estimate therapeutic index ▪ Expand adverse event data ▪ Evaluate additional dosing groups ▪ Expand target modulation and biomarker data ▪ Quality of life measures	▪ Quality of life comparisons ▪ Comparative costs

MTD, Maximum tolerated dose; *DLT*, dose-limiting toxicity; *PK/PD*, pharmacokinetic/pharmacodynamic.

TABLE 17-2 Standard Phase I Dose Escalation Scheme

Number of Patients with DLT at a Given Dose Level	Escalation Decision Rule
0 out of 3	Enter three patients at the next dose level.
≥2	Dose escalation will be stopped. This dose level will be declared the maximally administered dose (highest dose administered). Three additional patients will be entered at the next lowest dose level if only three patients were treated previously at that dose.
1 out of 3	Enter at least three more patients at this dose level. ▪ If none of these three patients experiences DLT, proceed to the next dose level. ▪ If one or more of this group suffer DLT, then dose escalation is stopped, and this dose is declared the maximally administered dose. Three additional patients will be entered at the next lowest dose level if only three patients were treated previously at that dose.
≤1 out of 6 at highest dose level below the maximally administered dose	This is generally the recommended phase 2 dose (MTD). At least six patients must be entered at the recommended phase 2 dose.

MTD, Maximum tolerated dose; *DLT*, dose-limiting toxicity.
From National Cancer Institute: Cancer Therapy Evaluation Program: http://ctep.cancer.gov/protocolDevelopment/templates_applications.htm.

Fibonacci method of dose escalation is used, wherein the dose is escalated 100%, 67%, 50%, 40%, and then 33% of the previous dose as the dosing cohorts increase.[7,11] Similar to starting at too low of a dose, if the escalations are too conservative, more patients receive a suboptimal dose; conversely, if the escalations are too rapid, more patients are at risk for significant toxicity and the accuracy of the MTD is compromised. Additionally, interdosing cohorts can be added during the study period if more refined escalation or de-escalation is found to be necessary.

Although the phase I MTD approach works well for traditional cytotoxic chemotherapeutics, it may be irrelevant for molecularly targeted drugs, and phase I trials designed to determine the BOD may be more relevant for so-called "static" agents.[8,12,13] Trials evaluating the BOD require validated assays that measure target effect in serial tumor samples and/or a surrogate tissue or fluid that documents activity at the molecular level. One example would be measuring γ-H2AX in tumor or surrogate normal tissues after use of a DNA-damaging agent.[14,15] This is a marker of double-stranded DNA breaks and has proved effective in both molecularly targeted and traditional agent evaluation. The depiction in Figure 17-1 shows the immunofluorescent measurement of γ-H2AX in canine lymphoma after treatment with topotecan, illustrating its use as a marker of the drug's biologic effect and PD readout. Classically, studies of inhibition of c-kit phosphorylation in canine mast cell tumors provided the rationale for approval of tyrosine kinase inhibitors (toceranib phosphate and masitinib).[16,17] Such pharmacodynamic modulation studies are increasingly important endpoints of phase I and II designs and now more commonly required as proof of mechanism for drug approval.

Phase II Trials (Activity/Efficacy Trials)

Several good reviews have outlined phase II trial design.[4,18-20] The primary goal of phase II trials is, using the MTD or BOD established in phase I, to identify the clinical or biologic activity in defined patient populations (e.g., tumors with a particular histology, tumors with a particular molecular target) and inform the decision to embark on a larger pivotal phase III trial. The traditional phase II design (phase IIA), the single-arm, open-label phase II trial, is a nonrandomized nonblind activity assessment of a novel

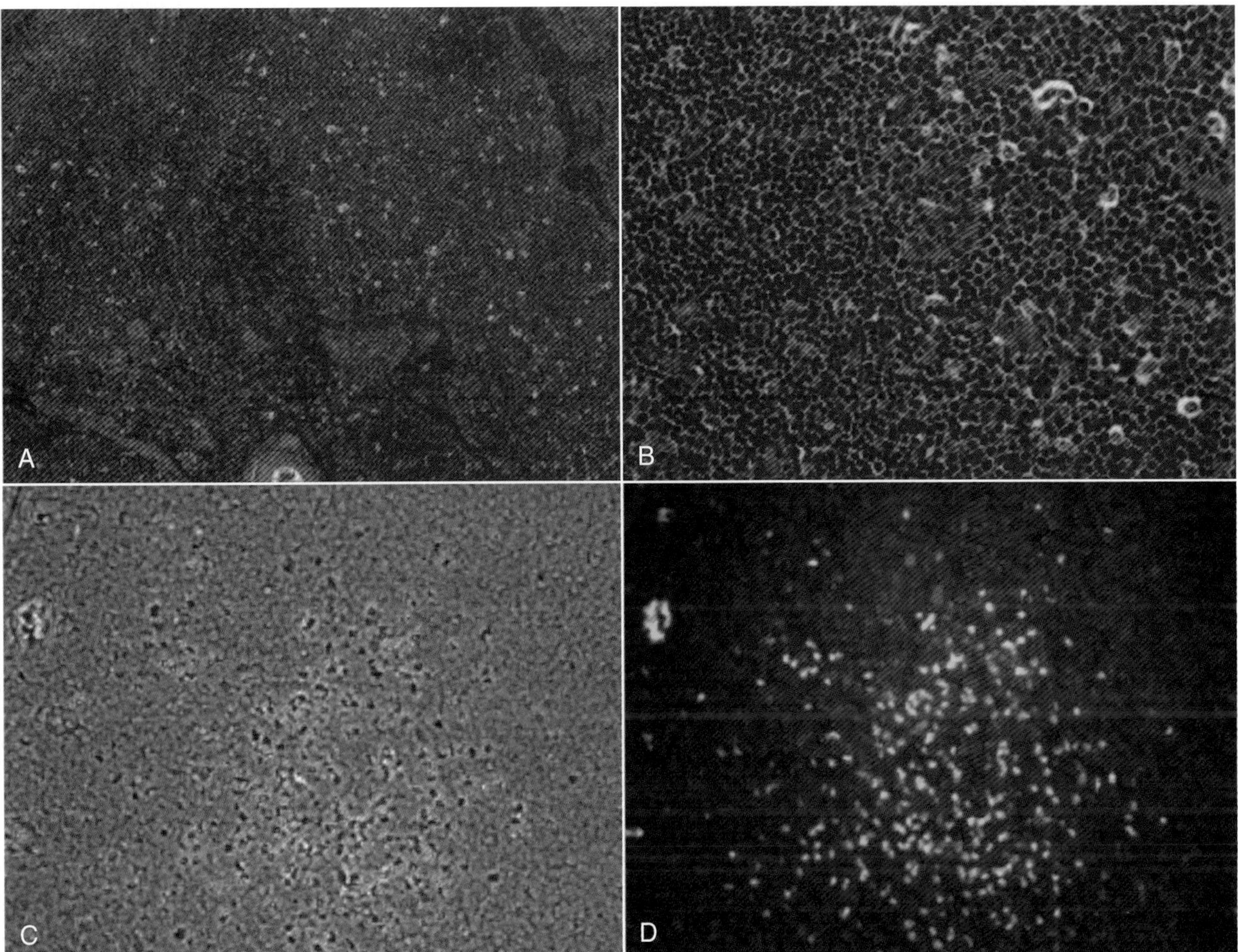

FIGURE 17-1 γ-H2AX phosphorylation is evident after treatment with topotecan in a dog with lymphoma. A biopsy was taken of a patient tumor (canine lymphoma) after administration with topotecan and histopathologic and immunofluorescent analysis performed. **A,** Hematoxylin and eosin (H&E) staining at 10×. **B,** H&E staining at 40×. **C,** Immunofluorescent image in black and white of same patient sample. **D,** Immunofluorescent staining of γ-H2AX phosphorylation with nuclei staining in blue (Dapi) and γ-H2AX in green. γ-H2AX phosphorylation is an intracellular pharmacodynamic (PD) readout of exposure to a DNA damaging agent.

drug or therapeutic modality that lacks a control group or uses historic controls that are prone to bias (selection, population drift, and stage migration bias).[4,18,19] Simplistically, at least 9 to 14 patients with the same histology or molecular target are treated with the investigational drug to test the null hypothesis of insufficient efficacy.[21] Assuming the likelihood of spontaneous regression is less than 5% and expecting at least a 25% response rate for the agent to be clinically useful, with a p less than 0.05 (type I [α] error; false positive) and a power of 0.8 (type II [β] error; false negative), if no responses are observed after the initial cases, the study ends. If a response is noted in one of the cases, the accrual is increased to 31 patients to establish a more accurate response rate.

If you expect a less robust response rate (e.g., 5% to 20%), the initial accrual number must be increased.[22] Sample-size impact on study power calculations will be outlined in a subsequent section. Some have opined that the leading cause of drug failure in later phase development is our overdependence on these unpredictable single-arm, uncontrolled phase II trials in oncology and that, as such, they should be avoided to ensure phase III trial resources are not wasted because of the results of poorly designed phase II trials.[23] It used to be considered that the consequence of type I error (false positive) was less deleterious than that of type II error (false negative) because false-positive trials are likely to be repeated, whereas false-negative trials would result in the abandonment of a potentially active treatment.[24] The goals of comparative oncology modeling can help minimize type II error by mechanistically defining activity of novel agents through more detailed PK-PD studies. In today's environment, however, with an abundance of novel drugs to be evaluated, false-positive results are just as serious because they tie up patient and financial resources. With this in mind, the ideal phase II design would be randomized (e.g., between more than one new investigational drug in the pipeline), blinded, and controlled; modifications of this type applied to standard phase II design are discussed subsequently (controlled phase II or phase IIB trials).[25]

Endpoints of Activity/Efficacy

Since the primary goal of phase II trials is assessment of activity/efficacy, endpoints used to evaluate response are critical to the design. With traditional cytotoxic chemotherapeutics, response criteria are fairly straightforward because size or volume is used to assess response according to several published methodologies (e.g., Response Evaluation Criteria in Solid Tumors [RECIST], World

Health Organization [WHO]).[26-28] These measurements are both repeatable and have criteria that are strictly defining. It is readily evident that such criteria may not be appropriate for newer molecular-targeted agents that are more likely to be cytostatic rather than cytotoxic and result in stabilization of disease rather than in measurable regression.[29,30] In such cases, temporal measures such as progression-free survival (PFS) or time to progression (TTP) are appropriate endpoints; however, these often take too long to mature for timely phase II trials.[31] Alternatively, an adequate compromise could be progression-free rate (PFR) at predetermined time points. Again, comparative oncology models may more expediently define TTP or PFR due to compressed progression times in our veterinary patients. These measures can also more accurately define response in the minimal residual disease (MRD) setting such as trials interrogating novel adjuvant therapies for canine osteosarcoma (OSA) in the postamputation setting. This will be expanded on in future sections.

Secondary endpoints that may be evaluated in phase II trials include QOL assessments, comparative cost of therapy, days of hospitalization, and more detailed adverse event evaluations. Importantly, phase II trials serve to expand our knowledge of the cumulative or long-term toxicities associated with new agents that may not be observed in short-term phase I trials designed to elucidate acute toxicity. An example of this in the veterinary literature involved a combined phase I/II trial simultaneously investigating the safety of liposome-encapsulated doxorubicin (LED) while comparing its activity with native doxorubicin in cats with vaccine-associated sarcomas.[32] Unexpectedly, the MTD established for LED in the acute phase I component of the trial was found to result in delayed and dose-limiting nephrotoxicity after long-term follow-up in the phase II component of the trial. Such discoveries are key to defining an agent's therapeutic window with repeated administrations.

New clinical trial concepts have entered into use in great part due to a recent initiative of the Food and Drug Administration (FDA) to allow for "preclinical studies to provide evidence necessary to support the safety of administering new compounds to humans."[33] These are known as phase 0 trials, and they precede the traditional trials defined previously.[34,35] The role of phase 0 in cancer drug development is for biomarker and assay development/validation and evaluation of target modulation.[33] Phase 0 trials allow for the systematic de-prioritization of investigational agents that exhibit excessive toxicity or fail to show expected biologic effects and are used to direct dose selection for future studies.[33] They represent first-in-species trials, usually of a small number of patients, and utilize lower and likely subtherapeutic drug doses. Comparative oncology trials allow the unique opportunity to answer the preclinical questions required within these trials. Phase 0 trials are "proof of concept" studies, and PD effects are measured within target tissues, such as the tumor itself.[34,35] These trials can also define surrogate markers of target effect, therapeutic response, or metabolites in surrogate tissues or fluids, such as blood or urine. PK data are also a hallmark of phase 0 trial designs. Biologic endpoints such as PK/PD analysis allow for a much broader understanding of new drug mechanism, therefore informing phase I/II trial design.

Phase III Trials (Pivotal/Confirming Trials)

It has been suggested that if phase II trials are "learning" trials, phase III trials are "confirming" trials.[2,19,36] These larger, randomized, blind, and controlled trials have the goal of comparing a new drug or combination with standard-of-care therapies. They are often performed by large co-operative groups, which ensures greater case accrual, and FDA pivotal trials require multiinstitutional involvement. True phase III trials have not been common in veterinary medicine because of their size and expense, but this culture is changing with a broader focus on veterinary oncology drug development and approval. An example of a multicenter phase III trial would be the randomized comparison of liposome-encapsulated cisplatin (SPI-77) versus standard-of-care carboplatin in dogs with appendicular OSA.[37] No difference was observed between treatment groups, and SPI-77 did not show an activity advantage, despite allowing five times the MTD of native cisplatin to be delivered in a liposome-encapsulated form.[37] This helps define the application of phase III efforts in veterinary oncology.

Additionally, there are a number of pivotal veterinary oncology clinical trials that have directly impacted how we treat patients today. Chemotherapy as an adjunct treatment has improved survival in many pets with cancer. This is highlighted in a disease such as canine OSA, in which disease-free survival (DFS) postamputation alone is just 4 months but, with the addition of chemotherapy (cisplatin, carboplatin, or doxorubicin), improves median survival to approximately 1 year.[38-42] Although a number of clinical trials have been performed with various schedules and regimens of delivery, all highlight the importance of treatment with chemotherapy in the micrometastatic minimal residual disease setting. These are treatment trials, wherein most studies compare groups to historic controls, but many are prospective in nature to more accurately detect a difference in treatment protocols if one exists. Another definitive example of clinical trials with high clinical impact were those comparing the inclusion of doxorubicin in multiagent chemotherapy protocols for dogs and cats with lymphoma versus COP (cyclophosphamide, vincristine, and prednisone) or single-agent therapy alone.[43-48] It was evidenced by a number of protocols that doxorubicin administration contributed significantly to improved survival over those protocols without it, therefore securing its place as the single most efficacious agent against lymphoma.[47,48] More recent pivotal trials have included the registration of the first approved veterinary oncology agents, two tyrosine kinase inhibitors (TKIs; Palladia, Pfizer; Kinavet, AB Sciences) for the treatment of mast cell tumors.[16,17,49,50] TKIs showed improvement in PFS over placebo controls, and these trials define the process for expanding future efforts in veterinary oncology drug approval.

Sample Size and Power

The overriding function of clinical research is to provide a definitive answer to a clinical question. However, it is rarely that simple. It is possible that once complete, clinical trial conclusions may be incorrect based on chance or design error. Chance error results when an erroneous inference is drawn from a study sample group that is not actually representative of an entire patient population. Accounting for this potential error is essential in prospective clinical trial design, and its first critical step is to articulate the study hypothesis.[51] Type I or α error (false positive) occurs if an investigator rejects the null hypothesis when it is actually true.[36,52] This is also referred to as the study's level of significance. Type II or β error (false negative) occurs when one fails to reject the null hypothesis when it is actually incorrect.[36,52] Type I and II errors are due to chance and cannot be avoided completely, although steps can be taken to reduce their potential impact by increasing sample size and augmenting study design or measurements.

Power is the ultimate measure of a clinical trial's results and also must be prospectively controlled. Power is defined as $1-\beta$, the probability of correctly rejecting the null in the sample if the actual effect in the population is equal to (or greater than) the effect size.[36,52] Power is governed by sample size, with the goal being to enroll enough patients to accurately allow for a difference to be seen between groups. Power is irrelevant if the results are statistically significant, but if not, it is important to ensure the study had adequate numbers to detect a difference between groups. If a study to detect the difference between two cancer treatments is designed with an α of 0.05, then the principal investigator (PI) has set 5% as the maximum chance of incorrectly rejecting the null hypothesis if it is true. This is the level of doubt the PI is willing to accept when statistical tests are used to compare the two treatments. If β is set at 0.10, the PI is willing to accept a 10% chance of missing an association of a given effect if it exists. This represents a power of 0.90 ($1-\beta$), or a 90% chance of finding an association of that size or greater. α and β levels are determined prior to trial initiation, and their set points are based on the importance of avoiding either a false-positive or a false-negative result.

Randomization

Bias is introduced error in clinical research. One of the main ways to minimize bias is through the use of randomization. Randomization is the process of assigning research participants to a group within a clinical trial by chance instead of choice.[2,36,52] Groups include either the investigational group, those to receive the study drug, or the control group, those to receive a placebo (or comparator drug). Each participant enrolling in a trial has an equal chance of receiving the study drug, and the goal is to balance the groups based on participant characteristics (e.g., age, stage of disease, previous treatments) that may influence a response to therapy.[2,36,52] At the end of the study, if bias is reduced by randomization, then the result (positive or negative) is more likely to be true. Although this is the ideal way to conduct clinical trials, it is still uncommon in veterinary oncology trials. Unfortunately, in veterinary medicine, historic rather than active controls have been used for comparison of new therapies all too often. It is common in oncology trials to also blind participants so that patients, or in our case clients, do not know which treatment group their pet is in. Blinded or true active comparator trials, although rare in veterinary oncology due in part to limited funding, are becoming more frequent as regulatory registration trials ultimately require them.

Reducing bias in clinical trials is an integral concept within trial design. Stratification is a concept used often in human oncology trials and is gaining headway in veterinary oncology trial design as well.[36,52,53] This allows for grouping of patients based on known prognostic factors. For example, this might include the stratification of dogs with lymphoma by clinical stage or T- versus B-cell immunophenotype with the goal of creating equal numbers of each within a treatment group. One of the main benefits of stratification is that it can prevent potential bias from *known* prognostic factors. For example, a treatment cohort may be doing comparatively poorly because the majority of dogs in that cohort had T-cell lymphoma. However, a difficulty with stratification is that the more prognostic factors are controlled, the less power the study has, and thus the need to increase sample size considerably. Randomization to treatment groups should be performed after stratification.

Phase IV Trials (Postregistration Trials)

Once a drug has been granted a license or registered for a specific label use by the appropriate regulatory body (e.g., the FDA), postregistration phase IV trials may be performed to gain more information on adverse events, long-term risks, off-label benefits, and the economic impact of the agent in the marketplace.[54] Essentially, phase IV trials investigate the drug more widely than do the clinical trials used for registration. They may also involve treatment of special populations (e.g., the elderly, pediatric patients, or individuals with renal or hepatic dysfunction).[4] The body of data on PK generated from postregistration trials is used to inform decisions on dose in special populations. Productivity and economic differences of one treatment over another, mostly due to insurance reimbursement requirements on the human side, are also a consideration in data collection and evaluation in phase IV clinical trials.

Good Manufacturing Practice/ Good Clinical Practice Criteria

When designing clinical trials it is key to define provisions that create uniformity and consistency in clinical research. Their primary intent is to ensure the safety of trial materials and participants and the integrity of clinical data. Such provisions determine good manufacturing practice (GMP) and good clinical practice (GCP). GMP principles ensure the safe manufacture and testing of pharmaceutical drugs, biologics, and medical devices by outlining aspects of production that can impact the quality of a product. GCP guidelines were devised by the International Conference on Harmonization (ICH) to protect the rights and safety of human patients in clinical trials.[36,55]

GCP includes standards on how clinical trials should be designed and conducted, defines the roles and responsibilities of trial sponsors and clinical research investigators, and monitors the reporting of trial data.[55] It requires the use of a standardized clinical protocol and strict documentation of procedures and adherence to that protocol. GCP also establishes guidelines for oversight by external bodies, such as the Institutional Review Board (IRB) and the Data Safety and Monitoring Board (DSMB).[55] The IRB serves as an independent ethics committee that has the power to approve, disapprove, or ask for modifications to planned study protocols. IRBs traditionally were institutional entities involved with in-house clinical trial oversight but now have grown in scope and purpose. IRBs must include at least one nonscientist and a noninstitutional member known as a *community member.* If a clinical trial includes a vulnerable population, then the IRB must include an expert in the needs and specialties of this group. The IRB reviews protocol ethics, informed consent, and possible conflicts of interest and provides scientific review of study protocol and results.[36,55] IRB review and approval occur both prior to study initiation and periodically within the conduct of a clinical trial to ensure ethical standards are being met throughout the trial process.

The DSMB (sometimes called a Data Monitoring Committee) is a third-party panel of experts consisting of at least one statistician and is populated by clinicians expert in the field of research or drug of study.[36,56] In long-term and high-impact studies an ethicist and/or a patient advocate representative may also serve on the DSMB. The purpose of the DSMB is to ensure the safety of participants, the validity of data, and the appropriate termination of studies for which significant benefits or risks have been uncovered or if it appears that the trial cannot be concluded successfully. The main role of the DSMB is to oversee serious adverse events (SAE) and their management to ensure patient safety.[56] However, the DSMB also reviews interim study results to determine if an overwhelming benefit is evident in either the study or the control arm or if it is unlikely the study will answer the proposed study aim. The latter results if interim data reveal continuance is unlikely to produce a statistically significant result, and the study will then be terminated prematurely. It is important for all safety monitoring to be contemporaneous, including disclosure to the FDA of SAEs in real time. GCP compliance is necessary for FDA registration trials in both veterinary and human oncology drug development. Oversight of GMP and GCP provisions are provided by the FDA (http://www.fda.gov), and in the European Union (EU), oversight is provided by the European Medicines Agency (EMA; http://www.ema.europa.eu).

Effectiveness versus Efficacy Definitions

A key distinction in phase III or comparativeness trials is that data may be obtained within the context of randomized clinical trials (RCTs) or from effectiveness studies in the "real world." The differences between the two types of study design have implications for the data that can be obtained and the interpretation of the resultant findings. Because RCTs are designed to assess the safety and efficacy of pharmaceuticals and because the study design of RCTs emphasizes study validity over generalizability, the applicability of data collected from them are limited.[36] The data may not be valid in more heterogeneous patients encountered in actual clinical practice and may be inaccurate because of strict protocol requirements or inclusion/exclusion criteria. Effectiveness studies, in which treatments are studied under real-world conditions, remedy some of these limitations.[36] Generalizability to actual users is enhanced in effectiveness designs, but data may be biased in other ways. An efficacy study asks the question, "Does the drug work?" Whereas an effectiveness study asks the question "Does the drug help the targeted general population?" Some refer to this efficacy research as type I research (bench to bedside) and effectiveness research as type II (bedside to curbside) research. Generally, a RCT that determines efficacy occurs under ideal conditions while long-term effectiveness studies, which can be prospective or on occasion either metaanalyses or retrospective, define the overall impact of a drug. Another important element of effectiveness studies may be pharmacoeconomics or cost analyses. A cost-benefit analysis weighs factors such as actual cost of medication, number or lives saved, minimization or exacerbation of hospital stays or doctor's visits, and QOL measures and computes their individual and societal expense. Once these outcome measures are studied and calculated, then comparisons between agents, new and old, can be made.[57-59] Measures of effectiveness reflect the actual effects of a drug or an intervention on a population or disease state over time.

Regulatory Oversight

The FDA is the regulatory body of the U. S. government that oversees the activities of the drug and pharmaceutical industry.[36,60,61] The FDA provides oversight for drug development primarily through written guidances, which describe rules and requirements for quality control and conduct. FDA guidances include oversight of drug standards, including chemistry, manufacturing, and control (CMC); preclinical animal toxicology; documentary requirements for investigational new drug (INDs) and new drug applications (NDAs); and ethics of clinical trials. It is responsible for reviewing clinical trial protocol designs and data, namely to evaluate safety and effectiveness of new drugs or biologics. In 1997 the FDA moved beyond its traditional approval paradigm by creating the FDA Modernization Act.[61] It necessitates PK bridging studies for new populations (e.g., pediatric PK studies) and allows for one adequate and well-controlled clinical investigation by "confirmatory evidence" comprising PK or PK/PD data to lead to drug approval. This emphasizes the importance of exposure and mechanism studies to more accurately determine the safety and effectiveness of novel drugs, especially targeted agents or ones evaluated in special populations.[62] FDA guidances are increasingly based on clinical pharmacology and the impact of this is felt most pertinently in oncology drug development.

FDA drug development is a multistep process that defines interaction between the FDA, the drug sponsor, and their discovery and clinical teams. The result of this process, if successful, is FDA approval. It involves a preclinical testing phase (IND requirements for CMC, animal testing, design of phase I clinical studies), IND evaluation, and NDA review, and marketing.[2] On the human side, due to recent concerns about safety and drug withdrawals (e.g., Vioxx in 2004, Avastin for breast cancer in 2011), the FDA is attempting to improve and expedite the process of drug development through a number of initiatives. The most innovative are the Critical Path Initiative (2004), end-of-phase 2a (EOP2a) meeting (2004), and model-based drug development (2005) (physiologically based PK [PBPK], 2009).[63] Various aspects of these efforts include biomarker development, bioinformatics focus, decrease of late phase II failures, and development of public/private partnerships or consortia.

Veterinary Registration Trials

Veterinary drug development follows the same critical regulatory steps described above but oversight is provided by the Center for Veterinary Medicine (FDA-CVM), and in the case of biologics, by the U.S. Department of Agriculture (USDA). Prior to 2007 with the conditional approval of ONCEPT (melanoma treatment vaccine, Merial), all cancer drugs used in veterinary medicine were originally developed for humans and not approved for use in animals. Cancer chemotherapeutics are used in an "extra-label" manner as allowed by the Animal Medicinal Drug Use Clarification Act of 1994. The last few years have seen significant gains in veterinary oncology product development with the approval of toceranib phosphate (Palladia, Pfizer), masitinib (Kinavet (US)/Masivet (EU/ROW), AB Science) and ONCEPT (Merial). Palladia and Kinavet are both receptor TKIs and are approved for use in the treatment of recurrent or inoperable grade II or III mast cell tumors with or without regional lymph node involvement.[16,17,49,64,65] Palladia was developed by SUGEN as SU11654, a sister compound to SU11248 later approved for human patients as Sutent. ONCEPT is a xenogeneic tyrosinase DNA vaccine indicated for dogs with stage II or stage III oral canine melanoma.[66,67] Registration trials for these agents involved safety and efficacy defining in multicenter clinical trials under GCP conditions. Postmarket analysis (phase IV) for each is still ongoing. However, their approvals have defined the process for future veterinary oncology product development for years to come.

Consortia

One of the most exciting achievements in veterinary oncology over the last decade has been the development of successful and collaborative consortia groups that are purposed to perform multicenter clinical trials and prospective tumor biospecimen repository collections. Consortia infrastructures allow larger scale clinical trials and provide the voice for collective advocacy in veterinary and comparative oncology. Their success is an example of the growing importance of the study of tumor and clinical biology. Some of these efforts are profiled here.

Comparative Oncology Trials Consortium

The Comparative Oncology Trials Consortium (COTC) is an active network of 20 academic comparative oncology centers (https://ccrod.cancer.gov/confluence/display/CCRCOPWeb/Comparative+Oncology+Trials+Consortium), centrally managed by the National Institutes of Health–National Cancer Institute's Comparative Oncology Program (NCI-COP), that functions to design and execute clinical trials in dogs with cancer to assess novel therapies.[68,69] The goal of this effort is to answer biologic questions geared to inform the development path of these agents for use in human cancer patients. COTC trials are pharmacokinetically and pharmacodynamically rich with the product of this work directly integrated into the design of current human early and late phase clinical trials. They are focused to answer mechanism of action (MOA) questions and define dose-toxicity and dose-response relationships. They can be designed to compare varying schedules and routes of drug administration, validate target biology, model clinical standard operating procedures (SOPs), and assess biomarkers. The COTC has also led the way for outlining proposed regulatory oversight of comparative oncology trials and established the first DSMB for client-owned animal clinical trials. Additionally, within this effort, the COTC PD Core was created. The COTC PD Core is a virtual laboratory of assays and services, including pathology, immunohistochemistry, immunocytochemistry, flow cytometry, genomics, proteomics, cell culture, PKs, and cell biology designed to support COTC clinical trial biologic endpoints.[70] As of 2011, the COTC has completed nine clinical trials and has been successful in promoting the utility of comparative oncology modeling within the drug development community.[69,71]

Animal Clinical Investigation

Animal Clinical Investigation (ACI; www.animalci.com) is a privately organized and run specialty network of veterinary hospitals that designs, conducts, and reports clinical studies for the animal health industry. ACI trials emphasize oncology drug development but have recently expanded to include other medical conditions, including inflammatory and metabolic disease, cardiovascular disease, and arthritis. ACI provides multisite, pivotal, or nonpivotal studies and commercialization support to help define effective novel veterinary therapeutics. It is the first example of a commercial clinical research organization (CRO) in veterinary medicine. Over 30 clinical trials have been conducted through this network over the last 10 years.[72,73]

Canine Comparative Oncology and Genomics Consortium

The Canine Comparative Oncology and Genomics Consortium (CCOGC; www.ccogc.net) is an informal collaboration of veterinary and medical oncologists, pathologists, surgeons, geneticists, and molecular and cellular biologists with a common interest in the comparative study of canine and human genomics and cancer. The goals of the CCOGC are to facilitate partnerships and collaborations focused on the problem of cancer in dogs. Early priorities included advocacy for the field of comparative oncology, the development of a mechanism to share reagents and resources in the community, and the development of a biospecimen repository. The repository houses tumor tissue, normal tissues, serum, plasma, peripheral blood mononuclear cell preparations, genomic DNA, RNA, and urine samples. Seven leading veterinary schools across the United States are currently acting as collection sites to populate this repository. Histologies were selected for collection due to their importance to the field of veterinary and comparative oncology and include lymphoma, melanoma, OSA, hemangiosarcoma (HSA), mast cell tumors, soft tissue sarcomas, and pulmonary tumors. As of 2011 the CCOGC has collected 1600 of 3000 anticipated samples. The repository will serve as a seminal resource for the research community to acquire tissues for target biology studies, as well as its mechanism for prospective collections of unique samples. Future efforts will focus on dissemination of these tissues.

Current Challenges and Opportunities in Oncology Drug Development

Oncology drug development is a difficult and costly process. It is estimated that only 5% to 10% of drugs entering phase I oncology clinical trials ultimately are approved by the FDA, with a cost of between 0.8 and 1.7 billion dollars per drug accrued through the development process.[57] The most prevalent cause of cancer drug failure is toxicity or inactivity. For every 1000 oncology agents in development, only 40% transition from preclinical studies to phase I, 75% from phase I to phase II, 60% from phase II to phase III, and 55% from phase III to approval.[57] This means that for every 1000 preclinical candidates, only 99 new drugs will reach the clinic. Oncology has one of the poorest records for drug development, with success rates more than three times lower than those for cardiovascular drugs. A recent review of the human literature revealed that the 2003-2010 phase III oncology failure rate was 34%, a real challenge as late-phase failures are extremely costly in time, expense, patient morbidity, and mortality. Although the highest success rate was also surprisingly low, 68% for autoimmune therapies, this highlights the need for new clinical trial approaches and models for oncology (outlined subsequently) and other fields as well.[59]

New Trial Designs

Alternative "accelerated titration" dose escalation strategies for phase I trials have been suggested.[2-4] These include (1) two-stage designs, wherein single-patient cohorts are used initially and dose is increased by a factor of 2 until a grade II toxicity occurs, and the second stage then involves more traditional three-patient cohorts and acceleration strategies; (2) within-patient escalation, wherein the same patient gets a higher dose on subsequent treatments until a DLT is observed (this may mask cumulative toxicity, however); (3) escalations based on PK parameters; (4) escalations based on target modification (if known); and (5) continuous reassessment methods using Bayesian methods (see subsequent section).[7] In the end, it is always a tradeoff of risk versus benefit; however, rapid accelerations are less likely to deny efficacious dosing to someone with a fatal disease.[3]

Adaptive Trial Designs and Stopping Rules

Adaptive trial designs allow investigators to modify trials while they are ongoing based on newly acquired data and, in some cases, taking into account data generated in other trials or past trials.

Stopping Rules

Stopping rules, which are rules that terminate a clinical trial earlier than originally projected or within a predetermined adaptive trial design, can be applied to randomized phase II or phase III trials. Several methods and variations have been extensively reviewed.[19,36,74-76] Stopping rules are designed to protect treatment subjects from unsafe drugs, to hasten the general availability of superior drugs as soon as sufficient evidence has been collected, and to help ensure the transfer of resources and patients to alternative trials. Trials are stopped for three reasons: the investigational treatment is clearly better than the control, the investigational treatment is clearly worse than the control (less activity or more toxicity), or the investigation's therapy is not likely to be better (so-called "stopping for futility" or "futility analysis"). The methods by which stopping rules are applied usually involve some type of interim analysis that looks at the data (by a blinded individual or DSMB) generated so far and makes a determination based on predetermined rules. The interim data are often analyzed for conditional power, which is the probability of the final study result demonstrating statistical significance in the primary efficacy endpoint, conditional on the current data observed so far, and a specific assumption about the pattern of the data to be observed in the remainder of the study.[75,76] If a study is designed up front to involve conditional power calculations of interim data, the rules for early termination are sometimes referred to as *stochastic curtailing.*

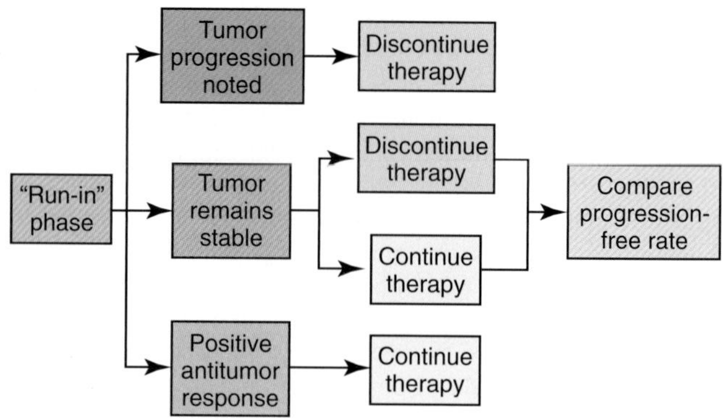

FIGURE 17-2 Generalized schema for a randomized discontinuation trial (RDT) design. *(Adapted from Stadler WM: The randomized discontinuation trial: A phase II design to assess growth-inhibitory agents,* Mol Cancer Ther *6(4):1180-1185, 2007, with permission.)*

Bayesian (Continuous Learning) Adaptive Designs

Adaptive trial designs can be used not only to stop trials early but also to adapt trials with respect to changing the randomization weight to better performing treatment arms, adding new treatment arms, dropping poorly performing arms, or extending accrual beyond the original target when more information is needed. With the availability of advanced computational techniques, a new statistical methodology, the Bayesian approach, was developed that makes statistical inferences that focus on the probability that a hypothesis is true given the available evidence.[75,76]

Traditionally, a *frequentist* approach to statistics is applied to clinical trials in which parameters are fixed and not subject to future probabilities. In contrast, Bayesian trials use available patient outcome information, including biomarkers that accumulate data related to outcome (if available and validated), and even historic information or results from other relevant trials.[77-79] The Bayesian approach uses this information to adapt the current trial design continually based on newly informed probabilities. Bayesian designs are intrinsically adaptive and data driven, which allows inferences to depend less on the original study design.[19] Bayesian approaches can be incorporated into the trial at the beginning or can be used to monitor clinical trials originally designed with frequentist statistical methods. An example that illustrates the utility of the Bayesian approach involves interim analysis applied to a randomized phase II trial of neoadjuvant epidermal growth factor receptor 2 (HER2/neu)–positive breast cancer.[80] In this trial initially designed to enter 164 patients (based on the frequentist approach to power), a Bayesian approach was used to perform an interim analysis after 34 patients were enrolled; 67% of patients in the investigational treatment arm experienced complete responses compared with 25% in the standard treatment arm. The Bayesian predictive probability of statistical significance if 164 patients were accrued, based on the data available from these 34 patients, was calculated to be 95%, and the trial was stopped and the drug moved to phase III early due to these promising results.

Randomized Discontinuation Trials

This phase II design was proposed for evaluating the efficacy of newer targeted agents that are thought to have disease-stabilizing activity (cytostatic) in contrast to disease-regression activity of more traditional cytotoxic chemotherapeutics. Several reviews of this trial design are recommended.[81-83] Trials that evaluated growth-inhibiting agents in tumors with a variable natural history seem ideally suited for randomized discontinuation trials (RDTs) because the "no treatment effect" is hard to control in these cases. In essence, these trials serve to enrich and homogenize the static agent for those patients likely to benefit from it. RDTs involve a two-stage trial design, wherein the first stage involves a "run-in" phase in which all patients receive the cytostatic agent under investigation (Figure 17-2). At the end of the run-in phase, assessment of disease response is made. If a response is noted, the subject continues on the investigational drug, whereas if progression (or excess toxicity) is noted, the subject is removed from trial and allowed to receive alternative treatment. Those patients who meet stable disease criteria enter the second stage of the RDT and are randomized to continue on the investigational drug or placebo (the discontinuation arm). Then, at predetermined times, follow-up determinations are made. Endpoints in stage 2 of the trial at these follow-up intervals are "stable or better" versus "progression." Time-to-event measures may be applied as well (e.g., PFS, TTP), although this takes more time to complete. If a subject progresses in the second stage, the code can be broken, and if that subject is in the placebo group, the investigational drug can be reinstituted. Therefore there are two ways for RDTs to be stopped: there are a substantial number of objective responses noted in the run-in phase, making a second stage unnecessary, or the number of subjects progressing in the second stage differs statistically between the treatment and placebo groups. It becomes intuitive that the length of the run-in phase is critical to RDTs: if it is too long, some initially responding patients progress during the late stage of the run-in and are missed (therefore increasing subject numbers); if it is too short, insufficient enrichment occurs (not enough time for nonresponders to progress) and the randomization might as well have been done at the outset. Therefore it pays to have some preliminary ideas as to the natural history of the disease. The two major advantages of RDTs are that all subjects receive the drug up front so that every patient is given a chance to respond to the drug (something that is popular with patients [or companion animal owners]) and enrichment of likely responders may increase power and decrease subject numbers. Potential disadvantages of RDTs include the ethics of discontinuation (but the design can allow reinstitution), the potential for a carry-over effect of the drug after discontinuation (unlikely for most targeted agents), and failure to detect short duration activity (but this would likely be a clinically irrelevant duration anyway). RDTs can be improved by combining other modifications of clinical trials, such as interim analysis and Bayesian analysis, and by using active controls. For purposes of illustration, an RDT in veterinary medicine that the author has considered would be the investigation of a cytostatic agent in dogs with pulmonary metastatic OSA. All dogs would enter the run-in phase, receive the cytostatic drug for 4 weeks, and then be evaluated for response. From what we already know about the natural history of OSA in dogs, most (probably 80%) of dogs that did not receive treatment would progress in that period. Those that were stable at 4 weeks, however, would be randomized to drug continuation or discontinuation (placebo) and followed with monthly reevaluations. This would ensure all dogs had a chance to respond to the drug and enrich the population likely to respond, and a positive result would be clinical response noted in the run-in phase or a statistical difference in PFR between groups in the second stage.

Personalized Medicine

Advancements in genomic, proteomic, and epigenetic profiling have created new opportunities to tailor cancer treatments to individual patient and tumor molecular characteristics; this field is known as personalized or molecular-based medicine. The goals of personalized medicine approaches include improving outcomes by revealing disease drivers, toxicity, susceptibilities, and resistance profiles unique to the individual patient. Molecular profiling approaches have been employed to stratify and prescribe therapies for human oncology patients. The most successful examples to date have been in the identification of oncogenic mutations such as HER2/neu (EGFR2) in breast cancer and *bcr-abl* in chronic myelogenous leukemia and the prescription of monoclonal antibodies (trastuzumab, Herceptin) and TKIs (imatinib, Gleevec) against these key pathways (also the basis for Bayesian approaches previously mentioned).[84-86] Veterinary oncology has also benefited from molecular-based approaches, most notably in the targeting of *c-kit* mutations in canine mast cell tumors (toceranib and masitinib).[87,88] TKIs (toceranib and masitinib) have shown clinical utility against macroscopic disease and have been approved by the FDA for use in this setting. Although both agents are nonselective inhibitors that also have activity against other key pathways (e.g., vascular endothelial growth factor receptor [VEGFR] for toceranib), their approval marks an important step forward in veterinary tumor biology-based therapeutics and sets the stage for future-directed research in other histologies.

The field of personalized medicine expands beyond patient prescription to also include the study of patient pharmacogenomics and pharmacometabolics, the genetic variation of response and metabolism of novel agents or medications. These include the study of individual patient single nucleotide polymorphisms (SNPs) in key metabolic pathways (cytochrome p450) and the measurement of metabolites in blood and urine. An example of this in veterinary oncology is the use of multidrug resistance gene 1 *(MDR1)* mutation analysis in certain herding breeds (e.g., collies and shelties) prior to initiating *MDR1* substrate chemotherapeutic agents (e.g., doxorubicin and vincristine).

Newer personalized medicine approaches based on complex mathematical algorithms have been created that include a broader base of tumor characteristics to define potential treatments. Although exciting, these techniques require prospective tumor biopsies and the extent of clinical benefit (improvement in outcome) from these time-consuming and costly techniques is yet unproved. Publishing the canine genome and the advent of high throughput technologies have enabled the field of veterinary oncology to describe canine cancer biology and characterize potential therapeutic targets more globally.[89] This creates the opportunity for personalized medicine investigations in the dog to inform novel therapy development for both veterinary and human oncology patients using these algorithmic approaches. In addition, strong cancer breed predilections support "breed-based" genetic approaches that may uncover oncogenic pathways and targets more easily and inform discovery and application of personalized medicine strategies. Many challenges remain as to the best ways to collect tissues, define applicable targets, prioritize single- or combinational-agent therapies, or measure the effects of predictive algorithms. Personalized medicine modeling in veterinary cancers may help advance the field through the address of these questions over the next 5 to 10 years.

Clinical Trial Ethics

There are key ethical standards employed in clinical trial design, and it is the goal of all clinicians to ensure standards are met when offering a trial to a client or enrolling a patient within a clinical trial. Many clinical trials provide partially or fully funded care for eligible pets with cancer. This is important because traditional veterinary oncology treatments, surgery, chemotherapy, and radiation therapy, are expensive and costs are prohibitive for some clients. Clinical trial enrollment may present an opportunity to help some clients who may not have the financial means to pursue treatment or receive care for their pet. Clinical trials can also provide treatment to those dogs or cats that have progressed in the face of traditional therapies. When all medical options are described to clients as far as care for their pet's disease, some may choose clinical trials in order to make an impact for future pets or people with cancer. This altruism (by proxy) drives the decision-making process for many caregivers.

Informed consent is required for all patients to enroll in a clinical trial. This consent is a written acknowledgment, created by a trial's principal investigators and signed by a client, of the possible positive and conversely adverse effects (known or unknown) of an investigational agent.[36,90] Goals for clinical trials must be clearly outlined so true informed consent (or assent as it is referred to in pediatric clinical trials) can be obtained. Informed consent defines a trial's purpose and the requirements for the client to return with their pet for future follow-up procedures/appointments. It ensures the relationship of all parties is clear to those involved. Although adverse events outside of those described are always possible, informed consent ensures that clients understand that in many trials the outcome/side effects are as yet unknown. Ethical considerations also require rigorous informed consent of study procedures, especially in biologically intensive trials, because repeated invasive procedures or even serial imaging may result in the false perception of a stronger therapeutic intent.[34,91] In academic human oncology centers, the goal is for all patients to be enrolled on clinical trials and this is an objective we should strive for in veterinary oncology as well.

Since the treatment of pet animals with cancer is purely a client-driven choice, there are no true "standards of care" in veterinary oncology. Although there are proven active regimes for the care of common cancers in dogs (i.e., cyclophosphamide, hydroxydaunorubicin (doxorubicin), vincristine [Oncovin], and prednisone [CHOP]-based chemotherapy in lymphoma, platinum or anthracyclines in OSA), these therapies are not required. Therefore veterinary and comparative oncology trials can offer investigational therapies in naïve disease. For clients, the main drivers of the decision to seek investigational trials are the costs or toxicities associated with traditional cytotoxic drugs and the lack of significantly effective available treatments. Clinical trials can randomize patients to placebo arms if there is an interest in comparing a novel therapy

Box 17-1 Suggested "Elements of Consent" to Include in Informed Client Consent Documents

1. Purpose of research
2. Expected duration of participation
3. Description of procedures
4. Possible discomforts and risks
5. Possible benefits
6. Alternative treatment (or alternative to participation)
7. Extent of confidentiality of records
8. Compensation or therapy for injuries or adverse events
9. Contact person for the study
10. Voluntary participation and right to withdraw
11. Termination of participation by the principal investigator
12. Unforeseen risks
13. Financial obligations
14. Hospital review committee contact person

Modified with permission from Morris Animal Foundation: www.morrisanimalfoundation.org.

to no therapy. Although, as in human trials, informed consent must clearly state the inclusion of a placebo arm, the protocol design may include an allowance for crossover to study drug or traditional therapies either at a defined interval or in documented progressive disease. Requirements for early stopping rules can also alleviate some of these ethical concerns when overt drug inactivity or activity is evident.[92] Box 17-1 defines the suggested elements that should be included in any clinical trial informed consent document.[1]

Many regulatory safeguards have been put in place to promote the welfare and interests of animals used in biomedical and clinical research. Protocols to use animal subjects in clinical research must be approved by institutional Animal Care and Use Committees (ACUC), and these bodies are also involved in oversight of research study conduct to ensure ethical standards are maintained. Some veterinary hospitals also have Clinical Review Boards that function similarly to human IRBs as described previously. Although clinical trials do have the potential to provide a therapeutic benefit for patients, early phase trials are used to assess the acute and chronic toxicities of novel drugs. In some cases, pet dogs are receiving "first in dog" drugs and adverse events are expected, with grade 5 events (fatality) possible. Although this would be predicted to reflect what is seen in an aged and ill cancer population, it is an important element to be detailed in informed consent. The grading and reporting of adverse events in VCOG-CTCAE version 1.1 clinical trials include uniform common toxicity criteria for adverse events, and ethical care includes treatment for any such events.[10] Clients also have the option to withdraw their pet from a clinical trial at any time without penalty. All of these provisions are designed to ensure safety for trial participants and the ethical conduct of clinical research. This field will continue to grow and evolve along with the scope of veterinary clinical oncology.

Conclusions

Clinical trials are an important research discipline to improve care and outcome for cancer patients in both human and veterinary oncology. Steps should be made to ensure study aims are achievable within a crafted study design and protocol. Rules governing design are prospective and involve questions of dose and schedule selection, toxicity, activity, and comparison to known effective therapies. Statistical expertise is also necessary to ensure appropriate clinical trial design. Regulatory oversight of veterinary oncology trials is increasing, and new approval of veterinary oncology agents will emphasize these processes over the next decade. Comparative oncology trials also are key to the inclusion of pet animals in the evaluation of novel anticancer therapeutics, imaging strategies, and medical devices. Consortia groups will continue to advocate and advance the use and utility of veterinary oncology clinical trials. The field of veterinary oncology will continue to grow through the proper use and design of both traditional and novel clinical trials.

REFERENCES

1. Vail DM: Cancer clinical trials: development and implementation, *Vet Clin North Am Small Anim Pract* 37:1033–1057, 2007.
2. Teicher BA, Andrews PA: *Anticancer drug development guide : preclinical screening, clinical trials, and approval*, Humana Press, 2004, Totowa, NJ.
3. Potter DM: Phase I studies of chemotherapeutic agents in cancer patients: a review of the designs, *J Biopharm Stat* 16:579–604, 2006.
4. Kummar S, Gutierrez M, Doroshow JH, et al: Drug development in oncology: classical cytotoxics and molecularly targeted agents, *Br J Clin Pharmacol* 62:15–26, 2006.
5. Khanna C, Lindblad-Toh K, Vail D, et al: The dog as a cancer model, *Nat Biotechnol* 24:1065–1066, 2006.
6. Paoloni M, Khanna C: Translation of new cancer treatments from pet dogs to humans, *Nat Rev Cancer* 8:147–156, 2008.
7. Le Tourneau C, Lee JJ, Siu LL: Dose escalation methods in phase I cancer clinical trials, *J Natl Cancer Inst* 101:708–720, 2009.
8. Bria E, Di Maio M, Carlini P, et al: Targeting targeted agents: open issues for clinical trial design, *J Exp Clin Cancer Res* 28:66, 2009.
9. Brunetto AT, Kristeleit RS, de Bono JS: Early oncology clinical trial design in the era of molecular-targeted agents, *Future Oncol* 6:1339–1352, 2010.
10. Vail D: Veterinary Co-operative Oncology Group—Common Terminology Criteria for Adverse Events (VCOG-CTCAE) following chemotherapy or biological antineoplastic therapy in dogs and cats v1.1, *Vet Comp Oncol* 10:1–30, 2011.
11. Piantadosi S: *Clinical trials: a methodologic perspective.* 2005, Wiley and Sons.
12. Hoekstra R, Verweij J, Eskens FA: Clinical trial design for target specific anticancer agents, *Invest New Drugs* 21:243–250, 2003.
13. Parulekar WR, Eisenhauer EA: Phase I trial design for solid tumor studies of targeted, non-cytotoxic agents: theory and practice, *J Natl Cancer Inst* 96:990–997, 2004.
14. Redon CE, Nakamura AJ, Zhang YW, et al. Histone gammaH2AX and poly(ADP-ribose) as clinical pharmacodynamic biomarkers, *Clin Cancer Res* 16:4532–4542, 2010.
15. Kinders RJ, Hollingshead M, Lawrence S, et al: Development of a validated immunofluorescence assay for gammaH2AX as a pharmacodynamic marker of topoisomerase I inhibitor activity, *Clin Cancer Res* 16:5447–5457, 2010.
16. London CA: Tyrosine kinase inhibitors in veterinary medicine, *Top Companion Anim Med* 24:106–112, 2009.
17. London CA, Malpas PB, Wood-Follis SL, et al: Multi-center, placebo-controlled, double-blind, randomized study of oral toceranib phosphate (SU11654), a receptor tyrosine kinase inhibitor, for the treatment of dogs with recurrent (either local or distant) mast cell tumor following surgical excision, *Clin Cancer Res* 15:3856–3865, 2009.
18. Gray R, Manola J, Saxman S, et al: Phase II clinical trial design: methods in translational research from the Genitourinary Committee at the Eastern Cooperative Oncology Group, *Clin Cancer Res* 12:1966–1969, 2006.

19. Lee JJ, Feng L: Randomized phase II designs in cancer clinical trials: current status and future directions, *J Clin Oncol* 23:4450–4457, 2005.
20. Brown SR, Gregory WM, Twelves CJ, et al: Designing phase II trials in cancer: a systematic review and guidance, *Br J Cancer* 105:194–199, 2011.
21. Simon R: Optimal two-stage designs for phase II clinical trials, *Control Clin Trials* 10:1–10, 1989.
22. Willan AR, Pinto EM: The value of information and optimal clinical trial design, *Stat Med* 24:1791–1806, 2005.
23. Michaelis LC, Ratain MJ: Phase II trials published in 2002: a cross-specialty comparison showing significant design differences between oncology trials and other medical specialties, *Clin Cancer Res* 13:2400–2405, 2007.
24. Ocana A, Tannock IF: When are "positive" clinical trials in oncology truly positive? *J Natl Cancer Inst* 103:16–20, 2011.
25. Mandrekar SJ, Sargent DJ: Randomized phase II trials: time for a new era in clinical trial design, *J Thorac Oncol* 5:932–934, 2010.
26. Eisenhauer EA, Therasse P, Bogaerts J, et al: New response evaluation criteria in solid tumours: revised RECIST guideline (version 1.1), *Eur J Cancer* 45:228–247, 2009.
27. Jaffe CC: Measures of response: RECIST, WHO, and new alternatives, *J Clin Oncol* 24:3245–3251, 2006.
28. Gomez-Roca C, Koscielny S, Ribrag V, et al: Tumour growth rates and RECIST criteria in early drug development, *Eur J Cancer* 47(17):2512–2516, 2011.
29. Rasmussen F: RECIST and targeted therapy, *Acta Radiol* 50:835–836, 2009.
30. Rosen MA: Use of modified RECIST criteria to improve response assessment in targeted therapies: challenges and opportunities, *Cancer Biol Ther* 9:20–22, 2010.
31. Gutierrez ME, Kummar S, Giaccone G: Next generation oncology drug development: opportunities and challenges, *Nat Rev Clin Oncol* 6:259–265, 2009.
32. Poirier VJ, Thamm DH, Kurzman ID, et al: Liposome-encapsulated doxorubicin (Doxil) and doxorubicin in the treatment of vaccine-associated sarcoma in cats, *J Vet Intern Med* 16, 726–731, 2002.
33. Kinders R, Parchment RE, Ji J, et al: Phase 0 clinical trials in cancer drug development: from FDA guidance to clinical practice, *Mol Interv* 7:325–334, 2007.
34. Kummar S, Kinders R, Rubinstein L, et al: Compressing drug development timelines in oncology using phase '0' trials, *Nat Rev Cancer* 7:131–139, 2007.
35. Murgo AJ, Kummar S, Rubinstein L, et al: Designing phase 0 cancer clinical trials, *Clin Cancer Res* 14, 3675–3682, 2008.
36. Hulley SB, Cummings SR, Browner WS, et al: *Designing clinical research*. Philadelphia, 2007, Lippincott Williams & Wilkins.
37. Vail DM, Kurzman ID, Glawe PC, et al: STEALTH liposome-encapsulated cisplatin (SPI-77) versus carboplatin as adjuvant therapy for spontaneously arising osteosarcoma (OSA) in the dog: a randomized multicenter clinical trial, *Cancer Chemother Pharmacol* 50:131–136, 2002.
38. Berg J, Gebhardt MC, Rand WM: Effect of timing of postoperative chemotherapy on survival of dogs with osteosarcoma, *Cancer* 79:1343–1350, 1997.
39. Kurzman ID, MacEwen EG, Rosenthal RC, et al: Adjuvant therapy for osteosarcoma in dogs: results of randomized clinical trials using combined liposome-encapsulated muramyl tripeptide and cisplatin, *Clin Cancer Res* 1:1595–1601, 1995.
40. Phillips B, Powers BE, Dernell WS, et al: Use of single-agent carboplatin as adjuvant or neoadjuvant therapy in conjunction with amputation for appendicular osteosarcoma in dogs, *J Am Anim Hosp Assoc* 45:33–38, 2009.
41. Thompson JP, Fugent MJ: Evaluation of survival times after limb amputation, with and without subsequent administration of cisplatin, for treatment of appendicular osteosarcoma in dogs: 30 cases (1979-1990), *J Am Vet Med Assoc* 200:531–533, 1992.
42. Vail DM, MacEwen EG: Spontaneously occurring tumors of companion animals as models for human cancer, *Cancer Invest* 18:781–792, 2000.
43. Sorenmo K, Overley B, Krick E, et al: Outcome and toxicity associated with a dose-intensified, maintenance-free CHOP-based chemotherapy protocol in canine lymphoma: 130 cases, *Vet Comp Oncol* 8:196–208, 2010.
44. Chun R: Lymphoma: which chemotherapy protocol and why? *Top Companion Anim Med* 24:157–162, 2009.
45. Hosoya K, Kisseberth WC, Lord LK, et al: Comparison of COAP and UW-19 protocols for dogs with multicentric lymphoma, *J Vet Intern Med* 21:1355–1363, 2007.
46. Moore AS, Cotter SM, Rand WM, et al: Evaluation of a discontinuous treatment protocol (VELCAP-S) for canine lymphoma, *J Vet Intern Med* 15:348–354, 2001.
47. Beaver LM, Strottner G, Klein MK: Response rate after administration of a single dose of doxorubicin in dogs with B-cell or T-cell lymphoma: 41 cases (2006-2008), *J Am Vet Med Assoc* 237:1052–1055, 2010.
48. Valerius KD, Ogilvie GK, Mallinckrodt CH, et al: Doxorubicin alone or in combination with asparaginase, followed by cyclophosphamide, vincristine, and prednisone for treatment of multicentric lymphoma in dogs: 121 cases (1987-1995), *J Am Vet Med Assoc* 210:512–516, 1997.
49. Hahn KA, Ogilvie G, Rusk T, et al: Masitinib is safe and effective for the treatment of canine mast cell tumors, *J Vet Intern Med* 22:1301–1309, 2008.
50. Hahn KA, Richardson RC, Teclaw RF, et al: Is maintenance chemotherapy appropriate for the management of canine malignant lymphoma? *J Vet Intern Med* 6:3–10, 1992.
51. Gallo C, Perrone F: Clinical trial design in oncology: statistical power, *Lancet Oncol* 5:760–761, 2004.
52. Friedman LM, Furberg C, DeMets DL, et al: *Fundamentals of clinical trials*, New York, 2010, Springer.
53. Fey MF: Clinical trial design in oncology: selection of patients, *Lancet Oncol* 5:760, 2004.
54. Lonning PE: Strength and weakness of phase I to IV trials, with an emphasis on translational aspects, *Breast Cancer Res* 10(suppl 4):S22, 2008.
55. Zon R, Meropol NJ, Catalano RB, et al: American Society of Clinical Oncology Statement on minimum standards and exemplary attributes of clinical trial sites, *J Clin Oncol* 26:2562–2567, 2008.
56. McLemore MR: The role of the data safety monitoring board: why was the Avastin phase III clinical trial stopped? *Clin J Oncol Nurs* 10:153–154, 2006.
57. DiMasi JA, Grabowski HG: Economics of new oncology drug development, *J Clin Oncol* 25:209–216, 2007.
58. Milne CP, Kaitin KI, Dimasi JA: Mandatory comparator trials for therapeutically similar drugs: an assessment of the facts, *Am J Ther* 14:231–234, 2007.
59. Biotechnology Industry Organization (BIO): *Late-stage clinical success rates*. BIO CEO & Investor Conference, New York, February 15, 2011.
60. Kaitin KI, Melville A, Morris B: FDA advisory committees and the new drug approval process, *J Clin Pharmacol* 29:886–890, 1989.
61. Rossen BR: FDA's proposed regulations to expand access to investigational drugs for treatment use: the status quo in the guise of reform, *Food Drug Law J* 64:183–223, 2009.
62. Karsdal MA, Henriksen K, Leeming DJ, et al: Biochemical markers and the FDA Critical Path: how biomarkers may contribute to the understanding of pathophysiology and provide unique and necessary tools for drug development, *Biomarkers* 14:181–202, 2009.
63. Woodcock J, Woosley R: The FDA critical path initiative and its influence on new drug development, *Annu Rev Med* 59:1–12, 2008.
64. Pryer NK, Lee LB, Zadovaskaya R, et al: Proof of target for SU11654: inhibition of KIT phosphorylation in canine mast cell tumors, *Clin Cancer Res* 9:5729–5734, 2003.

65. Hahn KA, Legendre AM, Shaw NG, et al: Evaluation of 12- and 24-month survival rates after treatment with masitinib in dogs with nonresectable mast cell tumors, *Am J Vet Res* 71:1354–1361, 2010.
66. Bergman PJ, McKnight J, Novosad A, et al: Long-term survival of dogs with advanced malignant melanoma after DNA vaccination with xenogeneic human tyrosinase: a phase I trial, *Clin Cancer Res* 9:1284–1290, 2003.
67. Liao JC, Gregor P, Wolchok JD, et al: Vaccination with human tyrosinase DNA induces antibody responses in dogs with advanced melanoma, *Cancer Immun* 6:8, 2006.
68. Gordon I, Paoloni M, Mazcko C, et al: The Comparative Oncology Trials Consortium: using spontaneously occurring cancers in dogs to inform the cancer drug development pathway, *PLoS Med* 6:e1000161, 2009.
69. Paoloni MC, Tandle A, Mazcko C, et al: Launching a novel preclinical infrastructure: comparative oncology trials consortium directed therapeutic targeting of TNFalpha to cancer vasculature, *PLoS One* 4:e4972, 2009.
70. Paoloni M, Lana S, Thamm D, et al: The creation of the Comparative Oncology Trials Consortium Pharmacodynamic Core: Infrastructure for a virtual laboratory, *Vet J* 185:88–89, 2010.
71. Paoloni MC, Mazcko C, Fox E, et al: Rapamycin pharmacokinetic and pharmacodynamic relationships in osteosarcoma: A comparative oncology study in dogs, *PLoS One* 5:e11013, 2010.
72. Rusk A, Cozzi E, Stebbins M, et al: Cooperative activity of cytotoxic chemotherapy with antiangiogenic thrombospondin-I peptides, ABT-526 in pet dogs with relapsed lymphoma, *Clin Cancer Res* 12:7456–7464, 2006.
73. Rusk A, McKeegan E, Haviv F, et al: Preclinical evaluation of antiangiogenic thrombospondin-1 peptide mimetics, ABT-526 and ABT-510, in companion dogs with naturally occurring cancers, *Clin Cancer Res* 12:7444–7455, 2006.
74. Whitehead J: Stopping clinical trials by design, *Nat Rev Drug Discov* 3:973–977, 2004.
75. Betensky RA: Conditional power calculations for early acceptance of H0 embedded in sequential tests, *Stat Med* 16:465–477, 1997.
76. Lachin JM: A review of methods for futility stopping based on conditional power, *Stat Med* 24:2747–2764, 2005.
77. Berry DA: Decision analysis and Bayesian methods in clinical trials, *Cancer Treat Res* 75:125–154, 1995.
78. Biswas S, Liu DD, Lee JJ, et al: Bayesian clinical trials at the University of Texas M. D. Anderson Cancer Center, *Clin Trials* 6:205–216, 2009.
79. Rosner GL, Berry DA: A Bayesian group sequential design for a multiple arm randomized clinical trial, *Stat Med* 14:381–394, 1995.
80. Buzdar AU, Ibrahim NK, Francis D, et al: Significantly higher pathologic complete remission rate after neoadjuvant therapy with trastuzumab, paclitaxel, and epirubicin chemotherapy: results of a randomized trial in human epidermal growth factor receptor 2-positive operable breast cancer, *J Clin Oncol* 23:3676–3685, 2005.
81. Stadler W: Other paradigms: randomized discontinuation trial design, *Cancer J* 15:431–434, 2009.
82. Stadler WM: The randomized discontinuation trial: a phase II design to assess growth-inhibitory agents, *Mol Cancer Ther* 6:1180–1185, 2007.
83. Rosner GL, Stadler W, Ratain MJ: Randomized discontinuation design: application to cytostatic antineoplastic agents, *J Clin Oncol* 20, 4478–4484, 2002.
84. Kindler T, Breitenbuecher F, Marx A, et al: Sustained complete hematologic remission after administration of the tyrosine kinase inhibitor imatinib mesylate in a patient with refractory, secondary AML, *Blood* 101:2960–2962, 2003.
85. McKeage K, Perry CM: Trastuzumab: a review of its use in the treatment of metastatic breast cancer overexpressing HER2, *Drugs* 62:209–243, 2002.
86. Sawyers CL, Hochhaus A, Feldman E, et al: Imatinib induces hematologic and cytogenetic responses in patients with chronic myelogenous leukemia in myeloid blast crisis: results of a phase II study, *Blood* 99:3530–3539, 2002.
87. Hahn KA, Ogilvie G, Rusk T, et al: Masitinib is safe and effective for the treatment of canine mast cell tumors, *J Vet Intern Med* 22: 1301–1309, 2002.
88. London CA, et al: Spontaneous canine mast cell tumors express tandem duplications in the proto-oncogene c-kit, *Exp Hematol* 27:689–697, 1999.
89. Lindblad-Toh K, Galli SJ, Yuuki T, et al: Genome sequence, comparative analysis and haplotype structure of the domestic dog, *Nature* 438:803–819, 2005.
90. Sullivan R: Clinical trial design in oncology: protocol design, *Lancet Oncol* 5:759, 2004.
91. Kimmelman J, Nalbantoglu J: Faithful companions: a proposal for neurooncology trials in pet dogs, *Cancer Res* 67: 4541–4544, 2007.
92. Pater J, Goss P, Ingle J, et al: The ethics of early stopping rules, *J Clin Oncol* 23:2862–2863; author reply 2863-2864, 2005.

Tumors of the Skin and Subcutaneous Tissues

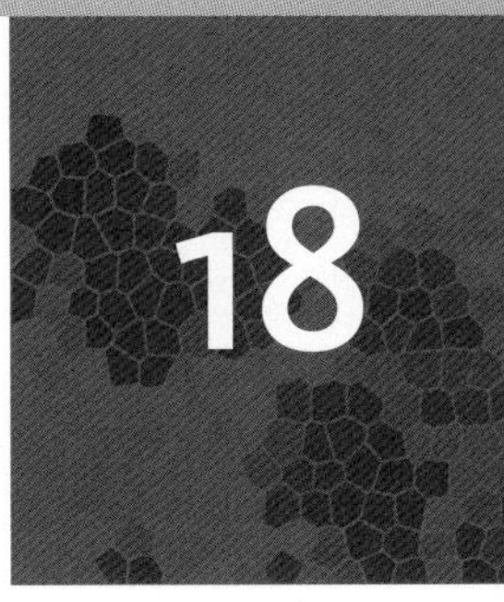

Marlene L. Hauck

Incidence

The overall incidence of tumors of the skin and subcutaneous tissues of dogs and cats is difficult to determine due to inconsistency of reporting, particularly with tumors of the subcutaneous tissues. If one considers only those tumors determined to be of "skin" origin, the percentage of biopsy specimens in this category has been reported to be 25.5% to 43%.[1-6] Of these skin tumors, between 20% and 40% are malignant.[2,3] In a survey of neoplasms in the California counties of Alameda and Contra Costa, performed from 1963 until 1966, the estimated incidence of skin and connective tissue tumors was 150.4/100,000 dogs.[4] If one considers only nonmelanoma skin tumors, the incidence is calculated at 90.4/100,000 dogs.

This same study places the incidence of skin and connective tissue tumors in cats at 51.7/100,000 cats.[4] In one report, skin tumors were 9.6% of all feline biopsy or necropsy accessions; however, skin tumors account for 29.6% of all cancer.[5] Other studies report a similar percentage of tumors arising from the skin, from 19.3%[6] to 21%.[7] Disregarding basal cell tumors (BCTs), the percentage of skin tumors that are malignant is much higher in cats than dogs, with studies reporting from 69.7%[6] to 82%.[5]

The relative prevalence of the most common tumor types in dogs and cats can be determined from multiple studies.[1,2,7-14] In dogs, the numbers are based on a fairly large number of surveys of skin tumor types from across the globe, totaling almost 9000 skin tumor submissions to various pathology services. The data for the prevalence of the most common tumors of dogs are presented in Table 18-1. The overall prevalence of lipomas and sebaceous adenomas is likely higher than reported as a result of the bias present in samples submitted for histopathologic evaluation. The data on the prevalence of feline tumors are compiled from four studies with a total of 1225 feline skin tumors and are presented in Table 18-2.[5,6,9,15] In cats, the top four tumor types of the skin and subcutaneous tissues are consistently BCTs, mast cell tumors, squamous cell carcinoma (SCC), and fibrosarcoma. These four tumor types make up on average approximately 70% of all feline skin tumors.

The remainder of this chapter will focus on SCCs, BCTs, glandular skin tumors, and additional assorted primary tumors of the skin, ears, and digits. Mast cell tumors, melanomas, cutaneous lymphomas, and soft tissue sarcomas will be addressed separately in corresponding chapters of this text.

Etiology

Physical Factors

Ionizing radiation and thermal injury have been reported to increase the risk of skin cancer in many species. A recent epidemiologic study on the incidence of cancer in human burn victims demonstrated no increased risk of the development of skin cancer when compared to the general population, however.[16] Ultraviolet (UV) radiation has long been known to cause neoplastic transformation in the skin and is a major contributor to rising rates of skin cancer of all subtypes in humans.[17] Evidence for the role of UV irradiation in the development of skin tumors in cats and dogs is primarily epidemiologic in nature[18-20] and supported by case reports on dogs diagnosed with a spectrum of sunlight-induced lesions.[21,22]

The association between SCC development and solar exposure of skin in light-colored cats has been established epidemiologically. Dorn and colleagues calculated that a white cat in California had a 13.4-fold increased risk of developing SCC, and 143 of the 149 cases of nonoral SCC in this study occurred on the head or neck.[18] Similar results were found in a case series of nasal planum or pinnal SCC in cats: of the 61 cats, 58 were white or partially white in color and all but three spent time outdoors.[23]

Viral Factors

The ability to induce neoplastic transformation in mucosal infections of papillomaviruses of humans is well established. Papillomaviruses are only able to replicate in terminally differentiated cells; therefore infection of the keratinocyte can stimulate increased proliferation and terminal differentiation.[24] Neoplastic transformation arises from the viral effects on cell proliferation, integration into the genome, and interaction of papilloma viral proteins with cellular proteins, particularly the destabilization of p53 by viral protein E6 and the inhibition of pRB by viral protein E7.[25] This disruption in p53 can result in increased levels of p16 protein, which is detectable with immunohistochemistry (IHC).[26] The association between papillomavirus infection and cutaneous SCC in humans is primarily epidemiologic in nature—organ transplant recipients and immunosuppressed individuals have an increased rate of cutaneous papillomavirus infection and increased risk of SCC development.[27,28]

The association between canine oral papillomavirus and the development of oral papillomas has been studied since the 1950s.[29] The association between viral infection and the development of SCC has evolved from a combination of evidence, including the detection of canine papillomavirus in oral and cutaneous SCCs and the induction of cutaneous SCC in 10 beagles—out of 4500 vaccinated—with a live oral papillomavirus vaccine.[30-32] Canine oral papillomavirus has also been detected in multiple cases of cutaneous SCC.[31] A novel papillomavirus with malignant potential was cloned from a dog with footpad papillomas.[33] Dogs persistently infected with this novel virus developed invasive and metastatic SCC.[34] Several additional novel canine papillomaviruses were detected in SCC from a variety of locations, including four cutaneous tumors.[35]

TABLE 18-1 Skin Tumor Incidence in Dogs*

TUMOR TYPE	OVERALL (NO.)	OVERALL (%)
Mast cell tumor	1494	16.8
Lipoma	758	8.5
Histiocytoma	752	8.4
Perianal gland adenoma	692	7.8
Sebaceous gland hyperplasia/adenoma	577	6.5
Squamous cell carcinoma	531	6.0
Melanoma	500	5.6
Fibrosarcoma	478	5.4
Basal cell tumor	445	5.0
Malignant peripheral nerve sheath tumor	381	4.3
Papilloma	251	2.8
Sweat gland adenocarcinoma	101	1.1
Sebaceous adenocarcinoma	42	0.5
Miscellaneous	1899	21.3
TOTAL	8901	100

*Overall incidence of the most common canine skin tumors as determined from the collation of 10 worldwide studies.

TABLE 18-2 Skin Tumor Incidence In Cats*

TUMOR TYPE	OVERALL (NO.)	OVERALL (%)
Basal cell tumor	282	23.02
Mast cell tumor	202	16.49
Squamous cell carcinoma	127	10.37
Fibrosarcoma	219	17.88
Apocrine adenoma	41	3.35
Lipoma	40	3.27
Hemangiosarcoma	35	2.86
Sebaceous adenoma	34	2.78
Fibroma	33	2.69
Hemangioma	21	1.71
Melanoma	21	1.71
Malignant fibrous histiocytoma	9	0.73
Miscellaneous	124	10.12
TOTAL	1225	100

*Relative incidence of the most common skin tumors in cats collated from three studies.

Case reports support the correlation between papillomavirus infection and the development of invasive SCC, including lesions of mixed histology.[32,36,37] Similar to the epidemiologic studies in immunosuppressed humans, a case report of a patient on ongoing chemotherapy developing cutaneous papillomavirus infection and multiple papillomas supports the necessity of immunosuppression in allowing persistent infection of papillomavirus.[38] Susceptibility to infection may also depend on the breed.[39,40] Recently, a dog with multiple viral plaques developed more than 20 invasive cutaneous SCC over a 3-year period, with no evidence of underlying immunosuppression.[41] A novel papillomavirus was sequenced from these lesions.

In cats, papillomaviruses are associated with viral plaques and feline fibropapillomas (sometimes referred to as *feline sarcoids*).[42,43] Papillomavirus can be detected with IHC in the majority of feline viral plaques, and as these plaques progress to SCC, the ability to detect papillomavirus antigens decreases.[44] However, when polymerase chain reaction (PCR) is used to amplify papillomavirus DNA, up to 76% of "UV-protected" SCCs are positive in comparison with 42% of SCCs in regions exposed to UV irradiation.[26] In humans, it has been suggested that UV exposure and papillomavirus infection may act as co-factors in the development of SCC. A large retrospective study tested for the presence of papillomavirus in 126 SCCs, SCCs in situ, or Bowen's in situ carcinoma (BISC) in 84 cats.[45] These investigators found no correlation between likelihood of papillomavirus infection and UV exposure. A novel feline papillomavirus has been sequenced from three feline BISC lesions.[46] A total of 25% of the 73 cutaneous lesions were positive for papillomavirus by PCR. Human papillomaviruses 5, 21, and 38 were identified in approximately half of the virus-positive cats. A second study evaluated the levels of p16 in 60 cats; tissues tested were comprised of 14 viral plaques, 14 BISC, 18 invasive SCCs, and 14 trichoblastomas (controls).[26] Eleven of the invasive SCCs were solar-induced, and seven were classified as non–solar-induced tumors. P16 protein levels were compared to the trichoblastomas and solar-induced SCC and were found to be elevated in all viral plaques, Bowenoid tumors, and non–solar invasive SCC, which is consistent with the presence of papillomavirus infection. Taken together, these data support the possibility of feline papillomaviruses' role in the development of SCC in cats.

Immune Status

Immunosuppressed humans have a greatly increased risk of skin cancer, whereas organ transplant recipients have up to 100-fold increased risk for development of SCC.[47] Although this may reflect susceptibility to persistent papillomavirus infection in some instances, it is also thought to reflect loss of normal immune surveillance, with resulting lack of an immune response against early neoplasia. A case report of the development of multiple cutaneous hamartomas and SCC in situ in a dog receiving long-term immunosuppressive therapy with prednisone and cyclosporine also demonstrated positive staining for papillomavirus antigens.[48] Interestingly, the lesions persisted and new lesions developed, even after discontinuation of the drug therapy. The successful use of immune stimulants for early cancer lesions such as imiquimod for carcinoma in situ supports the role of the immune system in controlling skin cancer. The ability of the immune system of dogs to cause regression of histiocytomas and papillomas also illustrates the role of immune surveillance in veterinary patients.[49]

Genetic Abnormalities in Skin Cancer

Cancer is a genetic disease (see Chapter 1, Section A). The accumulation of multiple alterations in critical genes is usually necessary for full neoplastic transformation. An understanding of the genetic abnormalities, including both genetic and epigenetic modifications in a particular cancer type, allows for the formulation of therapeutics to circumvent these critical mutations and their pathways. The accumulation of such genetic data is only beginning in veterinary oncology. The discovery of activating mutations in the stem cell factor receptor, c-KIT, in canine mast cell tumors and the subsequent successful targeting of this mutation with tyrosine kinase inhibitors (TKIs) is the first step in applying this approach in veterinary oncology. Current understanding of mutations present in the most common forms of skin cancer, and their role in either tumorigenesis or prognosis/response to treatment is presented according to tumor type.

Basal Cell Carcinomas

In humans, basal cell carcinomas (BCCs) are thought to arise from critical mutations in the hedgehog signaling pathway.[50] Very little genetic evaluation of BCTs has been performed in veterinary medicine. However, one study demonstrated a reciprocal translocation in a canine BCT: t(10;35).[51] In the dog, chromosome 10 contains the gene *GLI1*, which is the effector transcription factor of the hedgehog signaling cascade. Two aberrant karyotypes were found in feline BCTs: trisomy E3 and monosomy E3, although the significance of these findings are unknown.[52,53] IHC for p53 in five feline BCTs were negative.[54] Likewise, IHC evaluation for the presence of the apoptotic regulatory proteins Bcl-2 and Bax showed 23 of 24 tumors expressed Bcl-2, only 7 of the BCTs expressed Bax.[55] Interestingly, Bcl-2 staining is considered specific for human BCC.[56]

Squamous Cell Carcinomas

The genetic abnormalities responsible for the development of cutaneous SCCs are incompletely understood in human oncology. One common finding is mutations in p53. A proposed pathway of sequentially necessary mutations was proposed by Burnworth et al.[57] In addition, several genetic changes in cutaneous SCCs have been suggested to be of prognostic value in humans with this disease.

There are a number of studies evaluating p53 in canine and feline cutaneous SCCs. When p53 is present in the wild-type form, its short half-life prevents detection of the protein with IHC. The presence of a detectable form of the p53 protein correlates with mutations within the coding sequence. A series of three IHC studies of p53 in canine cutaneous SCCs revealed that 29.5%, or 19 of 65 tumors studied, were positive for p53 overexpression.[31,54,58] Interestingly, two of six cutaneous papillomas were also positive for p53 expression by IHC.[31] Detectable expression is even more prevalent in feline cutaneous SCCs, with 19 of 40 cutaneous SCCs (47.5%) positive for p53 expression in three studies.[53,54,59] In addition, feline actinic keratosis was also found to be highly positive for p53 expression (11 of 14 cases), whereas BISC lesions were less commonly positive (4 of 22 cases).[60] These studies have raised questions as to the relative roles of papillomavirus infection and UV irradiation in the development of different subtypes of feline SCCs because both mechanisms of tumorigenesis can result in increased identification of p53.

Several studies evaluated changes in selected protein expression with IHC. For example, immunohistochemical staining of p27, a protein thought important in maintaining cells in G0, showed SCCs to have much lower levels than benign cutaneous neoplasms.[61] β-Catenin is a protein responsible for normal skin homeostasis. When dysregulated, β-catenin can be oncogenic. A study of β-catenin expression in normal skin and benign and malignant tumors demonstrated nuclear presence of this protein, representing pathway activation, in 100% of the trichoepithelioma and pilomatricoma; no nuclear expression was found in any of the other malignant tumors or normal skin.[62] This finding led the authors to suggest a role for aberrantly activated β-catenin in the formation of tumors of the hair follicle. Evaluation for the presence of cyclin D1 and cyclin A, which are proteins important in the regulation of the cell cycle, demonstrated that cyclin A was present in 90% of feline SCCs and 44% of canine SCCs. Cyclin D1 was rarely expressed in skin tumors of any type.[54] Staining for these proteins in normal skin and benign tumors showed rare or weak staining. The investigators suggested a role for cyclin A in the regulation of proliferation and neoplastic transformation in cutaneous SCCs.

The syndrome of renal cystadenocarcinoma and nodular dermatofibrosis (RCND) deserves mention because this disease often presents to the veterinarian as the result of the manifestation of multiple firm cutaneous nodules. Although first described as a genetic disease in the mid-1980s, it was not until 2003 that the causative mutation in the *Birt-Hogg-Dubé (BHD)* gene was described.[63,64] The *BHD* gene codes for the tumor suppressor protein folliculin, and mutations in this gene are thought to lead to loss of function.[65] Although mostly seen in German shepherd dogs, this syndrome has been reported in Alsatians as well.[66]

Identification of the driver mutations underlying neoplastic transformation in the skin will be key to optimizing the use of drugs that target these pathways and avoiding unwanted cutaneous side effects. The use of pathway-specific drugs may have unanticipated effects in the skin. Sorafenib, a TKI of Raf and vascular endothelial growth factor/platelet-derived growth factor receptor (VEGF/PDGFR), has been associated with the rapid development of actinic keratosis and invasive SCCs in humans.[67,68] As better understanding of these pathways and their role in normal skin homeostasis develops, it may be possible to prevent these types of unintended consequences.

Pathologic Classification of Skin Tumors

Skin tumors arise from the epidermis and associated structures. For ease of use, these tumors are divided based on their differentiation into specific subelements of the skin.[69] Some histologies are divided into benign and malignant forms, based on known clinical and histologic predictors of behavior. In other tumor types, such clear-cut division may not be possible.

The World Health Organization (WHO) classification system of tumor-node-metastasis can be applied to skin tumors in the clinical setting.[70] Box 18-1 describes the application of this staging system to skin tumors. Location is also prognostic for particular tumor types; for example, melanomas of the oral cavity are often malignant, which differs from the expected behavior of a melanoma of haired skin, so this information should be included in the clinical description of the tumor at presentation.

History and Clinical Signs

Tumors of the skin are often noticed by pet owners and brought to their veterinarian's attention. The biologic history of these masses can be quite variable. Self-trauma or secondary infection may cause a patient to be presented for evaluation by their veterinarian. Ultimately, however, it is critical to remember that physical inspection cannot definitively determine whether a lesion is benign or malignant. Cytology or histopathology is necessary to diagnose any skin tumor.

Diagnostic Techniques and Work-Up

The evaluation of a skin tumor is generally similar to the evaluation for any solid tumor. A complete history can be very informative.

Box 18-1 Clinical Stages (TNM) of Canine or Feline Tumors of Epidermal or Dermal Origin

Primary Tumor

T0	No evidence of tumor
Tis	Carcinoma in situ
T1	Tumor <2 cm maximum diameter, superficial or exophytic
T2	Tumor 2-5 cm maximum diameter or with minimal invasion irrespective of size
T3	Tumor >5 cm maximum diameter or with invasion of the subcutis, irrespective of size
T4	Tumor invading other structures, such as fascia, muscle, bone, or cartilage

Simultaneous tumors are recorded by number, with the highest T category selected and the total number indicated in parentheses, for example, T2 (3). Successive tumors are classified independently.

Regional Lymph Nodes (RLN)

N0	No evidence of RLN involvement
N1	Movable ipsilateral nodes
N1a	Nodes considered non-metastatic
N1b	Nodes considered metastatic
N2	Movable contralateral or bilateral nodes
N2a	Nodes considered nonmetastatic
N2b	Nodes considered metastatic
N3	Fixed nodes

Distant Metastasis

M0	No evidence of distant metastasis
M1	Distant metastasis detected—specify site(s)

Careful elucidation of the length of duration, rate of growth, and any clinical signs associated with the tumor may be helpful in differentiating benign from malignant masses. There are two steps in the clinical evaluation of any patient with a mass: diagnosis and staging. Diagnosis of many cutaneous and subcutaneous masses can be achieved with fine-needle aspiration and cytology or direct impression cytology of a lesion. Cytology is an inexpensive and relatively noninvasive means of diagnosing many common benign skin tumors, such as lipomas or sebaceous adenomas. For lesions that appear malignant or are nondiagnostic on cytology, histopathology is necessary. In addition to confirming a diagnosis, histopathology yields useful information on the grade of some tumors such as mast cell tumors or the malignant behavior of a tumor on the tissue level, such as vascular and lymphatic invasion. Other characteristics such as degree of differentiation, nuclear morphology, and percentage of necrosis may be helpful with certain tumor types.

The type of biopsy performed is usually dictated by the location. Where wide surgical excision is feasible without undue morbidity, the biopsy can be combined with a therapeutic procedure. However, in most instances, the biopsy is a diagnostic test. The author's preference for a biopsy of a skin or subcutaneous mass is multiple punch biopsies or an incisional biopsy. These techniques allow the procurement of a sufficiently large piece of tissue for an accurate diagnosis and, where applicable, grading of the tumor. In addition, advanced histopathologic techniques such as IHC for evaluation of prognostic markers can also be performed. Molecular tests such as PCR can be carried out on formalin-fixed tissues as well.

Staging involves determination of the extent of disease locally, regionally, and distantly. Assessment of primary tumor size with measurement of the longest diameter is the first step in the staging process. For large, infiltrative, or fixed masses, local assessment may require advanced imaging such as a computed tomography (CT) scan or magnetic resonance imaging (MRI) to accurately determine tumor size and extent. One study demonstrated that the use of advanced local imaging techniques increased the stage of the primary tumor in 69% of patients.[71] Regional staging involves the assessment of the draining lymph node(s). Determination of the draining node can be difficult for some locations, so evaluation of all nodes in the region may be necessary. Metastatic lymph nodes may be a normal size and consistency on palpation. Conversely, large, firm nodes may be reactive in response to an infection or inflammatory process. Aspiration and cytologic examination by an experienced clinical pathologist is critical for the assessment of regional lymph nodes for evidence of metastasis. Despite careful evaluation of a cytology sample, it is possible to miss metastatic disease. In cases of questionable cytologic results, histopathologic evaluation of the lymph node is recommended.

Evaluation of the patient for distant metastatic disease prior to histopathologic confirmation of a neoplastic process is based on the degree of suspicion that the mass is malignant, as well as the desires and financial limitations of the owner. After confirmation of a malignant process, additional staging for detection of distant metastatic disease and evaluation of overall suitability for proposed treatments are indicated. Such staging may include chest radiographs, abdominal ultrasound, and/or additional tests as indicated by the tumor type or clinical findings.

Treatment and Prognosis for Specific Tumor Types

Given their external location, the primary treatment option to achieve local control of most skin and subcutaneous tumors is surgery. For benign masses, marginal excision may be adequate to achieve long-term control. For malignant tumors, adequate surgical excision requires a margin of normal tissue around the neoplasm. In order for a pathologist to determine if excision is complete, all surgical margins must be identified, with surgical ink or sutures, for correct reporting of margins to occur (see Chapter 9).[72] The surgeon or clinician must properly prepare the sample to allow the pathologist to report all critical information, including margin evaluation. A more complete discussion of this topic is reviewed by Kamstock et al.[72]

Likewise, in order to accurately report tumor grade in those tumors for which a grading scheme has been validated, a pathologist needs a reasonably sized piece of tissue to evaluate. Needle core or Tru-Cut biopsies often yield limited amounts of tissue and should only be used on those tumors for which they are the sole option.

The most common cutaneous and subcutaneous tumors, melanomas, mast cell tumors, and soft tissue sarcomas, are discussed in Chapters 19, 20, and 21, respectively. The remainder of this chapter will cover the additional skin tumors, focusing on those with malignant behavior.

Epithelial Tumors

Tumors of the Primitive Follicular Epithelium

The term *basal cell tumor* (BCT) was used for many years to include BCCs, basal cell epithelioma, trichoblastoma, and solid-cystic ductular sweat gland adenomas and adenocarcinomas. As pathologists' abilities to differentiate these tumors on the basis of keratin and other membrane markers has progressed, trichoblastomas and solid-cystic ductular sweat gland tumors are no longer considered "basal cell" tumors. As a consequence, older studies that reported high rates of BCT, particularly in cats, may not be reflective of diagnostic patterns today.[73] These related tumor types are believed to arise from stem cells in the outer follicular root sheath, displaying variable differentiation, although the origin for all tumors in this category cannot be absolutely identified. Basosquamous cell carcinoma is a tumor with characteristics of both BCCs and SCCs. Immunohistochemically, basosquamous cell carcinomas are more closely related to BCCs and will be discussed in this section. Trichoepitheliomas are a more differentiated form of the trichoblastoma. The most appropriate nomenclature and classification schema for this group of tumors remain controversial. Tumor types will be presented as categorized in the Armed Forces Institute of Pathology publication on the histologic classification of skin tumors.[69]

Basal Cell Carcinomas

The true incidence of BCCs in both dogs and cats is unknown. The different tumors previously categorized as BCTs are difficult to distinguish histologically and cytologically—both the category of tumor and differentiating benign lesions from malignant. On cytology, BCTs can contain inflammatory cells, squamous cells, sebaceous epithelial cells, melanin, and melanophages, and cells can express the criteria of malignancy. Well-differentiated fibroblasts, reactive fibroblasts, and mast cells may also be present on cytologic examination.[74] The inability to distinguish the subtypes on cytology has led to the suggestion these tumors be called *cutaneous basilar epithelial neoplasms* when evaluated by cytology alone.[75]

Based on histopathologic evaluation, tumors sometimes can be grossly differentiated based on growth pattern.[76] The epithelial membrane glycoprotein BerEP4 is highly specific for BCCs versus SCCs or cystic-solid ductular tumors in the diagnosis of BCC in humans.[56] Cytokeratin 8 (CAM 5.2) is used with human tumors to identify tumors with sweat gland epithelial differentiation and has been used to differentiate a BCC from a solid-cystic ductular tumor in a dog.[75] However, validation of these immunohistochemical markers in a larger veterinary population remains to be performed.

BCCs are thought to be rare in dogs. In two studies reporting BCCs or basal cell epithelioma (the benign variant), the incidence ranged from 5.5% to 8.4% of all skin tumors; however, it is unclear if trichoblastomas were included in these populations.[10,11] Breeds reported to be at increased risk for BCCs included cocker spaniels and poodles in one study; however, another study reported no breed predispositions. Clinically, these tumors present as plaques or nodules, often darkly pigmented. The overlying skin may be alopecic and intact or ulcerated. In dogs, the median age of patients was reported to be 9 years; however, dogs of all ages may be affected[10,11] (Figure 18-1). There are three recognized histologic subtypes: solid, keratinizing, and clear cell.[76]

In dogs, BCCs are considered a low-grade malignancy. Although there are reports of local recurrence of this tumor after surgical excision, no reports of metastasis in the dog could be found. The application of morphometric analysis of cell nuclei has been reported to be useful in differentiating BCCs potentially able to recur from those that are not likely to recur.[77]

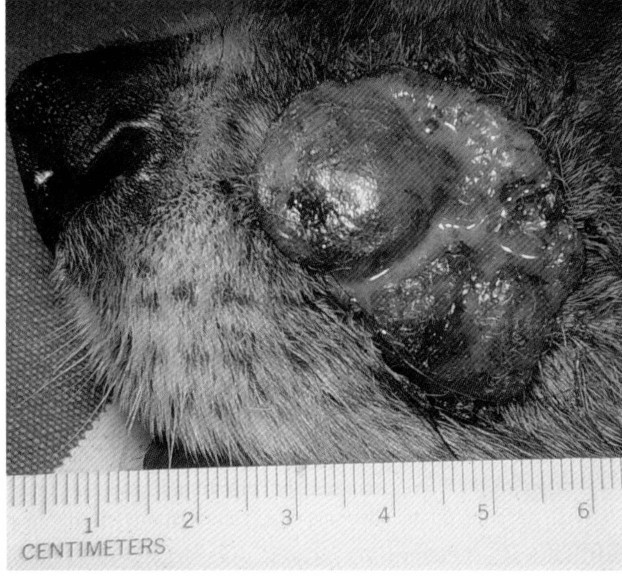

FIGURE 18-1 Large basal cell carcinoma on the muzzle of a dog.

In cats, BCCs are now thought to be rare, with many of the tumors previously diagnosed as BCTs actually falling into the categories of solid-cystic apocrine ductular adenoma (approximately 60%) and trichoblastoma (approximately 40%).[78] However, given the preponderance of the literature referring to "basal cell tumors" in cats, this group of tumors will be discussed here, realizing the population is actually mixed. These tumors comprise some of the most common solid tumors in cats, second only to mammary tumors in one large study.[79] They represent 10% to 26% of feline skin tumors.[5,9,79,80] These are tumors of middle-aged cats, with a reported mean age of 9.6 to 10.8 years.[5,6,80] Although one study reported a predisposition to BCT in Siamese cats, other studies did not find breed differences. BCCs can appear anywhere on the body but may have a predilection for the head and neck. BCC can appear pigmented and resemble a melanoma (Figure 18-2).

Clinically, the majority of tumors classified as BCT appear benign in their behavior. Based on the presence of stromal invasion, vascular invasion (five tumors), necrosis, high mitotic index, and lymph node metastasis (one tumor), 10 of 97 feline BCTs were considered malignant in one study.[79] A case report presented a cat with four concurrent BCTs,[81] and there are two cases in the literature deemed malignant BCCs based on the presence of lymphatic vascular invasion in one cat and the presence of pulmonary metastatic disease in the second.[82] Nucleomorphometric analysis was able to predict recurrence in one study of 24 cats with BCCs.[83] Overall, the likelihood of metastasis with BCCs in cats appears low.

Treatment for BCCs is wide surgical excision, which often results in long-term control. Although the data are limited, radiation therapy has been used to treat this tumor, along with subsequent doxorubicin chemotherapy.[82] The impact from these treatment options on survival is unknown.

Basosquamous Cell Carcinomas

Histologically, basosquamous cell tumors have characteristics of both SCCs and BCCs. Clinically, these tumors are indistinguishable

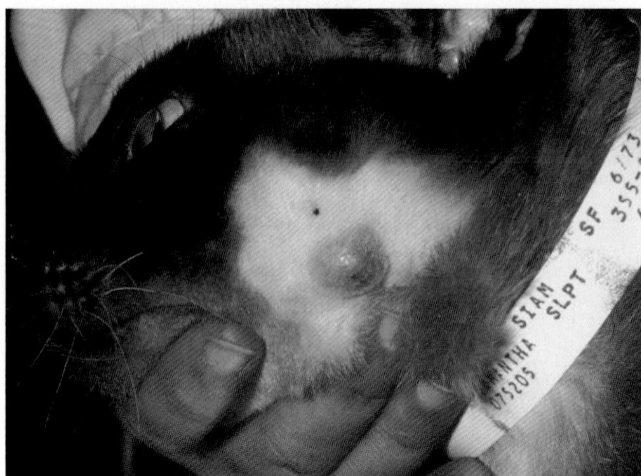

FIGURE 18-2 Firm, circumscribed, pigmented basal cell tumor (likely an apocrine ductal adenoma or a trichoblastoma) on the face of cat.

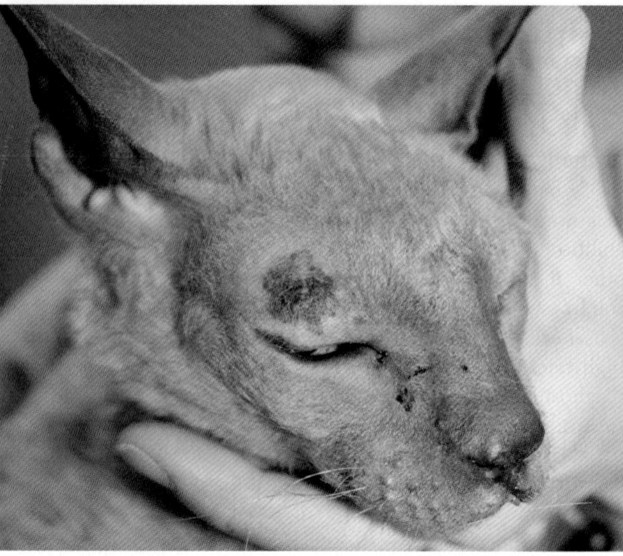

FIGURE 18-3 Plaquelike lesion of Bowen's in situ carcinoma on the head of a cat. Multiple such lesions may be present on the patient. *(Courtesy Dr. Rodney Rosychuk.)*

from both BCCs and SCCs. The true incidence and clinical behavior of these tumors in dogs and cats are unknown.

Papillomas

Papillomas are benign epidermal proliferative lesions that are often associated with papillomavirus infection.[34] They are considered rare in the cat and dog.[84] Papillomas typically have an exophytic growth pattern. Another benign variant is the inverted papilloma, which grows into the subcutaneous tissue rather than externally. Cutaneous papillomas are typically found in younger dogs, with an average age of 3.2 years[37] (see Figures 1-9 to 1-11). Surgical excision can be curative, and some of these lesions will spontaneously regress.[85] In patients with multiple lesions, azithromycin has been shown to be effective.[86]

In cats, a particular type of papilloma, the fibropapilloma, is seen. These tumors demonstrate a proliferation of mesenchymal cells covered by hyperplastic epithelium.[43] Evaluation for papillomavirus demonstrated an apparent nonproductive infection of the mesenchymal cells.[87] It has been suggested these feline tumors are more similar to equine sarcoids than papillomas.

Squamous Cell Carcinoma in Situ

SCC in situ is defined as a carcinoma that has not penetrated the basement membrane of the epithelium. When it appears in multiple sites, it is also known as Bowen's carcinoma, Bowenoid carcinoma in situ (BISC), and multicentric papillomavirus-induced SCC. This disease is seen primarily in cats, with only a few reports in dogs.[5,48,88-90] Actinic keratosis is the name typically used for SCC in situ that arises as a consequence of UV exposure.[76] Differentiation of actinic keratosis from BISC is based on location and histopathologic appearance.

Clinically, SCC in situ can present as erosions of the epidermis, proliferations, or crusted plaques. They may be painful on palpation. BISC lesions can occur anywhere on the body—both haired and unhaired skin, areas with and without sun exposure (Figure 18-3). Solitary lesions are unusual.[5,89] Actinic keratosis, on the other hand, occurs in lightly haired skin with UV exposure and can occur as a solitary lesion. It is typically accompanied by solar elastosis and fibrosis of the skin, consistent with the effects of chronic UV exposure.[76] By definition, carcinoma in situ is not yet invasive, and thus metastasis has not occurred. However, left untreated, carcinoma in situ can progress to invasive carcinoma and put the patient at risk for metastasis. Patients with BISC typically will continue to develop new lesions over time, but metastasis appears to be uncommon.[5,48,88-90]

Many treatment approaches are effective for SCC in situ. Surgical excision is the treatment of choice for most lesions. Median disease-free interval and survival in 39 cats treated with surgical excision were 594 days and 675 days, respectively.[23] Imiquimod cream (5%) has been reported to be effective in treating BISC in 12 cats, with 5 of the cats having at least one lesion undergoing a complete response to treatment.[89] Most cats were treated with daily application, although some were treated three times per week. The author's institution has found palliative radiation to be effective in controlling these lesions for at least 8 months. Photodynamic therapy is also very effective in the treatment of Bowen's disease in humans and cats, with reported response rates up to 100%.[91-93] Clinical stage of the tumor was prognostic for survival. Strontium-90 plesiotherapy in 14 cats with SCC in situ of the nasal planum resulted in 14 complete responses with no recurrences and an overall survival time of more than 3000 days.[94] As expected, metastasis appears rare in cats with SCC in situ/actinic keratosis—in 61 cats with SCC of the nasal planum and pinnae, only one cat eventually developed metastasis to the regional lymph node, at the same time as recurrence of the primary tumor.[23]

One study on the use of 13-cis-retinoic acid for SCC in situ did not demonstrate clinical efficacy in cats with BISC or SCC.[95] Etretinate showed some promise for the treatment of SCC in situ, as well as invasive SCC, but this drug is no longer available.[96]

Squamous Cell Carcinomas

SCCs are malignant tumors of the epidermis in which the cells demonstrate differentiation to squamous cells (keratinocytes).[97] These tumors typically occur in cats older than 10 years of age and at a median age of 10 to 11 years in dogs.[5,37,97] There is a predilection for cats to develop these tumors on their heads, particularly in lightly haired areas of white cats[5] (Figure 18-4) This predilection reflects the role of UV light in the induction of many of these

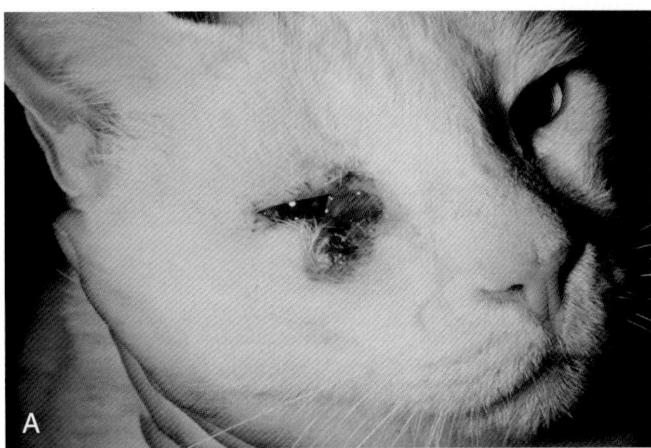

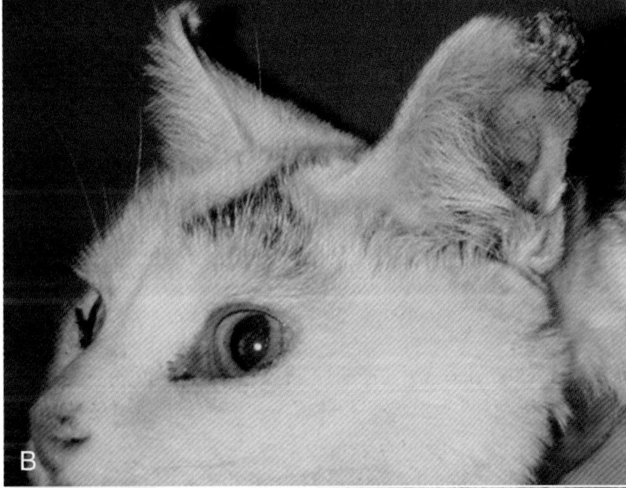

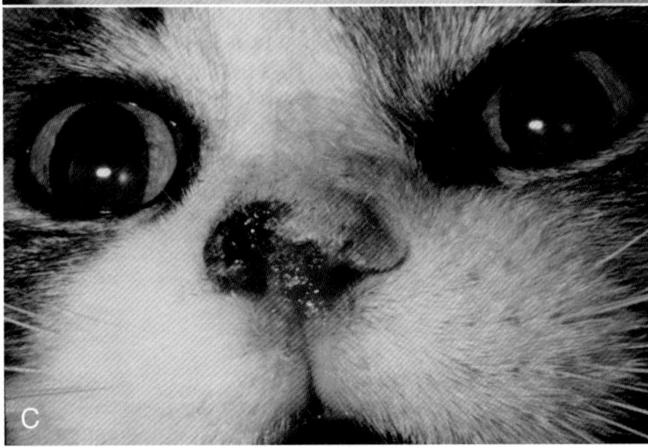

FIGURE 18-4 **A,** Squamous cell carcinoma of the lower eyelid of a white cat. This is a fairly advanced lesion characterized by local invasion and ulceration. **B,** Squamous cell carcinoma of the sparsely haired pinna of a cat. **C,** Squamous cell carcinoma of the nasal planum of a cat.

tumors. A decreased risk has been reported in Siamese, Himalayan, and Persian breeds.[5,84] There may be a predisposition for the development of nasal planum SCCs in Labradors and golden retrievers.[98] Bloodhounds, Bassett hounds, and standard poodles may be predisposed to develop cutaneous SCCs.[97]

Clinical presentation of cutaneous SCCs can be highly variable. Cutaneous SCCs can appear plaquelike to papillary, from crateriform to fungiform[76] (Figure 18-5). They may be erythemic, ulcerated, or covered with a crust.[84] Paraneoplastic hypercalcemia has been reported in three cats with cutaneous SCCs—two with aural tumors and one with multiple cutaneous tumors.[99,100] Metastasis at the time of death was present in 6 of 15 cats with invasive SCC of the nasal planum—organs involved included mandibular (6) and retropharyngeal (1) lymph nodes and lungs (1).[101] Metastasis in dogs with cutaneous SCCs appears very uncommon, with a literature review only disclosing four cases of distant metastasis: three to lung, liver, and bone in dogs that had received a bone marrow transplant and one to bone in a dog with a cutaneous SCC.[34,102] Four of 17 dogs with SCCs of the nasal planum had regional metastasis to the mandibular lymph nodes.[98] Metastasis to distant sites was not reported.

Treatment for cutaneous SCCs is primarily surgical when feasible. Wide surgical excision results in long-term control in both dogs and cats, given the low incidence of metastatic disease. In a series of 61 cats treated with surgery, radiation, and cryosurgery, surgery resulted in the longest median disease-free interval at 594 days, although many of these cats may not have had invasive disease.[23] Complete surgical excision of nasal planum SCCs in dogs resulted in long-term control in four of six dogs—the two dogs that suffered recurrence had incomplete resections.[103] (Also see Chapter 23, Section A.)

In cats, tumors of the nasal planum can be effectively treated with external-beam radiation therapy, strontium-90 plesiotherapy, and proton therapy.[94,101,104,105] Definitive radiation therapy (orthovoltage, 10 × 4 Gy) yielded a 60% 1-year survival in 90 cats treated with this modality.[101] This study also found that histologic stage was predictive of progression-free survival (PFS)—stage T1 tumors had an 85% 1-year survival rate, whereas the stage T3 tumor had a 45.5% 1-year survival rate. Proton radiation therapy to 15 cats with a dose equivalent to 40 Gy yielded 9 complete responses and 5 partial responses. One cat did not respond at all.[105] The PFS rate at one year was 64%, with a median survival of 946 days. Plesiotherapy with strontium-90 in 49 cats with invasive SCCs of the nasal planum had an overall response rate of 98%, with 88% (43 cats) having a complete response.[94] Median dose delivered in the single treatment administered to these cats was 128 Gy. Ten of 35 cats in this study developed a recurrence; median time to recurrence was 308 days. Median PFS was 1710 days, and the median overall survival was 3076 days. In a series of 15 cats treated by fractionated plesiotherapy with strontium-90, the 13 cats that achieved a complete remission had no recurrences at a median follow-up time of 652 days.[104]

Unlike in cats, radiation therapy does not appear to be effective for the treatment of nasal planum SCCs in dogs. In a group of four dogs treated with radiation alone to gross disease, only one achieved a durable remission.[98] In this same study, seven additional dogs were treated with a combination of surgery and radiation—all seven dogs had a recurrence at a median interval of 9 weeks. Eight dogs treated with either orthovoltage (six dogs) or implants of radon-222 (two dogs) experienced local recurrence in another case series.[106]

There are few data on the use of chemotherapy to treat cutaneous SCCs in dogs and cats. Intralesional carboplatin/sterile sesame oil injected into nasal planum SCCs in cats did show significant activity, with a complete response rate of 73% and a 55% PFS rate at 1 year.[107] Two dogs with metastatic SCCs were treated with cisplatin. One dog with metastatic cutaneous SCC (axillary lymph node, lung) had a marked reduction in the number and size of the lung nodules, as well as a partial response of the axillary mass following cisplatin chemotherapy. However, the patient progressed approximately 4.5 months after starting treatment. The other dog had a complete and durable response of multiple lesions (>22 months).[108] Bleomycin has demonstrated short-lived clinical

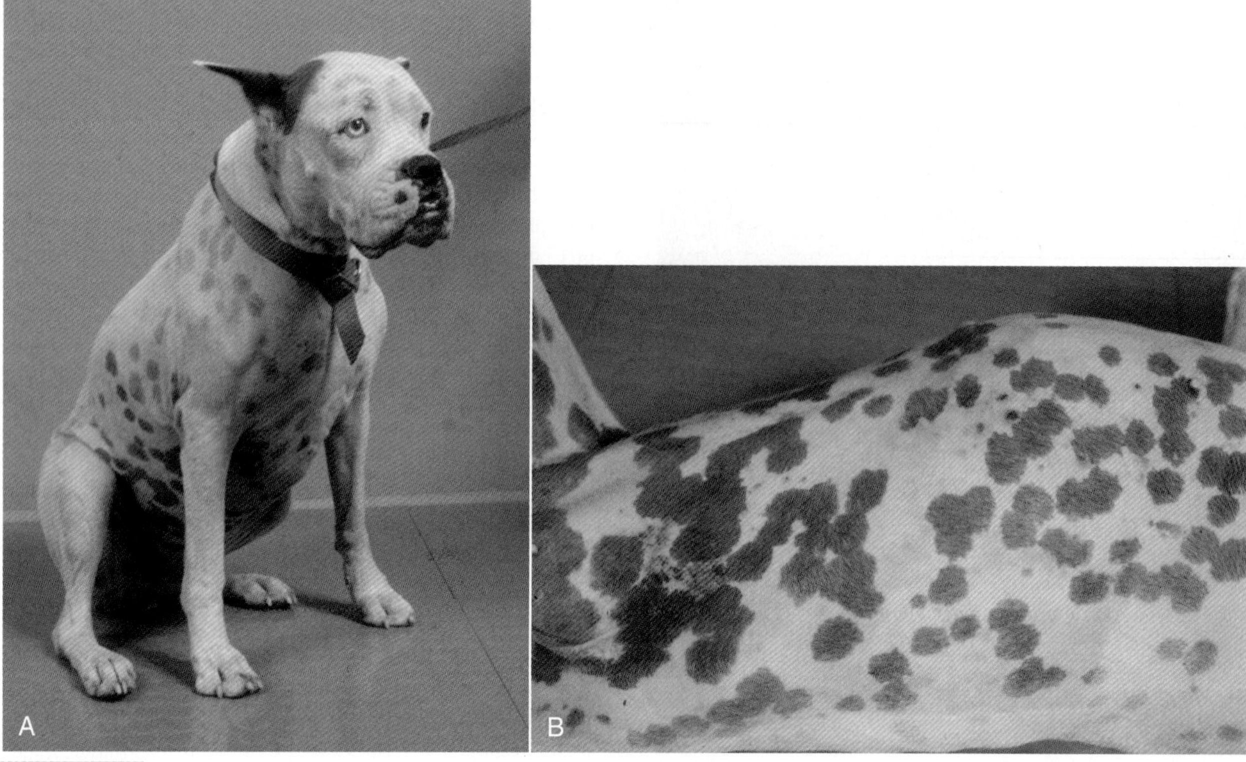

FIGURE 18-5 **A,** Wholebody photograph of a white boxer with cutaneous squamous cell carcinoma. **B,** Skin of ventral abdomen illustrating squamous cell carcinoma tracking in unpigmented regions of the skin.

activity in both dogs and cats.[109] Two dogs with SCCs were treated with actinomycin-D: one dog had stable disease after one dose and the second dog had a partial response and received a total of six doses.[110] Mitoxantrone treatment resulted in a response in 4 of 9 dogs with SCCs in one study, but only 4 of 32 cats with SCCs responded to treatment with mitoxantrone.[111,112]

Tumors with Adnexal Differentiation

There are a number of tumors that arise from the hair follicle, and the majority of these are benign. Treatment for these benign tumors is adequate surgical excision. Characteristics unique to these tumors are discussed individually.

Infundibular Keratinizing Acanthomas

Infundibular keratinizing acanthomas (IKAs) are benign tumors considered common in dogs. No reports of these tumors were found in cats. Previous names for this tumor include intracutaneous cornifying epithelioma (ICE), intracutaneous keratinizing epithelioma, keratoacanthoma, and squamous papilloma.[84] Peak incidence is from 4 to 9 years of age, but IKAs can occur in dogs younger than 4 years of age as well.[113] Nordic breeds (particularly Norwegian elkhounds), Belgian sheepdogs, Lhasa Apso, German shepherd dogs, terriers, and other breeds appear to be at increased risk for the development of these tumors, and a dog may have multiple tumors.[113-116] They occur most commonly on the back, neck, sides of thorax, tail, and limbs/shoulders. They may have a central pore communicating with the surface. Rupture of these masses can allow keratinized tissue into the adjacent dermis and incite a marked inflammatory response. When surgical excision is not feasible, isotretinoin therapy at a dose of 1.7 to 3.7 mg/kg/day had an effect in three of seven dogs treated, with one complete response and two dogs with partial improvement.[115]

Tricholemmoma

Tricholemmoma is a rare, benign tumor of dogs.[117,118] Gross appearance is a well-encapsulated mass in dermis or subcutaneous tissue. There may be hair loss in the overlying skin. The most common location appears to be the head.[113] Surgical excision is the treatment of choice.

Trichoblastoma

Trichoblastoma is the new designation for what were previously called *basal cell tumors* (BCTs) in the dog and the *spindle cell variant BCTs* in the cat.[84] Histologically, this tumor shows differentiation to the hair germ of the developing hair follicle. Breeds apparently at increased risk of developing trichoblastomas include poodles and setters.[113] It is considered a common tumor in the dog and cat. In one large review of follicular tumors and tumorlike lesions presenting to a veterinary teaching hospital, trichoblastomas comprised 25.6% of the samples in the 308 canine follicular lesions (approximately 2% of the skin biopsies overall), and 26% of the samples in the 50 follicular lesions from cats (1.5% of all skin biopsies).[113] Mean age at diagnosis in this population was approximately 7 years for dogs and 10 years for cats. In dogs, the most common sites for trichoblastomas are the head and neck; in cats, these tumors can be found on the head, neck, limbs, and trunk. Although there are at least six subtypes of trichoblastomas—ribbon, medusoid, trabecular, spindle, granular cell, and clear cell—all appear benign in their behavior and adequate surgical excision is the treatment of choice.[84,119]

Trichoepitheliomas

Trichoepitheliomas are benign tumors and demonstrate differentiation into all segments of the hair follicle.[69] Trichoepitheliomas appear to be uncommon tumors in both dogs and cats and comprise approximately 4% of the diagnoses in the retrospective study of follicular tumors and tumorlike lesions.[113] In dogs, their most common sites of occurrence were the limbs, neck, and back. Breeds predisposed to this tumor include Bassett hounds, coonhounds, English springer spaniels, and setters.[113,120] Persian cats may also be predisposed. Basset hounds and English springer spaniels may present with multiple tumors. Trichoepitheliomas are dermal in origin but can extend into the subcutis. Their surface can be ulcerated or alopecic. Surgical excision is the best treatment, except in cases with a multicentric presentation.[120]

Malignant Trichoepithelioma

The malignant version of the trichoepithelioma is differentiated on the basis of invasion into the surrounding tissues and lymphatic involvement. It is also known as *matrical carcinoma* and may be difficult to differentiate from a malignant pilomatrixoma.[121] The mitotic index is usually much higher in the malignant trichoepithelioma when compared to the benign counterpart.[69] The few cases presented in reference texts were highly metastatic to the regional lymph node and lungs.[120] The locally invasive nature of some trichoepitheliomas may also represent a lower grade malignant trichoepithelioma.[121] No information on response to therapy beyond surgical excision was found in the literature. Wide surgical excision appears necessary to prevent recurrence.[120]

Pilomatricomas

Pilomatricomas are benign follicular tumors that demonstrate only matrical differentiation.[69] Alternative names for these tumors include the necrotizing and calcifying epitheliomas of Malherbe and pilomatrixomas. These tumors are considered uncommon, representing 13% of the follicular lesions in one study and approximately 1% of all skin biopsies.[113] They are rare in the cat, with only one case out of 898 skin biopsies found in a literature review. Breed predispositions reported include the Kerry blue terrier, soft-coated Wheaton terrier, Bouvier des Flandres, standard poodle, Old English sheepdog, Bichon Frise, and Airedale terrier, among others.[122] The most common locations are the neck, back, and trunk, with an average age of 6.5 years. These tumors present as well-circumscribed masses and may be very firm due to ossification.[121,122] Treatment of choice is adequate surgical excision.

Malignant Pilomatricomas

Malignant pilomatricomas are thought to be rare, although a recent report suggests they may be more common than previously appreciated: of 13 pilomatricomas diagnosed in a 2-year period, 4 were malignant.[123] No reports of malignant pilomatricomas were found in cats. Defining a pilomatricoma as malignant can be difficult because some appear very like their benign counterpart on initial histologic evaluation.[124] Invasion into underlying tissues, particularly bone, may be a reasonable indicator of potential malignant behavior in the absence of a malignant appearance on histopathology.[123-125] A recent review of several published cases demonstrated their highly metastatic nature, with documented spread to lungs, bone, lymph node, mammary gland, or skin in 11 of the 12 dogs in this series—the last dog had no follow-up information available.[123] There is one report of the use of surgery followed by radiation therapy to control a recurrent malignant pilomatricoma, which prevented local recurrence until 14 months later, when diffuse pulmonary metastasis was documented.[124] No reports on the activity or efficacy of chemotherapy for the treatment of malignant pilomatricoma in dogs were found.

Tumors of Glandular Origin

Sebaceous Hyperplasia, Sebaceous Adenoma, Sebaceous Ductal Adenoma, and Sebaceous Epithelioma

Sebaceous hyperplasia, sebaceous adenoma, sebaceous ductal adenoma, and sebaceous epithelioma are very common in the dog and rare in the cat, and the division between these tumors may be "arbitrary."[84] A review of 172 tumors of the sebaceous gland revealed a preponderance of female representation with sebaceous hyperplasia and an overrepresentation of miniature schnauzers, beagles, poodles, and cocker spaniels.[126,127] Coonhounds, Nordic breeds, and some terriers may also be predisposed to develop benign sebaceous tumors.[128] Limbs, trunk, and eyelids were the most common locations. Although these tumors can occur even in young dogs, peak occurrence is from 7 to 13 years of age.

Sebaceous epitheliomas may recur locally, and lymphatic metastasis has been reported anecdotally. Because lymphatic invasion may occasionally be found at the margin of sebaceous epitheliomas, they are sometimes considered a low-grade malignancy rather than benign.[69] A recent report of distant metastases (lung, central nervous system) from a recurrent sebaceous epithelioma confirms their malignant potential.[129] In general, adequate surgical excision is the preferred treatment.

Sebaceous Gland Carcinomas

Sebaceous gland carcinomas are uncommon in the dog and cat.[84] They are more common in the intact male dog.[128] They most frequently occur on the head, and the Cavalier King Charles spaniel, cocker spaniel, and terrier breeds are at increased risk of developing these tumors. Sebaceous gland carcinomas tend to be low-grade malignancies, with metastasis beyond the lymph node found only in one report.[130,131] This patient had widespread metastasis, with bone, skin, and lung involvement. They are typically found on the head and neck in dogs and on the head, thorax, and perineum in cats.[128] The most common finding of malignancy is local infiltration. The only reported treatment for these tumors is wide surgical excision.

Apocrine Gland Adenomas and Solid-Cystic Apocrine Ductal Adenomas

Apocrine gland adenomas are considered fairly common in the dog, although they are not common in the cat. These tumors may be fluid filled. Apocrine ductal adenomas are firm on palpation. Feline apocrine gland adenomas have a high predilection for the head.[132] Solid-cystic apocrine ductal adenomas were previously designated as BCTs. These benign tumors are appropriately treated with adequate surgical excision.

Apocrine Gland Carcinomas

Apocrine sweat gland tumors are relatively uncommon in dogs (overall 1.1% of all skin tumors) and perhaps a bit more common in cats (overall 3% of all skin tumors). In dogs, the median age for diagnosis of these tumors is 9 years, with the majority of tumors occurring between 6 and 11 years of age.[133] The front legs were the most common site for dogs. Golden retrievers and Treeing Walker coonhounds may be predisposed to the development of apocrine gland adenocarcinomas.[132,134] In a series of apocrine gland tumors, 40 of 44 in dogs were considered malignant on histopathologic examination and 8 of 10 in cats.[134] In cats, the tumors occurred from 6 to 17 years of age, and no breed or sex predilections were identified. The most common locations for this tumor in cats are the head, limbs, and abdomen.[132] In both species, most lesions are solitary. In addition to the nodular tumors, apocrine gland carcinomas may present as erosive and inflammatory skin disease. This presentation is sometimes designated as an "inflammatory carcinoma."[132]

Local invasion of apocrine gland carcinomas is common, with 66% of tumors demonstrating invasion of the capsule and/or stroma and 11% invading the vasculature.[133] In another series of cases, 22.5% had invasion of the lymphatic system.[134] Grossly, there were no distinguishing features to differentiate benign from malignant lesions. Despite the high incidence of local invasion, the rate of distant metastasis in these two case series was low, with only two dogs developing local recurrence/continued growth (4%) and one developing distant metastatic disease to the lungs (2%). This is distinctly different from the high metastatic rate seen with apocrine gland carcinomas of the anal sac. In general, optimal treatment consists of wide surgical excision of these tumors, although the author has seen several of these tumors develop distant metastatic disease. No reports on the efficacy of radiation or chemotherapy for the treatment of apocrine gland carcinomas of the skin were found.

Eccrine Adenomas and Carcinomas

Eccrine adenomas and carcinomas are tumors of the sweat glands of the foot pads. They are considered rare in dogs and cats, and no reports on clinical behavior or outcome were found. Treatment is wide surgical excision.[84]

Neuroendocrine Carcinomas

Neuroendocrine carcinomas are also known as Merkel cell carcinomas. Merkel cells are thought to be part of the mechanoreceptor in the skin. Recent studies in human Merkel cell tumors have demonstrated a role for the Merkel cell polyomavirus in the development of these tumors.[135] Although a highly malignant tumor in humans, most case reports in veterinary medicine suggest a more benign clinical course.[136,137] There is a single case report in a cat with multiple recurrences and the development of pulmonary metastases, suggesting a more malignant behavior can be seen.[138] A similar case in a dog reported multiple skin masses with widespread metastasis in the abdomen.[139] An additional canine case report described a dog with multiple (six) lesions that progressed with carboplatin and doxorubicin chemotherapy, as well as with metronomic chemotherapy treatment.[140] A recent evaluation of two canine neuroendocrine carcinomas demonstrated expression of β-catenin or E-cadherin, which are proteins whose loss predicts a more malignant behavior in humans.[141] However, there was expression of chromogranin-A, neurone-specific enolase, S100, and c-KIT (which is also expressed in human neuroendocrine carcinomas). Current treatment recommendations reflect the generally benign behavior of these tumors and consist of wide surgical excision. The efficacy of chemotherapy for treatment of more widespread tumors is unknown, as is the effect of c-KIT-targeted TKI.

Renal Cystadenocarcinoma and Nodular Dermatofibrosis

A syndrome of renal cystadenocarcinoma and nodular dermatofibrosis has been described in German shepherd dogs and Alsatians (see Chapter 29).[63,66] These dogs have multiple firm, haired masses distributed over their bodies. On histopathologic examination, these nodules are dense, irregular collagen. They typically do not result in clinical problems unless they cause lameness or otherwise disrupt normal function. Surgical removal is indicated in these instances. Most of these dogs will die from renal failure or progressive renal cystadenocarcinoma, on average 3 years after initial detection of the dermatofibrosis.[142] There are no known effective treatments for the renal cysts or bilateral renal adenocarcinomas. A recent case report of nodular dermatofibrosis in an Australian cattle dog without any evidence at necropsy of renal cysts or adenocarcinomas reveals the possibility of a nonlethal version of this syndrome.[143]

Tumors of the Ear Canal

Ceruminous glands are modified apocrine glands found in the external ear canal. Benign and malignant tumors arising from these glands are the most common tumor types in the ear. Additional tumor types that have been reported include SCCs, undifferentiated carcinomas, BCCs, fibromas, papillomas, hemangiosarcomas (HSAs), mast cell tumors, melanomas, sebaceous gland tumors, ceruminous gland cysts, and histiocytomas.[144-147] Inflammatory polyps are also found in dogs and more commonly in cats.

In the largest published series of tumors of the ear canal, the 33 benign tumors diagnosed in dogs were comprised of polyps (8), papillomas (6), sebaceous gland adenomas (5), BCTs (5), ceruminous gland adenomas (4), and histiocytomas (2) and single cases of plasmacytoma, melanoma, and fibroma. The 8 benign feline tumors were polyps (4), ceruminous gland adenomas (3), and one papilloma.[147]

In this same series, the relative frequencies of malignant tumors in 48 dogs consisted of 23 ceruminous gland adenocarcinomas, 9 undifferentiated carcinomas, 8 SCCs, 3 round cell tumors, 2 sarcomas, 2 malignant melanomas, and a single case of HSA. In cats, the most common malignant tumor was also ceruminous gland adenocarcinomas, with 22 cases, followed by SCCs (20), carcinomas of undetermined origin (13), and one case of sebaceous gland adenocarcinoma.

Most tumors of the ear canal are diagnosed due to the mass effect, which may result in clinical signs such as chronic otitis or partial deafness. Occasionally, patients may present for pain on opening of the mouth or neurologic signs, but this is more common with malignant tumors.[147] The role of chronic otitis in the development of these tumors is an area of ongoing discussion.

Ceruminous Gland Adenomas and Cysts

Ceruminous gland adenomas and cysts are benign tumors of the ceruminous gland. On gross appearance, they are typically exophytic and pedunculated, although they can also be ulcerated.[148] Cats with ceruminous gland adenomas are slightly younger than those patients presenting with malignant tumors; in dogs, both lesions present around 9 years of age.[147,148] Cocker spaniels and poodles appear predisposed to the development of these tumors. Treatment of choice is adequate surgical excision.

Ceruminous gland cysts can be found in cats. These are darkly pigmented, sessile masses that are usually smaller than 5 mm in diameter and can be multiple.[146] If necessary, these can be surgically excised.

Ceruminous Gland Adenocarcinomas

Ceruminous gland adenocarcinomas are the most common malignant tumors of the ear canal in both dogs and cats. In dogs, it has been reported that cocker spaniels and German shepherd dogs are at increased risk.[148] Malignant ceruminous gland tumors are more common than benign tumors in cats; however, there is conflicting information on whether malignant or benign tumors are more common in the dog.[148,149]

Ceruminous gland adenocarcinomas have metastatic potential, and full staging is recommended prior to treatment. Local invasion, even through the cartilage of the ear canal, can occur. CT is indicated to better delineate the extent of local invasion prior to surgery. Skull radiographs revealed lysis of the bulla in 13 of 27 dogs with malignant tumors of the ear canal and sclerosis of the bulla in 8. In the cats with malignant tumors, 5 of 27 had lysis of the bulla on skull radiographs and 5 had sclerosis of the bulla.[147] Thirty dogs had regional lymph nodes evaluated cytologically for evidence of metastasis, and only one dog tested positive. In contrast, 5 of 56 cats had cytologic evidence of metastasis to the mandibular (4) or superficial cervical (1) node. Three of 35 dogs radiographed with malignant ear tumors had evidence of pulmonary metastasis at the time of diagnosis, and one had a lytic scapular lesion. Of the 32 cats evaluated for pulmonary metastasis, none had evidence on chest radiographs.[147] However, these tumors have an increased metastatic potential over time—in a series of seven patients (dogs and cats) evaluated for metastasis after radiation therapy, three had spread: one to a lymph node, one to the lungs, and one to abdominal organs.[150] A staging scheme derived from the one used in humans has been proposed for primary tumors of the ear canal (Box 18-2).[150]

The primary modality of treatment of tumors of the ear canal is complete surgical excision. This is best accomplished with a total ear canal ablation (TECA) and lateral bulla osteotomy.[151,152] Recurrence was significantly lower in both dogs and cats treated with this surgical approach, compared to those treated with a lateral ear canal resection: seven dogs treated with TECA had no recurrences and a median follow-up of 36 months; of four dogs treated with lateral ear canal resection, three recurred with a median follow-up time of 4 months. Of 16 cats treated with TECA/lateral bulla osteotomy, the recurrence rate was 25% with a median disease-free interval of 42 months. The six cats treated with a lateral ear canal resection had a recurrence rate of 66.7% and median disease-free interval of 10 months. A second case series of 18 cats treated with TECA for ceruminous gland adenocarcinomas was equally encouraging. Median survival for cats undergoing TECA for malignant tumors was 50.3 months, statistically equivalent to the median survivals for cats with nonneoplastic diseases (33.7 and 24.3 months).[153] Five of these cats developed local recurrence. None of the 18 cats had evidence of metastasis at the time of surgery. Radiation therapy also appears effective for the treatment of ceruminous gland adenocarcinomas.[150] Treatment of six cats and five dogs with orthovoltage, 48 Gy in 12 4-Gy fractions, resulted in an estimated mean PFS of 39.5 months. Six of these patients had previous surgery. One year PFS was 56%.

Several prognostic factors that have been determined for ceruminous gland adenocarcinomas are presented in Table 18-3. In cats, a grading scheme failed to be prognostic for survival, but a mitotic index of 2 or less predicted improved survival. A correlation between mitotic index and tumor grade was also noted in a series of patients treated with radiation therapy, although the small sample size precluded further evaluation for prognostic significance.[150] The overriding conclusion from the series of studies regarding treatment for ceruminous gland adenocarcinomas is that long-term survival is possible with appropriate local therapy.

Box 18-2 Proposed Staging Scheme for Primary Tumors of the Ear Canal

T1	Tumor confined to the external or horizontal ear canal
T2	Tumor extending beyond the tympanic membrane
T3	Tumor extending beyond the middle ear/bone destruction

Data from Theon AP, Barthez PY, Madewell BR, et al: Radiation therapy of ceruminous gland carcinomas in dogs and cats, *J Am Vet Med Assoc* 205:566–569, 1994.

Tumors of the Digit

The most common clinical signs in dogs with digital tumors are the presence of a mass and/or lameness. These dogs tend to be older, with a median age of 10 years.[156,157] A review of three retrospective studies totaling 362 malignancies on the relative frequency of different malignancies in the digit of the dog revealed that SCC is the most common, with 171 tumors (47.2%), followed by malignant melanoma, with 86 cases (23.8%).[156-158] Interestingly, approximately 3% of dogs with digital SCC demonstrated involvement of multiple digits. These patients are typically large breed dogs with black skin and haircoat[159] (Figure 18-6). Breeds with this syndrome include standard poodles, black Labradors, giant schnauzers, Gordon setters, and Rottweilers. Additional breeds that may be predisposed to digital SCC include the dachshund and flat coat retriever.[158]

Table 18-3 Prognostic Factors for Primary Tumors of the Ear Canal

Prognostic Factor		Species	Median Survival Months	Reference
Mitoses per high power field	≤2	Feline	≈180	153
	≥3		≈12	
Extension beyond the ear canal	No	Canine	30	147
	Yes		5.9	
Presence of neurologic signs	No	Feline	15.5	147
	Yes		1.5	
Histology	Ceruminous gland adenocarcinoma	Feline	49	147
	Squamous cell carcinoma		3.8	
	Cancer of unknown origin		5.7	
Extension beyond the ear canal	No	Feline	21.7	147
	Yes		4	

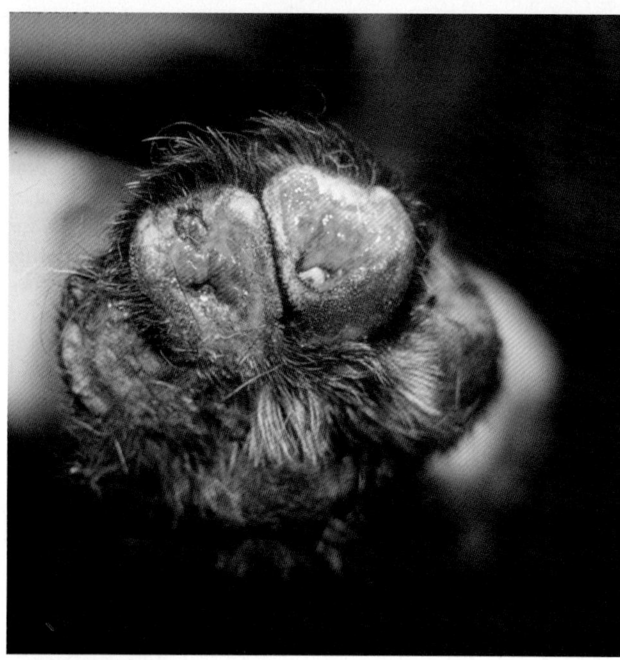

FIGURE 18-6 Paw of a dog with multiple, digital squamous cell carcinomas.

Scottish terriers were overrepresented in the dogs with digital malignant melanomas. The remainder of the tumors were comprised of 48 soft tissue sarcomas (13.3%); 28 mast cell tumors (7.7%); 12 osteosarcomas (OSAs;3.3%); 4 round cell sarcomas; 3 adenocarcinomas; 2 malignant adnexal tumors; 2 HSAs; 2 plasmacytomas and 1 dog each with lymphoma, chondrosarcoma, giant cell tumor of bone, and synovial cell sarcoma. Similar results were found for malignant tumors of feline digits.[160] In a series of 60 digital malignancies, 15 (25%) were SCC, 14 were fibrosarcoma (23.3%), 13 cases of adenocarcinoma (21.6%) were diagnosed, and there were 5 cases each of OSA and HSA. There were also 4 cases of mast cell tumor, 2 cases each of giant cell tumor of bone and malignant fibrous histiocytoma, and 1 sarcoma of unknown origin. There may be a predilection for tumor development in the front feet. Two of the cats with fibrosarcoma and 4 of the cats with adenocarcinoma had involvement of multiple digits. Primary SCC of the digit has also been reported to affect adjacent toes.[161] Malignant melanoma has also been diagnosed on feline digits.[162]

A number of nonneoplastic masses can also be found on the digit. In addition to the malignancies listed previously, pyogranulomatous inflammations, epithelial inclusion cysts, intracutaneous cornifying epitheliomas, IKAs, keratoacanthomas, benign adnexal tumors, histiocytomas, hemangiomas, BCTs, intraosseous epidermoid cysts, infiltrating lipomas, fibromas, papillomas, hamartomas, trichoblastomas, keratomas, cysts, and plasmacytomas have been diagnosed on canine digits.[156,158] It is clinically important that the diagnosis of digital masses is apparently difficult because a review among pathologists demonstrated an approximately 20% rate of disagreement in the diagnosis on amputated digits, with 75% of the changes in diagnosis being clinically significant.[163] In particular, the differentiation between SCC and IKA is apparently problematic. In cats, the nonneoplastic mass lesions included inflammatory masses, hemangiomas, and a BCT.[160]

One key difference in the evaluation of digital masses in cats is the clinical syndrome of digital metastasis with primary pulmonary carcinomas. In a series of 64 cats with digital carcinomas, 87.5% of the lesions represented metastasis from primary lung tumors, whereas only 8 had primary SCC of the digit.[161] These tumors were able to be differentiated based on histopathologic staining characteristics, as well as cell morphology. In this series of cases, median survival of cats with digital metastatic lesions was only 4.9 weeks, whereas cats with primary digital SCC had a median survival of 29.5 weeks.

Digital tumors can metastasize and thus require appropriate staging at initial evaluation.[155-158] In dogs with digital SCC, 8.8% (5/57) had evidence of metastasis at the time of presentation and an additional 23.2% (23/99) went on to develop metastasis. Bone lysis was very common in these patients, with 80.7% (46/57) showing lysis on radiographs. Dogs with malignant melanomas had a higher percentage presenting with metastatic disease, with 12/43 (28%) having either regional or distant metastasis. An additional 25 of 65 dogs (38.5%) developed metastasis at a later time. Nine dogs (21%) had evidence of bone invasion on radiographs, whereas 14/14 dogs in a separate study had histologic evidence of bone invasion.[164] Additional digital tumors that developed metastatic disease include one dog with OSA, one dog diagnosed with a keratoacanthoma (considered likely to be a well-differentiated SCC), and one dog with a malignant adnexal tumor. It is important to note these are minimum estimates of metastatic rates because not all dogs were fully staged or necropsied.

Of eight cats with digital SCC, three of six had evidence of bone invasion and one cat had metastasis to the draining lymph node.[161] Only three cats had chest radiographs, none of which demonstrated pulmonary metastasis. Of the five reported feline cases of digital malignant melanoma, four developed metastasis to lymph node, lung, bone, and vertebrae.[162]

Treatment reports for digital tumors are primarily limited to surgery, which is the only treatment modality that has been shown to improve outcome.[157] In the majority of cases, wide surgical excision can be accomplished with a toe amputation. However, a limb amputation may be necessary for larger tumors involving more of the foot. For SCC of the digit, reported 1-year survival rates range from 50% to 83% and reported 2-year survival rates from 18% to 62%.[156-158] When divided by site of origin, dogs with SCC arising from the subungual epithelium had a significantly improved survival in comparison with dogs with SCC from other sites on the digit. Dogs with a subungual SCC had 1- and 2-year survival rates of 95% and 74%, respectively, whereas dogs with SCC at other digital sites had 1- and 2-year survival rates of 60% and 40%, respectively.[156] Median survival times for cats with digital SCC are reported from 73 days to 29.5 weeks.[160,161]

Dogs with digital malignant melanoma had similar survival times as dogs with digital SCC. One-year survival rates for these patients ranged from 42% to 57%, and 2-year survival rates from 13% to 36%.[155-158,164] Of five cats diagnosed with digital malignant melanoma, survival times ranged from 0 to 577+ days, with four of the five cats developing metastatic disease.[162]

The possible roles of radiation therapy and chemotherapy remain to be elucidated for the treatment of malignant digital tumors in the dog and cat. The high metastatic rate in dogs with digital malignant melanoma clearly suggests that adjuvant treatment should be considered. A recent paper evaluated the use of a xenogeneic (murine) tyrosinase vaccine in dogs with digital melanoma.[165] Fifty-seven of the 58 dogs had surgical excision of their primary tumor prior to treatment with the vaccination. Three dogs had received adjuvant chemotherapy, and two dogs had received radiation therapy. Sixteen dogs (27%) had regional or distant metastasis at the time of presentation. The overall median survival time from the time of digit amputation was 476 days, with a 1- and 2-year survival rate of 63% and 32%, respectively. This study did identify the presence of metastatic disease as a negative prognostic factor. Distant metastatic disease carried a worse prognosis than metastasis to regional lymph nodes. This finding was interesting because evaluation of prognostic factors on overall survival in dogs with digital neoplasia, including tumor stage and the presence or absence of metastatic disease, resulted in no useful prognostic factors aside from surgery in an earlier study.[157] The implication of the earlier finding was that surgery is beneficial, even in dogs with metastatic disease. The smaller number of dogs (10) in this earlier study may have contributed to the lack of statistical significance.

In summary, complete resection of malignant digital tumors can result in long-term survival. Additional consideration to adjuvant treatment for possible metastatic disease should be considered in patients with malignant melanomas.

REFERENCES

1. Pakhrin B, Kang MS, Bae IH, et al: Retrospective study of canine cutaneous tumors in Korea, *J Vet Sci* 8:229–236, 2007.
2. Priester WA: Skin tumors in domestic animals. Data from 12 United States and Canadian colleges of veterinary medicine, *J Natl Cancer Inst* 50:457–466, 1973.
3. MacVean DW, Monlux AW, Anderson PS Jr, et al: Frequency of canine and feline tumors in a defined population, *Vet Pathol* 15:700–715, 1978.
4. Dorn CR, Taylor DO, Schneider R, et al: Survey of animal neoplasms in Alameda and Contra Costa Counties, California. II. Cancer morbidity in dogs and cats from Alameda County, *J Natl Cancer Inst* 40:307–318, 1968.
5. Miller MA, Nelson SL, Turk JR, et al: Cutaneous neoplasia in 340 cats, *Vet Pathol* 28:389–395, 1991.
6. Carpenter JL, Andrews LK, Holzworth J: Tumors and tumor-like lesions, In Holzworth J, editor: *Diseases of the cat: Medicine and surgery*, Philadephia, 1987, WB Saunders.
7. Brodey RS: Canine and feline neoplasia, *Adv Vet Sci Comp Med* 14:309–354, 1970.
8. Finnie JW, Bostock DE: Skin neoplasia in dogs, *Aust Vet J* 55:602–604, 1979.
9. Bostock DE: Neoplasia of the skin and mammary glands in dogs and cats. In Kirk RW, editor: *Current veterinary therapy small animal practice*, Philadelphia, 1977, WB Saunders.
10. Rothwell TL, Howlett CR, Middleton DJ, et al: Skin neoplasms of dogs in Sydney, *Aust Vet J* 64:161–164, 1987.
11. Kaldrymidou H, Leontides L, Koutinas AF, et al: Prevalence, distribution and factors associated with the presence and the potential for malignancy of cutaneous neoplasms in 174 dogs admitted to a clinic in northern Greece, *J Vet Med A Physiol Pathol Clin Med* 49:87–91, 2002.
12. Ladds PW, Kraft H, Sokale A, et al: Neoplasms of the skin of dogs in tropical Queensland, *Aust Vet J* 60:87–88, 1983.
13. Mukaratirwa S, Chipunza J, Chitanga S, et al: Canine cutaneous neoplasms: prevalence and influence of age, sex and site on the presence and potential malignancy of cutaneous neoplasms in dogs from Zimbabwe, *J S Afr Vet Assoc* 76:59–62, 2005.
14. Er JC, Sutton RH: A survey of skin neoplasms in dogs from the Brisbane region, *Aust Vet J* 66:225–227, 1989.
15. Jorger K: [Skin tumors in cats. Occurrence and frequency in the research material (biopsies from 1984-1987) of the Institute for Veterinary Pathology, Zurich], *Schweiz Arch Tierheilk* 130:559–569, 1988.
16. Mellemkjaer L, Holmich LR, Gridley G, et al: Risks for skin and other cancers up to 25 years after burn injuries, *Epidemiology* 17:668–673, 2006.
17. Narayanan DL, Saladi RN, Fox JL: Ultraviolet radiation and skin cancer, *Int J Dermatol* 49:978–986, 2010.
18. Dorn CR, Taylor DO, Schneider R: Sunlight exposure and risk of developing cutaneous and oral squamous cell carcinomas in white cats, *J Natl Cancer Inst* 46:1073–1078, 1971.
19. Nikula KJ, Benjamin SA, Angleton GM, et al: Ultraviolet radiation, solar dermatosis, and cutaneous neoplasia in beagle dogs, *Radiat Res* 129:11–18, 1992.
20. Hargis AM, Thomassen RW, Phemister RD: Chronic dermatosis and cutaneous squamous cell carcinoma in the beagle dog, *Vet Pathol* 14:218–228, 1977.
21. Madewell BR, Conroy JD, Hodgkins EM: Sunlight-skin cancer association in the dog: a report of three cases, *J Cutan Pathol* 8:434–443, 1981.
22. Knowles DP, Hargis AM: Solar elastosis associated with neoplasia in two dalmations, *Vet Pathol* 23:512–514, 1986.
23. Lana SE, Ogilvie GK, Withrow SJ, et al: Feline cutaneous squamous cell carcinoma of the nasal planum and the pinnae: 61 cases, *J Am Anim Hosp Assoc* 33:329–332, 1997.
24. Munday JS, Kiupel M: Papillomavirus-associated cutaneous neoplasia in mammals, *Vet Pathol* 47:254–264, 2010.
25. zur Hausen H: Human papillomavirus & cervical cancer, *Indian J Med Res* 130:209, 2009.
26. Munday JS, Gibson I, French AF: Papillomaviral DNA and increased p16CDKN2A protein are frequently present within feline cutaneous squamous cell carcinomas in ultraviolet-protected skin, *Vet Dermatol* 22:360–366, 2011.
27. Stockfleth E, Ulrich C, Meyer T, et al: Skin diseases following organ transplantation–risk factors and new therapeutic approaches, *Transplant Proc* 33:1848–1853, 2001.
28. Stockfleth E, Nindl I, Sterry W, et al: Human papillomaviruses in transplant-associated skin cancers, *Dermatol Surg* 30:604–609, 2004.
29. Chambers VC, Evans CA: Canine oral papillomatosis. I. Virus assay and observations on the various stages of the experimental infection, *Cancer Res* 19:1188–1195, 1959.
30. Bregman CL, Hirth RS, Sundberg JP, et al: Cutaneous neoplasms in dogs associated with canine oral papillomavirus vaccine, *Vet Pathol* 24:477–487, 1987.
31. Teifke JP, Lohr CV, Shirasawa H: Detection of canine oral papillomavirus-DNA in canine oral squamous cell carcinomas and p53 overexpressing skin papillomas of the dog using the polymerase chain reaction and non-radioactive in situ hybridization, *Vet Microbiol* 60:119–130, 1998.
32. Stokking LB, Ehrhart EJ, Lichtensteiger CA, et al: Pigmented epidermal plaques in three dogs, *J Am Anim Hosp Assoc* 40:411–417, 2004.
33. Yuan H, Ghim S, Newsome J, et al: An epidermotropic canine papillomavirus with malignant potential contains an E5 gene and establishes a unique genus, *Virology* 359:28–36, 2007.
34. Goldschmidt MH, Kennedy JS, Kennedy DR, et al: Severe papillomavirus infection progressing to metastatic squamous cell carcinoma in bone marrow-transplanted X-linked SCID dogs, *J Virol* 80:6621–6628, 2006.
35. Zaugg N, Nespeca G, Hauser B, et al: Detection of novel papillomaviruses in canine mucosal, cutaneous and in situ squamous cell carcinomas, *Vet Dermatol* 16:290–298, 2005.
36. Watrach AM, Small E, Case MT: Canine papilloma: progression of oral papilloma to carcinoma, *J Natl Cancer Inst* 45:915–920, 1970.
37. Schwegler K, Walter JH, Rudolph R: Epithelial neoplasms of the skin, the cutaneous mucosa and the transitional epithelium in dogs: an immunolocalization study for papillomavirus antigen, *Zentral Veterinarmed A* 44:115–123, 1997.
38. Lucroy MD, Hill FI, Moore PF, et al: Cutaneous papillomatosis in a dog with malignant lymphoma following long-term chemotherapy, *J Vet Diagn Invest* 10:369–371, 1998.
39. Campbell KL, Sundberg JP, Goldschmidt MH, et al: Cutaneous inverted papillomas in dogs, *Vet Pathol* 25:67–71, 1988.

40. Shimada A, Shinya K, Awakura T, et al: Cutaneous papillomatosis associated with papillomavirus infection in a dog, *J Compar Pathol* 108:103–107, 1993.
41. Munday JS, O'Connor KI, Smits B: Development of multiple pigmented viral plaques and squamous cell carcinomas in a dog infected by a novel papillomavirus, *Vet Dermatol* 22:104–110, 2011.
42. Sundberg JP, Van Ranst M, Montali R, et al: Feline papillomas and papillomaviruses, *Vet Pathol* 37:1–10, 2000.
43. Schulman FY, Krafft AE, Janczewski T: Feline cutaneous fibropapillomas: clinicopathologic findings and association with papillomavirus infection, *Vet Pathol* 38:291–296, 2001.
44. Wilhelm S, Degorce-Rubiales F, Godson D, et al: Clinical, histological and immunohistochemical study of feline viral plaques and bowenoid in situ carcinomas, *Vet Dermatol* 17:424–431, 2006.
45. O'Neill SH, Newkirk KM, Anis EA, et al: Detection of human papillomavirus DNA in feline premalignant and invasive squamous cell carcinoma, *Vet Dermatol* 22:68–74, 2011.
46. Lange CE, Tobler K, Markau T, et al: Sequence and classification of FdPV2, a papillomavirus isolated from feline Bowenoid in situ carcinomas, *Vet Microbiol* 137:60–65, 2009.
47. Moloney FJ, Comber H, O'Lorcain P, et al: A population-based study of skin cancer incidence and prevalence in renal transplant recipients, *Br J Dermatol* 154:498–504, 2006.
48. Callan MB, Preziosi D, Mauldin E: Multiple papillomavirus-associated epidermal hamartomas and squamous cell carcinomas in situ in a dog following chronic treatment with prednisone and cyclosporine, *Vet Dermatol* 16:338–345, 2005.
49. Cockerell GL, Slauson DO: Patterns of lymphoid infiltrate in the canine cutaneous histiocytoma, *J Compar Pathol* 89:193–203, 1979.
50. Epstein EH: Basal cell carcinomas: attack of the hedgehog, *Nat Rev Cancer* 8:743–754, 2008.
51. Mayr B, Wallner A, Reifinger M, et al: Reciprocal translocation in a case of canine basal cell carcinoma, *J Small Anim Pract* 39:96–97, 1998.
52. Ortner BM, Reifinger GL: Monosomy E3 in a feline basal cell tumour, *J Small Anim Pract* 36:400–401, 1995.
53. Mayr B, Ortner W: Trisomy E3 in a feline basal cell tumour, *J Small Anim Pract* 36:400–401, 1995.
54. Murakami Y, Tateyama S, Rungsipipat A, et al: Immunohistochemical analysis of cyclin A, cyclin D1 and P53 in mammary tumors, squamous cell carcinomas and basal cell tumors of dogs and cats, *J Vet Med Sci* 62:743–750, 2000.
55. Madewell BR, Gandour-Edwards R, Edwards BF, et al: Bax/bcl-2: cellular modulator of apoptosis in feline skin and basal cell tumours, *J Compar Pathol* 124:115–121, 2001.
56. Swanson PE, Fitzpatrick MM, Ritter JH, et al: Immunohistologic differential diagnosis of basal cell carcinoma, squamous cell carcinoma, and trichoepithelioma in small cutaneous biopsy specimens, *J Cutan Pathol* 25:153–159, 1998.
57. Burnworth B, Arendt S, Muffler S, et al: The multi-step process of human skin carcinogenesis: a role for p53, cyclin D1, hTERT, p16, and TSP-1, *Eur J Cell Biol* 86:763–780, 2007.
58. Teifke JP, Lohr CV: Immunohistochemical detection of P53 overexpression in paraffin wax-embedded squamous cell carcinomas of cattle, horses, cats and dogs, *J Compar Pathol* 114:205–210, 1996.
59. Nasir L, Krasner H, Argyle DJ, et al: Immunocytochemical analysis of the tumour suppressor protein (p53) in feline neoplasia, *Cancer Lett* 155:1–7, 2000.
60. Favrot C, Welle M, Heimann M, et al: Clinical, histologic, and immunohistochemical analyses of feline squamous cell carcinoma in situ, *Vet Pathol* 46:25–33, 2009.
61. Sakai H, Yamane T, Yanai T, et al: Expression of cyclin kinase inhibitor p27(Kip1) in skin tumours of dogs, *J Compar Pathol* 125:153–158, 2001.
62. Bongiovanni L, Malatesta D, Brachelente C, et al: beta-catenin in canine skin: immunohistochemical pattern of expression in normal skin and cutaneous epithelial tumours, *J Compar Pathol* 145:138–147, 2011.
63. Lium B, Moe L: Hereditary multifocal renal cystadenocarcinomas and nodular dermatofibrosis in the German shepherd dog: macroscopic and histopathologic changes, *Vet Pathol* 22:447–455, 1985.
64. Lingaas F, Comstock KE, Kirkness EF, et al: A mutation in the canine BHD gene is associated with hereditary multifocal renal cystadenocarcinoma and nodular dermatofibrosis in the German Shepherd dog, *Hum Mol Genet* 12:3043–3053, 2003.
65. Hasumi H, Baba M, Hong SB, et al: Identification and characterization of a novel folliculin-interacting protein FNIP2, *Gene* 415:60–67, 2008.
66. Suter M, Lott-Stolz G, Wild P: Generalized nodular dermatofibrosis in six Alsatians, *Vet Pathol* 20:632–634, 1983.
67. Hong DS, Reddy SB, Prieto VG, et al: Multiple squamous cell carcinomas of the skin after therapy with sorafenib combined with tipifarnib, *Arch Dermatol* 144:779–782, 2008.
68. Kwon EJ, Kish LS, Jaworsky C: The histologic spectrum of epithelial neoplasms induced by sorafenib, *J Am Acad Dermatol* 61:522–527, 2009.
69. Goldschmidt MH, Dunstan RW, Stannard AA, et al: Histological classification of epithelial and melanocytic tumors of the skin. In Schulman FY, editor: *Worldwide reference for comparative oncology*, ed 2, Washington, 1998, Armed Forces Institute for Pathology.
70. Owen LN: *TNM classification of tumors in domestic animals*, Geneva, 1980, World Health Organization.
71. Hahn KA, Lantz GC, Salisbury SK, et al: Comparison of survey radiography with ultrasonography and x-ray computed tomography for clinical staging of subcutaneous neoplasms in dogs, *J Am Vet Med Assoc* 196:1795–1798, 1990.
72. Kamstock DA, Ehrhart EJ, Getzy DM, et al: Recommended guidelines for submission, trimming, margin evaluation, and reporting of tumor biopsy specimens in veterinary surgical pathology, *Vet Pathol* 48:19–31, 2011.
73. Gross TL, Ihrke PJ, Walder EJ, et al: *Skin diseases of the dog and cat: Clinical and histopathologic diagnosis*, ed 2. Ames, Iowa, 2005, Blackwell Science Ltd.
74. Stockhaus C, Teske E, Rudolph R, et al: Assessment of cytological criteria for diagnosing basal cell tumours in the dog and cat, *J Small Anim Pract* 42:582–586, 2001.
75. Bohn AA, Wills T, Caplazi P: Basal cell tumor or cutaneous basilar epithelial neoplasm? Rethinking the cytologic diagnosis of basal cell tumors, *Vet Clin Pathol* 35:449–453, 2006.
76. Gross TL, Ihrke PJ, Walder EJ, et al: Epidermal tumors. In Gross TL, Ihrke PJ, Walder EJ, et al, editors: *Skin diseases in the dog and cat: clinical and histopathologic diagnosis*, Ames, Iowa, 2005, Blackwell Science Ltd.
77. Simeonov R, Simeonova G: Comparative morphometric analysis of recurrent and nonrecurrent canine basal cell carcinomas: a preliminary report, *Vet Clin Pathol* 39:96–98, 2010.
78. Gross TL, Ihrke PJ, Walder EJ, et al: Sweat gland tumors. In Gross TL, Ihrke PJ, Walder EJ, et al, editors: *Skin diseases of the dog and cat: clinical and histopathologic diagnosis*, ed 2, Ames, Iowa, 2005, Blackwell Science Ltd.
79. Carpenter JL, Andrews LK, Holzworth J: Tumors and tumor-like lesions. In Holzworth J, editor: *Diseases of the cat: medicine and surgery*, Philadelphia, 1987, WB Saunders.
80. Diters RW, Walsh KM: Feline basal cell tumors: A review of 124 cases, *Vet Pathol* 21:51–56, 1984.
81. Fehrer SL, Lin SH: Multicentric basal cell tumors in a cat, *J Am Vet Med Assoc* 189:1469–1470, 1986.
82. Day DG, Couto CG, Weisbrode SE, et al: Basal cell carcinoma in two cats, *J Am Anim Hosp Assoc* 30:265–269, 1994.
83. Simeonov R, Simeonova G: Nucleomorphometric analysis of feline basal cell carcinomas, *Res Vet Sci* 84:440–443, 2008.
84. Goldschmidt MH, Hendrick MJ: Tumors of the skin and soft tissues, In Meuten DJ, editor: *Tumors in domestic animals*, ed 4, Ames, Iowa, 2002, Iowa State Press.

85. Debey BM, Bagladi-Swanson M, Kapil S, et al: Digital papillomatosis in a confined Beagle, *J Vet Diagn Invest* 13:346–348, 2001.
86. Yagci BB, Ural K, Ocal N, et al: Azithromycin therapy of papillomatosis in dogs: a prospective, randomized, double-blinded, placebo-controlled clinical trial, *Vet Dermatol* 19:194–198, 2008.
87. Teifke JP, Kidney BA, Lohr CV, et al: Detection of papillomavirus-DNA in mesenchymal tumour cells and not in the hyperplastic epithelium of feline sarcoids, *Vet Dermatol* 14:47–56, 2003.
88. Baer KE, Helton K: Multicentric squamous cell carcinoma in situ resembling Bowen's disease in cats, *Vet Pathol* 30:535–543, 1993.
89. Gill VL, Bergman PJ, Baer KE, et al: Use of imiquimod 5% cream (Aldara) in cats with multicentric squamous cell carcinoma in situ: 12 cases (2002-2005), *Vet Comp Oncol* 6:55–64, 2008.
90. Gross TL, Brimacomb BH: Multifocal intraepidermal carcinoma in a dog histologically resembling Bowen's disease, *Am J Dermatopathol* 8:509–515, 1986.
91. Braathen LR, Szeimies RM, Basset-Seguin N, et al: Guidelines on the use of photodynamic therapy for nonmelanoma skin cancer: An international consensus. International Society for Photodynamic Therapy in Dermatology, 2005, *J Am Acad Dermatol* 56:125–143, 2007.
92. Buchholz J, Wergin M, Walt H, et al: Photodynamic therapy of feline cutaneous squamous cell carcinoma using a newly developed liposomal photosensitizer: preliminary results concerning drug safety and efficacy, *J Vet Intern Med* 21:770–775, 2007.
93. Peaston AE, Leach MW, Higgins RJ: Photodynamic therapy for nasal and aural squamous cell carcinoma in cats, *J Am Vet Med Assoc* 202:1261–1265, 1993.
94. Hammond GM, Gordon IK, Theon AP, et al: Evaluation of strontium Sr 90 for the treatment of superficial squamous cell carcinoma of the nasal planum in cats: 49 cases (1990-2006), *J Am Vet Med Assoc* 231:736–741, 2007.
95. Evans AG, Madewell BR, Stannard AA: A trial of 13-cis-retinoic acid for treatment of squamous cell carcinoma and preneoplastic lesions of the head in cats, *Am J Vet Res* 46:2553–2557, 1985.
96. Marks SL, Song MD, Stannard AA, et al: Clinical evaluation of etretinate for the treatment of canine solar-induced squamous cell carcinoma and preneoplastic lesions, *J Am Acad Dermatol* 27:11–16, 1992.
97. Goldschmidt MH, Shofer FS: Squamous cell carcinoma. In *Skin tumors of the dog and cat*. Oxford, 1998, Reed Educational and Professional Publishing Ltd.
98. Lascelles BD, Parry AT, Stidworthy MF, et al: Squamous cell carcinoma of the nasal planum in 17 dogs, *Vet Rec* 147:473–476, 2000.
99. Klausner JS, Bell FW, Hayden DW, et al: Hypercalcemia in two cats with squamous cell carcinomas, *J Am Vet Med Assoc* 196:103–105, 1990.
100. Savary KC, Price GS, Vaden SL: Hypercalcemia in cats: A retrospective study of 71 cases (1991-1997), *J Vet Intern Med* 14:184–189, 2000.
101. Theon AP, Madewell BR, Shearn VI, et al: Prognostic factors associated with radiotherapy of squamous cell carcinoma of the nasal plane in cats, *J Am Vet Med Assoc* 206:991–996, 1995.
102. Jonsson L, Gustafsson PO: Bone-metastasizing squamous-cell carcinoma of the skin in a dog, *J Small Anim Pract* 14:159–165, 1973.
103. Lascelles BD, Henderson RA, Seguin B, et al: Bilateral rostral maxillectomy and nasal planectomy for large rostral maxillofacial neoplasms in six dogs and one cat, *J Am Anim Hosp Assoc* 40:137–146, 2004.
104. Goodfellow M, Hayes A, Murphy S, et al: A retrospective study of (90)Strontium plesiotherapy for feline squamous cell carcinoma of the nasal planum, *J Feline Med Surg* 8:169–176, 2006.
105. Fidel JL, Egger E, Blattmann H, et al: Proton irradiation of feline nasal planum squamous cell carcinomas using an accelerated protocol, *Vet Radiol Ultrasound* 42:569–575, 2001.
106. Thrall DE, Adams WM: Radiotherapy of squamous cell carcinomas of the canine nasal plane, *Vet Radiol* 23:193–195, 1982.
107. Theon AP, VanVechten MK, Madewell BR: Intratumoral administration of carboplatin for treatment of squamous cell carcinomas of the nasal plane in cats, *Am J Vet Res* 57:205–210, 1996.
108. Himsel CA, Richardson RC, Craig JA: Cisplatin chemotherapy for metastatic squamous cell carcinoma in two dogs, *J Am Vet Med Assoc* 189:1575–1578, 1986.
109. Buhles WC Jr, Theilen GH: Preliminary evaluation of bleomycin in feline and canine squamous cell carcinoma, *Am J Vet Res* 34:289–291, 1973.
110. Hammer AS, Couto CG, Ayl RD, et al: Treatment of tumor-bearing dogs with actinomycin D, *J Vet Intern Med* 8:236–239, 1994.
111. Ogilvie GK, Obradovich JE, Elmslie RE, et al: Efficacy of mitoxantrone against various neoplasms in dogs, *J Am Vet Med Assoc* 198:1618–1621, 1991.
112. Ogilvie GK, Moore AS, Obradovich JE, et al: Toxicoses and efficacy associated with administration of mitoxantrone to cats with malignant tumors, *J Am Vet Med Assoc* 202:1839–1844, 1993.
113. Abramo F, Pratesi F, Cantile C, et al: Survey of canine and feline follicular tumours and tumour-like lesions in central Italy, *J Small Anim Pract* 40:479–481, 1999.
114. Stannard AA, Pulley LT: Intracutaneous cornifying epithelioma (keratoacanthoma) in the dog: a retrospective study of 25 cases, *J Am Vet Med Assoc* 167:385–388, 1975.
115. White SD, Rosychuk RA, Scott KV, et al: Use of isotretinoin and etretinate for the treatment of benign cutaneous neoplasia and cutaneous lymphoma in dogs, *J Am Vet Med Assoc* 202:387–391, 1993.
116. Goldschmidt MH, Schofer FS: *Intracutaneous cornifying epithelioma. Skin tumors of the dog and cat*, Oxford, 1998, Reed Educational and Professional Publishing Ltd.
117. Diters RW, Goldschmidt MH: Hair follicle tumors resembling tricholemmomas in six dogs, *Vet Pathol* 20:123–125, 1983.
118. Walsh KM, Corapi WV: Tricholemmomas in three dogs, *J Compar Pathol* 96:115–117, 1986.
119. Sharif M, Reinacher M: Clear cell trichoblastomas in two dogs, *J Vet Med A Physiol Pathol Clin Med* 53:352–354, 2006.
120. Goldschmidt MH, Schofer FS: *Trichoepithelioma. Skin tumors of the dog and cat*, Oxford, 1998, Reed Educational and Professional Publishing Ltd, pp 115–124.
121. Gross TL, Ihrke PJ, Walder EJ, et al: *Follicular tumors. Skin diseases of the dog and cat: clinical and histopathologic diagnosis*, ed 2, Ames, Iowa, 2005, Blackwell Science Ltd, pp 604–640.
122. Goldschmidt MH, Schofer FS: *Pilomatrixoma. Skin tumors of the dog and cat*, Oxford, 1998, Reed Educational and Professional Publishing Ltd, pp 125–130.
123. Carroll EE, Fossey SL, Mangus LM, et al: Malignant pilomatricoma in 3 dogs, *Vet Pathol* 47:937–943, 2010.
124. Johnson RP, Johnson JA, Groom SC, et al: Malignant pilomatrixoma in an old english sheepdog, *Can Vet J* 24:392–394, 1983.
125. Jackson K, Boger L, Goldschmidt M, et al: Malignant pilomatricoma in a soft-coated Wheaten Terrier, *Vet Clin Pathol* 39:236–240, 2010.
126. Scott DW, Anderson WI: Canine sebaceous gland tumors: a retrospective analysis of 172 cases, *Canine Practice* 15:19–27, 1990.
127. Strafuss AC: Sebaceous gland adenomas in dogs, *J Am Vet Med Assoc* 169:640–642, 1976.
128. Goldschmidt MH, Schofer FS: *Sebaceous tumors. Skin tumors of the dog and cat*, Oxford, 1998, Reed Educational and Professional Publishing Ltd.
129. Bettini G, Morini M, Mandrioli L, et al: CNS and lung metastasis of sebaceous epithelioma in a dog, *Vet Dermatol* 20:289–294, 2009.
130. Case MT, Bartz AR, Bernstein M, et al: Metastasis of a sebaceous gland carcinoma in the dog, *J Am Vet Med Assoc* 154:661–664, 1969.
131. Strafuss AC: Sebaceous gland carcinoma in dogs, *J Am Vet Med Assoc* 169:325–326, 1976.

132. Goldschmidt MH, Schofer FS: *Apocrine gland tumors. Skin tumors of the dog and cat*, Oxford, 1998, Reed Educational and Professional Publishing Ltd, pp 80–95.
133. Simko E, Wilcock BP, Yager JA: A retrospective study of 44 canine apocrine sweat gland adenocarcinomas, *Can Vet J* 44:38–42. 2003.
134. Kalaher KM, Anderson WI, Scott DW: Neoplasms of the apocrine sweat glands in 44 dogs and 10 cats, *Vet Rec* 127:400–403, 1990.
135. Chang Y, Moore PS: Merkel cell carcinoma: A virus-induced human cancer, *Annu Rev Pathol* 7:123–144, 2012.
136. Konno A, Nagata M, Nanko H: Immunohistochemical diagnosis of a Merkel cell tumor in a dog, *Vet Pathol* 35:538–540, 1998.
137. Bagnasco G, Properzi R, Porto R, et al: Feline cutaneous neuroendocrine carcinoma (Merkel cell tumour): clinical and pathological findings, *Vet Dermatol* 14:111–115, 2003.
138. Patnaik AK, Post GS, Erlandson RA: Clinicopathologic and electron microscopic study of cutaneous neuroendocrine (Merkel cell) carcinoma in a cat with comparisons to human and canine tumors, *Vet Pathol* 38:553–556, 2001.
139. Glick AD, Holscher MA, Crenshaw JD: Neuroendocrine carcinoma of the skin in a dog, *Vet Pathol* 20:761–763, 1983.
140. Joiner KS, Smith AN, Henderson RA, et al: Multicentric cutaneous neuroendocrine (Merkel cell) carcinoma in a dog, *Vet Pathol* 47:1090–1094, 2010.
141. Gil da Costa RM, Rema A, Pires MA, et al: Two canine Merkel cell tumours: immunoexpression of c-KIT, E-cadherin, beta-catenin and S100 protein, *Vet Dermatol* 21:198–201, 2010.
142. Moe L, Lium B: Hereditary multifocal renal cystadenocarcinomas and nodular dermatofibrosis in 51 German shepherd dogs, *J Small Anim Pract* 38:498–505, 1997.
143. Gardiner DW, Spraker TR: Generalized nodular dermatofibrosis in the absence of renal neoplasia in an Australian Cattle Dog, *Vet Pathol* 45:901–904, 2008.
144. Scott DW: External ear disorders, *J Am Anim Hosp Assoc* 16:426–433, 1980.
145. Legendre AM, Krahwinkel DJ: Feline ear tumors, *J Am Anim Hosp Assoc* 17:1035–1037, 1981.
146. Rogers KS: Tumors of the ear canal, *Vet Clin North Am Small Anim Pract* 18:859–868, 1988.
147. London CA, Dubilzeig RR, Vail DM, et al: Evaluation of dogs and cats with tumors of the ear canal: 145 cases (1978-1992), *J Am Vet Med Assoc* 208:1413–1418, 1996.
148. Goldschmidt MH, Schofer FS: *Ceruminous gland tumors. Skin tumors of the dog and cat*, Oxford, 1998, Reed Educational and Professional Publishing Ltd, pp 96–102.
149. Moisan PG, Watson GL: Ceruminous gland tumors in dogs and cats: a review of 124 cases, *J Am Anim Hosp Assoc* 32:448–452, 1996.
150. Theon AP, Barthez PY, Madewell BR, et al: Radiation therapy of ceruminous gland carcinomas in dogs and cats, *J Am Vet Med Assoc* 205:566–569, 1994.
151. Marino DJ, MacDonald JM, Matthiesen DT, et al: Results of surgery and long-term follow-up in dogs with ceruminous gland adenocarcinoma, *J Am Anim Hosp Assoc* 29:560–563, 1993.
152. Marino DJ, MacDonald JM, Matthiesen DT, et al: Results of surgery in cats with ceruminous gland adenocarcinoma, *J Am Anim Hosp Assoc* 30:54–58, 1994.
153. Bacon NJ, Gilbert RL, Bostock DE, et al: Total ear canal ablation in the cat: indications, morbidity and long-term survival, *J Small Anim Pract* 44:430–434, 2003.
154. Reference deleted in pages.
155. Aronsohn MG, Carpenter JL: Distal extremity melanocytic nevi and malignant melanoma in dogs, *J Am Anim Hosp Assoc* 26:605–612, 1990.
156. Marino DJ, Matthiesen DT, Stefanacci JD, et al: Evaluation of dogs with digit masses: 117 cases (1981-1991), *J Am Vet Med Assoc* 207:726–728, 1995.
157. Henry CJ, Brewer WG Jr, Whitley EM, et al: Canine digital tumors: A Veterinary Cooperative Oncology Group retrospective study of 64 dogs, *J Vet Intern Med* 19:720–724, 2005.
158. Wobeser BK, Kidney BA, Powers BE, et al: Diagnoses and clinical outcomes associated with surgically amputated canine digits submitted to multiple veterinary diagnostic laboratories, *Vet Pathol* 44:355–361, 2007.
159. Madewell BR, Pool RR, Theilen GH, et al: Multiple subungual squamous cell carcinomas in five dogs, *J Am Vet Med Assoc* 180:731–734, 1982.
160. Wobeser BK, Kidney BA, Powers BE, et al: Diagnoses and clinical outcomes associated with surgically amputated feline digits submitted to multiple veterinary diagnostic laboratories, *Vet Pathol* 44:362–365, 2007.
161. van der Linde-Sipman JS, van den Ingh tSGAM: Primary and metastatic carcinomas in the digits of cats, *Vet Q* 22:141–145, 2000.
162. Luna LD, Higginbotham ML, Henry CJ, et al: Feline non-ocular melanoma: a retrospective study of 23 cases (1991-1999), *J Feline Med Surg* 2:173–181, 2000.
163. Wobeser BK, Kidney BA, Powers BE, et al: Agreement among surgical pathologists evaluating routine histologic sections of digits amputated from cats and dogs, *J Vet Diagn Invest* 19:439–443, 2007.
164. Schultheiss PC: Histologic features and clinical outcomes of melanomas of lip, haired skin, and nail bed locations of dogs, *J Vet Diagn Invest* 18:422–425, 2006.
165. Manley CA, Leibman NF, Wolchok JD, et al: Xenogeneic murine tyrosinase DNA vaccine for malignant melanoma of the digit of dogs, *J Vet Intern Med* 25:94–99, 2011.

Melanoma

19

PHILIP J. BERGMAN, MICHAEL S. KENT, AND JAMES P. FARESE

Melanoma is a relatively common cancer of dogs, especially those with significant levels of skin pigmentation. Melanomas in cats are relatively rare. The most common location for canine malignant melanomas (CMMs) is the haired skin, in which they grossly appear to be small brown-to-black masses but can also appear as large, flat, and/or wrinkled masses.[1,2] Primary melanomas also can occur in the oral cavity, nail bed, footpad, eye, gastrointestinal tract, or mucocutaneous junction.[3] Ocular melanomas of dogs and cats represent a distinct clinical syndrome and are discussed in Chapter 31. Metastatic sites can be varied, including local draining lymph nodes, the lungs, liver, meninges, adrenals, and other miscellaneous sites.

Melanoma arises from melanocytes, which are the cells that generate pigment through the melanosome by a number of melanosomal glycoproteins. In humans, cutaneous melanoma can arise due to mutations induced by repeated, intense exposure to ultraviolet (UV) light (e.g., frequent tanning or working outdoors). Melanoma is currently the most rapidly increasing incident human cancer.[4] Significant recent research into the etiology of human melanoma suggests multiple causes that are independent of the aforementioned UV-associated mutagenesis.[5] Since most breeds of dogs have a hair coat that likely affords them protection from sunlight, UV-associated melanoma is less likely as a primary causative agent in the dog. However, pigment cells divide every time there is injury to the skin or if there is constant trauma (e.g., areas where dogs scratch or lick). Nevertheless, risk factors for canine melanoma are not well established.

The most common oral malignancy in the dog is melanoma.[2,3,6,7] Oral melanoma is most commonly diagnosed in Scottish terriers, golden retrievers, poodles, and dachshunds.[2,8] Oral melanoma is primarily a disease of older dogs without gender predilection but may be seen in younger dogs.[8-10] Additional oral tumor differentials include squamous cell carcinoma (SCC), fibrosarcoma, epulides/odontogenic tumors, and others.[2,3,7,11-13] Melanomas in the oral cavities of dogs are found in the following locations by order of decreasing frequency: gingiva, lips, tongue, and hard palate. Feline melanoma is relatively rare but appears to be malignant in most cases.[3,14-21]

Melanomas in dogs have extremely diverse biologic behaviors, depending on a large variety of factors. A thorough understanding of these factors helps the clinician to delineate in advance the appropriate staging, prognosis, and treatments. The primary factors that determine the biologic behavior of an oral melanoma in a dog are site, size, stage, and histologic parameters.[8-10,22,23] Unfortunately, even with a comprehensive understanding of all of these factors, there are melanomas that have an unreliable biologic behavior; thus there is a need for additional research into this relatively common, heterogeneous, and frequently extremely malignant tumor.

Pathology and Molecular Biology

Melanomas can be difficult to diagnose pathologically in some situations, especially anaplastic amelanotic melanomas, which can masquerade as soft tissue sarcomas.[24,25] Numerous investigators have attempted to increase the precision of identification of melanomas predominantly through immunohistochemical means.[25-29] This identification can be accomplished through the use of multiple immunohistochemical assays on suspected melanoma tissue or through the use of an immunohistochemical cocktail of antibodies. The use of PNL2 and tyrosinase, beyond the typical use of Melan A and S100, appears to hold particular promise.[30,31]

The molecular characterization of canine and feline melanomas remains comparatively attenuated compared to the more comprehensive evaluation of human melanomas.[32] *BRAF* is a member of the mitogen-activated protein kinase (MAPK) signaling pathway, which is commonly mutated in human cutaneous melanoma.[33] However, *BRAF* mutations are uncommon in canine oral malignant melanoma,[34] suggesting that certain canine and/or feline malignancies can have similar molecular signatures in addition to their already well-known clinical similarities in the context of resistance to chemotherapy and irradiation and similar variable sites of metastatic propensity. A number of investigators have reported a variety of molecular abnormalities or associations in canine and feline melanoma.[35-52]

Biologic Behavior and Prognostic Factors

The biologic behavior of canine oral melanoma is extremely variable and best characterized based on anatomic site, size, stage, and histologic parameters. On divergent ends of the spectrum would be a low-grade 0.5-cm haired-skin melanoma, which is highly likely to be cured with simple surgical extirpation, in comparison to a 5.0-cm high-grade malignant oral melanoma with a poor-to-grave prognosis. Similar to the development of a rational staging, prognostic, and therapeutic plan for any tumor, two primary questions must be answered: what is the local invasiveness of the tumor and what is the metastatic propensity? The answers to these questions will determine the prognosis and appropriate therapies.

The anatomic site of melanoma is highly, although not completely, predictive of local invasiveness and metastatic propensity. Melanomas involving the haired-skin that are not in proximity to mucosal margins often behave in a benign manner.[1,3] Surgical extirpation is often curative, but histopathologic examination is imperative for delineation of margins, as well as a description of cytologic features. The use of Ki67 immunohistochemistry (IHC) has been reported to more reliably predict potential malignant behavior compared to classic histology for cutaneous melanoma.[53]

Oral and/or mucosal melanoma has been considered an extremely malignant tumor with a high degree of local invasiveness and high metastatic propensity.[2,8-10,22,54] This biologic behavior is similar to human oral and/or mucosal melanoma.[3,55] Two recent studies have called this dogma into question and suggest benign oral melanomas can occur more frequently than previously published.[56,57] Caution is necessary when assessing histopathologic descriptions, suggesting a benign course for oral melanoma. The first author has managed approximately 20 dogs over the last 7 years presenting with florid systemic metastases with an original histopathologic report, suggesting an expectation for a benign clinical course based on a high degree of differentiation. Similar to cutaneous melanoma, Ki67 appears to hold prognostic importance in canine oral melanoma as well.[58]

Anatomic sites of intermediate prognostic significance between the generally benign-acting haired-skin and the often malignant and metastatic oral/mucosal melanomas in dogs include the digit and footpad. Dogs with melanoma of the digits without lymph node or distant metastasis treated with digit amputation are reported to have a median survival time (MST) of approximately 12 months, with 42% to 57% alive at 1 year and 11% to 13% alive at 2 years.[59,60] Unfortunately, metastasis from digit melanoma at presentation is reported to be 30% to 40%,[59,61] and the aforementioned outcomes with surgery suggest that subsequent distant metastasis is common even when no overt metastasis is found at presentation or digit amputation. The prognosis for dogs with melanoma of the footpad has not been thoroughly established; the first author (PJB) has found this anatomic site to be anecdotally similar in metastatic propensity and prognosis to digit melanoma. Interestingly, human acral lentiginous melanoma (plantar surface of the foot, palms of the hand and digit) has an increased propensity for metastasis.[62]

A thorough review of prognostic factors in canine melanocytic neoplasms has been recently published.[63] This review took a regimented, systematic approach to analyzing published reports to date in order to identify those factors that appear to be repeatable and statistically defensible, while also identifying areas in which additional work is necessary due to incomplete data. For those veterinary clinicians and/or researchers interested in canine melanoma, this publication cannot be more strongly recommended. Tables 1 and 2 from this report are particularly useful in estimating prognosis for a specific patient and subsequent identification of the most logical treatment options.

Size and Stage

For dogs with oral melanoma, primary tumor size has been found to be prognostic. The World Health Organization (WHO) staging scheme for dogs with oral melanoma is based on size and metastasis and is summarized in Box 19-1. MacEwen and colleagues reported MSTs for dogs with oral melanoma treated with surgery to be approximately 17 to 18 months, 5 to 6 months, and 3 months for stage I, II, and III disease, respectively.[9] More recent reports suggest stage I oral melanoma treated with conventional therapies, including surgery, radiation, and/or chemotherapy, have MSTs of approximately 12 to 14 months, with most dogs dying of distant metastatic disease rather than local recurrence.[64,65] Other investigators have found dogs with stage I oral melanoma to have median progression-free survival (PFS) times of 19 months, similar to the original MacEwen et al report.[66]

Box 19-1 Traditional World Health Organization (WHO) TNM-Based Staging Scheme for Dogs with Oral Melanoma

T: Primary Tumor
T1 Tumor ≤2 cm in diameter
T2 Tumor 2-4 cm in diameter
T3 Tumor >4 cm in diameter

N: Regional Lymph Nodes
N0 No evidence of regional node involvement
N1 Histologic/cytologic evidence of regional node involvement
N2 Fixed nodes

M: Distant Metastasis
M0 No evidence of distant metastasis
M1 Evidence of distant metastasis

Stage I = T1 N0 M0
Stage II = T2 N0 M0
Stage III = T2 N1 M0 or T3 N0 M0
Stage IV = Any T, any N, and M1

Staging

The staging of dogs with melanoma is relatively straightforward. A minimum database should include a thorough history and physical examination, complete blood and platelet count, biochemical profile, urinalysis, three-view thoracic radiographs, and local lymph node aspiration with cytology, whether lymphadenomegaly is present or not. Williams and Packer reported that approximately 70% of dogs with oral malignant melanoma had local lymph node metastasis when lymphadenomegaly was present, but more importantly, approximately 40% had local lymph node metastasis when no lymphadenomegaly was present.[67] Additional considerations should be made for abdominal compartment testing (e.g., abdominal ultrasound) in all cases of CMM, especially in cases with moderate-to-high metastatic anatomic sites such as the oral cavity, feet, or mucosal surface of the lips, because melanoma metastasizes to the abdominal lymph nodes, liver, adrenal glands, and other sites.

The use of sentinel lymph node mapping and lymphadenectomy is of diagnostic, prognostic, and clinical benefit in human melanoma.[68] Relatively few investigations have been reported to date for sentinel lymph node mapping and/or excision for dogs with malignancies,[69-73] and we strongly encourage additional investigation in this area. Furthermore, the use of novel staging modalities such as gallium citrate scintigraphy is also encouraged.[74]

Treatment

Surgical Aspects

Surgery continues to be the most effective local treatment modality for melanoma, and early detection is often necessary for a successful outcome. Tumors in the caudal aspect of the oral cavity are often large by the time they are diagnosed relative to rostral tumors; therefore it is more difficult to obtain complete surgical excision. Gross characteristics of melanomas raise suspicion for the

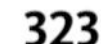

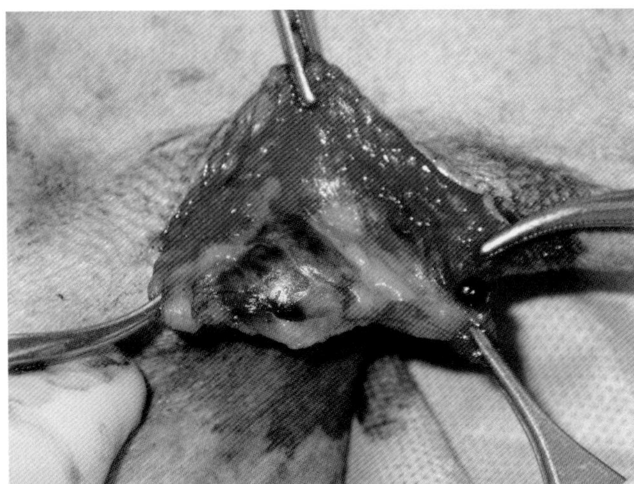

FIGURE 19-1 Excisional biopsy being performed on the popliteal lymph node from the dog in Figure 19-6. Note the effaced node overtaken with pigmented cells and the smaller nodule within the lymphatic vessel slightly distal to the node (toward the right in the photograph).

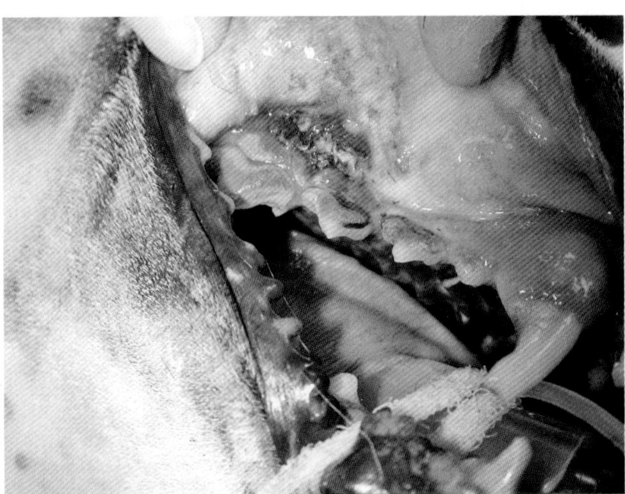

FIGURE 19-2 Local recurrence following incomplete resection and postoperative radiation of a gingival melanoma above the right carnassial tooth (caudal is to the left and the right canine tooth can be seen in the lower right-hand corner). When first treated, the mass was reportedly less than 1 cm diameter and wide resection (i.e., partial maxillectomy) was not performed.

diagnosis, and pigmented melanomas can be easily confirmed via fine needle aspiration and cytology. In dogs, small (<2 cm), mobile, well-circumscribed, slow-growing cutaneous melanomas tend to be benign and easily excisable, whereas large, poorly defined, ulcerated, and rapidly growing tumors can make surgical excision difficult. In the latter example, incisional biopsy and IHC can be an important part of the diagnostic work-up, particularly if the mass is nonpigmented and the diagnosis of melanoma is in question. In cases for which lymph node cytology results are equivocal (e.g., difficulty distinguishing between melanophages and melanoma cells), lymph nodes should be surgically excised and submitted for histopathologic evaluation (which includes IHC). Enlarged lymph nodes are often associated with metastasis, particularly with advanced tumors or tumors of high grade, and nodal effacement is common (Figure 19-1).

Benign cutaneous tumors are typically completely excised with 1-cm skin margins (and ideally one fascial plane deep). Partial mandibulectomy and maxillectomy are usually required for complete removal of oral melanomas arising from the gingiva or from other oral mucosa in close proximity to bone.[75] A common error is to "shave off" a gingival mass simply because bone invasion is not observed. Due to the close proximity of the gingiva to the underlying bone, this approach typically leaves residual microscopic disease that leads to local recurrence (Figure 19-2). Advanced imaging (i.e., computed tomography [CT] scans or magnetic resonance imaging [MRI]) is critical for assessment of tumor extent and potential bone involvement. It is also helpful in the detection of enlarged regional lymph nodes (e.g., medial retropharyngeal nodes) that are difficult to palpate.

Some tumors do occur in mucosal areas that are not adjacent to bone (e.g., buccal mucosa) or originate in the lip (Figure 19-3) or tongue (Figure 19-4) and are amenable to excision of the soft tissues only. The location of the tumor dictates the type of partial maxillectomy (i.e., premaxillary, unilateral rostral, central, or caudal) that is required. Complete excision of oral tumors has been shown to significantly impact prognosis.[76] Dogs with tumor cells extending to the peripheral margin were 3.6 times more likely to die from tumor-related causes compared to dogs for which margins were

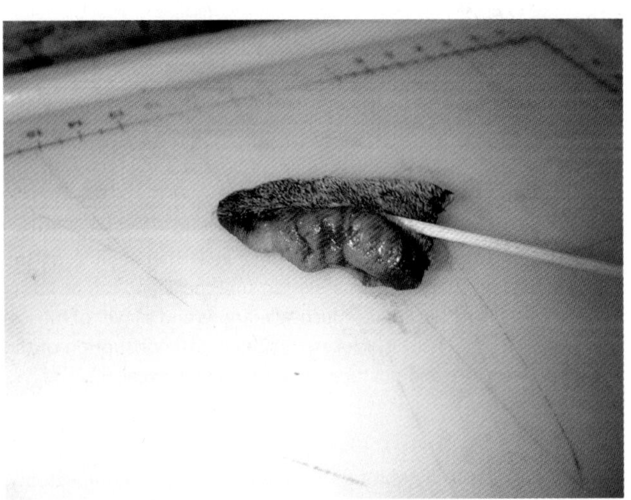

FIGURE 19-3 Amelanotic melanoma involving the rostral aspect of the right lip; 1- to 2-cm margins resulted in complete excision.

considered complete. In that same study, dogs with tumors caudal to premolar number three (PM3) were 4.3 times more likely to die from tumor-related causes compared to dogs with tumors located rostral to PM3.

For small caudal tumors lateral to the dental arcade (Figure 19-5), an oral approach provides enough exposure/access for complete excision; however, large tumors of the caudal maxilla or small tumors that extend medial to the dental arcade are best treated via a combined dorsal and intraoral approach.[77] The combined approach maximizes the surgeon's ability to obtain wide margins on tumors involving the caudal hard palate and inferior orbit. For small, superficial melanomas associated with the mandible, partial mandibulectomy is typically sufficient[78]; however, for large tumors that show evidence of intramedullary extension, consideration

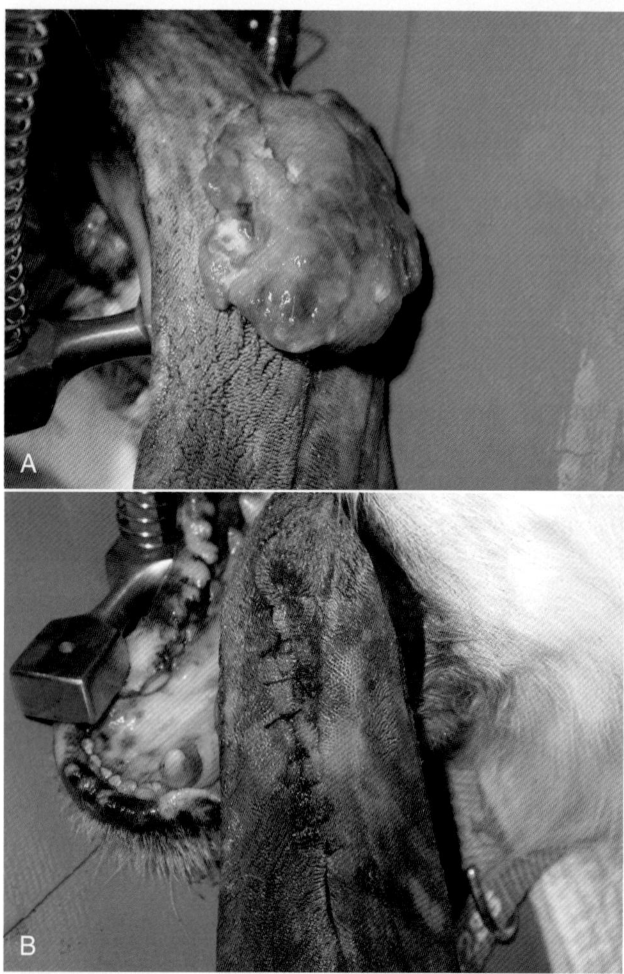

FIGURE 19-4 **A,** Lingual melanoma near the midline of the tongue of a dog. These masses are often superficial and can be easily excised with 1- to 2-cm lingual mucosal margins and a layer of muscle fibers deep to the mass. **B,** Closure results in little disruption of the lingual architecture and postoperative function is excellent.

should be given to a subtotal or complete hemimandibulectomy. Local recurrence rates vary from 22% following mandibulectomy to 48% after maxillectomy[75,79] and the MST for dogs treated with surgery alone varies from 150 to 318 days, with 1-year survival rates less than 35%.[28,75,76,78-81]

There are few objective data available to guide decision making for surgical margin width. Given the invasive nature of malignant melanomas, wide margins (2 to 3 cm) are optimal whenever possible; however, for oral lesions, wide margins are often not possible due to the limited amount of surrounding normal tissues. In the author's experience, 1 to 2 cm margins are usually adequate for complete excision of malignant tumors with well-defined borders (Figures 19-5 and 19-6). As with any oral tumor, inspection of the gross tumor borders must be interpreted along with diagnostic imaging to determine resectability and resection lines. Wider margins are usually possible with digital melanomas because digit amputation can often be performed at a level several joints above the proximal extent of the tumor.

With the widespread access to advanced imaging and improvements in surgical techniques (e.g., combined dorsal and intraoral approach for caudal maxillary tumors) and surgical oncologic

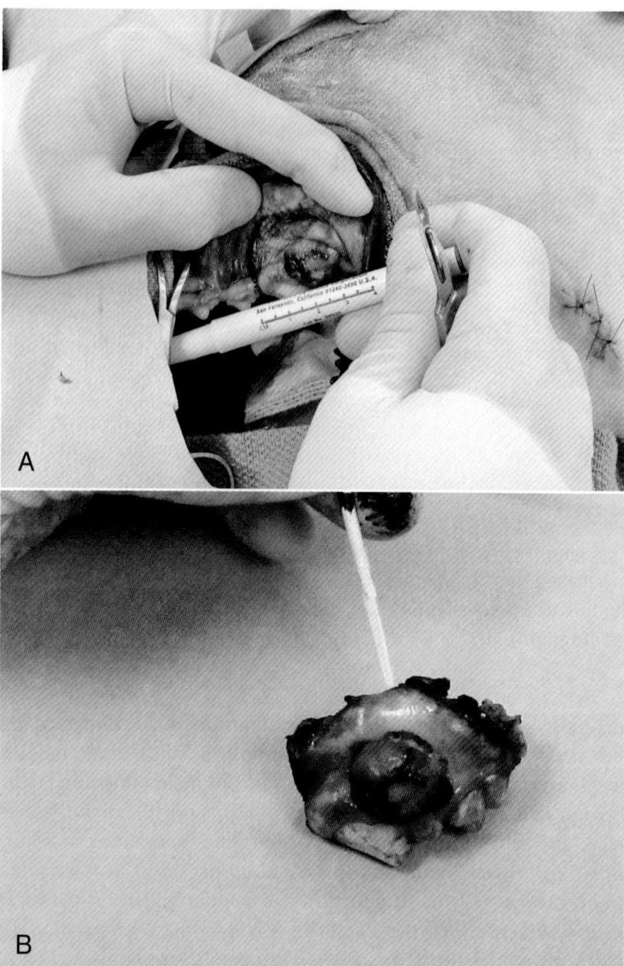

FIGURE 19-5 **A,** Intraoperative photograph of a melanoma confined to the lateral aspect of the caudal dental arcade. Surgical margin width in this case is approximately 1.5 cm around the cranial, dorsal, and caudal borders of the tumor. The incision along the hard palate was made just medial to the dental arcade. **B,** Surgical margins are inked with a green surgical ink and histopathologic assessment showed complete margins.

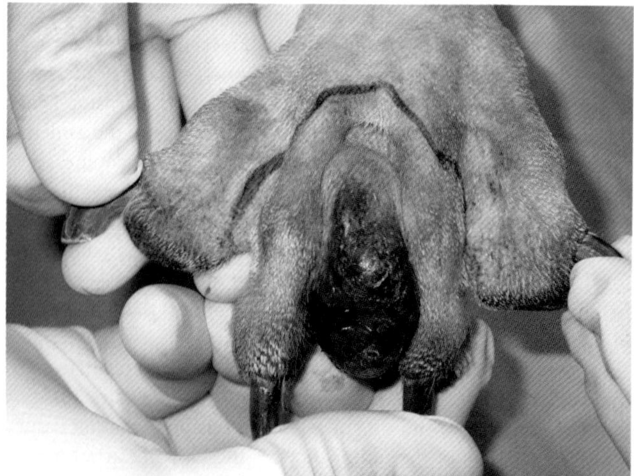

FIGURE 19-6 Malignant melanoma in the webbing between digits 3 and 4 (same dog as in Figure 19-1). Surgical margins were between 1 and 2 cm beyond the tumor edge. Excision was complete in this case.

training, complete tumor excision is more likely to be achieved. The surgical goals should be driven by the tumor stage, its location, and the surgeon's ability to perform a wide resection in locations where surgery is difficult (e.g., large caudal tumors). Unplanned or limited attempts at excision should not be made because the first chance to operate is the best chance to achieve tumor-free margins. For patients that undergo surgical excision, quality of life is usually very good and most dogs resume eating in the first day or two following surgery. Further, owner satisfaction with functional and cosmetic results following mandibulectomy and maxillectomy is high.[82] The functional outcome of single digit amputation is excellent and partial foot amputations (requiring excision of more than one digit; see Figure 19-6) are also tolerated very well and result in a good functional outcome.[83]

For tumors that are not amenable to wide excision or result in incomplete margins via histopathologic assessment, the combination of surgery and radiation or surgery plus adjuvant therapy should be considered. Historically, surgery has not been recommended when metastatic disease has been documented (e.g., a positive lymph node is discovered during tumor staging). However, the role of adjuvant therapy (chemotherapy or immunotherapy) in conjunction with cytoreductive surgery is being investigated for human metastatic melanoma and such approaches are now being explored in dogs (covered elsewhere in this chapter).[84-86]

Radiation Therapy

Radiation therapy plays an important role in the management and treatment of canine and feline oral melanomas. As with most tumor types, radiation therapy is used for the purpose of achieving local or regional control of the tumor. Radiation therapy has been described as both a primary and adjuvant therapy and both hypofractionated and definitive protocols have been used (Table 19-1).[87-92]

Melanoma is thought to be a relatively radioresistant tumor type often necessitating a higher dose in each fraction to achieve local control, although this point is somewhat controversial.[93] Most protocols used in dogs and cats have pursued higher dose per fraction protocols accordingly, although the relative radiosensitivity of melanoma in companion animal species has not been determined.

Hypofractionated protocols have the advantage of fewer treatments with fewer anesthetic episodes, lower cost, and less time commitment for the owner. These protocols in general also result in less severe acute effects. The main disadvantage of hypofractionated protocols is a lower overall and biologic equivalent dose, which results in lower rates of local control and an increased risk for late side effects. For a discussion of side effects, see the section on radiation side effects later in this chapter and in Chapter 12.

When planning a radiation field, most clinicians will choose to treat both the oral component of the disease and the regional lymph nodes, including the mandibular and medial retropharyngeal lymph nodes due to the high rate of metastasis to these sites.

Treatment planning can be done manually or can be planned by computer to allow a more conformal and homogeneous dose distribution with better sparing of normal tissues. Most studies have reported using at least a 2-cm margin around the tumor bed or surgical incision site. The field can be shaped by using manual blocking or, if available at the treating facility, a multileaf collimator (Figure 19-7).

Outcomes of Dogs and Cats Treated with Radiation Therapy for Oral Melanoma

The reported range of partial and complete responses to radiation therapy are 25% to 31% and 51% to 69%, respectively, yielding an overall response rate of 82% to 94%.[87,90,92] When treating gross disease, responses are generally rapid, and dramatic decreases in tumor volume can be seen within several weeks of starting therapy (Figure 19-8). PFS has been reported to range from 5 to 7.9 months.[89,90] Reported recurrence rates after radiotherapy vary and are confounded by different radiation protocols and adjuvant therapies used in these studies. Proulx et al reported a local recurrence rate of 26% when treating microscopic disease after incomplete surgical resection and radiotherapy and 45% for dogs treated with radiotherapy for macroscopic disease.[90]

The reported MSTs for dogs treated with radiotherapy range from 5.3 to 11.9 months (see Table 19-1).[87,90-92] The majority of these studies are retrospective and use a variety of radiotherapy equipment, protocols, and adjuvant therapies, making it difficult to determine an ideal treatment regimen. Reported protocols include 2 to 4 Gy fractions daily for 12 to 19 treatments, 4 Gy per fraction 3

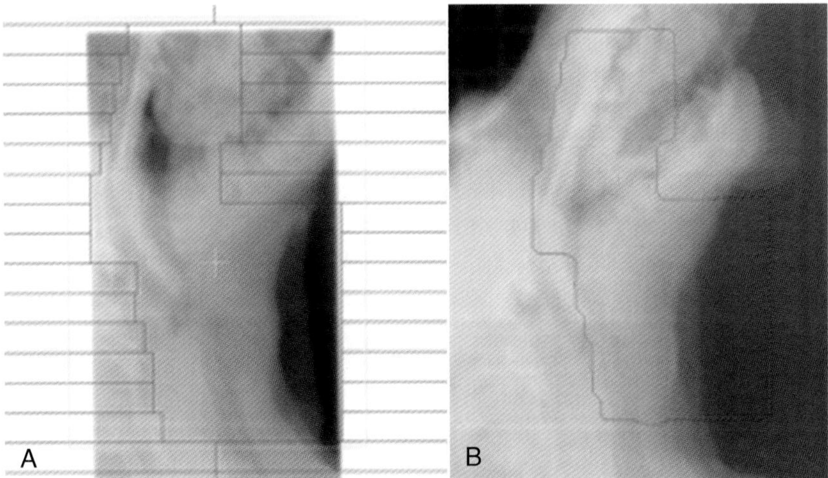

FIGURE 19-7 Multileaf collimator plan for a dog with an oral melanoma **(A)** and a portal image taken of the same dog **(B).** The outlined red area is the exposed field for the radiotherapy plan. A second wider exposure was taken to be able to view the surrounding anatomy and allow adjustment of the patient to ensure the correct anatomic area was treated. This plan was designed to cover the primary tumor, as well as the submandibular and medial retropharyngeal lymph nodes.

TABLE 19-1 Published Studies on the Treatment of Oral Melanoma with Radiation Therapy

Study (Year Published)	Species (No.)	Source and Dose of Radiation	Outcomes	Chemotherapy
Bateman et al (1994)[87]	Canine (18)	Cobalt-60: 24 Gy in three 8-Gy fractions once weekly.	One dog died during treatment, 9/18 had a complete response, 5/18 had a partial response, 3 had no response, MST: 7.9 months.	
Blackwood et al (1996)[88]	Canine (36)	4 MV linear accelerator (n = 29), 250 kVp orthovoltage unit (n = 1), combination of the two machines (n = 4), 36 Gy in four 9 Gy once weekly fractions.	25/36 dogs had a complete response, 9/36 had a partial response, overall MST not reported (range 5 to 213 weeks), MST for dogs that died of tumor-related causes: 21 weeks.	
Theon et al (1997)[89]	Canine (38)	Cobalt-60: 48 Gy in twelve 4-Gy fractions three times weekly.	PFS: 7.9 months, MST: not reported.	
Proulx et al (2003)[90]	Canine (140)	Cobalt-60: 36 Gy in four 9-Gy fractions once weekly (n = 54); 30 Gy in three 10-Gy fractions once weekly (n = 69), or 45.6-57 Gy in twelve to nineteen 2-4-Gy fractions (n = 17).	Median time to first event (metastasis, local recurrence, or death): 5.0 months, MST: 7.0 months.	80 dogs received chemotherapy (carboplatin [n = 60], cisplatin [n = 3], melphalan [n = 17]). Chemotherapy did not impact time to first event or survival.
Freeman et al (2003)[91]	Canine (39)	Cobalt-60 and 4 MV linear accelerator: 36 Gy in six 6-Gy fractions once weekly.	MST: 363 days.	Dogs received cisplatin (10-30 mg/m^2 IV) or carboplatin (90 mg/m^2 IV) chemotherapy 60 minutes before radiation delivery.
Farrelly et al (2004)[18]	Feline (5)	Cobalt-60: 24 Gy in three 8-Gy fractions once weekly.	One complete response, two partial responses, MST: 146 days.	Two cats received chemotherapy, one received carboplatin, one carboplatin and mitoxantrone, and one was treated with a DNA-based vaccine. One cat had additional radiation after initial failure.
Murphy et al (2005)[92]	Canine (28)	4 MV linear accelerator: 36 Gy in 4 once weekly fractions.	No chemotherapy group MST: 307 days. Chemotherapy-treated group MST: 286 days.	No chemotherapy given to 13. 15 received carboplatin chemotherapy (300 mg/m^2 IV every 21 days).

MST, Median survival time; *PFS,* progression-free survival; *IV,* intravenous.

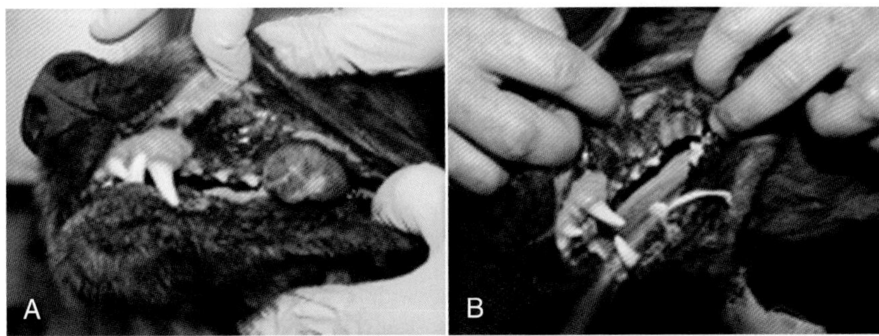

FIGURE 19-8 A dog with an oral melanoma treated with an 8 Gy per fraction once weekly protocol on the first day of therapy **(A)** and before the fourth and final fraction of radiotherapy **(B).** This dog went on to have a complete response.

times weekly for 4 weeks, 8 Gy per fraction once weekly for 3 treatments, and 9 Gy per fraction once weekly for 4 fractions.

Farrelly et al reported five cats that were treated with radiotherapy for oral melanoma.[18] There was one complete response and two partial responses with a MST of 146 days. One cat was treated with carboplatin, and one cat was treated with carboplatin and mitoxantrone, in addition to the radiation protocol. Another cat in this study was given a DNA-based vaccine as adjuvant to radiation.

Combining Chemotherapy with Radiation Therapy

There are conflicting data regarding the efficacy of chemotherapy used concurrently or in the adjuvant setting, and there is no clear evidence that chemotherapy decreases the risk of metastasis or local recurrence or that it extends MSTs. Published studies have reported on dogs receiving carboplatin, intralesional cisplatin, intravenous cisplatin, and melphalan.[90-92,94-97]

Freeman et al reported on 39 dogs with incompletely resected oral melanoma that were treated with either cisplatin (10 to 30 mg/m^2 IV) or carboplatin (90 mg/m^2 IV) given once weekly approximately 1 hour before receiving radiation therapy.[91] The radiation protocol consisted of 6 once-weekly 6 Gy fractions. They reported a MST of 11.9 months. Fifteen percent of the dogs had local recurrence, with a reported median time to metastasis of 10.2 months. Although this is among the longest survival times reported, the majority of dogs had stage T1 (56.4%) or stage T2 (35.9%) tumors prior to surgery, which may have biased their findings for longer survival times, making this result less applicable to the general population of dogs presenting with oral melanoma.

Proulx et al retrospectively looked at dogs treated with a variety of radiation protocols in which 60 dogs received no chemotherapy and 80 dogs received a chemotherapy protocol consisting of carboplatin (n = 60), cisplatin (n = 3), or melphalan (n = 17).[90] They found that chemotherapy treatment had no significant impact on either time to first event or overall survival. The mean dose of carboplatin used in this study was 225 mg/m^2 IV, which is lower than the dose most often used in this species.[95] This lower dose may have contributed to the lack of statistical differences in delaying time to metastasis or recurrence and impact on overall survival.

Murphy et al retrospectively evaluated a series of 28 dogs that received once weekly 8 Gy fractions to a total dose of 32 Gy.[92] Fifteen dogs in this study received 300 mg/m^2 IV of carboplatin every 21 days for a median of 3 doses, although chemotherapy dose reductions were allowed on subsequent doses if toxicity was found on the initial dose. Thirteen dogs received no chemotherapy with a MST of 307 days, and the 15 dogs that were treated with chemotherapy had an overall MST of 286 days. These numbers were not significantly different. The use of chemotherapy also did not reduce the proportion of dogs that died from metastasis. The dose of carboplatin in this study was chosen to decrease the risk of toxicity seen in another report that evaluated the use of carboplatin alone in dogs with melanoma in which dogs over 15 kg received 350 mg/m^2 IV, and several of the dogs experienced significant toxicity requiring hospitalization, although the dose used was higher than the dose used in the Proulx study.[90,96]

Some concerns have been raised that using radiotherapy and chemotherapy concurrently can increase systemic side effects. Hume et al reported on 65 dogs treated with concurrent carboplatin and a definitive course of radiation therapy; six of these dogs were diagnosed with an oral melanoma.[97] Carboplatin was administered at 200 to 300 mg/m^2 IV. Dogs with oral melanoma in this study were prescribed 4 Gy per fraction delivered on Mondays, Wednesdays, and Fridays for a total dose of 48 Gy. They found that 21% developed grade 3 or 4 neutropenia, 20% developed grade 3 or 4 thrombocytopenia, and 10% developed grade 3 to 5 gastrointestinal toxicity according to the Veterinary Cooperative Oncology Group—Common Terminology Criteria for Adverse Events (VCOG-CTAE), version 1.0.[98] Further, five of the dogs did not complete the radiation course and seven had delays in radiation therapy due to illness.

Radiation-Associated Prognostic Factors

Several possible prognostic factors have been identified that affect radiation treatment outcomes in dogs diagnosed with malignant oral melanoma. These factors must be viewed with caution because some of the data are conflicting and most are derived from retrospective case series without the use of control groups.

Proulx et al reported outcomes from a total of 140 dogs treated with radiation and identified that dogs without radiologic evidence of bone destruction were found to have longer times to first event and longer overall survival times than dogs with radiographically evident bone changes.[90] Destruction of underlying bone can be evaluated by using survey radiographs or by CT scan with greater sensitivity. Underlying bony involvement has been reported in up to 92% of dogs with melanoma (Figure 19-9).[91]

The size of an oral tumor also affects prognosis, but more studies need to be conducted to confirm that size is a prognostic factor for dogs undergoing irradiation. Theon et al analyzed a series of 105 dogs with oral tumors treated with 4 Gy per fraction of radiation on an alternate day basis to a total dose of 48 Gy.[89] Thirty-eight dogs in this report were diagnosed with oral melanoma. They found a

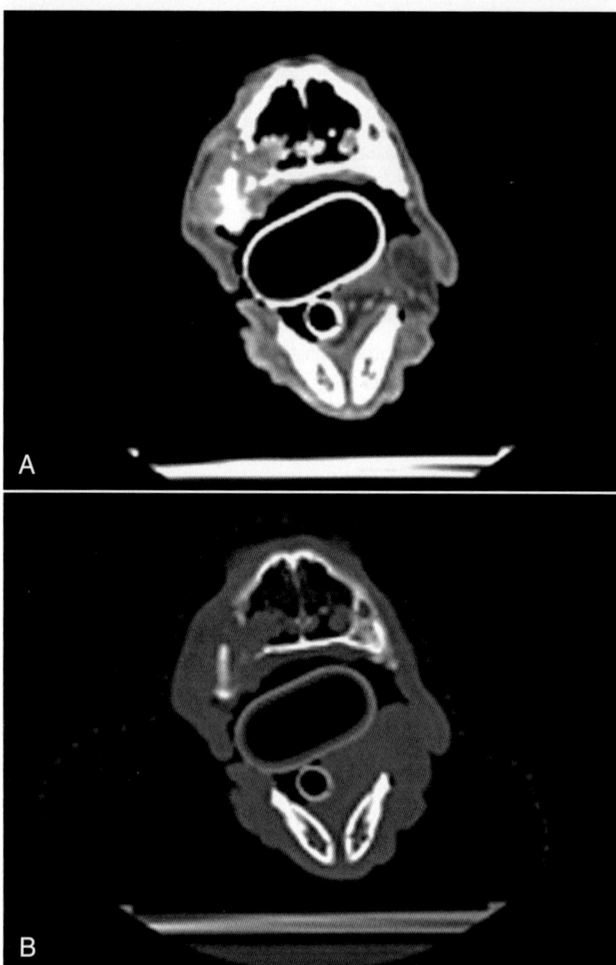

FIGURE 19-9 **A,** Postcontrast axial computed tomography (CT) image of a dog with a maxillary oral melanoma. Note the heterogeneously contrast enhancing soft tissue mass. **B,** Precontrast axial image at the same level as the image in **A.** Note the bone destruction of the maxillary bone and the invasion of the soft tissue mass into the nasal cavity.

median PFS of 7.9 months. Dogs from this group diagnosed with T1 stage lesions had a median PFS of 11.3 months, whereas dogs with stage T2 and T3 lesions had a median PFS of 6.0 and 6.7 months, respectively. They also found that distant metastasis as opposed to local failure of radiation was the major cause of first failure event. Blackwood et al also found that dogs with smaller oral melanomas treated with a 9 Gy per fraction once weekly protocol delivered over a 4-week period did better than dogs with larger tumors.[88] Dogs with tumors less than 5 cm^3 were more likely to achieve a complete response. Further, the volume of the tumor affected median overall survival with a MST of 86 weeks for dogs with tumors less than 5 cm^3 compared to 16 weeks for dogs with tumors between 5 and 15 cm^3 and 20.5 weeks for dogs with tumors greater than 15 cm^3 in size. Proulx et al found that tumor size affected times to first event, pulmonary metastasis, and death.[90] These studies contrast the findings of Bateman et al, who did not find an association of stage of the oral melanoma and response to radiation therapy or survival times.[87]

The role of vascular endothelial growth factor (VEGF) in the radiation response of melanoma has been incompletely evaluated. Several studies have found that dogs with oral melanoma have higher plasma VEGF concentrations than normal control dogs.[43,99] In a preliminary study looking at plasma VEGF levels in a variety of tumor types treated with hypofractionated radiotherapy, the four dogs diagnosed with melanoma had the highest mean plasma VEGF levels of all tumor types, although no significant changes in VEGF levels were noted over the course of treatment.[99] This same group also evaluated the effect that VEGF levels had on patient outcome.[100,101] In a group of 39 dogs, 6 of which were diagnosed with melanoma, it was also found that VEGF levels did not significantly increase over the course of radiotherapy. However, dogs with higher plasma VEGF levels treated with hypofractionated protocols had a shorter time to treatment failure and a shorter median survival.

Side Effects of Radiation Therapy

Side effects of radiation therapy are a major concern of owners and can impact a patient's quality of life. Prolonged side effects are particularly important to take into account when the goal of radiotherapy is palliative in nature (i.e., to improve quality of life). The severity and scope of radiation side effects and the type seen depend on several factors, including the total dose of radiation given, the dose per fraction, and the volume of tissue in the radiation field. Higher total radiation doses delivered in smaller dose per fractions tend to produce worse acute effects, whereas higher dose per fraction will increase the risk of late effects occurring. Newer treatment machines and computerized treatment planning have helped limit the volume of normal tissue that is irradiated, which in turn limits the area where these acute effects are seen. Side effects are generally broken down into acute and late effects. A standardized radiation scoring system for acute and late effects on oral mucosa and bone have been published by the Veterinary Radiation Therapy Oncology Group (VRTOG).[102] Acute radiation effects on the oral cavity range from injected mucous membranes (grade 1) to patchy mucositis without evidence of pain (grade 2) to confluent fibrinous mucositis requiring the use of analgesics to ulceration, hemorrhage, and necrosis (grade 3). These can be seen on the gingival surfaces, tongue, or buccal mucosa.[102] Although grade 3 toxicity is possible, most studies have not reported high-grade toxicity with either definitive or palliative protocols.[87-89] The worst clinical signs associated with acute effects generally occur toward the end or just after the completion of radiotherapy and heal within 1 to 2 weeks given that the oral mucosa tends to heal rapidly.

Skin effects can also be seen with dry and moist desquamation possible. Most studies have reported these side effects to be minimal and to resolve quickly after completion of the radiation course. Other skin side effects reported include permanent alopecia in the radiation field and skin fibrosis.[89]

Bone necrosis is a reported late side effect of radiation therapy and probably is a greater risk in hypofractionated protocols. Blackwood et al reported three cases of bone necrosis in a series of 36 dogs treated with a hypofractionated protocol; two required surgical debridement.[88] Theon et al also reported 7.6% of dogs developed bone necrosis and fistula formation in a series of oral tumors treated with a curative-intent protocol.[89]

Another possible late effect is a radiation-induced tumor. In order for a tumor to be classified as likely being radiation induced the following criteria are applied: (1) the tumor developed in an area that was previously irradiated, (2) an adequate period of time has passed since initial irradiation to allow for new tumor formation, (3) preirradiation evaluation revealed normal bone in cases in which the second tumor is of bone origin, and (4) histologic diagnosis of a second, different malignant tumor was confirmed at the site of initial irradiation.[103]

In dogs with oral melanoma treated with radiation therapy, most patients do not survive long enough for radiation-induced tumors to become a significant issue, but as more effective systemic adjuvant therapies become available, this becomes a concern. Sarcomas are thought to be the most common radiation-induced tumor, although Theon et al did report on a gingival SCC forming within a radiation field 36 months after radiation treatment.[89]

Salvage procedures using flaps for the surgical repair of radiation late effects have been described in dogs, although they are more likely to result in complications than the surgical flaps used in the surgical treatment of an area treated with preoperative radiotherapy or in flaps exposed to radiation in the immediate postoperative period.[104]

Radiation therapy is an effective modality used to achieve local-regional control for oral melanoma with minimal side effects in dogs and cats. Until more effective treatments to control and treat metastatic disease become available and the effectiveness of lower dose per fraction protocols are better studied, hypofractionated protocols will likely remain the most commonly used radiation protocols in veterinary medicine.

Treatments Other than Surgery and Radiation

Other modalities reported for local tumor control as case reports and/or case series have included intralesional cisplatin implants, intralesional bleomycin with electronic pulsing, and others, but widespread use has not been reported to date.[105-108]

In dogs with melanoma in the aforementioned anatomic sites predicted to have a moderate-to-high metastatic propensity or dogs with cutaneous melanoma with a high tumor score and/or increased proliferation index through increased Ki67 expression, the use of systemic therapies is warranted due to the high risk for metastasis. Rassnick and colleagues reported an overall response rate of 28% using carboplatin for dogs with malignant melanoma.[96] Unfortunately, only one dog had a minimally durable complete response (approximately 150 days), and the rest were nondurable partial responses. Similarly, Boria et al reported an 18% response rate and MST of 119 days with cisplatin and piroxicam in canine oral melanoma.[109] Other reports using single-agent dacarbazine, melphalan, or doxorubicin suggest poor or absent activity.[110-113] More recently and importantly, two studies suggest that chemotherapy plays an insignificant role in the adjuvant treatment of canine melanoma.[65,99] Although it can be argued that the studies performed to date that evaluate the activity of chemotherapy in an adjuvant setting for canine melanoma have been suboptimal due to a variety of reasons, the extensive human literature in this specific setting also suggests melanoma is an extremely chemotherapy-resistant tumor.[114] It is clear that new approaches to the systemic treatment of this disease are desperately needed.

One potential therapeutic avenue that has not been reported to date in canine or feline melanoma is the use of cyclooxygenase-2 (COX-2) inhibitors. A number of authors have investigated the expression of COX-2 in canine melanoma and have found positive correlations of COX-2 expression to proliferation and survival.[115-117] Studies investigating the clinical responsiveness of canine melanoma to COX-2 inhibitors (and potential correlation to COX-2 expression) are encouraged.

Immunotherapy represents one logical systemic therapeutic strategy for melanoma. A variety of immunotherapeutic strategies for the treatment of human melanoma have been reported previously, with typically poor outcomes due to a lack of breaking tolerance. Immunotherapy targets and strategies to date in canine melanoma have used autologous tumor cell vaccines (with or without transfection with immunostimulatory cytokines and/or melanosomal differentiation antigens), allogeneic tumor cell vaccines transfected with interleukin 2 (IL-2) or granulocyte-macrophage colony-stimulating factor (GM-CSF), liposomal-encapsulated nonspecific immunostimulators (e.g., L-MTP-PE), intralesional Fas ligand DNA, small interfering RNA (siRNA) against the survivin and/or *Bcl-2* genes, bacterial super-antigen approaches with GM-CSF or IL-2 as immune adjuvants, PEGylated tumor-necrosis factor α (TNF-α), suicide gene therapy, adenovector CD40 ligand, and finally, canine dendritic cell vaccines loaded with melanosomal differentiation antigens.[9,118-132] Although these approaches have produced some clinical antitumor responses, the methodologies for the generation of these products are expensive, time consuming, sometimes dependent on patient tumor samples being established into cell lines, and fraught with the difficulties of consistency, reproducibility, and other quality control issues. Furthermore, we are just beginning to more fully understand the native immune dysregulation potentially induced by the malignancy through increased T regulatory (Treg) cells, which suppress antitumor responses[133,134] (see also Chapter 13).

The advent of DNA vaccination circumvents many of the previously encountered hurdles in vaccine development. DNA is relatively inexpensive and simple to purify in large quantities. The gene coding for the antigen of interest is cloned into a bacterial expression plasmid with a constitutively active promoter. The plasmid is introduced into the skin or muscle with an intradermal or intramuscular injection. Once in the skin or muscle, professional antigen-presenting cells, particularly dendritic cells, are able to present the transcribed and translated antigen in the proper context of major histocompatibility complex and co-stimulatory molecules. Although DNA vaccines have induced immune responses to viral proteins, vaccinating against tissue-specific self-proteins on cancer cells is clearly a more difficult problem. One way to induce immunity against a tissue-specific differentiation antigen on cancer cells is to vaccinate with xenogeneic (different species) antigen or DNA that is homologous to the cancer antigen. As illustrated in Figure 19-10, vaccination with DNA-encoding cancer differentiation antigens is ineffective when self-DNA is used, but tumor immunity can be induced by orthologous DNA from another species.[135]

Tyrosinase is a melanosomal glycoprotein, essential in melanin synthesis, and routinely found to be overexpressed in a wide variety of melanomas across species.[31,136-139] Immunization with xenogeneic human DNA-encoding tyrosinase family proteins induced antibodies and cytotoxic T-cells against syngeneic B16 melanoma cells in C57BL/6 mice, but immunization with mouse tyrosinase-related DNA did not induce detectable immunity.[140] In particular, xenogeneic DNA vaccination induced tumor protection from syngeneic melanoma challenge and autoimmune hypopigmentation. Thus xenogeneic DNA vaccination could break tolerance against a self-tumor differentiation antigen, inducing antibody, T-cell, and antitumor responses.

Dogs with stage I to III locoregionally controlled CMM inclusive across all xenogeneic vaccine studies to date have a Kaplan-Meier (KM) MST of more than 1075 days (median not yet reached), whereas those dogs with stage I to III CMM without local tumor control have a KM MST of 553 days ($p = 0.0002$). The KM MST for stage II to IV dogs on the phase I trials of human tyrosinase (huTyr), murine GP75 (muGP75), and murine tyrosinase (muTyr) are 389,

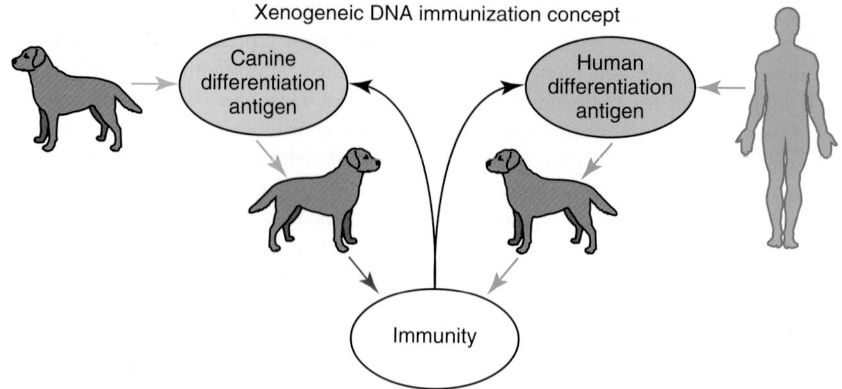

FIGURE 19-10 Cartoon outlining the xenogeneic DNA vaccination concept.

153, and 224 days, respectively. The KM MST for stage II to IV dogs treated with 50 μg muTyr, 100/400/800 μg human GM-CSF, or combination muTyr/human GM-CSF are 242, 148, and more than 900 days (median not reached), respectively. For dogs that received any melanoma vaccine except for dogs on the muTyr ± GM-CSF trial (i.e., huTyr, muTyr, and muGP75), the KM MST for stages I, II, III, and IV CMM was more than 939 days (median not reached with 92.8% survival), more than 908 days (median not reached, 79% alive at 1 year, 63% alive at 2 years), more than 1646 days (median not reached; 77%, 65%, and 57% alive at 1, 2, and 3 years, respectively), and 239 days (40.5% and 18.8% alive at 1 and 2 years, respectively).[141,142] The results from dogs vaccinated with huTyr were published in 2003.[143]

We investigated the humoral responses of dogs receiving huTyr as a potential explanation for the long-term survival seen in some of the dogs on this study. Utilizing standard enzyme-linked immunosorbent assay (ELISA) with mammalian expressed purified huTyr protein as the target of interest, we have found three of nine dogs with twofold to fivefold postvaccinal humoral responses compared to preimmune sera. We have confirmed these findings utilizing a flow-cytometric–based assay of prevaccinal and postvaccinal sera in permeabilized human SK-Mel melanoma cells expressing endogenous huTyr. Interestingly, the three dogs with postvaccinal anti-huTyr humoral responses are dogs with unexpected long-term tumor control.[144] Co-investigators have also determined that normal dogs receiving the huTyr-based melanoma vaccine develop Ag-specific interferon-γ (IFN-γ) T-cells.[145]

The results of these trials demonstrate that xenogeneic DNA vaccination in CMM (1) is safe, (2) causes dogs to develop specific anti-Tyr immune responses, (3) is potentially therapeutic in stage II/III locoregionally controlled disease, and (4) is an attractive candidate for further evaluation in an adjuvant, minimal residual disease phase II setting for CMM. Based on these preliminary studies, a multiinstitutional safety and efficacy trial for U.S. Drug Administration (USDA) licensure in dogs with locally controlled stage II/III oral melanoma was initiated in 2006 with granting of conditional licensure in 2007. Results of this trial documented a statistically significant improvement in survival for vaccinates compared to historic controls,[85] and a full licensure for the huTyr-based canine melanoma vaccine from USDA-Centers for Veterinary Biology (CVB) was received in 2009. Subsequently, we have investigated the efficacy of local tumor control and use of muTyr-based DNA vaccination in dogs with digit melanoma. These investigations have found an improvement in survival compared to historic outcomes with digit amputation only and also documented a decreased prognosis for dogs with advanced stage disease and/or increased time from digit amputation to the start of vaccination.[146]

A similar approach has been used in human patients with metastatic melanoma in the minimal residual disease setting. Although no clinical response data are available since these patients did not have measurable disease, several phase I trials of xenogeneic DNA vaccines have been completed. Across studies of tyrosinase and gp100 DNA immunization, approximately 40% of patients develop quantifiable CD8+ T-cell responses to the syngeneic human target antigen.[147-149] Two additional exciting new approaches that appear to confer a survival benefit in human metastatic melanoma include the use of the anti-CTLA-4 antibody, ipilimumab (Yervoy, Bristol-Myers Squibb), and the selective BRAF inhibitors, vemurafenib (Zelboraf, Genentech) and dabrafenib (GSK2118436, GlaxoSmith-Kline), in patients who are BRAF V600 mutation positive.[150-152]

CMM strongly appears to be a more clinically faithful therapeutic model for human melanoma when compared to more traditional mouse systems because both human and canine diseases are chemoresistant, are radioresistant, share similar metastatic phenotypes/site selectivity, and occur spontaneously in an outbred, immunocompetent scenario. It is hoped in the future that this same vaccine also plays a role in the treatment of melanoma in other species (e.g., horses, cats, humans) due to its xenogeneic origins[139] and in melanoma prevention once the genetic determinants of melanoma risk in dogs are further defined. The xenogeneic DNA vaccine platform holds promise for investigations with other antigen targets. To this end, we have recently completed a phase I study of murine CD20 DNA vaccination in dogs with B-cell non-Hodgkin's lymphoma. We also have phase I and phase II studies initiating shortly, utilizing murine CD20 and rat HER2 DNA vaccination.

REFERENCES

1. Goldschmidt MH: Pigmented lesions of the skin, *Clin Dermatol* 12(4):507–514, 1994.
2. Goldschmidt MH: Benign and malignant melanocytic neoplasms of domestic animals, *Am J Dermatopathol* 7(Suppl):203–212, 1985.
3. Smith SH, Goldschmidt MH, McManus PM: A comparative review of melanocytic neoplasms, *Vet Pathol* 39(6):651–678, 2002.
4. Leiter U, Garbe C: Epidemiology of melanoma and nonmelanoma skin cancer: the role of sunlight, *Adv Exp Med Biol* 624:89–103, 2008.

5. Ragnarsson-Olding BK: Spatial density of primary malignant melanoma in sun-shielded body sites: a potential guide to melanoma genesis, *Acta Oncol* 50(3):323–328, 2011.
6. Todoroff RJ, Brodey RS: Oral and pharyngeal neoplasia in the dog: a retrospective survey of 361 cases, *J Am Vet Med Assoc* 175(6):567–571, 1979.
7. Wallace J, Matthiesen DT, Patnaik AK: Hemimaxillectomy for the treatment of oral tumors in 69 dogs, *Vet Surg* 21(5):337–341, 1992.
8. Hahn KA, DeNicola DB, Richardson RC, et al: Canine oral malignant melanoma: prognostic utility of an alternative staging system, *J Small Anim Pract* 35(5):251–256, 1994.
9. Macewen EG, Patnaik AK, Harvey HJ, et al: Canine oral melanoma: comparison of surgery versus surgery plus Corynebacterium parvum, *Cancer Invest* 4(5):397–402, 1986.
10. Harvey HJ, Macewen EG, Braun D, et al: Prognostic criteria for dogs with oral melanoma, *J Am Vet Med Assoc* 178(6):580–582, 1981.
11. Bradley RL, Macewen EG, Loar AS: Mandibular resection for removal of oral tumors in 30 dogs and 6 cats, *J Am Vet Med Assoc* 184(4):460–463, 1984.
12. Harvey HJ: Oral tumors, *Vet Clin North Am Small Anim Pract* 15(3):493–500, 1985.
13. Kosovsky JK, Matthiesen DT, Marretta SM, et al: Results of partial mandibulectomy for the treatment of oral tumors in 142 dogs, *Vet Surg* 20(6):397–401, 1991.
14. Schobert CS, Labelle P, Dubielzig RR: Feline conjunctival melanoma: histopathological characteristics and clinical outcomes, *Vet Ophthalmol* 13(1):43–46, 2010.
15. Planellas M, Pastor J, Torres MD, et al: Unusual presentation of a metastatic uveal melanoma in a cat, *Vet Ophthalmol* 13(6):391–394, 2010.
16. Munday JS, French AF, Martin SJ: Cutaneous malignant melanoma in an 11-month-old Russian blue cat, *N Z Vet J* 59(3):143–146, 2011.
17. Morges MA, Zaks K: Malignant melanoma in pleural effusion in a 14-year-old cat, *J Feline Med Surg* 13(7):532–535, 2011.
18. Farrelly J, Denman DL, Hohenhaus AE, et al: Hypofractionated radiation therapy of oral melanoma in five cats, *Vet Radiol Ultrasound* 45(1):91–93, 2004.
19. Grahn BH, Peiffer RL, Cullen CL, et al: Classification of feline intraocular neoplasms based on morphology, histochemical staining, and immunohistochemical labeling, *Vet Ophthalmol* 9(6):395–403, 2006.
20. Patnaik AK, Mooney S: Feline melanoma: a comparative study of ocular, oral, and dermal neoplasms, *Vet Pathol* 25(2):105–112, 1988.
21. Luna LD, Higginbotham ML, Henry CJ, et al: Feline non-ocular melanoma: a retrospective study of 23 cases (1991-1999), *J Feline Med Surg* 2(4):173–181, 2000.
22. Bostock DE: Prognosis after surgical excision of canine melanomas, *Vet Pathol* 16(1):32–40, 1979.
23. Spangler WL, Kass PH: The histologic and epidemiologic bases for prognostic considerations in canine melanocytic neoplasia, *Vet Pathol* 43(2):136–149, 2006.
24. Smedley RC, Lamoureux J, Sledge DG, et al: Immunohistochemical diagnosis of canine oral amelanotic melanocytic neoplasms, *Vet Pathol* 48(1):32–40, 2011.
25. Choi C, Kusewitt DF: Comparison of tyrosinase-related protein-2, S-100, and Melan A immunoreactivity in canine amelanotic melanomas, *Vet Pathol* 40(6):713–718, 2003.
26. Berrington AJ, Jimbow K, Haines DM: Immunohistochemical detection of melanoma-associated antigens on formalin-fixed, paraffin-embedded canine tumors, *Vet Pathol* 31(4):455–461, 1994.
27. Koenig A, Wojcieszyn J, Weeks BR, et al: Expression of S100a, vimentin, NSE, and melan A/MART-1 in seven canine melanoma cells lines and twenty-nine retrospective cases of canine melanoma, *Vet Pathol* 38(4):427–435, 2001.
28. Ramos-Vara JA, Beissenherz ME, Miller MA, et al: Retrospective study of 338 canine oral melanomas with clinical, histologic, and immunohistochemical review of 129 cases, *Vet Pathol* 37(6):597–608, 2000.
29. Sandusky GEJ, Carlton WW, Wightman KA: Immunohistochemical staining for S100 protein in the diagnosis of canine amelanotic melanoma, *Vet Pathol* 22(6):577–581, 1985.
30. Giudice C, Ceciliani F, Rondena M, et al: Immunohistochemical investigation of PNL2 reactivity of canine melanocytic neoplasms and comparison with Melan A, *J Vet Diagn Invest* 22(3):389–394, 2010.
31. Ramos-Vara JA, Miller MA: Immunohistochemical identification of canine melanocytic neoplasms with antibodies to melanocytic antigen PNL2 and tyrosinase: comparison with Melan A, *Vet Pathol* 48(2):443–450, 2011.
32. Palmieri G, Capone M, Ascierto ML, et al: Main roads to melanoma, *J Transl Med* 7:86, 2009.
33. Bollag G, Hirth P, Tsai J, et al: Clinical efficacy of a RAF inhibitor needs broad target blockade in BRAF-mutant melanoma, *Nature* 467(7315):596–599, 2010.
34. Shelly S, Chien MB, Yip B, et al: Exon 15 BRAF mutations are uncommon in canine oral malignant melanomas, *Mamm Genome* 16(3):211–217, 2005.
35. Roels S, Tilmant K, Ducatelle R: p53 expression and apoptosis in melanomas of dogs and cats, *Res Vet Sci* 70(1):19–25, 2001.
36. Roels SL, van Daele AJ, van Marck EA, et al: DNA ploidy and nuclear morphometric variables for the evaluation of melanocytic tumors in dogs and cats, *Am J Vet Res* 61(9):1074–1079, 2000.
37. Modiano JF, Ritt MG, Wojcieszyn J: The molecular basis of canine melanoma: pathogenesis and trends in diagnosis and therapy, *J Vet Intern Med* 13(3):163–174, 1999.
38. Ritt MG, Or J, Wojcieszyn J, et al: Sustained nuclear localization of p21/WAF-1 upon growth arrest induced by contact inhibition, *Cancer Lett* 158(1):73–84, 2000.
39. Han JI, Kim DY, Na KJ: Dysregulation of the Wnt/beta-catenin signaling pathway in canine cutaneous melanotic tumor, *Vet Pathol* 47(2):285–291, 2010.
40. Stell AJ, Dobson JM, Scase TJ, et al: Evaluation of variants of melanoma-associated antigen genes and mRNA transcripts in melanomas of dogs, *Am J Vet Res* 70(12):1512–1520, 2009.
41. Thamm DH, Huelsmeyer MK, Mitzey AM, et al: RT-PCR-based tyrosine kinase display profiling of canine melanoma: IGF-1 receptor as a potential therapeutic target, *Melanoma Res* 20(1):35–42, 2010.
42. Kent MS, Collins CJ, Ye F: Activation of the AKT and mammalian target of rapamycin pathways and the inhibitory effects of rapamycin on those pathways in canine malignant melanoma cell lines, *Am J Vet Res* 70(2):263–269, 2009.
43. Taylor KH, Smith AN, Higginbotham M, et al: Expression of vascular endothelial growth factor in canine oral malignant melanoma, *Vet Comp Oncol* 5(4):208–218, 2007.
44. Murua EH, Gunther K, Richter A, et al: Absence of ras-gene hot-spot mutations in canine fibrosarcomas and melanomas, *Anticancer Res* 24(5A):3027–3028, 2004.
45. Dincer Z, Jasani B, Haywood S, et al: Metallothionein expression in canine and feline mammary and melanotic tumours, *J Comp Pathol* 125(2-3):130–136, 2001.
46. Stiles J, Bienzle D, Render JA, et al: Use of nested polymerase chain reaction (PCR) for detection of retroviruses from formalin-fixed, paraffin-embedded uveal melanomas in cats, *Vet Ophthalmol* 2(2):113–116, 1999.
47. Mayr B, Eschborn U, Schleger W, et al: Cytogenetic studies in a canine malignant melanoma, *J Comp Pathol* 106(3):319–322, 1992.
48. Mayr B, Schaffner G, Reifinger M, et al: N-ras mutations in canine malignant melanomas, *Vet J* 165(2):169–171, 2003.
49. Mayr B, Reifinger M, Grohe D, et al: Cytogenetic alterations in feline melanoma, *Vet J* 159(1):97–100, 2000.
50. Mayr B, Wilhelm B, Reifinger M, et al: Absence of p21 WAF1 and p27 kip1 gene mutations in various feline tumours, *Vet Res Commun* 24(2):115–124, 2000.
51. Sulaimon SS, Kitchell BE: The basic biology of malignant melanoma: molecular mechanisms of disease progression and comparative aspects, *J Vet Intern Med* 17(6):760–772, 2003.

52. Murakami A, Mori T, Sakai H, et al: Analysis of KIT expression and KIT exon 11 mutations in canine oral malignant melanomas, *Vet Comp Oncol* 9(3):219–224, 2011.
53. Laprie C, Abadie J, Amardeilh MF, et al: MIB-1 immunoreactivity correlates with biologic behaviour in canine cutaneous melanoma, *Vet Dermatol* 12(3):139–147, 2001.
54. Millanta F, Fratini F, Corazza M, et al: Proliferation activity in oral and cutaneous canine melanocytic tumours: correlation with histological parameters, location, and clinical behaviour, *Res Vet Sci* 73(1):45–51, 2002.
55. Vail DM, Macewen EG: Spontaneously occurring tumors of companion animals as models for human cancer, *Cancer Invest* 18(8):781–792, 2000.
56. Esplin DG: Survival of dogs following surgical excision of histologically well-differentiated melanocytic neoplasms of the mucous membranes of the lips and oral cavity, *Vet Pathol* 45(6):889–896, 2008.
57. Spangler WL, Kass PH: The histologic and epidemiologic bases for prognostic considerations in canine melanocytic neoplasia, *Vet Pathol* 43(2):136–149, 2006.
58. Bergin IL, Smedley RC, Esplin DG, et al: Prognostic evaluation of Ki67 threshold value in canine oral melanoma, *Vet Pathol* 48(1):41–53, 2011.
59. Henry CJ, Brewer WG Jr, Whitley EM, et al: Canine digital tumors: a veterinary cooperative oncology group retrospective study of 64 dogs, *J Vet Intern Med* 19(5):720–724, 2005.
60. Wobeser BK, Kidney BA, Powers BE, et al: Diagnoses and clinical outcomes associated with surgically amputated canine digits submitted to multiple veterinary diagnostic laboratories, *Vet Pathol* 44(3):355–361, 2007.
61. Marino DJ, Matthiesen DT, Stefanacci D, et al: Evaluation of dogs with digit masses: 117 cases (1981-1991), *J Am Vet Med Assoc* 207:726–728, 1995.
62. Piliang MP: Acral lentiginous melanoma, *Clin Lab Med* 31(2):281–288, 2011.
63. Smedley RC, Spangler WL, Esplin DG, et al: Prognostic markers for canine melanocytic neoplasms: a comparative review of the literature and goals for future investigation, *Vet Pathol* 48(1):54–72, 2011.
64. Freeman KP, Hahn KA, Harris FD, et al: Treatment of dogs with oral melanoma by hypofractionated radiation therapy and platinum-based chemotherapy (1987-1997), *J Vet Intern Med* 17(1):96–101, 2003.
65. Proulx DR, Ruslander DM, Dodge RK, et al: A retrospective analysis of 140 dogs with oral melanoma treated with external beam radiation, *Vet Radiol Ultrasound* 44(3):352–359, 2003.
66. Theon AP, Rodriguez C, Madewell BR: Analysis of prognostic factors and patterns of failure in dogs with malignant oral tumors treated with megavoltage irradiation, *J Am Vet Med Assoc* 210(6):778–784, 1997.
67. Williams LE, Packer RA: Association between lymph node size and metastasis in dogs with oral malignant melanoma: 100 cases (1987-2001), *J Am Vet Med Assoc* 222(9):1234–1236, 2003.
68. Leong SP, Accortt NA, Essner R, et al: Impact of sentinel node status and other risk factors on the clinical outcome of head and neck melanoma patients, *Arch Otolaryngol Head Neck Surg* 132(4):370–373, 2006.
69. Herring ES, Smith MM, Robertson J: Lymph node staging of oral and maxillofacial neoplasms in 31 dogs and cats, *J Vet Dent* 19(3):122–126, 2002.
70. Nwogu CE, Kanter PM, Anderson TM: Pulmonary lymphatic mapping in dogs: use of technetium sulfur colloid and isosulfan blue for pulmonary sentinel lymph node mapping in dogs, *Cancer Invest* 20(7-8):944–947, 2002.
71. Yudd AP, Kempf JS, Goydos JS, et al: Use of sentinel node lymphoscintigraphy in malignant melanoma, *Radiographics* 19(2):343–353, 1999.
72. Wells S, Bennett A, Walsh P, et al: Clinical usefulness of intradermal fluorescein and patent blue violet dyes for sentinel lymph node identification in dogs, *Vet Comp Oncol* 4(2):114–122, 2006.
73. Suga K, Karino Y, Fujita T, et al: Cutaneous drainage lymphatic map with interstitial multidetector-row computed tomographic lymphography using iopamidol: preliminary results, *Lymphology* 40(2):63–73, 2007.
74. Liuti T, de Vos J, Bosman T, et al: 67Gallium citrate scintigraphy to assess metastatic spread in a dog with an oral melanoma, *J Small Anim Pract* 50(1):31–34, 2009.
75. Wallace J, Matthiesen DT, Patnaik AK: Hemimaxillectomy for the treatment of oral tumors in 69 dogs, *Vet Surg* 21(5):337–341, 1992.
76. Schwarz PD, Withrow SJ, Curtis CR, et al: Partial maxillary resection as a treatment for oral cancer in 61 Dogs, *J Am Anim Hosp Assoc* 27:617–624, 1991.
77. Lascelles BD, Thomson MJ, Dernell WS, et al: Combined dorsolateral and intraoral approach for the resection of tumors of the maxilla in the dog, *J Am Anim Hosp Assoc* 39(3):294–305, 2003.
78. Schwarz PD, Withrow SJ, Curtis CR, et al: Mandibular resection as a treatment for oral cancer in 81 dogs, *J Am Anim Hosp Assoc* 27:601–610, 1991.
79. Kosovsky JK, Matthiesen DT, Marretta SM, et al: Results of partial mandibulectomy for the treatment of oral tumors in 142 dogs, *Vet Surg* 20(6):397–401, 1991.
80. Harvey HJ, MacEwen EG, Braun D, et al: Prognostic criteria for dogs with oral melanoma, *J Am Vet Med Assoc* 178(6):580–582, 1981.
81. Kurzman ID, MacEwen EG, Rosenthal RC, et al: Adjuvant therapy for osteosarcoma in dogs: results of randomized clinical trials using combined liposome-encapsulated muramyl tripeptide and cisplatin, *Clin Cancer Res* 1:1595–1601, 1995.
82. Fox LE, Geoghegan SL, Davis LH, et al: Owner satisfaction with partial mandibulectomy or maxillectomy for treatment of oral tumors in 27 dogs, *J Am Anim Hosp Assoc* 33:25–31, 1997.
83. Liptak JM, Dernell WS, Rizzo SA, et al: Partial foot amputation in 11 dogs, *J Am Anim Hosp Assoc* 41(1):47–55, 2005.
84. Bergman PJ, Wolchok JD: Of mice and men (and dogs): Development of a xenogeneic DNA vaccine for canine oral malignant melanoma, *Cancer Therapy* 6:817–826, 2008.
85. Grosenbaugh DA, Leard AT, Bergman PJ, et al: Safety and efficacy of a xenogeneic DNA vaccine encoding for human tyrosinase as adjunctive treatment for oral malignant melanoma in dogs following surgical excision of the primary tumor, *Am J Vet Res* 72(12):1631–1638, 2011.
86. Morton DL: Cytoreductive surgery and adjuvant immunotherapy in the management of metastatic melanoma, *Tumori* 87(4):S57-S59, 2001.
87. Bateman KE, Catton PA, Pennock PW, et al: 0-7-21 radiation therapy for the treatment of canine oral melanoma, *J Vet Intern Med* 8(4):267–272, 1994.
88. Blackwood L, Dobson JM: Radiotherapy of oral malignant melanomas in dogs, *J Am Vet Med Assoc* 209(1):98–102, 1996.
89. Theon AP, Rodriguez C, Madewell BR: Analysis of prognostic factors and patterns of failure in dogs with malignant oral tumors treated with megavoltage irradiation, *J Am Vet Med Assoc* 210(6):778–784, 1997.
90. Proulx DR, Ruslander DM, Dodge RK, et al: A retrospective analysis of 140 dogs with oral melanoma treated with external beam radiation, *Vet Radiol Ultrasound* 44(3):352–359, 2003.
91. Freeman KP, Hahn KA, Harris FD, et al: Treatment of dogs with oral melanoma by hypofractionated radiation therapy and platinum-based chemotherapy (1987-1997), *J Vet Intern Med* 17(1):96–101, 2003.
92. Murphy S, Hayes AM, Blackwood L, et al: Oral malignant melanoma: the effect of coarse fractionation radiotherapy alone or with adjuvant carboplatin therapy, *Vet Comp Oncol* 3(4):222–229, 2005.

93. Khan N, Khan MK, Almasan A, et al: The evolving role of radiation therapy in the management of malignant melanoma, *Int J Radiat Oncol Biol Phys* 80(3):645–654, 2011.
94. Theon AP, Madewell BR, Moore AS, et al: Localized thermo-cisplatin therapy: a pilot study in spontaneous canine and feline tumours, *Int J Hyperthermia* 7(6):881–892, 1991.
95. Bergman PJ, MacEwen EG, Kurzman ID, et al: Amputation and carboplatin for treatment of dogs with osteosarcoma: 48 cases (1991 to 1993), *J Vet Intern Med* 10(2):76–81, 1996.
96. Rassnick KM, Ruslander DM, Cotter SM, et al: Use of carboplatin for treatment of dogs with malignant melanoma: 27 cases (1989-2000), *J Am Vet Med Assoc* 218(9):1444–1448, 2001.
97. Hume KR, Johnson JL, Williams LE: Adverse effects of concurrent carboplatin chemotherapy and radiation therapy in dogs, *J Vet Intern Med* 23(1):24–30, 2009.
98. Veterinary Co-operative Oncology Group—Common Terminology Criteria for Adverse Events (VCOG-CTCAE) following chemotherapy or biological antineoplastic therapy in dogs and cats v1.0, *Vet Comp Oncol* 2(4):195–213, 2004.
99. Wergin MC, Ballmer-Hofer K, Roos M, et al: Preliminary study of plasma vascular endothelial growth factor (VEGF) during low- and high-dose radiation therapy of dogs with spontaneous tumors, *Vet Radiol Ultrasound* 45(3):247–254, 2004.
100. Wergin MC, Kaser-Hotz B: Plasma vascular endothelial growth factor (VEGF) measured in seventy dogs with spontaneously occurring tumours, *In Vivo* 18(1):15–19, 2004.
101. Wergin MC, Roos M, Inteeworn N, et al: The influence of fractionated radiation therapy on plasma vascular endothelial growth factor (VEGF) concentration in dogs with spontaneous tumors and its impact on outcome, *Radiother Oncol* 79(2):239–244, 2006.
102. Ladue T, Klein MK: Toxicity criteria of the veterinary radiation therapy oncology group, *Vet Radiol Ultrasound* 42(5):475–476, 2001.
103. Cahan WG, Woodard HQ: Sarcoma arising in irradiated bone; report of 11 cases, *Cancer* 1(1):3–29, 1948.
104. Seguin B, McDonald DE, Kent MS, et al: Tolerance of cutaneous or mucosal flaps placed into a radiation therapy field in dogs, *Vet Surg* 34(3):214–222, 2005.
105. Kitchell BE, Brown DM, Luck EE, et al: Intralesional implant for treatment of primary oral malignant melanoma in dogs, *J Am Vet Med Assoc* 204(2):229–236, 1994.
106. Theon AP, Madewell BR, Moore AS, et al: Localized thermo-cisplatin therapy: a pilot study in spontaneous canine and feline tumours, *Int J Hyperthermia* 7(6):881–892, 1991.
107. Spugnini EP, Dragonetti E, Vincenzi B, et al: Pulse-mediated chemotherapy enhances local control and survival in a spontaneous canine model of primary mucosal melanoma, *Melanoma Res* 16(1):23–27, 2006.
108. Rassnick KM, Ruslander DM, Cotter SM, et al: Use of carboplatin for treatment of dogs with malignant melanoma: 27 cases (1989-2000), *J Am Vet Med Assoc* 218(9):1444–1448, 2001.
109. Boria PA, Murry DJ, Bennett PF, et al: Evaluation of cisplatin combined with piroxicam for the treatment of oral malignant melanoma and oral squamous cell carcinoma in dogs, *J Am Vet Med Assoc* 224(3):388–394, 2004.
110. Page RL, Thrall DE, Dewhirst MW, et al: Phase I study of melphalan alone and melphalan plus whole body hyperthermia in dogs with malignant melanoma, *Int J Hyperthermia* 7(4):559–566, 1991.
111. Ogilvie GK, Reynolds HA, Richardson RC, et al: Phase II evaluation of doxorubicin for treatment of various canine neoplasms, *J Am Vet Med Assoc* 195(11):1580–1583, 1989.
112. Aigner K, Hild P, Breithaupt H, et al: Isolated extremity perfusion with DTIC: an experimental and clinical study, *Anticancer Res* 3(2):87–93, 1983.
113. Murphy S, Hayes AM, Blackwood L, et al: Oral malignant melanoma: the effect of coarse fractionation radiotherapy alone or with adjuvant carboplatin therapy, *Vet Comp Oncol* 3(4):222–229, 2005.
114. O'Day S, Boasberg P: Management of metastatic melanoma 2005, *Surg Oncol Clin N Am* 15(2):419–437, 2006.
115. Martinez CM, Penafiel-Verdu C, Vilafranca M, et al: Cyclooxygenase-2 expression is related with localization, proliferation, and overall survival in canine melanocytic neoplasms, *Vet Pathol* 48(6):1204–1211, 2011.
116. Pires I, Garcia A, Prada J, et al: COX-1 and COX-2 expression in canine cutaneous, oral and ocular melanocytic tumours, *J Comp Pathol* 143(2-3):142–149, 2010.
117. Paglia D, Dubielzig RR, Kado-Fong HK, et al: Expression of cyclooxygenase-2 in canine uveal melanocytic neoplasms, *Am J Vet Res* 70(10):1284–1290, 2009.
118. Alexander AN, Huelsmeyer MK, Mitzey A, et al: Development of an allogeneic whole-cell tumor vaccine expressing xenogeneic gp100 and its implementation in a phase II clinical trial in canine patients with malignant melanoma, *Cancer Immunol Immunother* 55(4):433–442, 2006.
119. Hogge GS, Burkholder JK, Culp J, et al: Preclinical development of human granulocyte-macrophage colony-stimulating factor-transfected melanoma cell vaccine using established canine cell lines and normal dogs, *Cancer Gene Ther* 6(1):26–36, 1999.
120. Macewen EG, Kurzman ID, Vail DM, et al: Adjuvant therapy for melanoma in dogs: results of randomized clinical trials using surgery, liposome-encapsulated muramyl tripeptide, and granulocyte macrophage colony-stimulating factor, *Clin Cancer Res* 5(12):4249–4258, 1999.
121. Bianco SR, Sun J, Fosmire SP, et al: Enhancing antimelanoma immune responses through apoptosis, *Cancer Gene Ther* 10(9):726–736, 2003.
122. Dow SW, Elmslie RE, Willson AP, et al: In vivo tumor transfection with superantigen plus cytokine genes induces tumor regression and prolongs survival in dogs with malignant melanoma, *J Clin Invest* 101(11):2406–2414, 1998.
123. Gyorffy S, Rodriguez-Lecompte JC, Woods JP, et al: Bone marrow-derived dendritic cell vaccination of dogs with naturally occurring melanoma by using human gp100 antigen, *J Vet Intern Med* 19(1):56–63, 2005.
124. Helfand SC, Soergel SA, Modiano JF, et al: Induction of lymphokine-activated killer (LAK) activity in canine lymphocytes with low dose human recombinant interleukin-2 in vitro, *Cancer Biother* 9(3):237–244, 1994.
125. Mayayo SL, Prestigio S, Maniscalco L, et al: Chondroitin sulfate proteoglycan-4: a biomarker and a potential immunotherapeutic target for canine malignant melanoma, *Vet J* 190(2):e26–e30, 2011.
126. Moriyama M, Kano R, Maruyama H, et al: Small interfering RNA (siRNA) against the survivin gene increases apoptosis in a canine melanoma cell line, *J Vet Med Sci* 72(12):1643–1646, 2010.
127. Watanabe Y, Kano R, Maruyama H, et al: Small interfering RNA (siRNA) against the Bcl-2 gene increases apoptosis in a canine melanoma cell line, *J Vet Med Sci* 72(3):383–386, 2010.
128. Thamm DH, Kurzman ID, Clark MA, et al: Preclinical investigation of PEGylated tumor necrosis factor alpha in dogs with spontaneous tumors: phase I evaluation, *Clin Cancer Res* 16(5):1498–1508, 2010.
129. Finocchiaro LM, Fiszman GL, Karara AL, et al: Suicide gene and cytokines combined nonviral gene therapy for spontaneous canine melanoma, *Cancer Gene Ther* 15(3):165–172, 2008.
130. Finocchiaro LM, Glikin GC: Cytokine-enhanced vaccine and suicide gene therapy as surgery adjuvant treatments for spontaneous canine melanoma, *Gene Ther* 15(4):267–276, 2008.
131. Gil-Cardeza ML, Villaverde MS, Fiszman GL, et al: Suicide gene therapy on spontaneous canine melanoma: correlations between in vivo tumors and their derived multicell spheroids in vitro, *Gene Ther* 17(1):26–36, 2010.
132. von Euler H, Sadeghi A, Carlsson B, et al: Efficient adenovector CD40 ligand immunotherapy of canine malignant melanoma, *J Immunother* 31(4):377–384, 2008.

133. Horiuchi Y, Tominaga M, Ichikawa M, et al: Relationship between regulatory and type 1 T cells in dogs with oral malignant melanoma, *Microbiol Immunol* 54(3):152–159, 2010.
134. Tominaga M, Horiuchi Y, Ichikawa M, et al: Flow cytometric analysis of peripheral blood and tumor-infiltrating regulatory T cells in dogs with oral malignant melanoma, *J Vet Diagn Invest* 22(3):438–441, 2010.
135. Guevara-Patino JA, Turk MJ, Wolchok JD, et al: Immunity to cancer through immune recognition of altered self: studies with melanoma, *Adv Cancer Res* 90:157–177, 2003.
136. Bouchard B, Vijayasaradhi S, Houghton AN: Production and characterization of antibodies against human tyrosinase, *J Invest Dermatol* 102(3):291–295, 1994.
137. Bouchard B, Del MV, Jackson IJ, et al: Molecular characterization of a human tyrosinase-related-protein-2 cDNA. Patterns of expression in melanocytic cells, *Eur J Biochem* 219(1-2):127–134, 1994.
138. Cangul IT, van Garderen E, van der Poel HJ, et al: Tyrosinase gene expression in clear cell sarcoma indicates a melanocytic origin: insight from the first reported canine case, *APMIS* 107(11):982–988, 1999.
139. Phillips JC, Lembcke LM, Noltenius CE, et al: Evaluation of tyrosinase expression in canine and equine melanocytic tumors, *Am J Vet Res* 73(2):272–278, 2012.
140. Weber LW, Bowne WB, Wolchok JD, et al: Tumor immunity and autoimmunity induced by immunization with homologous DNA, *J Clin Invest* 102(6):1258–1264, 1998.
141. Bergman PJ, Camps-Palau MA, McKnight JA, et al: Development of a xenogeneic DNA vaccine program for canine malignant melanoma at the Animal Medical Center, *Vaccine* 24:4582–4585, 2006.
142. Bergman PJ: Cancer immunotherapy, *Vet Clin North Am Small Anim Pract* 40(3):507–518, 2010.
143. Bergman PJ, McKnight J, Novosad A, et al: Long-term survival of dogs with advanced malignant melanoma after DNA vaccination with xenogeneic human tyrosinase: a phase I trial, *Clin Cancer Res* 9:1284–1290, 2003.
144. Liao JC, Gregor P, Wolchok JD, et al: Vaccination with human tyrosinase DNA induces antibody responses in dogs with advanced melanoma, *Cancer Immun* 6:8, 2006.
145. Goubier A, Fuhrmann L, Forest L, et al: Superiority of needle-free transdermal plasmid delivery for the induction of antigen-specific IFNgamma T cell responses in the dog, *Vaccine* 26:2186–2190, 2008.
146. Manley CA, Leibman NF, Wolchok JD, et al: Xenogeneic murine tyrosinase DNA vaccine for malignant melanoma of the digit of dogs, *J Vet Intern Med* 25(1):94–99, 2011.
147. Wolchok JD, Yuan J, Houghton AN, et al: Safety and immunogenicity of tyrosinase DNA vaccines in patients with melanoma, *Mol Ther* 15:2044–2050, 2007.
148. Yuan J, Ku GY, Gallardo HF, et al: Safety and immunogenicity of a human and mouse gp100 DNA vaccine in a phase I trial of patients with melanoma, *Cancer Immun* 9:5, 2009.
149. Ginsberg BA, Gallardo HF, Rasalan TS, et al: Immunologic response to xenogeneic gp100 DNA in melanoma patients: comparison of particle-mediated epidermal delivery with intramuscular injection, *Clin Cancer Res* 16(15):4057–4065, 2010.
150. Postow MA, Callahan MK, Wolchok JD: The antitumor immunity of ipilimumab: (T cell) memories to last a lifetime? *Clin Cancer Res* 18(7):1821–1823, 2012.
151. Chapman PB, Hauschild A, Robert C, et al: Improved survival with vemurafenib in melanoma with BRAF V600E mutation, *N Engl J Med* 364(26):2507–2516, 2011.
152. Ribas A, Flaherty KT: BRAF targeted therapy changes the treatment paradigm in melanoma, *Nat Rev Clin Oncol* 8(7):426–433, 2011.

Mast Cell Tumors 20

Cheryl A. London and Douglas H. Thamm

The neoplastic proliferation of mast cells referred to as a *mast cell tumor* (MCT; histiocytic mastocytoma, mast cell sarcoma) represents the most commonly encountered cutaneous tumor in the dog and the second most common cutaneous tumor in the cat.[1-5] Systemic forms of the disease are often referred to as *mastocytosis.* Canine and feline forms of the disease will be considered separately in this chapter because many differences exist with regard to histologic type, biologic behavior, therapy, and prognosis.

Canine Mast Cell Tumors

Biology of Canine Mast Cells

Mast cell precursors leave the bone marrow and migrate to various tissues throughout the body where they undergo differentiation into mature mast cells with their characteristic cytoplasmic granules, which stain metachromatically with Giemsa and toluidine blue.[6] These granules contain a number of bioactive substances, including heparin, histamine, preformed tumor necrosis factor-α (TNF-α), and several proteases.[6] The nature and composition of mast cell granules are highly influenced by the microenvironment in which the mast cells mature. For example, in dogs, mast cells in the gastrointestinal (GI) tract express primarily chymase, whereas mast cells in the skin express both chymase and tryptase.[7] When stimulated, mast cells can rapidly produce a variety of proteases (chymase, tryptase), cytokines (TNF-α, interleukin-6 [IL-6]), chemokines (CCL2, CXCL1), growth factors (vascular endothelial growth factor [VEGF], basic fibroblast growth factor [bFGF]), and lipid mediators (prostaglandin D_2 [PGD_2], leukotriene C_4 [LTC_4]).[6] Through this process, mast cells participate in several biologic activities, including wound healing, induction of innate immune responses, antiparasite activity, and modulation of reaction to insect and spider venoms.[6,8]

Normal canine mast cells can be generated from bone marrow–derived hematopoietic precursors.[9,10] These cells, known as *canine bone marrow–derived mast cells* (cBMMCs), have been used to characterize the functional properties of mast cells in this species. As with normal human mast cells, their differentiation requires the presence of the growth factor stem cell factor (SCF) and can be influenced by the presence of other cytokines.[9,10] When stimulated, these cells rapidly release histamine, monocyte chemotactic protein-1 (MCP-1), TNF-α, and tryptase, and they produce several additional cytokines and chemokines, including IL-3, IL-13, granulocyte-macrophage colony-stimulating factor (GM-CSF), and macrophage inflammatory protein 1α (MIP1α).[9,10] Interestingly, the cBMMCs are extremely sensitive to chemical degranulation, which may help to explain why dogs exhibit such a high degree of hypersensitivity to several chemical agents, including polysorbate 80, Cremophor EL, and doxorubicin.[9] The function of cBMMCs can be modulated by cytokines, steroids, and nonsteroidal antiinflammatory drugs (NSAIDs).[9-11]

Incidence and Risk Factors

MCTs represent the most common cutaneous tumor in the dog, accounting for between 16% and 21% of all cutaneous tumors.[1,3,5,12] Although MCTs are primarily a disease of older dogs (mean age approximately 8 to 9 years), they have also been reported in younger dogs and there is no apparent gender predilection.[1,3,5,13] Most tumors occur in mixed breeds; however, several breeds are at an increased risk for MCTs, including dogs of bulldog descent (Boxers, Boston terriers, English bulldogs, pugs), Labrador and golden retrievers, cocker spaniels, schnauzers, Staffordshire terriers, beagles, Rhodesian ridgebacks, Weimaraners, and Shar-Peis.[1,5,14-16] The increased incidence of MCTs in certain breeds suggests the possibility of an underlying genetic cause,[15] and studies are ongoing to identify these putative genetic risk factors. Interestingly, although dogs of bulldog ancestry are at higher risk for MCT development, it is generally accepted that MCTs in these dogs are more likely to behave in a benign fashion.[1] Additionally, it was recently demonstrated that pugs may develop multiple MCTs that behave in a benign fashion.[17] In contrast, anecdotal evidence suggests that Shar-Peis develop MCTs that may be more biologically aggressive. Spontaneously regressing MCTs in young animals have been described in cats, pigs, horses, and humans. Multiple cutaneous MCTs that regressed within 27 weeks were reported in a 3-week-old Jack Russell terrier.[18] This syndrome of spontaneous regression in young animals may indicate a hyperplastic or dysplastic syndrome rather than a true neoplastic lesion.

The etiology of MCTs in the dog is for the most part unknown. Historically, MCTs have been associated with chronic inflammation or the application of skin irritants; however, the epidemiology of disease in dogs does not support the role of a topical carcinogen.[19-21] Unequivocal evidence is lacking for a viral etiology, although MCTs have been transplanted to very young or immunocompromised laboratory dogs using tumor cell tissues and rarely by cell-free extracts.[22-24] No C-type or other identifiable virus particles have been observed, and no epidemiologic evidence exists to suggest horizontal transmission. Chromosomal fragile site expression, a phenomenon thought to genetically predispose humans to develop certain tumors, was shown to be increased in Boxers with MCTs.[25] However, the control population for this study was young, non–tumor-bearing Boxers, and the increased expression of chromosomal fragile sites may be due to this age difference.

The genetic changes that predispose dogs to MCTs are incompletely understood. Alterations in the *p53* tumor suppressor pathway have been identified in some canine MCTs,[26-28] but *p53* sequencing in a limited number of cases has revealed no mutations.[29] Perturbations in expression of the proteins p21 and p27, which are cyclin-dependent kinase inhibitors (CDKIs) that contribute to regulation of the cell cycle, have been identified in many canine MCTs.[30] Cytosolic receptors for estrogen and progesterone have also been detected in canine MCTs.[31] Their role in the etiopathogenesis of MCT is poorly understood, but evidence exists that estrogen and progesterone may influence mast cell function.[32] One European study reported that female dogs with MCTs had a more favorable prognosis with chemotherapy.[33] Although the majority of studies performed in the United States have failed to detect such an association, the relatively higher frequency of intact females present in the European population may have allowed the effect of sex hormones to have a greater statistical impact on biologic behavior.

Perhaps the best-described molecular abnormality in canine MCT involves the receptor tyrosine kinase (RTK), KIT. KIT is expressed normally on a variety of cells, including hematopoietic stem cells, melanocytes, and mast cells, among others.[34-36] The ligand for KIT, SCF, induces KIT dimerization, subsequent phosphorylation, and generation of intracellular signaling that promotes the proliferation, differentiation, and maturation of normal mast cells.[34-36] SCF is essential for the differentiation of mature mast cells from CD34+ hematopoietic stem cells in vitro, and inhibition of KIT signaling induces apoptosis of cBMMCs.[10,35,36] KIT expression has been demonstrated on canine MCTs, and aberrant cytoplasmic localization of KIT in MCTs may be associated with dysregulated KIT function.[37-40] A significant proportion of canine MCTs possess mutations in the *c-kit* gene involving either the juxtamembrane domain (exons 11 and 12) or extracellular domain (exons 8 and 9).[41-45] These mutations result in SCF-independent activation of KIT and subsequent unregulated KIT signal transduction.[43,44] In dogs, activating *c-kit* mutations appear to be present in 25% to 30% of intermediate-grade and high-grade MCTs, and evidence suggests that they are linked to increased risk of local recurrence, metastasis, and a worse prognosis.[41,44,46-48] The reason for the high rate of *c-kit* mutations in dog MCTs is unknown; however, it is clear that these mutations are not germline in nature.

History and Clinical Signs

The vast majority of MCTs in dogs occur in the dermis and subcutaneous tissue,[5,49] and most are solitary in nature, although 11% to 14% of dogs present with multiple lesions.[50-52] Approximately 50% of cutaneous MCTs occur on the trunk and perineal region, 40% on the limbs, and 10% on the head and neck.[20,53,54] MCTs have also been reported to occur on other sites, including the conjunctiva, salivary gland, nasopharynx, larynx, oral cavity, ureter, and spine.[55-59] A visceral form of MCT, often referred to as *disseminated* or *systemic mastocytosis,* has also been documented, although it is usually preceded by an aggressive primary lesion.[60-64] Infiltration of abdominal lymph nodes, spleen, liver, and bone marrow is commonly observed in the setting of visceral disease, and pleural/peritoneal effusions containing neoplastic mast cells have been documented. A case series of dogs with primary GI MCTs was recently reported in which most dogs presented with vomiting, diarrhea, and melena. Only 40% of the dogs were alive at 30 days after first admission, and fewer than 10% were alive at 6 months.[28]

It is important to note that cutaneous MCTs have an extremely varied range of clinical appearances, and they are sometimes inadvertently mistaken for nonneoplastic lesions. Well-differentiated MCTs tend to be solitary, small, slow-growing tumors that may have been present for several months. They are not typically ulcerated, but overlying hair may be lost. Undifferentiated MCTs tend to be rapidly growing, ulcerated lesions that cause considerable irritation and attain a large size. Surrounding tissues may become inflamed and edematous. Small satellite nodules may develop in surrounding tissues. Tumors of intermediate differentiation fill the spectrum between these two extremes. A subcutaneous form of MCT that is soft and fleshy on palpation is often misdiagnosed clinically as a lipoma (Figure 20-1).

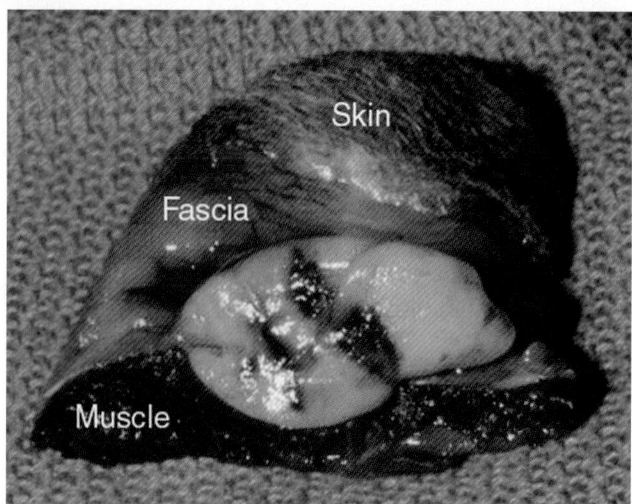

FIGURE 20-1 Subcutaneous MCT from the shoulder of a dog. This mass was originally misdiagnosed as a lipoma based on palpation alone. Note tumor extension through fascia and muscle. Wide surgical excision to include deep muscle layer is necessary to achieve complete ("clean") surgical margins.

The history and clinical signs of dogs with MCTs may be complicated by signs attributable to the release of histamine, heparin, and other vasoactive amines from mast cell granules. Occasionally, mechanical manipulation during examination of the tumor results in degranulation and subsequent erythema and wheal formation in surrounding tissues. This phenomenon has been referred to as *Darier's sign* (Figure 20-2)[51] and can also occur spontaneously; dog owners may describe the tumor as increasing and decreasing in size. GI ulceration has been documented in 35% to 83% of dogs with MCTs that underwent necropsy.[65,66] Histamine released from MCT granules is thought to act on parietal cells via H_2 receptors, resulting in increased hydrochloric acid secretion. Plasma histamine concentrations have been shown to be high in dogs with MCTs, and there is preliminary information that monitoring of plasma histamine concentrations may be useful in assessing disease progression.[67] These dogs also have decreased concentrations of plasma gastrin, which is normally released by antral G-cells in response to increased gastric hydrochloric acid concentrations, acting as a negative feedback loop. Dogs with substantial MCT burden (i.e., large tumors, metastatic disease, systemic disease) are much more likely to present with clinical signs related to the release of mast cell mediators. These may include vomiting, diarrhea, fever, peripheral edema, and, rarely, collapse.

Perioperative degranulation of MCTs and subsequent release of histamine and other less-characterized vasoactive substances may also result in potentially life-threatening hypotensive events during surgery. It is thought that prostaglandins in the D series secreted by tumor cells may mediate the hypotensive effects observed in humans with mast cell diseases.[68,69] Coagulation abnormalities, also reported in dogs with MCTs, are likely due to heparin release from mast cell granules.[63,70] Although clinical evidence of hemorrhage is not typically associated with this phenomenon, localized hemorrhage at the time of surgery as the result of degranulation following

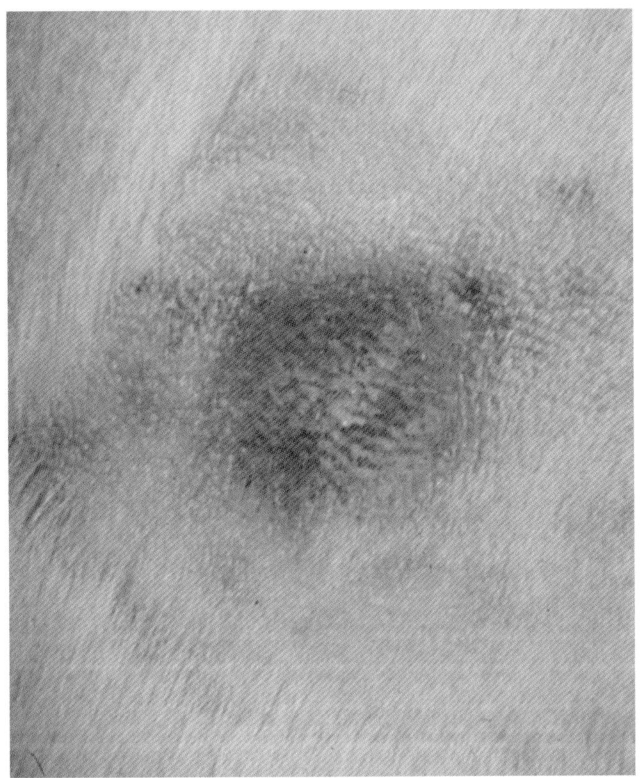

FIGURE 20-2 Erythema and wheal formation occurred in surrounding skin following manipulation of this cutaneous MCT. This phenomenon, resulting from the release of vasoactive amines from mast cell granules, is known as *Darier's sign*.

tumor manipulation can be a serious complication, even in the presence of normal presurgical coagulation parameters.

Prognostic Factors

A discussion of prognostic factors associated with canine MCTs will precede sections on diagnosis and treatment because steps followed in those sections are predicated on the presence or absence of these prognostic factors. Table 20-1 lists factors known to be predictive of biologic behavior and clinical outcome in dogs with MCTs. It is important to note that no one factor is entirely predictive of biologic behavior; thus all prognostic indicators should be taken into consideration when evaluating a patient.

Histologic grade is considered the most consistent and reliable prognostic factor available for dogs with MCTs, although it will not predict the behavior of every tumor.[14,49,71,72] Several investigators have applied histologic grading systems to canine MCTs based on degree of differentiation (Table 20-2). The number grades used in these studies are at odds. Therefore, for the sake of clarity, the three differentiation groups should be simply referred to as undifferentiated (high) grade, intermediate grade, and well-differentiated (low) grade. Table 20-3 lists the relative distribution of MCT grades encountered in larger series. Survival following surgical excision based on grade is presented in Table 20-4. The vast majority of dogs with well-differentiated tumors (80% to 90%) and approximately 75% of dogs with intermediate-grade tumors experience long-term survival following complete surgical excision.[50,71,74-77] Metastatic rates for undifferentiated tumors range from 55% to 96%, and most dogs with these tumors die of their disease within 1 year.[49,78] The majority disseminate first to local lymph nodes, then to the spleen

TABLE 20-1 Prognostic Factors for Mast Cell Tumors in Dogs

FACTOR	COMMENT
Histologic grade	Strongly predictive of outcome. Dogs with undifferentiated tumors typically die of their disease following local therapy alone, whereas those with well-differentiated tumors are usually cured with appropriate local therapy.
Clinical stage	Stages 0 and I, confined to the skin without local lymph node or distant metastasis, have a better prognosis than higher-stage disease.
Location	Subungual, oral, and other mucous membrane sites are associated with more high-grade tumors and worse prognosis. Preputial and scrotal tumors are also associated with a worse prognosis. Subcutaneous tumors may have a better prognosis. Visceral or bone marrow disease usually carries a grave prognosis.
Cell proliferation rate	MI, relative frequency of AgNORs, percentage of PCNA, or Ki67 immunopositivity are predictive of postsurgical outcome.
Growth rate	MCTs that remain localized and are present for prolonged periods of time (months or years) without significant change are usually benign.
DNA ploidy	There is a trend toward shorter survival times and higher-stage disease in dogs with aneuploid tumors.
Microvessel density	Increased microvessel density is associated with higher grade, a higher degree of invasiveness, and a worse prognosis.
Recurrence	Local recurrence following surgical excision may carry a more guarded prognosis.
Systemic signs	The presence of systemic illness (e.g., anorexia, vomiting, melena, GI ulceration) may be associated with higher-stage disease.
Age	Older dogs may have shorter median DFIs when treated with RT than younger dogs.
Breed	MCTs in Boxers (and potentially other brachycephalic breeds) tend to be low or intermediate grade and are thus associated with a better prognosis.
Sex	Male dogs had a shorter survival time than female dogs when treated with chemotherapy.
Tumor size	Large tumors may be associated with a worse prognosis following surgical removal and/or RT.
c-kit mutation	The presence of an activating mutation in the *c-kit* gene is associated with a worse prognosis.

MI, Mitotic index; *AgNORs,* argyrophilic nucleolar organizer regions; *PCNA,* proliferating cell nuclear antigen; *MCTs,* mast cell tumors; *GI,* gastrointestinal; *DFIs,* disease-free intervals; *RT,* radiation therapy.

TABLE 20-2 Histologic Classification of Mast Cell Tumors in Dogs

GRADE	BOSTOCK GRADING	PATNAIK GRADING	MICROSCOPIC DESCRIPTION
Anaplastic, undifferentiated (high grade)	1	3	Highly cellular, undifferentiated cytoplasmic boundaries, irregular size and shape of nuclei, frequent mitoses, sparse cytoplasmic granules.
Intermediate grade	2	2	Cells closely packed with indistinct cytoplasmic boundaries, nucleus-to-cytoplasmic ratio lower than anaplastic, infrequent mitoses, more granules than anaplastic.
Well differentiated (low grade)	3	1	Clearly defined cytoplasmic boundaries with regular, spheric, or ovoid nuclei; mitoses rare or absent; cytoplasmic granules large, deep staining, and abundant.

TABLE 20-3 Relative Frequency of Canine Mast Cell Tumors by Histologic Grade

INVESTIGATOR	DOGS (NO.)	HIGH GRADE (%)	INTERMEDIATE GRADE (%)	LOW GRADE (%)
Hottendorf[20]	300	19	27	54
Bostock[49]	114	39	26	34
Patnaik[14]	83	20	43	36
Simoes[72]	87	22	40	38

TABLE 20-4 Survival Times of Dogs with Surgically Treated Mast Cell Tumors According to Histologic Grade*

INVESTIGATOR	DOGS (NO.)	PERCENT ALIVE	MONTHS POSTSURGERY	MEDIAN SURVIVAL TIME (WEEKS)
Bostock[49]				
Low grade	39	79	7	NR
Intermediate grade	30	37	7	NR
High grade	45	15	7	NR
Patnaik[14]				
Low grade	30	83	48	NR
Intermediate grade	36	44	48	NR
High grade	17	6	48	NR
Bostock[73]				
Low grade	19	90	NR	>40†
Intermediate grade	16	75		>36
High grade	15	27		13
Murphy[71]				
Low grade	87	100	12	>80†
Intermediate grade	199	92	12	>80
High grade	54	46	12	40
Simoes[72]				
Low grade	33	91	20	NR
Intermediate grade	35	71	20	NR
High grade	19	42	20	NR

NR, Not reported.

*Unclear in these studies if death due to metastasis or local recurrence.

†Medians not reached at the time of last follow-up (i.e., >50% alive).

and liver. Other visceral organs may be involved; however, lung involvement is infrequent. Neoplastic mast cells may be observed in the bone marrow and peripheral blood in cases of widespread systemic dissemination.[63]

The current histopathologic grading system does not detect a small percentage (15% to 30%) of those well-differentiated or intermediately differentiated MCTs that result in the death of affected dogs; this is complicated by the fact that there is disagreement in tumor grading among pathologists. In one study, there was significant variation among pathologists in grading a specific set of MCTs ($p < 0.001$), although this was found to be less so if all pathologists strictly employed the system described by Patnaik.[14,79,80] Recently, an attempt was made to develop a new grading system that would separate tumors into high or low grade based on one of four features identified on histopathologic evaluation.[81] In this setting, tumors would be classified as high grade if they possessed (1) at least seven mitotic figures/10 HPF, (2) at least three multinucleated cells/10 HPF, (3) at least three bizarre nuclei/10 HPF, or (4) karyomegaly. In a series of 95 dogs evaluated by both the Patnaik system and this alternative system, the alternative system was somewhat better at predicting which dogs would be more likely to die of disease[81]; however, further validation of this new two-tiered system will be necessary to determine whether it is truly better than the more commonly used Patnaik three-tiered system for predicting the biologic behavior of MCTs.

Several markers of proliferation have been evaluated to assist in determining whether an MCT is likely to behave in a more aggressive manner.[47,72,82-90] Ki67 is a protein found in the nucleus, the levels of which appear to correlate with cell proliferation. In one study, the mean number of Ki67-positive nuclei was significantly higher for dogs that died of MCTs than for those that survived.[83] In another study, the Ki67 score was used to divide intermediate-grade MCTs into two groups with markedly different expected survival times.[84] Silver colloid staining of paraffin-embedded sections can be used to determine the relative presence of argyrophilic nucleolar organizer regions (AgNORs), another surrogate marker of proliferation. These have been correlated with histologic grade and postsurgical outcome.[72,73] In a study of 50 dogs with cutaneous MCTs, the AgNOR frequency was as predictive or more predictive of biologic behavior than histologic grade.[73] Finally, proliferating cell nuclear antigen (PCNA), another indicator of cell proliferation, has been used to determine the biologic behavior of MCTs, although this is probably not as reliable as the other markers.[72,73,91] The previously discussed markers of proliferation all require the use of special stains. In contrast, the mitotic index (MI), or number of mitoses/10 HPF in hematoxylin and eosin (H&E) sections, has been used to assess the biologic behavior of canine MCTs.[92] In one study, those dogs with tumors possessing an MI of 5 or lower had a median survival time (MST) of 80 months, compared to 3 months for those possessing an MI of more than 5, suggesting that the MI is a strong predictor of overall survival for dogs with MCTs. Additional studies have also found a role for MI in MCT prognosis.[81,90,92-95]

Other cellular assessments have been employed to evaluate the biologic behavior of MCT. A study of DNA ploidy determined by flow cytometric analysis suggested a trend toward shorter survival and higher clinical stage of disease in aneuploid tumors compared to diploid tumors.[96] Recent studies have found a correlation between intratumor microvessel density and invasiveness, mitotic rate, and prognosis[82,97] and a correlation between nuclear characteristics (assessed by computerized morphometry) and outcome and grade.[98,99] The potential role of KIT dysregulation in MCT prognosis was investigated by assessing KIT immunohistochemical staining patterns on histopathologic specimens.[100] Three distinct patterns were identified: membrane, focal/stippled, and diffuse cytoplasmic staining. Although there was some evidence that dogs with diffuse cytoplasmic KIT staining patterns did not live as long as those with other patterns, no group reached an MST and most dogs in each of the KIT staining groups evaluated experienced extremely long survival times postsurgery.[100] In contrast, the presence of *c-kit*–activating mutations has been associated with a higher rate of local recurrence, metastasis, and death from disease, suggesting that KIT dysregulation confers a more aggressive phenotype to MCTs.[41,46,47] Finally, investigators have attempted to correlate histologic grading of MCTs with a combined Ki67/PCNA/AgNOR/KIT immunohistochemical scoring.[101] No significant correlation was found for KIT staining and MCT grade, but high Ki67/PCNA/AgNOR scores all did correlate positively with tumor grade (i.e., higher scores for higher grade). This suggests that proliferation indices increase with increasing grade and are ultimately reflected in the eventual biologic behavior of the tumor.

Tumor location has been investigated as a potential prognostic indicator.[50,102-108] Tumors in the preputial/inguinal area, subungual (nailbed) region (Figure 20-3), and other mucocutaneous sites, including the oral cavity and perineum, have been associated historically with aggressive behavior. Two reports did not show a negative prognosis for tumors occurring in the inguinal and perineal

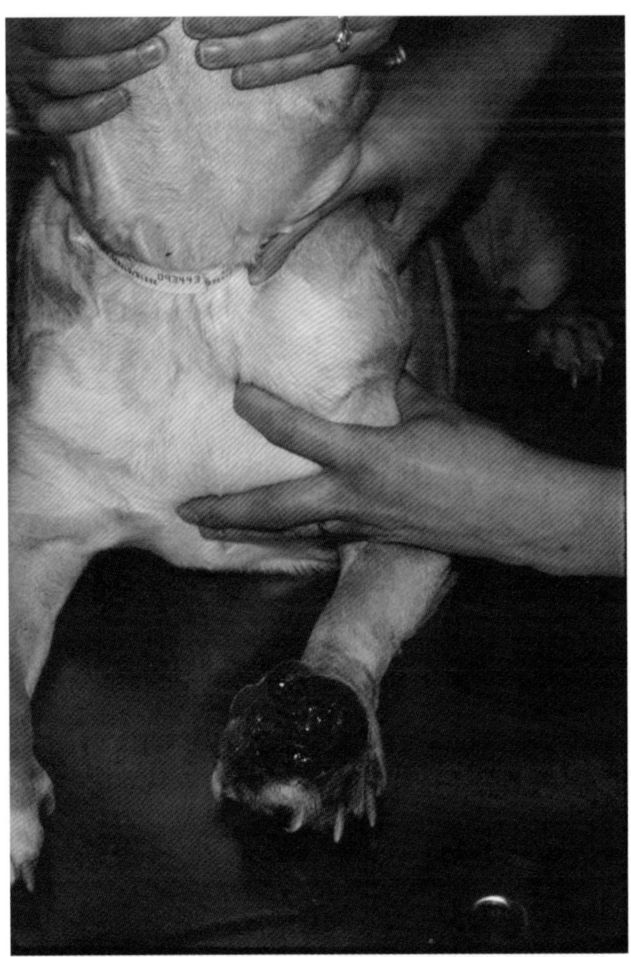

FIGURE 20-3 Subungual undifferentiated MCT in an English bulldog. As with some MCTs in this location, early lymph node metastasis has occurred.

region; however, when preputial and scrotal regions were specifically evaluated, they were indeed associated with a poorer prognosis.[106,107] Approximately 50% to 60% of dogs with MCTs located in the muzzle present with regional lymph node metastasis.[108,109] Interestingly, this does not necessarily indicate a worse long-term prognosis because the MST for dogs with metastatic disease was 14 months.[108] MCTs that originate in the viscera (GI tract, liver, spleen) or bone marrow carry a grave prognosis.[62,63] Recent data indicate that MCTs arising in the subcutaneous tissues have a favorable prognosis, with extended survival time and low rates of recurrence and metastasis. In one study of 306 dogs with subcutaneous MCTs, metastasis occurred in 4% of dogs and 8% experienced local recurrence.[95] The estimated 2- and 5-year survival probabilities were 92% and 86%, respectively. Decreased survival was linked to MI higher than 4, infiltrative growth pattern, and presence of multinucleation. Finally, conjunctival MCTs were found to have a good prognosis, with 15/32 dogs disease free at a mean of 21.4 months postsurgery; no dogs in this study died of MCT-related disease.[110]

Clinical stage, represented in Table 20-5, is also predictive of outcome.[33,49,96,105,111] There is controversy regarding the effect of multiple MCTs on prognosis, and as such, this part of the staging scheme may not accurately correlate with outcome. Several studies indicate that there is no difference in outcome between patients with a single cutaneous MCT and those with multiple MCTs,[50,112-114] whereas others have suggested an inferior outcome in dogs with multiple tumors.[94,115] It is uncertain at this time whether this phenomenon represents an atypical form of metastasis or multiple, unrelated tumors arising independently, although one study demonstrated a clonal origin for two distant cutaneous tumors arising over years.[116] The effect of lymph node metastasis on prognosis is also somewhat controversial. In two studies, the presence of mast cells in the regional lymph node was a negative prognostic factor for survival and disease-free interval (DFI)[113,117]; however, an additional study revealed that dogs with intermediately differentiated MCTs and lymph node metastasis treated with radiation therapy (RT) postsurgery achieved long-term survival.[118] Other studies have shown that dogs with intermediately differentiated MCT with lymph node metastasis may have a good prognosis if the affected lymph node is removed and adjuvant chemotherapy is administered.[113,114,119] For poorly differentiated tumors, the presence of metastatic disease resulted in an MST of 194 days compared to 503 days for dogs with no metastasis.[78] For these dogs, treatment of the lymph node improved survival time (240 days) compared to those dogs whose lymph nodes were not treated (42 days).[78] As with all cases, clinical judgment regarding lymph node metastasis is probably important. A dog with an effaced enlarged lymph node will be more likely to fail therapy when compared to a dog with a lymph node that is not clinically enlarged but has cytologic evidence of metastasis.

Several miscellaneous factors have been linked to prognosis in dogs with MCTs. Certain breeds of dogs such as Boxers, pugs, and dogs of bulldog descent appear to develop MCTs that often behave in a more benign fashion.[1,17,49] Recent rapid growth has been associated with a worse outcome. For example, in one study, 83% of dogs with tumors present for longer than 28 weeks prior to surgery survived for at least 30 weeks, compared to only 25% of dogs with tumors present for less than 28 weeks.[49] Systemic signs of anorexia, vomiting, melena, widespread erythema, and edema associated with vasoactive substances from mast cell degranulation are more commonly associated with visceral forms of MCT and carry a more guarded prognosis.[50,63,64] In 16 cases of visceral MCTs, an MST of 90 days was reported and all dogs with follow-up died of their disease.[103] Local tumor ulceration, erythema, or pruritus has been associated with a worse prognosis in some studies.[50,113] Finally, recurrence of MCT following surgical excision has also been associated with a more guarded prognosis.[113] Thus appropriate aggressive therapy at the time of first presentation, rather than at the time of recurrence, may improve the long-term prognosis in patients with MCTs.

TABLE 20-5 World Health Organization Clinical Staging System for Mast Cell Tumors

STAGE	DESCRIPTION
0	One tumor incompletely excised from the dermis, identified histologically, without regional lymph node involvement 1. Without systemic signs 2. With systemic signs
I	One tumor confined to the dermis, without regional lymph node involvement 1. Without systemic signs 2. With systemic signs
II	One tumor confined to the dermis, with regional lymph node involvement 1. Without systemic signs 2. With systemic signs
III	Multiple dermal tumors; large, infiltrating tumors with or without regional lymph node involvement 1. Without systemic signs 2. With systemic signs
IV	Any tumor with distant metastasis, including blood or bone marrow involvement

Diagnostic Technique and Work-Up

MCTs are initially diagnosed on the basis of fine-needle aspiration (FNA) cytology. The Romanowsky or rapid hematologic-type stains used in most practices will suffice. Mast cells appear as small to medium-sized round cells with abundant, small, uniform cytoplasmic granules that stain purplish red (metachromatic; see Figures 7-2 and 7-5).[1,120] A small percentage of MCTs have granules that do not stain readily, giving them an epithelial or macrophage-like appearance that has often been referred to as a "fried-egg" appearance (see Figure 7-2). In these cases, a Wright-Giemsa or toluidine blue stain will often reveal granules; however, histologic assessment may ultimately be necessary. Highly anaplastic, agranular MCTs can sometimes be challenging to definitively diagnose by routine light microscopy. Immunohistochemical techniques have been applied in an attempt to differentiate these from other anaplastic round cell tumors. MCTs are vimentin positive, and the majority are tryptase and CD117 (KIT) positive.[37,121-123] Other markers that could potentially be useful include chymase, MCP-1, and IL-8.[9,10]

Historically, complete staging has included a minimum database (complete blood count [CBC], serum biochemistry profile), a buffy coat smear to document peripheral mastocytosis, cytologic assessment of regional lymph nodes, abdominal ultrasound (US) with cytologic assessment of spleen or liver if warranted, thoracic radiographs, and bone marrow aspiration cytology. It is now likely that

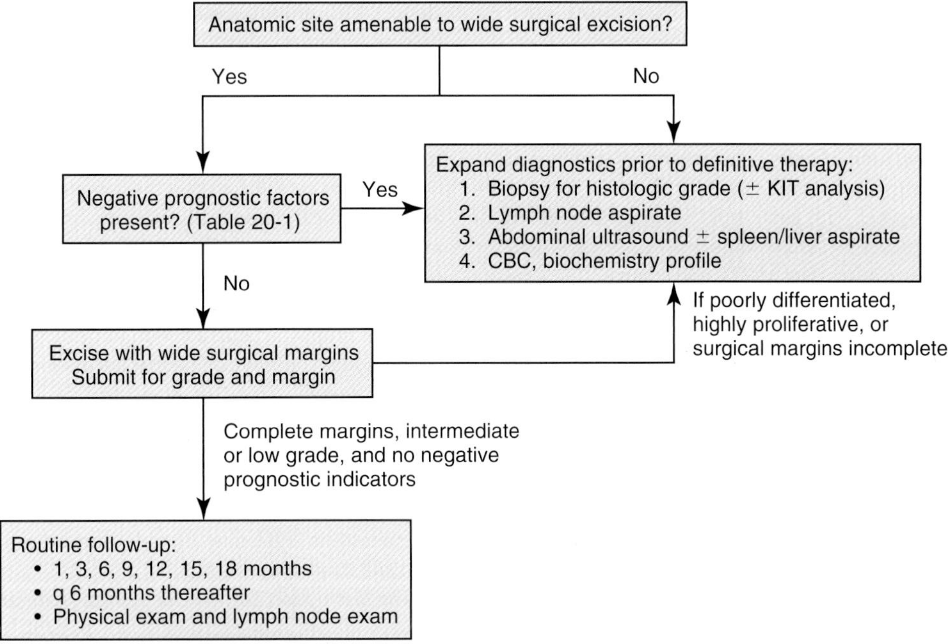

FIGURE 20-4 Suggested diagnostic steps for canine cutaneous MCTs.

an extensive work-up is not necessary for dogs with MCTs that do not exhibit the previously discussed negative prognostic factors. Figure 20-4 illustrates the diagnostic steps and the order in which they are pursued in the authors' practice. If the MCT is in a location amenable to wide surgical excision and no negative prognostic indicators are present (see Table 20-1), no further tests other than the minimum database and FNA of the regional lymph node (if possible) are performed prior to wide surgical excision. FNA cytology is not sufficient to grade MCT; thus histologic assessment following excision is strongly recommended to provide guidance regarding necessary further diagnostics and therapeutics.

If the tumor presents at a site that is not amenable to wide surgical excision (e.g., distal extremity) or if negative prognostic factors exist in the history or physical examination, ancillary diagnostics to further stage the disease are recommended prior to definitive therapy. An incisional/needle biopsy may be performed at this point for determination of histologic grade. The minimum staging that is advisable in those cases requiring presurgical staging consists of a minimum database, FNA cytology of the regional lymph node (even if normal size), and abdominal US. With respect to cytologic evaluation of lymph nodes, definitive criteria for metastatic disease can be challenging if mast cells are present in low numbers because mast cells are normally found in lymph nodes and their numbers can be increased in the presence of infection and ulceration, which are sometimes observed in MCTs. For example, in 56 healthy beagle dogs, approximately 24% of lymph node aspirates contained mast cells (range of 1 to 16 mast cells/slide, mean of 6.4 cells/slide).[124] Therefore an occasional solitary mast cell is not indicative of metastasis; rather, clustering and aggregates are more worrisome (Figure 20-5).[111] Surgical removal of a cytologically suspicious lymph node for histologic assessment may be necessary to accurately determine whether mast cells present in the lymph node truly represent metastatic disease. Abdominal US is now considered an important diagnostic test for the evaluation of dogs with potentially aggressive MCTs. Although FNA cytology of structurally normal livers or spleens is generally unrewarding,[125,126] the presence of negative

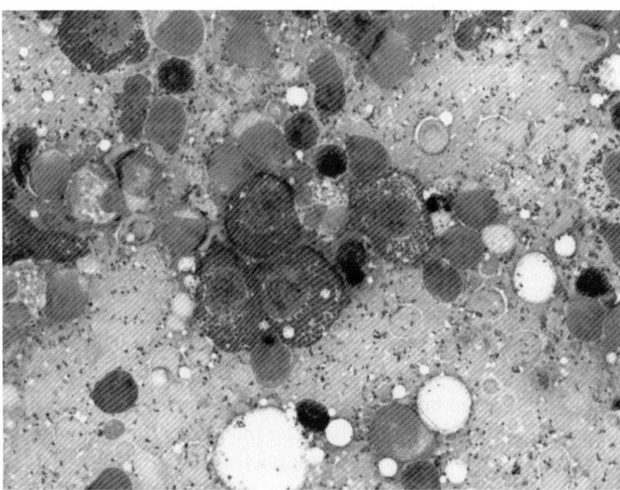

FIGURE 20-5 Regional lymph node aspirate from a dog with a cutaneous MCT. Note the clustering of mast cells in a background of lymphocytes that is more indicative of true metastasis.

prognostic indicators (e.g., metastatic lymph node, clinical signs) is sufficient justification to perform cytologic evaluation of these organs even if they appear normal on US.[127]

Thoracic radiographs rarely demonstrate metastasis; however, it is reasonable to procure them prior to an expensive or invasive procedure to rule out occult cardiopulmonary disease that could complicate anesthesia or unrelated disease processes (e.g., primary lung tumor). Occasionally, thoracic lymphadenopathy may be observed as a result of MCT metastasis. Knowledge of the extent of MCT margins prior to surgery, usually accomplished by digital palpation and occasionally local radiographs, can be enhanced with the use of diagnostic US or computed tomography (CT). Dogs bearing cutaneous MCTs or soft tissue sarcomas had the extent of local tumor margins upgraded in 19% and 65% of cases when imaged by US and CT, respectively.[128] Such information allows more appropriate planning of definitive surgery or RT. The cost effectiveness of such a study depends on the location of the tumor and whether wide excision is technically simple or difficult.

With respect to evaluation of buffy coat smears for evidence of systemic mast cell disease, peripheral mastocytosis (1 to 90 mast cells/μL) is reported in dogs with acute inflammatory disease (in particular, parvoviral infections), inflammatory skin disease, regenerative anemias, neoplasia other than MCTs, and trauma.[129-131] One study revealed that peripheral mastocytosis is actually more likely to occur and may be more dramatic in dogs with diseases other than MCTs.[130] Therefore this test is no longer routinely performed in the staging of MCT patients. In a report evaluating 157 dogs with MCTs, the incidence of bone marrow infiltration at initial staging was only 2.8%.[132] Although the presence of bone marrow involvement is indicative of systemic mast cell disease, it is usually easier to find evidence of systemic involvement in other organs (liver, spleen).[63] This is in contrast to dogs that present with visceral MCTs, in which 37% of buffy coat smears are positive for mast cells and 56% of bone marrow aspirates reveal mast cell dissemination[103]; however, these constitute a small minority of all MCT cases. Therefore, with the exception of the extremely rare case of primary mastocytic leukemia,[133,134] involvement of marrow or peripheral blood in the absence of disease in regional lymph node or abdominal organs is unlikely.[132]

Treatment

Treatment decisions are predicated on the presence or absence of negative prognostic factors and on the clinical stage of disease. In tumors localized to the skin in areas amenable to wide excision, surgery is the treatment of choice. Historically, surgical excision to include a 3-cm margin of surrounding normal tissue has been recommended for MCT. More recently, evidence exists that 1- to 2-cm lateral margins may be sufficient for complete excision of many MCTs, particularly those that are lower grade and small.[135,136] Indeed, in 100 dogs with 115 resectable MCTs (primarily intermediate and low grade), no local recurrence or metastasis was noted for greater than 2 years following excision with lateral histologic margins of 10 mm or larger and deep histologic margins of 4 mm or larger.[76] It should be noted that these microscopic, formalin-fixed margin parameters may not accurately reflect margin size at surgery: tissue shrinkage (up to 30% for cutaneous tissues) can occur subsequent to formalin fixation.[137-139] Considering that the majority of naïve dermal MCTs encountered in practice are intermediate- or low-grade tumors, it can be said that most MCTs can be cured with surgery alone, provided the site is amenable to adequate surgical resection. The quality of the deep margin is as important as that of the lateral margins, and it is recommended that one uninvolved fascial plane deep to the tumor be removed in continuity with the tumor. If necessary, muscle layers may also be removed deep to the tumor. All surgical margins should be evaluated histologically for completeness of excision. It is recommended that tumors in areas not amenable to wide surgical margins, such as distal extremities, be evaluated by biopsy to determine histologic grade prior to definitive therapy.

If a distal extremity MCT is low or intermediate grade and complete excision is not achievable, four primary therapy options exist. The most aggressive option is amputation; however, although wide margins are guaranteed, it results in the least functional outcome and is generally not recommended given the availability of other effective therapies. The second option is external-beam RT alone, which produces varying control rates in the literature when used as a primary therapy; doses between 40 and 50 Gy result in 1-year control rates of approximately 50%.[105,140-145]

The third and, in the authors' opinion, the ideal option for low- or intermediate-grade MCTs in areas where wide surgical excision is not possible is a combination of surgery and RT. The veterinary literature has established that the complementary use of surgery to achieve clinical stage 0 disease (i.e., microscopically incomplete margins) and external-beam RT is associated with long-term control. Two-year control rates of 85% to 95% can be expected for low- or intermediate-grade stage 0 tumors.[105,117,146-148] Some authors advocate prophylactic irradiation of cytologically negative regional lymph nodes (prophylactic nodal irradiation [PNI]).[114,117,118,149] Due to the generally low risk of postsurgical metastasis in low- to intermediate-grade tumors, PNI is probably unwarranted in this group of patients, and at least one study has demonstrated no advantage in terms of disease-free or overall survival when PNI is employed in this group of dogs[148]; however, in MCTs at high risk for metastasis, PNI may provide improvement in outcome over local site irradiation only.[114,149]

The last option for low- or intermediate-grade MCTs in areas where wide surgical excision is not possible is a combination of surgery and chemotherapy (discussed later). There are now several published studies that have demonstrated a low rate of recurrence in dogs with incompletely excised MCTs that receive some form of chemotherapy postsurgery.[150,151] Although not considered optimal, this approach can be used in cases in which RT is unavailable or unaffordable. Regardless of the local therapy chosen, dogs with low- and intermediate-grade tumors should be reevaluated regularly for local recurrence and possible metastasis. Local site and regional lymph node evaluation, complete physical examination, and aspiration of any new cutaneous masses or enlarged lymph nodes are performed at these intervals. More complete staging, including abdominal US, should be included if the dog has an MCT with negative prognostic indicators.

For cases in which planned curative excisional surgery is unsuccessful and histologic margins are incomplete, further local therapy is warranted. A second excision of the surgical scar with additional wide margins should be performed if possible (Figure 20-6) or adjuvant RT can be used in cases in which re-excision is not an option. Not all MCTs with surgically incomplete margins will recur; in some studies, only 20% to 30% of MCTs with histologically confirmed incomplete margins recurred.[84,152] Although recurrence rates vary by study, several studies have demonstrated increased recurrence rates and/or decreased overall survival in dogs with incompletely resected MCTs.[28,71,73,113] Figure 20-7 summarizes the treatment recommendations for clinical stage 0 and I, histologically low- or intermediate-grade MCTs. Alternative local therapies for MCTs have been reported and include hyperthermia in combination with RT,[153] intralesional brachytherapy,[154,155] photodynamic therapy,[156,157] intralesional corticosteroids,[158] cryotherapy, and electrochemotherapy.[159-161] Although some have advocated the use of intralesional deionized water at the site of an incompletely removed MCT, clinical data indicate that this approach is not effective at preventing local recurrence and should therefore not be used.[162-167] It is important to note that none of these alternative local therapies are as thoroughly investigated, clinically effective, or practical as surgery, RT, or a combination of the two. Finally, despite its common use, there is no information available to suggest that adjuvant corticosteroid therapy is beneficial in cases of individual intermediate-grade MCTs that have been either excised completely or treated with local RT postsurgery.

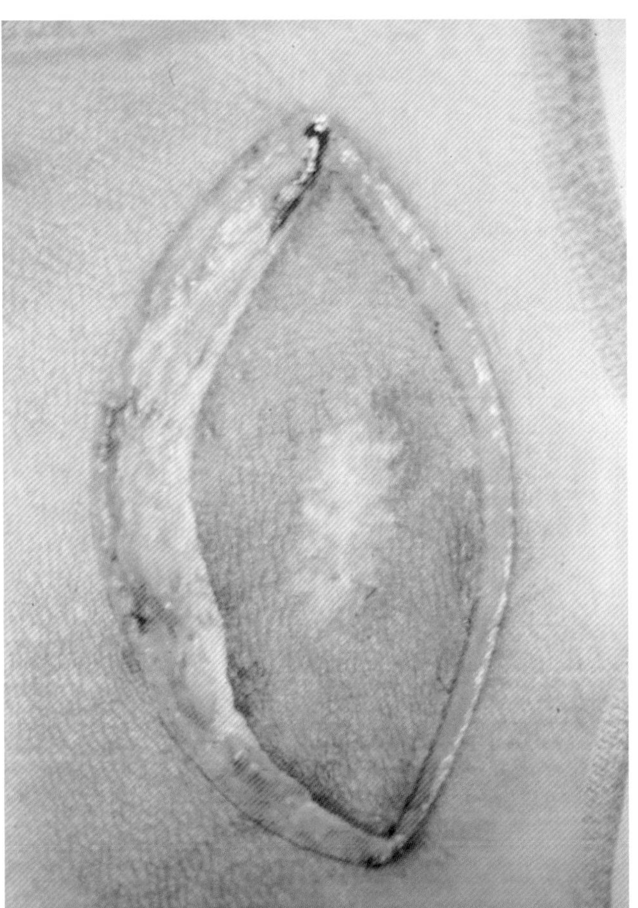

FIGURE 20-6 Re-excision of an MCT from the skin of a golden retriever. The first surgery resulted in incomplete surgical margins; thus 3-cm margins were taken around and deep to the previous incision and the entire sample was again submitted for margin analysis by the pathologist.

The treatment of anaplastic or undifferentiated MCTs remains a frustrating undertaking. This designation includes dogs with intermediate-grade tumors with regional or distant metastasis or high proliferative activity as assessed by MI or special stains, as well as those arising from a mucous membrane or mucocutaneous junction. There is some evidence to suggest that intermediate-grade tumors with only regional node involvement have a better prognosis than high-grade tumors.[108,114] In the authors' opinion, until convincing evidence exists, such tumors should be treated as if they have a high capacity for metastasis. Figure 20-8 summarizes the treatment recommendations for high-grade MCTs. The long-term prognosis for such dogs is less favorable because regional and distant metastases are more likely.

Poorly differentiated and metastatic MCT will, in most instances, progress to kill the dog in the absence of effective postsurgical intervention. Systemic adjuvant therapy should be offered in such cases in an attempt to decrease the likelihood of systemic involvement, or at least potentially improve DFIs. Corticosteroids such as prednisone have been reported for many years in preclinical or anecdotal settings to be of some benefit.[168-172] Although corticosteroids can inhibit canine MCT proliferation and induce tumor cell apoptosis in vitro,[173] they may also contribute to apparent antitumor response by decreasing peritumoral edema and inflammation. The Veterinary Cooperative Oncology Group (VCOG) studied the efficacy of single-agent systemic prednisone therapy for intermediate- and high-grade canine MCTs.[172] Of 21 dogs receiving 1 mg/kg daily by mouth (PO), only one complete response (CR) and four partial responses (PR) were noted, and these were short-lived, lasting only a few weeks in the majority of cases. More recent studies have reported 70% to 75% response rates; however, tumors were excised or irradiated following short-term prednisone treatment, thus duration of response was not evaluable.[145,171] A recent study found that response of MCT to corticosteroids was dependent on expression of the glucocorticoid receptor; those dogs with tumors that expressed low levels of this receptor had MCTs that were resistant to prednisolone therapy.[174] These data suggest that

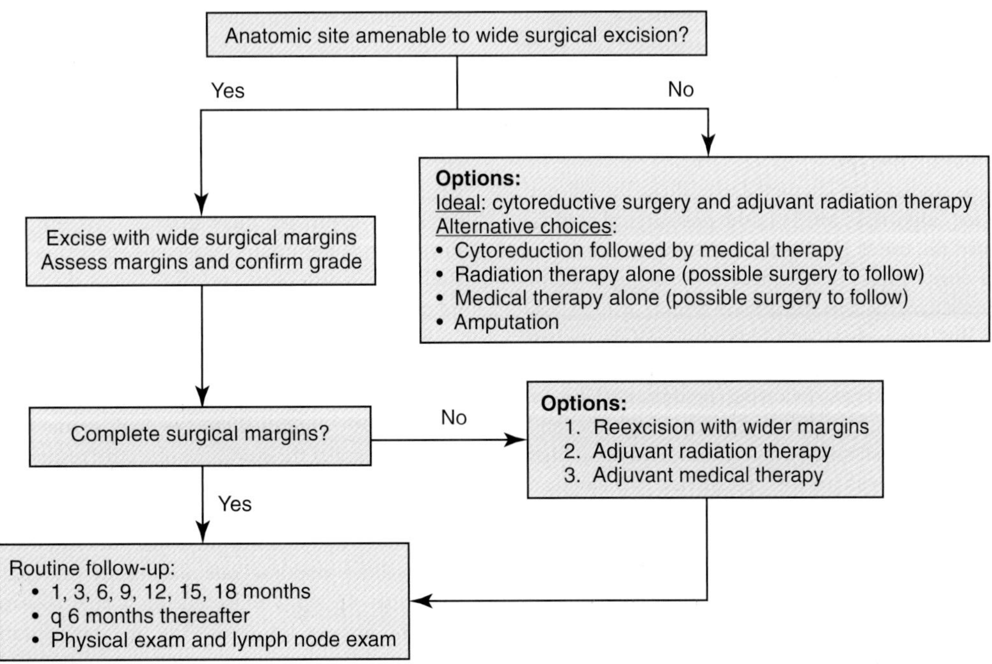

FIGURE 20-7 Suggested treatment approach for clinical stage 0 and stage I low- or intermediate-grade canine MCTs.

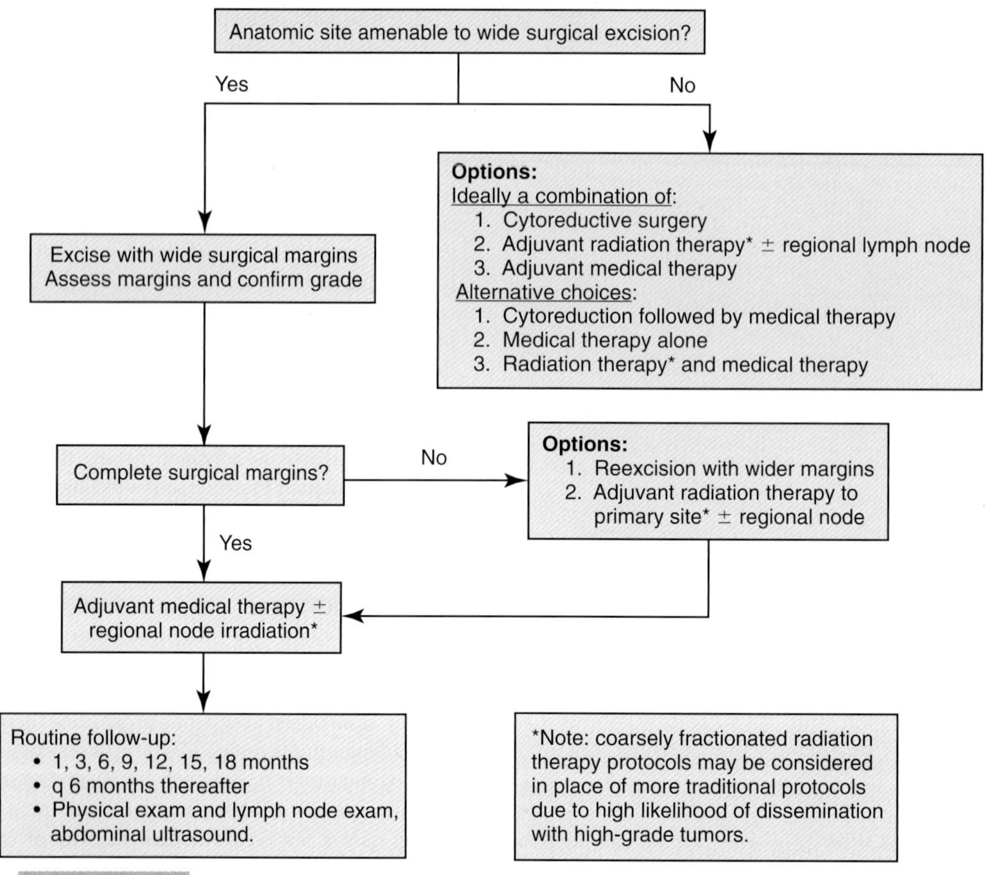

FIGURE 20-8 Suggested treatment approach for high-grade, biologically aggressive canine MCTs.

a subset of MCT may indeed benefit from corticosteroid therapy if there is adequate expression of the glucocorticoid receptor.

Recently, a number of studies have evaluated the response rates of measurable canine MCT to various cytotoxic chemotherapy drugs and protocols (Table 20-6).* Objective response rates as high as 64% have been reported, and accumulating evidence suggests that multiagent protocols may confer a higher response rate than single-agent therapy.† It is important to note that in most instances, the response of a bulky MCT to any chemotherapy protocol tends to be short-lived, stressing the need for local control of disease prior to institution of adjuvant therapy.

A few single-arm studies have attempted to evaluate the efficacy of chemotherapy for "high-risk" MCTs in the postsurgical setting. One study evaluated the use of postoperative prednisone and vinblastine (VBL) for dogs with MCT considered to be at high risk for metastasis (node-positive, mucous membrane origin, or high histologic grade). In this study, dogs with high-grade MCTs had an MST of 1374 days.[114] A second study reported 70% 1- and 2-year disease-free survival percentages following prednisone/VBL in high-grade MCT.[184] A combination of prednisone, lomustine, and VBL has been used for residual microscopic disease in dogs at high risk for dissemination. Dogs with microscopic disease had a median progression-free survival time of 35 weeks and an overall survival of 48 weeks.[177] Combination therapy using cyclophosphamide, VBL, and prednisone also yielded promising results in the microscopic residual disease setting for dogs considered at high risk of recurrence or metastasis. The reported progression-free and overall survival times were 865 days and more than 2092 days, respectively.[119] Most of the studies described used a dose of 2 mg/m^2 VBL; although there is now information suggesting that dogs may tolerate higher doses,[185-187] it remains to be seen if dose escalation of VBL will translate into improved efficacy.

As previously discussed, virtually all canine mast cell neoplasms express the KIT RTK, and a large minority of canine MCTs (20% to 40%, depending on the study) possess a mutation in the *c-kit* gene, which renders the KIT protein constitutively active.[41,44,48,188] New, orally available molecules have been developed that inhibit signaling through KIT called *small molecule TKIs.* The two veterinary-approved TKIs in this class are toceranib (Palladia, Pfizer) and masitinib (Masivet/Kinavet, AB Science); limited studies have also been performed with the human KIT inhibitor imatinib (Gleevec, Novartis).

Following encouraging *in vitro* and early-phase clinical trials,[45,189,190] a multicenter, placebo-controlled, double-blind, randomized study of toceranib was performed in dogs with recurrent or metastatic intermediate- or high-grade MCT.[191] During the blinded phase of the study, the objective response rate in toceranib-treated dogs (n = 86) was 37.2% (7 CR, 25 PR) versus 7.9% (5 PR) in placebo-treated dogs. When all 145 dogs that received toceranib were analyzed, including those that switched from placebo to drug, the objective response rate was 42.8% (21 CR, 41 PR), with an additional 16 dogs experiencing stable disease for an overall biologic activity of 60%. The median duration of objective response and time to tumor progression were 12.0 and 18.1 weeks, respectively. Interestingly, dogs whose MCT harbored activating

*References 33, 113, 119, 175, 177-182.

†References 33, 113, 119, 177, 181, 183.

TABLE 20-6 Response to Medical Therapy in Measurable Canine Mast Cell Tumors

AGENT(S)	TREATED (NO.)	CR (%)	PR (%)	ORR (%)	MEDIAN RESPONSE DURATION	REFERENCE
Prednisone	25	4	16	20	NR	172
Vincristine	27	0	7	7	NR	179
Vinblastine*	51	0-4	12-23	12-27	23-77 days	185
Lomustine (CCNU)	21	6	38	44	79 days†	178
Prednisone/VBL	17	33	13	47	154 days	113
P/C/V	11	18%	45	63	74 days	119
COP-HU	17	23	35	59	53 days	33
Prednisone/VBL/CCNU	37	24	32	57	30 weeks	177
Prednisone/VBL/CCNU	17	29	35	64	141 days/66 days (CR/PR)	182
BCG/hCG	46	14	14	29	NR	175b
Calcitriol	10	10	30	40	74-90 days	183
Hydroxyurea	46	4	24	28	46 days (for PRs)	175
Prednisone/chlorambucil	21	14	24	38	533 days	181

CR, Complete response; *PR*, partial response; *ORR*, overall response rate; *NR*, not reported; *VBL*, vinblastine; *P/C/V*, prednisone/cyclophosphamide/vinblastine; *COP-HU*, cyclophosphamide, vincristine, prednisone, hydroxyurea; *BCG/hCG*, Bacillus Calmette-Guérin/human chorionic gonadotropin.

*Two different dosages/schedules evaluated.

†Excludes patient that experienced a CR, euthanized without evidence of disease after 440 days.

mutations in the *c-kit* gene were roughly twice as likely to respond to toceranib as those with wild-type *c-kit* (69% versus 37%). GI toxicity, in the form of inappetence, weight loss, diarrhea, and occasionally vomiting or melena, was the most common adverse effect and was generally manageable with symptomatic therapy, drug holidays, and dosage reductions as necessary. Other adverse effects reported include mild-to-moderate leukopenia and occasional muscle pain.[191] Recent clinical experience with toceranib suggests that equivalent antitumor activity and reduced adverse effects may be observed if dosages lower than the label dosage are employed. A dosage of 2.5 to 2.75 mg/kg every other day or 3 days per week (Monday, Wednesday, Friday) is currently utilized by many.[192,193]

A clinical trial of similar design was recently completed with masitinib in dogs with recurrent or unresectable MCT.[194] This study demonstrated significantly improved time to progression in masitinib-treated versus placebo-treated dogs, and outcome again was improved in dogs with MCTs harboring activating *c-kit* mutations. Subsequent follow-up of patients treated with long-term masitinib identified an increased number of patients with long-term disease control compared to those treated with placebo (40% versus 15% alive at 2 years),[195] underscoring the potential for long-term disease stabilization to be an acceptable and clinically meaningful outcome in patients treated with this class of agent. GI adverse effects (vomiting or diarrhea) were most common but were mild in the majority of cases and self-limiting. Myelosuppression was also observed and was mild in most cases. A small percentage of dogs developed a protein-losing nephropathy leading to edema. Increases in urea and creatinine were observed in some dogs, and hemolytic anemia was observed rarely.[194]

Finally, small studies have evaluated the efficacy of imatinib for the treatment of measurable canine MCTs.[196-198] Imatinib was well tolerated, and objective antitumor responses were observed in dogs with both *c-kit* mutant and wild-type MCTs. It is important to note that no studies have yet been performed in dogs with MCTs to assess the pharmacokinetics of imatinib; thus current dosing recommendations are based on observed clinical activity, not pharmacokinetic and pharmacodynamic relationships.

At this time, there are only a few published studies regarding the safety and efficacy of combination therapy with KIT inhibitors and standard forms of therapy such as RT or cytotoxic chemotherapy, and evidence of benefit when used in the postoperative setting has yet to be demonstrated. One recent clinical trial evaluated a combination of toceranib and VBL in dogs with measurable MCTs. Significant reductions in VBL dosage and frequency were necessary because of additive myelosuppression resulting in a maximally tolerated dose of VBL of 1.6 mg/m^2 every other week in combination with toceranib given every other day.[199] Nevertheless, encouraging biologic activity (71% objective response rate) was observed despite the necessary dosage reductions, indicating that future evaluation of this combination regimen is warranted. Finally, another study investigated the combination of toceranib, prednisone, and hypofractionated RT in dogs with nonresectable and/or metastatic MCT.[192] The overall response rate (ORR) was 76.4%, with 58.8% of dogs achieving CR and 17.6% PR. The overall MST was not reached, and the median follow-up was 374 days. The combination of hypofractionated RT and toceranib was well tolerated and demonstrated efficacy in the majority of dogs, indicating that this may be a viable treatment option for nonresectable MCT.

Novel medical approaches that may hold promise for the future treatment of MCT include histone deacetylase inhibitors,[200-202] heat shock protein 90 (HSP90) inhibitors,[203,204] retinoids,[205-207] TNF-related apoptosis-inducing ligand (TRAIL),[208] and polo-like kinase-1 inhibitors.[209]

Ancillary therapy to address the systemic effects of mast cell mediators is sometimes warranted in dogs with MCTs. Minimizing the effects of histamine release can be accomplished by administering the H_1 blockers diphenhydramine (2 to 4 mg/kg PO twice a day [BID]) or chlorpheniramine (0.22 to 0.5 mg/kg three times a day [TID]) and the H_2 blockers cimetidine (4 to 5.5 mg/kg PO TID), famotidine (0.5 to 1 mg/kg BID), or ranitidine (2 mg/kg BID). Omeprazole (0.5 to 1 mg/kg daily), a proton pump inhibitor, may be more effective, particularly in bulky mast cell disease. These agents are generally used in the setting of gross disease, particularly those cases in which (1) systemic signs are present, (2) the tumor is likely to be entered or manipulated at surgery (i.e., cytoreductive surgery), or (3) treatment is undertaken where gross disease will remain and degranulation is likely to occur in situ (e.g., RT or medical therapy for tumors that are not cytoreduced). For cases with active evidence of gastric or duodenal ulceration, the addition of sucralfate (0.5 to 1.0 g PO TID) and occasionally misoprostol (2 to 4 μg/kg PO TID) to histamine blockers is prudent. Some experimental data suggest that the use of H_1 and H_2 blockers could also be beneficial for the prevention or resolution of histamine-mediated wound breakdown,[32,210,211] but this has not been systematically evaluated. The use of protamine sulfate, a heparin antagonist, has been mentioned by some for use in cases of severe hemorrhage.[104]

Feline Mast Cell Tumors

Unlike MCTs in the dog, which are primarily cutaneous/subcutaneous in nature, MCTs in the cat typically occur in three distinct syndromes, although there is some overlap among them. These syndromes are cutaneous MCT, splenic/visceral mast cell disease, and intestinal MCT. The etiology of feline MCTs is currently unknown and appears unrelated to viral infection.[212] However, it is now evident that feline MCTs also possess somatic activating mutations in *c-kit*.[213-215] In one study, 42/62 (67%) of cutaneous and splenic/visceral MCT had *c-kit* mutations that were primarily present in exons 8 (28/62) and 9 (15/62), both of which encode the fifth immunoglobulin domain of KIT. Similar to the canine juxtamembrane domain mutations, these feline *c-kit* mutations induce ligand-independent activation of KIT, which can be inhibited by imatinib in vitro.[215]

The granules present in feline MCTs stain blue with Giemsa and purple with toluidine blue.[1,2,4] As in the dog, granules present in feline mast cells contain vasoactive substances, such as heparin and histamine.[2,216] In culture, feline mast cells express surface-bound immunoglobulins and are capable of secreting histamine, heparin, and probably other vasoactive compounds when appropriately stimulated.[216] Feline mast cells also have phagocytic capability and can endocytose erythrocytes in both experimental models and clinical samples.[217] Complications associated with degranulation of MCT can also occur in the cat, including coagulation disorders, GI ulceration, and anaphylactoid reactions.[2,218,219] Since the biologic behavior of the three feline MCT syndromes is different, they will be described individually.

Cutaneous Feline Mast Cell Tumors

MCTs represent the second most common cutaneous tumor in the cat, accounting for approximately 20% of cutaneous tumors in this species in the United States.[2,4,12] The incidence of MCTs in cats appears to have increased dramatically since 1950.[2] Interestingly, MCTs appear to occur much less frequently in the United Kingdom than in the United States, accounting for only 8% of all cutaneous tumors.[1] The typical feline cutaneous MCT is a solitary, raised, firm, well-circumscribed, hairless, dermal nodule between 0.5 and 3 cm in diameter.[2,4,220,221] They are often white in appearance, although a pink erythematous form is occasionally encountered. Approximately 20% are multiple, although one series reported multiple lesions in the majority of cases.[1] Superficial ulceration is present in approximately one-fourth of cases. Other clinical forms that have been described include a flat pruritic plaquelike lesion similar in appearance to eosinophilic plaques and discrete subcutaneous nodules.

Two distinct types of cutaneous MCTs in the cat have been reported (Table 20-7): (1) the more typical mastocytic MCT, histologically similar to MCTs in dogs, and (2) the less common histiocytic MCTs, with morphologic features characteristic of histiocytic mast cells, that may regress spontaneously over a period of 4 to 24 months.[221,222] An overall mean age of 8 to 9 years is reported for cats with MCTs; however, the mastocytic and histiocytic forms occur at mean ages of 10 and 2.4 years, respectively.[2,4,220] Siamese cats appear to be predisposed to development of MCTs of both histologic types.[2,4,220-222] The distinct histiocytic form of MCTs in cats is reported to occur primarily in young (<4 years of age) Siamese cats, including two related litters.[222] In contrast to these reports, Siamese cats were not more likely to develop the histiocytic form of MCT than the mastocytic form in another series of cases.[4] Earlier studies reported a male predilection for development of MCT[219,220]; however, larger, more recent series have failed to confirm such a predilection.[2,4]

The mastocytic form can be further subdivided on histologic appearance into two categories, previously referred to as *compact* (representing 50% to 90% of all cases) and *diffuse* (histologically anaplastic), which may be of prognostic significance.[2,222,223] Well-differentiated compact tumors tend to behave in a benign manner, and metastasis is uncommon.[220,224,225] In contrast, anaplastic tumors may have a high MI and marked cellular and nuclear pleomorphism, with infiltration into the subcutaneous tissues.[221] These tumors have been reported as behaving in a more malignant manner with metastasis to lymph nodes and the abdomen, although a more recent study evaluated pleomorphic cutaneous MCTs from 15 cats and found that the majority were behaviorally benign; only one cat was euthanized due to disease progression.[226]

Unlike in the dog, the head and neck are the most common site for MCTs in the cat, followed by the trunk, limbs, and

TABLE 20-7 Histologic Classification of Mast Cell Tumors in Cats

TYPE	SUBTYPE	MICROSCOPIC DESCRIPTION
Mastocytic	Compact (well-differentiated)	Homogeneous cords and nests of slightly atypical mast cells with basophilic round nuclei, ample eosinophilic cytoplasm, and distinct cell borders. Eosinophils conspicuous in only half of cases.
	Diffuse (anaplastic)	Less discrete, infiltrated into subcutis. Larger nuclei (>50% cell diameter), 2-3 mitoses/HPF. Marked anisocytosis, including mononuclear and multinucleated giant cells. Eosinophils more commonly observed.
Histiocytic		Sheets of histiocyte-like cells with equivocal cytoplasmic granularity. Accompanied by randomly scattered lymphoid aggregates and eosinophils. Granules lacking in some reports, others report granules readily demonstrable.

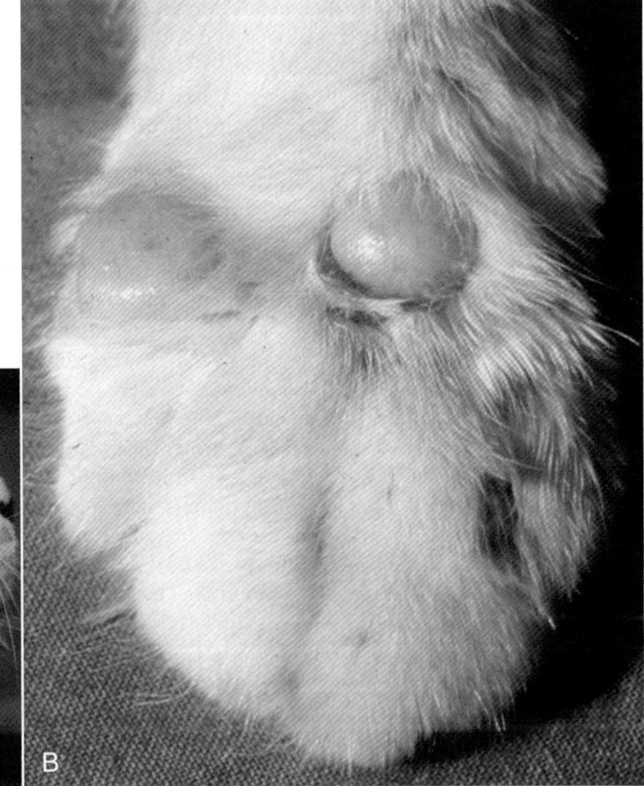

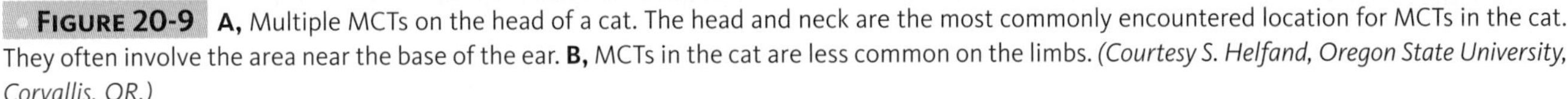

FIGURE 20-9 **A,** Multiple MCTs on the head of a cat. The head and neck are the most commonly encountered location for MCTs in the cat. They often involve the area near the base of the ear. **B,** MCTs in the cat are less common on the limbs. *(Courtesy S. Helfand, Oregon State University, Corvallis, OR.)*

miscellaneous sites (Figure 20-9).[2,4,220] Tumors on the head often involve the pinnae near the base of the ear. They rarely occur in the oral cavity. Intermittent pruritus and erythema are common, and self-trauma or vascular compromise may result in ulceration. Darier's sign, which is the erythema and wheal formation following mechanical manipulation of the tumor, has been reported in the cat.[219] Affected cats are usually otherwise healthy. The spontaneously regressing histiocytic form of cutaneous MCTs usually presents as multiple, nonpruritic, firm, hairless, pink, and sometimes ulcerated subcutaneous nodules (Figure 20-10).[4,222]

As with canine tumors, most feline MCTs are usually easily diagnosed by cytologic examination of fine needle aspirates. In contrast, the uncommon histiocytic form of feline MCTs is more challenging to diagnose both by FNA and histopathology.[221,222] Mast cells may comprise only 20% of the cells present, with the majority being sheets of histiocytes that lack distinct cytoplasmic granules and accompanied by randomly scattered lymphoid aggregates and eosinophils. In contrast, one report readily demonstrated metachromatic granules in seven cases of the histiocytic subtype. These tumors can be initially misdiagnosed as granulomatous nodular panniculitis or deep dermatitis.

Cats with cutaneous MCTs should be evaluated for evidence of additional tumors, as well as potential splenic involvement by abdominal US, because one study found that some cats with multiple cutaneous MCTs also had splenic disease.[224] In addition, a minimum database is recommended, along with careful examination of local lymph nodes for evidence of lymphadenopathy. Interestingly, unlike dogs, cats rarely exhibit evidence of circulating mast cells on buffy coat smears when healthy or ill from non–mast cell-related causes.[227] In contrast, one study demonstrated that 43% of cats with mast cell disease have positive buffy coats, although most of these cats tended to have the splenic/visceral form of the disease.[228]

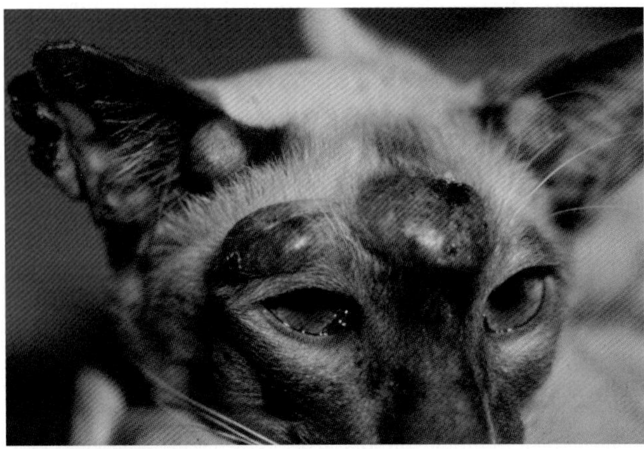

FIGURE 20-10 Histiocytic MCTs on the head of a young Siamese cat. This form of MCTs in cats typically regress spontaneously, as was the case in the cat pictured here. *(Courtesy Dr. K. Moriello, University of Wisconsin-Madison.)*

Feline MCTs are usually positive for vimentin, α-1 antitrypsin, and KIT.[229,230] Although the histologic grading system described for canine MCT has provided no prognostic information for the cat in several series and is not used,[220,231] tumors with a high MI appear to be at greatest risk for local recurrence and metastasis, suggesting that this histopathologic feature may be useful for predicting biologic behavior.[221,226] A more recent study evaluated the prognostic value of histologic and immunohistochemical features in feline cutaneous MCTs. Multiplicity of lesions, pleomorphic phenotype, KIT immunoreactivity score, MI, and Ki67 index correlated with an unfavorable outcome, although MI was the strongest predictive variable.[232]

The definitive treatment for cutaneous feline MCT is surgical excision. In a series of 32 cats with cutaneous MCTs, five tumors recurred following surgical excision, although none of the cats in this study died of disease. Completeness of excision and histopathologic factors such as nuclear pleomorphism and MI were not associated with tumor recurrence.[225] In a more recent series of cats with MCTs of the eyelids, local tumor control in 19/23 cats was achieved with surgery alone and another 3 cats experienced control with surgery plus RT or cryotherapy, resulting in an MST of 945 days.[233] Despite the fact that only 50% of the tumors were completely removed, only one cat developed disseminated cutaneous tumors and no cats developed metastatic disease to the lymph nodes or abdomen. Other reports have demonstrated local recurrence rates following excision between 0% and 24%.[2,220,221,224,226] These data suggest that most cutaneous feline MCTs are behaviorally benign, and wide surgical margins may not be as critical in the cat as in the dog. Frequency of systemic spread following surgical excision varies from 0% to 22%, although those that metastasize are more likely to be anaplastic tumors.[220,221,224-226] Therefore, for histologically anaplastic tumors or those with a high MI more likely to recur postsurgery or to metastasize, a more aggressive approach similar to that utilized for canine MCTs may be prudent.[226,234] Following biopsy confirmation, conservative resection or a "wait and see" approach may be taken with the histiocytic form in young cats with multiple masses because these may spontaneously regress.[2,4,222]

RT may be considered for tumors that are incompletely excised. In one study of feline cutaneous MCT, a 98% control rate was achieved with strontium-90 irradiation, with an MST of greater than 3 years.[235] Limited information exists concerning the utility of chemotherapy in cats with MCTs. It is generally believed that feline MCTs are less responsive to prednisone than their canine counterparts; biologic activity of corticosteroids in cats with the histiocytic variant was found to be equivocal.[222] Objective responses to lomustine (CCNU) have been reported in cats.[236,237] Of 20 cats with cutaneous MCTs, 10 exhibited CR (n = 2) or PR (n = 8) to lomustine.[237] The authors have observed evidence of clinical activity in cats treated with prednisone and VBL as well. Some investigators have utilized a combination of prednisone and chlorambucil to treat metastatic or multiple tumors. This is generally well tolerated, although its effectiveness is not known.

Biologic activity of imatinib has been observed in cats with MCTs expressing activating mutations in *c-kit,* although the responses were all partial in nature.[214,215,238] Studies in healthy cats have demonstrated that masitinib may be safe to administer to clinically normal cats, and plasma concentrations associated with MCT inhibitory activity are likely achievable. Cats should be monitored very closely for neutropenia, proteinuria, and increases in creatinine.[239,240] Neither masitinib nor toceranib have been formally evaluated in cats with MCTs.

Splenic/Visceral Feline Mast Cell Tumors

MCTs represent the most common differential for splenic disease in cats, accounting for 15% of submissions in a series of 455 pathologic specimens.[241] This disease primarily affects older animals (mean age 10 years) with no sex or breed predilection.[2,224,241] The majority of cats with splenic MCTs do not have a history of cutaneous MCTs, although recent evidence suggests that some cats with multiple cutaneous MCTs may also have splenic involvement.[224] Although the spleen is the primary site affected by this disease, other organs may also be involved.[2,218] Necropsy data on 30 cats with splenic MCTs revealed dissemination in the following organs in decreasing order of frequency: liver (90%), visceral lymph nodes (73%), bone marrow (40%), lung (20%), and intestine (17%).[2] Up to one-third of cases have peritoneal and pleural effusions rich in eosinophils and mast cells.[2,218] Peripheral blood mastocytosis has been reported in 40% to 100% of cases with peripheral mast cell counts up to 32,000 cells/μL.[2,228] In one clinical report of 43 cases, 23% had bone marrow involvement.[218]

Cats with splenic MCTs may present with signs of systemic illness, including vomiting, anorexia, and weight loss.[2,218] Dyspnea may be evident if pleural effusion is present. Abdominal palpation usually reveals a markedly enlarged spleen and/or liver. Other common differential diagnoses for splenomegaly in the cat include lymphoma, myeloproliferative disease, accessory spleen, hemangiosarcoma, hyperplastic nodules, and splenitis.[241] Clinical signs associated with the release of mast cell mediators, such as GI ulceration, hemorrhage, hypotensive shock, and labored breathing, may also be noted. Cats with suspected splenic MCTs should undergo a standard work-up, including a minimum database, as well as abdominal US and thoracic radiographs. FNA cytology is usually diagnostic for splenic MCTs, as is evaluation of thoracic or abdominal fluid. Anemia is a common hematologic finding, with eosinophilia less likely to be observed.[2,218] In one report of 43 cats with splenic MCT, 90% had an abnormal coagulation profile, although this did not appear to be clinically significant.[218] Hyperglobulinemia has also been reported in cats with splenic MCTs, the cause of which remains unknown.

Splenectomy is the treatment of choice for cats with splenic MCTs, even if other organ involvement is noted. Pretreatment with H_1 and H_2 blockers prior to therapy is indicated; intraoperative death may occur due to the release of mast cell mediators. Two gross forms of splenic involvement are possible: a diffuse, smooth form and a less common nodular form (Figure 20-11).[125,242] Surprisingly, even in the face of significant bone marrow and peripheral blood involvement, long-term survival with good quality of life is the norm following splenectomy, with MSTs from 12 to 19 months reported,[2,218,243-245] although one recent study reported an MST of only 132 days following splenectomy.[246] Anorexia, significant weight loss, and male gender were found to be negative prognostic indicators in one study.[218] Although peripheral mastocytosis usually does not completely resolve, it usually declines significantly and cats experience good quality of life for long periods of time. Cats should be followed postoperatively with buffy coat smears because a rise in the number of mast cells in the periphery may indicate disease progression. Adjunctive chemotherapy with prednisone, VBL, lomustine, and/or chlorambucil has been attempted in a limited number of cases, but it is not clear if these therapies are clinically valuable. As discussed previously, recent data indicate that cats with MCTs may respond to the KIT inhibitor imatinib if activating mutations in *c-kit* are present.[214,215]

Feline Intestinal Mast Cell Tumor

Intestinal MCT is the third most common primary intestinal tumor in cats after lymphoma and adenocarcinoma.[2] No breed or gender predilection is known. Older cats appear to be at risk, with a mean

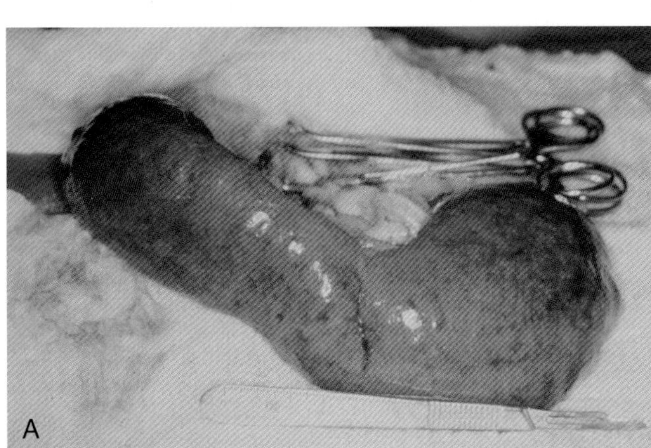

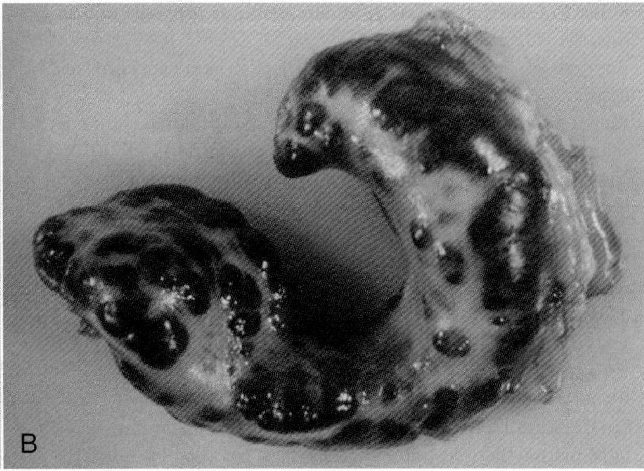

FIGURE 20-11 **A,** Diffuse massive splenomegaly in a cat with splenic mast cell disease. **B,** The less common nodular form of splenic MCT in a cat.

age of 13 years; however, cats as young as 3 years have been reported.[247] Most cats have a history of vomiting, diarrhea, and anorexia, and a solitary palpable abdominal mass is usually evident on physical examination.[2,247] Intestinal MCT more commonly involves the small intestine (equally divided between duodenum, jejunum, and ileum), with colonic involvement reported in less than 15% of cases; lesions can be solitary or multiple.[2,247,248] Diarrhea with or without hematochezia is commonly observed with the intestinal form, and fever may be present. Affected cats may have been ill for several months. Metastasis is common with this disease; thus enlarged mesenteric lymph nodes and/or hepatomegaly may be noted on physical examination. A peritoneal effusion may be present, and this often contains mast cells and eosinophils. Diagnosis is usually made by FNA of the mass or involved organs; mast cells from intestinal lesions are often less differentiated than those of skin tumors and cytoplasmic granules may be less prominent, making diagnosis challenging in certain cases. Cats with intestinal MCTs should be staged with a minimum database, thoracic radiographs, and abdominal US, which may be required to determine the extent of intestinal involvement and presence of visceral dissemination. Buffy coat smear may also be performed, although unlike splenic MCT, peripheral mastocytosis is rarely associated with intestinal MCT and only two reports of peripheral eosinophilia exist in the literature.[247]

Intestinal MCTs in cats often have a poor prognosis[2,247,248] because metastasis is commonly found at the time of diagnosis and many cats either die or are euthanized soon after they are diagnosed. Surgery is the treatment of choice, and wide surgical margins are necessary (5 to 10 cm) because the tumor typically extends histologically well beyond the obvious gross disease.[2,247] Recently, a variant of feline intestinal MCT, termed *sclerosing MCT,* was described in 50 cats.[248] Metastatic disease to the lymph nodes and/or liver was present in 23/36 cases evaluated. Of the 25 cases with clinical follow-up information, 23 died or were euthanized within 2 months of diagnosis, supporting the aggressive nature of this disease. Limited information exists regarding the use of chemotherapy for feline intestinal MCTs, although anecdotal responses to lomustine and chlorambucil have been reported. Recently, two cats exhibited objective responses (one CR, one PR) following treatment with lomustine, suggesting that this agent may be useful in cats with intestinal MCTs.[237] The role of KIT inhibitors in the treatment of this disease is not yet known.

Comparative Aspects of Mast Cell Tumors

Neoplastic diseases of mast cells are considered rare in humans and present as three main clinical entities.[176,249-252] Cutaneous mastocytosis, also known as *urticaria pigmentosa,* is a benign disease in which mast cell infiltration is confined to the skin. It primarily occurs in young children and usually regresses spontaneously before progression into adulthood. Systemic mastocytosis (SM) occurs primarily in adults and includes four major subtypes: (1) indolent SM, the most common form involving mainly skin and bone marrow that does not progress to aggressive disease; (2) a unique subcategory termed *SM with an associated non–mast cell clonal hematologic disease;* (3) aggressive SM, usually presenting without skin lesions; and (4) mast cell leukemia, probably representing the rarest variant of human leukemias. Finally, rare localized extracutaneous MCTs (either benign or malignant) have been reported. Dysregulation of KIT is also found commonly in human neoplastic mast cell diseases and is primarily driven by a point mutation in exon 17 of *c-kit* that induces ligand-independent activation.[250,253] More recently, mutations have also been identified in exons 8 to 11, most of which are also activating.[250,253]

Treatment of the benign human mast cell disorders is primarily focused on supportive therapy, including H_1 and H_2 antagonists, and topical or systemic therapy with corticosteroids. Unfortunately, there is no good therapy for cases of aggressive mastocytosis or mast cell leukemia. Treatment with interferon-α (IFN-α) and/or cladribine is often used, although response rates are typically low.[249,253] Most of the currently available small molecule KIT inhibitors, including imatinib, nilotinib, and dasatinib, have not been effective in treating human mastocytosis.[253] This may in part be due to the fact that inhibiting phosphorylation of KIT-expressing activating exon 17 mutations is extremely challenging. More recently, the protein kinase C inhibitor, midostaurin, has demonstrated activity in human mast cell disease.[253]

REFERENCES

1. Bostock DE: Neoplasms of the skin and subcutaneous tissues in dogs and cats, *Br Vet J* 142:1-19, 1986.
2. Carpenter JL, Andrews LK, Holzworth J: Tumors and tumor-like lesions. In Holzworth J, editor: *Diseases of the cat: medicine and surgery*, Philadelphia, 1987, WB Saunders.
3. Finnie JW, Bostock DE: Skin neoplasia in dogs, *Aust Vet J* 55:602-604, 1979.

4. Miller MA, Nelson SL, Turk JR, et al: Cutaneous neoplasia in 340 cats, *Vet Pathol* 28:389-395, 1991.
5. Rothwell TL, Howlett CR, Middleton DJ, et al: Skin neoplasms of dogs in Sydney, *Aust Vet J* 64:161-164, 1987.
6. Kumar V, Sharma A: Mast cells: emerging sentinel innate immune cells with diverse role in immunity, *Mol Immunol* 48:14-25, 2010.
7. Noviana D, Mamba K, Makimura S, et al: Distribution, histochemical and enzyme histochemical characterization of mast cells in dogs, *J Mol Histol* 35:123-132, 2004.
8. Metz M, Piliponsky AM, Chen CC, et al: Mast cells can enhance resistance to snake and honeybee venoms, *Science* 313:526-530, 2006.
9. Lin TY, London CA: A functional comparison of canine and murine bone marrow derived cultured mast cells, *Vet Immunol Immunopathol* 114:320-334, 2006.
10. Lin TY, Rush LJ, London CA: Generation and characterization of bone marrow-derived cultured canine mast cells, *Vet Immunol Immunopathol* 113:37-52, 2006.
11. Lin TY, London CA: Characterization and modulation of canine mast cell derived eicosanoids, *Vet Immunol Immunopathol* 135:118-127, 2010.
12. Brodey RS: Canine and feline neoplasia, *Adv Vet Sci Comp Med* 14:309-354, 1970.
13. Brodey RS, Riser WH: Canine osteosarcoma. A clinicopathologic study of 194 cases, *Clin Orthop* 62:54-64, 1969.
14. Patnaik AK, Ehler WJ, MacEwen EG: Canine cutaneous mast cell tumor: morphologic grading and survival time in 83 dogs, *Vet Pathol* 21:469-474, 1984.
15. Peters JA: Canine mastocytoma: excess risk as related to ancestry, *J Natl Cancer Inst* 42:435-443, 1969.
16. White CR, Hohenhaus AE, Kelsey J, et al: Cutaneous MCTs: Associations with spay/neuter status, breed, body size, and phylogenetic cluster, *J Am Anim Hosp Assoc* 47:210-216, 2011.
17. McNiel EA, Prink AL, O'Brien TD: Evaluation of risk and clinical outcome of mast cell tumours in pug dogs, *Vet Comp Oncol* 4:2-8, 2004.
18. Davis BJ, Page R, Sannes PL, et al: Cutaneous mastocytosis in a dog, *Vet Pathol* 29:363-365, 1992.
19. Dunn TB, Patter H: A transplantable mast cell neoplasm in the mouse, *J Natl Cancer Inst* 18:587-601, 1957.
20. Hottendorf GH, Nielsen SW: Pathologic survey of 300 extirpated canine mastocytomas, *Zentralbl Veterinarmed A* 14:272-281, 1967.
21. Peterson SL: Scar-associated canine mast cell tumor, *Canine Pract* 12:23-29, 1985.
22. Bowles CA, Kerber WT, Rangan SRS, et al: Characterization of a transplantable, canine, immature mast cell tumor, *Cancer Res* 32:1434-1441, 1972.
23. Lombard LS, Moloney JB: Experimental transmission of mast cell sarcoma in dogs, *Fed Proc* 18:490-495, 1959.
24. Nielson SW, Cole CR: Homologous transplantation of canine neoplasms, *Am J Vet Res* 27:663-672, 1961.
25. Stone JM, Jacky PB, Prieur DJ: Chromosomal fragile site expression in boxer dogs with mast cell tumors, *Am J Med Genetics* 40:223-229, 1991.
26. Ginn PE, Fox LE, Brower JC, et al: Immunohistochemical detection of p53 tumor-suppressor protein is a poor indicator of prognosis for canine cutaneous mast cell tumors, *Vet Pathol* 37:33-39, 2000.
27. Jaffe MH, Hosgood G, Taylor HW, et al: Immunohistochemical and clinical evaluation of p53 in canine cutaneous mast cell tumors, *Vet Pathol* 37:40-46, 2000.
28. Ozaki K, Yamagami T, Nomura K, et al: Mast cell tumors of the gastrointestinal tract in 39 dogs, *Vet Pathol* 39:557-564, 2002.
29. Mayr B, Reifinger M, Brem G, et al: Cytogenetic, ras, and p53: studies in cases of canine neoplasms (hemangiopericytoma, mastocytoma, histiocytoma, chloroma), *J Hered* 90:124-128, 1999.
30. Wu H, Hayashi T, Inoue M: Immunohistochemical expression of p27 and p21 in canine cutaneous mast cell tumors and histiocytomas, *Vet Pathol* 41:296-299, 2004.
31. Elling H, Ungemach FR: Sexual hormone receptors in canine mast cell tumour cytosol, *J Comp Pathol* 92:629-630, 1982.
32. Macy DW: Canine and feline mast cell tumors: Biologic behavior, diagnosis, and therapy, *Sem Vet Med Surg (Sm Anim)* 1:72-83, 1986.
33. Gerritsen RJ, Teske E, Kraus JS, et al: Multi-agent chemotherapy for mast cell tumours in the dog, *Vet Q* 20:28-31, 1998.
34. Galli SJ, Zsebo KM, Geissler EN: The kit ligand, stem cell factor, *Adv Immunol* 55:1-95, 1994.
35. Roskoski R Jr: Structure and regulation of Kit protein-tyrosine kinase—the stem cell factor receptor, *Biochem Biophys Res Commun* 338:1307-1315, 2005.
36. Roskoski R Jr: Signaling by Kit protein-tyrosine kinase—the stem cell factor receptor, *Biochem Biophys Res Commun* 337:1-13, 2005.
37. Kiupel M, Webster JD, Kaneene JB, et al: The use of KIT and tryptase expression patterns as prognostic tools for canine cutaneous mast cell tumors, *Vet Pathol* 41:371-377, 2004.
38. London CA, Kisseberth WC, Galli SJ, et al: Expression of stem cell factor receptor (c-kit) by the malignant mast cells from spontaneous canine mast cell tumours, *J Comp Pathol* 115:399-414, 1996.
39. Morini M, Bettini G, Preziosi R, et al: C-kit gene product (CD117) immunoreactivity in canine and feline paraffin sections, *J Histochem Cytochem* 52:705-708, 2004.
40. Reguera MJ, Rabanal RM, Puigdemont A, et al: Canine mast cell tumors express stem cell factor receptor, *Am J Dermatopathol* 22:49-54, 2000.
41. Downing S, Chien MB, Kass PH, et al: Prevalence and importance of internal tandem duplications in exons 11 and 12 of c-kit in mast cell tumors of dogs, *Am J Vet Res* 63:1718-1723, 2002.
42. Jones CL, Grahn RA, Chien MB, et al: Detection of c-kit mutations in canine mast cell tumors using fluorescent polyacrylamide gel electrophoresis, *J Vet Diagn Invest* 16:95-100, 2004.
43. Letard S, Yang Y, Hanssens K, et al: Gain-of-function mutations in the extracellular domain of KIT are common in canine mast cell tumors, *Mol Cancer Res* 6:1137-1145, 2008.
44. London CA, Galli SJ, Yuuki T, et al: Spontaneous canine mast cell tumors express tandem duplications in the proto-oncogene c-kit, *Exp Hematol* 27:689-697, 1999.
45. London CA, Hannah AL, Zadovoskaya R, et al: Phase I dose-escalating study of SU11654, a small molecule receptor tyrosine kinase inhibitor, in dogs with spontaneous malignancies, *Clin Cancer Res* 9:2755-2768, 2003.
46. Webster JD, Yuzbasiyan-Gurkan V, Kaneene JB, et al: The role of c-KIT in tumorigenesis: evaluation in canine cutaneous mast cell tumors, *Neoplasia* 8:104-111, 2006.
47. Webster JD, Yuzbasiyan-Gurkan V, Thamm DH, et al: Evaluation of prognostic markers for canine mast cell tumors treated with vinblastine and prednisone, *BMC Vet Res* 4:32, 2008.
48. Zemke D, Yamini B, Yuzbasiyan-Gurkan V: Mutations in the juxtamembrane domain of c-KIT are associated with higher grade mast cell tumors in dogs, *Vet Pathol* 39:529-535, 2002.
49. Bostock DE: The prognosis following surgical removal of mastocytomas in dogs, *J Small Anim Pract* 14:27-41, 1973.
50. Mullins MN, Dernell WS, Withrow SJ, et al: Evaluation of prognostic factors associated with outcome in dogs with multiple cutaneous mast cell tumors treated with surgery with and without adjuvant treatment: 54 cases (1998-2004), *J Am Vet Med Assoc* 228:91-95, 2006.
51. Tams TR, Macy DW: Canine mast cell tumors, *Comp Cont Ed Pract Vet* 27:259-263, 1981.
52. Van Pelt DR, Fowler JD, Leighton FA: Multiple cutaneous mast cell tumors in a dog: A case report and brief review, *Can Vet J* 27:259-263, 1986.
53. Cohen D, Reif SS, Brodey RS: Epidemiological analysis of the most prevalent sites and types of canine neoplasia observed in a veterinary hospital, *Cancer Res* 34:2859-2868, 1974.
54. Thamm DH, Vail DM: Mast cell tumors. In Withrow SJ, MacEwen EG, editors: *Small animal clinical oncology*, ed 3, Philadelphia, 2001, WB Saunders, pp 261-282.

55. Crowe DT, Goodwin MA, Greene CE: Total laryngectomy for laryngeal mast cell tumor in a dog, *J Am Anim Hosp Assoc* 22:809-816, 1986.
56. Iwata N, Ochiai K, Kadosawa T, et al: Canine extracutaneous mast-cell tumours consisting of connective tissue mast cells, *J Comp Pathol* 123:306-310, 2000.
57. Moore LE, Garrett LD, Debey B, et al: Spinal mast cell tumor in a dog, *J Am Anim Hosp Assoc* 38:67-70, 2002.
58. Patnaik AK, MacEwen EG, Black AP, et al: Extracutaneous mast-cell tumor in the dog, *Vet Pathol* 19:608-615, 1982.
59. Steffey M, Rassnick KM, Porter B, et al: Ureteral mast cell tumor in a dog, *J Am Anim Hosp Assoc* 40:82-85, 2004.
60. Davies AP, Hayden DW, Klausner JS, et al: Noncutaneous systemic mastocytosis and mast cell leukemia in a dog: case report and literature review, *J Am Anim Hosp Assoc* 17:361-368, 1981.
61. Lester SL, McGonigle LF, McDonald GK: Disseminated anaplastic mastocytoma with terminal mastcythemia in a dog, *J Am Anim Hosp Assoc* 17:355-360, 1981.
62. Takahashi T, Kadosawa T, Nagase M, et al: Visceral mast cell tumors in dogs: 10 cases (1982-1997), *J Am Vet Med Assoc* 216:222-226, 2000.
63. O'Keefe DA, Couto CG, Burke-Schwartz C, et al: Systemic mastocytosis in 16 dogs, *J Vet Intern Med* 1:75-80, 1987.
64. Pollack MJ, Flanders JA, Johnson RC: Disseminated malignant mastocytoma in a dog, *J Am Anim Hosp Assoc* 27:435-440, 1991.
65. Fox LE, Rosenthal RC, Twedt DC, et al: Plasma histamine and gastrin concentrations in 17 dogs with mast cell tumors, *J Vet Intern Med* 4:242-246, 1990.
66. Howard EB, Sawa TR, Nielsen SW, et al: Mastocytoma and gastroduodenal ulceration. Gastric and duodenal ulcers in dogs with mastocytoma, *Pathol Vet* 6:146-158, 1969.
67. Ishiguro T, Kadosawa T, Takagi S, et al: Relationship of disease progression and plasma histamine concentrations in 11 dogs with mast cell tumors, *J Vet Intern Med* 17:194-198, 2003.
68. Roberts LJ II, Sweetman BJ, Lewis RA, et al: Increased production of prostaglandin D2 in patients with systemic mastocytosis, *N Engl J Med* 303:1400-1484, 1980.
69. Scott HW, Parris WCV, Sandidge PC, et al: Hazards in operative management of patients with systemic mastocytosis, *Ann Surg* 197:507-514, 1983.
70. Hottendorf GH, Nielsen SW, Kenyon AJ: Canine mastocytoma: I. Blood coagulation time in dogs with mastocytoma, *Pathol Vet* 2:129-141, 1965.
71. Murphy S, Sparkes AH, Smith KC, et al: Relationships between the histological grade of cutaneous mast cell tumours in dogs, their survival and the efficacy of surgical resection, *Vet Rec* 154:743-746, 2004.
72. Simoes JP, Schoning P, Butine M: Prognosis of canine mast cell tumors: a comparison of three methods, *Vet Pathol* 31:637-647, 1994.
73. Bostock DE, Crocker J, Harris K, et al: Nucleolar organiser regions as indicators of post-surgical prognosis in canine spontaneous mast cell tumours, *Br J Cancer* 59:915-918, 1989.
74. Michels GM, Knapp DW, DeNicola DB, et al: Prognosis following surgical excision of canine cutaneous mast cell tumors with histopathologically tumor-free versus nontumor-free margins: a retrospective study of 31 cases, *J Am Anim Hosp Assoc* 38:458-466, 2002.
75. Seguin B, Leibman NF, Bregazzi VS, et al: Clinical outcome of dogs with grade-II mast cell tumors treated with surgery alone: 55 cases (1996-1999), *J Am Vet Med Assoc* 218:1120-1123, 2001.
76. Weisse C, Shofer FS, Sorenmo K: Recurrence rates and sites for grade II canine cutaneous mast cell tumors following complete surgical excision, *J Am Anim Hosp Assoc* 38:71-73, 2002.
77. Schultheiss PC, Gardiner DW, Rao S, et al: Association of histologic tumor characteristics and size of surgical margins with clinical outcome after surgical removal of cutaneous mast cell tumors in dogs, *J Am Vet Med Assoc* 238:1464-1469, 2011.
78. Hume CT, Kiupel M, Rigatti L, et al: Outcomes of dogs with grade 3 mast cell tumors: 43 cases (1997-2007), *J Am Anim Hosp Assoc* 47:37-44, 2011.
79. Northrup NC, Harmon BG, Gieger TL, et al: Variation among pathologists in histologic grading of canine cutaneous mast cell tumors, *J Vet Diagn Invest* 17:245-248, 2005.
80. Northrup NC, Howerth EW, Harmon BG, et al: Variation among pathologists in the histologic grading of canine cutaneous mast cell tumors with uniform use of a single grading reference, *J Vet Diagn Invest* 17:561-564, 2005.
81. Kiupel M, Webster JD, Bailey KL, et al: Proposal of a 2-tier histologic grading system for canine cutaneous mast cell tumors to more accurately predict biological behavior, *Vet Pathol* 48:147-155, 2011.
82. Preziosi R, Sarli G, Paltrinieri M: Prognostic value of intratumoral vessel density in cutaneous mast cell tumors of the dog, *J Comp Pathol* 130:143-151, 2004.
83. Abadie JJ, Amardeilh MA, Delverdier ME: Immunohistochemical detection of proliferating cell nuclear antigen and Ki-67 in mast cell tumors from dogs, *J Am Vet Med Assoc* 215:1629-1634, 1999.
84. Scase TJ, Edwards D, Miller J, et al: Canine mast cell tumors: correlation of apoptosis and proliferation markers with prognosis, *J Vet Intern Med* 20:151-158, 2006.
85. Seguin B, Besancon MF, McCallan JL, et al: Recurrence rate, clinical outcome, and cellular proliferation indices as prognostic indicators after incomplete surgical excision of cutaneous grade II mast cell tumors: 28 dogs (1994-2002), *J Vet Intern Med* 20(4):933-940, 2006.
86. Webster JD, Yuzbasiyan-Gurkan V, Miller RA, et al: Cellular proliferation in canine cutaneous mast cell tumors: associations with c-KIT and its role in prognostication, *Vet Pathol* 44:298-308, 2007.
87. Maglennon GA, Murphy S, Adams V, et al: Association of Ki67 index with prognosis for intermediate-grade canine cutaneous mast cell tumours, *Vet Comp Oncol* 6:268-274, 2008.
88. Ozaki K, Yamagami T, Nomura K, et al: Prognostic significance of surgical margin, Ki-67 and cyclin D1 protein expression in grade II canine cutaneous mast cell tumor, *J Vet Med Sci* 69:1117-1121, 2007.
89. Sakai H, Noda A, Shirai N, et al: Proliferative activity of canine mast cell tumours evaluated by bromodeoxyuridine incorporation and Ki-67 expression, *J Comp Pathol* 127:233-238, 2002.
90. Thompson JJ, Yager JA, Best SJ, et al: Canine subcutaneous mast cell tumors: cellular proliferation and KIT expression as prognostic indices, *Vet Pathol* 48:169-181, 2011.
91. Kravis LD, Vail DM, Kisseberth WC, et al: Frequency of argyrophilic nucleolar organizer regions in fine-needle aspirates and biopsy specimens from mast cell tumors in dogs, *J Am Vet Med Assoc* 209:1418-1420, 1996.
92. Romansik EM, Reilly CM, Kass PH, et al: Mitotic index is predictive for survival for canine cutaneous mast cell tumors, *Vet Pathol* 44:335-341, 2007.
93. Elston L, Sueiro FA, Cavalcanti J, et al: The importance of the mitotic index as a prognostic factor for canine cutaneous mast cell tumors - a validation study, *Vet Pathol* 46:362-365, 2009.
94. Preziosi R, Sarli G, Paltrinieri M: Multivariate survival analysis of histological parameters and clinical presentation in canine cutaneous mast cell tumours, *Vet Res Commun* 31:287-296, 2007.
95. Thompson JJ, Pearl DL, Yager JA, et al: Canine subcutaneous mast cell tumor: characterization and prognostic indices, *Vet Pathol* 48:156-168, 2011.
96. Ayl RD, Couto CG, Hammer AS, et al: Correlation of DNA ploidy to tumor histologic grade, clinical variables, and survival in dogs with mast cell tumors, *Vet Pathol* 29:386-390, 1992.
97. Patruno R, Arpaia N, Gadaleta CD, et al: VEGF concentration from plasma-activated platelets rich correlates with microvascular density and grading in canine mast cell tumour spontaneous model, *J Cell Mol Med* 13:555-561, 2009.
98. Strefezzi Rde F, Xavier JG, Catao-Dias JL: Morphometry of canine cutaneous mast cell tumors, *Vet Pathol* 40:268-275, 2003.

99. Strefezzi Rde F, Xavier JG, Kleeb SR, et al: Nuclear morphometry in cytopathology: a prognostic indicator for canine cutaneous mast cell tumors, *J Vet Diagn Invest* 21:821-825, 2009.
100. Webster JD, Kiupel M, Kaneene JB, et al: The use of KIT and tryptase expression patterns as prognostic tools for canine cutaneous mast cell tumors, *Vet Pathol* 41:371-377, 2004.
101. Bergman PJ, Craft DM, Newman SJ, et al: Correlation of histologic grading of canine mast cell tumors with Ki67/PCNA/AgNOR/c-Kit scores: 38 cases (2002-2003), *Vet Comp Oncol* 2:98, 2004.
102. Moriello KA, Rosenthal RC: Clinical approach to tumors of the skin and subcutaneous tissues, *Vet Clin North Am Small Anim Pract* 20:1163-1190, 1990.
103. O'Keefe DA: Canine mast cell tumors, *Vet Clin North Am Sm Anim Pract* 20:1105-1115, 1990.
104. Richardson RC, Rebar AH, Elliott GS: Common skin tumors of the dog: A clinical approach to diagnosis and treatment, *Comp Cont Ed Pract Vet* 6:1080-1086, 1984.
105. Turrel JM, Kitchell BE, Miller LM, et al: Prognostic factors for radiation treatment of mast cell tumor in 85 dogs, *J Am Vet Med Assoc* 193:936-940, 1988.
106. Cahalane AK, Payne S, Barber LG, et al: Prognostic factors for survival of dogs with inguinal and perineal mast cell tumors treated surgically with or without adjunctive treatment: 68 cases (1994-2002), *J Am Vet Med Assoc* 225:401-408, 2004.
107. Sfiligoi G, Rassnick KM, Scarlett JM, et al: Outcome of dogs with mast cell tumors in the inguinal or perineal region versus other cutaneous locations: 124 cases (1990-2001), *J Am Vet Med Assoc* 226:1368-1374, 2005.
108. Hillman LA, Garrett LD, de Lorimier LP, et al: Biological behavior of oral and perioral mast cell tumors in dogs: 44 cases (1996-2006), *J Am Vet Med Assoc* 237:936-942, 2010.
109. Gieger TL, Theon AP, Werner JA, et al: Biologic behavior and prognostic factors for mast cell tumors of the canine muzzle: 24 cases (1990-2001), *J Vet Intern Med* 17:687-692, 2003.
110. Fife M, Blocker T, Fife T, et al: Canine conjunctival mast cell tumors: a retrospective study, *Vet Ophthalmol* 14:153-160, 2011.
111. Krick EL, Billings AP, Shofer FS, et al: Cytological lymph node evaluation in dogs with mast cell tumours: association with grade and survival, *Vet Comp Oncol* 7:130-138, 2009.
112. Murphy S, Sparkes AH, Blunden AS, et al: Effects of stage and number of tumours on prognosis of dogs with cutaneous mast cell tumours, *Vet Rec* 158:287-291, 2006.
113. Thamm DH, Mauldin EA, Vail DM: Prednisone and vinblastine chemotherapy for canine mast cell tumor–41 cases (1992-1997), *J Vet Intern Med* 13:491-497, 1999.
114. Thamm DH, Turek MM, Vail DM: Outcome and prognostic factors following adjuvant prednisone/vinblastine chemotherapy for high-risk canine mast cell tumour: 61 cases, *J Vet Med Sci* 68:581-587, 2006.
115. Kiupel M, Webster JD, Miller RA, et al: Impact of tumour depth, tumour location and multiple synchronous masses on the prognosis of canine cutaneous mast cell tumours, *J Vet Med A Physiol Pathol Clin Med* 52:280-286, 2005.
116. Zavodovskaya R, Chien MB, London CA: Use of kit internal tandem duplications to establish mast cell tumor clonality in 2 dogs, *J Vet Intern Med* 18:915-917, 2004.
117. LaDue T, Price GS, Dodge R, et al: Radiation therapy for incompletely resected canine mast cell tumors, *Vet Radiol Ultrasound* 39:57-62, 1998.
118. Chaffin K, Thrall DE: Results of radiation therapy in 19 dogs with cutaneous mast cell tumor and regional lymph node metastasis, *Vet Radiol Ultrasound* 43:392-395, 2002.
119. Camps-Palau MA, Leibman NF, Elmslie R, et al: Treatment of canine mast cell tumours with vinblastine, cyclophosphamide and prednisone: 35 cases (1997-2004), *Vet Comp Oncol* 5:156-167, 2007.
120. Clinkenbeard KD: Diagnostic cytology: Mast cell tumors, *Comp Cont Ed Pract Vet* 13:1697-1704, 1991.
121. Mederle O, Mederle N, Bocan EV, et al: VEGF expression in dog mastocytoma, *Rev Med Chir Soc Med Nat Iasi* 114:185-188, 2010.
122. Rabanal RH, Fondevila DM, Montane V, et al: Immunocytochemical diagnosis of skin tumours of the dog with special reference to undifferentiated types, *Res Vet Sci* 47:129-133, 1989.
123. Sandusky GE, Carlton WW, Wightman KA: Diagnostic immunohistochemistry of canine round cell tumors, *Vet Pathol* 24:495-499, 1987.
124. Bookbinder PF, Butt MT, Harvey HJ: Determination of the number of mast cells in lymph node, bone marrow, and buffy coat cytologic specimens from dogs, *J Am Vet Med Assoc* 200:1648-1650, 1992.
125. Sato AF, Solano M: Ultrasonographic findings in abdominal mast cell disease: a retrospective study of 19 patients, *Vet Radiol Ultrasound* 45:51-57, 2004.
126. Stefanello D, Valenti P, Faverzani S, et al: Ultrasound-guided cytology of spleen and liver: a prognostic tool in canine cutaneous mast cell tumor, *J Vet Intern Med* 23:1051-1057, 2009.
127. Book AP, Fidel J, Wills T, et al: Correlation of ultrasound findings, liver and spleen cytology, and prognosis in the clinical staging of high metastatic risk canine mast cell tumors, *Vet Radiol Ultrasound* 52:548-554, 2011.
128. Hahn KA, Lantz GC, Salisbury SK: Comparison of survey radiography with ultrasonography and X-ray computed tomography for clinical staging of subcutaneous neoplasms in dogs, *J Am Vet Med Assoc* 196:1795-1798, 1990.
129. Cayatte SM, McManus PM, Miller WH Jr, et al: Identification of mast cells in buffy coat preparations from dogs with inflammatory skin diseases, *J Am Vet Med Assoc* 206:325-326, 1995.
130. McManus PM: Frequency and severity of mastocytemia in dogs with and without mast cell tumors: 120 cases (1995-1997), *J Am Vet Med Assoc* 215:355-357, 1999.
131. Stockham SL, Basel DL, Schmidt DA: Mastocytemia in dogs with acute inflammatory diseases, *Vet Clin Pathol* 15:16-21, 1986.
132. Endicott MM, Charney SC, McKnight JA, et al: Clinicopathological findings and results of bone marrow aspiration in dogs with cutaneous mast cell tumours: 157 cases (1999-2002), *Vet Comp Oncol* 5:31-37, 2007.
133. Plier ML, MacWilliams PS: Systemic mastocytosis and mast cell leukemia. In Feldman BF, Zinkl JG, Jain NC, editors: *Schalm's veterinary hematology*, ed 5, Philadelphia, 2000, Lippincott Williams & Wilkins.
134. Hikasa Y, Morita T, Futaoka Y, et al: Connective tissue-type mast cell leukemia in a dog, *J Vet Med Sci* 62:187-190, 2000.
135. Simpson AM, Ludwig LL, Newman SJ, et al: Evaluation of surgical margins required for complete excision of cutaneous mast cell tumors in dogs, *J Am Vet Med Assoc* 224:236-240, 2004.
136. Fulcher RP, Ludwig LL, Bergman PJ, et al: Evaluation of a two-centimeter lateral surgical margin for excision of grade I and grade II cutaneous mast cell tumors in dogs, *J Am Vet Med Assoc* 228:210-215, 2006.
137. Johnson RE, Sigman JD, Funk GF, et al: Quantification of surgical margin shrinkage in the oral cavity, *Head Neck* 19:281-286, 1997.
138. Kerns MJ, Darst MA, Olsen TG, et al: Shrinkage of cutaneous specimens: formalin or other factors involved? *J Cutan Pathol* 35:1093-1096, 2008.
139. Reimer SB, Seguin B, DeCock HE, et al: Evaluation of the effect of routine histologic processing on the size of skin samples obtained from dogs, *Am J Vet Res* 66:500-505, 2005.
140. Allan GS, Gilette EL: Response of canine mast cell tumors to radiation, *J Natl Cancer Inst* 63:691-694, 1979.
141. Gillette EL: Indications and selection of patients for radiation therapy, *Vet Clin North Am Small Anim Pract* 4:889-896, 1974.
142. Gillette EL: Radiation therapy of canine and feline tumors, *J Am Anim Hosp Assoc* 12:359-362, 1976.
143. Gillette EL: Veterinary radiotherapy, *J Am Vet Med Assoc* 157:1707-1712, 1976.
144. McClelland RB: The treatment of mastocytomas in dogs, *Cornell Vet* 54:517-519, 1964.

145. Dobson J, Cohen S, Gould S: Treatment of canine mast cell tumours with prednisolone and radiotherapy, *Vet Comp Oncol* 2:132-141, 2004.
146. al-Sarraf R, Mauldin GN, Patnaik AK, et al: A prospective study of radiation therapy for the treatment of grade 2 mast cell tumors in 32 dogs, *J Vet Intern Med* 10:376-378, 1996.
147. Frimberger AE, Moore AS, LaRue SM, et al: Radiotherapy of incompletely resected, moderately differentiated mast cell tumors in the dog: 37 cases (1989-1993), *J Am Anim Hosp Assoc* 33:320-324, 1997.
148. Poirier VJ, Adams WM, Forrest LJ, et al: Radiation therapy for incompletely excised grade II canine mast cell tumors, *J Am Anim Hosp Assoc* 42:430-434, 2006.
149. Hahn KA, King GK, Carreras JK: Efficacy of radiation therapy for incompletely resected grade-III mast cell tumors in dogs: 31 cases (1987-1998), *J Am Vet Med Assoc* 224:79-82, 2004.
150. Hosoya K, Kisseberth WC, Alvarez FJ, et al: Adjuvant CCNU (lomustine) and prednisone chemotherapy for dogs with incompletely excised grade 2 mast cell tumors, *J Am Anim Hosp Assoc* 45:14-18, 2009.
151. Davies DR, Wyatt KM, Jardine JE, et al: Vinblastine and prednisolone as adjunctive therapy for canine cutaneous mast cell tumors, *J Am Anim Hosp Assoc* 40:124-130, 2004.
152. Misdorp W: Incomplete surgery, local immunostimulation, and recurrence of some tumour types in dogs and cats, *Vet Q* 9:279-286, 1987.
153. Lagoretta RA, Denman DL, Kelley MC, et al: Use of hyperthermia and radiotherapy in treatment of a large mast cell sarcoma in a dog, *J Am Vet Med Assoc* 193:1545-1548, 1988.
154. Theon AP, Madewell BR, Castro J: High dose-rate remote afterloading brachytherapy: Preliminary results in canine and feline cutaneous and subcutaneous tumors, *Proc Annu Conf Vet Cancer Soc* 23:109-110, 1993.
155. Northrup NC, Roberts RE, Harrell TW, et al: Iridium-192 interstitial brachytherapy as adjunctive treatment for canine cutaneous mast cell tumors, *J Am Anim Hosp Assoc* 40:309-315, 2004.
156. Frimberger AE, Moore AS, Cincotta L, et al: Photodynamic therapy of naturally occurring tumors in animals using a novel benzophenothiazine photosensitizer, *Clin Cancer Res* 4:2207-2218, 1998.
157. Tanabe S, Yamaguchi M, Iijima M, et al: Fluorescence detection of a new photosensitizer, PAD-S31, in tumour tissues and its use as a photodynamic treatment for skin tumours in dogs and a cat: a preliminary report, *Vet J* 167:286-293, 2004.
158. Rogers KS: Common questions about diagnosing and treating canine mast cell tumors, *Vet Med* 88:246-250, 1993.
159. Spugnini EP, Vincenzi B, Baldi F, et al: Adjuvant electrochemotherapy for the treatment of incompletely resected canine mast cell tumors, *Anticancer Res* 26:4585-4589, 2006.
160. Spugnini EP, Vincenzi B, Citro G, et al: Evaluation of cisplatin as an electrochemotherapy agent for the treatment of incompletely excised mast cell tumors in dogs, *J Vet Intern Med* 25:407-411, 2011.
161. Kodre V, Cemazar M, Pecar J, et al: Electrochemotherapy compared to surgery for treatment of canine mast cell tumours, *In Vivo* 23:55-62, 2009.
162. Neyens IJ, Kirpensteijn J, Grinwis GC, et al: Pilot study of intraregional deionised water adjunct therapy for mast cell tumours in dogs, *Vet Rec* 154:90-91, 2004.
163. Grier RL, Di Guardo G, Schaffer CB, et al: Mast cell tumor destruction by deionized water, *Am J Vet Res* 51:1116-1120, 1990.
164. Grier RL, DiGuardo G, Myers R, et al: Mast cell tumour destruction in dogs by hypotonic solution, *J Small Anim Pract* 36:385-388, 1995.
165. Jaffe MH, Hosgood G, Kerwin SC, et al: The use of deionized water for the treatment of canine cutaneous mast cell tumors, *Vet Cancer Soc Newsl* 22:9-10, 1998.
166. Jaffe MH, Hosgood G, Kerwin SC, et al: Deionised water as an adjunct to surgery for the treatment of canine cutaneous mast cell tumours, *J Small Anim Pract* 41:7-11, 2000.
167. Brocks BA, Neyens IJ, Teske E, et al: Hypotonic water as adjuvant therapy for incompletely resected canine mast cell tumors: a randomized, double-blind, placebo-controlled study, *Vet Surg* 37:472-478, 2008.
168. Asboe-Hanson G: The mast cell: Cortisone action on connective tissue, *Proc Soc Exp Biol Med* 80:677-679, 1952.
169. Bloom F: Effect of cortisone on mast cell tumors (mastocytoma) of the dog, *Proc Soc Exp Biol Med* 80:651-654, 1952.
170. Brodey RS, McGrath JT, Martin JE: Preliminary observations on the use of cortisone in canine mast cell sarcoma, *J Am Vet Med Assoc* 123:391-393, 1953.
171. Stanclift RM, Gilson SD: Evaluation of neoadjuvant prednisone administration and surgical excision in treatment of cutaneous mast cell tumors in dogs, *J Am Vet Med Assoc* 232:53-62, 2008.
172. McCaw DL, Miller MA, Ogilvie GK, et al: Response of canine mast cell tumors to treatment with oral prednisone, *J Vet Intern Med* 8:406-408, 1994.
173. Takahashi T, Kadosawa T, Nagase M, et al: Inhibitory effects of glucocorticoids on proliferation of canine mast cell tumor, *J Vet Med Sci* 59:995-1001, 1997.
174. Matsuda A, Tanaka A, Amagai Y, et al: Glucocorticoid sensitivity depends on expression levels of glucocorticoid receptors in canine neoplastic mast cells, *Vet Immunol Immunopathol* 144:321-328, 2011.
175. Rassnick KM, Al-Sarraf R, Bailey DB, et al: Phase II open-label study of single-agent hydroxyurea for treatment of mast cell tumours in dogs, *Vet Comp Oncol* 8:103-111, 2010.
175b. Henry CJ, Downing S, Rosenthal RC, et al: Evaluation of a novel immunomodulator composed of human chorionic gonadotropin and bacillus Calmette-Guerin for treatment of canine mast cell tumors in clinically affected dogs, *Am J Vet Res* 68:1246–1251, 2007.
176. Valent P, Arock M, Akin C, et al: The classification of systemic mastocytosis should include mast cell leukemia (MCL) and systemic mastocytosis with a clonal hematologic non-mast cell lineage disease (SM-AHNMD), *Blood* 116:850-851, 2010.
177. Cooper M, Tsai X, Bennett P: Combination CCNU and vinblastine chemotherapy for canine mast cell tumours: 57 cases, *Vet Comp Oncol* 7:196-206, 2009.
178. Rassnick KM, Moore AS, Williams LE, et al: Treatment of canine mast cell tumors with CCNU (lomustine), *J Vet Intern Med* 13:601-605, 1999.
179. McCaw DL, Miller MA, Bergman PJ, et al: Vincristine therapy for mast cell tumors in dogs, *J Vet Intern Med* 11:375-378, 1997.
180. Grant IA, Rodriguez CO, Kent MS, et al: A phase II clinical trial of vinorelbine in dogs with cutaneous mast cell tumors, *J Vet Intern Med* 22:388-393, 2008.
181. Taylor F, Gear R, Hoather T, et al: Chlorambucil and prednisolone chemotherapy for dogs with inoperable mast cell tumours: 21 cases, *J Small Anim Pract* 50:284-289, 2009.
182. Rassnick KM, Bailey DB, Russell DS, et al: A phase II study to evaluate the toxicity and efficacy of alternating CCNU and high-dose vinblastine and prednisone (CVP) for treatment of dogs with high-grade, metastatic or nonresectable mast cell tumours, *Vet Comp Oncol* 8:138-152, 2010.
183. Malone EK, Rassnick KM, Wakshlag JJ, et al: Calcitriol (1, 25-dihydroxycholecalciferol) enhances mast cell tumour chemotherapy and receptor tyrosine kinase inhibitor activity in vitro and has single-agent activity against spontaneously occurring canine mast cell tumours, *Vet Comp Oncol* 8:209-220, 2010.
184. Hayes A, Adams V, Smith K, et al: Vinblastine and prednisolone chemotherapy for surgically excised grade III canine cutaneous mast cell tumours, *Vet Comp Oncol* 5:168-176, 2007.
185. Rassnick KM, Bailey DB, Flory AB, et al: Efficacy of vinblastine for treatment of canine mast cell tumors, *J Vet Intern Med* 22:1390-1396, 2008.
186. Vickery KR, Wilson H, Vail DM, et al: Dose-escalating vinblastine for the treatment of canine mast cell tumour, *Vet Comp Oncol* 6:111-119, 2008.

187. Singh J, Rana JS, Sood N, et al: Clinico-pathological studies on the effect of different anti-neoplastic chemotherapy regimens on transmissible venereal tumours in dogs, *Vet Res Commun* 20:71-81, 1996.
188. Ma Y, Longley BJ, Wang X, et al: Clustering of activating mutations in c-KIT's juxtamembrane coding region of canine mast cell neoplasms, *J Invest Dermatol* 112:165-170, 1999.
189. Liao AT, Chien MB, Shenoy N, et al: Inhibition of constitutively active forms of mutant kit by multitargeted indolinone tyrosine kinase inhibitors, *Blood* 100:585-593, 2002.
190. Pryer NK, Lee LB, Zadovaskaya R, et al: Proof of target for SU11654: inhibition of KIT phosphorylation in canine mast cell tumors, *Clin Cancer Res* 9:5729-5734, 2003.
191. London CA, Malpas PB, Wood-Follis SL, et al: Multi-center, placebo-controlled, double-blind, randomized study of oral toceranib phosphate (SU11654), a receptor tyrosine kinase inhibitor, for the treatment of dogs with recurrent (either local or distant) mast cell tumor following surgical excision, *Clin Cancer Res* 15:3856-3865, 2009.
192. Carlsten KS, London CA, Haney S, et al: Multicenter, prospective trial of hypofractionated radiation therapy plus toceranib for unresectable canine mast cell tumors, *J Vet Intern Med* 26:135-141, 2012.
193. London C, Mathie T, Stingle N, et al: Preliminary evidence for biologic activity of toceranib phosphate (Palladia) in solid tumours, *Vet Comp Oncol* Epub ahead of print, 2011.
194. Hahn KA, Ogilvie G, Rusk T, et al: Masitinib is safe and effective for the treatment of canine mast cell tumors, *J Vet Intern Med* 22:1301-1309, 2008.
195. Hahn KA, Legendre AM, Shaw NG, et al: Evaluation of 12- and 24-month survival rates after treatment with masitinib in dogs with nonresectable mast cell tumors, *Am J Vet Res* 71:1354-1361, 2010.
196. Isotani M, Ishida N, Tominaga M, et al: Effect of tyrosine kinase inhibition by imatinib mesylate on mast cell tumors in dogs, *J Vet Intern Med* 22(4):985-958, 2008.
197. Marconato L, Bettini G, Giacoboni C, et al: Clinicopathological features and outcome for dogs with mast cell tumors and bone marrow involvement, *J Vet Intern Med* 22(4):1001-1007, 2008.
198. Yamada O, Kobayashi M, Sugisaki O, et al: Imatinib elicited a favorable response in a dog with a mast cell tumor carrying a c-kit c.1523A>T mutation via suppression of constitutive KIT activation, *Vet Immunol Immunopathol* 142:101-106, 2011.
199. Robat C, London C, Bunting L, et al: Safety evaluation of combination vinblastine and toceranib phosphate (Palladia) in dogs: a phase I dose-finding study, *Vet Comp Oncol* Epub ahead of print, 2011.
200. Kisseberth WC, Murahari S, London CA, et al: Evaluation of the effects of histone deacetylase inhibitors on cells from canine cancer cell lines, *Am J Vet Res* 69:938-945, 2008.
201. Lin TY, Fenger J, Murahari S, et al: AR-42, a novel HDAC inhibitor, exhibits biologic activity against malignant mast cell lines via down-regulation of constitutively activated Kit, *Blood* 115:4217-4225, 2010.
202. Nagamine MK, Sanches DS, Pinello KC, et al: In vitro inhibitory effect of trichostatin A on canine grade 3 mast cell tumor, *Vet Res Commun* 35:391-399, 2011.
203. Lin TY, Bear M, Du Z, et al: The novel HSP90 inhibitor STA-9090 exhibits activity against Kit-dependent and -independent malignant mast cell tumors, *Exp Hematol* 36:1266-1277, 2008.
204. London CA, Bear MD, McCleese J, et al: Phase I evaluation of STA-1474, a Prodrug of the novel HSP90 inhibitor Ganetespib, in dogs with spontaneous cancer, *PLoS One* 6:e27018, 2011.
205. Pinello KC, Nagamine M, Silva TC, et al: In vitro chemosensitivity of canine mast cell tumors grades II and III to all-trans-retinoic acid (ATRA), *Vet Res Commun* Epub ahead of print, 2009.
206. Ohashi E, Miyajima N, Nakagawa T, et al: Retinoids induce growth inhibition and apoptosis in mast cell tumor cell lines, *J Vet Med Sci* 68:797-802, 2006.
207. Miyajima N, Watanabe M, Ohashi E, et al: Relationship between retinoic acid receptor alpha gene expression and growth-inhibitory effect of all-trans retinoic acid on canine tumor cells, *J Vet Intern Med* 20:348-354, 2006.
208. Elders RC, Baines SJ, Catchpole B: Susceptibility of the C2 canine mastocytoma cell line to the effects of tumor necrosis factor-related apoptosis-inducing ligand (TRAIL), *Vet Immunol Immunopathol* 130:11-16, 2009.
209. Peter B, Gleixner KV, Cerny-Reiterer S, et al: Polo-like kinase-1 as a novel target in neoplastic mast cells: demonstration of growth-inhibitory effects of small interfering RNA and the Polo-like kinase-1 targeting drug BI 2536, *Haematologica* 96:672-680, 2011.
210. Kenyon AJ, Ramos L, Michaels EB: Histamine-induced suppressor macrophage inhibits fibroblast growth and wound healing, *Am J Vet Res* 44:2164-2166, 1983.
211. Huttunen M, Hyttinen M, Nilsson G, et al: Inhibition of keratinocyte growth in cell culture and whole skin culture by mast cell mediators, *Exp Dermatol* 10:184-192, 2001.
212. Saar C, Opitz M, Lange W, et al: Mastzellenreitkulose bei katzen, *Berl Munch Tierarztl Wochenschr* 82:438-444, 1969.
213. Hadzijusufovic E, Peter B, Rebuzzi L, et al: Growth-inhibitory effects of four tyrosine kinase inhibitors on neoplastic feline mast cells exhibiting a Kit exon 8 ITD mutation, *Vet Immunol Immunopathol* 132:243-250, 2009.
214. Isotani M, Tamura K, Yagihara H, et al: Identification of a c-kit exon 8 internal tandem duplication in a feline mast cell tumor case and its favorable response to the tyrosine kinase inhibitor imatinib mesylate, *Vet Immunol Immunopathol* 114:168-172, 2006.
215. Isotani M, Yamada O, Lachowicz JL, et al: Mutations in the fifth immunoglobulin-like domain of kit are common and potentially sensitive to imatinib mesylate in feline mast cell tumours, *Br J Haematol* 148:144-153, 2009.
216. Mohr FC, Dunston SK: Culture and initial characterization of the secretory response of neoplastic cat mast cells, *Am J Vet Res* 53:820-828, 1992.
217. Antognoni MT, Spaterna A, Lepri E, et al: Characteristic clinical, haematological and histopathological findings in feline mastocytoma, *Vet Res Commun* 27(suppl 1):727-730, 2003.
218. Feinmehl R, Matus R, Mauldin GN, et al: Splenic mast cell tumors in 43 cats (1975-1992), *Proc Annu Conf Vet Cancer Soc* 12:50, 1992.
219. Macy DW, Reynolds HA: The incidence, characteristics, and clinical management of skin tumors of cats, *J Am Anim Hosp Assoc* 17:1026-1034, 1981.
220. Buerger RG, Scott DW: Cutaneous mast cell neoplasia in cats: 14 cases (1975-1985), *J Am Vet Med Assoc* 190:1440-1444, 1987.
221. Wilcock BP, Yager JA, Zink MC: The morphology and behavior of feline cutaneous mastocytomas, *Vet Pathol* 23:320-324, 1986.
222. Chastain CB, Turk MA, O'Brien D: Benign cutaneous mastocytomas in two litters of Siamese kittens, *J Am Vet Med Assoc* 193:959-960, 1988.
223. Holzinger EA: Feline cutaneous mastocytomas, *Cornell Vet* 63:87-93, 1973.
224. Litster AL, Sorenmo KU: Characterisation of the signalment, clinical and survival characteristics of 41 cats with mast cell neoplasia, *J Feline Med Surg* 8:177-183, 2006.
225. Molander-McCrary H, Henry CJ, Potter K, et al: Cutaneous mast cell tumors in cats: 32 cases (1991-1994), *J Am Anim Hosp Assoc* 34:281-284, 1998.
226. Johnson TO, Schulman FY, Lipscomb TP, et al: Histopathology and biologic behavior of pleomorphic cutaneous mast cell tumors in fifteen cats, *Vet Pathol* 39:452-457, 2002.
227. Garrett LD, Craig CL, Szladovits B, et al: Evaluation of buffy coat smears for circulating mast cells in healthy cats and ill cats without mast cell tumor-related disease, *J Am Vet Med Assoc* 231:1685-1687, 2007.
228. Skeldon NC, Gerber KL, Wilson RJ, et al: Mastocytaemia in cats: prevalence, detection and quantification methods, haematological

associations and potential implications in 30 cats with mast cell tumours, *J Feline Med Surg* 12:960-966, 2010.

229. Rodriguez-Carino C, Fondevila D, Segales J, et al: Expression of KIT receptor in feline cutaneous mast cell tumors, *Vet Pathol* 46:878-883, 2009.
230. Fondevila D, Rabanal R, Ferrer L: Immunoreactivity of canine and feline mast cell tumors, *Schweiz Arch Tierheilk* 132:409-484, 1990.
231. Buss MS, Mollander H, Potter K, et al: Predicting survival and prognosis in cats with cutaneous mastocytomas of varying histological grade, *Proc Annu Conf Vet Cancer Soc* 16:56-57, 1996.
232. Sabattini S, Bettini G: Prognostic value of histologic and immunohistochemical features in feline cutaneous mast cell tumors, *Vet Pathol* 47:643-653, 2010.
233. Montgomery KW, van der Woerdt A, Aquino SM, et al: Periocular cutaneous mast cell tumors in cats: evaluation of surgical excision (33 cases), *Vet Ophthalmol* 13:26-30, 2010.
234. Lepri E, Ricci G, Leonardi L, et al: Diagnostic and prognostic features of feline cutaneous mast cell tumours: a retrospective analysis of 40 cases, *Vet Res Commun* 27(suppl 1):707-709, 2003.
235. Turrel JM, Farrelly J, Page RL, et al: Evaluation of strontium 90 irradiation in treatment of cutaneous mast cell tumors in cats: 35 cases (1992-2002), *J Am Vet Med Assoc* 228:898-901, 2006.
236. Rassnick KM, Gieger TL, Williams LE, et al: Phase I evaluation of CCNU (lomustine) in tumor-bearing cats, *J Vet Intern Med* 15:196-199, 2001.
237. Rassnick KM, Williams LE, Kristal O, et al: Lomustine for treatment of mast cell tumors in cats: 38 cases (1999-2005), *J Am Vet Med Assoc* 232:1200-1205, 2008.
238. Lachowicz JL, Post GS, Brodsky E: A phase I clinical trial evaluating imatinib mesylate (Gleevec) in tumor-bearing cats, *J Vet Intern Med* 19:860-864, 2005.
239. Bellamy F, Bader T, Moussy A, et al: Pharmacokinetics of masitinib in cats, *Vet Res Commun* 33(8):831-837, 2009.
240. Daly M, Sheppard S, Cohen N, et al: Safety of masitinib mesylate in healthy cats, *J Vet Intern Med* 25:297-302, 2011.
241. Spangler WL, Culbertson MR: Prevalence and type of splenic diseases in cats: 455 cases (1985-1991), *J Am Vet Med Assoc* 201:773-776, 1992.
242. Hanson JA, Papageorges M, Girard E, et al: Ultrasonographic appearance of splenic disease in 101 cats, *Vet Radiol Ultrasound* 42:441-445, 2001.
243. Guerre R, Millet P, Groulade P: Systemic mastocytosis in a cat: remission after splenectomy, *J Small Anim Pract* 20:769-772, 1979.
244. Liska WD, MacEwen EG, Zaki FA, et al: Feline systemic mastocytosis: A review and results of splenectomy in seven cases, *J Am Anim Hosp Assoc* 15:589-597, 1979.
245. Schulman A: Splenic mastocytosis in a cat, *California Vet* 17:17-18, 1987.
246. Gordon SS, McClaran JK, Bergman PJ, et al: Outcome following splenectomy in cats, *J Feline Med Surg* 12:256-261, 2010.
247. Bortnowski HB, Rosenthal RC: Gastrointestinal mast cell tumors and eosinophilia in two cats, *J Am Anim Hosp Assoc* 28:271-275, 1992.
248. Halsey CH, Powers BE, Kamstock DA: Feline intestinal sclerosing mast cell tumour: 50 cases (1997-2008), *Vet Comp Oncol* 8:72-79, 2010.
249. Arock M, Valent P: Pathogenesis, classification and treatment of mastocytosis: state of the art in 2010 and future perspectives, *Exp Rev Hematol* 3:497-516, 2010.
250. Bodemer C, Hermine O, Palmerini F, et al: Pediatric mastocytosis is a clonal disease associated with D816V and other activating c-KIT mutations, *J Invest Dermatol* 130:804-815, 2010.
251. Horny HP, Sotlar K, Valent P: Mastocytosis: state of the art, *Pathobiology* 74:121-132, 2007.
252. Valent P, Akin C, Escribano L, et al: Standards and standardization in mastocytosis: consensus statements on diagnostics, treatment recommendations and response criteria, *Eur J Clin Invest* 37:435-453, 2007.
253. Ustun C, Deremer DL, Akin C: Tyrosine kinase inhibitors in the treatment of systemic mastocytosis, *Leuk Res* 35(9):1143-1152, 2011.

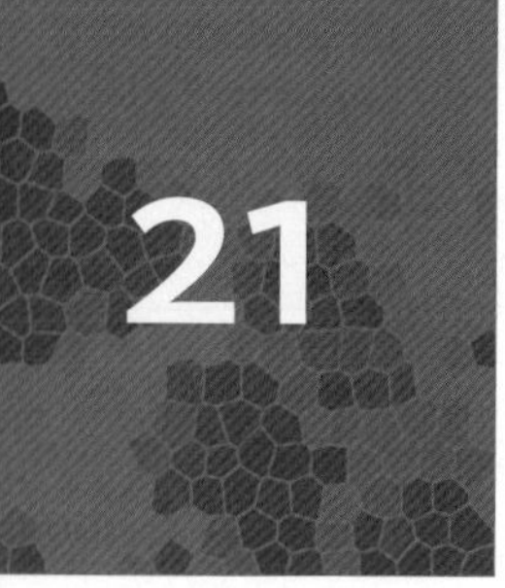

21 Soft Tissue Sarcomas

Julius M. Liptak and Lisa J. Forrest

Incidence and Risk Factors

Soft tissue sarcomas are a heterogeneous population of mesenchymal tumors that comprise 15% and 7% of all skin and subcutaneous tumors in the dog and cat, respectively.[1] The annual incidence of soft tissue sarcomas in companion animals is about 35 per 100,000 dogs at risk and 17 per 100,000 cats at risk.[2] In dogs, sarcomas have been associated with radiation, trauma, foreign bodies, orthopedic implants, and the parasite *Spirocerca lupi*.[3-9]

Most soft tissue sarcomas are solitary tumors in middle-aged to older dogs and cats. There is no specific breed or sex predilection for soft tissue sarcomas with the possible exception of synovial cell sarcomas in dogs. Earlier reports indicate a slight male predilection[10,11]; however, in a recent study, males and females were equally represented.[12] Another exception is the occurrence of rhabdomyosarcoma in young dogs.[13] Soft tissue sarcomas tend to be overrepresented in large breed dogs.

Pathology and Natural History*

Soft tissue sarcomas are a heterogeneous group of tumors whose classification is based on similar pathologic appearance and clinical behavior. Sarcomas arise from mesenchymal tissues and have features similar to the cell type of origin (Table 21-1). These tumors originate in connective tissues, including muscle, adipose, neurovascular, fascial, and fibrous tissue, and can give rise to benign and malignant entities. Only malignant soft tissue sarcomas will be covered in this chapter. Malignant neoplasms in this category include fibrosarcoma, peripheral nerve sheath tumor (PNST; also known as malignant schwannoma, neurofibrosarcoma, or hemangiopericytoma), myxosarcoma, undifferentiated sarcoma, liposarcoma, malignant fibrous histiocytoma, and rhabdomyosarcoma (Table 21-2).[14,15] The term *soft tissue sarcoma* generally excludes those tumors of hematopoietic or lymphoid origin. Hemangiosarcoma (covered briefly here), mast cell sarcoma, oral sarcoma, osteosarcoma, and chondrosarcoma are covered separately in other chapters. Feline sarcomas and vaccine-associated sarcomas are covered in a separate section at the end of this chapter.

Soft tissue sarcomas may arise from any anatomic site in the body, although skin and subcutaneous sites are most common. Soft tissue sarcomas have the following important common features with regard to their biologic behavior:

- They tend to appear as pseudoencapsulated soft-to-firm tumors but have poorly defined histologic margins or infiltrate through and along fascial planes, and they are locally invasive.
- Local recurrence after conservative surgical excision is common.
- Sarcomas tend to metastasize hematogenously in up to 20% of cases.
- Regional lymph node metastasis is unusual (except for synovial cell sarcoma).[10]
- Histopathologic grade is predictive of metastasis, and resected tumor margins predict local recurrence.[16]
- Measurable or bulky (>5 cm in diameter) tumors generally have a poor response to chemotherapy and radiation therapy (RT).

Soft tissue sarcomas present a diagnostic challenge. Many of these tumors have histologic patterns with overlapping features not only among themselves but also with a variety of other neoplasms with different histogenesis. The development of immunocytochemical procedures, the availability of monoclonal antibodies and polyclonal antibodies to various tissue markers, and tissue microarray technology have improved diagnosis of soft tissue sarcomas in human pathology and, to a limited degree, in veterinary pathology.[12,17-22]

The histologic nomenclature for some sarcomas may vary from pathologist to pathologist. Before the initiation of the appropriate therapy for the treatment of soft tissue sarcomas, it is necessary to know the histologic type, size, site, and grade and the stage of disease. Histologic grading (e.g., low, intermediate, or high or I, II, III) is assigned after histologic characterization from adequate biopsy specimens (Table 21-3).

Specific Tumor Types

Soft tissue sarcoma is a collective term used to describe a number of different types of tumors with similar histologic features and biologic behavior. The histogenesis of soft tissue sarcomas is controversial and may be difficult to differentiate on the basis of routine histologic and immunohistochemical analysis. Some pathologists have recommended the use of a more generic term such as soft tissue sarcoma or *spindle cell tumor of canine soft tissue* because of the difficulty in differentiating tumors such as fibrosarcoma, PNST, and hemangiopericytoma.[23] Moreover, histologic distinction of tumor type is not clinically important because most soft tissue sarcomas have a similar biologic behavior (i.e., locally aggressive with a low-to-moderate distant metastatic rate). Some types of soft tissue sarcomas covered briefly in this chapter are hemangiosarcomas, lymphangiosarcomas, and synovial cell sarcomas, which are atypical because their biologic behavior is different with a higher rate and different distribution of metastasis.

Tumors of Fibrous Origin

Nodular Fasciitis (Fibromatosis, Pseudosarcomatous Fibromatosis)

Nodular fasciitis is a benign nonneoplastic lesion arising from the subcutaneous fascia or superficial portions of the deep fascia in

*Tables 21-1 and 21-3 and general pathology description courtesy Dr. Barbara Powers, Colorado State University.

TABLE 21-1 Histiogenic Classification and Metastatic Potential of Canine Soft Tissue Sarcomas

TISSUE OF ORIGIN	BENIGN	MALIGNANT	PRIMARY SITES	METASTATIC POTENTIAL	METASTATIC SITES
Fibrous tissue	Fibroma	Fibrosarcoma	Extremity and oral cavity	Low-to-moderate*	Lungs
Nervous tissue	—	PNST	Extremity	Low-to-moderate*	Lungs
Myxomatous tissue	Myxoma	Myxosarcoma	Extremity and joints	Low-to-moderate	Lungs
Adipose tissue	Lipoma	Liposarcoma	Extremity and ventrum ± abdominal or thoracic cavity	Low-to-moderate	Lungs ± liver, spleen, bone
Skeletal muscle	Rhabdomyoma	Rhabdomyosarcoma	Tongue, larynx, heart, and urinary bladder	Low-to-moderate	Lungs ± liver, spleen, kidneys
Smooth muscle	Leiomyoma	Leiomyosarcoma†	Gastrointestinal ± spleen, liver, vulva and vagina, and subcutaneous tissue	Moderate	Lymph nodes, liver ± spleen, kidneys, peritoneum
Synovial tissue	Synovioma	Synovial cell sarcoma†	Joints	Moderate-to-high*	Lymph nodes and lungs
Histiocytic cells	Histiocytoma	Histiocytic sarcoma†	Extremity	Moderate-to-high	Lymph nodes ± lungs, spleen, liver, kidneys
Lymph vessels	Lymphangioma	Lymphangiosarcoma†	Extremity	Moderate	Lymph nodes
Blood vessels	Hemangioma	Hemangiosarcoma†	Spleen, heart, liver ± skin, muscle, bone, kidneys, and retroperitoneum	High	Lungs, liver, lymph nodes, distant dermal sites

PNST, Peripheral nerve sheath tumor.

*Dependent on histologic grade.

†Atypical soft tissue sarcoma with higher metastatic rate of metastasis to regional lymph node.

TABLE 21-2 Types of Soft Tissue Sarcoma

TYPE OF SARCOMA	TUMORS
Soft tissue sarcoma	Fibrosarcoma PNST* Liposarcoma Myxosarcoma Malignant mesenchymoma
Other soft tissue sarcoma	Leiomyosarcoma Rhabdomyosarcoma Synovial cell sarcoma Lymphangiosarcoma
Non–soft tissue sarcoma	Histiocytic sarcoma Hemangiosarcoma Osteosarcoma Chondrosarcoma Melanoma Lymphosarcoma (lymphoma)

Tumors listed under "Soft tissue sarcoma" have similar biologic behavior characterized by local aggression and low-to-moderate metastatic potential. Tumors listed under "Other soft tissue sarcoma" are atypical soft tissue sarcomas because of different location (e.g., leiomyosarcoma and synovial cell sarcoma) or higher metastatic rate (leiomyosarcoma, rhabdomyosarcoma, lymphangiosarcoma ± synovial cell sarcoma). Some sarcomas not considered as soft tissue sarcomas are discussed in this chapter because of similarities in location to other soft tissue sarcomas (e.g., histiocytic sarcoma and dermal hemangiosarcoma).[133]

PNST, Peripheral nerve sheath tumor.

*PNSTs include tumors previously classified as hemangiopericytoma, malignant schwannoma, and neurofibrosarcoma.

TABLE 21-3 Soft Tissue Sarcoma Grading System

SCORE	DIFFERENTIATION	MITOSIS*	NECROSIS
1	Resembles normal adult mesenchymal tissue	0-9	None
2	Specific histologic subtype	10-19	<50% necrosis
3	Undifferentiated	>20	>50% necrosis

Grade I: Cumulative score of ≤4 for the three categories.

Grade II: Cumulative score of 5-6.

Grade III: Cumulative score of ≥7.

*Mitosis is calculated as the number of mitotic figures/10 HPF.

dogs. These lesions are usually nodular, poorly circumscribed, and very invasive.[24] Histologically, nodular fasciitis is characterized by large plump or spindle-shaped fibroblasts in a stromal network of variable amounts of collagen and reticular fibers with scattered lymphocytes, plasma cells, and macrophages.[24] The morphologic and pathologic characteristics of nodular fasciitis can result in these lesions being misdiagnosed as fibrosarcoma. Infantile desmoid-type fibromatosis is a variant of nodular fasciitis and is characterized by fibroblast proliferation with a dense reticular fiber network and mucoid material.[25] Wide excision of both nodular fasciitis and infantile desmoid-type fibromatosis lesions is usually curative.[26] Local recurrence is possible with incomplete resection. These tumors do not metastasize.[24]

Fibrosarcoma

Most fibrosarcomas arise from the skin, subcutaneous tissue, or oral cavity and represent malignant fibroblasts. Tumors can be well differentiated, exhibiting spindle-shaped tumor cells with scant cytoplasm. The more anaplastic tumor is very cellular with closely packed spindle-shaped fibroblasts showing many mitotic figures and marked cellular pleomorphism.[27] Tumors tend to occur in older dogs and cats with no breed or sex predilection; however, one reference states a higher predilection in golden retrievers and Doberman Pinschers.[28] A unique form, histologically low-grade, yet biologically high-grade fibrosarcoma, is seen in the oral cavity and has a tendency to grow quite large and invade deeper structures, including bone. Metastasis can be seen in up to 20% of the cases.[19] Metastasis is rare, but these tumors are infiltrative, with microscopic tumor cells invading along fascial planes, and often recur after surgical excision.

Tumors of the Peripheral Nerves

Peripheral Nerve Sheath Tumor (Neurofibrosarcoma, Malignant Schwannoma, Hemangiopericytoma)

The PNSTs are malignant tumors of nerve sheath origin and have been referred to as neurofibrosarcoma, malignant schwannoma, and hemangiopericytoma. The confusion regarding hemangiopericytoma is the fact that blood vessel pericyte origin has yet to be proven in dogs. Most hemangiopericytomas will have features of nerve sheath tumors histologically.[27] Malignant PNSTs will stain positive with S-100 and vimentin, indicating peripheral nerve origin.[29]

Regardless of the nomenclature, these tumors can occur anywhere in the body. A PNST may involve nerves away from the brain or spinal cord (peripheral group), or they may involve nerves immediately adjacent to the brain or spinal cord (root group) or the brachial or lumbosacral plexus (plexus group).[30] The true peripheral form is much more treatable than the plexus or root form. Despite appearing encapsulated at surgery, these tumors are similar to fibrosarcomas and occur as poorly defined tumors without histologic encapsulation. Most of the tumors are adherent to deeper tissues and may infiltrate underlying fascia, muscle, and skin. Although these tumors are considered malignant, they have a modest metastatic rate. As with fibrosarcomas, local recurrence for PNSTs is common following conservative surgery. They tend to grow slowly and can range in size from 0.5 cm to over 10 to 12 cm in diameter. In some cases, they can easily be confused with lipomas on initial clinical examination.[27]

PNSTs located in the proximal axial region may result in the compression of nerves. The vast majority of cases will show signs of unilateral lameness, muscle atrophy, paralysis, and pain.[30] They can invade the spinal cord, and about 50% will invade the cord if a grade III tumor is diagnosed.[30] However, local disease usually limits survival before metastasis occurs.

Histiocytic Disorders

The reader is referred to Chapter 33, Section F, for a complete discussion of histiocytic disorders because the biology, nomenclature, and management of this collection of benign and malignant conditions continue to evolve. Malignant fibrous histiocytoma as a histopathologic diagnosis, however, is considered to be more consistent with soft tissue sarcomas in general and is managed with guidelines discussed later in this chapter.

Tumors of Adipose Tissue

Lipoma

Lipomas are benign tumors of adipose tissue. Variants of lipomas have been reported and include angiolipoma and angiofibrolipoma.[31] Lipomas are relatively common in older dogs, especially in subcutaneous locations, and are rarely symptomatic. Lipomas can also occur in the thoracic cavity, abdominal cavity, spinal canal, and vulva and vagina of dogs and can cause clinical abnormalities secondary to either compression or strangulation.[32-40] Parosteal and infiltrative lipomas have been rarely reported and these tumors can have a more aggressive behavior despite their benign histologic appearance.[41-46] Marginal resection is recommended for lipomas that interfere with normal function; however, the majority are asymptomatic and do not require surgical intervention. Lipomas can be differentiated from liposarcomas based on morphologic and histologic appearance. Histologically, lipomas have indistinct nuclei and cytoplasm resembling normal fat, whereas liposarcomas are characterized by increased cellularity, distinct nuclei, and abundant cytoplasm with one or more droplets of fat.[38] Surgical resection is usually curative, but local recurrence has been reported.[39]

Intermuscular Lipoma

Intermuscular lipomas are a variant of the subcutaneous lipoma and are located in the intermuscular region of the caudal thigh of dogs, particularly between the semitendinosus and semimembranosus muscles (Figure 21-1).[47] Clinically, intermuscular lipomas appear as a slow-growing, firm, and fixed mass in the caudal thigh region and may occasionally cause lameness.[47] Cytologic analysis of fine-needle aspirates is usually diagnostic. The recommended treatment is surgical resection, involving blunt dissection and digital extrusion, and placement of either a Penrose or negative-suction drain. Seromas are a common complication in dogs in which a

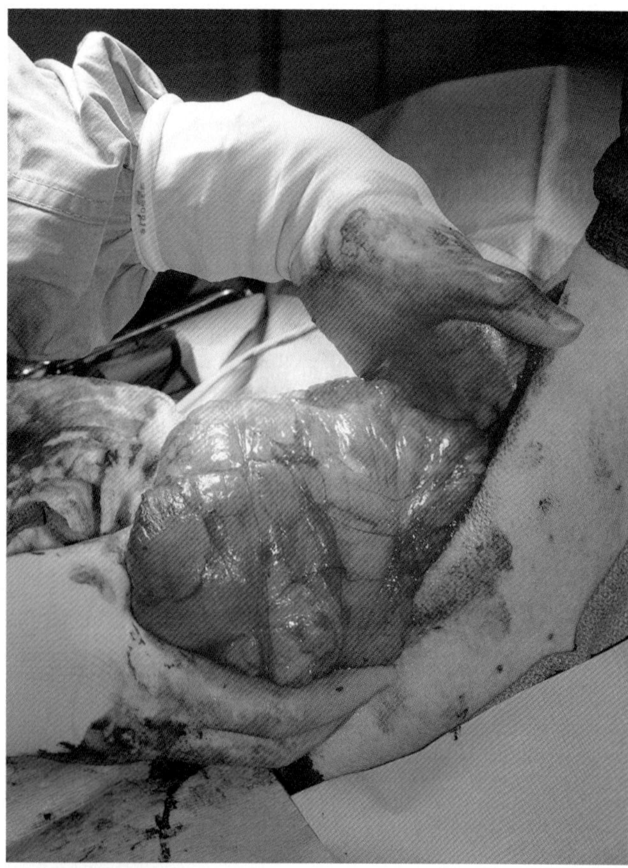

FIGURE 21-1 An intramuscular lipoma arising from between the semitendinosus and semimembranosus muscles. Surgical dissection and removal was curative.

drain is not used. The prognosis is excellent with no recurrence reported in 11 dogs following surgical removal.[47]

Infiltrative Lipoma

Infiltrative lipomas are uncommon tumors composed of well-differentiated adipose cells without evidence of anaplasia. These tumors cannot be readily distinguished from the more common simple lipoma by cytology or small biopsy specimens. They are considered "benign" and do not metastasize. However, infiltrative lipomas are locally aggressive and commonly invade adjacent muscle, fascia, nerve, myocardium, joint capsule, and even bone.[42,48,49] Computed tomography (CT) is used to better delineate these tumors; however, they do not contrast enhance and differentiating infiltrative lipomas from normal fat is problematic.[47] One retrospective analysis of 16 cases reported a 4:1 female-to-male ratio.[44] Aggressive treatment, including amputation, may be necessary for local control. RT can be considered either alone or in combination with surgical excision.[46]

Liposarcoma

Liposarcomas are uncommon malignant tumors originating from lipoblasts in older dogs.[50] Liposarcomas apparently do not arise from malignant transformation of lipomas. Specific causes are not known, but foreign body–associated liposarcoma has been reported in one dog.[5] There is no breed or sex predilection.[50] They are commonly reported in subcutaneous locations, especially along the ventrum and extremities, but can also occur in other primary sites such as bone and the abdominal cavity. Liposarcomas are differentiated from lipomas based on morphologic appearance and cytologic characteristics. Liposarcomas are usually firm and poorly circumscribed. They are locally invasive with a low metastatic potential. Metastatic sites include the lungs, liver, spleen, and bone.[27,50]

The prognosis for liposarcoma is good with appropriate surgical management. The median survival time (MST) following wide surgical excision is 1188 days; this is significantly better than either marginal excision or incisional biopsy, which have MSTs of 649 days and 183 days, respectively (Figure 21-2).[50] Liposarcoma is histologically classified as well-differentiated, myxoid, round cell (or poorly differentiated), pleomorphic, or dedifferentiated. This classification scheme has clinical and prognostic importance in humans because pleomorphic liposarcomas have a high metastatic rate, myxoid liposarcomas are more likely to metastasize to extrapulmonary soft tissue structures, and well-differentiated liposarcomas are unlikely to metastasize.[51-53] In a retrospective study in dogs, histologic subtype was not prognostic, but metastatic disease was more common in dogs with pleomorphic liposarcomas.[50]

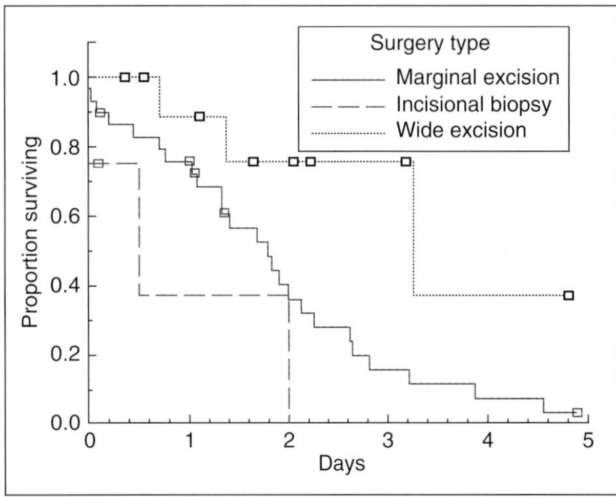

FIGURE 21-2 Kaplan-Meier survival curve of 56 dogs with liposarcoma treated with either incisional biopsy, marginal resection, or wide excision. The median survival time (MST) is significantly longer, at 1188 days, following wide surgical resection than less aggressive techniques. *(Reprinted with permission from Baez JL, Hendrick MJ, Shofer FS, et al: Liposarcomas in dogs: 56 cases (1989-2000),* J Am Vet Med Assoc *224:887, 2004.)*

Tumors of Smooth Muscle

Leiomyoma and Leiomyosarcoma

Leiomyomas and leiomyosarcomas are tumors arising from smooth muscle cells. The gastrointestinal (GI) tract is most commonly affected, but other primary sites include the spleen, liver, genitourinary tract, retroperitoneal space, vessel wall, and subcutaneous tissue.[54-57] Paraneoplastic syndromes associated with smooth muscle tumors, particularly GI leiomyomas and leiomyosarcomas, include hypoglycemia, nephrogenic diabetes insipidus, and secondary erythrocytosis.[55,58-61]

Leiomyomas are benign and usually small, localized, and well encapsulated. Leiomyomas of the vagina and vulva are often pedunculated, protrude from the vulva, and are hormonally dependent. Ovariohysterectomy is recommended in the management of dogs with vulval or vaginal leiomyomas.

Leiomyosarcomas are malignant tumors with a moderate metastatic potential, depending on the primary site.[55,62] The metastatic rate for dogs with hepatic leiomyosarcoma is apparently 100% but is approximately 50% for other primary intraabdominal sites and 0% for dermal smooth muscle tumors.[55,61,63,64] Regional lymph nodes, mesentery, and liver are the most common metastatic sites for GI leiomyosarcoma, although other sites include the spleen, kidneys, and peritoneum.[55,61-64]

Leiomyosarcoma is the second most common GI tumor in dogs and has a predilection for the jejunum and cecum, but any region of the GI tract can be affected from the esophagus to the rectum.[55,61-63,65] An immunohistochemical review of previously diagnosed GI leiomyomas and leiomyosarcomas has resulted in the vast majority of these tumors being reclassified as GI stromal tumors (GISTs) or GI stromal-like tumors.[66,67] Leiomyosarcomas have strong immunoreactivity to actin and desmin and rarely stain positively with c-kit, CD34, or S-100 protein. In contrast, true GISTs are consistently associated with mutations of the tyrosine kinase receptor gene *c-kit* and will have strong immunoreactivity to c-kit and CD34 proteins with variable reactivity to actin, desmin, and S-100 protein.[62,65-67] The GI stromal-like tumors have an identical immunohistochemical profile to GISTs, except they do not express c-kit.[66]

Older dogs are more commonly affected and there is no sex or breed predisposition.[55,61-63] In contrast, there is a male predisposition for GI leiomyomas and these tumors have a predilection for the stomach rather than the jejunum and cecum.[62,68] Presenting signs can include inappetence, weight loss, vomiting, diarrhea, polyuria, polydipsia, anemia, and hypoglycemia.[55,61-63]

Surgical resection is the recommended treatment for dogs with leiomyosarcomas. Intestinal perforation with localized to diffuse peritonitis is relatively common in dogs with GI leiomyosarcoma and is reported in up to 50% of cases.[61] Local tumor control is good following complete resection, but recurrence has been reported following incomplete resection of a gastric leiomyoma and cutaneous leiomyosarcomas.[64,66,68]

Prolonged survival and possibly cure has been reported following surgery in dogs with gastrointestinal leiomyosarcoma and GIST tumors.[54,55,59,67] Prognostic factors in humans with GIST include tumor size, metastasis, and histologic criteria such as tumor necrosis, number of mitotic figures, and proliferating cell nuclear antigen (PCNA) index[69]; however, prognostic factors have not been investigated in dogs with leiomyosarcoma. The MST for dogs with GI leiomyosarcoma and GIST surviving the immediate postoperative period is up to 37.4 months, with 1-, 2-, and 3-year survival rates of 75% to 83%, 62% to 67%, and 60%, respectively.[55,61,63,66,67] In addition, metastasis did not have a negative impact on survival time in one report with a 21.7 month MST for dogs with documented metastasis at the time of surgery.[61] However, other investigators have found metastasis significantly decreases survival time.[63] The MST is 8 months for dogs with splenic leiomyosarcoma, and all dogs with hepatic leiomyosarcoma in one series had evidence of metastasis at initial surgery and were euthanized.[55]

Tumors of Skeletal Muscle

Rhabdomyosarcoma

Rhabdomyosarcomas are rare malignant tumors originating from myoblasts or primitive mesenchymal cells capable of differentiating into striated muscle cells.[70] In dogs, rhabdomyosarcomas are most frequently reported to arise from skeletal muscle of the tongue, larynx, myocardium, and urinary bladder. They are locally invasive with a low-to-moderate metastatic potential. Metastatic sites include the lungs, liver, spleen, kidneys, and adrenal glands.[70]

Rhabdomyosarcomas are histologically classified as embryonal, botryoid, alveolar, and pleomorphic. The histologic diagnosis of rhabdomyosarcoma is difficult and immunohistochemical staining for vimentin, skeletal muscle actin, myoglobin, myogenin, and myogenic differentiation (MyoD) may be required for definitive diagnosis.[71] Embryonal rhabdomyosarcomas have a predilection for the head and neck region of older dogs, such as the tongue, oral cavity, and larynx. In contrast, botryoid rhabdomyosarcoma commonly arises in the urinary bladder of young, female large breed dogs with Saint Bernard dogs possibly being overrepresented in one data set.[70] Botryoid tumors are characterized by their grapelike appearance. The histologic classification scheme for rhabdomyosarcoma has prognostic significance in humans, but this has not been investigated in dogs. In humans, botryoid rhabdomyosarcoma has a good prognosis, embryonal rhabdomyosarcoma has an intermediate prognosis, and alveolar rhabdomyosarcoma has a poor prognosis.[70,72]

Rhabdomyosarcomas, particularly those involving the extremities, have a high rate of metastasis in humans; major metastatic sites include the lungs, lymph nodes, and bone marrow. The metastatic potential and prognosis in dogs with rhabdomyosarcoma have not been determined because it is rarely diagnosed and even more rarely treated with curative intent. However, disease-free and overall survival times have been encouraging in the few dogs treated with surgical resection with or without RT and chemotherapy.[73-77] In humans, in contrast to many other types of soft tissue sarcomas, multimodality treatment with surgery, RT, and chemotherapy has significantly improved survival rates, particularly in children with embryonal and botryoid rhabdomyosarcoma.[51,53,72]

Tumors of Vascular and Lymphatic Tissue

Lymphangiosarcoma

Lymphangiosarcomas are rare tumors seen in young dogs and cats that arise from lymphatic endothelial cells.[27,78,79] They are usually soft, cystic-like, and edematous, usually occurring in the subcutis (Figure 21-3).[27] In most cases, clinical signs are associated with extensive edema and drainage of lymph through the skin or a cystic mass. Aspiration may reveal a fluid-filled mass. Histopathologically, these tumors resemble normal endothelial cells and may be confused with hemangiosarcomas because of the vascular channels; however, red blood cells are not seen.[27] Lymphangiosarcomas tend to have a moderate-to-high metastatic potential.[80] In a single case report, a dog treated with surgery that had local recurrence had a complete response following doxorubicin chemotherapy with no evidence of recurrence or metastasis 9 months after remission.[81]

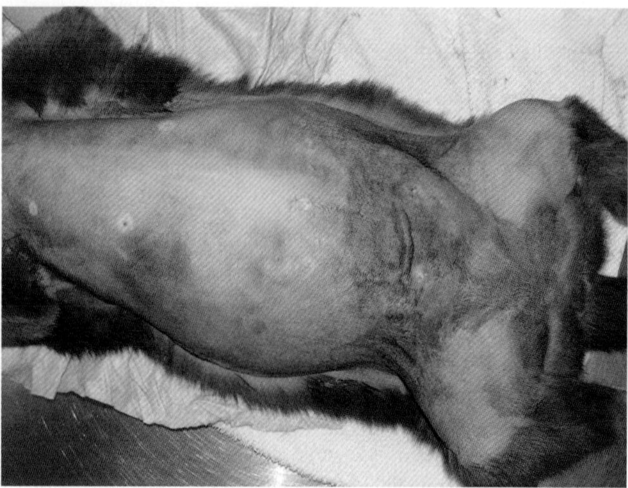

FIGURE 21-3 Lymphangiosarcoma of the ventral abdomen in a male cat. These tumors are often subcutaneous, soft and edematous, and with poorly defined margins.

Hemangioma

Hemangiomas and hemangiosarcomas (HSAs) are tumors of vascular endothelial origin. Hemangioma is a benign tumor that can occur in a variety of sites, including skin, liver, spleen, kidneys, bone, tongue, and heart.[82-84] Dermal hemangiomas may be induced by ultraviolet (UV) light in short-haired dogs with poorly pigmented skin.[27] Despite their benign biologic behavior, hemangiomas can cause severe anemia secondary to tumor-associated blood loss.[82,84] In humans, hemangiomas can spontaneously regress or be responsive to intralesional corticosteroids, but this has not been observed in dogs.[27] Complete surgical resection is usually curative.

Hemangiosarcoma

HSAs are highly malignant tumors. The most common primary sites in cats and dogs involve visceral organs, especially the spleen, right atrial appendage, and liver.[24] Other primary sites include the skin, pericardium, lung, kidneys, oral cavity, muscle, bone, genitourinary tract, and peritoneum and retroperitoneum.[24,85] A thorough review of HSAs is presented in Chapter 33, Section A. The discussion here is limited to dermal and subcutaneous HSAs. Primary dermal HSAs have a predilection for light-haired or poorly pigmented skin on the ventral abdomen and preputial region of dogs, particularly those confined to the dermis, and solar radiation has been proposed as a cause of dermal HSAs in dogs.[86]

Canine cutaneous HSAs are clinically staged according to depth of involvement with stage I tumors confined to the dermis, stage II tumors extending into subcutaneous tissue, and stage III HSAs

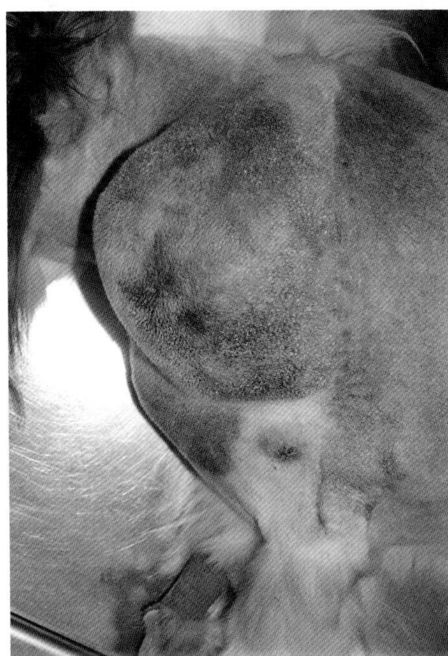

FIGURE 21-4 A dog with a subcutaneous hemangiosarcoma invading into the underlying musculature of the thoracic limb (stage III) with a typical bruised appearance. Local tumor control is more difficult in these cases and the prognosis is worse for dogs with higher grade dermal hemangiosarcoma if logoregional tumor control is not achieved.

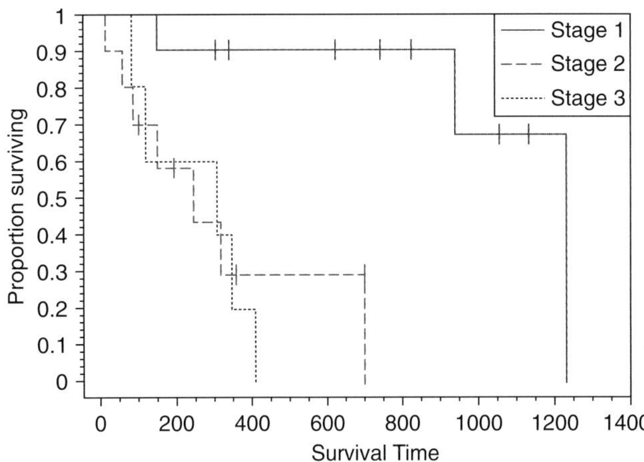

FIGURE 21-5 Kaplan-Meier survival curve for dogs with stage I (cutaneous), stage II (subcutaneous), and stage III (muscle) hemangiosarcoma. *(Reprinted with permission from Ward H, Fox LE, Calderwood-Mays MB, et al: Cutaneous hemangiosarcoma in 25 dogs: A retrospective study,* J Vet Intern Med *8:345, 1994.)*

involving the underlying muscle (Figure 21-4).[86] Stage II and III dermal HSAs are typically large and poorly circumscribed and have a bruised appearance that can be mistaken for a traumatic hematoma. The recommended treatment is wide surgical resection and adjuvant doxorubicin.[87] Doxorubicin-based chemotherapy protocols have been investigated in dogs with nonresectable stage II and III cutaneous HSAs, with approximately 40% of dogs showing a measurable response with a median response duration of 53 days.[88] Treatment with doxorubicin-based chemotherapy protocols may downstage dogs with large subcutaneous and intramuscular HSAs and thus decrease the size of the tumor, allowing for complete surgical excision.[88]

Clinical staging provides prognostic information on the success of local treatment, metastatic potential, and survival time. Dogs with stage I dermal HSAs have a complete surgical resection rate of 78%, 30% metastatic rate with all metastases occurring in distant dermal sites, and a MST of 780 days.[86] In contrast, dogs with stage II and III hypodermal HSAs have a complete surgical resection rate of only 23%, principally because these tumors are larger and less well circumscribed; are 60% metastatic to lungs, regional lymph nodes, and distant dermal sites; and have a significantly lower MST of 172 to 307 days (Figure 21-5).[86] For dogs with aggressive local control (using adequate surgery with or without RT) of subcutaneous or intramuscular HSA, the use of adjuvant doxorubicin results in encouraging survival times. The median disease-free interval (DFI) and survival time for dogs with subcutaneous and intramuscular HSAs treated with surgery and doxorubicin are 1553 and 1189 days and 266 and 273 days, respectively.[87]

Feline cutaneous HSAs are usually solitary tumors in older cats, with a mean age of 11.5 to 12.5 years and males possibly being overrepresented.[89,90] Unlike cutaneous hemangiomas, which have no site predilection, cutaneous HSAs occur primarily in poorly pigmented skin, particularly the skin of the pinna, head, and ventral abdomen and subcutaneous tissue of the inguinal region.[89-91] Local tumor control is poor following surgical resection, with local recurrence reported in 50% to 80% of cases at a median of 420 days postoperatively.[89-91] Metastasis has been reported but occurs less frequently than in dogs with dermal and hypodermal HSAs.[89-91] The MST of greater than 1460 days for cats treated with wide surgical resection is significantly better than the MST of 60 days reported for untreated cats with cutaneous HSAs.[90]

Tumors of Synovial Tissue

Synovial Cell Sarcoma

Synovial cell sarcomas are malignant tumors arising from synoviocytes of the joint capsule and tendon sheath. The two types of synoviocytes are type A synoviocytes, which are phagocytic and resemble macrophages, and type B synoviocytes, which are fibroblastic.[92] Synovial cell sarcomas have been classified as monophasic or biphasic, depending on the proportion of malignant epithelial (synovioblastic) and mesenchymal (fibroblastic) cells within the tumor. However, this classification scheme was adopted from human medicine and is probably not applicable in small animals because of the rarity of epithelial cells in canine synovial cell sarcomas.[92] To add further confusion to the nomenclature, synovial cell sarcomas and histiocytic sarcomas are often considered to be different types of joint tumors, but both may originate from synovial cells, with synovial cell sarcomas arising from type B synoviocytes and histiocytic sarcomas arising from type A synoviocytes. Expression of CD18 does not differentiate between the macrophages (or type A synoviocytes) and dendritic antigen-presenting cell (APC) lineage of histiocytic cells (P.F. Moore, personal communication). Recent immunohistochemical evidence, however, indicates that periarticular histiocytic sarcomas do arise from subsynovial dendritic APCs and not type A synoviocytes (P.F. Moore, unpublished data). Rare canine synovial myxomas have been reported. They were most common in large breed middle-aged dogs[93] and were reported most often at the stifle or a digit and may be confused with the more common synovial cell sarcoma.

The diagnosis of synovial cell sarcoma is controversial and immunohistochemistry (IHC) is recommended to differentiate synovial cell sarcomas from other types of joint tumors.[12,94,95] The immunohistochemical panel should include vimentin and cytokeratin for synovial cell sarcoma, CD18 for histiocytic sarcoma, and actin for malignant fibrous histiocytoma.[94] However, other investigators have questioned the value of IHC in the diagnosis of synovial cell sarcoma.[95] Synovial cell sarcomas are histologically graded from I to III based on criteria such as nuclear pleomorphism, mitotic figures, and necrosis, and this grading scheme provides prognostic information.[12]

Synovial cell sarcomas are locally aggressive with a moderate-to-high metastatic potential, depending on histologic grade.[12] Up to 32% of dogs with synovial cell sarcomas have evidence of metastatic disease at diagnosis and 54% by the time of euthanasia.[10,12] Regional lymph nodes and lungs are the most common metastatic sites.[12] Synovial cell sarcomas have a greater metastatic potential and a higher incidence of lymph node metastasis compared to typical soft tissue sarcomas. Synovial cell sarcomas are rare in cats, but feline and canine synovial cell sarcomas are similar in terms of histologic appearance, biologic behavior, and distribution of metastatic lesions.[96]

In dogs, synovial cell sarcomas usually occur in large breeds, with a predisposition for flat-coated and golden retrievers. Middle-aged dogs are most commonly affected, and there is no sex predilection. Synovial cell sarcomas usually involve the larger joints, particularly the stifle, elbow, and shoulder, but any joint can be affected. Lameness is the most common presenting complaint and can be confused with other orthopedic conditions.[12] Radiographic features of synovial cell sarcomas in dogs include periarticular soft tissue swelling and bone invasion, ranging from an ill-defined periosteal reaction to multifocal punctate osteolytic lesions, involving bones on either side of the joint.[12,92] Bone involvement is rare in cats.[96] Limb amputation is recommended for treatment of the local tumor because local tumor recurrence is significantly lower compared to marginal or wide resection.[12,95] Local tumor recurrence following limb amputation, known as stump recurrence, occurs at a relatively higher rate than other types of tumors for which limb amputation is commonly performed.[12] Thus the level of amputation should be as proximal as possible to minimize the risk of local tumor recurrence, such as forequarter amputation for synovial cell sarcomas of the thoracic limb and coxofemoral disarticulation or hemipelvectomy for synovial cell sarcomas of the pelvic limb. The role of adjuvant therapy is unknown, but synovial cell sarcomas in humans are more responsive to chemotherapy agents such as anthracyclines and ifosfamide than many other types of soft tissue sarcomas.[51] Doxorubicin-based chemotherapy protocols may be warranted in dogs with nonmetastatic grade III synovial cell sarcomas.[12,97]

Prognostic factors in dogs with synovial cell sarcoma include clinical stage, histologic grade, and extent of surgical treatment. Dogs with evidence of lymph node or lung metastasis at diagnosis have a MST of less than 6 months compared to 36 months or greater if there is no evidence of metastasis.[12] The MST for dogs treated with limb amputation is 850 days, which is significantly better than the 455 days reported following marginal resection.[95] Finally, the MST for dogs with grade III synovial cell sarcomas is 7 months and significantly worse than either grade I or II synovial cell sarcomas, with MSTs greater than 48 months and 36 months, respectively.[12] In one study comparing canine joint tumors, the metastatic rate and MST for dogs with synovial cell sarcoma was 25% and 31.8 months, 0% and 30.7 months for dogs with synovial myxoma, 91% and 5.3 months for dogs with histiocytic sarcoma, and 100% and 3.5 months for dogs with other types of periarticular sarcomas.[94]

Tumors of Uncertain Histogenesis

Myxosarcoma

Myxosarcomas are neoplasms of fibroblast origin with an abundant myxoid matrix composed of mucopolysaccharides. These rare tumors occur in middle-aged or older dogs and cats. The majority are subcutaneous tumors of the trunk or limbs,[27] but there are reports of myxosarcomas arising from the heart, eye, and brain.[98-100] These tumors tend to be infiltrative growths with ill-defined margins.[27]

Malignant Mesenchymoma

Malignant mesenchymomas are rare soft tissue sarcomas comprising a fibrous component with two or more different varieties of other types of sarcoma.[24] Malignant mesenchymomas have been reported in the lungs, thoracic wall, liver, spleen, kidney, digits, and soft tissue.[101-106] They have a slow rate of growth and can grow very large. Metastasis has been reported.[105,106] The outcome for dogs with splenic mesenchymomas is better than other types of splenic sarcomas, with a MST of 12 months and a 1-year survival rate of 50%.[101]

History and Clinical Signs

Soft tissue sarcomas generally present as a slow-growing mass anywhere in the body. Rapid tumor growth, intratumoral hemorrhage, or necrosis can be seen in some cases. Symptoms are directly related to site of involvement and tumor invasiveness. However, one exception is tumor hypoglycemia, which has been reported in dogs with smooth muscle tumors.[59,107] There is marked variability in the physical features of soft tissue sarcoma, but they are generally firm and adherent (fixed) to skin, muscle, or bone. Often, soft tissue sarcomas can be soft and lobulated, mimicking lipomas.

Intraabdominal tumors often compress the GI tract and patients may present with vomiting, diarrhea, and melena. A mass may be palpable, and weight loss and anorexia is common. Leiomyosarcomas are seen most commonly in the GI tract, spleen, and urogenital tract. GI leiomyosarcomas generally result in intestinal obstruction and may cause intestinal perforation leading to peritonitis.[61] Rhabdomyosarcomas, seen in young dogs and involving the bladder, present with signs of hematuria, dysuria, and rarely, hypertrophic osteopathy.[108,109]

PNSTs, involving the brachial or lumbosacral plexus, usually result in pain, lameness, muscle atrophy, and eventual paralysis. These tumors generally are located axially and are difficult to palpate, making early diagnosis difficult because patients do not present with clinical signs until the tumors are quite large and there is significant lameness and muscle atrophy.

Diagnostic Techniques and Work-Up

Fine-needle aspiration (FNA) is recommended to exclude other differentials (e.g., abscesses, cysts, or mast cell tumors [MCTs]). However, cytologic evaluation of FNA may not be sufficient for definitive diagnosis because false-negative results can occur because of nonrepresentative samples subject to variable degrees of necrosis and poor exfoliation of cells in comparison to epithelial and round cell tumors.[24] In one study in which FNA was performed on soft tissue sarcomas from 40 dogs, 15% of dogs were incorrectly diagnosed and a further 23% were nondiagnostic.[110] Biopsy methods for definitive preoperative diagnosis of soft tissue sarcomas include needle-core, punch, incisional, or excisional biopsies. The biopsy should be planned and positioned so that the biopsy tract can be included in the curative-intent treatment, whether it be surgery with or without RT, without increasing the surgical dose or size of the radiation field. Excisional biopsies are *not* recommended because they are rarely curative and the subsequent surgery required to achieve complete histologic margins is often more aggressive than surgery following core or incisional biopsies, resulting in additional morbidity and treatment costs. Furthermore, multiple attempts at resection, including excisional biopsy, prior to definitive therapy have a negative impact on survival time in dogs with soft tissue sarcomas.[111]

Diagnostic tests performed for work-up and clinical staging depend on the type of soft tissue sarcoma, especially with atypical forms (e.g., HSAs, histiocytic sarcomas, lymphangiosarcomas, and synovial cell sarcomas), but usually involve routine hematologic and serum biochemical blood tests, three-view thoracic radiographs, and regional imaging of the soft tissue sarcoma. Blood tests are usually within the normal reference range for most dogs with soft tissue sarcomas; however, there are some notable exceptions. Hematologic abnormalities such as anemia and thrombocytopenia are relatively common in dogs with disseminated histiocytic sarcomas and HSAs.[24,112,113] Hypoglycemia has been reported in dogs with intraabdominal leiomyomas and leiomyosarcomas.[55,58,59,107] Excessive production of insulin-like growth factor II has been implicated as the cause of hypoglycemia in humans with mesenchymal tumors and this has also been demonstrated in one dog with a gastric leiomyoma.[114-116]

Imaging studies of the local tumor may be required for planning of the surgical approach or RT if the tumor is fixed to underlying structures or located in an area that may make definitive treatment difficult, such as the pelvic region. Three-dimensional (3D) imaging techniques such as CT and magnetic resonance imaging (MRI) are particularly useful for staging local disease.[117] Other imaging modalities for staging of the local tumor include survey radiographs, ultrasonography, angiography, and nuclear scintigraphy.

Diagnostic tests for staging of metastatic disease include thoracic radiographs, abdominal ultrasonography or advanced imaging, and FNA or biopsy of the regional lymph nodes. Three-view thoracic radiographs should be performed prior to definitive treatment because the lungs are the most common metastatic site for typical soft tissue sarcomas.[16] Lymph node metastasis is uncommon. FNA or biopsy of regional lymph nodes should be performed in dogs with clinically abnormal lymph nodes, high-grade (III) soft tissue sarcomas, or atypical soft tissue sarcomas having a high rate of metastasis to regional lymph nodes, such as HSAs, histiocytic sarcomas, lymphangiosarcomas, synovial cell sarcomas, leiomyosarcomas, and possibly rhabdomyosarcomas.* Abdominal imaging is recommended for the assessment of metastasis to intraabdominal organs, especially the lymph nodes, spleen, and liver, in animals with suspected intraabdominal neoplasia (e.g., GI leiomyosarcoma or splenic sarcoma) or advanced stage and high-grade pelvic limb soft tissue sarcoma.

Clinical Staging

A modified staging system has been described for soft tissue sarcomas in dogs.[24] The American Joint Committee on Cancer (AJCC) staging system currently used in humans with soft tissue sarcomas has been substantially modified from the original staging system, on which the modified animal staging system is based. The most important change to the AJCC staging system is categorization of local disease, with less emphasis on tumor size, which is an arbitrary assignment, and greater emphasis on depth of invasion.[51,120] A superficial tumor is defined as a soft tissue sarcoma located above the superficial fascia and that does not invade the fascia, whereas a deep tumor is located deep to the superficial fascia, invades the fascia, or both.[108] Based on the current AJCC staging system, an updated modified staging system for animals is summarized in Box 21-1. The stage grouping takes into account both clinical staging criteria (TNM staging system) and histologic grade. The original and updated staging systems for animals with soft tissue sarcomas have not been investigated and the prognostic significance of either of these systems is unknown.

*References 12, 55, 61-63, 86, 118, 119.

Treatment

There are over 20 different histologic subtypes of soft tissue sarcomas described in dogs, but the vast majority of these subtypes have a very similar biologic behavior characterized by locally aggressive invasiveness and a low-to-moderate metastatic potential depending on histologic grade.[16] Local tumor control is the most important consideration in the management of soft tissue sarcomas because of their locally aggressive behavior. As such, surgical resection is the principal treatment for dogs with soft tissue sarcomas. RT also plays an important role in local tumor control, especially for incompletely resected and unresectable soft tissue sarcomas. However, definitive treatment options depend on histologic subtype (especially for atypical soft tissue sarcomas such as HSAs, histiocytic sarcomas, and lymphangiosarcomas), tumor location, clinical stage, histologic grade, and completeness of surgical margins.[24,121] A strategy for managing dogs with typical soft tissue sarcomas is presented in Figure 21-6.

Surgery

Soft tissue sarcomas are locally aggressive tumors that grow along paths of least resistance and invade surrounding tissue, resulting in the formation of a pseudocapsule of compressed viable tumor cells.[24] The pseudocapsule gives the false impression of a well-encapsulated tumor. However, surgical removal of the encapsulated mass without adequate margins will result in incomplete resection and a high risk of local tumor recurrence.[16] The minimum recommended margins for surgical resection are 3 cm lateral to the tumor and one fascial layer deep to the tumor (Figure 21-7).[121,122] Biopsy tracts and any areas of fixation, including bone and fascia, should be resected en bloc with the tumor using the recommended surgical margins. Radical surgery such as limb amputation or hemipelvectomy may be required to achieve adequate surgical margins and local tumor control. Alternatively, planned multimodal therapy with marginal surgical excision and postoperative RT may be limb sparing and reduce patient morbidity.

The resected tumor should be pinned out to the original dimensions to prevent shrinkage during formalin fixation (Figure 21-8)[123]; the lateral and deep margins should be inked to aid in histologic identification of surgical margins; and any areas of concern should be tagged with suture material, inked in a different color, or submitted separately for specific histologic assessment. Surgical margins and tumor grade are important in determining the need and type of further treatment. For instance, tumor grade is important in deciding whether a soft tissue sarcoma resected with complete but

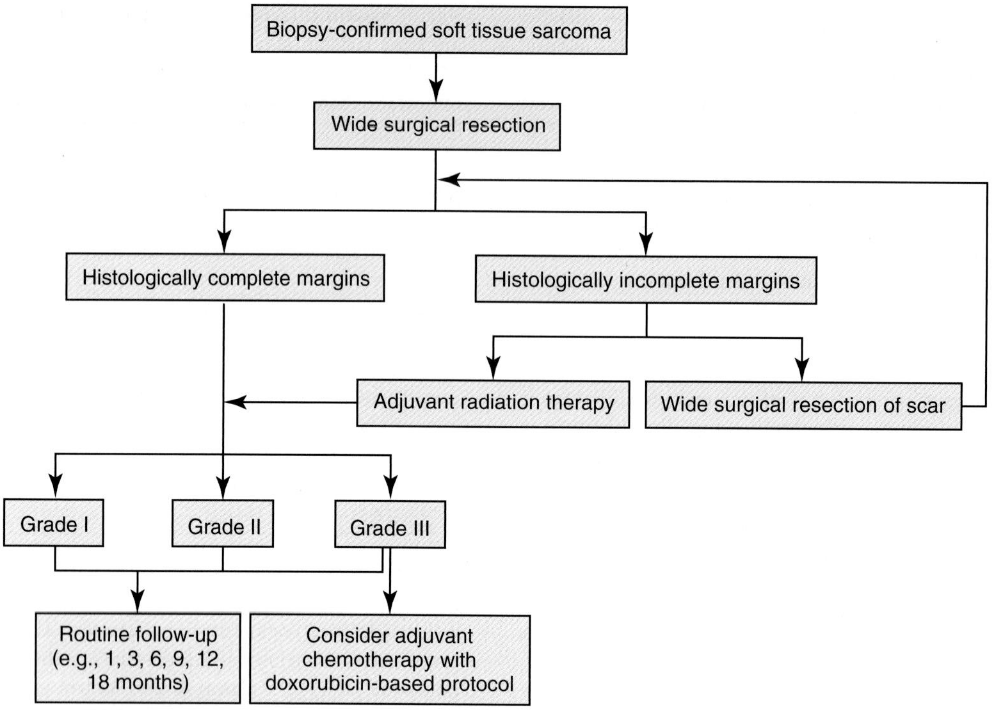

FIGURE 21-6 Suggested algorithm for the treatment of soft tissue sarcomas in dogs.

Box 21-1 Modified Staging System for Canine Soft Tissue Sarcomas

Modified Staging System for Soft Tissue Sarcomas

Primary Tumor (T)

- T1 Tumor ≤5 cm in diameter at greatest dimension
  - T1a Superficial tumor
  - T1b Deep tumor
- T2 Tumor >5 cm in diameter at greatest dimension
  - T2a Superficial tumor
  - T2b Deep tumor

Regional Lymph Nodes (N)

- N0 No regional lymph node metastasis
- N1 Regional lymph node metastasis

Distant Metastasis (M)

- M0 No distant metastasis
- M1 Distant metastasis

Stage Grouping	Tumor (T)	Nodes (N)	Metastasis (M)	Grade
I	Any T	N0	M0	I-II
II	T1a-1b, T2a	N0	M0	III
III	T2b	N0	M0	III
IV	Any T	N1	Any M	I-III
	Any T	Any N	M1	I-III

close surgical margins (i.e., 1 to 3 mm) will require further local treatment because surgical margins may be adequate with a low-grade soft tissue sarcoma but not with a high-grade soft tissue sarcoma.[121,122]

The first surgery provides the best opportunity for local tumor control as the management of incompletely resected tumors increases patient morbidity and treatment costs, increases the risk of further local tumor recurrences, and decreases survival time.[111,121,124-128] Traditionally, if a soft tissue sarcoma had been incompletely resected, then the surgical scar was managed with either a second aggressive surgery or RT because the entire surgical wound was considered contaminated and neoplastic.[121] However,

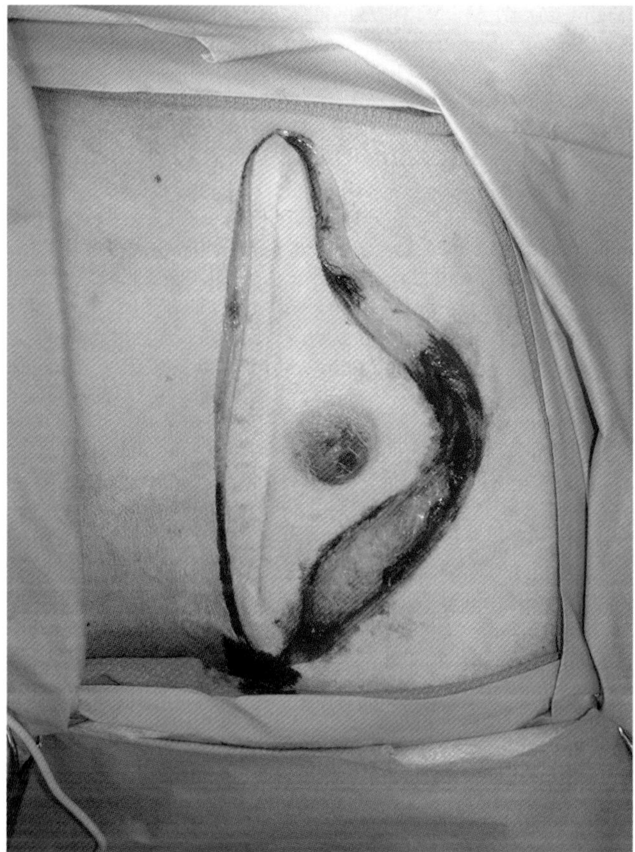

FIGURE 21-7 Intraoperative image of a dog with a recurrent soft tissue sarcoma. The soft tissue sarcoma is being resected with 3-cm margins around the recurrent tumor and previous scar because both are considered contaminated. Deep margins are one fascial layer.

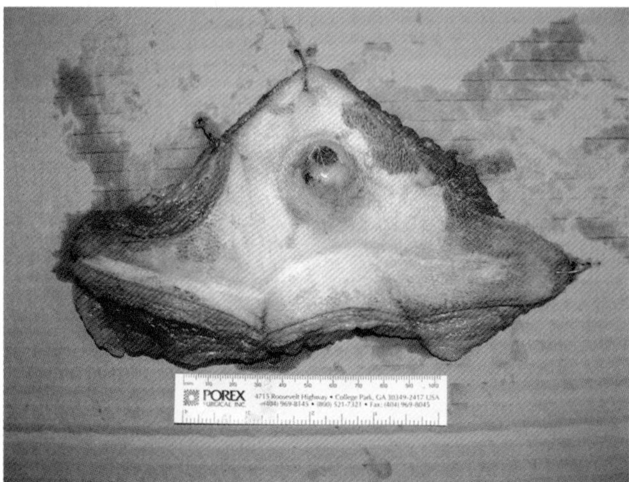

FIGURE 21-8 Following surgical resection, the lateral and deep margins should be inked (yellow ink was used in this case) to assist in identification of the margins histologically and pinned out on cardboard to prevent sample shrinkage during formalin fixation.

recent evidence suggests that this may not necessarily be true and a more conservative approach may be employed, particularly for low-grade soft tissue sarcomas. In one study, histologic evidence of residual tumor was identified in only 22% of 39 dogs with incompletely excised tumors.[129] Following excision of the surgical scar in these dogs with 0.5- to 3.5-cm margins, the local recurrence rate was 15%.[129] In a study of 104 canine soft tissue sarcomas managed with surgery alone in nonreferral practices, fewer than 10% were excised with 3-cm margins and local tumor recurrence was reported in 28% of dogs.[130] In a similar pathologic study, 75% of 139 canine subcutaneous soft tissue sarcomas were incompletely excised and the local tumor recurrence rate was significantly associated with histologic grade, with local tumor recurrence reported in only 7% of dogs with grade I soft tissue sarcomas compared to 34% and 75% of dogs with grade II and III tumors, respectively.[131] This was further supported by another study in which 11% of 35 dogs with low-grade soft tissue sarcomas of the extremities (below the elbow and stifle) had local tumor recurrence following marginal excision.[132] Thus, based on this evidence, dogs with incompletely excised soft tissue sarcomas, especially grade I and perhaps grade II tumors, can be managed with either active surveillance (i.e., frequent observation for local tumor recurrence and appropriate treatment if the tumor recurs) or a staging surgery. Staging surgery is a decision-making surgery. The surgical scar is excised with minimal margins (0.5 to 1.0 cm) with the aim being to determine if there is histologic evidence of residual tumor cells.[129] If there is no evidence of tumor cells, then no further treatment is required and these dogs should be monitored regularly for local tumor recurrence. If there is evidence of residual tumor cells, then wide resection of the surgical scar should be performed with the same margins recommended for primary soft tissue sarcomas, 3 cm lateral to the tumor and one fascial layer deep to the tumor,[117,121,126,127] or the entire surgical scar should be irradiated.[126,127] Surgery is preferred to RT for management of incompletely resected soft tissue sarcomas in humans because local tumor control is better with repeat surgical resection than adjunctive RT alone.[126,127] Another option for the management of dogs with incompletely excised soft tissue sarcomas may include metronomic (i.e., low-dose continuous) chemotherapy. The administration of piroxicam and low-dose cyclophosphamide in 30 dogs with incompletely excised soft tissue sarcomas resulted in a significantly prolonged DFI when compared to a nonrandomized control group of 85 dogs with incompletely excised soft tissue sarcomas and no metronomic chemotherapy.[133] Additional studies are needed to confirm this treatment alternative.

Surgery and Radiation Therapy

RT can be used as an adjunct to surgery following either planned marginal resection or unplanned incomplete resection. Marginal surgical resection combined with full-course postoperative RT is an attractive alternative to limb amputation for extremity soft tissue sarcoma (Figure 21-9). This multimodality approach requires additional planning and expense but preserves the limb and limb function. Surgery involves completely removing all grossly visible tumor and then marking the lateral, proximal, and distal extents of the surgical field with radiopaque clips to assist in planning of RT. Migration of the radiopaque clips has been reported but does not significantly influence the planned radiation field.[134]

RT should be started a minimum of 7 days postoperatively to minimize the risk of radiation-induced complications with the surgical wound, such as delayed healing and dehiscence.[135] Full-course fractionated protocols are recommended with reported schedules including 3.0- to 4.2-Gy fractions on a Monday-to-Friday or Monday-Wednesday-Friday schedule for a total dose of 42 to 63 Gy.[136,137] The optimal fractionation and total dose schemes for canine soft tissue sarcoma have not been determined, but cumulative doses greater than 50 Gy are recommended, and local tumor control is better with higher cumulative doses.[136] Acute side effects of RT such as moist desquamation are relatively mild and transient.[137]

Local tumor control and survival time are excellent when incompletely resected soft tissue sarcomas are treated with postoperative RT. The median time to local recurrence is 700 days to more than 798 days, with local tumor recurrence reported in 5% to 30% of dogs by 1 year and 16% to 60% of dogs in the long term (Figure 21-10).[111,136-140] The overall MST for incompletely resected nonoral soft tissue sarcomas treated with postoperative RT is 2270 days with 2-, 4-, and 5-year survival rates of 87%, 81%, and 76%, respectively (Figure 21-11).[136,137]

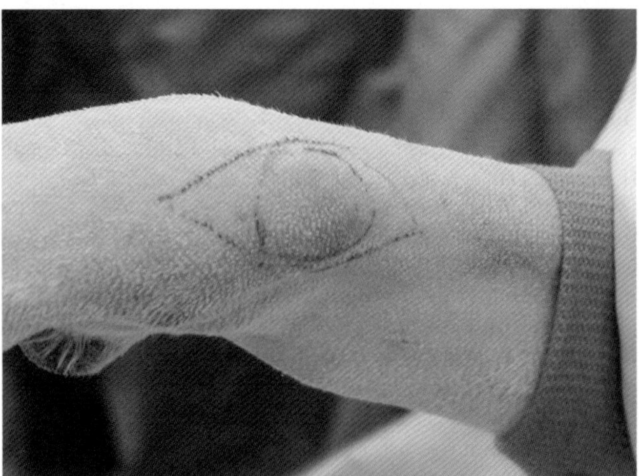

FIGURE 21-9 Planned marginal resection of a soft tissue sarcoma in a dog. Marginal resection followed by full-course postoperative radiation therapy (RT) provides excellent local tumor control and preserves both the limb and limb function. RT should not involve the limb circumferentially to preserve both lymphatic and venous drainage of the distal extremity. If close but clean margins were obtained for a grade I soft tissue sarcoma, observation alone may be an acceptable alternative.

Radiation Therapy

RT can be employed along with surgery in the treatment of soft tissue sarcomas with a curative intent, either preoperatively or postoperatively, or as a sole treatment for pain palliation. Radiotherapy alone as a single modality treatment using doses of 50 Gy resulted in 1-year tumor control rates of 50% that dropped to 33% at 2 years.[141] Measurable and palpable (i.e., macroscopic) soft tissue sarcomas are resistant to long-term control with conventional doses of irradiation alone (40 to 48 Gy).[142,143] Although one study reported a 30% complete response rate with RT alone,[144] these tumors do not rapidly regress after radiation, or if there is significant tumor shrinkage, it is not a durable response. As a single modality, RT is generally considered palliative with control defined as a slowly regressing or stable-in-size tumor mass. Palliative radiation, with 4 fractions of 8 Gy for a total dose of 32 Gy, has recently been investigated with similar results to full-course radiation with a 50% response rate in 16 dogs with measurable soft tissue sarcomas, median time to progression of 155 days, and a MST of 309 days.[145]

Inadequate durable tumor control using RT as a single modality resulted in the development of combination therapies using RT with hyperthermia and surgery, yielding superior control rates.* Current results of therapeutic clinical studies in dogs demonstrate that RT is the best treatment for incompletely resected soft tissue sarcomas.[15,136,137,149]

Although higher doses of irradiation will have higher control rates, the chances of normal tissue complications will also increase. In some studies, hyperthermia combined with irradiation showed promise for improved control versus irradiation alone and may also decrease the time to recurrence.[144,146,147] The median duration of local control with RT plus hyperthermia is 750 days and significantly greater than the 350 days with RT alone. Difficulty in homogeneous heating of large tumors limits the routine use of

*References 15, 136, 137, 144, 146-149.

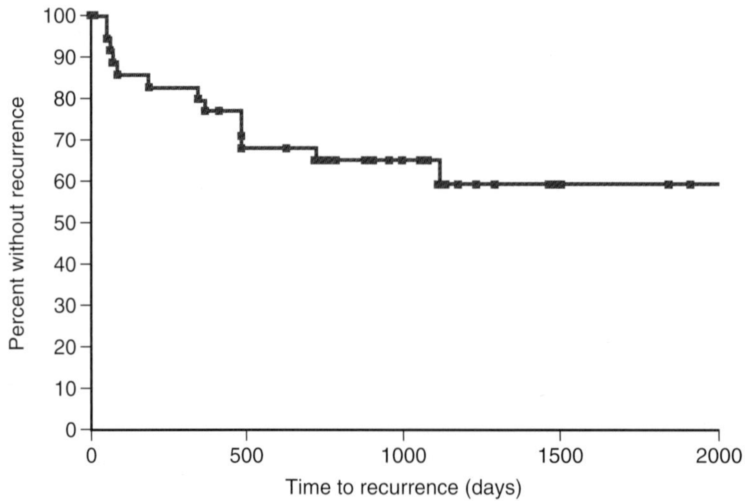

FIGURE 21-10 Kaplan-Meier curve for time to local tumor recurrence in 35 dogs treated with surgery (incomplete resection) and postoperative radiation therapy (RT). *(Reprinted with permission from Forrest LJ, Chun R, Adams WM, et al: Postoperative radiotherapy for canine soft tissue sarcoma,* J Vet Intern Med *14:578, 2000.)*

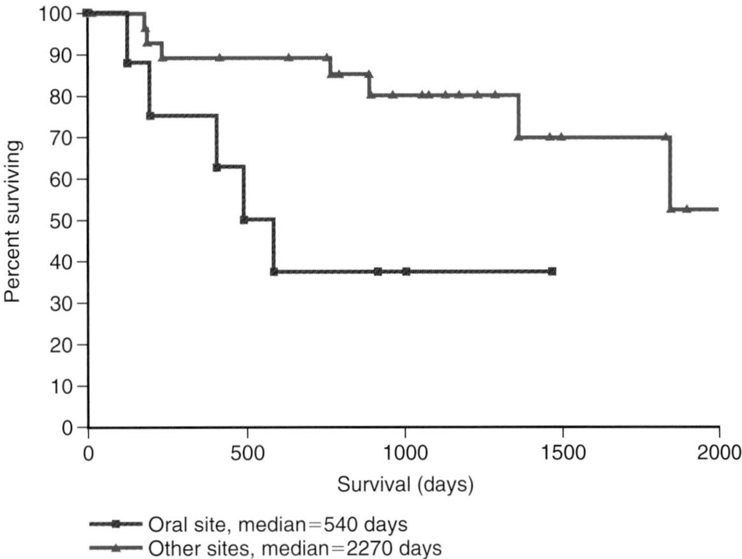

FIGURE 21-11 Kaplan-Meier survival curve of 35 dogs treated with surgery (incomplete resection) and postoperative RT after soft tissue sarcomas of oral sites were separated from other locations. *(Reprinted with permission from Forrest LJ, Chun R, Adams WM, et al: Postoperative radiotherapy for canine soft tissue sarcoma,* J Vet Intern Med *14:578, 2000.)*

hyperthermia for treating soft tissue sarcoma in conjunction with radiation. Addition of whole-body hyperthermia does not improve response rate when compared to RT and local hyperthermia and may have increased the risk for metastasis.[148] The response rate and survival time in dogs treated with irradiation and hyperthermia may be predicted with dynamic contrast-enhanced MRI of soft tissue sarcomas before and after the first hyperthermia.[150]

As mentioned previously, the combination of radiation and surgery provides long-term local control. Postoperative irradiation may be utilized if surgical removal is incomplete and further surgery is not feasible. Irradiation of microscopic tumors after excision is generally superior to radiation of measurable tumors. Control rates for adjuvant radiation after histologically incomplete resection of soft tissue sarcomas are 80% to 95% at 1 year and 72% to 91% at 2 years, with an expected 3-year and 5-year survival rate of 68% to 76%, respectively.[136,137,151] Dogs with soft tissue sarcomas with a mitotic rate greater than 9/10 HPF were more likely to have local tumor recurrence and shorter survival times in one study of 39 dogs treated with orthovoltage and doxorubicin as a radiation sensitizer.[151] Although not statistically significant, dogs with hemangiopericytoma had a 3-year survival rate of 92% in one retrospective study.[136]

Preoperative RT is becoming commonplace in veterinary oncology. The rationale and advantage of administering RT prior to surgery are that (1) the radiation field is smaller because, after surgery, the entire surgical site must be included in the field and this may contribute to local toxicity; (2) a large number of peripheral tumor cells are inactivated (with reduced contamination of the surgical site); and (3) tumor reduction may make surgical resection less difficult.[15,152-154] In a study of 112 human patients with soft tissue sarcomas, it was noted that there was no significant difference between preoperative or postoperative radiotherapy in terms of relapse-free survival, local control, or overall survival. However, wound complications were significantly more frequent in preoperative radiotherapy patients.[154] A subsequent review supported these findings.[155] Lower doses of preoperative radiotherapy (less than 50 Gy) are used to reduce the risk of surgical complications. The therapeutic goal of preoperative radiotherapy is to eradicate the microscopic tumor cells at the peripheral margins. Generally, preoperative radiotherapy is reserved for initially inoperable tumors as an alternative to radical surgery.

Chemotherapy

The role of chemotherapy in the management of dogs with soft tissue sarcoma is not yet known. The metastatic rate for cutaneous soft tissue sarcoma is grade dependent and varies from less than 15% for grade I and II soft tissue sarcoma to 41% for grade III soft tissue sarcoma.[16] Metastasis often occurs late in the course of disease, with a median time to metastasis of 365 days,[16] and this may minimize the beneficial effects of postoperative chemotherapy on the development of metastatic disease. However, there are clinical situations in which postoperative chemotherapy should be considered, including dogs with grade III soft tissue sarcoma, metastatic disease, intraabdominal soft tissue sarcoma (e.g., leiomyosarcoma and splenic sarcoma), and histologic subtypes with a higher rate of metastasis, such as histiocytic sarcomas, hypodermal HSAs (stage II or III), synovial cell sarcomas, rhabdomyosarcomas, and lymphangiosarcomas.[24,88,156-159]

Doxorubicin-based protocols, either alone or in combination with cyclophosphamide, have shown the most promise in dogs with soft tissue sarcoma with an overall response rate of 23%.[160] The need to combine cyclophosphamide with doxorubicin is debatable because single-agent doxorubicin has been shown to be equally as effective in the management of dogs with HSAs as doxorubicin combined with either cyclophosphamide or cyclophosphamide and vincristine.[161] Mitoxantrone, a chemotherapeutic drug related to doxorubicin, has a variable effect against soft tissue sarcomas in dogs, with the response rate varying from 0% in 6 dogs to 33% in 12 dogs.[162,163] Ifosfamide has also shown some potential with a complete response rate of 15% (2 dogs) in 13 dogs with solid sarcomas of the skin, bladder, and spleen.[164] Doxorubicin and ifosfamide are the most effective single agents in the management of soft tissue sarcoma in humans, but response rates are less than 30% and metaanalyses show single- and multiple-agent chemotherapy protocols do not significantly increase overall survival times compared to surgery alone.[165,166] A similar finding of no improvement in survival times has been reported in dogs with grade III soft tissue sarcomas treated with surgery alone compared to those treated with surgery and adjuvant doxorubicin.[167]

Postoperative systemic chemotherapy has also been shown to significantly improve disease-free survival times, but not overall survival time, in humans with soft tissue sarcomas, regardless of histologic grade.[165,166] Adjuvant chemotherapy has not shown the same effect on local tumor control in dogs with soft tissue sarcomas,[167] but metronomic and local chemotherapy protocols may be effective in decreasing the rate of local tumor recurrence and improving DFIs in dogs with soft tissue sarcomas. Metronomic chemotherapy with piroxicam and low-dose cyclophosphamide significantly prolongs DFI in a small group of dogs with incompletely excised soft tissue sarcomas.[133] Local release of cisplatin from a biodegradable polymer implanted into the surgical bed of incompletely resected soft tissue sarcomas may also decrease the risk of local tumor recurrence, with a 31% rate of local tumor recurrence in 32 dogs at a median of greater than 640 days postoperatively.[168]

Prognosis

The prognosis for dogs with soft tissue sarcoma is good. Local tumor control is often the most challenging aspect of managing soft tissue sarcomas.[16,110] Local tumor recurrence rates following either surgery alone or surgery and RT varies from 7% to 32%.[110,111,138,167,169] Poor prognostic factors for local tumor control include large tumor size, incomplete surgical margins, and high histologic tumor grade.[16] In one study of 75 dogs, the local tumor recurrence rate following incomplete resection was 28% and 11 times more likely than soft tissue sarcomas resected with complete margins (Figure 21-12).[16] Tumor size has been reported to have a negative effect on local tumor control[16] but probably influences the ability to achieve complete resection rather than having a direct effect on local tumor recurrence. Furthermore, tumor size has not been identified as a prognostic factor in other studies[110,138,169] and does not influence local tumor control in dogs treated with surgery and adjuvant RT or RT alone.[141,146,169,170] Management of recurrent soft tissue sarcomas is usually more difficult than management of primary tumors, which emphasizes the need for an aggressive approach initially. Curative-intent treatment of recurrent soft tissue sarcomas often requires a more aggressive approach, resulting in increased treatment-related morbidity, whereas the DFI is shorter, the metastatic rate higher, and survival times are decreased in comparison to dogs with naïve tumors.[110,121,124-128] Local tumor recurrence is still possible after either complete resection or incomplete resection combined with adjunctive RT.[16,136,137] Consequently, examination of the treatment site is recommended at regular intervals, such as monthly for the first 3 months, then every 3 months for the first 12 months, and then every 6 months thereafter.[121] The median time to local tumor recurrence was 368 days in one report of 75 dogs with soft tissue sarcomas, which emphasizes the need for long-term follow-up in these cases.[16]

The overall metastatic rate in dogs with soft tissue sarcoma varies from 8% to 17% with a median time to metastasis of 365 days.[16,136,137] Factors that increase the risk of metastatic disease include histologic grade, number of mitotic figures, percentage of tumor necrosis, and local tumor recurrence. As mentioned previously, the metastatic rate for dogs with grade I or II soft tissue sarcomas is less than 15% compared to 41% to 44% for grade III soft tissue sarcomas.[16,167] Metastasis is 5 times more likely when tumors have a mitotic rate of 20 or more mitotic figures/10 HPF compared to fewer than 20 mitotic figures/10 HPF.[16]

The MST for dogs with soft tissue sarcoma ranges from 1416 days following surgery alone to 2270 days with surgery and adjunctive RT.[16,136,137] Overall, up to 33% of dogs eventually die of

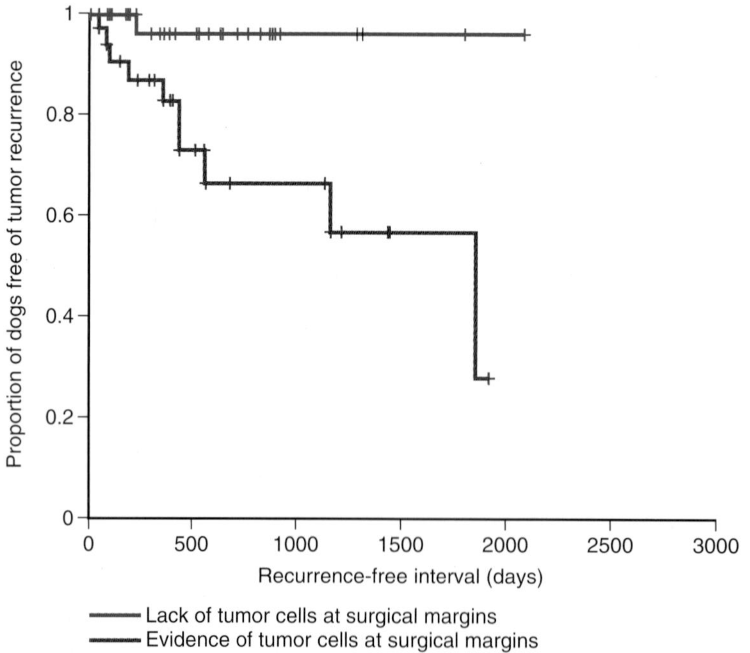

FIGURE 21-12 Kaplan-Meier curve for disease-free interval (DFI) in 39 dogs with complete surgical removal of soft tissue sarcomas and 36 dogs with incomplete surgical margins. *(Reprinted with permission from Kuntz CA, Dernell WS, Powers BE, et al: Prognostic factors for surgical treatment of soft-tissue sarcomas in dogs: 75 cases (1986-1996),* J Am Vet Med Assoc *211:1147, 1997.)*

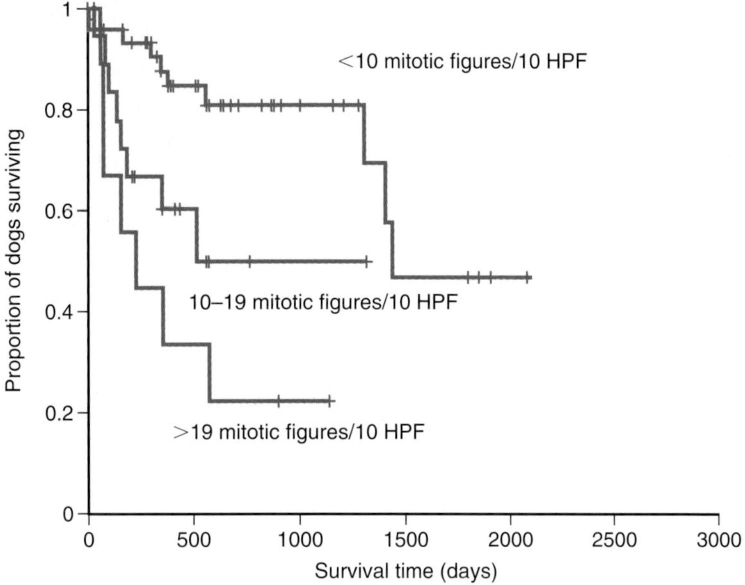

FIGURE 21-13 Kaplan-Meier survival curve for 75 dogs with soft tissue sarcomas based on mitotic rates. *(Reprinted with permission from Kuntz CA, Dernell WS, Powers BE, et al: Prognostic factors for surgical treatment of soft-tissue sarcomas in dogs: 75 cases (1986-1996),* J Am Vet Med Assoc *211:1147, 1997.)*

tumor-related causes.[16] Tumor-related deaths in dogs with soft tissue sarcoma is 2.8 times more likely with greater than 10% tumor necrosis and 2.6 times more likely with a mitotic rate of 20 or more mitotic figures/10 HPF.[16] The MSTs for dogs with 10 or fewer, 10 to 19, and 20 or more mitotic figures/10 HPF is 1444 days, 532 days, and 236 days, respectively (Figure 21-13).[16] The prognosis for specific subtypes of soft tissue sarcoma are discussed separately earlier in this chapter in the section on specific tumor types.

Feline Sarcomas and Vaccine-Associated Sarcomas

Epidemiology and Risk Factors

The following events are linked to the development of postvaccinal sarcomas in the cat. The prevalence of feline rabies led to the enactment of a law requiring rabies vaccinations for cats in Pennsylvania in 1987.[171] In addition, two changes in vaccines occurred in the mid-1980s: development of a killed rabies vaccine licensed for subcutaneous administration and a killed vaccine for feline leukemia virus (FeLV). Two pathologists, M. J. Hendrick and M. H. Goldschmidt, and their colleagues at the University of Pennsylvania School of Veterinary Medicine were the first to recognize the increased incidence of reactions and formation of sarcomas at sites of rabies vaccinations.[172-174] Epidemiologic studies have shown a strong association between the administration of inactivated feline vaccines, such as FeLV and rabies, and subsequent development of soft tissue sarcoma at vaccine sites.[172-176] Additionally, some authors report reaction to vaccines was additive and this increased the likelihood of sarcoma development with multiple vaccines given at the same site simultaneously.[175] The development of soft tissue sarcoma at sites of vaccine administration of FeLV or rabies is believed by some to be as high as 1/1000,[177,178] whereas others report a prevalence between 1 and 3.6/10,000 cases.[176,179,180]

The time to tumor development postvaccination has been reported to be 4 weeks to 10 years and is associated with a robust inflammatory reaction around the tumor.[176] Adjuvant-containing vaccines have been proposed to be more likely to cause a vaccine site reaction and/or develop into a soft tissue sarcoma.[176] However, two large epidemiologic studies did not provide evidence that aluminum-containing vaccines pose a greater risk.[165,182] Thus it remains unclear whether nonadjuvant vaccines are safer. A multicenter study of cats in the United States and Canada found that no single vaccine manufacturer or vaccine type had a higher or lower association with the development of soft tissue sarcoma.[182] Additionally, vaccine practices such as needle gauge, syringe reuse, use and shaking of multidose vials, mixing vaccines in a single syringe, and syringe type had no role in the development of tumors.[182]

The hypothesis that postvaccination inflammatory reactions lead to uncontrolled fibroblast and myofibroblast proliferation and eventual tumor formation either alone or along with immunologic factors is a popular theory.[183-188] The thought that inflammation precedes tumor development is supported by histologic identification of transition zones from inflammation to sarcoma and microscopic foci of sarcoma located in areas of granulomatous inflammation. A similar phenomenon of intraocular sarcoma development exists in cats after trauma or chronic uveitis.[189-191]

Growth factors regulate the cellular events involved in granulation tissue formation and wound healing. When these factors are added to fibroblast cultures, the cells develop a neoplastic phenotype. Immunohistochemical identification and localization of growth factors and their receptors are being investigated in vaccine-associated sarcomas. Through immunohistochemical study of growth factors and their receptors, Hendrick has found that vaccine-associated sarcomas are immunoreactive for platelet-derived growth factor (PDGF), epidermal growth factor (EGF) and its receptors, and transforming growth factor-β (TGF-β). Conversely, non–injection-site fibrosarcomas are negative or faintly positive.[192,193] Hendrick also found that lymphocytes in vaccine-associated sarcomas are positive for PDGF, but lymphocytes in non–injection-site fibrosarcomas and normal lymph nodes are negative.[192] Regional macrophages also stain positively for PDGF receptor (PDGFR). Neoplastic cells that are closest to lymphocytes in these tumors have the strongest staining for PDGFR, which has led to a hypothesis that lymphocytes in vaccine-associated sarcomas may secrete PDGF, recruit macrophages, and lead to fibroblast proliferation.[192,193] The expression of *C-jun,* a proto-oncogene coding for the transcriptional protein AP-1, has also been examined in vaccine-associated sarcomas. *C-jun* was found to be strongly positive in vaccine-associated sarcomas and not expressed in non–injection-site fibrosarcomas.[192,193] It appears that FeLV and the feline sarcoma virus are not involved in the pathogenesis of feline vaccine-associated sarcomas. Using immunohistochemical analysis and polymerase chain reaction (PCR) techniques, FeLV was not detected in vaccine-associated sarcomas.[194]

p53 mutations have been evaluated in feline vaccine-associated sarcomas.[195-198] *p53* is a tumor suppressor gene that encodes a nuclear protein critical in the regulation of the cell cycle. Normal or wild-type *p53* will increase in response to DNA damage resulting in cell arrest at the G1 interphase, allowing for DNA repair before replication or apoptosis if damage is irreparable. Cells lacking normal *p53* proceed through the cell cycle unregulated, leading to aberrant clones and possible malignancy.[186] Anti-*p53* antibodies have immunoreactivity in feline sarcomas and may play a role in predicting clinical outcome.[198]

Recent papers continue to link growth factors with development of vaccine-associated sarcomas in cats. Continued immunohistochemical probing of feline vaccine-associated sarcomas document expression of growth-regulating proteins: p53 protein, basic fibroblast growth factor β (bFGF-β), and TGF-α.[198] Researchers recently concluded that PDGF and its receptor play an important role in the in vitro growth of vaccine-associated sarcoma cell lines, both alone and in the presence of chemotherapeutic agents. Furthermore, they found that a signal transduction inhibitor, imatinib mesylate, inhibits the PDGF-dependent cell growth in a dose-dependent manner.[199]

The term *vaccine-associated sarcoma* has been used interchangeably with injection-site sarcoma because sarcomas arising at sites of injections other than vaccines, such as lufenuron and microchips, have been reported.[200-202] Vaccine-associated sarcoma has been used in this chapter because of the overwhelming prevalence of vaccines as a cause of these injection-site sarcomas.

Pathology

There are many similarities between the histologic subtypes and biologic behavior of soft tissue sarcomas in cats and dogs. The three principal exceptions in cats are vaccine-associated sarcomas, virally induced multicentric fibrosarcoma, and the relative rarity of PNST, synovial cell sarcoma, and histiocytic sarcoma.[188,203] There are significant differences between vaccine-associated sarcoma and non–vaccine-associated sarcoma. Tumors that develop after vaccination are typically mesenchymal in origin and include fibrosarcomas, rhabdomyosarcomas, malignant fibrous histiocytomas, undifferentiated sarcomas, and extraskeletal osteosarcomas and chondrosarcomas.[192,204,205] Vaccine-associated sarcomas have histologic features consistent with a more aggressive biologic behavior than non–vaccine-associated sarcomas, such as marked nuclear and cellular pleomorphism, increased tumor necrosis, high mitotic activity, and the presence of a peripheral inflammatory cell infiltrate consisting of lymphocytes and macrophages.[187,192,206] In a series of 91 cats with histologically confirmed and graded vaccine-associated sarcomas, the prevalence of high-grade lesions was substantially higher than reported in dogs,[16] with 59% of cats diagnosed with grade III tumors and only 5% with grade I tumors.[207] Microscopically, areas

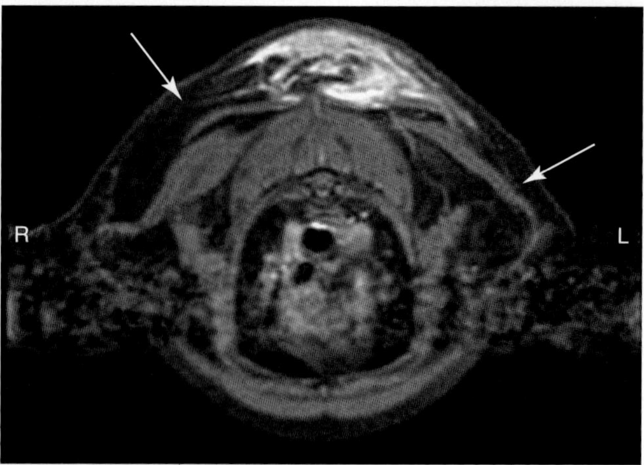

FIGURE 21-14 Contrast-enhanced magnetic resonance imaging (MRI) of a cat with a vaccine-associated sarcoma. Note the fingerlike projections of the tumor *(arrows).*

of transition between inflammation and tumor development are frequently observed in cats with vaccine-associated sarcoma.[161,192,208] The macrophages in these peripheral inflammatory cell infiltrates often contain a bluish-gray foreign material that has been identified as aluminum and oxygen by electron probe x-ray microanalysis.[188] Aluminum hydroxide is one of several adjuvants used in currently available feline vaccines.[188] Injection-site sarcomas are histologically similar to mesenchymal tumors arising in the traumatized eyes of cats, which suggests a common pathogenesis of inflammation and the development of soft tissue sarcomas in these cats.[190-193] The presence of inflammatory cells, fibroblasts, and myofibroblasts in and adjacent to vaccine-associated sarcomas supports this hypothesis.[24,209,210]

Diagnosis and Work-Up

The diagnostic techniques and clinical staging tests recommended for cats with suspected vaccine-associated sarcoma are similar to those described in dogs earlier in this chapter. Advanced imaging such as contrast-enhanced CT or MRI is recommended for local staging of the tumor because these 3D-imaging modalities provide essential information for proper planning of surgery and/or RT (Figure 21-14).[188] The volume of tumor based on contrast-enhanced CT is approximately twice the volume measured using calipers during physical examination.[185] Accurate pretreatment knowledge of the extent of disease is important because vaccine-associated sarcomas are very invasive, are frequently located in areas in which regional anatomy can complicate an aggressive surgical approach (e.g., interscapular area, body wall, and proximal pelvic limb), and have a high rate of local tumor recurrence, especially if incompletely resected. Excisional biopsy of a suspected vaccine-associated sarcoma is not recommended because the risk of local tumor recurrence is increased, and DFI and survival time are significantly decreased.[211,212]

Treatment

The Vaccine-Associated Feline Sarcoma Task Force has recommended that masses at vaccination sites be treated if the mass is still evident 3 or more months after vaccination, is larger than 2 cm in diameter, or is increasing in size more than 4 weeks after vaccine administration.[188] Vaccine-associated sarcomas are very invasive tumors, and aggressive treatment is required, with both wide

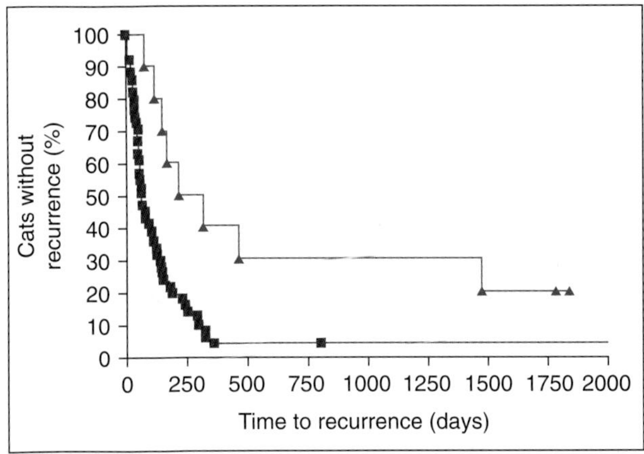

FIGURE 21-15 Kaplan-Meier curve for time to first local tumor recurrence in 47 cats with vaccine-associated sarcomas treated by referring veterinarians *(squares)* compared to 14 cats treated at referral institutions *(triangles)*. *(Reprinted with permission from Hershey AE, Sorenmo KU, Hendrick MJ, et al: Prognosis for presumed feline vaccine-associated sarcoma after excision: 61 cases (1986-1996),* J Am Vet Med Assoc *216:58, 2000.)*

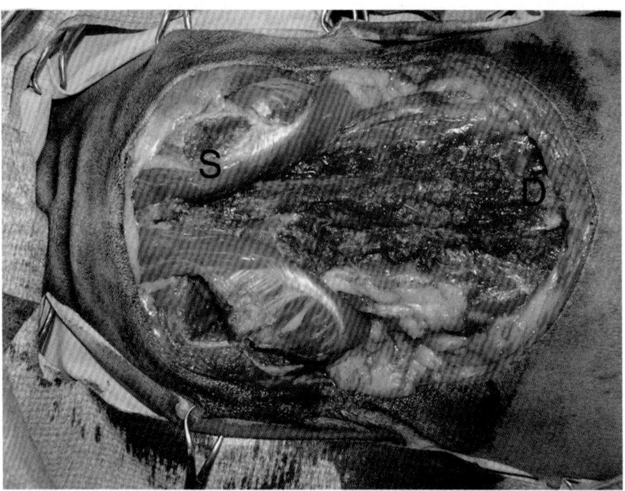

FIGURE 21-16 Aggressive resection of vaccine-associated sarcomas is required for prolonged local tumor control. In this cat, the vaccine-associated sarcoma was resected with 5-cm margins, including the dorsal spinous processes *(D)*. The scapulae *(S)* were spared because the tumor could be resected with two fascial planes without involving the scapula.

surgical resection and full-course RT, to achieve adequate local control.

Surgery

Vaccine-associated sarcomas are poorly encapsulated tumors with extension and infiltration along fascial planes.[213,214] The Vaccine-Associated Feline Sarcoma Task Force has recommended surgical resection with a minimum of 2-cm margins both lateral and deep to the tumor.[188] Marginal resection or excisional biopsy should not be attempted. The median DFI and survival time are significantly decreased with marginal resection, with an increased number of surgical interventions, and if surgery is performed by nonreferral surgeons (Figure 21-15).[205,211,212] The median time to first recurrence following marginal resection is 79 days compared to 325 to 419 days for wide resection or radical surgery.[212] In addition, the median time to first recurrence is only 66 days when the first surgery is performed at a nonreferral institution compared to 274 days at referral institutions.[211] Inadequate biopsy planning, preoperative staging, and/or attempts at first surgery will result in an increase in tumor margins and may make further surgical treatment impossible. The first attempt at surgical management of cats with vaccine-associated sarcomas should be performed by a referral surgeon with experience in aggressive resection, especially in the interscapular and pelvic regions, to increase the chance of a successful outcome.[185]

Similar to dogs with soft tissue sarcomas, biopsy tracts and any areas of fixation, including bone and fascia, should be resected en bloc with the tumor. In cats with vaccine-associated sarcomas, wide surgical resection of tumors located in the interscapular region will often involve excision of dorsal spinous processes and perhaps the dorsal aspect of the scapula (Figure 21-16), whereas thoracic or body wall resection is often required for truncal tumors.[211,212] Limb amputation or hemipelvectomy is usually required to achieve adequate surgical margins and local tumor control for vaccine-associated sarcomas located on the extremity.

Local tumor control is still disappointing with curative-intent surgery. Despite attempting aggressive surgery with 2- to 3-cm lateral margins and one fascial layer for deep margins, complete resection is achieved in less than 50% of cats.[211,212] Furthermore, overall 1- and 2-year disease-free rates are only 35% and 9%, respectively.[211] Median DFI and survival time are both greater than 16 months following complete histologic resection and significantly better than incompletely resected tumors. Local tumor control is improved for extremity vaccine-associated sarcomas, presumably because the lateral and deep surgical margins achieved with limb amputation are superior to other locations.[211] However, aggressive surgery is possible in other locations with good results. Chest wall and body resection, using a minimum of 3-cm margins, was well tolerated in six cats and local tumor recurrence was not reported in any of these cats at a minimum of 12 months postoperatively.[215]

A more aggressive surgical approach is recommended because of the low rate of complete resection and subsequent poor local tumor control, with surgical excision using 2 to 3 cm. This recommendation is based on a study of 91 cats with vaccine-associated sarcoma in various locations, including interscapular, trunk, and extremity, treated with surgery alone using 5-cm lateral margins and two fascial planes for deep margins.[207] Major surgical complications were reported in 11% of cats. Wound dehiscence following excision of interscapular tumors was the most common complication.[207] Complete histologic resection was achieved in 97% of cats and local tumor recurrence was reported in only 14% of cats.[207] These findings are supported by an earlier study of 57 cats treated with 4- to 5-cm lateral margins and one fascial layer for deep margins in which complete histologic excision was achieved in 95% of cats.[216] These results suggest that extrapolation from the surgical management of canine soft tissue sarcomas and the recommendations of the Vaccine-Associated Feline Sarcoma Task Force are inadequate for the surgical treatment of feline vaccine-associated sarcomas and better rates of complete surgical resection and local tumor control can be achieved using a more aggressive surgical approach.

Surgery and Radiation Therapy

As a result of the high rate of local tumor recurrence following wide surgical resection with 3-cm margins, full-course RT is highly recommended in the management of cats with vaccine-associated sarcoma.[205,217-220] The timing of surgery and RT is controversial. The advantages of preoperative radiation include greater antitumor effect because of a smaller population of resistant hypoxic cells as blood supply to the tumor is not disturbed; a smaller radiation field because, after surgery, the entire surgical site must be included in the field; reduction in tumor size, which facilitates surgical resection; and decreased risk of disseminating tumor cells during surgery.[153] The principal disadvantage of preoperative RT is the increased risk of surgical complications, such as wound dehiscence.[153] Postoperative RT may provide better tumor control because RT is more effective against microscopic disease than gross tumor and does not delay definitive surgery.[153] However, surgery increases the size of the radiation field and the population of radioresistant hypoxic tumor cells by altering the local blood supply, and there is a risk of tumor cells repopulating in the interval between surgery and the start of RT.[153,205]

In two studies investigating preoperative RT, local tumor recurrence was reported in 40% to 45% of cats at a median of 398 to 584 days postoperatively.[217,219] In both studies, complete resection significantly improved the time to local recurrence, with a 700- to 986-day median DFI for completely excised tumors and 112- to 292-day median DFI for tumors resected with incomplete margins. However, despite the prolonged interval to local tumor recurrence, complete resection following preoperative RT does not appear to improve local control rates because local tumor recurrence was reported in 42% of 59 cats with complete margins and 32% of 33 cats with incomplete margins.[219]

The outcome following postoperative RT is similar to preoperative RT. In one study, local tumor recurrence was reported in 41% of 76 cats at a median of 405 days postoperatively.[217] In another study investigating the effects of chemotherapy in cats treated with surgery and postoperative RT, local tumor recurrence occurred in 28% of 25 cats with a median time to first recurrence not reached in cats treated with surgery and RT alone and 661 days in cats also treated with doxorubicin.[218] In a recent study of 46 cats treated with surgery and curative-intent postoperative RT, the median progression-free interval (PFI) was 37 months with 1- and 2-year progression-free rates of 63% and 60%, respectively.[219] In comparison, 27 cats treated with postoperative palliative coarse fractionation protocols had a median PFI of 10 months and a MST of 24 months.[219] Importantly, RT should start 10 to 14 days postoperatively as DFI and survival time decreases as the interval between surgery and starting RT increases.[205] Local tumor recurrence does not influence survival time and, regardless of the timing of RT relative to surgery, survival data are encouraging with MSTs of 600 to 1300 days and 1-, 2-, and 3-year survival rates of 86%, 44% to 71%, and 28% to 68%, respectively.[205,217,218,220]

Local tumor control is still disappointing with 28% to 45% of tumors recurring after multimodality treatment with surgery and RT.[205,217-220] The radiation field used in these studies typically included a minimum of 3-cm margins around the tumor or surgical scar. The majority of tumors recur within the radiation field, although tumors have been reported to recur outside the radiation field.[218] Similar to surgery alone, a more aggressive approach may be warranted to improve local tumor control, such as higher radiation doses, larger radiation fields, and more aggressive surgical resections.

Radiation Therapy

Although RT alone is rarely effective for the management of cats and dogs with measurable soft tissue sarcomas, RT may have a role in the palliative setting for cats with large and unresectable vaccine-associated sarcomas. In a pilot study of 10 cats with vaccine-associated sarcomas, 7 cats achieved partial responses and 2 cats had complete responses following treatment with liposomal doxorubicin as a radiation sensitizer and irradiation with a median of 5 fractions of 4 Gy for a total dose of 20 Gy; however, PFIs were not durable (median of 117 days).[221]

Chemotherapy

The role of chemotherapy in the management of cats with vaccine-associated sarcoma remains undefined. Metastasis has been reported in 0% to 26% of cats with vaccine-associated sarcomas, despite the aggressive histologic appearance and prevalence of high-grade lesions in these tumors, with a median time to metastasis of 265 to 309 days.* Injection-site sarcoma cell lines have shown in vitro sensitivity at clinically relevant doses to doxorubicin, mitoxantrone, vincristine, and paclitaxel.[222,223] Clinically, partial and complete responses to doxorubicin, either alone or in combination with cyclophosphamide, have been reported in 39% to 50% of cats with gross tumors, but these responses are often short-lived with a median duration of 84 to 125 days.[224,225] However, MSTs are significantly prolonged in cats that respond to chemotherapy with 242 days for responders and 83 days for nonresponders.[224] Furthermore, MSTs are significantly increased for cats with gross residual disease following surgical excision and treated with postoperative RT and chemotherapy with a MST of 29 months compared to 5 months for cats treated with surgery and postoperative RT.[220]

Postoperative chemotherapy has minimal impact on survival in cats treated with curative-intent surgery and RT.[207,216-218,225] Chemotherapy may, however, have beneficial effects on local tumor control and time to local tumor recurrence. Doxorubicin and liposome-encapsulated doxorubicin significantly prolong the DFI following surgery, with a median DFI of 393 days for cats receiving chemotherapy and 93 days for those in which chemotherapy was not administered (Figure 21-17).[225] The completeness of surgical margins may be a confounding factor in this analysis because the median DFI was greater than 449 days in cats with complete surgical margins compared to 281 days following incomplete resection.[225] Carboplatin was associated with an insignificant but numerically superior median DFI of greater than 986 days in cats treated with preoperative RT and surgery.[219] Other studies have shown no effect of adjunctive chemotherapy on either local tumor control or survival time.[217,218]

Novel treatments such as electrochemotherapy and immunotherapy are also being investigated with some encouraging results. In one study, cats with high-grade soft tissue sarcomas were treated either intraoperatively or postoperatively with intratumoral bleomycin followed by 8 biphasic pulses of up to 1300 V/cm.[226] The median time to local tumor recurrence in the control (surgery only) group was 4 months compared to 12 months for cats treated intraoperatively and 19 months for cats treated postoperatively. Of further interest, the metastatic rate was only 1.7%.[226]

Immunotherapy, using recombinant viruses expressing interleukin-2 (IL-2), has shown some promise in improving local tumor control rates in cats with vaccine-associated sarcomas. Following surgical resection and iridium-based RT, the 1-year local tumor recurrence rate was 61% in cats receiving no adjunctive treatment, 39% in cats administered human IL-2 using a vaccinia virus vector, and 28% with feline IL-2 using a canary pox virus vector.[227] In a phase I trial, two doses of intratumoral feline IL-2,

*References 205, 207, 211, 212, 216, 217, 219.

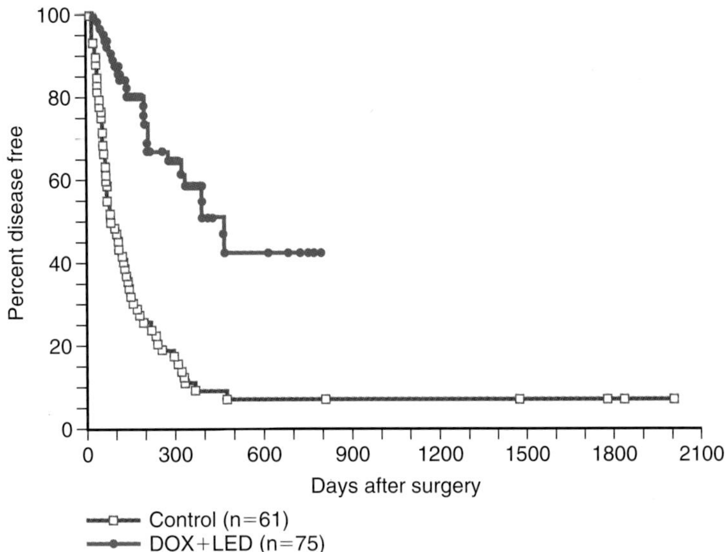

FIGURE 21-17 Kaplan-Meier curve for disease-free interval (DFI) in 75 cats with vaccine-associated sarcomas treated with surgery and postoperative chemotherapy (liposome-encapsulated doxorubicin or doxorubicin) or surgery alone (historic control). *(Reprinted with permission from Poirier VJ, Thamm DH, Kurzman ID, et al: Liposome-encapsulated doxorubicin (Doxil) and doxorubicin in the treatment of vaccine-associated sarcomas in cats,* J Vet Intern Med *16:726, 2002.)*

interferon γ (IFN-γ), and granulocyte-macrophage colony-stimulating factor (GM-CSF) followed by magnetofection prior to surgical resection resulted in a 1-year local recurrence rate of 24%.[228] In another phase I trial by the same research group, 2 doses of intratumoral GM-CSF followed by magnetofection prior to surgical resection resulted in a 1-year local recurrence rate of 50% and minimal treatment-related toxicities.[229] Other immunotherapeutic agents such as IL-12 and acemannan have been investigated with less favorable results.[230-232]

Prognosis

It has become clear that the prognosis for cats with vaccine-associated sarcomas treated with surgical excision alone, using traditional recommendations, can be poor with respect to tumor control, especially when the first surgery is marginal and multiple surgeries are employed as the method of treatment. However, long-term survival, even in the face of multiple recurrences, is the norm with this disease. The median time to first recurrence was 2 months for cats treated by conservative surgery (referring veterinarian) and 9 months for those cats treated by more aggressive surgery (referral institution); the overall survival time was 19 months.[212] Another study of single modality surgical excision reported an overall DFI of 10 months, which increased to longer than 16 months when excision was complete.[211] The prognosis with surgery alone is improved with aggressive surgical excision using 5-cm lateral margins and two fascial layers for deep margins.[207] A recent study looked at 3D histologic margins in 48 cats with vaccine-associated sarcomas and evaluated the predictive value of histologic margins and tumor grading on local recurrence.[233] Tumor margins were noninfiltrated in 32 cats and the remaining 16 cases had infiltrated margins. Overall, 6/32 (19%) tumors with noninfiltrated margins and 11/16 (69%) with infiltrated margins had tumor recurrence. Tumors with infiltrated margins recurred about 10 times more frequently compared to tumors with noninfiltrated margins.[233] The degree of infiltration of tumor margins may provide an indication for the need for adjuvant RT following surgical excision.

Outcomes are improved when cats with vaccine-associated sarcomas are treated with multimodality therapy, especially following surgical excision with less aggressive intent. Optimal outcome occurs when cats are treated aggressively initially and not after multiple failed resections.[220] The combination of radiotherapy either preoperatively or postoperatively has improved the DFI and overall survival time in cats with vaccine-associated sarcomas. DFI and MSTs range from 13 to 37 months and 23 to 43 months, respectively.[205,215-218] Injection-site sarcomas are locally invasive; however, approximately 15% to 24% will metastasize to the lungs or other sites.[207,208,212,216,217] Continued research into the treatment of vaccine-associated sarcomas is needed because there is room for improvement in outcomes.

Prognostic factors were investigated in one study of 42 cats with surgically resected nonvisceral soft tissue sarcomas, including 8 cats with presumed vaccine-associated sarcomas.[234] The overall MST was 608 days. The margins of excision lateral and deep to the tumor were not reported, but excision was incomplete in 74% of cats and local tumor recurrence was reported in 62% of cats. The median time to recurrence was 261 days and the MST in cats with local tumor recurrence was 576 days. Metastasis was suspected in 14% of cats and the MST in cats with suspected metastasis was 562 days. Prognostic factors included tumor size and histologic type. Cats with soft tissue sarcomas smaller than 2 cm in diameter had a MST of 643 days, which was significantly longer than the 558 days for cats with tumors 2 to 5 cm in diameter and 394 days for cats with soft tissue sarcomas larger than 5 cm in diameter. The MSTs for cats with fibrosarcoma (640 days) and PNST (645 days) were significantly better than for cats with malignant fibrous histiocytoma (290 days). Tumor location and injection-site versus non–injection-site sarcomas were not prognostic factors in this study.[234] Although these results are encouraging, the rates of incomplete excision and local tumor recurrence suggest that a more aggressive surgical approach and multimodal therapy with adjuvant RT should also be considered for cats with non–vaccine-associated sarcomas.

In two studies, one with 57 cats with vaccine-associated sarcomas treated primarily with wide surgical excision (4- to 5-cm lateral margins and one fascial layer for deep margins)[216] and the other with 91 cats treated with aggressive surgery alone (5-cm lateral margins and two fascial layers for deep margins),[207] prognostic factors for survival included histologic grade, local tumor recurrence, and distant metastasis. Local tumor recurrence was reported in 39% of the cats and was not associated with tumor diameter, tumor location, or histologic grade.[216] The MST for cats with local tumor recurrence was 365 to 499 days compared to 1098 to 1461 days for cats without local tumor recurrence.[207,216] The MST for cats without distant metastasis was 929 to 1528 days compared to 165 to 388 days for the 20% to 21% of cats that developed distant metastasis.[207,216] Furthermore, distant metastasis was more likely in cats with grade III sarcomas, suggesting that chemotherapy should be considered for cats with high-grade vaccine-associated sarcomas.[216]

Prevention

The recommendations on preventing vaccine-associated sarcomas in cats are controversial. These include changing the sites of vaccine administration, decreasing the use of polyvalent vaccines, using nonadjuvanted vaccines, avoiding the use of aluminum-based adjuvants, and increasing the interval between vaccinations.[24,178,235,236]

The Vaccine-Associated Feline Sarcoma Task Force has recommended that no vaccine be administered in the interscapular region, rabies vaccines be administered in the distal aspect of the right pelvic limb, FeLV vaccines be administered in the distal aspect of the left pelvic limb, and all other vaccines be administered in the right shoulder.[24] The location of each injection, the type of vaccine, and the manufacturer and serial number of the vaccine should be documented in the patient records. These recommendations are intended to provide epidemiologic information rather than prevent vaccine-associated sarcomas. Vaccines should be administered into the distal, rather than mid to proximal, aspects of the limb to aid in earlier detection and increase the chance of achieving complete resection. Subcutaneous and intramuscular administration can both cause local inflammatory reactions and result in the development of vaccine-associated sarcomas.[24] Subcutaneous administration is preferred to intramuscular injection because vaccine-associated sarcomas developing from subcutaneous sites are more readily palpable and diagnosed earlier in the course of disease. The Vaccine-Associated Feline Sarcoma Task Force has recommended that masses at vaccination sites be treated if the mass is evident 3 or more months after vaccination, is larger than 2 cm in diameter, or is increasing in size more than 4 weeks after vaccine administration.[185] Unfortunately, feline vaccine-associated sarcomas are still occurring at sites not recommended by the Vaccine-Associated Feline Sarcoma Task Force and are often difficult to cure with surgery and RT.[237]

Traditionally, annual boosters have been recommended for most vaccines in cats. The U.S. Department of Agriculture–Animal Plant Health Inspection Service (USDA-APHIS) does not require duration of immunity studies for licensing of vaccines. However, if a duration of immunity study has not been performed, the USDA-APHIS requires that vaccine labels include a recommendation for annual revaccination.[188] Recently, vaccine practices have been questioned by the profession and this has been supported by duration of immunity studies. The duration of immunity for a single commercially available inactivated, adjuvanted combination of feline panleukopenia, herpesvirus, and calicivirus is greater than 7 years with persistent antibodies against all three viruses for more than 3 years.[238,239] Local and state requirements often mandate annual rabies boosters, despite a duration of immunity of at least 3 years, because of the significant public health concern of rabies infection.[188] The Vaccine-Associated Feline Sarcoma Task Force has recommended that the administration of vaccines is a medicinal procedure and vaccination protocols should be customized for individual cats.[188] A vaccine should not be administered until the medical importance and zoonotic potential of the infectious agent, risk of exposure, and legal requirements have been considered and balanced against the risk of vaccine-associated sarcomas and other adverse effects.[188]

Comparative Aspects

In general, soft tissue sarcomas have a similar pathologic appearance, clinical presentation, and behavior in humans and animals. However, a higher incidence is seen in young people as opposed to young companion animals, with the exception of rhabdomyosarcoma, which is seen in young dogs. The distribution of soft tissue sarcoma in humans is similar to animals. In humans, 43% are in the extremities, with two-thirds occurring in the lower limb, and 34% are intraperitoneal, with 19% visceral in origin and 15% retroperitoneal. Soft tissue sarcomas of the trunk occur in 10% of human patients, and the remaining 13% occur at other sites. Metastasis is generally hematogenous and appears to be more common in human soft tissue sarcoma than in dogs, which may partially be explained by the higher numbers of nerve sheath tumors (with lower metastatic rate) seen in the dog.

Most sarcomas recognized in humans are also diagnosed in animals, although the specific incidences may vary markedly. There are many more histologic subtypes recognized in humans, which are often site dependent. With the exception of benign smooth muscle tumors and subcutaneous lipomas, there is little evidence that these lesions arise from their mature (differentiated) tissue counterparts. One current theory is that switching on a set of genes that programs mesenchymal differentiation in any mesenchymal cell may give rise to any type of mesenchymal tumor. Common subtypes of soft tissue sarcomas seen in the extremities of humans are liposarcomas, malignant fibrous histiosarcomas, synovial cell sarcomas, and fibrosarcomas. In the retroperitoneal location, liposarcomas and leiomyosarcomas are the most common histotypes noted in humans. The most common subtype noted viscerally are GISTs. Overall, leiomyosarcoma is the most common genitourinary sarcoma. Ten percent to 15% of all sarcomas occur in children, and the subtypes most commonly represented are rhabdomyosarcomas, Ewing's sarcoma, and primitive neuroectodermal tumors.

Prognostic variables in humans include clinical stage, histologic grade, necrosis, site, size, lymph node involvement, and aggressiveness of surgery or radiation. The histopathologic grading system used and shown to be predictive for metastasis in dogs is a grading system adopted from human pathology that is also predictive for survival.[24] Additionally, it appears that histologic grade is the predominant predictor of early recurrence, whereas tumor size plays a more important role for late recurrence. It is unclear whether age plays a prognostic role in human soft tissue sarcoma.

Surgical treatment is the mainstay of therapy for soft tissue sarcoma in the control of local disease. However, aggressive surgical resection combined with RT and chemotherapy, used before or after resection, allows effective limb-sparing treatment in 90% of patients. Amputation is reserved for patients with unresectable tumors, no evidence of metastasis, and the potential for good long-term rehabilitation. Local recurrence is greater in those patients undergoing limb-sparing therapies as compared to amputation; however, there is no difference in disease-free survival between the two groups. Since size is a prognostic factor for both local recurrence and metastasis, the recommended treatment is different. In patients with tumors smaller than 5 cm, complete surgical resection with 1-cm margins is usually sufficient. Larger lesions are treated with a combination of therapies, including chemotherapy and RT. RT techniques include external-beam RT and/or brachytherapy. Because half the human patients develop distant metastasis, despite local control, adjuvant chemotherapy is often used (doxorubicin alone or in combination with other chemotherapeutics). Ifosfamide is currently the most active salvage agent for patients who have failed doxorubicin-based protocols. Metaanalysis of combination therapy for soft tissue sarcoma reports a disease-free survival of 52% and an overall survival of 57% with a median follow-up of 9.4 years. Permanent local control with the first treatment is related to long-term survival. High-risk soft tissue sarcoma patients are treated with combined chemoradiation prior to surgical resection. The chemotherapy protocol often used is doxorubicin, ifosfamide, mesna, and dacarbazine. Local and systemic toxicity included expected wound-healing complications. In human patients with metastatic disease, combination chemotherapy produces response rates of 20%, and most patients are candidates for investigational agents.

REFERENCES

1. Theilen GH, Madewell BR: Tumors of the skin and subcutaneous tissues. In Theilen GH, Madewell BR, editors: *Veterinary cancer medicine*, Philadelphia, 1979, Lea & Febiger.
2. Dorn ER: Epidemiology of canine and feline tumors, *J Am Anim Hosp Assoc* 12:307–312, 1976.
3. Hardy WD: The etiology of canine and feline tumors, *J Am Anim Hosp Assoc* 12:313–334, 1976.
4. Madewell BR, Theilen GH: Etiology of cancer in animals. In Theilen GH, Madewell BR, editors: *Veterinary cancer medicine*, Philadelphia, 1979, Lea & Febiger, pp 13–25.
5. McCarthy PE, Hedlund CS, Veazy RS, et al: Liposarcoma associated with a glass foreign body in a dog, *J Am Vet Med Assoc* 209:612–614, 1996.
6. Thrall DE, Goldschmidt MH, Biery DN: Malignant tumor formation at the site of previously irradiated acanthomatous epulides in four dogs, *J Am Vet Med Assoc* 178:127–132, 1981.
7. Johnstone PA, Laskin WB, DeLuca AM, et al: Tumors in dogs exposed to experimental intraoperative radiotherapy, *Int J Radiat Oncol Biol Phys* 34:853–857, 1996.
8. Barnes M, Duray P, DeLuca A, et al: Tumor induction following intraoperative radiotherapy: late results of the National Cancer Institute canine trials, *Int J Radiat Oncol Biol Phys* 19:651–660, 1990.
9. Sinibaldi K, Rosen H, Liu SK, et al: Tumors associated with metallic implants in animals, *Clin Orthop* 118:257–266, 1976.
10. McGlennon NJ, Houlton JEF, Gorman NT: Synovial cell sarcoma-a review, *J Small Anim Pract* 29:139–152, 1988.
11. Murray JA: Synovial sarcoma, *Orthop Clin North Am* 8:963–972, 1977.
12. Vail DM, Powers BE, Getzy DM, et al: Evaluation of prognostic factors for dogs with synovial cell sarcoma: 36 cases (1986-1991), *J Am Vet Med Assoc* 205:1300–1307, 1994.
13. Kim DY, Hodgin EC, Cho DY, et al: Juvenile rhabdomyosarcomas in two dogs, *Vet Pathol* 33:447–450, 1996.
14. Duda RB: Review: Biology of mesenchymal tumors, *Cancer J* 7:52–62, 1994.
15. Thrall DE, Gillette EL: Soft-tissue sarcomas, *Semin Vet Med Surg Small Anim* 10:173–179, 1995.
16. Kuntz CA, Dernell WS, Powers BE, et al: Prognostic factors for surgical treatment of soft-tissue sarcomas in dogs: 75 cases (1986-1996), *J Am Vet Med Assoc* 21:1147–1151, 1997.
17. Ordonez NG: Immunocytochemistry in the diagnosis of soft tissue sarcomas, *Cancer Bull* 45:13–23, 1993.
18. Madewell BR, Munn RJ: The soft tissue sarcomas: Immunohistochemical and ultrastructural distinctions, *ACVIM Proc* 9:717–720, 1991.
19. Ciekot P, Powers B, Withrow S, et al: Histologically low-grade, yet biologically high-grade, fibrosarcoma of the mandible and maxilla in dogs: 25 cases (1982–1991), *J Am Vet Med Assoc* 204:610–615, 1994.
20. Zhang P, Brooks JS: Modern pathological evaluation of soft tissue sarcoma specimens and its potential role in soft tissue sarcoma research, *Curr Treat Options Oncol* 5:441–450, 2004.
21. Hogendoorn PC, Collin F, Daugaard S, et al: Pathology and Biology Subcommittee of the EORTC Soft Tissue and Bone Sarcoma Group. Changing concepts in the pathological basis of soft tissue and bone sarcoma treatment, *Eur J Cancer* 40:1644–1654, 2004.
22. Nilbert M, Engellau J: Experiences from tissue microarray in soft tissue sarcomas, *Acta Orthop Scand Suppl* 75:29–34, 2004.
23. Dennis MM, McSporran KD, Bacon NJ, et al: Prognostic factors for cutaneous and subcutaneous soft tissue sarcomas in dogs, *Vet Pathol* 48:73–84, 2011.
24. MacEwen EG, Powers BE, Macy D, et al: Soft tissue sarcomas. In Withrow SJ, MacEwen EG, editors: *Small animal clinical oncology*, Philadelphia, 2001, Saunders.
25. Cook JL, Turk JR, Pope ER, et al: Infantile desmoid-type fibromatosis in an Akita puppy, *J Am Anim Hosp Assoc* 34:291–294, 1998.
26. Gwin RM, Gelatt KN, Peiffer RL: Ophthalmic nodular fasciitis in the dog, *J Am Vet Med Assoc* 170:611–614, 1977.
27. Goldschmidt MH, Hendrick MJ: Tumors of the skin and soft tissue. In Meuten DJ, editor: *Tumors in domestic animals*, Ames, Iowa, 2002, Iowa State Press.
28. Goldschmidt MH, Shofer FS: *Skin tumors of the dog and cat*. Oxford, 1998, Butterworth Heinemann.
29. Chijiwa K, Uchida K, Tateyama S: Immunohistochemical evaluation of canine peripheral nerve sheath tumors and other soft tissue sarcomas, *Vet Pathol* 41:307–318, 2004.
30. Brehm D, Steinberg H, Haviland J, et al: A retrospective evaluation of 51 cases of peripheral nerve sheath tumors in the dog, *J Am Anim Hosp Assoc* 31:349–359, 1995.
31. Liggett AD, Frazier KS, Styler EL: Angiolipomatous tumors in dogs and a cat, *Vet Pathol* 39:286–289, 2002.
32. Brodey RS, Rozel JF: Neoplasms of the canine uterus, vagina, vulva: a clinicopathologic survey of 90 cases, *J Am Vet Med Assoc* 151:1294–1307, 1967.
33. Woolfson JM, Dulisch ML, Tams TR: Intrathoracic lipoma in a dog, *J Am Vet Med Assoc* 185:1007–1009, 1984.
34. Anderson SM, Lippincott CL: Intrathoracic lipoma in a dog, *Calif Vet* 43:9, 1989.
35. Umphlet RC, Vicini DS, Godshalk CP: Intradural-extramedullary lipoma in a dog, *Compend Contin Educ Pract Vet* 11:1192, 1989.
36. McLaughlin R, Kuzma AB: Intestinal strangulation caused by intra-abdominal lipomas in a dog, *J Am Vet Med Assoc* 199:1610–1611, 1991.
37. Plummer SB, Bunch SE, Khoo LH, et al: Tethered spinal cord and an intradural lipoma associated with a meningocele in a Manx-type cat, *J Am Vet Med Assoc* 203:1159–1161, 1993.
38. Head KW, Else RW, Dubielzig RR: Tumors of the alimentary tract. In Meuten DJ, editor: *Tumors in domestic animals*, Ames, Iowa, 2002, Iowa State Press.
39. Mayhew PD, Brockman DJ: Body cavity lipomas in six dogs, *J Small Anim Pract* 43:177–181, 2002.
40. Gibbons SE, Straw RC: Intra-abdominal lipoma in a dog, *Aust Vet Pract* 33:86, 2003.
41. Gleiser CA, Jardine JH, Raulston GL, et al: Infiltrating lipomas in the dog, *Vet Pathol* 16:623–624, 1979.

42. McChesney AE, Stephens LC, Lebel J, et al: Infiltrative lipoma in dogs, *Vet Pathol* 17:316–322, 1980.
43. Doige CE, Farrow CS, Presnell KR: Parosteal lipoma in a dog, *J Am Anim Hosp Assoc* 16:87, 1980.
44. Bergman PJ, Withrow SJ, Straw RC, et al: Infiltrative lipoma in dogs: 16 cases (1981-1992), *J Am Vet Med Assoc* 205:322–324, 1994.
45. McEntee MC, Page RL, Mauldin GN, et al: Results of irradiation of infiltrative lipoma in 13 dogs, *Vet Radiol Ultrasound* 41:554–556, 2000.
46. McEntee MC, Thrall DE: Computed tomographic imaging of infiltrative lipoma in 22 dogs, *Vet Radiol Ultrasound* 42:221–225, 2001.
47. Thomson MJ, Withrow SJ, Dernell WS, et al: Intermuscular lipomas of the thigh region in dogs: 11 cases, *J Am Anim Hosp Assoc* 35:165–167, 1999.
48. Kramek BA, Spackman CJA, Hayden DW: Infiltrative lipoma in three dogs, *J Am Vet Med Assoc* 186:81–82, 1985.
49. Frazier KS, Herron AJ, Dee JF, et al: Infiltrative lipoma in a stifle joint, *J Am Anim Hosp* 29:81–83, 1993.
50. Baez JL, Hendrick MJ, Shofer FS, et al: Liposarcomas in dogs: 56 cases (1989-2000), *J Am Vet Med Assoc* 224:887–891, 2004.
51. Brennan MF, Singer S, Maki RG, et al: Soft tissue sarcoma. In DeVita RT, Hellman S, Rosenberg SA, editors: *Cancer: Principles and practice of oncology*, Philadelphia, 2008, Lippincott Williams & Wilkins.
52. Chang HR, Hajdu SI, Collin C, et al: The prognostic value of histologic subtypes in primary extremity liposarcoma, *Cancer* 64:1514–1520, 1989.
53. Choong PFM, Pritchard DJ: Common malignant soft-tissue tumors. In Simon MA, Springfield D, editors: *Surgery for bone and soft-tissue tumors*, Philadelphia, 1998, Lippincott-Raven.
54. Bruecker KA, Withrow SJ: Intestinal leiomyosarcomas in six dogs, *J Am Anim Hosp Assoc* 24:281, 1988.
55. Kapatkin AS, Mullen HS, Matthiesen DT, et al: Leiomyosarcoma in dogs: 44 cases (1983-1988), *J Am Vet Med Assoc* 201:1077–1079, 1992.
56. Callanan JJ, McCarthy GM, McAllister H: Primary pulmonary artery leiomyosarcoma in an adult dog, *Vet Pathol* 37:663–664, 2000.
57. Miller MA, Ramos-Vara JA, Dickerson MF, et al: Uterine neoplasia in 13 cats, *J Vet Diagn Invest* 15:515–522, 2003.
58. Leifer CE, Peterson ME, Matus RE, et al: Hypoglycemia associated with nonislet cell tumor in 13 dogs, *J Am Vet Med Assoc* 186:53–55, 1985.
59. Bagley RS, Levy JK, Malarkey DE: Hypoglycemia associated with intra-abdominal leiomyoma and leiomyosarcoma in six dogs, *J Am Vet Med Assoc* 208:69–71, 1996.
60. Sato K, Hikasa Y, Morita T, et al: Secondary erythrocytosis associated with high plasma erythropoietin concentrations in a dog with cecal leiomyosarcoma, *J Am Vet Med Assoc* 220:486–490, 2002.
61. Cohen M, Post GS, Wright JC: Gastrointestinal leiomyosarcoma in 14 dogs, *J Vet Intern Med* 17:107–110, 2003.
62. Frost D, Lasota J, Miettinen M: Gastrointestinal stromal tumors and leiomyomas in the dog: a histopathologic, immunohistochemical, and molecular genetic study of 50 cases, *Vet Pathol* 40:42–54, 2003.
63. Crawshaw J, Berg J, Sardinas JC, et al: Prognosis for dogs with nonlymphomatous, small intestinal tumors treated by surgical excision, *J Am Anim Hosp Assoc* 34:451–456, 1998.
64. Liu SM, Mikaelian I: Cutaneous smooth muscle tumors in the dog and cat, *Vet Pathol* 40:685–692, 2003.
65. Larock RG, Ginn PE: Immunohistochemical staining characteristics of canine gastrointestinal stromal tumors, *Vet Pathol* 34:303–311, 1997.
66. Maas CP, ter Haar G, van der Gaag I, et al: Reclassification of small intestinal and cecal smooth muscle tumors in 72 dogs: clinical, histologic, and immunohistochemical evaluation, *Vet Surg* 36:302–313, 2007.
67. Russell KN, Mehler SJ, Skorupski KA, et al: Clinical and immunohistochemical differentiation of gastrointestinal stromal tumors from leiomyosarcomas in dogs: 42 cases (1990-2003), *J Am Vet Med Assoc* 230:1329–1333, 2007.
68. Kerpsack SJ, Birchard SJ: Removal of leiomyomas and other noninvasive masses from the cardiac region of the canine stomach, *J Am Anim Hosp Assoc* 30:500, 1994.
69. Kontogianni K, Demonakou M, Kavantzas N, et al: Prognostic predictors of gastrointestinal stromal tumors: a multi-institutional analysis of 102 patients with definition of a prognostic index, *Eur J Surg Oncol* 29:548–556, 2003.
70. Cooper BJ, Valentine BA: Tumors of muscle. In Meuten DJ, editor: *Tumors in domestic animals*, Ames, Iowa, 2002, Iowa State Press.
71. Kobayashi M, Sakai H, Hirata A, et al: Expression of myogenic regulating factors, myogenin and MyoD, in two canine botryoid rhabdomyosarcomas, *Vet Pathol* 41:275–277, 2004.
72. Russell HV, Pappo AS, Nuchtern JG, et al: Solid tumors of childhood. In DeVita RT, Hellman S, Rosenberg SA, editors: *Cancer: principles and practice of oncology*, Philadelphia, 2008, Lippincott Williams & Wilkins.
73. Senior DF, Lawrence DT, Gunison C, et al: Successful treatment of botryoid rhabdomyosarcoma in the bladder of a dog, *J Am Anim Hosp Assoc* 29:386, 1993.
74. Block G, Clarke K, Salisbury SK, et al: Total laryngectomy and permanent tracheostomy for treatment of laryngeal rhabdomyosarcoma in a dog, *J Am Anim Hosp Assoc* 31:510–513, 1995.
75. Lascelles BDX, McInnes E, Dobson JM, et al: Rhabdomyosarcoma of the tongue in a dog, *J Small Anim Pract* 39:587–591, 1998.
76. Ueno H, Kadosawa T, Isomura H, et al: Perianal rhabdomyosarcoma in a dog, *J Small Anim Pract* 43:217–220, 2002.
77. Takiguchi M, Watanabe T, Okada H, et al: Rhabdomyosarcoma (botryoid sarcoma) of the urinary bladder in a Maltese, *J Small Anim Pract* 43:269–271, 2002.
78. Kelly WR, Wilkinson GT, Allen PW: Canine angiosarcoma (lymphangiosarcoma): A case report, *Vet Pathol* 18:224–227, 1981.
79. Walsh K, Abbott DP: Lymphangiosarcoma in two cats, *J Comp Pathol* 94:611–614, 1984.
80. Diessler ME, Castellano MC, Massone AR, et al: Cutaneous lymphangiosarcoma in a young dog: clinical, anatomopathological and lectin histochemical description, *J Vet Med A Physiol Pathol Clin Med* 50:452–456, 2003.
81. Itoh T, Mikawa K, Mikawa M, et al: Lymphangiosarcoma in a dog treated with surgery and chemotherapy, *J Vet Med Sci* 66:197–199, 2004.
82. Widmer WR, Carlton WW: Persistent hematuria in a dog with renal hemangioma, *J Am Vet Med Assoc* 197:237–239, 1990.
83. Mott JCP, McAnulty JF, Darien DL, et al: Nephron sparing by partial median nephrectomy for treatment of renal hemangioma in a dog, *J Am Vet Med Assoc* 208:1274–1276, 1996.
84. Schoofs SH: Lingual hemangioma in a puppy: a case report and literature review, *J Am Anim Hosp Assoc* 33:161–165, 1997.
85. Liptak JM, Dernell WS, Ehrhart EJ, et al: Retroperitoneal sarcomas in dogs: 14 cases (1992-2002), *J Am Vet Med Assoc* 224:1471–1477, 2004.
86. Ward H, Fox LE, Calderwood-Mays MB, et al: Cutaneous hemangiosarcoma in 25 dogs: a retrospective study, *J Vet Intern Med* 8:345–346, 1994.
87. Bulakowski EJ, Philibert JC, Siegel S, et al: Evaluation of outcome associated with subcutaneous and intramuscular hemangiosarcoma treated with adjuvant doxorubicin in dogs: 21 cases (2001-2006), *J Am Vet Med Assoc* 233:122–128, 2008.
88. Wiley JL, Rook KA, Clifford CA, et al: Efficacy of doxorubicin-based chemotherapy for non-resectable canine subcutaneous haemangiosarcoma, *Vet Comp Oncol* 8:221–233, 2010.
89. Miller MA, Ramos JA, Kreeger JM: Cutaneous vascular neoplasia in 15 cats: clinical, morphologic, and immunohistochemical studies, *Vet Pathol* 29:329–336, 1992.

90. McAbee KP, Ludwig LL, Bergman PJ, et al: Feline cutaneous hemangiosarcoma: a retrospective study of 18 cases (1998-2003), *J Am Anim Hosp Assoc* 41:110–116, 2005.
91. Scavelli TD, Patnaik AK, Mehlhall CJ, et al: Hemangiosarcoma in the cat: retrospective evaluation of 31 surgical cases, *J Am Vet Med Assoc* 187:817–819, 1985.
92. Pool RR, Thompson KG: Tumors of joints. In Meuten DJ, editor: *Tumors in domestic animals*, Ames, Iowa, 2002, Iowa State Press.
93. Craig LE, Krimer PM, Cooley AJ: Canine synovial myxoma: 39 cases, *Vet Pathol* 47(5):931–936, 2010.
94. Craig LE, Julian ME, Ferracone JD: The diagnosis and prognosis of synovial tumors in dogs: 35 cases, *Vet Pathol* 39:66–73, 2002.
95. Fox DB, Cook JL, Kreeger JM, et al: Canine synovial cell sarcoma: a retrospective assessment of described prognostic criteria in 16 cases (1994-1999), *J Am Anim Hosp Assoc* 38:347–355, 2002.
96. Liptak JM, Withrow SJ, Macy DW, et al: Metastatic synovial cell sarcoma in two cats, *Vet Comp Oncol* 2:164–170, 2004.
97. Tilmant LL, Gorman NT, Ackerman N, et al: Chemotherapy of synovial cell sarcoma in a dog, *J Am Vet Med Assoc* 188:530–532, 1986.
98. Foale RD, White RA, Harley R, et al: Left ventricular myxosarcoma in a dog, *J Small Anim Pract* 44:503–507, 2003.
99. Briggs OM, Kirberger RM, Goldberg NB: Right atrial myxosarcoma in a dog, *J S Afr Vet Assoc* 68:144–146, 1997.
100. Richter M, Stankeova S, Hauser B, et al: Myxosarcoma in the eye and brain in a dog, *Vet Ophthalmol* 6:183–189, 2003.
101. Spangler WL, Culbertson MR, Kass PH: Primary mesenchymal (nonangiomatous/nonlymphomatous) neoplasms occurring in the canine spleen: anatomic classification, immunohistochemistry, and mitotic activity correlated with patient survival, *Vet Pathol* 31:37–47, 1994.
102. McDonald RK, Helman RG: Hepatic malignant mesenchymoma in a dog, *J Am Vet Med Assoc* 188:1052–1053, 1986.
103. Hahn KA, Richardson RC: Use of cisplatin for control of metastatic malignant mesenchymoma and hypertrophic osteopathy in a dog, *J Am Vet Med Assoc* 195:351–353, 1989.
104. Carpenter JL, Dayal Y, King NW, et al: Distinctive unclassified mesenchymal tumor of the digit of dogs, *Vet Pathol* 28:396–402, 1991.
105. Watson AD, Young KM, Dubielzig RR, et al: Primary mesenchymal or mixed-cell-origin lung tumors in four dogs, *J Am Vet Med Assoc* 202:968–970, 1993.
106. Robinson TM, Dubielzig RR, McAnulty JF: Malignant mesenchymoma associated with an unusual vasoinvasive metastasis in a dog, *J Am Anim Hosp Assoc* 34:295–299, 1998.
107. Beaudry D, Knapp D, Montgomery T, et al: Hypoglycemia in four dogs with smooth muscle tumors, *J Vet Intern Med* 9:415–418, 1995.
108. Pletcher JM, Dalton L: Botryoid rhabdomyosarcoma in the urinary bladder of a dog, *Vet Pathol* 18:695–697, 1981.
109. Kuwamura M, Yoshida H, Yamate J, et al: Urinary bladder rhabdomyosarcoma (sarcoma botryoides) in a young Newfoundland dog, *J Vet Med Sci* 60:619–621, 1998.
110. Baker-Gabb M, Hunt GB, France MP: Soft tissue sarcomas and mast cell tumours in dogs: clinical behaviour and response to surgery, *Aust Vet J* 81:732–738, 2003.
111. Postorino NC, Berg RJ, Powers BE, et al: Prognostic variables for canine hemangiopericytoma: 50 cases (1979-1984), *J Am Anim Hosp Assoc* 24:501–509, 1988.
112. Spangler WL, Kass PH: Splenic myeloid metaplasia, histiocytosis, and hypersplenism in the dog (65 cases), *Vet Pathol* 36:583–593, 1999.
113. Skorupski KA, Clifford CA, Paoloni MC, et al: CCNU for the treatment of dogs with histiocytic sarcoma, *J Vet Intern Med* 21:121–126, 2007.
114. LeRoith D, Clemmons D, Nissley P, et al: Insulin-like growth factors in health and disease, *Ann Intern Med* 116:854–862, 1992.
115. Cryer P: Glucose homeostasis and hypoglycemia. In Wilson J, Foster D, editors: *Williams textbook of endocrinology*, Philadelphia, 1992, Saunders.
116. Boari A, Venturoli M, Minuto F: Non-islet-cell tumor hypoglycemia in a dog associated with high levels of insulin-like growth factor II, *World Small Animal Vet Assoc Cong Proc* 17:678, 1992.
117. Sugiura H, Takahashi M, Katagiri H, et al: Additional wide resection of malignant soft tissue tumors, *Clin Orthop* 394:201–210, 2002.
118. Affolter VK, Moore PF: Canine cutaneous and systemic histiocytosis: reactive histiocytosis of dermal dendritic cells, *Am J Dermatopathol* 22:40–48, 2000.
119. Affolter VK, Moore PF: Localized and disseminated histiocytic sarcoma of dendritic cell origin in dogs, *Vet Pathol* 39:74–83, 2002.
120. Greene FL, Page DL, Fleming ID, et al: *AJCC cancer staging manual*, New York, 2002, Springer.
121. Dernell WS, Withrow SJ, Kuntz CA, et al: Principles of treatment for soft tissue sarcoma, *Clin Tech Small Anim Pract* 13:59–64, 1998.
122. Banks TA, Straw RC, Withrow SJ, et al: Prospective study of canine soft tissue sarcoma treated by wide surgical excision: quantitative evaluation of surgical margins, *Vet Cancer Soc Proc* 23:21, 2003.
123. Reimer SB, Séguin B, DeCock HE, et al: Evaluation of the effect of routine histologic processing on the size of skin samples obtained from dogs, *Am J Vet Res* 66:500–505, 2005.
124. Ramanathan RC, A'Hern R, Fisher C, et al: Prognostic index for extremity soft tissue sarcomas with isolated local recurrence, *Ann Surg Oncol* 8:278–289, 2001.
125. Stojadinovic A, Leung DHY, Hoos A, et al: Analysis of the prognostic significance of microscopic margins in 2,084 localized primary adult soft tissue sarcomas, *Ann Surg* 235:424–434, 2002.
126. Zagars GK, Ballo MT, Pisters PWT, et al: Prognostic factors for patients with localized soft-tissue sarcoma treated with conservative surgery and radiation therapy: an analysis of 1225 patients, *Cancer* 97:2530–2543, 2003.
127. Zagars GK, Ballo MT, Pisters PWT, et al: Surgical margins and reresection in the management of patients with soft tissue sarcoma using conservative surgery and radiation therapy, *Cancer* 97:2544–2553, 2003.
128. Eilber FC, Rosen G, Nelson SD, et al: High-grade extremity soft tissue sarcomas: factors predictive of local recurrence and its effect on morbidity and mortality, *Ann Surg* 237:218–226, 2003.
129. Bacon NJ, Dernell WS, Ehrhart N, et al: Evaluation of primary re-excision after inadequate resection of soft tissue sarcomas in dogs: 41 cases (1999-2004), *J Am Vet Med Assoc* 230:548–554, 2007.
130. Chase D, Bray J, Ide A, et al: Outcome following removal of canine spindle cell tumours in first opinion practice: 104 cases, *J Small Anim Pract* 50:568–574, 2009.
131. McSporran KD: Histologic grade predicts recurrence for marginally excised canine subcutaneous soft tissue sarcomas, *Vet Pathol* 46:928–933, 2009.
132. Stefanello D, Morello E, Roccabianca P, et al: Marginal excision of low-grade spindle cell sarcoma of canine extremities: 35 dogs (1996-2006), *Vet Surg* 37:461–465, 2008.
133. Elmslie RE, Glawe P, Dow SW: Metronomic chemotherapy with cyclophosphamide and piroxicam effectively delays tumor recurrence in dogs with incompletely resected soft tissue sarcomas, *J Vet Intern Med* 22:1373–1379, 2008.
134. McEntee MC, Samii VF, Walsh P, et al: Postoperative assessment of surgical clip position in 16 dogs with cancer: a pilot study, *J Am Anim Hosp Assoc* 40:300–308, 2004.
135. Henry CJ, Stoll MR, Higginbotham ML, et al: Effect of timing of radiation initiation on post-surgical wound healing in dogs, *Vet Cancer Soc Proc* 23:52, 2003.
136. Forrest LJ, Chun R, Adams WM, et al: Postoperative radiotherapy for canine soft tissue sarcoma, *J Vet Intern Med* 14:578–582, 2000.
137. McKnight JA, Mauldin GN, McEntee MC, et al: Radiation treatment of incompletely resected soft-tissue sarcomas in dogs, *J Am Vet Med Assoc* 217:205–210, 2000.

138. Graves GM, Bjorling DE, Mahaffey E: Canine hemangiopericytoma: 23 cases (1967-1984), *J Am Vet Med Assoc* 192:99–102, 1988.
139. Atwater SW, LaRue SM, Powers BE, et al: Adjuvant radiation therapy of soft-tissue sarcomas in dogs, *Vet Cancer Soc Proc* 12:41, 1992.
140. Mauldin GN, Meleo KA, Burk RL: Radiation therapy for the treatment of incompletely resected soft tissue sarcomas in dogs: 21 cases, *Vet Cancer Soc Proc* 13:111, 1993.
141. McChesney SL, Withrow SJ, Gillette EL, et al: Radiotherapy of soft tissue sarcomas in dogs, *J Am Vet Med Assoc* 194:60–63, 1989.
142. Hilmas DE, Gillett EL: Radiotherapy of spontaneous fibrous connective-tissue sarcomas in animals, *J Natl Cancer Inst* 56:365–368, 1976.
143. Banks WC, Morris E: Results of radiation treatment of naturally occurring animal tumors, *J Am Vet Med Assoc* 166:1063–1064, 1975.
144. Richardson RC, Anderson VL, Voorhees WD, et al: Irradiation-hyperthermia in canine hemangiopericytomas: Large-animal model for therapeutic response, *J Natl Cancer Inst* 73:1187–1194, 1984.
145. Lawrence J, Forrest L, Adams W, et al: Four-fraction radiation therapy for macroscopic soft tissue sarcomas in 16 dogs, *J Am Anim Hosp Assoc* 44:100–108, 2008.
146. McChesney-Gillette S, Dewhirst MW, Gillette EL, et al: Response of canine soft tissue sarcomas to radiation or radiation plus hyperthermia: a randomized phase II study, *Int J Hyperthermia* 8:309–320, 1992.
147. Brewer WG, Turrel JM: Radiotherapy and hyperthermia in the treatment of fibrosarcomas in the dog, *J Am Vet Med Assoc* 181:146–150, 1982.
148. Thrall D, Prescott D, Samulski T, et al: Radiation plus local hyperthermia versus radiation plus the combination of local and whole-body hyperthermia in canine sarcomas, *Int J Radiation Oncol Biol Phys* 34:1087–1096, 1996.
149. Mauldin GN: Soft tissue sarcomas, *Vet Clin North Am Small Anim Pract* 27:139–148, 1997.
150. Viglianti BL, Lora-Michiels M, Poulson JM, et al: Dynamic contrast-enhanced magnetic resonance imaging as a predictor of clinical outcome in canine spontaneous soft tissue sarcomas treated with thermoradiotherapy, *Clin Cancer Res* 15:4993–5001, 2009.
151. Simon D, Ruslander DM, Rassnick KM, et al: Orthovoltage radiation and weekly low dose of doxorubicin for the treatment of incompletely excised soft-tissue sarcomas in 39 dogs, *Vet Rec* 160:321–326, 2007.
152. Kalnicki S, Bloomer W: *Radiation therapy in the treatment of bone and soft tissue sarcomas*, Philadelphia, 1992, Saunders.
153. MacLeod DA, Thrall DE: The combination of surgery and radiation in the treatment of cancer. A review, *Vet Surg* 18:1–6, 1989.
154. Cheng EY, Dusenbery KE, Winters MR, et al: Soft tissue sarcomas: preoperative versus postoperative radiotherapy, *J Surg Oncol* 61:90–99, 1996.
155. Strander H, Turesson I, Cavallin-Stahl E: A systematic overview of radiation therapy effects in soft tissue sarcomas, *Acta Oncol* 42:516–531, 2003.
156. Rassnick KM, Moore AS, Russel DS, et al: Phase II, open-label trial of single-agent CCNU in dogs with previously untreated histiocytic sarcoma, *J Vet Intern Med* 24:1528–1531, 2010.
157. Skorupski KA, Rodriguez CO, Krick EL, et al: Long-term survival in dogs with localized histiocytic sarcoma treated with CCNU as an adjuvant to local therapy, *Vet Comp Oncol* 7:139–144, 2009.
158. Klahn SL, Kitchell BE, Dervisis NG: Evaluation and comparison of outcomes in dogs with periarticular and nonperiarticular histiocytic sarcoma, *J Am Vet Med Assoc* 239:90–96, 2011
159. Rassnick KM: Medical management of soft tissue sarcomas, *Vet Clin North Am Small Anim Pract* 33:517–531, 2003.
160. Ogilvie GK, Reynolds HA, Richardson RC, et al: Phase II evaluation of doxorubicin for treatment of various canine neoplasms, *J Am Vet Med Assoc* 195:1580–1583, 1989.
161. Ogilvie GK, Powers BE, Mallinckrodt CH, et al: Surgery and doxorubicin in dogs with hemangiosarcoma, *J Vet Intern Med* 6:379–384, 1996.
162. Ogilvie GK, Obradovich JE, Elmslie RE, et al: Efficacy of mitoxantrone against various neoplasms in dogs, *J Am Vet Med Assoc* 198:1618–1621, 1991.
163. Henry CJ, Buss MS, Potter KA, et al: Mitoxantrone and cyclophosphamide combination chemotherapy for the treatment of various canine malignancies, *J Am Anim Hosp Assoc* 35:236–239, 1999.
164. Rassnick KM, Frimberger AE, Wood CA, et al: Evaluation of ifosfamide for treatment of various canine neoplasms, *J Vet Intern Med* 14:271–276, 2000.
165. Sarcoma Meta-Analysis Collaboration: Adjuvant chemotherapy for localised resectable soft-tissue sarcoma of adults: meta-analysis of individual data, *Lancet* 350:1647–1654, 1997.
166. Komdeur R, Hoekstra HJ, van den Berg E, et al: Metastasis in soft tissue sarcomas: prognostic criteria and treatment perspectives, *Cancer Metastasis Rev* 21:167–183, 2002.
167. Selting KA, Powers BE, Thompson LJ, et al: Outcome of dogs with high-grade soft tissue sarcomas treated with and without adjuvant doxorubicin chemotherapy: 39 cases (1996-2004), *J Am Vet Med Assoc* 227:1442–1448, 2005.
168. Dernell WS, Withrow SJ, Straw RC, et al: Intracavitary treatment of soft tissue sarcomas in dogs using cisplatin in a biodegradable polymer, *Anticancer Res* 17:4499–4505, 1997.
169. Bostock DE, Dye MT: Prognosis after surgical excision of canine fibrous connective tissue sarcomas, *Vet Pathol* 17:581–588, 1980.
170. Evans SM: Canine hemangiopericytoma: a retrospective analysis of response to surgery and orthovoltage radiation, *Vet Radiol* 28:13–16, 1987.
171. Hauck M: Feline injection site sarcomas, *Vet Clin North Am Small Anim Pract* 33:553–557, 2003.
172. Hendrick MJ, Goldschmidt MH, Shofer FS, et al: Postvaccinal sarcomas in the cat: epidemiology and electron probe microanalytical identification of aluminum, *Cancer Res* 52:5391–5394, 1992.
173. Hendrick MJ, Goldschmidt MH: Do injection site reactions induce fibrosarcomas in cats? *J Am Vet Med Assoc* 199:968, 1991.
174. Hendrick MJ, Shofer FS, Goldschmidt MH, et al: Comparison of fibrosarcomas that developed at vaccination sites and at nonvaccination sites in cats: 239 cases (1991-1992), *J Am Vet Med Assoc* 205:1425–1429, 1994.
175. Kass PH, Barnes WG, Spangler WL, et al: Epidemiologic evidence for a causal relation between vaccination and fibrosarcoma tumorigenesis in cats, *J Am Vet Med Assoc* 203: 396–405, 1993.
176. Macy DW, Hendrick MJ: The potential role of inflammation in the development of postvaccinal sarcomas in cats, *Vet Clin North Am Small Anim Pract* 26:103–109, 1996.
177. Lester S, Clemett T, Burt A: Vaccine site-associated sarcomas in cats: clinical experience and a laboratory review (1982-1993), *J Am Anim Hosp Assoc* 32:91–95, 1996.
178. Hendrick MJ, Kass PH, McGill LD, et al: Postvaccinal sarcomas in cats, *J Natl Cancer Inst* 86:341–343, 1994.
179. Coyne MJ, Reeves NCP, Rosen DK, et al: Estimated prevalence of injection sarcomas in cats during 1992, *J Am Vet Med Assoc* 210:249–251, 1997.
180. Gober GM, Kass PH: World Wide Web-based survey of vaccination practices, postvaccinal reactions, and vaccine site-associated sarcomas in cats, *J Am Vet Med Assoc* 220:1477–1482, 2002.
181. Reference deleted in pages.
182. Kass PH, Spangler WL, Hendrick MJ, et al: Multicenter case-control study of risk factors associated with development of injection-site sarcomas in cats, *J Am Vet Med Assoc* 223:1283–1292, 2003.
183. Hendrick MJ: Feline injection-site sarcomas, *Cancer Invest* 17:273–274, 1999.
184. Dubielzig RR, Hawkins KL, Miller PE: Myofibroblastic sarcoma originating at the site of rabies vaccination in a cat, *J Vet Diagn Invest* 5:637–638, 1993.

185. McEntee MC, Page RL: Feline injection-site sarcomas, *J Vet Intern Med* 15:176–182, 2001.
186. McNiel EA: Vaccine-associate sarcomas in cats: a unique cancer model, *Clin Orthop* 382:21–27, 2001.
187. Séguin B: Injection site sarcomas in cats, *Clin Tech Small Anim Pract* 17:168–173, 2002.
188. Morrison WB, Starr RM: Injection-site Feline Sarcoma Task Force: Injection-site feline sarcomas, *J Am Vet Med Assoc* 218:697–702, 2001.
189. Peiffer RL, Monticello T, Bouldin TW: Primary ocular sarcomas in the cat, *J Small Anim Pract* 29:105, 1988.
190. Dubielzig RR, Everitt J, Shadduck JA, et al: Clinical and morphologic features of post-traumatic ocular sarcomas in cats, *Vet Pathol* 27:62–65, 1990.
191. Hakanson N, Forrester SD: Uveitis in the dog and cat, *Vet Clin North Am Small Anim Pract* 20:715–735, 1990.
192. Hendrick MJ, Brooks JJ: Postvaccinal sarcomas in the cat: histology and immunohistochemistry, *Vet Pathol* 31:126–129, 1994.
193. Hendrick MJ: Feline injection-site sarcomas: current studies on pathogenesis, *J Am Vet Med Assoc* 213:1425–1426, 1998.
194. Ellis JA, Jackson ML, Bartsch RC, et al: Use of immunohistochemistry and polymerase chain reaction for detection of oncornaviruses in formalin-fixed, paraffin-embedded fibrosarcomas from cats, *J Am Vet Med Assoc* 209:767–771, 1996.
195. Mayr B, Reifinger M, Alton K, et al: Novel p53 tumour suppressor mutations in cases of spindle cell sarcoma, pleomorphic sarcoma and fibrosarcoma in cats, *Vet Res Comm* 22:249–255, 1998.
196. Mayr B, Blauesnsteiner J, Edlinger A, et al: Presence of p53 mutations in feline neoplasms, *Res Vet Sci* 68:63–70, 2000.
197. Hershey AE, Dubielzig RR, Padilla ML, et al: Aberrant p53 expression in feline vaccine-associated sarcomas and correlation with prognosis, *Vet Pathol* 42:805–811, 2005.
198. Nieto A, Sánchez MA, Martínez E, et al: Immunohistochemical expression of p53, fibroblast growth factor-b and transforming growth factor-α in feline injection-site sarcomas, *Vet Pathol* 40:651–658, 2003.
199. Katayama R, Huelsmeyer MK, Marr AK, et al: Imatinib mesylate inhibits platelet-derived growth factor activity and increases chemosensitivity in feline injection-site sarcoma, *Cancer Chemother Pharmacol* 54:25–33, 2004.
200. Esplin DG, Bigelow M, McGill LD, et al: Fibrosarcoma at the site of a lufenuron injection in a cat, *Vet Cancer Soc Newsletter* 23:8, 1999.
201. Daly MK, Saba CF, Crochik SS, et al: Fibrosarcoma adjacent to the site of microchip implantation in a cat, *J Feline Med Surg* 10:202–205, 2008.
202. Carminato A, Vascellari M, Marchioro W, et al: Microchip-associated fibrosarcoma in a cat, *Vet Dermatol* 22(6):565–569, 2011.
203. Moore PF, Affolter VK: Canine and feline histiocytic diseases. In Ettinger SJ, Feldman EC, editors: *Textbook of veterinary internal medicine*, St Louis, 2005, Elsevier Saunders.
204. Heldmann E, Anderson MA, Wagner-Mann C: Feline osteosarcoma: 145 cases (1990-1995), *J Am Anim Hosp Assoc* 36:518–521, 2000.
205. Cohen M, Wright JC, Brawner WR, et al: Use of surgery and electron beam irradiation, with or without chemotherapy, for treatment of injection-site sarcomas in cats: 78 cases (1996-2000), *J Am Vet Med Assoc* 219:1582–1589, 2001.
206. Doddy FD, Glickman LT, Glickman NW, et al: Feline fibrosarcomas at vaccination sites and nonvaccination sites, *J Comp Pathol* 114:165–174, 1996.
207. Phelps HA, Kuntz CA, Milner RJ, et al: Radical excision with five-centimeter margins for treatment of feline injection-site sarcomas: 91 cases (1998-2002), *J Am Vet Med Assoc* 239:97–106, 2011.
208. Esplin DG, McGill LD, Meininger AC, et al: Postvaccination sarcomas in cats, *J Am Vet Med Assoc* 202:1245–1247, 1993.
209. Madewell BR, Griffey SM, McEntee MC, et al: Feline injection-site fibrosarcoma: an ultrastructural study of 20 tumors (1996-1999), *Vet Pathol* 38:196–202, 2001.
210. Couto SS, Griffey SM, Duarte PC, et al: Feline injection-site fibrosarcoma: morphologic distinctions, *Vet Pathol* 39:33–41, 2002.
211. Davidson EB, Gregory CR, Kass PH: Surgical excision of soft tissue fibrosarcomas in cats, *Vet Surg* 26:265–269, 1997.
212. Hershey AE, Sorenmo KU, Hendrick MJ, et al: Prognosis for presumed feline injection-site sarcoma after excision: 61 cases (1986-1996), *J Am Vet Med Assoc* 216:58–61, 2000.
213. Brown NO, Patnaik AK, Mooney S, et al: Soft tissue sarcomas in the cat, *J Am Vet Med Assoc* 173:744–749, 1978.
214. Kahler S: Collective effort needed to unlock factors related to feline injection site sarcomas, *J Am Vet Med Assoc* 202:1551–1554, 1993.
215. Lidbetter DA, Williams FA, Krahwinkel DJ, et al: Radical lateral body-wall resection for fibrosarcoma with reconstruction using polypropylene mesh and a caudal superficial epigastric axial pattern flap: a prospective clinical study of the technique and results in 6 cats, *Vet Surg* 31:57–64, 2002.
216. Romanelli G, Marconato L, Olivero D, et al: Analysis of prognostic factors associated with injection-site sarcomas in cats: 57 cases (2001-2007), *J Am Vet Med Assoc* 232:1193–1199, 2008.
217. Cronin K, Page RL, Spodnick G, et al: Radiation therapy and surgery for fibrosarcoma in 33 cats, *Vet Radiol Ultrasound* 39:51–56, 1998.
218. Bregazzi VS, LaRue SM, McNiel E, et al: Treatment with a combination of doxorubicin, surgery, and radiation versus surgery and radiation alone for cats with injection-site sarcomas: 25 cases (1995-2000), *J Am Vet Med Assoc* 218:547–550, 2001.
219. Kobayashi T, Hauck ML, Dodge R, et al: Preoperative radiotherapy for injection-site sarcoma in 92 cats, *Vet Radiol Ultrasound* 43:473–479, 2002.
220. Eckstein C, Guscetti F, Roos M, et al: A retrospective analysis of radiation therapy for treatment of feline vaccine-associated sarcoma, *Vet Comp Oncol* 7:54–68, 2009.
221. Kleiter M, Tichy A, Willmann M, et al: Concomitant liposomal doxorubicin and daily palliative radiation therapy in advanced feline soft tissue sarcomas, *Vet Radiol Ultrasound* 51:349–355, 2010.
222. Williams LE, Banerji N, Klausner JS, et al: Establishment of two injection-site feline sarcoma cell lines and determination of in vitro chemosensitivity to doxorubicin and mitoxantrone, *Am J Vet Res* 62:1354–1357, 2001.
223. Banerji N, Li X, Klausner JS, et al: Evaluation of in vitro chemosensitivity of injection-site feline sarcoma cell lines to vincristine and paclitaxel, *Am J Vet Res* 63:728–732, 2002.
224. Barber LG, Sorenmo KU, Cronin KL, et al: Combined doxorubicin and cyclophosphamide chemotherapy for nonresectable feline fibrosarcoma, *J Am Anim Hosp Assoc* 36:416–421, 2000.
225. Poirier VJ, Thamm DH, Kurzman ID, et al: Liposome-encapsulated doxorubicin (Doxil) and doxorubicin in the treatment of injection-site sarcomas in cats, *J Vet Intern Med* 16:726–731, 2002.
226. Spugnini EP, Baldi A, Vincenzi B, et al: Intraoperative versus postoperative electrochemotherapy in high grade soft tissue sarcomas: a preliminary study in a spontaneous feline model, *Cancer Chemother Pharmacol* 59:375–381, 2007.
227. Jourdier TM, Moste C, Bonnet MC, et al: Local immunotherapy of spontaneous feline fibrosarcomas using recombinant poxviruses expressing interleukin 2 (IL2), *Gene Ther* 10:2126–2132, 2003.
228. Jahnke A, Hirschberger J, Fischer C, et al: Intra-tumoral gene delivery of feIL-2, feIFN-gamma and feGM-CSF using magnetofection as a neoadjuvant treatment option for feline fibrosarcoma: a phase I trial, *J Vet Med A Physiol Pathol Clin Med* 54:599–606, 2007.
229. Hüttinger C, Hirschberger J, Jahnke A, et al: Neoadjuvant gene delivery of feline granulocyte-macrophage colony-stimulating factor using magnetofection for the treatment of feline fibrosarcomas: a phase I trial, *J Gene Med* 10:655–667, 2008.
230. Kent EM: Use of an immunostimulant as an aid in treatment and management of fibrosarcoma in three cats, *Fel Pract* 21:13, 1993.
231. King GK, Yates KM, Greenlace PG, et al: The effect of acemannan immunostimulant in combination with surgery and radiation

therapy on spontaneous canine and feline fibrosarcomas, *J Am Anim Hosp Assoc* 31:439–447, 1995.

232. Quintin-Colonna F, Devauchelle P, Fradelizi D, et al: Gene therapy of spontaneous canine melanoma and feline fibrosarcoma by intratumoral administration of histoincompatible cells expressing human interleukin-2, *Gene Ther* 3:1104–1112, 1996.
233. Giudice C, Stefanello D, Sala M, et al: Feline injection-site sarcoma: recurrence, tumour grading and surgical margin status evaluated using the three-dimensional histological technique, *Vet J* 186:84–88, 2010.
234. Dillon CJ, Mauldin GN, Baer KE: Outcome following surgical removal of nonvisceral soft tissue sarcomas in cats: 42 cases (1992-2000), *J Am Vet Med Assoc* 227:1955–1957, 2005.
235. Macy DW: Current understanding of vaccination site-associated sarcomas in the cat, *J Feline Med Surg* 1:15–21, 1999.
236. Martano M, Morello E, Buracco P: Feline injection-site sarcoma: past, present and future perspectives, *Vet J* 1888:136–141, 2011.
237. Shaw SC, Kent MS, Gordon IK, et al: Temporal changes in characteristics of injection-site sarcomas in cats: 392 cases (1990-2006), *J Am Vet Med Assoc* 234:376–380, 2009.
238. Scott FW, Geissinger CM: Duration of immunity in cats vaccinated with an inactivated feline panleukopenia, herpesvirus, and calicivirus vaccine, *Fel Pract* 25:12, 1997.
239. Scott FW, Geissinger CM: Long-term immunity in cats vaccinated with an inactivated trivalent vaccine, *Am J Vet Res* 60:652–658, 1999.

Cancer of the Gastrointestinal Tract

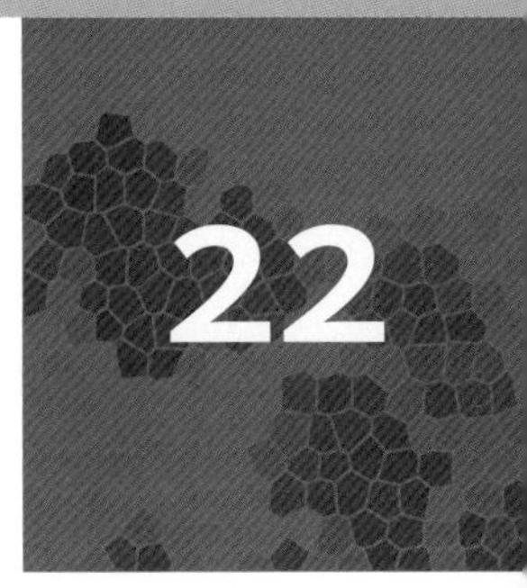

SECTION A
Oral Tumors

JULIUS M. LIPTAK AND STEPHEN J. WITHROW

Incidence and Risk Factors

Collectively, oral cancer accounts for 6% to 7% of canine cancer and is the fourth most common cancer overall.[1,2] In the cat, it accounts for 3% of all cancers.[3] Oropharyngeal cancer is 2.6 times more common in dogs than cats, and male dogs have a 2.4 times greater risk of developing oropharyngeal malignancy compared to female dogs.[4,5] A male sex predisposition has also been reported for dogs with malignant melanoma and tonsillar squamous cell carcinoma (SCC).[6,7] Dog breeds with the highest risk of developing oropharyngeal cancer include the cocker spaniel, German shepherd dog, German shorthaired pointer, Weimaraner, golden retriever, Gordon setter, miniature poodle, Chow Chow, and Boxer.[6,8,9] In one study, German shepherd dogs and Boxers had a decreased risk of developing oral melanoma.[9]

In dogs, the most common malignant oral tumors are, in descending order, malignant melanoma, SCC, and fibrosarcoma,[10-21] although in other studies SCC is more common than malignant melanoma.[2] SCC is the most common oropharyngeal cancer in cats, followed by fibrosarcoma, which accounts for 13% of feline oral tumors.[3] Other malignant oral tumors in dogs include osteosarcoma, chondrosarcoma, anaplastic sarcoma, multilobular osteochondrosarcoma, intraosseous carcinoma, myxosarcoma, hemangiosarcoma, lymphoma, mast cell tumor, and transmissible venereal tumor.[10-24] Tumors or tumorlike lesions of unusual sites, types, and biologic behavior (e.g., tonsillar SCC, tongue, malignancy of young dogs, viral papillomatosis, canine and feline eosinophilic granuloma complex, epulis, inductive fibroameloblastoma, and nasopharyngeal polyps) will be covered at the end of this chapter. A general summary of the common oral tumors is found in Table 22-1.

Pathology and Natural Behavior

The oral cavity is a very common site for a wide variety of malignant and benign cancers. Although most cancers are fairly straightforward histologically, some have confusing nomenclature or extenuating circumstances that warrant discussion.

Malignant Melanoma

In comparison to other malignant oral tumors, malignant melanoma tends to occur in smaller body weight dogs. Cocker spaniel, miniature poodle, Anatolian sheepdog, Gordon setter, Chow Chow, and golden retriever are overrepresented breeds.[9] A male predisposition has been reported,[7] but this is not consistent.[9] The mean age at presentation is 11.4 years.[9] Malignant melanoma occurs in cats but is uncommon.[25]

Malignant melanoma can present a confusing histopathologic picture if the tumor or the biopsy section does not contain melanin, and amelanotic melanomas represent one-third of all cases. A histopathologic diagnosis of undifferentiated or anaplastic sarcoma or even epithelial cancer should be viewed with suspicion for possible reclassification as melanoma. Melan A is an immunohistochemical stain with a moderate sensitivity and specificity for the diagnosis of melanoma in dogs and can be used to differentiate melanoma from other poorly differentiated oral tumors and may be helpful in differentiation.[9]

Melanoma of the oral cavity is a highly malignant tumor with frequent metastasis to the regional lymph nodes and then the lungs.[7,26,27] The metastatic rate is site, size, and stage dependent and reported in up to 80% of dogs.* The World Health Organization (WHO) clinical staging system for oral tumors in dogs may have prognostic significance in dogs with oral melanoma (Table 22-2).[7,26,31,36-38] Malignant melanoma is a highly immunogenic tumor, and molecular and immunomodulatory approaches to treatment are active areas of research.[33,34,39-47] A review of the biology and molecular mechanisms of canine melanoma development and progression is provided in Chapter 19.[48,49]

Squamous Cell Carcinoma

SCC is the most common oral tumor in cats and the second most common in dogs.[1,3,18-21] In cats, the risk of developing oral SCC is significantly increased by over 3.5-fold with the use of flea collars and high intake of either canned food in general or canned tuna fish specifically.[50] Exposure to household smoke increases the risk of oral SCC by twofold in cats,[50] and although this was not statistically significant, smoke exposure is associated with a significant increase in expression of *p53* in SCC lesions compared to cats with oral SCC not exposed to environmental smoke.[51] For this reason, mutations of *p53* may be involved in the development and progression of smoke-related oral SCC in cats.

SCC frequently invades bone in both cats and dogs, and bone invasion is usually severe and extensive in the cat. Increased tumor expression of parathyroid hormone–related protein in cats with oral SCC may play a role in bone resorption and tumor invasion.[52] Paraneoplastic hypercalcemia has also been reported in two cats with oral SCC.[53] Metastasis in the cat is rare and the true incidence is unknown because so few cats have had their local disease controlled; thus an accurate estimate of the metastatic potential has not been confirmed. The metastatic rate for non–tonsillar SCC in dogs

*References 7, 10, 18, 19, 26-35.

TABLE 22-1 Summary of Common Oral Tumors in the Dog and Cat*

	CANINE				FELINE	
	MALIGNANT MELANOMA	SCC	FIBROSARCOMA	ACANTHOMATOUS AMELOBLASTOMA	SCC	FIBROSARCOMA
Frequency	30%-40%	17%-25%	8%-25%	5%	70%-80%	13%-17%
Median age (years)	12	8-10	7-9	8	10-12	10
Sex Predisposition	None-Male	None	Male	None	None	None
Animal size	Smaller	Larger	Larger	None	—	—
Site predilection	Gingival, buccal, and labial mucosa	Rostral mandible	Maxillary gingiva and hard palate	Rostral mandible	Tongue, pharynx, and tonsils	Gingiva
Lymph node metastasis	Common (41%-74%)	Rare (<40%) Tonsil SCC up to 73%	Occasional (9%-28%)	None	Rare	Rare
Distant metastasis	Common (14%-92%)	Rare (<36%)	Occasional (0%-71%)	None	Rare	Rare (<20%)
Gross appearance	Pigmented (67%) or amelanotic (33%), ulcerated	Red, cauliflower, ulcerated	Flat, firm, ulcerated	Red, cauliflower, ulcerated	Proliferative, ulcerated	Firm
Bone involvement	Common (57%)	Common (77%)	Common (60%-72%)	Common (80%-100%)	Common	Common
Surgery response	Fair to good	Good	Fair to good	Excellent	Poor	Fair
Local recurrence	0%-59%	0%-50%	31%-60%	0%-11%		
MST	5-17 months	9-26 months	10-12 months	>28-64 months	45 days	
1-year survival rate	21%-35%	57%-91%	21%-50%	72%-100%	<10%	
Radiation response	Good	Good	Poor to fair	Excellent	Poor	Poor
Response rate	83%-94%	—	—	—		
Local recurrence	11%-27%	31%-42%	32%	8%-18%		
MST	4-12 months	16-36 months	7-26 months	37 months	90 days	
1-year survival rate	36%-71%	72%	76%	>85%		
Best treatment	Surgery and/or radiation ± chemotherapy ± immunotherapy	Surgery and/or radiation	Surgery and/or radiation	Surgery	Surgery and radiation ± sensitizer	Surgery and/or radiation
Prognosis	Fair to good	Good-excellent	Good	Excellent	Poor-fair	Fair
MST	<36 months	26-36 months	18-26 months	>64 months	14 months	
Cause of death	Distant disease	Local or distant disease	Local disease	Rarely tumor related	Local disease	Local disease

SCC, Squamous cell carcinoma; *MST,* Mean survival time.

*References 11-21, 28-32, 37, 53, 57-60, 78, 84-86, 104-111.

TABLE 22-2 Clinical Staging (TNM) of Oral Tumors in Dogs and Cats

Clinical Staging System for Oral Tumors	
Primary Tumor (T)	
Tis	Tumor in situ
T1	Tumor <2 cm in diameter at greatest dimension
T1a	Without evidence of bone invasion
T1b	With evidence of bone invasion
T2	Tumor 2-4 cm in diameter at greatest dimension
T2a	Without evidence of bone invasion
T2b	With evidence of bone invasion
T3	Tumor >4 cm in diameter at greatest dimension
T3a	Without evidence of bone invasion
T3b	With evidence of bone invasion
Regional Lymph Nodes (N)	
N0	No regional lymph node metastasis
N1	Movable ipsilateral lymph nodes
N1a	No evidence of lymph node metastasis
N1b	Evidence of lymph node metastasis
N2	Movable contralateral lymph nodes
N2a	No evidence of lymph node metastasis
N2b	Evidence of lymph node metastasis
N3	Fixed lymph nodes
Distant Metastasis (M)	
M0	No distant metastasis
M1	Distant metastasis [specify site(s)]

STAGE GROUPING	TUMOR (T)	NODES (N)	METASTASIS (M)
I	T1	N0, N1a, N2a	M0
II	T2	N0, N1a, N2a	M0
III	T3	N0, N1a, N2a	M0
	Any T	N1b	M0
IV	Any T	N2b, N3	M0
	Any T	Any N	M1

Data from Owen LN: *TNM classification of tumors in domestic animals,* Geneva, 1980, WHO.

is approximately 20%,[32] but the metastatic risk is site dependent—the rostral oral cavity has a low metastatic rate and the caudal tongue and tonsil have a high metastatic potential.

Fibrosarcoma

Oral fibrosarcoma is the second most common oral tumor in cats and the third most common in dogs.[1,3,18-21,54] In dogs, oral fibrosarcoma tends to occur in large breed dogs, particularly golden and Labrador retrievers; at a younger age, with a median of 7.3 to 8.6 years; and with a possible male predisposition. Oral fibrosarcoma will often look surprisingly benign histologically and, even with large biopsy samples, the pathologist can find it difficult to differentiate fibroma from low-grade fibrosarcoma. This syndrome, which is common on the hard palate (Figure 22-1) and maxillary arcade between the canine and carnassial teeth of large-breed dogs, has been termed *histologically low-grade but biologically high-grade fibrosarcoma.*[54] Even with a biopsy result suggesting fibroma or low-grade fibrosarcoma, the treatment should be aggressive, especially if the cancer is rapidly growing, recurrent, or invading bone.

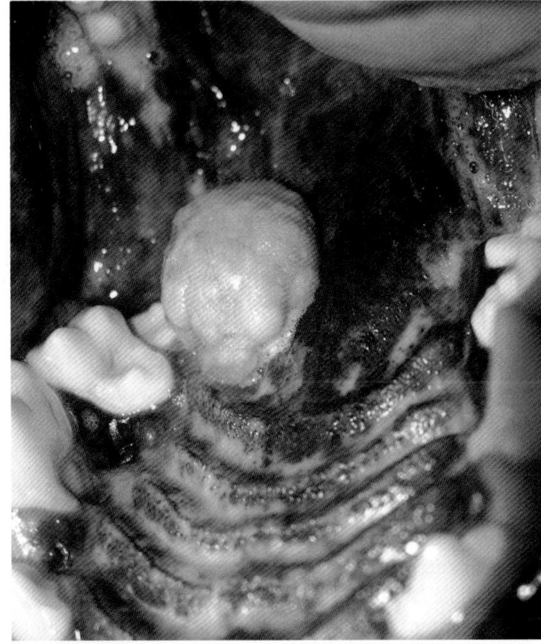

FIGURE 22-1 A histologically low-grade but biologically high-grade fibrosarcoma in the palate of a golden retriever. The tumor appears circumscribed and benign, but aggressive surgical resection and possibly postoperative radiation therapy (RT) are required for local tumor control.

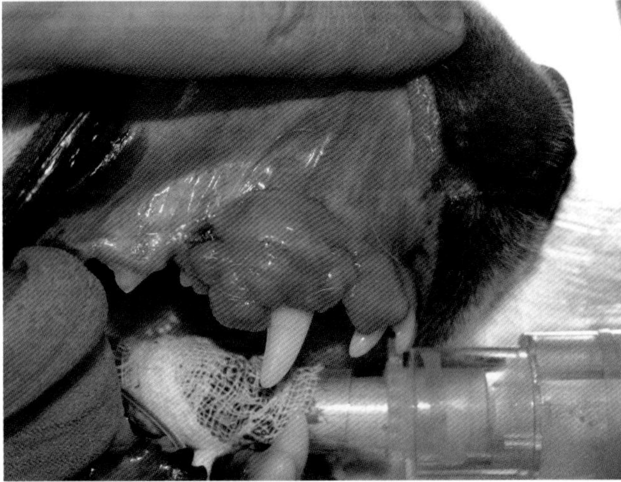

FIGURE 22-2 Typical appearance of a peripheral odontogenic fibroma. The mass is firmly adhered to the underlying bone but does not invade bone. Conservative resection with cautery was curative in this dog.

Fibrosarcoma is locally invasive but metastasizes to the lungs and occasionally regional lymph nodes in less than 30% of dogs.[10,18-21,32]

Epulides

Epulides are benign gingival proliferations arising from the periodontal ligament and appear similar to gingival hyperplasia (Figure 22-2). Three types of epulides have previously been described in the dog: acanthomatous, fibromatous, and ossifying.[56-58] However, the terminology for these tumors has changed; acanthomatous epulis is now termed *acanthomatous ameloblastoma* and peripheral odontogenic fibroma is the preferred nomenclature for fibrous and ossifying epulides.[59]

Peripheral Odontogenic Fibroma

Epulides are relatively common in dogs but rare in cats. Multiple epulides have been described in cats with 50% of cases occurring in cats younger than 3 years.[55] The mean age at presentation for dogs with peripheral odontogenic fibromas is 8 to 9 years, and a male predisposition has been reported in one study.[57,58] Peripheral odontogenic fibromas are slow-growing, firm masses that are usually covered by intact epithelium. They have a predilection for the maxilla rostral to the third premolar teeth.[58,59]

Acanthomatous Ameloblastoma

Acanthomatous ameloblastoma has an aggressive local behavior and frequently invades bone of the underlying mandible or maxilla. Shetland and Old English sheepdogs are predisposed.[57,58] The mean age at presentation is 7 to 10 years, and a sex predisposition is unlikely with three studies reporting conflicting results.[57,60,61] The rostral mandible is the most common site.[60] They do not metastasize. *Acanthomatous ameloblastoma* is the preferred term, but some pathologists will refer to these tumors by their previous terminology of *acanthomatous epulis* or *adamantinoma.*[56]

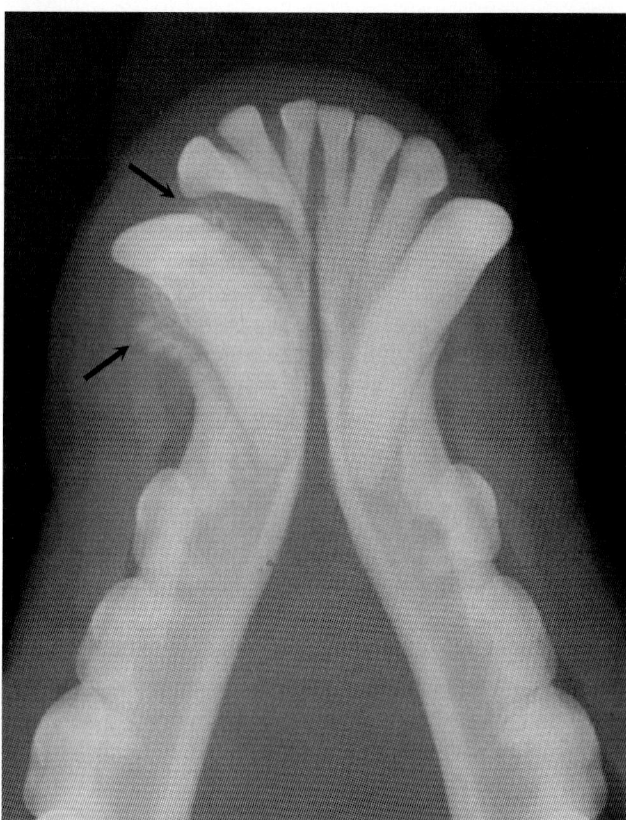

FIGURE 22-3 An intraoral radiograph of the rostral mandible of a dog with an acanthomatous ameloblastoma. Note the bone lysis and loosening of the incisor teeth.

History and Clinical Signs

Most cats and dogs with oral cancer present with a mass in the mouth noticed by the owner. Cancer in the caudal pharynx, however, is rarely seen by the owner, and the animal will present for signs of increased salivation, exophthalmos or facial swelling, epistaxis, weight loss, halitosis, bloody oral discharge, dysphagia or pain on opening the mouth, or occasionally cervical lymphadenopathy (especially SCC of the tonsil).[18-21,62] Loose teeth, especially in an animal with generally good dentition, should alert the clinician to possible underlying neoplastic bone lysis (Figure 22-3), especially in the cat.[63] Although paraneoplastic syndromes associated with oral tumors are rare, hypercalcemia has been reported in two cats with oral SCC[51] and hyperglycemia in a cat with a gingival vascular hamartoma.[64]

Diagnostic Techniques and Work-Up

The diagnostic evaluation for oral cancers is critical due to the wide ranges of cancer behavior and therapeutic options available. If the tumor is suspected of being malignant, thoracic radiographs and lymph node cytologic assessment can be performed prior to biopsy. The most likely cancers to metastasize visibly on thoracic radiographs at the time of diagnosis are melanoma and SCC of the caudal oral, pharyngeal, and tonsillar area. Most animals will require a short general anesthesia for careful palpation, regional imaging, and a biopsy.

Cancers that are adherent to bone, other than peripheral odontogenic fibromas, should have regional radiographs taken under general anesthesia. Regional radiographs include open mouth, intraoral, oblique lateral, and ventrodorsal or dorsoventral projections.[65] Bone lysis is not radiographically evident until 40% or more of the cortex is destroyed (Figure 22-4). However, apparently normal radiographs do not exclude bone invasion. This evaluation will assist in determining clinical staging information and the extent of resection when surgery is indicated. Computed tomography (CT) or magnetic resonance imaging (MRI) can be a very valuable staging tool, especially for evaluation of bone invasion and possible tumor extension into the nasal cavity or in the caudal pharynx and orbit, and is preferred to regional radiographs when available (Figure 22-5).[66]

Regional lymph nodes should be carefully palpated for enlargement or asymmetry. However, caution should be exercised when making clinical judgments of whether neoplastic involvement of regional lymph nodes is present. Lymph node size is not an accurate predictor of metastasis. In one study of 100 dogs with oral melanoma, 40% of dogs with normal-sized lymph nodes had metastasis and 49% of dogs with enlarged lymph nodes did not have metastasis.[27] The regional lymph nodes include the mandibular, parotid, and medial retropharyngeal lymph nodes; however, the parotid and medial retropharyngeal lymph nodes are normally not palpable.[67] Furthermore, only 55% of 31 cats and dogs with metastasis to the regional lymph nodes had metastasis to the mandibular lymph node.[68] Lymphoscintigraphy or contrast-enhanced ultrasonography can be used to detect the sentinel lymph nodes and guide lymph node aspirates.[69] Lymph node aspiration should be performed in all animals with oral tumors, regardless of the size or degree of fixation of the lymph nodes.[27,68] En bloc resection of the regional lymph nodes has been described and, although the therapeutic benefit of this approach is unknown, it may provide valuable staging information.[67,68] Based on these diagnostic steps, oral tumors are then clinically staged according to the WHO staging scheme (see Table 22-2).[36]

The last step, under the same anesthesia, is a large incisional biopsy. Cytologic touch or aspiration preparations of oral tumors

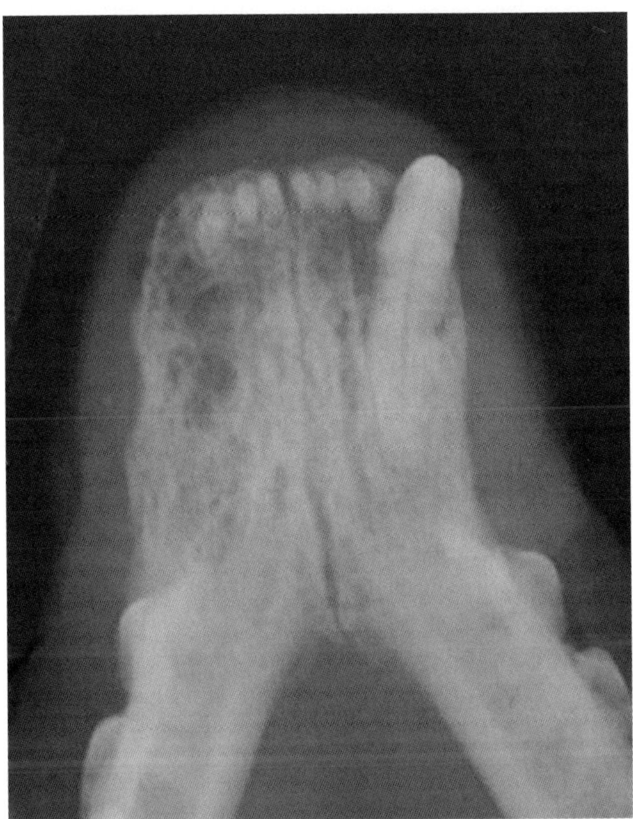

FIGURE 22-4 An intraoral radiograph of the rostral mandible of a cat with a SCC. Note the extensive, ill-defined bone lysis that is very common in cats with this type of tumor.

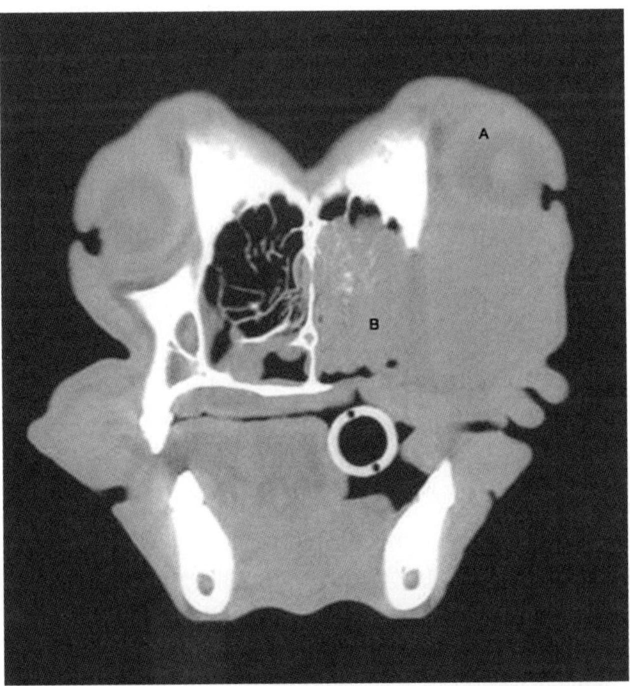

FIGURE 22-5 A CT image of a dog with a maxillary fibrosarcoma. Advanced imaging allows better planning of surgery and radiation therapy (RT) because the extent of bone involvement and extension into the nasal cavity is often much greater than can be appreciated grossly.

are usually not rewarding because of the necrosis and inflammation that commonly accompanies these cancers. Dogs with exophytic or ulcerated masses will generally tolerate a deep wedge or core punch biopsy without general anesthesia. Biopsy is recommended to differentiate benign from malignant disease, for owners basing their treatment options on prognosis, and when other treatment modalities such as radiation therapy (RT) arc being considered. Oral cancers are commonly infected, inflamed, or necrotic, and it is important to obtain a large specimen. Electrocautery may distort the specimen and should only be used for hemostasis after blade incision or punch biopsy. Large samples of healthy tissue at the edge and center of the lesion will increase the diagnostic yield, but care must be taken not to contaminate normal tissue, which cannot be removed with surgery or included in the radiation field. Biopsies should always be performed from within the oral cavity and not through the lip to avoid seeding tumor cells in normal skin and compromising curative-intent surgical resection. For small lesions (e.g., epulides, papillomas, or small labial mucosal melanoma), curative-intent resection (excisional biopsy) may be undertaken at the time of initial evaluation. For more extensive disease, waiting for biopsy results to accurately plan treatment is strongly encouraged.

Therapy

Surgery

Surgery and RT are the most common treatments used for the local control of oral tumors. Surgical resection is the most economic, expeditious, and curative treatment. The type of oral surgery depends on tumor histology and location. Except for peripheral odontogenic fibromas, most oral tumors have some underlying bone involvement and surgical resection should include bony margins to increase the likelihood of local tumor control. More aggressive surgeries such as mandibulectomy, maxillectomy, and orbitectomy are generally well tolerated by cats and dogs. These procedures are indicated for all aggressive and/or invasive oral tumors, particularly lesions with extensive bone invasion, with poor sensitivity to RT, or that are too large for cryosurgery (Tables 22-3 and 22-4).[11-21,70-73] Margins of at least 2 cm are necessary for malignant cancers such as SCC, malignant melanoma, and fibrosarcoma in the dog. If possible, SCC in the cat should be treated with surgical margins greater than 2 cm because of high local recurrence rates. Bone reconstruction following bony resection has been described but is rarely necessary.[13,74-76] Rostral and segmental resections (e.g., mandibulectomy and maxillectomy) may be sufficient for benign lesions and rostral SCC in dogs. Rim resections with a biradial oscillating saw, in which the ventral cortex of the mandible is preserved, may be possible for small benign tumors localized to the alveolar margin of the mandible (Figure 22-6).[77] Larger resections, including hemimandibulectomy, hemimaxillectomy, orbitectomy, and radical maxillectomy, are necessary for more aggressive tumors, especially fibrosarcoma, and malignant tumors with a more caudal location.[11-21,70-72] Although these large resections carry some morbidity, owner satisfaction with the cosmetic and functional outcomes is in excess of 85%.[11-21,71,73,78] Cosmesis is usually very good following most mandibulectomy and maxillectomy procedures (Figure 22-7) but can be challenging with aggressive bilateral rostral mandibulectomies and radical maxillectomies.[11-21,70-72] Blood loss and hypotension are the most common intraoperative complications, particularly during caudal or aggressive maxillectomy procedures.[19,71] Postoperative complications include incisional dehiscence, epistaxis, increased salivation, mandibular drift

TABLE 22-3 Various Mandibulectomies

MANDIBULECTOMY PROCEDURE	INDICATIONS	COMMENTS
Unilateral rostral	Lesions confined to rostral hemimandible; not crossing midline	Most common tumor types are squamous cell carcinoma and adamantinoma that do not require removal of entire affected bone; tongue may lag to resected side. 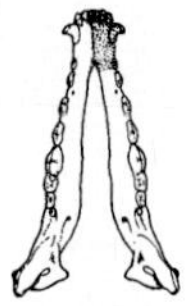
Bilateral rostral	Bilateral rostral lesions crossing the symphysis	Tongue will be "too long," and some cheilitis of chin skin will occur; has been performed as far back as PM4 but preferably at PM1. 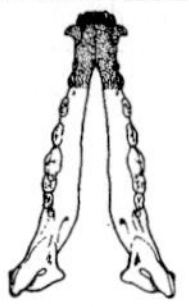
Vertical ramus	Low-grade bony or cartilaginous lesions confined to vertical ramus	These tumors are variously called *chondroma rodens* or *multilobular osteosarcoma;* temporomandibular joint may be removed; cosmetics and function are excellent. 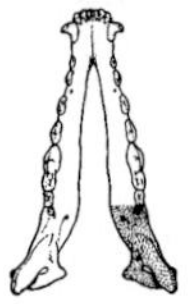
Complete unilateral	High-grade tumors with extensive involvement of horizontal ramus or invasion into medullary canal of ramus	Usually reserved for aggressive tumors; function and cosmetics are good. 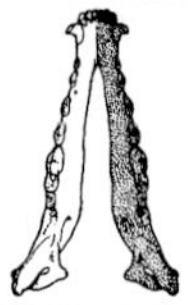
Segmental	Low-grade midhorizontal ramus cancer, preferably not into medullary cavity	Poor choice for highly malignant cancer in medullary cavity because growth along mandibular artery, vein, and nerve is common. 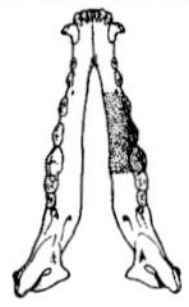

TABLE 22-4 Various Maxillectomies

MAXILLECTOMY PROCEDURE	INDICATIONS	COMMENTS
Unilateral rostral	Lesions confined to hard palate on one side	One-layer closure. 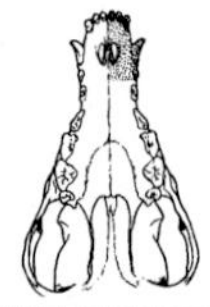
Bilateral rostral	Bilateral lesions of rostral hard palate	Needs viable buccal mucosa on both sides for flap closure. 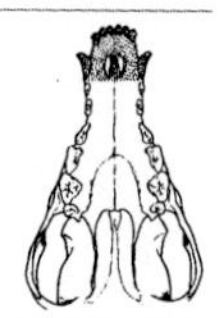
Lateral	Laterally placed midmaxillary lesions	Single-layer closure if small defect, two-layer if large. 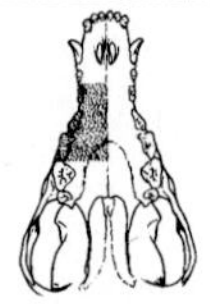
Bilateral	Bilateral palatine lesions	High rate of closure dehiscence because lip flap rarely reaches from side to side; may result in permanent oronasal fistula. 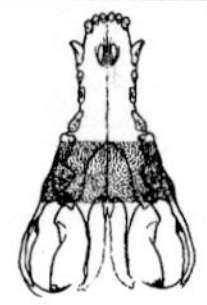

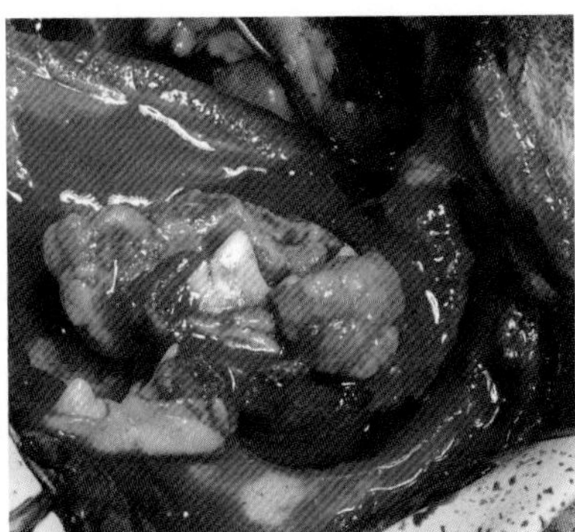

FIGURE 22-6 A rim resection has been performed for removal of an acanthomatous ameloblastoma with 1-cm margins. Note that the ventral cortex of the mandible has been preserved. Preservation of the ventral cortex prevents the development of mandibular drift and malocclusion.

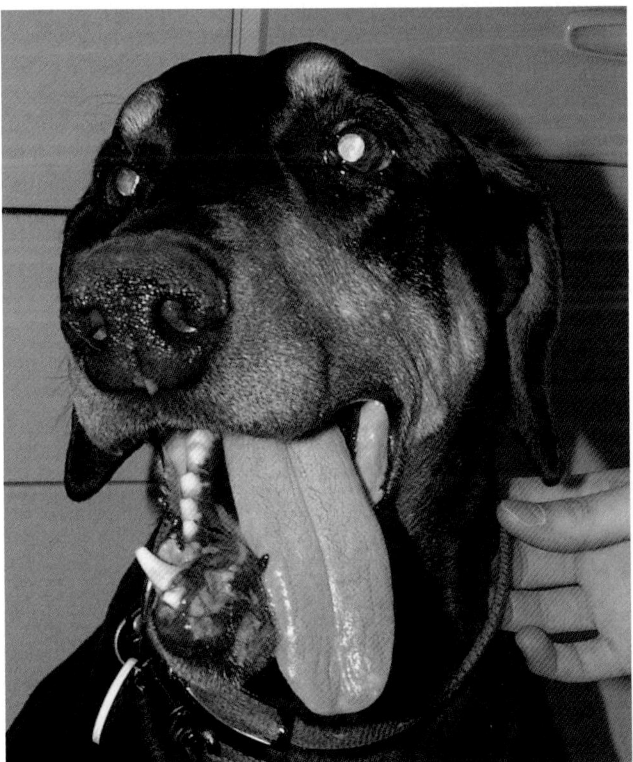

FIGURE 22-7 The typical appearance of a dog 6 months postoperatively after subtotal unilateral mandibulectomy for an osteosarcoma. The tongue will often hang out and the remaining hemimandible will drift towards the resected side.

and malocclusion, and difficulty prehending food, particularly after bilateral rostral mandibulectomy caudal to the second premolar teeth.[13-21,53,71] Elastic training, consisting of an orthodontic elastic rubber chain between an orthodontic button on the lingual aspect of the intact mandible tooth and buccal aspect of the maxillary fourth premolar tooth, has been described to maintain occlusion and prevent mandibular drift following mandibulectomy in dogs.[79] Enteral feeding tubes are not usually required following oral surgery in dogs; however, they are recommended for cats treated with any type of mandibulectomy because eating can be difficult for 2 to 4 months following surgery.[53,78]

Local disease control is the goal of treatment for most animals with oral tumors. Regional lymph node resection has been described in cats and dogs; although it adds to clinical staging information, its effectiveness in controlling local and metastatic disease is unknown.[67,68]

Cryosurgery may be indicated for lesions less than 2 cm in diameter that are fixed or minimally invasive into bone. Larger lesions should generally be surgically resected. More extensive lesions in bone will often result in a fracture (mandible) or oronasal fistula (maxilla) if aggressively frozen. Cancer of soft tissue only should be surgically excised and not frozen.

Radiation Therapy

RT can be effective for locoregional control of oral tumors. RT can be used as a primary treatment, with either palliative or curative intent, or as an adjunct for incompletely resected tumors or tumors with an aggressive local behavior, such as oral fibrosarcoma. Malignant melanoma, canine oral SCC, and some benign tumors, such as the acanthomatous ameloblastoma, are known to be radiation responsive, and RT should be considered in the primary treatment of these tumors.[31-33,80,81] For canine oral SCC, dental tumors, and fibrosarcoma, daily and alternate day protocols have been described consisting of 2.7 Gy to 4.2 Gy per fraction with a total dose ranging from 48 Gy to 57 Gy.[32,82] Tumor control is better for smaller benign and malignant lesions (T1 and T2 tumors) treated with radiation alone.[31,32,80] Local tumor control and survival time may be improved by combining RT with surgery and/or chemotherapy, especially for tumors considered radiation resistant, such as canine oral fibrosarcoma and feline oral SCC.[53,83-88] Radiation sensitizers, such as etanidazole and gemcitabine, may improve response rates in cats with oral SCC, and platinum drugs have been used as radiation sensitizers in dogs with oral melanoma.[28,37,84,87,88] However, gemcitabine is not recommended as a radiosensitizer in cats because of significant hematologic and local tissue toxicities.[89]

Oral melanoma is moderately responsive to coarse fractionation protocols. Four different hypofractionated radiation protocols have been described: (1) three weekly 8- to 10-Gy fractions for a total dose of 24 to 30 Gy,[30,37] (2) four weekly fractions of 9 Gy for a total dose of 36 Gy,[31,37] (3) six weekly 6-Gy fractions for a total dose of 36 Gy,[28] and (4) eight weekly 6-Gy fractions for a total dose of 48 Gy.[90] In humans, the effect of total radiation dose is controversial, but fraction size does have an impact on response rates. Doses greater than 4 Gy per fraction are recommended as response rates are significantly better with fractions greater than 8 Gy compared to less than 4 Gy.[91] However, in one study of dogs with oral melanoma comparing two hypofractionated protocols of 9 to 10 Gy per fraction to a fully fractionated protocol of 2 to 4 Gy per fraction, there were no significant differences in either local recurrence rates or survival time.[37] Coarse fractionation of oral melanoma has also been described in five cats with limited success, including one complete response and two partial responses.[25]

Acute effects are common but self-limiting. These include alopecia and moist desquamation, oral mucositis, dysphagia, and ocular changes, such as blepharitis, conjunctivitis, keratitis, and uveitis.[32,80,92-94] The acute effects of coarse fractionation are less than experienced with the full-course protocols used for oral SCC and dental tumors and usually resolve rapidly.[31] Late complications are rare, occurring in less than 5% of cases, but can include permanent alopecia, skin fibrosis, bone necrosis and oronasal fistula formation, development of a second malignancy within the radiation field, keratoconjunctivitis sicca, cataract formation, xerostomia, and retinal atrophy.[32,61,80,95] Orthovoltage radiation may be associated with a higher incidence of second malignancies and bone necrosis than megavoltage irradiation.[32,61,80]

Hyperthermia offers no advantage over cryosurgery or surgery if it is used alone. In fact, bone penetration is less reproducible with heat versus cold treatment. Hyperthermia at moderate temperatures (42 to 43°C) has been used as an adjunct to irradiation.[29,96,97]

Chemotherapy

The major problem with most oral tumors is control of local disease. However, chemotherapy is indicated for some tumors with higher metastatic potential, especially oral melanoma in dogs and tonsillar SCC in cats and dogs. Expression of cyclooxygenase 2 (COX-2) has been noted in feline oral SCC[98]; however, nonsteroidal antiinflammatory drugs (NSAIDs) such as piroxicam have not been effective in the management of this disease in cats in preliminary studies.[99] Piroxicam does appear to have some effect against oral SCC in dogs,[100] and response rate is improved when piroxicam is combined with either cisplatin or carboplatin.[101,102] Liposome-encapsulated cisplatin is not effective in cats with oral SCC,[103] but mitoxantrone, in combination with RT, has shown some potential in a limited number of cats with good local responses and durable remission.[85,86]

The platinum drugs show the most promise, albeit modest, in treating dogs with oral melanoma, including intralesional cisplatin[104] and systemic carboplatin.[105] Measurable responses to melphalan have also been reported.[106]

Malignant melanoma is a highly immunogenic tumor. The use of immunomodulatory agents is an emerging and exciting approach for the adjunctive management of dogs with oral melanoma. A thorough discussion of the immunotherapeutic approach to management of canine melanoma is provided in Chapter 19.

Prognosis

Clinical series of over 500 dogs with various oral malignancies treated with either mandibulectomy or maxillectomy have been described.[11-21,70-72] The majority of cases were treated with surgery alone. Unfortunately, the methods of reporting and outcome results vary with each paper, but an attempt to combine cases by tumor type and outcome is shown in Tables 22-5 and 22-6. Overall, the lowest rates of local tumor recurrence and best survival times are reported in dogs with acanthomatous ameloblastoma and SCC, whereas fibrosarcoma and malignant melanoma are associated with the poorest results.[11-21] Most of these reports suggest that histologically complete resection, smaller diameter, and a rostral location are favorable prognostic factors. In two studies of 142 dogs treated with either mandibulectomy or maxillectomy, tumor-related deaths were 10 to 21 times more likely with malignant tumors, up to 5 times more likely with tumors located caudal to the canine teeth, and 2 to 4 times more likely following incomplete resection.[20,21] Rostral locations are usually detected at an earlier stage and are more likely to be resectable with complete surgical margins. Local tumor recurrence is more frequent following incomplete resection, with 15% to 22% and 62% to 65% of tumors recurring following complete and incomplete excision, respectively.[20,21] Recurrent disease negatively impacts survival time because further treatment is more difficult and the response to treatment is poorer.[35] Fibrosarcoma continues to have an unacceptable local recurrence rate and needs to be addressed with wider resections or other adjuvant therapies, such as postoperative radiation.[82] On the other hand, melanoma is controlled locally in 75% of cases, but metastatic disease requires more effective adjuvant therapy, such as RT, chemotherapy, or immunotherapy.

For dogs treated with megavoltage radiation, tumor type and tumor size are important factors in local tumor control for both benign and malignant oral tumors. As noted previously,

TABLE 22-5 Postoperative Outcome After Mandibulectomy for Different Tumor Types*

Tumor Type	Number	Local Recurrence (%)	Median Survival Time (Months)	1-Year Survival Rate (%)
Malignant melanoma	81	0-40	7-17	21
Squamous cell carcinoma	74	0-23	9-26	80-91
Fibrosarcoma	58	31-60	11-12	23-50
Osteosarcoma	144	15-44	6-18	35-71
Acanthomatous ameloblastoma	116	0-3	>28-64	98-100

*References 11-21, 57-60, 124-126.

TABLE 22-6 Postoperative Outcome After Maxillectomy for Different Tumor Types*

Tumor Type	Number	Local Recurrence (%)	Median Survival Time (Months)	1-Year Survival Rate (%)
Malignant melanoma	37	21-48	5-10	27
Squamous cell carcinoma	13	29-50	19	57
Fibrosarcoma	33	33-57	10-12	21-50
Osteosarcoma	50	27-100	4-10	17-27
Acanthomatous ameloblastoma	30	0-11	>26-30	72-100

*References 11-21, 56-58, 119-121.

acanthomatous ameloblastoma and SCC in dogs are radiation sensitive. Local recurrence is reported in 30% of oral tumors regardless of treatment, but recurrence is a function of tumor size. Compared to small tumors (T1: <2-cm diameter), recurrence is 3 times more likely in T2 tumors (2- to 4-cm diameter) and up to 8 times more likely in T3 tumors (>4-cm diameter).[32,80] Tumor size is also associated with survival in dogs with malignant oral tumors, with 3-year progression-free survival (PFS) rates of 55%, 32%, and 20% for T1, T2, and T3 tumors, respectively.[32]

Malignant Melanoma

The prognosis for dogs with oral melanoma is guarded. Metastatic disease is the most common cause of death with metastasis to the lungs reported in 14% to 67% of dogs.* Surgery or RT can provide good local control, but strategies to manage the high metastatic potential such as chemotherapy and immunotherapy require further investigation.

Surgery is the most common treatment for management of the local tumor. The local tumor recurrence rate varies from 22% following mandibulectomy to 48% after maxillectomy.[7,18,19] The median survival time (MST) for dogs with malignant melanoma treated with surgery alone varies from 150 to 318 days with 1-year survival rates less than 35%.† Regardless, tumor control and survival time are significantly better when surgery is included in the treatment plan.[38] In comparison, the MST for untreated dogs with oral melanoma is 65 days.[35] Variables known to have prognostic significance in dogs treated with surgery alone or in combination with other modalities include tumor size, clinical stage, and ability of the first treatment to achieve local control.‡ Dogs with tumors less than 2-cm in diameter have a MST of 511 days compared to 164 days for dogs with tumors greater than 2-cm diameter or lymph node metastasis.[33] MSTs are significantly shorter for dogs with recurrent oral malignant melanomas compared to dogs with previously untreated oral melanomas.[26,35]

Oral melanoma is responsive to hypofractionated RT protocols. Response rates are excellent with 83% to 100% of tumors responding and a complete response observed in up to 70% of melanomas.[28,30-32,90] Local recurrence is reported in 15% to 26% of dogs experiencing a complete response with a median time to local recurrence of 139 days.[28,30-32] Progressive local disease was observed in all dogs that did not achieve a complete response in one study.[30] The most common cause of death is metastasis and this is reported in 58% of dogs with a median time of metastasis of 311 days.[28] The MST for dogs treated with RT is 211 to 363 days, with a 1-year survival rate of 36% to 48% and a 2-year survival rate of 21%.[28,30-32,37] Local tumor control and survival time are significantly improved with rostral tumor location, smaller tumor volume, no radiographic evidence of bone lysis, and postoperative irradiation of microscopic disease.[31,32,37] The risk factors associated with poor outcomes in dogs with melanoma include nonrostral location, bone lysis, and macroscopic disease, and in one series of 140 dogs with oral melanoma, the MST was 21 months if none of these risk factors were present compared to a MST of 11 months with one risk factor, 5 months with two risk factors, and 3 months with all three risk factors.[37] Tumor size is important with median PFS for dogs with T1 oral melanomas of 19 months compared to less than 7 months for T2 and T3 tumors.[32] Hypofractionated RT has also been described in five cats with oral melanoma, resulting in a 60% response rate and MST of 146 days (range: 66 to 224 days).[25]

Chemotherapy or immunotherapy is indicated in the adjunctive management of dogs with oral melanoma because of the high metastatic risk. A thorough discussion of malignant melanoma and its prognosis following definitive treatment with surgery, RT, chemotherapy, and/or immunomodulatory agents is provided in Chapter 19.

The location of malignant melanoma may also have some prognostic significance. Melanomas of the lip and tongue have a lower metastatic rate and survival is more dependent on local control of the tumor. In one series of 60 dogs with oral melanomas at various sites treated with combinations of surgery, RT, chemotherapy, and immunotherapy, the MST for dogs with lip melanomas was 580 days and was not reached and greater than 551 days for dogs with tongue melanomas.[7] In comparison, the MST was 319 days for maxillary melanomas and 330 days for melanomas of the hard palate.[7]

In another study, only 5% of 64 dogs with well-differentiated melanomas of the mucous membranes of the lips and oral cavities treated with surgery alone had died from tumor-related reasons with an overall MST of 34 months.[109] This improved prognosis may reflect the location of these lesions (lip compared to oral cavity) or the degree of differentiation. Nuclear atypia and mitotic index has also been shown to be prognostic in dogs with oral malignant melanomas.[110]

Squamous Cell Carcinoma

Canine Oral Squamous Cell Carcinoma

The prognosis for dogs with oral SCC is good, particularly for rostral tumor locations. Local tumor control is usually the most important challenge, although metastasis to the regional lymph nodes is reported in up to 10% of dogs and to the lungs in 3% to 36% of dogs.[32] In contrast, SCC of the tonsils and base of the tongue are highly metastatic, with metastasis reported in up to 73% of dogs, and locoregional recurrence is common.[111-113] Surgery and RT can both be used for locoregional control of oral SCC in dogs. Photodynamic therapy has also been reported with fair-to-good results in 11 dogs with smaller oral SCC.[114]

Surgery is the most common treatment for non-tonsillar SCC.[11] Following mandibulectomy, the local recurrence rate is 10% and the MST varies from 19 to 26 months with a 91% 1-year survival time.[18] In comparison, the local recurrence rate is 29% after maxillectomy with a MST of 10 to 19 months and a 1-year survival rate of 57%.[19] The higher local control and survival rates with mandibular resections probably result because the rostral mandible is the most common location for oral SCC in dogs, and complete surgical resection is more likely for rostral locations.

Full-course RT, either alone or as an adjunct following incomplete surgical resection, is also a successful treatment modality for the management of oral SCC in dogs.[32,115,116] The local tumor recurrence rate is 31%. The MST for RT alone is 15 to 16 months and increases to 34 months when combined with surgery.[115,116] In one series of 39 dogs with oral SCC, the overall median PFS time was 36 months with 1- and 3-year PFS rates of 72% and 55%, respectively.[32] Local tumor control was more successful with smaller lesions; the median PFS time for T1 tumors (<2-cm diameter) was not reached and greater than 68 months compared to 28 months for T2 tumors (2- to 4-cm diameter) and 8 months for dogs with T3 tumors (>4-cm diameter).[32] Additional favorable prognostic factors for dogs receiving orthovoltage irradiation include rostral tumor location, maxillary SCC, and young age.[115] Younger age is

*References 7, 10, 18, 19, 26-35.

†References 7, 9, 18-21, 26, 34, 35, 58.

‡References 7, 26, 28, 29, 31-35.

also favorable for dogs treated with megavoltage radiation (< 9 years of age—1080 days; > 9 years of age—315 days).[116]

Chemotherapy is indicated for dogs with metastatic disease, dogs with bulky disease, and when owners decline surgery and RT. However, as the metastatic potential of oral SCC in dogs is relatively low, the role of chemotherapy in minimizing the risk of metastatic disease is unknown. In a series of 17 dogs treated with piroxicam alone, the response rate was 17%, with one complete response and two partial responses.[100] The median progression-free interval for dogs responding to piroxicam was 180 days and significantly longer than the 102 days for dogs with stable disease.[100] The outcome is better when piroxicam is combined with either cisplatin or carboplatin. In a series of nine dogs treated with piroxicam and cisplatin, the overall MST was 237 days, with the 56% of dogs responding to this chemotherapy protocol having a significantly better outcome than nonresponders with a MST of 272 days compared to 116 days.[101] However, renal toxicity was reported in 41% of dogs in this study and such toxicities limit the clinical usefulness of this protocol. In another small series of seven dogs with T3 oral SCC treated with piroxicam and carboplatin, a complete response was observed in 57% of dogs and this response was sustained in all dogs at the median follow-up time of 534 days.[102] Novel therapies under investigation include the combination of intralesional bleomycin and feline interleukin-12 (IL-12) DNA with translesional electroporation.[107]

Feline Oral Squamous Cell Carcinoma

The prognosis for cats with oral SCC is poor.[14,62,117,118] There is no known effective treatment that consistently results in durable control or survival. Local control is the most challenging problem. In one series of 52 cats, the 1-year survival rate was less than 10%, with MSTs of 3 months or less for surgery alone, surgery and RT, RT and low-dose chemotherapy, or RT and hyperthermia.[62] However, 42% of these cats had SCC involving the tongue, pharynx, or tonsils. In another series of 54 cats treated in general practice, the MST was 44 days with a 9.5% 1-year survival rate.[119] The oncologic outcome may be better for cats with mandibular SCC. The MST for seven cats treated with a combination of mandibulectomy and RT was 14 months with a 1-year survival rate of 57%.[53] Local recurrence was the cause of failure in 86% of these cats between 3 to 36 months after therapy. In another series of 22 cats treated with mandibulectomy alone, the median disease-free interval (DFI) was 340 days.[78] Tumor location and extent of resection had prognostic importance with a MST of 911 days for rostral tumors, 217 days following hemimandibulectomy, and 192 days when more than 50% of the mandible was resected.[78] Expansile, blastic, and discrete lesions are often more resectable than invasive, lytic, and ill-defined lesions in the experience of the authors. The use of esophagostomy or gastrostomy tubes may be necessary to provide supplemental nutrition in these cats for up to 4 months postoperatively.[78]

RT alone is generally considered ineffective in the management of cats with oral SCC. In nine cats treated with an accelerated radiation protocol (14 fractions of 3.5 Gy delivered twice daily for 9 days), the overall MST was 86 days and, although not significant, the MST for cats with a complete response was 298 days.[81] The combination of RT with radiation sensitizers or chemotherapy improves response rates and survival times. Using the same accelerated radiation protocol with carboplatin resulted in a MST of 163 days in 14 cats.[88] Intratumoral etanidazole, a hypoxic cell sensitizer, resulted in a 100% partial response rate in nine cats completing the RT course with a median decrease in tumor size of 70% and a MST of 116 days.[84] Gemcitabine was used at low doses as a radiation sensitizer in eight cats with oral SCC with an overall response rate of 75%, including two cats with complete responses, for a median duration of 43 days and a MST of 112 days.[87] However, gemcitabine is not recommended as a radiosensitizer in cats because of significant hematologic and local tissue toxicities.[89] The combination of RT with mitoxantrone holds some promise because, in two series of 18 cats, a complete response was observed in 73% with a median duration of response of 138 to 170 days and an MST of 184 days.[85,86] Palliative radiation protocols, consisting of 8 Gy fractions on days 0, 7, and 21, are not recommended because of poor disease control and radiation-induced adverse effects.[120] Localized irradiation with strontium-90 may be effective for selected cats with very superficial disease.[121]

Chemotherapy appears ineffective in the management of cats with oral SCC. No responses were observed in 18 cats treated with liposome-encapsulated cisplatin or 13 cats treated with piroxicam.[99,103] In one study, the administration of a NSAID improved survival times in cats with oral SCC.[119]

Fibrosarcoma

The prognosis for dogs with oral fibrosarcoma is guarded. These are locally aggressive tumors and local control is more problematic than metastasis. Metastasis is reported to the regional lymph nodes in 19% to 22% of dogs and to the lungs in up to 27% of dogs.[18,19,32] Multimodality treatment of local disease appears to afford the best survival rates, with combinations of surgery and RT or RT and hyperthermia.[29,78]

Surgery is the most common treatment for oral fibrosarcoma. The median DFI for five cats treated with mandibulectomy was 859 days.[78] Following mandibulectomy, local recurrence is reported in 59% of dogs with a MST of 11 months and a 1-year survival rate of 50%.[18] The outcome is similar following maxillectomy, with local recurrence in 40% of dogs and a MST of 12 months.[19] One-year survival rates rarely exceed 50% with surgery alone.[11-21] The combination of surgery and RT provides the best opportunity to control local disease.

Oral fibrosarcomas are considered radiation resistant.[83,122,123] The mean survival time of 17 dogs treated with RT alone was only 7 months.[83] RT combined with regional hyperthermia improved local control rates to 50% at 1 year in a series of 10 cases.[29] When RT is used as an adjunct to surgical resection, local tumor recurrence was reported in 32% of dogs overall and the MST increased to 18 to 26 months with a 1-year PFS rate of 76%.[32,82] A smaller tumor size improves the outcome following RT, with a median PFS time of 45 months for dogs with T1 tumors compared to 31 months and 7 months for T2 and T3 tumors, respectively.[32]

Osteosarcoma

Osteosarcoma of axial sites is less common than appendicular osteosarcoma and represents approximately 25% of all cases.[124] Of the axial osteosarcomas, the mandible and maxilla are involved in 27% and 16% to 22% of cases, respectively.[124,125] The prognosis for dogs with oral osteosarcoma is better than appendicular osteosarcoma because of an apparent lower metastatic potential.[119] A female sex predisposition has been reported.[124]

The outcome following mandibulectomy alone is variable with MSTs of 14 to 18 months and 1-year survival rates of 35% to 71%.[18,124,126] In 20 dogs treated with mandibulectomy alone, the cause of death was local recurrence in 15% of dogs and metastatic disease in 35% of dogs.[18] Following maxillectomy, the MST varies from 5 to 10 months with a 1-year survival rate of 17% to 27% and local tumor recurrence in 83% to 100% of dogs.[19,124] The majority of dogs with maxillary osteosarcoma die as a result of local tumor recurrence with metastasis not reported in any dogs in two studies.[106,125]

Local tumor control is the most challenging problem and resecting oral osteosarcomas with complete surgical margins is imperative. In one study of 60 dogs with osteosarcoma of the skull, including the mandible and maxilla, the median DFI and survival times were not reached at greater than 1503 days following complete excision and significantly better than incomplete resection with a median DFI of 128 days and a MST of 199 days.[127] The combination of surgery with either RT or chemotherapy did not improve the outcome in dogs with incompletely resected tumors, highlighting the necessity for an aggressive surgical approach. These results are supported by another study of 45 dogs with axial osteosarcoma in which favorable prognostic factors included complete surgical excision, mandibular location, and smaller body weight dogs.[125] Chemotherapy's role in the management of dogs with axial osteosarcoma is unknown but should be evaluated.

Epulides

Peripheral Odontogenic Fibroma

The prognosis for dogs with peripheral odontogenic fibromas is excellent following treatment with either surgery or rarely RT. These are benign tumors and metastasis has not been reported; hence local tumor control is the principal goal of therapy. For peripheral odontogenic fibromas, the local tumor recurrence rate following surgical resection without bone removal varies from 0% to 17%.[57,128] RT is also effective with a 3-year PFS rate of 86%.[80] However, full-course RT is usually not required because these tumors can be adequately managed with simple surgical resection.[57] Local recurrence is common in cats with multiple epulides and is reported in 73% of 11 cats 3 months to 8 years after surgical resection.[55]

Acanthomatous Ameloblastoma

Surgery or RT is also used in the management of dogs with acanthomatous ameloblastoma. Mandibulectomy or maxillectomy is required for surgical resection of acanthomatous ameloblastomas because of frequent bone invasion by this benign tumor. Local recurrence rates following bone-removing surgery are less than 5%.* Megavoltage RT, consisting of an alternate day protocol of 4 Gy per fraction to a total of 48 Gy, results in a 3-year PFS rate of 80% in dogs with acanthomatous ameloblastomas.[80] The overall local recurrence rate with RT varies from 8% to 18% in two studies of 39 dogs and recurrence was 8 times more likely with T3 tumors compared to T1 and T2 tumors.[61,80] The majority of tumors recur within the radiation field, which suggests a higher radiation dose may be required to achieve higher rates of local tumor control, particularly for tumors greater than 4 cm in diameter.[80] Other complications associated with RT include malignant transformation in 5% to 18% of dogs and bone necrosis in 6% of dogs.[61,80] Intralesional bleomycin has been described in four dogs, and a complete response was observed in all dogs and was sustained for a minimum of 1 year with no local recurrence.[129]

Selected Sites or Cancer Conditions in the Oral Cavity

Tonsillar Squamous Cell Carcinoma

Tonsillar SCC is 10 times more common in animals living in urban versus rural areas, implying an etiologic association with environmental pollutants.[130] Primary tonsillar cancer is often SCC. Lymphoma can affect the tonsils but is usually accompanied by generalized lymphadenopathy and is often bilateral. Other cancers, especially malignant melanoma, can metastasize to the tonsils. Cervical lymphadenopathy is a common presenting sign, even with very small primary tonsillar cancers. Fine-needle aspirates of the regional lymph nodes or excisional biopsy of the tonsil will confirm the diagnosis. Thoracic radiographs are positive for metastasis in 10% to 20% of cases at presentation. In spite of disease apparently confined to the tonsil, this disease is considered systemic at diagnosis in over 90% of cats and dogs. Simple tonsillectomy is almost never curative but probably should be done bilaterally due to the high percentage of bilateral disease.[10] Cervical lymphadenectomy, especially if the regional lymph nodes are large and fixed, is rarely curative and should be considered diagnostic only. Regional RT of the pharyngeal region and cervical lymph nodes is capable of controlling local disease in over 75% of the cases; however, survival still remains poor with 1-year survival rates of only 10%.[111,113] Local tumor control and survival times were significantly improved in one study of 22 dogs with tonsillar SCC when RT was combined with a variety of different chemotherapy drugs.[113] Cause of death is local disease early and systemic disease (usually lung metastasis) later. To date, no known effective chemotherapeutic agents exist for canine or feline SCC, although cisplatin, carboplatin, doxorubicin, vinblastine, and bleomycin have been used with limited success.[113,131] In one study of 44 dogs with tonsillar SCC treated with surgery, RT, and/or chemotherapy, the MST was 179 days and dogs presenting with either anorexia or lethargy had a significantly shorter survival time.[132]

Tongue

Cancer confined to the tongue is rare. In one study, 54% of tongue lesions were neoplastic and 64% of these were malignant.[133] White dogs appear to be at higher risk for SCC, even though lack of pigment would not seem to be as much a problem as it is in other more exposed areas of the body (e.g., nose, eyelids, and ears).[134] Other reported breed predilections include Chow Chow and Chinese Shar-Pei for malignant melanoma; poodle, Labrador retriever, and Samoyed for SCC; border collie and golden retriever for hemangiosarcoma and fibrosarcoma; and cocker spaniel for plasma cell tumors.[133] The most common cancer of the canine tongue is SCC, accounting for approximately 50% of cases, followed by granular cell myoblastoma, malignant melanoma, mast cell tumor, fibrosarcoma, adenocarcinoma, neurofibrosarcoma, leiomyosarcoma, hemangiosarcoma and hemangioma, rhabdomyoma and rhabdomyosarcoma, myxoma, and lipoma.[133-135] Feline tongue tumors are usually SCCs, and most are located on the ventral surface near the frenulum. Presenting signs are similar to other oral tumors. Ulceration is common with SCC.

Under general anesthesia, the tongue may be biopsied with a wedge incision and closed with horizontal mattress sutures. Biopsies are necessary to differentiate malignant tumors from nonneoplastic lesions such as eosinophilic granuloma, inflammatory disease, and calcinosis circumscripta. Ultrasonography can be useful in delineating the margins of tongue masses to determine surgical resectability.[136] Regional lymph nodes should be aspirated for staging purposes and three-view thoracic radiographs evaluated for lung metastasis.

Surgical resection is recommended, whereas RT is reserved for melanomas, inoperable cancer, or tumors metastatic to the regional lymph nodes. Partial glossectomy of up to 60% of the tongue has been recommended for unilateral tumors not crossing the midline

*References 11, 13, 18, 19, 57, and 60.

or tumors confined to the rostral mobile portion of the tongue. However, 54% of canine tongue tumors are located in the midline or are bilaterally symmetrical, which limits the ability to achieve complete surgical resection.[112] Recently, 50% to 100% resection or avulsion of the tongue was reported in five dogs with minimal postoperative problems, which suggests more aggressive resections may be possible without compromising quality of life.[137] Feeding tubes are recommended for enteral nutrition during postoperative recovery but, in the long term, eating and drinking are usually only mildly impaired and good hydration and nutrition can be maintained postoperatively.[134,137] Hypersalivation is the most common complaint following aggressive resections.[137] Thermoregulation can be a problem in hot and humid environments. Grooming in cats will be compromised and may result in poor hair-coat hygiene.

The prognosis for tongue tumors depends on the site, type, and grade of cancer.[134] Tongue SCCs in dogs are graded from I (least malignant) to III (most malignant) based on histologic features such as degree of differentiation and keratinization, mitotic rate, tissue and vascular invasion, nuclear pleomorphism, and scirrhous reaction.[134] The MST for dogs with grade I tongue SCC is 16 months following surgical resection, which is significantly better than the MSTs of 4 and 3 months reported for grade II and III SCC, respectively.[134] The 1-year survival rate is 50% following complete surgical resection and approaches 80% with complete histologic resection of low-grade SCC.[134] Cancer in the rostral (mobile) tongue has a better prognosis possibly because rostral lesions are detected at an earlier stage, the caudal tongue may have richer lymphatic and vascular channels to allow metastasis, and rostral tumors are easier to resect with wide margins. Long-term control of feline tongue tumors is rarely reported with 1-year survival rates for tongue SCC less than 25%.

Granular cell myoblastoma is a curable cancer.[138] These cancers may look large and invasive but are almost always removable by conservative and close margins (Figure 22-8). Permanent local control rates exceed 80%. They may recur late, but serial surgeries are usually possible. Metastasis is rare with this cancer. Local control in four of five tongue melanomas was obtained by surgery, and the metastatic rate was less than 50% in this small series.[117] In another series of dogs with tongue melanoma, the MST was not reached and was greater than 551 days.[7] The biologic behavior of other tongue cancers is generally unknown due to the rarity of these conditions.[117]

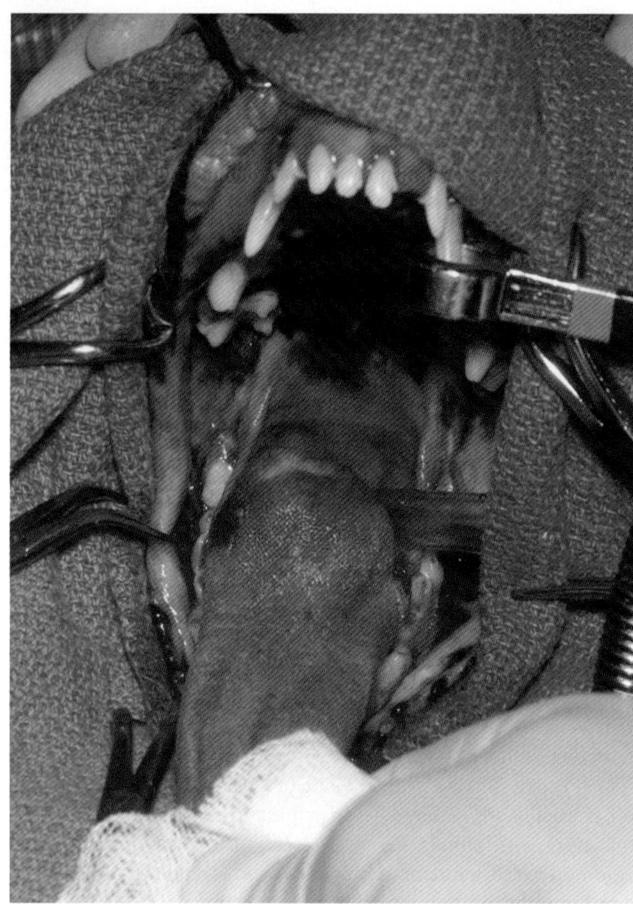

FIGURE 22-8 This large granular cell myoblastoma was easily removed surgically. The dog had a recurrence 2 years postoperatively, which was resected again, and the dog is tumor-free 3 years after the second surgery.

Undifferentiated Malignancy of Young Dogs

Undifferentiated malignancy is seen in dogs under 2 years of age (range: 6 to 22 months).[139] Most dogs are large breeds and there is no sex predilection. The disease is manifest by a rapidly growing mass in the area of the hard palate, upper molar teeth, maxilla, and/or orbit. Biopsies reveal an undifferentiated malignancy of undetermined histiogenesis. The majority of dogs present with metastasis to the regional lymph nodes and distant sites beyond the head and neck. An effective treatment has not been identified, although chemotherapy would be necessary considering the high metastatic rate. Most dogs are euthanatized within 30 days of diagnosis due to progressive and uncontrolled tumor growth.

Papillary SCC has been reported to occur in the oral cavity of very young dogs (2 to 5 months of age). Treatment recommendations include complete surgical resection or surgical cytoreduction and curettage followed by radiation (40 Gy in 20 fractions). Using this latter combination therapy, no dog had metastasis and long-term control was achieved in all dogs for periods up to 4 years.[140]

Multilobular Osteochondrosarcoma

Multilobular osteochondrosarcoma is an infrequently diagnosed bony and cartilaginous tumor that usually arises from the canine skull, including the mandible, maxilla, hard palate, orbit, and calvarium.[23,24] Histologically, these tumors are characterized by multiple lobules with a central cartilaginous or bone matrix surrounded by a thin layer of spindle cells.[23,24] On imaging, multilobular osteochondrosarcoma is characterized by a typical "popcorn" appearance (Figure 22-9). Surgery is recommended for management of the local tumor, although there are anecdotal reports that multilobular osteochondrosarcoma may also be responsive to RT. The overall rate of local recurrence following surgical resection is 47% to 58% and depends on completeness of surgical resection and histologic grade.[23,24] The median DFI for completely resected multilobular osteochondrosarcoma is 1332 days and significantly better than the 330 days reported for incompletely excised tumors.[24] In terms of tumor grade, the local recurrence rate for grade III tumors is 78% and significantly worse than the recurrence rates of 30% and 47% for grade I and II multilobular osteochondrosarcoma, respectively.[24] This tumor has a moderate metastatic potential (usually to the lung), which is grade dependent, but usually occurs late in the

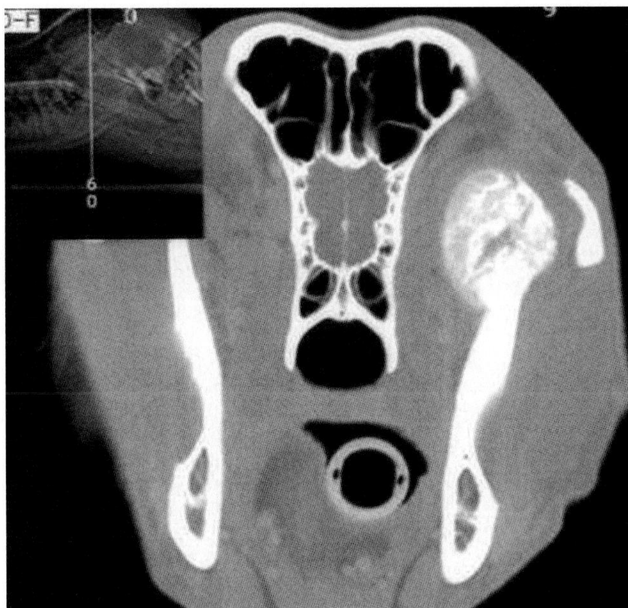

FIGURE 22-9 A CT image of a multilobular osteochondrosarcoma of the vertical ramus of the mandible. Note the characteristic "popcorn" appearance of the mass. Following resection of the vertical ramus, this dog was tumor-free 3 years after surgery.

course of disease. Metastasis is reported in up to 58% of dogs with the median time to metastasis of 426 to 542 days.[23,24] Metastasis is significantly more likely following incomplete surgical resection, with a 25% metastatic rate in completely excised tumors and 75% following incomplete resection.[24] Tumor grade also has a significant impact on metastatic rate with metastasis reported in 78% of grade III multilobular osteochondrosarcoma compared to 30% of grade I and 60% of grade II tumors.[24] There is no known effective chemotherapy treatment for metastatic disease, but survival times greater than 12 months have been reported with pulmonary metastasectomy because of the slow-growing nature of this tumor.[24] The overall MST is 21 months and is grade dependent, with reported MSTs of 50 months, 22 months, and 11 months for grade I, II, and III tumors, respectively.[23,24] Tumor location also has prognostic significance because the outcome for dogs with mandibular multilobular osteochondrosarcoma is significantly better with a MST of 1487 days compared to 587 days for these tumors at other sites.[24]

Viral Papillomatosis

Viral papillomatosis is horizontally transmitted by a DNA viral agent (papovavirus) from dog to dog.[141] Affected animals are generally young. The lesions appear wartlike and are generally multiple in the oral cavity, pharynx, tongue, or lips. A biopsy can be performed if necessary, but visual examination is usually diagnostic. Most patients never suffer any significant side effects of this disease, although an occasional dog will have such marked involvement as to require surgical or cryosurgical cytoreduction in order to permit swallowing. The majority of patients will undergo a spontaneous regression of disease within 4 to 8 weeks. For resistant cases, an immunodeficiency etiology is suggested and a wide variety of treatments have been attempted, including crushing lesions in situ to "release" viral antigens and using several immunomodulators, including autogenous vaccines, interleukins, levamisole, thiabendazole, imiquimod, and L-MTP-PE.[142] However, these methods are seldom required or effective. Furthermore, autogenous vaccines are not recommended because malignant skin tumors have been reported at the site of inoculation.[56] The prognosis is usually excellent.

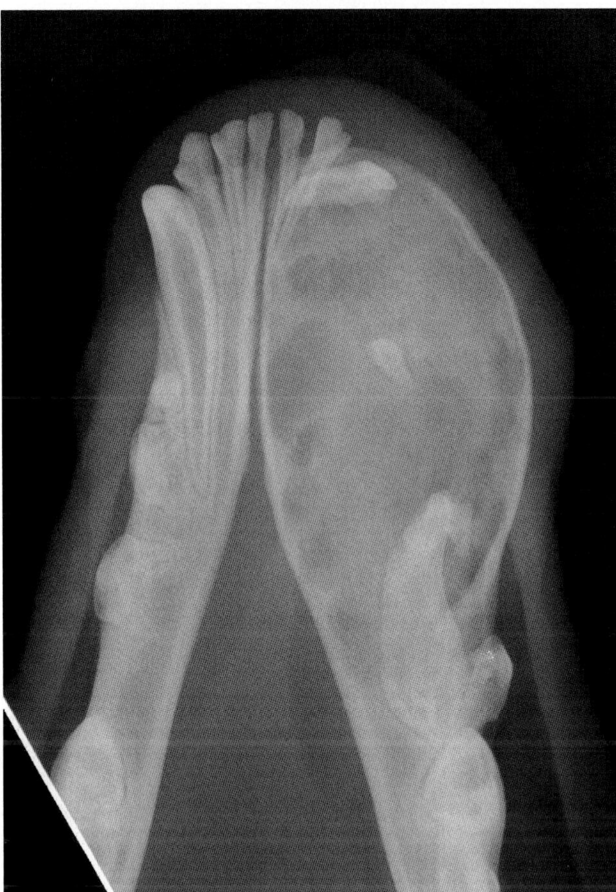

FIGURE 22-10 An intraoral radiograph of the rostral mandible in a dog with an ameloblastoma. Note the smooth expansile mandibular mass. The tumor was curetted and filled with cancellous bone graft and the dog was tumor-free 1 year after surgery.

Odontogenic Tumors

Odontogenic tumors originate from epithelial cells of the dental lamina and account for up to 2.4% of all feline oral tumors.[3] They are broadly classified into two groups depending on whether the tumors are able to induce a stromal reaction.[143] Inductive odontogenic tumors include ameloblastic fibroma, dentinoma, and ameloblastic, complex, and compound odontomas. Ameloblastomas and calcifying epithelial odontogenic tumors are examples of noninductive odontogenic tumors.[143]

Inductive fibroameloblastoma is the most common odontogenic tumor in cats, usually occurs in cats less than 18 months of age, and has a predilection for the region of the upper canine teeth and maxilla.[3,56,143-145] Radiographically the tumor site shows variable degrees of bone destruction, production, and expansion of the mandibular or maxillary bones (Figure 22-10). Teeth deformity is common. Smaller lesions are treated with surgical debulking and cryosurgery or premaxillectomy. Larger lesions will respond to radiation. Local treatment needs to be aggressive, but control rates are good and metastasis has not been reported.[3,56]

Odontomas are benign tumors arising from the dental follicle during the early stages of tooth development.[146] Odontomas induce both enamel and dentin within the tumor. Odontomas have a similar biologic behavior to ameloblastomas.

Dentigerous cysts are nonneoplastic, circumscribed cystic lesions originating from islands of odontogenic epithelium.[143] They contain one or more teeth embedded in the cyst wall. Radiographs show a characteristic radiolucent halo surrounding the nonerupted tooth originating at the cementoenamel junction and enveloping the crown of the tooth.[65] Odontogenic cysts may represent an early stage of malignant epithelial tumors.[143] Surgical treatment is recommended, consisting of surgical removal of nonerupted teeth and the cyst lining with possible cancellous bone grafting, to prevent local tumor recurrence.[65]

Eosinophilic Granulomas

Eosinophilic Granulomas in Dogs

Canine oral eosinophilic granulomas affect young dogs (1 to 7 years of age) and may be heritable in the Siberian husky and Cavalier King Charles spaniel.[147-149] It is histologically similar to the feline disease, with eosinophils and granulomatous inflammation predominating. The granulomas typically occur on the lateral and ventral aspects of the tongue. They are raised, frequently ulcerated, and may mimic more malignant cancers in gross appearance. Treatment with corticosteroids or surgical excision is generally curative, although spontaneous regression may occur. Local recurrences are uncommon.

Eosinophilic Granuloma in the Cat

Eosinophilic granuloma, a condition also known as rodent ulcer or indolent ulcer, occurs more commonly in female cats with a mean age of 5 years.[150-153] The etiology is unknown. Any oral site is at risk, but it is most common on the upper lip near the midline (Figure 22-11). The history is usually that of a slowly progressive (months to years) erosion of the lip. Biopsies are often necessary to differentiate the condition from true cancers.

Various treatments are proposed, including (in order of author preference): oral prednisone at 1 to 2 mg/kg twice a day (BID) for 30 days or subcutaneous methylprednisolone acetate* at 20 mg/cat every 2 weeks, megestrol acetate,† hypoallergenic diets, RT, surgery, immunomodulation, or cryosurgery. The prognosis for complete and permanent recovery is fair, although rare cases may undergo spontaneous regression.

Nasopharyngeal Polyps in Cats

Nasopharyngeal polyps are nonneoplastic, inflammatory masses originating from either the middle ear or eustachian tube and can extend into the external ear canal or nasopharynx.[154,155] Young cats are usually affected, with a mean age of 13.6 months in one series of 31 cats.[154,156] The cause is unknown, but a viral etiology and congenital abnormality of the branchial arches have been suggested.[155] Clinical signs include sneezing, change in voice, swallowing problems, rhinitis, and difficulty in breathing. Firm, fleshy masses can be seen or palpated in the caudal pharynx or above the soft palate. Occasionally, masses can be visualized in the external ear canal.[157,158] Radiographs or advanced imaging of the skull may reveal fluid or tissue in the tympanic bullae.[159] Traction on the stalk of the inflammatory polyp, either through the oral cavity or external ear canal depending on accessibility, is recommended for initial treatment of inflammatory polyps. However, recurrences have been reported in four of eight cats treated with this method alone.[154] A ventral bulla osteotomy is recommended for cats with either recurrent inflammatory polyps or evidence of tympanic bulla involvement on skull imaging. Less than 4% of cats have recurrence of inflammatory polyps following bulla osteotomy.[154,158,160]

*Depo-Medrol, Upjohn.

†Ovaban, Schering.

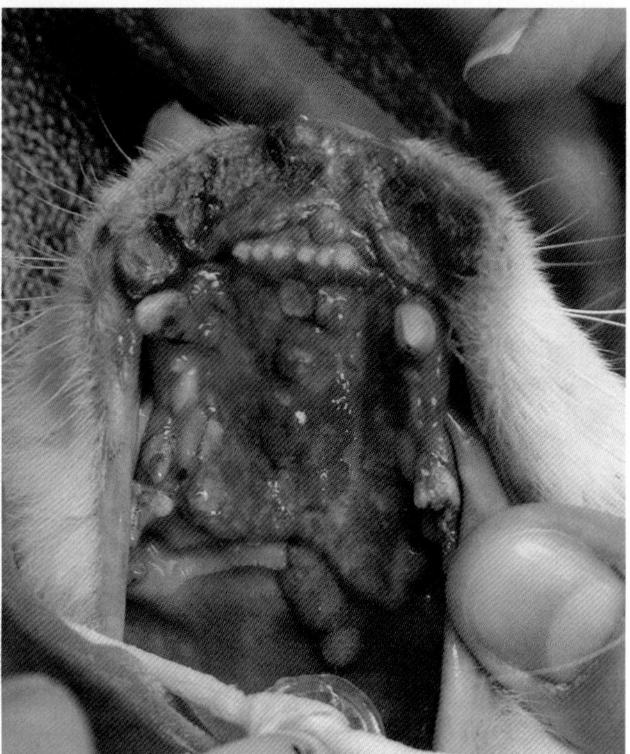

FIGURE 22-11 An extensive eosinophilic granuloma in a cat involving the lips and hard palate. These lesions can appear aggressive and similar to malignant oral tumors such as squamous cell carcinomas (SCCs). An incisional biopsy is often required to differentiate this benign nonsurgical disease from malignant diseases.

Comparative Aspects[161]

SCC accounts for the vast majority of oral cancer in humans. Oral tumors are associated with alcohol and tobacco use and usually occur in patients over 40 years old. Patients with oral cancer have an increased risk of developing esophageal and lung cancer. Tumors are staged similar to animals and clinical stage influences both treatment options and prognosis.

Surgery and RT are the only options that provide the opportunity for a cure. Surgery and radiation are occasionally combined, especially since neither modality is likely to achieve a cure rate greater than 70% when used as sole therapy. Chemotherapy has a limited role for control of local disease but has shown promise, often in combination with radiation, for advanced-stage cancer.

Prognosis is strongly correlated to histologic grade, stage, and site. Metastasis, particularly to the regional lymph nodes, is more frequent with tonsillar and pharyngeal SCC and larger sized tumors. Tumors of the pharynx and caudal tongue are associated with a worse prognosis than cancers of the rostral tongue and oral cavity because of the higher incidence of nodal metastasis and difficulty in controlling disease once it has spread beyond the primary site.

REFERENCES

1. Hoyt RF, Withrow SJ: Oral malignancy in the dog, *J Am Anim Hosp Assoc* 20:83, 1984.
2. Bronden LB, Eriksen T, Kristensen AT: Oral malignant melanomas and other head and neck neoplasms in Danish dogs: data from the Danish Veterinary Cancer Registry, *Acta Vet Scand* 51:54, 2009.
3. Stebbins KE, Morse CC, Goldschmidt MH: Feline oral neoplasia: a ten year survey, *Vet Pathol* 26:121, 1989.
4. Dorn CR, Taylor DON, Frye FL, et al: Survey of animal neoplasms in Alameda and Contra Costa Counties, California. I. Methodology and description of cases, *J Natl Cancer Inst* 40:295, 1968.
5. Dorn CR, Taylor DON, Schneider R, et al: Survey of animal neoplasms in Alameda and Contra Costa Counties, California. II. Cancer morbidity in dogs and cats from Alameda County, *J Natl Cancer Inst* 40:307, 1968.
6. Cohen D, Brodey RS, Chen SM: Epidemiologic aspects of oral and pharyngeal neoplasms in the dog, *Am J Vet Res* 25:1776, 1964.
7. Kudnig ST, Ehrhart N, Withrow SJ, et al: Survival analysis of oral melanoma in dogs, *Vet Cancer Soc Proc* 23:39, 2003.
8. Dorn CR, Priester WA: Epidemiologic analysis of oral and pharyngeal cancer in dogs, cats, horses and cattle, *J Am Vet Med Assoc* 169:1202, 1976.
9. Ramos-Vara JA, Beissenherz ME, Miller MA, et al: Retrospective study of 338 canine oral melanomas with clinical, histologic, and immunohistochemical review of 129 cases, *Vet Pathol* 37:597, 2000.
10. Todoroff RJ, Brodey RS: Oral and pharyngeal neoplasia in the dog: a retrospective survey of 361 cases, *J Am Vet Med Assoc* 175:567, 1979.
11. Withrow SJ, Holmberg DL: Mandibulectomy in the treatment of oral cancer, *J Am Anim Hosp Assoc* 19:273, 1983.
12. Withrow SJ, Nelson AW, Manley PA, et al: Premaxillectomy in the dog, *J Am Anim Hosp Assoc* 21:49, 1985.
13. White RAS, Gorman NT, Watkins SB, et al: The surgical management of bone-involved oral tumours in the dog, *J Small Anim Pract* 26:693, 1985.
14. Bradley RL, MacEwen EG, Loar AS: Mandibular resection for removal of oral tumors in 30 dogs and 6 cats, *J Am Vet Med Assoc* 184:460, 1984.
15. Salisbury SK, Richardson DC, Lantz GC: Partial maxillectomy and premaxillectomy in the treatment of oral neoplasia in the dog and cat, *Vet Surg* 15:16, 1986.
16. Salisbury SK, Lantz GC: Long-term results of partial mandibulectomy for treatment of oral tumors in 30 dogs, *J Am Anim Hosp Assoc* 24:285, 1988.
17. White RAS: Mandibulectomy and maxillectomy in the dog: long-term survival in 100 cases, *J Small Anim Pract* 32:69, 1991.
18. Kosovsky JK, Matthiesen DT, Marretta SM, et al: Results of partial mandibulectomy for the treatment of oral tumors in 142 dogs, *Vet Surg* 20:397, 1991.
19. Wallace J, Matthiesen DT, Patnaik AK: Hemimaxillectomy for the treatment of oral tumors in 69 dogs, *Vet Surg* 21:337, 1992.
20. Schwarz PD, Withrow SJ, Curtis CR, et al: Mandibular resection as a treatment for oral cancer in 81 dogs, *J Am Anim Hosp Assoc* 27:601, 1991.
21. Schwarz PD, Withrow SJ, Curtis CR, et al: Partial maxillary resection as a treatment for oral cancer in 61 dogs, *J Am Anim Hosp Assoc* 27:617, 1991.
22. Richardson RC: Canine transmissible venereal tumor, *Compend Contin Educ Pract Vet* 3:951, 1981.
23. Straw RC, LeCouteur RA, Powers BE, et al: Multilobular osteochondrosarcoma of the canine skull: 16 cases (1978-1988), *J Am Vet Med Assoc* 195:1764, 1989.
24. Dernell WS, Straw RC, Cooper MF, et al: Multilobular osteochondrosarcoma in 39 dogs: 1979-1993, *J Am Anim Hosp Assoc* 34:11, 1998.
25. Farrelly J, Denman DL, Hohenhaus AE, et al: Hypofractionated radiation therapy of oral melanoma in five cats, *Vet Radiol Ultrasound* 45:91, 2004.
26. Overley B, Goldschmidt M, Shofer F, et al: Canine oral melanoma: a retrospective study, *Vet Cancer Soc Proc* 21:43, 2001.
27. William LE, Packer RA: Association between lymph node size and metastasis in dogs with oral malignant melanoma: 100 cases (1987-2001), *J Am Vet Med Assoc* 222:1234, 2003.
28. Freeman KP, Hahn KA, Harris FD, et al: Treatment of dogs with oral melanoma by hypofractionated radiation therapy and platinum-based chemotherapy (1987-1997), *J Vet Intern Med* 17:96, 2003.
29. Brewer WG, Turrel JM: Radiotherapy and hyperthermia in the treatment of fibrosarcomas in the dog, *J Am Vet Med Assoc* 181:146, 1982.
30. Bateman KE, Catton PA, Pennock PW, et al: Radiation therapy for the treatment of canine oral melanoma, *J Vet Intern Med* 8:267, 1994.
31. Blackwood L, Dobson JM: Radiotherapy of oral malignant melanomas in dogs, *J Am Vet Med Assoc* 209:98, 1996.
32. Théon AP, Rodriguez C, Madewell BR: Analysis of prognostic factors and patterns of failure in dogs with malignant oral tumors treated with megavoltage irradiation, *J Am Vet Med Assoc* 210:778, 1997.
33. MacEwen EG, Patnaik AK, Harvey HJ, et al: Canine oral melanoma: comparison of surgery versus surgery plus Corynebacterium parvum, *Cancer Invest* 4:397, 1986.
34. MacEwen EG, Kurzman ID, Vail DM, et al: Adjuvant therapy for melanoma in dogs: results of randomized clinical trials using surgery, liposome-encapsulated muramyl tripeptide and granulocyte-macrophage colony-stimulating factor, *Clin Cancer Res* 5:4249, 1999.
35. Harvey HJ, MacEwen GE, Braun D, et al: Prognostic criteria for dogs with oral melanoma, *J Am Vet Med Assoc* 178:580, 1981.
36. Owen LN: *TNM classification of tumors in domestic animals*, Geneva, 1980, WHO.
37. Proulx DR, Ruslander DM, Dodge RK, et al: A retrospective analysis of 140 dogs with oral melanoma treated with external beam radiation, *Vet Radiol Ultrasound* 44:352, 2003.
38. Hahn KA, DeNicola DB, Richardson RC, et al: Canine oral malignant melanoma: prognostic utility of an alternative staging system, *J Small Anim Pract* 35:251, 1994.
39. Moore AS, Theilen GH, Newell AD, et al: Preclinical study of sequential tumor necrosis factor and interleukin 2 in the treatment of spontaneous canine neoplasms, *Cancer Res* 51:233, 1991.
40. Elmslie RE, Dow SW, Potter TA: Genetic immunotherapy of canine oral melanoma, *Vet Cancer Soc Proc* 14:111, 1994.
41. Elmslie RE, Potter TA, Dow SW: Direct DNA injection for the treatment of malignant melanoma, *Vet Cancer Soc Proc* 15:52, 1995.
42. Dow SW, Elmslie RE, Willson AP, et al: In vivo tumor transfection with superantigen plus cytokine genes induces tumor regression and prolongs survival in dogs with malignant melanoma, *J Clin Invest* 101:2406, 1998.
43. Hogge G, Burkholder J, Culp J, et al: Development of human granulocyte-macrophage colony-stimulating factor-transfected tumor cell vaccines for the treatment of spontaneous cancer, *Human Gene Ther* 9:1851, 1998.
44. Quintin-Colonna F, Devauchelle P, Fradelizi D, et al: Gene therapy of spontaneous canine melanoma and feline fibrosarcoma by intratumoral administration of histoincompatible cells expressing human interleukin-2, *Gene Ther* 3:1104, 1996.
45. Bergman PJ, Camps-Palau MA, McKnight JA, et al: Development of a xenogeneic DNA vaccine program for canine malignant melanoma with prolongation of survival in dogs with locoregionally controlled stage II-III disease, *Vet Cancer Soc Proc* 23:40, 2003.
46. Bergman PJ, McKnight J, Novosad A, et al: Long-term survival of dogs with advanced malignant melanoma after DNA vaccination with xenogeneic human tyrosinase: a phase I trial, *Clin Cancer Res* 9:1284, 2003.

47. Bergman PJ, Camps-Palau MA, McKnight JA, et al: Phase I & IB trials of murine tyrosinase ± human GM-CSF DNA vaccination in dogs with advanced malignant melanoma, *Vet Cancer Soc Proc* 24:55, 2004.
48. Modiano JF, Ritt MG, Wojcieszyn J: The molecular basis of canine melanoma: pathogenesis and trends in diagnosis and therapy, *J Vet Intern Med* 13:163, 1999.
49. Sulaimon SS, Kitchell BE: The basic biology of malignant melanoma: molecular mechanisms of disease progression and comparative aspects, *J Vet Intern Med* 17:760, 2003.
50. Bertone ER, Snyder LA, Moore AS, et al: Environmental and lifestyle risk factors for oral squamous cell carcinoma in domestic cats, *J Vet Intern Med* 17:557, 2003.
51. Snyder LA, Bertone ER, Jakowski RM, et al: p53 expression and environmental tobacco smoke exposure in feline oral squamous cell carcinoma, *Vet Pathol* 41:209, 2004.
52. Martin CK, Tannehill-Gregg SH, Wolfe TD, et al: Bone-invasive oral squamous cell carcinoma in cats: pathology and expression of parathyroid hormone-related protein, *Vet Pathol* 48:302, 2011.
53. Hutson CA, Willauer CC, Walder EJ, et al: Treatment of mandibular squamous cell carcinoma in cats by use of mandibulectomy and radiotherapy: seven cases (1987-1989), *J Am Vet Med Assoc* 201:777, 1992.
54. Ciekot PA, Powers BE, Withrow SJ, et al: Histologically low grade yet biologically high grade fibrosarcomas of the mandible and maxilla of 25 dogs (1982-1991), *J Am Vet Med Assoc* 204:610, 1994.
55. Colgin LMA, Schulman FY, Dubielzig RR: Multiple epulides in 13 cats, *Vet Pathol* 38:227, 2001.
56. Dubielzig RR: Proliferative dental and gingival disease of dogs and cats, *J Am Anim Hosp Assoc* 18:577, 1982.
57. Bjorling DE, Chambers JN, Mahaffey EA: Surgical treatment of epulides in dogs: 25 cases (1974-1984), *J Am Vet Med Assoc* 190:1315, 1987.
58. Yoshida K, Yanai T, Iwasaki T, et al: Clinicopathological study of canine oral epulides, *J Vet Med Sci* 61:897, 1999.
59. Fiani N, Vertstraete FJ, Kass PH, et al: Clinicopathologic characterization of odontogenic tumors and focal fibrous hyperplasia in dogs: 152 cases (1995-2005), *J Am Vet Med Assoc* 238:495, 2011.
60. White RAS, Gorman NT: Wide local excision of acanthomatous epulides in the dog, *Vet Surg* 18:12, 1989.
61. Thrall DE: Orthovoltage radiotherapy of acanthomatous epulides in 39 dogs, *J Am Vet Med Assoc* 184:826, 1984.
62. Reeves NCP, Turrel JM, Withrow SJ: Oral squamous cell carcinoma in the cat, *J Am Anim Hosp Assoc* 29:438, 1993.
63. Madewell BR, Ackerman N, Sesline DH: Invasive carcinoma radiographically mimicking primary bone cancer in the mandibles of two cats, *J Am Vet Radiol Soc* 27:213, 1976.
64. Padgett SL, Tillson DM, Henry CJ, et al: Gingival vascular hamartoma with associated paraneoplastic hyperglycemia in a kitten, *J Am Vet Med Assoc* 210:914, 1997.
65. Dhaliwal RS, Kitchell BE, Marretta SM: Oral tumors in dogs and cats. Part I. Diagnosis and clinical signs, *Compend Contin Educ Pract Vet* 20:1011, 1998.
66. Gendler A, Lewis JR, Reetz JA, et al: Computed tomographic features of oral squamous cell carcinoma in cats: 18 cases (2002-2008), *J Am Vet Med Assoc* 236:319, 2010.
67. Smith MM: Surgical approach for lymph node staging of oral and maxillofacial neoplasms in dogs, *J Am Anim Hosp Assoc* 31:514, 1995.
68. Herring ES, Smith MM, Robertson JL: Lymph node staging of oral and maxillofacial neoplasms in 31 dogs and cats, *J Vet Dent* 19:122, 2002.
69. Lurie DM, Seguin B, Verstraete FJ, et al: Contrast-assisted ultrasound for sentinel node detection in canine head and neck neoplasia, *Invest Radiol* 41:415, 2006.
70. Kirpensteijn J, Withrow SJ, Straw RC: Combined resection of the nasal planum and premaxilla in three dogs, *Vet Surg* 23:341, 1994.
71. Lascelles BD, Thomson MJ, Dernell WS, et al: Combined dorsolateral and intraoral approach for the resection of tumors of the maxilla in the dog, *J Am Anim Hosp Assoc* 39:294, 2003.
72. Lascelles BDX, Henderson RA, Seguin B, et al: Bilateral rostral maxillectomy and nasal planectomy for large rostral maxillofacial neoplasms in six dogs and one cat, *J Am Anim Hosp Assoc* 40:137, 2004.
73. Fox LE, Geoghegan SL, Davis LH, et al: Owner satisfaction with partial mandibulectomy or maxillectomy for treatment of oral tumors in 27 dogs, *J Am Anim Hosp Assoc* 33:25, 1997.
74. Boudrieau RJ, Tidwell AS, Ullman SL, et al: Correction of mandibular nonunion and malocclusion by plate fixation and autogenous cortical bone grafts in two dogs, *J Am Vet Med Assoc* 204:774, 1994.
75. Boudrieau RJ, Mitchell SL, Seeherman H: Mandibular reconstruction of a partial hemimandibulectomy in a dog with severe malocclusion, *Vet Surg* 33:119, 2004.
76. Bracker KE, Trout NJ: Use of a free cortical ulnar autograft following en bloc resection of a mandibular tumor, *J Am Anim Hosp Assoc* 36:76, 2000.
77. Arzi B, Verstraete FJ: Mandibular rim excision in seven dogs, *Vet Surg* 39:226, 2010.
78. Northrup NC, Selting KA, Rassnick KM, et al: Outcomes of cats with oral tumors treated with mandibulectomy, *J Am Anim Hosp Assoc* 42:350, 2006.
79. Bar-Am Y, Verstraete FJM: Elastic training for the prevention of mandibular drift following mandibulectomy in dogs: 18 cases (2005-2008), *Vet Surg* 39:574, 2010.
80. Théon AP, Rodriguez C, Griffey S, et al: Analysis of prognostic factors and patterns of failure in dogs with periodontal tumors treated with megavoltage irradiation, *J Am Vet Med Assoc* 210:785, 1997.
81. Fidel JL, Sellon RK, Houston RK, et al: A nine-day accelerated radiation protocol for feline squamous cell carcinoma, *Vet Radiol Ultrasound* 48:482, 2007.
82. Forrest LJ, Chun R, Adams WM, et al: Postoperative radiation therapy for canine soft tissue sarcoma, *J Vet Intern Med* 14:578, 2000.
83. Thrall DE: Orthovoltage radiotherapy of oral fibrosarcomas in dogs, *J Am Vet Med Assoc* 172:159, 1981.
84. Evans SM, LaCreta F, Helfand S, et al: Technique, pharmacokinetics, toxicity, and efficacy of intratumoral etanidazole and radiotherapy for treatment of spontaneous feline oral squamous cell carcinoma, *Int J Radiat Oncol Biol Phys* 20:703, 1991.
85. Personal Communication: LaRue SM, Vail DM, Ogilvie GK, et al: Shrinking-field radiation therapy in combination with mitoxantrone chemotherapy for the treatment of oral squamous cell carcinoma in the cat, *Vet Cancer Soc Proc* 11:99, 1991.
86. Ogilvie GK, Moore AS, Obradovich JE, et al: Toxicoses and efficacy associated with administration of mitoxantrone to cats with malignant tumor, *J Am Vet Med Assoc* 202:1839, 1993.
87. Jones PD, de Lorimier LP, Kitchell BE, et al: Gemcitabine as a radiosensitizer for nonresectable feline oral squamous cell carcinoma, *J Am Anim Hosp Assoc* 39:463, 2003.
88. Fidel J, Lyons J, Tripp C, et al: Treatment of oral squamous cell carcinoma with accelerated radiation therapy and concomitant carboplatin in cats, *J Vet Intern Med* 25:504, 2011.
89. LeBlanc AL, LaDue TA, Turrel JM, et al: Unexpected toxicity following use of gemcitabine as a radiosensitizer in head and neck carcinomas: a Veterinary Radiation Therapy Oncology Group pilot study, *Vet Radiol Ultrasound* 45:466, 2004.
90. Turrel JM: Principles of radiation therapy. In Thielen GH, Madewell BR, editors: *Veterinary cancer medicine*, Philadelphia, 1987, Lea & Febiger.
91. Overgaard J, Overgaard M, Hansen PV, et al: Some factors of importance in the radiation treatment of malignant melanoma, *Radiother Oncol* 5:183, 1986.

92. Roberts SM, Lavach SD, Severin GA, et al: Ophthalmic complications following megavoltage irradiation of the nasal and paranasal cavities in dogs, *J Am Vet Med Assoc* 190:43, 1987.
93. Jamieson VE, Davidson MG, Naisse MP, et al: Ocular complications following cobalt 60 radiotherapy of neoplasms in the canine head region, *J Am Anim Hosp Assoc* 27:51, 1991.
94. LaRue SM, Gillette EL: Radiation therapy. In Withrow SJ, MacEwen EG, editors: *Small animal clinical oncology*, Philadelphia, 2001, Saunders.
95. Thrall DE, Goldschmidt MH, Biery DN: Malignant tumor formation at the site of previously irradiated acanthomatous epulides in four dogs, *J Am Vet Med Assoc* 178:127, 1981.
96. Gillette EL, McChesney SL, Dewhirst MW, et al: Response of canine oral carcinomas to heat and radiation, *Int J Radiat Oncol Biol Phys* 13:1861, 1987.
97. Dewhirst MW, Sim DA, Forsyth K, et al: Local control and distant metastases in primary canine malignant melanomas treated with hyperthermia and/or radiotherapy, *Int J Hyperthermia* 1:219, 1985.
98. Hayes A, Scase T, Miller J, et al: COX-1 and COX-2 expression in feline oral squamous cell carcinoma, *J Comp Pathol* 135:93, 2006.
99. DiBernardi L, Dore M, Davis JA, et al: Study of feline oral squamous cell carcinoma: potential target for cyclooxygenase inhibitor treatment, *Prostaglandins Leukot Essent Fatty Acids* 76:245, 2007.
100. Schmidt BR, Glickman NW, DeNicola DB, et al: Evaluation of piroxicam for the treatment of oral squamous cell carcinoma in dogs, *J Am Vet Med Assoc* 218:1783, 2001.
101. Boria PA, Murry DJ, Bennett PF, et al: Evaluation of cisplatin combined with piroxicam for the treatment of oral malignant melanoma and oral squamous cell carcinoma in dogs, *J Am Vet Med Assoc* 224:388, 2004.
102. de Vos JP, Burm AGD, Focker BP, et al: Piroxicam and carboplatin as a combination treatment of canine oral non-tonsillar squamous cell carcinoma: a pilot study and a literature review of a canine model of human head and neck squamous cell carcinoma, *Vet Comp Oncol* 3:16, 2005.
103. Fox LE, Rosenthal RC, King RR, et al: Use of cis-bis-neodecanoato-trans-R,R-1,2-diaminocyclohexane platinum (II), a liposomal cisplatin analogue, in cats with oral squamous cell carcinoma, *Am J Vet Res* 61:791, 2000.
104. Kitchell BE, Brown DM, Luck EE, et al: Intralesional implant for treatment of primary oral malignant melanoma in dogs, *J Am Vet Med Assoc* 204:229, 1994.
105. Rassnick KM, Ruslander DM, Cotter SM, et al: Use of carboplatin for treatment of dogs with malignant melanoma: 27 cases (1989-2000), *J Am Vet Med Assoc* 218:1444, 2001.
106. Page RL, Thrall DE, Dewhirst MW, et al: Phase I study of melphalan alone and melphalan plus whole body hyperthermia in dogs with malignant melanoma, *Int J Hyperthermia* 7:559, 1991.
107. Reed SD, Fulmer A, Buckholz J, et al: Bleomycin/interleukin-12 electrochemogenetherapy for treating naturally occurring spontaneous neoplasms in dogs, *Cancer Gene Ther* 17:571, 2010.
108. Spugnini EP, Dragonetti E, Vincenzi B, et al: Pulse-mediated chemotherapy enhances local control and survival in a spontaneous canine model of primary mucosal melanoma, *Melanoma Res* 16:23, 2006.
109. Esplin DG: Survival of dogs following surgical excision of histologically well-differentiated melanocytic neoplasms of the mucous membranes of the lips and oral cavity, *Vet Pathol* 45:889, 2008.
110. Spangler WL, Kass PH: The histologic and epidemiologic bases for prognostic considerations in canine melanocytic neoplasia, *Vet Pathol* 43:136, 2006.
111. MacMillan R, Withrow SJ, Gillette EL: Surgery and regional irradiation for treatment of canine tonsillar squamous cell carcinoma: retrospective review of eight cases, *J Am Anim Hosp Assoc* 18:311, 1982.
112. Beck ER, Withrow SJ, McChesney AE, et al: Canine tongue tumors: a retrospective review of 57 cases, *J Am Anim Hosp Assoc* 22:525, 1986.
113. Brooks MB, Matus RE, Leifer CE, et al: Chemotherapy versus chemotherapy plus radiotherapy in the treatment of tonsillar squamous cell carcinoma in the dog, *J Vet Intern Med* 2:206, 1988.
114. McCaw DL, Pope ER, Payne JT, et al: Treatment of canine oral squamous cell carcinomas with photodynamic therapy, *Br J Cancer* 82:1297, 2000.
115. Evans SM, Shofer F: Canine oral nontonsillar squamous cell carcinoma, *Vet Radiol* 29:133, 1988.
116. LaDue-Miller T, Price S, Page RL, et al: Radiotherapy for canine non-tonsillar squamous cell carcinoma, *Vet Radiol Ultrasound* 37:74, 1996.
117. Bostock DE: The prognosis in cats bearing squamous cell carcinoma, *J Small Anim Pract* 13:119, 1972.
118. Cotter SM: Oral pharyngeal neoplasms in the cat, *J Am Anim Hosp Assoc* 17:917, 1981.
119. Hayes AM, Adams VJ, Scase TJ, et al: Survival of 54 cats with oral squamous cell carcinoma in United Kingdom general practice, *J Small Anim Pract* 48:394, 2007.
120. Bregazzi VS, LaRue SM, Powers BE, et al: Response of feline oral squamous cell carcinoma to palliative radiation therapy, *Vet Radiol Ultrasound* 42:77, 2001.
121. Nagata K, Selting KA, Cook CR, et al: 90Sr therapy for oral squamous cell carcinoma in two cats, *Vet Radiol Ultrasound* 52:114, 2011.
122. Hilmas DE, Gillette EL: Radiotherapy of spontaneous fibrous connective-tissue sarcomas in animals, *J Natl Cancer Inst* 56:365, 1976.
123. Creasey WA, Phil D, Thrall DE: Pharmacokinetic and anti-tumor studies with the radiosensitizer misonidazole in dogs with spontaneous fibrosarcomas, *Am J Vet Res* 43:1015, 1982.
124. Heyman SJ, Diefenderfer DL, Goldschmidt MH, et al: Canine axial skeletal osteosarcoma: a retrospective study of 116 cases (1986 to 1989), *Vet Surg* 21:304, 1992.
125. Hammer AS, Weeren FR, Weisbrode SE, et al: Prognostic factors in dogs with osteosarcomas of the flat and irregular bones, *J Am Anim Hosp Assoc* 31:321, 1995.
126. Straw RC, Powers BE, Klausner J, et al: Canine mandibular osteosarcoma: 51 cases (1980-1992), *J Am Anim Hosp Assoc* 32:257, 1996.
127. Kazmierski KJ, Dernell WS, Lafferty MH, et al: Osteosarcoma of the canine head: a retrospective study of 60 cases, *Vet Cancer Soc Proc* 22:30, 2002.
128. Bostock DE, White RAS: Classification and behaviour after surgery of canine epulides, *J Comp Pathol* 97:197, 1987.
129. Yoshida K, Watarai Y, Sakai Y, et al: The effect of intralesional bleomycin on canine acanthomatous epulis, *J Am Anim Hosp Assoc* 34:457, 1998.
130. Reif JS, Cohen D: The environmental distribution of canine respiratory tract neoplasms, *Arch Environ Health* 22:136, 1971.
131. Buhles WC, Theilan GH: Preliminary evaluation of bleomycin in feline and canine squamous cell carcinomas, *Am J Vet Res* 34:289, 1973.
132. Mas A, Blackwood L, Cripps P, et al: Canine tonsillar squamous cell carcinoma: a multicentre retrospective review of 44 clinical cases, *J Small Anim Pract* 52:359, 2011.
133. Dennis MM, Ehrhart N, Duncan CG, et al: Frequency of and risk factors associated with lingual lesions in dogs: 1,196 cases (1995-2004), *J Am Vet Med Assoc* 228:1533, 2006.
134. Carpenter LG, Withrow SJ, Power BE, et al: Squamous cell carcinoma of the tongue in 10 dogs, *J Am Anim Hosp Assoc* 29:17, 1993.
135. Brodey RS: A clinical and pathologic study of 130 neoplasms of the mouth and pharynx in the dog, *Am J Vet Res* 21:787, 1960.
136. Solano M, Penninck DG: Ultrasonography of the canine, feline and equine tongue: normal findings and case history reports, *Vet Radiol Ultrasound* 37:206, 1996.

137. Dvorak LD, Beaver DP, Ellison GW, et al: Major glossectomy in dogs: a case series and proposed classification system, *J Am Anim Hosp Assoc* 40:331, 2004.
138. Turk MAM, Johnson GC, Gallina AM: Canine granular cell tumour (myoblastoma): a report of four cases and review of the literature, *J Small Anim Pract* 24:637, 1983.
139. Patnaik AK, Lieberman PH, Erlandson RA, et al: A clinicopathologic and ultrastructural study of undifferentiated malignant tumors of the oral cavity in dogs, *Vet Pathol* 23:170, 1986.
140. Ogilvie GK, Sundberg JP, O'Banion MK, et al: Papillary squamous cell carcinoma in three young dogs, *J Am Vet Med Assoc* 192:933, 1988.
141. Norris AM, Withrow SJ, Dubielzig RR: Oropharyngeal neoplasms. In Harvey CE, editor: *Oral disease in the dog and cat: veterinary dentistry*, Philadelphia, 1985, Saunders.
142. Calvert CA: Canine viral and transmissible neoplasias. In Greene CE, editor: *Clinical microbiology and infectious diseases of the dog and cat*, Philadelphia, 1984, Saunders.
143. Poulet FM, Valentine BA, Summers BA: A survey of epithelial odontogenic tumors and cysts in dogs and cats, *Vet Pathol* 29:369, 1992.
144. Dubielzig RR, Adams WM, Brodey RS: Inductive fibroameloblastoma, an unusual dental tumor of young cats, *J Am Vet Med Assoc* 174:720, 1979.
145. Dernell WS, Hullinger GH: Surgical management of ameloblastic fibroma in the cat, *J Small Anim Pract* 35:35, 1994.
146. Figueiredo C, Barros HM, Alvares LC, et al: Composed complex odontoma in a dog, *Vet Med Small Anim Clin* 69:268, 1974.
147. Potter KA, Tucker RD, Carpenter JL: Oral eosinophilic granuloma of Siberian huskies, *J Am Anim Hosp Assoc* 16:595, 1980.
148. Madewell BR, Stannard AA, Pulley LT, et al: Oral eosinophilic granuloma in Siberian husky dogs, *J Am Vet Med Assoc* 177:701, 1980.
149. Bredal WP, Gunnes G, Vollset I, et al: Oral eosinophilic granuloma in three Cavalier King Charles spaniels, *J Small Anim Pract* 37:499, 1996.
150. Scott DW: Chapter 11: Disorders of unknown or multiple origin, *J Am Anim Hosp Assoc* 16:406, 1980.
151. McClelland RB: X-ray therapy in labial and cutaneous granulomas in cats, *J Am Vet Med Assoc* 125:469, 1954.
152. MacEwen EG, Hess PW: Evaluation of effect of immunomodulation on the feline eosinophilic granuloma complex, *J Am Anim Hosp Assoc* 23:519, 1987.
153. Song MD: Diagnosing and treating feline eosinophilic granuloma complex, *Vet Med* December:1141, 1994.
154. Kapatkin AS, Matthiesen DT, Noone KE, et al: Results of surgery and long-term follow-up in 31 cats with nasopharyngeal polyps, *J Am Anim Hosp Assoc* 26:387, 1990.
155. Kudnig ST: Nasopharyngeal polyps in cats, *Clin Tech Small Anim Pract* 17:174, 2002.
156. Bradley RL, Noone KE, Saunders GK, et al: Nasopharyngeal and middle ear polypoid masses in five cats, *Vet Surg* 14:141, 1985.
157. Harvey CE, Goldschmidt MH: Inflammatory polypoid growths in the ear canal of cats, *J Small Anim Pract* 19:669, 1978.
158. Faulkner JE, Budsberg SC: Results of ventral bulla osteotomy for treatment of middle ear polyps in cats, *J Am Anim Hosp Assoc* 26:496, 1990.
159. Parker NR, Binnington AG: Nasopharyngeal polyps in cats: three case reports and a review of the literature, *J Am Anim Hosp Assoc* 21:473, 1985.
160. Trevor PB, Martin RA: Tympanic bulla osteotomy for treatment of middle ear disease in cats: 19 cases (1984-1991), *J Am Vet Med Assoc* 202:123, 1993.
161. Mendenhall WM, Riggs CE, Cassissi NJ: Treatment of head and neck cancers. In DeVita RT, Hellman S, Rosenberg SA, editors: *Cancer: Principles and practice of oncology*, Philadelphia, 2005, Lippincott Williams & Wilkins.

SECTION B
Salivary Gland Cancer

STEPHEN J. WITHROW

Incidence and Risk Factors

Primary salivary gland cancer is rare in the dog and cat. Most cases are reported in older patients (10 to 12 years of age), and no specific breed or sex predilection has been determined in dogs.[1-3] The Siamese cat may be at higher risk than other breeds, with male cats being affected twice as often as female cats.[4]

Pathology

The vast majority of salivary cancers are adenocarcinomas, but a wide range of specific histologic types including osteosarcoma, mast cell tumor, sebaceous carcinoma, oncocytoma, and malignant fibrous histiocytoma have been reported.[1,5-9] They can arise from major (parotid, mandibular, sublingual, zygomatic) or minor accessory glands throughout the oral cavity. Of 245 submissions of salivary tissue for histologic diagnosis in both species, 30% were neoplastic.[3] Benign salivary gland tumors, including pleomorphic adenoma, are rare in animals[10,11] compared to humans. The mandibular gland is most commonly affected.[3,4] Malignancies are variably locally invasive, and metastasis to regional lymph nodes is common (39% for cats and 17% for dogs).[4,12] Distant metastasis has been reported (16% for cats and 8% for dogs at presentation) but may be slow to develop.[4,13] Benign lipomatous infiltration of the canine salivary gland has also been reported, and surgical excision was curative in all treated cases.[14,15]

History and Clinical Signs

Symptoms are nonspecific and generally include halitosis, dysphagia, exophthalmus, or a unilateral, firm, painless swelling of the upper neck (mandibular and sublingual), base of the ear (parotid), upper lip or maxilla (zygomatic), or mucous membrane of the lip or tongue (accessory salivary tissue). Major differential diagnoses are mucoceles, abscesses, salivary gland infarction, sialadenitis, lymphoma, or reactive or metastatic lymphadenopathy.[3,16]

Diagnostic Techniques and Work-Up

Fine-needle aspiration (FNA) cytology of masses in these locations should help differentiate noncancer diseases from cancer. Regional radiographs will usually be normal but may reveal periosteal reaction on adjacent bones or displacement of surrounding structures. CT imaging may be helpful in determining extent of disease and infiltration into surrounding structures. Needle core or wedge biopsies will usually be necessary to make a definitive diagnosis.

Therapy

When possible, aggressive surgical removal should be performed. Unfortunately, many lesions are extracapsular and widely extensive throughout the regional area, which contains numerous vital structures. However, complete extirpation of the ipsilateral neck can be performed with good functional outcome. The primary clinical impairment after a "radical" neck resection is the inability to blink the eye, which can be managed with a tarsorrhaphy or eye drops. If this surgery can be performed to the level of microscopic residual disease and RT is planned postoperatively, this complication is acceptable.

Postoperative RT resulted in good local control and prolonged survival in three reported cases.[6] Chemotherapy for salivary gland adenocarcinoma has been largely unreported.

Prognosis

The prognosis for salivary gland cancer is generally unknown. Clinical experience on a limited number of cases would indicate that aggressive local resection (usually histologically incomplete) followed by adjuvant radiation can attain permanent local control and long-term survival.[4,17] Incomplete removal will invariably result in local recurrence.[2] Histologic grade was not prognostic for outcome, whereas advanced stage was a negative prognosticator.[4] Median survival for 24 dogs and 30 cats treated with surgical resection with or without adjuvant radiation was 550 and 516 days, respectively.[4] The prognosis for long-term survival for cats is worse than for dogs.[4,18] Another report of six dogs with salivary carcinoma treated with surgery alone had a median survival of only 74 days, and all six dogs developed pulmonary metastasis.[19]

Comparative Aspects[20]

Salivary gland tumors are more common in older humans than in animals and account for 4% of head and neck neoplasms. The parotid gland is most commonly affected. A wide variety of benign and malignant neoplasms are recognized. Treatment is with surgical excision, and radiation is utilized for inoperable disease or after incomplete removal. Five-year survival usually exceeds 75% but depends on stage and histologic type.

REFERENCES

1. Koestner A, Buerger L: Primary neoplasms of the salivary glands in animals compared to similar tumors in man, *Pathol Vet* 2:201–226, 1965.
2. Carberry CA, Glanders JA, Harvey HJ, et al: Salivary gland tumors in dogs and cats: a literature and case review, *J Am Anim Hosp Assoc* 24:561–567, 1988.
3. Spangler WL, Culbertson MR: Salivary gland disease in dogs and cats: 245 cases (1985-1988), *J Am Vet Med Assoc* 198:465–469, 1991.
4. Hammer A, Getzy D, Ogilvie G, et al: Salivary gland neoplasia in the dog and cat: survival times and prognostic factors, *J Am Vet Med Assoc* 37:478–482, 2001.
5. Thomsen BV, Myers RK: Extraskeletal osteosarcoma of the mandibular salivary gland in a dog, *Vet Pathol* 36:71–73, 1999.
6. Carberry CA, Flanders JA, Anderson WI, et al: Mast cell tumor in the mandibular salivary gland in a dog, *Cornell Vet* 77:362–366, 1987.
7. Sozmen M, Brown PJ, Eveson JW: Sebaceous carcinoma of the salivary gland in a cat, *J Vet Med A Physiol Pathol Clin Med* 49:425–427, 2002.
8. Perez-Martinez C, Garcia Fernandez RA, Reyes Avila LE, et al: Malignant fibrous histiocytoma (giant cell type) associated with a malignant mixed tumor in the salivary gland of a dog, *Vet Pathol* 37:350–353, 2000.
9. Brocks BA, Peeters ME, Kimpfler S: Oncocytoma in the mandibular salivary gland of the cat, *J Feline Med Surg* 10:188–191, 2008.
10. Boydell P, Pike R, Crossley D, et al: Sialadenosis in dogs, *J Am Vet Med Assoc* 216:872–874, 2000.
11. Canapp SO Jr, Cohn LA, Maggs DJ, et al: Xerostomia, xerophthalmia, and plasmacytic infiltrates of the salivary glands (Sjögren's-like syndrome) in a cat, *J Am Vet Med Assoc* 218:59–65, 2001.
12. Mazzullo G, Sfacteria A, Ianelli N, et al: Carcinoma of the submandibular salivary glands with multiple metastases in a cat, *Vet Clin Pathol* 34:61–64, 2005.
13. Sozmen M, Brown PJ, Eveson JW: Salivary duct carcinoma in five cats, *Comp Path* 121:311–319, 1999.
14. Kitshoff AM, Millward IR, Williams JH, et al: Infiltrative angiolipoma of the parotid salivary gland in a dog, *J S Afr Vet Assoc* 81:258–261, 2010.
15. Brown PJ, Lucke VM, Sozmen M, et al: Lipomatous infiltration of the canine salivary gland, *J Small Anim Pract* 28:234–236, 1997.
16. McGill S, Lester N, McLachlan A, et al: Concurrent sialocele and necrotizing sialadenitis in a dog, *J Small Anim Pract* 50:151–156, 2009.
17. Evans SM, Thrall DE: Postoperative orthovoltage radiation therapy of parotid salivary gland adenocarcinoma in three dogs, *J Am Vet Med Assoc* 182:993–994, 1983.
18. Volmer C, Benal Y, Caplier F, et al: Atypical vimentin expression in a feline salivary gland adenocarcinoma with widespread metastases, *J Vet Med Sci* 71:1681–1684, 2009.
19. Hahn KA, Nolan ML: Surgical prognosis for canine salivary gland neoplasms, *Proc Annu Conf Am Coll Vet Radiol Vet Cancer Soc* 1997.
20. Mendehall WM, Riggs CE, Cassisi NJ: Cancer of the head and neck, section 2. In DeVita VT, editor: *Cancer: principles and practice of oncology*, ed 7, Philadelphia, 2005, Lippincott Williams & Wilkins.

SECTION C

Esophageal Cancer

STEPHEN J. WITHROW

Incidence and Risk Factors

Cancer of the esophagus is very rare and accounts for less than 0.5% of all cancer in the dog and cat.[1] Sarcomas, secondary to *Spirocerca lupi* infestation, have been reported in indigenous areas (Africa, Israel, and the southeastern United States).[2-5] No cause is known for the more common carcinomas. Most animals are older, and no gender or breed predilection is evident.

Pathology and Natural Behavior

The more commonly reported histologic types include SCC, leiomyosarcoma, fibrosarcoma, and osteosarcoma. Rarely, benign neoplasms such as leiomyoma, adenomatous polyp,[6] and plasmacytoma may be encountered, especially in the area of the terminal esophagus and cardia.[7-10] Paraesophageal tumors such as thymic, heart base, or thyroid may also invade the esophagus.[1] In cats, SCCs are usually seen in females and are located in the middle third of the esophagus just caudal to the thoracic inlet.[10-13] Most esophageal cancers are locally invasive, and metastasis is to draining lymph nodes, direct extension, or hematogenously to distant sites.

History and Clinical Signs

Signs other than those of general debilitation and weight loss include pain on swallowing, dysphagia, and regurgitation of undigested food. Pneumonia, secondary to aspiration, may also be noted. Hypertrophic osteopathy has been reported, especially with *Spirocerca lupi*–induced sarcomas.[2,4] *Spirocerca* usually affects the caudal thoracic esophagus and can be associated with thoracic spondylitis and a microcytic hypochromic anemia and a neutrophilia.[3,4]

Diagnostic Techniques and Work-Up

It is generally evident from the history that the patient is suffering from a partial or complete upper gastrointestinal (GI) obstruction. Plain radiographs may reveal retention of gas within the esophageal lumen, a mass, or esophageal dilatation proximal to the cancer. A positive-contrast esophagogram with or without fluoroscopy will generally reveal a stricture or mass lesion in the lumen. Esophagoscopy allows visualization of the lesion, which is frequently ulcerated. Several biopsies should be taken because necrosis and inflammation are often prominent. The risk of esophageal perforation during the biopsy is generally minimal. Leiomyomas appear as circumscribed submucosal masses, with a normal and freely movable mucosa making endoscopic biopsy unrewarding. Advanced imaging such as CT or MRI may be helpful to determine extent of the lesion, especially when minimal mucosal involvement is evident on endoscopic evaluation.

Open surgical biopsy via thoracotomy or cervical exploration is another option to obtain tissue for a diagnosis. *Spirocerca lupi* ova may be detected in the feces.[3]

Therapy

Therapy for malignant cancer of the esophagus is difficult at best because of the advanced stage of disease in most cases.[14] Intrathoracic resections are further complicated by poor exposure, lengthy resections, tension on the anastomosis, and unique healing problems of the thoracic esophagus. Low-grade leiomyosarcomas can be marginally excised with successful outcomes. They generally do not invade the mucosa and the muscular defect in the esophageal wall can be plicated with good postoperative function.[15] For lesions in the caudal esophagus or cardia, gastric advancement through the diaphragm can be considered but carries a high complication rate, including reflux esophagitis.

Various procedures to partially replace the resected esophagus have been described, including microvascular transfer of colon or small bowel, but clinical reports on their use in the cancer patient are lacking.[16-18] Chemotherapy has rarely been attempted. RT for the cervical esophagus can be attempted but is of limited value for the intrathoracic esophagus because of the poor tolerance of surrounding normal tissues such as the lung and heart. Short-term palliation can be achieved via esophagotomy or gastrostomy tubes. Benign leiomyomas of the esophagus or cardia can be approached via thoracotomy or celiotomy.[9]

Prognosis

Except for benign lesions,[7,8] lymphoma, or low-grade leiomyosarcoma,[15] the prognosis for esophageal tumors (primarily carcinomas) is very poor for cure or palliation due to poor resection options and high metastatic rate. One report describes a series of six dogs treated with partial esophagectomy for esophageal sarcomas associated with *Spirocerca*. Five of the six also received doxorubicin, and the median survival was 267 days.[19]

Comparative Aspects[20]

Esophageal cancer (principally SCC) is rare in humans but still accounts for 7000 deaths per year in the United States. Marked geographic variance in worldwide incidence implies numerous environmental influences on development, including tobacco, alcohol, hot food, and nitrosamines.

Most esophageal cancers have extensive local tumor growth and lymph node involvement precluding curative treatment. Combinations or single use of surgery, radiation, and chemotherapy have resulted in 5-year survivals of less than 20% of the more common advanced-stage disease. A variety of palliative bypass procedures for inoperable disease are also performed (esophagogastrostomy, intraluminal intubation, dilatation, and feeding gastrostomies).

REFERENCES

1. Ridgeway RL, Suter PF: Clinical and radiographic signs in primary and metastatic esophageal neoplasms of the dog, *J Am Vet Med Assoc* 174:700–704, 1979.
2. Bailey WS: Spirocerca lupi: a continuing inquiry, *J Parasitol* 58:3–22, 1972.
3. Ranen E, Lavy E, Aizenbert I, et al: Spirocercosis-associated esophageal sarcomas in dogs: a retrospective study of 17 cases (1997-2003), *Vet Parasitol* 119:209–221, 2004.
4. Dvir E, Kirberger RM, Mukorera V, et al: Clinical differentiation between dogs with benign and malignant spirocercosis, *Vet Parasitol* 155:80–88, 2008.
5. Lindsay N, Kirberger R, Williams M: Imaging diagnosis—spinal cord chondrosarcoma associated with spirocercosis in a dog, *Vet Radiol Ultrasound* 51:614–616, 2010.
6. Gibson CJ, Parry NM, Jakowski RM, et al: Adenomatous polyp with intestinal metaplasia of the esophagus (Barrett esophagus) in a dog, *Vet Pathol* 47:116–119, 2010.
7. Culbertson R, Branam JE, Rosenblatt LS: Esophageal/gastric leiomyoma in the laboratory beagle, *J Am Vet Med Assoc* 183:1168–1171, 1983.
8. Hamilton TA, Carpenter JL: Esophageal plasmacytoma in a dog, *J Am Vet Med Assoc* 204:1210–1211, 1994.
9. Rolfe DS, Twedt DC, Seim HB: Chronic regurgitation or vomiting caused by esophageal leiomyoma in three dogs, *J Am Anim Hosp Assoc* 30:425–430, 1994.
10. Carpenter JL, Andrews LN, Holzworth J: Tumor and tumor-like lesion. In Holzworth J, editor: *Diseases of the cat*, Philadelphia, 1987, WB Saunders.
11. Cotchin E: Neoplasms in cats, *Proc R Soc Med* 45:671, 1952.
12. Gualtieri M, Monzeglio MG, Di Giancamillo M: Oesophageal squamous cell carcinoma in two cats, *J Small Anim Pract* 40:79–83, 1999.
13. Shinozuka J, Nakayama H, Suzuki M, et al: Esophageal adenosquamous carcinoma in a cat, *J Vet Med Sci* 63:91–93, 2001.
14. McCaw D, Pratt M, Walshaw R: Squamous cell carcinoma of the esophagus in a dog, *J Am Anim Hosp Assoc* 16:561–563, 1980.
15. Farese JP, Bacon NJ, Ehrhart NP, et al: Oesophageal leiomyosarcoma in dogs: surgical management and clinical outcome of four cases, *Vet Comp Oncol* 6:31–38, 2008.
16. Gregory CR, Gourley IM, Bruyette DS, et al: Free jejunal segment for treatment of cervical esophageal stricture in a dog, *J Am Vet Med Assoc* 193:230–232, 1988.
17. Kuzma AB, Holmberg DL, Miller CW, et al: Esophageal replacement in the dog by microvascular colon transfer, *Vet Surg* 18:439–445, 1989.
18. Straw RC, Tomlinson JL, Constantinescu G, et al: Use of a vascular skeletal muscle graft for canine esophageal reconstruction, *Vet Surg* 16:155–156, 1987.

19. Ranen E, Shamir MH, Shahar R, et al: Partial esophagectomy with single layer closure for treatment of esophageal sarcomas in 6 dogs, *Vet Surg* 33:428–434, 2004.
20. Posner MC, Forastiere AA, Minsky BD: Cancer of the esophagus. In DeVita VT, Hellman S, Rosenberg SA, editors: *Cancer: principles and practice of oncology*, ed 7, Philadelphia, 2005, Lippincott Williams & Wilkins.

SECTION D
Exocrine Pancreatic Cancer

STEPHEN J. WITHROW

Incidence and Risk Factors

Cancer of the exocrine pancreas is very rare (<0.5% of all cancers) in the dog and the cat.[1,2] Older female dogs and spaniels have been described as being at higher risk.[3-5] Experimentally, N-ethyl-N′-nitro-N-nitrosoguanidine has been shown to induce pancreatic duct adenocarcinoma when administered intraductally in dogs.[6]

Pathology and Natural Behavior

Almost all cancers of the pancreas are epithelial and most are adenocarcinoma of ductular or acinar origin. Nodular hyperplasia is a common asymptomatic finding in older dogs or cats. "Benign" pancreatic pseudocysts and adenomas have been diagnosed by ultrasonography or surgery in dogs and cats.[2,7] In the vast majority of cases, malignant cancer has metastasized to regional or distant sites before a diagnosis can be made.[1,4,8]

History and Clinical Signs

The history and clinical signs of exocrine pancreatic cancer are vague and nonspecific and may mimic or be accompanied by pancreatitis. Weight loss and anorexia (marked in cats), paraneoplastic alopecia in cats,[9,10] vomiting, rare associated diabetes mellitus,[11] abdominal distension due to mass effect or abdominal effusions secondary to tumor implantation on the peritoneum (i.e., carcinomatosis; common in cats), icterus (with common bile duct obstruction), and depression are common symptoms. Alternatively, patients may present for symptoms of metastatic disease.

Diagnostic Techniques and Work-Up

Most hematologic and biochemical evaluations are nonspecific but may include mild anemia, hyperglycemia, neutrophilia, and bilirubinemia (if occluding the common bile duct.).[1,2] Elevations of serum amylase and lipase are inconsistent.[12] In extreme cases, signs of pancreatic insufficiency may be exhibited.[13] Positive-contrast upper GI radiographs may reveal slowed gastric emptying and occasionally compression or invasion of the duodenum.

Ascites may be a clinical sign and, when present, may reveal malignant cells on cytologic examination (carcinomatosis). Flow cytometry can be considered to help distinguish malignant from nonmalignant abdominal effusions. In the dog, most tumors are not palpable through the abdominal wall. In the cat, late stage, large palpable masses may be present.

Ultrasonography should be a useful diagnostic tool for localization of the primary tumor, documentation, and aspiration of fluid, as well as metastasis to liver and regional lymph nodes.[14] A large (>2 cm), apparently single mass is suggestive of pancreatic cancer versus nodular hyperplasia in cats.[15] The utility of advanced imaging such as CT and MRI has not been documented for pancreatic tumors in veterinary patients. At present, most diagnoses are made at exploratory laparotomy.

Therapy

Most non–islet cell carcinomas of the pancreas are metastatic (regional lymph nodes and liver) or locally and extensively invasive at the time of diagnosis. If the liver, peritoneal cavity, or draining lymph nodes are positive for tumor, aggressive surgery should generally not be performed. Complete pancreatectomy or pancreaticoduodenectomy (Whipple's procedure) has been described in humans and dogs,[16] but it carries a high operative morbidity and mortality without significant cure rates. Palliative GI bypass (gastrojejunostomy) is a short-term option if bowel obstruction is imminent. Radiation and chemotherapy have shown limited value in humans and animals. Occasionally, uncomfortable effusions from carcinomatosis can be diminished with systemic or intracavitary chemotherapy (see Chapter 11); however, the palliative response tends to be short lived.

Prognosis

The outlook for this disease in animals is very poor due to its critical location and advanced stage at diagnosis. One-year survival after diagnosis, regardless of treatment, has not been reported.

Comparative Aspects[17]

Pancreatic exocrine carcinoma accounts for more than 27,000 deaths per year in the United States. Most patients have disease progression beyond the pancreas at the time of initial diagnosis. Seventy-five percent are located in the head of the pancreas and the remainder in the body and tail. Direct extension to duodenum, bile duct, and stomach, as well as common metastasis to lymph node and liver, make treatment difficult.

When possible, pancreaticoduodenectomy (Whipple's procedure) or complete pancreatectomy are the treatments of choice. However, operative mortality ranges from 5% to 30%. Palliative bypass of the biliary tree and duodenum is commonly performed for inoperable lesions.

Traditional external beam RT is generally palliative rather than curative. Intraoperative and interstitial radiation are being explored as means for high-dose delivery to the tumor while sparing normal radiosensitive structures.[18,19] Chemotherapy alone (especially the taxols and gemcitabine) or in combination with radiation or surgery has demonstrated some improvement in quality of life, yet only very modest improvements in survival. Overall, 5-year survival for all patients remains less than 5%.

REFERENCES

1. Davenport D: Pancreatic carcinoma in twenty dogs and five cats, Personal communication.
2. Seaman RL: Exocrine pancreatic neoplasia in the cat: a case series, *J Am Anim Hosp Assoc* 40:238–245, 2004.
3. Kircher CH, Nielsen SW: Tumours of the pancreas, *Bull WHO* 53:195–202, 1976.

4. Anderson NV, Johnson KH: Pancreatic carcinoma in the dog, *J Am Vet Med Assoc* 150:286–295, 1967.
5. Brown PJ, Mason KV, Merrett DJ, et al: Multifocal necrotizing steatitis associated with pancreatic carcinoma in three dogs, *J Small Anim Pract* 35:129–132, 1994.
6. Kamano T, Azuma N, Katami A, et al: Preliminary observation on pancreatic duct adenocarcinoma induced by intraductal administration of N1-ethyl-N′-nitro-N-nitrosoguanidine in dogs, *Jpn J Cancer Res* 79:1–4, 1988.
7. VanEnkevort BA, O'Brien RT, Young KM: Pancreatic pseudocysts in 4 dogs and 2 cats: ultrasonographic and clinicopathologic findings, *J Vet Intern Med* 13:309–313, 1999.
8. Chang SC, Liao JW, Lin YC, et al: Pancreatic acinar cell carcinoma with intracranial metastasis in a dog, *J Vet Med Sci* 69:91–93, 2007.
9. Tasker S, Griffon DJ, Nuttall TJ, et al: Resolution of paraneoplastic alopecia following surgical removal of a pancreatic carcinoma in a cat, *J Small Anim Pract* 40:16–19, 1999.
10. Brooks DG, Campbell KL, Dennis JS, et al: Pancreatic paraneoplastic alopecia in three cats, *J Am Anim Hosp Assoc* 30:557–563, 1994.
11. Kipperman BS, Nelson RW, Griffey SM, et al: Diabetes mellitus and exocrine pancreatic neoplasia in two cats with hyperadrenocorticism, *J Am Anim Hosp Assoc* 28:415–418, 1992.
12. Quigley KA, Jackson MI, Haines DM: Hyperlipasemia in 6 dogs with pancreatic or hepatic neoplasia: evidence for tumor lipase production, *Vet Clin Pathol* 30:114–120, 2001.
13. Bright JM: Pancreatic adenocarcinoma in a dog with a maldigestion syndrome, *J Am Vet Med Assoc* 187:420–421, 1985.
14. Bennett PF, Hahn KA, Toal RL, et al: Ultrasonographic and cytopathological diagnosis of exocrine pancreatic carcinoma in the dog and cat, *J Am Anim Hosp Assoc* 37:466–473, 2001.
15. Hecht S, Penninck DG, Keating JH: Imaging findings in pancreatic neoplasia and nodular hyperplasia in 19 cats, *Vet Radiol Ultrasound* 48:45–50, 2007.
16. Cobb LF, Merrell RC: Total pancreatectomy in dogs, *J Surg Res* 37:235–240, 1984.
17. Yeo CJ, Yeo TP, Hruban RH, et al: Cancer of the pancreas. In DeVita VT, Hellman S, Rosenberg SA, editors: *Cancer: principles and practice of oncology*, Philadelphia, 2005, Lippincott Williams & Wilkins.
18. Ahmadu-Suka F, Gillette EL, Withrow SJ, et al: Pathologic response of the pancreas and duodenum to experimental intraoperative irradiation, *Int J Radiat Oncol Biol Phys* 14:1197–1204, 1988.
19. Dobelbower RR, Konski AA, Merrick HW, et al: Intraoperative electron beam radiation therapy (IOEBRT) for carcinoma of the exocrine pancreas, *Int J Radiat Oncol Biol Phys* 20:113–119, 1991.

SECTION E

Gastric Cancer

Stephen J. Withrow

Incidence and Risk Factors

Gastric cancer is more common than esophageal cancer but still accounts for less than 1% of all malignancies. No definitive etiology is known, although long-term administration of nitrosamines may induce carcinomas in dogs.[1] Several articles have described a high incidence of gastric carcinoma in related Belgian shepherds, Norwegian lundehunds, and Dutch Tervueren shepherd dogs, implying a genetic mechanism in development of this disease.[2-5] The average age of affected carcinoma patients is 8 years, with a 2.5:1 male-to-female ratio.[6,7] Males are also more commonly affected with gastric lymphoma than females.[8] Leiomyomas tend to occur in very old dogs (average age 15 years).[9,10] Chronic gastritis, *Helicobacter,* and common descent have been implicated in feline gastric cancer.[11,12]

Pathology and Natural Behavior

Adenocarcinoma accounts for 70% to 80% of cancer of the canine stomach.[13] It is often scirrhous (firm and white on the serosal surface) and has been termed *linitis plastica* (leather bottle) because of its firm and nondistensible texture. Lesions can be diffusely infiltrative, expansile (often with a central crater and ulceration), or may look more polypoid.[14] Other reported malignancies include leiomyosarcoma,[15] lymphoma,[8] mast cell tumor,[16] extramedullary plasmacytoma,[17,18] and fibrosarcoma. GI stromal tumors (GISTs) have been described in the GI tract of the dog, with 20% occurring in the stomach, and were likely previously classified as leiomyomas.[19-21] In humans and in approximately 50% of cases in dogs, GISTs express CD117 (c-kit), a tyrosine kinase receptor, and mutations in c-kit likely play a role in tumorigenesis of this cancer.[19] In one series, one-third of GISTs in dogs had metastasized at the time of diagnosis.[19] Adenocarcinoma will frequently spread to regional lymph nodes (70% to 80% at necropsy) followed by liver and lung.[2,7,12,16] An unusual occurrence of metastasis of gastric adenocarcinomas to the testes has been reported in three dogs.[22] Adenocarcinomas have been described as diffuse or interstitial, but little clinical significance can be associated with these variants.[7,23] The tumor antigen C2-O-sLe(X) is unregulated in canine gastric carcinoma and may play a role in the metastatic potential.[24] Benign lesions are generally leiomyomas, hypertrophic gastropathy, hamartomas,[25] or adenomas.[10,26-31] Feline gastric adenocarcinoma is rare, and the stomach is the least commonly affected GI site in the cat.[31,32] Lymphoma is the most common gastric tumor in the cat and may be solitary or one component of systemic involvement. Most cats with gastric lymphoma are negative for feline leukemia virus (FeLV).

History and Clinical Signs

The most common history is one of progressive vomiting (often blood tinged or "coffee grounds" in nature), anorexia, and weight loss. The weight loss may be a result of poor digestion, loss of protein and blood from an ulcer, or generalized tumor cachexia. Duration of symptoms is from weeks to many months.

Diagnostic Techniques and Work-Up

Routine laboratory tests and noncontrast radiographs are generally not diagnostic. Hypoglycemia may be a paraneoplastic syndrome associated with leiomyomas or leiomyosarcomas.[33,34] A microcytic hypochromic anemia is common. Occult blood in the feces may be detected. Liver "enzymes" may be elevated because of hepatic metastasis or obstruction of the common bile duct. Elevated gastrin levels are occasionally detected.[5,35] Thoracic radiographs are only rarely positive for metastasis at the time of initial presentation.

Positive- or double-contrast gastric radiographs may reveal a mass lesion extending into the lumen (Figure 22-12). Ulceration is also a common sign. Delayed gastric emptying, poor motility, or delayed adherence of contrast material to an ulcerated tumor may also be detected. Fluoroscopy may aid in determining motility alterations. Ultrasonography may also be a useful imaging modality in concert with fine-needle or needle core biopsy.[36,37] Ultrasound was of diagnostic utility in 27% of dogs with gastric adenocarcinoma of gastric lymphoma.[38] Malignancies tend to be sessile, and adenocarcinoma tends to occur most commonly on the lesser

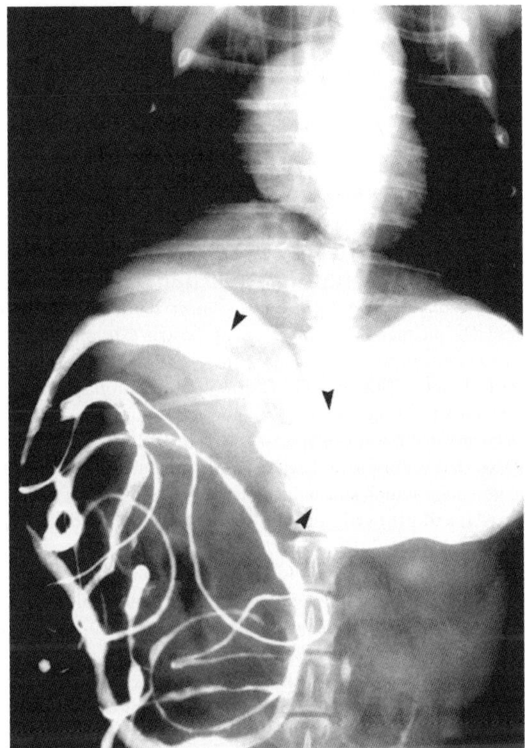

FIGURE 22-12 Ventrodorsal view of a dog with gastric cancer. Note the filling defect and partial outflow obstruction of gastric antrum and pylorus.

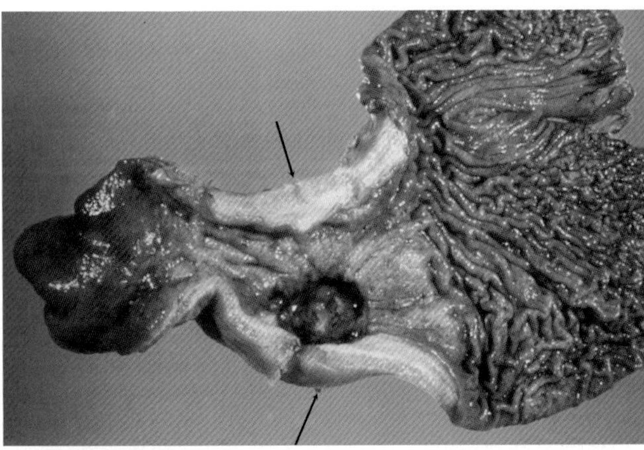

FIGURE 22-13 Gross specimen of the stomach from a dog with gastric adenocarcinoma. Note the large ulcer and fibrous thickening of stomach wall in area of gastric antrum *(arrows)*. This patient had metastasis to regional lymph nodes and liver.

curvature and gastric antrum (Figure 22-13). Benign lesions may be pedunculated or well circumscribed. Leiomyomas often occur at the cardia and will grow into the lumen as a smooth circumscribed mass.[10]

Gastroscopy with a flexible endoscope will generally reveal larger lesions that can be biopsied.[39,40] Several "large" samples should be taken because most gastric tumors have superficial necrosis, inflammation, and ulceration. Endoscopic biopsies were more likely to detect gastric lymphoma than intestinal lymphoma in cats.[41] In some patients, the gastric lesions are submucosal only, making endoscopic biopsy difficult. False-negative biopsies through the gastroscope are common. Open surgical biopsy is the most definitive method of diagnosis. For suspected GIST tumors, a CD117 immunohistochemical stain should be applied for confirmation.

Therapy

Except for lymphoma, surgery is the most common form of treatment for gastric cancer. As with esophageal cancer, curative resection is complicated by advanced stage disease in a difficult operative area (lesser curvature, antrum, and pylorus) with a frequently debilitated patient. At the time of surgery, a careful evaluation of liver and regional lymph nodes should be made to adequately stage the cancer. Lymph node metastasis can be quite varied, and all abdominal lymph nodes should be examined. If the cancer is felt to be localized to the stomach at laparotomy, a curative resection may be attempted. If possible, wide partial gastrectomy or antrectomy followed by a gastroduodenostomy (Billroth I) should be performed because of the increased morbidity associated with more extensive surgery such as gastrectomy and gastrojejunostomy (Billroth II).[42,43] Lesions requiring biliary bypass and very extensive surgery (complete gastrectomy) are generally too advanced to make these procedures worthwhile in terms of survival. For obstructive lesions felt to be inoperable for cure or for those that are metastatic, it is possible to perform a palliative gastrojejunostomy to allow passage of food into the intestine, although this procedure may be associated with significant postoperative mobidity.[42]

Leiomyomas are usually discrete, solitary lesions in the area of the cardia. They are not premalignant but can cause symptoms because of a mass effect. They can be easily "shelled out" via a midline laparotomy, gastrotomy, and submucosal removal or via intercostal thoracotomy if the side of the lesion can be clearly delineated.[10] In humans, GIST tumors may be responsive to inhibitors of c-Kit (e.g., toceranib, imatinib). The recent development of these agents in veterinary oncology could theoretically have efficacy for this tumor.

RT is rarely utilized due to the poor radiation tolerance of surrounding normal tissue (liver and intestine). Nonresectable lymphoma may be dramatically reduced with lower doses of irradiation than required for other tumors. No effective chemotherapy is known for adenocarcinoma.

Lymphoma may be excised if localized but does not generally respond well to conventional chemotherapy, although several exceptions exist in cats with gastric lymphoma (see Chapter 32, Section B).[8,44] The need for postoperative chemotherapy after "complete" resection of lymphoma is unknown.

Prognosis

The prognosis for most malignant gastric cancer is poor. Even if surgery can be performed, most patients are dead within 6 months as a result of recurrent or metastatic cancer.[3,11,45-49] In a series of 24 dogs undergoing pylorectomy and gastroduodenostomy, the perioperative mortality was 24% with a MST of 33 days. Preoperative weight loss was a negative indicator of outcome.[43] Few adenocarcinoma patients are operable for cure, and the short-term morbidity with radical resection can be high. Of 17 dogs treated with surgery for gastric adenocarcinoma, the median survival was 2 months.[11] Rare cases have survived as long as 3 years.[3] Palliation via bypass can be achieved for 1 to 6 months. The median survival for seven dogs with gastric leiomyosarcoma that lived at least 2 weeks postoperatively was 1 year.[15] Another paper suggested median survivals for GI leiomyosarcomas, or GISTs, of 8 to 12 months.[21] The hypoglycemia seen with some smooth muscle tumors is reversible after tumor resection. Patients with benign lesions can be cured with complete surgical excision.[10,50,51] Gastric extramedullary plasmacytomas appear to carry an excellent prognosis with surgery and chemotherapy. GI mast cell tumors were usually metastatic to regional nodes, and fewer than 10% of patients survived 6 months.[16-18]

Comparative Aspects[52]

Gastric cancer is the sixth most common cause of cancer death in humans. Adenocarcinoma constitutes over 90% of all malignant gastric cancer. Multiple socioeconomic, geographic, and environmental factors are associated with risk of tumor development. *Helicobacter* has been associated with the development of human gastric carcinoma and lymphoma but has not been correlated with carcinogenesis in the dog or cat, even though the organism is prevalent in the species.

Most lesions will be firm, ulcerative, and located in the antrum or lower third of the stomach, as in the dog. Most lesions are detected late in the course of disease and have direct tumor extension to surrounding organs, lymph node metastasis, or systemic metastasis, as with the dog.

Treatment is with surgical resection when possible or with less effective radiation and chemotherapy. Five-year survival for all patients is less than 10%, with a 30% survival for patients deemed operatively to have "localized" disease.

REFERENCES

1. Sasajima K, Kawachi T, Sano T, et al: Esophageal and gastric cancers with metastasis induced in dogs by N-ethyl-N′-nitro-N nitrosoguanidine, *J Natl Cancer Inst* 58:1789–1794, 1977.
2. Scanziani E, Giusti AM, Gualtieri M, et al: Gastric carcinoma in the Belgian shepherd dog, *J Small Anim Pract* 32:465–469, 1991.
3. Fonda D, Gualtieri M, Scanziani E: Gastric carcinoma in the dog: a clinicopathological study of 11 cases, *J Small Anim Pract* 30:353–360, 1989.
4. Lubbes D, Mandigers PJ, Heuven HC, et al: Incidence of gastric carcinoma in Dutch Tervueren shepherd dogs born between 1991 and 2002, *Tijdschrift voor Diergeneeskunde* 134:606–610, 2009.
5. Qvigstad G, Kolbjornsen O, Skancke E, et al: Gastric neuroendocrine carcinoma with atrophic gastritis in the Norwegian lundehund, *J Comp Pathol* 139:194–201, 2008.
6. Sautter JH, Hanlon GF: Gastric neoplasms in the dog: a report of 20 cases, *J Am Vet Med Assoc* 166:691–696, 1975.
7. Patnaik AK, Hurvitz AI, Johnson GE: Canine gastric adenocarcinoma, *Vet Pathol* 15:600–607, 1978.
8. Couto CG, Rutgers HC, Sherding RG, et al: Gastrointestinal lymphoma in 20 dogs, *J Vet Intern Med* 3:73–78, 1989.
9. Patnaik AK, Hurvitz AI, Johnson GF: Canine gastrointestinal neoplasms, *Vet Pathol* 14:547–555, 1977.
10. Kerpsack SJ, Birchard SJ: Removal of leiomyomas and other noninvasive masses from the cardiac region of the canine stomach, *J Am Anim Hosp Assoc* 30:500–504, 1994.
11. Dennis MM, Bennett N, Ehrhart EJ: Gastric adenocarcinoma and chronic gastritis in two related Persian cats, *Vet Pathol* 43:358–362, 2006.
12. Bridgeford EC, Marini RP, Feng Y, et al: Gastric Helicobacter species as a cause of feline gastric lymphoma: a viable hypothesis, *Vet Immunol Immunopathol* 123:106–113, 2008.
13. Swann HM, Holt DE: Canine gastric adenocarcinoma and leiomyosarcoma: a retrospective study of 21 cases (1986-1999) and literature review, *J Am Anim Hosp Assoc* 38:157–164, 2002.
14. Murray M, Robinson PB, McKeating FJ, et al: Primary gastric neoplasia in the dog: a clinicopathological study, *Vet Rec* 91:474–479, 1972.
15. Kapatkin AS, Mullen HS, Matthiesen DT, et al: Leiomyosarcoma in dogs: 44 cases (1983-1988), *J Am Vet Med Assoc* 201:1077–1079, 1992.
16. Ozaki K, Yamagami T, Nomura K, et al: Mast cell tumors of the gastrointestinal tract in 39 dogs, *Vet Pathol* 39:557–564, 2002.
17. Brunnert SR, Dee LA, Herron AJ, et al: Gastric extramedullary plasmacytoma in a dog, *J Am Vet Med Assoc* 200:1501–1502, 1992.
18. Zikes CD, Spielman B, Shapiro W, et al: Gastric extramedullary plasmacytoma in a cat, *J Vet Intern Med* 12:381–383, 1998.
19. Frost D, Lasota J, Miettinen M: Gastrointestinal stromal tumors and leiomyomas in the dog: a histopathologic, immunohistochemical, and molecular genetic study of 50 cases, *Vet Pathol* 40:42–54, 2003.
20. Carrasco V, Canfran S, Rodriguez-Franco F, et al: Canine gastric carcinoma: immunohistochemical expression of cell cycle proteins (p53, p21, and p16) and heat shock proteins (Hsp27 and Hsp70), *Vet Pathol* 48:322–329, 2011.
21. Russell KN, Mehler SJ, Skorupski KA, et al: Clinical and immunohistochemical differentiation of gastrointestinal stromal tumors from leiomyosarcomas in dogs: 42 cases (1990-2003), *J Am Vet Med Assoc* 230:1329–1333, 2007.
22. Esplin DG, Wilson SR: Gastrointestinal adenocarcinomas metastatic to the testes and associated structures in three dogs, *J Am Anim Hosp Assoc* 34:287–290, 1998.
23. Lingeman CH, Garner FM, Taylor DON: Spontaneous gastric adenocarcinomas of dogs: a review, *J Natl Cancer Inst* 47:137–149, 1971.
24. Janke L, Carlson CS, St Hill CA: The novel carbohydrate tumor antigen C2-O-sLe x is upregulated in canine gastric carcinomas, *Vet Pathol* 47:455–461, 2010.
25. Smith TJ, Baltzer WI, Ruaux CG, et al: Gastric smooth muscle hamartoma in a cat, *J Feline Med Surg* 12:334–337, 2010.
26. Walter MC, Goldschmidt MH, Stone EA, et al: Chronic hypertrophic pyloric gastropathy as a cause of pyloric obstruction in the dog, *J Am Vet Med Assoc* 186:157–161, 1985.
27. Kipnis RM: Focal cystic hypertrophic gastropathy in a dog, *J Am Vet Med Assoc* 173:182–184, 1978.
28. Happe RP, Van Der Gaag W, Wolvekamp THC, et al: Multiple polyps of the gastric mucosa in two dogs, *J Small Anim Pract* 18:179–189, 1977.
29. Culbertson R, Branam JE, Rosenblatt LS: Esophageal/gastric leiomyoma in the laboratory beagle, *J Am Vet Med Assoc* 183:1168–1172, 1983.
30. Hayden DW, Nielsen SW: Canine alimentary neoplasia, *Zentralbl Veterinarmed A* 20:1–22, 1973.
31. Brodey RS: Alimentary tract neoplasms in the cat: a clinicopathologic survey of 46 cases, *Am J Vet Res* 27:74–80, 1966.
32. Turk MAM, Gallina AM, Russell TS: Nonhematopoietic gastrointestinal neoplasia in cats: a retrospective study of 44 cases, *Vet Pathol* 18:614–620, 1981.
33. Bagley RS, Levy JK, Malarkey DE: Hypoglycemia associated with intra-abdominal leiomyoma and leiomyosarcoma in six dogs, *J Am Vet Med Assoc* 208:69–71, 1996.
34. Beaudry D, Knapp DW, Montgomery T, et al: Hypoglycemia in four dogs with smooth muscle tumors, *J Vet Intern Med* 9:415–418, 1995.
35. de Brito Galvao JF, Pressler BM, Freeman LJ, et al: Mucinous gastric carcinoma with abdominal carcinomatosis and hypergastrinemia in a dog, *J Am Anim Hosp Assoc* 45:197–202, 2009.
36. Rivers BJ, Walter PA, Johnston GR, et al: Canine gastric neoplasia: utility of ultrasonography in diagnosis, *J Am Anim Hosp Assoc* 33:144–155, 1997.
37. Beck C, Slocombe RF, O'Neill T, et al: The use of ultrasound in the investigation of gastric carcinoma in a dog, *Aust Vet J* 79:332–334, 2001.

38. Leib MS, Larson MM, Panciera DL, et al: Diagnostic utility of abdominal ultrasonography in dogs with chronic vomiting, *J Vet Intern Med* 24:803–808, 2010.
39. Lecoindre P, Chevallier M: Findings on endoultrasonographic (EUS) and endoscopic examination of gastric tumours of dogs, *Eur J Comp Gastroenterol* 2:21–28, 1997.
40. Kubiak K, Jankowski M, Nicpon J, et al: Gastroscopy in diagnosing gastric tumors in dogs, *Medycyna Weterynaryjna* 60:836–838, 2004.
41. Evans SE, Bonczynski JJ, Broussard JD, et al: Comparison of endoscopic and full-thickness biopsy specimens for diagnosis of inflammatory bowel disease and alimentary tract lymphoma in cats, *J Am Vet Med Assoc* 229:1447–1450, 2006.
42. Beaumont PR: Anastomotic jejunal ulcer secondary to gastrojejunostomy in a dog, *J Am Anim Hosp Assoc* 17:133–137, 1981.
43. Eisele J, McClaran JK, Runge JJ, et al: Evaluation of risk factors for morbidity after pylorectomy and gastroduodenostomy in dogs, *Vet Surg* 39:261–267, 2010.
44. MacEwen EG, Mooney S, Brown NO, et al: Management of feline neoplasms. In Holzworth J, editor: *Diseases of the cat*, vol. 1, Philadelphia, 1987, WB Saunders.
45. Olivieri M, Gosselin Y, Sauvageau R: Gastric adenocarcinoma in a dog: six-and-one-half month survival following partial gastrectomy and gastroduodenostomy, *J Am Anim Hosp Assoc* 20:78–82, 1984.
46. Elliott GS, Stoffregen DA, Richardson DC, et al: Surgical, medical, and nutritional management of gastric adenocarcinoma in a dog, *J Am Vet Med Assoc* 185:98–101, 1984.
47. Walter MC, Matthiesen DT, Stone EA: Pylorectomy and gastroduodenostomy in the dog: technique and clinical results in 28 cases, *J Am Vet Med Assoc* 187:909–914, 1985.
48. McDonald AE: Primary gastric carcinoma of the dog: review and case report, *Vet Surg* 3:70–73, 1978.
49. Sellon RK, Bissonnette K, Bunch SE: Long-term survival after total gastrectomy for gastric adenocarcinoma in a dog, *J Vet Intern Med* 10:333–335, 1996.
50. Rolfe DS, Twedt DC, Seim HB: Chronic regurgitation or vomiting caused by esophageal leiomyoma in three dogs, *J Am Anim Hosp Assoc* 30:425–430, 1994.
51. Beck JA, Simpson DS: Surgical treatment of gastric leiomyoma in a dog, *Aust Vet J* 77:161–162, 1999.
52. Pisters PW, Kelsen DP, Powel SM, et al: Cancer of the stomach. In DeVita VT, Hellman S, Rosenberg SA, editors: *Cancer: principles and practice of oncology*, ed 7, Philadelphia, 2005, Lippincott Williams & Wilkins.

SECTION F

Hepatobiliary Tumors

Julius M. Liptak

Incidence and Risk Factors

Primary hepatic tumors are uncommon and account for less than 1.5% of all canine tumors and 1.0% to 2.9% of all feline tumors, but up to 6.9% of nonhematopoietic tumors in cats.[1-4] Metastasis to the liver from nonhepatic neoplasia is more common and occurs 2.5 times more frequently than primary liver tumors in dogs, particularly from primary cancer of the spleen, pancreas, and GI tract.[1,2] Primary hepatobiliary tumors are more common than metastatic disease in cats.[4] The liver can also be involved in other malignant processes, such as lymphoma, malignant histiocytosis, and systemic mastocytosis.[2,3] Nodular hyperplasia is a relatively common diagnosis in older dogs but is benign and probably does not represent a preneoplastic lesion.[4]

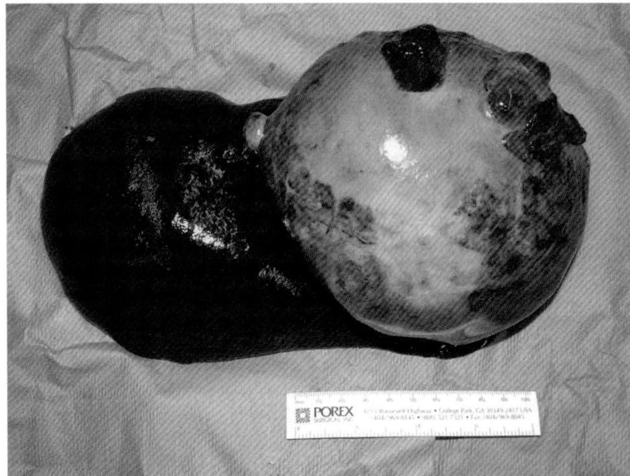

Figure 22-14 A solitary hepatic leiomyosarcoma with classic massive liver tumor morphology.

Table 22-7 Morphologic Types of Canine Hepatic Tumors

	Massive (%)	Nodular (%)	Diffuse (%)
Hepatocellular carcinoma	53-84	16-25	0-19
Bile duct carcinoma	37-46	0-46	17-54
Neuroendocrine tumor	0	33	67
Sarcoma	36	64	0

There are four basic categories of primary malignant hepatobiliary tumors in cats and dogs: hepatocellular, bile duct, neuroendocrine (or carcinoid), and mesenchymal.[4] Malignant tumors are more common in dogs, whereas benign tumors occur more frequently in cats.[2-8] There are three morphologic types of these primary hepatic tumors: massive, nodular, and diffuse (Table 22-7).[5] Massive liver tumors are defined as a large, solitary mass confined to a single liver lobe (Figure 22-14); nodular tumors are multifocal and involve several liver lobes (Figure 22-15); and diffuse involvement may represent the final spectrum of neoplastic disease with multifocal or coalescing nodules in all liver lobes or diffuse effacement of the hepatic parenchyma (Figure 22-16).[4,5]

The prognosis for cats and dogs with liver tumors is determined by histology and morphology. The prognosis is good for massive hepatocellular carcinoma (HCC) and benign tumors because complete surgical resection is possible and their biologic behavior is relatively nonaggressive.[7-11] In contrast, the prognosis is poor for cats with any type of malignant tumor, dogs with malignant tumors other than massive HCC, and cats and dogs with nodular and diffuse liver tumors because metastasis is more common.[2-14]

Pathology and Natural Behavior

Hepatocellular Tumors

Hepatocellular tumors include HCC, hepatocellular adenoma (or hepatoma), and hepatoblastoma.[4] Hepatoblastoma is a rare tumor of primordial hepatic stem cells and has only been reported in one dog.[15] Hepatocellular adenoma is usually an incidental finding and

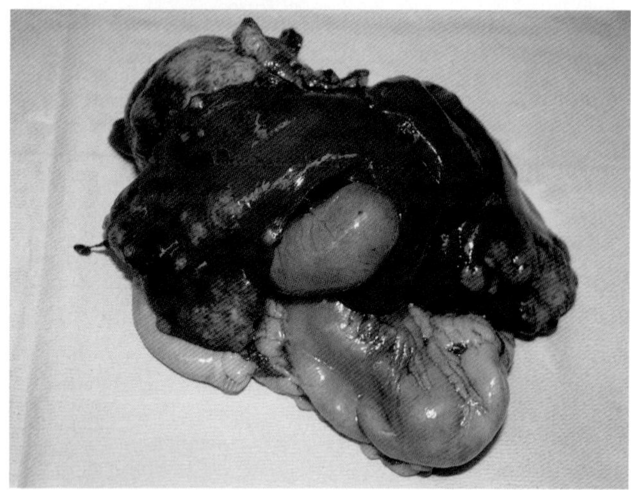

FIGURE 22-15 Nodular morphologic appearance of a bile duct carcinoma in a cat.

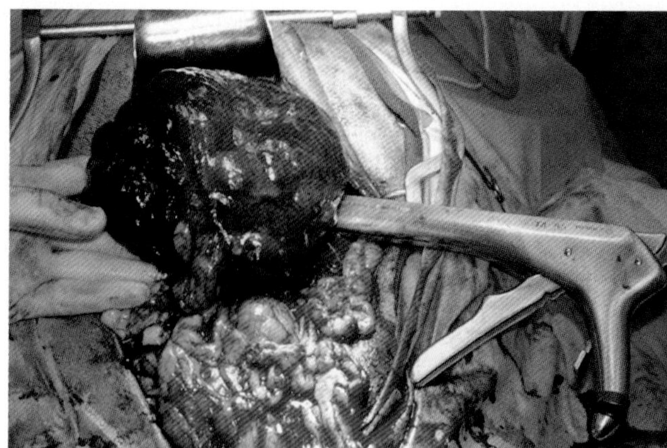

FIGURE 22-17 Liver lobectomy of a massive hepatocellular carcinoma using a thoracoabdominal surgical stapling device.

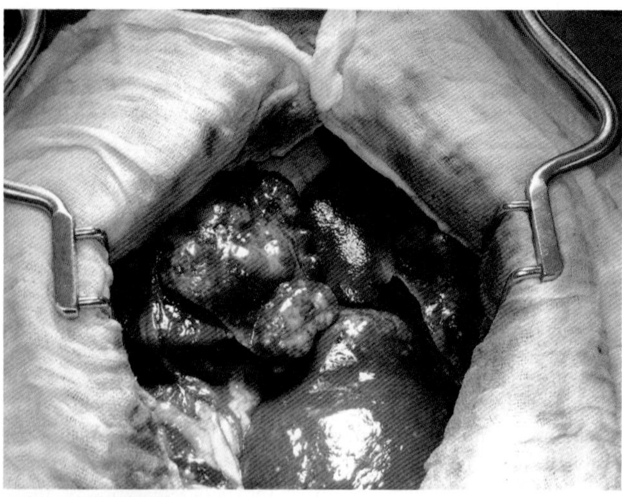

FIGURE 22-16 Diffuse morphologic appearance in a dog with a bile duct carcinoma.

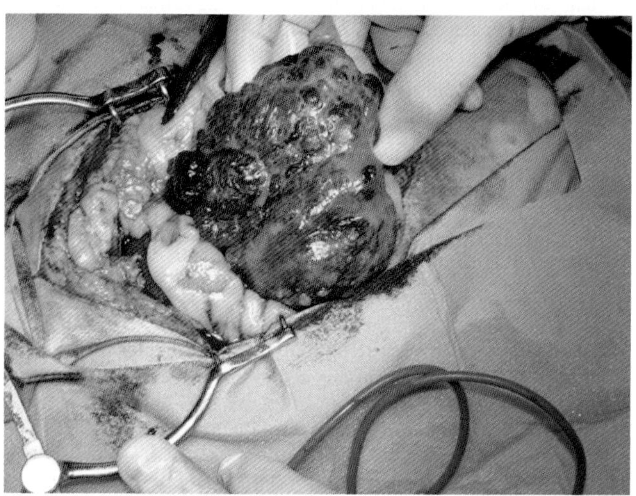

FIGURE 22-18 Intraoperative image of a bile duct cystadenoma in a cat. Surgical resection was curative in this cat.

rarely causes clinical signs.[2] Of the hepatocellular tumors, hepatocellular adenoma is more common in cats and HCC occurs more frequently in dogs.[2,5,6]

HCC is the most common primary liver tumor in dogs, accounting for 50% of cases, and second most common in cats.[2-8] Etiologic factors implicated in the development of HCC in humans include infection with hepatitis virus B or C and cirrhosis.[16] A viral etiology has also been demonstrated in woodchucks but not in cats or dogs, and cirrhosis is rare in dogs with HCC.[6-9] In one study, 20% of dogs with HCC were diagnosed with additional tumors although most were benign and endocrine in origin.[5]

A breed and sex predisposition has not been confirmed in dogs with HCC, but miniature schnauzers and male dogs are overrepresented in some studies.[5,9,11,17] Morphologically, 53% to 83% of HCCs are massive (Figure 22-17), 16% to 25% are nodular, and up to 19% are diffuse.[2,5] The left liver lobes, which include the left lateral and medial lobes and papillary process of the caudate lobe, are involved in over two-thirds of dogs with massive HCC.[5,9-11] Metastasis to regional lymph nodes, peritoneum, and lungs is more common in dogs with nodular and diffuse HCC.[2,5,9] Other metastatic sites include the heart, kidneys, adrenal glands, pancreas, intestines, spleen, and urinary bladder.[2,5,9] The metastatic rate varies from 0% to 37% for dogs with massive HCCs and 93% to 100% for dogs with nodular and diffuse HCCs.[2,5-11]

Bile Duct Tumors

Bile Duct Adenoma (Biliary Cystadenoma)

There are two types of bile duct tumors in cats and dogs: bile duct adenoma and carcinoma.[2,5-8,12,13,18-22] Bile duct adenomas are common in cats, accounting for more than 50% of all feline hepatobiliary tumors, and are also known as biliary or hepatobiliary cystadenomas due to their cystic appearance (Figure 22-18).[6-8,18-20] Male cats may be predisposed.[18,20] Bile duct adenomas usually do not cause clinical signs until they reach a large size and compress adjacent organs.[18-20] There is an even distribution between single and multiple lesions.[6-8,18-20] Malignant transformation has been reported in humans and anaplastic changes have been observed in some feline adenomas.[6,18]

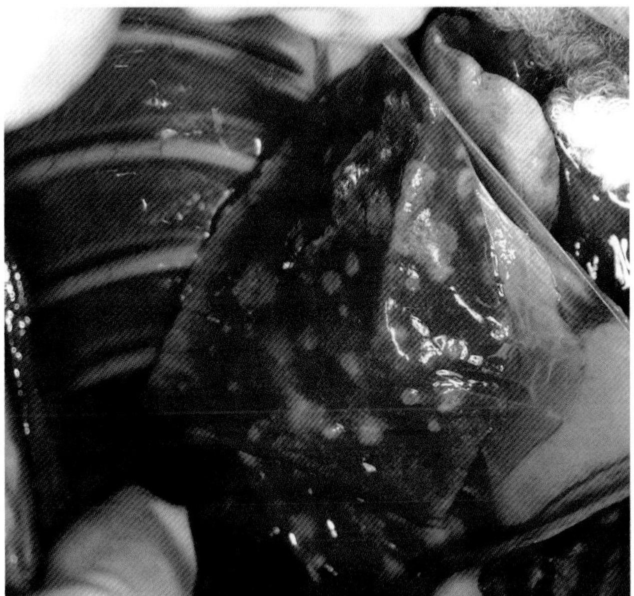

FIGURE 22-19 Lung metastasis in the cat with bile duct carcinoma depicted in Figure 22-15. This cat also had diffuse peritoneal metastasis.

Bile Duct Carcinoma (Cholangiocarcinoma)

Bile duct carcinoma is the most common malignant hepatobiliary tumor in cats and the second most common in dogs.[2,5-8] Bile duct carcinomas account for 22% to 41% of all malignant liver tumors in dogs.[5,23] In humans, trematode infestation, cholelithiasis, and sclerosing cholangitis are known risk factors for bile duct carcinoma.[24] Trematodes may also be involved in the etiology of bile duct carcinoma in cats and dogs, but they are unlikely to be a major contributor because bile duct carcinomas also occur in geographic regions outside the normal distribution of trematodes.[4,8,13]

A predilection for Labrador retrievers has been proposed.[13] A sex predisposition has been reported for female dogs.[5,12,17] In cats, however, the sex predisposition is conflicting, with both male and female cats reported to be predisposed.[6-8] The distribution of morphologic types of bile duct carcinoma is similar to HCC, with 37% to 46% massive, up to 54% nodular (see Figure 22-15), and 17% to 54% diffuse.[2,5,12,13] Bile duct carcinomas can be intrahepatic, extrahepatic, or within the gall bladder.[2,5-8,12,13] Intrahepatic carcinomas are more common in dogs,[5,12,13] whereas an equal distribution of intrahepatic and extrahepatic tumors to extrahepatic predominance has been reported in cats.[6-8] Solid and cystic (or cystadenocarcinoma) bile duct carcinomas have been reported, but this distinction does not influence either treatment or prognosis.[12] Bile duct carcinoma of the gall bladder is rare in both species.[2,5-8,12,13]

Bile duct carcinomas have an aggressive biologic behavior. Metastasis is common in dogs, with up to 88% metastasizing to the regional lymph nodes and lungs (Figure 22-19)—other sites include the heart, spleen, adrenal glands, pancreas, kidneys, and spinal cord.[2,5,12,13] In cats, diffuse intraperitoneal metastasis and carcinomatosis occur in 67% to 80% of cases.[6-8]

Neuroendocrine Tumors

Neuroendocrine tumors, also known as carcinoids, are rare in cats and dogs.[2,5-8,25] These tumors arise from neuroectodermal cells and are histologically differentiated from carcinomas with the use of silver stains.[3,14] Neuroendocrine hepatobiliary tumors are usually intrahepatic, although extrahepatic tumors have been reported in the gall bladder.[14,21,22,25] Carcinoids tend to occur at a younger age than other primary hepatobiliary tumors.[5,14] Morphologically, carcinoids are nodular in 33% and diffuse in the remaining 67% of cases.[5,14] Primary hepatic neuroendocrine tumors have an aggressive biologic behavior with frequent involvement of more than one liver lobe and metastasis to the regional lymph nodes, peritoneum, and lungs in cats and dogs.[5,14,25] Other metastatic sites include the heart, spleen, kidneys, adrenal glands, and pancreas.[14]

Sarcomas

Primary and nonhematopoietic hepatic sarcomas are rare in cats and dogs.[2,5-8,24] The most common primary hepatic sarcomas are hemangiosarcoma, leiomyosarcoma (see Figure 22-14), and fibrosarcoma, with hemangiosarcoma the most frequently diagnosed primary hepatic sarcoma in cats and leiomyosarcoma the most common in dogs.* The liver is a common site for metastatic hemangiosarcoma in dogs, whereas only 4% to 6% of hemangiosarcomas occur primarily in the liver.[28,29] Other primary hepatic sarcomas include rhabdomyosarcoma, liposarcoma, osteosarcoma, and malignant mesenchymoma.[2-8] The liver, with lungs, lymph nodes, spleen, and bone marrow, is commonly involved in dogs with disseminated histiocytic sarcoma.[30,31] Benign mesenchymal tumors such as hemangiomas are rare.[2-8] There are no known breed predispositions, although a male predilection has been reported.[5] Diffuse morphology has not been reported with massive and nodular types accounting for 36% and 64% of sarcomas, respectively.[5,24] Hepatic sarcomas have an aggressive biologic behavior, with metastasis to the spleen and lungs reported in 86% to 100% of dogs.[5,24]

Other Primary Hepatic Tumors

Myelolipoma is a benign hepatobiliary tumor in cats.[3,4] Histologically, myelolipomas are composed of well-differentiated adipose tissue intermixed with normal hematopoietic elements.[4] Chronic hypoxia has been proposed as an etiologic factor because myelolipomas have been reported in liver lobes entrapped in diaphragmatic herniae.[4] Myelolipomas can be either single or multifocal.[4]

History and Clinical Signs

Hepatobiliary tumors are symptomatic in approximately 50% of cats and 75% of dogs, especially in animals with malignant tumors.[1-15] The most common presenting signs are nonspecific, such as inappetence, weight loss, lethargy, vomiting, polydipsia-polyuria, and ascites.[1-15] Weakness, ataxia, and seizures are uncommon and may be caused by hepatic encephalopathy, paraneoplastic hypoglycemia, or central nervous system metastasis.[5,9,32] Icterus is more common in dogs with extrahepatic bile duct carcinomas and diffuse neuroendocrine tumors.[2,5,12] Hemoperitoneum secondary to rupture of massive HCC has been reported in two dogs.[33] However, these symptoms rarely assist in differentiating primary and metastatic liver tumors from nonneoplastic hepatic diseases.[3] Physical examination findings can be equally unrewarding. A cranial abdominal mass is palpable in up to three-quarters of cats and dogs with liver tumors, although palpation can be misleading because hepatic enlargement may be either absent in nodular and diffuse forms of liver tumors or missed due to the location of the liver in the cranial abdominal cavity deep to the costal arch.[1-15]

*References 2, 5-8, 24, 26-29.

Diagnostic Techniques and Work-Up

Laboratory Tests

Hematologic and serum biochemical abnormalities are usually nonspecific. Leukocytosis, anemia, and thrombocytosis are common in dogs with liver tumors.[1-14] Leukocytosis is probably caused by inflammation and necrosis associated with large liver masses.[9,10] Anemia is usually mild and nonregenerative.[5,11] The cause of anemia is unknown, although anemia of chronic disease, inflammation, red blood cell sequestration, microangiopathic destruction, and iron deficiency may be involved.[34] Thrombocytosis, defined as a platelet count greater than $500 \times 10^3/\mu L$, is seen in approximately 50% of dogs with massive HCC.[11] Proposed causes of thrombocytosis include anemia, iron deficiency, inflammatory cytokines, and paraneoplastic production of thrombopoietin.[35-37] Anemia and thrombocytopenia are relatively common in dogs with primary and metastatic hepatic hemangiosarcomas.[3] Prolonged coagulation times (e.g., increased prothrombin time, thrombin time, and activated partial thromboplastin time) and specific clotting factor abnormalities (e.g., decreased factor VIII:C and increased factor VIII:RA and fibrinogen degradation products) have been identified in dogs with hepatobiliary tumors, although these are rarely clinically relevant.[38]

Liver enzymes are commonly elevated in dogs with hepatobiliary tumors (Table 22-8). Increased activity of liver enzymes probably reflects hepatocellular damage or biliary stasis and is not specific for hepatic neoplasia.[4] There is also no correlation between the degree of hepatic involvement and magnitude of liver enzyme alterations.[4,11] The type of liver enzyme abnormalities may provide an indication of the type of tumor and differentiate primary and metastatic liver tumors.[39] Alkaline phosphatase (ALP) and alanine transferase (ALT) are commonly increased in dogs with primary hepatic tumors, whereas aspartate aminotransferase (AST) and bilirubin are more consistently elevated in dogs with metastatic liver tumors.[1,39] Furthermore, an AST-to-ALT ratio less than 1 is consistent with HCC or bile duct carcinoma, whereas a neuroendocrine tumor or sarcoma is more likely when the ratio is greater than 1.[5] In general, however, liver enzyme elevations are not specific for the diagnosis of hepatobiliary diseases.[41] Other changes in the serum biochemical profile in dogs with hepatic tumors may include hypoglycemia, hypoalbuminemia, hyperglobulinemia, and increased preprandial and postprandial bile acids.[1,2,5,9-14] Hypoglycemia is a paraneoplastic syndrome reported secondary to hepatic adenoma and management is described in more detail in Chapter 5. In contrast to dogs, azotemia is often present in cats with hepatobiliary tumors and may be the only biochemical abnormality, although liver enzyme abnormalities, especially ALT, AST, and total bilirubin, are also common and are significantly higher in cats with malignant tumors.[6-8]

α-Fetoprotein, an oncofetal glycoprotein, is used in the diagnosis, monitoring response to treatment, and prognostication of HCC in humans.[16] In dogs, serum levels of α-fetoprotein are increased in 75% of HCC and 55% of bile duct carcinomas.[42,43] However, α-fetoprotein has limited value in the diagnosis and treatment monitoring of canine HCC as serum levels of α-fetoprotein are also increased in other types of liver tumors, such as bile duct carcinoma and lymphoma, and nonneoplastic hepatic disease.[43,44] Hyperferritinemia is common in dogs with histiocytic sarcoma and immune-mediated hemolytic anemia (IMHA); thus, once IMHA has been excluded, serum ferritin levels may be useful in differentiating histiocytic sarcoma from other causes of liver disease.[45]

Table 22-8 Common Clinicopathologic Abnormalities in Cats and Dogs with Hepatobiliary Tumors

Parameter	Cat (%)	Dog (%)
Leukocytosis		54-73
Anemia		27-51
Hypoalbuminemia		52-83
Increased ALP	10-64	61-100
Increased ALT	10-78	44-75
Increased AST	15-78	56-100
Increased GGT	78	39
Increased total bilirubin	33-78	18-33
Increased serum bile acids	67	50-75

ALP, Alkaline phosphatase; *ALT,* alanine transferase; *AST,* aspartate aminotransferase; *GGT,* γ-glutamyltransferase.

Imaging

Radiographs, ultrasonography, and advanced imaging can be used for the diagnosis, staging, and surgical planning of cats and dogs with hepatobiliary tumors. A cranial abdominal mass, with caudal and lateral displacement of the stomach, is frequently noted on abdominal radiographs of cats and dogs with massive liver tumors.[10,11,17] Mineralization of the biliary tree is a rare finding in dogs with bile duct carcinoma.[4] Sonographic examination is recommended because these radiographic findings are not specific for the diagnosis of a hepatic mass and do not provide information on the relationship of the hepatic mass with regional anatomic structures.

Abdominal ultrasonography is the preferred method for identifying and characterizing hepatobiliary tumors in cats and dogs.[20,46-50] Sonographic examination is useful in determining the presence of a hepatic mass and defining the tumor as massive, nodular, or diffuse[46-50] and, in the case of cats, whether the tumor is cystic or not.[20] If focal, the size and location of the mass and its relationship with adjacent anatomic structures, such as the gall bladder or caudal vena cava, can be assessed.[20,46-50] Tumor vascularization can be determined using Doppler imaging techniques.[4] The ultrasonographic appearance of hepatobiliary tumors varies and does not correlate with histologic tumor type.[20,46-50] However, contrast-enhanced ultrasonography is useful in differentiating malignant tumors from benign lesions.[51-53]

Ultrasound-guided FNA or needle core biopsy of hepatic masses is a useful, minimally invasive technique to obtain cellular or tissue samples for diagnostic purposes.[47-50] A coagulation profile is recommended prior to hepatic biopsy because mild-to-moderate hemorrhage is the most frequent complication, occurring in approximately 5% of cases.[47-50] A correct diagnosis is obtained in up to 60% of hepatic aspirates and 90% of needle core biopsies.[47-50,54] More invasive techniques, such as laparoscopy and open keyhole approaches, can also be used for the biopsy and staging of cats and dogs with suspected liver tumors. In humans, laparoscopy is recommended for local staging as up to 20% of cases do not proceed with open surgery because of either nodular or diffuse tumors or unresectable disease.[55] However, for solitary and massive hepatic masses, surgical resection can be performed without a preoperative biopsy because

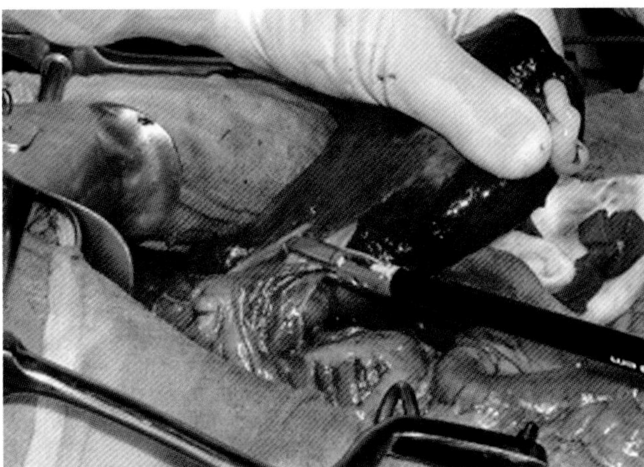

FIGURE 22-20 Liver lobectomy using a bipolar vessel sealant device. *(Courtesy Univ. Prof. Dr. Gilles Dupré, University of Vienna, College of Veterinary Medicine.)*

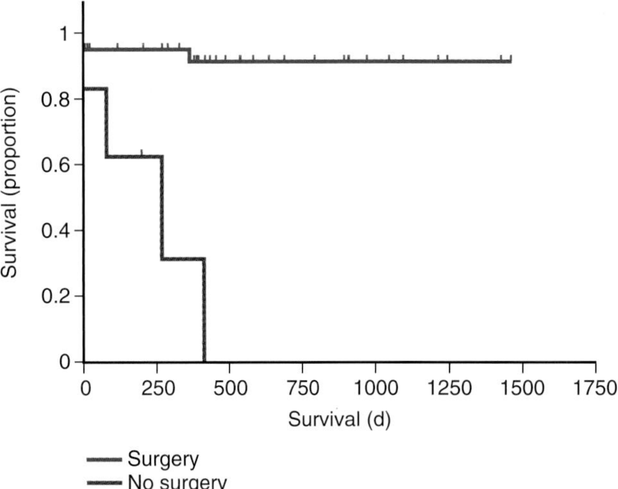

FIGURE 22-21 Kaplan-Meier survival curve for dogs with massive hepatocellular carcinoma. The median survival time (MST) for dogs with surgically resected tumors is significantly better than dogs not treated with curative-intent liver lobectomy. *(Reprinted with permission from Liptak JM, Dernell WS, Monnet E, et al: Massive hepatocellular carcinoma in dogs: 48 cases (1992-2002),* J Am Vet Med Assoc *225:1225, 2004.)*

both diagnosis and treatment can be achieved in a single procedure.

Advanced imaging techniques, such as CT and MRI, are preferred in humans for the diagnosis and staging of liver tumors.[16] Unlike ultrasonography, imaging appearance may provide an indication of tumor type.[16] Furthermore, CT and MRI are more sensitive for the detection of small hepatic lesions and determining the relationship of liver masses with adjacent vascular and soft tissue structures.[16] The use of advanced imaging in cats and dogs with hepatobiliary tumors has not been evaluated.

Imaging is also important for the staging of cats and dogs with liver tumors. Local extension and regional metastasis can be assessed with abdominal ultrasonography, CT, MRI, or laparoscopy. The sonographic and sometimes gross appearance of nodular hyperplasia and metastatic disease is similar. In two studies, 25% to 36% of dogs with ultrasonographically detectable focal hepatic lesions were diagnosed with nodular hyperplasia.[47,56] Biopsy of such lesions is recommended prior to definitively diagnosing metastatic disease and excluding animals from curative-intent surgery.[57] Although rare at the time of diagnosis, three-view thoracic radiographs or advanced imaging techniques should be assessed for evidence of lung metastasis prior to treatment.

Therapy and Prognosis

Hepatocellular Tumors

Liver lobectomy is recommended for cats and dogs with any hepatic tumor that has a massive morphologic appearance, particularly HCC. Surgical techniques for liver lobectomy include finger fracture, mass ligation, mattress sutures, bipolar vessel sealant devices, and surgical stapling.[58] Mass ligation is not recommended for large dogs, tumors involving either the central or right liver divisions, or tumors with a wide base.[58] The finger-fracture technique, involving blunt dissection through hepatic parenchyma and individual ligation of bile ducts and vessels, is acceptable for smaller lesions. Surgical staplers or bipolar vessel sealant devices are preferred for liver lobectomy because operative time is shorter with fewer complications (Figure 22-20).[11,58] A hilar dissection technique may be required for larger tumors extending to the hilus of the liver lobe because adequate margins may not be achievable with a surgical stapler.[59] Advanced imaging and intraoperative ultrasonography may provide information on the relationship of right-sided and central liver tumors with the caudal vena cava prior to liver lobectomy. Right-sided liver tumors can be excised even if intimately associated with the caudal vena cava, with or without an ultrasonic aspirator, but the surgeon should be very familiar with the course of the caudal vena cava through the hepatic parenchyma. En bloc resection of the caudal vena cava with a right-sided HCC has been reported.[60] In one report of 42 dogs with massive HCC treated with liver lobectomy, the intraoperative mortality rate was 4.8% and the complication rate was 28.6%.[11] Complications include hemorrhage, vascular compromise to adjacent liver lobes, and transient hypoglycemia and reduced hepatic function.[4,11,58]

Prognostic factors in dogs with massive HCC include surgical treatment, side of liver involvement, ALT and AST activity, and ratios of ALP-to-AST and ALT-to-AST.[11] The MST for 42 dogs with massive HCC following liver lobectomy was not reached after more than 1460 days of followup because the majority of dogs were either still alive or died of diseases unrelated to their liver tumor (Figure 22-21).[11] In comparison, the MST of 270 days was significantly decreased for six dogs managed conservatively and these dogs were 15.4 times more likely to die of tumor-related causes than dogs treated surgically.[11] Right-sided liver tumors, involving either the right lateral lobe or caudate process of the caudate lobe, had a poorer prognosis because intraoperative death was more likely due to caudal vena cava trauma during surgical dissection.[11] There was no difference in survival time if dogs with right-sided massive HCC survived surgery.[11] Increased ALT and AST were associated with a poor prognosis, which may reflect more severe hepatocellular injury secondary to either large tumor size or more aggressive biologic behavior.[11]

The prognosis for dogs with massive HCC is good. Local tumor recurrence is reported in 0% to 13% of dogs with massive HCC following liver lobectomy.[10,11] Metastasis to other regions of the liver and lungs has been documented in 0% to 37% of dogs, but metastasis is rare in recent clinical reports and most deaths are unrelated to HCC.[5,10,11]

In contrast, the prognosis for dogs with nodular and diffuse HCC is poor. Surgical resection is usually not possible due to involvement of multiple liver lobes. Treatment options for nodular and diffuse HCC in humans include liver transplantation or minimally invasive procedures for regional control, such as ablation or embolization.[16] Bland embolization and chemoembolization have been reported with moderate success in the palliation of four dogs with HCC.[61,62] The role of radiation and chemotherapy in the management of HCC is largely unknown. RT is unlikely to be effective as the canine liver cannot tolerate cumulative doses greater than 30 Gy.[4,16] Hepatocellular carcinoma is considered chemoresistant in humans because response rates are usually less than 20%.[4,16] The poor response to systemic chemotherapy is probably a result of rapid development of drug resistance due to either the role of hepatocytes in detoxification or expression of P-glycoprotein, a cell membrane efflux pump associated with multidrug resistance.[4] However, single-agent gemcitabine has been investigated in dogs with unresectable HCC with encouraging results.[63] Novel treatment options currently being investigated in human medicine include immunotherapy, hormonal therapy with tamoxifen, and antiangiogenic agents.[16]

Bile Duct Tumors

Bile duct adenomas can present as either single (e.g., massive) or multifocal lesions. Liver lobectomy is recommended for cats with single bile duct adenoma (cystadenoma) or multifocal lesions confined to one to two lobes.[6-8,18-20] The prognosis is very good following surgical resection with resolution of clinical signs and no reports of local recurrence or malignant transformation.[8,18,19]

Liver lobectomy is also recommended for cats and dogs with massive bile duct carcinoma. However, survival time has been poor in cats and dogs treated with liver lobectomy because the majority have died within 6 months due to local recurrence and metastatic disease.[8,64] There is no known effective treatment for cats and dogs with nodular or diffuse bile duct carcinomas because these lesions are not amenable to surgical resection and other treatments are often not successful.

Neuroendocrine Tumors

Carcinoids have an aggressive biologic behavior and are usually not amenable to surgical resection because solitary lesions and massive morphology are rare.[5,14] The efficacy of RT and chemotherapy is unknown. Prognosis is poor because metastasis to the regional lymph nodes, peritoneum, and lungs occurs in 93% of dogs and usually early in the course of disease.[5,14]

Sarcomas

Liver lobectomy can be attempted for solitary and massive sarcomas. However, prognosis is poor because metastatic disease is often present at the time of surgery.[5,24] Chemotherapy has not been investigated in the treatment of primary hepatic sarcomas, although, similar to other solid sarcomas, response rates are likely to be poor. Doxorubicin-based protocols and ifosfamide have shown some promise with sarcomas in other locations and warrant consideration for cats and dogs with primary hepatic sarcomas.[65,66]

Other Primary Hepatic Tumors

Surgical resection with liver lobectomy is recommended for cats with primary hepatic myelolipoma, and the prognosis is excellent with prolonged survival time and no reports of local recurrence.[4]

Comparative Aspects

Hepatocellular carcinoma is one of the most common malignancies in humans as a result of viral infections with hepatitis viruses B and C and cirrhosis induced by alcohol consumption and other disease.[16] A number of paraneoplastic syndromes have been described including hypoglycemia, erythrocytosis, and hypercalcemia.[16] Ultrasonography is considered a good screening imaging modality, but advanced imaging with contrast-enhanced CT or MRI is preferred to determine the location, size, and extent of hepatic lesions.[16] Other tests include serum α-fetoprotein, serologic tests for hepatitis B and C viruses, and histologic confirmation with core liver biopsies.[16] Unlike HCC in dogs, the morphology of HCC in humans is often nodular or diffuse, which makes definitive treatment more problematic. Treatment options depend on the stage of disease and include surgery (e.g., liver lobectomy and liver transplantation), local ablative therapies (e.g., cryosurgery, ethanol or acetic acid injection, and microwave or radiofrequency ablation), regional therapies (e.g., transarterial chemotherapy, embolization, chemoembolization, or RT), and systemic treatment with chemotherapy or immunotherapy.[16] Response rates to single- and multiple-agent chemotherapy protocols are less than 25%, and chemotherapy is no longer recommended for human patients with HCC.[16]

Bile duct carcinomas are rare and, similar to cats and dogs, often associated with a poor prognosis.[26] Risk factors include primary sclerosing cholangitis, the liver flukes *Opisthorchis viverrini* and *Clonorchis sinensis* in endemic areas of Southeast Asia and China, and cholelithiasis.[26] Surgical resection is preferred but, because of the high rate of local or regional recurrence, adjuvant treatment with RT or chemotherapy is recommended.[26] However, because of the rarity of this tumor, studies supporting the efficacy of these adjuvant treatments are lacking. Papillary histology, extrahepatic location, and complete resection are favorable prognostic factors in humans with bile duct carcinomas.[67]

REFERENCES

1. Strombeck DR: Clinicopathologic features of primary and metastatic neoplastic disease of the liver in dogs, *J Am Vet Med Assoc* 173:267, 1978.
2. Cullen JM, Popp JA: Tumors of the liver and gall bladder. In Meuten DJ, editor: *Tumors in domestic animals*, ed 4, Ames, Iowa, 2002, Iowa State Press.
3. Hammer AS, Sikkema DA: Hepatic neoplasia in the dog and cat, *Vet Clin North Am Small Anim Pract* 25:419, 1995.
4. Thamm DH: Hepatobiliary tumors. In Withrow SJ, MacEwen EG, editors: *Small animal clinical oncology*, ed 3, Philadelphia, 2001, WB Saunders.
5. Patnaik AK, Hurvitz AI, Lieberman PH: Canine hepatic neoplasms: a clinicopathological study, *Vet Pathol* 17:553, 1980.
6. Patnaik AK: A morphologic and immunohistochemical study of hepatic neoplasms in cats, *Vet Pathol* 29:405, 1992.
7. Post G, Patnaik AK: Nonhematopoietic hepatic neoplasms in cats: 21 cases (1983-1988), *J Am Vet Med Assoc* 201:1080, 1992.
8. Lawrence HJ, Erb HN, Harvey HJ: Nonlymphomatous hepatobiliary masses in cats: 41 cases (1972 to 1991), *Vet Surg* 23:365, 1994.
9. Patnaik AK, Hurvitz AI, Lieberman PH, et al: Canine hepatocellular carcinoma, *Vet Pathol* 18:427, 1981.
10. Kosovsky JE, Manfra-Marretta S, Matthiesen DT, et al: Results of partial hepatectomy in 18 dogs with hepatocellular carcinoma, *J Am Anim Hosp Assoc* 25:203, 1989.
11. Liptak JM, Dernell WS, Monnet E, et al: Massive hepatocellular carcinoma in dogs: 48 cases (1992-2002), *J Am Vet Med Assoc* 225:1225, 2004.

12. Patnaik AK, Hurvitz AI, Lieberman PH, et al: Canine bile duct carcinoma, *Vet Pathol* 18:439, 1981.
13. Hayes HM, Morin MM, Rubenstein DA: Canine biliary carcinoma: epidemiological comparisons with man, *J Comp Pathol* 93:99, 1983.
14. Patnaik AK, Lieberman PH, Hurvitz AI, et al: Canine hepatic carcinoids, *Vet Pathol* 18:439, 1981.
15. Shiga A, Shirota K, Shida T, et al: Hepatoblastoma in a dog, *J Vet Med Sci* 59:1167, 1997.
16. Bartlett DL, Carr BI, Marsh JW: Cancer of the liver. In DeVita VT, Hellman S, Rosenberg SA, editors: *Cancer: principles and practice of oncology*, Philadelphia, 2005, Lippincott Williams & Wilkins.
17. Evans SM: The radiographic appearance of primary liver neoplasia in dogs, *Vet Radiol* 28:192, 1987.
18. Adler R, Wilson DW: Biliary cystadenomas of cats, *Vet Pathol* 32:415, 1995.
19. Trout NJ, Berg J, McMillan MC, et al: Surgical treatment of hepatobiliary cystadenomas in cats: five cases (1988-1993), *J Am Vet Med Assoc* 206:505, 1995.
20. Nyland TG, Koblik PD, Tellyer SE: Ultrasonographic evaluation of biliary cystadenomas in cats, *Vet Radiol Ultrasound* 40:300, 1999.
21. Willard MD, Dunstan RW, Faulkner J: Neuroendocrine carcinoma of the gall bladder in a dog, *J Am Vet Med Assoc* 192:926, 1988.
22. Morrell CN, Volk MV, Mankowski JL: A carcinoid tumor in the gallbladder of a dog, *Vet Pathol* 39:756, 2002.
23. Trigo FJ, Thompson H, Breeze RG, et al: The pathology of liver tumors in the dog, *J Comp Pathol* 92:21, 1982.
24. Kapatkin AS, Mullen HS, Matthiesen DT, et al: Leiomyosarcoma in dogs: 44 cases (1983-1988), *J Am Vet Med Assoc* 201:1077, 1992.
25. Patnaik AK, Lieberman PH, Erlandson RA, et al: Hepatobiliary neuroendocrine carcinoma in cats: a clinicopathologic, immunohistochemical, and ultrastructural study of 17 cases, *Vet Pathol* 42:331, 2005.
26. Bartlett DL, Ramanathan RK, Deutsch M: Cancer of the biliary tree. In DeVita VT, Hellman S, Rosenberg SA, editors: *Cancer: principles and practice of oncology*, ed 7, Philadelphia, 2005, Lippincott Williams & Wilkins.
27. Scavelli TD, Patnaik AK, Mehlhaff CJ, et al: Hemangiosarcoma in the cat: retrospective evaluation of 31 surgical cases, *J Am Vet Med Assoc* 187:817–819, 1985.
28. Brown NO, Patnaik AK, MacEwen EG: Canine hemangiosarcoma: retrospective analysis of 104 cases, *J Am Vet Med Assoc* 186:56–58, 1985.
29. Srebernik N, Appleby EC: Breed prevalence and sites of haemangioma and haemangiosarcoma in dogs, *Vet Rec* 129:408–409, 1991.
30. Affolter VK, Moore PF: Canine cutaneous and systemic histiocytosis: reactive histiocytosis of dermal dendritic cells, *Am J Dermatopathol* 22:40, 2000.
31. Affolter VK, Moore PF: Localized and disseminated histiocytic sarcoma of dendritic cell origin in dogs, *Vet Pathol* 39:74, 2002.
32. Leifer CE, Peterson ME, Matus RE, et al: Hypoglycemia associated with nonislet cell tumor in 13 dogs, *J Am Vet Med Assoc* 186:53, 1985.
33. Arohnson MG, Dubiel B, Roberts B, et al: Prognosis for acute nontraumatic hemoperitoneum in the dog: a retrospective analysis of 60 cases (2003-2006), *J Am Anim Hosp Assoc* 45:72, 2009.
34. Rogers KS: Anemia. In Ettinger SJ, Feldman EC, editors: *Textbook of veterinary internal medicine*, ed 5, Philadelphia, 2000, WB Saunders.
35. Helfand SC: Platelets and neoplasia, *Vet Clin North Am Small Anim Pract* 18:131, 1988.
36. Baatout S: Interleukin-6 and megakaryocytopoiesis: an update, *Ann Hematol* 73:157, 1996.
37. Jelkmann W: The role of the liver in the production of thrombopoietin compared with erythropoietin, *Eur J Gastroenterol Hepatol* 13:791, 2001.
38. Badylak SF, Dodds WJ, van Vleet JF: Plasma coagulation factor abnormalities in dogs with naturally occurring hepatic disease, *Am J Vet Res* 44:2336, 1983.
39. McConnell MF, Lumsden JH: Biochemical evaluation of metastatic liver disease in the dog, *J Am Anim Hosp Assoc* 19:173, 1983.
40. Reference deleted in pages.
41. Center SA, Slater MR, Manwarren T, et al: Diagnostic efficacy of serum alkaline phosphatase and γ-glutamyltransferase in dogs with histologically confirmed hepatobiliary disease: 270 cases (1980-1990), *J Am Vet Med Assoc* 201:1258, 1992.
42. Lowseth LA, Gillett NA, Chang IY, et al: Detection of serum α-fetoprotein in dogs with hepatic tumors, *J Am Vet Med Assoc* 199:735, 1991.
43. Yamada T, Fujita M, Kitao S, et al: Serum alpha-fetoprotein values in dogs with various hepatic diseases, *J Vet Med Sci* 61:657, 1999.
44. Hahn KA, Richardson RC: Detection of serum alpha-fetoprotein in dogs with naturally occurring malignant neoplasia, *Vet Clin Pathol* 24:18, 1995.
45. Friedrichs KR, Thomas C, Plier M, et al: Evaluation of serum ferritin as a tumor marker for canine histiocytic sarcoma, *J Vet Intern Med* 24:904, 2010.
46. Feeney DA, Johnston GR, Hardy RM: Two-dimensional, gray-scale ultrasonography for assessment of hepatic and splenic neoplasia in the dog and cat, *J Am Vet Med Assoc* 184:68, 1984.
47. Vörös K, Vrabély T, Papp L, et al: Correlation of ultrasonographic and pathomorphological findings in canine hepatic diseases, *J Small Anim Pract* 32:627, 1991.
48. Newell SM, Selcer BA, Girard E, et al: Correlations between ultrasonographic findings and specific hepatic disease in cats: 72 cases (1985-1997), *J Am Vet Med Assoc* 213:94, 1998.
49. Leveille R, Partington BP, Biller DS, et al: Complications after ultrasound-guided biopsy of abdominal structures in dogs and cats: 246 cases (1984-1991), *J Am Vet Med Assoc* 203:413, 1993.
50. Barr F: Percutaneous biopsy of abdominal organs under ultrasound guidance, *J Small Anim Pract* 36:105, 1995.
51. O'Brien RT, Iani M, Matheson J, et al: Contrast harmonic ultrasound of spontaneous liver nodules in 32 dogs, *Vet Radiol Ultrasound* 45:547, 2004.
52. Kutara K, Asano K, Kito A, et al: Contrast harmonic imaging of canine hepatic tumors, *J Vet Med Sci* 68:433, 2006.
53. Nakamura K, Takagi S, Sasaki N, et al: Contrast-enhanced ultrasonography for characterization of canine focal liver lesions, *Vet Radiol Ultrasound* 51:79, 2010.
54. Roth L: Comparison of liver cytology and biopsy diagnoses in dogs and cats: 56 cases, *Vet Clin Pathol* 30:35, 2001.
55. D'Angelica M, Fong Y, Weber S, et al: The role of staging laparoscopy in hepatobiliary malignancy: prospective analysis of 401 cases, *Ann Surg Oncol* 10:183, 2003.
56. Cuccovillo A, Lamb CR: Cellular features of sonographic target lesions of the liver and spleen in 21 dogs and a cat, *Vet Radiol Ultrasound* 43:275, 2002.
57. Stowater JL, Lamb CR, Schelling SH: Ultrasonographic features of canine hepatic nodular hyperplasia, *Vet Radiol* 31:268, 1990.
58. Martin RA, Lanz OI, Tobias KM: Liver and biliary system. In Slatter DH, editor: *Textbook of small animal surgery*, ed 3, Philadelphia, 2003, WB Saunders.
59. Covey JL, Degner DA, Jackson AH, et al: Hilar liver resection in dogs, *Vet Surg* 38:104, 2009.
60. Seki M, Asano K, Ishigaki K, et al: En block resection of a large hepatocellular carcinoma involving the caudal vena cava in a dog, *J Vet Med Sci* 73(5):693–696, 2011.
61. Weisse C, Clifford CA, Holt D, et al: Percutaneous arterial embolization and chemoembolization for treatment of benign and malignant tumors in three dogs and a goat, *J Am Vet Med Assoc* 221:1430, 2002.
62. Cave TA, Johnson V, Beths T, et al: Treatment of unresectable hepatocellular adenoma in dogs with transarterial iodized oil and chemotherapy with and without an embolic agent: a report of two cases, *Vet Comp Oncol* 1:191, 2003.

63. Elpiner A, Brodsky E, Hazzah T, et al: Single agent gemcitabine chemotherapy in dogs with hepatocellular carcinoma, *Vet Comp Oncol* 9(4):260–268, 2011.
64. Fry PD, Rest JR: Partial hepatectomy in two dogs, *J Small Anim Pract* 34:192, 1993.
65. Ogilvie GK, Powers BE, Mallinckrodt CH, et al: Surgery and doxorubicin in dogs with hemangiosarcoma, *J Vet Intern Med* 10:379, 1996.
66. Rassnick KM, Frimberger AE, Wood CA, et al: Evaluation of ifosfamide for treatment of various canine neoplasms, *J Vet Intern Med* 14:271, 2000.
67. Chung C, Bautista N, O'Connell TX: Prognosis and treatment of bile duct carcinoma, *Am Surg* 64:921, 1998.

SECTION G
Intestinal Tumors

KIM A. SELTING

Incidence and Risk Factors

Reports vary, but overall intestinal tumors are rare in dogs and cats.[1-3] In a survey of insured dogs in the United Kingdom, a standardized incidence rate of 210/100,000 dogs was reported for alimentary tumors. This accounted for 8% of all tumor submissions.[4] Incidence of feline digestive neoplasia in a South African survey comprised 13.5% of all tumors, which likely included oral tumors.[5] In the United States, a query of over 300,000 cat submissions to the Veterinary Medical Database (VMDB) found 8% to relate to cancer and less than 1% (13% of the cancer cases) to be intestinal neoplasia.[6] Less than 1% of over 10,000 dogs submitted for necropsy at one institution were diagnosed with intestinal adenocarcinoma, which agrees with other reports.[2,7,8] Regarding specific tumor types, lymphoma comprises nearly 30% of all feline tumors and 6% of all canine tumors and is the most common intestinal tumor in most reports.[2,9-11] Adenocarcinoma is the second most frequent tumor in both species, with mast cell tumors in cats and leiomyosarcomas or GISTs in dogs next.

As with many cancers, incidence of intestinal neoplasia increases in older dogs and cats. Mean ages of affected cats for small and large intestinal neoplasia generally range between 10 and 12 years, and increasing risk after age 7 has been reported.[2,6,12-20] Dogs are also usually middle aged or older, with mean ages most often between 6 and 9 years, possibly older (12 years) for dogs with leiomyosarcoma.[11,21-24] Some earlier studies of feline lymphoma report younger median ages, most likely a result of a larger percentage of FeLV-positive cats in the study population.[25,26]

There is a slight sex predilection for males to develop intestinal tumors in some studies for both dogs and cats. Many studies report a near equal incidence among male and female dogs,[24,27-29] although one study did find 76% of dogs with intestinal adenocarcinoma to be male.[30] Males also appear overrepresented in smooth muscle tumors, comprising 82% of GI leiomyomas[31] and 76% of dogs with leiomyosarcoma.[23] Additionally, 90% of dogs with GI lymphoma were male.[22] Furthermore, there is a slight male predominance in nonlymphomatous small intestinal tumors in dogs.[11,32,33]

In cats, there also is a predominance of males in some studies,[17,34] with males equaling or only slightly exceeding females in others,* although three of four cats with large granular lymphoma were female.[14]

Siamese cats are 1.8 times more likely to develop intestinal neoplasia.[6] Siamese cats are overrepresented in studies of intestinal adenocarcinoma, up to eight times greater than other breeds, suggesting a predisposition for this disease.[2,6,15,32,38] Although small numbers of Siamese cats are included in many series of feline intestinal lymphoma, one study did show a significant overrepresentation.[13] Otherwise, there is no breed predilection for intestinal lymphoma in cats.

In dogs, few studies of intestinal neoplasia report an overrepresentation of specific breeds. Large breed dogs in general constituted most cases in a series of smooth muscle tumors.[28] Collies and German shepherd dogs are overrepresented in some reports for intestinal tumors, especially adenocarcinoma and rectal carcinoma and polyps.[21,39] It is interesting to note, however, that in 104 benign and malignant tumors diagnosed in a cohort of military working dogs (German shepherd dogs and Belgian Malinois), only one (a leiomyosarcoma) was intestinal.[40] Mast cell tumors have been reported primarily in Maltese, among other miniature breeds. Although these reports came from Japan where small breeds are popular, over 50% of reported cases in two series were in Maltese dogs, with a male predominance.[41,42]

With the exception of retroviral influence on the development of feline lymphoma, there are no known etiologic organisms or chemical agents that reliably contribute to the development of spontaneously occurring intestinal neoplasia in dogs and cats. There is a known association of FeLV and feline immunodeficiency virus (FIV) with feline lymphoma. Older cats with intestinal lymphoma are usually negative for FeLV on serology, although evaluation of feline intestinal lymphoma by polymerase chain reaction (PCR) for the long terminal repeat region and immunohistochemistry (IHC) for gp70 antigen has shown some tumors to be positive for viral DNA, even when seronegative for FeLV p27 antigen. For intestinal lymphoma, PCR was more often positive than IHC.[43,44] These results suggest FeLV exposure in the development of lymphoma in some cats serologically negative for FeLV, and they support PCR as the most useful of these tests for identifying possible occult, latent, replication-deficient, or partial genome virus infection in tissue. With younger cats more often IHC positive and IHC correlating well with seropositivity, PCR may identify cats with lymphoma that have been exposed to FeLV but are seronegative.[43] There is no association between retroviral infection and nonlymphomatous intestinal neoplasia in cats, with most cats testing negative for FeLV and/or FIV serologically.[15,32]

In other species, type-A retrovirus particles have been found in a metastatic intestinal adenocarcinoma in a boa, and cytomegalovirus has been associated with GI epithelial masses in macaque monkeys infected with simian immunodeficiency virus.[45,46]

Helicobacter pylori infection is associated with increased risk of gastric cancer in humans, although no such association has been confirmed in domestic animals. Concurrent lymphoma and *Helicobacter* infection has been reported in a cat, but causal association was not proved.[47] Multiple gastroduodenal adenocarcinomas and a rectal adenoma were found in a cougar with concurrent *Helicobacter*-like organisms and spirochetes.[48] Some cats shed *Helicobacter* species in the feces and thus may represent normal flora rather than pathogens.[49]

Finally, lymphoma (although not specifically intestinal) has been reported in a dog 4 weeks after initiation of cyclosporine and ketoconazole therapy for anal furunculosis.[50] There is an

*References 12, 13, 15, 16, 18-20, 25, 26, 35-37.

association between cyclosporine use in human transplant patients and the development of lymphoma.

Pathology and Natural Behavior

Epithelial, mesenchymal, neuroendocrine, and discrete/round cell neoplasias can all be found in the intestinal tract. In both cats and dogs, lymphoma is the most common type of small intestinal neoplasia, followed by adenocarcinoma. Subtypes of feline intestinal lymphoma include lymphocytic, lymphoblastic, epitheliotropic, and large granular lymphocyte (LGL) types. Because of advances in novel targeted receptor tyrosine kinase inhibitors (TKIs) in human medicine, characteristics of GISTs have also been reported in dogs. Other tumors include leiomyosarcoma in both dogs and cats, carcinoids in dogs, and mast cell tumors in cats. There are scattered case reports of uncommon tumors, such as extramedullary plasmacytoma, extraskeletal osteosarcoma, and hemangiosarcoma. Although most small intestinal neoplasia is malignant in dogs, most rectal tumors are benign polyps, adenomas, or carcinoma in situ[29,51] (Figure 22-22).

Most alimentary adenocarcinoma in cats is found in the small intestine.[1,30,37] However, the colon and rectum are a more common site in dogs.[7,8] Of colorectal adenocarcinomas, the rectum is a more common site than the colon.[52] The cecum is more likely to develop leiomyosarcoma or GIST than adenocarcinoma.[8,23] Histologic descriptors for carcinoma of the intestine include adeno- (forming glands), mucinous (>50% mucin), signet ring (>50% of cells have intracellular mucin), and undifferentiated or solid (no evidence of gland formation).[7] Grossly, colorectal adenocarcinomas may demonstrate a pedunculated (especially in the distal rectum), cobblestone (middle rectum), or annular (middle rectum) appearance, which may relate to behavior and prognosis[8,52,53] (Figure 22-23).

Adenomatous polyps are found in the rectum of dogs, and carcinoma in situ is found in both the colon and rectum. Most lesions are solitary, although multiple and diffuse lesions can be seen and are associated with increased recurrence rates.[29] In cats, polyps are more common in the duodenum.

The term *carcinoid* refers to tumors that arise from the diffuse endocrine system rather than the intestinal epithelium, despite histologic similarity to carcinomas. Carcinoid cells arise from enterochromaffin cells of the intestinal mucosa and contain secretory granules that may contain substances such as 5-hydroxytryptamine (serotonin), secretin, somatostatin, and gastrin, among others.[7] IHC for cytokeratin and for secretory substances such as serotonin may be positive, and serum concentration of serotonin has been documented at 10 times the normal range in one dog with a carcinoid.[54] Described in many species, carcinoids may occur in both the large and the small intestines and frequently metastasize to the liver.[2,8,54] Carcinoids may follow an aggressive and debilitating clinical course.[54]

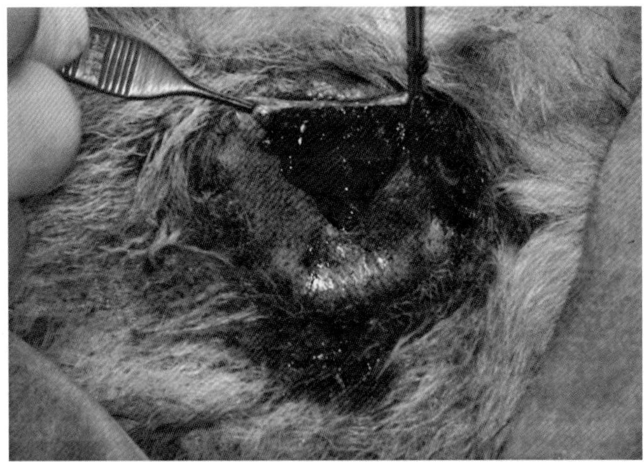

FIGURE 22-22 Cobblestone appearance to a rectal adenocarcinoma. Dogs with this tumor type live an average of 12 months following surgical excision.[52] *(Courtesy Dr. Eric Pope, Ross University, College of Veterinary Medicine.)*

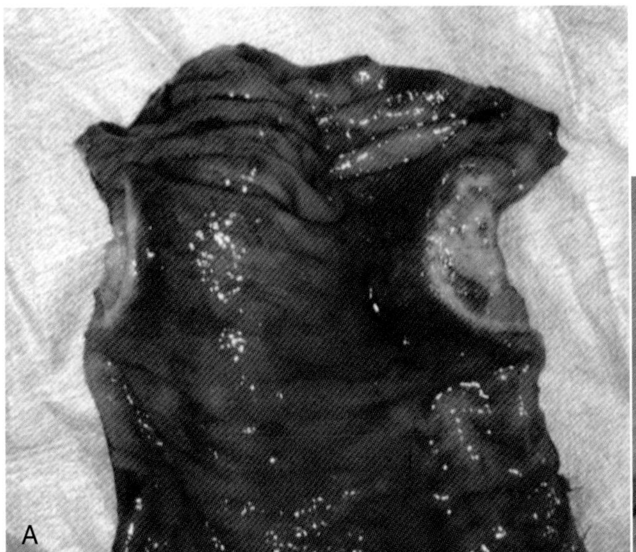

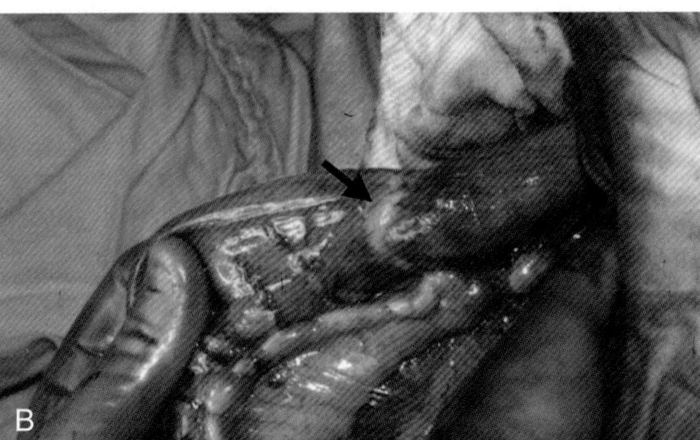

FIGURE 22-23 An annular form of clonic adenocarcinoma causing a stricture. The thick band of tissue **(B)** creating the stricture is seen on cross-section **(A)**. In one study, dogs with this type of tumor survived an average of only 1.6 months.[52] *(Courtesy Dr. Eric Pope, Ross University, College of Veterinary Medicine.)*

GISTs are well documented in humans and have been reported in dogs.[55] These nonlymphoid tumors of mesenchymal origin were originally diagnosed as leiomyosarcomas and some but not all were leiomyomas. Histologically, GISTs are highly cellular mesenchymal tumors that do *not* show ultrastructural characteristics consistent with smooth muscle differentiation. GISTs are thought to arise from multipotential stem cells phenotypically similar to interstitial cells of Cajal, driven by activating mutations of Kit. These cells regulate intestinal motility via an autonomic pacemaker effect. Although these cells can differentiate into smooth muscle cells if deprived of Kit, GISTs are a discrete clinical entity from leiomyosarcoma.[56] GISTs are distinguished by high vimentin immunoreactivity, low alpha smooth muscle actin reactivity, CD117 (Kit) reactivity, and a site predilection for the large intestine (compared to the stomach for leiomyoma).[31,57] Activating mutations were identified in Kit exon 11 encoding the juxtamembrane domain in two of four cases examined.[31] CD117 reactivity is considered a major diagnostic criteria and in many studies is used to distinguish GISTs from leiomyosarcomas.[58,59] When stratified as such, 28 of 42 leiomyosarcomas in dogs were reclassified as GISTs and only 2 of the 28 cases of GIST metastasized (7%). These investigators also found that GISTs were significantly more likely to occur in the large intestine, specifically the cecum, and leiomyosarcomas in the stomach and small intestine.[58] Considering these findings, the incidence of true leiomyosarcoma is likely low because many previously reported cases may have actually been GISTs. Leiomyomas occur more commonly in the stomach but have also been reported in the esophagus, small intestine, and colorectum.[31]

Intestinal lymphoma in dogs occurs in the stomach and small intestine equally and more often in both of these sites than the large intestine. Lesions are typically diffuse, and neoplastic cells infiltrate the submucosa and lamina propria. Additional visceral and systemic involvement may be seen.

Intestinal lymphoma in cats was originally thought to be predominantly of B-cell origin, resulting from its origin in Peyer's patches and germinal centers; however, some reports suggest that the incidence of T-cell lymphoma may equal or exceed that of B-cell lymphoma.[20,34,44] IHC and PCR for antigen receptor rearrangement (PARR) can be useful in identifying predominant immunophenotype and clonality, as well as distinguishing lymphoma from severe inflammation.[60,61] There is no clear association between the presence of FeLV antigens in tissue and clonality (B-cell versus T-cell).[44] Incidence of feline intestinal lymphoma appears to have increased over the past 2 decades to an extent that may exceed that attributed to an aging cat population.[62] Within a diagnosis of intestinal lymphoma, subtype also impacts behavior. In one series, cats with lymphocytic/small cell lymphoma experienced a 69% complete remission rate with prednisone and chlorambucil for a MST of nearly 2 years, whereas cats with lymphoblastic lymphoma had only an 18% complete remission rate with combination chemotherapy for a MST of less than 3 months. Cats with lymphoblastic lymphoma were more likely to have a palpable abdominal mass and require surgery for intestinal obstruction than cats with lymphocytic lymphoma.[35]

Other unique subsets of feline intestinal lymphoma include epitheliotropic and LGL lymphoma. Most of these cats are serologically negative for FeLV. Immunohistochemical evaluation of feline epitheliotropic lymphoma shows these tumors to be strictly T-cell in origin and 80% small/lymphocytic.[34,63] In one study, although great overlap of values occurred, there was a significantly greater percentage of intraepithelial lymphocytes in neoplastic compared to normal cats and inflammatory bowel disease cases. The determination of epitheliotropism depends on the pathologist's interpretation. As with epitheliotropic cutaneous lymphoma, microabscesses are often seen. Intraepithelial lymphocytes are richer in villous than crypt epithelium, suggesting that this diagnosis may be reliably made with endoscopic biopsies. This disease may represent a continuum from inflammatory bowel disease.[34]

By contrast, LGL lymphoma of the intestine (also called globule leukocyte and granulated round cell tumor) often has a rapidly progressive and fatal course.[64,65] These tumors are distinguished by heterogeneous cytoplasmic granules (azurophilic on cytology and eosinophilic on histopathology with routine hematoxylin and eosin [H&E] staining) and are commonly seen in the intestinal tract (especially jejunum), occasionally with leukemic cells.[66,67] Perforin-like immunoreactivity has been demonstrated and may help distinguish these from other lymphomas.[14]

Extramedullary plasmacytoma (EMP) refers to solitary tumors with no evidence of systemic multiple myeloma. Case reports of GI EMP in dogs and cats exist, though uncommon. In one series, one-fourth of EMPs were found in the digestive system, most in the mouth.[68] One case report in a dog with EMP of the colon and rectum was associated with monoclonal gammopathy.[69] Another uncommon tumor type is extraskeletal osteosarcoma, which has been reported in the duodenum of a cat. This cat had no evidence of metastasis at diagnosis but did well for only 4 months after surgery when clinical signs recurred and the cat died.[70] Three of 55 extraskeletal and 145 total cases of feline osteosarcoma were of intestinal origin.[71] A series of four cats was reported with intestinal hemangiosarcoma arising from four different locations within the intestines, with none surviving greater than 1 week.[72] Finally, one dog was diagnosed with ganglioneuroma of the rectum and experienced long-term survival following surgical resection.[73]

Intestinal mast cell tumors are cited as the third most common tumor following lymphoma and adenocarcinoma in cats, but incidence and behavior are poorly reported. They have been confused with carcinoids but are distinct.[12] They may present as an eosinophilic enteritis, and conversely, eosinophilic enteritis may mimic intestinal tumors.[74,75] Intestinal sclerosing mast cell tumor in the cat is a potentially aggressive variant characterized by moderate-to-abundant dense stromal tissue, marked eosinophilic infiltrates, and some cases with tryptase and c-kit immunoreactivity. Ultrasonographic changes were transmural, and tumors were most commonly located in the small intestine. Outcome was reported for 25 of 50 cats, and survival was less than 2 months for 23/25; however, outcome was unknown for the remaining 25 cats.[76] In dogs, intestinal mast cell tumors occur primarily in the stomach and small intestine, are typically poorly granulated, and are often immunohistochemically positive for toluidine blue, c-kit, and tryptase. Mucosal mast cells may be structurally distinct from cutaneous mast cells.[41]

When tumors of the GI system metastasize, sites of predilection in decreasing frequency include mesenteric lymph nodes (especially adenocarcinoma), liver (especially leiomyosarcoma), mesentery, omentum, spleen, kidney, bone, peritoneum/carcinomatosis, and lung.[11,32,37,53] Interestingly, metastasis from intestinal adenocarcinoma was discovered in three dogs initially presented for testicular masses.[77] One dog was presented for multiple cutaneous masses that suggested round cell or epithelial malignancy on cytology but for which IHC confirmed epithelial origin. A primary small intestinal adenocarcinoma with additional visceral metastasis was identified at necropsy.[78] Lymphoma is often a systemic disease, and one-fourth of dogs and four-fifths of cats with GI lymphoma will have concurrent involvement of other organs.[13,22]

Molecular Aspects

With an increasing armamentarium of molecular diagnostics, insights as to the pathogenesis, progression, and prognosis of tumors are constantly emerging. Cellular adhesion and invasion (e.g., Tenascin-C,[51,79] versica, hyaluronan,[80] β-catenin, and E-cadherin[81-83]), stromal remodeling, and alterations in tumor suppressor genes (e.g., *p53*[81,83-85]) may play a role in the development and progression of intestinal neoplasia. The importance of the relationship between a tumor cell and its stroma should not be overlooked. Although molecular markers/targets likely play an important role in intestinal tumors, the utility of these in diagnostics, prognostication, and therapy in companion animal species, with the exception of GIST and CD117 expression, is limited until further interrogations characterize their importance and provide avenues for their utility.[55]

Measures of cellular proliferation include markers such as argyrophilic nucleolar organizer regions (AgNORs). In feline intestinal lymphoma, AgNORs did not correlate with remission rate or duration or with survival time.[19]

COX enzymes are responsible for prostaglandin synthesis, and COX-2 is overexpressed in many head/neck and genitourinary tumors, creating a possible therapeutic target. COX-2 has been identified in both benign and malignant small intestinal and colorectal epithelial tumors in dogs, although the number of positive cells varies and in some studies was very low.[86,87] Additionally, one study found no COX-2 staining in 13 intestinal tumors in cats.[88] COX inhibitors are thus of questionable value in treating intestinal tumors.

History and Clinical Signs

The duration of clinical signs prior to presentation typically averages 6 to 8 weeks but can range from less than 1 day to several months.[11,22,23] Clinical signs include (in varying order of frequency): weight loss, diarrhea, vomiting, and anorexia and less frequently melena, anemia, and hypoglycemia (with smooth muscle tumors).* Clinical signs often relate to location of the tumor within the GI tract. Proximal lesions more commonly result in vomiting, small intestinal lesions in weight loss, and large bowel lesions in hematochezia and tenesmus.[30,32] Although carcinoids may secrete endocrine substances, clinical signs do not always reflect hypersecretion.[7] Dogs and cats may present with clinical signs relating to intestinal obstruction, such as anorexia, weight loss, and vomiting. Although uncommon, perforation and septic peritonitis can occur.[34] Smooth muscle tumors are located within the muscular layer of the intestines and not within the lumen and evidence of GI bleeding is often absent, but anemia and melena have been reported.[23,24]

Paraneoplastic Syndromes

One dog was presented for alopecia and *Cheyletiella* infection within 2 months of euthanasia for abdominal carcinomatosis from intestinal carcinoma. The neoplasia was not identified with abdominal ultrasound at the original work-up, but immunosuppression resulting from an underlying neoplasia was thought to lead to opportunistic *Cheyletiella* infection. While pruritus resolved with ivermectin therapy, alopecia persisted, suggesting paraneoplastic origin.[89] Neutrophilic leukocytosis (in one dog associated with monocytosis and eosinophilia) has been reported in dogs with rectal tumors. Resolution or improvement of hematologic abnormalities occurred following treatment for adenomatous rectal polyps.[90,91] Hypereosinophilia and eosinophilic tumor infiltrates have been reported in a cat and several dogs with intestinal T-cell lymphoma; the suggested cause was IL-5 secretion by the neoplastic lymphocytes.[92-94] Extramedullary plasmacytoma may lead to a hyperviscosity syndrome resulting from overproduction of immunoglobulin.[95]

Erythrocytosis managed with periodic phlebotomy was related to a cecal leiomyosarcoma in a 14-year-old dog. The diagnosis was made at postmortem 2 years later, and erythropoietin mRNA and protein were isolated from tumor cells, suggesting ectopic erythropoietin production as the cause of the erythrocytosis.[96] Hypoglycemia is also reported with intestinal smooth muscle tumors as a paraneoplastic syndrome.[97] Nephrogenic diabetes insipidus has also been documented in one dog with intestinal leiomyosarcoma.[98]

*References 2, 11, 15, 25, 27, 34, 35, 38.

Diagnostic Techniques and Work-Up

Physical Examination

An abdominal mass may be palpated on initial examination in approximately 20% to 40% of dogs with lymphoma[22,27] and 20% to 50% of dogs with nonlymphomatous solid intestinal tumors.[11,30,32] Pain and fever were reported in 20% of dogs with lymphoma in one report.[22] Digital rectal examination may identify masses or annular strictures due to rectal tumors or polyps in as high as 63% of dogs.[30,52]

Abdominal masses are also often readily palpated in cats with both lymphoma and adenocarcinoma. Approximately 50% of cats with nonlymphomatous tumors will be presented with a palpable mass.[15,32] Abnormal abdominal palpation is common in cats with lymphoma with up to 86% having a palpable mass.[16,34] Dehydration is also common, occurring in 30% to 60% of cats with nonlymphomatous tumors.[15,32]

Clinical Pathology

Complete Blood Count

Anemia is common in dogs and cats with intestinal tumors and is often not characterized but may occur in conjunction with melena and elevated blood urea nitrogen (BUN). Anemia affects nearly 40% of dogs in most studies and as low as 15% but up to 70% of cats.* Leukogram changes are also common including leukocytosis in 25% to 70% of dogs and 40% of cats.[11,15,24,32] Left shift may be seen as well as monocytosis in some patients.[32,34]

Chemistry Profile

Biochemical abnormalities are similar between dogs and cats with intestinal tumors. As a result of malabsorption, hypoproteinemia may be present in one-fourth to one-third of patients.† Other common abnormalities include elevated liver enzymes, specifically alkaline phosphatase in 15% to 33% of dogs and up to 85% of cats with nonlymphomatous neoplasia.[11,24,30,32,34] In one series a high cholesterol was seen in 41% of cats with nonlymphomatous tumors.[32] An elevated blood urea nitrogen has been reported in 13% of dogs and 30% of cats with intestinal adenocarcinoma.[11,15] This may be a result of concurrent renal insufficiency or intestinal bleeding due to the tumor or of dehydration. While some cats may have hyperglycemia,[32] smooth muscle tumors can cause up to 55%

*References 11, 16, 23, 24, 30, 32, 34.

†References 11, 15, 16, 24, 27, 30.

of patients to be hypoglycemic as a result of insulin-like growth factor secretion.[23] Dogs may also have increased amylase and electrolyte disturbances,[30] and patients with lymphoma may be hypercalcemic.[16]

Serum alpha 1-acid glycoprotein (AGP), an acute phase reactant protein, may be increased in cats with cancer but lacks specificity and prognostic relevance.[99,100]

Cytology and Histopathology

As with other anatomic sites, cytology of the intestinal tract can help differentiate among major tumor types. Additionally, lymphocyte accumulations can be tested using PARR for clonality. If amplification of variable regions in the genome of lymphocytes using PARR reveals monotony consistent with a clonal expansion, then a diagnosis of lymphoma can be confirmed. This test can be performed using either stained or unstained slides from ultrasound-guided aspirates.[60,101] PARR may detect clonal expansions not yet evident (as lymphoma) on histopathology of the same sample.[102] Because of reported eosinophilia with intestinal lymphoma and reports of mast cell tumor with concurrent small T-cell lymphoma in cats, it may be challenging to distinguish between the two.[103] Despite concerns of complications following surgery in cats with intestinal lymphoma for the purpose of obtaining diagnostic samples for histopathology or for resection of a mass, the risk of perioperative dehiscence appears to be low.[104]

Imaging

Plain and Contrast Abdominal Radiographs

In dogs and cats with intestinal lymphoma, concurrent enlargement of liver, spleen, and/or mesenteric lymph nodes may be seen.[22] Plain abdominal radiographs may reveal an abdominal mass in approximately 40% of both dogs and cats, although some reports are higher for solid tumor types and lower for lymphoma.* Intestinal lymphoma may be more difficult to identify on plain radiography because of other organ involvement, peritoneal effusion, or diffuse intestinal lesions. An obstructive pattern may also be seen on plain radiographs, with incidence ranging from 10% to 75%.[11,24,30,32] Other abnormalities may include poor serosal detail and thickened stomach wall.[16]

Contrast radiography, although used less following advances in ultrasound, has often been used to evaluate patients with signs of primary GI disease. Contrast radiography can help rule in or out an obstruction, localize a tumor, and view areas of the GI tract that are difficult to image with ultrasonography because of gas accumulation (Figure 22-24). Contrast radiographs may reveal filling defects in approximately half the cats and dogs with GI neoplasia.[32] In dogs with GI lymphoma, all 12 dogs examined had abnormal contrast series.[22] In one series, 87% of cats with intestinal adenocarcinoma showed evidence of partial or complete obstruction.[15]

Thoracic Radiographs

Thoracic radiographs are critical to the complete evaluation of the cancer patient. For dogs with nonlymphomatous intestinal tumors, yield is low with very few patients presenting with pulmonary metastasis.[11] This may be due to a bias in reporting because many reports detail outcome of treatment and patients with metastatic disease may not receive treatment. In fact, many case series report no evidence of metastasis on initial evaluation for solid tumors of the intestine in dogs.[11,23,24,30,32] In cats, 2 of 14 cats in one series and no cats in another had pulmonary nodules at initial evaluation.[15,32]

*References 11, 15, 16, 22, 24, 32.

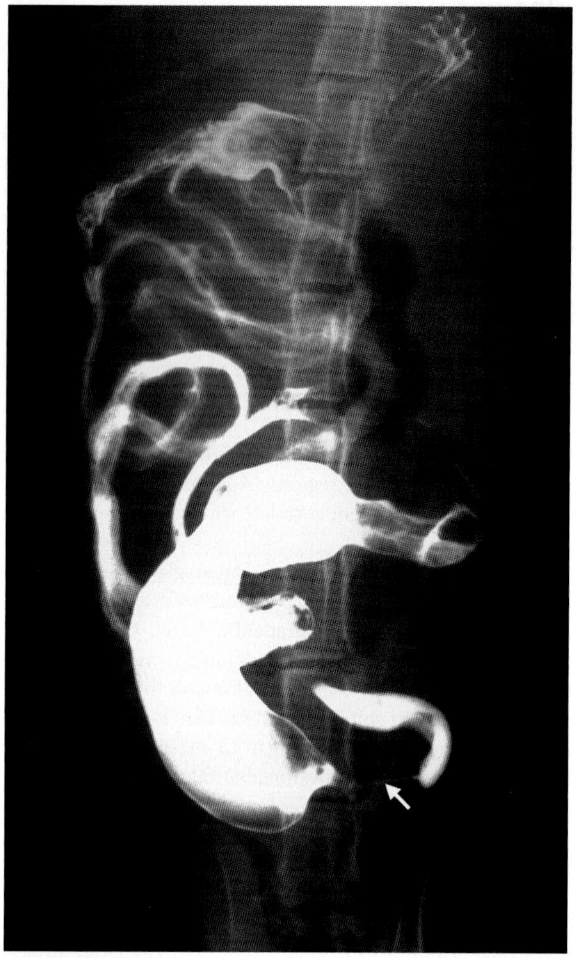

FIGURE 22-24 The arrow indicates an obstructing tumor on contrast radiography. The thin trail of barium is all that will pass through the lumen of the tumor and the obstruction is evidenced by the dilated segment of small bowel adjacent and oral to the tumor. *(Courtesy Dr. Jimmy Lattimer, University of Missouri, College of Veterinary Medicine.)*

For cats and dogs with lymphoma, enlarged sternal or perihilar lymph nodes, pleural effusion, or diffuse interstitial changes may be seen.[16,22]

Abdominal Ultrasound

Ultrasound allows noninvasive localization of the tumor and identification of other sites of metastasis/involvement. It also can guide needle aspiration or needle biopsy or assist in treatment planning. Ultrasound is a more sensitive diagnostic test than radiographs for identifying a mass.[11,23,28,105] Ultrasound is also less time consuming than contrast radiography, and the increased use, availability, and operator skill for the former has diminished the need for the latter.

Ultrasound findings in dogs and cats with intestinal neoplasia most consistently include bowel wall thickening and loss of normal wall layers.[30,105,106] Degree of thickening, distribution of lesion(s), and symmetry are also used to help differentiate neoplasia from nonneoplastic disease.[107] Intestinal lymphoma in dogs more often results in long segments of involved bowel and either a solitary mass or diffusely thickened bowel loops with thickening of the muscularis propria in cats.[35,106,108] Adenocarcinoma in cats has been described as having mixed echogenicity and was asymmetric in

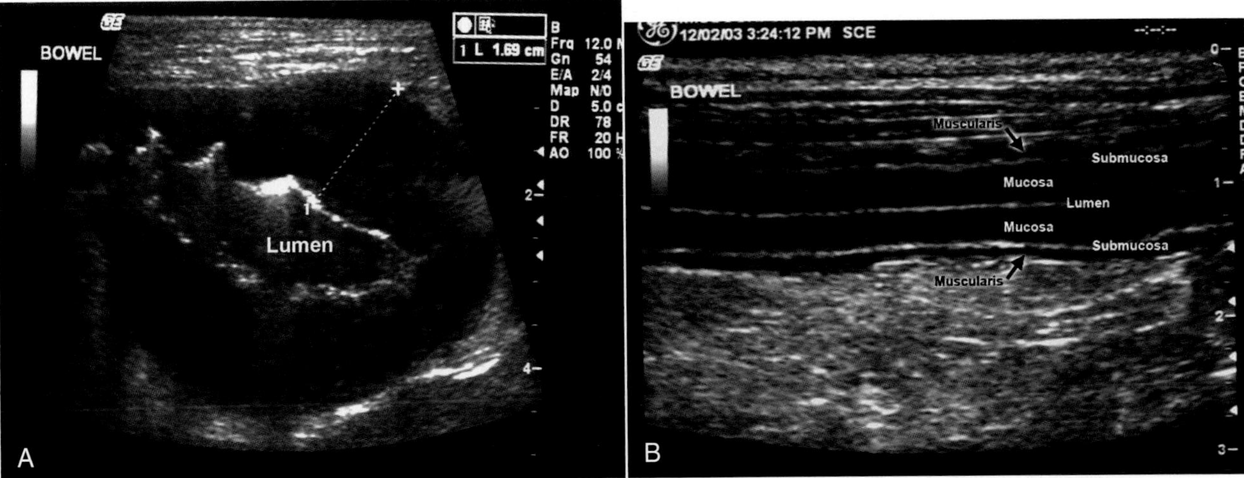

FIGURE 22-25 A cross-sectional ultrasound image of a segment of small intestine with lymphoma **(A)** is compared to a longitudinal view of a segment of normal small intestine **(B)**. Note that the clearly defined intestinal layers in the normal tissue are completely effaced in the tumor tissue. A loss of layering is strongly supportive of neoplasia. The diseased bowel is also markedly thickened, suggesting neoplasia. *(Courtesy Dr. Stephanie Essman, University of Missouri, College of Veterinary Medicine.)*

three of five cats.[105] In one study, two-thirds of dogs with intestinal adenocarcinoma had hypoechoic tumors, and most had decreased motility. Masses averaged 4-cm long with a median wall thickness of 1.2 cm.[8,30] Mast cell tumors have an eccentric appearance with alteration but not loss of wall layering, commonly involving the muscularis propria.[103] Smooth muscle tumors are characteristically large (median diameter 4.8 cm) and anechoic/hypoechoic, and a muscular layer origin may be identified. Leiomyomas may have a smooth contour.[28]

Ultrasound has also proven useful in differentiating neoplastic from nonneoplastic intestinal disease. Dogs with tumors have significantly thicker intestinal walls, and 99% have a loss of wall layering compared to a maintenance of wall layering in 88% of dogs with nonneoplastic disease (Figure 22-25). In fact, dogs with a loss of wall layering are more than 50 times more likely to have a tumor than enteritis. Additionally, dogs with walls thicker than 1 cm are nearly 4 times as likely to have a tumor, and those with focal lesions are nearly 20 times as likely.[106] Nevertheless, possible differential diagnoses include fungal (Pythiosis and histoplasmosis) masses that can mimic neoplasia.[107] Lymphadenopathy can also be seen with both neoplasia (lymphoma and solid tumors), as well as with infectious or inflammatory bowel disease. In general, neoplasia exhibits more dramatic thickening with loss of wall layering and greater lymph node enlargement, as well as more frequent focal lesions than nonneoplastic intestinal disease.[107]

In a series of 14 cats with carcinomatosis, 3 of which were a result of small intestinal tumors (2 carcinomas and 1 lymphoma), the hallmark ultrasonographic finding (100% of cats) was the presence of masses in the double sheet portion of peritoneum that connects the visceral and parietal portions. All cats also had free peritoneal fluid.[36]

Endoscopy and Laparoscopy

Minimally invasive methods of collecting tissues to aid in diagnosis are increasingly used. Endoscopic findings in dogs with intestinal lymphoma include an irregular cobblestone or patchy erythematous appearance to the duodenal mucosa and poor distensibility and elasticity of the duodenal wall.[27]

Significant interobserver variation may occur in the interpretation of biopsy samples. In one study, blinded pathologists assigned a degree of mucosal cellular infiltrate as severe as neoplasia in five clinically normal research dogs.[109] Interobserver variation is likely to be more pronounced with small tissue samples and this is a limitation of these less invasive approaches.

Exploratory Laparotomy

When noninvasive or minimally invasive diagnostics fail to confirm a diagnosis, an exploratory laparotomy may be indicated for a dog or cat with persistent signs of GI disease. Benefits include direct visualization of all abdominal viscera and the ability to collect full thickness biopsies of all segments of intestines and other viscera. Patients with resectable solid tumors may be both diagnosed and treated in one procedure with resection and anastomosis. In a series of dogs with GI lymphoma, endoscopic biopsies were sometimes difficult to interpret because of lymphoplasmacytic infiltrate, but biopsies obtained by laparotomy confirmed the diagnosis in all cases undergoing surgery.[22] It should be noted that carcinomatosis should not always be seen as an indication for euthanasia (Figure 22-26). Following removal of the primary intestinal adenocarcinoma, two cats with malignant effusion lived 4.5 and 28 months after surgery.[15]

Therapy and Prognosis

Surgery

With the exception of lymphoma, surgical resection is the primary treatment for intestinal tumors. As long as severe extraserosal invasion and/or adhesions do not complicate the surgical approach, complete excision is often possible. For dogs and cats without evidence of local or distant metastasis, long-term survival is possible, although some tumors may later metastasize. Overall, the 1-year survival rate is approximately 40% for dogs with solid small intestinal tumors.[11] For cats with adenocarcinoma, approximately 50% will metastasize to the local lymph nodes, 30% to the peritoneal cavity (carcinomatosis), and 20% or less to the lungs.[2,32,37] Dogs have similar rates of metastasis to lymph nodes for both adenocarcinoma

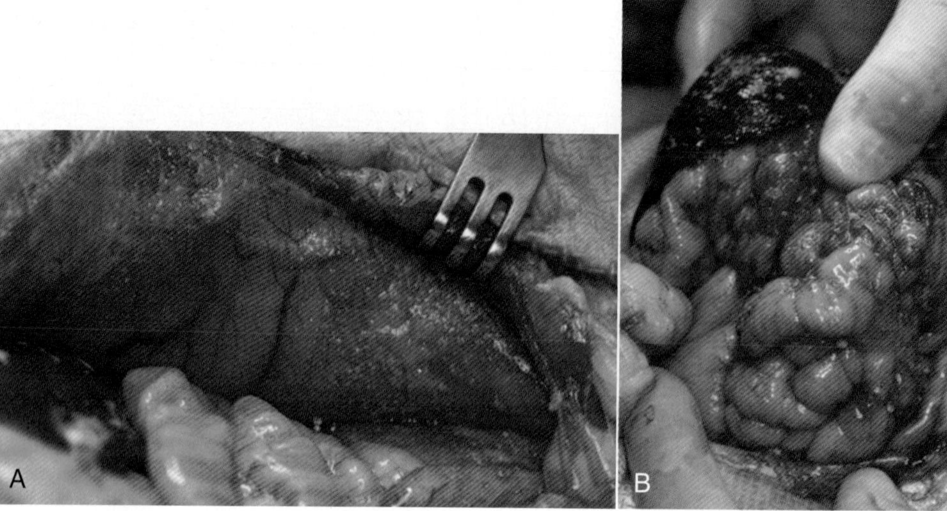

FIGURE 22-26 Carcinomatosis discovered at exploratory laparotomy. Note the irregular peritoneal surface instead of a normal glossy appearance **(A)** and the multiple serosal implants **(B)**. *(Courtesy Dr. F. A. Mann, University of Missouri, College of Veterinary Medicine.)*

and leiomyosarcoma, although liver is usually the second most frequent site.[8,11,32] Perioperative mortality can approach 30% to 50% as a result of sepsis, peritonitis, or owner decision for euthanasia when nonresectable tumors are present.[11,23]

The benefit of surgery is questionable for dogs with intestinal mast cell tumors. In two case series, most dogs died within the first month. Only 2 of 49 dogs (combined total for two series, almost all GI) lived past 180 days and prednisone was not helpful in most cases.[41,42]

Various surgical techniques have been used to treat small and large intestinal tumors. For dogs with colorectal adenocarcinoma, local excision via anal approach and rectal prolapse (when amenable) or other methods yielded a median survival of 2 to almost 4 years compared to 15 months for stool softeners alone[52,110-112]; colorectal plasmacytomas and polyps also fare well with MSTs of 15 months and 2 years or more, respectively, following surgical excision.[39,113] This is in contrast to small intestinal adenocarcinoma in which 12 days mean survival was reported without treatment, and a mean survival of only 114 days for dogs with surgical resection, though others report 7 and 10 months.[11,30,32] Regarding surgical techniques for resection and anastomosis of small intestine, stapling techniques have been shown to be equivalent to hand suturing.[114] Dogs with leiomyosarcoma who survive the perioperative period fare somewhat better with MSTs of 1.1 and almost 2 years.[23,24] One case series found the median postoperative survival for 28 dogs with GIST to be approximately 38 months (1 year if postoperative deaths were included) versus 8 months for 10 dogs with leiomyosarcoma, although the difference was not statistically significant.[58] Additionally, another study found no difference between GIST and leiomyosarcoma with 1-year survival of approximately 80%.[59] Colostomy use has been reported to aid in management of dogs with nonresectable rectal tumors. In one report, skin excoriation was the most common complication, but colostomy bags were managed for up to 7 months.[115]

Transrectal endoscopic removal of benign canine rectal tumors that would have otherwise required rectal pull-through surgery or pubic osteotomy afforded five of six dogs significant improvement in quality of life, with three dogs cured.[116] Standard treatment with surgery yields a 41% recurrence of clinical signs, and 18% of dogs experienced transition to malignancy with tumor recurrence.[29] Surgical removal of duodenal polyps in cats typically also affords a cure.[17]

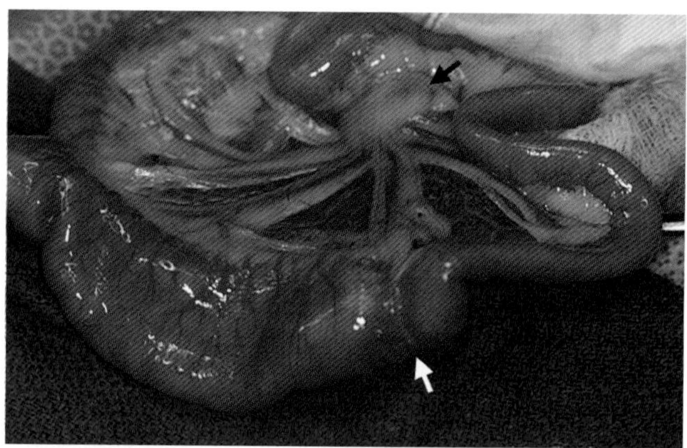

FIGURE 22-27 Intestinal obstruction as a result of adenocarcinoma *(white arrow)*. Note the distension of the jejunum oral to the mass as compared to the normal diameter aboral to the mass. There is also an enlarged lymph node *(black arrow)*. *(Courtesy Dr. Eric Pope, Ross University, College of Veterinary Medicine.)*

In cats with small intestinal adenocarcinoma, there is significant perioperative risk, but cats that live beyond 2 weeks may experience long-term control with surgery alone (Figure 22-27). In two series, all cats that did not have their tumors resected were euthanized or died within 2 weeks of surgery.[15,32] One-half of cats in one report and all cats in another that had their tumors resected died within 2 weeks of surgery, and 4 of 11 died within 2 months in another of complications or nontumor causes.[15,32,37] For the remaining cats that survived 2 weeks beyond surgery, mean survival was 15 months, although only 20 weeks in another report (median 5 weeks).[15,38]

In cats with large intestinal neoplasia, survival following surgery alone was approximately 3.5 months for lymphoma, 4.5 months for adenocarcinoma, and 6.5 months for mast cell tumor. Adjuvant

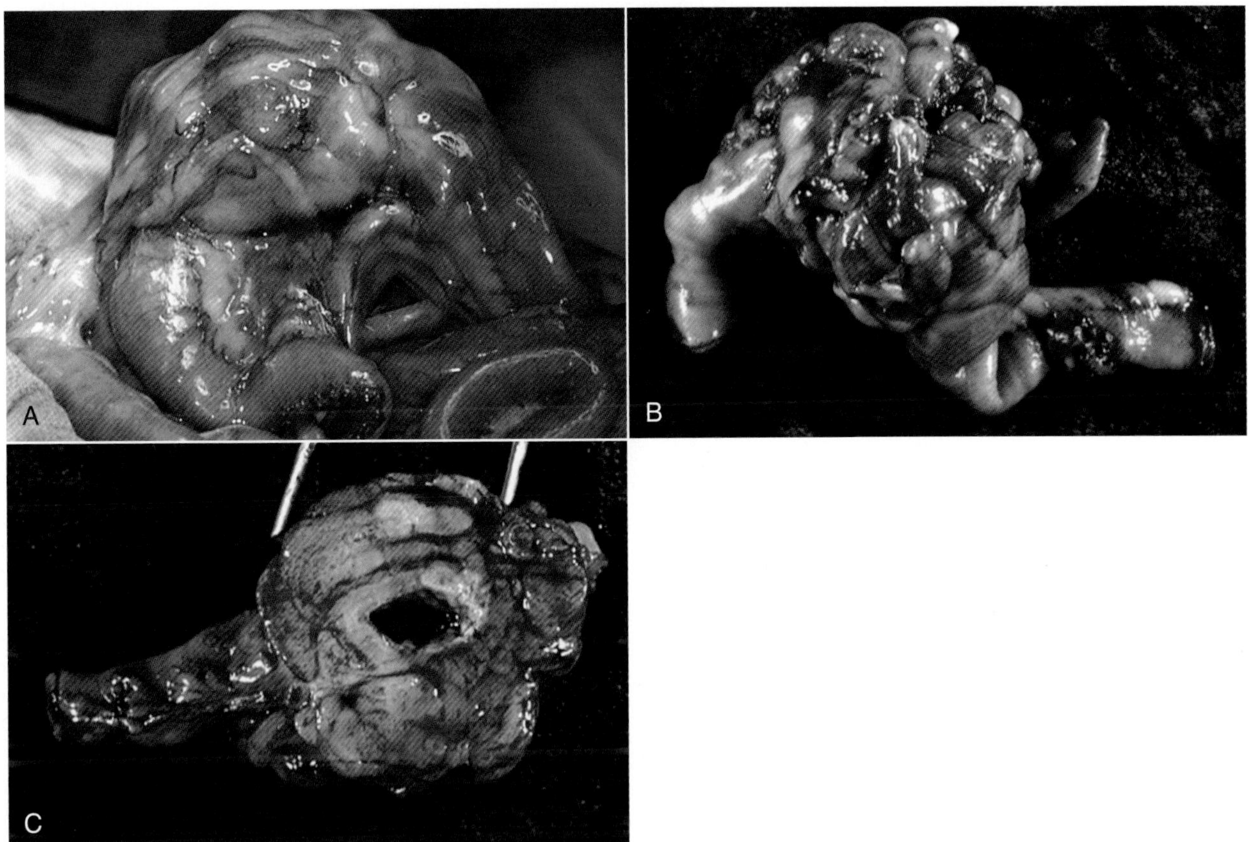

FIGURE 22-28 Intestinal lymphoma in a dog **(A)**. The specimen is shown after resection and anastomosis **(B)** and on cross-section **(C)** to illustrate the marked thickening of the bowel wall. *(Courtesy Dr. Eric Pope, Ross University, College of Veterinary Medicine.)*

chemotherapy improved survival for cats with adenocarcinoma but not for cats with lymphoma.[18]

Lymphoma is treated primarily with chemotherapy, except when intestinal perforation or the need for a biopsy necessitates surgery (Figure 22-28). Surgery and chemotherapy did not improve survival compared to chemotherapy alone for cats with alimentary lymphoma.[20] In cats with LGL lymphoma of the intestines, few attempts at therapy have been reported in the literature. Chemotherapy induced partial or complete remission in some cats, but MST was only 57 days.[64] One cat did well for over a year following surgical resection until the tumor recurred.

Chemotherapy

No randomized studies exist to confirm or deny any benefit of adjuvant chemotherapy following resection of epithelial intestinal tumors in dogs and cats. The benefit of adjuvant chemotherapy in humans is questionable, although current fluorouracil-based regimens are often considered to be the standard of care. One retrospective study in cats with colonic adenocarcinoma did show a significant survival advantage for cats receiving adjuvant doxorubicin, with a median survival of 280 days with and 56 days without chemotherapy.[18] For carcinomatosis, intracavitary therapy may be helpful with carboplatin for cats or cisplatin or 5-fluorouracil (5-FU) for dogs.[117] When attempted, adjuvant chemotherapy typically includes doxorubicin in veterinary medicine. Two dogs with leiomyosarcoma received adjuvant chemotherapy following surgical resection. One had metastasis at surgery and died 4 months later, and the other was lost at over 2 years, but there were several other dogs in that series that were long lived that did not receive chemotherapy.[23] Two dogs with adenocarcinoma also received chemotherapy following surgery and both survived over 17 months.[30]

In dogs with GI lymphoma, of the eight dogs treated in one report, all were euthanized by 14 weeks.[22] In cats with intestinal lymphoma, MST is typically 6 to 9 months, although many studies comment that a subset of cats did very well, living over 2 years.[16,25,35] This may relate to histologic subtype because cats with lymphocytic lymphoma (75% of cases, 70% to 90% response rate, approximately 2-year MST with chlorambucil and prednisone) fared vastly better than those with lymphoblastic lymphoma (25% of cases, <20% response rate, 2.7-month MST with multiagent chemotherapy).[35,63] General treatment of feline lymphoma is discussed elsewhere (see Chapter 33, Section B), but treatment regimens reported typically include vincristine, doxorubicin, prednisone, and cyclophosphamide for lymphoblastic lymphoma and chlorambucil and prednisone for cats with lymphocytic lymphoma.[35]

A reduction in the size and clinical signs of rectal polyps in eight dogs was noted following piroxicam therapy, either orally or in suppository form. Clinical response did not relate to whether there was inflammation associated with the tumor.[91]

Radiation Therapy

Because of concern for toxicity to surrounding abdominal viscera, the ability to often completely excise intestinal tumors for adequate local control, and the inability to reliably irradiate the same tissue each day because intestines are mobile, RT is seldom used in the treatment of intestinal tumors.

Prognostic Factors

Intestinal perforation does not appear to be a negative prognostic factor for leiomyosarcoma because dogs surviving the perioperative period enjoyed prolonged survival in one series.[23] For colorectal tumors, treatment is prognostic with local excision significantly better than palliative care. Gross appearance, although not statistically examined, may determine outcome because dogs with annular, obstructing masses survived a mean of 1.6 months; nodular or cobblestone masses 12 months; and single, pedunculated masses 32 months.[52]

For nonlymphomatous small intestinal tumors in dogs, metastasis at the time of surgery resulted in significantly shorter survival times (3 months versus 15 months). One-year survival for dogs with lymph node metastasis was 20% as compared to 67% without.[11] In another study, however, dogs with and without visceral metastasis from leiomyosarcoma survived equally long following surgical resection (21 months).[23] In one study, males fared significantly better than females for small intestinal adenocarcinoma, although the number of females was small.[30]

The strongest prognostic factor for cats with intestinal lymphoma is response to treatment. Cats achieving a complete resolution of clinical signs typically fare significantly better than those that do not.[20,118] For cats with epitheliotropic lymphoma, those that did not achieve remission (euthanized within 3.5 months) had a worse survival than those that achieved remission (median 11 months).[34] For 103 cats with lymphoma, 28 of which were intestinal, negative prognostic factors were FeLV positivity (median survival 3 months if positive, 17 months if negative for early stage disease, not prognostic for advanced stages) and advanced stage of disease.[26] FeLV status did not affect outcome in other studies.[20,25] For large intestinal neoplasia, cats with surgery for lymphoma fared equally poorly with and without adjuvant chemotherapy (median survival of just over 3 months in both groups). Cats with adenocarcinoma, however, survived significantly longer if they were treated with subtotal colectomy (138 days versus 68 days with mass excision), received postoperative doxorubicin (280 days with versus 56 days without), and had negative lymph nodes at surgery (259 days negative versus 49 days positive).[18]

Comparative Aspects

Although cancer of the large intestine and rectum is well characterized in humans, small intestinal neoplasia is rare. Theories for this discrepancy include more rapid small intestinal transit time as compared to the large intestine (creating less contact time for carcinogens), dilution of carcinogens with fluid as compared to solid stool, differences in pH, relative lack of bacteria to allow transformation of procarcinogens, presence of detoxifying enzymes, and increased presence of immunoglobulin A promoting local immunosurveillance of damaged cells as a result of increased lymphocytes in the small intestine. Intake of red meat, salt-cured foods, and fat are associated with an increased risk of small intestinal neoplasia, although tobacco and alcohol use were not.[119] This is in contrast to veterinary medicine where in cats and sometimes dogs, malignant neoplasia is more common in the small than the large intestine. This may reflect differences in physiology, diet, or genetics among species. The difference in species may also be a matter of proportion in that humans develop a large number of colorectal cancers as a result of diet and genetic influences. As in animals, tumors of the small intestine of humans are usually malignant. Diagnostic evaluation is similar to that described in animals, although advanced imaging such as CT is more often used. Most diagnoses are made at surgery and 5-year survival rates average just over 20%.[119]

In contrast to the rarity of small bowel neoplasia, large bowel/colorectal cancer is one of the most frequently diagnosed cancers in both men and women. Risk factors include genetic predisposition/familial history, tobacco and alcohol intake, advanced age, and predisposing medical conditions, among others. Colorectal cancer development may further be influenced by intake of red meat (especially fried), low-fiber and/or high-fat diet, obesity, fecal pH, and fecal mutagens. Among genetic risk factors, polymorphism in colonic enzymes and mutations leading to familial adenomatous syndromes are uncommon but are important as models of carcinogenesis. In most familial polyposis syndromes, the adenomatous polyposis coli (APC) gene is mutated. The multistage progression from benign polyp to carcinoma is well understood and underscores the importance of early detection.[120] In contrast, hereditary nonpolyposis colon cancer (HNPCC) develops without known premalignant polyps. It is inherited via autosomal dominance with high penetration and is characterized by microsatellite instability.[121]

Severe celiac disease in humans is associated with an increased risk of lymphoma. Progression to lymphoma from inflammatory bowel disease (IBD), especially in cats, has been postulated but not confirmed. Two of 97 cats with lymphoma had a history of IBD in a population of cats examined for comparison to a group of cats with IBD at one institution during the same time period.[122]

The most clinically important aspects of comparative oncology when considering intestinal neoplasia in humans are the use of COX inhibitors in treatment, the prevention of colorectal neoplasia, and the use of TKIs. In people, KIT mutations in GI stromal tumors have led to the use of imatinib mesylate, a TKI that inhibits KIT.[123] This illustrates the notion of therapy directed at the molecular defect rather than the histologic diagnosis. KIT is mutated in some canine GISTs, and thus TKIs may benefit this population as well.

COX inhibition by NSAIDs will decrease the incidence of colorectal cancer and decrease mortality by 40% to 50%.[124] Among the proposed mechanisms of action, prostaglandin production is thought to be related to tumor progression and therefore inhibition leads to cancer prevention. Additionally, non-COX pathways include inhibition of transcription factors and induction of nuclear hormone receptors that lead to cellular differentiation.[124] Interestingly, a recent retrospective study found a significantly reduced incidence of cancer in dogs with a history of NSAID use (71% reduced risk).[125]

Therapy in humans is similar to that in companion animals. Surgical resection is the primary mode of therapy, with adjuvant targeted or traditional chemotherapy in many cases, especially if patients present with lymph node metastasis or unresectable disease. Transanal endoscopic resection is used when possible for rectal tumors, and this technique has been performed with some success in dogs. TKIs may improve prognosis for unresectable and metastatic GISTs.[123] Adjuvant chemotherapy is used in colon cancer, with 5-FU–based combinations providing the best control often in combination with a platinum agent, with some studies showing decreased local recurrence but not increased overall survival.[126] RT is used primarily for areas of the GI tract that are not very mobile, such as the stomach and rectum.

REFERENCES

1. Cotchin E: Some tumours of dogs and cats of comparative veterinary and human interest, *Vet Rec* 71(45):1040–1050, 1959.

2. Patnaik AK, Liu SK, Johnson GF: Feline intestinal adenocarcinoma, *Vet Pathol* 13:1–10, 1976.
3. Engle GG, Brodey RS: A retrospective study of 395 feline neoplasms, *J Am Anim Hosp Assoc* 5:21–31, 1969.
4. Dobson JM, Samuel S, Milstein H, et al: Canine neoplasia in the UK: estimates of incidence rates from a population of insured dogs, *J Small Anim Pract* 43(6):240–246, 2002.
5. Bastianello SS: A survey of neoplasia in domestic species over a 40-year period from 1935 to 1974 in the republic of South Africa. V. Tumours occurring in the cat, *Onderstepoort J Vet Res* 50:105–110, 1983.
6. Rissetto K, Villamil JA, Selting KA, et al: Recent trends in feline intestinal neoplasia: an epidemiologic study of 1,129 cases in the veterinary medical database from 1964 to 2004, *J Am Anim Hosp Assoc* 47:28–36, 2011.
7. Head KW, Else RW, Dubielzig RR: Tumors of the intestines. In Meuten DJ, editor: *Tumors in domestic animals*, ed 4, Ames, Iowa, 2002, Iowa State Press.
8. Patnaik AK, Hurvitz AI, Johnson GF: Canine intestinal adenocarcinoma and carcinoid, *Vet Pathol* 17:149–163, 1980.
9. Dorn CR, Taylor DON, Schneider R, et al: Survey of animal neoplasms in Alameda and Contra Costa Counties, California. II. Cancer morbidity in dogs and cats from Alameda County, *J Natl Cancer Inst* 40:307–318, 1968.
10. Veterinary Cancer Registry, www.vetcancerregistry.com. Searched March 2005, by permission from Dr. Steve Steinberg.
11. Crawshaw J, Berg J, Sardinas JC, et al: Prognosis for dogs with nonlymphomatous, small intestinal tumors treated by surgical excision, *J Am Anim Hosp Assoc* 34:451–456, 1998.
12. Alroy J, Leav I, DeLellis RA, et al: Distinctive intestinal mast cell neoplasms of domestic cats, *Lab Invest* 33(2):159–167, 1975.
13. Gabor LJ, Malik R, Canfield PJ: Clinical and anatomical features of lymphosarcoma in 118 cats, *Aust Vet J* 76(11):725–732, 1998.
14. Kariya K, Konno A, Ishida T: Perforin-like immunoreactivity in four cases of lymphoma of large granular lymphocytes in the cat, *Vet Pathol* 34:156–159, 1997.
15. Kosovsky JE, Matthiesen DT, Patnaik AK: Small intestinal adenocarcinoma in cats: 32 cases (1978-1985), *J Am Vet Med Assoc* 192(2):233–235, 1988.
16. Mahony OM, Moore AS, Cotter SM, et al: Alimentary lymphoma in cats: 28 cases (1988-1993), *J Am Vet Med Assoc* 207(12):1593–1598, 1995.
17. MacDonald JM, Mullen HS, Moroff SD: Adenomatous polyps of the duodenum in cats: 18 cases (1985-1990), *J Am Vet Med Assoc* 202(4):647–651, 1993.
18. Slaweinski MJ, Mauldin GE, Mauldin GN, et al: Malignant colonic neoplasia in cats: 46 cases (1990-1996), *J Am Vet Med Assoc* 211:878–881, 1997.
19. Rassnick KM, Mauldin GN, Moroff SD, et al: Prognostic value of argyrophilic nucleolar organizer region (AgNOR) staining in feline intestinal lymphoma, *J Vet Intern Med* 13:187–190, 1999.
20. Zwahlen CH, Lucroy MD, Kraegel SA, et al: Results of chemotherapy for cats with alimentary malignant lymphoma: 21 cases (1993-1997), *J Am Vet Med Assoc* 213:1144–1149, 1998.
21. Patnaik AK, Hurvitz AI, Johnson GF: Canine gastrointestinal neoplasms, *Vet Pathol* 14:547–555, 1977.
22. Couto CG, Rutgers HC, Sherding RG, et al: Gastrointestinal lymphoma in 20 dogs: a retrospective study, *J Vet Intern Med* 3:73–78, 1989.
23. Cohen M, Post GS, Wright JC: Gastrointestinal leiomyosarcoma in 14 dogs, *J Vet Intern Med* 17:107–110, 2003.
24. Kapatkin AS, Mullen HS, Matthiesen DT, et al: Leiomyosarcoma in dogs: 44 cases (1983-1988), *J Am Vet Med Assoc* 201(7):1077–1079, 1992.
25. Jeglum KA, Whereat A, Young K: Chemotherapy of lymphoma in 75 cats, *J Am Vet Med Assoc* 190(2):174–178, 1987.
26. Mooney SC, Hayes AA, MacEwen EG, et al: Treatment and prognostic factors in lymphoma in cats: 103 cases (1977-1981), *J Am Vet Med Assoc* 194(5):696–699, 1989.
27. Miura T, Maruyama H, Sakai M, et al: Endoscopic findings on alimentary lymphoma in 7 dogs, *J Vet Med Sci* 66(5):577–580, 2004.
28. Myers NC, Penninck DG: Ultrasonographic diagnosis of gastrointestinal smooth muscle tumors in the dog, *Vet Radiol Ultrasound* 35(5):391–397, 1994.
29. Valerius KD, Powers BE, McPherron MA, et al: Adenomatous polyps and carcinoma *in situ* of the canine colon and rectum: 34 cases (1982-1994), *J Am Anim Hosp Assoc* 33:156–160, 1997.
30. Paoloni MC, Penninck DG, Moore AS: Ultrasonographic and clinicopathologic findings in 21 dogs with intestinal adenocarcinoma, *Vet Radiol Ultrasound* 43(6):562–567, 2002.
31. Frost D, Lasota J, Miettinen M: Gastrointestinal stromal tumors and leiomyomas in the dog: a histopathologic, immunohistochemical, and molecular genetic study of 50 cases, *Vet Pathol* 40:42–54, 2003.
32. Birchard SJ, Couto CG, Johnson S: Nonlymphoid intestinal neoplasia in 32 dogs and 14 cats, *J Am Anim Hosp Assoc* 22:533–537, 1986.
33. Wolf JC, Ginn PE, Homer B, et al: Immunohistochemical detection of p53 tumor suppressor gene protein in canine epithelial colorectal tumors, *Vet Pathol* 34:394–404, 1997.
34. Carreras JK, Goldschmidt M, Lamb M, et al: Feline epitheliotropic intestinal malignant lymphoma: 10 cases (1997-2000), *J Vet Intern Med* 17:326–331, 2003.
35. Fondacaro JV, Richter KP, Carpenter JL, et al: Feline gastrointestinal lymphoma: 67 cases (1988-1996), *Eur J Comp Gastroenterol* 4(2):5–11, 1999.
36. Monteiro CB, O'Brien RT: A retrospective study on the sonographic findings of abdominal carcinomatosis in 14 cats, *Vet Radiol Ultrasound* 45(6):559–564, 2004.
37. Cribb AE: Feline gastrointestinal adenocarcinoma: a review and retrospective study, *Can Vet J* 29:709–712, 1988.
38. Turk MAM, Gallina AM, Russell TS: Nonhematopoietic gastrointestinal neoplasia in cats: a retrospective study of 44 cases, *Vet Pathol* 18:614–620, 1981.
39. Seiler RJ: Colorectal polyps of the dog: a clinicopathologic study of 17 cases, *J Am Vet Med Assoc* 174:72–75, 1979.
40. Peterson MR, Frommelt RA, Dunn DG: A study of the lifetime occurrence of neoplasia and breed differences in a cohort of German Shepherd Dogs and Belgian Malinois military working dogs that died in 1992, *J Vet Intern Med* 14:140–145, 2000.
41. Ozaki K, Yamagami T, Nomura K, et al: Mast cell tumors of the gastrointestinal tract in 39 dogs, *Vet Pathol* 39:557–564, 2002.
42. Takahashi T, Kadosawa T, Nagase M, et al: Visceral mast cell tumors in dogs: 10 cases (1982-1997), *J Am Vet Med Assoc* 216:222–226, 2000.
43. Jackson ML, Haines DM, Meric SM, et al: Feline leukemia virus detection by immunohistochemistry and polymerase chain reaction in formalin-fixed, paraffin-embedded tumor tissue from cats with lymphosarcoma, *Can J Vet Res* 57:269–276, 1993.
44. Jackson ML, Wood SL, Misra V, et al: Immunohistochemical identification of B and T lymphocytes in formalin-fixed, paraffin-embedded feline lymphosarcomas: relation to feline leukemia virus status, tumor site, and patient age, *Can J Vet Res* 60:199–204, 1996.
45. Oros J, Lorenzo H, Andrada M, et al: Type A-like retroviral particles in a metastatic intestinal adenocarcinoma in an emerald tree boa (*Corallus caninus*), *Vet Pathol* 41:515–518, 2004.
46. Hendricks-Hutto E, Anderson DC, Mansfield KG: Cytomegalovirus-associated discrete gastrointestinal masses in macaques infected with the simian immunodeficiency virus, *Vet Pathol* 41:691–695, 2004.
47. Fry DR, Slocombe RF, Beck C: Gastric lymphoma associated with the presence of helicobacter in a cat, *Aust Vet Pract* 33(3):126–131, 2003.
48. Yamazaki Y, Aono I, Ohya T, et al: Gastroduodenal adenocarcinomas and rectal adenoma in a cougar (*Felis concolor*) infected with *Helicobacter*-like organisms and spirochetes, *J Vet Med Sci* 64(2):149–153, 2002.

49. Fox JG, Shen Z, Xu S, et al: *Helicobacter marmotae* sp. nov. isolated from livers of woodchucks and intestines of cats, *J Clin Microbiol* 40(7):2513–2519, 2002.
50. Blackwood L, German AJ, Stell AJ, et al: Multicentric lymphoma in a dog after cyclosporine therapy, *J Small Anim Pract* 45:259–262, 2004.
51. Mukaratirwa S, de Witte E, van Ederen AM, et al: Tenascin expression in relation to stromal tumour cells in canine gastrointestinal epithelial tumours, *J Comp Path* 129:137–146, 2003.
52. Church EM, Mehlhaff CJ, Patnaik AK: Colorectal adenocarcinoma in dogs: 78 cases (1973-1984), *J Am Vet Med Assoc* 191(6):727–730, 1987.
53. Prater MR, Flatland B, Newman SJ, et al: Diffuse annular fusiform adenocarcinoma in a dog, *J Am Anim Hosp Assoc* 36:169–173, 2000.
54. Sako T, Uchida E, Okamoto M, et al: Immunohistochemical evaluation of a malignant intestinal carcinoid in a dog, *Vet Pathol* 40:212–215, 2003.
55. Gillespie V, Baer K, Farrelly J, et al: Canine gastrointestinal stromal tumors: immunohistochemical expression of CD34 and examination of prognostic indicators including proliferation markers Ki67 and AgNOR, *Vet Pathol* 48:283, 2011.
56. Miettinen M, Majidi M, Lasota J: Pathology and diagnostic criteria of gastrointestinal stromal tumors (GISTs): a review, *Eur J Cancer* 38 Suppl 5:S39–S51, 2002.
57. LaRock RG, Ginn PE: Immunohistochemical staining characteristics of canine gastrointestinal stromal tumors, *Vet Pathol* 34:303–311, 1997.
58. Russell KN, Mehler SJ, Skorupski KA, et al: Clinical and immunohistochemical differentiation of gastrointestinal stromal tumors from leiomyosarcomas in dogs: 42 cases (1990-2003), *J Am Vet Med Assoc* 230(9):1329–1333, 2007.
59. Maas CPHJ, Haar G, van der Gaag I, et al: Reclassification of small intestinal and cecal smooth muscle tumors in 72 dogs: clinical, histologic, and immunohistochemical evaluation, *Vet Surg* 36(4):302–313, 2007.
60. Waly NE, Gruffydd-Jones TJ, Stokes CR, et al: Immunohistochemical diagnosis of alimentary lymphomas and severe intestinal inflammation in cats, *J Comp Pathol* 133(4):253–260, 2005.
61. Kiupel M, Smedley RC, Pfent C, et al: Diagnostic algorithm to differentiate lymphoma from inflammation in feline small intestinal biopsy samples, *Vet Pathol* 48(1):212–222, 2011.
62. Louwerens M, London CA, Pedersen NC, et al: Feline lymphoma in the post-feline leukemia virus era, *J Vet Intern Med* 19(3):329–335, 2005.
63. Stein TJ, Pellin M, Steinberg H, et al: Treatment of feline gastrointestinal small-cell lymphoma with chlorambucil and glucocorticoids, *J Am Anim Hosp Assoc* 46(6):413–417, 2010.
64. Snead ECR: Large granular intestinal lymphosarcoma and leukemia in a dog, *Can Vet J* 48(8):848–851, 2007.
65. Krick EL, Little L, Patel R, et al: Description of clinical and pathological findings, treatment and outcome of feline large granular lymphocyte lymphoma (1996-2004), *Vet Comp Oncol* 6(2):102–110, 2008.
66. Wellman ML, Hammer AS, DiBartola SP, et al: Lymphoma involving large granular lymphocytes in cats: 11 cases (1982-1991), *J Am Vet Med Assoc* 201(8):1265–1269, 1992.
67. McEntee MF, Horton S, Blue J, et al: Granulated round cell tumor of cats, *Vet Pathol* 30:195–203, 1993.
68. Platz SJ, Breuer W, Pfleghaar S, et al: Prognostic value of histopathological grading in canine extramedullary plasmacytomas, *Vet Pathol* 36:23–27, 1999.
69. Trevor PB, Saunders GK, Waldron DR, et al: Metastatic extramedullary plasmacytoma of the colon and rectum in a dog, *J Am Vet Med Assoc* 203(3):406–409, 1993.
70. Stimson EL, Cook WT, Smith MM, et al: Extraskeletal osteosarcoma in the duodenum of a cat, *J Am Anim Hosp Assoc* 36:332–336, 2000.
71. Heldmann E, Anderson MA, Wagner-Mann C: Feline osteosarcoma: 145 cases (1990-1995), *J Am Anim Hosp Assoc* 36:518–521, 2000.
72. Sharpe A, Cannon MJ, Lucke VM, et al: Intestinal haemangiosarcoma in the cat: clinical and pathological features of four cases, *J Small Anim Pract* 41(9):411–415, 2000.
73. Reimer ME, Reimer MS, Saunders GK, et al: Rectal ganglioneuroma in a dog, *J Am Anim Hosp Assoc* 35:107–110, 1999.
74. Howl JH, Peterson MG: Intestinal mast cell tumor in a cat: presentation as eosinophilic enteritis, *J Am Anim Hosp Assoc* 31:457–461, 1995.
75. Regnier A, Delverdier M, Dossin O: Segmental eosinophilic enteritis mimicking intestinal tumors in a dog, *Canine Practice* 21(6):25–29, 1996.
76. Halsey CHC, Powers BE, Kamstock DA: Feline intestinal sclerosing mast cell tumour: 50 cases (1997-2008), *Vet Comp Oncol* 8(1):72–79, 2010.
77. Esplin DG, Wilson SR: Gastrointestinal adenocarcinomas metastatic to the testes and associated structures in three dogs, *J Am Anim Hosp Assoc* 34:287–290, 1998.
78. Juopperi TA, Cesta M, Tomlinson L, et al: Extensive cutaneous metastases in a dog with duodenal adenocarcinoma, *Vet Clin Pathol* 32:88–91, 2003.
79. Mukaratirwa S, Gruys E, Nederbragt H: Relationship between cell proliferation and tenascin-C expression in canine gastrointestinal tumours and normal mucosa, *Res Vet Sci* 76:133–138, 2004.
80. Mukaratirwa S, van Ederen AM, Gruys E, et al: Versican and hyaluronan expression in canine colonic adenomas and carcinomas: relation to malignancy and depth of tumour invasion, *J Comp Path* 131:259–270, 2004.
81. McEntee MF, Brenneman KA: Dysregulation of beta-catenin is common in canine sporadic colorectal tumors, *Vet Pathol* 36:228–236, 1999.
82. Restucci B, Martano M, De Vico G, et al: Expression of E-cadherin, beta-catenin and APC protein in canine colorectal tumours, *Anticancer Res* 29(8):2919–2925, 2009.
83. Aresu L, Pregel P, Zanetti R, et al: E-cadherin and β-catenin expression in canine colorectal adenocarcinoma, *Res Vet Sci* 89(3):409–414, 2010.
84. Gamblin RM, Sagartz JE, Couto CG: Overexpression of p53 tumor suppressor protein in spontaneously arising neoplasms of dogs, *Am J Vet Res* 58(8):857–863, 1997.
85. Mayr B, Reifinger M: Canine tumour suppressor gene p53 mutation in a case of anaplastic carcinoma of the intestine, *Acta Vet Hung* 50(1):31–35, 2002.
86. Knottenbelt C, Mellor D, Nixon C, et al: Cohort study of COX-1 and COX-2 expression in canine rectal and bladder tumours, *J Small Anim Pract* 47(4):196–200, 2006.
87. McEntee MF, Cates JM, Neilsen N: Cyclooxygenase-2 expression in spontaneous intestinal neoplasia of domestic dogs, *Vet Pathol* 39:428–436, 2002.
88. Beam SL, Rassnick KM, Moore AS, et al: An immunohistochemical study of cyclooxygenase-2 expression in various feline neoplasms, *Vet Pathol* 40:496–500, 2003.
89. Muller A, Guaguere E, Degorce-Rubiales F: Cheyletiellosis associated with a bowel carcinoma in an old dog, *Prat Medic Chirurg* 37(5):405–406, 2002.
90. Thompson JP, Christopher MM, Ellison GW, et al: Paraneoplastic leukocytosis associated with a rectal adenomatous polyp in a dog, *J Am Vet Med Assoc* 201(5):737–738, 1992.
91. Knottenbelt CM, Simpson JW, Tasker S, et al: Preliminary clinical observations on the use of piroxicam in the management of rectal tubulopapillary polyps, *J Small Anim Pract* 41(9):393–397, 2000.
92. Barrs VR, Beatty JA, McCandlish IA, et al: Hypereosinophilic paraneoplastic syndrome in a cat with intestinal T cell lymphosarcoma, *J Small Anim Practice* 43:401–405, 2002.
93. Ozaki K, Yamagami T, Nomura K, et al: T-cell lymphoma with eosinophilic infiltration involving the intestinal tract in 11 dogs, *Vet Pathol* 43(3):339–344, 2006.

94. Marchetti V, Benetti C, Citi S, et al: Paraneoplastic hypereosinophilia in a dog with intestinal T-cell lymphoma, *Vet Clin Pathol* 34(3):259–263, 2005.
95. Jackson MW, Helfand SC, Smedes SL, et al: Primary IgG secreting plasma cell tumor in the gastrointestinal tract of a dog, *J Am Vet Med Assoc* 204(3):404–406, 1994.
96. Sato K, Hikasa Y, Morita T, et al: Secondary erythrocytosis associated with high plasma erythropoietin concentrations in a dog with cecal leiomyosarcoma, *J Am Vet Med Assoc* 220(4):486–490, 2002.
97. Bagley RS, Levy JK, Malarkey DE: Hypoglycemia associated with intra-abdominal leiomyoma and leiomyosarcoma in six dogs, *J Am Vet Med Assoc* 208(1):69–71, 1996.
98. Cohen M, Post GS: Nephrogenic diabetes insipidus in a dog with intestinal leiomyosarcoma, *J Am Vet Med Assoc* 215(12):1818–1820, 1999.
99. Selting KA, Ogilvie GK, Lana SE, et al: Serum Alpha 1-acid glycoprotein concentrations in healthy and tumor-bearing cats, *J Vet Intern Med* 14(5):503–506, 2000.
100. Correa SS, Mauldin GN, Mauldin GE, et al: Serum Alpha 1-acid glycoprotein concentration in cats with lymphoma, *J Am Anim Hosp Assoc* 37:153–158, 2001.
101. Avery PR, Avery AC: Molecular methods to distinguish reactive and neoplastic lymphocyte expansions and their importance in transitional neoplastic states, *Vet Clin Pathol* 33(4):196–207, 2004.
102. Kaneko N, Yamamoto Y, Wada Y, et al: Application of polymerase chain reaction to analysis of antigen receptor rearrangements to support endoscopic diagnosis of canine alimentary lymphoma, *J Vet Med Sci* 71(5):555–559, 2009.
103. Laurenson MP, Skorupski KA, Moore PF, et al: Ultrasonography of intestinal mast cell tumors in the cat, *Vet Radiol Ultrasound* 52(3):330–334, 2011.
104. Smith AL, Wilson AP, Hardie RJ, et al: Perioperative complications after full-thickness gastrointestinal surgery in cats with alimentary lymphoma, *Vet Surg* 40, 849–852, 2011.
105. Rivers BJ, Walter PA, Feeney DA, et al: Ultrasonographic features of intestinal adenocarcinoma in five cats, *Vet Radiol* 38(4):300–306, 1997.
106. Penninck DG, Smyers B, Webster CRL, et al: Diagnostic value of ultrasonography in differentiating enteritis from intestinal neoplasia in dogs, *Vet Radiol Ultrasound* 44(5):570–575, 2003.
107. Gaschen L: Ultrasonography of small intestinal inflammatory and neoplastic diseases in dogs and cats, *Vet Clin North Am Small Anim Pract* 41(2):329–344, 2011.
108. Zwingenberger AL, Marks SL, Baker TW, et al: Ultrasonographic evaluation of the muscularis propria in cats with diffuse small intestinal lymphoma or inflammatory bowel disease, *J Vet Intern Med* 24(2):289–292, 2010.
109. Willard MD, Jergens AE, Duncan RB, et al: Interobserver variation among histopathologic evaluations of intestinal tissues from dogs and cats, *J Am Vet Med Assoc* 220:1177–1182, 2002.
110. Danova NA, Robles-Emanuelli JC, Bjorling DE: Surgical excision of primary canine rectal tumors by an anal approach in twenty-three dogs, *Vet Surg* 35(4):337–340, 2006.
111. Morello E, Martano M, Squassino C, et al: Transanal pull-through rectal amputation for treatment of colorectal carcinoma in 11 dogs, *Vet Surg* 37(5):420–426, 2008.
112. Swiderski J, Withrow S: A novel surgical stapling technique for rectal mass removal: a retrospective analysis, *J Am Anim Hosp Assoc* 45(2):67–71, 2009.
113. Kupanoff PA, Popovitch CA, Goldschmidt MH: Colorectal plasmacytomas: a retrospective study of nine dogs, *J Am Anim Hosp Assoc* 42(1):37–43, 2006.
114. Coolman BR, Ehrhart N, Pijanowski G, et al: Comparison of skin staples with sutures for anastomosis of the small intestine in dogs, *Vet Surg* 29:293–302, 2000.
115. Hardie EM, Gilson SD: Use of colostomy to manage rectal disease in dogs, *Vet Surg* 26(4):270–274, 1997.
116. Holt PE, Durdey P: Transanal endoscopic treatment of benign canine rectal tumours: preliminary results in six cases (1992 to 1996), *J Small Anim Prac* 40:423–427, 1999.
117. Moore AS, Kirk C, Cardona A: Intracavitary cisplatin chemotherapy experience with six dogs, *J Vet Intern Med* 5(4):227–231, 1991.
118. Malik R, Gabor LJ, Foster SF, et al: Therapy for Australian cats with lymphosarcoma, *Aust Vet J* 79:808–817, 2001.
119. Coit DG: Cancer of the small intestine. In DeVita VT, Hellman S, Rosenberg SA, editors: *Cancer: principles and practice of oncology*, ed 6, Philadelphia, 2001, Lippincott Williams & Wilkins.
120. Skibber JM, Minsky BD, Hoff PM: Cancer of the colon. In DeVita VT, Hellman S, Rosenberg SA, editors: *Cancer: principles and practice of oncology*, ed 6, Philadelphia, 2001, Lippincott Williams & Wilkins.
121. Squire JA, Whitmore GF, Phillips RA: Genetic basis of cancer. In Tannock IF, Hill RP, editors: *The basic science of oncology*, ed 3, New York, 1998, McGraw-Hill.
122. Hart JR, Shaker E, Patnaik AK, et al: Lymphocytic-plasmacytic enterocolitis in cats: 60 cases (1988-1990), *J Am Anim Hosp Assoc* 30:505–514, 1994.
123. Sawaki A, Yamao K: Imatinib mesylate acts in metastatic or unresectable gastrointestinal stromal tumor by targeting KIT receptors- a review, *Cancer Chemother Pharmacol* 54(suppl 1):S44–S49, 2004.
124. Peek RM: Prevention of colorectal cancer through the use of COX-2 selective inhibitors, *Cancer Chemother Pharmacol* 54(suppl 1):S50–S56, 2004.
125. Personal communication: Oberthaler K, Shofer F, Bowden A, et al: Chemoprevention using NSAIDs in dogs: A preliminary epidemiological survey, Proceedings 24th annual conference of the Veterinary Cancer Society, p 3.
126. Anonymous: Adjuvant chemotherapy for localised colon cancer. Fluorouracil + folinic acid for node-positive, non-metastatic disease, *Prescrire Int* 20(113):46–49, 2011.

SECTION H

Perianal Tumors

Michelle M. Turek and Stephen J. Withrow

The perianal area of dogs contains several glands and structures from which tumors may develop. Perianal, or circumanal, glands are located in the dermis in a circular fashion around the anus and are also scattered in areas on the prepuce, tail, pelvic limbs, and trunk.[1] These are commonly referred to as *hepatoid glands* as a result of their cellular morphologic resemblance to hepatocytes and are considered nonsecretory, sebaceous glands in the adult dog.[1-3] The anal sacs represent blind cutaneous diverticula that are located on each side of the anus at the four o'clock and eight o'clock positions. Located in the connective tissue surrounding these diverticula are distinct apocrine sweat glands that empty their secretions into the lumen of the anal sacs. The most frequently observed tumors of this region in dogs include perianal sebaceous adenomas, perianal sebaceous adenocarcinomas, and apocrine gland adenocarcinomas of the anal sac (Table 22-9).

Because cats do not have glands analogous to the perianal sebaceous glands in the dog, perianal adenoma and perianal adenocarcinoma are uncommonly recognized in this species. Apocrine gland adenocarcinoma of the anal sac occurs rarely in the cat.[4-10]

Incidence and Risk Factors

Perianal adenomas (circumanal, hepatoid tumors) represent the majority, 58% to 96%, of canine perianal tumors.[1,11] Development

TABLE 22-9 Perianal Tumors in Dogs

	PERIANAL GLAND		ANAL SAC
	BENIGN	MALIGNANT	MALIGNANT
Cell type	Sebaceous	Sebaceous	Apocrine
Tumor type	Perianal adenoma	Perianal adenocarcinoma	Anal sac adenocarcinoma
Frequency	Common in intact males, very rare in females	Rare	Low frequency
Hormonal factors	Male: Usually intact male, testosterone dependent Female: Ovariohysterectomized (i.e., lack of estrogen)*	None	None
Location and appearance	Superficial hairless perineum; single, multiple, or diffuse; may be on prepuce or tail head	Usually single; may be invasive; often ulcerated.	Subcutaneous at 4 or 8 o'clock, firm and fixed; primary tumor may be small with nodal metastasis.
Paraneoplastic syndromes	None	None (very rarely hypercalcemia).	25%-50% have hypercalcemia.
Metastatic pattern	None	First to regional nodes, then to distant sites; metastasis rate up to 50%, especially with multiple local recurrences.	Common to regional lymph nodes and then to distant sites.
Special work-up	None; cytology may have difficulty distinguishing between benign and malignant	Abdominal imaging (radiographs and/or ultrasound) with focus on caudal abdomen; thoracic radiographs.	Abdominal imaging (radiographs and/or ultrasound); thoracic radiographs; serum calcium levels and renal function.
Treatment	Castration, conservative surgical removal†	Wide excision of primary tumor and lymphadenectomy if lymph nodes involved; postoperative radiotherapy for residual microscopic disease; radiation or chemotherapy if inoperable; castration of little benefit.	Wide excision of primary tumor and lymphadenectomy if lymph nodes involved; consider postoperative radiotherapy to primary site and to regional lymph nodes, as well as chemotherapy.
Prognosis	Excellent, less than 10% recurrence rate if castrated	Fair to good (tumors <5 cm do well); recurrence is common but may take many months and several surgeries can be done.	Fair; good in some cases (appears to depend on stage and treatment).

*If multiple, recurrent, or large (male-like), consider testosterone secretion from adrenal glands; Cushing's signs may or may not be present.

†Estrogens will cause regression but carry risk of bone marrow suppression. Adenomas will respond to radiation therapy, but surgery is cheaper, faster, and safer. Electrochemotherapy and cryosurgery have been reported.

and progression of these benign tumors appear to be sex hormone–dependent, with growth stimulated by androgenic hormones and depressed by estrogenic hormones.[1,12,13] The older, intact male is at high risk.[1,11,12] The mean reported age is 10 years.[11] A high incidence of associated testicular interstitial cell tumors has been reported for males with adenomas, supporting testosterone production as a cause.[12] However, a true cause-and-effect relationship has not been clarified since interstitial cell tumors are a common incidental finding in non–adenoma-bearing, older intact males. Perianal adenomas in the female occur almost exclusively in ovariohysterectomized animals in which low levels of estrogen do not suppress tumor growth. Rarely, testosterone secretion from the adrenal glands, occasionally accompanied by signs of hyperadrenocorticism, may stimulate perianal adenoma formation in the female.[14,15] Cocker spaniels, beagles, bulldogs, and Samoyeds may be predisposed.[1,12]

Perianal adenocarcinoma, a malignant tumor of the perianal glands, occurs much less frequently than its benign counterpart, representing only 3% to 21% of all tumors in this region.[1,11] Average age of affected dogs is 11 years.[11,16] Tumors occur in castrated or intact males, as well as in females, implying no hormonal dependency; however, this does not preclude earlier hormonal initiation.[12,16] Large-breed males appear to be overrepresented.[16]

Apocrine gland adenocarcinoma of the anal sacs occurs at relatively low frequency in the dog, representing 17% of perianal malignancies and 2% of all skin and subcutaneous tumors.[11,17] A breed survey of a large cohort of British dogs with anal sac adenocarcinoma suggests that spaniels, in particular English cocker spaniels, are at increased risk.[18] Earlier reports suggested a female predilection[11,19-21]; however, approximately equal sex distribution has been shown in multiple larger series.[18,22-24] In male dogs, it has been proposed that neutering may be associated with increased incidence of anal sac apocrine gland adenocarcinoma.[18] The average age of dogs diagnosed with this disease is 9 to 11 years.[11,19,20,22-26] Dogs as young as 5 years have been reported,[19,20,23,25,27] suggesting that evaluation of the perineum and palpation of the anal sacs should be a routine part of the physical examination in every adult dog.[23] Benign tumors of the anal sac are very rare.

Anal gland apocrine gland adenocarcinoma occurs rarely in the cat, representing 0.5% of all feline skin and subcutaneous neoplasms.[7] Median age of affected cats is 12 years, although animals as young as 6 years have been reported.[7,10] Siamese cats may be at higher risk.[7]

Pathology and Natural Behavior

Almost any tumor can occasionally affect the perianal region, including lymphoma, soft tissue sarcoma, SCC, melanoma, leiomyoma, transmissible venereal tumor, and mast cell tumor. However, the most common tumors in the dog are those that arise from the sebaceous glands of the perineum. The histologic distinction between perianal adenoma and adenocarcinoma may not always be clear, and clinically there may be an intermediate condition called *invasive perianal adenoma,* which may look benign microscopically, yet be moderately invasive in the patient.

Perianal adenomas follow a benign clinical course. The tumors are slow-growing, and although local disease may be extensive, metastasis does not occur.[1,11,12]

Perianal adenocarcinoma is generally associated with a low rate of metastasis (15%) at the time of original diagnosis.[16] It has been suggested that metastasis is most likely to develop later in the course of disease as the primary tumor becomes larger and more invasive.[16] The most frequent site of metastasis is the regional sublumbar and pelvic lymph nodes, including the iliac, hypogastric, and sacral nodes.[1,16] Distant metastases may rarely affect lungs, liver, kidney, and bone.[12,16] These tumors tend to be more rapidly growing, fixed, and firmer than the more common benign perianal adenomas.

Anal sac apocrine gland adenocarcinoma in the dog is distinct from perianal sebaceous gland adenocarcinoma clinically and histologically. Usually, only one anal sac is affected; however, bilateral tumors can occur.[19,20,25,28] The metastatic potential of this tumor is well established with most reports identifying about 50% metastasis (range 46% to 96%) at the time of initial presentation.[11,20-26,28] Regional sublumbar lymph nodes and pelvic nodes are by far the most common sites of metastasis early in the course of disease.[22-26,28] The primary anal sac tumor may be as small as 0.5 cm, with greatly enlarged metastatic nodes. Distant metastatic sites, including lungs, liver, spleen, bone, and, less commonly, heart, adrenal glands, pancreas, kidneys, and/or the mediastinum, may rarely develop later.[11,19,20,22-25] The association between anal sac apocrine gland adenocarcinoma and paraneoplastic hypercalcemia of malignancy, mediated by tumor secretion of parathyroid hormone–related peptide,[29-31] has been well documented.* Incidence of hypercalcemia is approximately 27% based on an analysis of 113 dogs with anal sac adenocarcinoma.[23] Along with lymphoma, plasma-ionized calcium concentrations tend to be higher with this tumor than with other types of neoplasia.[34]

The pathogenesis of canine perianal tumors is not known. In a large study evaluating tumor growth characteristics of 240 perianal gland tumors, cell proliferation and apoptosis were quantified by proliferating cell nuclear antigen (PCNA) staining and microscopic detection of apoptotic corpuscles.[35] An increase in both parameters was observed in malignant lesions compared to benign ones.[35] Various other immunohistochemical studies have attempted to elucidate possible molecular mechanisms involved in canine perianal gland tumorigenesis. Using a single polyclonal antihuman antibody, nuclear *p53* accumulation was detected in 50% (8 of 16) of perianal sebaceous gland adenocarcinomas in one study, suggesting that expression of a mutated *p53* tumor suppressor protein may play a role.[36] Discordant results were reported in another study in which *p53* reactivity was found in none of 11 perianal gland adenocarcinomas and in only a small percentage of adenomas.[37] In the same tumor samples, *Mdm2* expression was observed in both adenomas and adenocarcinomas.[37] A study that evaluated androgen receptor expression found no difference between perianal adenomas and their malignant counterparts; the authors concluded that the mechanism by which androgens may influence carcinogenesis is still unknown.[38] Finally, another proposed mediator of tumor growth or evolution is growth hormone. Growth hormone was detected immunohistochemically in 96% (23 of 24) of perianal adenomas and 100% (5 of 5) of perianal sebaceous gland adenocarcinomas.[39] With respect to anal sac adenocarcinoma, expression of E-cadherin, a protein known to mediate adhesion and communication between cells and the extracellular matrix, was evaluated in tumor biopsies from dogs using a polyclonal antihuman antibody that has been validated for use in canines.[26] E-cadherin expression correlated with the presence of metastasis and shorter survival time, suggesting that it may play a role in tumor progression.[26] *p53* expression has been detected immunohistochemically in a low-to-moderate proportion of anal gland adenocarcinoma tissue biopsies; however, no clinical implications have come from these findings.[36] A recent genetic analysis study in English cocker spaniels showed an association between tumor development and major histocompatibility complex haplotype (DLA-DQB1 allele), suggesting that a genetic factor may play a role in tumor development in this at-risk breed.[40]

The biologic behavior of anal sac apocrine gland adenocarcinoma in the cat has not been clearly defined. Most reports suggest that it is a locally invasive disease associated with a moderate-to-high risk of tumor recurrence following surgery.[5-8,10] The rate of metastasis is variable between studies ranging from low to high.[6,7,10] Described sites of metastasis include sublumbar lymph nodes, liver, diaphragm, and lungs.[6,7,10] Paraneoplastic hypercalcemia is not a common complication of this disease in cats.[7,10] Bilateral tumors have not been reported.

History and Clinical Signs

The history for benign perianal adenoma is that of a slow-growing (over months to years) mass or masses that are nonpainful and usually asymptomatic. These may be single, multiple, or diffuse (similar to generalized hyperplasia or hypertrophy of the perianal tissue; Figure 22-29).[1] Most occur on the hairless skin area around the anus, although they may extend to haired regions and can develop on the prepuce, scrotum, or tail head (stud tail or "caudal tail gland").[1] Benign lesions may ulcerate and become infected but are rarely adherent or fixed to deeper structures.[1] They are usually fairly well circumscribed, on average 0.5 to 3 cm in diameter, and elevated from the perineum.[1]

The male perianal adenocarcinoma may look similar to adenomas but tends to grow more rapidly, be more firm, become ulcerated, adhere to underlying tissues, recur following conservative surgery, and generally be larger than its benign counterpart.[16] Obstipation, dyschezia, or perianal pain/irritation can be seen with larger masses.[16] Rarely, signs are related to obstruction of the pelvic canal by lymph node metastasis. Tumors can be multiple.[16] Castrated males with new or recurrent perianal tumors should raise

*References 20-23, 25-28, 32-34.

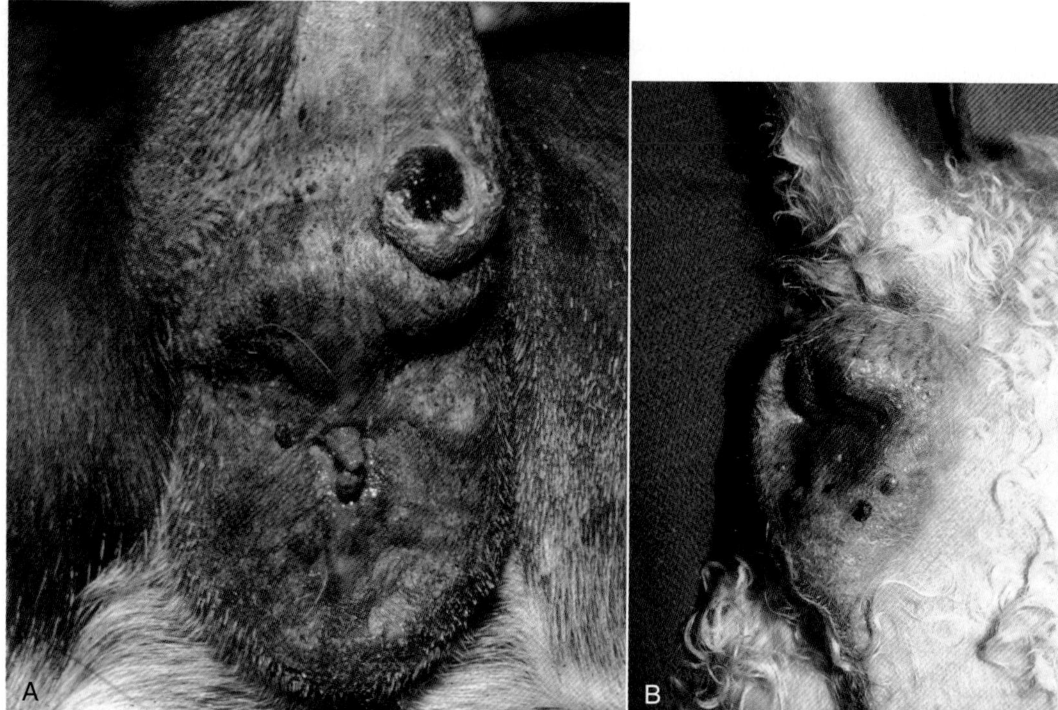

FIGURE 22-29 **A,** Typical small and ulcerated perianal adenoma can be seen at 1 o'clock. Treatment with castration and cryosurgery was curative. **B,** Diffuse 360-degree involvement of the perianal region with perianal adenoma. Aggressive resection or cryosurgery should not be performed; instead, castration, a waiting period of several months for partial regression, and the local treatment for residual disease were applied.

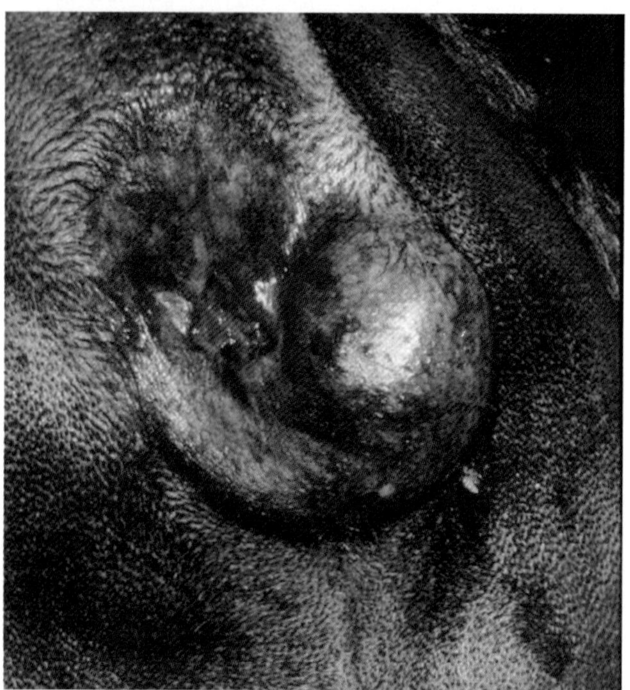

FIGURE 22-30 An anal sac adenocarcinoma in a female dog. Note the typical 4 o'clock position.

the suspicion for malignant rather than benign disease because adenocarcinomas are not hormonally dependent.

Clinical signs of dogs with anal sac adenocarcinoma are often referable to either the presence of the primary mass (perianal discomfort, swelling [Figure 22-30], bleeding; scooting),

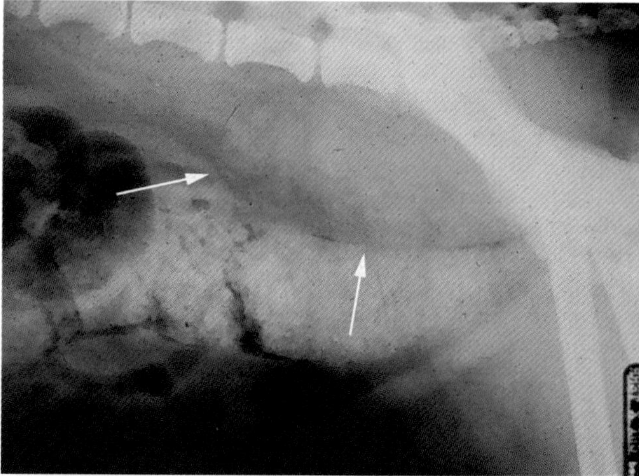

FIGURE 22-31 Lateral radiograph of the caudal abdomen in a male dog with anal sac adenocarcinoma. Note the metastatic involvement of sublumbar/iliac lymph nodes *(arrows)* and downward displacement of large bowel.

to obstruction of the pelvic canal by regional nodal metastasis (tenesmus, constipation [Figure 22-31]), or to hypercalcemia (polyuria, polydipsia; anorexia; lethargy; vomiting).[22,23] In as many as 39% of dogs, the primary tumor can be an incidental finding on physical examination.[23] Rarely, regional bone metastasis or direct extension of tumor from sublumbar lymph nodes into the lumbar vertebrae with associated pain or fracture may be seen.

In cats, the most common history and clinical signs associated with anal sac adenocarcinoma are related to the presence of local disease. Like dogs, cats may be presented for tenesmus, constipation, scooting, presence of a mass, hemorrhagic discharge, or excessive grooming of the perineal area.[6-8,10] Lethargy and/or inappetence may be secondary to severe constipation.[5] Not all cats present with clinical signs, and tumors can be detected incidentally during a routine physical examination.[7] Clinicians should recognize anal sac adenocarcinoma as a distinct clinical entity in the cat and include it as a differential diagnosis for animals with anal sac disease.[7] It is not uncommon for anal sac adenocarcinoma to be misdiagnosed as an anal sac abscess based on the presence of a mass, ulceration, or a fistulous tract in the perineal region.[7]

Diagnostic Techniques and Work-Up

In the intact male with suspected perianal adenoma, a routine geriatric work-up prior to anesthesia is desirable. Thoracic radiographs to evaluate for lung metastasis may not be cost effective unless indicated for other cardiopulmonary evaluation given the benign biologic behavior of these tumors. Evaluation of regional lymph node size is indicated if one suspects perianal adenocarcinoma based on signalment (neutered male), recurrent disease, or physical examination characteristics of malignancy. Ultrasonographic evaluation of regional lymph nodes is a superior staging tool in comparison to plain radiography which can both underestimate and overestimate lymph node disease.[41] Although distant metastasis is uncommon, thoracic radiographs to evaluate for lung metastasis are recommended in dogs with perianal adenocarcinoma. FNA and cytology to differentiate benign from malignant tumors in the male can be unrewarding, although they are helpful in ruling out other forms of cancer or mass development. Tissue biopsy is necessary to make the distinction in most cases, and the most important histologic criteria supporting a diagnosis of perianal sebaceous gland adenocarcinoma is invasiveness of tumor cells into surrounding tissue.[42] Disorderly arrangement of cells, increased nuclear pleomorphism, and increased numbers of mitotic figures also favor a diagnosis of malignancy.[42] The use of monoclonal antibodies, MAbs4A9 and 1A10, developed against a canine mammary cell line and screened for reactivity with perianal adenocarcinoma, has been proposed as a diagnostic tool to help distinguish benign perianal tumors from adenocarcinoma when routine light microscopy is not conclusive.[43] Clinical validation is needed to confirm the utility of this approach.

Since dogs with anal sac adenocarcinoma may present with signs unrelated to perianal disease (i.e., polyuria, polydipsia due to hypercalcemia), assessment of animals with suspicious clinical signs requires a careful rectal examination, including palpation of the anal sacs and evaluation for possible regional lymphadenopathy. Definitive diagnosis must be made cytologically or histologically, but a strong presumption of anal sac adenocarcinoma can be made for animals in which rectal examination identifies the presence of a firm and discrete mass in the area of the anal sac. This tumor has a characteristic cytologic appearance and is made up of polyhedral cells that have uniform round nuclei and light blue-gray, slightly granular cytoplasm. Features of malignancy may be subtle. In addition to suggesting the presence of cancer in the anal sacs, FNA is valuable for ruling out infection or inflammatory disease of the anal sac. The clinician should be aware that anal sac tumors can become secondarily infected or inflamed. Staging of disease includes thoracic radiographs for rare detection of pulmonary or mediastinal involvement. Abdominal radiographs may reveal regional lymphadenopathy in advanced cases (see Figure 22-31). Ultrasonographic evaluation of regional lymph nodes is a superior staging evaluation because plain radiography can both underestimate and overestimate lymph node disease.[41] A recent study evaluating sonographic features of abdominal lymph nodes found that alterations in shape, contour, cavitation, echogenicity and parenchymal uniformity do not reliably distinguish neoplastic from benign nodes. The only significant difference identified between neoplastic and benign lymph nodes was size.[44] Ultrasound also allows for evaluation of other possible sites of abdominal metastasis, particularly liver and spleen. Advanced imaging, including CT and MRI, may yield a more complete assessment of abdominal involvement.[45] In rare instances, pulmonary metastasis can be present without obvious regional lymph node disease. Lameness or bone pain should be evaluated with radiography and/or nuclear scintigraphy to rule out bone metastasis. Work-up also includes complete blood count, serum chemistry panel, and urinalysis. Hypercalcemia of malignancy can result in renal damage, which may modify prognosis and anesthetic risk. Medical management of hypercalcemia or impaired renal function may be necessary prior to surgery (see Chapter 5).

Careful rectal examination should be performed on all dogs with perianal tumors to detect the clinical degree of fixation prior to surgery, the probability of resection, and the risk of postoperative complications, particularly incontinence, although this is very rare with even aggressive unilateral resection. It is also important to palpate for the presence of enlarged sacral lymph nodes located along the ventral surface of the vertebrae because these are not easily detectable by ultrasound due to their position in the caudal pelvic canal.

Similarly to dogs, feline anal sac adenocarcinoma can be diagnosed cytologically and histologically. Complete staging of this tumor in cats includes thoracic radiographs to evaluate for pulmonary metastasis and abdominal imaging.[4-6,8] Abdominal ultrasound is more sensitive than radiography for detection of metastasis involving abdominal organs or lymph nodes. Positive immunoreactivity with anticytokeratin monoclonal antibody, CAM 5.2, was recently reported in a series of 12 cats with anal sac adenocarcinoma.[7]

Therapy and Prognosis

Due to the hormonal dependence of perianal adenomas, the vast majority of these tumors will regress (at least partially) following castration, and recurrence is uncommon.[12] Surgery is recommended in males with ulcerated tumors or recurrence, as well as in females with typical small and focal masses.[12] For diffuse or large benign lesions situated on or in the anal sphincter, castration followed by an observation period of several months to allow reduction in tumor volume may permit safer and easier mass removal. This will only be effective for benign lesions that are hormone dependent. Over 90% of male dogs will be cured with castration and mass removal.[1,12] Adenomas can be excised with minimal margins. In addition to standard surgical techniques, mass removal can be achieved using cryosurgery or carbon dioxide laser, which should only be used for focal lesions less than 1 to 2 cm in diameter.[46,47] Use of either of these techniques precludes evaluation of the surgical margins for completeness of excision, which may be acceptable for benign masses; however, as the most consistent criterion for malignancy is invasiveness, lack of margin assessment is not without risk. Hyperthermia and RT have also been used successfully.[48,49] The cost, added morbidity, and limited availability of these techniques make them a poor alternative to standard blade excision. Electrochemotherapy has been recently described[50,51] and consists of intratumoral injections of chemotherapy (cisplatin and/or bleomycin in recent reports) followed by local delivery of electric pulses to potentiate drug uptake. Treatments are delivered in one or two weekly sessions. Based on limited studies, the reported overall response rate is greater than 90%, with 65% complete responses.[50,51] Smaller tumors (<5 cm) generally respond better than larger tumors.[50,51] Larger tumors are more likely to develop local complications, including focal necrosis, erythema, and inflammation.[50,51] Systemic effects are not reported.[50,51] Castration and surgical excision remain the treatments of choice for adenomas. Adenomas may also regress following estrogen therapy; however, its use is contraindicated by the risk of myelosuppression. Cyclosporin is reported to have had a palliative effect in a single dog with multiple ulcerated perianal adenomas and a measurable reduction in tumor size was observed.[52]

Perianal sebaceous gland adenocarcinoma is more locally invasive than its benign counterpart and generally does not respond to castration.[12] Aggressive surgical removal with adequate margins is indicated. Removal of one-half or more of the anal sphincter is possible with only rare transient loss of continence. Recurrent disease becomes more difficult to resect. Unfortunately, most perianal adenocarcinomas are not suspected or known until after a conservative resection, which contaminates further tissue planes and can make the second resection problematic. Due to common local recurrence, this tumor is difficult to cure and may require numerous palliative resections over several years. Preoperative diagnosis of malignancy (i.e., incisional biopsy) and more aggressive initial resection should improve local control and should be strongly encouraged. The utility of postsurgical RT should also improve local control; however, data for this approach are lacking. The use of electrochemotherapy has been reported in a small series of dogs.[51] Although the study suggested a favorable outcome in the adjuvant setting, additional clinical studies are needed for validation of the efficacy of the approach.[51]

In a series of 41 dogs with perianal adenocarcinoma, stage of tumor had a significant influence on DFI and overall survival (Figure 22-32).[16] Tumors less than 5 cm in diameter (T2) were associated with 2-year tumor control rates in excess of 60%, suggesting that surgical removal of these masses at an early stage is relatively successful with respect to disease control. Fifteen percent of dogs had evidence of metastasis at the time of diagnosis, which related negatively to survival (see Figure 22-32).[16] MST for dogs with lymph node or distant metastasis was 7 months; however, aggressive treatment was not attempted in five of six cases.[16] If present, regional lymph node metastasis may be excised. Large nodal volume is not a contraindication to caudal abdominal exploratory and lymphadenectomy because some nodes "shell out" readily, whereas others are invasive. Enlarged lymph nodes should be considered for removal, especially if they are causing obstruction of the pelvic canal. The use of radiation and/or chemotherapy, including actinomycin D, has been reported anecdotally, but their role in local or distant control is largely undefined.[16,53,54] Controlled clinical trials have not been performed. It has been suggested that nuclear size measured by computer-assisted image analysis in cytologic tumor samples may correlate with biologic behavior in this tumor type.[55]

Apocrine gland adenocarcinoma of the anal sac is generally locally invasive, and aggressive surgical excision is recommended. Recurrence rate is high after marginal surgery alone.[20,22] Complete resection of large perianal malignancies is difficult due to proximity to the rectum and poor definition of perineal tissue to define an adequate margin. Metastasis is present at the time of diagnosis in approximately 50% to 80% of cases,[19,20,22,23,25] with regional lymph nodes being the most common site.

Enlarged lymph nodes should be considered for removal, especially if they are causing obstruction of the pelvic canal or contributing to hypercalcemia. Radiation and/or chemotherapy may be used adjuvantly or as the sole treatment.[22-25,28]

Large-scale studies controlled for tumor stage and treatment are lacking in dogs with anal sac adenocarcinoma. There is discordance in the outcome and prognosis reported in the literature. Earlier small studies suggest a MST of 6 to 12 months.[20,22,27] This is in contrast to recent reports in which the MST ranges from 16 to 18 months.[23,24] These later studies involve larger groups of dogs (113

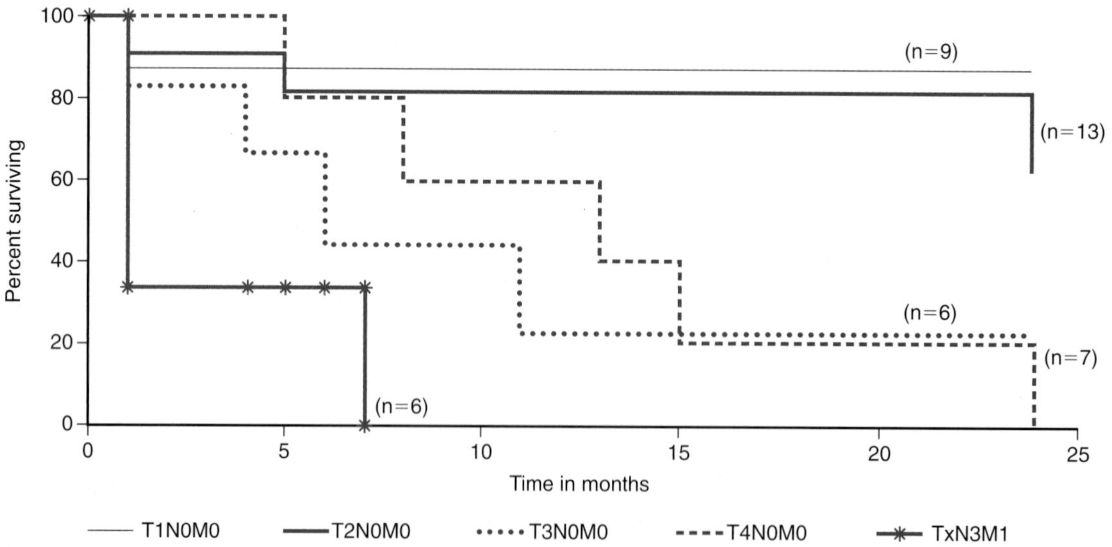

FIGURE 22-32 Survival duration in 41 male dogs with perianal adenocarcinoma based on stage. Note that dogs with small tumors (T1 or T2) without lymph node involvement will do well after aggressive removal of the primary tumor. T1 = tumor <2 cm, T2 = tumor 2-5 cm, T3 = tumor >5 cm, T4 = tumor invading other structures, such as fascia, muscle, or bone; N0 = no evidence of regional lymph node involvement, N3 = fixed lymph nodes; M0 = no evidence of distant metastasis, M1 = distant metastasis detected.

dogs and 80 dogs, respectively).[23,24] However, there is variability in stage of disease and treatment in the study populations that leads to difficulty accurately predicting the prognosis of individual dogs with this tumor type. Negative prognostic indicators gleaned from these and other studies include increasing primary tumor size,[23,24] presence of lymph node metastasis,[24] presence of distant metastasis,[23,24,26] advanced clinical stage,[24] nonpursuit of surgery,[23] treatment with chemotherapy alone,[23] and lack of any therapy at all.[24] In one study, extirpation of involved sublumbar lymph nodes in dogs without distant metastasis correlated with improved survival compared to animals in which nodal metastases were not removed.[24] E-cadherin expression detected immunohistochemically in tumor biopsies has also been suggested to directly correlate with survival.[26] These prognostic variables should be confirmed in controlled clinical trials.

Although chemotherapy and RT are generally considered standard adjuvant treatment options for anal sac adenocarcinoma, the role of these modalities alone or in combination is not well defined. Chemotherapy is theoretically indicated given the high rate of metastasis. Chemotherapeutics with demonstrated antitumor activity in the gross disease setting include carboplatin, cisplatin, and actinomycin D.[22,24,52] Other drugs reported in the adjuvant setting include mitoxantrone and melphalan.[25,28] Gross tumor responses have not been described for these agents when used alone, and their true role in combination therapies is not known. Toceranib phosphate, a TKI, has been associated with modest tumor responses with median response durations of 19 to 25 weeks in a series of 33 dogs with multiple prior failed therapies.[56] This antitumor effect may be mediated through inhibition of the platelet-derived growth factor receptor β (PDGFR-β) based on immunoreactivity of tumor biopsies to anti-PDGFR antibody.[57] Controlled clinical trials are needed to determine the role of toceranib in the treatment of anal sac adenocarcinoma. Adjuvant electrochemotherapy using cisplatin is reported in a single dog following an incomplete primary tumor excision.[58]

The optimal combination of therapies for anal sac adenocarcinoma is not known. In three clinical studies with controlled treatment regimes, MSTs ranged from 17 to 31 months.[24,25,28] A study of 14 dogs that underwent surgical excision and melphalan chemotherapy reported an overall MST of 20 months (95% CI, 11.6 to 28.4 months).[28] Seven dogs had known nodal metastasis at the time of diagnosis, and nodal metastasis was not prognostic for survival in this small study. A significant relationship between a modified clinical staging scheme and survival was found in a study of 50 dogs treated prospectively according to a predetermined management algorithm.[24] Treatment included various combinations of surgery, carboplatin chemotherapy, and hypofractionated (9 Gy × 4 weekly fractions) RT. Fifteen dogs had sublumbar lymphadenopathy and/or distant metastasis at the time of treatment. MST was 17 months (95% CI, 7 to 27 months). Toxicity associated with the treatment was not reported. The third study utilized a standardized RT protocol with concurrent chemotherapy in a cohort of 15 dogs.[25] Dogs were treated with combination surgery (primary tumor ± metastatic lymph nodes), curative-intent radiation (3.2 Gy × 15 daily fractions for a total dose of 48 Gy) to the primary tumor site and regional lymph node beds, and mitoxantrone chemotherapy. Seven dogs had lymph node metastasis at diagnosis. Median event-free survival was 9 months (range: 2.5 to 35 months), and overall survival was 31 months (range: 5 to 47 months). Measurable responses were observed in bulky metastatic lymph nodes. The relative importance of radiation versus mitoxantrone chemotherapy is not clear from this study. Without more rigorously controlled clinical trials, strong statements about the "best" treatment and prognosis are difficult to support. In a case series of five dogs selected for resectability of metastatic lymph nodes, a MST of 20 months was achieved with surgery alone.[59] One dog underwent repeated lymph node debulking surgeries and survived for 54 months. Another dog survived 18 months following omentalization of cystic sublumbar lymph node metastasis for palliation of tenesmus and dysuria.[60] Taken together, these findings of prolonged survival, despite varying tumor stages and varying treatments, strongly suggest the need for prospective, controlled clinical trials to elucidate any benefits of treatment modalities, such as radiation, chemotherapy, molecular-targeted drugs, and their combinations. Identification of reliable prognostic criteria predictive of outcome or treatment response is also needed. It has been suggested in a small study using computer-assisted analysis that nuclear size of tumor cells may correlate with biologic behavior; nuclear size parameters were larger in metastatic anal gland adenocarcinomas than in nonmetastatic tumors.[61] Further validation of this approach is needed before it can be considered clinically useful. Finally, when short-term palliation is the therapeutic goal, treatment options include surgery, palliative RT, chemotherapy and/or toceranib, even though efficacy of these approaches has not been definitively established.

Curative-intent RT of the perineal and pelvic regions is associated with self-limiting, acute radiation effects, including mild-to-severe moist desquamation, colitis, and perineal discomfort lasting 2 to 4 weeks posttherapy. Radiation prescriptions should be designed to minimize the risk of late effects, including rectal stricture or perforation. Two studies have demonstrated that radiation doses of less than 3 Gy per fraction should be used to minimize this risk.[62,63] In the only report of standardized curative-intent RT for anal sac adenocarcinoma,[25] none of the side effects were reported as life-threatening, and all dogs maintained reasonable quality of life as assessed by owners. Chronic complications included tenesmus and narrow stool, diarrhea, and rectal stricture. The daily radiation dose in this study was 3.2 Gy. Future studies should be designed with daily radiation doses of less than 3 Gy to reduce the risk of chronic complications.

There is discordance in the data reported regarding the prognostic significance of hypercalcemia of malignancy accompanying anal sac adenocarcinoma. Hypercalcemia has generally been associated with shorter survival[20,23]; however, other studies have not supported this finding.[22,25,26,28] Complete or near-complete removal of the tumor results in reversal of hypercalcemia. Return of hypercalcemia after therapy usually signals recurrence or metastasis.

Prognosis associated with feline anal sac adenocarcinoma has not been clearly established and some reports are conflicting. Local recurrence after surgical resection appears relatively common. The reported rate of metastasis is variable. In a study involving 39 cats that underwent incisional biopsy or tumor resection, survival time ranged from 0 to 23 months.[7] Eighty-five percent of cats succumbed to local disease or presumptive metastasis. MST in this group was 3 months; 1- and 2-year survival rates were 19% and 0%, respectively.[7] This is in contrast to a recent retrospective study of 23 cats that reported a median DFI and survival time of over 300 days.[10] The role of chemotherapy and RT is not known. A short-lived partial response to carboplatin was reported in a cat with recurrent anal sac adenocarcinoma.[8] In another report, outcome following concurrent adjuvant curative-intent RT (48 Gy) and chemotherapy (carboplatin) resulted in local recurrence and/or metastatic disease within 6 months of treatment in two cats.[6] In both cases, RT was well tolerated with minimal acute effects.[6] Although these survival data are not encouraging, more studies are needed to determine the true role of radiation and chemotherapy in this disease. Based on individual cases of long-term survival, it has been suggested that early detection and completeness of excision may positively impact outcome.[6,7]

Comparative Aspects[64-66]

No similar hormonally dependent perianal disease state exists in humans. The most common cancer of the anal margin is squamous cell (epidermoid) carcinoma. These tumors arise from the junction of haired skin and mucous membrane of the anal canal. Risk of developing cancer in this location is positively correlated with sexual activity, and most tumors are associated with human papillomavirus infection. Precancerous changes (dysplasia) in the epithelium of the anal canal may precede tumor development. Regional lymph nodes are the most common site of metastasis. Previously considered a surgical disease requiring a permanent colostomy, improved outcomes have been achieved with definitive chemoradiation. The standard approach to therapy is concomitant radiation and chemotherapy using 5-FU and mitomycin C. Surgery is reserved for locally recurrent or persistent disease. Mean 5-year disease-free survival and overall survival are 60% and 75%, respectively. Size and degree of invasion of the primary tumor, regional lymph node involvement, and presence of distant metastases are important prognostic factors. Identification of biomarkers that may serve as predictors of outcome or targets for therapy is being explored.

REFERENCES

1. Nielsen SW, Aftosmis J: Canine perianal gland tumors, *J Am Vet Med Assoc* 144:127–135, 1964.
2. Esplin DG, Wilson SR, Hullinger GA: Squamous cell carcinoma of the anal sac in five dogs, *Vet Pathol* 40:332–334, 2003.
3. Maita K, Ishida K: Structure and development of the perianal gland of the dog, *Jpn J Vet Sci* 37:349–356, 1975.
4. Chun R, Jakovljevic S, Morrison WB, et al: Apocrine gland adenocarcinoma and pheochromocytoma in a cat, *J Am Anim Hosp Assoc* 33:33–36, 1997.
5. Mellanby RJ, Foale R, Friend E, et al: Anal sac adenocarcinoma in a Siamese cat, *J Feline Med Surg* 4:205–207, 2002.
6. Elliott JW, Blackwood L: Treatment and outcome of four cats with apocrine gland carcinoma of the anal sac and review of the literature, *J Feline Med Surg* 13:712–717, 2011.
7. Shoieb AM, Hanshaw DM: Anal sac gland carcinoma in 64 cats in the United Kingdom (1995-2007), *Vet Pathol* 46:677–683, 2009.
8. Wright ZM, Fryer JS, Calise DV: Carboplatin chemotherapy in a cat with a recurrent anal sac apocrine gland adenocarcinoma, *J Am Anim Hosp Assoc* 46:66–69, 2010.
9. Parry NMA: Anal sac gland carcinoma in a cat, *Vet Pathol* 43:1008–1009, 2006.
10. Personal communication: Cavanaugh R, Bacon N, Schallberger S, et al: Biologic behavior and clinical outcome of cats with anal sac adenocarcinoma: a Veterinary Society of Surgical Oncology retrospective study of 23 cats, *Vet Cancer Soc Proc* 28:63, 2008.
11. Berrocal A, Vos JH, van den Ingh TS, et al: Canine perineal tumours, *J Vet Med Ser A* 36:739–749, 1989.
12. Wilson GP, Hayes HM: Castration for treatment of perianal gland neoplasms in the dog, *J Am Vet Med Assoc* 174(12):1301–1303, 1979.
13. Chaisiri N, Pierrpoint CG: Steroid-receptor interaction in a canine anal adenoma, *J Small Anim Pract* 20:405–416, 1979.
14. Dow SW, Olson PN, Rosychuk RA, et al: Perianal adenomas and hypertestosteronemia in a spayed bitch with pituitary-dependent hyperadrenocorticism, *J Am Vet Med Assoc* 192:1439–1441, 1988.
15. Hill KE, Scott-Montrieff CR, Koshko MA, et al: Secretion of sex hormones in dogs with adrenal dysfunction, *J Am Vet Med Assoc* 226:556–561, 2005.
16. Vail DM, Withrow SJ, Schwarz PD, et al: Perianal adenocarcinoma in the canine male: a retrospective study of 41 cases, *J Am Anim Hosp Assoc* 26:329 334, 1990.
17. Goldschmidt MH, Shofer FS: *Skin tumors of the dog and cat*, Oxford, UK, 1992, Pergamon Press.
18. Polton GA, Mowat V, Lee HC, et al: Breed, gender and neutering status of British dogs with anal sac gland carcinoma, *Vet Comp Oncol* 4(3):125–131, 2006.
19. Goldschmidt MH, Zoltowski C: Anal sac gland adenocarcinoma in the dog: 14 cases, *J Small Anim Pract* 22:119–128, 1981.
20. Ross JT, Scavelli TD, Matthiesen DT, et al: Adenocarcinoma of the apocrine glands of the anal sac in dogs: a review of 32 cases, *J Am Anim Hosp Assoc* 27:349–355, 1991.
21. Meuten DJ, Cooper BJ, Capen CC, et al: Hypercalcemia associated with an adenocarcinoma derived from the apocrine glands of the anal sac, *Vet Pathol* 18:454–471, 1981.
22. Bennett PF, DeNicola DB, Bonney P, et al: Canine anal sac adenocarcinomas: clinical presentation and response to therapy, *J Vet Intern Med* 16:100–104, 2002.
23. Williams LE, Gliatto JM, Dodge RK, et al: Carcinoma of the apocrine glands of the anal sac in dogs: 113 cases (1985-1995), *J Am Vet Med Assoc* 223:825–831, 2003.
24. Polton GA, Brearley MJ: Clinical stage, therapy, and prognosis in canine anal sac gland carcinoma, *J Vet Intern Med* 21:274–280, 2007.
25. Turek MM, Forrest LJ, Adams WM, et al: Postoperative radiotherapy and mitoxantrone for anal sac adenocarcinoma in the dog: 15 cases (1991-2001), *Vet Comp Oncol* 1(2):94–104, 2003.
26. Polton GA, Brearley MJ, Green LM, et al: Expression of E-cadherin in canine anal sac gland carcinoma and its association with survival, *Vet Comp Oncol* 5(4):232–238, 2007.
27. White RAS, Gorman NT: The clinical diagnosis and management of rectal and pararectal tumours in the dog, *J Small Anim Pract* 28:87–107, 1987.
28. Emms SG: Anal sac tumours of the dog and their response to cytoreductive surgery and chemotherapy, *Aust Vet J* 83(6):340–343, 2005.
29. Rosol TJ, Capen CC, Danks JA, et al: Identification of parathyroid hormone-related protein in canine apocrine adenocarcinoma of the anal sac, *Vet Pathol* 27:89–95, 1990.
30. Gröne A, Werkmeister JR, Steinmeyer CL, et al: Parathyroid hormone-related protein in normal and neoplastic canine tissues: immunohistochemical localization and biochemical extraction, *Vet Pathol* 31:308–315, 1994.
31. Mellanby RJ, Craig R, Evans H, et al: Plasma concentrations of parathyroid hormone-related protein in dogs with potential disorders of calcium metabolism, *Vet Rec* 159:833–838, 2006.
32. Hause WR, Stevenson S, Meuten DJ, et al: Pseudohyperparathyroidism associated with adenocarcinomas of anal sac origin in four dogs, *J Am Anim Hosp Assoc* 17:373–379, 1981.
33. Meuten DJ, Segre GV, Capen CC, et al: Hypercalcemia in dogs with adenocarcinoma derived from apocrine glands of the anal sac, *Lab Invest* 48(4):428–434, 1983.
34. Messinger JS, Windham WR, Ward CR: Ionized hypercalcemia in dogs: a retrospective study of 109 cases (1998-2003), *J Vet Intern Med* 23:514–519, 2009.
35. Martins AMCRPF, Vasques-Peyser A, Torres LN, et al: Retrospective-systematic study and quantitative analysis of cellular proliferation and apoptosis in normal, hyperplastic and neoplastic perianal glands in dogs, *Vet Comp Oncol* 6(2):71–79, 2008.
36. Gamblin RM, Sagartz JE, Couto CG: Overexpression of p53 tumor suppressor protein in spontaneously arising neoplasms of dogs, *Am J Vet Res* 58(8):857–863, 1997.
37. Nakano M, Taura Y, Inoue M: Protein expression of Mdm2 and p53 in hyperplastic and neoplastic lesions of the canine circumanal gland, *J Comp Path* 132:27–32, 2005.

38. Pisani G, Millanta F, Lorenzi D, et al: Androgen receptor expression in normal, hyperplastic and neoplastic hepatoid glands in the dog, *Res Vet Sci* 81:231–236, 2006.
39. Petterino C, Martini M, Castagnaro M: Immunohistochemical detection of growth hormone (GH) in canine hepatoid gland tumors, *J Vet Med Sci* 66(5):569–572, 2004.
40. Aguirre-Hernandez J, Polton G, Kennedy LJ, et al: Association between anal sac gland carcinoma and dog leukocyte antigen-DQB1 in the English Cocker Spaniel, *Tissue Antigens* 76:476–481, 2010.
41. Llabrés-Díaz FJ: Ultrasonography of the medial iliac lymph nodes in the dog, *Vet Radiol Ultrasound* 45(2):156–165, 2004.
42. Stannard AA, Pulley LT: Tumors of the skin and soft tissues. In Moulton JE, editor: *Tumors in domestic animals*, Berkeley, 1978, University of California Press.
43. Ganguly A, Wolfe LG: Canine perianal gland carcinoma-associated antigens defined by monoclonal antibodies, *Hybridoma* 25(1):10–14, 2006.
44. De Swarte M, Alexander K, Rannou B, et al: Comparison of sonographic features of benign and neoplastic deep lymph nodes in dogs, *Vet Radiol Ultrasound* 52:451–456, 2011.
45. Personal communication: Anderson C, Fidel J, Sellon R: Comparison of abdominal ultrasound and magnetic resonance imaging for detection of abdominal lymphadenopathy in dogs with metastatic anal sac gland adenocarcinoma, *Vet Cancer Soc Proc* 30:124, 2010.
46. Liska WD, Withrow SJ: Cryosurgical treatment of perianal gland adenomas in the dog, *J Am Anim Hosp Assoc* 14:457–463, 1978.
47. Shelley BA: Use of the carbon dioxide laser for perianal and rectal surgery, *Vet Clin North Am Small Anim Pract* 32:621–637, 2002.
48. Grier RL, Brewer WG, Theilen GH: Hyperthermic treatment of superficial tumors in cats and dogs, *J Am Vet Med Assoc* 177(3): 227–233, 1980.
49. Gillette EL: Veterinary radiotherapy, *J Am Vet Med Assoc* 157(11):1707–1712, 1970.
50. Tozon N, Kodre V, Sersa G, et al: Effective treatment of perianal tumors in dogs with electrochemotherapy, *Anticancer Res* 25:839–846, 2005.
51. Spugnini EP, Dotsinsky I, Mudrov N, et al: Biphasic pulses enhance bleomycin efficacy in a spontaneous canine perianal tumor model, *J Exp Clin Cancer Res* 26(4):483–487, 2007.
52. Park C, Yoo JH, Kim HJ, et al: Cyclosporine treatment of perianal gland adenoma concurrent with benign prostatic hyperplasia in a dog, *Can Vet J* 51:1279–1282, 2010.
53. Hammer AS, Couto CG, Ayl RD, et al: Treatment of tumor-bearing dogs with actinomycin D, *J Vet Intern Med* 8(3):236–239, 1994.
54. Bley CR, Stankeova S, Sumova A, et al: Metastases of perianal gland carcinoma in a dog: palliative tumor therapy, *Schweiz Arch Tierheilkd* 145(2):89–94, 2003.
55. Simeonov R, Simeonova G: Computer-assisted nuclear morphometry in the cytological evaluation of canine perianal adenocarcinomas, *J Comp Path* 139:226–230, 2008.
56. London C, Mathie T, Stingle N, et al: Preliminary evidence for biologic activity of toceranib phosphate (Palladia) in solid tumours, *Vet Comp Oncol* Epub ahead of print, 2011.
57. Brown RJ, Newman SJ, Durtschi DC, et al: Expression of PDGFR-β and kit in canine anal sac apocrine gland adenocarcinoma using tissue immunohistochemistry, *Vet Comp Oncol* 10(1):74–79, 2012.
58. Spugnini EP, Dotsinsky I, Mudrov N, et al: Adjuvant electrochemotherapy for incompletely excised anal sac carcinoma in a dog, *In Vivo* 22:47–50, 2008.
59. Hobson HP, Brown MR, Rogers KS: Surgery of metastatic anal sac adenocarcinoma in five dogs, *Vet Surg* 35:267–270, 2006.
60. Hoelzler MG, Bellah JR, Donofro MC: Omentalization of cystic sublumbar lymph node metastases for long-term palliation of tenesmus and dysuria in a dog with anal sac adenocarcinoma, *J Am Vet Med Assoc* 219(12):1729–1731, 2001.
61. Simeonov R, Simeonova G: Quantitative analysis in spontaneous canine anal sac gland adenomas and carcinomas, *Res Vet Sci* 85:559–562, 2008.
62. Anderson CR, McNiel EA, Gillette EL, et al.: Late complications of pelvic irradiation in 16 dogs, *Vet Radiol Ultrasound* 43(2):187–192, 2002.
63. Arthur JJ, Kleiter MM, Thrall DE: Characterization of normal tissue complications in 51 dogs undergoing definitive pelvic region irradiation, *Vet Radiol Ultrasound* 49(1):85–89, 2008.
64. Lampejo T, Davanagh D, Clark J: Prognostic biomarkers in squamous cell carcinoma of the anus: a systematic review, *Br J Cancer* 103:1858–1869, 2010.
65. Chan E, Kachnic LA, Thomas CR Jr: Anal cancer: Progress on combined-modality and organ preservation, *Curr Prob Cancer* 33:302–326, 2009.
66. Shia J: An update on tumors of the anal canal, *Arch Pathol Lab Med* 134:1601–1611, 2010.

23 Tumors of the Respiratory System

SECTION A
Cancer of the Nasal Planum

STEPHEN J. WITHROW

Incidence and Risk Factors

Cancer of the nasal planum is uncommon in the dog and relatively common in the cat. The development of squamous cell carcinoma (SCC) has been correlated with ultraviolet (UV) light exposure and lack of protective pigment.[1] One paper suggests a papillomavirus may be involved in feline SCC development.[2] Classically, it is seen in older, lightly pigmented cats.

Pathology and Natural Behavior

By far the most common cancer is SCC. Depending on when the biopsy is performed, the tumors may be reported as carcinoma in situ, superficial SCC (<2 mm deep), or deeply infiltrative SCC. They may be very locally invasive but only rarely metastasize.

Other cancers reported in the nasal planum are lymphoma, fibrosarcoma, hemangioma, melanoma, mast cell tumor, fibroma, and eosinophilic granuloma. Immune-mediated disease may manifest as erosive or crusty lesions on the nose, but it is rarely proliferative, and other sites on the body usually are affected. Immune-mediated disease probably is not a contributing factor in tumor development.

History and Clinical Signs

Invasive SCC usually is preceded by a protracted course of disease (months to years) that progresses through the following stages (Figure 23-1): crusting and erythema, superficial erosions and ulcers (carcinoma in situ or early SCC), and, finally, deeply invasive, erosive lesions. In cats SCC usually originates on the cornified external surface of the nasal planum, whereas in dogs it often occurs in the mucous membrane of the nostril or the external planum. Associated lesions on the eyelid, preauricular skin, and ear pinna may be seen in cats if these sites lack protective pigment. Patients often have been treated with corticosteroids or topical ointments, with minimal response.

Diagnostic Techniques and Work-Up

For erosive or proliferative lesions, a deep wedge biopsy may be done to determine the degree of invasion and the histologic type of disease. These biopsies require a brief general anesthetic because of the sensitivity of the nasal planum. Hemorrhage can be temporarily profuse and usually requires one or two deep sutures to appose the edges. Cytologic scrapings and superficial biopsies are of little value because they frequently reveal only inflammation, which may accompany both cancer and noncancerous conditions. Lymph nodes are rarely involved except in very advanced disease, and thoracic radiographs are almost invariably negative for metastasis. Regional radiographs generally are unrewarding. Computed tomography (CT) and magnetic resonance imaging (MRI) have proved to be valuable staging tool in dogs with SCC of the nostril. They can help define the posterior extent of the tumor and guide the posterior level of resection or the posterior extent of the radiation field.

Therapy

Limiting exposure to the sun or tattooing to add pigment protection may prevent or arrest the course of the preneoplastic disease. Topical sunscreens are easily licked off and rarely help. Maintaining the tattoo is very difficult when inflammation and ulceration are present because it is rapidly removed by macrophages. Even under the best of circumstances, tattooing must be repeated regularly and reports of success are anecdotal. Attempts to increase epithelial differentiation with synthetic derivatives of vitamin A generally have been unsuccessful for advanced disease but may be of help in reversing or limiting the growth of preneoplastic lesions.[3,4]

SCC and probably other neoplasms as well fall into two general categories: superficial, minimally invasive disease versus deeply infiltrating disease. Superficial cancers can be managed effectively by almost any method, including cryosurgery, lasers,[5,6] photodynamic therapy,[7-9] intralesional carboplatin chemotherapy,[10] intralesional carboplatin combined with radiation therapy (RT),[11] hyperthermia, and irradiation alone.[12-19] A distinct disadvantage with these techniques is the inability to obtain a surgical margin by which to document the adequacy of treatment. RT, in particular, which would have the greatest chance of preserving the cosmetic appearance of the nose, has had poor local control rates for larger and more invasive SCC in the dog but is more effective treating SCC of the nasal planum in the cat.[14,15,20] Expectations for radiation with other tumor types must be extrapolated from results achieved in more conventional sites.

In the cat, invasive cancer of the nasal planum can be completely excised with an acceptable cosmetic result.[21] The nasal planum is removed with a 360-degree skin incision that also transects the underlying turbinates (Figure 23-2). A single cutaneous purse-string suture of 3-0 nylon is placed to pull the skin into an open circle (1 cm in diameter) around the airways. The purse-string suture must not be pulled too tight or it may heal across the

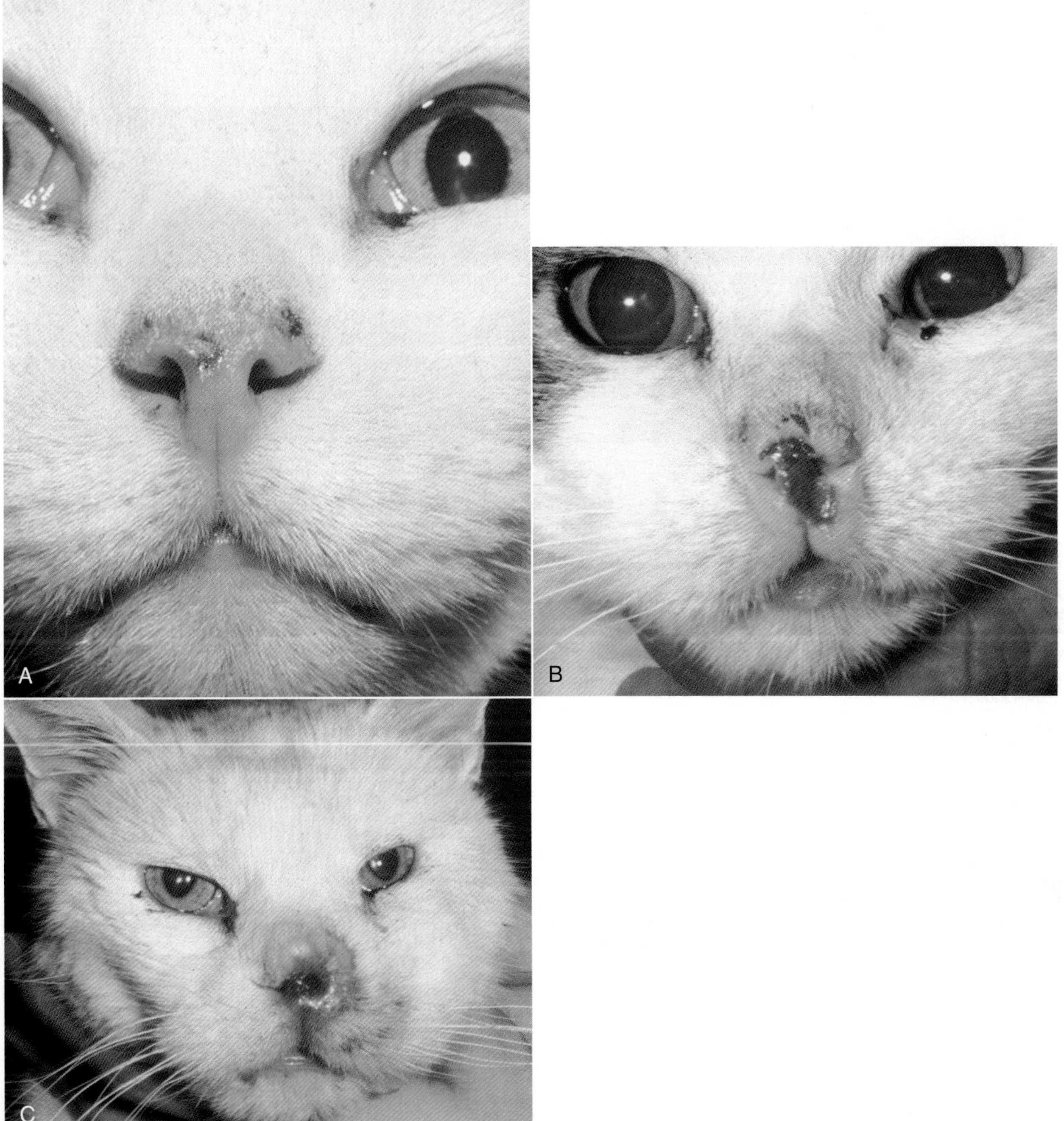

FIGURE 23-1 **A,** Crusting and erythema on the nose of a white cat. The condition had been slowly progressive for 8 months, and 6 months later, the lesion was confirmed through biopsy as carcinoma in situ. **B,** A cat with an invasive SCC that has caused some erosion of the nasal planum but is still confined to the nasal planum. Nosectomy was curative. **C,** This cat had a 2-year history of progressive nasal ulceration and deformity. The nasal planum is markedly deformed, and the surrounding skin up to the eyelids is swollen and infiltrated with SCC. Even nosectomy would not be curative. Note the concomitant eyelid lesions, which were carcinoma in situ.

airways. The site subsequently crusts and scabs over. The scab is removed at suture removal (this often requires sedation or anesthesia), and healing of the skin with two patent airways ("nostrils") is complete by 1 month. An occasional problem with "nosectomy" is stricture of the combined nasal orifice. This can be frustrating and has been variously managed with wide skin excision and removal of the nasal septum rostrally, laser ablation, rubber stents, or permanent placement of a stainless steel intraluminal expansile stent.[22] Functional and cosmetic results are good in the cat (Figure 23-3), and fair to good in the dog[23,24] (Figure 23-4). This procedure probably is the treatment of choice for invasive lesions that have not spread extensively to the lip or surrounding skin. The author has found that adjuvant RT has been successful if the margins of removal are incomplete. Combined removal of the premaxilla and nasal planum has been reported in the dog with extensive, invasive lesions.[23,25,26]

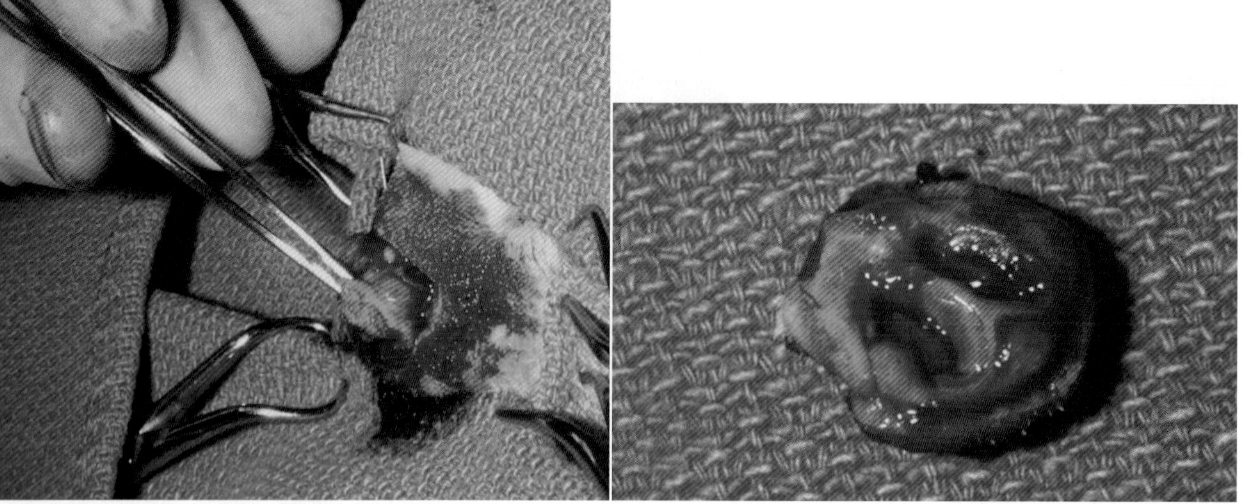

FIGURE 23-2 Operative view of resected nasal planum in a cat with invasive carcinoma that was confined to the nasal planum.

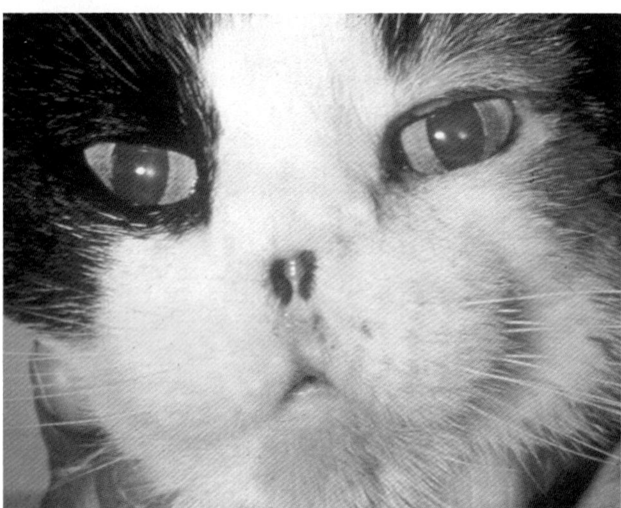

FIGURE 23-3 One-year postoperative view of a cat after nosectomy for SCC. Note the well-healed skin around patent airways. This cat remains free of disease 28 months after surgery.

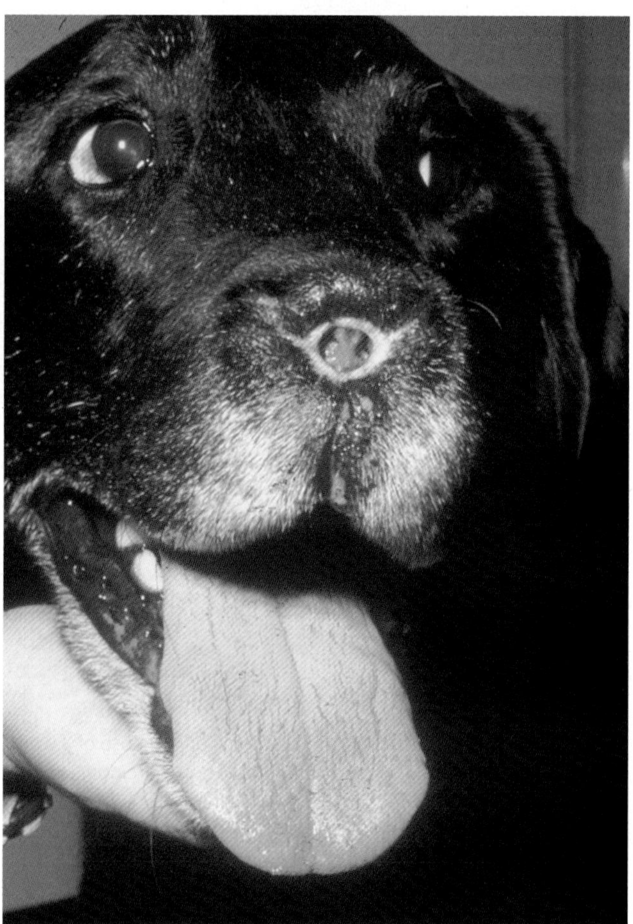

FIGURE 23-4 Two-year postoperative view of a dog after nasal planum resection for SCC.

Prognosis

The outlook for SCC is good for early, noninvasive disease. However, the development of new sites of neoplasia on other areas of the planum after localized treatment is common because the underlying causes are not reversed.[27] Later-stage disease can be cured with aggressive surgery but is poorly responsive to most other treatments.[20,21,25] More than 80% of cats with invasive SCC of the nasal planum treated with wide resection (nosectomy) are free of recurrent disease at 1 year.[5,21] Newer reports of proton irradiation[16] and irradiation with intralesional chemotherapy[11] suggest control rates in cats exceeding 60%. Strontium (Sr) 90 plesiotherapy can achieve 75% complete response (CR) rates for superficial SCC, and retreatment is possible. In a study of nosectomy (with or without removal of the pinnae) in 38 cats, the median survival time (MST) exceeded 22 months.[5] Photodynamic therapy can be effective in treating cats with SCC of the nose, but the lesions must be small and minimally invasive for a good result.[7-9] In dogs, the local recurrence rate after nosectomy is low.[20,26] Delayed lymph node metastasis (longer than 1 year after surgery) in dogs with SCC has been successfully treated with lymphadenectomy. Because SCC rarely metastasizes from the nasal planum, even untreated animals with advanced cancer can live a long time, albeit with an ulcerated and deforming cancer.

Comparative Aspects[28]

As in the cat, cancer of the human nasal skin and nasal vestibule (anterior entrance to the nasal cavity) may be induced by exposure to UV light. Lack of protective pigment is also a contributing factor in humans. SCC of the vestibule is treated with irradiation (interstitial or external beam) or surgery. Surgery generally involves resection of the nasal skin and cartilage, followed by reconstruction using composite ear skin and cartilage, nasolabial flaps, or a prosthesis. Local control generally is good.

REFERENCES

1. Hargis AM: A review of solar-induced lesions in domestic animals, *Comp Cont Ed Pract Vet* 3:287–294, 1981.
2. Munday JS, Dunowska M, De Grey S: Detection of two different papillomaviruses within a feline cutaneous squamous cell carcinoma: case report and review of the literature, *N Z Vet J* 57:248–251, 2009.
3. Evans AG, Madewell BR, Stannard AA: A trial of 13-cis-retinoic acid for treatment of squamous cell carcinoma and preneoplastic lesions of the head in cats, *Am J Vet Res* 46:2553–2557, 1985.
4. Marks SL, Song MD, Stannard AA, et al: Clinical evaluation of etretinate for the treatment of canine solar-induced squamous cell carcinoma and preneoplastic lesions, *J Am Acad Dermatol* 27:11–16, 1992.
5. Lana SE, Ogilvie GK, Withrow SJ, et al: Feline cutaneous squamous cell carcinoma of the nasal planum and the pinnae: 61 cases, *J Am Anim Hosp Assoc* 33:329–332, 1997.
6. Olivieri L, Nardini G, Pengo G, et al: Cutaneous progressive angiomatosis on the muzzle of a dog, treated by laser photocoagulation therapy, *Vet Dermatol* 21:517–521, 2010.
7. Peaston AE, Leach MW, Higgins RJ: Photodynamic therapy for nasal and aural squamous cell carcinoma in cats, *J Am Vet Med Assoc* 202:1261–1265, 1993.
8. Ferreira I, Rahal SC, Rocha NS, et al: Hematoporphyrin-based photodynamic therapy for cutaneous squamous cell carcinoma in cats, *Vet Dermatol* 20:174–178, 2009.
9. Bexfield NH, Stell AJ, Gear RN, et al: Photodynamic therapy of superficial nasal planum squamous cell carcinomas in cats: 55 cases, *J Vet Intern Med/Am Coll Vet Int Med* 22:1385–1389, 2008.
10. Théon AP, Madewell BR, Shearn VI, et al: Prognostic factors associated with radiotherapy of squamous cell carcinoma of the nasal plane in cats, *J Am Vet Med Assoc* 206:991–996, 1995.
11. de Vos JP, Burm GO, Focker BP: Results from the treatment of advanced stage squamous cell carcinoma of the nasal planum in cats, using a combination of intralesional carboplatin and superficial radiotherapy: a pilot study, *Vet Comp Oncol* 2:75–81, 2004.
12. Grier RL, Brewer WG, Theilen GH: Hyperthermic treatment of superficial tumors in cats and dogs, *J Am Vet Med Assoc* 177:227–233, 1980.
13. Shelley BA, Bartels KE, Ely RW, et al: Use of the neodymium:yttrium-aluminum-garnet laser for treatment of squamous cell carcinoma of the nasal planum in a cat, *J Am Vet Med Assoc* 201:756–758, 1992.
14. Carlisle CH, Gould S: Response of squamous cell carcinoma of the nose of the cat to treatment with x-rays, *Vet Radiol* 23:186–192, 1982.
15. Thrall DE, Adams WM: Radiotherapy of squamous cell carcinomas of the canine nasal plane, *Vet Radiol* 23:193–195, 1982.
16. Fidel JL, Egger E, Blattmann H, et al: Proton irradiation of feline nasal planum squamous cell carcinoma using an accelerated protocol, *Vet Radiol Ultrasound* 42:569–575, 2001.
17. Trivillin VA, Heber EM, Rao M, et al: Boron neutron capture therapy (BNCT) for the treatment of spontaneous nasal planum squamous cell carcinoma in felines, *Radiat Environ Biophys* 47:147–155, 2008.
18. Goodfellow M, Hayes A, Murphy S, et al: A retrospective study of (90)Strontium plesiotherapy for feline squamous cell carcinoma of the nasal planum, *J Feline Med Surg* 8:169–176, 2006.
19. Hammond GM, Gordon IK, Theon AP, et al: Evaluation of strontium Sr 90 for the treatment of superficial squamous cell carcinoma of the nasal planum in cats: 49 cases (1990-2006), *J Am Vet Med Assoc* 231:736–741, 2007.
20. Lascelles BD, Parry AT, Stidworthy MF, et al: Squamous cell carcinoma of the nasal planum in 17 dogs, *Vet Rec* 147:473–476, 2000.
21. Withrow SJ, Straw RC: Resection of the nasal planum in nine cats and five dogs, *J Am Anim Hosp Assoc* 26:219–222, 1990.
22. Novo RE, Kramek B: Surgical repair of nasopharyngeal stenosis in a cat using a stent, *J Am Anim Hosp Assoc* 35:251–256, 1999.
23. Gallegos J, Schmiedt CW, McAnulty JF: Cosmetic rostral nasal reconstruction after nasal planum and premaxilla resection: technique and results in two dogs, *Vet Surg* 36:669–674, 2007.
24. Thomson M: Squamous cell carcinoma of the nasal planum in cats and dogs, *Clin Tech Small Anim Pract* 22:42–45, 2007.
25. Lascelles BD, Henderson RA, Sequin B, et al: Bilateral rostral maxillectomy and nasal planectomy for large rostral maxillofacial neoplasms in six dogs and one cat, *J Am Anim Hosp Assoc* 40:137–146, 2004.
26. Kirpensteijn J, Withrow SJ, Straw RC: Combined resection of the nasal planum and premaxilla in three dogs, *Vet Surg* 23:341–346, 1994.
27. Théon AP, VanVechten MK, Madewell BR: Intratumoral administration of carboplatin for treatment of squamous cell carcinomas of the nasal plane in cats, *Am J Vet Res* 57:205–210, 1996.
28. Aasi SZ, Leffell DJ: Cancer of the skin. In DeVita VT, et al, editors: *Cancer: principles and practices of oncology*, Philadelphia, 2005, Lippincott-Raven.

SECTION B
Nasosinal Tumors

MICHELLE M. TUREK AND SUSAN E. LANA

Canine Nasosinal Tumors

Incidence and Risk Factors

Tumors of the nasal cavity and paranasal sinuses account for approximately 1% of all neoplasms in dogs.[1] The average age of dogs with this disease is approximately 10 years, although canine patients as young as 9 months have been reported.[2,3] Medium-to-large breeds may be more commonly affected.[2] A slight male predilection has been suggested.[2,4] It has been speculated, but is unproved, that dolichocephalic breeds (long-nosed) or dogs living in urban environments, with resultant nasal filtering of pollutants, may be at higher risk for developing nasal cancer.[4-6] Exposure to environmental tobacco smoke has been associated with an increased risk of nasal cancer in a group of dogs in one study,[7] but the same was not true in another.[6] Indoor exposure to fossil fuel combustion products, such as those produced by coal or kerosene heaters, may contribute to the suggested environmental component of this cancer.[6]

Pathology and Natural Behavior

Carcinomas, including adenocarcinoma, SCC, and undifferentiated carcinoma represent nearly two-thirds of canine intranasal tumors.[8] Sarcomas (usually fibrosarcoma, chondrosarcoma, osteosarcoma, and undifferentiated sarcoma) comprise the bulk of the remaining cancers.[9] Both carcinomas and sarcomas are characterized by progressive local invasion. The metastatic rate is generally considered low at the time of diagnosis but may be as high as 40% to 50% at the time of death, which is usually attributable to the primary disease rather than metastatic lesions.[2] The most common sites of metastasis are the regional lymph nodes and the lungs.[2,9,10] Less common sites include bones, kidneys, liver, skin, and brain.[11-14]

Rare tumors of the nasosinal region in dogs include round cell tumors, such as lymphoma (unlike in cats, in which this is a common nasal tumor); mast cell tumors; and transmissible venereal cancer. Other malignancies include hemangiosarcoma, melanoma, neuroendocrine carcinoma, nerve sheath tumor, neuroblastoma, fibrous histiocytoma, multilobular osteochondrosarcoma, hamartoma, rhabdomyosarcoma, and leiomyosarcoma.[2,15-28] The biologic behavior of these less common malignancies is not well defined. Benign lesions such as polyps, fibromas, dermoid cysts, and angiomatous proliferation can also be seen.

A number of studies have attempted to elucidate possible molecular mechanisms associated with canine nasosinal tumorigenesis. In one study using a single polyclonal antihuman antibody, nuclear *p53* accumulation was detected in nearly 60% of nasal adenocarcinomas (11 of 19), which suggests that overexpression of a mutated *p53* tumor suppressor protein may play a role.[29] Cyclooxygenase-2 (COX-2) expression has been detected to varying degrees in most nasosinal epithelial tumors sampled[30-33] and in normal paratumoral respiratory epithelium and stromal tissue.[33] In a recent study, epidermal growth factor receptor (EGFR) expression and vascular endothelial growth factor (VEGF) expression were detected in over 50% and 90% of the 24 nasal carcinomas evaluated, respectively.[34] All tumors expressed either EGFR or VEGFR, but there was no association between the immunoreactivity for each protein.[34] Expression of peroxisome proliferator-activated receptor γ (PPAR-γ), a nuclear receptor involved in glucose metabolism and fatty acid storage, has also been shown in canine nasal carcinomas.[35] The authors of that study suggested that expression patterns may differ in tumor tissue compared to normal nasal epithelium.[35] The role of these proteins in carcinogenesis is not clear, and further investigation is needed before clinical relevancy can be determined. Evaluation of the inflammatory infiltrate in 31 canine nasal carcinomas revealed an abundance of neutrophils and macrophages, which were present in greater numbers than in normal canine mucosa.[36] Plasma cells were also detected in the majority of tumors but varied in number compared to normal tissue. T-lymphocytes were detected less commonly, in lower numbers than in the normal mucosa, and predominately at the periphery of the tumors. Activity of matrix metalloproteinase-2 (MMP-2) in nasal adenocarcinomas was negligible in one small study.[37]

History and Clinical Signs

Although many intranasal diseases will have overlapping clinical signs, a strong suspicion of cancer is appropriate for older animals with an intermittent and progressive history of unilateral (initially) epistaxis or mucopurulent discharge (or both). The average duration of clinical signs prior to diagnosis is 2 to 3 months[1,38]; these most commonly include epistaxis, bloody or mucopurulent nasal discharge, facial deformity due to bone erosion and subcutaneous extension of tumor, unwillingness to open the mouth, sneezing, dyspnea or stertorous breathing, exophthalmus, and ocular discharge as a result of mechanical obstruction of the nasolacrimal duct.[2,8,38] Differential diagnoses for animals with these clinical signs include fungal (*Aspergillus* sp.) or bacterial rhinitis, idiopathic nonspecific rhinitis (usually lymphoplasmacytic), rare nasal parasites, bleeding disorders, hypertension, foreign body, trauma, and developmental anomalies (e.g., cystic Rathke's clefts).[39-41] If facial deformity is present, the diagnosis is almost always cancer[42,43]; however, aspergillosis, sporotrichosis, and a rare, benign condition, angiomatous proliferation of the nasal cavity, also can cause facial deformity. Dogs with epistaxis and concurrent clinical signs of systemic disease, including lethargy, inappetence, weight loss, hemorrhage at extranasal sites and concurrent neurologic disease, are more likely to have nonneoplastic systemic disorders such as bleeding disorders, hypertension, and tick-borne or bacterial infections.[43,44]

Clinical signs can be temporarily alleviated by a variety of symptomatic treatments, including antibiotics, steroids, and nonsteroidal antiinflammatory drugs (NSAIDs).[38] An initial response to these treatments should not diminish the index of suspicion for neoplasia in older dogs with clinical signs consistent with cancer.[38]

On rare occasions, animals with tumors involving the caudal region of the nasal cavity may have only neurologic signs (e.g., seizures, acute blindness, behavior change, paresis, circling, and obtundation) caused by direct invasion of the cranial vault.[45] However, absence of neurologic signs does not rule out tumor extension into the cranial vault because most dogs with nasal tumors that extend beyond the cribriform plate do not exhibit neurologic signs.

Diagnosis and Staging

A definitive diagnosis of nasosinal cancer requires a tissue biopsy, even though diagnostic imaging and historic information can be highly suggestive. Coagulation disorders must be ruled out before biopsy because bleeding during the procedure is to be expected. Attention should be paid to the platelet count, appropriate clotting at venipuncture sites, and the presence of hematuria, retinal hemorrhage, or petechial hemorrhages. A clotting profile (prothrombin time [PT], activated partial thromboplastin time [APTT]), bleeding time, or activated clotting time (ACT) can also be done.

The superior imaging value of CT and MRI over conventional radiographs for canine nasal disease, including neoplasia, is well documented.[3,23,39,46-52] Cross-sectional imaging provides improved anatomic detail, which allows accurate determination of the extent of tumor (staging) and localization of nasal cavity abnormalities (Figure 23-5).[3,23,39,46-53] It also facilitates evaluation of the integrity of the cribriform plate and identification of potential tumor extension into the cranial vault, which are important prognostic criteria. Although, in general, MRI allows for better resolution of soft tissue structures, a recent study showed no clinically relevant benefit to using MRI over CT to evaluate nasal tumors that do not extend into the cranial vault.[49] CT enables better visualization of lysis of bones bordering the nasal cavity, which is important for accurate radiation treatment planning. It has been proposed that tumor signal intensity on MRI may help distinguish sarcomas from carcinomas,[50] although this application requires further validation before it can be used clinically. Both modalities are useful for imaging nasal tumors, although CT is used more commonly than MRI due to its lower cost in most facilities, wider availability, and usefulness for computer planning of radiation treatments.

Certain CT or MRI findings have been correlated with a diagnosis of cancer in dogs with nasal disease.[23,39,53] None of these, alone or in combination, is definitive for neoplasia.[23,39,53] These findings include bony destruction (e.g., ethmoid bones, cribriform plate, and the bones surrounding the nasal cavities), destruction of the sphenoid sinus, abnormal soft tissue in the retrobulbar space, nasopharyngeal invasion, hyperostosis of the lateral maxilla, and patchy areas of increased density within abnormal soft tissue opacity.[23,53] It

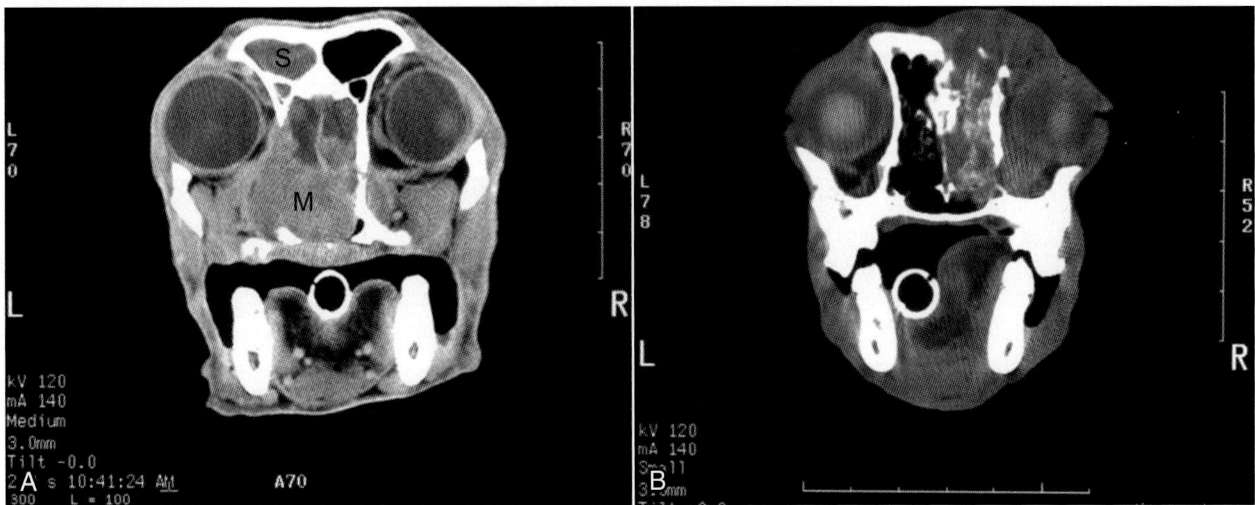

FIGURE 23-5 **A,** Contrast-enhanced CT image of a dog with nasosinal cancer taken in the transverse plane at the level of the orbit and the olfactory bulb of the brain. Note the contrast-enhancing mass *(M)* in the nasopharynx, which is causing erosion of the frontal and palatine bones. The tumor has invaded the left retroorbital space and the cranial vault, resulting in deviation of the falx cerebri. Non–contrast-enhancing material in the left frontal sinus *(S)* suggests accumulation of nasal exudates. **B,** Non–contrast-enhanced CT image of a dog with nasosinal cancer taken in the transverse plane at the level of the orbit. Note the soft tissue attenuating mass in the right nasal cavity. Erosion of the frontal bone has allowed the tumor to extend into the subcutaneous tissues on the dorsum of the head; erosion of the palatine bone has allowed invasion of the right retroorbital space.

is important to recognize that detection of a mass in the nasal cavity of a dog is not specific for a diagnosis of neoplasia.[23] Idiopathic inflammatory disease and fungal infections can present in this manner.[23]

Conventional radiography can still have a place in the diagnostic work-up of dogs suspected of having nasal tumors. Despite the inherent limitation of tissue superimposition, the sensitivity of radiography in detecting major nasal cavity abnormalities in dogs with nasal tumors is comparable to that of CT or MRI when tumors are sufficiently advanced to cause clinical signs.[46,52,54] Certain radiographic signs have been correlated with a positive predictive value for neoplasia.[55] These include the presence of a soft tissue opacity, loss of turbinate detail affecting the entire ipsilateral nasal cavity, invasion of bones surrounding the nasal cavity, and soft tissue/fluid opacities within the ipsilateral frontal sinus (Figure 23-6).[55] As is true for CT and MRI changes, no radiographic sign is definitively diagnostic for neoplasia.[52,55] Nasal radiography therefore represents an easily accessible and less costly screening procedure that can guide further diagnostics, including biopsy, additional imaging, or both.[52,56] Standard radiographs taken under anesthesia include lateral, dorsoventral (DV), frontal sinus, and open-mouth oblique views. The most informative views are the open-mouth DV oblique view (to show the caudal nasal cavity and cribriform plate) and the isolated nasal cavity exposure with the film placed in the mouth and exposed in the DV plane.

A tissue biopsy should be obtained while the patient is under anesthesia for diagnostic imaging. Suitable samples can be acquired by a variety of techniques.[57,58] These include vigorous nasal flushing to dislodge mass lesions, transnostril blind biopsy using cup forceps or a bone curette, fiberoptic-guided biopsy, fine-needle aspiration (FNA) or punch biopsy of facial deformities, rhinotomy, and transnostril aspiration and core biopsy (Figure 23-7). Transnostril aspiration and core biopsy involves passing either a punch biopsy needle or a large bore (3 to 5 mm) plastic cannula into the nasal cavity through the nostril and directing it to the tumor (Figure 23-8).[57] With any transnostril technique, it is important to avoid penetrating the cribriform plate. The biopsy instrument should be marked with tape or cut off at a length that ensures that the instrument does not penetrate farther than the distance from the tip of the naris to the medial canthus of the eye (Figure 23-9). Mild-to-moderate hemorrhage is to be expected and subsides within several minutes. It is important to ensure the integrity and inflation of the endotracheal tube cuff during any of these procedures. If hemorrhage is severe, the ipsilateral carotid artery can be permanently ligated, but this is rarely indicated.[59] Inadequate biopsy size or sampling outside the region of the tumor may preclude an accurate diagnosis. Further testing may be necessary when clinical and histologic findings are incongruent. In cases in which imaging results are suggestive of an aggressive process yet histopathologic changes are consistent with nonspecific inflammatory disease, a surgical biopsy obtained by rhinotomy may be required for definitive diagnosis.[3,23]

Attempts at nasal washing and fluid retrieval for cytologic examination generally have been unrewarding and are not recommended as the sole means of diagnosis.[1] Brush cytology also has been described, but it often is not diagnostic.[60] Rhinoscopy can be used to visualize the nasal cavity, if necessary, and to guide biopsy, although samples collected in this manner often are small and superficial.[61]

Multiple staging systems for canine nasosinal neoplasia have been proposed on the basis of local tumor extent and bony erosion (Table 23-1).[4,63-65,67] The least clinically relevant is the World Health Organization (WHO) staging method because no correlation has been found between primary tumor extent and prognosis using this system.[38,65,67,68] The prognostic significance of the other staging systems remains controversial. A recent review of 94 dogs with

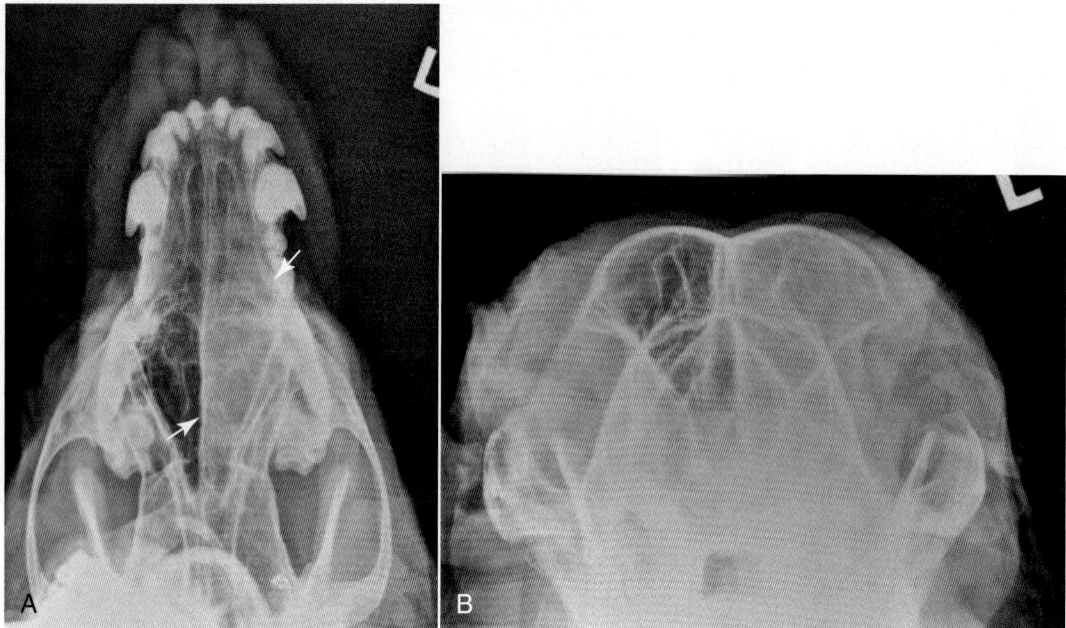

FIGURE 23-6 Radiographs of a dog with an intranasal anaplastic carcinoma. **A,** In this open mouth ventrodorsal view of the maxilla, note the asymmetry from side to side. A soft tissue opacity in the left nasal cavity *(arrows)* suggests the presence of a space-occupying mass. **B,** Rostral-caudal skyline view of the frontal sinuses. A soft tissue opacity in the left frontal sinus suggests extension of tumor or obstructive rhinitis. *(Courtesy Dr. David Jimenez.)*

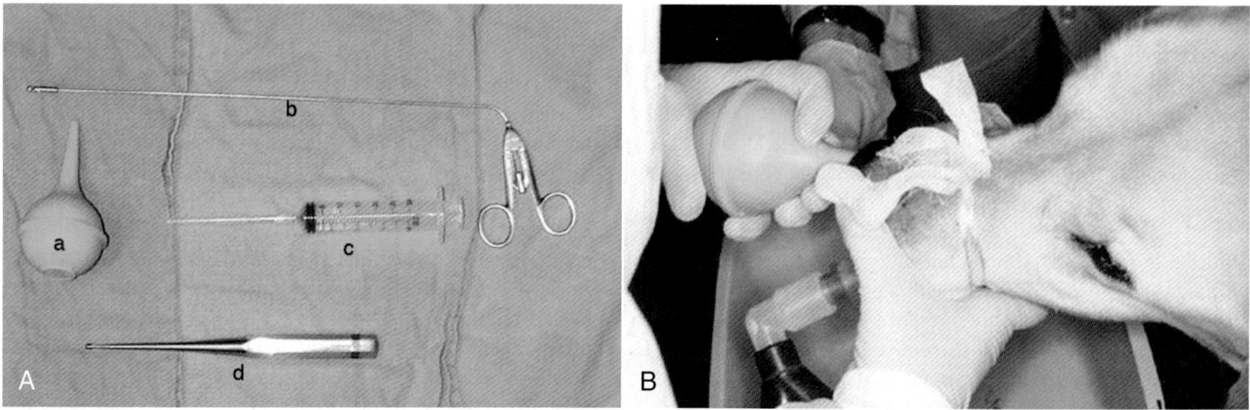

FIGURE 23-7 **A,** Several techniques can be used to procure tissue biopsy material from dogs with nasal tumors. A bulb syringe *(a)* can be used to flush out tumor material, or a biopsy forceps *(b)*, plastic cannula *(c)*, or bone curette *(d)* can be inserted through the nostril. **B,** To flush biopsy tissue in an anesthetized dog with an endotracheal tube, the contralateral passage is occluded and flushing pressure is created with a saline-filled bulb syringe; the tissue is flushed back through the nasopharynx and out the mouth into a collection bowl.

nasal tumors treated with definitive RT showed that the CT-based Adams staging system and its recently modified version in which stage 4 represents cribriform plate involvement alone correlate with disease outcome.[65] Prognostic significance improved when CT findings were combined with histologic category.[65]

Regional lymph node cytology is positive for metastasis in as many as 10% to 24% of cases and is most commonly associated with carcinoma.[10,38,66,68] Enlarged regional (mandibular and superficial cervical) lymph nodes should be sampled for cytology to differentiate between a reactive process and metastasis. Thoracic radiographs usually are negative for metastasis at initial presentation.[1,2,10,38]

Hematologic and biochemical findings generally are noncontributory in dogs with nasosinal tumors. In rare cases, paraneoplastic erythrocytosis and hypercalcemia have been documented.[69-71]

Treatment and Prognosis

Therapy is directed primarily at control of local disease, which usually manifests in a relatively advanced stage in a critical location near the brain and eyes (Figure 23-10). Without treatment, the MST

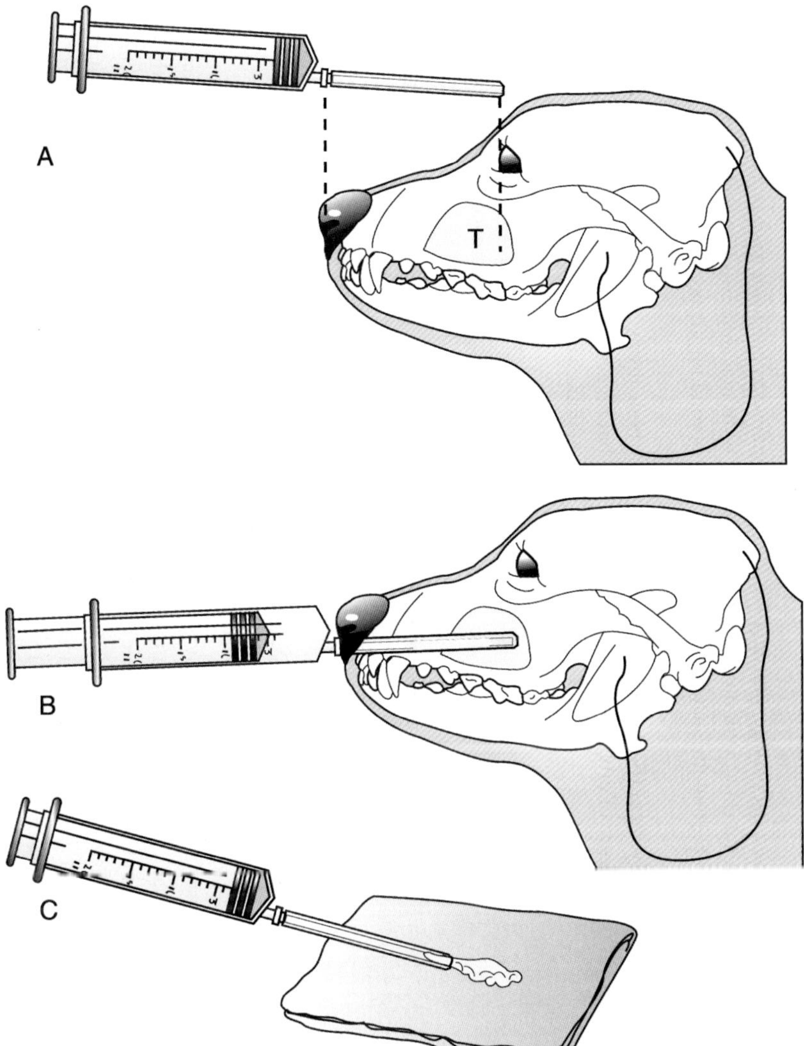

FIGURE 23-8 **A,** A caudally situated tumor *(T)* in a dog. To avoid injury to the brain, the plastic cannula for the core aspirate has been shortened so that it extends no deeper than the medial canthus of the eye. **B,** The cannula is introduced into the nasal cavity through the nares. Slight resistance usually is felt as the tumor is entered. Negative pressure is applied as the cannula is redirected at various angles. **C,** Tissue and blood are expelled onto a gauze sponge, where blood is separated from tissue. The tissue is submitted for histologic evaluation.

of dogs with nasal carcinoma is 95 days as reported in a retrospective case series of 139 dogs.[38] Prognosis of dogs with epistaxis appears worse than in dogs without epistaxis (MST 88 days versus 224 days).[38] Bone invasion occurs early, with nasosinal neoplasia, and curative surgery is virtually impossible. Although surgical removal by means of rhinotomy has been recommended, a high rate of morbidity without significant extension of life greatly limits the utility of this procedure as a sole form of treatment.[1,8,10,72,73] The median survival time after surgery is approximately 3 to 6 months, similar to that reported for no treatment.[1,10,72,73] In one study, surgery in conjunction with low-energy orthovoltage irradiation provided the best clinical outcome, MST, compared to other treatment modalities[74]; however, more recent reports have not supported this finding (Table 23-2).[13,75]

RT using high-energy megavoltage (MeV) equipment (cobalt source or linear accelerator) as the sole treatment modality has become the therapy of choice for canine nasosinal tumors (Table 23-3; see also Table 23-2). It has the advantage of treating the entire nasal cavity, including bone, and its use has been associated with the greatest improvement in survival. Although surgical removal of the tumor before MeV irradiation has not been shown to improve clinical outcome,[10,74,83] controlled studies have not been done for this combination. MST after MeV irradiation with curative intent (i.e., full-course or definitive radiation) alone ranges from 8 to 19.7 months.* The 1- and 2-year survival rates range from 43% to 68% (1 year) and 11% to 44% (2 years).[63,64,76-78,86] Doses of 42 to 54 Gy are usually delivered in 10 to 18 treatments of 3- to 4.2-Gy fractions over 2 to 4 weeks to the nasal cavity and frontal sinuses as dictated by imaging.[63-65,74,77-79] True statistical comparisons between reports are not possible because of inconsistencies in methodology (even within individual reports) with respect to total dose, fraction number, dose per fraction, treatment schedules, use of CT staging, use of computerized treatment planning, response monitoring, and statistical assessment. Furthermore, differences in tumor type and tumor stage also affect patient outcome.[65] CT-based computerized

*References 63-65, 76-79, 83-86.

TABLE 23-1 Staging Systems for Canine Nasosinal Neoplasia

World Health Organization (WHO)[62]	Théon[63]	Adams[64]	Modified Adams[65]
Staging System			
T: Primary Tumor **T0** No evidence of tumor **T1** Tumor ipsilateral, minimal or no bone destruction **T2** Tumor bilateral and/or moderate bone destruction **T3** Tumor invading neighboring tissue *N: Regional Lymph Nodes (RLN)* **N1** No evidence of RLN involvement **N2** Movable ipsilateral nodes **N3** Fixed nodes *M: Distant Metastasis* **M1** No evidence of distant metastasis **M2** Distant metastasis detected (including nodes)	*Stage 1* Unilateral or bilateral neoplasm confined to the nasal passage without extension into the frontal sinuses *Stage 2* Bilateral neoplasm extending into the frontal sinuses with erosion of any bone of the nasal passage	*Stage 1* Confined to one nasal passage, paranasal sinus, or frontal sinus, with no bone involvement beyond turbinates *Stage 2* Any bone involvement (beyond turbinates), but no evidence of orbit/subcutaneous/submucosal mass *Stage 3* Orbit involved, or subcutaneous or submucosal mass *Stage 4* Extension into nasopharynx or (osteolysis of) cribriform plate	*Stage 1* Confined to one nasal passage, paranasal sinus. or frontal sinus, with no bone involvement beyond turbinates *Stage 2* Any bone involvement (beyond turbinates), but no evidence of orbit/subcutaneous/submucosal mass *Stage 3* Orbit involved, or nasopharyngeal or subcutaneous or submucosal mass *Stage 4* Tumor-causing lysis of the cribriform plate
Clinical Relevance			
Primary tumor stage (T value) not useful in predicting clinical outcome in any study where it was evaluated.	Predicted risk of relapse when applied to radiographic findings: Stage 2 tumors were 2.3 times more likely to relapse than stage 1 tumors.[63]	Predicted relapse-free interval and survival on CT findings: Stage 1 and 2 tumors had improved clinical outcomes (median relapse-free interval 615 days; median survival 745 days) compared to stage 3 and 4 tumors (median relapse-free interval 745 days; median survival 315 days).[64] Predicted shorter DFI and survival in stage 4 dogs in an expanded cohort.[65] Predicted DFI and survival in a study of palliative RT (stage 1 and 2 more than stage 3 and 4).[66]	Based on CT findings: Predicted shorter DFI and survival in stage 4. Stronger association with outcome than original Adams stage 4. Cribriform involvement had the shortest survival (median 6.7 months). Stage 1 had the longest median survival (23.4 months).[65]

CT, Computed tomography; *DFI,* disease-free interval; *RT,* radiation therapy.

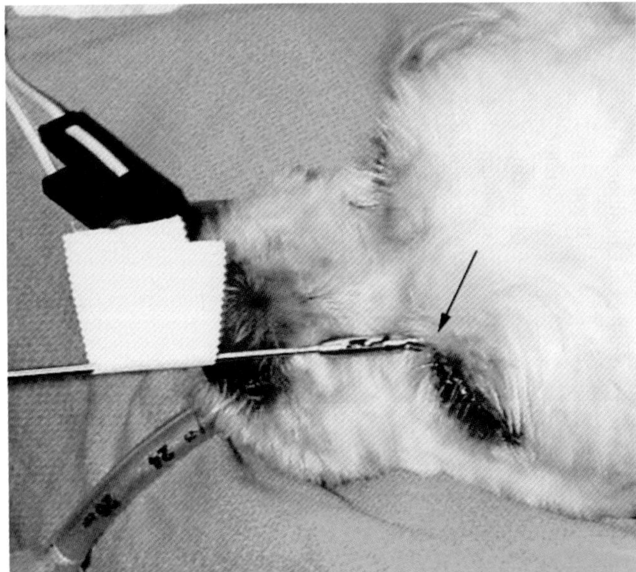

FIGURE 23-9 Regardless of the biopsy technique chosen, any instrument that is passed through the naris must be measured; it also should be marked with tape or cut off at a length that ensures that the instrument does not penetrate farther than the distance from the tip of the naris to the medial canthus of the eye. This ensures that the instrument does not pass through a potentially compromised cribriform plate.

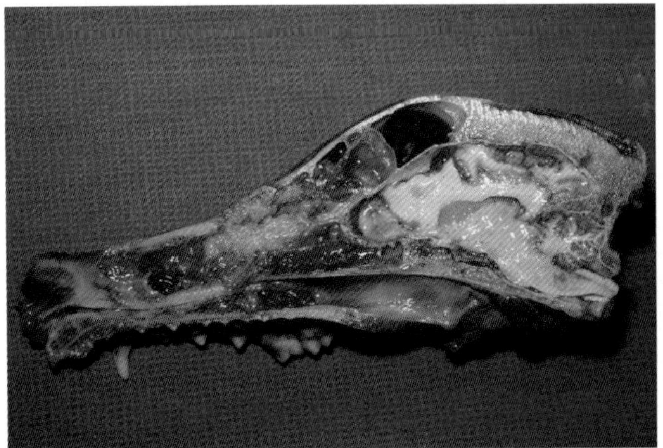

FIGURE 23-10 Cross-section of a dog's skull with a typical intranasal carcinoma. Note the middle to caudal position of the tumor in the nasal cavity, the erosion of the dorsal nasal bones, the dark mucus in the frontal sinus secondary to obstruction, and the proximity of the tumor to the cribriform plate. Complete surgical resection is impossible.

treatment planning can greatly enhance normal tissue sparing while ensuring optimized dose distribution within the tumor. The MST ranges from 11 to 19.7 months in dogs treated with CT-staged, computer-planned MeV irradiation to a minimum of 41 Gy.* As computer-based radiation planning becomes more advanced in veterinary medicine, it follows that clinical outcomes may continue to improve.[66]

*References 64, 65, 76-79, 84, 86.

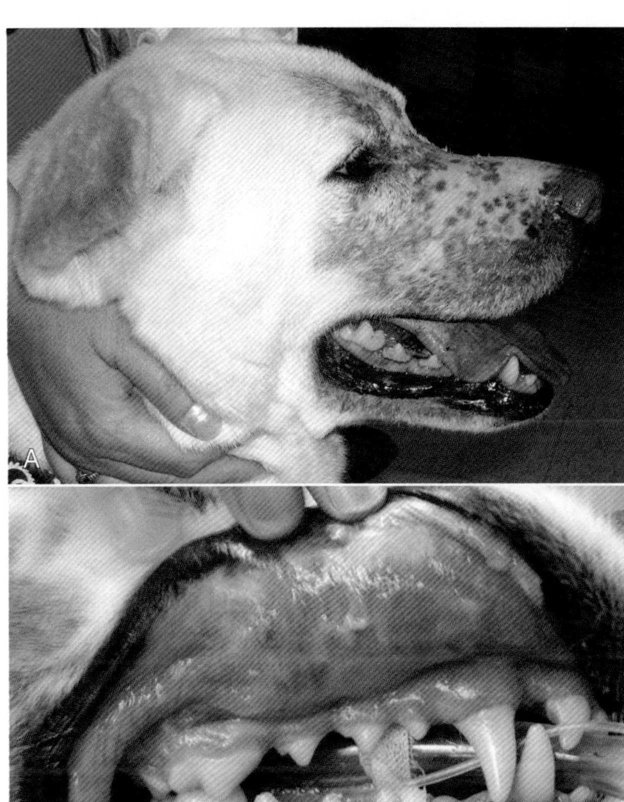

FIGURE 23-11 Potential acute effects of radiation therapy (RT) in dogs. **A,** Resolving desquamation one month after definitive RT for a nasal tumor. Note the hair loss in the radiation field. **B,** Oral mucositis on the last day of a definitive radiation protocol. Note the yellowish material on inner aspect of the upper lip. This represents dead epithelium that is being shed from the mucosa.

RT can induce normal tissue complications in the radiation treatment field (see Chapter 12). Acute and late toxicities affect rapidly and slowly renewing tissues, respectively, and depend on daily dose to the tissue, total dose, overall treatment time, and volume of tissue treated.[87] The severity of side effects can therefore vary among protocols and also between individuals on the same treatment schedule, depending on the tissues included in the radiation field. Acute toxicities associated with definitive, full-course irradiation of nasosinal tumors typically involve the oral cavity (oral mucositis), eye (keratoconjunctivitis and blepharitis), nasal cavity (rhinitis), and skin (desquamation) (Figure 23-11).[63,64,76,79,88] Acute effects develop during the course of RT and resolve within 2 to 8 weeks after treatment.[63,64,76,88] Oral antibiotics, pain medication, and/or ocular medication including artificial tears may be needed to support the patient during this period. Rarely, temporary esophagostomy or gastrostomy tube feedings may be indicated if oral mucositis is severe in order to maintain adequate nutritional intake.

Late radiation effects, although less common than acute effects, are more detrimental and long lasting. Their development should be prevented, if possible, with thoughtful radiation treatment planning. Tissues that may be affected include the ocular lens (cataracts), cornea (keratitis, atrophy, keratoconjunctivitis sicca),

TABLE 23-2 Summary of Selected Articles on Treatment of Nasosinal Tumors in Dogs (No Treatment or Definitive Radiation)

	Rassnick et al[38]	Adams et al[74]	Northrup et al[13]	Théon et al[63]	McEntee et al[76]	Adams et al[64]	Lana et al[77]	Adams et al[78]	Adams et al[78] (Historic Controls)	Adams[65]	Lawrence[79]
Number of dogs	139	67	42	77	27	21	13	13	40	94	31 (IMRT)/ 36 (2D RT)
Adjuvant Treatment											
Surgery	None	41/67	42/42	21/77*	6/27	None	None	11/13 post-RT	None	None	None
Chemotherapy	None	None	None	None	None	14/21†	13/13‡	None	None	None	None
Survival											
Median (months)	3.2	8.1	7.4	12.6	12.8	14.3	19.3	47.7	19.7	10.83	14
1 year/2 year (%)	12/2	38/30	37/17	60/25	59/22	60/36	81/39	76/69	68/44	NA	NA
Dose (Gy)											
Mean	0	43									
Median	0		48	48	41-54	42	49.5	42	42	42 (range 42-57)	42
Number of fractions	0	5-10	12	12	10-12	9-10	15	10	10	10 (range 10-19)	10
Radiation source	NA	Variable	Orthovoltage (low energy)	Cobalt	Cobalt	Cobalt	6 MeV linear accelerator	Cobalt	Cobalt	Cobalt or 4 MeV linear accelerator	Tomotherapy/ cobalt
Prognostic indicators/ conclusions	Epistaxis associated with shorter survival	SX + low energy, no advantage if SX + high energy	SX + low energy less effective than reported by Adams[38]; resolution of clinical signs favorable for survival; facial deformity not favorable for survival	SX did not affect outcome; SA > CA	SX did not affect outcome; SA = CA	Immunomodulator did not affect outcome		Post-SX complications include rhinitis (bacterial or fungal), osteomyelitis, fistula		Cribriform involvement associated with shortest clinical outcome; histologic category (anaplastic CA, undifferentiated CA, SCC) not favorable for survival	IMRT resulted in bilateral ocular-sparing compared to 2D historic controls

*Measurable disease remained in all dogs after the surgical procedure.

†Immunotherapy given using liposome-encapsulated MTP-PE.

‡Slow-release formulation of cisplatin given as chemotherapy.

IMRT, Intensity-modulated radiation therapy; *2D,* 2-dimensional; *RT,* radiation therapy; *NA,* not applicable; *SX,* surgery; *SA,* sarcoma; *CA,* carcinoma; *SCC,* squamous cell carcinoma.

TABLE 23-3 Summary of Selected Articles Describing Palliative Radiation Therapy for Nasosinal Tumors in Dogs

	MELLANBY ET AL[80]	GEIGER ET AL[81]	BUCHHOLZ ET AL[66]	BELSHAW ET AL[33]	MARUO ET AL[82]
Number of dogs	56	48	38	42	63
Adjuvant Treatment					
Surgery	None	None	None	None	None
Chemotherapy	None	None	None	None	None
Survival					
Median (months)	7	4.9	10.1	6.7	6.4
1 year/2 year (%)	45/15	25/9	NA	NA	25/8
Total dose (Gy)	36	Median 24 (range 16-40)	Median 32 (range 24-30)	34-36	32 (range 10-40)
Number of fractions	4	Median 4 (range 2-5)	Median 5 (range 4-10)	4	4
Dose/fraction (Gy)	9	Median 8 (range 4-10)	Median 6 (range 3-8)	9 (range 8.5-9)	8 (range 5-10)
Treatment schedule	Every 7 days	Every 7 days or daily	Every 7 days, biweekly, or daily	Every 7 days	Every 7 days
Radiation source	4 MeV linear accelerator	Cobalt or linear accelerator	6 MeV linear accelerator	4 MeV linear accelerator	4 MeV linear accelerator
Prognostic indicators/ conclusions	95% of dogs experienced improvement of clinical signs.	66% of dogs had complete resolution of clinical signs for a median duration of 120 days; complete resolution of clinical signs predicted favorable survival; clinical signs present for <90 days before diagnosis associated with higher risk of relapse.	Adams stage prognostic for outcome; 100% of dogs had resolution of clinical signs; clinical outcome may be improved with better treatment planning.	COX-2 expression did not correlate with survival.	Improvement of clinical signs in 84% of dogs.

NA, Not applicable; *COX-2*, cyclooxygenase-2.

anterior uvea (uveitis), retina (hemorrhage and degeneration), neuronal tissue (brain necrosis, causing neurologic changes and/or seizures, and optic nerve degeneration), bone (osteonecrosis), and skin (fibrosis).* Late complications develop months to years after therapy and are generally irreversible. The most commonly observed clinically relevant late effects in dogs treated with definitive RT for nasosinal tumors are those affecting ocular structures.[68,76] Late ocular changes in the dog typically occur 6 to 9 months following RT and most often include keratoconjunctivitis sicca, cataract formation, and blindness in the irradiated eye if radiation doses are not limited.[79] Other late effects are rare.

Overall, although most dogs with nasosinal neoplasia experience a favorable tumor response to RT, the long-term prognosis is poor (see Table 23-2). Even when treated with a definitive (curative-intent) radiation protocol, most dogs die or are euthanized as a result of local disease progression. An investigation of treatment failure patterns following full-course MeV irradiation showed that the median duration of local control in 24 dogs was 312 days.[92] Marked tumor regression (90% reduction in size) was observed using CT in 46% of cases and was associated with a longer duration of local control than that seen in dogs in which tumor response to radiation was less favorable (389 versus 161 days).[92] Most of the dogs in that series experienced local progressive disease, which affirms the need for more effective treatment strategies.

The following approaches have been investigated in an attempt to improve local control .

1. Full-course preoperative RT *followed* by surgical exenteration of residual or recurrent disease showed promise in a small series of dogs (n = 13), with a MST of 47 months compared to 19 months for dogs treated with radiation alone (see Table 23-2).[78] The combination treatment was associated with an increased incidence of late effects, including rhinitis (bacterial and fungal), osteomyelitis, and fistula formation.[78] A larger group of dogs must be treated in this manner to confirm these findings.
2. A logical and intuitive approach to improve local control is to increase radiation dose. This has been investigated using a boost technique in one study in which the total radiation dose was escalated to 57 Gy without an increase in overall treatment time. The treatment proved too toxic with respect to acute effects and resulted in radiation-related deaths in one-third of evaluated dogs.[88] It appears that normal tissue tolerance may not allow dose escalation within standard overall treatment times using conventional radiation planning and delivery techniques.
3. The use of radiosensitizers in conjunction with ionizing radiation has been reported. A Veterinary Radiation Therapy Oncology Group (VRTOG) pilot study described the use of gemcitabine as a radiosensitizer for nasosinal carcinoma.[93] Gemcitabine was given intravenously at a dosage of 50 mg/m^2 twice weekly before daily RT. The authors reported significant hematologic toxicity (neutropenia) and local acute tissue complications associated with this dose and schedule. In another report, low-dose cisplatin (7.5 mg/m^2 given intravenously every other day) administered in conjunction with full-course RT was well tolerated and did not appear to cause an increase in acute or late radiation effects.[84] The efficacy of this approach with respect to improvement of clinical outcome is not known. A combination of radiation and cisplatin, administered intramuscularly throughout therapy using a slow-release polymer system (open cell polylactic acid polymer impregnated with platinum [OPLA-Pt]), has been shown to be well tolerated; however, survival times were similar to those in other studies that used RT alone (MST: 474 days).[77]
4. The goal of RT is to deliver the maximum radiation dose to the tumor while limiting the dose to surrounding normal tissues to their tolerance level.[94] Currently, in veterinary medicine, maximally optimized radiation delivery is most widely achieved through the use of conventional computerized treatment planning that allows the use of multiple treatment fields directed at the patient from different angles, with differential weighting of beams, and beam shape modulators to tailor the distribution of radiation dose to each patient as much as possible. Even with the development of more advanced planning systems (i.e., 3-dimensional [3D] versus 2-dimensional [2D]), these conventional methods have limitations that prevent escalation of the radiation dose without also increasing complications.[88]

A potential solution to this challenge is the rapidly emerging technology called intensity-modulated RT (IMRT). IMRT achieves conformal distribution of radiation dose to the tumor while sparing sensitive normal tissues.[79,95-98] Multiple radiation fields of nonuniform beam intensity are delivered with the goal of distributing the radiation dose among larger volumes of normal tissue. This results in modest (tolerable) doses to normal tissues and integration of the multiple beams into a higher total dose throughout the volume of the tumor. IMRT treatment plans are generated by "automated optimization" in which the computer itself determines the optimal nonuniform radiation exposure that must be delivered to give the desired conformal dose pattern.

Through specialized software, the delivery of IMRT is achieved by using a large number of beams of varying radiation intensity that are modulated spatially and temporally.[95] Modulation of beam intensity is realized using a multileaf collimator, which is a collimator that is made of multiple leaves that move rapidly and independently under computer control, customizing beam shape and intensity to the patient. As a result, IMRT has the potential to achieve a much higher degree of target conformity and normal tissue sparing than conventional (2D or 3D conformal) treatment-planning techniques.[79,95-97] The complex shape of nasosinal tumors and the surrounding critical structures, including eyes and brain, provide a strong rationale for application of IMRT with this tumor type. RT-related morbidity can be significantly reduced in dogs with nasosinal tumors when IMRT is used.[79,96] A recent clinical study compared radiation-induced ocular toxicity in dogs with nasal tumors treated with IMRT to that of historical controls treated with conventional 2D RT.[79] IMRT reduced the radiation dose delivered to the eyes and resulted in bilateral ocular sparing. This was in contrast to profound ocular morbidity observed in the historical control group. MSTs for both groups were similar. Paramount to the success of highly conformal RT is precise daily patient positioning.[95] Millimeter variation in patient setup can result in underdosing of the tumor or overdosing of normal tissues. A recent study suggested that daily setup variation associated with conventional nonrigid immobilization techniques used in veterinary RT may be insufficient to ensure high-quality IMRT delivery over a multiple-week course of treatment for nasal tumors.[98] In that study, daily image guidance was necessary to ensure daily setup precision. Rigid immobilization techniques (head and cranial body fixation devices) have been developed for veterinary patients[99-102] and, in conjunction with daily image guidance, permit successful implementation of highly conformal therapy.[98,99] Image-guided RT (IGRT) refers to the use of "on-board" imaging, most commonly CT, integrated into IMRT delivery units. Advanced IGRT systems, such as Varian's

*References 63, 64, 76, 79, 88-91.

Trilogy, Tomotherapy, and CyberKnife, are in use at select veterinary RT facilities,[98,99,103] and availability is growing. IMRT/IGRT provides the theoretical opportunity for tumor dose escalation without increasing the number of radiation treatments and overall treatment time. This in principle could translate into improved tumor control.[97] A newly emerging application of IMRT/IGRT in veterinary medicine is stereotactic RT (SRT). SRT refers to the delivery of high-dose (ablative) radiation in a single dose or a few fractions.[104] The treatment is delivered with extreme accuracy, and the dose is pinpointed to the tumor, minimizing the effect on nearby organs. This technique is optimally suited for small, well-defined tumor targets, although the advancement of radiation delivery technology has allowed for successful application in larger tumors.[104] The high degree of precision is achieved by delivering many (up to hundreds) irregular subfields using specialized software and sophisticated multileaf collimation to create a complex intensity pattern.[104] SRT fractionation schedules usually involve daily treatment for 1 to 3 days, which has obvious practical advantages compared to conventionally fractionated schedules that take weeks to complete. SRT requires highly reproducible patient immobilization, high-fidelity image guidance and an intensity modulated radiation beam to achieve extreme precision.[104] Nasal tumors provide an excellent rationale for use of SRT; however, efficacy with respect to tumor control and survival rates associated with this hypofractionated treatment has not yet been proved. Initial experiences in dogs with nasal tumors include treatment with doses up to 30 Gy delivered in three fractions or in single fraction treatments of up to 15 Gy.[105,106] Toxicity and tumor control data are preliminary but appear favorable.[105,106] Despite the multiple apparent advantages of IMRT and SRT, the high financial costs and logistical challenges associated with optimal use of this technology must be balanced. Controlled clinical trials that rigorously examine normal tissue effects and tumor responses are needed to validate superiority of IMRT/IGRT to conventional RT in veterinary medicine.

In contrast to curative-intent radiation protocols, treatment schedules that are less intensive can be used to palliate tumor-related clinical signs. The goal of palliative radiation is to improve quality of life without aiming to maximize tumor sterilization. Most palliative protocols involve coarse fractionated treatments (6 to 9 Gy) delivered weekly or biweekly.[33,66,80-82] The result of this approach is temporary improvement of clinical signs in 66% to 100% of dogs and limited morbidity associated with acute side effects.[66,80-82] The reported median duration of control of clinical signs ranges from 120 to 300 days.[66,81] Acute toxicities affecting the oral mucosa and skin are generally mild and short lived.[66,80-82] A multiinstitutional retrospective study reported development of chronic ocular toxicities in 13% of 39 dogs that had at least one eye irradiated.[81] Reported MSTs range from 146 days to 300 days.[33,66,80-82] Tumor stage (Adams stage I) and duration of clinical signs (>90 days) have been correlated with longer survival in cases receiving this type of radiation.[66,81] While true statistical comparisons between studies are not possible because of inconsistencies in methodology, the best clinical outcome in terms of duration of resolution of clinical signs and survival (approximately 300 days for both) is reported in a study of 38 dogs in which radiation treatment planning was performed using CT-staging and 3D-conformal computerized treatment planning software.[66] In contrast to other studies, radiation delivery was planned using standardized dose and volume specifications ensuring uniform tumor dose distributions. The authors suggested that sophisticated radiation treatment planning in canine nasal tumor patients treated palliatively may result in more favorable clinical outcomes than previously reported.[66]

A recent report suggested that some dogs with recurrent nasal tumors can experience a second clinical remission following reirradiation of the tumor.[107] The study evaluated a selected cohort of nine dogs in which the median time to tumor progression after a first full course of RT was 513 days. The first course of radiation delivered a median of 50 Gy in a median of 18 fractions. The median total dose used in the second protocol was 36 Gy, delivered in approximately 2-Gy fractions. The overall MST for this small, selection-biased cohort of dogs was 927 days (95% confidence interval [CI] 423 days to 1767 days). All dogs developed one or more late effects involving the skin, eyes, and nasal cavity. Late effects in seven of the nine dogs were considered mild and did not affect quality of life. Severe late effects were reported in two dogs, and both had sudden blindness that led to euthanasia. The authors concluded that there is a population of canine nasal tumor patients (i.e., those with slowly progressive tumors) that will benefit from reirradiation. Further work is needed to refine time-dose prescriptions to minimize radiation-induced late effects. Conformal techniques such as IMRT could play a role in this setting to limit morbidity.

Chemotherapy is used rarely as a sole therapy for canine nasosinal tumors. Treatment with cisplatin alone has been shown to benefit some dogs.[108] A clinical response rate of 27%, including one radiographically confirmed complete remission, was reported in a small series of 11 dogs.[108] All of the dogs experienced alleviation of clinical signs, and the MST was 5 months. Another report evaluated a combination chemotherapy protocol of doxorubicin, carboplatin, and oral piroxicam in eight dogs with advanced nasal tumors.[109] A clinical response rate of 75% was observed, including 4 CRs confirmed by CT imaging. All dogs experienced resolution of clinical signs, and the protocol was well tolerated. MST in these eight dogs was 210 days (range 150 days to 960 days). These preliminary results are favorable, but the case number is small and more dogs need to be treated in this manner to confirm these findings.

Other therapeutic approaches to nasal tumors that have been investigated include proton-beam therapy, brachytherapy, immunotherapy, cryotherapy, and photodynamic therapy (PDT). Charged particles like protons have a well-defined tissue range and sharp dose fall off, which could potentially be exploited for conformal tumor targeting and normal tissue sparing.[110] A small clinical trial involving nine dogs with nasal tumors treated with proton-beam therapy resulted in tumor responses and survival times similar to those reported for MeV irradiation.[110] Acute effects of the skin and eyes were pronounced in some dogs, and 50% of dogs developed radiation-induced cataracts. Due to limited availability of proton irradiators, this technology is unlikely to be optimized for use in dogs. Intracavitary radiation using radioactive isotopes (brachytherapy) has been evaluated after surgical removal of nasosinal tumors in dogs.[111,112] Potential problems associated with this type of radiation include dose distribution and radiation exposure to personnel. The question of whether brachytherapy improves survival over traditional external-beam radiation has not been answered. Immunotherapy and cryosurgery have not improved survival times.[1,113] A recent case report described the use of image-guided cryotherapy in the treatment of a rapidly recurrent nasal carcinoma that resulted in long-term tumor control and survival.[114] The authors suggested that further investigation of this technique may be warranted for the management of focal residual or recurrent nasal tumors. Reports evaluating PDT have been published; however, results are too preliminary to draw any conclusions.[115,116]

When all treatments fail to control epistaxis, unilateral or bilateral carotid artery ligation can palliate the symptoms in dogs for up to 3 months or longer without damage to the brain.[58]

The importance of prognostic factors in the treatment of canine nasosinal tumors remains controversial. Negative predictors of survival from various studies include age (>10 years),[68] epistaxis,[38] duration of clinical signs,[81] advanced local tumor stage,[63-66,68] metastatic disease,[10,68] histologic subtype (carcinoma, particularly squamous cell or undifferentiated),[63,65,74] and failure to achieve resolution of clinical signs.[81] An analysis of 94 dogs with varying subtypes of nasal carcinoma or sarcoma treated with curative RT at three veterinary facilities was recently performed.[65] A correlation was demonstrated between clinical outcome and the original Adams tumor staging scheme,[64] as well as the modified Adams tumor system.[65] Based on these findings, dogs with cribriform plate involvement as determined by CT imaging have the shortest disease-free survival (DFS) and overall survival (OS). This subset of dogs had a median DFS of 3.8 months and a median OS of almost 7 months, compared to dogs with unilateral tumors without bone involvement in which DFS and OS were 6.5 and 23 months, respectively. The study also showed that prognosis varied based on histologic category. When grouped together, dogs with anaplastic carcinoma, undifferentiated carcinoma, and SCC had a shorter DFS. There was no effect on clinical outcome when all carcinomas were compared with all sarcomas. The statistically strongest association with clinical outcome was made when clinical stage was combined with histologic findings.

A major pitfall of many veterinary studies with respect to assessment of treatment efficacy in canine nasosinal cancer is the evaluable endpoint. Tumor response and time to tumor progression are the most representative measures of treatment efficacy. Regular diagnostic imaging, ideally CT or MRI, would be required to allow accurate determination of these endpoints. Due to high costs associated with imaging and the need for anesthesia, follow-up is rarely done in this manner. Analyzing the return of clinical signs as an indication of tumor recurrence is problematic since similar signs can result from rhinitis secondary to therapy (radiation and/or surgery) or residual tumor.[117] Assessment of the survival time, as is commonly done in most veterinary nasosinal cancer studies, may be biased by the use of additional treatments on suspicion of progressive disease and by the decision for euthanasia, which can vary greatly from one pet owner to another. Furthermore, inconsistencies in methodology between studies and even within individual reports, as well as lack of controlled studies, are other limitations that have prevented the informed development of the optimal treatment approach to nasosinal tumors in dogs.

Feline Nasosinal Tumors

Nasal and sinus cavity tumors in the cat are malignant in more than 90% of the histologically diagnosed cases. They occur in an older population of cats with a mean age reported between 9 and 10 years.[118-120] In general, these tumors are locally invasive and associated with a low metastatic rate at the time of diagnosis.[119,121]

Clinical signs related to nasosinal tumors in cats overlap with those of other causes of chronic nasal disease.[118,120] These include nasal discharge, upper respiratory tract dyspnea, sneezing, epistaxis, facial swelling, ocular discharge, and weight loss.[118-120,122-124] Although each of these signs can occur with both neoplasia and rhinitis, in some reports, certain signs are more commonly associated with neoplasia such as unilateral discharge or epistaxis,[118] whereas in others, the character of the clinical signs does not distinguish the underlying cause.[120] The median duration of clinical signs prior to diagnosis is several months, and many cats will experience temporary alleviation of clinical signs with use of antibiotics and or glucocorticosteroids.[118-120] Differential diagnoses for chronic nasal signs include chronic rhinitis, infectious rhinitis, foreign body, nasal polyp, nasopharyngeal stenosis, and trauma.

Lymphoma is the most commonly diagnosed tumor type in the feline nasal cavity and sinuses followed by epithelial neoplasms (carcinoma, adenocarcinoma, SCC). Less frequently reported tumor types include sarcomas (fibrosarcoma, osteosarcoma, chondrosarcoma), mast cell tumor, melanoma, plasmacytoma, olfactory neuroblastoma, and benign lesions such as nasal hamartoma, chondroma, and neurofibroma.[118-120,125,126]

Diagnostic principles are similar to those in the dog. A tissue sample is required to make a definitive diagnosis of cancer in most cases. DeLorenzi et al evaluated cytology from squash preparations obtained from endoscopic biopsies of nasopharyngeal masses in cats and found that cytologic results were in good agreement with histopathology with an overall accuracy of 90%.[127] However, distinguishing lymphoma from lymphoid inflammatory disease was not as accurate and histopathologic confirmation was recommended.[127] Another study evaluated the histopathologic and cytologic features of nasal lymphoma in 50 cases. These authors found that 91% of cases were classified as immunoblastic lymphoma according to the National Institutes of Health (NIH) working formulation. The majority of cases were B-cell (68%) and 20% were T-cell, with 12% having a mixed population of B- and T-cells.[125]

Radiographs of the nasal cavity have been reported as a diagnostic tool in cats with both chronic rhinitis and nasal neoplasia. Although no radiographic sign is entirely specific for neoplasia, findings with the highest predictive value for cancer include displacement of midline structures, unilateral changes such as soft tissue opacity and loss of turbinate detail, and evidence of bone invasion.[128] Similarly, as CT scan becomes a common imaging tool, reports of the characteristic findings of scans from cats with sinonasal disease of all etiologies have been published.[129-131] One retrospective assessment of CT imaging in 62 cats with nasosinal disease showed that, although certain findings such as osteolysis of paranasal bones, extension of disease into the orbit of facial soft tissues, the presence of a space-occupying mass, and turbinate destruction may suggest a CT diagnosis of neoplasia over rhinitis, nasal biopsy is necessary for confirmation.[129] Another study evaluated the clinical characteristics and CT findings in 43 cats and found that those with neoplasia were significantly more likely to have unilateral lysis of the ethmoturbinates as well as dorsal and lateral maxilla, lysis of the vomer bone and ventral maxilla, and unilateral soft tissue or fluid in the sphenoid recess, frontal sinus, or retrobulbar space. Interestingly, in that study population, cribriform plate lysis was not significantly associated with neoplasia.[130] In another report describing CT findings in cats with confirmed fungal rhinitis, they found that some of the features overlap with those seen in neoplasia patients, including older age at the time of diagnosis, soft tissue mass, and osteolysis. Although these studies confirm the utility of CT scan determining extent of disease, no one group of features replaces histopathology for definitive diagnosis.

Even though the metastatic rate of feline nasosinal cancer at the time of diagnosis is reportedly low, any enlarged regional lymph nodes should be evaluated cytologically to differentiate a reactive process from metastasis. In a recent report of 123 cases of feline nasosinal cancer, 21 cats had regional lymphadenopathy. None showed cytologic evidence of metastasis.[119]

As in the dog, RT continues to be the predominant local therapy of choice for this disease. Reports of treatment for feline nonlymphoma nasosinal tumors are few, and case numbers are small.[121,132] In the largest published study, 16 cats with nonlymphoproliferative

TABLE 23-4 Summary of Selected Reports Describing Clinical Outcomes for Nasosinal Tumors in Cats

	TAYLOR ET AL[122]	HANEY ET AL[124]	SFILIGOI ET AL[123]
Number of cats	69, stage unknown	97, stage 1 disease	19, stage 1 disease
Treatment			
Chemotherapy	69	18	NA
Chemotherapy protocol	COP	Multiagent	
Radiation	NA	19	NA
Total dose		Median 32, Gy range 10-57	
Both	NA	60	19
Total RT dose (Gy)		Median 30 (range 15-48)	Median 42 (range 22-48)
Chemotherapy		Multiagent	Multiagent
Response			
OOR	93%	70%	89%
CR/PR	73%/20%	53%/18%	NR
Survival			
Median (days)		172	
RT		456	
Chemotherapy	140	117	
Both		174	955
If CR achieved	749	536	NR
If PR achieved	54	120	NR
Distant disease at time of death	NR	10/79 (13%)	3/19 (16%)
Prognostic indicators/ conclusions	Chemotherapy is effective for nasal LSA, and cats achieving a complete remission have a significantly longer survival.	Histopathologic grade, cribriform lysis, and treatment type did not significantly impact survival. Total RT dose >32 Gy improved survival; achieving CR improved survival.	Cribriform plate destruction negatively influenced survival; distant disease still occurs in a small number of patients.

NA, Not applicable; *COP,* cytoxan, oncovin, prednisone; *RT,* radiation therapy; *OOR,* overall response, *CR,* complete response, *PR,* partial response, *NR,* not reported; *LSA,* lymphosarcoma.

neoplasms were treated using a definitive course of radiation to a total dose of 48 Gy. The therapy was well tolerated, and MST was 12 months with 44% and 16% of cats alive at 1 and 2 years, respectively.[121] In another report of radiation treatment for nonlymphoproliferative tumors, this time treated using a coarse fractionation regime, results showed that the protocol was well tolerated, with a median survival of almost 13 months and a 63% 1-year survival rate reported.[132]

Recent reports of feline nasal and nasal pharyngeal lymphoma treated with radiation and/or chemotherapy indicate the potential for long-term survival (Table 23-4).[122-125,133] Although treatment protocols vary between reports, in general, overall response rate for feline nasal lymphoma is high, between 70% and 90%. The inclusion of RT appears to enhance overall survival with median survival for combination therapy ranging from 174 to 955 days.[123,124] Interestingly, systemic failure of disease at nonnasal sites is also reported in 13% to 16% of cases, indicating that a combination of RT and chemotherapy may be warranted in some patients. However, the timing of such treatment remains to be determined (concurrent versus sequential), as does which patients are at highest risk for local failure. Furthermore, improved radiation treatment planning along with optimized radiation treatment schedules and doses may prove to ameliorate local control rates and reduce the risk of systemic failure without the addition of chemotherapy.

Comparative Aspects[134]

In humans, cancer of the nasal cavity and paranasal sinuses is classified with other cancers of the upper aerodigestive tract under the all-encompassing title, tumors of the head and neck. Tumors of four anatomically defined regions are included: nasal cavity and paranasal sinuses, nasopharynx, oral cavity, and oropharynx. The majority of tumors affecting these sites are SCCs (head and neck SCC [HNSCC]). However, a large variety of histologically distinct cancers can develop in the nasal cavity and paranasal sinuses, including adenocarcinoma, esthesioneuroblastoma, lymphoma, melanoma, angiosarcoma, and tumors of connective tissues.

Tumors specifically of the nasal cavity and paranasal sinuses are rare in humans and represent the smallest proportion of head and neck cancers, with a yearly risk of 1 in every 100,000 people. They generally affect persons between the ages of 45 and 85 years old and are twice as common in males as females. The etiologic factors for the disease are predominantly environmental and workplace in nature and include exposure to wood, textile, and leather dusts, as well as flour, nickel, chromium, and radium. Other factors associated with increased risk for all head and neck cancers include smoking and alcohol use, which may have an additive effect.

Tumors at this site are locally invasive. They are typically advanced at the time of diagnosis because lesions in this area can go undetected for extended periods of time and clinical signs can mimic those of infectious or inflammatory disease. The likelihood of lymph node metastasis at the time of diagnosis is low—reportedly between 10% and 15%, depending on the location of the primary tumor.

Surgery and RT are the mainstay of curative treatment when considered possible, based on stage and location of disease. Chemotherapy can be useful in an adjuvant setting, but it is not curative when used alone. Both radiation and surgery have advantages and disadvantages as primary therapies. Overall, survival at 5 years is approximately 60% and 30% for nasal cavity and parasinal tumors, respectively. More favorable prognoses are associated with smaller lesions in which complete surgical resection is achievable. The main form of treatment failure is local recurrence, which is caused by incomplete local control of advanced tumors in many cases. When adequate margins cannot be obtained, surgery and radiation are often combined.

The role of chemotherapy in cancer of the nasal cavity and paranasal sinuses is not clear because these cases are usually reported in conjunction with other head and neck tumors. Active chemotherapy agents include the taxanes, 5-fluorouracil (5-FU), and the platinum drugs. Several studies have reported improved local control and, in some cases, improved overall survival in treatment protocols that combine traditional fractionated radiation and chemotherapy; however, the toxicity may also be increased. The optimal case selection, chemotherapy agents, and radiation schedule has yet to be defined.

Clinical trials of targeted therapies for head and neck cancer have been done and most involve EGFR antagonists. Cetuximab (Erbitux), a chimeric (mouse/human) monoclonal antibody against EGFR, has been shown to improve locoregional control and survival when used as a radiation sensitizer in people with HNSCC undergoing RT with curative intent. It has been approved by the Food and Drug Administration (FDA) for this indication, as well as for use as a single agent in patients whose cancer has progressed on platinum-containing therapy. Positive results associated with cetuximab have had a significant impact on the standard of care for advanced HNSCC. The subset of patients who might benefit from these types of treatments will need to be identified in order to maximize their use and improve outcome for this disease.

REFERENCES

1. MacEwen EG, Withrow SJ, Patnaik AK: Nasal tumors in the dog: retrospective evaluation of diagnosis, prognosis, and treatment, *J Am Vet Med Assoc* 170:45–48, 1977.
2. Patnaik AK: Canine sinonasal neoplasms: Clinicopathological study of 285 cases, *J Am Anim Hosp Assoc* 25:103–114, 1989.
3. Lefebvre J, Kuehn NJ, Wortinger A: Computed tomography as an aid in the diagnosis of chronic nasal disease in dogs, *J Small Anim Pract* 46:280–285, 2005.
4. Strunzi H, Hauser B: Tumors of the nasal cavity, *Bull World Health Organ* 53:257–263, 1976.
5. Reif JS, Cohen D: The environmental distribution of canine respiratory tract neoplasms, *Arch Environ Health* 22:136–140, 1971.
6. Bukowski JA, Wartenberg D: Environmental causes for sinonasal cancers in pet dogs, and their usefulness as sentinels of indoor cancer risk, *J Toxicol Environ Health* 54:579–591, 1998.
7. Reif JS, Bruns C, Lower KS: Cancer of the nasal cavity and paranasal sinuses and exposure to environmental tobacco smoke in pet dogs, *Am J Epidemiol* 147:488–492, 1998.
8. Madewell BR, Priester WA, Gillette EL, et al: Neoplasms of the nasal passages and paranasal sinuses in domesticated animals as reported by 13 veterinary colleges, *Am J Vet Res* 851–856, 1976.
9. Patnaik AK, Lieberman PH, Erlandson RA, et al: Canine sinonasal skeletal neoplasms: Chondrosarcomas and osteosarcomas, *Vet Pathol* 21:475–482, 1984.
10. Henry CJ, Brewer WG, Tyler JW, et al: Survival in dogs with nasal adenocarcinoma: 64 cases (1981-1995), *J Vet Intern Med* 12:436–439, 1998.
11. Hahn KA, Matlock CL: Nasal adenocarcinoma metastatic to bone in two dogs, *J Am Vet Med Assoc* 197(4):491–494, 1990.
12. Hahn KA, McGavin MD, Adams WH: Bilateral renal metastases of nasal chondrosarcoma in a dog, *Vet Pathol* 34:352–355, 1997.
13. Northrup NC, Etue SM, Ruslander DM, et al: Retrospective study of orthovoltage radiation therapy for nasal tumors in 42 dogs, *J Vet Intern Med* 15:183–189, 2001.
14. Snyder MK, Lipitz L, Skorupski KA et al: Secondary intracranial neoplasia in the dog: 177 cases (1986-2003), *J Vet Intern Med* 22:172–177, 2008.
15. Kaldrymidou E, Papaioannou N, Poutahidis T, et al: Malignant lymphoma in nasal cavity and paranasal sinuses of a dog, *J Vet Med A Physiol Pathol Clin Med* 47(8):457–462, 2000.
16. Naganobu K, Ogawa H, Uchida K, et al: Mast cell tumor in the nasal cavity of a dog, *J Vet Med Sci* 62(9):1009–1011, 2000.
17. Weir EC, Pond MJ, Duncan JR, et al: Extragenital occurrence of transmissible venereal tumor in the dog: literature review and case reports, *J Am Anim Hosp Assoc* 14:532–536, 1978.
18. Perez J, Bautista MJ, Carrasco L, et al: Primary extragenital occurrence of transmissible venereal tumors: three case reports, *Can Pract* 19(1):7–10, 1994.
19. Ginel PJ, Molleda JM, Novales M, et al: Primary transmissible venereal tumour in the nasal cavity of a dog, *Vet Rec* 136:222–223, 1995.
20. Papzoglou LG, Koutinas AF, Plevraki AG, et al: Primary intranasal transmissible venereal tumour in the dog: a retrospective study of six spontaneous cases, *J Vet Med A Physiol Pathol Clin Med* 48(7):391–400, 2001.
21. Patnaik AK: Canine sinonasal neoplasms: soft tissue tumors, *J Am Anim Hosp Assoc* 25:491–497, 1989.
22. Patnaik AK, Ludwig LL, Erlandson RA: Neuroendocrine carcinoma of the nasopharynx in a dog, *Vet Pathol* 39:496–500, 2002.
23. Miles MS, Dhaliwal RS, Moore MP, et al: Association of magnetic resonance imaging findings and histologic diagnosis in dogs with nasal disease: 78 cases (2001-2004), *J Am Vet Med Assoc* 232:1844–1849, 2008.
24. Hicks DG, Fidel JL: Intranasal malignant melanoma in a dog, *J Am Anim Hosp Assoc* 42:472–476, 2006.
25. Ueno H, Kobayashi Y, Yamada K: Olfactory esthesioneuroblastoma treated with orthovoltage radiotherapy in a dog, *Aust Vet J* 85:271–275, 2007.
26. Kitagawa M, Okada M, Yamamura H, et al: Diagnosis of olfactory neuroblastoma in a dog by magnetic resonance imaging, *Vet Rec* 159:288–289, 2006.
27. LeRoith T, Binder EM, Graham AH, et al: Respiratory epithelial adenomatoid hamartoma in a dog, *J Vet Diagn Invest* 21:918–920, 2009.
28. Fujita M, Takaishi Y, Yasuda D, et al: Intranasal hemangiosarcoma in a dog, *J Vet Med Sci* 70:525–528, 2008.
29. Gamblin FM, Sagartz JE, Guillermo C: Overexpression of p53 tumor suppressor protein in spontaneously arising neoplasms of dogs, *Am J Vet Res* 58(8):857–863, 1997.
30. Kleiter MK, Malarkey DE, Ruslander DE, et al: Expression of cyclooxygenase-2 in canine epithelial nasal tumors, *Vet Radiol Ultrasound* 45(3):255–260, 2004.

31. Borzacchiello G, Paciello O, Papparella S: Expression of cyclooxygenase-1 and -2 in canine nasal carcinomas, *J Comp Pathol* 131(1):70–76, 2004.
32. Impellizeri JA, Esplin DG: Expression of cyclooxygenase-2 in canine nasal carcinomas, *Vet J* 176:408–410, 2008.
33. Belshaw Z, Constantio-Casas F, Brearley MJ, et al: COX-2 expression and outcome in canine nasal carcinomas treated with hypofractionated radiotherapy, *Vet Comp Oncol* 9:141–148, 2010.
34. Shiomitsu K, Johnson CL, Malarkey DE, et al: Expression of epidermal growth factor receptor and vascular endothelial growth factor in malignant canine epithelial nasal tumours, *Vet Comp Oncol* 7:106–114, 2009.
35. Paciello O, Borzacchiello G, Varricchio E, et al: Expression of peroxisome proliferator-activated receptor gamma (PPAR-γ) in canine nasal carcinomas, *J Vet Med A Physiol Pathol Clin Med* 54:406–410, 2007.
36. Vanherberghen M, Day MJ, Delvaux F, et al: An Immunohistochemical study of the inflammatory infiltrate associated with nasal carcinoma in dogs and cats, *J Comp Pathol* 141:17–26, 2009.
37. Nakaichi M, Yunuki T, Okuda M, et al: Activity of matrix metalloproteinase-2 (MMP-2) in canine oronasal tumors, *Res Vet Sci* 82:271–279, 2007.
38. Rassnick KM, Goldkamp CE, Erb HN, et al: Evaluation of factors associated with survival in dogs with untreated nasal carcinomas: 139 cases (1993-2003), *J Am Vet Med Assoc* 229:401–406, 2006.
39. Saunders JH, Van Bree H, Gielen I, et al: Diagnostic value of computed tomography in dogs with chronic nasal disease, *Vet Radiol Ultrasound* 44(4):409–413, 2003.
40. Burrow RD: A nasal dermoid sinus in an English bull terrier, *J Small Anim Pract* 45(11):572–574, 2004.
41. Beck JA, Hunt GB, Goldsmid SE, et al: Nasopharyngeal obstruction due to cystic Rathke's clefts in two dogs, *Aust Vet J* 77:94–96, 1999.
42. Lobetti RG: A retrospective study of chronic nasal disease in 75 dogs, *J S Afr Vet Assoc* 80:224–228, 2009.
43. Strasser JL, Hawkins EC: Clinical features of epistaxis in dogs: a retrospective study of 35 cases (1999-2002), *J Am Anim Hosp Assoc* 41:179–184, 2005.
44. Bissett SA, Drobatz KJ, McKnight A, et al: Prevalence, clinical features, and causes of epistaxis in dogs: 176 cases (1996-2001), *J Am Vet Med Assoc* 231:1843–1850, 2007.
45. Smith MO, Turrel JM, Bailey CS, et al: Neurologic abnormalities as the predominant signs of neoplasia of the nasal cavity in dogs and cats: Seven cases (1973-1986), *J Am Vet Med Assoc* 195:242–245, 1989.
46. Thrall DE, Robertson ID, McLeod DA, et al: A comparison of radiographic and computed tomographic findings in 31 dogs with malignant nasal cavity tumors, *Vet Radiol* 30:59–66, 1989.
47. Park RD, Beck ER, LeCouteur RA: Comparison of computed tomography and radiography for detecting changes induced by malignant nasal neoplasia in dogs, *J Am Vet Med Assoc* 201:1720–1724, 1992.
48. Codner EC, Lurus AG, Miller JB, et al: Comparison of computed tomography with radiography as a noninvasive diagnostic technique for chronic nasal disease in dogs, *J Am Vet Med Assoc* 202:1106–1110, 1993.
49. Drees R, Forrest LJ, Chappell R: Comparison of computed tomography and magnetic resonance imaging for the evaluation of canine intranasal neoplasia, *J Small Anim Pract* 50:334–340, 2009.
50. Avner A, Dobson JM, Sales JI, et al: Retrospective review of 50 canine nasal tumours evaluated by low-field magnetic resonance imaging, *J Small Anim Pract* 49:233–239, 2008.
51. Agthe P, Caine AR, Gear RNA, et al: Prognostic significance of specific magnetic resonance imaging features in canine nasal tumours treated by radiotherapy, *J Small Anim Pract* 50:641–648, 2009.
52. Petite AFB, Dennis R: Comparison of radiography and magnetic resonance imaging for evaluating the extent of nasal neoplasia in dogs, *J Small Anim Pract* 47:529–536, 2006.
53. Burk RL: Computed tomographic imaging of nasal disease in 100 dogs., *Vet Radiol Ultrasound* 33(3):177–180, 1992.
54. Gibbs C, Lane JG, Denny HR: Radiological features of intra-nasal lesions in the dog: A review of 100 cases, *J Small Anim Pract* 20:515–535, 1979.
55. Russo M, Lamb CR, Jakovljevic S: Distinguishing rhinitis and nasal neoplasia by radiography, *Vet Radiol Ultrasound* 41(2):118–124, 2000.
56. Forrest LJ, Thrall DE: Oncologic applications of diagnostic imaging techniques, *Vet Clin North Am Small Anim Pract* 25(1):185–205, 1995.
57. Withrow SJ, Susaneck SJ, Macy DW, et al: Aspiration and punch biopsy techniques for nasal tumors, *J Am Anim Hosp Assoc* 21:551–554, 1985.
58. Rudd RG, Richardson DC: A diagnostic and therapeutic approach to nasal disease in dogs, *Compend Contin Educ Pract Vet* 7:103–112, 1985.
59. Clendenin MA, Conrad MC: Collateral vessel development after chronic bilateral common carotid artery occlusion in the dog, *Am J Vet Res* 40:1244, 1979.
60. Clercx C, Wallon J, Gilbert S, et al: Imprint and brush cytology in the diagnosis of canine intranasal tumours, *J Small Anim Pract* 37:423–427, 1996.
61. Lent SEF, Hawkins EC: Evaluation of rhinoscopy and rhinoscopy-assisted mucosal biopsy in diagnosis of nasal disease in dogs: 199 cases (1985-1989), *J Am Vet Med Assoc* 201:1425–1429, 1992.
62. Owen LN: *TNM Classification of tumors in domestic animals*, Geneva, 1980, World Health Organization.
63. Theon AP, Madewell BR, Harb MF, et al: Megavoltage irradiation of neoplasms of the nasal and paranasal cavities in 77 dogs, *J Am Vet Med Assoc* 202:1469–1475, 1993.
64. Adams WM, Miller PE, Vail DM, et al: An accelerated technique for irradiation of malignant canine nasal and paranasal sinus tumors, *Vet Radiol Ultrasound* 39:475–481, 1998.
65. Adams WM, Kleiter MM, Thrall DE, et al: Prognostic significance of tumor histology and computed tomographic staging for radiation treatment response of canine nasal tumors, *Vet Radiol Ultrasound* 50:330–335, 2009.
66. Buchholz J, Hagen R, Leo C, et al: 3D conformal radiation therapy for palliative treatment of canine nasal tumors, *Vet Radiol Ultrasound* 50:679–683, 2009.
67. Kondo Y, Matsunaga S, Mochizuki M, et al: Prognosis of canine patients with nasal tumors according to modified clinical stages based on computed tomography: a retrospective study, *J Vet Med Sci* 70:207–212, 2008.
68. LaDue TA, Dodge R, Page RL, et al: Factors influencing survival after radiotherapy of nasal tumors in 130 dogs, *Vet Radiol Ultrasound* 40:312–317, 1999.
69. Couto CF, Boudrieau RJ, Zanjani ED: Tumor-associated erythrocytosis in a dog with nasal fibrosarcoma, *J Vet Intern Med* 3:183–185, 1989.
70. Wilson RB, Bronstad DC: Hypercalcemia associated with nasal adenocarcinoma in a dog, *J Am Vet Med Assoc* 182:1246–1247, 1983.
71. Anderson GM, Lane I, Fischer J, et al: Hypercalcemia and parathyroid hormone-related protein in a dog with undifferentiated nasal carcinoma, *Can Vet J* 40:341–342, 1999.
72. Laing EJ, Binnington AG: Surgical therapy of canine nasal tumors: a retrospective study (1982-1986), *Can Vet J* 29:809–813, 1988.
73. Holmberg DL, Fries C, Cockshutt J, et al: Ventral rhinotomy in the dog and cat, *Vet Surg* 18:446–449, 1989.
74. Adams WM, Withrow SJ, Walshaw R, et al: Radiotherapy of malignant nasal tumors in 67 dogs, *J Am Vet Med Assoc* 191:311–315, 1987.
75. Evans SM, Goldschmidt M, McKee LJ, et al: Prognostic factors and survival after radiotherapy for intranasal neoplasms in dogs: 70 cases (1974-1985), *J Am Vet Med Assoc* 194:1460–1463, 1989.

76. McEntee MC, Page RL, Heidner GL, et al: A retrospective study of 27 dogs with intranasal neoplasms treated with cobalt radiation, *Vet Radiol Ultrasound* 32:135–139, 1991.
77. Lana SE, Dernell WS, Lafferty MS, et al: Use of radiation and a slow-release cisplatin formulation for treatment of canine nasal tumors, *Vet Radiol Ultrasound* 45:1–5, 2004.
78. Adams WM, Bjorling DE, McAnulty JF, et al: Outcome of accelerated radiotherapy alone or accelerated radiotherapy followed by exenteration of the nasal cavity in dogs with intranasal neoplasia: 53 cases (1993-2002), *J Am Vet Med Assoc* 227:936–941, 2005.
79. Lawrence JA, Forrest LJ, Turek MM, et al: Proof of principle of ocular sparing in dogs with sinonasal tumors treated with intensity-modulated radiation therapy, *Vet Radiol Ultrasound* 51:561–570, 2010.
80. Mellanby RJ, Stevenson RK, Herrtage ME, et al: Long-term outcome of 56 dogs with nasal tumours treated with four doses of radiation at intervals of seven days, *Vet Rec* 151:253–257, 2002.
81. Geiger T, Rassnick K, Siegel S, et al: Palliation of clinical signs in 48 dogs with nasal carcinomas treated with coarse-fraction radiation therapy, *J Am Anim Hosp Assoc* 44:116–123, 2008.
82. Maruo T, Shida T, Fukuyama Y, et al: Retrospective study of canine nasal tumor treated with hypofractionated radiotherapy, *J Vet Med Sci* 73:193–197, 2011.
83. Morris JS, Dunn KJ, Dobson JM, et al: Effects of radiotherapy alone and surgery and radiotherapy on survival of dogs with nasal tumours, *J Small Anim Pract* 35:567–573, 1994.
84. Nadeau M, Kitchell BE, Rooks RL, et al: Cobalt radiation with or without low-dose cisplatin for treatment of canine naso-sinus carcinomas, *Vet Radiol Ultrasound* 45(4):362–367, 2004.
85. Yoon JH, Feeney DA, Jessen CR, et al: External-beam Co-60 radiotherapy for canine nasal tumors: a comparison of survival by treatment protocol, *Res Vet Sci* 84:140–149, 2008.
86. Hunley DW, Mauldin GN, Shiomitsu K, et al: Clinical outcome in dogs with nasal tumors treated with intensity-modulated radiation therapy, *Can Vet J* 51:293–300, 2010.
87. Hall EJ, Giaccia AJ: Time, dose, and fractionation in radiotherapy. In Hall EJ, et al, editors: *Radiobiology for the radiologist*, ed 6, Philadelphia, 2006, Lippincott Williams & Wilkins.
88. Thrall DE, McEntee MC, Novotney C: A boost technique for irradiation of malignant canine nasal tumors, *Vet Radiol Ultrasound* 34(4):295–300, 1993.
89. Jamieson VE, Davidson MG, Nasisse MP, et al: Ocular complications following cobalt 60 radiotherapy of neoplasms in the canine head region, *J Am Anim Hosp Assoc* 27:51–55, 1991.
90. Ching SV, Gillette SM, Powers BE, et al: Radiation-induced ocular injury in the dog: a histological study, *Int J Radiation Oncology Biol Phys* 19:321–328, 1990.
91. Roberts SM, Lavach JD, Severin GA, et al: Ophthalmic complications following megavoltage irradiation of the nasal and paranasal cavities in dogs, *J Am Vet Med Assoc* 100:43–47, 1987.
92. Thrall DE, Heidner GL, Novotny CA, et al: Failure patterns following cobalt irradiation in dogs with nasal carcinoma, *Vet Radiol Ultrasound* 34(2):126–133, 1993.
93. LeBlanc AK, LaDue TA, Turrel JM, et al: Unexpected toxicity following use of gemcitabine as a radiosensitizer in head and neck carcinomas: a veterinary radiation therapy oncology group pilot study, *Vet Radiol Ultrasound* 45(5):466–470, 2004.
94. McEntee MC: Veterinary radiation therapy: Review and current state of the art, *J Am Anim Hosp Assoc* 42:94–109, 2006.
95. Hong TS, Ritter MA, Tome WA, et al: Intensity-modulated radiation therapy: emerging cancer treatment technology, *Br J Cancer* 92:1819–1824, 2005.
96. Vaudaux C, Schneider U, Kaser-Hotz B: Potential for intensity-modulated radiation therapy to permit dose escalation for canine nasal cancer, *Vet Radiol Ultrasound* 48:475–481, 2007.
97. Guttierrez AN, Deveau M, Forrest LJ, et al: Radiobiological and treatment planning study of a simultaneously integrated boost for canine nasal tumors using helical tomotherapy, *Vet Radiol Ultrasound* 48:594–602, 2007.
98. Deveau MA, Gutierrez AN, Mackie TR, et al: Dosimetric impact of daily setup variations during treatment of canine nasal tumors using intensity-modulated radiation therapy, *Vet Radiol Ultrasound* 51:90–96, 2010.
99. Harmon J, Van Ufflen D, LaRue S: Assessment of a radiotherapy patient cranial immobilization device using daily on-board kilovoltage imaging, *Vet Radiol Ultrasound* 50:230–234, 2009.
100. Rohrer Bley C, Blattmann H, Roos M, et al: Assessment of a radiotherapy patient immobilization device using single plane port radiographs and a remote computed tomography scanner, *Vet Radiol Ultrasound* 44:470–475, 2003.
101. Kippenes H, Gavin PR, Sande RD, et al: Comparison of the accuracy of positioning devices for radiation therapy of canine and feline head tumors, *Vet Radiol Ultrasound* 41:371–376, 2000.
102. Kent MS, Gordon IK, Benavides I, et al: Assessment of the accuracy and precision of a patient immobilization device for radiation therapy in canine head and neck tumors, *Vet Radiol Ultrasound* 50:550–554, 2009.
103. Forrest LJ, Mackie TR, Ruchala K, et al: The utility of megavoltage computed tomography images from a helical tomotherapy system for setup verification purposes, *Int J Radiat Oncol Biol Phys* 60:1639–1644, 2004.
104. Martin A, Gaya A: Stereotactic body radiotherapy: A review, *Clin Oncol* 22:157–172, 2010.
105. Personal Communication: Custis J, Harmon J, Ryan S, et al: Stereotactic radiation therapy for the treatment of canine nasal tumors, *Vet Cancer Soc Proc* 30:46, 2010.
106. Personal Communication: Charney S, Witten M, Ettinger S, et al: Cyber knife radiosurgery for irradiation of tumors in dogs and cats, *Vet Cancer Soc Proc* 30:97, 2010.
107. Bommarito DA, Kent MS, Selting KA, et al: Reirradiation of recurrent canine nasal tumors, *Vet Radiol Ultrasound* 52:207–212, 2011.
108. Hahn KA, Knapp DW, Richardson RC, et al: Clinical response of nasal adenocarcinoma to cisplatin chemotherapy in 11 dogs, *J Am Vet Med Assoc* 200:355–357, 1992.
109. Langova V, Mutsaers AJ, Phillips B, et al: Treatment of eight dogs with nasal tumours with alternating doses of doxorubicin and carboplatin in conjunction with oral piroxicam, *Aust Vet J* 82:676–680, 2004.
110. Mayer-Stankeova S, Fidel J, Wergin MC, et al: Proton spot scanning radiotherapy of spontaneous canine tumors, *Vet Radiol Ultrasound* 50:314–318, 2009.
111. White R, Walker M, Legendre AM, et al: Development of brachytherapy technique for nasal tumors in dogs, *Am J Vet Res* 51:1250–1256, 1990.
112. Thompson JP, Ackerman N, Bellah JR, et al: 192Iridium brachytherapy, using an intracavitary afterload device, for treatment of intranasal neoplasms in dogs, *Am J Vet Res* 53:617–622, 1992.
113. Withrow SJ: Cryosurgical therapy for nasal tumors in the dog, *J Am Anim Hosp Assoc* 18:585–589, 1982.
114. Murphy SM, Lawrence JA, Schmiedt CW, et al: Image-guide transnasal cryoablation of a recurrent nasal adenocarcinoma in a dog, *J Small Anim Pract* 52:329–333, 2011.
115. Lucroy MD, Long KR, Blaik MA, et al: Photodynamic therapy for the treatment of intranasal tumors in 3 dogs and 1 cat, *J Vet Intern Med* 17:727–729, 2003.
116. Osaki T, Takagi S, Hoshino Y, et al: Efficacy of antivascular photodynamic therapy using benzoporphyrin derivative monoacid ring A (BPD-MA) in 14 dogs with oral and nasal tumors, *J Vet Med Sci* 71:125–132, 2009.
117. Thrall DE, Harvey CE: Radiotherapy of malignant nasal tumors in 21 dogs, *J Am Vet Med Assoc* 183:663–666, 1983.
118. Henderson SM, Bradley K, Day MJ, et al: Investigation of nasal disease in the cat—a retrospective study of 77 cases, *J Feline Med Surg* 6:245–257, 2004.

119. Mukaratirwa S, van der Linde-Sipman JS, Gruys E: Feline nasal and paranasal sinus tumors: clinicopathological study, histomorphological description and diagnostic immunohistochemistry of 123 cases, *J Feline Med Surg* 3:235–245, 2001.
120. Demko, JL, Cohn LA: Chronic nasal discharge in cats: 75 cases (1993-2004), *J Am Vet Med Assoc* 230:1032–1037, 2007.
121. Theon AP, Peaston AE, Madewell BR, et al: Irradiation of nonlymphoproliferative neoplasms of the nasal cavity and paranasal sinuses in 16 cats, *J Am Vet Med Assoc* 204:78–83, 1994.
122. Taylor SS, Goodfellow MR, Browne WJ, et al: Feline extranodal lymphoma: response to chemotherapy and survival in 110 cats, *J Small Anim Pract* 50:584–592, 2009.
123. Sfiligoi G, Theon AP, Kent MS: Response of nineteen cats with nasal lymphoma to radiation therapy and chemotherapy, *Vet Radiol Ultrasound* 48:388–393, 2007.
124. Haney SM, Beaver L, Turrel J, et al: Survival analysis of 97 cats with nasal lymphoma: a multi institutional retrospective study (1986-2006), *J Vet Intern Med* 23:287–294, 2009.
125. Little L, Patel R, Goldschmidt M: Nasal and nasopharyngeal lymphoma in cats: 50 cases (1989-2005), *Vet Pathol* 44:885–892, 2007.
126. Greci V, Mortellaro CM, Olivero D, et al: Inflammatory polyps of the nasal turbinates of cats: an argument for designation of feline mesenchymal nasal hamartoma, *J Feline Med Surg* 13:213–219, 2011.
127. DeLorenzi D, Bertoncello D, Bottero E: Squash preparation cytology from nasopharyngeal masses in the cat: cytological results and histological correlations in 30 cases, *J Feline Med Surg* 10:55–60, 2008.
128. Lamb CR, Richbell S, Mantis P: Radiographic signs in cats with nasal disease, *J Feline Med Surg* 5(4):227–235, 2003.
129. Schoenborn WC, Wisner ER, Kass PP, et al: Retrospective assessment of computed tomographic imaging of feline sinonasal disease in 62 cats, *Vet Radiol Ultrasound* 44(2):185–195, 2003.
130. Tromblee TC, Jones JC, Etue AE, et al: Association between clinical characteristics, computed tomography characteristics, and histologic diagnosis for cats with sinonasal disease, *Vet Radiol Ultrasound* 47:241–248, 2006.
131. Karnik K, Riechle JK, Fischetti AJ, et al: Computed tomographic findings of fungal rhinitis and sinusitis in cats, *Vet Radiol Ultrasound* 50:65–68, 2009.
132. Mellanby RJ, Herrtage ME, Dobson JM: Long-term outcome of eight cats with non-lymphoproliferative nasal tumours treated by megavoltage radiotherapy, *J Feline Med Surg* 4:77–81, 2002.
133. Elmslie RE, Ogilvie GK, Gillette EL, et al: Radiotherapy with and without chemotherapy for localized lymphoma in 10 cats, *Vet Radiol* 32:277–280, 1991.
134. Mendenhall WM, Werning JW, Pfister DG: Cancer of the head and neck. In DeVita VT, Lawrence TS, Rosenberg SA, editors: *Cancer: Principles and practice of oncology*, Philadelphia, 2008, Lippincott Williams & Wilkins.

SECTION C

Cancer of the Larynx and Trachea

STEPHEN J. WITHROW

Incidence and Risk Factors

Cancer in either the larynx or the trachea is rare in dogs and cats.[1,2] Young patients with active osteochondral ossification sites are at higher risk for benign tracheal osteocartilaginous tumors, which grow in synchrony with the rest of the musculoskeletal system.[1,3] Laryngeal oncocytomas also appear to occur in younger mature dogs.[4,5] No breed or gender predilection is known for either site.

Pathology and Natural Behavior

Reported canine laryngeal tumors include rhabdomyoma (oncocytoma), osteosarcoma, extramedullary plasmacytoma,[4,6] chondrosarcoma, osteosarcoma, undifferentiated carcinoma, fibrosarcoma, granular cell tumor, mast cell tumor, adenocarcinoma, and SCC.[7-10] Rhabdomyomas in the dog may be large, are minimally invasive, and do not appear to metastasize.[4,5,11,12] A 6-month-old dog with a laryngeal cyst has been reported.[13] Most other laryngeal tumors are very locally invasive and have a significant metastatic potential. Feline laryngeal neoplasms most commonly are lymphomas, although SCC and adenocarcinoma have been reported.[2,8,10,14,15] Benign tracheal tumors and cysts in cats are rare.[2,14,16]

Reported tracheal cancer includes lymphoma, chondrosarcoma, histiocytic sarcoma, adenocarcinoma, and SCC.[17,18] Tracheal leiomyomas and polyps have also been reported.[19-21] Several reports of benign tracheal osteochondral tumors exist in the literature.[3,22] These lesions grow from the cartilaginous rings and are composed of cancellous bone capped by cartilage. They may reflect a malfunction of osteogenesis rather than true cancer and are benign.[22] The larynx and trachea may be secondarily invaded by neoplasms such as lymphoma and thyroid adenocarcinoma.

History and Clinical Signs

Patients with laryngeal tumors usually have a progressive change in voice or bark, exercise intolerance, or dysphagia. Patients with tracheal tumors usually have coughing and exercise intolerance. Because osteochondral lesions of young dogs grow at the same rate as the rest of the skeleton, symptoms become most noticeable during the skeletal growth spurt.

Diagnostic Techniques and Work-Up

Laryngeal tumors usually can be biopsied under direct visualization. Small samples or cytology alone may yield false negative results.[2] Regional radiographs may reveal the general location of the lesion, but CT images will yield more precise localization.[23]

Tracheal tumors offer more of a diagnostic challenge but can be biopsied with the use of fiberoptic instruments or a rigid bronchoscope (Figure 23-12, *A*). Alternatively, open surgical biopsy, often coupled with excision, can be performed. Plain radiographs or a tracheogram may reveal a mass narrowing the lumen (Figure 23-12, *B*). CT or MRI may aid localization of the lesion.[23]

Therapy

Benign laryngeal cancers such as rhabdomyomas and cysts can be removed successfully with preservation of function.[4,11-13,16] Temporary tracheostomy will provide short-term relief of upper airway obstruction and is well tolerated in dogs and some cats.[24] Complete laryngectomy with a permanent tracheostomy is another option used in humans, but it has had limited use in veterinary medicine.[11,25-29] Depending on their suspected radioresponsiveness, invasive cancers can be treated with irradiation to better preserve laryngeal function. Radiation should control lymphoma or

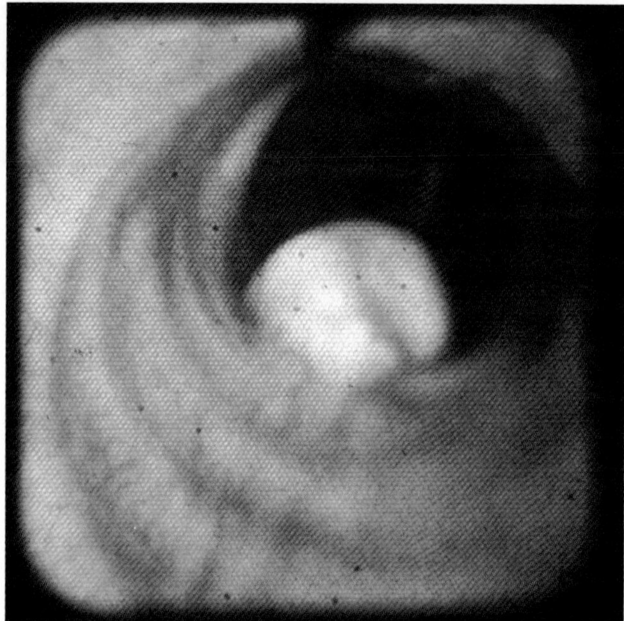

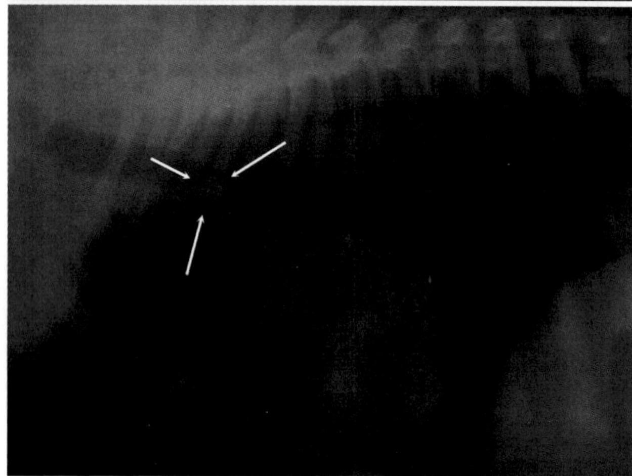

FIGURE 23-12 **A,** Fiberoptic view of tracheal osteochondroma in a 5-month-old dog. **B,** Lateral thoracic radiograph of the dog in **A.**

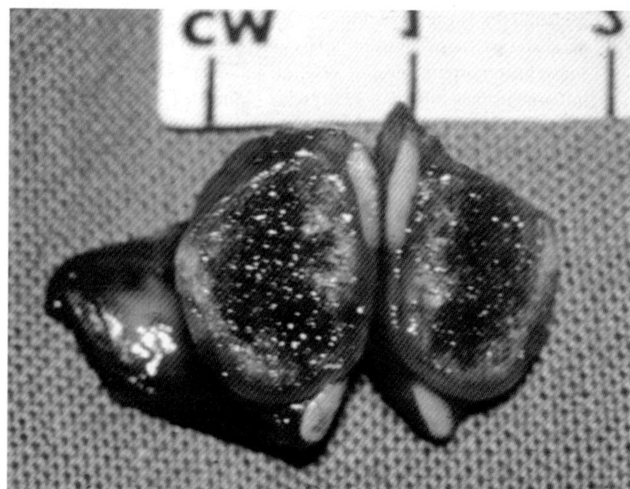

FIGURE 23-13 Resected tumor and associated tracheal cartilage rings of the dog in Figure 23-12. The tumor is bisected and has the typical appearance of cancellous bone with a cartilaginous cap. The patient recovered uneventfully from surgery and survived for longer than 5 years, when it was lost to follow-up.

plasmacytoma in the dog or cat larynx or trachea. Chemotherapy, with or without surgery, may also be effective.[6,30]

Tracheal tumors should be treated with resection, especially benign osteochondral tumors (Figure 23-13).[3,31] Full thickness removal with end-to-end anastomosis can easily be performed on up to three or four rings. Experimentally, up to 50% of tracheal length has been removed with successful closure.[32] Intraluminal stents may provide temporary palliation.

Phototherapy via bronchoscopy has been used successfully in humans for small lesions (carcinoma in situ or early carcinoma), but these lesions are only rarely recognized in the dog or cat.

Prognosis

Benign lesions of the trachea and larynx have a good prognosis if they can be resected.[16] Most dogs with resectable rhabdomyomas live longer than 1 year and may be presumed cured.[4,11,12] Long-term outcomes may be expected with treatment of extramedullary plasmacytomas or granular cell tumors.[6,9] Very limited information is available for the malignancies because very few have been treated and reported.[10,17] In one study in cats, the MST for 27 cats with a variety of laryngeal and tracheal lesions was 5 days and only 7% were alive at 1 year.[2]

Comparative Aspects[33]

Laryngeal cancer is common in humans (2% of all cancers) and is related to smoking and alcohol consumption. The lesion is nearly always SCC. Earlier detection prompted by voice changes makes treatment more feasible. In humans, the disease appears to progress through stages of development from dysphagia, to carcinoma in situ, to minimally invasive carcinoma, to invasive carcinoma. Of patients with carcinomas, 60% have local disease only, 30% have regional nodal metastasis, and 10% have distant metastasis. The disease is treated with surgery (partial or complete laryngectomy) or irradiation. Local control and cure rates are good to excellent.

Tracheal cancer independent of lung cancer is very rare in humans.

REFERENCES

1. Brown MR, Rogers KS: Primary tracheal tumors in dogs and cats, *Comp Pract Vet* 25:854–860, 2003.
2. Jakubiak MJ, Siedlecki CT, Zenger E, et al: Laryngeal, laryngotracheal, and tracheal masses in cats: 27 cases (1998-2003), *J Am Anim Hosp Assoc* 41:310–316, 2005.
3. Withrow SJ, Holmberg DL, Doige CE, et al: Treatment of a tracheal osteochondroma with an overlapping end-to-end tracheal anastomosis, *J Am Anim Hosp Assoc* 14:469–473, 1978.
4. Meuten DJ, Calderwood-Mays MB, Dillman RC, et al: Canine laryngeal rhabdomyoma, *Vet Pathol* 22:533–539, 1985.
5. Pass DA, Huxtable CR, Cooper BJ, et al: Canine laryngeal oncocytomas, *Vet Pathol* 17:672–677, 1980.
6. Hayes AM, Gregory SP, Murphy S, et al: Solitary extramedullary plasmacytoma of the canine larynx, *J Small Anim Pract* 48:288–291, 2007.

7. Wheeldon EB, Suter PF, Jenkins T: Neoplasia of the larynx in the dog, *J Am Vet Med Assoc* 180:642–647, 1982.
8. Saik JE, Toll SL, Diters RW, et al: Canine and feline laryngeal neoplasia: a 10-year survey, *J Am Anim Hosp Assoc* 22:359–365, 1986.
9. Rossi G, Tarantino C, Taccini E, et al: Granular cell tumour affecting the left vocal cord in a dog, *J Comp Pathol* 136:74–78, 2007.
10. Carlisle CH, Biery DN, Thrall DE: Tracheal and laryngeal tumors in the dog and cat: literature review and 13 additional patients, *Vet Radiol* 32:229–235, 1991.
11. Henderson RA, Powers RD, Perry L: Development of hypoparathyroidism after excision of laryngeal rhabdomyosarcoma in a dog, *J Am Vet Med Assoc* 198:639–643, 1991.
12. Calderwood-Mays MB: Laryngeal oncocytoma in two dogs, *J Am Vet Med Assoc* 185:677–679, 1984.
13. Cuddy LC, Bacon NJ, Coomer AR, et al: Excision of a congenital laryngeal cyst in a five-month-old dog via a lateral extraluminal approach, *J Am Vet Med Assoc* 236:1328–1333, 2010.
14. Vasseur PB: Laryngeal adenocarcinoma in a cat, *J Am Anim Hosp Assoc* 17:639–641, 1981.
15. Sheaffer KA, Dillon AR: Obstructive tracheal mass due to an inflammatory polyp in a cat, *J Am Anim Hosp Assoc* 32:431–434, 1996.
16. Rudorf H, Lane JG, Brown PJ, et al: Ultrasonographic diagnosis of a laryngeal cyst in a cat, *J Small Anim Pract* 40:275–277, 1999.
17. Evers P, Sukhiani HR, Sumner-Smith G, et al: Tracheal adenocarcinoma in two domestic shorthaired cats, *J Small Anim Pract* 35:217–220, 1994.
18. Bell R, Philbey AW, Martineau H, et al: Dynamic tracheal collapse associated with disseminated histiocytic sarcoma in a cat, *J Small Anim Pract* 47:461–464, 2006.
19. Byran RD, Frame RW, Kier AB: Tracheal leiomyoma in a dog, *J Am Vet Med Assoc* 178:1069–1070, 1981.
20. Black AP, Liu S, Randolph JF: Primary tracheal leiomyoma in a dog, *J Am Vet Med Assoc* 179:905–907, 1981.
21. Hendricks JC, O'Brien JA: Tracheal collapse in two cats, *J Am Vet Med Assoc* 187:418–419, 1985.
22. Carb A, Halliwell WH: Osteochondral dysplasias of the canine trachea, *J Am Anim Hosp Assoc* 17:193–199, 1981.
23. Stadler K, Hartman S, Matheson J, et al: Computed tomographic imaging of dogs with primary laryngeal or tracheal airway obstruction, *Vet Radiol Ultrasound* 52(4):377–384, 2011.
24. Guenther-Yenke CL, Rozanski EA: Tracheostomy in cats: 23 cases (1998-2006), *J Feline Med Surg* 9:451–457, 2007.
25. Nelson AW: Upper respiratory system. In Slatter DH, editor: *Textbook of small animal surgery*, Philadelphia, 1993, WB Saunders.
26. Harvey CE: Speaking out, *J Am Anim Hosp Assoc* 22:568, 1986.
27. Crowe DT, Goodwin MA, Greene CE: Total laryngectomy for laryngeal mast cell tumor in a dog, *J Am Anim Hosp Assoc* 22:809–816, 1986.
28. Block G, Clarke K, Salisbury SK, et al: Total laryngectomy and permanent tracheostomy for treatment of laryngeal rhabdomyosarcoma in a dog, *J Am Anim Hosp Assoc* 31:510–513, 1995.
29. Salisbury SK: Aggressive cancer surgery and aftercare. In Morrison WB, editor: *Cancer in dogs and cats: medical and surgical management*, Baltimore, 1998, Williams & Wilkins.
30. Schneider PR, Smith CW, Feller DL: Histiocytic lymphosarcoma of the trachea in the cat, *J Am Anim Hosp Assoc* 15:485–487, 1979.
31. Pearson GR, Lane JG, Holt PE, et al: Chondromatous hamartomas of the respiratory tract in the dog, *J Small Anim Pract* 28:705–712, 1987.
32. Nelson AW: Lower respiratory system. In Slatter DH, editor: *Textbook of small animal surgery*, Philadelphia, 1993, WB Saunders.
33. Mendenhall WM, Riggs CE, Cassisi NJ: Treatment of head and neck cancers. In DeVita VT, et al, editors: *Cancer: principles and practices of oncology*, Philadelphia, 2005, Lippincott-Raven.

SECTION D
Pulmonary Neoplasia

Robert B. Rebhun and William T.N. Culp

Incidence and Risk Factors

Lung cancer is the leading cause of cancer-related human deaths worldwide, but primary lung cancer remains relatively uncommon in pet dogs and cats. The incidence of primary lung cancer in pet dogs and cats presenting for necropsy is less than 1%.[1-4] Incidence rates in pet dogs range from 4.2 per 10,000 dogs per year in the United States to 15 per 100,000 dogs per year in the United Kingdom.[5,6] In contrast, the incidence of pulmonary neoplasia was 8.8% in a closed colony of "normal" beagles and was dominated by a high incidence of pulmonary tumors in dogs dying after the median lifespan of 13.6 years.[7]

The average age of pet dogs diagnosed with primary lung tumors is approximately 11 years,[1,8] with the exception of anaplastic carcinomas that occur at an average age of 7.5 years.[9] The Boxer, Doberman, Australian shepherd, Irish setter, and Bernese Mountain dog breeds are possibly overrepresented.[1,8,10] The average age of cats with pulmonary tumors is 12 to 13 years.[3,9,11] No breed or gender predisposition has been reported in cats with the possible exception of Persian cats.[4]

In people, the risk of developing primary lung cancer is strongly associated with smoking, but no such definitive risk factors have been identified in the pet population. Urban living and secondhand smoke exposure have both been implicated as potential causes of lung cancer in dogs but are yet to be clearly demonstrated.[12,13] An increased risk of lung cancer was found in dogs with increased amounts of anthracosis, suggesting an association between inhalation of polluted air and lung cancer.[14] Cytologic analysis of bronchoalveolar lavage fluid also revealed increased anthracosis in dogs that had been exposed to passive tobacco smoke when compared to dogs without a history of exposure.[15] In the experimental setting, laboratory dogs trained to smoke cigarettes through a tracheostoma (in the presence or absence of asbestos exposure) did develop lung cancer at a higher rate than control dogs.[16,17] Experimentally induced exposure to radiation such as that found in plutonium also significantly increases the occurrence of lung cancer when inhaled as an aerosol in research dogs.[18,19]

Pathology and Natural Behavior

Pulmonary tumors can arise from any tissue in the lung but most commonly originate from epithelium of the airways or alveolar parenchyma. Tumors derived from epithelium of large airways are typically located near the hilus, whereas parenchymally derived tumors tend to be peripherally located. However, the most recent WHO guidelines on classification of pulmonary neoplasms largely classify lung tumors of domestic animals by histologic pattern and not by site of origin.[10]

Approximately 85% of canine lung tumors are bronchoalveolar in origin, whereas adenocarcinoma, adenosquamous carcinoma, and SCC collectively comprise the remaining 13% to 15% of primary lung tumors.[7,8] Adenocarcinoma represents 60% to 70% of feline lung tumors, whereas bronchoalveolar carcinoma, SCC, and adenosquamous carcinoma are less common.[4,10,11] Small cell carcinoma represents approximately 25% of human pulmonary neoplasms but rarely occurs in the dog or cat.

Lung tumors can spread by local invasion or hematogenous and lymphatic routes, resulting in locoregional spread to other areas of the lung or lymph nodes or distant metastasis. Intrapulmonary metastases are believed to occur through vascular and lymphatic invasion or intra-airway seeding. Seventy-one percent of canine pulmonary malignant tumors had evidence of local vascular or lymphatic invasion, and 23% had distant metastasis beyond hilar lymph nodes.[8] SCC and anaplastic carcinomas have metastatic rates that exceed 50% and 90% of cases, respectively, and thus are believed to be more likely to metastasize than adenocarcinoma or bronchoalveolar carcinoma.[3]

Metastasis is common in the cat, with a metastatic rate of 76% in feline patients with pulmonary tumors.[4,11] The incidence of lymph node metastasis and the incidence of intrathoracic metastasis are equivalent at 30% of patients, whereas extrathoracic metastases occurred in only 16% of cats. Metastasis to bone or the nervous system is not uncommon in dogs or cats. Metastasis to the digits is a common and well-described clinical phenomenon in cats.[20]

Distinguishing poorly differentiated primary lung tumors from metastatic carcinoma can occasionally provide a diagnostic challenge. Immunohistochemistry using antibodies directed against thyroid transcription factor-1, cytokeratin, or vimentin may be useful in differentiating primary lung tumors from metastatic disease.[21-23] Antibodies against CD18 may also be useful for differentiating pulmonary tumors of histiocytic origin.[24]

Clinical Signs and Physical Examination Findings

Veterinary patients will often be diagnosed with a primary pulmonary tumor incidentally during a routine geriatric screen.[1,7,25] Up to 30% of cases of primary pulmonary tumors will be diagnosed without the presence of clinical signs.[25] The most common clinical sign reported in dogs with pulmonary neoplasia is coughing, which is noted in 52% to 93% of dogs.[1,25-28] Other clinical signs that have been recorded include dyspnea (6% to 24%), lethargy (12% to 18%), anorexia (13%), weight loss (7% to 12%), hemoptysis (3% to 9%) and lameness likely secondary to hypertrophic osteopathy (4%).[25-27]

The clinical signs in cats are similar to dogs; however, the occurrence of these signs is variable and gastrointestinal signs may be noted as well.[29,30] As in dogs, signs referable to the respiratory tract are common, with dyspnea (24% to 65%), cough (29% to 53%), tachypnea (14%), and hemoptysis (10%) being noted regularly.[29,30] Nonspecific signs such as lethargy and anorexia can be seen in 24% to 43% and 19% to 71% of cats, respectively.[30,31] Vomiting/regurgitation and diarrhea are seen in approximately 19% of cats with primary pulmonary neoplasia.[29,30]

Abnormal physical examination findings consistent with pulmonary neoplasia are often not seen.[25] Increased bronchovesicular sounds may be auscultated in dogs with extensive pulmonary involvement.[26] As pulmonary effusion can occur in many cases, dull lung and heart sounds may also be noted.[25,29,30] Metastasis to the nervous system has been reported in several cases of primary pulmonary tumors, and neurologic abnormalities can be diagnosed on physical examination.[31-34]

Lameness can occur in dogs and cats associated with primary pulmonary neoplasia for a variety of reasons. Hypertrophic osteopathy is a paraneoplastic syndrome that has been most commonly associated with primary and metastatic lung tumors, although other malignant and nonmalignant diseases have resulted in hypertrophic osteopathy.[27,35-39] The disease is characterized by periosteal new bone formation at a site distant to the primary tumor. Lameness may improve with removal of the lung tumor.[35,38]

Several reports of cats with concurrent pulmonary neoplasia and digital metastasis can be found in the veterinary literature; this phenomenon has been noted with both pulmonary adenocarcinoma and SCC.[4,20,40-43] Of 36 cats with metastatic bronchogenic carcinoma to the digit, all were presented for lameness and none were presented for respiratory signs.[43] The authors of that study concluded that thoracotomy with lung lobectomy and digital amputation should not be recommended because nonrespiratory disease often progressed and metastatic lesions in other digits resulted in continued lameness.[43] The MST for cats undergoing digital amputation alone was only 67 days.[43]

Diagnostic Techniques and Work-Up

Clinical Laboratory Findings

A complete blood count (CBC) and serum chemistry panel are unlikely to signal a clinician to the presence of a pulmonary mass. Nonspecific changes in these diagnostics have been reported in veterinary cases, and routine blood tests are often within normal limits.[11,43] These diagnostics, however, are essential to the preanesthetic and overall evaluation of a patient undergoing treatment for a pulmonary neoplasm.

The presence of pleural effusion at diagnosis is less common in dogs than cats. When pleural effusion is noted, a sample should be obtained via thoracocentesis. The pleural fluid tends to be a clear or blood-tinged modified transudate.[25,29] Thirty percent (26/86) of cats in one study were noted to have pleural effusion, and thoracocentesis was performed in 13; fluid analysis was diagnostic for a primary lung tumor in 12/13 cats.[11] However, in a separate feline study, fluid analysis was diagnostic for a malignant effusion secondary to a malignant neoplasm in only 1/8 cases.[29] Of three dogs with pleural effusion in one study, one was diagnosed with carcinoma based on evaluation of fluid obtained by thoracocentesis.[25]

Bronchoalveolar lavage (BAL) and transtracheal washes have been advocated as a method of diagnosing pulmonary neoplasia.[25,44-46] In a series of cases that underwent BAL to aid in the diagnosis of respiratory tract diseases, 14 carcinomas were identified. Of those 14 cases, the BAL was definitive, supportive, or not helpful in eight, four, and two cases, respectively.[45] Transtracheal washes have been less successful; in one study, in six dogs with confirmed primary pulmonary neoplasia, none of the washes yielded neoplastic cells.[25]

The majority of pulmonary tumors are diagnosed on thoracic radiographs (see Chapter 6). When evaluating 277 canine cases from two large case series, 83% of pulmonary tumors were viewed on thoracic radiographs.[25,27] In cats with primary pulmonary tumors, 67% to 91% will have radiographic evidence of solitary or multiple pulmonary masses on thoracic radiographs.[11,30]

Several studies have evaluated tumor location and number within the lungs.[1,26,27] In a series of 210 dogs with primary pulmonary tumors, tumor location was determined in 191 cases.[27] Of the total dogs in that study, 53.8% were found in a single lung lobe and 37.1% were found in multiple lung lobes.[27] Only 2 dogs were found to have a tumor in multiple lobes in a smaller study of 15 total dogs; of the 17 affected lobes in that study, 13 were on the right and 4 were on the left.[26] Of 29 dogs with primary pulmonary tumors in

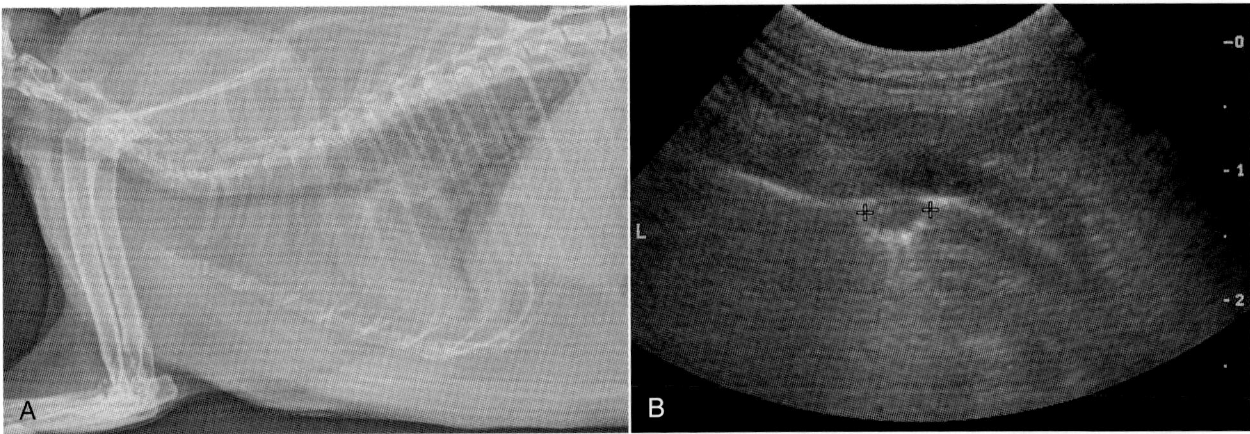

FIGURE 23-14 **A,** Right lateral radiograph. **B,** Ultrasound image of a pulmonary carcinoma in the left caudal lung lobe of a cat.

a separate study, the side of the tumor was recorded in 26 with 13 left-sided and 13 right-sided tumors.[1] One study has reported that clinical signs were not noted until the pulmonary tumor grew to at least 3 cm in size.[7]

In a study of 86 cats with primary pulmonary neoplasia, the location was determined in all cases.[11] Tumors were left-sided in 26 cats, right-sided in 27 cats, and bilateral in 33 cats.[11] In 45 cats, the tumors were found in a single lung lobe and the right and left caudal lobes were more commonly diagnosed with pulmonary tumors (34) versus the right and left cranial (9) and right middle lung lobes (2), which was likely the result of increased tissue at risk in caudal lobes.[11] Nineteen cats in one study were found to have a single lung lobe affected, whereas two cats had multiple lesions.[30] Of 17 cats in a separate study, all single lesions were left-sided; however, 10/17 had multiple lesions (both right- and left-sided).[29]

The radiographic pattern of primary pulmonary neoplasia has been variably reported in dogs and cats. Four radiographic patterns were described in a study evaluating 41 cats with primary pulmonary tumors: focal, localized, diffuse, and normal.[47] In the focal group, 65% demonstrated solitary masses and 35% demonstrated multiple masses.[47] Of the cases with focal (solitary and multiple) and localized masses, 17 were on the right side and 20 were on the left side.[47]

Thoracic ultrasound may be employed to assess pulmonary neoplasia or to obtain a sample of tissue via FNA or pretreatment biopsy (Figure 23-14). The ultrasonographic appearance of pulmonary neoplasia has been described in several studies.[48-50] Pulmonary masses may be hypoechoic or may exhibit variable echogenicity, and tumors are generally considered to have both a lack of discernable bronchi and normal branching vessels.[48,49]

Thoracic CT scans are gaining popularity for the preoperative assessment of pulmonary neoplasia and many clinicians feel this diagnostic is a necessity (Figure 23-15). Recently, the CT findings of primary lung tumors were described.[51] Several characteristics of solitary lung tumors were noted with CT in a majority of cases; 17/18 were well circumscribed, 16/19 were located in a cranial or caudal lobe, and 14/18 were located in the center to periphery of the lobe.[51] Internal mineralization was an uncommon finding being diagnosed in only 3/19 cases.[51]

Thoracic CT has been shown to be more accurate than thoracic radiographs in the assessment of tracheobronchial lymph node metastasis.[28] In 14 dogs diagnosed with primary pulmonary tumors, the accuracy of CT to determine tracheobronchial lymph node metastasis was 93% compared with 57% for thoracic radiography.[28] Additionally, five dogs deemed to be free of pulmonary metastasis with thoracic radiographs were found to have pulmonary metastasis with CT.[28]

In a study evaluating the assessment of pulmonary metastatic disease in 18 dogs (two of which had bronchoalveolar carcinoma) by thoracic radiography and CT, only 9% of CT-detected pulmonary nodules were noted on thoracic radiographs.[52] CT was able to detect pulmonary nodules down to approximately 1 mm in size, whereas thoracic radiography required a size of 7 to 9 mm for detection.[51] Overall, CT was significantly more sensitive than thoracic radiography in the identification of pulmonary nodules.[52,53]

Fine-Needle Aspiration

FNA of a pulmonary mass may be performed prior to lung lobectomy to attempt to obtain a cytologic diagnosis. FNA is often performed with ultrasound or CT guidance; however, blind aspirates have been reported.[11,50,54,55] Sedation is generally required to prevent iatrogenic trauma during the aspiration process. In dogs, preoperative FNA with cytology has resulted in a diagnosis in 38% to 90% of cases in which it is performed.[25-27] Diagnosis of primary pulmonary neoplasia in cats is reportedly higher, with 80% to 100% of cases being diagnosed by FNA and cytology.[11,30,54]

A pretreatment biopsy (biopsy performed prior to definitive therapy) can be performed prior to lung lobectomy, although the clinical relevance is questionable.[56] If there is suspicion that a pulmonary neoplasm is not a primary lesion (i.e., either metastatic or systemic neoplasia such as lymphoma), a pretreatment biopsy may be considered; however, if the eventual goal is to treat the pulmonary tumor by lung lobectomy, a pretreatment biopsy is not necessary. Multiple techniques for performing a pretreatment biopsy have been described, including utilizing a biopsy needle, bronchoscopic biopsy, keyhole incision with staple application, and thoracoscopy.*

To perform a pretreatment biopsy with a biopsy needle, sedation or anesthesia is required. Additionally, the use of ultrasound, fluoroscopic, or CT guidance is recommended to improve the targeting of the lesion and decrease the chance of iatrogenic trauma to normal structures.[50,55-56] In a study of dogs and cats undergoing CT-guided tissue core biopsy of intrathoracic lesions (including

*References 11, 25, 27, 46, 55-57.

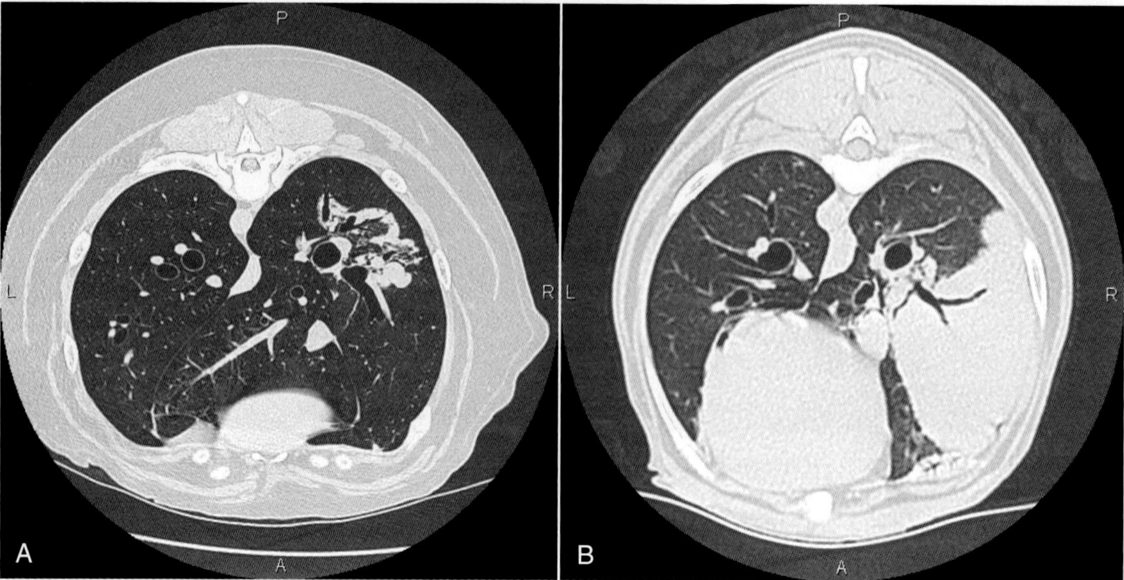

FIGURE 23-15 Transverse CT scan images of a right caudal lung lobe histiocytic sarcoma **(A)** in a 9-year-old Bernese Mountain dog and a right caudal pulmonary carcinoma **(B)** in a 10-year-old Fox terrier.

pulmonary tumors), the accuracy of diagnosis for the biopsy technique was 92% and the sensitivity for neoplasia was 80%.[55] A procedural complication rate of 43% was reported in that cohort; pulmonary hemorrhage and pneumothorax were seen in 30% and 27% of cases, respectively.[55]

Bronchoscopic biopsy has been performed in dogs and cats with pulmonary neoplasia with mixed success.[11,27] Findings that have been reported during bronchoscopic examination in veterinary patients with primary pulmonary neoplasia include narrowing of bronchi, mucosal erosions, and mucosal swelling and hyperemia.[58] In one series of cats, 5/7 cases were successfully diagnosed by means of endoscopic bronchiolar brushing.[11]

A keyhole lung biopsy technique has been described for non-neoplastic lung disease.[46] For this technique, a small thoracotomy (3 to 7 cm) was performed and a surgical stapler was applied across the lung lobe to seal vessels and small airways.[46] Thoracoscopy is a minimally invasive surgical option that may be utilized to obtain a pretreatment biopsy.[59] In a study describing the use of thoracoscopy to determine the cause of pleural effusion, biopsies of several suspicious intrathoracic lesions were performed.[60] In 8/18 cases, neoplasia was the cause of the pleural effusion, although the number of primary pulmonary tumors resulting in pleural effusion was unknown.[60] Performing a biopsy with thoracoscopy allowed for sufficient sample acquisition and the opportunity to perform an exploration of the thoracic cavity.[60]

Treatment

Surgery is the treatment of choice for primary pulmonary tumors. The surgical approach to a pulmonary tumor is clinician dependent, but certain overarching criteria exist. For unilateral tumors, a lateral thoracotomy or median sternotomy may be performed. Thoracoscopic lung lobectomy can be considered if the mass is deemed to be peripherally located and is in a suitable location. If nodules in multiple lobes are found bilaterally and the goal is to remove all gross disease, a median sternotomy should be performed.

Both partial and complete lung lobectomies have been described, and the elected technique is based on the location of the tumor. In general, a complete lung lobectomy should be performed; however, partial lung lobectomy may be an option for small tumors located in a peripheral position on the lung lobe. A cuff of normal tissue should be removed with the tumor to increase the chance of obtaining a wide margin.

Partial and complete lung lobectomies are generally performed with either a suturing method or the use of a surgical stapler. When performing a partial lung lobectomy with the suture method, the area to be removed is delineated by placing crushing forceps proximal to the lesion.[61] A continuous overlapping suture can then be placed proximal to the clamps.[61] For complete lung lobectomy utilizing suture ligation, the pulmonary artery and vein are individually ligated, and the bronchi are oversewn to prevent air leakage. Pneumonectomy can be performed when indicated.[62]

Several studies have evaluated the use of stapling equipment for lung lobectomy.[26,63,64] In a study of 37 dogs and cats undergoing resection of pulmonary lesions (67% were neoplastic) by surgical staples, the complications were minimal and the surgery was determined to be safe, fast, and efficient.[63] Use of surgical staplers is considered by many to be the technique of choice for partial and complete lung lobectomy (Figure 23-16).

Thoracoscopy is being employed more commonly for both diagnostic and treatment purposes. Thoracoscopy can be utilized to localize pulmonary lesions and to obtain biopsies.[59,60] Additionally, thoracoscopic lung lobectomy and thoracoscopic-assisted lung lobectomy have been recently described in several reports.[65-67] In one study of nine dogs with pulmonary neoplasia (seven metastatic and two primary), successful thoracoscopic lung lobectomy was performed in five cases.[65] Cases that were deemed to be good candidates for thoracoscopic removal in that study included those with small masses located away from the hilus. Caudal lung lobectomy was determined to be easier than cranial lung lobectomy; however, both were performed successfully.[65] Conversion from a thoracoscopic technique to an open procedure was most commonly performed because of poor operative vision.[65] One-lung ventilation should be considered in cases of thoracoscopic lung lobectomy to improve visualization.[65,66,68]

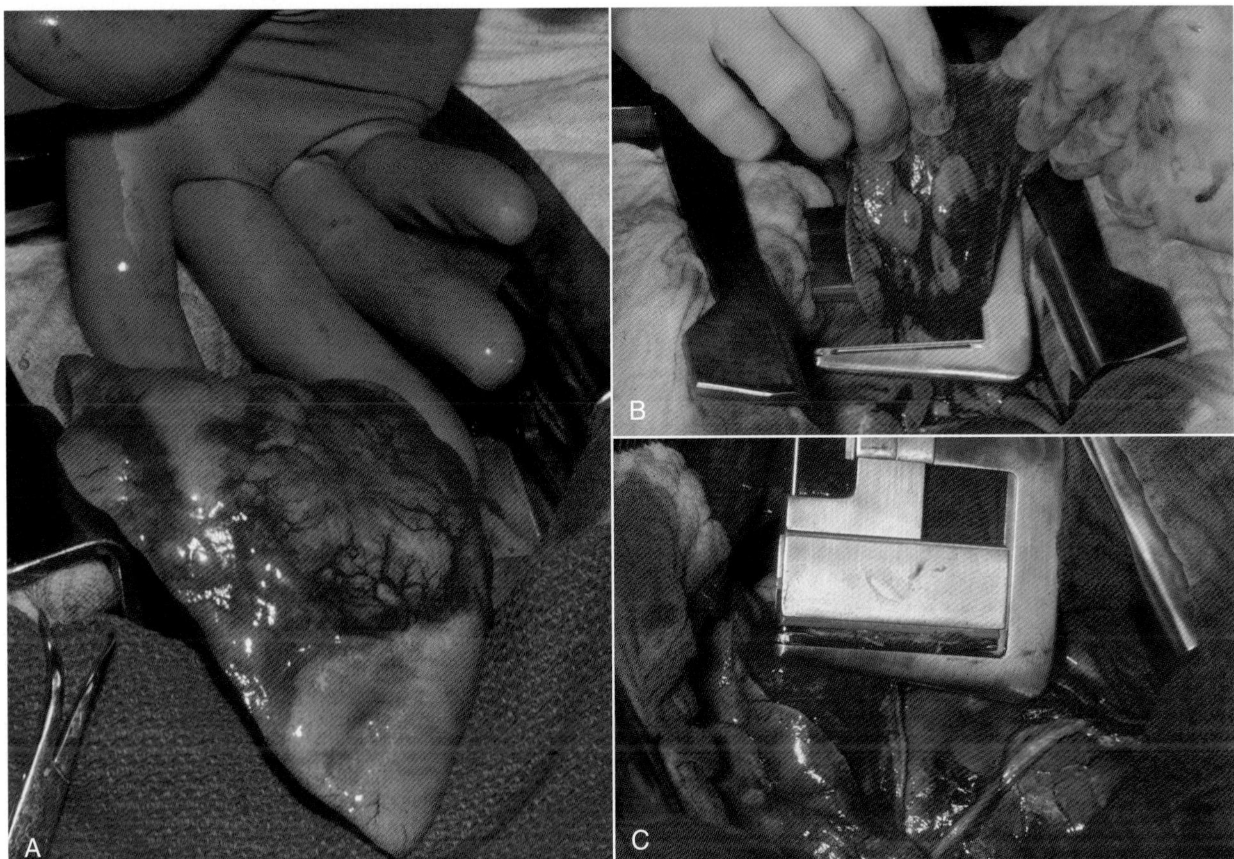

FIGURE 23-16 **A,** Operative view of lung cancer. Note the typical raised lesion with superficial neovascularization. **B,** The lung lobe is lifted up, and surgical staples are placed at the level of the proximal mainstem bronchus. **C,** Firing the stapler releases a double row of B-shaped, stainless steel staples. The lung mass then is removed, and the instrument is released. The artery, vein, and bronchus are inspected for any small leaks, which are sutured.

Biopsy of hilar lymph nodes is recommended as a staging tool because metastatic disease to the lymph nodes significantly affects prognosis.[28] Lymph node biopsy is relatively easy to perform via a lateral thoracotomy, but the position of the lymph nodes during a median sternotomy increases the difficulty. In the largest thoracoscopic lung lobectomy study in veterinary patients to date, none of the hilar lymph nodes were biopsied; however, thoracoscopic lymph node biopsy is performed regularly in human patients.[65,69]

Cisplatin-based chemotherapy protocols are considered the standard of care for human patients that receive chemotherapy in the adjuvant or palliative setting.[70] Relatively little is known about the efficacy of chemotherapy treatment for pulmonary tumors in domestic animals; however, chemotherapy treatment has been largely unrewarding in the gross disease setting. Early clinical trials evaluating the safety and efficacy of doxorubicin in cancer-bearing pet dogs included one evaluable dog with papillary pulmonary adenocarcinoma that experienced progressive disease.[71] No responses were seen in three dogs with lung adenocarcinoma that were treated with mitoxantrone.[72] Minimal responses were reported in two dogs treated with vindesine, whereas two dogs treated with the combination of vindesine and cisplatin both experienced greater than 50% reduction in measurable disease.[26] Treatment with vinorelbine resulted in partial responses in two out of seven dogs with measurable bronchoalveolar carcinoma.[73] Three additional dogs with microscopic disease were treated with adjuvant vinorelbine in the microscopic disease setting and those patients achieved survival times of 113, 169, and greater than 730 days.[73] Pharmacokinetic studies in humans have concluded that vinorelbine treatment results in 300-fold higher concentration in the lung when compared to plasma, which is 3.4- to13.8-fold higher than lung concentrations of vindesine and vincristine, respectively.[74] Based on observed partial responses in dogs and pharmacokinetic data in humans, treatment with vinorelbine or cisplatin appears to hold the most promise.

Delivery of aerosolized chemotherapy or cytokines has been described and appears well tolerated in dogs with primary or metastatic pulmonary neoplasia. Complete and partial responses have been described in dogs treated with inhalational therapy for metastatic tumors, whereas stable or progressive disease was reported in dogs with primary lung tumors.[75,76]

Treatment with monoclonal antibodies or small-molecule tyrosine kinase inhibitors (TKIs) directed against cell signaling pathways has been shown to be beneficial in distinct subpopulations of human patients with non–small-cell lung cancer (NSCLC). Such targeted therapies are yet to be thoroughly examined in dogs with this disease. With the recent availability of receptor TKIs toceranib (Palladia) and masitinib (Kinavet) for use in veterinary patients, future interrogation of such therapeutics may be warranted. In a phase I study, monotherapy with toceranib resulted in stable disease for more than 10 weeks in the only dog with primary lung carcinoma.[77]

Malignant pleural effusions can be responsive to systemic chemotherapy, intrapleural chemotherapy, or a combination of both routes. Cisplatin, carboplatin, or mitoxantrone have been used successfully for this purpose, resulting in temporary palliation of clinical signs.[78-81] Sclerosing agents such as talc or tetracyclines have been also been used in a palliative setting.[82]

RT in physician-based medicine is most often reserved for tumors that are unresectable.[70] Elective nodal irradiation for locally advanced NSCLC of human patients has traditionally been recommended but is a current source of controversy. Technologies such as IMRT, gamma-knife, or tomotherapy can now be used to provide more precise delivery of radiation while sparing unaffected tissues, especially when used together with respiratory gating or breath-hold techniques. Use of such modalities in veterinary patients is now becoming more accessible but remains to be investigated in dogs and cats with lung tumors.

Interventional oncology is a specialty that utilizes minimally invasive, image-guided techniques to perform diagnostic and therapeutic procedures in the treatment of cancer. Interventional oncologic techniques for the treatment of primary pulmonary neoplasia have not been described in the veterinary literature; however, several treatment options exist in human medicine for pulmonary neoplasia.[83-86] These options are generally reserved for cases of pulmonary metastatic disease, cases of nonresectable pulmonary tumors, or patients in which surgery is contraindicated due to existing comorbidities.[84-87] Significant research and proper case selection would need to be performed before these techniques could be routinely performed in clinical veterinary patients.

Radiofrequency ablation (RFA) and regional chemotherapy administration are two interventional oncology techniques that have been reported in the treatment of pulmonary neoplasia. RFA is performed by placing an electrode within a tumor and generating heat; the heat results in coagulative necrosis in a defined region.[83,85,86] The goal is to produce a 360-degree region of necrosis around the tumor, with a 1-cm thick margin of normal tissue included.[83,85]

RFA has been performed in dogs with experimentally induced transmissible venereal tumor of the lung.[88] In this group of five dogs, RFA was applied percutaneously with CT guidance to 14 tumors. On harvest of the affected lung lobes, gross and histopathologic evaluations demonstrated complete thermal coagulation necrosis of all the lesions that had been treated; no viable tumor was identified in any dogs.[88]

Regional chemotherapy has been developed with the goal of increasing the efficacy of chemotherapy agents and decreasing systemic side effects.[89] Regional delivery allows for increased concentrations of chemotherapy to be delivered to the tumor by selective catheterization of the tumoral arterial supply.[89] Regional techniques involving the administration of chemotherapy into the bronchial arteries and pulmonary arteries have been described in several human studies.[87,89,90] Recently, a study demonstrated that significantly higher concentrations of chemotherapy agents (gemcitabine and carboplatin) were noted in pulmonary tissue that had been treated with regional techniques (selective pulmonary artery perfusion) as compared to the concentration after intravenous administration in an experimental model.[90] As stated previously, the indications for these treatments remain to be determined in veterinary patients.

Prognosis

Several studies have evaluated prognostic variables in both dogs and cats with primary pulmonary neoplasia (Table 23-5).*

*References 25, 27, 28, 30, 91, 92.

TABLE 23-5 Factors Associated with Survival Time for Pulmonary Tumors in Dogs and Cats

FACTOR	REFERENCE
Dogs	
Size >100 cm^3	26
TNM stage	25, 27, 92
Lymph node involvement	25, 27, 28
Clinical signs at diagnosis	25
Gross disease postoperatively	91
Histologic type	25, 26, 92
Involvement of entire lung lobe	26
Histologic grade	25
Cats	
Histologic grade	30

Dogs with clinical signs at the time of diagnosis have been found to have significantly shorter disease-free intervals (DFIs) and survival times versus those in which a pulmonary tumor was found incidentally.[25] Metastatic disease within the lymph nodes is also associated with a significantly decreased DFI and survival time in dogs.[25,27,28] In one study, dogs with well-differentiated tumors lived longer and had longer DFIs than dogs with moderately or poorly differentiated tumors.[25] Similarly, histologic grade is predictive of outcome in cats. The MST for cats undergoing surgical resection of pulmonary tumors was 2.5 months and 23 months for poorly differentiated and well differentiated tumors, respectively.[30]

One study evaluated the effect of several variables on remission and survival in dogs with primary lung tumors.[91] Dogs for which surgery was successful in rendering them free of macroscopic disease lived significantly longer than dogs that had gross disease postoperatively.[91] Factors significantly associated with remission included limited degree of primary tumor involvement, normal-sized lymph nodes, and lack of metastatic disease.[91] In a separate study of 15 dogs, trends for longer survival times were noted in dogs with adenocarcinoma versus SCC, in dogs with peripheral lesions versus lesions that involved an entire lobe, and in dogs with tumor volume smaller than 100 cm^3 when compared to dogs with tumor volume larger than 100 cm^3.[26]

Dogs without clinical signs at the time of diagnosis have a MST of 545 days versus 240 days in dogs with clinical signs.[25] Tumor stage (T) is also prognostic for MST, with T1 (solitary), T2 (multiple), and T3 (invasive into adjacent tissues) tumors having MSTs of 26 months, 7 months, and 3 months, respectively.[25] Dogs with lymph node metastasis had a MST of 1 month compared with dogs without lymph node involvement that survived for a median of 15 months.[25] In another study, dogs with lymph node enlargement diagnosed prior to surgery survived for a median time of 60 days, whereas dogs without lymph node enlargement had a MST of 285 days.[91] A similar finding was noted in a more recent study in which dogs with lymphadenopathy had MSTs of 126 days versus a MST that had not been reached in the dogs without lymphadenopathy.[28] In dogs for which a surgical remission could be achieved, the MST is 330 days versus 28 days in dogs that could not be rendered free of visible disease.[91] Although not statistically significant, the MST of dogs with SCC was 8 months and the MST of dogs with adenocarcinoma was 19 months in one study.[26] Finally, dogs with well-differentiated, moderately differentiated, and poorly differentiated lung tumors have MSTs of 790 days, 251 days, and 5 days, respectively.[25]

A recent study evaluated 42 dogs with primary lung tumors and based the prognostic evaluation on the WHO classification scheme.[89] In these cases, 34 tumors were determined to be carcinomas (26 papillary adenocarcinomas) and eight were determined to be sarcomas. Fourteen of the carcinomas and two of the sarcomas were T1N0M0. Dogs with papillary adenocarcinomas and a clinical stage of T1N0M0 had the best overall prognosis with an MST of 555 days; this survival time was significantly longer than dogs with any other tumor type or dogs with a worse clinical stage.[92] Dogs with other tumor types had a MST of 72 days.[92]

Comparative Aspects[70]

Lung cancer is the leading cause of cancer deaths in the United States and worldwide.[93] Approximately 85% of human lung cancers are NSCLCs, with the remainder being small-cell lung cancer. NSCLCs are comprised of three distinct histologic subtypes: SCC, adenocarcinoma, and large-cell lung cancer. Large airway origin tumors predominated in humans through the 1960s and were commonly associated with smoking cigarettes. Adenocarcinoma arising from the smaller airways now predominates in human patients, which is likely a result of changes to tobacco blends and the use of cigarette filters.[94]

If curative-intent resection can be performed, prognosis for human patients with NSCLC is largely dependent on stage, with 5-year survival rates greater than 60% to 70% for patients with stage I disease. Five-year survival rates are roughly 30% to 40%, 10% to 30%, and less than 5% for patients with stage II, stage III, and stage IV disease, respectively.[70]

Inherited cancer syndromes caused by germline *p53* mutations, retinoblastoma, EGFR, and other genes have been reported to increase the risk of lung cancer. Furthermore, an association between single-nucleotide polymorphism variations has been linked to lung carcinogenesis and may cooperate with nicotine exposure. DNA synthesis and repair genes may also play a role in the development and prognosis of lung cancer. Commonly acquired molecular abnormalities in human lung cancer include but are not limited to microsatellite instabilities, EGFR mutations, *p53* inactivation, RB inactivation, P16INK4a inactivation, allelic loss, and high telomerase activity. K-*ras* mutations have been found in up to 30% of human NSCLCs.[95] Close homology exists between canine and human K-*ras*. Interestingly, K-*ras* mutations were detected in 5 of 21 canine NSCLC specimens by direct sequencing. Further studies concluded that the frequency and type of mutations in canine NSCLC tissues more closely matched those for tumors from human nonsmokers with K-*ras* mutations than those for smokers.[8]

The FDA has approved the use of two EGFR-targeted molecules, gefitinib (Iressa, Astra Zeneca) and erlotinib (Tarceva, Genentech/Roche), in the second- and third-line treatment of human lung cancer. Gefitinib monotherapy confers substantial clinical benefit in terms of progression-free survival and overall survival in NSCLC patients with EGFR mutations. These mutations were commonly found in patients fitting the responsive profile observed in initial and subsequent clinical studies: specifically female, nonsmokers, Asian descent, and adenocarcinoma, which suggest a distinctive biology in this subgroup of individuals.[96]

Miscellaneous Lung Conditions

Canine Pulmonary Lymphomatoid Granulomatosis

Canine pulmonary lymphomatoid granulomatosis is a poorly understood disease occurring most commonly in young to middle-aged dogs with no breed or gender predilection.[97] The most common laboratory abnormalities occurring in seven cases included basophilia and leukocytosis. Lung lobe consolidation or large pulmonary granulomas and tracheobronchial lymph node enlargement are typically seen on thoracic radiographs. Transthoracic FNA is not often diagnostically rewarding. Differential diagnoses include heartworm granulomas, metastatic neoplasia, and primary lung tumors. Traditionally, a definitive diagnosis requires biopsy and histopathology. Characteristic histopathology often demonstrates angiocentric and angiodestructive infiltration of the pulmonary parenchyma by large lymphoreticular and plasmacytoid cells in addition to normal-appearing lymphocytes, eosinophils, and plasma cells. This infiltrate is typically centered around small-to-medium arteries and veins.

The etiology of this disease is not known but is suspected to be neoplastic or preneoplastic. A recent case report indicates evidence of clonality based on polymerase chain reaction testing for antigen-receptor rearrangements (PARR), but this finding needs to be investigated in a larger series of cases.[98] It is not known whether flow cytometry or PARR testing may improve the diagnostic power of FNA.

In a very limited number of cases, the response to chemotherapy is quite variable.[99,100] Of five dogs that were treated with cyclophosphamide, vincristine, and prednisone, three achieved a CR. The remaining dogs showed either worsening in clinical signs or progressed to lymphoid leukemia within 2 months. Dogs achieving a complete response were alive at 7, 12, and 32 months.

Histiocytic Sarcoma

Histiocytic sarcoma (HS) was originally reported in a series of 11 Bernese Mountain dogs and is believed to be inherited with a polygenic mode of inheritance in this breed[101,102] (see Chapter 33, Section F). *Histiocytic sarcoma* is currently the preferred term for identifying malignant tumors of antigen-presenting dendritic cell origin, whereas the original term *malignant histiocytosis* refers to the systemic (disseminated) form of the disease. Other breeds at risk include the Rottweiler, golden retriever, and flat-coated retriever. Dogs often present with respiratory signs but nonspecific presenting complaints of weight loss, lethargy, fever, and anorexia are also common. HS commonly metastasizes to lymph nodes, the kidneys, the liver, and the central nervous system. HS can occur in a hemophagocytic form, resulting in anemia, hypoalbuminemia, thrombocytopenia, and leukopenia. Paraneoplastic hypercalcemia can also occur with this disease. Dogs presenting with the hemophagocytic form of HS have a particularly poor prognosis, with hypoalbuminemia and thrombocytopenia being associated with a dismal prognosis.[103,104] In contrast to dogs with disseminated HS, dogs with localized HS that underwent surgical excision and adjuvant therapy with CCNU had a reported MST of 568 days.[105] Interestingly, 5 out of 16 dogs within that study had localized pulmonary lesions that were resected prior to therapy with CCNU.

REFERENCES

1. Brodey RS, Craig PH: Primary pulmonary neoplasms in the dog: a review of 29 cases, *J Am Vet Med Assoc* 147:1628–1643, 1965.

2. Nielsen SW, Horava A: Primary pulmonary tumors of the dog. A report of sixteen cases, *Am J Vet Res* 21:813–830, 1960.
3. Moulton JE, von Tscharner C, Schneider R: Classification of lung carcinomas in the dog and cat, *Vet Pathol* 18:513–528, 1981.
4. D'Costa S, Yoon B-I, Kim DY, et al: Morphologic and molecular analysis of 39 spontaneous feline pulmonary carcinomas, *Vet Pathol* DOI 10.1177103009858l1419529, 2011.
5. Dorn CR, Taylor DO, Frye FL, et al: Survey of animal neoplasms in Alameda and Contra Costa Counties, California. I. Methodology and description of cases, *J Natl Cancer Inst* 40:295–305, 1968.
6. Dobson JM, Samuel S, Milstein H, et al: Canine neoplasia in the UK: estimates of incidence rates from a population of insured dogs, *J Small Anim Pract* 43:240–246, 2002.
7. Hahn FF, Muggenburg BA, Griffith WC: Primary lung neoplasia in a beagle colony, *Vet Pathol* 33:633–638, 1996.
8. Griffey SM, Kraegel SA, Madewell BR: Rapid detection of K-ras gene mutations in canine lung cancer using single-strand conformational polymorphism analysis, *Carcinogenesis* 19:959–963, 1998.
9. Stunzi H, Head KW, Nielsen SW: Tumours of the lung, *Bull World Health Organ* 50:9–19, 1974.
10. Meuten DJ: *Tumors in domestic animals*, ed 4, Ames, Iowa, 2002, Iowa State University Press.
11. Hahn KA, McEntee MF: Primary lung tumors in cats: 86 cases (1979-1994), *J Am Vet Med Assoc* 211:1257–1260, 1997.
12. Reif JS, Cohen D: The environmental distribution of canine respiratory tract neoplasms, *Arch Environ Health* 22:136–140, 1971.
13. Reif JS, Dunn K, Ogilvie GK, et al: Passive smoking and canine lung cancer risk, *Am J Epidemiol* 135:234–239, 1992.
14. Bettini G, Morini M, Marconato L, et al: Association between environmental dust exposure and lung cancer in dogs, *Vet J* 186(3):364–369, 2009.
15. Roza MR, Viegas CA: The dog as a passive smoker: effects of exposure to environmental cigarette smoke on domestic dogs, *Nicotine Tob Res* 9:1171–1176, 2007.
16. Auerbach O, Hammond EC, Kirman D, et al: Effects of cigarette smoking on dogs. II. Pulmonary neoplasms, *Arch Environ Health* 21:754–768, 1970.
17. Humphrey EW, Ewing SL, Wrigley JV, et al: The production of malignant tumors of the lung and pleura in dogs from intratracheal asbestos instillation and cigarette smoking, *Cancer* 47:1994–1999, 1981.
18. Gillett NA, Stegelmeier BL, Kelly G, et al: Expression of epidermal growth factor receptor in plutonium-239-induced lung neoplasms in dogs, *Vet Pathol* 29:46–52, 1992.
19. Wilson DA, Mohr LC, Frey GD, et al: Lung, liver and bone cancer mortality after plutonium exposure in beagle dogs and nuclear workers, *Health Phys* 98:42–52, 2010.
20. van der Linde-Sipman JS, van den Ingh TS: Primary and metastatic carcinomas in the digits of cats, *Vet Q* 22:141–145, 2000.
21. Ramos-Vara JA, Miller MA, Johnson GC: Usefulness of thyroid transcription factor-1 immunohistochemical staining in the differential diagnosis of primary pulmonary tumors of dogs, *Vet Pathol* 42:315–320, 2005.
22. Bettini G, Marconato L, Morini M, et al: Thyroid transcription factor-1 immunohistochemistry: diagnostic tool and malignancy marker in canine malignant lung tumours, *Vet Comp Oncol* 7:28–37, 2009.
23. Burgess HJ, Kerr ME: Cytokeratin and vimentin co-expression in 21 canine primary pulmonary epithelial neoplasms, *J Vet Diagn Invest* 21:815–820, 2009.
24. Affolter VK, Moore PF: Localized and disseminated histiocytic sarcoma of dendritic cell origin in dogs, *Vet Pathol* 39:74–83, 2002.
25. McNiel EA, Ogilvie GK, Powers BE, et al: Evaluation of prognostic factors for dogs with primary lung tumors: 67 cases (1985-1992), *J Am Vet Med Assoc* 211:1422–1427, 1997.
26. Mehlhaff CJ, Leifer CE, Patnaik AK, et al: Surgical treatment of primary pulmonary neoplasia in 15 dogs, *J Am Anim Hosp Assoc* 20:5, 1984.
27. Ogilvie GK, Haschek WM, Withrow SJ, et al: Classification of primary lung tumors in dogs: 210 cases (1975-1985), *J Am Vet Med Assoc* 195:106–108, 1989.
28. Paoloni MC, Adams WM, Dubielzig RR, et al: Comparison of results of computed tomography and radiography with histopathologic findings in tracheobronchial lymph nodes in dogs with primary lung tumors: 14 cases (1999-2002), *J Am Vet Med Assoc* 228:1718–1722, 2006.
29. Barr F, Gruffydd-Jones TJ, Brown PJ, et al: Primary lung tumours in the cat, *J Small Anim Pract* 1987:11, 1987.
30. Hahn KA, McEntee MF: Prognosis factors for survival in cats after removal of a primary lung tumor: 21 cases (1979-1994), *Vet Surg* 27:307–311, 1998.
31. MacCoy DM, Trotter EJ, deLahunta A, et al: Pelvic limb paralysis in a young miniature pinscher due to metastatic bronchogenic adenocarcinoma, *J Am Anim Hosp Assoc* 1976:4, 1976.
32. Sorjonen DC, Braund KG, Hoff EJ: Paraplegia and subclinical neuromyopathy associated with a primary lung tumor in a dog, *J Am Vet Med Assoc* 180:1209–1211, 1982.
33. Moore JA, Taylor HW: Primary pulmonary adenocarcinoma with brain stem metastasis in a dog, *J Am Vet Med Assoc* 192:219–221, 1988.
34. Mori T, Yamagami T, Umeda M, et al: Small cell anaplastic carcinoma of the lung with cerebral metastasis in a dog, *J Vet Med Sci* 53:1129–1131, 1991.
35. Brodey RS: Hypertrophic osteoarthropathy in the dog: a clinicopathologic survey of 60 cases, *J Am Vet Med Assoc* 159:1242–1256, 1971.
36. Halliwell WH, Ackerman N: Botryoid rhabdomyosarcoma of the urinary bladder and hypertrophic osteoarthropathy in a young dog, *J Am Vet Med Assoc* 165:911–913, 1974.
37. Caywood DD, Kramek BA, Feeney DA, et al: Hypertrophic osteopathy associated with a bronchial foreign body and lobar pneumonia in a dog, *J Am Vet Med Assoc* 186:698–700, 1985.
38. Liptak JM, Monnet E, Dernell WS, et al: Pulmonary metastatectomy in the management of four dogs with hypertrophic osteopathy, *Vet Comp Oncol* 2:1–12, 2004.
39. Grillo TP, Brandao CV, Mamprim MJ, et al: Hypertrophic osteopathy associated with renal pelvis transitional cell carcinoma in a dog, *Can Vet J* 48:745–747, 2007.
40. Moore AS, Middleton DJ: Pulmonary adenocarcinoma in 3 cats with non-respiratory signs only, *J Small Anim Pract* 23(9):501–509, 1982.
41. Pollack M, Martin RA, Diters RW: Metastatic squamous cell carcinoma in multiple digits of a cat, *J Am Anim Hosp Assoc* 20:835–839, 1984.
42. Scott-Moncrieff JCGSE, Radovsky A, Blevins WE: Pulmonary squamous cell carcinoma with multiple digital metastases in a cat, *J Small Anim Pract* 30:696–699, 1989.
43. Gottfried SD, Popovitch CA, Goldschmidt MH, et al: Metastatic digital carcinoma in the cat: a retrospective study of 36 cats (1992-1998), *J Am Anim Hosp Assoc* 36:501–509, 2000.
44. Hawkins EC, DeNicola DB, Kuehn NF: Bronchoalveolar lavage in the evaluation of pulmonary disease in the dog and cat. State of the art, *J Vet Intern Med* 4:267–274, 1990.
45. Hawkins EC, DeNicola DB, Plier ML: Cytological analysis of bronchoalveolar lavage fluid in the diagnosis of spontaneous respiratory tract disease in dogs: a retrospective study, *J Vet Intern Med* 9:386–392, 1995.
46. Norris CR, Griffey SM, Walsh P: Use of keyhole lung biopsy for diagnosis of interstitial lung diseases in dogs and cats: 13 cases (1998-2001), *J Am Vet Med Assoc* 221:1453–1459, 2002.
47. PD K: Radiographic appearance of primary lung tumors in cats, *Vet Radiol* 27:8, 1986.
48. Schwarz LA, Tidwell AS: Alternative imaging of the lung, *Clin Tech Small Anim Pract* 14:187–206, 1999.
49. Reichle JK, Wisner ER: Non-cardiac thoracic ultrasound in 75 feline and canine patients, *Vet Radiol Ultrasound* 41:154–162, 2000.

50. Larson MM: Ultrasound of the thorax (noncardiac), *Vet Clin North Am Small Anim Pract* 39:733–745, 2009.
51. Marolf AJ, Gibbons DS, Podell BK, et al: Computed tomographic appearance of primary lung tumors in dogs, *Vet Radiol Ultrasound* 52:168–172, 2011.
52. Nemanic S, London CA, Wisner ER: Comparison of thoracic radiographs and single breath-hold helical CT for detection of pulmonary nodules in dogs with metastatic neoplasia, *J Vet Intern Med* 20:508–515, 2006.
53. Eberle N, Fork M, von Babo V, et al: Comparison of examination of thoracic radiographs and thoracic computed tomography in dogs with appendicular osteosarcoma, *Vet Pathol* DOI 10.1111/j.1476-5829.2010.00241.x, 2011.
54. Wood EF, O'Brien RT, Young KM: Ultrasound-guided fine-needle aspiration of focal parenchymal lesions of the lung in dogs and cats, *J Vet Intern Med* 12:338–342, 1998.
55. Zekas LJ, Crawford JT, O'Brien RT: Computed tomography-guided fine-needle aspirate and tissue-core biopsy of intrathoracic lesions in thirty dogs and cats, *Vet Radiol Ultrasound* 46:200–204, 2005.
56. Bauer TG: Lung biopsy, *Vet Clin North Am Small Anim Pract* 30:1207–1225, 2003.
57. Norris CR, Griffey SM, Samii VF, et al: Comparison of results of thoracic radiography, cytologic evaluation of bronchoalveolar lavage fluid, and histologic evaluation of lung specimens in dogs with respiratory tract disease: 16 cases (1996-2000), *J Am Vet Med Assoc* 218:1456–1461, 2001.
58. Venker-van Haagen AJVM, Heijn A et al: Bronchoscopy in small animal clinics: an analysis of the results of 228 bronchoscopies, *J Am Anim Hosp Assoc* 24:6, 1985.
59. Faunt KK, Jones BD, Turk JR, et al: Evaluation of biopsy specimens obtained during thoracoscopy from lungs of clinically normal dogs, *Am J Vet Res* 59:1499–1502, 1998.
60. Kovak JR, Ludwig LL, Bergman PJ, et al: Use of thoracoscopy to determine the etiology of pleural effusion in dogs and cats: 18 cases (1998-2001), *J Am Vet Med Assoc* 221:990–994, 2002.
61. Slatter DH: *Textbook of small animal surgery*, ed 3, Philadelphia, 2003, Saunders.
62. Liptak JM, Monnet E, Dernell WS, et al: Pneumonectomy, four case studies and a comparative review, *J Small Anim Prac* 45:441–447, 2004.
63. LaRue SM, Withrow SJ, Wykes PM: Lung resection using surgical staples in dogs and cats, *Vet Surg* 16:238–240, 1987.
64. Walshaw R: Stapling techniques in pulmonary surgery, *Vet Clin North Am Small Anim Pract* 24:335–366, 1994.
65. Lansdowne JL, Monnet E, Twedt DC, et al: Thoracoscopic lung lobectomy for treatment of lung tumors in dogs, *Vet Surg* 34:530–535, 2005.
66. Levionnois OL, Bergadano A, Schatzmann U: Accidental entrapment of an endo-bronchial blocker tip by a surgical stapler during selective ventilation for lung lobectomy in a dog, *Vet Surg* 35:82–85, 2006.
67. Dhumeaux MP, Haudiquet PR: Primary pulmonary osteosarcoma treated by thoracoscopy-assisted lung resection in a dog, *Can Vet J* 50:755–758, 2009.
68. Mosing M, Iff I, Moens Y: Endoscopic removal of a bronchial carcinoma in a dog using one-lung ventilation, *Vet Surg* 37:222–225, 2008.
69. Denlinger CE, Fernandez F, Meyers BF, et al: Lymph node evaluation in video-assisted thoracoscopic lobectomy versus lobectomy by thoracotomy, *Ann Thorac Surg* 89:1730–1735; discussion 1736, 2010.
70. DeVita VT, Lawrence TS, Rosenberg SA: *DeVita, Hellman, and Rosenberg's cancer: principles & practice of oncology*, ed 8, Philadelphia, 2008, Wolters Kluwer/Lippincott Williams & Wilkins.
71. Ogilvie GK, Reynolds HA, Richardson RC, et al: Phase II evaluation of doxorubicin for treatment of various canine neoplasms, *J Am Vet Med Assoc* 195:1580–1583, 1989.
72. Ogilvie GK, Obradovich JE, Elmslie RE, et al: Efficacy of mitoxantrone against various neoplasms in dogs, *J Am Vet Med Assoc* 198:1618–1621, 1991.
73. Poirier VJ, Burgess KE, Adams WM, et al: Toxicity, dosage, and efficacy of vinorelbine (Navelbine) in dogs with spontaneous neoplasia, *J Vet Intern Med* 18:536–539, 2004.
74. Chabner B, Longo DL: *Cancer chemotherapy and biotherapy: principles and practice*, ed 4, Philadelphia, 2006, Lippincott Williams & Wilkins.
75. Hershey AE, Kurzman ID, Forrest LJ, et al: Inhalation chemotherapy for macroscopic primary or metastatic lung tumors: proof of principle using dogs with spontaneously occurring tumors as a model, *Clin Cancer Res* 5:2653–2659, 1999.
76. Khanna C, Vail DM: Targeting the lung: preclinical and comparative evaluation of anticancer aerosols in dogs with naturally occurring cancers, *Curr Cancer Drug Targets* 3:265–273, 2003.
77. London CA, Hannah AL, Zadovoskaya R, et al: Phase I dose-escalating study of SU11654, a small molecule receptor tyrosine kinase inhibitor, in dogs with spontaneous malignancies, *Clin Cancer Res* 9:2755–2768, 2003.
78. Moore AS, Kirk C, Cardona A: Intracavitary cisplatin chemotherapy experience with six dogs, *J Vet Intern Med* 5:227–231, 1991.
79. Spugnini EP, Crispi S, Scarabello A, et al: Piroxicam and intracavitary platinum-based chemotherapy for the treatment of advanced mesothelioma in pets: preliminary observations, *J Exp Clin Cancer Res* 27:6, 2008.
80. Kelly J, Holmes EC, Rosen G: Mitoxantrone for malignant pleural effusion due to metastatic sarcoma, *Surg Oncol* 2:299–301, 1993.
81. Sparkes A, Murphy S, McConnell F, et al: Palliative intracavitary carboplatin therapy in a cat with suspected pleural mesothelioma, *J Feline Med Surg* 7:313–316, 2005.
82. Laing EJNA: Pleurodesis as a treatment for pleural effusion in the dog, *J Am Anim Hosp Assoc* 2:4, 1986.
83. Rose SC, Thistlethwaite PA, Sewell PE, et al: Lung cancer and radiofrequency ablation, *J Vasc Interv Radiol* 17:927–951; quiz 951, 2006.
84. Okuma T, Matsuoka T, Yamamoto A, et al: Frequency and risk factors of various complications after computed tomography-guided radiofrequency ablation of lung tumors, *Cardiovasc Intervent Radiol* 31:122–130, 2008.
85. Crocetti L, Lencioni R: Radiofrequency ablation of pulmonary tumors, *Eur J Radiol* 75:23–27, 2010.
86. Duncan M, Wijesekera N, Padley S: Interventional radiology of the thorax, *Respirology* 15:401–412, 2010.
87. Grootenboers MJ, Schramel FM, van Boven WJ, et al: Selective pulmonary artery perfusion followed by blood flow occlusion: new challenge for the treatment of pulmonary malignancies, *Lung Cancer* 63:400–404, 2009.
88. Ahrar K, Price RE, Wallace MJ, et al: Percutaneous radiofrequency ablation of lung tumors in a large animal model, *J Vasc Interv Radiol* 14:1037–1043, 2003.
89. Muller H, Guadagni S: Regional chemotherapy for carcinoma of the lung, *Surg Oncol Clin N Am* 17:895–917, 2008.
90. van Putte BP, Grootenboers M, van Boven WJ, et al: Selective pulmonary artery perfusion for the treatment of primary lung cancer: Improved drug exposure of the lung, *Lung Cancer* 65:208–213, 2009.
91. Ogilvie GK, Weigel RM, Haschek WM, et al: Prognostic factors for tumor remission and survival in dogs after surgery for primary lung tumor: 76 cases (1975-1985), *J Am Vet Med Assoc* 195:109–112, 1989.
92. Polton GA, Brearley MJ, Powell SM, et al: Impact of primary tumour stage on survival in dogs with solitary lung tumours, *J Small Anim Pract* 49:66–71, 2008.
93. Jemal A, Center MM, DeSantis C, et al: Global patterns of cancer incidence and mortality rates and trends, *Cancer Epidemiol Biomarkers Prev* 19:1893–1907, 2010.

94. Valaitis J, Warren S, Gamble D: Increasing incidence of adenocarcinoma of the lung, *Cancer* 47:1042–1046, 1981.
95. Westra WH, Slebos RJ, Offerhaus GJ, et al: K-ras oncogene activation in lung adenocarcinomas from former smokers. Evidence that K-ras mutations are an early and irreversible event in the development of adenocarcinoma of the lung, *Cancer* 72:432–438, 1993.
96. Pugh TJ, Bebb G, Barclay L, et al: Correlations of EGFR mutations and increases in EGFR and HER2 copy number to gefitinib response in a retrospective analysis of lung cancer patients, *BMC Cancer* 7:128, 2007.
97. Postorino NC, Wheeler SL, Park RD, et al: A syndrome resembling lymphomatoid granulomatosis in the dog, *J Vet Intern Med* 3:15–19, 1989.
98. Shimazaki T, Nagata M, Goto-Koshino Y, et al: A case of canine lymphomatoid granulomatosis with cutaneous lesions, *J Vet Med Sci* 72(8):1067–1069, 2010.
99. Berry CR, Moore PF, Thomas WP, et al: Pulmonary lymphomatoid granulomatosis in seven dogs (1976-1987), *J Vet Intern Med* 4:157–166, 1990.
100. Hatoya S, Kumagai D, Takeda S, et al: Successful management with CHOP for pulmonary lymphomatoid granulomatosis in a dog, *J Vet Med Sci* 73(4):527–530, 2011.
101. Rosin A, Moore P, Dubielzig R: Malignant histiocytosis in Bernese Mountain dogs, *J Am Vet Med Assoc* 188:1041–1045, 1986.
102. Padgett GA, Madewell BR, Keller ET, et al: Inheritance of histiocytosis in Bernese mountain dogs, *J Small Anim Pract* 36:93–98, 1995.
103. Moore PF, Affolter VK, Vernau W: Canine hemophagocytic histiocytic sarcoma: a proliferative disorder of CD11d+ macrophages, *Vet Pathol* 43:632–645, 2006.
104. Skorupski KA, Clifford CA, Paoloni MC, et al: CCNU for the treatment of dogs with histiocytic sarcoma, *J Vet Intern Med* 21:121–126, 2007.
105. Skorupski KA, Rodriguez CO, Krick EL, et al: Long-term survival in dogs with localized histiocytic sarcoma treated with CCNU as an adjuvant to local therapy, *Vet Comp Oncol* 7:139–144, 2009.

Tumors of the Skeletal System 24

NICOLE P. EHRHART, STEWART D. RYAN, AND TIMOTHY M. FAN

Osteosarcoma in Dogs

Incidence and Risk Factors

Osteosarcoma (OS) is the most common primary bone tumor in dogs, accounting for up to 85% of malignancies originating in the skeleton.[1-5] OS is estimated to occur in more than 10,000 dogs each year in the United States; however, this is probably an underestimation, since not all cases are confirmed or recorded.[6,7] The demographics of canine OS have been well reported.[1-5,8-19] It is largely a disease of middle-aged to older dogs, with a median age of 7 years. There is a large range in age of onset, with a reported case in a 6-month-old pup[20] and a small early peak in age frequency at 18 to 24 months.[13] Primary rib OS tends to occur in younger adult dogs with a mean age of 4.5 to 5.4 years.[21,22] OS is classically a cancer of large and giant breeds. In a review of 1462 cases of canine OS, dogs weighing more than 40 kg accounted for 29% of all cases and only 5% of their tumors occurred in the axial skeleton. Only 5% of OSs occur in dogs weighing less than 15 kg, but 59% of their tumors originated in the axial skeleton. Increasing weight and, more specifically, height appear to be the most predictive factors for the disease in the dog.[23] In the United States, the breeds most at risk for OS are Saint Bernard, Great Dane, Irish setter, Doberman pinscher, Rottweiler, German shepherd, and golden retriever; however, size seems to be a more important predisposing factor than breed.* A hereditary basis for the formation of OS has been suspected, based primarily on the (large) breed prevalence of the disease, as well as the subjective assessment of increased incidence in some related families. Males are reported to be slightly more frequently affected than females (1.1 to 1.5 : 1),† with the exception of the Saint Bernard, Rottweiler, and Great Dane and for dogs with primary OS of the axial skeleton (except rib and spine) in which affected females outnumber males.[2,22] However, in 1775 cases of canine OS of all sites treated at Colorado State University between 1978 and 2005, the male-to-female ratio was 1 : 1 (unpublished data, Colorado State University Animal Cancer Center [CSU-ACC] OS Database). Intact males and females were reported to have an increased risk for OS[23]; however, in the Rottweiler breed, male and female dogs that underwent gonadectomy before 1 year of age had an approximate one in four lifetime risk for bone sarcoma and were significantly more likely to develop bone sarcoma than dogs that were sexually intact.[24] There was a highly significant inverse dose-response relationship between duration of lifetime gonadal exposure and incidence rate of bone sarcoma independent of adult height or body weight.

*References 1, 2, 4, 8, 9, 13, 16, 18, 23.

†References 2, 3, 9, 12, 13, 15.

Approximately 75% of OSs occur in the appendicular skeleton, with the remainder occurring in the axial skeleton.[2,22] The metaphyseal region of long bones is the most common primary site, with front limbs affected twice as often as rear limbs, and the distal radius and proximal humerus are the two most common locations.[11] It is extremely rare for OSs to be located in bones adjacent to the elbow, although there is one report of 12 cases located at the proximal radius or distal humerus.[25] There was no prognostic difference in these cases as compared to more common appendicular sites. In the rear limbs, tumors are fairly evenly distributed between the distal femur, distal tibia, and proximal tibia, with the proximal femur a slightly less common site.[2] Primary OS distal to the antebrachiocarpal and tarsocrural joints is relatively rare in dogs.[26] In 116 cases of canine primary OS in the axial skeleton, it was reported that 27% were located in the mandible, 22% in the maxilla, 15% in the spine, 14% in the cranium, 10% in ribs, 9% in the nasal cavity or paranasal sinuses, and 6% in the pelvis.[22] Single reports of OS development in the os penis[27] and the patella[28] exist for the dog. Clinically documentable multicentric OS at the time of initial diagnosis occurs in less than 10% of all cases.[29] OS of extraskeletal sites is rare, but primary OS has been reported in mammary tissue, subcutaneous tissue, spleen, bowel, liver, kidney, testicle, vagina, eye, gastric ligament, synovium, meninges, and adrenal gland.[30-35]

Etiology

The etiology of canine OS is generally unknown. Some have speculated a viral cause because OS can occur in litter mates and may be experimentally induced by injecting OS cells into canine fetii.[36] However, an etiologic virus has not been isolated.

Physical Factors

A simplistic theory based on circumstantial evidence is that because OS tends to occur in major weight-bearing bones adjacent to late-closing physes and heavy dogs are predisposed, multiple minor trauma and subsequent injury to sensitive cells in the physeal region may occur. This may initiate the disease by inducing mitogenic signals, increasing the probability for the development of a mutant lineage. One in vitro study comparing the incidence of microdamage in cadaver radii of small- and large-breed dogs found no difference between the groups.[37] OS has been associated with metallic implants used for fracture repair, with chronic osteomyelitis, and with fractures in which no internal repair was used.[38-42] OS has also been reported at the site of a bone allograft used for fracture repair 5 years previous.[43] Exposure to ionizing radiation can induce OS.[35,44-52] In humans exposed to plutonium, 29% and 71% of the OSs were in the appendicular and axial skeleton, respectively, with the spine having the most tumors (36%). An almost identical distribution of plutonium-induced OS was reported for dogs injected with ^{239}Pu as young adults in experimental studies. This distribution of OS is quite different from the distributions of naturally occurring OS for both species and appears to be related to bone volume and turnover. Similar findings were seen for dogs injected with 226R (radium).[52] A distribution favoring bone marrow volume was seen for dogs exposed to strontium-90.[51] OS is a rare, late complication of radiation therapy (RT) in humans and dogs.[44,46,48-50] Three of 87 (3.4%) spontaneous tumor-bearing dogs treated for soft tissue sarcomas developed OS within the field of radiation.[44] In another experimental study, 21% of dogs undergoing intraoperative RT (>25 Gy) followed by external-beam RT to the vertebral column developed OS following treatment.[48] Secondary OS developed between 1.7 and 5 years after radiation in that study, and the authors speculated that high dose of radiation per fraction or total dose may predispose to this serious late effect of irradiation. OS was reported in 3% of 57 dogs irradiated for acanthomatous epulis of the oral cavity in another study.[46] Postirradiation OS in humans comprised approximately 2% to 4% of all OSs reviewed in two large series.[53,54]

OSs have been concurrently seen in dogs with bone infarcts, but it is not clear whether there is any causal relationship.[55-59] Bone infarcts are uncommon, are of unknown etiology, and may be identified as incidental findings by radiography. Bone infarcts are probably not associated with tumor emboli and appear to be more common in smaller breeds. A single report exists of OS occurrence secondary to a bone infarct caused by total hip arthroplasty.[60] A case of OS was also reported to be associated with osteochondritis dissecans in the humoral head,[61] and another report documents malignant transformation of an aneurysmal bone cyst.[62]

Genetic Factors

Ample evidence exists implicating the involvement of genetic and heritable factors for the development of OS in dogs. Currently, the most thoroughly described gene mutation that contributes to OS formation and/or progression in dogs is *p53*.[63-70] Initial studies performed in immortalized canine OS cell lines demonstrated that the functionality of the *p53* gene was defective based on the incapacity of *p53* to regulate appropriately the transcriptional expression of downstream target genes including *p21* and *mdm2* following genotoxic insult.[65] Furthermore, *p53* mRNA and protein were overexpressed in 60% of cell lines and correlated with the presence of missense point mutations within the DNA-binding domain.[65] Corroborating in vitro cell line studies, mutations in *p53* have also been demonstrated in dogs with spontaneously-arising OS. Several studies using either single-strand conformational polymorphism, polymerase chain reaction, or southern blotting, followed by nucleotide sequence analysis have identified missense mutations involving exons 4 to 8 of *p53* in 24% to 47% of all spontaneously arising OS samples.[63,67,69,70] In addition to exons 4 to 8, the entire gene sequence of *p53* has also been assessed by polymerase chain reaction (PCR) and single-strand conformational polymorphism from 59 spontaneously arising appendicular and axial OS samples.[64] In 41% of tumors, *p53* mutations were identified, with the majority of abnormalities being point mutations (74%), which resulted in an amino acid substitution, with a lesser percentage of mutations (26%) being deletions.[64] Finally, through the implementation of targeted microarray-based comparative genomic hybridization analysis of 38 canine OS cases, similar recurrent cytogenetic aberrations classically present in human OS samples were also identified in OS specimens collected from dogs, including loss of heterozygosity (LOH) of the *p53* gene in 18% of tumors.[71]

Substantiation for the presence of *p53* mutations in sporadic canine OS has also been documented by immunohistochemical studies because a hallmark of many *p53* mutations is enhanced protein stability of this normally labile protein, enabling detection of protein with methodologies such as immunohistochemistry (IHC).[72] In one study evaluating p53 protein expressions in 106 osteogenic tumors, a greater percentage of appendicular (84%) OSs overexpressed p53 protein in comparison with OSs arising from the axial skeleton (56%) and other non-OS bone tumors (20%).[68] Finally, loss of *p53* gene function in 167 osseous tumors has been characterized by p53 nuclear staining frequency and intensity expressed as a p53 index. Of 103 OS samples, 67% stained positively for p53 protein, and the p53 index was significantly greater in OS derived from the appendicular (n = 84) versus axial (n = 38) skeleton.[66] Interestingly, the p53 index of appendicular OS derived from Rottweilers was significantly higher than in Great Danes or other commonly affected breeds, supporting the notion that *p53* gene mutations may be associated with breed susceptibilities to OS development.[24]

Another tumor suppressor gene likely to be permissive for OS development is the *RB* gene. Based on investigations using five tumorigenic immortalized canine OS cell lines, the *RB* gene signaling pathway was found to be dysregulated with the persistence of hyperphosphorylated RB protein in the absence of mitogen stimulation. Despite apparent aberrant *RB* gene signaling, reduction in RB protein was identified in only one of five cell lines.[65] Corroborating these in vitro findings, the evaluation of 21 spontaneously arising OSs failed to identify gross *RB* gene alterations by Southern blotting, and protein expressions of RB were identified in all OS samples evaluated.[67]

Despite normal protein expression of RB in canine OS samples, the observed translational normalcy does not exclude the possibility for allelic deletion of the *RB* gene because prior studies in human OS samples have demonstrated that LOH at the *RB* gene locus does not absolutely correlate with inactivation of RB at the protein level.[73] Substantiating the possibility that *RB* gene may have allelic deletion in spontaneously arising canine OS, analysis of 38 OS samples with comparative genomic hybridization techniques identified copy number loss in 11/38 cases (29%), resulting in a correlative reduction or absence of RB protein expression in 62% of OS samples tested.[71] Based on these recent findings, it is probable that aberrations in the *RB* gene indeed participate in sporadic OS formation and/or progression in dogs.

In addition to *p53* and *RB* gene abnormalities, the phosphatase and tensin homolog *(PTEN)* tumor suppressor gene is suspected to participate in the genetic pathogenesis of canine OS. Original in vitro studies conducted with canine OS cell lines demonstrated that the majority of cell lines (60%) harbored mutations in *PTEN*, resulting in the absence of gene transcription and protein translation. Corroborating the cell line findings, expression of *PTEN* was either absent (n = 6) or variable (n = 4) in 15 spontaneously arising OS samples.[74] Further support for the loss of *PTEN* gene in canine OS pathogenesis has been the identification of specific recurrent chromosome copy number aberrations (CNAs) through targeted microarray-based comparative genomic hybridization studies.[71,75] In one study utilizing 38 OS samples derived from Rottweilers and golden retrievers, deletion of a chromosomal region (CFA 26q25), which encompasses the *PTEN* tumor suppressor gene locus, occurred in 42% of OS samples.[71] In a subsequent study analyzing 123 OS samples predominantly derived from Rottweilers, greyhounds, golden retrievers, and great Pyrenees, high-resolution comparative genomic hybridization studies similarly identified high recurrent copy number loss encompassing the *PTEN* gene in 30% of samples.[75] In addition to the *PTEN* gene, other genes identified by high-resolution comparative genome hybridization studies potentially involved in the genetic pathogenesis of OS included overexpression of *RHOC* and *RUNX2* and underexpression of *TUSC3*.[75]

A growing body of evidence in dogs supports breed-associated inheritance of OS, especially in Scottish deerhounds, Rottweilers, greyhounds, Great Danes, Saint Bernards, and Irish wolfhounds.[24,30,76-79] Many domestic dog breeds have narrow genetic diversity as a consequence of selective breeding practices; this has provided the opportunity to more clearly elucidate the heritability of OS in dogs. For Scottish deerhounds in particular, the reported incidence of OS formation is 15%,[76,77] and the narrow heritability in this breed was 0.69, indicating that 69% of the cause for OS development in Scottish deerhounds is due to heritable trait, likely a Mendelian major gene with dominant expression.[77] Further studies in Scottish deerhounds using a whole genome linkage approach have mapped a novel locus (OSA1) for OS formation in this breed to CFA34 and provide the opportunity to pinpoint specific candidate genes directly involved in OS etiology for this specific dog breed.

Molecular Factors

Because of the heterogeneous and chaotic nature of OS, it has been difficult to definitively ascribe specific molecular derangements responsible for the etiopathogenesis of OS.[80] Nonetheless, substantive progress has been achieved through experimental, preclinical, and comparative investigations to identify dysregulated intracellular signaling and cell survival pathways likely to participate in the pathogenesis of OS. Significantly, the identification and tumorigenic consequences of several putative pathways have been recently characterized not only in immortalized OS cell lines but also in spontaneously arising OS samples.

The *MET* proto-oncogene encodes a tyrosine kinase receptor that on ligation with hepatocyte growth factor (HGF) mediates multiple cellular functions, including cell scattering, motility, and proliferation. Given its biologic activities, excessive or dysregulated *MET* signaling in canine OS has been demonstrated to promote tumorigenic phenotypes in cell lines.[81-83] Furthermore, in a small pilot study with spontaneously arising OS samples, the expression of *MET* proto-oncogene was identified in the majority (5/7, 71%) of tumor specimens by northern blot analysis.[84] Additionally, a novel germline mutation that results in constitutive receptor phosphorylation and aberrant MET signaling has been identified primarily in the Rottweiler breed.[85] In a larger study of 59 primary OS samples, mRNA expressions for *MET* and HGF were detected by real-time PCR (RT-PCR) in all specimens and suggested the existence of a putative *MET*/HGF autocrine or paracrine feedback loop.[86] In a subset of OS samples, proteolytically activated HGF was identified in homogenized tumor lysates (n = 6) by western blot, and MET protein was expressed by 100% of tumors analyzed (n = 16) by IHC. Increased expression of *MET* mRNA correlated with regional lymph node metastases, supporting the participation of *MET* signaling for metastases and cell invasion.

The cellular effects of growth hormone (GH) are mediated through the hepatic production of insulin-like growth factor-1 (IGF-1). In osteoblasts, IGF-1 induces cell mitogenesis and protection from apoptosis, as well as promoting angiogenesis. Derived from experimental and preclinical investigations, aberrant or excessive IGF-1 signaling likely participates in OS pathogenesis. In three canine OS cell lines, the expression and functionality of the IGF-1/IGF-1 receptor (IGF-1R) signaling cascade has been reported.[87] In all cell lines, IGF-1R expression was confirmed by northern blot analysis and radioligand binding studies; however, despite uniform receptor expression, IGF-1–mediated promotion of anchorage independent growth and invasion appeared to be cell-line specific.[87] Furthermore, to validate IGF-1/IGF-1R as a molecular target, dogs treated with definitive surgery and systemic chemotherapy received a long-acting somatostatin analog (OncoLAR) in an adjuvant setting to attenuate the protumorigenic effects of IGF-1. Despite significant reductions in circulating IGF-1 concentrations, no clinical benefit was detected in dogs treated with OncoLAR compared to placebo.[88]

The proto-oncogene *erbB-2* encodes human epidermal growth factor receptor-2 (HER-2), which is a tyrosine kinase receptor capable of promoting cell transformation and growth. In both dogs and humans, the overexpression of HER2 protein as a result of gene amplification is a negative prognostic factor in mammary carcinoma; however, less clarity exists for the role of HER2 overexpression in OS.[89,90] To better characterize HER2 expressions in canine OS, one study evaluated *HER2* mRNA transcript and protein expressions in seven cell lines and 10 OS tumor specimens.[91] Based on RT-PCR, the majority of OS cell lines (6/7) and 40% of primary OS tumor samples overexpressed HER2. Similarly, the overexpression of HER2 protein was confirmed by IHC. Although not adequately powered, the results of the study suggested the possibility of HER2 overexpression as a negative prognostic factor for survival.

The mammalian target of rapamycin (mTOR) is an evolutionary conserved protein kinase downstream of Akt, which acts as a central hub for the integration of cellular signals induced by growth factors, nutrients, energy, and stress for the purposes of regulating cell cycle progression and growth. As such, aberrant signaling through the mTOR pathway contributes to growth, survival, and chemotherapy resistance in multiple tumor types. To characterize the functionality of the mTOR pathway in canine OS, one study using three canine OS cell lines investigated the expressions of mTOR and p70S6K, a downstream effector protein of mTOR.[92] Study results indicated that the mTOR pathway was active in canine OS cells, and phosphorylation of mTOR and p70S6K could be inhibited by rapamycin, resulting in apoptosis and reduced growth of OS cells in vitro. In a complementary phase I dose-escalation study to assess the feasibility of mTOR inhibition as a treatment strategy, the pharmacokinetics and pharmacodynamics of rapamycin were investigated in dogs with primary OS.[93] Results from the phase I trial demonstrated that biologically effective concentrations of rapamycin were safely obtainable in dogs and that modulation of mTOR target proteins by rapamycin was achievable within the bone tumor microenvironment.

The tropomyosin-related kinase *(Trk)* proto-oncogenes encode for high-affinity receptor tyrosine kinases (RTKs), including TrkA, B, and C. Specifically in osteoblasts, TrkA receptor binds nerve growth factor (NGF), resulting in cellular mitogenesis and the inhibition of apoptosis. To characterize the possible involvement of TrkA signaling in OS pathogenesis, one study investigated the expression of TrkA and the functional consequences of TrkA receptor ligation in OS cell lines and tumor samples.[94] All canine OS cell lines (n = 2) and the majority of primary OS tumors (10/15) and pulmonary metastatic lesions (9/12) expressed TrkA receptors. Additionally, although TrkA signaling did not induce OS cell mitogenesis, blockade of basal TrkA signaling with either a small molecule inhibitor or blocking antibody increased serum starvation-induced apoptosis. The inhibition studies suggest that TrkA signaling participates in OS cell survival and may serve as a novel druggable target.

Telomeres are highly conserved nucleoprotein complexes at the ends of linear chromosomes that safeguard against harmful recombination events. The maintenance of telomere length and thus prevention of cellular senescence is through the activity of telomerase, a ribonucleoprotein complex that catalyzes the addition of telomeric sequences to the 3′ ends of chromosomes. Telomerase endows cells with infinite replicative capacity, and given its protumorigenic potential, telomerase has been investigated in canine OS. In an exploratory study, telomerase activity was identified in 100% of OS cell lines (5/5) and in the majority of primary tumors (5/6, 83%).[95] In a larger corroborative study using 67 OS tumors, telomerase activity was identified in 73% of OS samples and supported the hypothesis that the majority of OSs possess the enzymatic machinery required for infinite replicative capacity.[96]

In addition to various growth and survival pathways that potentially contribute to OS pathogenesis, the ability of OS cells to interact with their immediate microenvironment found in bone and lung tissues likely influences OS progression and metastases. Tissue invasion and focal osteolysis are hallmark characteristics of OS, and local disease progression is promoted by several OS-associated proteins, including matrix metalloproteinases (MMPs), receptor activator of NF-κB ligand (RANKL), and lysosomal cathepsin K.[97-100] Similar to the ability of OS cells to invade local tissues, specific proteins have been identified to participate in the progression of canine OS metastases, including ezrin,[101] a cytoskeletal linker protein, as well as CXCR4,[102] a chemokine receptor.

Pathology and Natural Behavior

OS is a malignant mesenchymal tumor of primitive bone cells. These cells produce an extracellular matrix of osteoid, and the presence of tumor osteoid is the basis for the histologic diagnosis, differentiating OS from other sarcomas of bone. The histologic pattern may vary between tumors or even within the same tumor. Small biopsy samples of an OS may lead to misdiagnoses such as chondrosarcoma, fibrosarcoma, hemangiosarcoma, or simply reactive bone. These histologic diagnoses from small biopsies must be interpreted with caution. It is important to obtain a histologic analysis of the entire tumor following definitive excision to confirm the diagnosis. There are many histologic subclassifications of OS based on the type and amount of matrix and characteristics of the cells: osteoblastic, chondroblastic, fibroblastic, poorly differentiated, and telangiectatic OS (a vascular subtype). Alkaline phosphatase staining on histopathologic and aspiration cytology specimens has been shown to aid in differentiating OS pathologically from other connective tissue tumors.[103-105] In dogs, it has not been well established that there is a difference in the biologic behavior of the different histologic subclassifications; however, histologic grade, based on microscopic features, may be predictive for systemic behavior (metastasis).[106] Newer techniques (see previous section) designed to recognize molecular or genetic alterations are being evaluated to determine their potential use in predicting behavior of OS.[107] The degree of aneuploidy, as measured by flow cytometry, of primary and metastatic tumors is potentially indicative of biologic behavior.[80] OS has very aggressive local effects and causes lysis, production of bone, or both processes, which can occur concurrently (Figure 24-1). The local disease is usually attended by soft tissue swelling. Pathologic fracture of the affected bone can occur. Pathologic fracture at presentation in humans and dogs with OS does not necessarily preclude limb salvage and does not carry a worse prognosis than patients without fracture at presentation.[108-111] OS rarely will cross a joint surface. This confinement to the bone may be secondary to collagenase inhibitors limiting progression through synovium.[112,113]

Metastasis is very common and arises early in the course of the disease, although usually subclinically. Although less than 15% of dogs have radiographically detectable pulmonary or osseous metastasis at presentation, approximately 90% will die within 1 year (median survival time [MST]: 19 weeks) with metastatic disease, usually to the lungs, when amputation is the only treatment.[2,15] Metastasis via the hematogenous route is most common; however, on rare occasions, extension to regional lymph nodes may occur.[114] Although the lung is the most commonly reported site for metastasis, tumor spread to bones or other soft tissue sites occurs with some frequency.[115] An increase in the incidence of bone metastasis following systemic chemotherapy has also been documented in humans and is suspected in dogs.[116,117] Possible explanations for this change include a change in the behavior of this cancer independent of treatment; selective killing of metastatic cancer by chemotherapy in certain sites such as the lung, which allows metastasis in other sites to become clinically relevant; lung resection and chemotherapy have improved survival, and bone sites become clinically relevant; more sensitive detection methods, which allow previously undetectable metastases to be seen; or more complete and detailed necropsies compared to those performed previously, which identify asymptomatic metastatic sites. The concept of concomitant tumor resistance has been described in which animals harboring large primary tumors are resistant to the growth of smaller metastatic tumors by systemic angiogenic suppression.[118] Development and growth of metastatic lesions can be rapid after the removal of the primary tumor and consequent increase in angiogenic activity in animal OS models.[119] Suspected locoregional synchronous regional bone metastases (skip metastases) have also been reported.[120] Skip metastases in human patients are a rare (1% to 6%) presentation and have a poor prognosis.[121] Whole body magnetic resonance imaging (MRI) or positron emission tomography/computed tomography (PET/CT) imaging can aid in detection of occult skip metastases. Some differences in metastatic behavior have been observed based on the anatomic location of the primary OS site. For example, mandibular OS and, to a degree, other calvarium locations may have a less aggressive metastatic behavior, although contradictory evidence exists (see the later section on Therapy and Prognosis).[122,123]

There is a report of four cases of histologically confirmed OS that subsequently underwent spontaneous regression without tumor-specific treatment.[124] This phenomenon, while extremely rare, has also been reported in humans.

History and Clinical Signs

Dogs with OS of appendicular sites generally present with a lameness and swelling at the primary site. There may be a history of mild trauma just prior to the onset of lameness. This history can often lead to misdiagnosis as another orthopedic or soft tissue injury. The pain is likely due to microfractures or disruption of the periosteum induced by osteolysis of cortical bone with tumor extension from the medullary canal. The lameness worsens and a moderately firm-to-soft, variably painful swelling arises at the primary site. Dogs may present with acute, severe lameness associated with pathologic fractures, although pathologic fractures account for less than 3% of all fractures seen.[59] Large- and giant-breed dogs that present with lameness or localized swelling at metaphyseal sites should be evaluated with OS as a likely diagnosis.

The signs associated with axial skeletal OS are site dependent. Signs vary from localized swelling with or without lameness to

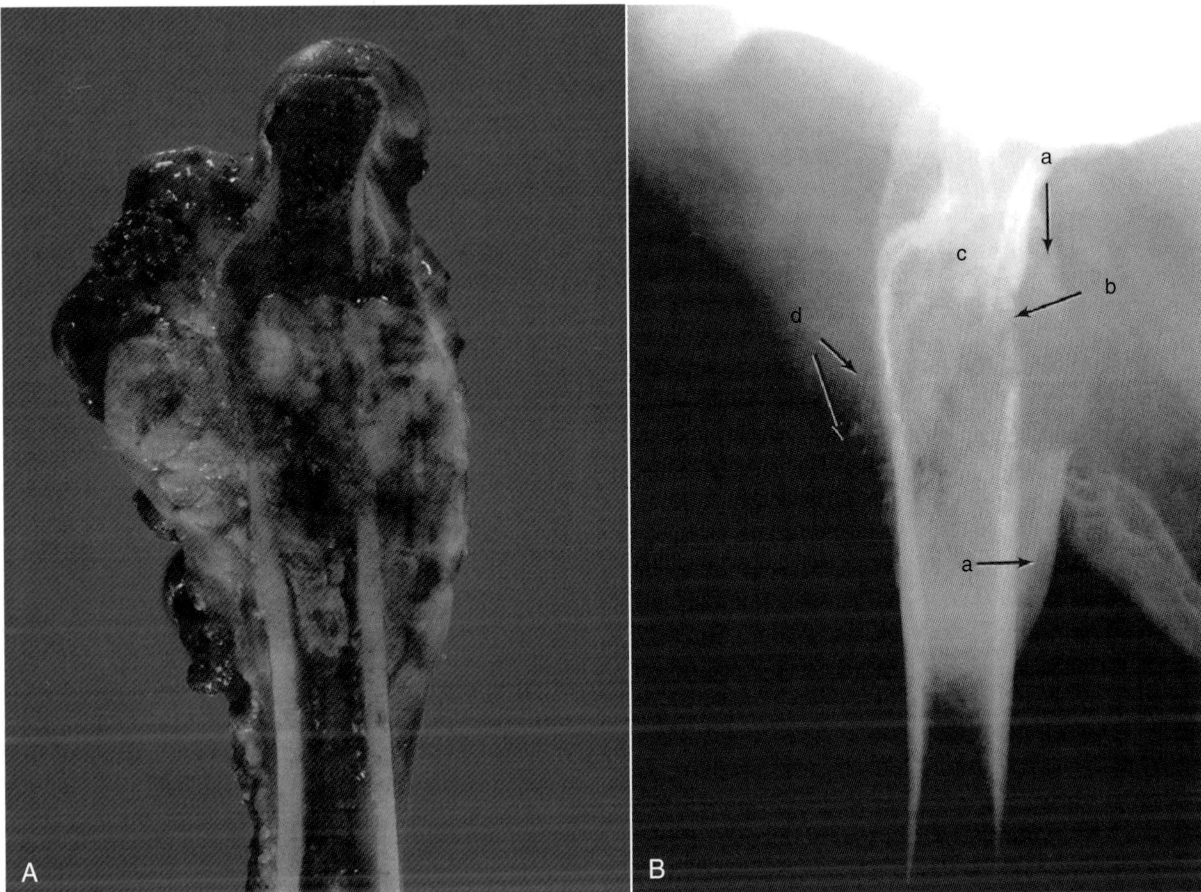

FIGURE 24-1 **A,** Gross, longitudinally split specimen of a proximal femoral OS lesion in a dog showing cortical destruction, soft tissue, and osteoid neoplastic components. **B,** Lateral radiograph of a proximal femoral OS lesion from the case in **A.** Radiographic features include *(a)* Codman's triangle, *(b)* cortical lysis, *(c)* loss of trabecular pattern in the metaphyses, and *(d)* tumor bone extension into the soft tissues in a sunburst pattern.

dysphagia (oral sites), exophthalmos and pain on opening the mouth (caudal mandibular or orbital sites), facial deformity and nasal discharge (sinus and nasal cavity sites), and hyperesthesia with or without neurologic signs (spinal sites). Dogs with tumors arising from ribs usually present because of a palpable, variably painful mass. Respiratory signs are not common even where the lesions have large intrathoracic components, and malignant pleural effusion is quite rare.

Dogs rarely have respiratory signs as the first clinical evidence of pulmonary metastasis; rather, their first signs are usually vague. With radiographically detectable pulmonary metastasis, dogs may remain asymptomatic for many months, but most dogs develop decreased appetites and nonspecific signs such as malaise within 1 month. Hypertrophic osteopathy may develop in dogs with pulmonary metastasis (see Chapter 5).

Systemic Alterations

Alterations in energy expenditure, protein synthesis, urinary nitrogen loss, and carbohydrate flux have been documented in dogs with OS, similar to results documented in humans with neoplasia. Changes were documented in resting energy expenditure and protein and carbohydrate metabolism in dogs with OS. These changes were evident even in dogs that did not have clinical signs of cachexia.[125] Systemic, metabolic derangements reported for dogs with OS include lower chromium and zinc levels, lower iron and iron-binding capacity, and increased ferritin levels as compared to normal dogs.[126] Hypercalcemia is extremely rare. The impact of these changes on patient treatment, response, or outcome is unknown.

Diagnostic Techniques and Work-Up

Radiology

Initial evaluation of the primary site involves interpretation of good quality radiographs taken in lateral and craniocaudal projections. Special views may be necessary for lesions occurring in sites other than in the appendicular skeleton. The overall radiographic abnormality of bone varies from mostly bone lysis to almost entirely osteoblastic or osteogenic changes (see Figure 24-1, *B*). There is an entire spectrum of changes between these two extremes, and the appearance of OS can be quite variable. There are some features, however, that are commonly seen. Cortical lysis is a feature of OS and may be severe enough to leave obvious areas of discontinuity of the cortex leading to pathologic fracture. There is often soft tissue extension with an obvious soft tissue swelling, and new bone (tumor or reactive bone) may form in these areas in a palisading pattern perpendicular or radiating from the axis of the cortex (i.e., "sunburst"). As tumor invades the cortex, the periosteum is elevated and new bone is laid down by the cambium layer providing a triangular-appearing deposition of dense new bone on the cortex at the periphery of the lesion. This periosteal new bone has been called "Codman's triangle," but this is not pathognomonic for OS. OS does not directly cross articular cartilage, and primary lesions usually remain monostotic. The tumors may extend into periarticular soft tissues, however, and adjacent bones are at risk because of extension through adjacent soft tissue structures. Other radiographic changes that can attend OS are loss of the fine trabecular pattern in the metaphysis, a vague transition zone at the periphery of the medullary extent of the lesion (rather than a sharp sclerotic margin), or areas of fine punctate lysis. Any one or combinations of these changes may be seen, depending on the size, histologic subtype, location, and duration of the lesion. The radiographic appearance of OS is similar to osteomyelitis, specifically of fungal etiology.[127] In cases in which the travel or clinical history might support the possibility of osteomyelitis, a biopsy with submission for histology and culture may be warranted.

Based on signalment, history, physical examination, and radiographic findings, a presumptive diagnosis of OS can be made. Differential diagnoses of lytic, proliferative, or mixed pattern aggressive bone lesions identified on radiographs include other primary bone tumors (chondrosarcoma, fibrosarcoma, hemangiosarcoma); metastatic bone cancer; multiple myeloma or lymphoma of bone; systemic mycosis with bony localization; bacterial osteomyelitis; and, albeit rare, bone cysts.

Other primary bone tumors are far less common but may be suspected, especially in dogs with unusual signalment or tumor location. Metastatic cancer can spread to bone from almost any malignancy. A careful physical examination is important, including a rectal examination, with special attention paid to the genitourinary system to help rule out the presence of a primary cancer. Dogs with a history of cancer in the past should have their original biopsy reviewed and should be restaged for the original disease. Common sites for metastatic bone cancer are lumbar and sacral vertebrae, pelvis, and diaphyses of long bones. There are usually other clues for the diagnosis of multiple myeloma, such as hyperproteinemia, and both multiple myeloma and lymphoma of bone are usually attended by radiographic lesions that are almost entirely lytic. Two classic radiographic appearances of myeloma bone lesions are described: "punched-out" areas of lysis or a generalized osteoporotic thinning of cortices.

Tissue Biopsy

A diagnosis of primary malignant bone tumor may be suggested by signalment, history, physical examination, and radiographic findings. Cytology has not been thought to be definitive for diagnosis; however, it may support the tentative diagnosis, and enough confidence in the diagnosis, combined with clinical features and radiographic appearance, may exist to facilitate a discussion of treatment options. Consistent cytologic criteria of OS has recently been described, and with repeated evaluations, dependent on experience, cytopathologists may be more definitive in making a diagnosis from cytology alone.[128,129] Alkaline phosphatase staining of cytologic samples has been shown to differentiate OS from other vimentin-positive tumors.[103] However, in most cases, a definitive diagnosis lies in procurement and interpretation of tissue for histopathology. With new treatments such as limb sparing (see subsequent sections), knowledge of the specific tumor type may avoid overextension or inappropriate treatment of bone tumors thought to be OS (e.g., chondrosarcoma, myeloma, or lymphoma). It is crucial to the success of a limb-sparing surgery that the biopsy procedure is planned and performed carefully with close attention to asepsis, hemostasis, and wound closure.[130] The skin incision for the biopsy must be small and placed so that it can be completely excised with the tumor at limb sparing without compromising the procedure. Transverse or large incisions must be avoided. It has been recommended that the surgeon who is to perform the definitive surgical procedure (especially if limb sparing) should be the person to perform the preoperative bone biopsy.[131]

Bone biopsy may be performed as an open incisional, closed needle (Figure 24-2), or trephine biopsy. The advantage of an open technique is that a large sample of tissue is procured, which presumably improves the likelihood of establishing an accurate histologic diagnosis. Unfortunately, this advantage may be outweighed by the disadvantages of an involved operative procedure and risk of postsurgical complications such as hematoma formation, wound breakdown, infection, local seeding of tumor, and pathologic fracture.[132,133] Although biopsy with a trephine yields a diagnostic accuracy rate of 93.8%, there is the increased risk of creating pathologic fracture when compared with using a smaller gauge needle.[134] This underscores some of the advantages of a closed biopsy using a Jamshidi bone marrow biopsy needle (Jamshidi bone marrow needle, American Pharmaseal Co, Valencia, CA; bone marrow biopsy needle, Sherwood Medical Co, St. Louis, MO) or similar type of needle. Jamshidi needle biopsy has an accuracy rate of 91.9% for detecting tumor versus other disorders and an 82.3% accuracy rate for diagnosis of specific tumor subtype.[135] Accuracy of diagnoses from needle core samples can depend on the pathologist's experience and comfort level with examining small samples. Histology reports indicating the presence of reactive bone should not rule out the presence of a primary bone tumor or other pathology, especially if the radiographic changes suggest tumor. In some cases, it can be very difficult to get the diagnosis by preoperative biopsy (i.e., repeated biopsy attempts yield "reactive bone") and yet the pathologist has no trouble identifying tumor when the entire specimen is available for histopathologic analysis (e.g., postamputation), This is likely a result of the heterogeneity of the tumor tissue itself and the large amount of reactive bone present within the tumor.

The biopsy site is selected carefully. Radiographs (two views) are reviewed, and the center of the lesion chosen for biopsy. Biopsy at the lesion periphery will often result in sampling the reactive bone surrounding the tumor growth without a resulting diagnosis.[135] The skin incision is made so the biopsy tract and any potentially seeded tumor cells can be completely removed at the time of definitive surgery. Care is used to avoid major nerves, vessels, and joint spaces. A 4-inch, 8- or 11-gauge needle is used. With the dog anesthetized, prepared, and draped for surgery, a small stab incision (2 to 3 mm) is made in the skin with a #11 scalpel blade. The bone needle cannula, with the stylet locked in place, is pushed through the soft tissue to the bone cortex. The stylet is removed, and the cannula is advanced through the bone cortex into the medullary cavity using a gentle twisting motion and firm pressure. The opposite cortex is not penetrated. The needle is removed, and the specimen is gently pushed out of the base of the cannula by inserting the probe into the cannula tip. One or two more samples can be obtained by redirecting the needle through the same skin incision so that samples of the transition zone may also be obtained. Ideal specimens should be 1 or 2 cm in length and not fragmented. Biopsy is repeated until solid tissue cores are obtained. Material for culture and cytology may be taken from the samples prior to fixation in 10% neutral buffered formalin. Diagnostic accuracy is improved when samples are evaluated by a pathologist thoroughly familiar with bone cancer. Fluoroscopy or advanced imaging (CT) can assist in obtaining needle-core biopsy samples of suspected bone lesions, especially for axial sites.[136]

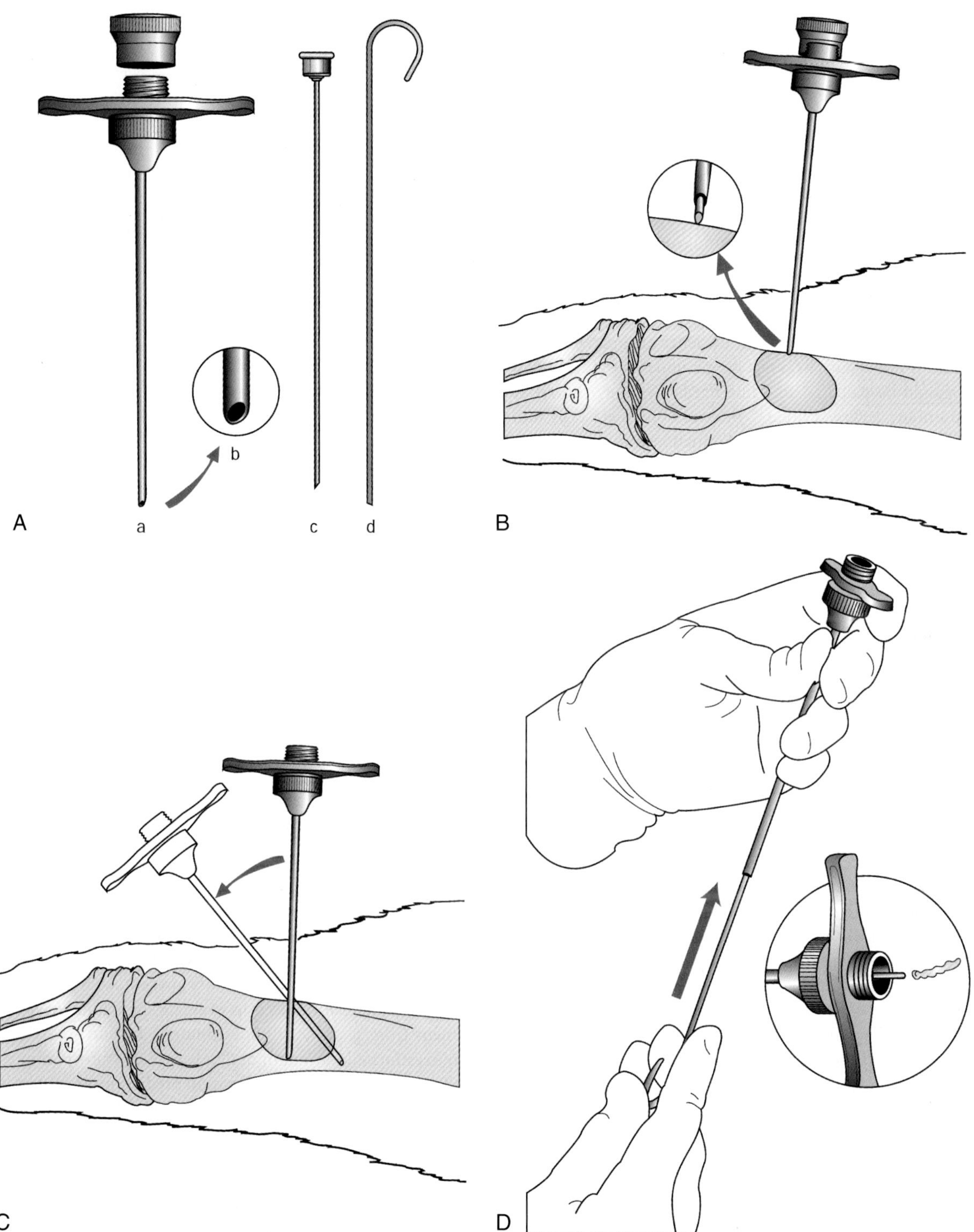

FIGURE 24-2 **A**, The Jamshidi bone biopsy needle: cannula and screw-on cap *(a)*, tapered point *(b)*, pointed stylet to advance cannula through soft tissues *(c)*, and probe to expel specimen from cannula *(d)*. **B,** With the stylet locked in place, the cannula is advanced through the soft tissue until bone is reached. The inset is a close-up view showing stylet against bone cortex. **C,** The stylet is removed, and the bone cortex penetrated with the cannula. The cannula is withdrawn, and the procedure repeated with redirection of the instrument to obtain multiple core samples. **D,** The probe is then inserted retrograde into the tip of the cannula to expel the specimen through the base *(inset)*. *(Reprinted with permission from Powers BE, LaRue SM, Withrow SJ, et al: Jamshidi needle biopsy for diagnosis of bone lesions in small animals,* J Am Vet Med Assoc *193:206–207, 1988.)*

After tumor removal (amputation or limb sparing), histology should be performed on a larger specimen to confirm the preoperative diagnosis. If the clinical and radiographic features are typical for OS, especially when there is little possibility of fungal or bacterial infection, confirmation of histologic diagnosis following surgical treatment of local disease (amputation or limb sparing) can be considered. Few diseases causing advanced destruction of the bone can be effectively treated without removal of the local disease. If the owners are willing to treat aggressively, surgical removal of local disease with biopsy submission following surgery may be acceptable.

Staging and Patient Assessment

Systemic Staging Examination for evidence of apparent spread of the disease is important. Regional lymph nodes, although rarely involved, should be palpated, and fine needle cytology should be performed on any enlarged node.[114] Sites of bone metastasis may be detected by a careful orthopedic examination with palpation of long bones and the accessible axial skeleton. Organomegaly may be detected by abdominal palpation. Usually, pulmonary metastases are undetectable by clinical examination, but careful thoracic auscultation is important to detect intercurrent cardiopulmonary disorders. High-detail thoracic radiographs should be taken during inspiration with the patient awake. Although some controversy exists,[137] it is still considered important by most oncologists to include three views: a ventrodorsal or a dorsoventral view and both right and left lateral views. OS pulmonary metastases are generally soft tissue dense and cannot be detected radiographically until the nodules are 6 to 8 mm in diameter. It is uncommon to detect pulmonary metastatic disease at the time of diagnosis (<10% of dogs). Advanced imaging (e.g., CT, MRI, PET/CT) may play a role in patient staging and is used to evaluate for pulmonary metastases and for evaluation of tumor vascularity, soft tissue and medullary involvement, metabolic or functional activity, and response to treatment.[138,139] Currently, published treatment recommendations and prognoses are based on the results of plain radiographs. As advanced imaging becomes more commonplace for staging dogs with OS, comparisons to previous protocols will be subject to stage-migration and lead-time bias because earlier diagnosis will result.[140]

Bone survey radiography has been useful in detecting dogs with second skeletal sites of OS.[29] Bone surveys include lateral radiographs of all bones in the body and a ventrodorsal projection of the pelvis using standard radiographic technique appropriate for the region radiographed. In one study, 171 dogs with primary bone tumors underwent radiographic bone surveys and thoracic radiography; at presentation, there was a higher yield in finding other sites of OS with radiographic bone survey (6.4%, 11 of 171 dogs) than with thoracic radiographs (4%, 7 of 171 dogs).[141] There are conflicting reports on the usefulness of nuclear scintigraphy (bone scan) (Figure 24-3) for clinical staging of dogs with OS.[142-146] Bone scintigraphy was used in one study to identify suspected second bone sites of OS in 14 of 25 dogs with appendicular primaries.[143] Seven of these lesions were biopsied and confirmed to be OS. Another study of 70 dogs with appendicular primary bone tumors resulted in only one scintigraphically detectable occult bone lesion.[142] In a third report, of 23 dogs with suspected skeletal neoplasia that were evaluated with scintigraphy and radiography, 4 dogs had second skeletal sites suspected to be neoplastic.[146] The suspicious site in one of these dogs was found on histologic evaluation to be normal bone. Another study found secondary sites considered highly suspect of bony metastasis in 7.8% of 399 cases; however, most suspected lesions were not subjected to histologic conformation.[144] Nuclear bone scan can be a useful tool for the detection and localization of bone metastasis in dogs presenting for vague lameness or signs such as back pain, and, although very sensitive, it is not specific for identifying sites of skeletal tumor. Any region of osteoblastic activity will be identified by this technique, including osteoarthritis and infection. Follow-up with high-detail radiographs of sites found suspicious on scintigraphy will generally help rule out nonneoplastic disease; however, definitive biopsy may be necessary.

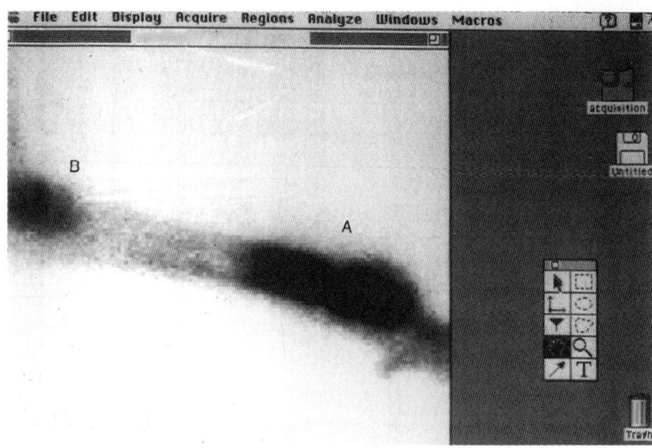

FIGURE 24-3 Scintigraphic view of a distal radial OS lesion in a dog following Tecnetium^{99M}-hydroxymethylene diphosphonate injection. *A*, Uptake within the tumor. *B*, Mild uptake within the elbow joint secondary to degenerative joint disease.

Surgical Staging A surgical staging system for sarcomas of the skeleton has been devised for humans.[147] This system is based on the histologic grade (G), the anatomic setting of the primary tumor (T), and regional or distant metastasis (M). There are three stages: stage I, the low-grade (G1) lesions without metastasis; stage II, the high-grade (G2) lesions without metastasis; and stage III, the lesion with regional or distant metastasis regardless of histologic grade. The stages are subdivided by the anatomic setting: *A* is intracompartmental (T1) and *B* is extracompartmental (T2). According to this system, most dogs with OS present with stage IIB disease. Scintigraphy can be used to evaluate the degree of bone involvement from a primary bone tumor.[148] In one study, scintigraphy overestimated the length of OS disease in limb-sparing patients by 30%, allowing for adequate margin prediction, preoperatively.[149] CT may be useful to plan surgery, especially for tumors located in the axial skeleton; however, one study reported that plain radiographs were as accurate as advanced imaging (CT, MRI) in predicting true length of tumor involvement.[150] In contrast, MRI was more accurate than plain radiographs or CT in predicting length of tumor involvement for appendicular canine OS in another study.[151] This could prove invaluable for limb-sparing patients, and further evaluation is warranted.

Patient Assessment The patient's overall health status requires careful assessment. Advancing years do not preclude treatment; however, prolonged anesthesia and chemotherapy may not be tolerated in dogs with organ compromise. Particular attention to the cardiovascular system is important. Coexisting cardiomyopathy or any degree of heart failure may lead to serious complications, particularly during fluid diuresis, anesthesia, or administration of certain chemotherapy agents. Electrocardiogram and echocardiogram should be performed on dogs in which the history or physical findings implicate a cardiac disorder. Renal function must be evaluated prior to administration of cisplatin. A minimum database should include a complete blood count (CBC), platelet count, serum biochemical analysis, and urinalysis.

Known or Suggested Prognostic Factors

Anatomic Location and Signalment

In a multiinstitutional study of 162 dogs with appendicular OS treated with amputation alone, dogs younger than 5 years of age had shorter survival than older dogs.[15] Additional studies have related large tumor size[13,152,153] and humerus location[154,155] to poor outcome. Large tumor size has been reported to be a negative prognostic factor for humans with OS.[156] For OS originating from flat bones, small dog size and completeness of excision were positive prognostic indicators.[157] Although there are differences in disease distribution and prevalence, documentation of improved survival for small dogs with OS is lacking.[158] A negative prognosis can also be predicted by a higher tumor grade and mitotic index, based on the results of one study.[106]

The biologic behavior for nonappendicular sites of OS appears to be similar (aggressive) with the exception of the mandible and possibly the rest of the calvarium.[122,123,159-162] OS affecting the head (mandible, maxilla, and skull) is locally aggressive but has a lower metastatic rate (37%) than appendicular OS.[162] Reported median disease-free intervals (DFIs) and survival times for skull OS are 191 days and 204 days, respectively. Dogs with OS of the mandible treated with mandibulectomy alone had a 1-year survival rate of 71% in one study.[122] In contrast, maxillary OSs have demonstrated a median survival of 5 months following maxillectomy.[159,160] A study evaluating response to treatment for orbital OS reported long-term survival following complete surgical excision.[163] Similar behavior is seen for OSs of flat bones in humans.[164] Median survival for rib OS lesions is reported to be 3 months for dogs treated with rib resection alone and 8 months for dogs treated with resection and adjuvant chemotherapy.[165-168] OS of the canine scapula has been reported to have a poor prognosis when treated with subtotal scapulectomy surgery and chemotherapy.[157,169,170] DFI and MST in dogs diagnosed with scapula OS was 210 days (range 118 to 245 days) and 246 days (range 177 to 651 days), respectively.[171] Use of adjunctive chemotherapy was prognostic for both increased DFI and survival. Limb function after subtotal scapulectomy is good to excellent.[171] Survival of dogs with OS distal to the antebrachiocarpal or tarsocrural joints was somewhat longer (median: 466 days) than survival of dogs with OSs of more common appendicular sites; however, OS in these sites is aggressive, with a high potential for metastasis.[26] Vertebral OS is uncommon; however, reported cases indicate aggressive local and systemic behavior.[22,172] In 15 dogs treated with a combination of surgery, radiation, and chemotherapy, the median survival was 4 months.[172] The biologic behavior of OS in other nonappendicular bone sites (e.g., pelvis) has not been thoroughly evaluated.

Extraskeletal OS is rare and most commonly affects visceral sites (gastrointestinal tract, spleen, liver, kidney, urinary bladder), skin or subcutaneous tissue, or mammary glands. Extraskeletal (soft tissue) OS sites also appear to have aggressive systemic behavior with a high metastatic rate. In one report, extraskeletal OS treated with surgery alone had a median survival of only 1 month, and a median survival of 5 months was obtained for cases treated with surgery and adjuvant chemotherapy.[31] In a larger study, soft tissue OSs were separated from mammary gland OSs; median survival of nonmammary gland soft tissue lesions was 1 month and mammary gland lesions 3 months following primarily surgical resection alone.[32] The major cause of death was local recurrence (92%) in the soft tissue OS cases and pulmonary metastasis (62.5%) in the mammary gland OS cases.

Dogs presented with stage III disease (measurable metastases) have a very poor prognosis.[115] MST of 90 dogs with stage III disease at presentation was 76 days, with a range of 0 to 1583 days. No significant differences in survival times on the basis of age, sex, breed, or primary site were observed. Dogs with bone metastases (132 days) had a longer survival time than dogs with lung (59 days) or lung and other soft tissue (19 days) metastases. Dogs with lymph node metastasis had short survivals with a median of only 57 to 59 days, compared to 318 days for dogs without nodal spread.[114,115] Dogs with stage III disease treated palliatively with RT and chemotherapy had a significantly longer survival time (130 days) than dogs in all other treatment groups.

Serum Alkaline Phosphatase Elevated alkaline phosphatase (AP) has been clearly associated with a poorer prognosis for dogs with appendicular OS in several studies.[114,154,173-175] A preoperative elevation of either total (serum) or the bone isoenzyme of AP (>110 U/L or 23 U/L, respectively) is associated with a shorter DFI and survival (Figure 24-4). Likewise, dogs that have elevated preoperative values that do not return to normal within 40 days following surgical removal of the primary lesion also develop earlier metastasis. One study substantiated the predictive nature of elevated preoperative AP levels; however, no association was found for elevated postoperative serum levels.[173]

Molecular, Genetic, and Immunologic Indices of Prognosis Although our understanding of the pathogenesis of OS remains incomplete, the availability of canine-specific reagents, as well as sequencing of the canine genome, has permitted the discovery of key molecular, genetic, and immunologic events that might participate in OS progression and metastases. With increased clarity for the critical events involved in directing OS biology, specific tumor- and host-associated characteristics have recently been identified as important factors that influence OS prognosis.

The expression of several molecular proteins, including ezrin, recepteur d'origine nantaise (RON), survivin, vascular endothelial growth factor (VEGF), and cyclooxygenase-2 (COX-2), has been reported to influence DFI and survival times in dogs.[101,176-179] Ezrin is a cellular protein belonging to the ERM (ezrin-radixin-moesin) family and serves as a physical and functional anchor site for cytoskeletal F-actin fibers. Because of ezrin's involvement in cytoskeletal remodeling, it has been demonstrated in murine preclinical models that ezrin is necessary for OS metastases.[101] Through the use of a canine tissue microarray with known clinical outcome data (n = 73), it was shown that the presence of high ezrin staining in primary tumors was associated with a significantly shorter median DFI compared to dogs with low primary tumor ezrin staining, 116 versus 188 days, respectively.

HGF receptor (MET) and RON are members of the *MET* proto-oncogene family of RTKs, and signaling through MET or RON promotes tumorigenesis and the formation of metastases. MET and RON are capable of heterodimerization with one another, resulting in cellular cross-talk that might alter the strength and duration of signal transduction, with resultant protumorigenic effects. Given the role of MET and RON in metastases, their expression in OS has been evaluated in dogs.[176] Through the use of a canine OS tissue array with linked outcome data (n = 105), expression of RON but not MET was prognostic for survival. Dogs with high RON expression in their primary tumors lived significantly shorter than dogs with absent, low, or intermediate RON expression.

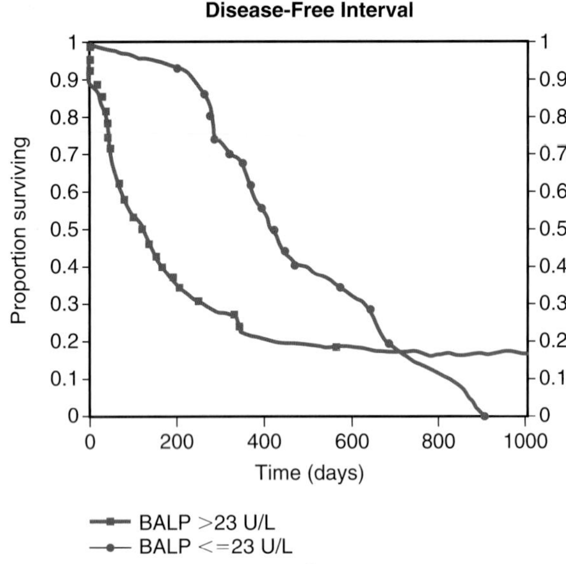

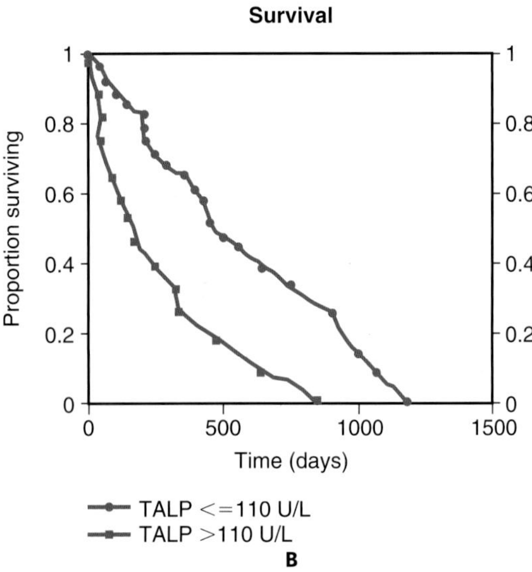

FIGURE 24-4 **A,** Disease-free interval (DFI) outcome of dogs treated for OS comparing bone alkaline phosphatase levels above and below 23 U/L preoperatively. **B,** Survival outcome of dogs treated for OS comparing serum alkaline phosphatase levels above and below 110 U/L preoperatively. *BALP,* Bone alkaline phosphatase; *TALP,* total alkaline phosphatase. *(Reprinted with permission from Erhart N, Dernell WS, Hoffmann WE, et al: Prognostic importance of alkaline phosphatase activity in serum from dogs with appendicular OS: 75 cases (1990-1996),* J Am Vet Med Assoc *213:1003, 1998.)*

Survivin is a small protein belonging to the inhibitor of apoptosis (IAP) family and participates in the processes of cell division, as well as apoptosis inhibition. As a dimer, survivin inhibits both caspase-dependent and caspase-independent mediated apoptosis, and its expression can promote tumorigenesis. Given survivin's antiapoptotic properties, its overexpression might provide a survival advantage to cancer cells and be associated with a negative prognosis. In a recent study, the expression of survivin was characterized in 67 primary OS samples with known outcome data.[178] Survivin expression was detected in the majority of tissue samples (65/67), and expression intensity was associated with DFIs. Dogs with primary tumors expressing low survivin immunoreactivity scores achieved significantly longer DFIs than dogs with high survivin immunoreactivity scores within the primary tumor, 331 and 173 days, respectively.

VEGF and the enzymatic activities of COX-2 serve as potent regulators of angiogenesis, and their independent expressions have been associated with a poorer prognosis for a variety of cancers. Angiogenesis is a necessary step for tumor growth and metastases; thus both VEGF and COX-2 have been investigated in dogs with OS.[177,179] In one study with 25 dogs treated with definitive surgery and systemic chemotherapy, baseline platelet-corrected serum VEGF concentrations were associated with DFI but not survival time.[179] Dogs with VEGF concentration in the lower 50 percentile achieved significantly longer DFIs than dogs with VEGF levels in the upper 50 percentile, 356 and 145 days, respectively. In another study, COX-2 expression was characterized in primary tumors derived from 44 dogs treated with amputation and doxorubicin.[177] Immunoreactivity for COX-2 was identified in 88% of primary tumors, although intratumoral COX-2 staining was variable and heterogeneous. A COX-2 immunoreactivity score, a product of stain intensity and percentage of positive cells, was potentially correlated with disease outcome. Dogs with primary tumors demonstrating strong stain intensity (n = 4) had a significantly shorter MST of 86 days in comparison with dogs with tumors staining negative (n = 10, MST: 423 days), poor (n = 19, MST: 399 days), or moderate (n = 11, MST: 370 days) for COX-2. However, given the small sample size of dogs with strong COX-2–staining intensity, the prognostic value of COX-2 expression in OS warrants a more thorough evaluation.

With the near complete sequencing of the canine genome and the commercial availability of canine-specific gene microarrays, it has become possible to characterize and validate specific tumor-associated genetic determinants associated with clinical outcomes and prognosis. In one gene expression profiling study, primary OS tissues were analyzed from two groups of dogs with different clinical outcomes, specifically dogs achieving DFIs either less than 100 days (n = 10) or greater than 300 days (n = 10) following uniform treatment with amputation and systemic chemotherapy.[107] Derived from microarray analysis and confirmed by RT-PCR, eight specific gene transcripts were significantly different between poor responders (<100 days) and good responders (>300 days). In dogs categorized as poor responders, six transcripts, including IGF-2 and alcohol dehydrogenase, were downregulated and two transcripts were upregulated in comparison to good responders. To better characterize the molecular pathways associated with the differentially expressed genes identified in microarray analysis, a broader systems approach was used to identify changes in groups of interacting genes or pathways that might contribute to metastatic progression or chemotherapy resistance. In general, pathway expression differences between good and poor responders involved oxidative phosphorylation, bone development, protein kinase A (PKA) signaling, cell adhesion, cytoskeletal remodeling, and immune response.

In a similar expression profiling study, prognostic gene profiles were derived from 32 primary OS tumors derived from two groups of dogs based on survival time.[180] Dogs surviving for less than 6 months or greater than 6 months were categorized as either poor or good responders, respectively. Gene profiling identified 51 gene transcripts to be differentially expressed; within the poor responder group, genes uniformly overexpressed were associated with biologic pathways involved in proliferation, drug resistance, and metastases. In addition to identifying differentially expressed genes and associated pathways between dogs categorized as good and poor responders, the findings from the study further substantiated the molecular pathway similarities shared between humans and dogs, including Wnt signaling, integrin signaling, and chemokine/cytokine signaling.

Finally, a highly impactful study was conducted that leveraged the more homogeneous genetic background of dogs diagnosed with OS to detect underlying and conserved gene expression patterns previously undetectable in historic canine and human gene microarray analysis.[181] By differential gene expression profiling of early passage immortalized OS cell lines derived from primary tumors, the investigators were able to identify gene signatures associated with G2/M transition and DNA damage checkpoint, as well as microenvironment interactions, which permitted the unbiased segregation of OS samples into distinct molecular subclassification and predicted outcome. Most significantly, the same genetic signatures identified in dogs, also allowed for prognostic molecular classification of human OS—powerfully underscoring the scientific merit derived from comparative oncologic studies.

Perturbations of the immune system are common among cancer patients, and regulatory T-cells (Tregs) and myeloid-derived suppressor cells have the capacity to attenuate effective antitumor immunity responses, with the potential to negatively impact prognosis. Tregs have been characterized in healthy and cancer-bearing dogs,[182-184] with some studies demonstrating that dogs with OS have increases in the percentage and absolute counts of circulating Tregs.[185] The clinical significance of Tregs on OS prognosis has recently been characterized in a study of 12 dogs treated uniformly with amputation and systemic chemotherapy.[185] Dogs with high (above mean) versus low (below mean) percentages of Tregs identified in blood or tumor tissue did not have differences in DFI or survival time. However, a high or low CD8/Treg ratio in the blood was associated with clinical outcomes because dogs with low CD8/Treg ratios (n = 6) were observed to have a significantly shorter survival time than dogs with high CD8/Treg ratios (n = 6).

In addition to Tregs and their potential prognostic value in OS, one study demonstrated that routine hemogram parameters, specifically lymphocyte and monocyte counts, can also predict clinical outcomes in dogs with OS.[155] In 69 dogs treated with amputation and systemic chemotherapy, baseline lymphocyte and monocyte counts were associated with DFIs. Shorter DFIs were observed in dogs (n = 69) initially presenting with relative lymphocytosis (≥1000 cells/μL) and relative monocytosis (≥400 cells/μL), and these original conclusions were further substantiated by a second population of OS dogs (n = 21) treated in an identical manner. Mechanistically, it was hypothesized that the association of relative monocytosis and reduced DFI could be the presence of myeloid-derived suppressor cells, a population of cells characterized by their ability to suppress antitumor immune response.

Therapy Directed at the Primary Tumor

Surgery

Table 24-1 provides an overview of surgical options for primary bone tumors based on anatomic site.

Amputation Amputation of the affected limb is the standard local treatment for canine appendicular OS. Even large- and giant-breed dogs usually function well after limb amputation, and most owners are pleased with their pets' mobility and quality of life after surgery.[210,211] Even moderate preexisting degenerative joint disease at the level found in most older, large-breed dogs is rarely a contraindication for amputation. Most dogs will readily compensate, and although the osteoarthritis may progress more rapidly in the three-legged dog, this rarely results in a clinical problem. Severe preexisting orthopedic or neurologic conditions may cause poor results in some cases, and careful preoperative examination is important. A complete forequarter amputation for forelimb lesions is generally recommended, as is a coxofemoral disarticulation amputation for hind leg lesions. This level of amputation ensures complete local disease removal and also results in a more cosmetic and functional outcome. For proximal femoral lesions, a complete amputation and en bloc acetabulectomy is recommended to obtain proximal soft tissue margins (Figure 24-5). Surgery alone must be considered palliative for OS because microscopic metastatic disease is present in the vast majority of cases at diagnosis, and amputation does not address these.

Limb-Sparing Surgery Although most dogs function well with amputation, in some dogs limb sparing would be preferred, such as dogs with severe preexisting orthopedic or neurologic disease or dogs with owners who absolutely will not permit amputation. Until recently, only a few reports of limb sparing in dogs, with limited follow-up, have appeared in the literature.[189-193] To date, more than 600 limb-sparing procedures have been performed at Colorado State University Animal Cancer Center (CSU-ACC). Limb function has generally been good to excellent in most dogs, and survival has not been adversely affected by removing the primary tumor with marginal resection.[194]

Suitable candidates for limb sparing include dogs with OS clinically and radiographically confined to the leg, dogs in which the primary tumor affects less than 50% of the bone (as determined radiographically), and dogs that are in otherwise good general health. Other criteria for consideration include absence of pathologic fracture, less than 360-degree involvement of soft tissues, and a firm/definable soft tissue mass versus an edematous lesion. Early in the development of limb-sparing procedures, many dogs treated at CSU-ACC received some form of preoperative treatment (i.e., primary or neoadjuvant intraarterial [IA] cisplatin, intravenous [IV] cisplatin, RT to the tumor bone, or a combination of radiotherapy with IV or IA cisplatin). Results from 21 dogs treated with RT alone given in large doses per fraction prior to limb sparing were unsatisfactory for preservation of life or limb.[191] Many of the dogs treated with two preoperative IA cisplatin doses 21 days apart, with the last treatment 21 days prior to surgery, showed marked decrease in the degree of vascularization of the tumor. This represented a high degree of induced tumor necrosis in the resected specimen, especially when combined with RT, and facilitated limb sparing.[193,212] Currently at CSU-ACC, case selection predetermines the use of local chemotherapy or preoperative downstaging for limb-sparing cases, and most dogs receive systemic carboplatin, doxorubicin, or combination therapy after surgery (see the later section on Systemic Adjuvant Therapy for Dogs with Osteosarcoma).

The most suitable patients for limb sparing are dogs with tumors in the distal radius or ulna because function following limb sparing and carpal arthrodesis is good. Arthrodesis of the scapulohumeral, coxofemoral, stifle, or tarsal joints following limb sparing generally results in only fair to poor function.[154] Resulting poor function, combined with a high complication rate, has generally led surgeons away from recommending limb sparing near these joints. Limb sparing is a complicated process and requires a coordinated team effort between surgical and medical oncologists, radiologists, pathologists, and technical staff. Several methods of limb sparing have been described, each with unique advantages and limitations.

TABLE 24-1 Surgical Treatment Options for Osteosarcoma by Site

SITE	TREATMENT OPTIONS	COMMENTS
Humerus, femur, tibia	Amputation Limb sparing in limited cases	Generally high complication rate for limb sparing[154] Diaphyseal locations amenable to intercalary allografts[186] Total hip sparing possible for proximal femoral lesions[187] Intraoperative extracorporeal radiation technique may apply[188]
Radius	Amputation Limb-sparing allograft[189-194] Endosteal prosthesis[187] Intercalary bone graft[186] Ulnar transposition[195,196] Bone transport osteogenesis[197-200] Pasteurized autograft[201,202] Extracorporeal intraoperative RT[188]	Can combine radius/ulna resection (graft radius only)
Ulna	Amputation Ulnectomy[204]	 Often does not require allograft reconstruction
Scapula	Amputation Scapulectomy[169,205]	Proximal lesions best; complete scapulectomy described
Pelvis	Pelvectomy with or without amputation[206]	Lateral portion of sacrum can be excised; may include body wall
Metacarpus/metatarsus	Amputation[25] Local resection[26]	 Limb-sparing function dependent on bone(s) involved
Mandible	Mandibulectomy[122]	Often requires total hemimandibulectomy Bilaterally limited to fourth premolar
Maxilla/orbit	Maxillectomy[207] Orbitectomy[208]	Limited by midline palate or cranial vault invasion Combined approach may assist exposure
Calvarium	Resection ± radiation	Resection dependent on venous sinus involvement
Vertebrae	Decompression (palliative) ± radiation/ chemotherapy[172]	Vertebrectomy techniques not well developed; limited local disease control
Rib	Rib resection[165,168,209]	Requires removal of additional cranial and caudal rib

RT, Radiation therapy.

The choice of limb-sparing method depends on several factors, including owner choice, patient personality, surgeon experience, and individual risk factors. At the CSU-ACC, owners are given a choice of limb-sparing procedures and informed about the risks and benefits of each method compared with amputation. A brief description of the surgical options for a distal radial location (most common) follows. In all cases, cephalosporin antibiotics are administered via IV immediately preoperatively, intraoperatively, and for 24 hours postoperatively. Meticulous aseptic technique is essential.

Allograft Limb Sparing For a distal radial site, the dog is placed in lateral or dorsal recumbency, with the affected limb uppermost. A skin incision is made on the dorsolateral aspect of the antebrachium from a point just distal to the elbow, to just proximal to the metacarpophalangeal joint. Any biopsy tracts are excised en bloc. Soft tissue is dissected to the level of the tumor pseudocapsule. Care is taken not to enter the tumor. The bone is cut with an oscillating bone saw 3 to 5 cm proximal to the proximal radiographic (or scintigraphic) margin of the tumor. Extensor muscles attached to the tumor pseudocapsule are transected at a level to maintain 2 to 3 cm soft tissue margins. The joint capsule is incised, keeping close to the proximal row of carpal bones. For tumors of the middiaphysis, tumor resection follows similar guidelines with the exception that an attempt to spare extensor and flexor muscle groups is undertaken so the joint (above and below) may be spared.[186] The ulna is sectioned sagittally with an osteotome, and the medial ulnar cortex adjacent to the tumor is removed en bloc with the radius. For tumors that have extension to the ulna (rare), the ulna is also cut with a bone saw, and the distal one-third or more is removed with the tumor. Care is taken to preserve as much vasculature as possible, especially on the palmar surface.

Large vessels associated with the tumor are ligated and divided. Surgical hemostatic staples (Surgiclip, United States Surgical Corp, New York) are very useful. The specimen is radiographed, then submitted for histologic evaluation, including assessment of completeness of surgical margins and percentage of tumor necrosis. In addition, a sample of bone marrow proximal to the resection level (radius) is obtained for histologic evaluation of marrow involvement. Intraoperative frozen section histology is used in humans to assess the adequacy of surgical resection of primary bone tumors during limb sparing.[213] Although this technique is being used in veterinary medicine, it is still considered somewhat unreliable for bone specimens.

A fresh-frozen cortical allograft is thawed in 1 L of an antibiotic and saline solution (Neomycin 1 g, polymyxin B 500,000 U, potassium penicillin 5,000,000 U), the articular cartilage is removed, the graft is cut to fit, and the medullary cavity reamed to remove fat and cellular debris.[214,215] The articular cartilage of the proximal carpal bones is removed, and the allograft is stabilized in

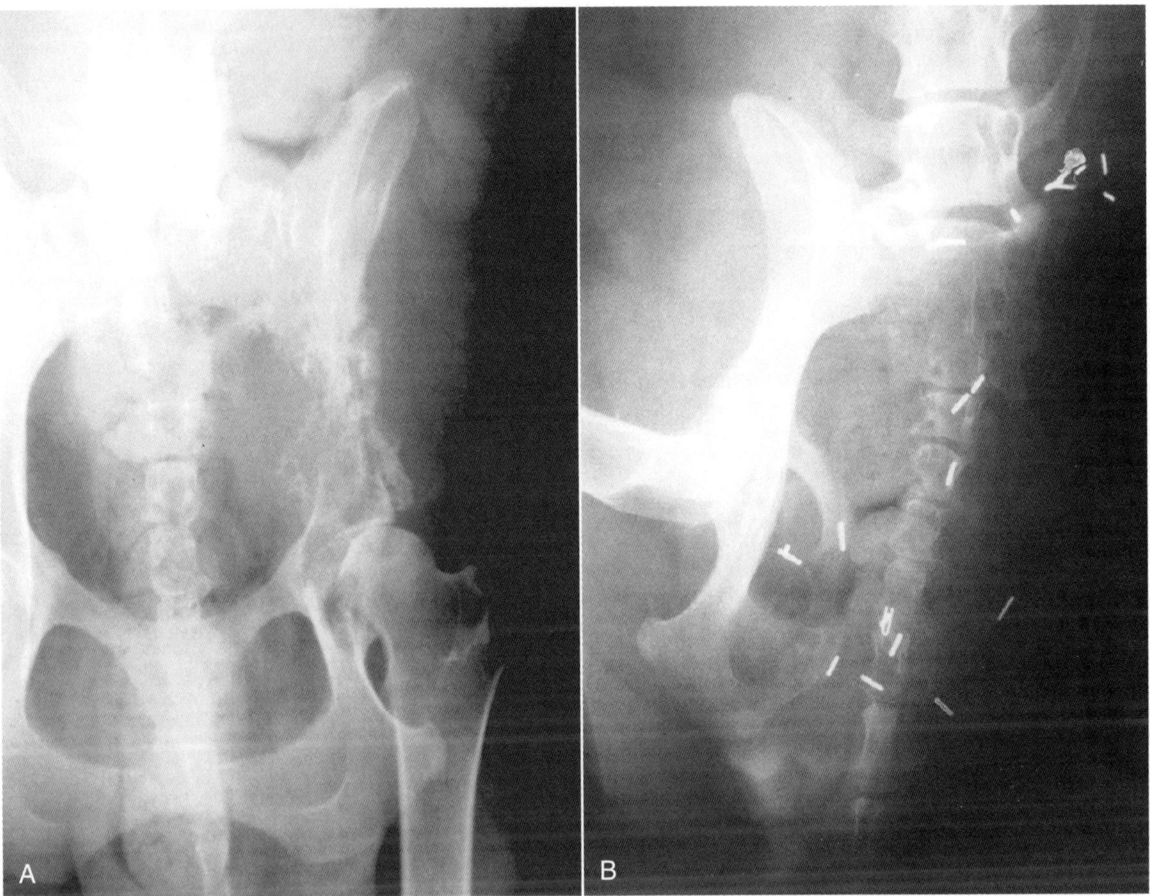

FIGURE 24-5 **A,** Ventrodorsal radiographic view of an OS of the ilium of a dog. **B,** Ventrodorsal radiographic view of the dog in **A** 3 years after hemipelvectomy and amputation followed by cisplatin chemotherapy.

compression using Association for the Study of Internal Fixation (ASIF/AO) principles. A dynamic compression plate with a minimum of three screws proximal and four screws distal to the graft is used; 3.5-mm broad locking plates of up to 22 hole size or a custom-designed limb salvage plate are appropriate in most cases, but for very large dogs, 4.5-mm narrow or broad plates are selected. The plate is fastened in the patient to the allograft with two or three screws, removed from the surgery site, and the medullary canal of the allograft is filled with polymethyl methacrylate (Palacos radiopaque bone cement, Smith & Nephew Richards, Inc., Memphis, TN) bone cement containing amikacin (1 g amikacin to 40 g of polymer powder). This provides support for the screws during revascularization of the graft and acts as a reservoir for antibiotics. The healing of the allograft is not significantly impeded by the presence of the cement and has been shown to significantly decrease the incidence of orthopedic failure, including allograft fracture and screw pullout.[216,217] The plate extends proximally in the host radius and distally to a level just proximal to the metacarpophalangeal joint (Figure 24-6). For intercalary limb spares, the plate extends proximally and distally to meet or exceed ASIF standards with the intent to spare joint motion.

The wound is thoroughly lavaged with saline, and it is at this point that local (polymer) chemotherapy may be implanted. A closed suction drain is inserted adjacent to the allograft, and the wound is closed. The leg is supported in a padded bandage. The drain is removed the day after surgery in most cases. It is most important to prevent self-mutilation (licking) after surgery, and Elizabethan collars should be used as necessary. No external coaptation is used and most dogs use the limb fairly well by 10 days after surgery. Postoperative foot swelling can be considerable but usually resolves by 2 weeks. Although decreased exercise is recommended for the first 4 to 6 weeks to allow soft tissues to heal, no exercise restriction need apply after this time. In fact, it is important that limb use is encouraged, even in early postoperative times, so that flexure contracture of the digits does not occur. Early weight bearing will often decrease the occurrence and incidence of postoperative swelling.

The advantages to allograft limb sparing include the absence of external fixation, and little owner involvement is required in the postoperative period aside from bandage changes in the first 2 weeks. The disadvantages are the high infection rate, potential for local recurrence, and the need for permanent internal hardware. Canine limb spare patients have an infection rate of approximately 40% and 50%. Once an infection occurs, it may be controlled with long-term antibiotic therapy but is rarely, if ever, resolved.[218] Infection may result in soft tissue defects from draining tracts, exposure of the plate or allograft, and hardware loosening. Revision surgeries, either for hardware complications or soft tissue reconstruction, are not uncommon. Additionally, amputation for catastrophic implant failure, local recurrence, or unmanageable infection is sometimes required.

Metal Endoprosthesis Limb Sparing. The metal endoprosthesis limb-sparing technique utilizes a commercially available metal endoprosthesis with a modified bone plate (Figure 24-7). The

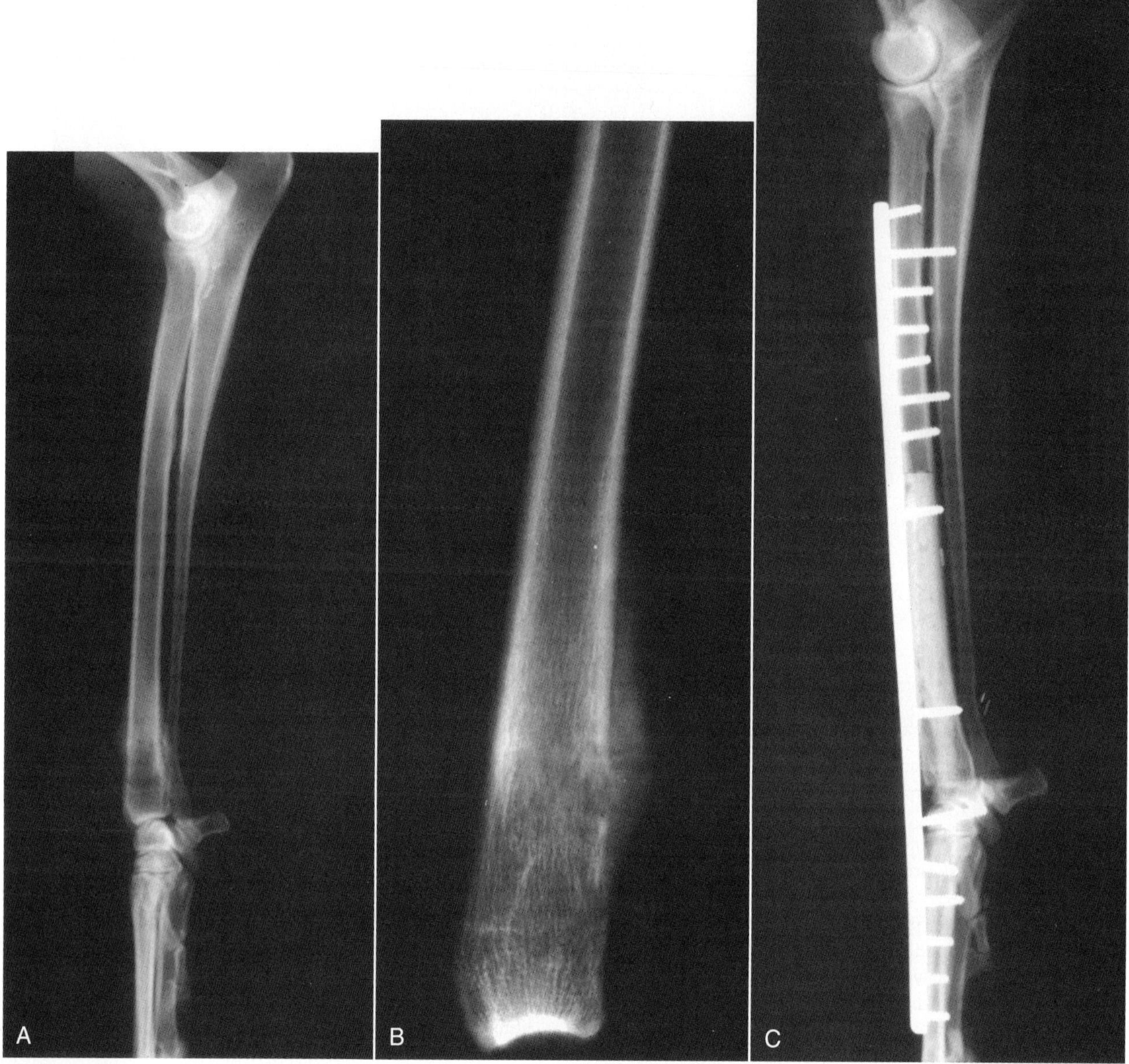

FIGURE 24-6 Limb sparing. **A,** Preoperative lateral radiograph of a distal radial OS lesion in a dog. **B,** Craniocaudal specimen radiograph following tumor resection of the case in **A. C,** Lateral postoperative radiograph following allograft placement and plate fixation of the case in **A** and **B.**

surgery is nearly identical to the procedure described earlier; however, instead of reconstruction with an allograft, the endoprosthesis is used to span the radial defect. A prospective comparison of complications between allograft limb sparing and metal endoprosthesis limb sparing was published in 2006.[187] No significant differences in the number of complications were noted between metal implants and allografts in the patient population studied. An endoprosthesis is an attractive alternative to cortical allografts for limb salvage of the distal aspect of the radius in dogs because surgical and oncologic outcomes are similar, but the endoprosthesis is an immediately available off-the-shelf implant that is not complicated by the bone harvesting and banking requirements associated with cortical allografts.

Pasteurized Tumoral Autograft. Two reports exist of a limb-sparing technique that involves removal of the segment of bone with the tumor and pasteurizing the bone segment at 65° C for 40 minutes, followed by reimplantation.[201,202] Limb function was good in 12 of 13 dogs with a 15% local recurrence, 31% infection, and 23% implant failure rate. The advantages of this method are that there is no need for an allograft, and anatomic apposition is excellent. The disadvantages are similar to the allograft technique in terms of complications; however, overall survival and disease-free progression were similar to other studies.

Longitudinal Bone Transport Osteogenesis. The longitudinal bone transport osteogenesis (BTO) technique for limb sparing has been reported in veterinary patients (Figure 24-8).[197,198] This

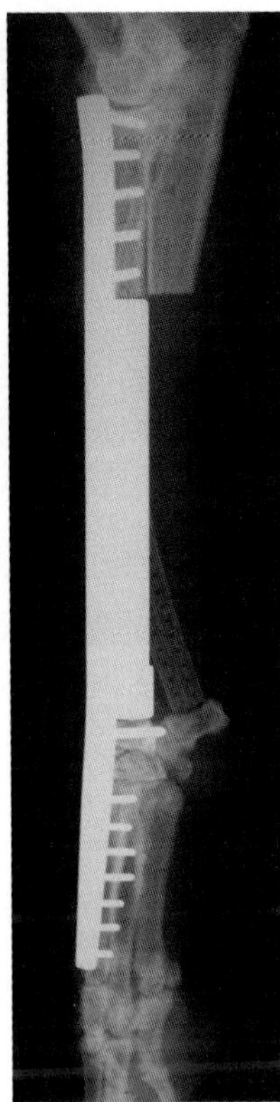

FIGURE 24-7 Lateral radiographic projection of a limb-sparing technique using a commercially available metal endoprosthesis with a modified bone plate in a dog with distal radial and ulnar OS. A limb-sparing plate spans host radius and metacarpus, connecting to the implant, which abuts the host radius proximally and the radial carpal bone distally. A negative suction drain has also been placed at the surgical site to decrease postoperative fluid accumulation.

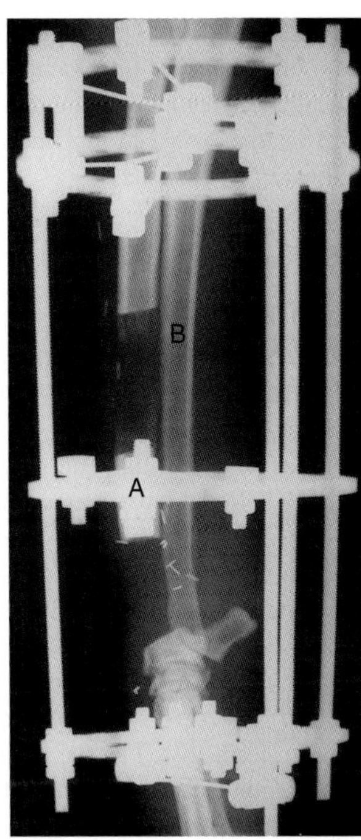

FIGURE 24-8 Lateral radiographic projection of a limb-sparing technique known as *longitudinal bone transport osteogenesis* (BTO). In this case, a distal radial OS was removed and BTO was accomplished using circular fixators and the principles of distraction osteogenesis to create bone in the defect remaining following tumor resection. Briefly, a longitudinal section of normal bone *(A)*, termed the *transport segment,* from the radius is osteotomized and attached to the transport ring, and the osteotomized bone segment is slowly transported into the defect at a rate of 1 mm per day. Distraction osteogenesis occurs in the trailing distraction pathway *(B).*

method utilizes Ilizarov (circular) fixators and the principles of distraction osteogenesis to create bone in the defect following tumor resection. Prior to surgery, a five- to six-ring circular fixator is constructed to allow one central ring (termed a *transport ring*) to move independently from the rest of the fixator. Following the same procedure for removal of the tumor and preparation of the radiocarpal bone described earlier, the circular fixator is placed on the limb and attached to the remaining radius using tensioned 1.6-mm diameter wires. A longitudinal section of normal bone (termed the *transport segment*) from the radius immediately proximal to the defect is osteotomized and attached to the transport ring with wires. Following a 3- to 7-day delay period, the osteotomized bone segment is slowly transported into the defect at a rate of 1 mm per day. Distraction osteogenesis occurs in the trailing distraction pathway. New bone continues to form longitudinally within the defect proximal to the transport segment for as long as the steady, slow distraction continues. When the transport segment reaches the radiocarpal bone (docking), the transport segment is compressed to the radiocarpal bone and heals to create an arthrodesis. The circular fixator remains on the limb while the newly formed bone remodels and the arthrodesis occurs. This technique is compatible with cisplatin, carboplatin, and combination chemotherapy.[197,199]

The advantages to BTO limb sparing are the lack of internal hardware; the low risk of infection due to the autologous, vascularized nature of the replacement bone; and the ability of the new bone tissue to remodel over time. Patients are typically weight bearing within the first 48 hours and once the incision is healed do not require exercise restriction. The disadvantage of the BTO procedure is the extensive client involvement needed to perform the daily distractions on the fixator and the extended amount of time the fixator remains on the limb. Double level longitudinal transport and translational transport of the ulna can significantly diminish the time required for distraction and have been used successfully in a case of limb salvage for a distal tibial OS.[200]

Ulna Transposition Limb Sparing. The vascularized ulna transposition technique uses the ipsilateral distal ulna as an autograft to reconstruct the distal radial defect by rotating the graft into position while preserving the caudal interosseous artery and vein.[195,196] Following excision of the tumor as described previously, two transverse osteotomies of the ulna are made. The distal osteotomy is performed at the level of the isthmus proximal to the facet that articulates with the radius. The proximal ulna osteotomy is performed 1 to 2 mm distal to the level of the radial osteotomy. Direct visualization of the caudal interosseous artery and vein allows these structures to be preserved during dissection of the autograft. The ulna graft is "rolled over" into the radial defect and fixed using a bone plate that extends from the proximal radius to the distal one-third of metacarpal IV (i.e., carpal arthrodesis).

Advantages to the ulna transposition technique are that there is no distant donor site morbidity; the replacement bone is autologous; and the graft is vascularized, making it less likely to get infected, and possibly speeding healing. The disadvantages to this technique are that the ulna transposition technique may be more prone to biomechanical complications in the postoperative period due to its smaller size relative to the radius and the need for permanent internal hardware.[195]

Nonsurgical Alternative Methods of Limb Salvage

Intraoperative Radiation Therapy and Extracorporeal Intraoperative Radiation Therapy

The extracorporeal intraoperative RT (IORT) technique for limb sparing has been utilized in a small number of canine OS patients,[188,219] as well as in human patients with extremity bone tumors.[220-222] This limb-salvage technique involves a surgical approach to the bone with osteotomy above or below the affected site (depending on the anatomic location of the tumor) and reflection of normal soft tissues from the tumor-affected bone. The neurovascular bundle, muscle, and skin are held away from the affected bone, and the tumor is pivoted from the site on the intact joint tissue. The patient is then transported to the radiation suite and a single dose of 70 Gy radiation is then directed to the tumor, taking care to spare the distracted neurovascular bundle. The irradiated bone is then anatomically replaced and surgical fixation of the osteotomy applied with dynamic compression plating, an interlocking nail system or a combination. One advantage of IORT for limb salvage over surgical limb salvage is that it can be used to preserve limb function in anatomic sites that are not amenable to reliable surgical limb salvage (e.g., proximal humerus).[154] Patients treated with IORT had good limb function in the immediate postoperative period; however, complications related to surgery or radiation led to implant revisions in 69% of cases within 5 to 9 months of initial surgery, including four amputations. Pathologic fracture of the irradiated bone was the most common complication. Additionally, local tumor recurrence occurred in four patients and infection in four patients. A modification of this technique includes complete temporary removal of diaphyseal tumors, performing extracorporeal radiation, and then reimplantation and stabilization. In situ radiation of distal femur and any tibial tumors can be performed without osteotomy. The disease-free and overall success rates for limb and joint salvage for extracorporeal IORT were 46% and 54%, respectively. The MST for dogs with appendicular sarcoma treated with limb- and joint-sparing extracorporeal IORT was 298 days (range: 116 to 1775 days).

A small case series of five distal radius IORT cases described joint sparing of the radiocarpal joint by avoiding transcarpal plating.[219] Radiocarpal joint function could not be preserved long term in any dog due to complications related to implant failure, deep tissue infection, and pathologic fracture that was treated by amputation or pancarpal plating. The IORT technique for limb salvage cannot be recommended currently due to the high complication rate associated with orthopedic implants and infection in irradiated bone.

Stereotactic Radiosurgery

Stereotactic radiosurgery (SRS) offers the ability to deliver high-dose RT to the tumor volume with relative sparing of the surrounding normal tissues by use of image guidance and a sharp drop off in dose intensity (Figure 24-9). In this respect, it is a refinement of the IORT technique that avoids the need for surgical exposure. A nonsurgical limb-salvage technique using SRS was developed at the University of Florida, and initial results were reported in 11 dogs.[223]

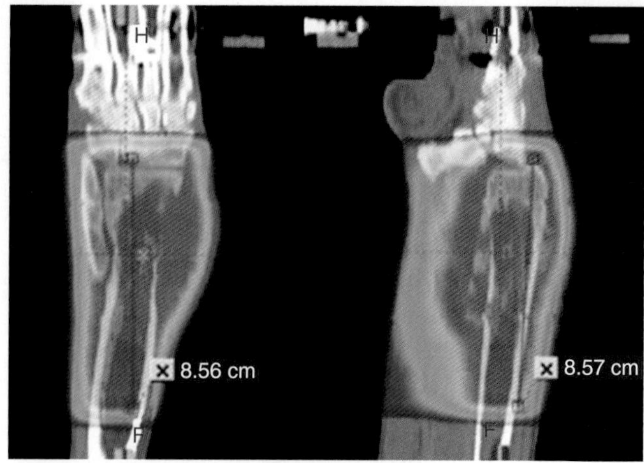

FIGURE 24-9 Dose color wash map of radiation distribution for SRT of distal radius OS lesion showing steep dose-gradient drop-off between tumor volume and normal tissues.

Adjuvant carboplatin chemotherapy was used in six dogs immediately prior to radiation treatment for its potential radiosensitization action in addition to its conventional cytotoxic qualities, and five dogs received radiosurgery alone. Five dogs developed pathologic fractures, and one dog developed infection. Acute effects to the skin were mild to moderate in most dogs. Limb use in the dogs that received SRS and chemotherapy was excellent. The reported overall median survival was 363 days in this series; however, the population size was small. Advantages of this technique include limb preservation for anatomic sites not amenable to reliable surgical limb salvage, the normal tissue-sparing effects of stereotactic RT (SRT) compared to conventional RT, no surgical procedures, and good-to-excellent limb function. Disadvantages of the technique include access to equipment that is not typically available to veterinarians and the high complication rate with postirradiation pathologic fracture. These initial results suggested that SRS could provide a viable nonsurgical limb-sparing alternative. Since the publication of this first report, other veterinary centers with linear accelerators capable of delivery of SRT have adapted the SRT limb-salvage technique.

At CSU, an SRT protocol using a Varian Trilogy linear accelerator was developed for treatment of canine extremity OS. The current SRT protocol utilizes a 3×12 Gy (total dose 36 Gy) SRT protocol with fractions delivered on consecutive days. Carboplatin chemotherapy is administered within 2 hours before or after the first or second SRT fraction. Standard adjuvant chemotherapy with either single-agent carboplatin or doxorubicin or combination chemotherapy is continued after SRT at 3 weeks interval for 4 to 6 cycles. We have seen two suspected cases of "radiation recall" skin effects associated with the use of doxorubicin, so care is recommended with use of this chemotherapeutic agent when used in conjunction with SRT. We recommend administration of pamidronate (a bisphosphonate) as soon as possible after diagnosis and ideally 24 to 72 hours before SRT. We do not recommend continued bisphosphonate therapy after SRT because there is no ongoing tumor-associated osteolysis or bone remodeling processes in the irradiated field based on histopathologic examination. Local tumor control has been excellent as assessed by static radiographic findings on serial evaluation, repeat scintigraphic imaging in a few cases, and decreases in urine N-telopeptide (NTx) levels. A mean percentage of tumor necrosis of greater than 90% has been

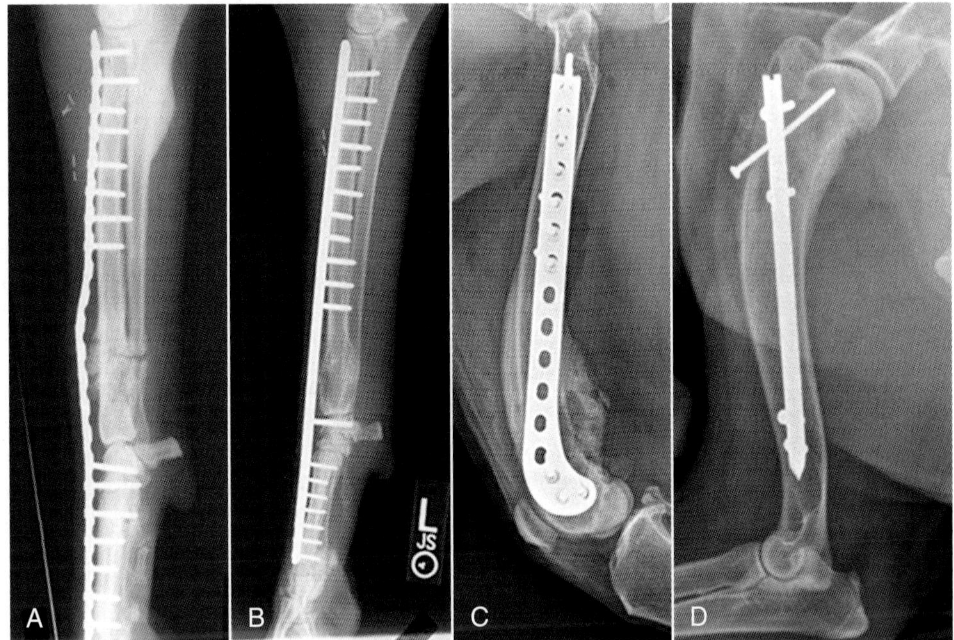

FIGURE 24-10 Radiographs of internal fixation after fracture **(A)** and preemptive stabilization **(B, C,** and **D)** for SRT limb-salvage cases with lytic lesions.

observed on 12 retrieved limb specimens collected at a variety of time points after SRT. Pathologic fracture has been the most frequent complication after SRT. This is due to the amount of preexisting tumor-associated osteolysis and postirradiation bone necrosis and the loss of dynamic bone remodeling and healing capacity after SRT. Smaller, more blastic lesions are better candidates for SRT limb salvage than larger, more lytic lesions. Pathologic fracture has been treated by internal fixation, external coaptation, or amputation. In more recent cases, preemptive stabilization has been used for more lytic tumors immediately after the third fraction of SRT to help prevent fracture (Figure 24-10). Using data in which surgical stabilization is employed when needed, the overall limb survival rate is 83%. The MST for the first 50 dogs treated with this SRT and adjuvant chemotherapy limb-salvage technique is 275 days, which is similar to reported survival times for amputation or surgical limb salvage and adjuvant chemotherapy. Further research into the potential beneficial roles for total radiation dose reduction and adjuvant therapies such as radioprotectant and other bisphosphonates and parathyroid hormone is indicated.

Isolation of Limb Circulation and Perfusion

Isolated limb perfusion with chemotherapy has been used in humans and dogs with sarcomas and melanomas as a sole treatment or to downstage local disease and allow limb sparing.[224-226] Isolated limb perfusion (ILP) allows delivery of high concentrations of chemotherapy, as well as delivery of compounds that are poorly tolerated systemically. Varying degrees of local toxicity are reportedly dependent on the drugs used. Successful use of ILP in canine OS has been reported.[224] One study determined that appendicular bone tumors have significantly higher interstitial fluid pressure and lower blood flow than do adjacent, unaffected soft tissues.[227] ILP may be a method to facilitate delivery of therapeutic drug concentrations to primary tumors for preoperative downstaging prior to limb salvage.

Systemic administration of ^{153}samarium ethylenediamine-tetramethylene phosphonate (^{153}Sm-EDTMP) is limited by systemic myelotoxicity (see Radioisotopes section later). In a study at CSU, ^{153}Sm-EDTMP (37 MBq/kg) was administered via ILP through the isolated limb circulation for 1 hour in nine dogs with primary OS of the appendicular skeleton 3 weeks prior to amputation to evaluate the potential for decreased systemic toxicity and to induce a clinically meaningful percentage of tumor necrosis prior to primary tumor removal. No systemic toxicity was observed. Despite good dosimetry to the lesion, the mean percent tumor necrosis was 27.6% (Std Dev ± 17.6%; range 3.4% to 56.4%), which was similar to mean percent tumor necrosis of 26.8% in untreated OS cases.[228] This low tumor necrosis percentage may be due to incomplete perfusion of the ^{153}Sm-EDTMP, the heterogeneous nature of OS, and the inability of the beta particles to exert a cytotoxic effect on the noncalcified regions of the tumor due to their short track length (3 mm). Future experiments should evaluate dose escalation in the perfused limb now that systemic safety has been demonstrated with the ILP technique.

Summary of Outcome Following Limb Salvage for Dogs with Osteosarcoma

There is no significant difference in survival rates for dogs treated with amputation and cisplatin compared to dogs treated with limb sparing and cisplatin.[194] Overall, limb function has been satisfactory, with approximately 80% of dogs experiencing good-to-excellent limb function.[16] Limb-sparing surgery is usually combined with some form of adjuvant therapy, and complications can arise in any or all phases of treatment (chemotherapy, radiation, or surgery). High-dose external-beam RT may complicate wound and bone healing and potentiate infection.[191] Moderate-dose external-beam radiation in combination with chemotherapy may, however, be useful for control of local disease, as indicated by percentage of tumor necrosis data.[193,228] The major complications related to limb-sparing surgery are recurrent local disease, allograft infection, and implant complications. In a review of 220 limb-sparing surgeries performed at CSU-ACC, the 1-year local recurrence-free rate determined by Kaplan-Meier life table analysis is over 76% with 60% alive at 1 year.[194]

In two case series, 40% and 47.5% of dogs, respectively, developed allograft infections.[194,229] The majority had their infections adequately controlled with systemic antibiotics with or without local antibiotics (antibiotic-impregnated polymethyl methacrylate beads).[218] Many of these dogs continued to have evidence of infection; however, their function was not severely affected. In severe and uncontrolled infections, allografts had to be removed and a small number of dogs required amputation. An unexpected finding has been that dogs with allograft infections experienced a statistically significant prolongation of overall survival times compared to dogs with limb sparing without infected allografts.[230] This finding has also been reported in humans with deep infections after limb-salvage surgery for OS.[231] A mouse model of OS examined the effects of infection on tumor angiogenesis and innate immunity and demonstrated that chronic localized bacterial infection could elicit significant systemic antitumor activity, depending on natural killer (NK) cells and macrophages.[232]

Surgery for Nonappendicular and Less Common Appendicular Sites of OS

Certain primary bone tumors of the pelvis can be removed by hemipelvectomy and, although these surgeries are difficult, function and cosmetic outcome have been excellent (see Figure 24-5).[206,233] Kramer et al provide an excellent review of the technique for hemipelvectomy and the surgical and oncologic factors to be considered with this surgery.[233] SRT has been used for long-term palliation of primary bone tumors arising from the pelvis. The total radiation dose that can be delivered to tumors in this location is limited by the dose tolerance of the colon, rectum, nerves, and perineum within the treatment field. A 5-fraction SRT protocol is used at CSU in preference to the 3-fraction protocol used for extremity OS to help spare these normal tissues. Concurrent administration of carboplatin during SRT for intrapelvic or pelvic tumors is avoided due to the increased frequency of complications observed.

Vertebral OS sites are the most difficult sites to adequately treat local disease. Techniques of complete vertebrectomy are not well established in veterinary medicine,[234] and surgery often is an attempt to decompress dogs with neurologic deficits or intractable pain and to obtain a diagnosis.[172] Present recommendations are to perform surgery in cases that require decompression (with or without stabilization) and institute RT (discussed later) and chemotherapy. SRT is an emerging treatment option for vertebral body tumors. RT likely plays a role in the treatment of OS of the vertebrae. In a series of 14 dogs with vertebral OS treated between 1986 and 1995, 12 had surgery to decompress the spinal cord, 7 were treated with OPLA-Pt implanted in a distant intramuscular site, and 11 were given IV cisplatin. Nine dogs were treated with fractionated external-beam RT. All dogs had surgery, RT, or both, and no dog was treated with chemotherapy alone. Four dogs improved neurologically, four dogs worsened, and six dogs remained the same. The median survival of 135 days after treatment was relatively short.[172] Local disease recurrence rather than metastasis was the usual cause of death.

A combination allograft and custom total joint arthroplasty has been described for successful limb salvage of a proximal femur OS.[235] An intraosseous transcutaneous amputation prosthesis (ITAP) for limb salvage has been described in a case series of four dogs for distal radius and distal tibia OS lesions.[236] A case report using an ITAP prosthesis for a traumatic distal tibia injury has also been reported.[237] The success of an ITAP prosthesis requires a biologic seal to be formed between the skin and the prosthesis to prevent the possibility of deep infection.

Bone tumors originating in proximal sites of the scapula can be successfully removed by partial scapulectomy (Figure 24-11).[169,171,205] Dogs function well with partial scapulectomy but take 1 to 3 months to improve. Seroma formation is common in the immediate postoperative period. Intensive postoperative physical therapy is important in these cases to regain normal function. Significant gait abnormalities may occur after complete scapulectomy by disarticulation at the scapulohumeral joint.[171] Small primary tumors of the ulna can be removed by partial ulnectomy, and reconstruction is rarely needed.[204] Tumors located in the metatarsal and metacarpal bones can be treated with local resections or partial foot amputation.[237a] Experience at our institution supports removal of a single bone or the central two bones in most dogs, with good functional outcome. In small dogs, removal of the medial or lateral two bones can result in normal function. Resection to this extent has not been attempted in larger dogs. Mandibulectomy and maxillectomy are appropriate surgeries for primary bone tumors of oral sites.[160,161,238,238a,239] In a survey of owners of dogs undergoing partial mandibulectomy or maxillectomy, 85% were satisfied with the outcome despite 44% citing difficulty in eating as a complication.[236] Tumors of periorbital sites can be removed by orbitectomy.[208] Rib tumors can be removed by thoracic wall resection, and the defect can be reconstructed with polypropylene mesh (Marlex mesh, CR Bard Inc, Billerica, MD) with plastic plates (Lubra plates, Lubra Co, Fort Collins, CO) for large defects or by muscle flap techniques.[165,167,168] Diaphragmatic advancement can be used for caudally located defects.

Radiation

At present, the role of RT for curative-intent local tumor control is still evolving in veterinary medicine. Currently, the most common role of RT in dogs with appendicular OS is for palliation of bone pain (see later section on Palliative Treatment: Primary and Metastatic Bone Cancer Pain). RT at relatively high total doses can cause considerable necrosis of primary OS in dogs and humans, either before limb salvage to downstage the primary tumor to improve the success of local disease control following removal or as a primary therapy for unresectable tumors.[191,193,240-242] As a primary therapy, an MST of 209 days was reported in 14 dogs with appendicular OS treated with fractionated high-dose radiation (median dose of 57 Gy) to the primary tumor and systemic chemotherapy for micrometastasis.[243] Similar results are seen in humans with extremity OS treated with high-dose radiation, with and without surgical stabilization.[220] The introduction of SRT has allowed delivery of high doses of radiation to the tumor volume with excellent local tumor control and relative sparing of the surrounding normal tissues.

Radioisotopes

The bone-seeking, beta emitter radioisotope, ^{153}Sm-EDTMP, has been used to treat primary OS and metastatic bone neoplasia in dogs and humans via systemic IV administration (see later section on Palliative Treatment: Primary and Metastatic Bone Pain). Radium-223 chloride (Alpharadin, Algeta ASA, Oslo), a high linear energy transfer (LET) alpha-emitting radioisotope, has been recently approved by the Food and Drug Administration (FDA) and European regulatory authorities for treatment of multifocal

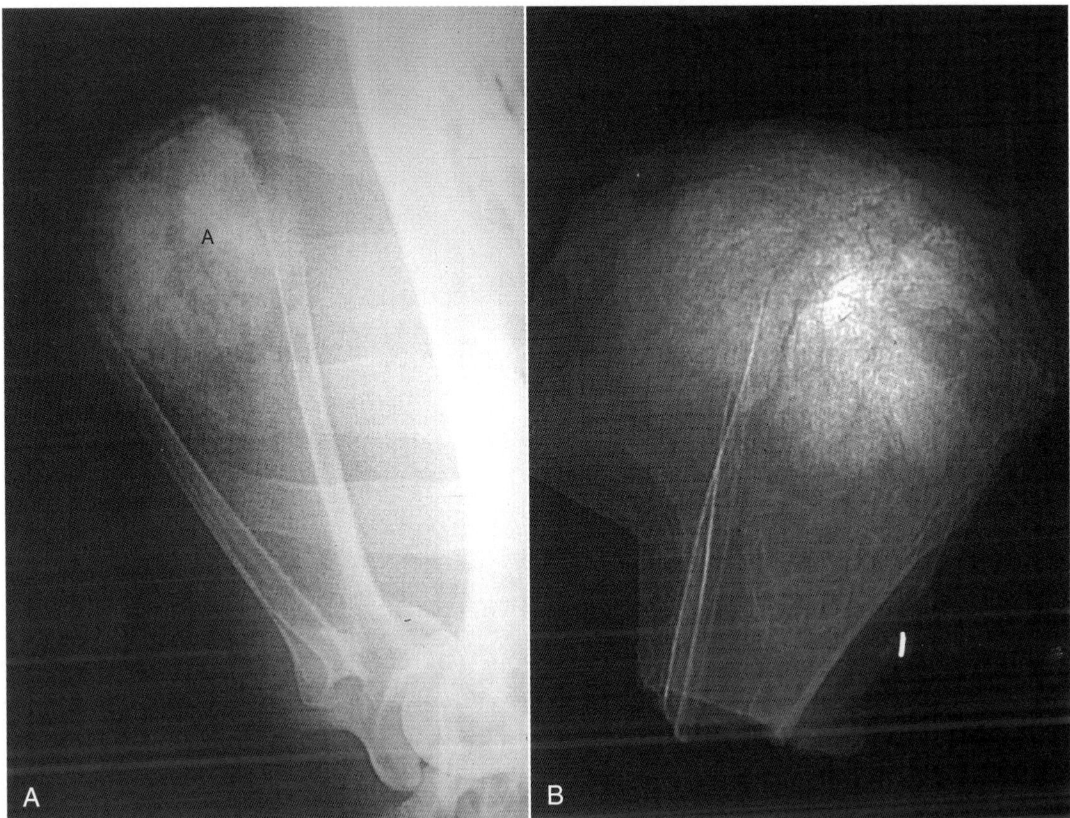

FIGURE 24-11 **A,** Preoperative radiograph (scapula technique) of an OS of the proximal scapula. **B,** Specimen radiograph of the case in **A** after partial scapulectomy.

metastatic bone cancer in men affected by hormone refractory prostate cancer.[244,245] Radium-223 chloride is a natural bone-seeking radioisotope that has been shown to prolong survival in patients with advanced prostate cancer in phase II and III clinical trials.[246] In acute and long-term repeat dose toxicity studies in normal beagles, the main side effect was temporary and reversible myelosuppression (leukocytopenia and thrombocytopenia). Radium-223 chloride was tolerated well when administered at 50 KBq/kg IV once per month for 6 consecutive months and at single doses up to 450 KBq/kg.

Systemic Adjuvant Therapy for Dogs with Osteosarcoma

For the most effective management of canine OS, multimodality therapy is required to address both local and metastatic disease. Although amputation and limb-sparing surgeries, as well as nonsurgical techniques such as SRT, have proved highly effective for local OS management, the ability to control the progression of OS metastases remains an urgent clinical challenge, and substantive improvements in DFIs and survival times await advances in systemic antimetastatic treatment options.

Systemic chemotherapy remains the backbone for the management of OS metastases, and it is improbable that the discovery of new chemotherapeutic agents or dose-intensification with existing agents will dramatically improve current clinical outcomes. The future of OS management will likely depend on combining conventional cytotoxic agents with targeted molecular therapeutics or immunomodulatory agents. As such, considerable research focus has been committed to discovering and validating new combination therapies for improving the long-term prognosis of canine OS. Current adjuvant chemotherapies, used singly or in combination with other cytotoxic agents, are discussed in the following section.

Chemotherapy

Table 24-2 provides an abbreviated summary of conventional chemotherapeutic agents used in the adjuvant setting, evaluated as single agents or in combination in at least 20 dogs. More detailed information regarding the studies highlighted in Table 24-2 is provided in the following section.

Cisplatin: Single Agent

Similar to its activity in an adjuvant or neoadjuvant setting for the treatment of pediatric OS, cisplatin has been demonstrated to improve survival in dogs with OS after amputation in several studies with small-to-modest patient population sizes.[16,189] In one report, 36 dogs received 2 treatments of cisplatin every 21 days at a dosage of 70 mg/m^2.[16] In approximately half of the dogs (group 1, n = 17), cisplatin was administered postoperative; for the remaining dogs (group 2, n=19), cisplatin was administered at diagnosis (preamputation) and again 21 days later immediately following amputation (perioperative). The median survival for group 1 (262 days; 1- and 2-year survival rates of 38% and 18%, respectively) was not significantly different from that of group 2 dogs (282 days; 1- and 2-year survival rates of 43% and 16%, respectively); suggesting that the administration of cisplatin in a neoadjuvant setting did not improve clinical outcomes. In a second study, 22 dogs with appendicular OS were treated with definitive surgery (amputation or

TABLE 24-2 Abbreviated Summary of Historic and Current Adjuvant Chemotherapy Protocols Derived from Studies with at least 20 Dogs*

DRUG	DOSE REGIMEN (NO.)	DISEASE FREE	SURVIVAL	COMMENTS
Cisplatin[16] (single agent)	70 mg/m^2 IV on 2 occasions, every 21 days (36)	Median 177-226 days	38%-43% at 1 year, 16%-18% at 2 years, median 262-282 days	No significant difference between survival data for dogs given cisplatin before amputation compared to those treated after amputation.
Cisplatin[189] (some dogs treated with limb sparing; single agent)	60 mg/m^2 IV on 1-6 occasions, every 21 days (22)	Not reported	45.5% at 1 year, 20.9 at 2 years, median 325 days	Apparent increase in treatment failures due to bone metastases.
SPI-77[247] (liposome-encapsulated cisplatin, single agent)	350 mg/m^2 IV every 21 days for 4 cycles (20)	Median 156 days	Median 333 days	Dramatic increase in cumulative cisplatin dosage without the need for diuresis.
Carboplatin[152] (single agent)	300 mg/m^2 every 21 days for 4 cycles (48)	Median 257 days	34.5% at 1 year, median 321 days	Well-tolerated with low incidence (<10%) of hematologic toxicity requiring dose delay.
Carboplatin[88] (comparator arm, single agent)	300 mg/m^2 every 21 days for 3 cycles (21)	Median 196 days	Median 230 days	Well-tolerated and safely combined with long-acting somatostatin analog.
Carboplatin[247] (comparator arm, single agent)	300 mg/m^2 every 21 days for 4 cycles (20)	Median 123 days	Median 207 days	Well-tolerated, with no patient requiring any treatment delays.
Carboplatin[248] (single agent)	Variable dosage and schedule (155)	Median 256 days	36.8% at 1 year, 18.7% at 2 years, median 307 days	Retrospective VCOG study inclusive of diverse patient and drug variables.
Carboplatin[249] (single agent)	300 mg/m^2 every 21 days for 4-6 cycles (65)	Median 137 days	36% at 1 year, 22% at 2 years, median 277 days	Well tolerated with <5% grade III or higher toxicity.
Lobaplatin[250] (single agent)	35 mg/m^2 every 21 days for 4 cycles (28)	1-year disease free survival rate of 21.8%	1-year overall survival rate of 31.8%	No need for diuresis with this platinum analog.
Doxorubicin[251] (single agent)	30 mg/m^2 every 2 weeks for 5 cycles (35)	Not reported	50.5% at 1 year, 9.7% at 2 years, median 366 days	Percentage necrosis of tumor predicted survival.
Doxorubicin[175] (comparator arm, single-agent)	30 mg/m^2 every 2 weeks for 5 cycles (303; comparator and BAY 12-9566)	Not reported	35% at 1 year, 17% at 2 years, median 8 months	Data not presented to allow segregation of placebo versus BAY 12-9566.
Doxorubicin and cisplatin[252] (concurrent combination)	Doxorubicin at 12.5-25 mg/m^2 followed in 2 hours by cisplatin at 60 mg/m^2 for 3 cycles (102)	Not reported	48% at 1 year, 28% at 2 years, median 345 days	Unacceptable toxicity with doxorubicin at 25 mg/m^2.
Doxorubicin and cisplatin[253] (concurrent combination)	Cisplatin at 50 mg/m^2 day 1 and doxorubicin at 15 mg/m^2 day 2 for 4 cycles (35)	Median 240 days	Median 300 days	Better tolerated protocol compared to reference 252.
Doxorubicin and carboplatin[254] (concurrent combination)	Carboplatin at 175 mg/m^2 on day 1 and doxorubicin at 15 mg/m^2 on day 2, every 21 days for 4 cycles (24)	Median 195 days	Median 235 days	The combination at these dosages was well tolerated in most cases.

VCOG, Veterinary Cooperative Oncology Group.

Table 24-2 Abbreviated Summary of Historic and Current Adjuvant Chemotherapy Protocols Derived from Studies with at least 20 Dogs (continued)

Drug	Dose Regimen (No.)	Disease Free	Survival	Comments
Doxorubicin and cisplatin[255] (alternating combination)	Doxorubicin at 30 mg/m^2, followed by cisplatin 60 mg/m^2 21 days later, every 3 weeks for 2 cycles (38)	Not reported	Median 300 days	Alternating combination well tolerated with no grade III or IV dose-limiting toxicities.
Doxorubicin and carboplatin[256] (alternating combination)	Carboplatin at 300 mg/m^2 on day 1 and doxorubicin at 30 mg/m^2 on day 21, alternating at 3-week intervals for 3 cycles for 6 total treatments (32)	Median 227 days	48% at 1 year, 18% at 2 years, median 320 days	Includes both amputation and limb-salvage therapies for the primary.
Doxorubicin and carboplatin[257] (alternating combination)	Carboplatin at 300 mg/m^2 on day 1 and doxorubicin at 30 mg/m^2 on day 21, alternating at 3-week intervals for 3 cycles for 6 total treatments (50)	Median 202 days	Median 258 days	Initial sequencing of carboplatin and doxorubicin not uniformly instituted.
Carboplatin and gemcitabine[258] (concurrent combination)	Carboplatin at 300 mg/m^2 then gemcitabine 2 mg/kg as a 20-minute infusion 4 hours post-carboplatin every 21 days for 4 cycles (50)	Median 203 days	29.5% at 1 year, 11.3% at 2 years, median 279 days	Well-tolerated protocol with low incidence of grade III or IV hematologic toxicity.

IV, Intravenous.

*Few of these protocols include sufficient numbers for adequate statistical power and fewer compare treatment protocols in a randomized prospective fashion. In addition, staging, inclusion, and response criteria vary considerably among protocols presented. Therefore evaluations of efficacy among protocols are subject to bias, making direct comparisons difficult and indeed precarious.

limb-sparing), and 1 week after surgical recovery began treatment with cisplatin at 60 mg/m^2 every 21 days for 1 to 6 treatment cycles.[189] The MST achieved by dogs receiving cisplatin was estimated to be 46.4 weeks, and 1- and 2-year survival rates were estimated to be 45.5% and 20.9%, respectively.

Despite the fact that some studies have documented cisplatin's antimetastatic effects at relatively low-dose intensities (50 mg/m^2 every 4 weeks), the recommended dose for cisplatin is 70 mg/m^2 body surface area, given intravenously every 3 weeks. Although cisplatin is relatively well tolerated, it is highly emetogenic and preemptive treatment with antiemetics such as maropitant should be recommended.[259,260] In addition to its emetogenic potential, a more serious side effect of cisplatin is the induction of nephrotoxicity. Therefore normal baseline renal function is essential prior to administration, and diuresis protocols must be performed concurrent with treatment. The diuresis protocol used most commonly involves a 4-hour pretreatment diuresis with 18.3 mL/kg/hr of 0.9% NaCl, followed by a 20-minute infusion of cisplatin diluted in a volume of 0.9% NaCl that will allow the same (18.3 mL/kg/hr) fluid infusion rate as the rate before diuresis. The cisplatin infusion is then followed by an additional 2 hours of diuresis with 18.3 mL/kg/hr of 0.9% NaCl.[261]

Carboplatin: Single Agent

Carboplatin is a second-generation platinum compound that is less nephrotoxic than cisplatin with comparable antitumor activity. Given its ease of administration, carboplatin has largely supplanted the use of cisplatin in the postoperative setting. In the first study reporting the tolerability and activity of carboplatin, 48 dogs with OS were treated with amputation and intent-to-treat with 4 doses of carboplatin (300 mg/m^2 every 21 days).[152] Carboplatin was well tolerated, with neutropenia being identified as the dose-limiting toxicity. For the entire study population (n = 48), the median DFI and survival time achieved was 257 and 321 days, respectively.

Despite the initial report of carboplatin's comparable activity to cisplatin,[152] two prospective randomized studies using single-agent carboplatin as a comparator arm demonstrated less impressive antimetastatic effects.[88,247] In one study, dogs were treated with a single neoadjuvant dose of carboplatin and amputation 7 days later, then received 2 additional treatments with carboplatin (300 mg/m^2) every 21 days. On completion of carboplatin, dogs were then randomized to receive either placebo (n = 21) or a long-acting somatostatin analog (n = 23).[88] For dogs treated with carboplatin and placebo, the median DFI and survival time achieved was 196 and 230 days, respectively. In a second study comparing the activity of a liposome-encapsulated cisplatin formulation (SPI-77) versus single-agent carboplatin, 40 dogs were treated with a single neoadjuvant dose of either SPI-77 (350 mg/m^2) or carboplatin (300 mg/m^2) 1 week prior to amputation, then received an additional 3 treatments of SPI-77 or carboplatin every 21 days.[247] No difference was identified between treatment groups, with dogs receiving single-agent carboplatin achieving median DFI and survival time of 123 and 207 days, respectively.

Two relatively large, retrospective studies have been conducted to substantiate the activity of carboplatin for managing pulmonary micrometastases.[248,249] In a study initiated by the Veterinary Cooperative Oncology Group (VCOG), 155 dogs treated with amputation and carboplatin (variable dosage and schedule) achieved median DFI and survival times of 256 and 307 days, respectively.[248] In a second retrospective investigation, 65 dogs undergoing amputation and subsequent carboplatin at a dosage of 300 mg/m^2 every 21 days for 4 to 6 treatment cycles achieved median DFI and survival time of 137 and 277 days, respectively.[249]

Lobaplatin: Single Agent

Lobaplatin, a third-generation platinum compound, has been investigated in the adjuvant setting for the treatment of canine OS. In a study of 28 dogs, lobaplatin at 35 mg/m^2 was administered as an IV bolus every 21 days for 4 treatments.[250] Lobaplatin was well tolerated, with a low incidence of vomiting. Transient and reversible hematologic toxicity manifested as neutropenia and thrombocytopenia were observed 7 to 10 days following lobaplatin administration. The 1-year survival percentage was reported to be 32%, which is comparable to what is achieved with cisplatin or carboplatin.

Doxorubicin: Single Agent

Doxorubicin is considered effective for delaying the development and progression of micrometastatic disease in dogs with OS. However, doxorubicin's antimetastatic effects are more definitively substantiated when administered every 2 weeks, rather than every 3 weeks. In one study, doxorubicin was given at a dosage of 30 mg/m^2 every 2 weeks for 5 treatments to 35 dogs with appendicular OSs in a neoadjuvant setting. Dogs were treated with 2 or 3 dosages of doxorubicin prior to amputation and continued to receive doxorubicin postsurgery for a total of 5 treatments.[251] The 1- and 2-year survival rates were 50.5% and 9.7%, respectively. In a second study evaluating the activity of an MMP inhibitor (BAY 12-9566), 303 dogs were treated with amputation and doxorubicin (30 mg/m^2 every 2 weeks for a total of 5 treatment cycles) and then randomized to receive daily oral placebo or BAY 12-9566.[175] No difference in survival time was identified between dogs receiving placebo or BAY 12-9566, and the MST for all 303 dogs was 8 months.

Doxorubicin/Cisplatin: Concurrent Combination

With the establishment of single-agent activity of doxorubicin and cisplatin for the management of canine OS in the postoperative setting, two studies were conducted to evaluate the tolerability and activity of doxorubicin/cisplatin combinations producing summation dose intensities of greater than one.[252,253,262] In one study, 102 dogs treated with combination doxorubicin/cisplatin either 2 or 10 days postamputation were evaluated.[252] Doxorubicin was administered at a dosage of 12.5-25 mg/m^2 during saline diuresis and before cisplatin administration. The dosage of cisplatin was 60 mg/m^2 and was given with 6-hour saline diuresis. Dogs received combination doxorubicin/cisplatin every 21 days for a total of 3 treatments. Unacceptable toxicity was associated with doxorubicin administered at 25 mg/m^2 in conjunction with cisplatin at 60 mg/m^2, which resulted in approximately 10% treatment-associated mortality. With the exclusion of deaths associated with therapy, dogs capable of tolerating the protocol achieved MST of 11 to 11.5 months, with 1-year, 2-year, and 3-year survival rates of 48%, 28%, and 18%, respectively. In a second, less dose-intense combination study, 35 dogs with appendicular OS underwent amputation and chemotherapy with cisplatin and doxorubicin every 21 days for up to 4 cycles.[253] Cisplatin was administered at a dosage of 50 mg/m^2 in conjunction with 6-hour saline diuresis, and doxorubicin was administered at a dosage of 15 mg/m^2 24 hours later. Of the original 35 dogs, only 16 patients completed all four treatment cycles. For all dogs, the median DFI and survival time achieved was 240 and 300 days, respectively.

Doxorubicin/Carboplatin: Concurrent Combination

Given the modest-to-severe toxicity associated with doxorubicin/cisplatin combination therapy, one study investigated if combination tolerability could be improved by replacing cisplatin with carboplatin. The rationale to use carboplatin was based on its comparable anticancer activities and improved side effect profile relative to cisplatin, which excludes the need for saline diuresis and minimizes the likelihood of severe emesis. Twenty-four dogs were treated with definitive surgery, followed by combination chemotherapy consisting of carboplatin (175 mg/m^2) administered on day one and followed by doxorubicin (15 mg/m^2) on day two.[254] Combination doxorubicin/carboplatin was administered every 21 days for a maximum of 4 treatment cycles. Nineteen dogs completed four treatment cycles, and the tolerability of the combination was good with mild gastrointestinal toxicity reported in approximately 50% of patients and rare frequency of grade III hematologic toxicity or greater. The median DFI and survival time achieved was 195 and 235 days, respectively, and not considered superior to historic single-agent studies.

Doxorubicin/Cisplatin: Alternating Combination

To minimize toxicosis associated with concurrent combination protocols with summation dose intensities greater than 1.0 but to still exploit differing mechanisms of action of two compounds, alternating two drug protocols has been investigated for canine OS. In one of the first alternating two drug protocols described, 38 dogs were treated with definitive surgery alone (n = 19) or with adjuvant chemotherapy (n = 19) alternating doxorubicin and cisplatin.[255] Doxorubicin (30 mg/m^2) was the first drug to be administered 14 days after surgery, and cisplatin (60 mg/m^2) was given 21 days later; treatment was repeated for a total of 4 treatments (2 doxorubicin and 2 cisplatin). For dogs treated with amputation alone, the MST was 175 days; whereas for dogs treated with amputation (n = 17) or complete resection (n = 2; rib OS) followed by alternating doxorubicin and cisplatin therapy, the MST was 300 days. The alternating combination of full-dose doxorubicin and cisplatin did not result in any grade III or IV dose-limiting toxicities and significantly improved survival time in comparison to amputation alone.

Doxorubicin/Carboplatin: Alternating Combination

The tolerability and activity of full-dose, alternating combinations with doxorubicin and carboplatin have been recently conducted. In one study, 32 dogs were treated with amputation or limb-sparing surgery, then subsequently treated with carboplatin (300 mg/m^2, or 10 mg/kg if <15 kg) and 21 days later received doxorubicin (30 mg/m^2, or 1.0 mg/kg if < 15 kg).[256] Dogs received up to 3 treatment cycles (3 carboplatin and 3 doxorubicin). Alternating carboplatin and doxorubicin therapy was well tolerated, and out of 88 doses of carboplatin and 82 doses of doxorubicin administered, only one grade III neutropenia, one grade III thrombocytopenia, and one grade III vomiting were recorded. The median DFI and survival times were 227 and 320 days, respectively; with 1- and 2-year survival rates being 48% and 18%, respectively.

In a second confirmatory study, 50 dogs were treated with amputation and 10 to 14 days postoperative received alternating combination chemotherapy with carboplatin (300 mg/m^2) and doxorubicin (30 mg/m^2) every 21 days for 3 cycles (3 carboplatin and 3 doxorubicin).[257] However, dogs were not standardized to receive carboplatin first and doxorubicin second; and of the 50 dogs, 30 received carboplatin first, and the remaining 20 dogs received doxorubicin as their initial treatment. Adverse toxicities, including grade III or IV hematologic toxicity in 18% of dogs, and grade III or IV gastrointestinal toxicity in 12% of dogs were recorded. The median DFI and survival time were 202 and 258 days, respectively.

Carboplatin/Gemcitabine: Concurrent Combination

Based on in vitro data demonstrating strong synergism between carboplatin and gemcitabine in canine OS cell lines at pharmacokinetically achievable concentrations and durations of exposure,[263] a prospective study was conducted to assess if combination chemotherapy with carboplatin and gemcitabine could improve clinical outcomes in dogs with OS.[258] Fifty dogs were treated with amputation, and 14 days postsurgery were treated first with carboplatin (300 mg/m^2) and then gemcitabine was administered as a 20-minute IV infusion 4 hours postcarboplatin administration. Dogs were treated every 21 days for up to 4 dosages of carboplatin and gemcitabine. The combination of carboplatin and gemcitabine was well-tolerated with 74% of patients receiving all 4 treatment cycles, and only 5 episodes of grade III or IV hematologic toxicity was recorded. The median DFI and survival time were 203 and 279 days, respectively; with 1- and 2-year survival rates being 29.5% and 11.3%, respectively.

Preliminary Agents

Satraplatin, by virtue of its lipophilicity, is a platinum drug formulation with high oral bioavailability. Given the advantages of novel oral drug formulations, the pharmacokinetics and tolerability of oral satraplatin was determined in tumor-bearing dogs in a phase I dose-escalation study.[264] Oral satraplatin was administered daily for 5 consecutive days every 3 to 4 weeks for up to a total of 4 treatment cycles. Dose-limiting toxicity was myelosuppression, with grade III and IV neutropenia and/or thrombocytopenia being documented with satraplatin doses equal to or greater than 35 mg/m^2/day for 5 consecutive days. Out of the 23 dogs enrolled in the phase I study, 12 dogs had a diagnosis of appendicular OS (6 micrometastatic and 6 gross macroscopic). In the six dogs receiving satraplatin in the adjuvant setting, the median DFI and survival time were 456 and 659 days, respectively. Based on these early findings derived from a small subset of dogs with OS, satraplatin should be investigated more formally for appendicular OS.

Immunotherapy

Harnessing and directing the immune system for controlling micrometastatic disease remains a highly desirable anticancer strategy. Despite the various forms of immunotherapies such as monoclonal antibodies and dendritic cell vaccines currently instituted for the treatment of metastatic tumor histologies in humans, only a few immunotherapy studies in dogs have been conducted as randomized, double-blind trials. The best documented and clinically effective immunotherapy trials for dogs with OS have evaluated the anticancer immune effects associated with the administration of liposome-encapsulated muramyl tripeptide-phosphatidylethanolamine (L-MTP-PE). Being a lipophilic derivative of muramyl dipeptide, a synthetic analog of a *Mycobacterium* cell wall component, L-MTP-PE has been demonstrated to augment canine alveolar macrophage tumoricidal properties as supported by enhanced cytotoxicity against OS cells in vitro.[265]

In an initial clinical study of 27 dogs, the single-agent activity of intravenously administered L-MTP-PE was assessed immediately following amputation. Dogs were treated twice weekly with either L-MTP-PE (n = 14) or empty liposomes (n = 13) for a duration of 8 weeks. Dogs receiving L-MTP-PE achieved a significant prolongation in median DFI compared to dogs treated with empty liposomes (168 versus 58 days). Similarly, the MST was significantly longer for dogs receiving L-MTP-PE than dogs treated with empty liposomes (222 versus 77 days).[266] Based on these comparisons, it was concluded that L-MTP-PE induced beneficial immunobiologic effects capable of delaying the progression of pulmonary micrometastatic disease.

After establishing the anticancer activity of single-agent L-MTP-PE when used in the adjuvant setting, two subsequent randomized, double-blind studies were conducted to determine the effectiveness of combining L-MTP-PE with cisplatin.[267] In trial 1, dogs underwent limb amputation and received cisplatin every 4 weeks for 4 treatments. On completion of cisplatin therapy, dogs (n = 25) without overt evidence of pulmonary metastases were randomized to receive either L-MTP-PE (n = 11) or empty liposomes (n = 14) twice a week for 8 consecutive weeks. Dogs receiving L-MTP-PE had a significantly longer MST in comparison to dogs treated with empty liposomes, 14.4 versus 9.8 months.

Unlike trial 1 in which the cisplatin and L-MTP-PE were administered serially, the study design of trial 2 sought to characterize the anticancer activities of concurrently administered cisplatin and L-MTP-PE. All dogs (n = 64) were treated with limb amputation and cisplatin every 3 weeks for 4 treatments. Within 24 hours following the first cisplatin treatment, dogs were randomized to concurrently receive either L-MTP-PE twice a week (n = 21), L-MTP-PE once a week (n = 21), or empty liposomes once a week (n = 22) for a duration of 8 weeks. Disappointingly, dogs receiving concurrent L-MTP-PE (twice or once weekly) and cisplatin failed to demonstrate any improvement in DFI or survival time when compared to dogs treated with concurrent empty liposome (once weekly) and cisplatin. The reported MSTs for L-MTP-PE and empty liposome groups were 10.3, 10.5, and 7.6 months, respectively.

Molecular-Targeted Therapies for Dogs with Osteosarcoma

Micrometastatic Adjuvant Setting

The molecular pathogenesis for OS remains incomplete; however, a growing body of scientific evidence supports the participatory role of several cell signaling pathways that promote OS growth and survival. One particular growth factor signaling cascade more thoroughly investigated in OS has been GH and IGF-1. The putative roles of GH and IGF-1 in OS pathogenesis is supported by several clinical observations in both humans and dogs. For pediatric OS, the peak incidence of OS development occurs during the adolescent growth spurt,[268] which coincides with the greatest circulating concentrations of GH and IGF-1. Similarly in dogs, large to giant skeletal size is a strong positive determinant for appendicular OS development. Given the central roles of GH and IGF-1 in skeletal growth and homeostasis, as well as their role in cell survival, it has been hypothesized that aberrant or excessive GH and IGF-1 signaling is likely involved in OS pathogenesis.[269] To investigate the biologic consequences of attenuating GH and IGF-1 autocrine and/or paracrine signaling in OS, a randomized clinical trial in 44 dogs with OS was conducted in which circulating IGF-1 concentrations were suppressed with the administration of a long-acting analog of somatostatin (OncoLAR).[88] All dogs were treated with amputation and carboplatin in combination with either OncoLAR (n = 23) or vehicle (n = 21). The administration of OncoLAR resulted in a 43% reduction in circulating IGF-1 concentrations in comparison to baseline values; however, disappointingly, the suppression in IGF-1 did not translate result in improved DFIs or overall survival times in comparison to dogs receiving vehicle.

Molecular therapies with the capacity to delay or inhibit the development of pulmonary metastases would dramatically improve current treatment outcomes. As such, novel anticancer agents have been designed to selectively inhibit obligate steps necessary for successful tumor cell invasion and metastasis. One specific strategy has been the inhibition of MMPs, which are proteolytic enzymes involved in local tissue invasion and metastases. Based on documented gelatinolytic activities of MMP-2 and MMP-9 in canine cell lines and OS samples,[97,99] it has been rationalized that specific inhibitors of MMP activity might have the potential to increase the metastasis-free period after amputation and systemic chemotherapy. As such, a prospective, double-blind, randomized, placebo-controlled clinical trial evaluating the adjuvant activity of a MMP-2 and -9 inhibitor (BAY 12-9566), was evaluated in dogs with OS.[175] Following amputation and doxorubicin therapy, dogs without radiographic evidence of pulmonary metastatic disease (n = 223) were randomized and treated with either BAY 12-9566 (10 mg/kg) or placebo control daily until clinical failure. The addition of BAY 12-9566 did not improve DFI or survival time in comparison to placebo control. Correlating with the absence of biologic effect, serum MMP-2 and -9 activities were not different between dogs receiving BAY 12-9566 or placebo.

Treating Gross Metastatic Disease

Surgery

Resection of pulmonary metastasis from OSs or other solid tumors has been reported in humans.[270] One report of 36 dogs treated with pulmonary metastasectomy for OS exists.[271] Lesions located subpleurally were gently lifted from the lung parenchyma by thumb forceps and a single pursestring of 2-0 or 3-0 polygalactin 910 (Vicryl, Ethicon, Sommerville, NJ) suture was tied around the base of normal tissue. Larger lesions located deeper in the lung parenchyma were removed by complete or partial lobectomy using surgical staples (TA30 or TA55, United States Surgical Corp, New York). No chemotherapy was given after these surgeries. Although the initial treatments varied between dogs, the MST of the entire group was 487 days. The median survival after pulmonary metastasectomy was 176 days (range 20 to 1495 days). The criteria established for case selection for pulmonary metastasectomy in order to maximize the probability of long survival periods are (1) primary tumor in complete remission, preferably for a long relapse-free interval (>300 days); (2) one or two nodules visible on plain thoracic radiographs; (3) cancer only found in the lung (negative bone scan); and perhaps (4) long doubling time (>30 days) with no new visible lesions within this time. Pulmonary metastasectomy can also be performed for palliative relief in dogs with hypertrophic osteopathy.[272] Thoracoscopic lung lobectomy has been described for removal of primary and metastatic lung tumors.[273]

Surgical intervention to treat metastatic skeletal lesions with limb-sparing surgery alone or combined with stereotactic RT have been used in a few selected cases at the authors' institution, but this is not routinely recommended. A whole body technetium bone scan or PET/CT scan with F-18 is strongly recommended to identify the complete extent of metastatic skeletal disease prior to any surgical intervention. A recent report describes the feasibility of aggressive cancer treatment consisting of fracture fixation and postoperative chemotherapy as a treatment option for dogs with fractures associated with primary OS.[108] Dogs with stage III OS with bone metastases without pulmonary metastases are reported to have longer survival times than dogs with pulmonary metastases.[115] With the increased availability of locking plates, intraoperative imaging and minimally invasive osteosynthetic techniques, stabilization of metastatic bone lesions or fractures is a palliative treatment option that may provide increased quality of life for selected patients and owners.

Chemotherapy and Receptor Tyrosine Kinase Inhibitors for Gross (Macroscopic) Osteosarcoma

The treatment of gross measurable OSs with conventional cytotoxic agents or RTK inhibitors remains unsatisfactory. In part, the ineffectiveness of systemic therapies to cytoreduce gross measurable OS lesions is due to the development of drug-resistant clones, in conjunction with unfavorable and altered drug biodistribution within large tumor microenvironments. Because formidable biologic barriers are operative within macroscopic tumors that favor cancer cell survival, the majority of studies demonstrate only marginal effectiveness of conventional cytotoxic agents or RTK inhibitors for the management of gross, measurable OS.

In one study, 45 dogs that had either developed gross metastatic OS following standard-of-care therapy (amputation and systemic chemotherapy) or diagnosed at presentation with metastatic OS were treated with single-agent chemotherapies, including cisplatin (n = 31), doxorubicin (n = 11), or mitoxantrone (n = 3).[274] Out of the 45 dogs treated, only 1 dog achieved a short-lived (21-day) partial response, findings which suggest that conventional cytotoxic agents that are effective in the adjuvant setting are not efficacious for managing macroscopic metastatic OS. In a second study evaluating the tolerability and anticancer activities of paclitaxel in dogs with measurable tumor burdens, two out of nine dogs with macroscopic pulmonary metastatic OS achieved a partial response, suggesting that inhibitors of microtubule depolymerization might have modest activity for the management of gross measurable OS lesions.[275]

In addition to cytotoxic agents, the RTK inhibitor, toceranib phosphate (Palladia), has recently demonstrated preliminary anticancer activity across a broad range of tumor histologies, including metastatic pulmonary OS. Targets of toceranib include several members of the split-kinase family such as VEGF receptor, platelet-derived growth factor (PDGF) receptor, and c-kit.[276] Based on toceranib's ability to inhibit multiple signaling pathways, its potential activity was evaluated in 23 dogs with measurable pulmonary OS metastases.[277] Toceranib was orally administered at a median dose 2.7 mg/kg (every other day or Monday/Wednesday/Friday) and resulted in a partial response rate of 4.3% (1/23 dogs) and stable disease rate of 43.5% (10/23 dogs).

Strategies to enhance the susceptibility of metastatic cancers to conventional chemotherapeutic agents have also been recently conducted. By virtue of their chromatin remodeling effects, histone deacetylase inhibitors (HDACi) used in combination with cytotoxic agents might enhance the nuclear accumulation of cytotoxic agents and improve therapeutic outcomes. Based on this premise, a phase I dose-escalation study combining valproic acid and doxorubicin was conducted in dogs with various spontaneous tumors to determine the tolerability and activity of this HDACi/chemotherapy combination.[278] Three dogs with macroscopic OS pulmonary metastases were treated with valproic acid and doxorubicin, with one dog achieving durable disease stabilization.

Investigational Therapies for Gross Metastatic Disease

Aerosol Drug Delivery

Because the pulmonary parenchyma has a large absorptive surface area and high blood flow, the administration of therapeutic agents directly to it remains a potential tractable and noninvasive method for localized and systemic drug delivery. Although the majority of clinical indications for aerosol drug delivery are the management of inflammatory airway pathologies (i.e., bronchitis), the ability of inhalation therapy to achieve high drug concentrations directly to the lungs with the minimization of systemic toxicities provides justification to test this method of drug delivery for the management of macroscopic pulmonary OS metastases in dogs.

Two studies have been conducted to evaluate the feasibility, tolerability, and anticancer activities of aerosolized cytotoxic therapies in dogs diagnosed with macroscopic pulmonary OS metastases.[279,280] In one study, six dogs with macroscopic pulmonary OS metastases were treated every 14 days for a total of 6 treatment cycles with inhalation doxorubicin, paclitaxel, or both.[279] Aerosolization therapy was well tolerated, with no dose-limiting hematologic or biochemical toxicity associated with inhalation therapy. However, in dogs treated with aerosolized doxorubicin, pulmonary histologic changes were identified at necropsy in some patients consisting of toxin-induced pneumonitis, multifocal interstitial fibrosis, alveolar histiocytosis, and type II pneumocyte proliferation. Measurable anticancer activity was documented in two dogs (partial remission) treated with inhalation doxorubicin and one dog (complete remission) treated with inhalation paclitaxel. The duration of complete remission in the one responder dog treated with inhalation paclitaxel was durable, lasting greater than 325 days.

In addition to doxorubicin and paclitaxel, aerosolized gemcitabine has also been evaluated in dogs with metastatic OSs. Although categorized as a pyrimidine antimetabolite that belongs to the nucleoside analog family, it was demonstrated in preclinical mouse OS xenograft models that the anticancer activity of aerosolized gemcitabine was mediated though the upregulation of Fas receptor expression on the surface of pulmonary metastatic OS cells.[281] Because lung epithelium basally expresses Fas ligand, the restoration of Fas receptor expression by OS cells would consequently render them susceptible to Fas receptor-/Fas ligand-mediated apoptosis. Based on this preclinical information, a comparative study with aerosolized gemcitabine was conducted in 20 dogs with macroscopic pulmonary OS metastases.[280] Dogs were treated twice weekly with inhalation gemcitabine and monitored for toxicity and anticancer activity. Aerosolized gemcitabine was well tolerated with no dose-limiting hematologic or biochemical toxicity reported and minimal histologic lung pathology following inhalation therapy. Mechanistic anticancer activities of aerosolized gemcitabine were supported by the identification of increases in percentage of necrosis, Fas receptor expression, and terminal deoxynucleotidyl transferase dUTP nick end labeling (TUNEL) positivity in macroscopic pulmonary OS metastatic lesions; however, clinically relevant tumor reductions, either partial or complete, were not achieved in any of the dogs treated.

Augmentation of Antitumor Immunity

Cytokines are cellular peptides, some of which actively aid or stimulate the immune system to recognize and attack cancer cells. Although numerous cytokines participate in shaping the strength, specificity, and longevity of antitumor immune responses, interleukin-2 (IL-2) is a critical cytokine necessary for stimulating the growth, differentiation, and survival of antigen-specific cytotoxic T-cells. Additional immune effects orchestrated by IL-2 include the facilitation of immunoglobulin production by B-cells, as well as the differentiation and proliferation of NK cells. Despite the pleiotropic and desirable antitumor immune activities of IL-2, its systemic administration has been clinically limited due to severe toxicities. As such, alternative delivery strategies have been investigated to attenuate IL-2–associated toxicities, yet maximize its potent immunomodulatory effects.

For the treatment of pulmonary metastases, the localized deposition of IL-2 or the preferential gene expression of IL-2 within the lung parenchyma has been investigated as a novel and effective treatment option in dogs with macroscopic OS metastases. Initial studies evaluated the antitumor activities of liposomal IL-2 when delivered directly to the pulmonary parenchyma in the form of inhalation therapy.[282] Dogs were nebulized with liposomal IL-2 daily for 30 days, and immunomodulatory effects of IL-2 were confirmed by increases in bronchoalveolar lavage effector cell numbers and lytic activities, with resultant complete regression of macroscopic pulmonary OS metastases in two of four dogs. The duration of complete regression was durable in responder dogs, lasting between 12 and 20 months. Alternatively to inhaled liposomal IL-2 delivery strategies, IV gene therapy as liposome-DNA complexes encoding IL-2 has also been investigated.[283] Based on its preferential accumulation and subsequent transgene expression within the lung parenchyma, the tolerability, immunomodulatory effects, and antitumor activity of IV liposome DNA complexes encoding IL-2 were evaluated in 20 dogs with chemotherapy-resistant macroscopic OS metastases. Following administration, the immunomodulatory effects of liposome DNA complexes were substantiated by the induction of fever, leukogram changes, monocyte activation, and increased NK cell activities. On completion of 12 consecutive weekly IV treatments with liposome DNA complexes, measurable responses were achieved in 3 out of 20 dogs, with one complete remission and two partial remissions.

Additional to IL-2 therapy, other investigations have evaluated alternative strategies for activating the immune system including the IV administration of a genetically-modified and attenuated bacterial species, *Salmonella typhimurium* (VNP20009).[284] Based on the premise that anaerobic bacteria have potential as novel immunomodulatory cancer therapeutics, a phase I dose escalation study was conducted with VNP20009 in 41 dogs with spontaneous cancers. Dose-limiting toxicity associated with VNP20009 administration included fever and vomiting, symptoms associated with systemic immune activation. Importantly, preferential tumor tissue tropism of VNP20009 was confirmed by gene transcription and bacterial culture techniques in a substantial proportion of tumor samples. In a subset of four dogs with macroscopic OS pulmonary metastases, one partial remission was achieved for a duration of 68 days.

Palliative Treatment: Primary and Metastatic Bone Cancer Pain

Bone Cancer Pain Physiology

Although pain is an evolutionarily conserved protective mechanism, its categorization can be differentiated based on temporal aspects (acute, chronic, or intermittent), intensity (mild, moderate, severe, or excruciating), and anatomic origin (somatic, visceral, or neuropathic). The sensation of pain is mediated by specialized afferent nerve endings, called *nociceptors,* that initiate sodium channel opening and subsequent neuronal depolarization events within small, myelinated Aδ and unmyelinated C fibers. Generated neuronal impulses are propagated through the dorsal horn of the spinal cord via the dorsal root ganglia, where they synapse with second-order neurons of the gray matter with subsequent modulation of impulse intensity. The resultant nociceptive information is carried to the brain via the spinothalamic tracts, where it can be integrated, processed, and recognized in multiple areas of the brain.[285]

The greatest density of afferent nociceptors responsible for pain-impulse generation is found at the periosteal surface and medullary cavity, specifically in bone. As such, malignant perturbations affecting these bone anatomic compartments are associated with intense pain.[286,287] In dogs with OS, the generation of bone cancer pain is attributed to two specific host responses. First, the invasive growth of malignant osteoblasts in the bone microenvironment results in the release of chemical mediators by nonneoplastic stromal cells, which in turn stimulate nociceptors and lead to the generation of painful sensations. Second, the genesis, maintenance, and exacerbation of bone cancer pain are directly attributed to dysregulated and pathologic osteoclastic bone resorption.[286,287] Based on these mechanisms of bone cancer pain generation, the most effective management of malignant osteolytic pain would combine the eradication of malignant osteoblasts in bone matrix and the inhibition of tumor-induced osteoclastic bone resorption.

Palliative Radiation Therapy

RT is considered the most effective treatment modality for the management of osteolytic bone pain in human cancer patients and likewise has been investigated and extensively applied to alleviating bone cancer pain in dogs diagnosed with OS. Mechanistically, the analgesic effects of ionizing radiation may be attributed to the induction of apoptosis in both malignant osteoblasts and resorbing osteoclasts,[288] and in dogs, these effects have been supported by percent tumor necrosis assessment.[193,228,289] As such, ionizing radiation reduces overall tumor burden and attenuates the degree of osteoclastic resorption within the focal OS microenvironment.

Multiple palliative radiation protocols have been evaluated and reported in the veterinary literature, with the majority of dosing schemes utilizing 2 to 4 individual treatments of 6 to 10 Gy fractions. Although variable and subjectively reported in these studies, the alleviation of bone cancer pain was achieved in the majority of OS dogs treated and ranged from 74% to 93%. Although the majority of dogs symptomatically improved following palliative RT, the median time interval of subjective pain alleviation was not durable and ranged from 53 to 130 days.[290-295] Because most conventional palliative radiation protocols only utilize 2 to 4 treatment fractions, the total cumulative radiation dose administered is relatively low (<32 Gy); therefore acute and late radiation toxicity is not a limiting factor for the majority of patients treated. This also may allow repetition of palliative radiation protocols in the same patient subsequent to return of pain as the tumor ultimately advances. Although megavoltage palliative RT appears effective when used as a single-agent treatment option for short-term pain management, some investigations suggest that the concurrent administration of IV systemic chemotherapy along with palliative radiation might enhance analgesic response rates and durations.[293] Systemic chemotherapy is indicated for the delay of micrometastatic disease development in dogs diagnosed with appendicular OS, thus the adjuvant institution of chemotherapy combined with palliative RT might have the dual benefit of improving local pain control and improving overall survival time through the delay of micrometastatic disease development.

Radiopharmaceuticals

^{153}Samarium is a radioisotope that undergoes gamma and beta decay, allowing for concurrent biodistribution tracking studies, as well as therapeutic ionizing radiation delivery within a 2- to 3-mm deposition radius. When ^{153}Samarium is conjugated to EDTMP, which is a bisphosphonate, the resultant compound ^{153}Sm-EDTMP preferentially concentrates in areas of increased osteoblastic activity and binds to exposed hydroxyapatite crystals.[296] By virtue of its osteotropism and defined radius of ionizing radiation deposition, ^{153}Sm-EDTMP is currently used as a radiopharmaceutical for the palliative treatment of multifocal, skeletal metastases in humans afflicted with breast or prostate carcinoma.[297]

Similar to humans diagnosed with skeletal malignant osteolysis, the use of ^{153}Sm-EDTMP has been investigated and reported for alleviating bone cancer pain in dogs with appendicular and axial OS.[298-301] In dogs treated with ^{153}Sm-EDTMP, the predicted radiation dose equivalent achieved within the immediate bone tumor microenvironment has been estimated to approximate 20 Gy,[298] although its intratumoral biodistribution is expected to be nonhomogeneous based on regional differences in reparative osteoblastic activities. Following IV ^{153}Sm-EDTMP administration, the majority (63% to 83%) of dogs with OS demonstrate improved lameness scores and activity levels, suggesting the achievement of pain palliation.[298-301] Despite clinical improvement in most dogs treated, the duration of pain alleviation has not been extensively documented but appears to approximate similar durations of pain control achieved with megavoltage teletherapy. In a small fraction (<5%) of treated dogs, ^{153}Sm-EDTMP has resulted in the complete involution of malignant skeletal lesions, resulting in durable pain alleviation and prolonged survival times. Overall, ^{153}Sm-EDTMP is well-tolerated; however, side effects associated with treatment include transient decreases in platelet and white blood cell counts as a consequence of beta energy deposition within the proximity of pluripotent marrow stem cells.[300]

Aminobisphosphonates

Aminobisphosphonates (NBPs) are synthetic analogs of inorganic pyrophosphate that were initially utilized for diagnostic purposes in bone scanning, based on their ability to preferentially adsorb to sites of active bone mineral remodeling. The pharmaceutical use of NBPs has gained wide acceptance in the therapy of human nonneoplastic bone resorptive disorders, such as osteoporosis and Paget's disease.[302] In addition to the management of these metabolic disorders, NBPs are considered first-line treatment for malignant skeletal osteolysis, including paraneoplastic hypercalcemia, multiple myeloma, and metastatic bone diseases in human cancer patients.[303,304]

The effective treatment of bone disorders by NBPs is attributed to their differential effect on bone resorption and bone mineralization. At concentrations safely obtainable in vivo, NBPs inhibit bone resorption without inhibiting the process of bone mineralization. Mechanistically, the bone protective effects exerted by NBPs are through the induction of osteoclast apoptosis, which results in the net attenuation of pathologic bone resorption.[305,306] Specifically, NBPs interfere with posttranslational prenylation of small guanosine triphosphate (GTP)-binding proteins, including Ras, Rho, and Rac,[307] and the disruption of these small GTP-binding proteins results in the failure of normal intracellular signaling and interaction with the extracellular matrix, thereby triggering osteoclast apoptosis.

Although NBPs are commercially available in different formulations, the effective management of tumor-induced hypercalcemia, osteolytic bone metastases of breast cancer, and osteolytic lesions of multiple myeloma appear to require the administration of IV NBP and at relatively high doses. Historically, pamidronate and zoledronate have been the two most commonly utilized IV NBP formulations in human oncology for their ability to decrease bone pain, improve quality of life, delay progression of the bone lesions, and decrease the frequency of malignant skeletal events.

Because OS is characterized by focal and aggressive malignant osteolysis, the investigation of NBPs has been a focus of clinical interest, and several studies have demonstrated the cytotoxic effects of NBPs against canine OS cell lines in vitro. In three independent studies, it was concluded that various NBPs, including alendronate, pamidronate, and zoledronate exerted dose- and time-dependent cytotoxicity in immortalized canine OS cell lines.[308-310] Although the in vitro studies were in agreement with the cytotoxic effects of NBPs on canine OS cell viability, the inhibitory concentration 50% (IC50) derived from the experiments varied among the studies. Nonetheless, the documented direct cytotoxic effects of NBPs on canine OS cell lines served as a springboard to rationally investigate the bone pain–alleviating effects of NBPs in dogs with OS.

The first reported description in the veterinary literature was the use of oral alendronate for the palliative management of two dogs with OS.[311] Based on the unexpectedly long survival times reported in this anecdotal study, the authors suggested that NBP therapy might have a role in managing canine malignant bone disorders. Given that IV NBPs have been historically used for the management of malignant osteolysis in humans, a prospective study principally evaluating the safety of IV pamidronate was conducted in 33 dogs diagnosed with primary and secondary skeletal tumors.[312] IV pamidronate (1.0 mg/kg diluted with 0.9% sodium chloride to a total volume of 250 ml) as a 2-hour constant rate infusion (CRI) every 28 days was well tolerated, and in a subset of dogs, the bone biologic and clinically relevant therapeutic effects of IV pamidronate were documented as significant reductions in urine NTx concentrations, increases in relative primary tumor bone mineral density (rBMD) as assessed by dual-energy x-ray absorptiometry (DEXA), and subjective pain alleviation.

Following the established safety of IV pamidronate in dogs with skeletal tumors, a second study of 43 dogs treated with IV pamidronate (comparing 1.0 mg/kg versus 2.0 mg/kg) was conducted to further characterize the biologic activity of pamidronate specifically for the management of appendicular OS-associated bone pain and pathologic bone resorption.[313] Overall, 12/43 (28%) OS-bearing dogs treated with single-agent IV pamidronate achieved pain alleviation for greater than 4 months. In addition to the subjective analgesic effects of pamidronate reported by pet owners, changes in urine NTx concentrations and DEXA-assessed rBMD correlated with therapeutic response.

Although original studies have focused on the palliative effects of pamidronate when used as a single-agent, a recent study has documented the synergistic activity of pamidronate when coupled with palliative RT in dogs with appendicular OS through the use of subjective and objective surrogate endpoints. In a prospective, double-blind, randomized, placebo-controlled clinical trial, dogs with appendicular OS were to receive palliative RT (8 Gy, days 1 and 2) plus 0.9% saline infusion or pamidronate once every 4 weeks for 3 treatments (12-week study).[314] Prior to initial palliative RT and subsequent to each IV treatment with either 0.9% saline or pamidronate, all dogs were evaluated by force plate gait analysis, urine NTx concentrations, numeric lameness evaluation, and owner quality-of-life questionnaires. Out of 17 dogs, 8 received 0.9% saline and 9 received IV pamidronate (1.0 mg/kg). The saline placebo group dogs experienced a significant increase in numeric lameness score between weeks 0 and 12, and pamidronate significantly lowered the lameness scores on week 12 compared to saline. In addition, dogs receiving pamidronate had a significantly greater vertical impulse and total stance time on weeks 4 through 12 compared to saline placebo-treated dogs. Based on these findings, the addition of pamidronate to palliative therapy appeared to improve limb function compared to palliative RT alone.

In another study evaluating the benefit of combining pamidronate with conventional therapies for managing bone cancer pain, a double-blind, placebo-controlled study of 50 dogs with OS receiving palliative radiation, doxorubicin, and either saline placebo or pamidronate was conducted.[315] The median pain-free interval for dogs receiving adjuvant pamidronate or saline was 76 days and 75 days, respectively. Despite the apparent lack of pet owner–perceived analgesia, dogs that received adjuvant pamidronate did demonstrate improved quality-of-life scores and more importantly, superior bone biologic effects representative of decreased malignant bone resorption at the level of the primary tumor. Collectively, the findings from this clinical trial suggest that adjuvant pamidronate may not subjectively improve analgesia when dogs are already receiving treatment with megavoltage radiation and doxorubicin but still exert beneficial bone biologic effects within the bone tumor microenvironment in dogs with OS.

Although the majority of palliative studies have documented the effects of pamidronate, other more potent IV NBPs for managing malignant bone pain have also been evaluated in dogs with skeletal tumors. Zoledronate possesses 100-fold greater antiresorptive potency in comparison with pamidronate and has the advantage of being safely administered over a shorter period of time than other NBPs. In one case report, the use of IV zoledronate administered every 28 days was effective for the long-term pain management of a dog diagnosed with OS affecting the distal radius.[316] In a larger study, the bone biologic effects of IV zoledronate were evaluated in dogs diagnosed with primary and secondary skeletal tumors.[317] In this study, zoledronate was administered at a dose of 0.25 mg/kg as a 15-minute CRI every 28 days and was well tolerated with no overt biochemical evidence of renal toxicity in patients receiving multiple monthly infusions. In 10 dogs with appendicular OS, 50% of dogs treated achieved pain alleviation for greater than 4 months and also demonstrated significant increases in rBMD. The observation for increased rBMD in conjunction with pain alleviation suggests that zoledronate inhibits local malignant osteolysis and the generation of pain within the immediate bone-tumor microenvironment.

Comparative Aspects

Animal models for the study of human diseases are important to our understanding of the mechanism and etiology of disease and for the development and refinement of therapeutic strategies. Spontaneously developing diseases in animal populations are particularly useful for study.[318-320] Canine OS has many similarities to human OS in terms of genetic similarities, clinical presentation, biologic behavior, and metastatic progression and has been shown through many studies to be a valuable comparative model for study (Table 24-3).[7,320] OS is more common in dogs than in humans; therefore case accrual is more rapid. Because disease progression is more rapid in dogs than in humans, results of novel treatment protocols can be reported earlier than those of similar trials in humans. Research costs for clinical trials in dogs are less compared to those in human clinical trials, and, from an animal welfare

TABLE 24-3 Comparison of Canine and Human Osteosarcoma Characteristics

VARIABLE	DOG	HUMAN
Incidence in United States	>10,000/year	1000/year
Mean age	7 years	14 years
Race/breed	Large or giant purebreds	None
Body weight	90% >20 kg	Heavy
Site	77% long bones Metaphyseal Distal radius > proximal humerus Distal femur > tibia	90% long bones Metaphyseal Distal femur > proximal tibia Proximal humerus
Etiology	Generally unknown	Generally unknown
Percentage clinically confined to the limb at presentation	80%-90%	80%-90%
Percentage histologically high grade	95%	85%-90%
DNA index	75% aneuploid	75% aneuploid
Recognized genetic and molecular alterations	*p53, RB, PTEN, c-Met,* GH, and IGF-1	*p53, RB,* RecQ Helicase, *c-Met,* GH, and IGF-1
Prognostic indicators[173,174]	Alkaline phosphatase	Alkaline phosphatase
Metastatic rate without chemotherapy	90% before 1 year	80% before 2 years
Metastatic sites	Lung > bone > soft tissue	Lung > bone > soft tissue
Improved survival with chemotherapy	Yes	Yes
Regional lymph node metastasis	<5%, negative prognostically	Poor prognosis

Modified with permission from Withrow SJ, Powers BE, Straw RC, et al: Comparative aspects of osteosarcoma: dog versus man, *Clin Orthop Relat Res* 270:159–167, 1991.

GH, Growth hormone; *IGF-1,* insulin-like growth factor-1.

standpoint, no disease is induced and dogs with cancer can potentially be helped through the course of the research.

OS is an uncommon cancer of humans affecting mainly children in their second decade of life and remains a very serious, aggressive solid tumor. Fortunately, there has been a great improvement in survival rates with the use of established multidrug adjuvant protocols. The long-term survival rate for human OS is presently 60%, which contrasts to the 20% expected 5-year survival rates of the early 1980s. A retrospective study of 648 human OS patients reported a mean survival of 3 years; however, this represented all cases at one institution since the 1970s and therefore improvements over time were not presented.[321] Factors that negatively affected outcome included older age, advanced local or systemic stage, axial location, larger size, and a lower percentage of necrosis following neoadjuvant treatment. The type of surgery (amputation or limb sparing) did not impact outcome, supporting the need for advancement of systemic medical therapy to impact survival. Limb-sparing programs are becoming more common, and many survivors of OS retain functional, pain-free limbs. In two reports, one from the United States[322] and one from Italy,[323,324] aggressive neoadjuvant chemotherapy resulted in limb-sparing success of 93.5% and 83%, respectively, and a projected 10-year survival of 93%.

Bone Surface Osteosarcoma

OS usually originates from elements within the medullary canal of bones (intraosseous OS); however, there are forms of this cancer that originate from the outside surface of bones. Periosteal OS is a high-grade form of surface OS and seems to arise from the periosteal surface but has invasive characteristics seen radiographically.[325] There is cortical lysis with extension of the tumor into the bone and surrounding soft tissues. These tumors are histologically similar to intraosseous OS and have similar aggressive biologic behavior.

In contrast, parosteal OS, or juxtacortical OS, arises from the periosteal surface of bones but appears less aggressive than periosteal OS both radiographically and in terms of biologic behavior. Parosteal OS is relatively uncommon and has a moderately well-circumscribed radiographic appearance. The tumors grow out from the periosteal side of a cortex and cortical lysis is usually very mild on radiographs. Histologically, these tumors look more benign compared to intraosseous or periosteal OS. These tumors contain well-differentiated cartilage, fibrous tissue, and bone with sparse regions of sarcoma cells adjacent to tumor osteoid. Histologic specimens must be evaluated carefully because it is often easy to miss the areas of tumor cells and misdiagnose the lesion as osteoma, chondroma, or reactive bone. These tumors generally do not invade the medullary canal and tend to grow out from the bone on broad pedicles. Diagnosis is based on typical histologic and radiographic findings.

Parosteal OS is usually slow growing but can induce pain at the local site. Metastases can occur, but the prognosis for long-term survival is much better than for intraosseous OS.[326,327] Control of parosteal OS can be achieved by en bloc resection of the tumor with the adjacent cortical bone. This has been reported for tumors of the zygomatic arch (Figure 24-12).[327] If full-thickness cortex needs to be removed for tumors on long bones, reconstruction may be performed using autogenous corticocancellous bone, such as a rib, ileal crest, or allogeneic cortical bone. A report described a surface OS without cortical destruction (similar to parosteal) that had an aggressive histology and biologic behavior.[328]

Other Primary Bone Tumors of Dogs

Primary bone tumors other than OS make up somewhere between 5% and 10% of bone malignancies in dogs. These tumors are chondrosarcomas, hemangiosarcomas, fibrosarcomas, lymphomas

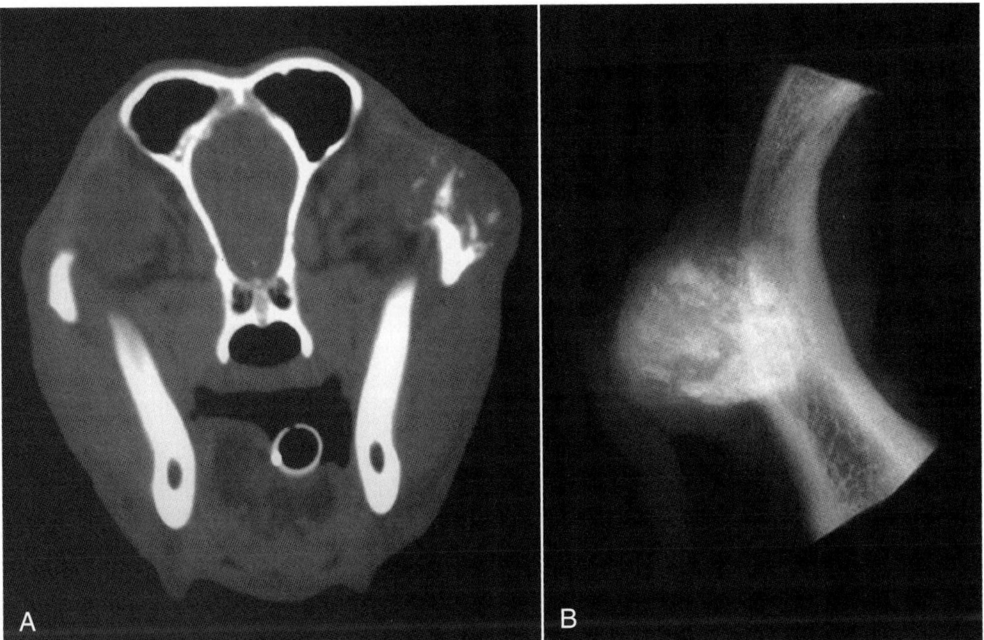

FIGURE 24-12 **A,** CT scan of a low-grade parosteal OS of the zygomatic arch in a dog. Low-grade primary bone tumors are often more radiodense and well circumscribed. **B,** Specimen radiograph of the case in **A** after zygomatic arch resection.

(see Chapter 32, Section A), and plasma cell tumors (see Chapter 32, Section D).

It can be difficult to distinguish chondroblastic OS from chondrosarcoma, fibroblastic OS from fibrosarcoma, and telangiectatic OS from hemangiosarcoma when only small amounts of biopsy tissue are evaluated.[135] This makes interpretation of older reports difficult in terms of trying to establish the true incidence of the different types of primary bone tumors. This also underscores the importance of evaluating the entire excised specimen to validate the preoperative biopsy. All too often a bone malignancy thought to be relatively low grade from preoperative biopsy is upgraded to a true OS once the histology of the surgical specimen is reviewed. This may change the prognosis and postsurgical treatment plan.

Chondrosarcoma

Chondrosarcoma is the second most common primary tumor of bone in humans and dogs and accounts for approximately 5% to 10% of all canine primary bone tumors.[2-5,329] Chondrosarcomas are characterized histologically by anaplastic cartilage cells that elaborate a cartilaginous matrix. There is a spectrum of degree of differentiation and maturation of the cells within and between each tumor. Histologic grading systems have been devised.[330] The etiology is generally unknown, although chondrosarcoma can arise in dogs with preexisting multiple cartilaginous exostosis.[331-333] In a clinicopathologic study of 97 dogs with chondrosarcoma, the mean age was 8.7 years (ranging from 1 to 15 years) and golden retrievers were at a higher risk of developing chondrosarcoma than any other breed.[334] There was no sex predilection, and 61% of the tumors occurred on flat bones. Chondrosarcoma can originate in the nasal cavity, ribs, long bones, pelvis, extraskeletal sites (such as the mammary gland, heart valves, aorta, larynx, trachea, lung, and omentum), vertebrae, facial bones, digits, and os penis.[35,330,334-341] The nasal cavity is the most common site for canine chondrosarcoma.[330,334]

Chondrosarcoma is generally considered to be slow to metastasize. Tumor location rather than histologic grade was prognostic in one study.[330] The reported median survival of dogs with nasal chondrosarcoma ranges from 210 days to 580 days with various treatments (RT, rhinotomy and RT, and rhinotomy alone; see Chapter 23, Section B).[334,342] Metastatic disease is not a reported feature of nasal chondrosarcoma in dogs. The reported median survival for dogs with rib chondrosarcoma varies widely.[21,167,330,343] Reports prior to 1992 contained few cases that were treated with intent to cure, but 15 dogs with rib chondrosarcoma treated with en bloc resection in a more recent study had a median survival of 1080 days.[165] The median survival for dogs with chondrosarcoma was 540 days in a study of five dogs treated with amputation alone.[334] Death was usually associated with metastatic disease. A reliable adjuvant chemotherapeutic agent is not known for canine chondrosarcoma. In humans, chondrosarcoma is considered a local disease, with a moderate rate of metastasis, which can be predicted by histologic grade. Aggressive surgical resection often results in long-term tumor control.[344] Although this tumor is generally considered resistant to standard RT, the authors have noted objective responses to coarse-fraction radiation protocols in a handful of cases in which surgery was not an option.

Hemangiosarcoma

Primary hemangiosarcoma of bone is rare and accounts for less than 5% of all bone tumors (see Chapter 33, Section A). This disease generally affects middle-aged to older dogs and can occur in dogs of any size. This is a highly metastatic tumor, and virtually all dogs affected will develop measurable metastatic disease within 6 months of diagnosis. Metastases can be widely spread throughout various organs such as lungs, liver, spleen, heart, skeletal muscles, kidney, brain, and bones. Dogs can present with multiple lesions, making it difficult to determine the site of primary disease. Histologically, hemangiosarcoma is composed of highly anaplastic mesenchymal cells, which are precursors to vascular endothelium. The cells are arranged in chords separated by a collagenous background and may appear to be forming vascular channels or sinuses. Cellular pleomorphism and numerous mitotic figures are features of this highly malignant disease. There is profound bone lysis, and the malignant cells aggressively invade adjacent normal structures. The lesion, however, may be confused with telangiectatic OS, especially if the diagnosis is based on small tissue samples. Often the dominant radiographic feature is lysis; however, hemangiosarcoma does not have an unequivocally unique radiographic appearance, and diagnosis is based on histology.

If hemangiosarcoma is diagnosed, the dog must be thoroughly staged with thoracic and abdominal films, bone survey radiography or bone scintigraphy, and ultrasonographic evaluation, particularly of the heart and abdominal organs. Right atrial hemangiosarcoma may be present without clinical or radiographic signs of pericardial effusion. The prognosis is poor, and even dogs with hemangiosarcoma clinically confined to one bony site have less than a 10% probability of surviving 1 year following complete excision. Cyclophosphamide, vincristine, and doxorubicin have been used in combination as an adjuvant protocol, and the reported median survival of dogs with nonskeletal hemangiosarcoma is 172 days.[345] In a patient population represented by a variety of primary tumor sites, doxorubicin as a single-agent adjuvant seemed to be as effective as the combination of drugs, with an MST of 172 days in patients in which all gross disease is surgically resected.[346] In a group of dogs with splenic hemangiosarcoma, L-MTP-PE resulted in a median survival of 277 days, compared to 143 days for dogs receiving empty liposomes.[347]

Fibrosarcoma

Primary fibrosarcoma is also a rare tumor of dogs and accounts for less than 5% of all primary bone tumors.[4] Unfortunately, the difficulty in distinguishing fibrosarcoma from fibroblastic OS histologically (especially from small tissue samples) renders study of this tumor difficult. In one report, 11 dogs thought to have fibrosarcoma were reevaluated after complete resection and the histologic diagnosis was changed to OS in 6 dogs.[348] Histologic characteristics of fibrosarcoma have been described as interwoven bundles of fibroblasts within a collagen matrix permeating cancellous and cortical bone but not associated with osteoid produced by the tumor cells. Host-derived new bone can be seen, however, especially at the periphery of the tumor.

Complete surgical resection of the primary lesion is recommended for dogs with fibrosarcoma clinically confined to the primary site. This treatment may be curative, although metastatic potential may be considerable. There is no good evidence that adjuvant chemotherapy is of any benefit in preventing metastatic disease. It has been postulated that primary fibrosarcoma of bone has a propensity to metastasize to such sites as the heart, pericardium, skin, and bones rather than lung.[348]

Multilobular Osteochondrosarcoma

Multilobular osteochondrosarcoma (MLO) is an uncommon tumor that generally arises from the skull of dogs.[349-351] Many names have been used to describe this disease, including chondroma rodens and multilobular osteoma. These tumors have a characteristic appearance on radiographs, CT, and MRI: generally the borders of the tumor are sharply demarcated with limited lysis of adjacent bone, and there is a coarse granular mineral density throughout (Figure 24-13).[352,353] However, there is one report of an MLO of the vertebra that did not have radiographic abnormalities.[354] Histologically, these tumors are composed of multiple lobules, each centered on a core of cartilaginous or bony matrix that is surrounded by a thin layer of spindle cells. A histologic grading system has been described.[350,351] These tumors have the potential to recur locally following incomplete resection, and metastasis can occur. In one report of 39 dogs, the median age of affected dogs was 8 years, the median weight was 29 kg, and there was no breed or sex predilection.[351] Slightly less than 50% of dogs had local tumor recurrence following resection at a median time of approximately 800 days. A little over half the dogs developed metastases after treatment; however, time to metastasis was prolonged with a median of 542 days. The MST was 800 days. Local tumor recurrence and metastasis after treatment appears to be predicted by histologic grade and the ability to obtain histologically complete resection. Local tumor excision with histologically complete surgical margins appears to offer a good opportunity for long-term tumor control, especially for low-grade lesions. When metastatic lesions are identified by thoracic radiography, dogs may remain asymptomatic for their lung disease for up to 1 year or more. The role of chemotherapy and RT in the management of MLO is not well defined.

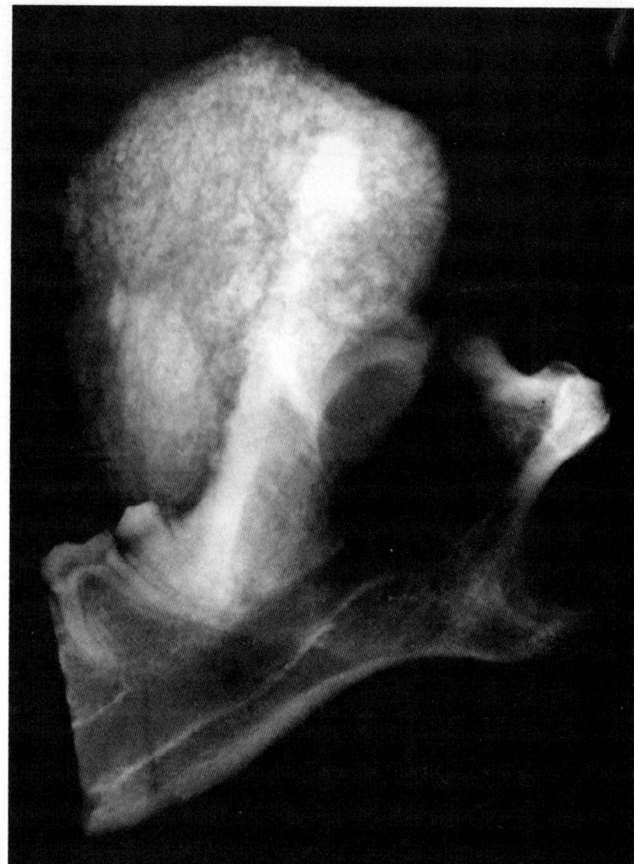

FIGURE 24-13 Specimen radiograph of a multilobular osteochondrosarcoma arising from the vertical ramus of the mandible in a dog. These tumors have a granular radiographic appearance often referred to as "popcorn ball."

Metastatic Tumors of Bone

Almost any malignant tumor can metastasize to bone via the hematogenous route. The lumbar vertebrae, femur, humerus, rib, and pelvis are common sites for cancer spread, possibly because these are predilection sites for bone metastasis from the common

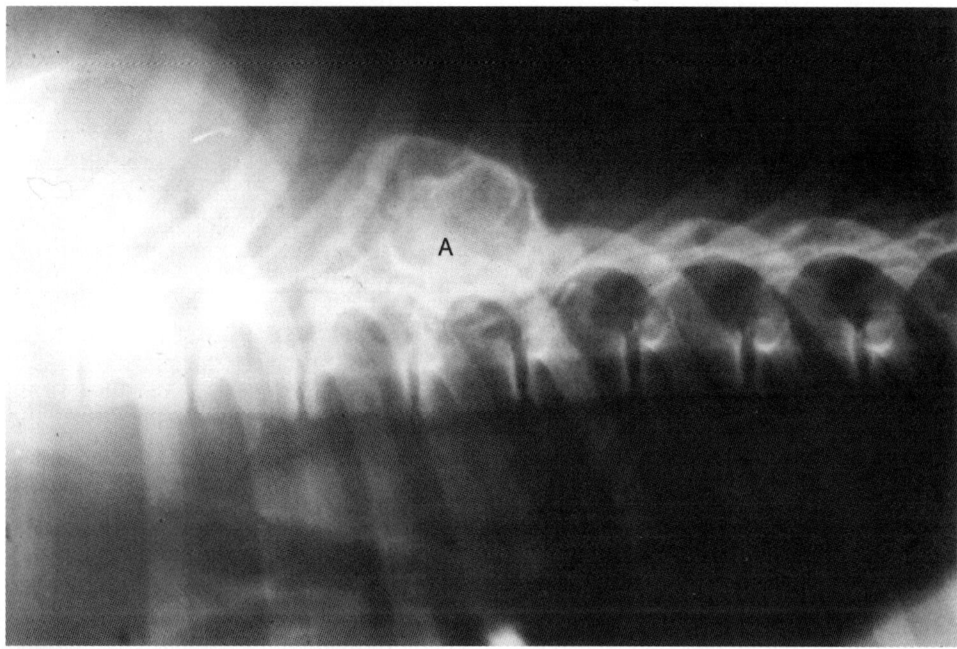

FIGURE 24-14 Lateral radiograph of a multiple cartilaginous exostosis lesion of the dorsal spinous process in a dog *(A)*.

urinogenital malignancies, such as prostate, bladder, urethral, and mammary cancer.[355,356] Metastatic lesions in long bones frequently affect the diaphysis, likely because of the proximity to a nutrient foramen. Nuclear scintigraphy is a sensitive technique to detect bone metastasis. A whole-skeleton bone scan is recommended when metastatic bone cancer is suspected because it is common for multiple sites of metastasis to be present, even if the patient is symptomatic for only one bone.

Benign Tumors of Bone

Osteomas

Osteomas are benign tumors of bone.[357] Radiographically, these are well-circumscribed, dense bony projections, which are usually not painful to palpation. Histologically, they are composed of tissue nearly indistinguishable from reactive bone. The diagnosis is made after considering the history and physical examination, as well as radiographic and histologic findings. The most important differential diagnosis is MLO when the lesion occurs on the skull. Treatment for osteoma is simple surgical excision, which is usually curative.

Multiple Cartilaginous Exostosis

Multiple cartilaginous exostosis (MCE) is considered a developmental condition of growing dogs. There is evidence that the etiology of this condition may have a heritable component.[332,358] The actual incidence of MCE is difficult to determine because affected dogs may show no signs and the diagnosis is often incidental. Lesions occur by the process of endochondral ossification when new bone is formed from a cartilage cap analogous to a physis. Lesions are located on bones, which form from endochondral ossification, and lesions stop growing at skeletal maturity. Malignant transformation of MCE lesions has been reported, but generally, they remain as unchanged, mature, bony projections from the surface of the bone from which they arose.[333]

Dogs typically present because of a nonpainful or moderately painful palpable mass on the surface of a bone or bones. The pain and lameness is thought to be due to mechanical interference of the mass with the overlying soft tissue structures. In the case of MCE of vertebral bodies, animals can present with clinical signs associated with spinal cord impingement. Radiographically, there is a bony mass on the surface of the affected bone, which has a benign appearance with fine trabecular pattern in the body of the mass (Figure 24-14). To obtain a histologic diagnosis, biopsy material must be collected so sections can include the cartilaginous cap and the underlying stalk of bone. Histologically, this cartilaginous cap gives rise to an orderly array of maturing bone according to the sequence of endochondral ossification. The cortical bone surfaces of the mass and the adjacent bone are confluent.[331] A strong presumptive diagnosis is made by evaluation of the physical findings, history, and radiographic findings.

Treatment involves conservative surgical excision, but this is only necessary if signs do not abate after the dog is skeletally mature. Because of the likelihood of a heritable etiology, affected dogs should not be bred. Owners should also be advised of the possibility of late malignant transformation. Dogs with a previous history of MCE should be carefully evaluated for bone malignancy if signs return later in life.

Bone Cysts

Cysts are rare, benign lesions of bone. The majority of the veterinary literature pertaining to bone cysts centers on several small series of cases or single case reports.[359-363] Affected animals are often young and present because of mild or moderate lameness; however, pathologic fracture can occur through cystic areas of long bones, leading to severe lameness. There appears to be a familial tendency in Doberman pinschers and Old English sheepdogs. The nomenclature in various reviews of canine bone cysts is confusing. By definition, a cyst is a fluid-filled sac lined by epithelium. The only true cyst of primary intraosseous origin is a simple bone cyst (SBC, or unicameral bone cyst). These lesions are usually in metaphyseal regions of long bones, and they can adjoin an open growth plate. Sometimes, however, unicameral bone cysts can be diaphyseal or epiphyseal. Neither the etiology nor the pathogenesis is known, but it is speculated that the lesions may be the result of trauma to the growth plate interfering with proper endochondral ossification. Others have theorized that with the rapid resorption and deposition of bone occurring in the metaphysis of a young animal, a cyst might develop if resorption is so rapid that a focus of loose fibrous tissue forms. The focus of fibrous tissue may then obstruct the thin-walled sinusoids, causing interstitial fluid to build up and form a cyst. The theory that appears to be partially substantiated is the synovial "rest" thesis. It is suggested that during fetal development a "rest" of synovial or perisynovial tissue becomes misplaced or incorporated into the adjacent osseous tissue. If this tissue remains or becomes functional, subsequent synovial secretion results in a cyst developing in the bone. Cysts have been described in bone just below articular cartilage (subchondral bone cysts or juxtacortical bone cysts).[361,362,364] In these, it has often been possible to demonstrate direct communication with the articular synovial membrane. Radiographically, SBCs are single or, more commonly, multilocular, sharply defined, centrally located, radiolucent defects in the medullary canal of long bones. Variable degrees of thinning of the cortex with symmetric bone "expansion" are often a feature of the radiographs (Figure 24-15). The diagnosis cannot be reliably made from interpretation of radiographs alone. Lytic OS can be misdiagnosed as SBC. Diagnosis of an SBC relies on the histologic finding of a thin, fibrous wall lined by flat to slightly plump layers of mesothelial or endothelial cells. Treatment consists of meticulous curettage and packing the space with autogenous bone graft.

Aneurysmal bone "cysts" (ABCs) are spongy, multiloculated masses filled with free-flowing blood. The walls of an ABC are rarely lined by epithelium, and the lesion is possibly an arteriovenous malformation. A proposed pathogenesis of ABCs is that a primary event such as trauma or a benign bone tumor occurs within the bone or periosteum. This event disrupts the vasculature, resulting in a rapidly enlarging lesion with anomalous blood flow, which damages the bone mesenchyme. The bone reacts by proliferating. As the vascular anomaly becomes stabilized, the reactive bone becomes more consolidated and matures. It is important to differentiate these lesions from OS or other malignant lesions of bone. The age of affected dogs ranges from 2 to 14 years, but it has been reported in a 6-month-old dog.[360] Treatment can be achieved by en bloc resection and reconstruction, but extensive curettage with packing of the defect with autogenous bone graft can be effective.

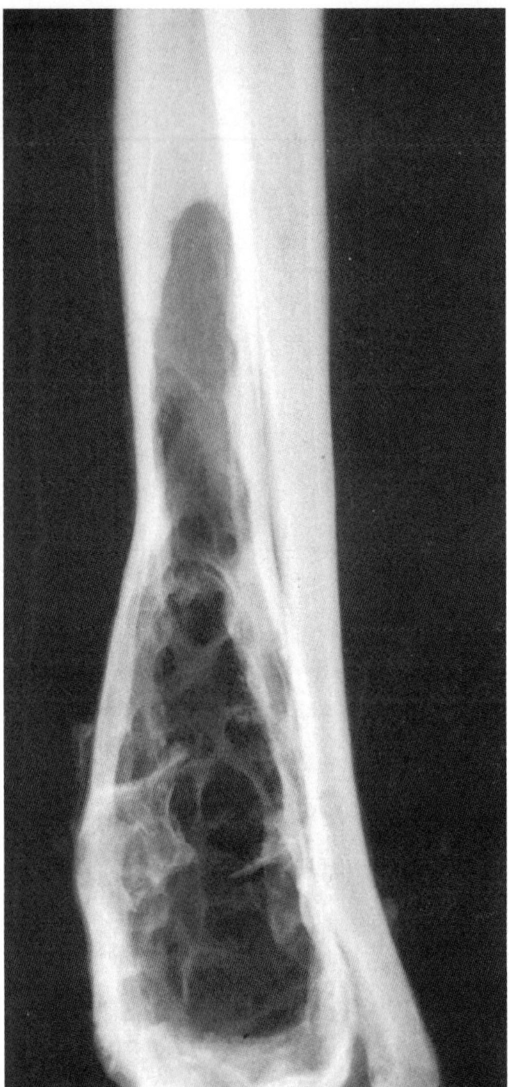

FIGURE 24-15 Lateral radiograph of a distal radial bone lesion histologically confirmed as a simple bone cyst (SBC). Typical radiographic features include a multilocular, sharply defined, centrally located radiolucency, without evidence of cortical destruction.

Primary Bone Tumors of Cats

Incidence and Risk Factors

Primary tumors involving the bones of cats are rare. An estimate of the incidence of all bone tumors in cats is 4.9 per 100,000.[365] Between 67% and 90% of bone tumors in cats are histologically malignant. OSs are the most common primary bone tumor in cats accounting for 70% to 80% of all primary malignant cancer of cats. Feline OS occurs in appendicular or axial skeletal sites and extraskeletal sites. OS occurs in appendicular long bones approximately twice as often as in axial skeleton sites.[366] However, in one study, 50 of 90 skeletal OS cases were appendicular and 40 of 90 were axial.[367] Axial OS originates most commonly in the skull (especially oral cavity) and pelvis but is also reported in the ribs and vertebrae. The disease in cats differs from that in dogs in that the primary lesions occur more often in hind limbs in cats (distal femur and proximal tibia) and the disease is reported to be far less metastatic than in dogs.[368] In a large feline OS case study, 56 of 146 cases were extraskeletal in origin, with the most commonly affected sites being those commonly used for vaccination: interscapular, dorsal lumbar, or thigh areas. Other locations included ocular/orbital, oral, intestinal, and mammary sites. No mention is made of any differences in the pathology of these tumors in comparison to skeletal sites.[367] There are case reports of feline extraskeletal OSs in the flank, liver, and duodenum.[369-371]

OS generally affects older cats (reported mean ages of 8.5,[366] 10,[368] 10.2,[368] and 10.7[372] years), but the age range of reported cases is large (1 to 20 years), so bone lesions in younger cats cannot be ruled out as OSs based on age criteria alone. The age at presentation for axial OS is greater than appendicular OS.[367] Conflicting reports on gender predisposition exist with either no difference between sexes or a slight male predisposition.[366-368,372] OS was reported to arise after a limb fracture was repaired with an intramedullary pin in one cat and following RT in another.[38]

MCE is a disease that occurs after skeletal maturity in cats. This is in contrast to dogs in which exostoses develop before closure of growth plates. Also, in contrast to dogs, the lesions seldom affect long bones, are rarely symmetric, and are probably of viral rather than familial origin. There does not appear to be any breed or sex predisposition, although early reports of this condition were in the Siamese.[373] Affected cats range in age from 1.3 to 8 years (mean 3.2 years).[374] Virtually all cats with MCEs will test positive for feline leukemia virus (FeLV) antigenemia. This disease has an aggressive natural behavior.

Pathology and Natural Behavior

The histologic characteristics of feline OS are similar to canine OS. OS of cats is composed of mesenchymal cells embedded in malignant osteoid. There may be a considerable amount of cartilage present, and osteoid may be scant. A feature of some feline OS cases is the presence of multinucleate giant cells, which may be numerous. Reactive host bone and remnants of host bone are often present in specimens. Tumors are seen to be invasive; however, some surrounding soft tissue may be compressed rather than infiltrated. There is often variation of the histologic appearance within the tumor, with some portions having a more fibrosarcomatous appearance and others more cartilaginous. Some authors have described subtypes that resemble those seen in dogs: chondroblastic, fibroblastic, and telangiectatic, as well as the giant cell variant. These histologic subtypes, however, do not appear to confer any prognostic predictive value.[375,376] OSs in cats are locally aggressive but have a low metastatic rate compared to canine OS. Feline OS can be of the juxtacortical type.

Osteochondroma may occur as a solitary lesion in cats, but there is a form that is multicentric (osteochondromatosis). The lesions are composed of hard, irregular exostoses with a fibrous and cartilaginous cap.[377] Endochondral ossification occurs from the cartilage cap, which extends to a variable thickness. This cap tends to blend with adjacent tissue, making its surgical removal difficult. Cats usually develop multiple sites of disease, and there is a potential for malignant transformation and metastasis. The presence of FeLV antigenemia is also a foreboding prognostic finding for these cats.

History and Clinical Signs

The most common signs of OS are lameness, swelling, and deformity, depending on the location of the lesion. The lesions may appear radiographically similar to the OS in dogs with mixed osteoblastic and osteolytic aggressive bone lesion with an ill-defined zone of transition between normal and tumor-affected bone; however, some cats have lesions arising from the periosteal surface (juxtacortical OS).[366] Tumors can reach a large size without evidence of severe clinical signs. It is rare for cats to have metastatic OS at presentation.

Cats with viral-associated MCE have rapidly progressing, conspicuous, hard swellings over affected sites causing pain and loss of function. Common sites for lesion development are the scapula, vertebrae, and mandible; however, any bone can become affected. Radiographically, the lesions are either sessile or pedunculated protuberances from bone surfaces with indistinct borders with the normal bone. There may be a loss of smooth contour with evidence of lysis, particularly if there is malignant transformation.

Diagnostic Work-Up

Both OS and MCE may be suspected, based on the radiographic appearance of the lesions and the FeLV status of the cat. Definitive diagnosis is made by histopathologic evaluation of properly collected biopsy tissue. Metastatic rates for cats with primary bone tumors are low compared to dogs (5% to 10% versus >90%), and three-view thoracic radiographs are recommended as part of the staging process. Presurgical evaluation with a CBC, chemistry profile, and urinalysis is recommended to rule out concurrent disease.

Therapy and Prognosis

Amputation is the recommended treatment for feline appendicular OS in which there are no clinically detectable metastatic lesions. Complete surgical excision of the primary tumor is prognostic for increased survival time, DFI, and recurrence-free interval.[372] Due to the low metastatic rate and prolonged MSTs of 24 to 44 months with amputation alone,[366,368] adjuvant chemotherapy is not indicated or recommended in cats, which is in contrast to the situation in dogs. No adjuvant therapy is known to be efficacious in extending survival time in cats. The MST for feline OS in axial sites (6.7 months) is lower than that of appendicular and extraskeletal OS sites.[367] This likely reflects the difficulty of achieving complete resection and local tumor control in these anatomic sites rather than a difference in biologic behavior. A combination of surgical resection and RT may be appropriate in these cases. SRT has been used in several cats for local tumor control in appendicular and axial sites.

Histologic grade, using a grading scheme that evaluates tumor vascular invasion, pleomorphism, mitotic index, and tumor matrix and cell necrosis, is prognostic for survival.[372] Specifically, tumors with high number of mitoses have a higher hazard ratio for decreased recurrence-free intervals. The metastatic potential of OS in cats (5% to 10%) is much less than for the same disease in dogs or humans. Reported anatomic sites for metastases are lung, kidney, liver, brain, and spleen. Cats with MCE have a guarded prognosis. Lesions may be removed surgically for palliation; however, local recurrences are common, or new, painful, debilitating lesions may occur. No reliably effective treatment is known for this condition in cats.

Fibrosarcoma, Chondrosarcoma, and Hemangiosarcoma

Non-OS primary bone tumors in cats are rare. Fibrosarcoma is the second most common primary bone tumor of cats.[375] Chondrosarcoma is reported to be next in terms of frequency, and hemangiosarcomas rarely involve bones of cats.[368] Little is known about the biologic behavior of these rare lesions. Aggressive surgical resection is the preferred treatment for these tumors. The metastatic rate is low; however, metastases have been seen in cats with chondrosarcoma and hemangiosarcoma.[368,376]

REFERENCES

1. Brodey RS, Mc GJ, Reynolds H: A clinical and radiological study of canine bone neoplasms. I, *J Am Vet Med Assoc* 134:53–71, 1959.
2. Brodey RS, Riser WH: Canine osteosarcoma: a clinicopathologic study of 194 cases, *Clin Orthop Relat Res* 62:54–64, 1969.
3. Brodey RS, Sauer RM, Medway W: Canine bone neoplasms, *J Am Vet Med Assoc* 143:471–495, 1963.
4. Dorfman SK, Hurvitz AI, Patnaik AK: Primary and secondary bone tumours in the dog, *J Small Anim Pract* 18:313–326, 1977.
5. Ling GV, Morgan JP, Pool RR: Primary bone tumors in the dog: a combined clinical, radiographic, and histologic approach to early diagnosis, *J Am Vet Med Assoc* 165:55–67, 1974.
6. Priester WA, McKay FW: The occurrence of tumors in domestic animals, *Natl Cancer Inst Monogr* 1–210, 1980.
7. Withrow SJ, Powers BE, Straw RC, et al: Comparative aspects of osteosarcoma: dog versus man, *Clin Orthop Relat Res* Sept(270): 159–168, 1991.

8. Alexander JW, Patton CS: Primary tumors of the skeletal system, *Vet Clin North Am Small Anim Pract* 13:181–195, 1983.
9. Brodey RS, Abt DA: Results of surgical treatment in 65 dogs with osteosarcoma, *J Am Vet Med Assoc* 168:1032–1035, 1976.
10. Jongeward SJ: Primary bone tumors, *Vet Clin North Am Small Anim Pract* 15:609–641, 1985.
11. Knecht CD, Priester WA: Musculoskeletal tumors in dogs, *J Am Vet Med Assoc* 172:72–74, 1978.
12. Misdorp W: Skeletal osteosarcoma: animal model: canine osteosarcoma, *Am J Pathol* 98:285–288, 1980.
13. Misdorp W, Hart AA: Some prognostic and epidemiologic factors in canine osteosarcoma, *J Natl Cancer Inst* 62:537–545, 1979.
14. Nielsen SW, Schroder JD, Smith DL: The pathology of osteogenic sarcoma in dogs, *J Am Vet Med Assoc* 124:28–35, 1954.
15. Spodnick GJ, Berg J, Rand WM, et al: Prognosis for dogs with appendicular osteosarcoma treated by amputation alone: 162 cases (1978-1988), *J Am Vet Med Assoc* 200:995–999, 1992.
16. Straw RC, Withrow SJ, Richter SL, et al: Amputation and cisplatin for treatment of canine osteosarcoma, *J Vet Intern Med* 5:205–210, 1991.
17. Tjalma RA: Canine bone sarcoma: estimation of relative risk as a function of body size, *J Natl Cancer Inst* 36:1137–1150, 1966.
18. Wolke RE, Nielsen SW: Site incidence of canine osteosarcoma, *J Small Anim Pract* 7:489–492, 1966.
19. Smith RL Sr: Osteosarcoma in dogs in the Brisbane area, *Aust Vet Pract* 18:97–100, 1988.
20. Phillips L, Hager D, Parker R, et al: Osteosarcoma with a pathologic fracture in a six-month-old dog, *Vet Radiol* 27:18–19, 1986.
21. Feeney DA, Johnston GR, Grindem CB, et al: Malignant neoplasia of canine ribs: clinical, radiographic, and pathologic findings, *J Am Vet Med Assoc* 180:927–933, 1982.
22. Heyman SJ, Diefenderfer DL, Goldschmidt MH, et al: Canine axial skeletal osteosarcoma. A retrospective study of 116 cases (1986 to 1989), *Vet Surg* 21:304–310, 1992.
23. Ru G, Terracini B, Glickman LT: Host related risk factors for canine osteosarcoma, *Vet J* 156:31–39, 1998.
24. Cooley DM, Beranek BC, Schlittler DL, et al: Endogenous gonadal hormone exposure and bone sarcoma risk, *Cancer Epidemiol Biomarkers Prev* 11:1434–1440, 2002.
25. Liptak JM, Dernell WS, Straw RC, et al: Proximal radial and distal humeral osteosarcoma in 12 dogs, *J Am Anim Hosp Assoc* 40:461–467, 2004.
26. Gamblin RM, Straw RC, Powers BE, et al: Primary osteosarcoma distal to the antebrachiocarpal and tarsocrural joints in nine dogs (1980-1992), *J Am Anim Hosp Assoc* 31:86–91, 1995.
27. Bleier T, Lewitschek HP, Reinacher M: Canine osteosarcoma of the penile bone, *J Vet Med A Physiol Pathol Clin Med* 50:397–398, 2003.
28. Lucroy MD, Peck JN, Berry CR: Osteosarcoma of the patella with pulmonary metastases in a dog, *Vet Radiol Ultrasound* 42:218–220, 2001.
29. LaRue SM, Withrow SJ, Wrigley RH: Radiographic bone surveys in the evaluation of primary bone tumors in dogs, *J Am Vet Med Assoc* 188:514–516, 1986.
30. Bech-Nielsen S, Haskins ME, Reif JS, et al: Frequency of osteosarcoma among first-degree relatives of St. Bernard dogs, *J Natl Cancer Inst* 60:349–353, 1978.
31. Kuntz CA, Dernell WS, Powers BE, et al: Extraskeletal osteosarcomas in dogs: 14 cases, *J Am Anim Hosp Assoc* 34:26–30, 1998.
32. Langenbach A, Anderson MA, Dambach DM, et al: Extraskeletal osteosarcomas in dogs: a retrospective study of 169 cases (1986-1996), *J Am Anim Hosp Assoc* 34:113–120, 1998.
33. Patnaik AK: Canine extraskeletal osteosarcoma and chondrosarcoma: a clinicopathologic study of 14 cases, *Vet Pathol* 27:46–55, 1990.
34. Ringenberg MA, Neitzel LE, Zachary JF: Meningeal osteosarcoma in a dog, *Vet Pathol* 37:653–655, 2000.
35. Thamm DH, Mauldin EA, Edinger DT, et al: Primary osteosarcoma of the synovium in a dog, *J Am Anim Hosp Assoc* 36:326–331, 2000.
36. Owen LN: Transplantation of canine osteosarcoma, *Eur J Cancer* 5:615–620, 1969.
37. Gellasch KL, Kalscheur VL, Clayton MK, et al: Fatigue microdamage in the radial predilection site for osteosarcoma in dogs, *Am J Vet Res* 63:896–899, 2002.
38. Bennett D, Campbell JR, Brown P: Osteosarcoma associated with healed fractures, *J Small Anim Pract* 20:13–18, 1979.
39. Sinibaldi K, Rosen H, Liu SK, et al: Tumors associated with metallic implants in animals, *Clin Orthop Relat Res* 257–266, 1976.
40. Stevenson S, Hohn RB, Pohler OE, et al: Fracture-associated sarcoma in the dog, *J Am Vet Med Assoc* 180:1189–1196, 1982.
41. Rosin A, Rowland GN: Undifferentiated sarcoma in a dog following chronic irritation by a metallic foreign body and concurrent infection, *J Am Anim Hosp Assoc* 17:593–598, 1981.
42. Knecht CD, Priester WA: Osteosarcoma in dogs: a study of previous trauma, fracture, and fracture fixation, *J Am Anim Hosp Assoc* 14:82–84, 1978.
43. Vasseur PB, Stevenson S: Osteosarcoma at the site of a cortical bone allograft in a dog, *Vet Surg* 16:70–74, 1987.
44. Gillette SM, Gillette EL, Powers BE, et al: Radiation-induced osteosarcoma in dogs after external beam or intraoperative radiation therapy, *Cancer Res* 50:54–57, 1990.
45. Lloyd RD, Taylor GN, Angus W, et al: Distribution of skeletal malignancies in beagles injected with 239Pu citrate, *Health Phys* 66:407–413, 1994.
46. McEntee MC, Page RL, Theon A, et al: Malignant tumor formation in dogs previously irradiated for acanthomatous epulis, *Vet Radiol Ultrasound* 45:357–361, 2004.
47. Miller SC, Lloyd RD, Bruenger FW, et al: Comparisons of the skeletal locations of putative plutonium-induced osteosarcomas in humans with those in beagle dogs and with naturally occurring tumors in both species, *Radiat Res* 160:517–523, 2003.
48. Powers BE, Gillette EL, McChesney SL, et al: Bone necrosis and tumor induction following experimental intraoperative irradiation, *Int J Radiat Oncol Biol Phys* 17:559–567, 1989.
49. Robinson E, Neugut AI, Wylie P: Clinical aspects of postirradiation sarcomas, *J Natl Cancer Inst* 80:233–240, 1988.
50. Tillotson C, Rosenberg A, Gebhardt M, et al: Postradiation multicentric osteosarcoma, *Cancer* 62:67–71, 1988.
51. White RG, Raabe OG, Culbertson MR, et al: Bone sarcoma characteristics and distribution in beagles fed strontium-90, *Radiat Res* 136:178–189, 1993.
52. White RG, Raabe OG, Culbertson MR, et al: Bone sarcoma characteristics and distribution in beagles injected with radium-226, *Radiat Res* 137:361–370, 1994.
53. Dahlin DC, Coventry MB: Osteogenic sarcoma: a study of six hundred cases, *J Bone Joint Surg Am* 49:101–110, 1967.
54. McKenna RJ, Schwinn CP, Higginbotham NL: Osteogenic sarcoma in children, *CA Cancer J Clin* 16:26–28, 1966.
55. Dubielzig RR, Biery DN, Brodey RS: Bone sarcomas associated with multifocal medullary bone infarction in dogs, *J Am Vet Med Assoc* 179:64–68, 1981.
56. Riser WH, Brodey RS, Biery DN: Bone infarctions associated with malignant bone tumors in dogs, *J Am Vet Med Assoc* 160:414–421, 1972.
57. Prior C, Watrous BJ, Penfold D: Radial diaphyseal osteosarcoma with associated bone infarction in a dog, *J Am Anim Hosp Assoc* 22:43–48, 1986.
58. Ansari MM: Bone infarcts associated with malignant sarcomas, *Comp Cont Ed Pract Vet* 3:367–370, 1991.
59. Boulay J, Wallace L, Lipowitz A: Pathologic fracture of long bones in the dog, *J Am Anim Hosp Assoc* 23:297–303, 1987.
60. Marcellin-Little DJ, DeYoung DJ, Thrall DE, et al: Osteosarcoma at the site of bone infarction associated with total hip arthroplasty in a dog, *Vet Surg* 28:54–60, 1999.

61. Holmberg BJ, Farese JP, Taylor D, et al: Osteosarcoma of the humeral head associated with osteochondritis dissecans in a dog, *J Am Anim Hosp Assoc* 40:246–249, 2004.
62. Barnhart MD: Malignant transformation of an aneurysmal bone cyst in a dog, *Vet Surg* 31:519–524, 2002.
63. Johnson AS, Couto CG, Weghorst CM: Mutation of the p53 tumor suppressor gene in spontaneously occurring osteosarcomas of the dog, *Carcinogenesis* 19:213–217, 1998.
64. Kirpensteijn J, Kik M, Teske E, et al: TP53 gene mutations in canine osteosarcoma, *Vet Surg* 37:454–460, 2008.
65. Levine RA, Fleischli MA: Inactivation of p53 and retinoblastoma family pathways in canine osteosarcoma cell lines, *Vet Pathol* 37:54–61, 2000.
66. Loukopoulos P, Thornton JR, Robinson WF: Clinical and pathologic relevance of p53 index in canine osseous tumors, *Vet Pathol* 40:237–248, 2003.
67. Mendoza S, Konishi T, Dernell WS, et al: Status of the p53, Rb and MDM2 genes in canine osteosarcoma, *Anticancer Res* 18:4449–4453, 1998.
68. Sagartz JE, Bodley WL, Gamblin RM, et al: p53 tumor suppressor protein overexpression in osteogenic tumors of dogs, *Vet Pathol* 33:213–221, 1996.
69. Setoguchi A, Sakai T, Okuda M, et al: Aberrations of the p53 tumor suppressor gene in various tumors in dogs, *Am J Vet Res* 62:433–439, 2001.
70. van Leeuwen IS, Cornelisse CJ, Misdorp W, et al: P53 gene mutations in osteosarcomas in the dog, *Cancer Lett* 111:173–178, 1997.
71. Thomas R, Wang HJ, Tsai PC, et al: Influence of genetic background on tumor karyotypes: evidence for breed-associated cytogenetic aberrations in canine appendicular osteosarcoma, *Chromosome Res* 17:365–377, 2009.
72. Levine AJ, Chang A, Dittmer D, et al: The p53 tumor suppressor gene, *J Lab Clin Med* 123:817–823, 1994.
73. Wadayama B, Toguchida J, Shimizu T, et al: Mutation spectrum of the retinoblastoma gene in osteosarcomas, *Cancer Res* 54:3042–3048, 1994.
74. Levine RA, Forest T, Smith C: Tumor suppressor PTEN is mutated in canine osteosarcoma cell lines and tumors, *Vet Pathol* 39:372–378, 2002.
75. Angstadt AY, Motsinger-Reif A, Thomas R, et al: Characterization of canine osteosarcoma by array comparative genomic hybridization and RT-qPCR: signatures of genomic imbalance in canine osteosarcoma parallel the human counterpart, *Genes Chromosomes Cancer* 50:859–874, 2011.
76. Phillips JC, Lembcke L, Chamberlin T: A novel locus for canine osteosarcoma (OSA1) maps to CFA34, the canine orthologue of human 3q26, *Genomics* 96:220–227, 2010.
77. Phillips JC, Stephenson B, Hauck M, et al: Heritability and segregation analysis of osteosarcoma in the Scottish deerhound, *Genomics* 90:354–363, 2007.
78. Urfer SR, Gaillard C, Steiger A: Lifespan and disease predispositions in the Irish Wolfhound: a review, *Vet Q* 29:102–111, 2007.
79. Rosenberger JA, Pablo NV, Crawford PC: Prevalence of and intrinsic risk factors for appendicular osteosarcoma in dogs: 179 cases (1996-2005), *J Am Vet Med Assoc* 231:1076–1080, 2007.
80. Fox MH, Armstrong LW, Withrow SJ, et al: Comparison of DNA aneuploidy of primary and metastatic spontaneous canine osteosarcomas, *Cancer Res* 50:6176–6178, 1990.
81. Liao AT, McCleese J, Kamerling S, et al: A novel small molecule Met inhibitor, PF2362376, exhibits biological activity against osteosarcoma, *Vet Comp Oncol* 5:177–196, 2007.
82. Liao AT, McMahon M, London C: Characterization, expression and function of c-Met in canine spontaneous cancers, *Vet Comp Oncol* 3:61–72, 2005.
83. MacEwen EG, Kutzke J, Carew J, et al: c-Met tyrosine kinase receptor expression and function in human and canine osteosarcoma cells, *Clin Exp Metastasis* 20:421–430, 2003.
84. Ferracini R, Angelini P, Cagliero E, et al: MET oncogene aberrant expression in canine osteosarcoma, *J Orthop Res* 18:253–256, 2000.
85. Liao AT, McMahon M, London CA: Identification of a novel germline MET mutation in dogs, *Anim Genet* 37:248–252, 2006.
86. Fieten H, Spee B, Ijzer J, et al: Expression of hepatocyte growth factor and the proto-oncogenic receptor c-Met in canine osteosarcoma, *Vet Pathol* 46:869–877, 2009.
87. MacEwen EG, Pastor J, Kutzke J, et al: IGF-1 receptor contributes to the malignant phenotype in human and canine osteosarcoma, *J Cell Biochem* 92:77–91, 2004.
88. Khanna C, Prehn J, Hayden D, et al: A randomized controlled trial of octreotide pamoate long-acting release and carboplatin versus carboplatin alone in dogs with naturally occurring osteosarcoma: evaluation of insulin-like growth factor suppression and chemotherapy, *Clin Cancer Res* 8:2406–2412, 2002.
89. Gorlick R, Huvos AG, Heller G, et al: Expression of HER2/erbB-2 correlates with survival in osteosarcoma, *J Clin Oncol* 17:2781–2788, 1999.
90. Scotlandi K, Manara MC, Hattinger CM, et al: Prognostic and therapeutic relevance of HER2 expression in osteosarcoma and Ewing's sarcoma, *Eur J Cancer* 41:1349–1361, 2005.
91. Flint AF, U'Ren L, Legare ME, et al: Overexpression of the erbB-2 proto-oncogene in canine osteosarcoma cell lines and tumors, *Vet Pathol* 41:291–296, 2004.
92. Gordon IK, Ye F, Kent MS: Evaluation of the mammalian target of rapamycin pathway and the effect of rapamycin on target expression and cellular proliferation in osteosarcoma cells from dogs, *Am J Vet Res* 69:1079–1084, 2008.
93. Paoloni MC, Mazcko C, Fox E, et al: Rapamycin pharmacokinetic and pharmacodynamic relationships in osteosarcoma: a comparative oncology study in dogs, *PLoS One* 5:e11013, 2010.
94. Fan TM, Barger AM, Sprandel IT, et al: Investigating TrkA expression in canine appendicular osteosarcoma, *J Vet Intern Med* 22:1181–1188, 2008.
95. Kow K, Bailey SM, Williams ES, et al: Telomerase activity in canine osteosarcoma, *Vet Comp Oncol* 4:184–187, 2006.
96. Kow K, Thamm DH, Terry J, et al: Impact of telomerase status on canine osteosarcoma patients, *J Vet Intern Med* 22:1366–1372, 2008.
97. Loukopoulos P, O'Brien T, Ghoddusi M, et al: Characterisation of three novel canine osteosarcoma cell lines producing high levels of matrix metalloproteinases, *Res Vet Sci* 77:131–141, 2004.
98. Barger AM, Fan TM, de Lorimier LP, et al: Expression of receptor activator of nuclear factor kappa-B ligand (RANKL) in neoplasms of dogs and cats, *J Vet Intern Med* 21:133–140, 2007.
99. Lana SE, Ogilvie GK, Hansen RA, et al: Identification of matrix metalloproteinases in canine neoplastic tissue, *Am J Vet Res* 61:111–114, 2000.
100. Schmit JM, Pondenis HC, Barger AM, et al: Cathepsin k expression and activity in canine osteosarcoma, *J Vet Intern Med* 26:126–134, 2012.
101. Khanna C, Wan X, Bose S, et al: The membrane-cytoskeleton linker ezrin is necessary for osteosarcoma metastasis, *Nat Med* 10:182–186, 2004.
102. Fan TM, Barger AM, Fredrickson RL, et al: Investigating CXCR4 expression in canine appendicular osteosarcoma, *J Vet Intern Med* 22:602–608, 2008.
103. Barger A, Graca R, Bailey K, et al: Use of alkaline phosphatase staining to differentiate canine osteosarcoma from other vimentin-positive tumors, *Vet Pathol* 42:161–165, 2005.
104. Neihaus SA, Locke JE, Barger AM, et al: A novel method of core aspirate cytology compared to fine-needle aspiration for diagnosing canine osteosarcoma, *J Am Anim Hosp Assoc* 47:317–323, 2011.
105. Britt T, Clifford C, Barger A, et al: Diagnosing appendicular osteosarcoma with ultrasound-guided fine-needle aspiration: 36 cases, *J Small Anim Pract* 48:145–150, 2007.
106. Kirpensteijn J, Kik M, Rutteman GR, et al: Prognostic significance of a new histologic grading system for canine osteosarcoma, *Vet Pathol* 39:240–246, 2002.

107. O'Donoghue LE, Ptitsyn AA, Kamstock DA, et al: Expression profiling in canine osteosarcoma: identification of biomarkers and pathways associated with outcome, *BMC Cancer* 10:506, 2010.
108. Bhandal J, Boston SE: Pathologic fracture in dogs with suspected or confirmed osteosarcoma, *Vet Surg* 40:423–430, 2011.
109. Kim MS, Lee SY, Lee TR, et al: Prognostic effect of pathologic fracture in localized osteosarcoma: a cohort/case controlled study at a single institute, *J Surg Oncol* 100:233–239, 2009.
110. Ebeid W, Amin S, Abdelmegid A: Limb salvage management of pathologic fractures of primary malignant bone tumors, *Cancer Control* 12:57–61, 2005.
111. Bacci G, Ferrari S, Longhi A, et al: Nonmetastatic osteosarcoma of the extremity with pathologic fracture at presentation: local and systemic control by amputation or limb salvage after preoperative chemotherapy, *Acta Orthop Scand* 74:449–454, 2003.
112. Kuettner KE, Pauli BU, Soble L: Morphological studies on the resistance of cartilage to invasion by osteosarcoma cells in vitro and in vivo, *Cancer Res* 38:277–287, 1978.
113. Brem H, Folkman J: Inhibition of tumor angiogenesis mediated by cartilage, *J Exp Med* 141:427–439, 1975.
114. Hillers KR, Dernell WS, Lafferty MH, et al: Incidence and prognostic importance of lymph node metastases in dogs with appendicular osteosarcoma: 228 cases (1986-2003), *J Am Vet Med Assoc* 226:1364–1367, 2005.
115. Boston SE, Ehrhart NP, Dernell WS, et al: Evaluation of survival time in dogs with stage III osteosarcoma that undergo treatment: 90 cases (1985-2004), *J Am Vet Med Assoc* 228:1905–1908, 2006.
116. Giuliano AE, Feig S, Eilber FR: Changing metastatic patterns of osteosarcoma, *Cancer* 54:2160–2164, 1984.
117. Bacci G, Avella M, Picci P, et al: Metastatic patterns in osteosarcoma, *Tumori* 74:421–427, 1988.
118. Kaya M, Wada T, Nagoya S, et al: Concomitant tumour resistance in patients with osteosarcoma: a clue to a new therapeutic strategy, *J Bone Joint Surg Br* 86:143–147, 2004.
119. Tsunemi T, Nagoya S, Kaya M, et al: Postoperative progression of pulmonary metastasis in osteosarcoma, *Clin Orthop* 407:159–166, 2003.
120. Moore GE, Mathey WS, Eggers JS, et al: Osteosarcoma in adjacent lumbar vertebrae in a dog, *J Am Vet Med Assoc* 217:1038–1040, 1008, 2000.
121. Sajadi KR, Heck RK, Neel MD, et al: The incidence and prognosis of osteosarcoma skip metastases, *Clin Orthop Relat Res* 92–96, 2004.
122. Straw R, Powers BE, Klausner J, et al: Canine mandibular osteosarcoma: 51 cases (1980-1992), *J Am Anim Hosp Assoc* 32:257–262, 1996.
123. Dickerson ME, Page RL, LaDue TA, et al: Retrospective analysis of axial skeleton osteosarcoma in 22 large-breed dogs, *J Vet Intern Med* 15:120–124, 2001.
124. Mehl ML, Withrow SJ, Seguin B, et al: Spontaneous regression of osteosarcoma in four dogs, *J Am Vet Med Assoc* 219:614–617, 2001.
125. Mazzaferro EM, Hackett TB, Stein TP, et al: Metabolic alterations in dogs with osteosarcoma, *Am J Vet Res* 62:1234–1239, 2001.
126. Kazmierski KJ, Ogilvie GK, Fettman MJ, et al: Serum zinc, chromium, and iron concentrations in dogs with lymphoma and osteosarcoma, *J Vet Intern Med* 15:585–588, 2001.
127. Wrigley RH: Malignant versus nonmalignant bone disease, *Vet Clin North Am Small Anim Pract* 30:315–347, vi–vii, 2000.
128. Reinhardt S, Stockhaus C, Teske E, et al: Assessment of cytological criteria for diagnosing osteosarcoma in dogs, *J Small Anim Pract* 46:65–70, 2005.
129. Samii VF, Nyland TG, Werner LL, et al: Ultrasound-guided fine-needle aspiration biopsy of bone lesions: a preliminary report, *Vet Radiol Ultrasound* 40:82–86, 1999.
130. Ehrhart N: Principles of tumor biopsy, *Clin Tech Small Anim Pract* 13:10–16, 1998.
131. Mankin HJ, Lange TA, Spanier SS: The hazards of biopsy in patients with malignant primary bone and soft-tissue tumors, *J Bone Joint Surg Am* 64:1121–1127, 1982.
132. deSantos LA, Murray JA, Ayala AG: The value of percutaneous needle biopsy in the management of primary bone tumors, *Cancer* 43:735–744, 1979.
133. Simon MA: Biopsy of musculoskeletal tumors, *J Bone Joint Surg Am* 64:1253–1257, 1982.
134. Wykes PM, Withrow SJ, Powers BE: Closed biopsy for diagnosis of long bone tumors: accuracy and results, *J Am Anim Hosp Assoc* 21:489–494, 1985.
135. Powers BE, LaRue SM, Withrow SJ, et al: Jamshidi needle biopsy for diagnosis of bone lesions in small animals, *J Am Vet Med Assoc* 193:205–210, 1988.
136. Vignoli M, Ohlerth S, Rossi F, et al: Computed tomography-guided fine-needle aspiration and tissue-core biopsy of bone lesions in small animals, *Vet Radiol Ultrasound* 45:125–130, 2004.
137. Barthez PY, Hornof WJ, Theon AP, et al: Receiver operating characteristic curve analysis of the performance of various radiographic protocols when screening dogs for pulmonary metastases, *J Am Vet Med Assoc* 204:237–240, 1994.
138. Picci P, Vanel D, Briccoli A, et al: Computed tomography of pulmonary metastases from osteosarcoma: the less poor technique: a study of 51 patients with histological correlation, *Ann Oncol* 12:1601–1604, 2001.
139. Waters DJ, Coakley FV, Cohen MD, et al: The detection of pulmonary metastases by helical CT: a clinicopathologic study in dogs, *J Comput Assist Tomogr* 22:235–240, 1998.
140. Eberle N, Fork M, von Babo V, et al: Comparison of examination of thoracic radiographs and thoracic computed tomography in dogs with appendicular osteosarcoma, *Vet Comp Oncol* 9:131–140, 2011.
141. Straw RC, Cook NL, LaRue SM, et al: Radiographic bone surveys, *J Am Vet Med Assoc* 195:1458, 1989.
142. Berg J, Lamb CR, O'Callaghan MW: Bone scintigraphy in the initial evaluation of dogs with primary bone tumors, *J Am Vet Med Assoc* 196:917–920, 1990.
143. Hahn KA, Hurd C, Cantwell HD: Single-phase methylene diphosphate bone scintigraphy in the diagnostic evaluation of dogs with osteosarcoma, *J Am Vet Med Assoc* 196:1483–1486, 1990.
144. Jankowski MK, Steyn PF, Lana SE, et al: Nuclear scanning with 99mTc-HDP for the initial evaluation of osseous metastasis in canine osteosarcoma, *Vet Comp Oncol* 1:152–158, 2003.
145. Lamb CR: Bone scintigraphy in small animals, *J Am Vet Med Assoc* 191:1616–1622, 1987.
146. Parchman MB, Flanders JA, Erb HN, et al: Nuclear medical bone imaging and targeted radiography for evaluation of skeletal neoplasms in 23 dogs, *Vet Surg* 18:454–458, 1989.
147. Enneking WF, Spanier SS, Goodman MA: A system for the surgical staging of musculoskeletal sarcoma, *Clin Orthop Relat Res* 106–120, 1980.
148. Lamb CR, Berg J, Bengtson AE: Preoperative measurement of canine primary bone tumors, using radiography and bone scintigraphy, *J Am Vet Med Assoc* 196:1474–1478, 1990.
149. Leibman NF, Kuntz CA, Steyn PF, et al: Accuracy of radiography, nuclear scintigraphy, and histopathology for determining the proximal extent of distal radius osteosarcoma in dogs, *Vet Surg* 30:240–245, 2001.
150. Davis GJ, Kapatkin AS, Craig LE, et al: Comparison of radiography, computed tomography, and magnetic resonance imaging for evaluation of appendicular osteosarcoma in dogs, *J Am Vet Med Assoc* 220:1171–1176, 2002.
151. Wallack ST, Wisner ER, Werner JA, et al: Accuracy of magnetic resonance imaging for estimating intramedullary osteosarcoma extent in pre-operative planning of canine limb-salvage procedures, *Vet Radiol Ultrasound* 43:432–441, 2002.
152. Bergman PJ, MacEwen EG, Kurzman ID, et al: Amputation and carboplatin for treatment of dogs with osteosarcoma: 48 cases (1991 to 1993), *J Vet Intern Med* 10:76–81, 1996.
153. Cho WH, Song WS, Jeon DG, et al: Differential presentations, clinical courses, and survivals of osteosarcomas of the proximal

humerus over other extremity locations, *Ann Surg Oncol* 17:702–708, 2010.
154. Kuntz CA, Asselin TL, Dernell WS, et al: Limb salvage surgery for osteosarcoma of the proximal humerus: outcome in 17 dogs, *Vet Surg* 27:417–422, 1998.
155. Sottnik JL, Rao S, Lafferty MH, et al: Association of blood monocyte and lymphocyte count and disease-free interval in dogs with osteosarcoma, *J Vet Intern Med* 24:1439–1444, 2010.
156. Brostrom LA, Strander H, Nilsonne U: Survival in osteosarcoma in relation to tumor size and location, *Clin Orthop Relat Res* 250–254, 1982.
157. Hammer AS, Weeren FR, Weisbrode SE, et al: Prognostic factors in dogs with osteosarcomas of the flat or irregular bones, *J Am Anim Hosp Assoc* 31:321–326, 1995.
158. Cooley DM, Waters DJ: Skeletal neoplasms of small dogs: a retrospective study and literature review, *J Am Anim Hosp Assoc* 33:11–23, 1997.
159. Wallace J, Matthiesen DT, Patnaik AK: Hemimaxillectomy for the treatment of oral tumors in 69 dogs, *Vet Surg* 21:337–341, 1992.
160. Schwarz PD, Withrow SJ, Curtis CR, et al: Partial maxillary resection as a treatment for oral cancer in 61 dogs, *J Am Anim Hosp Assoc* 27:616–624, 1991.
161. Kosovsky JK, Matthiesen DT, Marretta SM, et al: Results of partial mandibulectomy for the treatment of oral tumors in 142 dogs, *Vet Surg* 20:397–401, 1991.
162. Beckwith K, Eickhoff J, Dernell WS, et al: Osteosarcoma of the canine head: a retrospective analysis of 136 cases (1991-2008), *Veterinary Cancer Society*. San Diego, CA, 49, 2010.
163. Hendrix DV, Gelatt KN: Diagnosis, treatment and outcome of orbital neoplasia in dogs: a retrospective study of 44 cases, *J Small Anim Pract* 41:105–108, 2000.
164. Duffaud F, Digue L, Baciuchka-Palmaro M, et al: Osteosarcomas of flat bones in adolescents and adults, *Cancer* 88:324–332, 2000.
165. Pirkey-Ehrhart N, Withrow SJ, Straw RC, et al: Primary rib tumors in 54 dogs, *J Am Anim Hosp Assoc* 31:65–69, 1995.
166. Baines SJ, Lewis S, White RA: Primary thoracic wall tumours of mesenchymal origin in dogs: a retrospective study of 46 cases, *Vet Rec* 150:335–339, 2002.
167. Montgomery RD, Henderson RA, Powers RD, et al: Retrospective study of 26 primary thoracic wall tumors in dogs, *J Am Anim Hosp Assoc* 29:68–72, 1993.
168. Matthiesen DT, Clark GN, Orsher RJ, et al: En bloc resection of primary rib tumors in 40 dogs, *Vet Surg* 21:201–204, 1992.
169. Trout NJ, Pavletic MM, Kraus KH: Partial scapulectomy for management of sarcomas in three dogs and two cats, *J Am Vet Med Assoc* 207:585–587, 1995.
170. Norton C, Drenen CM, Emms SG: Subtotal scapulectomy as the treatment for scapular tumour in the dog: a report of six cases, *Aust Vet J* 84:364–366, 2006.
171. Montinaro V, Boston SE, Buracco P, et al: Evaluation of scapulectomy for primary bone tumors in 42 dogs: a Veterinary Society of Surgical Oncology (VSSO) retrospective study, *Vet Surg* 2012; Accepted for publication.
172. Dernell WS, Van Vechten BJ, Straw RC, et al: Outcome following treatment for vertebral tumors in 20 dogs, *J Am Anim Hosp Assoc* 36:245–251, 2000.
173. Garzotto CK, Berg J, Hoffmann WE, et al: Prognostic significance of serum alkaline phosphatase activity in canine appendicular osteosarcoma, *J Vet Intern Med* 14:587–592, 2000.
174. Ehrhart N, Dernell WS, Hoffmann WE, et al: Prognostic importance of alkaline phosphatase activity in serum from dogs with appendicular osteosarcoma: 75 cases (1990-1996), *J Am Vet Med Assoc* 213:1002–1006, 1998.
175. Moore AS, Dernell WS, Ogilvie GK, et al: Doxorubicin and BAY 12-9566 for the treatment of osteosarcoma in dogs: a randomized, double-blind, placebo-controlled study, *J Vet Intern Med* 21:783–790, 2007.
176. McCleese JK, Bear MD, Kulp SK, et al: Met interacts with EGFR and Ron in canine osteosarcoma, *Vet Comp Oncol* 2011.
177. Mullins MN, Lana SE, Dernell WS, et al: Cyclooxygenase-2 expression in canine appendicular osteosarcomas, *J Vet Intern Med* 18:859–865, 2004.
178. Shoeneman JK, Ehrhart EJ 3rd, Eickhoff JC, et al: Expression and function of survivin in canine osteosarcoma, *Cancer Res* 72:249–259, 2012.
179. Thamm DH, O'Brien MG, Vail DM: Serum vascular endothelial growth factor concentrations and postsurgical outcome in dogs with osteosarcoma, *Vet Comp Oncol* 6:126–132, 2008.
180. Selvarajah GT, Kirpensteijn J, van Wolferen ME, et al: Gene expression profiling of canine osteosarcoma reveals genes associated with short and long survival times, *Mol Cancer* 8:72, 2009.
181. Scott MC, Sarver AL, Gavin KJ, et al: Molecular subtypes of osteosarcoma identified by reducing tumor heterogeneity through an interspecies comparative approach, *Bone* 49:356–367, 2011.
182. Biller BJ, Elmslie RE, Burnett RC, et al: Use of FoxP3 expression to identify regulatory T cells in healthy dogs and dogs with cancer, *Vet Immunol Immunopathol* 116:69–78, 2007.
183. O'Neill K, Guth A, Biller B, et al: Changes in regulatory T cells in dogs with cancer and associations with tumor type, *J Vet Intern Med* 23:875–881, 2009.
184. Rissetto KC, Rindt H, Selting KA, et al: Cloning and expression of canine CD25 for validation of an anti-human CD25 antibody to compare T regulatory lymphocytes in healthy dogs and dogs with osteosarcoma, *Vet Immunol Immunopathol* 135:137–145, 2010.
185. Biller BJ, Guth A, Burton JH, et al: Decreased ratio of CD8+ T cells to regulatory T cells associated with decreased survival in dogs with osteosarcoma, *J Vet Intern Med* 24:1118–1123, 2010.
186. Liptak JM, Dernell WS, Straw RC, et al: Intercalary bone grafts for joint and limb preservation in 17 dogs with high-grade malignant tumors of the diaphysis, *Vet Surg* 33:457–467, 2004.
187. Liptak JM, Dernell WS, Ehrhart N, et al: Cortical allograft and endoprosthesis for limb-sparing surgery in dogs with distal radial osteosarcoma: a prospective clinical comparison of two different limb-sparing techniques, *Vet Surg* 35:518–533, 2006.
188. Liptak JM, Dernell WS, Lascelles BD, et al: Intraoperative extracorporeal irradiation for limb sparing in 13 dogs, *Vet Surg* 33:446–456, 2004.
189. Berg J, Weinstein MJ, Schelling SH, et al: Treatment of dogs with osteosarcoma by administration of cisplatin after amputation or limb-sparing surgery: 22 cases (1987-1990), *J Am Vet Med Assoc* 200:2005–2008, 1992.
190. LaRue SM, Withrow SJ, Powers BE, et al: Limb-sparing treatment for osteosarcoma in dogs, *J Am Vet Med Assoc* 195:1734–1744, 1989.
191. Thrall DE, Withrow SJ, Powers BE, et al: Radiotherapy prior to cortical allograft limb sparing in dogs with osteosarcoma: a dose response assay, *Int J Radiat Oncol Biol Phys* 18:1351–1357, 1990.
192. Vasseur P: Limb preservation in dogs with primary bone tumors, *Vet Clin North Am Small Anim Pract* 17:889–903, 1987.
193. Withrow SJ, Thrall DE, Straw RC, et al: Intra-arterial cisplatin with or without radiation in limb-sparing for canine osteosarcoma, *Cancer* 71:2484–2490, 1993.
194. Straw RC, Withrow SJ: Limb-sparing surgery versus amputation for dogs with bone tumors, *Vet Clin North Am Small Anim Pract* 26:135–143, 1996.
195. Pooya HA, Seguin B, Mason DR, et al: Biomechanical comparison of cortical radial graft versus ulnar transposition graft limb-sparing techniques for the distal radial site in dogs, *Vet Surg* 33:301–308, 2004.
196. Seguin B, Walsh PJ, Mason DR, et al: Use of an ipsilateral vascularized ulnar transposition autograft for limb-sparing surgery of the distal radius in dogs: an anatomic and clinical study, *Vet Surg* 32:69–79, 2003.
197. Ehrhart N: Longitudinal bone transport for treatment of primary bone tumors in dogs: technique description and outcome in 9 dogs, *Vet Surg* 34:24–34, 2005.

198. Tommasini M, Ehrhart N, Ferretti A, et al: Bone transport osteogenesis for limb salvage following resection of primary bone tumors: experience with 6 cases (1991-1996), *Vet Comp Orthop Traumatol* 23:43–51, 2000.
199. Ehrhart N, Eurell JA, Tommasini M, et al: Effect of cisplatin on bone transport osteogenesis in dogs, *Am J Vet Res* 63:703–711, 2002.
200. Rovesti GL, Bascucci M, Schmidt K, et al: Limb sparing using a double bone-transport technique for treatment of a distal tibial osteosarcoma in a dog, *Vet Surg* 31:70–77, 2002.
201. Buracco P, Morello E, Martano M, et al: Pasteurized tumoral autograft as a novel procedure for limb sparing in the dog: A clinical report, *Vet Surg* 31:525–532, 2002.
202. Morello E, Vasconi E, Martano M, et al: Pasteurized tumoral autograft and adjuvant chemotherapy for the treatment of canine distal radial osteosarcoma: 13 cases, *Vet Surg* 32:539–544, 2003.
203. Reference deleted in pages.
204. Straw RC, Withrow SJ, Powers BE: Primary osteosarcoma of the ulna in 12 dogs, *J Am Anim Hosp Assoc* 27:323–326, 1991.
205. Kirpensteijn J, Straw RC, Pardo AD, et al: Partial and total scapulectomy in the dog, *J Am Anim Hosp Assoc* 30:313–319, 1994.
206. Straw RC, Withrow SJ, Powers BE: Partial or total hemipelvectomy in the management of sarcomas in nine dogs and two cats, *Vet Surg* 21:183–188, 1992.
207. Lascelles BD, Thomson MJ, Dernell WS, et al: Combined dorsolateral and intraoral approach for the resection of tumors of the maxilla in the dog, *J Am Anim Hosp Assoc* 39:294–305, 2003.
208. O'Brien MG, Withrow SJ, Straw RC, et al: Total and partial orbitectomy for the treatment of periorbital tumors in 24 dogs and 6 cats: a retrospective study, *Vet Surg* 25:471–479, 1996.
209. VCOG: Retrospective study of 26 primary tumors of the osseous thoracic wall in dogs, *J Am Anim Hosp Assoc* 29:68–72, 1993.
210. Withrow SJ, Hirsch VM: Owner response to amputation of a pet's leg, *Vet Med Small Anim Clin* 74:332, 334, 1979.
211. Carberry CA, Harvey HJ: Owner satisfaction with limb amputation in dogs and cats, *J Am Anim Hosp Assoc* 23:227–232, 1987.
212. O'Brien MG, Withrow SJ, Straw RC: Recent advances in the treatment of canine appendicular osteosarcoma, *Comp Cont Ed Pract Vet* 15:613–616, 1993.
213. Meyer MS, Spanier SS, Moser M, et al: Evaluating marrow margins for resection of osteosarcoma. A modern approach, *Clin Orthop Relat Res* 170–175, 1999.
214. Morello E, Buracco P, Martano M, et al: Bone allografts and adjuvant cisplatin for the treatment of canine appendicular osteosarcoma in 18 dogs, *J Small Anim Pract* 42:61–66, 2001.
215. Tomford WW, Doppelt SH, Mankin HJ, et al: 1983 bone bank procedures, *Clin Orthop Relat Res* 15–21, 1983.
216. Straw RC, Powers BE, Withrow SJ, et al: The effect of intramedullary polymethylmethacrylate on healing of intercalary cortical allografts in a canine model, *J Orthop Res* 10:434–439, 1992.
217. Kirpensteijn J, Steinheimer D, Park RD, et al: Comparison of cemented and non-cemented allografts for limb sparing procedures in dogs with osteosarcoma of the distal radius, *Vet Comp Orthop Traumatol* 11:178–184, 1998.
218. Dernell WS, Withrow SJ, Straw RC, et al: Clinical response to antibiotic impregnated polymethyl methacrylate bead implantation of dogs with severe infections after limb sparing with allograft replacement-18 cases (1994-1996), *Vet Comp Orthop Traumatol* 11:94–99, 1998.
219. Boston SE, Duerr F, Bacon N, et al: Intraoperative radiation for limb sparing of the distal aspect of the radius without transcarpal plating in five dogs, *Vet Surg* 36:314–323, 2007.
220. Oya N, Kokubo M, Mizowaki T, et al: Definitive intraoperative very high-dose radiotherapy for localized osteosarcoma in the extremities, *Int J Radiat Oncol Biol Phys* 51:87–93, 2001.
221. Sakayama K, Kidani T, Fujibuchi T, et al: Definitive intraoperative radiotherapy for musculoskeletal sarcomas and malignant lymphoma in combination with surgical excision, *Int J Clin Oncol* 8:174–179, 2003.
222. Tsuboyama T, Toguchida J, Kotoura Y, et al: Intra-operative radiation therapy for osteosarcoma in the extremities, *Int Orthop* 24:202–207, 2000.
223. Farese JP, Milner R, Thompson MS, et al: Stereotactic radiosurgery for treatment of osteosarcomas involving the distal portions of the limbs in dogs, *J Am Vet Med Assoc* 225:1567–1572, 1548, 2004.
224. Van Ginkel RJ, Hoekstra HJ, Meutstege FJ, et al: Hyperthermic isolated regional perfusion with cisplatin in the local treatment of spontaneous canine osteosarcoma: assessment of short-term effects, *J Surg Oncol* 59:169–176, 1995.
225. Rossi CR, Pasquali S, Mocellin S, et al: Long-term results of melphalan-based isolated limb perfusion with or without low-dose TNF for in-transit melanoma metastases, *Ann Surg Oncol* 17:3000–3007, 2010.
226. Deroose JP, van Geel AN, Burger JW, et al: Isolated limb perfusion with TNF-alpha and melphalan for distal parts of the limb in soft tissue sarcoma patients, *J Surg Oncol* 2011.
227. Zachos TA, Aiken SW, DiResta GR, et al: Interstitial fluid pressure and blood flow in canine osteosarcoma and other tumors, *Clin Orthop Relat Res* 230–236, 2001.
228. Powers BE, Withrow SJ, Thrall DE, et al: Percent tumor necrosis as a predictor of treatment response in canine osteosarcoma, *Cancer* 67:126–134, 1991.
229. Withrow SJ, Liptak JM, Straw RC, et al: Biodegradable cisplatin polymer in limb-sparing surgery for canine osteosarcoma, *Ann Surg Oncol* 11:705–713, 2004.
230. Lascelles BD, Dernell WS, Correa MT, et al: Improved survival associated with postoperative wound infection in dogs treated with limb-salvage surgery for osteosarcoma, *Ann Surg Oncol* 12:1073–1083, 2005.
231. Jeys LM, Grimer RJ, Carter SR, et al: Post operative infection and increased survival in osteosarcoma patients: are they associated? *Ann Surg Oncol* 14:2887–2895, 2007.
232. Sottnik JL, U'Ren LW, Thamm DH, et al: Chronic bacterial osteomyelitis suppression of tumor growth requires innate immune responses, *Cancer Immunol Immunother* 59:367–378, 2010.
233. Kramer A, Walsh PJ, Seguin B: Hemipelvectomy in dogs and cats: technique overview, variations, and description, *Vet Surg* 37:413–419, 2008.
234. Chauvet AE, Hogge GS, Sandin JA, et al: Vertebrectomy, bone allograft fusion, and antitumor vaccination for the treatment of vertebral fibrosarcoma in a dog, *Vet Surg* 28:480–488, 1999.
235. Liptak JM, Pluhar GE, Dernell WS, et al: Limb-sparing surgery in a dog with osteosarcoma of the proximal femur, *Vet Surg* 34:71–77, 2005.
236. Fitzpatrick N, Smith TJ, Pendegrass CJ, et al: Intraosseous transcutaneous amputation prosthesis (ITAP) for limb salvage in 4 dogs, *Vet Surg* 40:909–925, 2011.
237. Drygas KA, Taylor R, Sidebotham CG, et al: Transcutaneous tibial implants: a surgical procedure for restoring ambulation after amputation of the distal aspect of the tibia in a dog, *Vet Surg* 37:322–327, 2008.
237a. Liptak JM, Dernell WS, Rizzo SA, et al: Partial foot amputation in 11 dogs, *J Am Anim Hosp Assoc* 41:47–55, 2005.
238. Fox LE, Geoghegan SL, Davis LH, et al: Owner satisfaction with partial mandibulectomy or maxillectomy for treatment of oral tumors in 27 dogs, *J Am Anim Hosp Assoc* 33:25–31, 1997.
238a. White RAS: Mandibulectomy and maxillectomy in the dog: long-term survival in 100 cases, *J Small Anim Pract* 32:69–74, 1991.
239. Withrow SJ, Holmberg DL: Mandibulectomy in the treatment of oral cancer, *J Am Anim Hosp Assoc* 19:273–286, 1983.
240. Gaitan-Yanguas M: A study of the response of osteogenic sarcoma and adjacent normal tissues to radiation, *Int J Radiat Oncol Biol Phys* 7:593–595, 1981.
241. Caceres E, Zaharia M, Valdivia S, et al: Local control of osteogenic sarcoma by radiation and chemotherapy, *Int J Radiat Oncol Biol Phys* 10:35–39, 1984.

242. Machak GN, Tkachev SI, Solovyev YN, et al: Neoadjuvant chemotherapy and local radiotherapy for high-grade osteosarcoma of the extremities, *Mayo Clinic Proc* 78:147–155, 2003.
243. Walter CU, Dernell WS, LaRue SM, et al: Curative-intent radiation therapy as a treatment modality for appendicular and axial osteosarcoma: a preliminary retrospective evaluation of 14 dogs with the disease, *Vet Comp Oncol* 3:1–7, 2005.
244. Liepe K: Alpharadin, a 223Ra-based alpha-particle-emitting pharmaceutical for the treatment of bone metastases in patients with cancer, *Curr Opin Investig Drugs* 10:1346–1358, 2009.
245. Nilsson S, Strang P, Ginman C, et al: Palliation of bone pain in prostate cancer using chemotherapy and strontium-89: a randomized phase II study, *J Pain Symptom Manage* 29:352–357, 2005.
246. Nilsson S, Franzen L, Parker C, et al: Bone-targeted radium-223 in symptomatic, hormone-refractory prostate cancer: a randomised, multicentre, placebo-controlled phase II study, *Lancet Oncol* 8:587–594, 2007.
247. Vail DM, Kurzman ID, Glawe PC, et al: STEALTH liposome-encapsulated cisplatin (SPI-77) versus carboplatin as adjuvant therapy for spontaneously arising osteosarcoma (OSA) in the dog: a randomized multicenter clinical trial, *Cancer Chemother Pharmacol* 50:131–136, 2002.
248. Phillips B, Powers BE, Dernell WS, et al: Use of single-agent carboplatin as adjuvant or neoadjuvant therapy in conjunction with amputation for appendicular osteosarcoma in dogs, *J Am Anim Hosp Assoc* 45:33–38, 2009.
249. Saam DE, Liptak JM, Stalker MJ, et al: Predictors of outcome in dogs treated with adjuvant carboplatin for appendicular osteosarcoma: 65 cases (1996-2006), *J Am Vet Med Assoc* 238: 195–206, 2011.
250. Kirpensteijn J, Teske E, Kik M, et al: Lobaplatin as an adjuvant chemotherapy to surgery in canine appendicular osteosarcoma: a phase II evaluation, *Anticancer Res* 22:2765–2770, 2002.
251. Berg J, Weinstein MJ, Springfield DS, et al: Results of surgery and doxorubicin chemotherapy in dogs with osteosarcoma, *J Am Vet Med Assoc* 206:1555–1560, 1995.
252. Berg J, Gebhardt MC, Rand WM: Effect of timing of postoperative chemotherapy on survival of dogs with osteosarcoma, *Cancer* 79:1343–1350, 1997.
253. Chun R, Garrett LD, Henry C, et al: Toxicity and efficacy of cisplatin and doxorubicin combination chemotherapy for the treatment of canine osteosarcoma, *J Am Anim Hosp Assoc* 41:382–387, 2005.
254. Bailey D, Erb H, Williams L, et al: Carboplatin and doxorubicin combination chemotherapy for the treatment of appendicular osteosarcoma in the dog, *J Vet Intern Med* 17:199–205, 2003.
255. Mauldin GN, Matus RE, Withrow SJ, et al: Canine osteosarcoma: treatment by amputation versus amputation and adjuvant chemotherapy using doxorubicin and cisplatin, *J Vet Intern Med* 2:177–180, 1988.
256. Kent MS, Strom A, London CA, et al: Alternating carboplatin and doxorubicin as adjunctive chemotherapy to amputation or limb-sparing surgery in the treatment of appendicular osteosarcoma in dogs, *J Vet Intern Med* 18:540–544, 2004.
257. Bacon NJ, Ehrhart NP, Dernell WS, et al: Use of alternating administration of carboplatin and doxorubicin in dogs with microscopic metastases after amputation for appendicular osteosarcoma: 50 cases (1999-2006), *J Am Vet Med Assoc* 232:1504–1510, 2008.
258. McMahon M, Mathie T, Stingle N, et al: Adjuvant carboplatin and gemcitabine combination chemotherapy postamputation in canine appendicular osteosarcoma, *J Vet Intern Med* 25:511–517, 2011.
259. de la Puente-Redondo VA, Tilt N, Rowan TG, et al: Efficacy of maropitant for treatment and prevention of emesis caused by intravenous infusion of cisplatin in dogs, *Am J Vet Res* 68:48–56, 2007.
260. Vail DM, Rodabaugh HS, Conder GA, et al: Efficacy of injectable maropitant (Cerenia) in a randomized clinical trial for prevention and treatment of cisplatin-induced emesis in dogs presented as veterinary patients, *Vet Comp Oncol* 5:38–46, 2007.
261. Ogilvie GK, Krawiec DR, Gelberg HB, et al: Evaluation of a short-term saline diuresis protocol for the administration of cisplatin, *Am J Vet Res* 49:1076–1078, 1988.
262. DeRegis CJ, Moore AS, Rand WM, et al: Cisplatin and doxorubicin toxicosis in dogs with osteosarcoma, *J Vet Intern Med* 17:668–673, 2003.
263. McMahon MB, Bear MD, Kulp SK, et al: Biological activity of gemcitabine against canine osteosarcoma cell lines in vitro, *Am J Vet Res* 71:799–808, 2010.
264. Selting KA, Wang X, Gustafson DL, et al: Evaluation of satraplatin in dogs with spontaneously occurring malignant tumors, *J Vet Intern Med* 25:909–915, 2011.
265. Kurzman ID, Shi F, Vail DM, et al: In vitro and in vivo enhancement of canine pulmonary alveolar macrophage cytotoxic activity against canine osteosarcoma cells, *Cancer Biother Radiopharm* 14:121–128, 1999.
266. MacEwen EG, Kurzman ID, Rosenthal RC, et al: Therapy for osteosarcoma in dogs with intravenous injection of liposome-encapsulated muramyl tripeptide, *J Natl Cancer Inst* 81:935–938, 1989.
267. Kurzman ID, MacEwen EG, Rosenthal RC, et al: Adjuvant therapy for osteosarcoma in dogs: results of randomized clinical trials using combined liposome-encapsulated muramyl tripeptide and cisplatin, *Clin Cancer Res* 1:1595–1601, 1995.
268. Savage SA, Mirabello L: Using epidemiology and genomics to understand osteosarcoma etiology, *Sarcoma* 2011:548151, 2011.
269. Polednak AP: Human biology and epidemiology of childhood bone cancers: a review, *Hum Biol* 57:1–26, 1985.
270. Downey RJ: Surgical treatment of pulmonary metastases, *Surg Oncol Clin N Am* 8:341, 1999.
271. O'Brien MG, Straw RC, Withrow SJ, et al: Resection of pulmonary metastases in canine osteosarcoma: 36 cases (1983-1992), *Vet Surg* 22:105–109, 1993.
272. Liptak JM, Monnet E, Dernell WS, et al: Pulmonary metastasectomy in the management of four dogs with hypertrophic osteopathy, *Vet Comp Oncol* 2:1–12, 2004.
273. Lansdowne JL, Monnet E, Twedt DC, et al: Thoracoscopic lung lobectomy for treatment of lung tumors in dogs, *Vet Surg* 34: 530–535, 2005.
274. Ogilvie GK, Straw RC, Jameson VJ, et al: Evaluation of single-agent chemotherapy for treatment of clinically evident osteosarcoma metastases in dogs: 45 cases (1987-1991), *J Am Vet Med Assoc* 202:304–306, 1993.
275. Poirier VJ, Hershey AE, Burgess KE, et al: Efficacy and toxicity of paclitaxel (Taxol) for the treatment of canine malignant tumors, *J Vet Intern Med* 18:219–222, 2004.
276. London CA, Hannah AL, Zadovoskaya R, et al: Phase I dose-escalating study of SU11654, a small molecule receptor tyrosine kinase inhibitor, in dogs with spontaneous malignancies, *Clin Cancer Res* 9:2755–2768, 2003.
277. London C, Mathie T, Stingle N, et al: Preliminary evidence for biologic activity of toceranib phosphate (Palladia) in solid tumours, *Vet Comp Oncol* 2011.
278. Wittenburg LA, Gustafson DL, Thamm DH: Phase I pharmacokinetic and pharmacodynamic evaluation of combined valproic acid/doxorubicin treatment in dogs with spontaneous cancer, *Clin Cancer Res* 16:4832–4842, 2010.
279. Hershey AE, Kurzman ID, Forrest LJ, et al: Inhalation chemotherapy for macroscopic primary or metastatic lung tumors: proof of principle using dogs with spontaneously occurring tumors as a model, *Clin Cancer Res* 5:2653–2659, 1999.
280. Rodriguez CO Jr, Crabbs TA, Wilson DW, et al: Aerosol gemcitabine: preclinical safety and in vivo antitumor activity in osteosarcoma-bearing dogs, *J Aerosol Med Pulm Drug Deliv* 23:197–206, 2010.

281. Koshkina NV, Kleinerman ES: Aerosol gemcitabine inhibits the growth of primary osteosarcoma and osteosarcoma lung metastases, *Int J Cancer* 116:458–463, 2005.
282. Khanna C, Anderson PM, Hasz DE, et al: Interleukin-2 liposome inhalation therapy is safe and effective for dogs with spontaneous pulmonary metastases, *Cancer* 79:1409–1421, 1997.
283. Dow S, Elmslie R, Kurzman I, et al: Phase I study of liposome-DNA complexes encoding the interleukin-2 gene in dogs with osteosarcoma lung metastases, *Hum Gene Ther* 16:937–946, 2005.
284. Thamm DH, Kurzman ID, King I, et al: Systemic administration of an attenuated, tumor-targeting Salmonella typhimurium to dogs with spontaneous neoplasia: phase I evaluation, *Clin Cancer Res* 11:4827–4834, 2005.
285. Portenoy RK: Treatment of cancer pain, *Lancet* 377:2236–2247, 2011.
286. Clohisy DR, Mantyh PW: Bone cancer pain, *Clin Orthop Relat Res* S279–S288, 2003.
287. Goblirsch MJ, Zwolak PP, Clohisy DR: Biology of bone cancer pain, *Clin Cancer Res* 12:6231s–6235s, 2006.
288. Goblirsch M, Mathews W, Lynch C, et al: Radiation treatment decreases bone cancer pain, osteolysis and tumor size, *Radiat Res* 161:228–234, 2004.
289. Withrow SJ, Powers BE, Straw RC, et al: Tumor necrosis following radiation therapy and/or chemotherapy for canine osteosarcoma, *Chir Organi Mov* 75:29–31, 1990.
290. Green EM, Adams WM, Forrest LJ: Four fraction palliative radiotherapy for osteosarcoma in 24 dogs, *J Am Anim Hosp Assoc* 38:445–451, 2002.
291. Knapp-Hoch HM, Fidel JL, Sellon RK, et al: An expedited palliative radiation protocol for lytic or proliferative lesions of appendicular bone in dogs, *J Am Anim Hosp Assoc* 45:24–32, 2009.
292. Mueller F, Poirier V, Melzer K, et al: Palliative radiotherapy with electrons of appendicular osteosarcoma in 54 dogs, *In Vivo* 19:713–716, 2005.
293. Ramirez O III, Dodge RK, Page RL, et al: Palliative radiotherapy of appendicular osteosarcoma in 95 dogs, *Vet Radiol Ultrasound* 40:517–522, 1999.
294. Bateman KE, Catton PA, Pennock PW, et al: 0-7-21 radiation therapy for the palliation of advanced cancer in dogs, *J Vet Intern Med* 8:394–399, 1994.
295. McEntee MC, Page RL, Novotney CA, et al: Palliative radiotherapy for canine appendicular osteosarcoma, *Vet Radiol Ultrasound* 34:367–370, 1993.
296. Holmes RA: [153Sm]EDTMP: a potential therapy for bone cancer pain, *Semin Nucl Med* 22:41–45, 1992.
297. Serafini AN: Samarium Sm-153 lexidronam for the palliation of bone pain associated with metastases, *Cancer* 88:2934–2939, 2000.
298. Aas M, Moe L, Gamlem H, et al: Internal radionuclide therapy of primary osteosarcoma in dogs, using 153Sm-ethylene-diamino-tetramethylene-phosphonate (EDTMP), *Clin Cancer Res* 5:3148s–3152s, 1999.
299. Barnard SM, Zuber RM, Moore AS: Samarium Sm 153 lexidronam for the palliative treatment of dogs with primary bone tumors: 35 cases (1999-2005), *J Am Vet Med Assoc* 230:1877–1881, 2007.
300. Lattimer JC, Corwin LA Jr, Stapleton J, et al: Clinical and clinicopathologic response of canine bone tumor patients to treatment with samarium-153-EDTMP, *J Nucl Med* 31:1316–1325, 1990.
301. Milner RJ, Dormehl I, Louw WK, et al: Targeted radiotherapy with Sm-153-EDTMP in nine cases of canine primary bone tumours, *J S Afr Vet Assoc* 69:12–17, 1998.
302. Lipton A: New therapeutic agents for the treatment of bone diseases, *Expert Opin Biol Ther* 5:817–832, 2005.
303. Coleman RE: Therapeutic use of bisphosphonates in oncology, *BMJ* 309:1233, 1994.
304. Coleman RE, McCloskey EV: Bisphosphonates in oncology, *Bone* 49:71–76, 2011.
305. Carano A, Teitelbaum SL, Konsek JD, et al: Bisphosphonates directly inhibit the bone resorption activity of isolated avian osteoclasts in vitro, *J Clin Invest* 85:456–461, 1990.
306. Hughes DE, Wright KR, Uy HL, et al: Bisphosphonates promote apoptosis in murine osteoclasts in vitro and in vivo, *J Bone Miner Res* 10:1478–1487, 1995.
307. Luckman SP, Hughes DE, Coxon FP, et al: Nitrogen-containing bisphosphonates inhibit the mevalonate pathway and prevent post-translational prenylation of GTP-binding proteins, including Ras, *J Bone Miner Res* 13:581–589, 1998.
308. Ashton JA, Farese JP, Milner RJ, et al: Investigation of the effect of pamidronate disodium on the in vitro viability of osteosarcoma cells from dogs, *Am J Vet Res* 66:885–891, 2005.
309. Farese JP, Ashton J, Milner R, et al: The effect of the bisphosphonate alendronate on viability of canine osteosarcoma cells in vitro, *In Vitro Cell Dev Biol Anim* 40:113–117, 2004.
310. Poirier VJ, Huelsmeyer MK, Kurzman ID, et al: The bisphosphonates alendronate and zoledronate are inhibitors of canine and human osteosarcoma cell growth in vitro, *Vet Comp Oncol* 1:207–215, 2003.
311. Tomlin JL, Sturgeon C, Pead MJ, et al: Use of the bisphosphonate drug alendronate for palliative management of osteosarcoma in two dogs, *Vet Rec* 147:129–132, 2000.
312. Fan TM, de Lorimier LP, Charney SC, et al: Evaluation of intravenous pamidronate administration in 33 cancer-bearing dogs with primary or secondary bone involvement, *J Vet Intern Med* 19:74–80, 2005.
313. Fan TM, de Lorimier LP, O'Dell-Anderson K, et al: Single-agent pamidronate for palliative therapy of canine appendicular osteosarcoma bone pain, *J Vet Intern Med* 21:431–439, 2007.
314. Ryan SD, Timbie JW, Haussler KK, et al: Randomized, placebo-controlled, clinical trial of radiation therapy with or without pamidronate for palliative treatment of canine appendicular osteosarcoma, *Vet Comp Oncol* 9:e1–e49, 2011.
315. Fan TM, Charney SC, de Lorimier LP, et al: Double-blind placebo-controlled trial of adjuvant pamidronate with palliative radiotherapy and intravenous doxorubicin for canine appendicular osteosarcoma bone pain, *J Vet Intern Med* 23:152–160, 2009.
316. Spugnini EP, Vincenzi B, Caruso G, et al: Zoledronic acid for the treatment of appendicular osteosarcoma in a dog, *J Small Anim Pract* 50:44–46, 2009.
317. Fan TM, de Lorimier LP, Garrett LD, et al: The bone biologic effects of zoledronate in healthy dogs and dogs with malignant osteolysis, *J Vet Intern Med* 22:380–387, 2008.
318. Vail DM, MacEwen EG: Spontaneously occurring tumors of companion animals as models for human cancer, *Cancer Invest* 18:781–792, 2000.
319. Rowell JL, McCarthy DO, Alvarez CE: Dog models of naturally occurring cancer, *Trends Mol Med* 17:380–388, 2011.
320. Withrow SJ, Wilkins RM: Cross talk from pets to people: translational osteosarcoma treatments, *ILAR J* 51:208–213, 2010.
321. Mankin HJ, Hornicek FJ, Rosenberg AE, et al: Survival data for 648 patients with osteosarcoma treated at one institution, *Clin Orthop Relat Res* 286–291, 2004.
322. Wilkins RM, Cullen JW, Camozzi AB, et al: Improved survival in primary nonmetastatic pediatric osteosarcoma of the extremity, *Clin Orthop Relat Res* 438:128–136, 2005.
323. Bacci G, Ferrari S, Bertoni F, et al: Long-term outcome for patients with nonmetastatic osteosarcoma of the extremity treated at the Istituto Ortopedico Rizzoli, according to the Istituto Ortopedico Rizzoli/osteosarcoma-2 protocol: an updated report, *J Clin Oncol* 18:4016–4027, 2000.
324. Bacci G, Ruggieri P, Bertoni F, et al: Local and systemic control for osteosarcoma of the extremity treated with neoadjuvant chemotherapy and limb salvage surgery: the Rizzoli experience, *Oncol Rep* 7:1129–1133, 2000.
325. Okada K, Unni KK, Swee RG, et al: High grade surface osteosarcoma: a clinicopathologic study of 46 cases, *Cancer* 85:1044–1054, 1999.

326. Banks WC: Parosteal osteosarcoma in a dog and a cat, *J Am Vet Med Assoc* 158:1412–1415, 1971.
327. Withrow SJ, Doige CE: En block resection of a juxtacortical and three intra-osseous osteosarcomas of the zygomatic arch in dogs, *J Am Anim Hosp Assoc* 16:867–872, 1980.
328. Moores AP, Beck AL, Baker JF: High-grade surface osteosarcoma in a dog, *J Small Anim Pract* 44:218–220, 2003.
329. Brodey RS, Misdorp W, Riser WH, et al: Canine skeletal chondrosarcoma: a clinicopathologic study of 35 cases, *J Am Vet Med Assoc* 165:68–78, 1974.
330. Sylvestre AM, Brash ML, Atilola MAO, et al: A case series of 25 dogs with chondrosarcoma, *Vet Comp Orthop Traumatol* 5:13–17, 1992.
331. Doige CE: Multiple cartilaginous exostoses in dogs, *Vet Pathol* 24:276–278, 1987.
332. Gee BR, Doige CE: Multiple cartilaginous exostoses in a litter of dogs, *J Am Vet Med Assoc* 156:53–59, 1970.
333. Doige CE, Pharr JW, Withrow SJ: Chondrosarcoma arising in multiple cartilaginous exostosis in a dog, *J Am Anim Hosp Assoc* 14:605–611, 1978.
334. Popovitch CA, Weinstein MJ, Goldschmidt MH, et al: Chondrosarcoma: a retrospective study of 97 dogs (1987-1990), *J Am Anim Hosp Assoc* 30:81–85, 1994.
335. Anderson WI, Carberry CA, King JM, et al: Primary aortic chondrosarcoma in a dog, *Vet Pathol* 25:180–181, 1988.
336. Flanders JA, Castleman W, Carberry CA, et al: Laryngeal chondrosarcoma in a dog, *J Am Vet Med Assoc* 190:68–70, 1987.
337. Greenlee PG, Liu SK: Chondrosarcoma of the mitral leaflet in a dog, *Vet Pathol* 21:540–542, 1984.
338. Southerland EM, Miller RT, Jones CL: Primary right atrial chondrosarcoma in a dog, *J Am Vet Med Assoc* 203:1697–1698, 1993.
339. Weller RE, Dagle GE, Perry RL, et al: Primary pulmonary chondrosarcoma in a dog, *Cornell Vet* 82:447–452, 1992.
340. Patnaik AK, Mattiesen DT, Zawie DA: Two cases of canine penile neoplasm: squamous cell carcinoma and mesenchymal chondrosarcoma, *J Am Anim Hosp Assoc* 24:403–406, 1988.
341. Aron DN, DeVreis R, Short CE: Primary tracheal chondrosarcoma in a dog: a case report with description of surgical and anesthetic techniques, *J Am Anim Hosp Assoc* 16:31–37, 1980.
342. Lana SE, Dernell WS, LaRue SM, et al: Slow release cisplatin combined with radiation for the treatment of canine nasal tumors, *Vet Radiol Ultrasound* 38:474–478, 1997.
343. Yamaguchi T, Toguchida J, Yamamuro T, et al: Allelotype analysis in osteosarcomas: Frequent allele loss on 3q, 13q, 17p, and 18q, *Cancer Res* 52:2419–2423, 1992.
344. Bjornsson J, McLeod RA, Unni KK, et al: Primary chondrosarcoma of long bones and limb girdles, *Cancer* 83:2105–2119, 1998.
345. Hammer AS, Couto CG, Filppi J, et al: Efficacy and toxicity of VAC chemotherapy (vincristine, doxorubicin, and cyclophosphamide) in dogs with hemangiosarcoma, *J Vet Intern Med* 5:160–166, 1991.
346. Ogilvie GK, Powers BE, Mallinckrodt CH, et al: Surgery and doxorubicin in dogs with hemangiosarcoma, *J Vet Intern Med* 10:379–384, 1996.
347. Vail DM, MacEwen EG, Kurzman ID, et al: Liposome-encapsulated muramyl tripeptide phosphatidylethanolamine adjuvant immunotherapy for splenic hemangiosarcoma in the dog: a randomized multi-institutional clinical trial, *Clin Cancer Res* 1:1165–1170, 1995.
348. Wesselhoeft-Ablin LA, Berg RJ, Schelling SH: Fibrosarcoma in the canine appendicular skeleton, *J Am Anim Hosp Assoc* 27:303–309, 1991.
349. Banks TA, Straw RC: Multilobular osteochondrosarcoma of the hard palate in a dog, *Aust Vet J* 82:409–412, 2004.
350. Straw RC, LeCouteur RA, Powers BE, et al: Multilobular osteochondrosarcoma of the canine skull: 16 cases (1978-1988), *J Am Vet Med Assoc* 195:1764–1769, 1989.
351. Dernell WS, Straw RC, Cooper MF, et al: Multilobular osteochondrosarcoma in 39 dogs: 1979-1993, *J Am Anim Hosp Assoc* 34:11–18, 1998.
352. Hathcock JT, Newton JC: Computed tomographic characteristics of multilobular tumor of bone involving the cranium in 7 dogs and zygomatic arch in 2 dogs, *Vet Radiol Ultrasound* 41:214–217, 2000.
353. Lipsitz D, Levitski RE, Berry WL: Magnetic resonance imaging features of multilobular osteochondrosarcoma in 3 dogs, *Vet Radiol Ultrasound* 42:14–19, 2001.
354. Stoll MR, Roush JK, Moisan PG: Multilobular tumour of bone with no abnormalities on plain radiography in a dog, *J Small Anim Pract* 42:453–455, 2001.
355. Cooley DM, Waters DJ: Skeletal metastasis as the initial clinical manifestation of metastatic carcinoma in 19 dogs, *J Vet Intern Med* 12:288–293, 1998.
356. Cornell KK, Bostwick DG, Cooley DM, et al: Clinical and pathologic aspects of spontaneous canine prostate carcinoma: a retrospective analysis of 76 cases, *Prostate* 45:173–183, 2000.
357. Johnson KA, Cooley AJ, Darien DL: Zygomatic osteoma with atypical heterogeneity in a dog, *J Comp Pathol* 114:199–203, 1996.
358. Chester DK: Multiple cartilaginous exostoses in two generations of dogs, *J Am Vet Med Assoc* 159:895–897, 1971.
359. Hunt GB, Malik R, Johnson KA: What is your diagnosis? Benign bone cyst in the distal portion of the left femur, *J Am Vet Med Assoc* 199:1071–1072, 1991.
360. Pernell RT, Dunstan RW, DeCamp CE: Aneurysmal bone cyst in a six-month-old dog, *J Am Vet Med Assoc* 201:1897–1899, 1992.
361. Basher AWP, Doige CE, Presnell KR: Subchondral bone cysts in a dog with osteochondrosis, *J Am Anim Hosp Assoc* 24:321–326, 1988.
362. Schrader SC, Burk RL, Liu SK: Bone cysts in two dogs and a review of similar cystic bone lesions in the dog, *J Am Vet Med Assoc* 182:490–495, 1983.
363. Biery DN, Goldschmidt M, Riser WH, et al: Bone cysts in the dog, *Vet Am Vet Radiol* 17:202–212, 1976.
364. Grabias S, Mankin H: Chondrosarcoma arising in histologically proved unicameral bone cyst, *J Bone Joint Surg* 56:1501–1503, 1973.
365. Dorn CR, Taylor DO, Schneider R, et al: Survey of animal neoplasms in Alameda and Contra Costa Counties, California. II. Cancer morbidity in dogs and cats from Alameda County, *J Natl Cancer Inst* 40:307–318, 1968.
366. Bitetto WV, Patnaik AK, Schrader SC, et al: Osteosarcoma in cats: 22 cases (1974-1984), *J Am Vet Med Assoc* 190:91–93, 1987.
367. Heldmann E, Anderson MA, Wagner-Mann C: Feline osteosarcoma: 145 cases (1990-1995), *J Am Anim Hosp Assoc* 36:518–521, 2000.
368. Turrel JM, Pool RR: Primary bone-tumors in the cat: a retrospective study of 15 cats and a literature-review, *Vet Radiol* 23:152–166, 1982.
369. Spugnini EP, Ruslander D, Bartolazzi A: Extraskeletal osteosarcoma in a cat, *J Am Vet Med Assoc* 219:60–62, 49, 2001.
370. Stimson EL, Cook WT, Smith MM, et al: Extraskeletal osteosarcoma in the duodenum of a cat, *J Am Anim Hosp Assoc* 36:332–336, 2000.
371. Dhaliwal RS, Johnson TO, Kitchell BE: Primary extraskeletal hepatic osteosarcoma in a cat, *J Am Vet Med Assoc* 222:340–342, 316, 2003.
372. Dimopoulou M, Kirpensteijn J, Moens H, et al: Histologic prognosticators in feline osteosarcoma: a comparison with phenotypically similar canine osteosarcoma, *Vet Surg* 37:466–471, 2008.
373. Pool RR, Carrig CB: Multiple cartilaginous exostoses in a cat, *Vet Pathol* 9:350–359, 1972.
374. Carpenter J, Andrews L, Holzworth J: Tumors and tumor-like lesions. In Holzworth J, editor: *Diseases of the cat: medicine and surgery*, Philadelphia, 1987, WB Saunders.
375. Liu SK, Dorfman HD, Patnaik AK: Primary and secondary bone tumours in the cat, *J Small Anim Pract* 15:141–156, 1974.
376. Quigley PJ, Leedale AH: Tumors involving bone in the domestic cat: a review of 58 cases, *Vet Pathol* 20:670–686, 1983.
377. Riddle WE Jr, Leighton RL: Osteochondromatosis in a cat, *J Am Vet Med Assoc* 156:1428–1430, 1970.

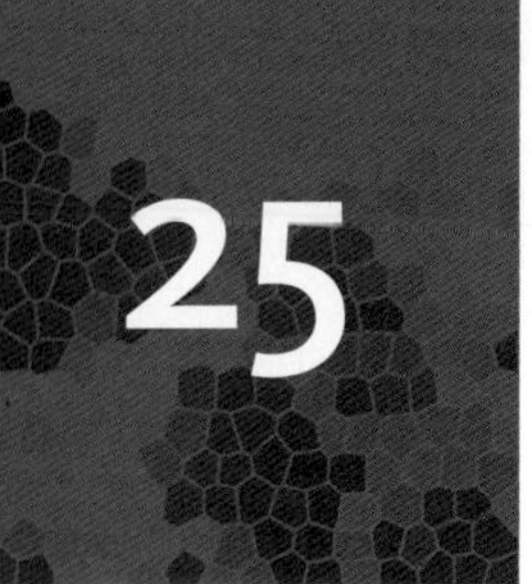

25 Tumors of the Endocrine System

KATHARINE F. LUNN AND RODNEY L. PAGE

Endocrine tumors may be classified as nonneoplastic hyperplasias, benign adenomas, or malignant carcinomas. These conditions represent points on a continuous spectrum of endocrine function-dysfunction. Nonneoplastic hyperplasia is the consequence of aberrant secretion of trophic hormones resulting in growth and increased function. Hyperplasia is often focal but not necessarily reversible when the inciting trophic factor is removed, illustrating the overlap between nonneoplastic and neoplastic endocrine disease.[1] Adenomas and carcinomas grow autonomously in the absence of trophic stimulation. Distinguishing between benign and malignant lesions can be challenging. In particular, the cellular morphologic features of adenomas and carcinomas are often similar, making cytologic samples, small biopsies, and even entire tumors difficult to accurately classify.[1] The clinical manifestations of endocrine tumors may be the result of growth, expansion, and metastasis of the tumor, producing traditional sequelae due to compression of normal tissue (adenoma), invasion and destruction of regional or systemic normal tissue function (carcinoma), secretion of hormones or hormone-like substances that produce signs of disease specific to the downstream tissue impact, and often a combination of these effects.

In this chapter, we will review the common endocrine tumors of dogs and cats. A discussion of endocrine neoplasia in ferrets is beyond the scope of this chapter; however, a thorough review is available for the interested reader.[2] Multiple endocrine neoplasia is not discussed here because it remains rarely reported in companion species.

Pathogenesis of Endocrine Tumors

Endocrine tissue is distinct from nonendocrine tissue in several ways that influence the pathogenesis of cancer. Endocrine glands normally expand in secretory capacity by an increased number of cells, increase in size and productivity of individual cells, or both, when the necessary stimulus is applied. They then return to a relatively quiescent state when the trophic substance is removed. Growth (cellular enlargement and division) and function (production of hormone) are therefore tightly linked and controlled by the same physiologic stimulus. Cells within endocrine organs are relatively stable. For example, the thyroid gland is expected to have only six to eight renewals in the lifespan of an adult human, dog, or mouse.[3] This low turnover rate (2.3 years in dogs) is associated with longer intermitotic intervals compared to many other cell types in nonendocrine tissues. Such quiescence may result in a lower mutation rate, although any mutations acquired may be retained for longer periods.[4] Prolonged stimulation of mutation-bearing endocrine tissue by a trophic substance may result in transformation. Clinically, this may be observed when longstanding hyperplasia ultimately progresses to neoplasia. In this situation, growth and function within the endocrine organ ultimately become independent of trophic hormone stimulation.

The orchestrated accumulation of somatic mutations leading to dedifferentiation from mature to anaplastic cells is considered the classic theory of carcinogenesis in thyroid tissue, and this area is where the majority of research has occurred.[5] Loss of tumor suppressor gene function, or oncogene activation, may lead to neoplasia. Only recently has a cancer stem cell theory of carcinogenesis emerged for endocrine neoplasia, in particular for thyroid neoplasia.[6-9] Although a cancer stem cell has not yet been isolated from human thyroid cancer tissue, the strong appearance of an epithelial-to-mesenchymal transition in the morphology of thyroid anaplastic carcinoma suggests the potential of cancer stem cells. Additional well-known pathways of carcinogenesis include the germline alterations predisposing to tumor development and conventional agents such as exposure to ionizing radiation or environmental exposures to endocrine disruptors and thyroid mimics.

Growth factors such as growth hormone (GH), insulin-like growth factors (IGFs), and epidermal growth factor (EGF) also play an integral role in the pathogenesis of endocrine neoplasia.[10] However, normally differentiated and neoplastic endocrine cells respond similarly to growth factor stimulation, and it is unlikely that any single growth factor can cause transformation of a cell. The role of growth factors within endocrine oncogenesis therefore is thought to be that of a tumor promoter, whereby growth factor–stimulated hyperplasia increases the probability of mutational events that may eventually release the cell from growth control.

Pituitary Tumors

Primary tumors of the pituitary gland can arise from several different cell types, including corticotrophs, somatotrophs, thyrotrophs, gonadotrophs, and lactotrophs. The clinical signs associated with these tumors depend on their size and their secretory properties. The most clinically important pituitary tumor in the dog is the corticotroph adenoma. This tumor produces chronically excessive amounts of adrenocorticotrophic hormone (ACTH) and is associated with clinical signs of hypercortisolism. In the cat, the most clinically significant pituitary tumor is the GH-secreting somatotroph adenoma, causing acromegaly and insulin-resistant diabetes mellitus.

Nonfunctional pituitary tumors become clinically significant when they are large enough to cause neurologic signs, including obtundation, stupor, behavioral changes, decreased appetite, gait abnormalities, seizures, blindness, and other cranial nerve abnormalities.[11-14] In one case series, pituitary tumors were the second most common type of secondary brain tumor, accounting for 25% of 177 cases.[15]

The pituitary gland may also be affected by secondary tumors, either through direct extension or by metastatic spread from a distant site.[1] Locally invasive or compressive primary or secondary pituitary tumors also have the potential to cause loss of pituitary function, resulting in hypothyroidism, hypocortisolism, gonadal atrophy, or central diabetes insipidus.[16]

Pituitary Corticotroph Tumors: Hypercortisolism (Hyperadrenocorticism or Cushing's Syndrome)

Pathogenesis

Hypercortisolism (HC), also termed *hyperadrenocorticism* or *Cushing's syndrome,* is a common endocrine disease of middle-aged and older dogs.[17] It is uncommon in cats. This clinical syndrome results from chronic exposure to excessive blood levels of glucocorticoids. Naturally occurring canine and feline HC are almost always either pituitary-dependent or a result of excessive glucocorticoid secretion from an adrenocortical tumor.[17,18]

HC in human medicine is differentiated into ACTH-dependent and ACTH-independent disease.[19] ACTH-dependent disease most commonly results from excessive ACTH secretion from a pituitary tumor but may also be caused by ectopic secretion of ACTH from an extrapituitary tumor or very rarely by ectopic secretion of corticotrophin-releasing hormone (CRH). There is only one clearly documented report of ectopic ACTH secretion in the dog,[20] which may reflect the fact that it is very difficult to prove this diagnosis.

Pituitary-dependent hypercortisolism (PDH) is the most common form of spontaneous HC in dogs and cats, accounting for 80% to 85% of cases in these species.[17,18,21,22] This disorder is a consequence of autonomous synthesis and secretion of ACTH from a pituitary tumor. The secretion of ACTH from the pituitary tumor is chronically excessive, leading to bilateral adrenal cortical hyperplasia and hypercortisolemia. The pituitary tumor is relatively insensitive to negative feedback by cortisol and there is also a loss of hypothalamic control over ACTH release because CRH secretion is suppressed by the chronic hypercortisolemia.[18]

Pituitary tumors that secrete ACTH are derived from pituitary corticotroph cells. Expression of several proteins and their receptors thought to be involved in the etiology of human pituitary tumors responsible for ACTH hypersecretion has been studied. Leukemia inhibitory factor and its receptor are expressed in canine pituitary adenoma samples, although no mutations were identified in the receptor that might account for autonomous ACTH production.[23,24] Dopamine and somatostatin receptor subtype expressions were evaluated in normal canine pituitary tissue and compared to adenomatous tissue. The type 2 dopamine receptor and somatostatin type 2 (SST2) receptor were most prevalent in canine pituitary tumors but expressed at low levels.

Pituitary tumors may be described as macrotumors or microtumors.[18] The latter distinction is derived from human medicine: microtumors are less than 1 cm in diameter and macrotumors are 1 cm or larger in diameter. The use of this size-based classification is controversial in veterinary medicine, at least partly due to variability in patient size and conformation.[12] Pituitary tumors may also be classified as noninvasive adenomas, invasive adenomas, or adenocarcinomas. The latter term is reserved for tumors in which there is demonstrated evidence of metastatic disease. Canine pituitary adenocarcinomas are uncommon. A recent study of 33 dogs with pituitary tumors, all of which underwent necropsy evaluation after brain imaging, revealed that 61% had a pituitary adenoma, 33% had an invasive adenoma, and 6% had an adenocarcinoma.[11]

ACTH-independent HC refers to disease of the adrenal cortex, including neoplasia, dysplasia, or hyperplasia. This will be referred to as adrenal-dependent hypercortisolism (ADH) in this chapter and will be discussed in the section on adrenal gland tumors.

Clinical Findings and Diagnostic Evaluation in Dogs

The majority of dogs with PDH are older than 9 years of age, and female dogs are slightly overrepresented. Breed predispositions have been noted in Dachshunds, terrier breeds, German shepherd dogs, and poodle breeds.[17,18] The onset of canine Cushing's syndrome is often slow, and the signs may progress slowly. Affected dogs are often not considered by their owners to be sick; they have a good appetite and do not show signs such as vomiting, diarrhea, coughing, or weight loss. Because spontaneous HC typically affects elderly dogs, the signs may initially be attributed to normal aging. The progress of the disorder is generally insidious, but eventually the owners of affected dogs seek veterinary care due to the frustration associated with signs such as polyuria, polydipsia, panting, and exercise intolerance.

The most common signs of canine HC are polyuria, polydipsia, polyphagia, abdominal enlargement, lethargy, panting, exercise intolerance, muscle weakness, alopecia, calcinosis cutis, thinning of the skin, and reproductive abnormalities.[17,18] These clinical signs are the result of the gluconeogenic, catabolic, immunosuppressive, and antiinflammatory effects of excessive circulating glucocorticoids. Glucose intolerance and insulin resistance have been shown to be common in dogs with HC,[25] and overt diabetes mellitus may develop in as many as 10% of these patients.[26] The catabolic effects of glucocorticoids result in thinning of the skin, poor wound healing, muscle wasting, and decreased bone density.[27] The antiinflammatory and immunosuppressive properties of glucocorticoids are responsible for the increased susceptibility to infections in dogs with hypercortisolemia.[17] This most often manifests as an increased incidence of urinary tract infections in canine patients. In one study, 46% of dogs with HC were found to have a urinary tract infection.[28]

More serious disorders associated with canine HC include hypertension and proteinuria.[17,29] These are particularly insidious because they may not initially be associated with overt clinical signs. If untreated, hypertension can damage end organs such as the eye, brain, and kidneys, leading to complications that may include blindness or glomerular disease. Over 80% of dogs with canine Cushing's syndrome were reported to be hypertensive in one case series.[30] Although uncommon, pulmonary thromboembolism is another potentially life-threatening complication of HC.[26,31]

Spontaneous HC is suspected when typical clinical signs are detected in a middle-aged or older dog that is not receiving exogenous glucocorticoid therapy. The diagnosis is further investigated when initial laboratory tests reveal classic abnormalities, including neutrophilia, monocytosis, lymphopenia, eosinopenia, thrombocytosis, elevated serum alkaline phosphatase levels, a mild increase in alanine aminotransferase, and elevated cholesterol. Urinalysis may demonstrate minimally concentrated, isosthenuric, or hyposthenuric urine. Ancillary tests recommended in dogs suspected to have HC include urine culture, blood pressure measurement, thoracic radiographs, and abdominal ultrasonography.[17,18,32]

The tests that are most commonly used to screen for the presence of spontaneous HC are the urine cortisol : creatinine ratio, the ACTH stimulation test, and the low-dose dexamethasone suppression test (LDDST). These tests should be reserved for patients in which there is clinical suspicion of HC. Due to space considerations, readers are directed to several excellent references for more in-depth discussion of the comparative aspects of these tests.[17,18,32,33] The urine cortisol : creatinine ratio is very sensitive, but specificity is low and it should not be used in patients with concurrent illnesses. The ACTH stimulation test has a lower sensitivity and higher specificity in comparison to the LDDST. The LDDST is highly sensitive and therefore less likely to give false-negative results. An additional advantage of this test is that it is capable of distinguishing between PDH and ADH in some cases.[17] For patients with typical clinical signs of HC and positive results on the ACTH stimulation test, further testing is generally performed to differentiate between pituitary and adrenal-dependent disease. These further tests are also necessary after positive results on the LDDST for those patients in which this test does not additionally confirm the presence of PDH. Differentiation tests that are commonly used include the high-dose dexamethasone suppression test (HDDST) and the measurement of endogenous ACTH levels.[17,32] In dogs with ADH, it is expected that endogenous ACTH levels will be low due to feedback inhibition of pituitary ACTH release by chronic hypercortisolemia. Patients with PDH would be expected to have elevated endogenous ACTH levels.[34-36]

The results of imaging studies, including ultrasonography, computed tomography (CT), or magnetic resonance imaging (MRI), may assist in differentiating between PDH and ADH.[17,18] Abdominal ultrasonography should not be used as a screening test for HC, and it should also not be used as the sole mechanism for discriminating between PDH and ADH; however, it can provide useful information.[35,37-40] The adrenals of patients with PDH are often bilaterally enlarged with increased thickness, and they typically maintain a normal shape and are homogeneous in echogenicity.[37] However, there can be overlap between adrenal gland measurements in normal dogs, dogs with nonadrenal disease, and dogs with HC. Adrenal gland asymmetry may also be detected in dogs with PDH due to nodular hyperplasia. In some cases, this appearance can be confused with adrenal neoplasia. To further complicate the diagnostic accuracy of abdominal ultrasonography, a small percentage of patients with HC may have concurrent PDH and ADH.[41] Bilateral adrenal tumors may also occur, including both functional or nonfunctional adrenocortical tumors and pheochromocytomas.[39,42-45] Thus ultrasound findings must always be interpreted concurrently with clinical findings and endocrine test results. Abdominal CT is used less commonly than ultrasonography to evaluate the adrenals, but CT findings may also assist in the discrimination between PDH and ADH.[46,47] This technique also demonstrates overlap between adrenal volume in dogs with PDH and dogs with nonadrenal disease and also confirms that dogs with PDH can have nodular adrenal lesions.[47]

Although 80% to 85% of dogs with spontaneous HC have PDH and almost all cases of PDH are due to the presence of a pituitary tumor, canine patients do not often show clinical signs directly referable to the local effects of the tumor.[17] The vast majority of cases are initially presented for veterinary care due to the typical clinical signs of HC, as described previously. Pituitary tumors may be detected by CT,[12,14] dynamic CT,[48,49] MRI,[12,14,50-53] or dynamic MRI[54]; however, these techniques are not routinely performed in all dogs that are diagnosed with PDH.[12] In most cases, the diagnosis is based on the presence of typical clinical signs and clinicopathologic changes of hypercortisolemia, together with the results of endocrine testing.[17]

As noted previously, brain imaging is not performed in the great majority of dogs with PDH, and most receive treatment to address adrenal hyperfunction rather than the pituitary tumor itself. This is most likely due to the fact that brain imaging and pituitary surgery or radiation therapy (RT) are not affordable or accessible to many clients. Although medical therapy for PDH (see later) has a long history of successful use, it is important to note that the pituitary lesion in dogs with PDH will progress over time. In a study of 13 dogs that underwent MRI evaluation of the brain at the time of diagnosis of PDH and before medical therapy was instituted, 8 of the dogs had a visible pituitary mass and none of the dogs had clinical signs of neurologic disease.[53] Four of the dogs showed enlargement of the pituitary tumor on MRI 1 year later, and a pituitary tumor was also detected in two dogs that did not have a visible mass on the initial MRI. Two of the 13 dogs had developed neurologic signs at the time of the 1-year follow-up MRI. A recent study evaluated diagnostic imaging findings in 157 dogs with PDH with and without neurologic signs.[14] Central nervous system (CNS)-specific signs such as circling, seizures, or ataxia were neither sensitive nor specific for predicting the presence of a pituitary macrotumor. However, signs such as lethargy, mental dullness, and decreased appetite were highly specific for detection of a pituitary macrotumor but not highly sensitive. Other studies have also documented that mentation and appetite changes are the most common signs associated with pituitary tumors.[13,55]

When considering brain imaging in dogs with PDH, several factors should be taken into account: 40% to 50% of dogs with PDH have tumors that are not visible on CT or MRI, and these dogs are unlikely to develop neurologic signs associated with the tumor; 15% to 25% of dogs with PDH are at risk for the development of neurologic signs due to the presence of an enlarging tumor, and these signs typically develop within 6 to 18 months of the diagnosis of PDH; brain imaging may be helpful in predicting dogs likely to develop neurologic signs in patients with PDH that initially have no signs directly attributable to the tumor[17]; and if RT is being considered, early treatment will likely improve prognosis.[13,56] It is also possible that measurement of plasma ACTH precursor concentrations could help in the selection of patients for brain imaging because it has been shown that pro-opiomelanocortin/pro-ACTH levels in plasma are correlated with pituitary tumor size in dogs with PDH.[57,58] However, plasma cortisol concentrations at baseline and 4 or 8 hours after administration of a low dose of dexamethasone do not appear to correlate with the development of neurologic signs.[14]

Treatment of Canine Pituitary-Dependent Hypercortisolism

Options for management of canine PDH include medical therapies that address adrenocortical hyperfunction, as well as direct treatment of the pituitary lesion through surgery or RT. The decision to treat patients with PDH should be guided by the patient's quality of life, the owner's wishes, and consideration of the risks of serious or life-threatening complications of the disease, such as neurologic signs, hypertension, recurrent infections, or thromboembolic disease. Some dogs with PDH have mild clinical signs and a good quality of life when initially diagnosed. There is no clear evidence that early treatment of these patients is necessary to improve long-term survival. Treatment of PDH is rarely an emergency, and more serious concurrent illnesses should be addressed first.

Surgery

Hypophysectomy is the treatment of choice for PDH in humans and can be successful in dogs.[59-61] A recent prospective study of 150 dogs that underwent transsphenoidal hypophysectomy for PDH gave 1-, 2-, 3-, and 4-year estimated survival rates of 84%, 76%, 72%, and 68%, respectively. Twelve dogs died postoperatively and 127 went into remission, with 32 of those dogs later experiencing a recurrence of disease. Complications included central diabetes insipidus in 53% of dogs undergoing remission and incomplete hypophysectomy in nine dogs. The overall success rate of transsphenoidal hypophysectomy was determined to be 65% in this study.[61] Unfortunately, this approach requires a high degree of specialized surgical skill and experience, and it is not readily available outside of one center in Europe.

Radiation Therapy

There are several reports of the successful use of radiation in the treatment of canine PDH.[13,56,62-64] Dow and colleagues treated six dogs with functional pituitary macrotumors with 40 Gy given in 10 equal fractions. Median survival was reported to be 743 days, neurologic signs resolved in all dogs, and ACTH levels remained high for at least 1 year after therapy.[62] Goossens et al used cobalt 60 RT to treat six dogs with PDH caused by a pituitary tumor that was detectable on MRI, and tumor size was significantly reduced in all cases. However, clinical signs of PDH were only adequately controlled in one dog.[63] Théon and Feldman evaluated the effects of megavoltage irradiation on pituitary tumors in 24 dogs with neurologic signs. Ten dogs experienced complete remission of neurologic signs, and another 10 dogs achieved partial remission. As in previous studies, these authors noted a correlation between relative tumor size and the severity of neurologic signs in dogs with pituitary tumors. They also noted a correlation between tumor size and remission of neurologic signs after pituitary irradiation, suggesting that early treatment of these tumors should improve prognosis, although control of ACTH secretion was unlikely.[56] A recent retrospective study of RT for the treatment of pituitary masses demonstrated significantly improved survival times and control of neurologic signs in 19 dogs that received RT, compared to 27 untreated control dogs with pituitary masses. Mean survival time in the treated group was 1405 days, compared to 551 days in the nonirradiated group. The 1-, 2-, and 3-year estimated survival rates were 93%, 87%, and 55% for the irradiated and 45%, 32%, and 25% for the nonirradiated dogs, respectively. Treated dogs with smaller tumors lived longer than those with larger tumors, again suggesting that early diagnosis and treatment of pituitary tumors are beneficial. Five of 14 dogs with PDH in this study were reported to show resolution of clinical signs of HC together with at least one normal ACTH stimulation test result after completion of RT.[13]

Most of the reports that document the use of RT for the treatment of pituitary tumors in dogs provide little detailed information regarding the progress of the clinical syndrome of HC in these patients.[13,56,62-64] Thus, although RT appears effective in controlling neurologic signs and increasing survival,[13] it is difficult to predict the endocrinologic outcome of RT for dogs with PDH.

Medical Therapy

A detailed review of medical therapy for PDH is beyond the scope of this chapter, and the information here should be regarded as a brief introduction. Readers are strongly encouraged to consult any of several excellent discussions of this subject before initiating medical therapy in any patient.[17,18] The two medications that are most commonly used to treat PDH in dogs are mitotane and trilostane. Other drugs such as ketoconazole, L-deprenyl, metyrapone, bromocriptine, and retinoic acid are used rarely and will not be discussed further in this chapter.

Mitotane (o,p′-DDD, Lysodren) is a potent adrenocorticolytic agent that is cytotoxic to the adrenal cortex, particularly the zona fasciculata and zona reticularis. Mitotane therapy is most commonly divided into a loading or induction phase that typically lasts between 5 and 9 days, followed by maintenance therapy. Patients should be monitored very closely during loading with mitotane, and this phase is regarded as being complete when the post-ACTH cortisol is less than 5 (or 4) μg/dL on an ACTH stimulation test. This usually coincides with a decrease in appetite or in polyuria/polydipsia in the patient, but not always. Thus an ACTH stimulation test should be performed as soon as the patient shows any change in clinical signs or within 5 to 7 days of starting mitotane, whichever occurs first. A typical induction dose of mitotane is 30 to 50 mg/kg day, and maintenance therapy with mitotane typically requires giving the initial induction dose weekly, although the exact dose depends on how the patient responded to the induction course. Thus a patient requiring 500 mg per day for induction will often be started on 500 mg weekly for maintenance, with the weekly dose typically divided between 2 to 4 days. The mitotane dose should always be divided when possible and given with food, and clients should be instructed to wear gloves when handling the medication. An ACTH stimulation test is typically performed 1 month after initiation of maintenance therapy and then several times a year thereafter. The frequency of testing will depend on the dog's clinical signs and the frequency with which dose adjustments are made. An alternate mitotane protocol has also been described for dogs with PDH. In contrast to the selective adrenocorticolysis protocol summarized earlier, which is designed to spare the zona glomerulosa, mitotane can also be used to achieve nonselective complete adrenocorticolysis. In this protocol, the medication is given at a higher dose for a fixed time period, and glucocorticoid and mineralocorticoid supplementation are started shortly after initiation of mitotane therapy and continued thereafter.[65] This approach may be preferred in dogs that relapse frequently on the selective protocol and in dogs with concurrent diabetes mellitus. It may also be less expensive in some patients. However, this protocol was reported to cause adverse effects requiring temporary cessation of therapy in 29% of dogs, and relapse occurred in 39% of dogs that underwent remission.[65] Thus the use of this protocol does not eliminate the need for careful long-term follow-up.

Trilostane (Vetoryl) is an orally active synthetic corticosteroid analog that competitively inhibits 3-β-hydroxysteroid dehydrogenase.[66] This enzyme is essential for synthesis of cortisol and other steroids such as corticosterone, androstenedione, and aldosterone. Trilostane has been used in Europe for several years for the management of canine PDH and recently was approved for use in the United States. Initial publications suggested a starting dose of trilostane of around 6 mg/kg once daily, with the first follow-up ACTH stimulation test performed at 10 to 14 days.[67] As more experience has been gained with this medication, it has become apparent that much lower starting doses may be effective and potentially associated with fewer adverse effects.[68,69] It is also appears that trilostane should be used twice daily in most dogs,[70] with a recent study suggesting a starting dose in the range of 0.2-1.1 mg/kg every 12 hours.[68] The response to trilostane is also monitored with ACTH stimulation testing, with the aim of achieving a post-ACTH cortisol value in the range of 1.5 to 5 μg/dL. Values slightly above this range are acceptable if the patient's clinical signs are well controlled.[66] It is recommended that the ACTH stimulation test be started 3 to 4

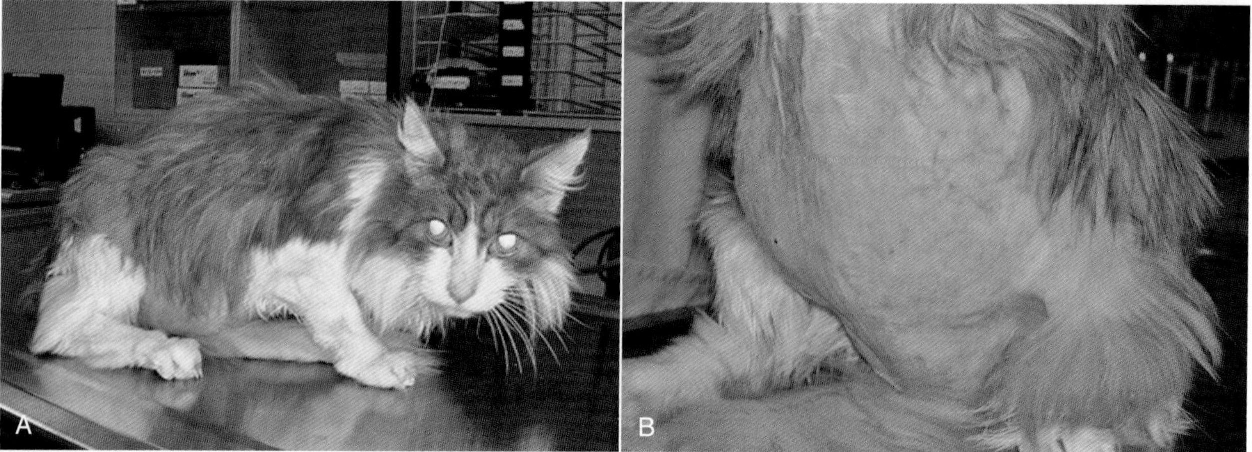

FIGURE 25-1 A 14-year-old male neutered domestic longhair cat with pituitary-dependent hypercortisolism. **A,** The patient appears weak, with muscle atrophy and an unkempt haircoat. **B,** The abdomen has a potbellied appearance with thinning of the skin.

hours after trilostane is given for dogs receiving twice daily therapy. Although most authors suggest performing the first ACTH stimulation test at 10 to 14 days, the reason for this is unclear because the results of this test generally continue to improve beyond 2 weeks, even when the dose is not changed.

Both mitotane and trilostane are highly effective for the treatment of canine PDH. A retrospective comparison of mitotane and trilostane in dogs with PDH demonstrated a median survival time (MST) of 662 days for trilostane and 708 days for mitotane.[71] It is important to note that both mitotane and trilostane can have adverse effects in dogs. Both medications can be associated with anorexia, vomiting, or diarrhea, and both can cause hypoadrenocorticism.[17,18,66] Trilostane therapy has also been associated with adrenal necrosis.[72,73] It should also be noted that the adrenal glands of dogs receiving mitotane therapy for PDH will become smaller over time, whereas the adrenal glands of dogs on trilostane therapy have been shown to increase in size by 6 weeks after initiation of therapy and may develop an irregular nodular ultrasonographic appearance after several months of therapy.[74]

In deciding whether to use trilostane or mitotane in a patient with PDH, the clinician should consider his or her own comfort level and experience with each medication and also the wishes of the client. A cost analysis should also be performed, including the cost of follow-up office visits and ACTH stimulation testing, as well as the cost of the medication itself. It is recommended that clinicians exercise caution in using compounded trilostane as any potential cost savings may be offset by the highly variable drug concentrations that have been detected within and between batches of medications obtained from compounding pharmacies.[75]

Feline Pituitary-Dependent Hypercortisolism

As noted previously, approximately 80% to 85% of cases of HC in the cat are due to pituitary disease.[17,21,22] However, Cushing's syndrome is considerably less common in cats than in dogs. The mean age of cats with PDH is reported to be around 10 years.[21] Feline HC is often associated with insulin-resistant diabetes mellitus, with signs of polyuria, polydipsia, polyphagia, and weight loss. Cats with HC often have a potbellied appearance due to hepatomegaly and muscle weakness, and they frequently have thin fragile skin that tears and bruises easily. Additional signs include lethargy, generalized muscle atrophy, weakness, alopecia, and an unkempt haircoat (Figure 25-1). On routine laboratory testing, elevated alkaline phosphatase is much less frequently detected in cats with HC compared to dogs. Cats may have elevated alanine aminotransferase, hypercholesterolemia, azotemia, and minimally concentrated urine. Hyperglycemia and glycosuria are expected in cats with concurrent diabetes mellitus. No consistent complete blood count (CBC) changes have been reported in cats with HC.[21,22]

Tests used to screen for spontaneous HC in cats include the urine cortisol:creatinine ratio, the ACTH stimulation test, and the LDDST. It is important to note that the details of these protocols differ between dogs and cats, and readers are directed to more complete references for further information.[21,22] The HDDST, endogenous ACTH levels, and abdominal ultrasound examination may be used to assist in differentiation of PDH from ADH in the cat.

Because PDH is relatively uncommon in the cat, there are few case series and case reports on which to base treatment recommendations.[76,77] Direct treatment of the pituitary tumor has been reported, with either surgical hypophysectomy or RT.[59,78-80] Surgical bilateral adrenalectomy has also been described and was considered the treatment of choice for some time.[81] However, these cats are often poor surgical candidates, they have poor healing ability, and complications are common. Laparoscopic adrenalectomy is potentially a better option for these patients because the incisions are much smaller and more likely to heal; however, this has not yet been reported in cats with PDH. Medical therapy with trilostane may be a reasonable option for these cats, based on the authors' experience and a small number of published cases.[82,83] This drug could be used as the sole therapy or to prepare cats for surgery or RT.

Pituitary Somatotroph Tumors (Feline Acromegaly)

Feline acromegaly is a disease of older cats resulting from chronic excessive GH secretion, usually from a functional somatotroph adenoma of the pars distalis of the pituitary gland.[84] Feline acromegaly has historically been regarded as a rare condition; however, recent findings suggest that it may be significantly underdiagnosed. In a study of 184 diabetic cats, 59 had markedly increased IGF-1 concentrations, and acromegaly was confirmed in 17 of 18 cats that

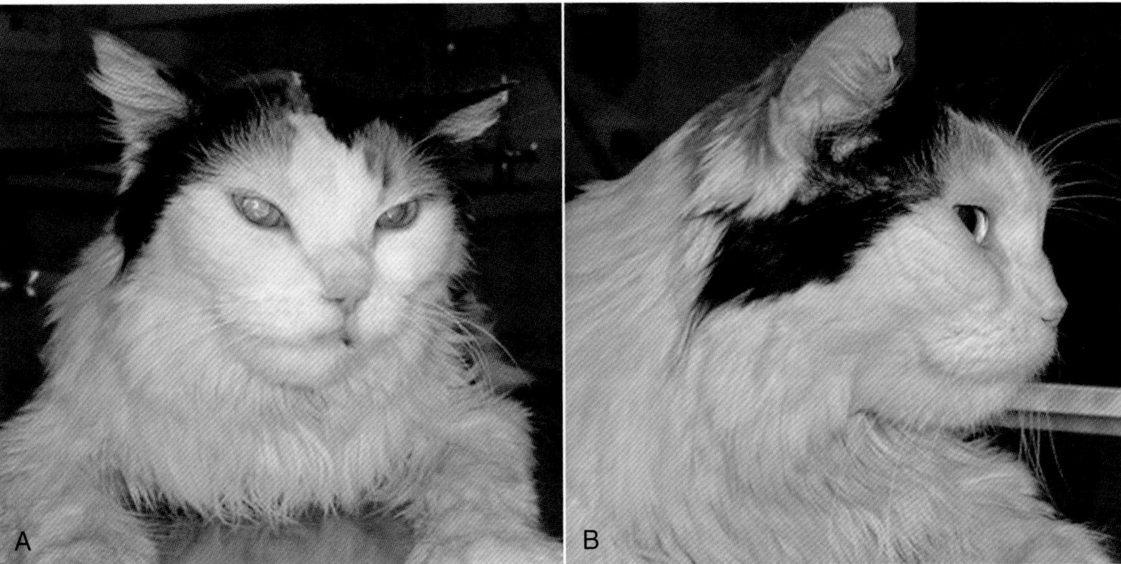

FIGURE 25-2 **A** and **B,** A 12-year-old female spayed domestic longhair cat with acromegaly due to a pituitary tumor. Note the broad forehead and large mandible.

were examined by CT, MRI, or necropsy.[85] These findings have prompted the suggestion that any cat with clinical features of acromegaly, including insulin resistance, should be screened for this disorder.[86]

Acromegaly is reported to be more common in male cats, with no apparent breed predilection, and most affected cats are middle-aged or older.[87] The typical history is of insulin-resistant diabetes mellitus, with affected cats requiring 10 to 20 units of insulin per dose or more, often with inadequate control of the diabetes. This insulin resistance is due to a GH-induced postreceptor defect in the action of insulin on target cells. Affected cats remain polyuric, polydipsic, and polyphagic and continue to gain weight. Most cats with poorly regulated diabetes mellitus will lose weight, and therefore weight gain in this situation is highly suggestive of feline acromegaly. The physical changes of acromegaly develop slowly and are often not noted by the owner until they are advanced. These changes may include enlarged feet, broadening of the face, protrusion of the mandible (Figure 25-2), increased spacing between the teeth, and abdominal enlargement.[85,87-90] Owners of affected cats also frequently note noisy or stertorous breathing or respiratory stridor.[85,89-91] Physical examination may reveal additional abnormalities, such as enlarged abdominal organs and cardiac murmurs, arrhythmias, or a gallop rhythm.[85,87,90]

Neurologic signs associated with the pituitary tumor appear to be generally uncommon but may be underrecognized or underreported. Lethargy, mental dullness, or impaired vision may occur but can often be subtle. Affected cats may also demonstrate signs of diabetic neuropathy or lameness, possibly due to acromegaly-associated arthopathy.[85,87] Additional complications of acromegaly may include cardiac disease and protein-losing nephropathy.[87]

Acromegaly is the result of excessive GH secretion from a pituitary gland tumor, and elevated GH levels have been reported in several cats with acromegaly.* Overlap between GH values in diabetic cats with and without acromegaly has also been noted.[93] An ovine GH assay has been validated for the diagnosis of feline acromegaly and is available in Europe.[94] This assay clearly differentiated between normal cats and cats with acromegaly. Unfortunately, at the time of writing, a feline GH assay was not reliably available in the United States.

The physical changes in patients with acromegaly are due to the anabolic effects of GH, which are mediated by peripherally synthesized IGF-1.[84] This hormone is predominantly produced in the liver, and levels of IGF-1 increase in the presence of chronically increased GH production. Because GH secretion may be pulsatile, even in some acromegalics, and because it has a short half-life, increased serum IGF-1 has been suggested to be a more sensitive test for acromegaly because it may reflect GH levels over the preceding 24 hours.[84,86] Serum IGF-1 values are widely reported in acromegalic cats.* A recent study confirmed that IGF-1 measurement is a useful screening test for feline acromegaly, with sensitivity and specificity of 84% and 92%, respectively.[89] There was no difference in serum IGF-1 concentrations among well-controlled diabetic cats, poorly controlled diabetic cats, and healthy cats.[89] The highest IGF-1 noted in a diabetic cat was 153 nM, with a normal reference range of 12-92 nM; thus there is some overlap between the IGF-1 values found in acromegalic cats and those found in poorly regulated diabetic cats. However, it is these authors' experience that IGF-1 levels in cats with acromegaly are usually at least twice the value of the high end of the reference range. Feline IGF-1 measurement is currently readily available to veterinarians in the United States, and this test should be considered in cats with diabetes mellitus that appear to be insulin resistant.[86]

The presence of a pituitary tumor can be demonstrated by either CT or MRI in cats with acromegaly, and both have been reported in the literature.† MRI is likely more sensitive than CT,[85] but both imaging modalities may reveal a normal pituitary in a cat with acromegaly, if the size of the mass is below the limit of detection.

Treatment options for acromegaly in human medicine include surgery, conventional external-beam RT, stereotactic RT (SRT), and

*References 63, 79, 85, 87, 91-96.

*References 79, 84, 85, 89, 91, 96-101.

†References 63, 79, 85, 87, 89, 95-100, 102.

medical therapy.[103-105] Some of these therapies are also used in feline patients, but not all are available and many have not been adequately evaluated in cats.

In humans, transsphenoidal surgery to remove the pituitary tumor is generally regarded as the treatment of choice[106]; however, there are only rare reports of the use of surgery for treatment of feline acromegaly.[79,96,99]

RT is rarely used as a first-line therapy in human medicine.[105] In contrast, RT is the treatment for feline acromegaly that is most widely reported in the veterinary literature.* Conventional fractionated RT is administered in multiple fractions typically spread over a period of weeks. Protocols range from 5 fractions given weekly to as many as 20 fractions given over a period of 4 weeks.[80,98,108] A recent study showed that RT improved diabetic control in 13 of 14 cats, although IGF-1 concentrations did not correlate with this improved control.[100] Improved control of diabetes mellitus has also been noted in other studies.†

There are few reports of long-term follow-up of acromegalic cats receiving RT; thus it is difficult to assess the risk of complications of this modality in this species. Published case reports and case series of cats receiving conventional RT suggest that short- and long-term adverse effects of this therapy are relatively uncommon.[80,100,107,108]

Disadvantages of RT as a treatment for feline acromegaly include cost, availability, and the necessity for repeated anesthetic events. The latter disadvantage can be lessened by the use of SRT (see Chapter 12). SRT is widely used in the treatment of pituitary tumors in human patients.[109] There is one case series in veterinary medicine in which cats with pituitary tumors received treatment with a linear accelerator-based modified radiosurgical approach.[101] Cats received a single large dose of radiation, but it was delivered in a nonconformal fashion. The technique was reported to be safe and effective. At Colorado State University (CSU), SRT is routinely used in the treatment of feline acromegaly, with promising results.[110] Cats typically receive 2 to 4 fractions of radiation administered over a period of up to 5 days. This offers considerable advantages in terms of owner time commitment and the risks of anesthesia and hospitalization in elderly diabetic cats.

Medical therapy for acromegaly is commonly used in humans, either as a first-line treatment or as an adjunct to surgery or RT. The classes of drugs used are somatostatin analogs, GH-receptor antagonists, and dopamine agonists.[103-106] GH-receptor antagonists have not been evaluated in cats, and dopamine agonists do not appear to be useful in this species.[111]

Somatostatin analogs, also termed *somatostatin receptor ligands* (SRLs), bind to somatostatin receptors, suppressing the release of GH from the pituitary gland. The medications are available as long- or short-acting preparations, and response to SRLs is assessed by measurement of IGF-1 and GH levels and tumor size and evaluation of clinical signs.[103] Octreotide has been evaluated in a small number of cats with acromegaly. In five cats, short-acting octreotide was used for up to 4 weeks, with no apparent improvement in GH levels.[87,92] However, a more recent study showed that GH levels were significantly decreased for up to 120 minutes postinjection in five cats with acromegaly that received a single dose of octreotide.[95] These studies used the short-acting form of octreotide and were performed over a very short time period without assessment of clinical response. A study is currently underway at CSU to evaluate the use of a long-acting octreotide preparation for the treatment of feline acromegaly.

For many cats with acromegaly, insulin therapy is the only treatment that is available or acceptable to the owner. In general, these patients should receive the amount of insulin that is necessary to control their diabetes, although adequate blood glucose regulation can be difficult to achieve in many cases. The use of home blood glucose monitoring, with close cooperation between the owner and veterinarian, is strongly recommended. The feeding of a low-carbohydrate diet may also be beneficial.[111] It should be expected that these patients will receive insulin doses in the range of 10 to 20 units per dose or more. Concurrent illnesses and complications of acromegaly and diabetes mellitus should also be addressed.

The short-term prognosis for cats diagnosed with acromegaly is generally fair to good, but the long-term prognosis is poor. Patients may succumb to cardiac or renal failure, neurologic disease, or complications of poorly regulated diabetes mellitus.[84] The median survival was reported to be 20.5 months in one case series.[87]

Adrenal Gland Neoplasia

The prevalence of primary adrenal gland tumors in the dog and cat is difficult to discern from the literature. A search of the Veterinary Medical Database from 1985 to 1996 revealed that primary adrenal tumors were reported in approximately 0.17% to 0.76% of pet dogs (representing 1% to 2% of all canine tumors) and 0.03% of cats (representing 0.2% of feline tumors).[112] However, this likely underestimates the true prevalence because gross pathologic or histopathologic records were not available for the majority of these patients. For dogs and cats undergoing necropsy or adrenal surgery, it appears that tumors of the adrenal cortex are more common than those of the medulla. A retrospective study of patients with adrenal tumors identified from surgical biopsies or necropsy during a 20-year period at the University of California, Davis (UC Davis), demonstrated that 195 (41%) of 472 neoplastic canine adrenal lesions were adrenocortical tumors (154 adenomas; 41 carcinomas), 151 (32%) were pheochromocytomas (84 benign; 67 malignant), and 126 (27%) were metastatic lesions.[113] Of 20 feline adrenal neoplastic lesions, 6 (30%) were adrenocortical tumors (3 adenoma; 3 carcinoma), 2 (10%) were pheochromocytomas (1 benign; 1 malignant), and 12 (60%) were metastatic lesions.[113] Less than half of these metastatic lesions were grossly visible at necropsy. Lymphoma was the most common cancer to spread to the adrenal glands in both species. Other metastatic tumors commonly identified in the dog included hemangiosarcoma, mammary carcinoma, histiocytic sarcoma, pulmonary carcinoma, and melanoma. Right and left adrenal glands were affected equally, as were the cortex and medulla. The only notable exception was that all metastatic melanomas were restricted to the adrenal medulla.[113]

A number of case series in the last decade have documented the outcome of adrenal surgery in dogs.[43,45,114,115] When the data from these cases are combined, a histopathologic diagnosis was reported for a total of 191 adrenal tumors, with 153 (80%) arising from the adrenal cortex and 33 (17%) from the medulla. The remaining tumors included two myelolipomas and one each of fibrosarcoma, lymphoma, and leiomyosarcoma. For the adrenocortical tumors that were further classified, 63 of 125 (50%) were carcinomas, 54 of 125 (43%) were adenomas, and 8 of 125 (6%) were described as hyperplastic lesions. It is important to note the bias inherent in these data because only dogs that underwent surgery are included.

Advanced imaging techniques such as ultrasonography, CT, and MRI have now greatly enhanced our ability to identify both clinical

*References 63, 80, 87, 90, 98, 100, 107, 108.

†References 63, 80, 87, 98, 107, 108.

and subclinical adrenal abnormalities,[38,43,116,117] and it appears that the adrenal gland is affected with neoplasia more commonly than was previously suspected. The ability to detect these adrenal lesions also leads to diagnostic dilemmas as the clinician attempts to elucidate whether the lesions arise from the cortex or medulla, whether they are functional or nonfunctional, and whether they are benign or malignant. Functional adrenal tumors may secrete cortisol, catecholamines, aldosterone, sex hormones, or steroid hormone precursors, and these may be associated with specific clinical and laboratory findings. Hormonal testing and imaging techniques are central to the diagnostic evaluation of these patients so that the most appropriate course of therapy can be pursued. Large adrenal masses may be detected on abdominal radiographs,[34,118,119] and the presence of mineralization suggests an adrenal tumor; however, this finding is not highly specific, and it cannot be used to differentiate between benign and malignant masses. The normal ultrasonographic appearance of canine adrenal glands has been described,[116,120] and there are many reports of the ultrasonographic appearance of adrenal lesions in dogs. Abdominal ultrasound examination is frequently used to detect metastatic disease and determine the local invasiveness of adrenal tumors. Ultrasonography has been reported to be 80% to 100% sensitive and approximately 90% specific for the detection of adrenal tumor invasion into the caudal vena cava.[43,45]

The CT appearance of both normal and abnormal canine adrenal glands has been described.[46,119,121-124] Contrast-enhanced CT has been shown to provide accurate preoperative evaluation of canine adrenal masses, with 92% sensitivity and 100% specificity for the detection of vascular invasion by adrenal tumors.[125] The MRI appearance of presumed normal canine adrenal glands has also been described,[126] but as yet there are few reports that document the systematic use of MRI for evaluation of adrenal lesions in dogs and cats. The characterization of adrenal lesions by imaging techniques has undergone recent significant advancement in human medicine. Malignant and benign lesions can frequently be differentiated using modalities such as contrast-enhanced ultrasound, CT densitometry, CT washout characteristics, chemical shift MRI, positron emission tomography (PET), and PET/CT.[127-130] Most of these techniques have yet to be explored in veterinary medicine.

Adrenocortical Tumors

Functional cortisol-secreting tumors of the adrenal cortex are responsible for 15% to 20% of canine and feline cases of naturally occurring HC, with PDH accounting for 80% to 85%.[17,18,21,22] In the necropsy and surgical biopsy data from UC Davis, adrenocortical adenomas were almost 4 times more common than carcinomas[113]; however, the functionality of these tumors was not assessed. A review of case reports of functional adrenocortical tumors in dogs suggests that approximately 60% of surgically removed tumors are carcinomas.* Adenomas are typically smaller, with tumors larger than 2 cm more likely to be carcinomas.[132] However, adenomas up to 6 cm have been reported.[17] On histopathologic examination, adenocarcinomas appear more likely to exhibit a trabecular growth pattern, peripheral fibrosis, capsular invasion, necrosis, and/or hemorrhage.[132] They are less likely to exhibit cytoplasmic vacuolization, extramedullary hematopoiesis, or fibrin thrombi. Approximately 20% of adrenocortical carcinomas locally invade into the phrenicoabdominal vein, with extension into the renal vein and/or caudal vena cava.[42,131] Intravascular invasion has the potential to cause severe and life-threatening intraabdominal or retroperitoneal hemorrhage.[45,133] Metastasis was identified in approximately 50% of dogs with adrenocortical carcinomas.[131,132] Although involvement of the liver and lungs is most common, other organs reported to be affected with metastases include the kidney, ovary, mesenteric lymph nodes, peritoneal cavity, and thyroid gland. In the absence of evidence of tumor invasion or metastasis, there are no consistent clinical, biochemical, or imaging findings that reliably distinguish between functional adrenocortical adenomas and carcinomas in dogs and cats. The cellular and molecular events underlying the development of canine adrenocortical tumors are unknown. Recent studies have demonstrated downregulation of ACTH receptors in cortisol-secreting adrenocortical carcinomas and ectopic expression of gastric-inhibitory polypeptide and vasopressin (2) receptor proteins in neoplastic zona fasciculata tissue from canine adrenocortical tumors.[134,135] The significance of these findings in tumorigenesis remains to be elucidated.

Dogs with PDH and dogs with ADH are similar in age, but almost 50% of dogs with ADH weigh more than 20 kg, compared to approximately 25% of dogs with PDH.[34] The historic features, physical changes, clinical signs, and basic laboratory findings in canine Cushing's syndrome are essentially the same in dogs with PDH and dogs with ADH and are described in the earlier section on Pituitary Corticotroph Tumors. Similar screening tests are used to confirm the diagnosis of HC; however, the sensitivity of the ACTH stimulation test for the diagnosis of ADH is only around 60%.[32] Thus the LDDST is a better screening test when ADH is suspected. Dogs with ADH fail to show suppression on the LDDST or the HDDST, and differentiation from PDH is generally determined by imaging studies, particularly abdominal ultrasound examination,[33] and measurement of endogenous ACTH levels.[34] Excessive secretion of glucocorticoids by a functional adrenocortical adenoma or adenocarcinoma occurs independent of pituitary control, with secondary atrophy of the normal adrenocortical cells in both the affected and contralateral adrenal glands. Unfortunately the functional atrophy of the contralateral adrenal gland is not always easily detected on abdominal ultrasonography.[39] This finding, termed *equivocal adrenal asymmetry,* is also observed in some dogs with PDH, associated with asymmetric hyperplasia of the glands.[37] The results of a recent ultrasound study of dogs with equivocal adrenal asymmetry suggested that a maximal dorsoventral thickness of the smaller gland of less than 5.00 mm was consistent with a diagnosis of ADH.[40]

Surgical adrenalectomy is the treatment of choice for dogs with ADH,* and surgical management is further addressed later. An early case series of dogs undergoing surgical removal of adrenocortical tumors revealed that 60% of patients were euthanized during surgery or died within 2 weeks.[131] In a more recent case series, the perioperative mortality has ranged from 19% to 28%.[17,42,43,136] In one series of 144 dogs undergoing surgical removal of a functional adrenocortical tumor, the prognosis was described as excellent for patients that survived 4 weeks postoperatively, with an average life expectancy of 3 years. Nine of 144 dogs were euthanized at the time of surgery, and 29 dogs died during surgery or immediately postoperatively.[17] Median survival times of 230 to 778 days have been reported for dogs undergoing adrenalectomy for adrenal carcinomas,[42,114,115] compared to a MST of 687.5 days for dogs with adenomas.[114] Laparoscopic adrenalectomy has been described for noninvasive adrenocortical carcinomas in a small number of dogs; further studies are needed to determine if this technique can reduce

*References 34, 42, 45, 114, 115, 131.

*References 42, 43, 114, 115, 131, 136.

the postoperative complications associated with conventional surgery.[137]

Medical therapy for ADH should be used when surgery is not a good option for the patient or client, or it may be used prior to adrenalectomy in patients that are significantly debilitated by HC. The primary options for medical therapy are mitotane and trilostane. Treatment with mitotane as an alternative to surgical adrenalectomy utilizes the drug as a true cytotoxic agent. Detailed protocols are readily available,[138] and clinicians should be aware that this approach typically requires higher doses of mitotane than those used in PDH[139] and that relapses are common. However, this treatment can be effective, with a mean survival of 16.4 months reported in a series of 32 dogs. Dogs without evidence of metastatic disease may show a better response to mitotane therapy.[140] Trilostane is not a cytotoxic drug, but it has been used to successfully manage patients with ADH,[68,69,141] including a small number of dogs with metastatic disease.[142] A recent retrospective study comparing trilostane and mitotane in dogs with ADH reported a median survival of 353 days with trilostane therapy compared to 102 days for mitotane. These survival times were not significantly different; however, this study did further confirm that survival times are significantly decreased in the presence of metastatic disease.[143]

Functional adrenocortical tumors in dogs and cats can also secrete one or more sex hormones, including androstenedione, progesterone, 17-hydroxyprogesterone, testosterone, and estradiol. These tumors may or may not secrete glucocorticoids, and some patients have been reported to show signs of HC in the absence of elevated cortisol levels on typical screening tests.[144-149] Signs of sex hormone excess appear uncommon in dogs with sex-hormone–secreting adrenal tumors but have been reported in a small number of cats.[150,151]

Aldosterone-secreting adrenocortical tumors have rarely been reported in dogs,[152-154] but there is increasing evidence that primary hyperaldosteronism (also termed *primary aldosteronism* or *Conn's syndrome*) may be an underrecognized condition in cats. In fact, it has been suggested to be the most common adrenocortical disorder in this species.[155] Affected cats are middle-aged or older, and the most common clinical sign is muscle weakness due to hypokalemia. Arterial hypertension is frequently detected in these patients and may be associated with ocular changes. Routine laboratory testing often reveals hypokalemia, but hypernatremia is uncommon, presumably due to intact water balance mechanisms in these patients. Some cats may also have evidence of concurrent renal disease. Plasma aldosterone can be measured in cats, and normal or elevated levels in the face of hypokalemia would be regarded as inappropriate. However, definitive diagnosis using aldosterone levels is difficult without the measurement of plasma renin activity and the calculation of an aldosterone : renin ratio.[156] Unfortunately, a plasma renin activity assay is not readily available to most clinicians. An oral fludrocortisone suppression test has recently been suggested to be a useful diagnostic test for feline hyperaldosteronism,[157] but the use of this tool has not yet been widely reported. Imaging of the adrenal glands is often performed in the evaluation of these patients,[158,159] and this may distinguish between unilateral and bilateral lesions and also reveal the presence of vascular invasion or metastatic disease. Most cats with hyperaldosteronism have an adrenal adenoma or carcinoma.[160] Bilateral adenomas have been reported,[160] and some cats have adrenal hyperplasia.[156] Adrenalectomy is the treatment of choice for cats with unilateral disease, and good outcomes have been reported for both adenomas and carcinomas, as well as for tumors associated with vena cava thrombosis.[160-163] Medical management with potassium supplementation, antihypertensive drugs, and the aldosterone antagonist spironolactone can give reasonable survival times in patients that are not surgical candidates.[156,160,161]

Adrenal Medullary Tumors

Chromaffin cells are part of the sympathetic nervous system and are present in the adrenal medulla and other locations throughout the body. Neoplastic chromaffin cells in the adrenal medulla give rise to pheochromocytomas, which are tumors that predominantly secrete catecholamines. Chromaffin cell tumors (termed *paragangliomas* or *extraadrenal pheochromocytomas*) can arise in other parts of the body, but these are rare in veterinary medicine. Pheochromocytomas are uncommon in dogs and rare in cats.[164,165] In past decades, the diagnosis of pheochromocytoma was most often made incidentally at necropsy,[166,167] but these tumors are now likely to be detected antemortem because advanced abdominal imaging techniques are routinely used in small animal patients. Pheochromocytomas are generally considered to be malignant tumors in dogs.[164] Metastasis is reported in up to 40% of affected dogs; sites include liver, spleen, lung, regional lymph nodes, bone, and CNS.[166-168] Vascular invasion by the tumor has been reported in as many as 82% of cases.[43,45,169] This finding is not specific for pheochromocytoma because vascular invasion can also occur with adrenocortical tumors.

Pheochromocytoma is usually diagnosed in older dogs,[164,167] and males may be overrepresented.[169] Catecholamine release by pheochromocytomas is typically episodic, and thus clinical signs may be intermittent and often absent at the time of physical examination. Signs may include weakness, episodic collapse, panting, anxiety, restlessness, exercise intolerance, decreased appetite, weight loss, polyuria, and polydipsia. Physical examination of dogs with pheochromocytoma may be normal due to the episodic nature of catecholamine release or may reveal tachypnea, panting, tachycardia, weakness, pallor, cardiac arrhythmias, or hypertension.[164,166,167] Some dogs have signs referable to an abdominal mass, and acute collapse may occur secondary to tumor rupture with abdominal or retroperitoneal bleeding.[133] There are no consistent abnormalities on the CBC, serum biochemistry profile, or urinalysis in dogs with pheochromocytomas.

Diagnostic imaging, particularly abdominal ultrasound examination, is central to the evaluation of patients with pheochromocytoma. In many dogs, evaluation for pheochromocytoma occurs after an adrenal mass is found when abdominal ultrasonography is performed for other reasons. In addition to revealing the presence of an adrenal tumor, abdominal ultrasonography may reveal metastatic disease and is sensitive and specific for detecting vascular invasion by adrenal tumors.[43,45] CT and MRI are the imaging modalities of choice for humans with pheochromocytomas, and early experience in canine patients has been encouraging.[170-172] Abdominal radiographs may reveal the presence of a large adrenal mass[166,170] but are generally less informative than ultrasound examination. Thoracic radiographs are recommended to evaluate the cardiovascular system and for detection of pulmonary metastases in any patient with a suspected adrenal tumor. There are rare reports of PET or nuclear scintigraphy imaging in dogs with pheochromocytomas.[173,174] Immunohistochemical staining for chromogranin A can distinguish pheochromocytomas from adrenocortical tumors on tissue obtained at surgery or necropsy.[175]

Plasma and urinary concentrations of catecholamines and their metabolites are routinely measured in humans for the diagnosis of pheochromocytoma.[164] Recent reports have suggested that urinary catecholamine and metanephrine to creatinine ratios hold promise as a diagnostic tool in dogs.[176-178] Plasma-free metanephrine and normetanephrines have also been evaluated in cats and dogs, with encouraging preliminary results.[165,179]

Surgery is the only definitive treatment for pheochromocytoma.[43,164,166,167,169] This should be performed by an experienced surgical and anesthesiology team because potentially life-threatening complications, including hypertension, hypotension, cardiac arrhythmias and hemorrage,[169] may occur during anesthetic induction and handling of the tumor. It has been shown that dogs receiving phenoxybenzamine, a noncompetitive α-adrenergic antagonist, prior to surgery are significantly more likely to survive adrenalectomy. Specifically, dogs that received this medication at doses ranging from 0.1 to 2.5 mg/kg every 12 hours, for a median period of 20 days, had a 13% mortality rate, compared to a mortality rate of 48% in dogs that did not receive this therapy.[169] Chemotherapy and RT have not been evaluated in dogs with pheochromocytoma. RT using ^{131}I-metaiodobenzylguanidine (^{131}I-MIBG) was recently reported in one case.[180]

The prognosis for dogs with pheochromocytoma is affected by tumor size, presence of metastases, and local invasion. A MST of 374 days has been reported after surgical treatment of pheochromocytoma,[114] and some dogs may survive for as long as 2 to 3 years.[167,181] Dogs without metastatic disease that survive the perioperative period appear to have a good prognosis.[164]

Surgical Management of Adrenal Tumors

Prior to adrenalectomy, every attempt should be made to determine whether an adrenal tumor is functional, whether there is evidence of metastatic disease, and whether there is vascular invasion. Patients suspected to have a pheochromocytoma should be treated preoperatively with phenoxybenzamine. If tachyarrhythmias are present, a β-blocker such as propranolol or atenolol may also be administered but should only be started after α-adrenergic blockade has been initiated to prevent unopposed α-adrenergic stimulation and severe hypertension.[164] Patients with HC due to ADH may be medically managed with trilostane or mitotane prior to surgery if they are significantly debilitated by their disease, although this is rarely necessary. The potential for intraoperative and postoperative complications associated with adrenalectomy is significant[182]; these cases are best managed by an experienced team, including a surgeon, anesthesiologist, internist, and critical care specialist. Particular concerns with pheochromocytomas include cardiovascular complications and hemorrhage, as noted previously. Patients with functional adrenocortical tumors are at risk for adrenocortical insufficiency, pulmonary thromboembolism, pancreatitis, renal failure, and wound dehiscence.* Protocols are available to guide the perioperative management of adrenalectomy patients.[17] At CSU, patients with pheochromocytoma are treated preoperatively with phenoxybenzamine as described earlier. Patients with functional adrenocortical tumors receive heparin and corticosteroid therapy during and after surgery. Postoperatively, an ACTH stimulation test is performed 24 to 48 hours after surgery, and electrolytes and blood glucose are measured frequently. The duration of prednisolone therapy and the necessity for mineralocorticoid supplementation are each determined on an individual case basis. For patients with adrenal tumors of unknown origin, preoperative phenoxybenzamine is recommended, and the protocol for functional adrenocortical tumors is followed, until postoperative ACTH stimulation test results and histopathology results are available to guide further management.

*References 17, 42, 43, 114, 131, 182.

The overall perioperative mortality rate for dogs undergoing adrenalectomy for all adrenal tumors is around 10% to 20%,[43,45,114,115] and MSTs of 690 to 953 days have been reported.[114,115] A number of investigators have evaluated prognostic factors and predictors of outcome in these patients. In two studies, the presence of caval tumor thrombus did not affect perioperative morbidity and mortality, although the long-term prognosis for dogs with an adrenocortical tumor may be poorer in the presence of a thrombus.[43] In contrast, a more recent study suggested that vein thrombosis was associated with a poorer prognosis.[115] In the latter study, vein thrombosis was associated with tumors with major axis length of 5 cm or larger, and the presence of metastases or tumor size of 5 cm or larger were both associated with a poorer prognosis.[115] Large tumors were also associated with increased perioperative mortality in a series of dogs undergoing elective or emergency adrenalectomy. The dogs in this report that had emergency surgery for acute adrenal bleeding experienced a 50% perioperative mortality rate.[45]

Incidental Adrenal Masses

Advances in abdominal imaging have led to the diagnostic dilemma of the incidental adrenal mass ("incidentaloma") in both human and veterinary medicine. When an incidental adrenal mass is identified in a dog or cat, a thorough history and physical examination, including blood pressure measurement and fundic examination, are indicated. Endocrinologic testing should be pursued to rule out a functional adrenocortical tumor. Given the high incidence of metastatic lesions in canine and feline adrenal glands, imaging of the thorax and abdomen should be performed to rule out another primary tumor. Aspiration cytology and ultrasound- or CT-guided biopsies are not routinely recommended for incidentalomas because of the high risk of complications and the inability to reliably differentiate benign and malignant lesions.[38,112] Adrenalectomy should be considered for masses that are functional, locally invasive, or larger than 2.5 cm in maximum dimension. Masses smaller than 2 cm with no evidence of hormonal activity should be monitored with abdominal ultrasonography. A suggested interval is to repeat the sonogram 1 month after the initial study and then after 2, 4, and 6 months, with further intervals determined by the appearance of the mass and the clinical status of the patient.[164]

Thyroid Gland Neoplasia in Dogs

Thyroid tumors account for 1.1% to 3.8% of all tumors in dogs.[183-185] In necropsy studies, it is estimated that 30% to 50% of canine thyroid tumors are benign adenomas.[183,186] A recent Veterinary Medical Database review reported that 90% of 545 canine thyroid cancers submitted to the database from veterinary teaching hospitals were carcinomas or adenocarcinomas, with 9.3% being adenomas.[185] Most adenomas are small, noninvasive, and clinically silent. Consequently, almost all canine thyroid masses associated with clinical signs are malignant.[184,187,188] Thyroid tumors of follicular cell origin are subclassified as papillary, follicular, compact (solid), or anaplastic. All subgroups stain positive for thyroglobulin and thyroid transcription factor-1.[189-191] Papillary carcinomas are most common in humans,[10,192] whereas follicular and compact forms are most common in dogs.[1,184,189,193] Medullary thyroid carcinomas, also called *parafollicular* or *C-cell carcinomas,* are relatively uncommon in both humans and dogs.[191] Positive immunohistochemical staining for calcitonin is the most accurate way to identify these tumors, but they also often stain positive for calcitonin gene-related peptide, thyroid transcription factor-1, chromogranin A, and neuron-specific enolase.[175,189-191,194]

The etiology of thyroid neoplasia in dogs is largely unknown. The molecular pathogenesis of thyroid neoplasia is best defined in humans.[5,7,10] The classic hypothesis involves a discrete series of mutations. Activation of receptor tyrosine kinases such as *RET* and *TRK* are common in papillary carcinomas, activating mutations in *RAS* are frequently identified in follicular carcinomas, and inactivation of *p53* is commonly seen in anaplastic carcinomas. Thyroid-stimulating hormone (TSH) or the TSH receptor may play a contributing role in carcinogenesis.[195] The TSH receptor in humans with thyroid neoplasia is frequently affected with either hyperfunctioning or silencing mutations. Canine thyroid tumors retain TSH receptors, and hypothyroid beagles that did not receive thyroid hormone supplementation had an increased incidence of thyroid tumors, presumably due to TSH trophic effects without feedback in the context of potential mutations.[196,197] Thyroid irradiation is associated with an increased incidence of thyroid tumors in all species, including humans, rodents, and dogs.[1,10,186,192] In dogs, one report identified a *p53* mutation in 1 of 23 primary thyroid carcinomas.[198] Another report confirmed trisomy 18 in a canine thyroid adenoma.[199]

Thyroid tumors typically arise in older dogs, with a median reported age of 9 to 11 years.[184,193,200-202] A sex predilection has not been reported. Predilection of breeds for thyroid tumors includes golden retrievers, beagles, Boxers, and Siberian huskies.[184,185] Familial medullary thyroid carcinoma has also been described in a family of dogs with an Alaskan malamute influence.[203] The right and left lobes are affected with equal frequency in canine thyroid tumors, and as many as 60% of patients will have bilateral involvement.[200,204] On rare occasions, ectopic thyroid tissue can give rise to tumors at the base of the tongue, cervical ventral neck, cranial mediastinum, and heart.[204-210] Up to 35% to 40% of dogs have visible metastatic disease at initial presentation, and as many as 80% will ultimately develop metastasis.[184,191,204,211] Metastatic potential is reported to increase when the primary tumor volume exceeds 23 cm^3 and approaches 100% when tumor volume exceeds 100 cm^3.[186] Bilateral tumors are 16 times more likely to metastasize than unilateral tumors.[200] The lungs and regional lymph nodes, including the retropharyngeal, cranial cervical, and mandibular lymph nodes, are affected most commonly, but a wide variety of tissues can be affected. Medullary carcinomas may have a lower metastatic potential than follicular and solid carcinomas.[191]

The majority of canine thyroid carcinomas are nonfunctional. Based on clinical signs and serum T_4 concentrations, approximately 60% of patients are euthyroid, 30% are hypothyroid secondary to destruction of the normal thyroid parenchyma, and 10% are hyperthyroid.[188,202,212-214] Most dogs are presented for a palpable ventral cervical mass.[184,191,193] Less common abnormalities include coughing, rapid breathing, dyspnea, dysphagia, dysphonia (change in bark), laryngeal paralysis, Horner's syndrome, and facial edema. Acute severe hemorrhage can occur secondary to invasion into the cervical vasculature.[215] In addition to clinical signs referable to the physical thyroid mass, dogs with hyperthyroidism frequently exhibit polyphagia, weight loss, muscle wasting, polyuria, and polydipsia.[188,212-214]

The differential diagnosis for a mass in the region of the thyroid gland in dogs includes abscesses or granulomas, salivary mucoceles, lymphatic metastasis from tonsillar squamous cell carcinoma, lymphoma, carotid body tumor, and sarcomas. In humans, thyroid cytology is very accurate for identifying thyroid tumors and distinguishing whether they are benign or malignant.[10,192] Accuracy of cytology in dogs with thyroid masses is reported to be problematic. In several reports, cytology confirms the mass to be of thyroid origin in only half of affected dogs, and definitive recognition of malignancy occurs less often.[184,188] Use of a needle without physical aspiration and thorough examination of the feathered edge may improve diagnostic accuracy. Malignant thyroid tumors have a higher vascular density than normal thyroid tissue and benign tumors,[202] and hemodilution is a common problem (see Chapter 6). This increased vascularity also adds significant risk to large core needle biopsy procedures.

Routine staging for dogs with thyroid carcinoma includes general health assessment with laboratory evaluation (CBC, serum biochemistry profile, and urinalysis), three-view thoracic radiographs, and cytologic or histologic evaluation of the mandibular lymph nodes. Cervical ultrasonography can be used to confirm if a mass is of thyroid origin and to assess invasiveness and vascularity.[216,217] The retropharyngeal and cranial cervical lymph nodes can also be examined for evidence of metastasis. The MRI and CT appearances of the normal canine thyroid have been described,[218,219] and these modalities are useful in the investigation of cervical masses in the dog and in the staging of thyroid carcinomas.[215,218,219] Scintigraphy using ^{99m}Tc-pertechnetate or, less commonly, radioactive iodine (^{123}I or ^{131}I) is performed primarily to identify local residual disease after surgery, ectopic tumors, or metastatic disease.* Most primary tumors are visualized, although the pattern of uptake is often heterogeneous. Metastatic disease is identified less consistently. To be visualized with scintigraphy, a thyroid tumor must be capable of trapping ^{99m}Tc-pertechnetate or trapping and organifying ^{123}I or ^{131}I. It may or may not be able to complete the remaining steps necessary for synthesis and secretion of functional thyroid hormone.

Treatment of canine thyroid carcinomas is dictated by the size of the mass, extent of invasion, presence or absence of gross metastatic disease, and any concurrent symptoms of thyrotoxicosis. Surgical excision provides the best outcome with the least morbidity when tumors are freely movable without extensive deep tissue invasion.[191,193,222] Thyroidectomy is not recommended when the tumor is not freely movable in all directions or extensively invades adjacent structures, including major vasculature, recurrent laryngeal nerves, the vagosympathetic trunk, the larynx, the trachea, or the esophagus. Extensive hemorrhage can result from the vascularity of the tumor, invasion into adjacent blood vessels, and local coagulopathies.[202] Other potential complications of thyroidectomy include hypocalcemia due to hypoparathyroidism if the parathyroid glands are removed, damage to the recurrent laryngeal nerve(s), and hypothyroidism after bilateral thyroidectomy.[193,223] According to limited, retrospective data sets, it was estimated that only 25% to 50% of thyroid carcinomas were mobile and amenable to surgery at the time of initial diagnosis.[191,193] Palpation under anesthesia and preoperative imaging are current general recommendations for surgical evaluation at the authors' institution, with some extracapsular extension and invasion considered acceptable. Median survival after thyroidectomy is around 3 years if the tumor is freely movable and 6 to 12 months if the tumor is more invasive.[191,193] Recently, a report describing resection of mobile, discrete bilateral thyroid tumors in a limited number of dogs suggested reasonable overall survival with persistent postoperative management of thyroid and parathyroid endocrinopathies.[224]

Nonresectable thyroid carcinomas may be managed with radiation as a primary therapy or as a means to achieve a surgical option. External-beam RT is used most commonly for dogs. One study evaluated definitive RT (48 Gy delivered in 4 Gy fractions on an alternate-day schedule) in 25 dogs with unresectable thyroid

*References 184, 200, 204, 217, 220, 221.

carcinomas and no visible metastasis.[200] Tumors either stabilized or decreased in size. The time to maximal tumor reduction ranged from 8 to 22 months in dogs whose tumors did respond. The progression-free survival rates were 80% at 1 year and 72% at 3 years. The first cause of treatment failure was local progression in three dogs, metastasis in four dogs, and concurrent local progression and metastasis in three dogs. Limited information exists regarding the use of definitive radiation in the adjuvant or neoadjuvant settings.[201,225] This same RT protocol described was evaluated in an additional eight dogs, seven of which had undergone incomplete thyroidectomy prior to irradiation.[201] Median survival was just over 2 years (range 1 to 3 years). None developed local recurrence, although four died from metastatic disease. Radiation-induced toxicoses to the larynx, trachea, and esophagus are usually well tolerated. Hypothyroidism may develop months to years after treatment.[200,225]

For dogs that present with gross metastatic disease, hypofractionated RT may still provide effective palliation of the primary tumor, due to a generally slow rate of progression in both the primary and metastatic lesions. In a study evaluating palliative RT as the sole treatment modality, 13 dogs received 36 Gy in four weekly 9 Gy fractions.[211] Complete or partial reduction of the primary tumor occurred in one and nine dogs, respectively. Local progression occurred in five dogs, 11 to 24 months after irradiation. Gross metastatic disease was present in five dogs at initial presentation and developed in an additional two dogs during the study. Overall median survival was around 22 months, with local and metastatic progression occurring equally in all dogs.

In humans with well-differentiated thyroid carcinoma, ^{131}I is routinely administered postoperatively to destroy occult microscopic local or metastatic carcinoma.[10,192] Experience with ^{131}I thyroid ablation in dogs is substantial, with two recent, relatively large clinical studies providing evidence of efficacy of ^{131}I for advanced unresectable, metastatic, or residual thyroid neoplasia.[226,227] Collectively, from all reports, over 80 dogs with stage II (2 to 5 cm diameter; fixed or unfixed), stage III (>5 cm diameter, fixed or unfixed), or stage IV metastatic thyroid carcinoma have received ^{131}I for the intent of managing tumor burden and clinical signs. MSTs for stage II and III patients exceed 2 years, and dogs with metastatic carcinoma experienced survival times of approximately 1 year. Such results are comparable to external-beam RT. Interestingly, similar survival times were noted in dogs that were hypothyroid, euthyroid, or hyperthyroid. Recommendations for ^{131}I dosimetry remain unresolved. Fatal myelosuppression was observed in three dogs in one report, although no specific dose-effect relationship was defined.[227] The biologic effect both on tumor and normal tissue is a complex function of ^{131}I uptake that depends on extent of the tumor burden, degree of organification and excretion of ^{131}I, bone marrow sensitivity, and administered dose of radiation. Dosing regimens are currently empiric in dogs but could be more carefully defined by administering a ^{131}I tracer for calculation of definitive dosing, as in humans. Until such time as dosing is individualized, the maximum dose administered should be 0.2 GBq/kg (5 mCi/kg), and bone marrow monitoring posttreatment is recommended. Additional doses may be administered if necessary, as determined by persistent hyperthyroidism or activity on posttreatment nuclear scans. Dogs receiving ^{131}I will require thyroid hormone supplementation.

Chemotherapy has been evaluated in dogs with thyroid tumors. Of those dogs treated with either doxorubicin or cisplatin, 30% to 50% demonstrated a partial response (>50% reduction in volume).[228,229] Individual responses have also been reported using mitoxantrone or actinomycin D.[230,231] Chemotherapy may be considered for dogs with large nonresectable primary tumors and/or gross metastatic disease.

Thyroid Gland Neoplasia in Cats

Hyperthyroidism (thyrotoxicosis) is the most common endocrine disorder in cats.[232,233] It is almost always caused by a primary thyroid abnormality that results in the production and secretion of excessive thyroxine (T_4) and triiodothyronine (T_3). Multinodular adenomatous hyperplasia is identified histologically in the majority of thyrotoxic cats.[1,232-234] Both thyroid lobes are affected in 70% to 90% of cases,[233-235] although they may be asymmetrically enlarged at the time of diagnosis. Malignant carcinomas are the least common cause of hyperthyroidism, occurring in only 1% to 3% of thyrotoxic cats.[1,232-234] Nonfunctional thyroid carcinomas are uncommon.[236,237] Feline thyroid carcinomas are more locally invasive than their benign counterparts, and their metastatic rate is up to 70%, with regional lymph nodes and lungs being affected most commonly.[238,239]

TSH from the pituitary regulates both the secretion of thyroid hormones and the proliferation of thyroid cells. The interaction of TSH with receptors on the surface of thyroid cells activates G protein-mediated cyclic adenosine monophosphate (cAMP) signal transduction pathways.[240] Some of the components of the TSH receptor-G protein-cAMP system have therefore been evaluated for changes that could result in feline hyperthyroidism. Decreased expression of the inhibitory subunit $G_{i\alpha}$ has been identified in adenomatous feline thyroid glands,[241] and a further study demonstrated that G_{i2} was decreased.[242] Mutations in the $G_{s\alpha}$ gene were also reported in 4 of 10 hyperthyroid cats evaluated.[243] Both of these changes could lead to stimulation of adenyl cyclase with the potential for increased levels of cAMP. However, a more recent study showed that ligand-stimulated activation of G proteins was the same in thyroid cell membranes obtained from hyperthyroid and euthyroid cats.[244] Therefore the role of alterations in inherent G(s) or G(i) activities in the pathogenesis of hyperthyroidism in cats remains unresolved. Mutations in the TSH receptor in hyperthyroid cats have been investigated and were not documented in early studies.[243,245] However, a more recent study that targeted hyperplastic or adenomatous thyroid nodules from 50 hyperthyroid cats detected a total of 11 different mutations in the TSH receptor gene.[246] Oncogene expression has also been evaluated in thyroid tissue from hyperthyroid cats. Overexpression of one or more *RAS* oncogenes was identified in adenomas and hyperplasias from 18 of 18 cats diagnosed with hyperthyroidism but not in adjacent normal thyroid tissue or in thyroid tissue from 14 unaffected cats.[247] In the same tumors that overexpressed *RAS*, Bcl-2 and p53 proteins were undetectable using immunohistochemistry.

Hyperthyroidism was not recognized as a clinical disorder in cats until 1979, yet currently it is estimated to affect as many as 1 out of every 300 cats.[232] This may reflect a true increase in incidence, heightened awareness and testing by veterinarians, or both. If there has been a true increased incidence, environmental factors may have contributed. Several risk factors have been associated with hyperthyroidism, including the consumption of commercially prepared canned cat food, indoor residence, use of cat litter, exposure to brominated flame retardants, and use of flea-control products, but none have been incriminated as a primary inciting cause.[248-253] The iodine content of cat food has also been suggested to play a role in the development of hyperthyroidism, but this relationship is unproven.[254]

Due to space constraints, only a brief overview of the clinical features, diagnosis, and treatment of feline hyperthyroidism will be presented here, with an emphasis on malignant thyroid tumors. The reader is directed to several excellent and detailed reviews of feline hyperthyroidism for additional information.[232,233]

Most hyperthyroid cats are older, with mean and median ages of 12 to 15 years.[234,255-257] The disease is rare in cats under 8 years of age.[232] There is no gender predilection, but Siamese and Himalayan breeds were found in one study to be at decreased risk.[248] The most common signs reported by owners include weight loss, polyphagia, polydipsia, polyuria, gastrointestinal signs (vomiting, diarrhea, increased stool production), and increased activity.[232,233,235,255] Additional abnormalities commonly identified on physical examination include the presence of a palpable thyroid nodule, cardiovascular abnormalities (tachycardia, heart murmur, gallop rhythm, premature beats), and poor hair coat. Hyperthyroidism may also contribute to hypertension in elderly cats.[258] Definitive diagnosis of hyperthyroidism is routinely based on an elevated serum total T_4 level.[235,255,259] Less than 10% of hyperthyroid cats will have a total T_4 level within the reference range. This is usually due to normal fluctuations in serum thyroid hormone concentrations and/or the presence of concurrent nonthyroidal illness.[259,260] If hyperthyroidism is suspected in a cat with a normal total T_4 level, total T_4 should be measured again in 1 to 2 weeks, particularly if the total T_4 is in the upper half of the reference range. Free T_4 measurement may also aid in the diagnosis of hyperthyroidism when total T_4 is within the reference range. However, this test should only be used in cats with clinical signs of hyperthyroidism in which the total T_4 is high-normal. Free T_4 concentrations can be high in cats with nonthyroidal illness,[259,261,262] and these patients would be expected to have low total T_4 values. Thus free T_4 should never be used as a screening test for hyperthyroidism. For those patients in which hyperthyroidism is suspected, but not confirmed by measurement of total or free T_4, additional tests have been used to confirm the diagnosis. These include thyroid scintigraphy (see later), the TSH stimulation test or the thyrotropin-releasing hormone (TRH) stimulation test (both of which are of limited utility[263,264]), or the triiodothyronine suppression test. The latter test can provide useful information but relies on significant owner and patient compliance.[265,266] Thyroid function tests cannot be used to differentiate benign and malignant tumors.

Staging for cats with hyperthyroidism should minimally include baseline CBC, serum biochemistry profile, urinalysis, and blood pressure measurement. Additional diagnostic tests that may be recommended include thoracic radiography, electrocardiography, and echocardiography.[235,267,268] ^{99m}Tc-pertechnetate scintigraphy is very useful for determining the anatomic extent of functional thyroid tissue and planning therapy, as well as for confirming the diagnosis.[257,269] Unilateral uptake occurs in cats with a solitary adenoma and atrophy of the normal contralateral gland. Bilateral uptake, even if asymmetric, is indicative of adenomatous hyperplasia. Thyroid scintigraphy is particularly useful for revealing the presence of ectopic thyroid tissue or multiple areas of hyperfunctioning thyroid tissue. In one study, these were present in 20% to 25% of hyperthyroid cats undergoing thyroid scintigraphy.[257] Metastatic disease due to thyroid carcinoma may be detected by scintigraphy,[235] and the pattern of uptake of radionuclide may be suggestive of the presence of malignant disease; however, two recent studies demonstrated that there are no scintigraphic findings that can definitively distinguish between benign and malignant thyroid disease in all hyperthyroid cats.[237,257]

Treatment options for feline hyperthyroidism include antithyroid drugs, surgical thyroidectomy, and radioactive iodine therapy. Methimazole is the most widely used antithyroid drug in North America.[270] Carbimazole is more widely used in Europe.[271] These are thioureylene drugs that inhibit thyroid hormone synthesis by interfering with oxidation of iodide, iodination of tyrosyl residues in thyroglobulin, and the coupling of iodotyrosines to iodothyronines.[233,270,271] These drugs are often used for assessing the effect of resolution of hyperthyroidism on renal function (see later) and preparing a cat for anesthesia and thyroidectomy. They are also frequently used as a long-term treatment modality, but it is important to note that they have no antitumor activity and no cytotoxic effect on thyroid follicular cells. Methimazole and carbimazole are both highly effective in lowering serum thyroid hormone concentrations and controlling hyperthyroidism. Carbimazole is converted to methimazole in the body, and a dose of 5 mg of carbimazole is considered to be equivalent to 3 mg of methimazole.[233] Methimazole is usually administered at a starting dose of 2.5 mg orally twice daily for 2 weeks. Based on clinical signs and serum T_4 levels, the dosage can be adjusted incrementally, with monitoring of serum T_4 concentrations. Once-daily administration of methimazole has been reported to be less effective,[272] but this approach can be successful in some cats, particularly those that need very low doses to control their disease. Carbimazole is usually administered 2 to 3 times daily, but a controlled-release formulation has recently been shown to be effective when administered once daily.[273] For cats that are difficult to medicate orally or that have gastrointestinal side-effects, methimazole compounded in pluronic lecithin organogel (PLO) can be applied topically to the pinna.[274-276] Transdermal carbimazole has also been shown to be effective.[277] Approximately 10% to 15% of patients treated with methimazole develop adverse effects, including lethargy, anorexia, vomiting, facial excoriations, hepatotoxicity, and blood dyscrasias.[232,233,270,278] Gastrointestinal side effects are often self-limiting or can be avoided by transdermal drug delivery. Blood dyscrasias are rare but most likely to occur within the first 3 months of treatment; therefore CBCs should be monitored most closely during that time. Medication should be discontinued in patients that experience facial excoriations, blood dyscrasias, or hepatotoxicity. Carbimazole or transdermal methimazole are likely to have the same effects and should therefore not be used in patients experiencing these adverse effects with oral methimazole. Other medical therapies that have been used to treat feline hyperthyroidism include ipodate and iopanoic acid[279,280]; however, these are unlikely to be effective for long-term therapy and are rarely used. A potentially interesting new development in the management of feline hyperthyroidism is the use of an iodine-restricted diet to control the disease.[281-283] At the time of writing, a feline prescription diet for the management of hyperthyroidism had been recently released, but no peer-reviewed manuscript was available for evaluation.

Definitive therapy for feline hyperthyroidism currently consists of surgical thyroidectomy or radioactive iodine. Surgical excision of the affected thyroid lobe(s) is an effective treatment.[234,284,285] Although the majority of cats have bilateral disease, this may be asymmetric and not apparent on palpation or surgical exploration. Thus thyroid scintigraphy is recommended before surgery in order to determine whether unilateral or bilateral thyroidectomy is necessary.[234] Intracapsular and extracapsular thyroidectomy techniques have been described.[284,286] Intracapsular techniques better preserve adjacent parathyroid tissue, whereas extracapsular ones more consistently remove all hyperplastic or neoplastic thyroid tissue. Hyperthyroid cats are often poor anesthetic candidates, and preoperative stabilization with oral antithyroid medications or β-adrenergic blockers should be considered. The most significant intraoperative complication of thyroidectomy in hyperthyroid cats may be cardiac dysrhythmias.[285] Otherwise, the surgery is not considered to be technically demanding.[234,285] Hypocalcemia due to transient hypoparathyroidism is the most commonly reported postoperative complication, with rates ranging from 6% to 15%.[234,285] Other potential complications include hypothyroidism and rarely, Horner's syndrome or laryngeal paralysis. All surgically excised tissue should be submitted for histopathology to rule out the presence of a thyroid carcinoma. Cats with thyroid carcinoma that undergo thyroidectomy usually experience improvement in their clinical signs, but most remain hyperthyroid or develop recurrent hyperthyroidism within a few months of surgery.[236,238] Cats with ectopic hyperplastic thyroid tissue are also at risk for postoperative recurrence of hyperthyroidism.[234] Radioactive iodine therapy is recommended for patients with thyroid carcinoma or ectopic hyperplastic thyroid tissue.

Radioactive iodine, or ^{131}I therapy, is often regarded as the treatment of choice for cats with hyperthyroidism, particularly those with bilateral thyroid hyperplasia, ectopic thyroid tissue, or thyroid carcinoma.[236-238,287,288] ^{131}I has a half-life of 8 days and emits both beta and gamma radiation.[233] Beta particles, which account for 80% of the tissue damage, travel a maximum of 2 mm in tissue and have an average path length of 400 μm. They therefore cause local destruction while sparing adjacent hypoplastic thyroid tissue, parathyroid glands, and other cervical structures. The dose of ^{131}I can be calculated from tracer kinetic studies,[289,290] but these are rarely performed. The administration of a fixed dose of ^{131}I is reported by some authors,[288,291] whereas others use doses that take into account variables, such as the number or size of thyroid nodules, patient body weight, severity of clinical signs, or magnitude of elevation in serum total T_4.[232,287,292,293] ^{131}I is usually administered by the subcutaneous route because it is effective, less stressful for the patient, and safer for personnel.[292] For cats with benign thyroid disease, ^{131}I doses typically range from 2.0 to 6.0 mCi based on clinical signs, serum T_4 concentration, and thyroid nodule size.[287] Using this dosing strategy, less than 5% of cats remain hyperthyroid or experience relapse of clinical signs. When this occurs, a second treatment is usually curative. The proportion of cats that develop persistent hypothyroidism requiring thyroid hormone supplementation varies among studies, and the risk of this has been suggested to be higher in cats with scintigraphic evidence of bilateral disease.[294] Cats with thyroid carcinomas usually have larger tumor burdens, and malignant cells trap and retain iodine less efficiently.[233,236] These cats are therefore treated with higher ablative doses of ^{131}I, in the range of 20 to 30 mCi.[232,233,236-238] In one large study of hyperthyroid cats treated with ^{131}I, median survival was reported to be 2 years, with survival rates at 1, 2, and 3 years of 89%, 72%, and 52%, respectively.[287] The most common causes of death or euthanasia were cancer or renal disease,[287] which is perhaps not surprising in this population of older cats. A more recent study reported a MST of 4 years for cats treated with ^{131}I, compared to 2 years for cats that were treated with methimazole.[256]

Ultrasound-guided percutaneous ethanol injection has also been evaluated as a treatment for feline hyperthyroidism. Cats with solitary adenomas have a good response, with resolution of clinical signs persisting for over 12 months.[295] This technique is not recommended for bilateral hyperplasia.[296] Ultrasound-guided percutaneous radiofrequency heat ablation has been shown to be ineffective for long-term control of hyperthyroidism.[297] Given the ready availability of permanent effective treatments for unilateral or bilateral disease, these alternative treatments are unlikely to be widely used.

Chronic kidney disease (CKD) is a relatively common problem in older cats, and therefore concurrent CKD and hyperthyroidism frequently occur in this population. The hyperthyroid state increases glomerular filtration rate (GFR)[298,299] and therefore decreases serum creatinine values. The implications of this are that hyperthyroid cats with normal serum creatinine values may in fact have concurrent "masked" CKD and that decline in renal function is a risk of all effective forms of treatment of feline hyperthyroidism, with some nonazotemic cats becoming azotemic, or the potential for worsening of preexisting azotemia.[293,298,300,301] This decline in renal function occurs within 1 month after treatment and appears to remain stable thereafter.[293,302] Measurement of pretreatment GFR may help to predict which cats will become azotemic after resolution of hyperthyroidism[293,301]; however, this is impractical for most patients. Unfortunately, no readily available clinical data can predict the effects of therapy on renal function in an individual cat.[303] For this reason, many clinicians recommend a therapeutic trial with methimazole prior to definitive therapy for feline hyperthyroidism.[303] This may have value in providing owners with information about the likely consequence of therapy for these cats, but regardless of the detected change in renal function, effective therapy for hyperthyroidism is still required in these patients. One recent study showed that the development of azotemia was not significantly associated with survival of cats treated for hyperthyroidism,[304] but the same group also demonstrated a significantly shorter survival time in cats with iatrogenic hypothyroidism that became azotemic after treatment compared with those that remained nonazotemic.[305]

Parathyroid Tumors

Parathyroid tumors are uncommon in dogs and rare in cats. These tumors arise from the chief cells and autonomously secrete parathyroid hormone (PTH), leading to hypercalcemia due to primary hyperparathyroidism. Hypercalcemia is the result of direct effects of PTH on bone and the kidneys and indirect effects on the intestine, mediated by vitamin D. Approximately 90% of dogs and cats with primary hyperparathyroidism have a single parathyroid mass,[306-312] with adenomas being most commonly diagnosed and cystadenoma, carcinoma, and hyperplasia diagnosed less frequently.[306-309,311-314] Two or more parathyroid masses may be found in some canine and feline patients, and they may not necessarily all be of the same histologic type. The presence of four hyperplastic parathyroid masses should prompt careful evaluation for causes of secondary hyperparathyroidism.

Primary hyperparathyroidism is most common in older dogs and cats, with reported mean ages of approximately 11 years in dogs[309,311] and 13 years in cats.[306] A breed predisposition has been reported in Keeshonden dogs[307,309,314,315] in which the disease appears to follow an autosomal dominant mode of inheritance, although the affected gene has not yet been identified in this breed.[314,315] It is not clear if there is a breed predilection in cats. The clinical signs of hyperparathyroidism result from hypercalcemia and include polyuria/polydipsia, weakness, lethargy, decreased appetite, weight loss, muscle wasting, vomiting, and trembling. It is not uncommon for owners to detect no clinical signs in affected dogs or cats, with hypercalcemia being diagnosed when blood is drawn for a routine health check or for investigation of an unrelated problem. However, it is also the case that signs can be subtle and are only recognized in retrospect after the hyperparathyroidism has been treated and the hypercalcemia has resolved. In a large case series, the most common clinical problems reported in dogs with hyperparathyroidism were related to the lower urinary tract, usually associated with urolithiasis or urinary tract infection.[309] Specific physical examination abnormalities are rare in dogs and cats, although a palpable parathyroid mass has been reported in a proportion of cats with hyperparathyroidism; the latter is an extremely rare finding in dogs.[308,309]

Hyperparathyroidism is usually diagnosed after finding hypercalcemia on a serum biochemistry profile, either as an incidental finding or when investigating a problem such as calcium oxalate urolithiasis, polyuria/polydipsia, or weakness. The presence of hypercalcemia should be verified by measuring serum ionized calcium, with appropriate careful sample handling.[316,317] There are many causes of hypercalcemia in dogs and cats,[318,319] and diagnostic tests may be performed to investigate several possible causes simultaneously. The reader is directed to Chapter 5 for a further discussion of the causes of hypercalcemia in dogs and cats. Hypercalcemia due to primary hyperparathyroidism is often accompanied by hypophosphatemia or serum inorganic phosphorus at the low end of the reference range. This finding is not pathognomonic for hyperparathyroidism and can be associated with humoral hypercalcemia of malignancy, but it can assist in ranking the differential diagnoses because vitamin D toxicosis and renal failure would both be expected to cause hyperphosphatemia. The diagnosis of hyperparathyroidism is confirmed by documenting an inappropriately high serum PTH level in the presence of ionized hypercalcemia. It is important to note that PTH is frequently within the reference range in patients with hyperparathyroidism, with 73% of cases reported to have a normal PTH in one large series.[309] A normal PTH in the face of hypercalcemia is an abnormal finding because PTH should be suppressed as calcium increases. The lack of suppression of PTH is indicative of loss of the normal negative feedback effects of calcium due to autonomous hormone secretion by hyperplastic or neoplastic parathyroid tissue. Ultrasound examination of the neck is commonly used in the diagnosis of hyperparathyroidism in dogs and cats[309,310,320,321] and is particularly useful for localizing parathyroid mass(es) prior to surgery or other ablative procedures. The normal sonographic appearance of canine parathyroid glands has been described,[322] and parathyroid masses as small as 3 mm in greatest diameter have been identified ultrasonographically.[309] Parathyroid scintigraphy and selective venous sampling to assess local PTH concentrations do not appear to be helpful in localizing hyperplastic or neoplastic parathyroid tissue.[320,323,324]

The management of hypercalcemia is further addressed in Chapter 5. Primary hyperparathyroidism in dogs and cats is usually associated with slowly progressing hypercalcemia, and the calcium elevation itself rarely requires emergency treatment. Hypercalcemia is a risk factor for renal failure. Mechanisms include altered glomerular capillary permeability, decreased renal blood flow, and mineralization of the kidneys. The risk of mineralization is increased when the calcium × phosphorus product exceeds 70. As noted previously, decreased or low-normal phosphorus often occurs in patients with hyperparathyroidism, thus decreasing the risk of renal mineralization. In fact, it appears that renal failure occurs rarely in dogs with primary hyperparathyroidism. In a large canine case series, it was found that mean blood urea nitrogen (BUN) and serum creatinine were both significantly lower in 210 dogs with primary hyperparathyroidism, compared with 200 control dogs.[309] In addition, 95% of the hyperparathyroid dogs had BUN and serum creatinine values within or below the reference range. This may partly be a result of the secondary nephrogenic diabetes insipidus that causes polyuria/polydipsia in these patients.

Definitive therapy for primary hyperparathyroidism requires removal of the hyperfunctioning gland(s). This is most commonly achieved by surgery in both dogs and cats; however, percutaneous ultrasound-guided ethanol ablation and percutaneous ultrasound-guided heat ablation are also well described in the dog.[311,325,326] The latter techniques may not be as widely available as surgery, and success likely depends on the experience of the operator.[311] In a retrospective comparison of surgery, ethanol ablation, and heat ablation, all three techniques performed well, but surgical parathyroidectomy had the highest success rate and lowest rate of complications.[311] Ultrasound examination of the neck is strongly recommended prior to surgery, and the surgeon should carefully evaluate all the parathyroid glands because approximately 10% of patients have masses in more than one gland. Up to three of the four parathyroid glands can be removed without risk of permanent hypoparathyroidism. Patients with involvement of all four glands present a dilemma, and it is important to ensure that hyperplasia in these cases is not secondary. If the hyperparathyroidism is believed to be primary, removal of all parathyroid tissue is required to control hypercalcemia, but this will necessitate life-long supplemental therapy. In human medicine, total parathyroidectomy may be followed by autotransplantation of one of the glands or may be accompanied by cryopreservation of parathyroid tissue.[327] These approaches have not been explored in veterinary medicine.

Hypocalcemia is a potential complication of surgical parathyroidectomy, ethanol ablation, or heat ablation. This happens because chronic hypercalcemia inhibits PTH secretion by the normal parathyroid glands and leads to parathyroid atrophy. It is logical to assume that the risk of this posttreatment complication increases with duration and severity of hypercalcemia; however, it is still difficult to predict whether an individual patient will become hypocalcemic. Thus it is recommended that serum ionized calcium levels be monitored at least twice daily for as long as 5 to 7 days after surgery or other ablative procedures. Hypocalcemia should be treated if the ionized calcium falls below 0.8 to 0.9 mmol/L, the total calcium is less than 8 to 9 mg/dL, or the patient has signs of tetany. Intravenous (IV) calcium salts are used for acute therapy for hypocalcemia; subcutaneous (SQ) administration should be avoided. Vitamin D and oral calcium are used for subacute and chronic therapy. Several excellent references are available regarding treatment of hypoparathyroidism.[312,328] In summary, 1,25-dihydroxyvitamin D_3 (calcitriol) is recommended for vitamin D supplementation because it has a rapid onset of action and a short half-life. This facilitates dose adjustments and reduces the risk of hypercalcemia. Oral calcium supplementation alone is not sufficient to treat hypoparathyroidism, and in fact this therapy can be gradually withdrawn once the calcium is stable because most maintenance diets contain an adequate amount of calcium. Calcitriol therapy can be started up to 24 hours prior to surgery or parathyroid ablation, if the risk of hypocalcemia is thought to be high. This allows the medication to reach therapeutic levels more quickly, but it will not necessarily prevent the development of hypocalcemia. When adjusting the dose of calcitriol, the goal is to maintain the calcium barely below the normal reference range rather than within normal. This reduces the risk of hypercalcemia and provides the stimulus for recovery of function of the remaining normal parathyroid glands. Once the serum calcium has been stable for at least 1 to 2 weeks in an outpatient, the dose of calcitriol can be gradually reduced, with careful monitoring. The time for return of normal parathyroid function is unpredictable, and therefore clients should expect frequent rechecks of the patient's calcium levels for several weeks to months after treatment of hyperparathyroidism.

The long-term prognosis after surgical or ablative treatment for hyperparathyroidism is very good. Metastatic disease is extremely rare, and the complication of hypocalcemia is generally amenable to medical therapy. A small number of patients may appear resistant to the postoperative management of hypocalcemia, and this may be the result of the "hungry bone syndrome" in which there is aggressive unregulated uptake of calcium by the bones. In human medicine, this syndrome has been managed with preoperative bisphosphonate administration[329] or the use of recombinant PTH.[330] Neither of these approaches has been used in veterinary medicine, and most patients will eventually respond to high doses of calcitriol and calcium supplementation. Less than 10% of dogs and cats treated for hyperparathyroidism will experience a recurrence of the disease.[308,312] If this occurs, a second surgery or ablative procedure should be performed. The short-term prognosis for dogs and cats that do not undergo definitive surgical or ablative therapy for hyperparathyroidism may still be favorable because the disease tends to be slowly progressive, clinical signs may be mild, and renal failure may be a less common outcome than previously suspected.[309]

Pancreatic Beta-Cell Tumors (Insulinomas)

Pancreatic beta-cell tumors are rare in humans and cats and uncommon in dogs.[331-333] These tumors are often functional, but the neoplastic beta-cells fail to appropriately inhibit insulin secretion at low blood glucose concentrations. Thus the hallmark of insulinoma is a normal or elevated blood insulin concentration in the presence of low blood glucose levels. A feline insulinoma was recently shown to demonstrate abnormal glucokinase and hexokinase expression.[332] These changes may contribute to enhanced glucose sensitivity and hence an abnormal insulin secretory response in insulinoma cells. Although the clinical signs of insulinoma result from hypoglycemia associated with unregulated insulin secretion, immunocytochemical analysis reveals that these tumors often produce many additional hormones, including glucagon, somatostatin, pancreatic polypeptide, GH, IGF-1, and gastrin.[332,334-338]

In humans, 90% of insulinomas are solitary and benign, and 5% to 10% are associated with multiple endocrine neoplasia type 1 (MEN1). Insulinomas in dogs are much more likely to be malignant, although morphologic classification into adenoma or adenocarcinoma does not consistently reflect the biologic behavior of these tumors.[331,336,339] Metastatic lesions are detected in approximately 50% of canine insulinomas, with the regional lymph nodes and liver most commonly affected. Pulmonary metastases are very rare in dogs.[337,340-344]

Beta-Cell Tumors in Dogs

The cellular and molecular events causing beta-cell tumors in dogs are unknown. Canine insulinomas have been shown to express somatostatin receptors, which may have implications for both diagnosis and therapy (see later).[345] Local production of GH and IGF-1 have also been demonstrated in canine insulinomas, with a higher level of expression of GH and IGF-1 mRNA in metastases compared to primary tumors.[338,346] It has been suggested that the locally produced hormones may have autocrine or paracrine effects on cell proliferation, and tumor growth and progression. Furthermore, it is speculated that locally produced somatostatin has inhibitory effects on insulinomas within the pancreas, but that these effects are decreased in metastases, leading to increased GH production.[346]

The World Health Organization (WHO) recommendations have been used to stage canine pancreatic tumors.[341] Thus clinical stage I tumors involve only the pancreas with no evidence of local or distant lymph node involvement and no distant metastasis (T1N0M0). Stage II tumors have lymph node involvement (T1N1M0), and stage III tumors have distant metastasis (T1N1M1 or T1N0M1). A recent study evaluated several clinicopathologic and morphologic criteria of canine insulinomas with the goal of establishing prognostic biomarkers for this tumor.[339] It was found that tumor size was predictive for disease-free interval (DFI) in a multivariate analysis, and Ki67 index, a marker of proliferation, was predictive for both DFI and survival time.

Canine insulinomas are most commonly reported in medium- and large-breed dogs, particularly Labrador retrievers, Golden retrievers, German shepherd dogs, German pointers, Irish setters, Boxers, and mixed breed dogs. Small-breed dogs can also be affected; West Highland white terriers appear overrepresented in some reports. Depending on the case series, the median reported age is 9 to 10 years, with a range of 3 to 15 years, and no sex predilection.[337,340-342,346,347]

The clinical signs of insulinoma result from the effects of hypoglycemia on the nervous system, which is termed *neuroglycopenia,* and these signs include weakness, ataxia, collapse, disorientation, behavioral changes, and seizures. Catecholamine release stimulated by low blood glucose levels may also cause muscle tremors, shaking, anxiety, and hunger. Clinical signs may be present for days to months and are often intermittent or episodic. They may be precipitated by fasting, exercise, excitement, or eating. Signs may be less pronounced with more chronic hypoglycemia, and patients may be clinically normal with significantly low blood glucose levels. Physical examination findings are usually otherwise unremarkable in these patients. A paraneoplastic peripheral neuropathy has been described in dogs with insulinoma. This appears to be rare, although subclinical neuropathies may be present and undetected.[348-352] Brain lesions associated with hypoglycemia have also been reported in rare cases.[353,354]

The diagnosis of insulinoma is confirmed by documenting hypoglycemia (blood glucose <60 mg/dL) with a concurrent normal or elevated serum insulin concentration. In some cases, it may be necessary to fast the patient, with careful monitoring, and repeat blood glucose measurements every 30 to 60 minutes. Once the blood glucose is less than 60 mg/dL, a serum sample should be submitted for concurrent insulin measurement. The presence of normal or high serum insulin concentration in the face of hypoglycemia is inappropriate and generally sufficient to confirm the diagnosis of insulinoma. This insulin-glucose pair should be performed more than once if the initial sample provides equivocal results.[355] The use of insulin : glucose or glucose : insulin ratios is not recommended because these do not improve diagnostic accuracy. Provocative testing is also rarely used in veterinary medicine because of risks, expense, and poor sensitivity.[342] Serum fructosamine and glycosylated hemoglobin concentrations can also be measured in dogs to support a suspicion of insulinoma.[356-359] Concentrations of these glycosylated proteins would be expected to be lower than normal in dogs with chronic hypoglycemia, although this is not necessarily pathognomonic for insulinoma.

Imaging studies are often used in the evaluation of insulinoma patients, particularly in preparation for surgical management. Thoracic and abdominal radiographs are usually unremarkable but are often obtained to investigate other potential causes of hypoglycemia. Abdominal ultrasonography is commonly performed but has been reported to clearly identify and localize a pancreatic mass in less than 50% of cases.[344,347,360,361] Abdominal ultrasonography is also used to identify metastatic lesions in dogs with insulinoma but has low sensitivity and specificity for this purpose. Thus, although abdominal ultrasonography is widely available and often used in the evaluation of patients with hypoglycemia, it cannot be used to rule in or rule out a diagnosis of insulinoma. In human medicine, endoscopic and intraoperative ultrasonography are used to identify small pancreatic tumors, but these techniques have yet to be reported in canine patients.[362]

CT findings have been reported in a small number of dogs with insulinoma.[361,363,364] In a study comparing ultrasound, CT, and single-photon emission CT (SPECT), CT was found to be the most sensitive technique, identifying 10 of 14 confirmed primary insulinomas. However, CT also identified a significant number of false-positive metastatic lesions.[361] The results of SPECT with ^{111}In-DTPA-D-Phe^{1}-octreotide have been reported in a total of 19 dogs with insulinoma, with an overall sensitivity of 50% for detection and correct localization of the primary tumor.[345,361] Enhanced CT techniques such as dynamic CT or dual-phase CT angiography hold promise for greater sensitivity of detection of insulinomas in dogs, but large-scale studies have yet to be reported in the veterinary literature.[363,364] Somatostatin receptor scintigraphy (SRS) is an important imaging modality in humans with pancreatic endocrine tumors, including insulinomas. Indium In-111 pentetreotide SRS has been reported in a total of six dogs with insulinoma, with positive results reported in five cases, although an accurate anatomic localization was only obtained in one case.[365,366] PET has been used in human patients to localize insulinomas when CT, MRI, and ultrasound are negative.[367] This modality has yet to be explored in canine insulinoma patients.

Therapy for canine insulinoma involves acute and chronic treatment of hypoglycemia and long-term management of the tumor. Acute treatment of hypoglycemia is accomplished through administration of intravenous dextrose, often as a slow bolus, followed by continuous rate infusion (CRI). This should be given with caution because this treatment can stimulate further unregulated insulin secretion and worsened hypoglycemia. A CRI of glucagon has also been used in the management of hyperinsulinemic-hypoglycemic crisis in a dog.[368]

Exploratory laparotomy is indicated in dogs with hypoglycemia and inappropriately elevated serum insulin concentrations, regardless of the results of abdominal imaging studies.[340-342,344,347] Blood glucose levels should be stabilized before surgery and monitored throughout the procedure. Surgery allows confirmation of the diagnosis of insulinoma, resection of primary and metastatic neoplasia, and staging of the disease. Details of the technique of partial pancreatectomy are described elsewhere.[182] The majority of canine insulinomas are visible or palpable at surgery, and tumors are identified in both lobes of the pancreas with equal frequency. Suspected metastatic lesions should be resected whenever possible, and the liver and regional lymph nodes should always be biopsied. Potential postoperative complications include pancreatitis, persistent hypoglycemia, transient hyperglycemia or diabetes mellitus, and exocrine pancreatic insufficiency.[187,331,342]

Medical treatment of insulinoma is used to stabilize patients preoperatively, as an alternate therapy if surgery is not possible, and in conjunction with surgical management. Medical therapies are primarily used to control hypoglycemia, but cytotoxic agents have also been used to destroy pancreatic beta-cells. Streptozocin (streptozotocin) is the chemotherapeutic drug that has been used most often, albeit infrequently, in dogs. Its use in dogs was historically limited by its nephrotoxicity,[331] but more recent reports suggest that the risk of nephrotoxicity is significantly reduced if the drug is given in combination with intensive saline diuresis.[369,370] Other side effects of this drug include vomiting during administration, diabetes mellitus, hypoglycemia, and mild hematologic changes.[369,370] The administration of streptozocin does not significantly increase the duration of normoglycemia in dogs with insulinoma compared with control dogs treated medically or surgically.[369] Although individual dogs have demonstrated reductions in tumor size or resolution of paraneoplastic neuropathy with streptozocin, it is still unclear if the risks of therapy outweigh the benefits of this treatment for dogs with insulinoma.

Strategies used to control hypoglycemia consist of dietary modification and medical therapy with prednisone, diazoxide, or octreotide. Excitement should be avoided in these patients, and exercise limited. Diets high in fat, protein, and complex carbohydrates should be fed in small, frequent meals, and simple sugars avoided.[331] Prednisone is used for its insulin-antagonizing, gluconeogenic, and glycogenolytic effects.[331] A starting dose of 0.25 mg/kg by mouth (PO) twice daily is recommended, with gradual dose increases as needed to control hypoglycemia.[331,342] Typical glucocorticoid side effects should be anticipated. Diazoxide is a nondiuretic benzothiadiazine that suppresses insulin release from beta-cells. It also stimulates hepatic gluconeogenesis and glycogenolysis and inhibits cellular uptake of glucose. Diazoxide is not cytotoxic and does not inhibit insulin synthesis. A starting dose of 5 mg/kg PO twice daily is recommended, and the dose can be gradually increased to 30 mg/kg PO twice daily if necessary.[331,342] Approximately 70% of canine insulinoma patients respond to diazoxide therapy.[331,340] Side effects are uncommon but may include ptyalism, vomiting, anorexia, and diarrhea.[331,342,371] The use of diazoxide has been limited by its cost and inconsistent availability. Octreotide is a somatostatin receptor ligand that inhibits synthesis and secretion of insulin by pancreatic beta-cells. It has been reported to alleviate hypoglycemia in up to 50% of dogs with insulinoma, although some may become refractory to treatment.[331,345] The suggested dose is 10 to 50 µg SQ 2 to 3 times daily, and side effects appear to be rare. In a more recent study, a single 50 µg dose of octreotide was administered to 12 dogs with insulinoma. Plasma insulin concentrations decreased significantly after administration of octreotide in dogs with insulinoma, but GH, ACTH, cortisol, and glucagon levels did not change and glucose levels increased.[372] These findings suggest that the use of octreotide warrants further investigation in canine patients with insulinoma, although the cost of the medication may be a significant impediment.

The prognosis for dogs with insulinomas is good in the short term but guarded to poor in the long term. Patients that undergo surgery followed by medical management are more likely to become euglycemic, remain euglycemic for longer periods, and have longer survival times compared to patients that receive only medical therapy.[344,347] MSTs following partial pancreatectomy range from 12 to 14 months over several different studies.[371] The prognosis following surgery depends on the clinical stage of the disease. Dogs in stage I have a longer DFI compared to dogs in stages II and III, with 50% of dogs in stage I free of hypoglycemia 14 months after surgery compared to less than 20% of dogs in stages II and III being free of hypoglycemia at this time.[341] Dogs in clinical stage III have a significantly shorter survival time than dogs in stages I and II, with approximately 50% of dogs with metastasis dead by 6 months.[341] A more recent retrospective study showed improved survival in dogs with insulinoma compared to earlier reports.[347] The authors reported a MST of 785 days for 19 dogs undergoing partial pancreatectomy, with a median DFI of 496 days. The subset of nine dogs that received surgery followed by medical therapy with prednisolone had a MST of 1316 days. For eight dogs receiving medical therapy alone, the MST was 196 days. When all the dogs that received medical therapy were considered as a group, the MST after institution of the medical treatment was 452 days.[347] These results lend strong support to the use of medical therapy in canine patients with insulinoma, particularly when clinical signs recur after surgery.

Beta-Cell Tumors in Cats

Compared to dogs, there are significantly fewer reports of insulinomas in cats. History, clinical signs, and biologic behavior in this species appear to be similar to those in the dog, and concurrent measurements of blood glucose and serum insulin concentrations are used to confirm the diagnosis. However, it is important to use an insulin assay that has been validated in cats. Siamese cats may be overrepresented,[371] but because the disease is rarely reported, firm conclusions on breed predisposition should not be drawn. Surgical management has been reported in feline patients, with survival times ranging from 1 to 32 months.[331,373-377] Medical therapy with dietary management and prednisolone have also been used in cats. Octreotide may also be considered, although there is little evidence to support its use, and no evidence to support the use of diazoxide or streptozotocin in this species.[331]

Gastrointestinal Endocrine Tumors

Gastrinoma

Gastrinomas are neuroendocrine tumors that secrete excessive amounts of gastrin. Zollinger-Ellison syndrome refers to the triad of a non–beta-cell neuroendocrine tumor in the pancreas, hypergastrinemia, and gastrointestinal ulceration. Gastrinomas are rare in dogs and very rare in cats.[378,379] Almost all reported gastrinomas in these species were identified in the pancreas, although there is one report of a duodenal gastrinoma in a dog.[380] In contrast, the majority of gastrinomas in humans arise in the duodenum, with fewer detected in the pancreas.[10] Although gastrin-producing G cells normally exist in the duodenum and gastric antrum, they are not present in the pancreas. The cell of origin for primary pancreatic gastrinomas is not known, but D cells (which secrete gastrin in the fetus and neonate) are the most likely candidates.[378,379] Gastrinomas are highly metastatic, with involvement of the liver, regional lymph nodes, spleen, peritoneum, small intestine, omentum, or mesentery identified in 85% of dogs and cats at the time of initial diagnosis.[378,379,381-383]

Gastrinomas are typically reported in middle-aged dogs and older cats.[378,379] No obvious breed or sex predilections have been identified. Clinical signs result from gastric acid hypersecretion and gastric mucosal hyperplasia.[378,379,381-389] The most common signs are vomiting and weight loss. Melena, abdominal pain, anorexia, hematemesis, hematochezia, and diarrhea may also occur. Physical examination findings range from unremarkable to a patient in hypovolemic shock due to perforation of an ulcer. Serum biochemistry profile, CBC, and urinalysis may demonstrate changes associated with protein loss and bleeding due to gastrointestinal ulceration or may reflect the consequences of severe or persistent vomiting or the presence of hepatic metastases. One case of common bile duct obstruction due to a duodenal gastrinoma has been reported in a dog.[380] Abdominal radiographs may be unremarkable unless gastrointestinal perforation has occurred. Contrast radiographs and abdominal ultrasound examination may show evidence of gastrointestinal ulceration and thickened pyloric antrum and gastric wall. Ultrasound examination may also reveal metastatic lesions in the liver or regional lymph nodes; however, the primary tumor in the pancreas is usually too small to be detected with this modality.[383] The results of techniques such as CT and MRI have not been widely reported in dogs and cats with gastrinomas. Endoscopy may reveal esophagitis with ulceration, gastric and duodenal ulceration, thickened gastric rugae, and hypertrophy of the pyloric antrum. The diagnosis may be supported by measuring basal serum gastrin levels or levels after provocative testing or by scintigraphy using radiolabeled pentetreotide.[390] Basal gastrin levels have been significantly elevated in dogs and cats with gastrinoma; however, gastrin levels can also be elevated in renal, hepatic, or gastric disease, and after therapy with antacids such as H_2-receptor antagonists and proton pump inhibitors.[391] Provocative testing has rarely been reported in veterinary medicine.[187,378,379]

Exploratory laparotomy is recommended for dogs and cats suspected to have a gastrinoma. Even though the majority of dogs and cats have visible metastasis at the time of initial diagnosis, surgical debulking will reduce gastrin secretory capacity and enhance the efficacy of medical therapy.[379] In addition, deep or perforated gastrointestinal ulcers can be identified and excised. Long-term medical management includes the use of proton pump inhibitors, H_2-receptor antagonists, and sucralfate.[384,388] Octreotide has been used in two dogs with success.[390,392] Survival times for dogs and cats with gastrinoma have ranged from 1 week to 26 months.[378,379,388]

Glucagonoma

Glucagonomas are rare in dogs and humans, and there are no case reports in cats.[10,378,379] These tumors are associated with a crusting dermatologic condition referred to as superficial necrolytic dermatitis, diabetic dermatopathy, hepatocutaneous syndrome, or necrolytic migratory erythema (NME). Other associated problems include hyperglycemia or overt diabetes mellitus, hypoaminoacidemia, and increased liver enzyme values. Lesions associated with NME include hyperkeratosis, crusting, ulceration and erosions of the footpads, mucocutaneous junctions, external genitalia, distal extremities, pressure points, and ventral abdomen.[187,378,379,393-397] Glucagonomas arise from alpha-cells in the pancreas and are sometimes detected on abdominal ultrasound examination or CT.[379,395,397] Plasma glucagon levels may be measured, and amino acid concentrations have also been evaluated in a small number of patients,[394-396] but the sensitivity and specificity of these diagnostic tests is unknown. Surgical resection or debulking is the treatment of choice for canine glucagonoma, but metastasis is common at the time of surgery, and prognosis is generally poor.[187,378,379,395] There are rare reports of the use of somatostatin analogs.[396,397] The dermatologic lesions of NME may improve after surgery or medical therapy, and lesions may also respond to treatment with amino acid infusions, oral protein supplementation (with protein powders or egg yolks), zinc, or essential fatty acids.[379] When NME is suspected, it is important to rule out liver disease because this is a more common cause of this dermatologic condition in dogs.

Intestinal Carcinoid

Intestinal carcinoid tumors are rare in dogs and cats. They arise from enterochromaffin cells that are found in a variety of locations; hence these tumors have been reported in several sites throughout the gastrointestinal tract, liver, gallbladder, and pancreas.[378,379,398-403] Clinical signs are generally associated with the anatomic location of the tumor; the physiologic effects of vasoactive substances released from the tumor were suspected in one dog with an intestinal carcinoid.[402] In general, the prognosis for these tumors is guarded because metastasis is common at the time of diagnosis.[379]

Surgical removal is recommended,[378] and there is a single case report describing adjuvant chemotherapy in a canine patient.[404]

REFERENCES

1. Capen CC: Tumors of the endocrine glands. In Meuten DJ, editor: *Tumors in domestic animals*, ed 4, Ames, Iowa, 2002, Iowa State Press.
2. Chen S: Advanced diagnostic approaches and current medical management of insulinomas and adrenocortical disease in ferrets (Mustela putorius furo), *Vet Clin North Am Exot Anim Pract* 13:439–452, 2010.
3. Coclet J, Foureau F, Ketelbant P, et al: Cell population kinetics in dog and human adult thyroid, *Clin Endocrinol (Oxf)* 31:655–665, 1989.
4. Williams D: General features of the origin and pathogenesis of endocrine tumors. In Mazzaferri EL, Samaan NA, editors: *Endocrine Tumors*. Cambridge, 1993, Blackwell Scientific.
5. Kondo T, Ezzat S, Asa SL: Pathogenetic mechanisms in thyroid follicular-cell neoplasia, *Nat Rev Cancer* 6:292–306, 2006.
6. Lin RY: New insights into thyroid stem cells, *Thyroid* 17:1019–1023, 2007.
7. Thomas D, Friedman S, Lin RY: Thyroid stem cells: lessons from normal development and thyroid cancer, *Endocr Relat Cancer* 15:51–58, 2008.
8. Lichtenauer UD, Beuschlein F: The tumor stem cell concept-implications for endocrine tumors? *Mol Cell Endocrinol* 300:158–163, 2009.
9. Klonisch T, Hoang-Vu C, Hombach-Klonisch S: Thyroid stem cells and cancer, *Thyroid* 19:1303–1315, 2009.
10. Wells J, Carling T, Udelsman R, et al: Cancer of the endocrine system. In DeVita J, Lawrence TS, Rosenberg SA, editors: *Cancer: principles & practice of oncology*, Philadelphia, 2008, Lippincott Williams & Wilkins.
11. Pollard RE, Reilly CM, Uerling MR, et al: Cross-sectional imaging characteristics of pituitary adenomas, invasive adenomas and adenocarcinomas in dogs: 33 cases (1988-2006), *J Vet Intern Med* 24:160–165, 2010.
12. Moore SA, O'Brien DP: Canine pituitary macrotumors, *Compend Contin Educ Vet* 30:33–41, 2008.
13. Kent MS, Bommarito D, Feldman E, et al: Survival, neurologic response, and prognostic factors in dogs with pituitary masses treated with radiation therapy and untreated dogs, *J Vet Intern Med* 21:1027–1033, 2007.
14. Wood FD, Pollard RE, Uerling MR, et al: Diagnostic imaging findings and endocrine test results in dogs with pituitary-dependent hyperadrenocorticism that did or did not have neurologic abnormalities: 157 cases (1989-2005), *J Am Vet Med Assoc* 231:1081–1085, 2007.
15. Snyder JM, Lipitz L, Skorupski KA, et al: Secondary intracranial neoplasia in the dog: 177 cases (1986-2003), *J Vet Intern Med* 22:172–177, 2008.
16. Goossens MM, Rijnberk A, Mol JA, et al: Central diabetes insipidus in a dog with a pro-opiomelanocortin-producing pituitary tumor not causing hyperadrenocorticism, *J Vet Intern Med* 9:361–365, 1995.
17. Feldman EC, Nelson RW: Canine hyperadrenocorticism (Cushing's syndrome). In Feldman EC, Nelson RW, editors: *Canine and feline endocrinology and reproduction*, ed 3, St. Louis, 2004, Saunders.
18. Melian C, Perez-Alenza MD, Peterson ME: Hyperadrenocorticism in dogs. In Ettinger SJ, Feldman EC, editors: *Textbook of veterinary internal medicine*, ed 7, St. Louis, 2010, Saunders Elsevier.
19. Newell-Price J, Bertagna X, Grossman AB, et al: Cushing's syndrome, *Lancet* 367:1605–1617, 2006.
20. Galac S, Kooistra HS, Voorhout G, et al: Hyperadrenocorticism in a dog due to ectopic secretion of adrenocorticotropic hormone, *Domest Anim Endocrinol* 28:338–348, 2005.
21. Graves TK: Hypercortisolism in cats (feline Cushing's syndrome). In Ettinger SJ, Feldman EC, editors: *Textbook of veterinary internal medicine*, ed 7, St. Louis, 2010, Saunders Elsevier.
22. Feldman EC, Nelson RW: Hyperadrenocorticism in cats (Cushing's syndrome). In Feldman EC, Nelson RW, editors: *Canine and feline endocrinology and reproduction*, ed 3, St. Louis, 2004, Saunders.
23. Hanson JM, Mol JA, Meij BP: Expression of leukemia inhibitory factor and leukemia inhibitory factor receptor in the canine pituitary gland and corticotrope adenomas, *Domest Anim Endocrinol* 38:260–271, 2010.
24. Hanson JM, Mol JA, Leegwater PA, et al: Expression and mutation analysis of Tpit in the canine pituitary gland and corticotroph adenomas, *Domest Anim Endocrinol* 34:217–222, 2008.
25. Peterson ME, Altszuler N, Nichols CE: Decreased insulin sensitivity and glucose-tolerance in spontaneous canine hyperadrenocorticism, *Res Vet Sci* 36:177–182, 1984.
26. Nichols R: Complications and concurrent disease associated with canine hyperadrenocorticism, *Vet Clin North Am Small Anim Pract* 27:309–320, 1997.
27. Behrend EN, Kemppainen RJ: Glucocorticoid therapy. Pharmacology, indications, and complications, *Vet Clin North Am Small Anim Pract* 27:187–213, 1997.
28. Forrester SD, Troy GC, Dalton MN, et al: Retrospective evaluation of urinary tract infection in 42 dogs with hyperadrenocorticism or diabetes mellitus or both, *J Vet Intern Med* 13:557–560, 1999.
29. Hurley KJ, Vaden SL: Evaluation of urine protein content in dogs with pituitary-dependent hyperadrenocorticism, *J Am Vet Med Assoc* 212:369–373, 1998.
30. Ortega TM, Feldman EC, Nelson RW, et al: Systemic arterial blood pressure and urine protein/creatinine ratio in dogs with hyperadrenocorticism, *J Am Vet Med Assoc* 209:1724–1729, 1996.
31. Johnson LR, Lappin MR, Baker DC: Pulmonary thromboembolism in 29 dogs: 1985-1995, *J Vet Intern Med* 13:338–345, 1999.
32. Behrend EN, Kemppainen RJ: Diagnosis of canine hyperadrenocorticism, *Vet Clin North Am Small Anim Pract* 31:985–1001, 2001.
33. Peterson ME: Diagnosis of hyperadrenocorticism in dogs, *Clin Tech Small Anim Pract* 22:2–11, 2007.
34. Reusch CE, Feldman EC: Canine hyperadrenocorticism due to adrenocortical neoplasia. Pretreatment evaluation of 41 dogs, *J Vet Intern Med* 5:3–10, 1991.
35. Gould SM, Baines EA, Mannion PA, et al: Use of endogenous ACTH concentration and adrenal ultrasonography to distinguish the cause of canine hyperadrenocorticism, *J Small Anim Pract* 42:113–121, 2001.
36. Rodriguez Pineiro MI, Benchekroun G, de Fornel-Thibaud P, et al: Accuracy of an adrenocorticotropic hormone (ACTH) immunoluminometric assay for differentiating ACTH-dependent from ACTH-independent hyperadrenocorticism in dogs, *J Vet Intern Med* 23:850–855, 2009.
37. Grooters AM, Biller DS, Theisen SK, et al: Ultrasonographic characteristics of the adrenal glands in dogs with pituitary-dependent hyperadrenocorticism: Comparison with normal dogs, *J Vet Intern Med* 10:110–115, 1996.
38. Besso JG, Penninck DG, Gliatto JM: Retrospective ultrasonographic evaluation of adrenal lesions in 26 dogs, *Vet Radiol Ultrasound* 38:448–455, 1997.
39. Hoerauf A, Reusch C: Ultrasonographic characteristics of both adrenal glands in 15 dogs with functional adrenocortical tumors, *J Am Anim Hosp Assoc* 35:193–199, 1999.
40. Benchekroun G, de Fornel-Thibaud P, Pineiro MIR, et al: Ultrasonography criteria for differentiating ACTH dependency from ACTH independency in 47 dogs with hyperadrenocorticism and equivocal adrenal asymmetry, *J Vet Intern Med* 24:1077–1085, 2010.
41. Greco DS, Peterson ME, Davidson AP, et al: Concurrent pituitary and adrenal tumors in dogs with hyperadrenocorticism: 17 cases (1978-1995), *J Am Vet Med Assoc* 214:1349–1353, 1999.

42. Anderson CR, Birchard SJ, Powers BE, et al: Surgical treatment of adrenocortical tumors: 21 cases (1990-1996), *J Am Anim Hosp Assoc* 37:93–97, 2001.
43. Kyles AE, Feldman EC, De Cock HE, et al: Surgical management of adrenal gland tumors with and without associated tumor thrombi in dogs: 40 cases (1994-2001), *J Am Vet Med Assoc* 223:654–662, 2003.
44. Morandi F, Mays JL, Newman SJ, et al: Imaging diagnosis–bilateral adrenal adenomas and myelolipomas in a dog, *Vet Radiol Ultrasound* 48:246–249, 2007.
45. Lang JM, Schertel E, Kennedy S, et al: Elective and emergency surgical management of adrenal gland tumors: 60 cases (1999-2006), *J Am Anim Hosp Assoc* 47:428–435, 2011.
46. Voorhout G, Stolp R, Lubberink AA, et al: Computed tomography in the diagnosis of canine hyperadrenocorticism not suppressible by dexamethasone, *J Am Vet Med Assoc* 192:641–646, 1988.
47. Bertolini G, Furlanello T, Drigo M, et al: Computed tomographic adrenal gland quantification in canine adrenocorticotroph hormone-dependent hyperadrenocorticism, *Vet Radiol Ultrasound* 49:449–453, 2008.
48. van der Vlugt-Meijer RH, Meij BP, van den Ingh TS, et al: Dynamic computed tomography of the pituitary gland in dogs with pituitary-dependent hyperadrenocorticism, *J Vet Intern Med* 17:773–780, 2003.
49. van der Vlugt-Meijer RH, Meij BP, Voorhout G: Dynamic helical computed tomography of the pituitary gland in healthy dogs, *Vet Radiol Ultrasound* 48:118–124, 2007.
50. Auriemma E, Barthez PY, van der Vlugt-Meijer RH, et al: Computed tomography and low-field magnetic resonance imaging of the pituitary gland in dogs with pituitary-dependent hyperadrenocorticism: 11 cases (2001-2003), *J Am Vet Med Assoc* 235:409–414, 2009.
51. Bertoy EH, Feldman EC, Nelson RW, et al: Magnetic resonance imaging of the brain in dogs with recently diagnosed but untreated pituitary-dependent hyperadrenocorticism, *J Am Vet Med Assoc* 206:651–656, 1995.
52. Duesberg CA, Feldman EC, Nelson RW, et al: Magnetic resonance imaging for diagnosis of pituitary macrotumors in dogs, *J Am Vet Med Assoc* 206:657–662, 1995.
53. Bertoy EH, Feldman EC, Nelson RW, et al: One-year follow-up evaluation of magnetic resonance imaging of the brain in dogs with pituitary-dependent hyperadrenocorticism, *J Am Vet Med Assoc* 208:1268–1273, 1996.
54. Zhao Q, Lee S, Kent M, et al: Dynamic contrast-enhanced magnetic resonance imaging of canine brain tumors, *Vet Radiol Ultrasound* 51:122–129, 2010.
55. Nelson RW, Ihle SL, Feldman EC: Pituitary macroadenomas and macroadenocarcinomas in dogs treated with mitotane for pituitary-dependent hyperadrenocorticism: 13 cases (1981-1986), *J Am Vet Med Assoc* 194:1612–1617, 1989.
56. Théon AP, Feldman EC: Megavoltage irradiation of pituitary macrotumors in dogs with neurologic signs, *J Am Vet Med Assoc* 213:225–231, 1998.
57. Bosje JT, Rijnberk A, Mol JA, et al: Plasma concentrations of ACTH precursors correlate with pituitary size and resistance to dexamethasone in dogs with pituitary-dependent hyperadrenocorticism, *Domest Anim Endocrinol* 22:201–210, 2002.
58. Granger N, de Fornel P, Devauchelle P, et al: Plasma pro-opiomelanocortin, pro-adrenocorticotropin hormone, and pituitary adenoma size in dogs with Cushing's disease, *J Vet Intern Med* 19:23–28, 2005.
59. Meij B, Voorhout G, Rijnberk A: Progress in transsphenoidal hypophysectomy for treatment of pituitary-dependent hyperadrenocorticism in dogs and cats, *Mol Cell Endocrinol* 197:89–96, 2002.
60. Meij BP, Voorhout G, van den Ingh TS, et al: Results of transsphenoidal hypophysectomy in 52 dogs with pituitary-dependent hyperadrenocorticism, *Vet Surg* 27:246–261, 1998.
61. Hanson JM, van 't HM, Voorhout G, et al: Efficacy of transsphenoidal hypophysectomy in treatment of dogs with pituitary-dependent hyperadrenocorticism, *J Vet Intern Med* 19:687–694, 2005.
62. Dow SW, Lecouteur RA, Rosychuk RAW, et al: Response of dogs with functional pituitary macroadenomas and macrocarcinomas to radiation, *J Small Anim Pract* 31:287–294, 1990.
63. Goossens MM, Feldman EC, Nelson RW, et al: Cobalt 60 irradiation of pituitary gland tumors in three cats with acromegaly, *J Am Vet Med Assoc* 213:374–376, 1998.
64. De Fornel P, Delisle F, Devauchelle P, et al: Effects of radiotherapy on pituitary corticotroph macrotumors in dogs: A retrospective study of 12 cases, *Can Vet J* 48:481–486, 2007.
65. den Hertog E, Braakman JC, Teske E, et al: Results of non-selective adrenocorticolysis by o,p′-DDD in 129 dogs with pituitary-dependent hyperadrenocorticism, *Vet Rec* 144:12–17, 1999.
66. Ramsey IK: Trilostane in dogs, *Vet Clin North Am Small Anim Pract* 40:269–283, 2010.
67. Neiger R, Ramsey I, O'Connor J, et al: Trilostane treatment of 78 dogs with pituitary-dependent hyperadrenocorticism, *Vet Rec* 150:799–804, 2002.
68. Feldman EC: Evaluation of twice-daily lower-dose trilostane treatment administered orally in dogs with naturally occurring hyperadrenocorticism, *J Am Vet Med Assoc* 238:1441–1451, 2011.
69. Vaughan MA, Feldman EC, Hoar BR, et al: Evaluation of twice-daily, low-dose trilostane treatment administered orally in dogs with naturally occurring hyperadrenocorticism, *J Am Vet Med Assoc* 232:1321–1328, 2008.
70. Alenza DP, Arenas C, Lopez ML, et al: Long-term efficacy of trilostane administered twice daily in dogs with pituitary-dependent hyperadrenocorticism, *J Am Anim Hosp Assoc* 42:269–276, 2006.
71. Barker EN, Campbell S, Tebb AJ, et al: A comparison of the survival times of dogs treated with mitotane or trilostane for pituitary-dependent hyperadrenocorticism, *J Vet Intern Med* 19:810–815, 2005.
72. Chapman PS, Kelly DF, Archer J, et al: Adrenal necrosis in a dog receiving trilostane for the treatment of hyperadrenocorticism, *J Small Anim Pract* 45:307–310, 2004.
73. Reusch CE, Sieber-Ruckstuhl N, Wenger M, et al: Histological evaluation of the adrenal glands of seven dogs with hyperadrenocorticism treated with trilostane, *Vet Rec* 160:219–224, 2007.
74. Ruckstuhl NS, Nett CS, Reusch CE: Results of clinical examinations, laboratory tests, and ultrasonography in dogs with pituitary-dependent hyperadrenocorticism treated with trilostane, *Am J Vet Res* 63:506–512, 2002.
75. Cook AK, Nieuwoudt CD, Longhofer SL: Evaluation of content of compounded trilostane products, *J Vet Intern Med* 24:684–685, 2010.
76. Nelson RW, Feldman EC, Smith MC: Hyperadrenocorticism in cats: seven cases (1978-1987), *J Am Vet Med Assoc* 193:245–250, 1988.
77. Watson PJ, Herrtage ME: Hyperadrenocorticism in six cats, *J Small Anim Pract* 39:175–184, 1998.
78. Meij BP, Voorhout G, Van Den Ingh TS, et al: Transsphenoidal hypophysectomy for treatment of pituitary-dependent hyperadrenocorticism in 7 cats, *Vet Surg* 30:72–86, 2001.
79. Meij BP, van der Vlugt-Meijer RH, van den Ingh TS, et al: Somatotroph and corticotroph pituitary adenoma (double adenoma) in a cat with diabetes mellitus and hyperadrenocorticism, *J Comp Pathol* 130:209–215, 2004.
80. Mayer MN, Greco DS, LaRue SM: Outcomes of pituitary tumor irradiation in cats, *J Vet Intern Med* 20:1151–1154, 2006.
81. Duesberg CA, Nelson RW, Feldman EC, et al: Adrenalectomy for treatment of hyperadrenocorticism in cats: 10 cases (1988-1992), *J Am Vet Med Assoc* 207:1066–1070, 1995.
82. Skelly BJ, Petrus D, Nicholls PK: Use of trilostane for the treatment of pituitary-dependent hyperadrenocorticism in a cat, *J Small Anim Pract* 44:269–272, 2003.

83. Neiger R, Witt AL, Noble A, et al: Trilostane therapy for treatment of pituitary-dependent hyperadrenocorticism in 5 cats, *J Vet Intern Med* 18:160–164, 2004.
84. Feldman EC, Nelson RW: Disorders of growth hormone. In Feldman EC, Nelson RW, editors: *Canine and feline endocrinology and reproduction*, ed 3, St. Louis, 2004, Saunders.
85. Niessen SJ, Petrie G, Gaudiano F, et al: Feline acromegaly: an underdiagnosed endocrinopathy? *J Vet Intern Med* 21:899–905, 2007.
86. Peterson ME: Acromegaly in cats: are we only diagnosing the tip of the iceberg? *J Vet Intern Med* 21:889–891, 2007.
87. Peterson ME, Taylor RS, Greco DS, et al: Acromegaly in 14 cats, *J Vet Intern Med* 4:192–201, 1990.
88. Hurty CA, Flatland B: Feline acromegaly: a review of the syndrome, *J Am Anim Hosp Assoc* 41:292–297, 2005.
89. Berg RI, Nelson RW, Feldman EC, et al: Serum insulin-like growth factor-1 concentration in cats with diabetes mellitus and acromegaly, *J Vet Intern Med* 21:892–898, 2007.
90. Niessen SJ: Feline acromegaly: an essential differential diagnosis for the difficult diabetic, *J Feline Med Surg* 12:15–23, 2010.
91. Norman EJ, Mooney CT: Diagnosis and management of diabetes mellitus in five cats with somatotrophic abnormalities, *J Feline Med Surg* 2:183–190, 2000.
92. Morrison SA, Randolph J, Lothrop CD Jr: Hypersomatotropism and insulin-resistant diabetes mellitus in a cat, *J Am Vet Med Assoc* 194:91–94, 1989.
93. Reusch CE, Kley S, Casella M, et al: Measurements of growth hormone and insulin-like growth factor 1 in cats with diabetes mellitus, *Vet Rec* 158:195–200, 2006.
94. Niessen SJ, Khalid M, Petrie G, et al: Validation and application of a radioimmunoassay for ovine growth hormone in the diagnosis of acromegaly in cats, *Vet Rec* 160:902–907, 2007.
95. Slingerland LI, Voorhout G, Rijnberk A, et al: Growth hormone excess and the effect of octreotide in cats with diabetes mellitus, *Domest Anim Endocrinol* 35:352–361, 2008.
96. Meij BP, Auriemma E, Grinwis G, et al: Successful treatment of acromegaly in a diabetic cat with transsphenoidal hypophysectomy, *J Feline Med Surg* 12:406–410, 2010.
97. Elliott DA, Feldman EC, Koblik PD, et al: Prevalence of pituitary tumors among diabetic cats with insulin resistance, *J Am Vet Med Assoc* 216:1765–1768, 2000.
98. Littler RM, Polton GA, Brearley MJ: Resolution of diabetes mellitus but not acromegaly in a cat with a pituitary macroadenoma treated with hypofractionated radiation, *J Small Anim Pract* 47:392–395, 2006.
99. Blois SL, Holmberg DL: Cryohypophysectomy used in the treatment of a case of feline acromegaly, *J Small Anim Pract* 49:596–600, 2008.
100. Dunning MD, Lowrie CS, Bexfield NH, et al: Exogenous insulin treatment after hypofractionated radiotherapy in cats with diabetes mellitus and acromegaly, *J Vet Intern Med* 23:243–249, 2009.
101. Sellon RK, Fidel J, Houston R, et al: Linear-accelerator-based modified radiosurgical treatment of pituitary tumors in cats: 11 cases (1997-2008), *J Vet Intern Med* 23:1038–1044, 2009.
102. Posch B, Dobson J, Herrtage M: Magnetic resonance imaging findings in 15 acromegalic cats, *Vet Radiol Ultrasound* 52:422–427, 2011.
103. Melmed S: Medical progress: Acromegaly, *N Engl J Med* 355:2558–2573, 2006.
104. Melmed S: Acromegaly pathogenesis and treatment, *J Clin Invest* 119:3189–3202, 2009.
105. Melmed S, Colao A, Barkan A, et al: Guidelines for acromegaly management: an update, *J Clin Endocrinol Metab* 94:1509–1517, 2009.
106. Manjila S, Wu OC, Khan FR, et al: Pharmacological management of acromegaly: a current perspective, *Neurosurg Focus* 29:E14, 2010.
107. Kaser-Hotz B, Rohrer CR, Stankeova S, et al: Radiotherapy of pituitary tumours in five cats, *J Small Anim Pract* 43:303–307, 2002.
108. Brearley MJ, Polton GA, Littler RM, et al: Coarse fractionated radiation therapy for pituitary tumours in cats: a retrospective study of 12 cases, *Vet Comp Oncol* 4:209–217, 2006.
109. Laws ER, Sheehan JP, Sheehan JM, et al: Stereotactic radiosurgery for pituitary adenomas: a review of the literature, *J Neurooncol* 69:257–272, 2004.
110. Lunn KF, LaRue SM: Endocrine function in cats after stereotactic radiosurgery treatment of acromegaly, *J Vet Intern Med* 23:698, 2009.
111. Abraham LA, Helmond SE, Mitten RW, et al: Treatment of an acromegalic cat with the dopamine agonist L-deprenyl, *Aust Vet J* 80:479–483, 2002.
112. Myers NC III: Adrenal incidentalomas. Diagnostic workup of the incidentally discovered adrenal mass, *Vet Clin North Am Small Anim Pract* 27:381–399, 1997.
113. Labelle P, De Cock HE: Metastatic tumors to the adrenal glands in domestic animals, *Vet Pathol* 42:52–58, 2005.
114. Schwartz P, Kovak JR, Koprowski A, et al: Evaluation of prognostic factors in the surgical treatment of adrenal gland tumors in dogs: 41 cases (1999-2005), *J Am Vet Med Assoc* 232:77–84, 2008.
115. Massari F, Nicoli S, Romanelli G, et al: Adrenalectomy in dogs with adrenal gland tumors: 52 cases (2002-2008), *J Am Vet Med Assoc* 239:216–221, 2011.
116. Widmer WR, Guptill L: Imaging techniques for facilitating diagnosis of hyperadrenocorticism in dogs and cats, *J Am Vet Med Assoc* 206:1857–1864, 1995.
117. Tidwell AS, Penninck DG, Besso JG: Imaging of adrenal gland disorders, *Vet Clin North Am Small Anim Pract* 27:237–254, 1997.
118. Penninck DG, Feldman EC, Nyland TG: Radiographic features of canine hyperadrenocorticism caused by autonomously functioning adrenocortical tumors: 23 cases (1978-1986), *J Am Vet Med Assoc* 192:1604–1608, 1988.
119. Voorhout G, Stolp R, Rijnberk A, et al: Assessment of survey radiography and comparison with X-ray computed-tomography for detection of hyperfunctioning adrenocortical tumors in dogs, *J Am Vet Med Assoc* 196:1799–1803, 1990.
120. Douglass JP, Berry CR, James S: Ultrasonographic adrenal gland measurements in dogs without evidence of adrenal disease, *Vet Radiol Ultrasound* 38:124–130, 1997.
121. Voorhout G: X-ray-computed tomography, nephrotomography, and ultrasonography of the adrenal glands of healthy dogs, *Am J Vet Res* 51:625–631, 1990.
122. Voorhout G, Rijnberk A, Sjollema BE, et al: Nephrotomography and ultrasonography for the localization of hyperfunctioning adrenocortical tumors in dogs, *Am J Vet Res* 51:1280–1285, 1990.
123. Emms SG, Wortman JA, Johnston DE, et al: Evaluation of canine hyperadrenocorticism, using computed tomography, *J Am Vet Med Assoc* 189:432–439, 1986.
124. Bertolini G, Furlanello T, De Lorenzi D, et al: Computed tomographic quantification of canine adrenal gland volume and attenuation, *Vet Radiol Ultrasound* 47:444–448, 2006.
125. Schultz RM, Wisner ER, Johnson EG, et al: Contrast-enhanced computed tomography as a preoperative indicator of vascular invasion from adrenal masses in dogs, *Vet Radiol Ultrasound* 50:625–629, 2009.
126. Llabres-Diaz FJ, Dennis R: Magnetic resonance imaging of the presumed normal canine adrenal glands, *Vet Radiol Ultrasound* 44:5–19, 2003.
127. Blake MA, Cronin CG, Boland GW: Adrenal imaging, *AJR Am J Roentgenol* 194:1450–1460, 2010.
128. Boland GW, Dwamena BA, Jagtiani Sangwaiya M, et al: Characterization of adrenal masses by using FDG PET: a systematic review and meta-analysis of diagnostic test performance, *Radiology* 259:117–126, 2011.
129. Sangwaiya MJ, Boland GW, Cronin CG, et al: Incidental adrenal lesions: accuracy of characterization with contrast-enhanced washout multidetector CT—10-minute delayed imaging protocol revisited in a large patient cohort, *Radiology* 256:504–510, 2010.

130. Friedrich-Rust M, Glasemann T, Polta A, et al: Differentiation between benign and malignant adrenal mass using contrast-enhanced ultrasound, *Ultraschall Med* 32:460–471, 2011.
131. Scavelli TD, Peterson ME, Matthiesen DT: Results of surgical treatment for hyperadrenocorticism caused by adrenocortical neoplasia in the dog: 25 cases (1980-1984), *J Am Vet Med Assoc* 189:1360–1364, 1986.
132. Labelle P, Kyles AE, Farver TB, et al: Indicators of malignancy of canine adrenocortical tumors: histopathology and proliferation index, *Vet Pathol* 41:490–497, 2004.
133. Whittemore JC, Preston CA, Kyles AE, et al: Nontraumatic rupture of an adrenal gland tumor causing intra-abdominal or retroperitoneal hemorrhage in four dogs, *J Am Vet Med Assoc* 219:329–333, 2001.
134. Galac S, Kars VJ, Klarenbeek S, et al: Expression of receptors for luteinizing hormone, gastric-inhibitory polypeptide, and vasopressin in normal adrenal glands and cortisol-secreting adrenocortical tumors in dogs, *Domest Anim Endocrinol* 39:63–75, 2010.
135. Galac S, Kool MM, Naan EC, et al: Expression of the ACTH receptor, steroidogenic acute regulatory protein, and steroidogenic enzymes in canine cortisol-secreting adrenocortical tumors, *Domest Anim Endocrinol* 39:259–267, 2010.
136. van Sluijs FJ, Sjollema BE, Voorhout G, et al: Results of adrenalectomy in 36 dogs with hyperadrenocorticism caused by adreno-cortical tumour, *Vet Q* 17:113–116, 1995.
137. Jimenez Pelaez M, Bouvy BM, Dupre GP: Laparoscopic adrenalectomy for treatment of unilateral adrenocortical carcinomas: technique, complications, and results in seven dogs, *Vet Surg* 37:444–453, 2008.
138. Kintzer PP, Peterson ME: Diagnosis and management of canine cortisol-secreting adrenal tumors, *Vet Clin North Am Small Anim Pract* 27:299–307, 1997.
139. Feldman EC, Nelson RW, Feldman MS, et al: Comparison of mitotane treatment for adrenal tumor versus pituitary-dependent hyperadrenocorticism in dogs, *J Am Vet Med Assoc* 200:1642–1647, 1992.
140. Kintzer PP, Peterson ME: Mitotane treatment of 32 dogs with cortisol-secreting adrenocortical neoplasms, *J Am Vet Med Assoc* 205:54–61, 1994.
141. Eastwood JM, Elwood CM, Hurley KJ: Trilostane treatment of a dog with functional adrenocortical neoplasia, *J Small Anim Pract* 44:126–131, 2003.
142. Benchekroun G, de Fornel-Thibaud P, Lafarge S, et al: Trilostane therapy for hyperadrenocorticism in three dogs with adrenocortical metastasis, *Vet Rec* 163:190–192, 2008.
143. Helm JR, McLauchlan G, Boden LA, et al: A comparison of factors that influence survival in dogs with adrenal-dependent hyperadrenocorticism treated with mitotane or trilostane, *J Vet Intern Med* 25:251–260, 2011.
144. Boord M, Griffin C: Progesterone secreting adrenal mass in a cat with clinical signs of hyperadrenocorticism, *J Am Vet Med Assoc* 214:666–669, 1999.
145. Rossmeisl JH Jr, Scott-Moncrieff JC, Siems J, et al: Hyperadrenocorticism and hyperprogesteronemia in a cat with an adrenocortical adenocarcinoma, *J Am Anim Hosp Assoc* 36:512–517, 2000.
146. Syme HM, Scott-Moncrieff JC, Treadwell NG, et al: Hyperadrenocorticism associated with excessive sex hormone production by an adrenocortical tumor in two dogs, *J Am Vet Med Assoc* 219:1725–1728, 1707–1728, 2001.
147. Hill KE, Scott-Moncrieff JC, Koshko MA, et al: Secretion of sex hormones in dogs with adrenal dysfunction, *J Am Vet Med Assoc* 226:556–561, 2005.
148. DeClue AE, Breshears LA, Pardo ID, et al: Hyperaldosteronism and hyperprogesteronism in a cat with an adrenal cortical carcinoma, *J Vet Intern Med* 19:355–358, 2005.
149. Briscoe K, Barrs VR, Foster DF, et al: Hyperaldosteronism and hyperprogesteronism in a cat, *J Feline Med Surg* 11:758–762, 2009.
150. Millard RP, Pickens EH, Wells KL: Excessive production of sex hormones in a cat with an adrenocortical tumor, *J Am Vet Med Assoc* 234:505–508, 2009.
151. Meler EN, Scott-Moncrieff JC, Peter AT, et al: Cyclic estrous-like behavior in a spayed cat associated with excessive sex-hormone production by an adrenocortical carcinoma, *J Feline Med Surg* 13:473–478, 2011.
152. Rijnberk A, Kooistra HS, van Vonderen IK, et al: Aldosteronoma in a dog with polyuria as the leading symptom, *Domest Anim Endocrinol* 20:227–240, 2001.
153. Behrend EN, Weigand CM, Whitley EM, et al: Corticosterone- and aldosterone-secreting adrenocortical tumor in a dog, *J Am Vet Med Assoc* 226:1662–1666, 2005.
154. Machida T, Uchida E, Matsuda K, et al: Aldosterone-, corticosterone- and cortisol-secreting adrenocortical carcinoma in a dog: case report, *J Vet Med Sci* 70:317–320, 2008.
155. Djajadiningrat-Laanen S, Galac S, Kooistra H: Primary hyperaldosteronism: expanding the diagnostic net, *J Feline Med Surg* 13:641–650, 2011.
156. Javadi S, Djajadiningrat-Laanen SC, Kooistra HS, et al: Primary hyperaldosteronism, a mediator of progressive renal disease in cats, *Domest Anim Endocrinol* 28:85–104, 2005.
157. Djajadiningrat-Laanen SC, Galac S, Cammelbeeck SE, et al: Urinary aldosterone to creatinine ratio in cats before and after suppression with salt or fludrocortisone acetate, *J Vet Intern Med* 22:1283–1288, 2008.
158. Moore LE, Biller DS, Smith TA: Use of abdominal ultrasonography in the diagnosis of primary hyperaldosteronism in a cat, *J Am Vet Med Assoc* 217:213–215, 2000.
159. Schulman RL: Feline primary hyperaldosteronism, *Vet Clin North Am Small Anim Pract* 40:353–359, 2010.
160. Ash RA, Harvey AM, Tasker S: Primary hyperaldosteronism in the cat: a series of 13 cases, *J Feline Med Surg* 7:173–182, 2005.
161. Flood SM, Randolph JF, Gelzer AR, et al: Primary hyperaldosteronism in two cats, *J Am Anim Hosp Assoc* 35:411–416, 1999.
162. MacKay AD, Holt PE, Sparkes AH: Successful surgical treatment of a cat with primary aldosteronism, *J Feline Med Surg* 1:117–122, 1999.
163. Rose SA, Kyles AE, Labelle P, et al: Adrenalectomy and caval thrombectomy in a cat with primary hyperaldosteronism, *J Am Anim Hosp Assoc* 43:209–214, 2007.
164. Herrera M, Nelson RW: Pheochromocytoma. In Ettinger SJ, Feldman EC, editors: *Textbook of veterinary internal medicine*, ed 7, St. Louis, 2010, Saunders Elsevier.
165. Wimpole JA, Adagra CF, Billson MF, et al: Plasma free metanephrines in healthy cats, cats with non-adrenal disease and a cat with suspected phaeochromocytoma, *J Feline Med Surg* 12:435–440, 2010.
166. Gilson SD, Withrow SJ, Wheeler SL, et al: Pheochromocytoma in 50 dogs, *J Vet Intern Med* 8:228–232, 1994.
167. Barthez PY, Marks SL, Woo J, et al: Pheochromocytoma in dogs: 61 cases (1984-1995), *J Vet Intern Med* 11:272–278, 1997.
168. Feldman EC, Nelson RW: Pheochromocytoma and multiple endocrine neoplasia. In Feldman EC, Nelson RW, editors: *Canine and feline endocrinology and reproduction*, ed 3, St. Louis, 2004, Saunders.
169. Herrera MA, Mehl ML, Kass PH, et al: Predictive factors and the effect of phenoxybenzamine on outcome in dogs undergoing adrenalectomy for pheochromocytoma, *J Vet Intern Med* 22:1333–1339, 2008.
170. Rosenstein DS: Diagnostic imaging in canine pheochromocytoma, *Vet Radiol Ultrasound* 41:499–506, 2000.
171. Hylands R: Veterinary diagnostic imaging. Malignant pheochromocytoma of the left adrenal gland invading the caudal vena cava, accompanied by a cortisol secreting adrenocortical carcinoma of the right adrenal gland, *Can Vet J* 46:1156–1158, 2005.

172. Spall B, Chen AV, Tucker RL, et al: Imaging diagnosis-metastatic adrenal pheochromocytoma in a dog, *Vet Radiol Ultrasound* 52:534–537, 2011.
173. Berry CR, DeGrado TR, Nutter F, et al: Imaging of pheochromocytoma in 2 dogs using p-[18F] fluorobenzylguanidine, *Vet Radiol Ultrasound* 3:183–186, 2002.
174. Head LL, Daniel GB: Scintigraphic diagnosis—an unusual presentation of metastatic pheochromocytoma in a dog, *Vet Radiol Ultrasound* 45:574–576, 2004.
175. Doss JC, Grone A, Capen CC, et al: Immunohistochemical localization of chromogranin A in endocrine tissues and endocrine tumors of dogs, *Vet Pathol* 35:312–315, 1998.
176. Kook PH, Boretti FS, Hersberger M, et al: Urinary catecholamine and metanephrine to creatinine ratios in healthy dogs at home and in a hospital environment and in 2 dogs with pheochromocytoma, *J Vet Intern Med* 21:388–393, 2007.
177. Kook PH, Grest P, Quante S, et al: Urinary catecholamine and metadrenaline to creatinine ratios in dogs with a phaeochromocytoma, *Vet Rec* 166:169–174, 2010.
178. Quante S, Boretti FS, Kook PH, et al: Urinary catecholamine and metanephrine to creatinine ratios in dogs with hyperadrenocorticism or pheochromocytoma, and in healthy dogs, *J Vet Intern Med* 24:1093–1097, 2010.
179. Gostelow R, Syme HM: Plasma free metanephrine and normetanephrine concentrations are elevated in dogs with pheochromocytoma, *J Vet Intern Med* 25:680–681, 2011.
180. Bommarito DA, Lattimer JC, Selting KA, et al: Treatment of a malignant pheochromocytoma in a dog using 131I metaiodobenzylguanidine, *J Am Anim Hosp Assoc* 47:e188–e194, 2011.
181. Gilson SD, Withrow SJ, Orton EC: Surgical treatment of pheochromocytoma: technique, complications, and results in six dogs, *Vet Surg* 23:195–200, 1994.
182. Matthiesen DT, Mullen HS: Problems and complications associated with endocrine surgery in the dog and cat, *Probl Vet Med* 2:627–667, 1990.
183. Brodey RS, Kelly DF: Thyroid neoplasms in the dog. A clinicopathologic study of fifty-seven cases, *Cancer* 22:406–416, 1968.
184. Harari J, Patterson JS, Rosenthal RC: Clinical and pathologic features of thyroid tumors in 26 dogs, *J Am Vet Med Assoc* 188:1160–1164, 1986.
185. Wucherer KL, Wilke V: Thyroid cancer in dogs: an update based on 638 cases (1995-2005), *J Am Anim Hosp Assoc* 46:249–254, 2010.
186. Leav I, Schiller AL, Rijnberk A, et al: Adenomas and carcinomas of the canine and feline thyroid, *Am J Pathol* 83:61–122, 1976.
187. Lurye JC, Behrend EN: Endocrine tumors, *Vet Clin North Am Small Anim Pract* 31:1083–1110, 2001.
188. Feldman EC, Nelson RW: Canine thyroid tumors and hyperthyroidism. In Feldman EC, Nelson RW, editors: *Canine and feline endocrinology and reproduction*, ed 3, St. Louis, 2004, Saunders.
189. Ramos-Vara JA, Miller MA, Johnson GC, et al: Immunohistochemical detection of thyroid transcription factor-1, thyroglobulin, and calcitonin in canine normal, hyperplastic, and neoplastic thyroid gland, *Vet Pathol* 39:480–487, 2002.
190. Leblanc B, Parodi AL, Lagadic M, et al: Immunocytochemistry of canine thyroid tumors, *Vet Pathol* 28:370–380, 1991.
191. Carver JR, Kapatkin A, Patnaik AK: A comparison of medullary thyroid carcinoma and thyroid adenocarcinoma in dogs: a retrospective study of 38 cases, *Vet Surg* 24:315–319, 1995.
192. Schlumberger MJ: Papillary and follicular thyroid carcinoma, *N Engl J Med* 338:297–306, 1998.
193. Klein MK, Powers BE, Withrow SJ, et al: Treatment of thyroid carcinoma in dogs by surgical resection alone: 20 cases (1981-1989), *J Am Vet Med Assoc* 206:1007–1009, 1995.
194. Patnaik AK, Lieberman PH: Gross, histologic, cytochemical, and immunocytochemical study of medullary thyroid carcinoma in sixteen dogs, *Vet Pathol* 28:223–233, 1991.
195. Garcia-Jimenez C, Santisteban P: TSH signalling and cancer, *Arq Bras Endocrinol Metabol* 51:654–671, 2007.
196. Verschueren CP, Rutteman GR, Vos JH, et al: Thyrotrophin receptors in normal and neoplastic (primary and metastatic) canine thyroid tissue, *J Endocrinol* 132:461–468, 1992.
197. Benjamin SA, Stephens LC, Hamilton BF, et al: Associations between lymphocytic thyroiditis, hypothyroidism, and thyroid neoplasia in beagles, *Vet Pathol* 33:486–494, 1996.
198. Devilee P, Van Leeuwen IS, Voesten A, et al: The canine p53 gene is subject to somatic mutations in thyroid carcinoma, *Anticancer Res* 14:2039–2046, 1994.
199. Reimann N, Nolte I, Bonk U, et al: Trisomy 18 in a canine thyroid adenoma, *Cancer Genet Cytogenet* 90:154–156, 1996.
200. Theon AP, Marks SL, Feldman ES, et al: Prognostic factors and patterns of treatment failure in dogs with unresectable differentiated thyroid carcinomas treated with megavoltage irradiation, *J Am Vet Med Assoc* 216:1775–1779, 2000.
201. Pack L, Roberts RE, Dawson SD, et al: Definitive radiation therapy for infiltrative thyroid carcinoma in dogs, *Vet Radiol Ultrasound* 42:471–474, 2001.
202. Kent MS, Griffey SM, Verstraete FJ, et al: Computer-assisted image analysis of neovascularization in thyroid neoplasms from dogs, *Am J Vet Res* 63:363–369, 2002.
203. Lee JJ, Larsson C, Lui WO, et al: A dog pedigree with familial medullary thyroid cancer, *Int J Oncol* 29:1173–1182, 2006.
204. Marks SL, Koblik PD, Hornof WJ, et al: 99mTc-pertechnetate imaging of thyroid tumors in dogs: 29 cases (1980-1992), *J Am Vet Med Assoc* 204:756–760, 1994.
205. Lantz GC, Salisbury SK: Surgical excision of ectopic thyroid carcinoma involving the base of the tongue in dogs: three cases (1980-1987), *J Am Vet Med Assoc* 195:1606–1608, 1989.
206. Ware WA, Hopper DL: Cardiac tumors in dogs: 1982-1995, *J Vet Intern Med* 13:95–103, 1999.
207. Almes KM, Heaney AM, Andrews GA: Intracardiac ectopic thyroid carcinosarcoma in a dog, *Vet Pathol* 45:500–504, 2008.
208. Bracha S, Caron I, Holmberg DL, et al: Ectopic thyroid carcinoma causing right ventricular outflow tract obstruction in a dog, *J Am Anim Hosp Assoc* 45:138–141, 2009.
209. Roth DR, Perentes E: Ectopic thyroid tissue in the periaortic area, cardiac cavity and aortic valve in a Beagle dog: a case report, *Exp Toxicol Pathol* 64(3):243–245, 2012.
210. Di Palma S, Lombard C, Kappeler A, et al: Intracardiac ectopic thyroid adenoma in a dog, *Vet Rec* 167:709–710, 2010.
211. Brearley MJ, Hayes AM, Murphy S: Hypofractionated radiation therapy for invasive thyroid carcinoma in dogs: a retrospective analysis of survival, *J Small Anim Pract* 40:206–210, 1999.
212. Bezzola P: Thyroid carcinoma and hyperthyroidism in a dog, *Can Vet J* 43:125–126, 2002.
213. Lawrence D, Thompson J, Layton AW, et al: Hyperthyroidism associated with a thyroid adenoma in a dog, *J Am Vet Med Assoc* 199:81–83, 1991.
214. Simpson AC, McCown JL: Systemic hypertension in a dog with a functional thyroid gland adenocarcinoma, *J Am Vet Med Assoc* 235:1474–1479, 2009.
215. Slensky KA, Volk SW, Schwarz T, et al: Acute severe hemorrhage secondary to arterial invasion in a dog with thyroid carcinoma, *J Am Vet Med Assoc* 223:649–653, 2003.
216. Wisner ER, Nyland TG: Ultrasonography of the thyroid and parathyroid glands, *Vet Clin North Am Small Anim Pract* 28:973–991, 1998.
217. Taeymans O, Peremans K, Saunders JH: Thyroid imaging in the dog: current status and future directions, *J Vet Intern Med* 21:673–684, 2007.
218. Taeymans O, Dennis R, Saunders JH: Magnetic resonance imaging of the normal canine thyroid gland, *Vet Radiol Ultrasound* 49:238–242, 2008.

219. Taeymans O, Schwarz T, Duchateau L, et al: Computed tomographic features of the normal canine thyroid gland, *Vet Radiol Ultrasound* 49:13–19, 2008.
220. Broome MR, Donner GS: The insensitivity of ^{99m}Tc pertechnetate for detecting metastases of a functional thyroid carcinoma in a dog, *Vet Radiol Ultrasound* 34:118–124, 1993.
221. Feeney DA, Anderson KL: Nuclear imaging and radiation therapy in canine and feline thyroid disease, *Vet Clin North Am Small Anim Pract* 37:799–821, 2007.
222. Itoh T, Kojimoto A, Nibe K, et al: Functional thyroid gland adenoma in a dog treated with surgical excision alone, *J Vet Med Sci* 69:61–63, 2007.
223. Radlinsky MG: Thyroid surgery in dogs and cats, *Vet Clin North Am Small Anim Pract* 37:789–798, 2007.
224. Tuohy JL, Worley DR, Withrow SJ: Outcome following simultaneous bilateral thyroid lobectomy for treatment of thyroid carcinoma in 15 dogs, *J Am Vet Med Assoc* 2012 (In Press).
225. Kramer RW, Price GS, Spodnick GJ: Hypothyroidism in a dog after surgery and radiation therapy for a functional thyroid adenocarcinoma, *Vet Radiol Ultrasound* 35:132–136, 1994.
226. Worth AJ, Zuber RM, Hocking M: Radioiodide (131I) therapy for the treatment of canine thyroid carcinoma, *Aust Vet J* 83:208–214, 2005.
227. Turrel JM, McEntee MC, Burke BP, et al: Sodium iodide I 131 treatment of dogs with nonresectable thyroid tumors: 39 cases (1990-2003), *J Am Vet Med Assoc* 229:542–548, 2006.
228. Jeglum KA, Whereat A: Chemotherapy of canine thyroid carcinoma, *Compend Contin Educ Vet* 5:96–98, 1983.
229. Fineman LS, Hamilton TA, de Gortari A, et al: Cisplatin chemotherapy for treatment of thyroid carcinoma in dogs: 13 cases, *J Am Anim Hosp Assoc* 34:109–112, 1998.
230. Ogilvie GK, Obradovich JE, Elmslie RE, et al: Efficacy of mitoxantrone against various neoplasms in dogs, *J Am Vet Med Assoc* 198:1618–1621, 1991.
231. Hammer AS, Couto CG, Ayl RD, et al: Treatment of tumor-bearing dogs with actinomycin D, *J Vet Intern Med* 8:236–239, 1994.
232. Feldman EC, Nelson RW: Feline hyperthyroidism (thyrotoxicosis). In Feldman EC, Nelson RW, editors: *Canine and feline endocrinology and reproduction*, ed 3, St. Louis, 2004, Saunders.
233. Mooney CT: Hyperthyroidism. In Ettinger SJ, Feldman EC, editors: *Textbook of veterinary internal medicine*, ed 7, St. Louis, 2010, Saunders Elsevier.
234. Naan EC, Kirpensteijn J, Kooistra HS, et al: Results of thyroidectomy in 101 cats with hyperthyroidism, *Vet Surg* 35:287–293, 2006.
235. Peterson ME, Kintzer PP, Cavanagh PG, et al: Feline hyperthyroidism: pretreatment clinical and laboratory evaluation of 131 cases, *J Am Vet Med Assoc* 183:103–110, 1983.
236. Guptill L, Scott-Moncrieff CR, Janovitz EB, et al: Response to high-dose radioactive iodine administration in cats with thyroid carcinoma that had previously undergone surgery, *J Am Vet Med Assoc* 207:1055–1058, 1995.
237. Hibbert A, Gruffydd-Jones T, Barrett EL, et al: Feline thyroid carcinoma: diagnosis and response to high-dose radioactive iodine treatment, *J Feline Med Surg* 11:116–124, 2009.
238. Turrel JM, Feldman EC, Nelson RW, et al: Thyroid carcinoma causing hyperthyroidism in cats: 14 cases (1981-1986), *J Am Vet Med Assoc* 193:359–364, 1988.
239. Cook SM, Daniel GB, Walker MA, et al: Radiographic and scintigraphic evidence of focal pulmonary neoplasia in three cats with hyperthyroidism: diagnostic and therapeutic considerations, *J Vet Intern Med* 7:303–308, 1993.
240. Peterson ME, Ward CR: Etiopathologic findings of hyperthyroidism in cats, *Vet Clin North Am Small Anim Pract* 37:633–645, 2007.
241. Hammer KB, Holt DE, Ward CR: Altered expression of G proteins in thyroid gland adenomas obtained from hyperthyroid cats, *Am J Vet Res* 61:874–879, 2000.
242. Ward CR, Achenbach SE, Peterson ME, et al: Expression of inhibitory G proteins in adenomatous thyroid glands obtained from hyperthyroid cats, *Am J Vet Res* 66:1478–1482, 2005.
243. Peeters ME, Timmermans-Sprang EP, Mol JA: Feline thyroid adenomas are in part associated with mutations in the G(s alpha) gene and not with polymorphisms found in the thyrotropin receptor, *Thyroid* 12:571–575, 2002.
244. Ward CR, Windham WR, Dise D: Evaluation of activation of G proteins in response to thyroid stimulating hormone in thyroid gland cells from euthyroid and hyperthyroid cats, *Am J Vet Res* 71:643–648, 2010.
245. Pearce SH, Foster DJ, Imrie H, et al: Mutational analysis of the thyrotropin receptor gene in sporadic and familial feline thyrotoxicosis, *Thyroid* 7:923–927, 1997.
246. Watson SG, Radford AD, Kipar A, et al: Somatic mutations of the thyroid-stimulating hormone receptor gene in feline hyperthyroidism: parallels with human hyperthyroidism, *J Endocrinol* 186:523–537, 2005.
247. Merryman JI, Buckles EL, Bowers G, et al: Overexpression of c-Ras in hyperplasia and adenomas of the feline thyroid gland: an immunohistochemical analysis of 34 cases, *Vet Pathol* 36:117–124, 1999.
248. Kass PH, Peterson ME, Levy J, et al: Evaluation of environmental, nutritional, and host factors in cats with hyperthyroidism, *J Vet Intern Med* 13:323–329, 1999.
249. Martin KM, Rossing MA, Ryland LM, et al: Evaluation of dietary and environmental risk factors for hyperthyroidism in cats, *J Am Vet Med Assoc* 217:853–856, 2000.
250. Edinboro CH, Scott-Moncrieff JC, Janovitz E, et al: Epidemiologic study of relationships between consumption of commercial canned food and risk of hyperthyroidism in cats, *J Am Vet Med Assoc* 224:879–886, 2004.
251. Olczak J, Jones BR, Pfeiffer DU, et al: Multivariate analysis of risk factors for feline hyperthyroidism in New Zealand, *N Z Vet J* 53:53–58, 2005.
252. Dye JA, Venier M, Zhu L, et al: Elevated PBDE levels in pet cats: sentinels for humans? *Environ Sci Technol* 41:6350–6356, 2007.
253. Wakeling J, Everard A, Brodbelt D, et al: Risk factors for feline hyperthyroidism in the UK, *J Small Anim Pract* 50:406–414, 2009.
254. Edinboro CH, Scott-Moncrieff JC, Glickman LT: Feline hyperthyroidism: potential relationship with iodine supplement requirements of commercial cat foods, *J Feline Med Surg* 12:672–679, 2010.
255. Broussard JD, Peterson ME, Fox PR: Changes in clinical and laboratory findings in cats with hyperthyroidism from 1983 to 1993, *J Am Vet Med Assoc* 206:302–305, 1995.
256. Milner RJ, Channell CD, Levy JK, et al: Survival times for cats with hyperthyroidism treated with iodine 131, methimazole, or both: 167 cases (1996-2003), *J Am Vet Med Assoc* 228:559–563, 2006.
257. Harvey AM, Hibbert A, Barrett EL, et al: Scintigraphic findings in 120 hyperthyroid cats, *J Feline Med Surg* 11:96–106, 2009.
258. Elliott J, Barber PJ, Syme HM, et al: Feline hypertension: clinical findings and response to antihypertensive treatment in 30 cases, *J Small Anim Pract* 42:122–129, 2001.
259. Peterson ME, Melian C, Nichols R: Measurement of serum concentrations of free thyroxine, total thyroxine, and total triiodothyronine in cats with hyperthyroidism and cats with nonthyroidal disease, *J Am Vet Med Assoc* 218:529–536, 2001.
260. Peterson ME, Graves TK, Cavanagh I: Serum thyroid hormone concentrations fluctuate in cats with hyperthyroidism, *J Vet Intern Med* 1:142–146, 1987.
261. Mooney CT, Little CJ, Macrae AW: Effect of illness not associated with the thyroid gland on serum total and free thyroxine concentrations in cats, *J Am Vet Med Assoc* 208:2004–2008, 1996.
262. Wakeling J, Moore K, Elliott J, et al: Diagnosis of hyperthyroidism in cats with mild chronic kidney disease, *J Small Anim Pract* 49:287–294, 2008.

263. Mooney CT, Thoday KL, Doxey DL: Serum thyroxine and triiodothyronine responses of hyperthyroid cats to thyrotropin, *Am J Vet Res* 57:987–991, 1996.
264. Tomsa K, Glaus TM, Kacl GM, et al: Thyrotropin-releasing hormone stimulation test to assess thyroid function in severely sick cats, *J Vet Intern Med* 15:89–93, 2001.
265. Peterson ME, Graves TK, Gamble DA: Triiodothyronine (T3) suppression test. An aid in the diagnosis of mild hyperthyroidism in cats, *J Vet Intern Med* 4:233–238, 1990.
266. Refsal KR, Nachreiner RF, Stein BE, et al: Use of the triiodothyronine suppression test for diagnosis of hyperthyroidism in ill cats that have serum concentration of iodothyronines within normal range, *J Am Vet Med Assoc* 199:1594–1601, 1991.
267. Bond BR, Fox PR, Peterson ME, et al: Echocardiographic findings in 103 cats with hyperthyroidism, *J Am Vet Med Assoc* 192:1546–1549, 1988.
268. Fox PR, Peterson ME, Broussard JD: Electrocardiographic and radiographic changes in cats with hyperthyroidism: comparison of populations evaluated during 1992-1993 vs. 1979-1982, *J Am Anim Hosp Assoc* 35:27–31, 1999.
269. Peterson ME, Becker DV: Radionuclide thyroid imaging in 135 cats with hyperthyroidism, *Vet Radiol Ultrasound* 25:23–27, 1984.
270. Peterson ME, Kintzer PP, Hurvitz AI: Methimazole treatment of 262 cats with hyperthyroidism, *J Vet Intern Med* 2:150–157, 1988.
271. Mooney CT, Thoday KL, Doxey DL: Carbimazole therapy of feline hyperthyroidism, *J Small Anim Pract* 33:228–235, 1992.
272. Trepanier LA, Hoffman SB, Kroll M, et al: Efficacy and safety of once versus twice daily administration of methimazole in cats with hyperthyroidism, *J Am Vet Med Assoc* 222:954–958, 2003.
273. Frenais R, Rosenberg D, Burgaud S, et al: Clinical efficacy and safety of a once-daily formulation of carbimazole in cats with hyperthyroidism, *J Small Anim Pract* 50:510–515, 2009.
274. Hoffman SB, Yoder AR, Trepanier LA: Bioavailability of transdermal methimazole in a pluronic lecithin organogel (PLO) in healthy cats, *J Vet Pharmacol Ther* 25:189–193, 2002.
275. Hoffmann G, Marks SL, Taboada J, et al: Transdermal methimazole treatment in cats with hyperthyroidism, *J Feline Med Surg* 5:77–82, 2003.
276. Sartor LL, Trepanier LA, Kroll MM, et al: Efficacy and safety of transdermal methimazole in the treatment of cats with hyperthyroidism, *J Vet Intern Med* 18:651–655, 2004.
277. Buijtels JJ, Kurvers IA, Galac S, et al: [Transdermal carbimazole for the treatment of feline hyperthyroidism], *Tijdschr Diergeneeskd* 131:478–482, 2006.
278. Trepanier LA: Pharmacologic management of feline hyperthyroidism, *Vet Clin North Am Small Anim Pract* 37:775–788, 2007.
279. Murray LA, Peterson ME: Ipodate treatment of hyperthyroidism in cats, *J Am Vet Med Assoc* 211:63–67, 1997.
280. Gallagher AE, Panciera DL: Efficacy of iopanoic acid for treatment of spontaneous hyperthyroidism in cats, *J Feline Med Surg* 13:441–447, 2011.
281. Melendez LD, Yamka RM, Burris PA: Titration of dietary iodine for maintaining normal serum thyroxine concentrations in hyperthyroid cats, *J Vet Intern Med* 25:683, 2011.
282. Melendez LM, Yamka RM, Forrester SD, et al: Titration of dietary iodine for reducing serum thyroxine concentrations in newly diagnosed hyperthyroid cats, *J Vet Intern Med* 25:683, 2011.
283. Yu S, Wedekind KJ, Burris PA, et al: Controlled level of dietary iodine normalizes serum total thyroxine in cats with naturally occurring hyperthyroidism, *J Vet Intern Med* 25:683–684, 2011.
284. Flanders JA: Surgical options for the treatment of hyperthyroidism in the cat, *J Feline Med Surg* 1:127–134, 1999.
285. Birchard SJ: Thyroidectomy in the cat, *Clin Tech Small Anim Pract* 21:29–33, 2006.
286. Padgett S: Feline thyroid surgery, *Vet Clin North Am Small Anim Pract* 32:851–859, 2002.
287. Peterson ME, Becker DV: Radioiodine treatment of 524 cats with hyperthyroidism, *J Am Vet Med Assoc* 207:1422–1428, 1995.
288. Chun R, Garrett LD, Sargeant J, et al: Predictors of response to radioiodine therapy in hyperthyroid cats, *Vet Radiol Ultrasound* 43:587–591, 2002.
289. Turrel JM, Feldman EC, Hays M, et al: Radioactive iodine therapy in cats with hyperthyroidism, *J Am Vet Med Assoc* 184:554–559, 1984.
290. Meric SM, Hawkins EC, Washabau RJ, et al: Serum thyroxine concentrations after radioactive iodine therapy in cats with hyperthyroidism, *J Am Vet Med Assoc* 188:1038–1040, 1986.
291. Meric SM, Rubin SI: Serum thyroxine concentrations following fixed-dose radioactive iodine treatment in hyperthyroid cats: 62 cases (1986-1989), *J Am Vet Med Assoc* 197:621–623, 1990.
292. Peterson ME: Radioiodine treatment of hyperthyroidism, *Clin Tech Small Anim Pract* 21:34–39, 2006.
293. Boag AK, Neiger R, Slater L, et al: Changes in the glomerular filtration rate of 27 cats with hyperthyroidism after treatment with radioactive iodine, *Vet Rec* 161:711–715, 2007.
294. Nykamp SG, Dykes NL, Zarfoss MK, et al: Association of the risk of development of hypothyroidism after iodine 131 treatment with the pretreatment pattern of sodium pertechnetate Tc 99m uptake in the thyroid gland in cats with hyperthyroidism: 165 cases (1990-2002), *J Am Vet Med Assoc* 226:1671–1675, 2005.
295. Goldstein RE, Long C, Swift NC, et al: Percutaneous ethanol injection for treatment of unilateral hyperplastic thyroid nodules in cats, *J Am Vet Med Assoc* 218:1298–1302, 2001.
296. Wells AL, Long CD, Hornof WJ, et al: Use of percutaneous ethanol injection for treatment of bilateral hyperplastic thyroid nodules in cats, *J Am Vet Med Assoc* 218:1293–1297, 2001.
297. Mallery KF, Pollard RE, Nelson RW, et al: Percutaneous ultrasound-guided radiofrequency heat ablation for treatment of hyperthyroidism in cats, *J Am Vet Med Assoc* 223:1602–1607, 2003.
298. Graves TK, Olivier NB, Nachreiner RF, et al: Changes in renal function associated with treatment of hyperthyroidism in cats, *Am J Vet Res* 55:1745–1749, 1994.
299. Becker TJ, Graves TK, Kruger JM, et al: Effects of methimazole on renal function in cats with hyperthyroidism, *J Am Anim Hosp Assoc* 36:215–223, 2000.
300. DiBartola SP, Broome MR, Stein BS, et al: Effect of treatment of hyperthyroidism on renal function in cats, *J Am Vet Med Assoc* 208:875–878, 1996.
301. Adams WH, Daniel GB, Legendre AM, et al: Changes in renal function in cats following treatment of hyperthyroidism using 131I, *Vet Radiol Ultrasound* 38:231–238, 1997.
302. van Hoek I, Lefebvre HP, Peremans K, et al: Short- and long-term follow-up of glomerular and tubular renal markers of kidney function in hyperthyroid cats after treatment with radioiodine, *Domest Anim Endocrinol* 36:45–56, 2009.
303. Riensche MR, Graves TK, Schaeffer DJ: An investigation of predictors of renal insufficiency following treatment of hyperthyroidism in cats, *J Feline Med Surg* 10:160–166, 2008.
304. Williams TL, Peak KJ, Brodbelt D, et al: Survival and the development of azotemia after treatment of hyperthyroid cats, *J Vet Intern Med* 24:863–869, 2010.
305. Williams TL, Elliott J, Syme HM: Association of iatrogenic hypothyroidism with azotemia and reduced survival time in cats treated for hyperthyroidism, *J Vet Intern Med* 24:1086–1092, 2010.
306. Kallet AJ, Richter KP, Feldman EC, et al: Primary hyperparathyroidism in cats: seven cases (1984-1989), *J Am Vet Med Assoc* 199:1767–1771, 1991.
307. Feldman EC, Nelson RW: Hypercalcemia and primary hyperparathyroidism. In Feldman EC, Nelson RW, editors: *Canine and feline endocrinology and reproduction*, ed 3, St. Louis, 2004, Saunders.
308. Barber PJ: Disorders of the parathyroid glands, *J Feline Med Surg* 6:259–269, 2004.

309. Feldman EC, Hoar B, Pollard R, et al: Pretreatment clinical and laboratory findings in dogs with primary hyperparathyroidism: 210 cases (1987-2004), *J Am Vet Med Assoc* 227:756–761, 2005.
310. Gear RN, Neiger R, Skelly BJ, et al: Primary hyperparathyroidism in 29 dogs: diagnosis, treatment, outcome and associated renal failure, *J Small Anim Pract* 46:10–16, 2005.
311. Rasor L, Pollard R, Feldman EC: Retrospective evaluation of three treatment methods for primary hyperparathyroidism in dogs, *J Am Anim Hosp Assoc* 43:70–77, 2007.
312. Feldman EC: Disorders of the parathyroid glands. In Ettinger SJ, Feldman EC, editors: *Textbook of veterinary internal medicine*, ed 7, St. Louis, 2010, Saunders Elsevier.
313. Cavana P, Vittone V, Capucchio MT, et al: Parathyroid adenocarcinoma in a nephropathic Persian cat, *J Feline Med Surg* 8:340–344, 2006.
314. Skelly BJ, Franklin RJ: Mutations in genes causing human familial isolated hyperparathyroidism do not account for hyperparathyroidism in Keeshond dogs, *Vet J* 174:652–654, 2007.
315. Goldstein RE, Atwater DZ, Cazolli DM, et al: Inheritance, mode of inheritance, and candidate genes for primary hyperparathyroidism in Keeshonden, *J Vet Intern Med* 21:199–203, 2007.
316. Schenck PA, Chew DJ: Prediction of serum ionized calcium concentration by use of serum total calcium concentration in dogs, *Am J Vet Res* 66:1330–1336, 2005.
317. Schenck PA, Chew DJ: Prediction of serum ionized calcium concentration by serum total calcium measurement in cats, *Can J Vet Res* 74:209–213, 2010.
318. Savary KC, Price GS, Vaden SL: Hypercalcemia in cats: a retrospective study of 71 cases (1991-1997), *J Vet Intern Med* 14:184–189, 2000.
319. Messinger JS, Windham WR, Ward CR: Ionized hypercalcemia in dogs: a retrospective study of 109 cases (1998-2003), *J Vet Intern Med* 23:514–519, 2009.
320. Feldman EC, Wisner ER, Nelson RW, et al: Comparison of results of hormonal analysis of samples obtained from selected venous sites versus cervical ultrasonography for localizing parathyroid masses in dogs, *J Am Vet Med Assoc* 211:54–56, 1997.
321. Sueda MT, Stefanacci JD: Ultrasound evaluation of the parathyroid glands in two hypercalcemic cats, *Vet Radiol Ultrasound* 41:448–451, 2000.
322. Liles SR, Linder KE, Cain B, et al: Ultrasonography of histologically normal parathyroid glands and thyroid lobules in normocalcemic dogs, *Vet Radiol Ultrasound* 51:447–452, 2010.
323. Matwichuk CL, Taylor SM, Daniel GB, et al: Double-phase parathyroid scintigraphy in dogs using technetium-99M-sestamibi, *Vet Radiol Ultrasound* 41:461–469, 2000.
324. Ham K, Greenfield CL, Barger A, et al: Validation of a rapid parathyroid hormone assay and intraoperative measurement of parathyroid hormone in dogs with benign naturally occurring primary hyperparathyroidism, *Vet Surg* 38:122–132, 2009.
325. Long CD, Goldstein RE, Hornof WJ, et al: Percutaneous ultrasound-guided chemical parathyroid ablation for treatment of primary hyperparathyroidism in dogs, *J Am Vet Med Assoc* 215:217–221, 1999.
326. Pollard RE, Long CD, Nelson RW, et al: Percutaneous ultrasonographically guided radiofrequency heat ablation for treatment of primary hyperparathyroidism in dogs, *J Am Vet Med Assoc* 218:1106–1110, 2001.
327. Moffett JM, Suliburk J: Parathyroid autotransplantation, *Endocr Pract* 17(Suppl 1):83–89, 2011.
328. Chew DJ, Nagode LA, Schenck PA: Treatment of hypoparathyroidism. In Bonagura JD, Twedt DC, editors: *Kirk's current veterinary therapy XIV*, St. Louis, 2009, Saunders Elsevier.
329. Lee IT, Sheu WH, Tu ST, et al: Bisphosphonate pretreatment attenuates hungry bone syndrome postoperatively in subjects with primary hyperparathyroidism, *J Bone Miner Metab* 24:255–258, 2006.
330. Mahajan A, Narayanan M, Jaffers G, et al: Hypoparathyroidism associated with severe mineral bone disease postrenal transplantation, treated successfully with recombinant PTH, *Hemodial Int* 13:547–550, 2009.
331. Feldman EC, Nelson RW: Beta-cell neoplasia: insulinoma. In Feldman EC, Nelson RW, editors: *Canine and feline endocrinology and reproduction*, ed 3, St. Louis, 2004, Saunders.
332. Jackson TC, Debey B, Lindbloom-Hawley S, et al: Cellular and molecular characterization of a feline insulinoma, *J Vet Intern Med* 23:383–387, 2009.
333. Batcher E, Madaj P, Gianoukakis AG: Pancreatic neuroendocrine tumors, *Endocr Res* 36:35–43, 2011.
334. Hawkins KL, Summers BA, Kuhajda FP, et al: Immunocytochemistry of normal pancreatic islets and spontaneous islet cell tumors in dogs, *Vet Pathol* 24:170–179, 1987.
335. Myers NC III, Andrews GA, Chard-Bergstrom C: Chromogranin A plasma concentration and expression in pancreatic islet cell tumors of dogs and cats, *Am J Vet Res* 58:615–620, 1997.
336. Minkus G, Jutting U, Aubele M, et al: Canine neuroendocrine tumors of the pancreas: a study using image analysis techniques for the discrimination of metastatic versus nonmetastatic tumors, *Vet Pathol* 34:138–145, 1997.
337. Madarame H, Kayanuma H, Shida T, et al: Retrospective study of canine insulinomas: eight cases (2005-2008), *J Vet Med Sci* 71:905–911, 2009.
338. Buishand FO, van Erp MG, Groenveld HA, et al: Expression of insulin-like growth factor-1 by canine insulinomas and their metastases, *Vet J* 191(3):334–340, 2012.
339. Buishand FO, Kik M, Kirpensteijn J: Evaluation of clinico-pathological criteria and the Ki67 index as prognostic indicators in canine insulinoma, *Vet J* 185:62–67, 2010.
340. Leifer CE, Peterson ME, Matus RE: Insulin-secreting tumor: diagnosis and medical and surgical management in 55 dogs, *J Am Vet Med Assoc* 188:60–64, 1986.
341. Caywood DD, Klausner JS, O'Leary TP, et al: Pancreatic insulin-secreting neoplasms: clinical, diagnostic, and prognostic features in 73 dogs, *J Am Anim Hosp Assoc* 24:577–584, 1988.
342. Steiner JM, Bruyette DS: Canine insulinoma, *Compend Contin Educ Vet* 18:13–25, 1996.
343. Trifonidou MA, Kirpensteijn J, Robben JH: A retrospective evaluation of 51 dogs with insulinoma, *Vet Q* 20(Suppl 1):S114–S115, 1998.
344. Tobin RL, Nelson RW, Lucroy MD, et al: Outcome of surgical versus medical treatment of dogs with beta cell neoplasia: 39 cases (1990-1997), *J Am Vet Med Assoc* 215:226–230, 1999.
345. Robben JH, Visser-Wisselaar HA, Rutteman GR, et al: In vitro and in vivo detection of functional somatostatin receptors in canine insulinomas, *J Nucl Med* 38:1036–1042, 1997.
346. Robben JH, Van Garderen E, Mol JA, et al: Locally produced growth hormone in canine insulinomas, *Mol Cell Endocrinol* 197:187–195, 2002.
347. Polton GA, White RN, Brearley MJ, et al: Improved survival in a retrospective cohort of 28 dogs with insulinoma, *J Small Anim Pract* 48:151–156, 2007.
348. Shahar R, Rousseaux C, Steiss J: Peripheral polyneuropathy in a dog with functional islet B-cell tumor and widespread metastasis, *J Am Vet Med Assoc* 187:175–177, 1985.
349. Braund KG, McGuire JA, Amling KA, et al: Peripheral neuropathy associated with malignant neoplasms in dogs, *Vet Pathol* 24:16–21, 1987.
350. Braund KG, Steiss JE, Amling KA, et al: Insulinoma and subclinical peripheral neuropathy in two dogs, *J Vet Intern Med* 1:86–90, 1987.
351. Schrauwen E: Clinical peripheral polyneuropathy associated with canine insulinoma, *Vet Rec* 128:211–212, 1991.
352. Van Ham L, Braund KG, Roels S, et al: Treatment of a dog with an insulinoma-related peripheral polyneuropathy with corticosteroids, *Vet Rec* 141:98–100, 1997.

353. Shimada A, Morita T, Ikeda N, et al: Hypoglycaemic brain lesions in a dog with insulinoma, *J Comp Pathol* 122:67–71, 2000.
354. Fukazawa K, Kayanuma H, Kanai E, et al: Insulinoma with basal ganglion involvement detected by magnetic resonance imaging in a dog, *J Vet Med Sci* 71:689–692, 2009.
355. Siliart B, Stambouli F: Laboratory diagnosis of insulinoma in the dog: a retrospective study and a new diagnostic procedure, *J Small Anim Pract* 37:367–370, 1996.
356. Thoresen SI, Aleksandersen M, Lonaas L, et al: Pancreatic insulin-secreting carcinoma in a dog: fructosamine for determining persistent hypoglycaemia, *J Small Anim Pract* 36:282–286, 1995.
357. Elliott DA, Nelson RW, Feldman EC, et al: Glycosylated hemoglobin concentrations in the blood of healthy dogs and dogs with naturally developing diabetes mellitus, pancreatic beta-cell neoplasia, hyperadrenocorticism, and anemia, *J Am Vet Med Assoc* 211:723–727, 1997.
358. Loste A, Marca MC, Perez M, et al: Clinical value of fructosamine measurements in non-healthy dogs, *Vet Res Commun* 25:109–115, 2001.
359. Mellanby RJ, Herrtage ME: Insulinoma in a normoglycaemic dog with low serum fructosamine, *J Small Anim Pract* 43:506–508, 2002.
360. Lamb CR, Simpson KW, Boswood A, et al: Ultrasonography of pancreatic neoplasia in the dog: a retrospective review of 16 cases, *Vet Rec* 137:65–68, 1995.
361. Robben JH, Pollak YW, Kirpensteijn J, et al: Comparison of ultrasonography, computed tomography, and single-photon emission computed tomography for the detection and localization of canine insulinoma, *J Vet Intern Med* 19:15–22, 2005.
362. Ekeblad S: Islet cell tumours, *Adv Exp Med Biol* 654:771–789, 2010.
363. Iseri T, Yamada K, Chijiwa K, et al: Dynamic computed tomography of the pancreas in normal dogs and in a dog with pancreatic insulinoma, *Vet Radiol Ultrasound* 48:328–331, 2007.
364. Mai W, Caceres AV: Dual-phase computed tomographic angiography in three dogs with pancreatic insulinoma, *Vet Radiol Ultrasound* 49:141–148, 2008.
365. Lester NV, Newell SM, Hill RC, et al: Scintigraphic diagnosis of insulinoma in a dog, *Vet Radiol Ultrasound* 40:174–178, 1999.
366. Garden OA, Reubi JC, Dykes NL, et al: Somatostatin receptor imaging in vivo by planar scintigraphy facilitates the diagnosis of canine insulinomas, *J Vet Intern Med* 19:168–176, 2005.
367. Sundin A, Garske U, Orlefors H: Nuclear imaging of neuroendocrine tumours, *Best Pract Res Clin Endocrinol Metab* 21:69–85, 2007.
368. Fischer JR, Smith SA, Harkin KR: Glucagon constant-rate infusion: a novel strategy for the management of hyperinsulinemic-hypoglycemic crisis in the dog, *J Am Anim Hosp Assoc* 36:27–32, 2000.
369. Moore AS, Nelson RW, Henry CJ, et al: Streptozocin for treatment of pancreatic islet cell tumors in dogs: 17 cases (1989-1999), *J Am Vet Med Assoc* 221:811–818, 2002.
370. Bell R, Mooney CT, Mansfield CS, et al: Treatment of insulinoma in a springer spaniel with streptozotocin, *J Small Anim Pract* 46:247–250, 2005.
371. Hess RS: Insulin-secreting islet cell neoplasia. In Ettinger SJ, Feldman EC, editors: *Textbook of veterinary internal medicine*, ed 7, St. Louis, 2010, Saunders Elsevier.
372. Robben JH, van den Brom WE, Mol JA, et al: Effect of octreotide on plasma concentrations of glucose, insulin, glucagon, growth hormone, and cortisol in healthy dogs and dogs with insulinoma, *Res Vet Sci* 80:25–32, 2006.
373. McMillan FD, Barr B, Feldman EC: Functional pancreatic islet cell tumor in a cat, *J Am Anim Hosp Assoc* 21:741–746, 1985.
374. O'Brien TD, Norton F, Turner TM, et al: Pancreatic endocrine tumor in a cat: clinical, pathological, and immunohistochemical evaluation, *J Am Anim Hosp Assoc* 26:453–457, 1990.
375. Hawks D, Peterson ME, Hawkins KL, et al: Insulin-secreting pancreatic (islet cell) carcinoma in a cat, *J Vet Intern Med* 6:193–196, 1992.
376. Kraje AC: Hypoglycemia and irreversible neurologic complications in a cat with insulinoma, *J Am Vet Med Assoc* 223:812–814, 2003.
377. Greene SN, Bright RM: Insulinoma in a cat, *J Small Anim Pract* 49:38–40, 2008.
378. Feldman EC, Nelson RW: Gastrinoma, glucagonoma, and other APUDomas. In Feldman EC, Nelson RW, editors: *Canine and feline endocrinology and reproduction*, ed 3, St. Louis, 2004, Saunders.
379. Ward CR: Gastrointestinal endocrine disease. In Ettinger SJ, Feldman EC, editors: *Textbook of veterinary internal medicine*, ed 7, St. Louis, 2010, Saunders Elsevier.
380. Vergine M, Pozzo S, Pogliani E, et al: Common bile duct obstruction due to a duodenal gastrinoma in a dog, *Vet J* 170: 141–143, 2005.
381. Shaw DH: Gastrinoma (Zollinger-Ellison syndrome) in the dog and cat, *Can Vet J* 29:448–452, 1988.
382. Green RA, Gartrell CL: Gastrinoma: a retrospective study of four cases (1985-1995), *J Am Anim Hosp Assoc* 33:524–527, 1997.
383. Simpson KW, Dykes NL: Diagnosis and treatment of gastrinoma, *Semin Vet Med Surg (Small Anim)* 12:274–281, 1997.
384. Brooks D, Watson GL: Omeprazole in a dog with gastrinoma, *J Vet Intern Med* 11:379–381, 1997.
385. Liptak JM, Hunt GB, Barrs VR, et al: Gastroduodenal ulceration in cats: eight cases and a review of the literature, *J Feline Med Surg* 4:27–42, 2002.
386. Fukushima R, Ichikawa K, Hirabayashi M, et al: A case of canine gastrinoma, *J Vet Med Sci* 66:993–995, 2004.
387. Fukushima U, Sato M, Okano S, et al: A case of gastrinoma in a Shih-Tzu dog, *J Vet Med Sci* 66:311–313, 2004.
388. Hughes SM: Canine gastrinoma: a case study and literature review of therapeutic options, *N Z Vet J* 54:242–247, 2006.
389. Diroff JS, Sanders NA, McDonough SP, et al: Gastrin-secreting neoplasia in a cat, *J Vet Intern Med* 20:1245–1247, 2006.
390. Altschul M, Simpson KW, Dykes NL, et al: Evaluation of somatostatin analogues for the detection and treatment of gastrinoma in a dog, *J Small Anim Pract* 38:286–291, 1997.
391. Dhillo WS, Jayasena CN, Lewis CJ, et al: Plasma gastrin measurement cannot be used to diagnose a gastrinoma in patients on either proton pump inhibitors or histamine type-2 receptor antagonists, *Ann Clin Biochem* 43:153–155, 2006.
392. Lothrop CD: Medical treatment of neuroendocrine tumors of the gastroenteropancreatic system with somatostatin. In Kirk RW, editor: *Current veterinary therapy X*, Philadelphia, 1989, Saunders.
393. Gross TL, O'Brien TD, Davies AP, et al: Glucagon-producing pancreatic endocrine tumors in two dogs with superficial necrolytic dermatitis, *J Am Vet Med Assoc* 197:1619–1622, 1990.
394. Allenspach K, Arnold P, Glaus T, et al: Glucagon-producing neuroendocrine tumour associated with hypoaminoacidaemia and skin lesions, *J Small Anim Pract* 41:402–406, 2000.
395. Langer NB, Jergens AE, Miles KG: Canine glucagonoma, *Compend Contin Educ Vet* 25:56–63, 2003.
396. Mizuno T, Hiraoka H, Yoshioka C, et al: Superficial necrolytic dermatitis associated with extrapancreatic glucagonoma in a dog, *Vet Dermatol* 20:72–79, 2009.
397. Oberkirchner U, Linder KE, Zadrozny L, et al: Successful treatment of canine necrolytic migratory erythema (superficial necrolytic dermatitis) due to metastatic glucagonoma with octreotide, *Vet Dermatol* 21:510–516, 2010.
398. Rossmeisl JH Jr, Forrester SD, Robertson JL, et al: Chronic vomiting associated with a gastric carcinoid in a cat, *J Am Anim Hosp Assoc* 38:61–66, 2002.
399. Morrell CN, Volk MV, Mankowski JL: A carcinoid tumor in the gallbladder of a dog, *Vet Pathol* 39:756–758, 2002.
400. Sako T, Uchida E, Okamoto M, et al: Immunohistochemical evaluation of a malignant intestinal carcinoid in a dog, *Vet Pathol* 40:212–215, 2003.

401. Lippo NJ, Williams JE, Brawer RS, et al: Acute hemobilia and hemocholecyst in 2 dogs with gallbladder carcinoid, *J Vet Intern Med* 22:1249–1252, 2008.
402. Tappin S, Brown P, Ferasin L: An intestinal neuroendocrine tumour associated with paroxysmal ventricular tachycardia and melaena in a 10-year-old boxer, *J Small Anim Pract* 49:33–37, 2008.
403. Baker SG, Mayhew PD, Mehler SJ: Choledochotomy and primary repair of extrahepatic biliary duct rupture in seven dogs and two cats, *J Small Anim Pract* 52:32–37, 2011.
404. Spugnini EP, Gargiulo M, Assin R, et al: Adjuvant carboplatin for the treatment of intestinal carcinoid in a dog, *In Vivo* 22:759–761, 2008.

26

Tumors of the Female Reproductive System

COREY F. SABA AND JESSICA A. LAWRENCE

Ovarian Tumors

Incidence

Ovarian tumors are uncommon in dogs and cats, resulting in part from the routine practice of ovariohysterectomy (OHE) in many areas of the world. The overall reported prevalence in dogs is 0.5% to 1.2%,[1-3] with an estimated prevalence of 6.25% in intact bitches.[4] Ovarian tumors are equally rare in cats, with a reported prevalence of 0.7% to 3.6% in intact queens.[5,6] These numbers are primarily derived from pathology surveys and likely overestimate the true incidence in the pet population. Breed predilections are also difficult to discern; however, German shepherd dogs, Boxers, Yorkshire terriers, poodles, and Boston terriers appear to be most commonly affected.[2,7,8] Aside from germ cell tumors and specifically teratomas, most ovarian tumors develop in older dogs (approximately 6 years of age and older).[2,7-9] Teratomas are often found in younger dogs (≤6 years of age).[7,8,10,11] Ovarian tumors have been reported in cats ranging from less than 1 year to 20 years (mean age: 6.7 years).[12-15]

Pathology and Natural Behavior

Canine Ovarian Tumors

Due to the complexity of the canine ovary, a variety of histologic tumor types may occur. Historically, canine ovarian tumors have been classified based on the World Health Organization (WHO) classification scheme for human ovarian tumors, with primary tumor types including epithelial tumors, germ cell tumors, sex cord stromal (gonadostromal) tumors, and mesenchymal tumors.[2,8,16,17] Recently, the human WHO classification system was revised to subdivide each of the aforementioned categories into histologic types based on morphologic similarities; the use of immunohistochemistry has aided in further differentiating ovarian tumors.[18] Attempts to recapitulate such classification schemes in dogs have been reported but are not routinely employed.[19,20]

Epithelial Tumors

Epithelial tumors arise from the outer surface of the ovary[9] and according to several reports are most common.[2,8,16] Malignant tumors outnumber benign tumors,[7,8,16] and larger size is suggestive of malignancy.[8,16] Malignant histologies include papillary adenocarcinomas, tubular adenocarcinomas, and undifferentiated carcinomas; benign tumors such as rete adenomas, papillary adenomas and cystadenomas also occur.[2,8,16] Reportedly, 48% of adenocarcinomas will metastasize, generally within the peritoneal cavity to the intraabdominal lymph nodes, omentum, and liver.[8] Direct tumor cell implantation and subsequent malignant effusion may also occur.[3,8] Although most are unilateral, bilateral epithelial ovarian tumors have been described.[8] Cysts in the contralateral ovary, as well as cystic endometrial hyperplasia, may also be found.

Epithelial ovarian tumors routinely express cytokeratin AE1/AE3 (CK AE1/AE3), vimentin, and desmin.[19,20] Although papillary adenocarcinomas also demonstrate placental alkaline phosphatase (PLAP) and cytokeratin 7 (CK 7) immunoreactivity, positive immunoreactivity appears to be less frequent in tubular adenocarcinomas.[19] Alpha fetoprotein (AFP),[19] S100,[19] and endothelin-A (ET-A)[21] are variably expressed. Faint to strong intracytoplasmic cyclooxygenase-2 (COX-2)[22] and endothelin-1 (ET-1)[21] immunoreactivity has been reported in 81% and 83% of canine ovarian carcinomas, respectively. Inhibin-α (INH-α), a glycopeptide synthesized in gonadal cells of the ovaries, inhibits pituitary secretion of follicle-stimulating hormone (FSH), and it has been described as a sensitive and specific marker for granulosa-theca cell tumor (GTCT).[23] Therefore epithelial tumor cells should not express INH-α, and demonstration of INH-α expression has resulted in reclassification of epithelial tumors as GTCT.[20]

Sex Cord Stomal Tumors

Sex cord stromal tumors, specifically GTCT, are also common and likely second in occurrence to epithelial tumors. Less common histologies include Sertoli-Leydig tumors, thecomas, and luteomas. These tumors arise from the specialized estrogen- and progesterone-producing gonadal stroma of the ovary and therefore have the potential to secrete these steroid hormones if functional.[3,4,8,16] The metastatic rate of GTCT is low, occurring in approximately 20% of cases.[3,8,9,16] Metastatic sites include sublumbar lymph nodes, pancreas, and lungs, with peritoneal carcinomatosis noted in some cases.[1,3,8,16] Although rare, thecomas and luteomas are for the most part considered benign.[8,16]

Although most sex cord stromal tumors are unilateral, bilateral tumors are possible, especially among Sertoli-Leydig tumors.[8] Concomitant cystic endometrial hyperplasia and cysts in the contralateral ovary appear common within this group.[8]

Solid, nest, cord, palisade, cystic, and spindle are the histologic patterns described for GTCT, and a mixture of these may exist within a single tumor.[8,19] GTCTs are generally vimentin,[19] S100,[19] and INH-α[20] positive, although one study has reported INH-α negative GTCT.[19] Variable expression of CK AE1/AE3,[20] CK 7,[20] and ET-A[21] has been described, and moderate-to-strong intracytoplasmic ET-1 immunoreactivity has been detected in 88% of canine GTCT.

Germ Cell Tumors

Germ cell tumors, including dysgerminomas, teratomas, and malignant teratomas (teratocarcinomas), arise from primordial germ cells of the ovary.[8,16,24] Concurrent cysts in the contralateral ovary and uterine abnormalities such as pyometra and cystic endometrial hyperplasia are common.[24]

Dysgerminomas, also known as *ovarian seminomas,* are most common in this group and arise from undifferentiated germ cells. Histologically, these tumors consist of a uniform population of cells resembling ovarian primordial germ cells.[3,8,16] Bilateral dysgerminomas have been reported; however, most are unilateral.[8,16,24] The reported metastatic rate is low (10% to 30%), with sites of metastasis including lymph nodes, liver, kidney, omentum, pancreas, and adrenal glands.[3,8,9,24-26]

Teratomas are composed of germ cells that undergo differentiation into at least two germinal cell layers and any combination of tissues can be seen. These tissues are usually well differentiated, and tissues from virtually any organ (excluding ovary or testis) may be present. Malignant teratomas are composed of predominantly immature, undifferentiated tissues resembling those of the embryo.[24] Metastasis has been noted in up to 50%. Although distant visceral metastasis can occur, peritoneal metastasis with carcinomatosis is most common.[8,9,24]

Germ cell tumors, specifically dysgerminomas, are vimentin positive and PLAP, CK 7, desmin, S100, CK AE1/AE3, and INH-α negative.[19]

Mesenchymal Tumors

Mesenchymal ovarian tumors are rare. Reported tumor types include hemangiosarcoma,[2,16] hemangioma,[16] and leiomyoma.[2,16] Behavior of this group is difficult to predict because information in the literature is sparse.

Miscellaneous

In addition to the various primary ovarian tumors, other differential diagnoses should be considered. These include ovarian cysts, paraovarian cysts, cystic rete tubules, vascular hamartomas, and adenomatous hyperplasia of the rete ovarii. Although rare, metastasis to the ovary has been reported in cases of mammary (especially inflammatory carcinoma),[27] intestinal, and pancreatic carcinoma, as well as lymphoma.[16]

Feline Ovarian Tumors

Reported feline ovarian tumor classifications include epithelial, germ cell, and sex cord stromal tumors. Although mesenchymal ovarian tumors have not been reported in cats, it seems plausible that they may occur. Ovarian involvement in cats with lymphoma has been documented.[15]

Sex cord stromal tumors are most common in cats, accounting for at least half of reported cases. They are often unilateral. Of these, GTCTs are most common and approximately 50% are malignant. Metastatic sites include the peritoneum, regional lymph nodes, omentum, diaphragm, kidney, spleen, liver, and lungs.[15] Luteomas, thecomas, and Sertoli-Leydig cell tumors are rare and typically benign.

Germ cell tumors are also rare in cats. Of these, dysgerminomas are most common.[15] They are generally considered benign, yet metastasis has been reported in 20% to 33% of cases.[15] Teratomas have been rarely documented.[15,28]

Epithelial tumors are perhaps the least common ovarian tumor in the cat. Cystadenomas and adenocarcinomas have been described. Metastasis to the lungs, liver, and abdominal peritoneum was seen in one case of ovarian adenocarcinoma.[15]

History and Clinical Signs

Canine Ovarian Tumors

History and clinical signs associated with canine ovarian tumors vary, depending on the tissue of origin. Although initially insidious, ovarian tumors grow to the point of being palpable and clinical signs are typically referable to a space-occupying abdominal mass (Figure 26-1).[9,29-31] Functional sex cord stromal tumors may produce one or multiple hormones, or they may be nonfunctional.[8,16,32] Sex cord stromal tumors that produce steroid hormones such as estrogen may cause vulvar enlargement, sanguineous vulvar discharge, persistent estrus, alopecia, and aplastic pancytopenia, whereas excessive progesterone production may cause cystic endometrial hyperplasia and pyometra.[3,8,9,16,30] Hyperadrenocorticism was reported in a dog with an ovarian-steroid tumor resembling a luteoma, and the associated clinical signs resolved following OHE.[33] Germ cell tumors have been associated with evidence of hormonal dysfunction, although they are most often associated with clinical signs referable to a space-occupying abdominal mass.[24]

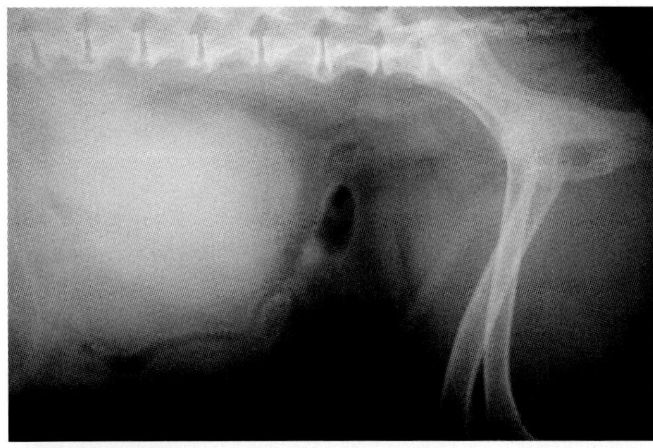

FIGURE 26-1 Right lateral caudal abdominal radiograph of a dog with an ovarian tumor. *(Courtesy Dr. T. Schwarz, University of Edinburgh.)*

Feline Ovarian Tumors

Ovarian tumors in cats also have an insidious onset and eventually grow to the point of being detectable by abdominal palpation. Signs referable to a space-occupying abdominal mass such as weight loss, lethargy, vomiting, ascites, and abdominal distension are often noted. GTCTs are most common, and they are generally functional, producing estrogen, progesterone, or testosterone. Clinical signs of hyperestrogenism, including persistent estrus, alopecia, and endometrial hyperplasia, have been reported.[15] Virilizing behavior secondary to a testosterone-producing thecoma of the ovarian stump was reported in a 6-year-old domestic shorthair cat.[34]

Diagnostic Techniques and Work-Up

Laboratory abnormalities attributable to ovarian tumors are generally not noted. However, hypercalcemia secondary to tumor production of parathyroid hormone–related peptide (PTH-rP) has been reported in a dog with ovarian adenocarcinoma.[31] Thoracic radiographs should be evaluated for evidence of metastatic disease. Abdominal imaging, specifically ultrasound, is useful in identifying ovarian masses and associated abdominal metastasis or uterine abnormalities (Figure 26-2). Ultrasonographic patterns include solid, solid with cystic component, and cystic. Malignant tumors are typically solid, whereas benign tumors are generally cystic with smooth borders. Concurrent uterine abnormalities such as pyometra and cystic endometrial hyperplasia may be detectable via ultrasound in up to 50% of dogs.[35] Because the risk of tumor seeding is high, transabdominal needle biopsies of ovarian tumors are not

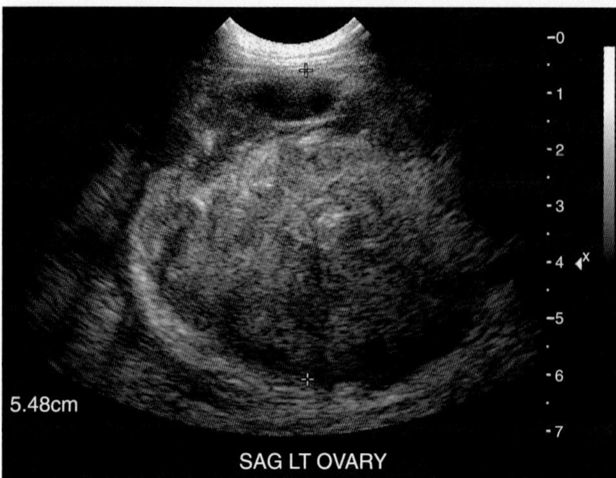

FIGURE 26-2 A large, irregularly shaped mixed echogenic left ovarian mass identified on abdominal ultrasound. The mass was histologically consistent with a granulosa cell tumor. *(Courtesy Dr. D. Jimenez, University of Georgia.)*

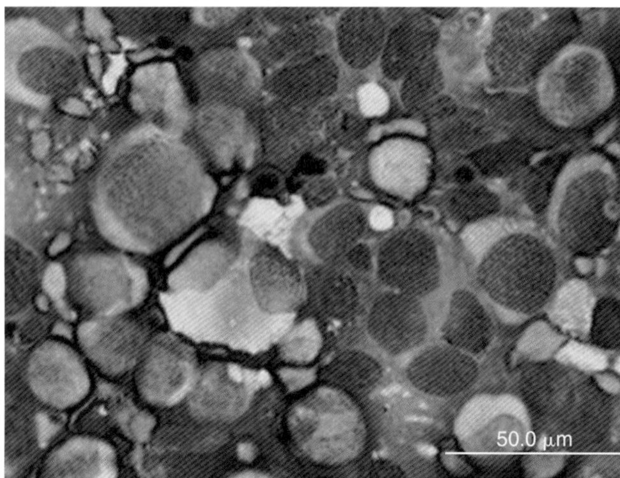

FIGURE 26-3 Ovarian dysgerminoma population of highly pleomorphic round cells. These cells have a scant amount of lightly basophilic cytoplasm and round to irregularly shaped nuclei with a coarsely granular to smudged chromatin pattern with occasional indistinct nucleoli. Binucleated and multinucleated cells are seen and occasional micronuclei are observed. There is moderate-to-marked anisocytosis and anisokaryosis. *(Courtesy Dr. M. Camus, University of Georgia.)*

recommended. If present, abdominal fluid may be safely collected, and cytologic evaluation of fluid often is suggestive of malignant effusions. In a series of 19 cases with a variety of ovarian tumors, cytologic diagnosis was consistent with histopathology in 94.7% (Figure 26-3).[2] Finally, if a functional tumor is suspected, evaluation of vaginal cytology for evidence of estrogen-induced cornification is also indicated.

Therapy

Complete OHE is the treatment of choice for most localized ovarian tumors. Standard oncologic surgical principles must be practiced to minimize tumor seeding of the abdominal cavity. A thorough exploration of the abdominal cavity with biopsy of any abnormalities is recommended for definitive diagnosis and to rule out metastatic lesions.[9]

Use of chemotherapy and/or radiation therapy in the treatment of ovarian tumors has not been widely investigated in veterinary medicine; therefore recommendations are difficult to make. Palliation of malignant effusions with intracavitary instillation of chemotherapeutics such as the platinum agents may be considered.[36] It is important to remember that the use of cisplatin is considered unsafe in cats.[37]

Prognosis

Prognosis for both dogs and cats with ovarian tumors is difficult to predict due to lack of evidence in the literature. Intuitively, it seems the prognosis is good with complete excision of benign or localized malignant tumors but poor with detection of metastatic disease.

Comparative Aspects

As in dogs, ovarian cancer in women includes tumors of epithelial, germ cell, or sex cord stromal origin. Epithelial tumors are most common and generally occur in postmenopausal women (median age: 60 years), whereas germ cell tumors are often diagnosed in younger women. An increased incidence of epithelial tumors has been noted in Caucasian women as compared to African-American women, and ovarian cancer risk (specifically epithelial tumors) appears lower in women who have had children, who have breastfed, or who have taken oral contraceptives. Although uncommon, germline mutations in the *BRCA1* or *BRCA2* genes have been identified in women with familial ovarian cancer. Such mutations also convey an increased risk of other cancers, specifically breast cancer.[38]

Epithelial ovarian tumors in women also resemble the canine counterpart in terms of biologic behavior. They typically metastasize locoregionally within the abdomen; however, distant metastasis may also occur. Patients are often asymptomatic until the disease spreads to the upper abdomen, and presenting symptoms, including abdominal discomfort, bloating, and ascites, are nonspecific. Approximately 70% of women present with advanced disease; as a result, epithelial ovarian cancer is the leading cause of gynecologic cancer mortality.[38]

Cytoreductive surgery and chemotherapy are preferred treatments in epithelial ovarian cancer patients. Even in cases with advanced disease, cytoreductive surgery appears beneficial. Removal of large, necrotic tumors with poor blood supply theoretically improves chemotherapy delivery. Platinum agents (primarily cisplatin) and taxanes are commonly used chemotherapeutic agents. Radiation therapy (RT) has fallen out of use in high-risk early stage patients because it has proven less effective and more toxic than platinum-containing chemotherapy regimens.[38]

Stage is the most important predictor of prognosis. The 5-year survival rate in patients with stage III, optimally debulked, gross residual disease is 20% to 30%.[38]

Uterine Tumors

Incidence

Uterine tumors are rare, accounting for 0.3% to 0.4%[6] and 0.29%[39] of all canine and feline tumors, respectively. Middle-aged to older animals are most commonly affected, although uterine carcinoma has been reported in dogs as young as 10 months.[40] No specific breed predilections have been reported.

Pathology and Natural Behavior

Benign mesenchymal tumors (leiomyomas) are most common in the canine uterus.[9,41-43] Other reported but rare uterine tumors include leiomyosarcoma, fibroma, fibrosarcoma, hemangiosarcoma, angiolipoleiomyoma, lymphoma, and lipoma.[41,44] Epithelial tumors are rarely reported but may occur in dogs.[42] Most epithelial tumors are malignant,[45] but benign histologies have been reported.[46]

Leiomyomas generally are slow growing, noninvasive, and not metastatic.[9] Grossly, they are difficult to distinguish from their malignant counterparts.[41] A syndrome characterized by multiple uterine leiomyomas, bilateral renal cystadenomas, and nodular dermatofibrosis has been characterized in German shepherd dogs.[47,48] This syndrome has been noted to have a hereditary component associated with a mutation in the canine *Birt-Hogg-Dube (BHD)* gene.[49]

A majority of studies suggest that adenocarcinoma is the most common tumor in the feline uterus.[15,39,50,51] Less common histologies include müllerian tumor (adenosarcoma), leiomyoma, leiomyosarcoma, rhabdomyosarcoma, fibrosarcoma, lymphoma, fibroma, hemangioma, and lipoma.[15,39,52-57] Metastasis to the cerebrum, eyes, ovaries, adrenal glands, lungs, liver, kidneys, bladder, colon, diaphragm, and regional lymph nodes has been reported.[15,39,50,58,59]

One study evaluating immunohistochemical reactivity of six feline endometrial adenocarcinomas suggests these tumors routinely express CK AE1/AE3, COX-2, E-cadherin, and β-catenin. Five of six tumors demonstrated expression of progesterone receptors, and infrequent vimentin and estrogen receptor staining was seen.[51]

History and Clinical Signs

Although it seems logical that uterine tumors occur in intact animals, it is important to note that these may arise from uterine stumps after incomplete OHE (Figure 26-4).[44] Clinical signs associated with uterine tumors are not commonly reported, and most are incidental findings.[9] However, in some cases, they grow large enough to produce abdominal distension and signs referable to a space-occupying abdominal mass. Abnormal estrus cycles, vaginal discharge, stranguria, constipation, pyometra, polyuria, polydipsia, vomiting, abdominal distension, and weight loss may also occur.*

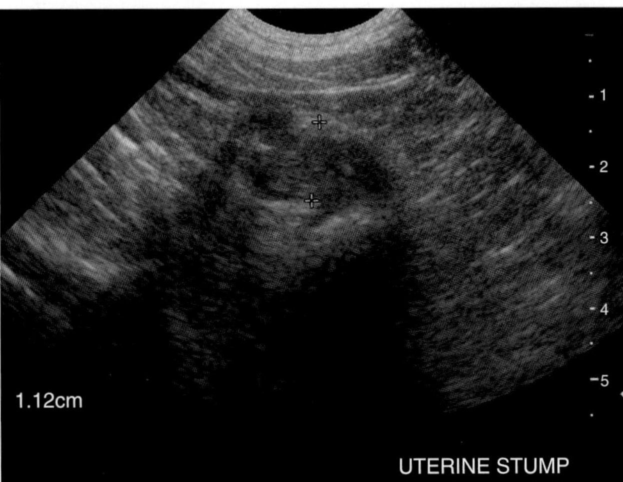

FIGURE 26-4 Irregular, hypoechoic mass at the uterine stump in a dog following ovariohysterectomy. *(Courtesy Dr. D. Jimenez, University of Georgia.)*

Diagnostic Therapeutics and Work-Up

Although abdominal imaging helps confirm the presence of an abdominal or uterine mass, histologic evaluation via complete surgical excision is required for definitive diagnosis. As a result, complete staging, including thoracic radiographs and abdominal ultrasound, should be considered prior to surgery to rule out the possibility of locoregional and distant metastasis.

Therapy

Complete OHE is the treatment of choice for uterine tumors. At the time of surgery, thorough examination of the abdominal cavity must be performed with biopsy of any suspected metastatic foci. Little is known about the role of chemotherapy.

Prognosis

As most uterine tumors in dogs are benign, surgery is often curative. The prognosis is also potentially good for completely excised, localized malignant tumors. However, the presence of metastatic disease warrants a grave prognosis.

Feline uterine adenocarcinomas have well-documented metastatic potential[39,50]; therefore the prognosis must be considered guarded.

Vaginal and Vulvar Tumors

Incidence

Vaginal and vulvar tumors account for 2.4% to 3%[43,60] of all canine tumors. Excluding skin tumors arising on the labia of the vulva, most are benign smooth muscle tumors (leiomyomas). These generally occur in middle-aged to older intact female dogs. Lipomas often occur in younger dogs ranging in age from 1 to 8 years (mean age: 6.3 years).[43,60]

Incidence rates are not available for the cat. Leiomyomas are reported most commonly, occurring in older intact queens.[15,61]

Pathology and Natural Behavior

Benign smooth muscle tumors including leiomyoma, fibroleiomyoma, fibroma, and polyps comprise approximately 83% of reported vaginal tumors.[9,60] The most common malignant tumor is leiomyosarcoma, and associated distant metastasis has been reported.[43,60] Other less common tumor types include lipoma, fibrous histiocytoma, benign melanoma, myxoma, myxofibroma, adenocarcinoma, hemangiosarcoma, osteosarcoma, epidermoid carcinoma, and, in endemic areas, transmissible venereal tumor (TVT).[60,62] Carcinomas arising from the bladder or urethra may manifest as vaginal masses near the urethral papilla, and any skin tumor (e.g., mast cell tumors) may develop on the labia of the vulva.[60]

Macroscopically, tumors of the vestibule or vagina are described as extraluminal or intraluminal.[9] Extraluminal tumors appear as slowly growing, well-encapsulated, perineal masses. Intraluminal tumors are attached to the vestibular or vaginal wall by a pedicle, and multiple tumors may occur.[9] In one study, all pedunculated or polypoid tumors were benign; however, it is important to note that definitive diagnosis requires histopathology.[60]

It has been suggested that vaginal leiomyomas may be hormone dependent, as most dogs with these tumors are intact at

*References 9, 15, 30, 39, 44, 45, 50.

diagnosis.[9,43,60] Furthermore, one study reported a recurrence rate of 0% in dogs undergoing OHE at the time of tumor removal, whereas 15% of dogs that were left intact experienced local recurrence.[9,60]

History and Clinical Signs

Presence of a mass protruding from the vulva is the most common clinical sign, although vaginal bleeding or discharge is often noted. Other clinical signs may include dysuria, hematuria, tenesmus, constipation, excessive vulvar licking, and dystocia.[9,60]

Lipomas are generally slow growing but eventually impinge on adjacent structures. These tumors can arise from the perivascular and perivaginal fat and lie within the pelvic canal and may attach to the tuber ischium. All lipomas are reported to be well circumscribed and relatively avascular.[60]

Concurrent cystic ovaries and mammary adenocarcinoma have also been reported in a cat with vaginal leiomyoma.[60]

Diagnostic Techniques and Work-Up

A presumptive diagnosis may be made based on patient signalment and tumor location, although definitive diagnosis requires histopathology. Vaginal and rectal palpation, vaginoscopic examination, and vaginal cytology are often the first steps performed in evaluation of vaginal and vulvar tumors. Retrograde vaginography or urethrocystography may also be used to help delineate the extent of the mass. For some tumor types (e.g., TVT), aspiration cytology of the tumor may be diagnostic; alternatively, incisional biopsy may be performed. Although most vaginal and vulvar tumors are benign, complete staging, including thoracic radiographs and thorough abdominal ultrasound, should be considered in cases in which malignancy is suspected (e.g., rapidly growing, nonpedunculated tumors) or confirmed.

Therapy

Surgical excision combined with OHE is the treatment of choice for most vaginal and vulvar tumors. For benign tumors, this is likely curative, and wide resections are not necessary, especially if OHE is performed. Intraluminal tumors can be removed easily by transecting the pedicle. A dorsal episiotomy may be performed if needed for adequate visualization and exposure.[9,60]

Surgical removal of extraluminal tumors also can be accomplished through a dorsal episiotomy. Because these tumors are often well encapsulated and poorly vascularized, blunt dissection generally removes them entirely. On rare occasions, a perineal approach or pelvic split may be required. Urethral catheterization prevents accidental damage to the urethra during tumor excision. Malignant, infiltrative vaginal neoplasms can be addressed with complete vulvovaginectomy and perineal urethrostomy in carefully selected cases. OHE is indicated in cases with multifocal disease because stable disease or regression may be obtained with hormone ablation.

Prognosis

For benign tumors, surgical excision and OHE are nearly always curative. The prognosis for malignant tumors must be considered guarded due to high rates of local recurrence and metastasis.[60] Surgery with OHE was curative in the one feline leiomyoma reported.

REFERENCES

1. Hayes A, Harvey HJ: Treatment of metastatic granulosa cell tumor in a dog, *J Am Vet Med Assoc* 174:1304–1306, 1979.
2. Sforna M, Brachelente C, Lepri E, et al: Canine ovarian tumours: a retrospective study of 49 cases, *Vet Res Commun* 27(Suppl 1):359–361, 2003.
3. Cotchin E: Canine ovarian neoplasms, *Res Vet Sci* 2:133–142, 1961.
4. Dow C: Ovarian abnormalities in the bitch, *J Comp Pathol* 70:59–69, 1960.
5. Cotchin E: Some tumours of dogs and cats of comparative veterinary and human interest, *Vet Rec* 71:1040–1054, 1959.
6. Brodey RS: Canine and feline neoplasia, *Adv Vet Sci Comp Med* 14:309–354, 1970.
7. Bertazzolo W, Dell'Orco M, Bonfanti U, et al: Cytological features of canine ovarian tumours: a retrospective study of 19 cases, *J Small Anim Pract* 45:539–545, 2004.
8. Patnaik AK, Greenlee PG: Canine ovarian neoplasms: a clinicopathologic study of 71 cases, including histology of 12 granulosa cell tumors, *Vet Pathol* 24:509–514, 1987.
9. Herron MA: Tumors of the canine genital system, *J Am Anim Hosp Assoc* 19:981–994, 1983.
10. Jergens AE, Knapp DW, Shaw DP: Ovarian teratoma in a bitch, *J Am Vet Med Assoc* 191:81–83, 1987.
11. Elena Gorman M, Bildfell R, Seguin B: What is your diagnosis? Peritoneal fluid from a 1-year-old female German Shepherd dog. Malignant teratoma, *Vet Clin Pathol* 39:393–394, 2010.
12. Gruys E, van Dijk JE: Four canine ovarian teratomas and a nonovarian feline teratoma, *Vet Pathol* 13:455–459, 1976.
13. Gelberg HB, McEntee K: Feline ovarian neoplasms, *Vet Pathol* 22:572–576, 1985.
14. Basaraba RJ, Kraft SL, Andrews GA, et al: An ovarian teratoma in a cat, *Vet Pathol* 35:141–144, 1998.
15. Stein BS: Tumors of the feline genital tract, *J Am Anim Hosp Assoc* 17:1022–1025, 1981.
16. Nielsen SW, Misdorp W, McEntee K: Tumours of the ovary, *Bull World Health Organ* 53:203–215, 1976.
17. Kennedy PC, Cullen JM, Edwards JF, et al: Tumors of the ovary. In *Histological classification of tumors of the genital system of domestic animals*, Washington, DC, 1998, AFIP.
18. McCluggage WG: Recent advances in immunohistochemistry in the diagnosis of ovarian neoplasms, *J Clin Pathol* 53:327–334, 2000.
19. Akihara Y, Shimoyama Y, Kawasako K, et al: Immunohistochemical evaluation of canine ovarian tumors, *J Vet Med Sci* 69:703–708, 2007.
20. Riccardi E, Grieco V, Verganti S, et al: Immunohistochemical diagnosis of canine ovarian epithelial and granulosa cell tumors, *J Vet Diagn Invest* 19:431–435, 2007.
21. Borzacchiello G, Mogavero S, Tortorella G, et al: Expression of endothelin-1 and endothelin receptor a in canine ovarian tumours, *Reprod Domest Anim* 45:e465–e468, 2010.
22. Borzacchiello G, Russo V, Russo M: Immunohistochemical expression of cyclooxygenase-2 in canine ovarian carcinomas, *J Vet Med A Physiol Pathol Clin Med* 54:247–249, 2007.
23. Pelkey TJ, Frierson HF Jr, Mills SE, et al: The diagnostic utility of inhibin staining in ovarian neoplasms, *Int J Gynecol Pathol* 17:97–105, 1998.
24. Greenlee PG, Patnaik AK: Canine ovarian tumors of germ cell origin, *Vet Pathol* 22:117–122, 1985.
25. Andrews EJ, Stookey JL, Helland DR, et al: A histopathological study of canine and feline ovarian dysgerminomas, *Can J Comp Med* 38:85–89, 1974.
26. Dehner LP, Norris HJ, Garner FM, et al: Comparative pathology of ovarian neoplasms. 3. Germ cell tumours of canine, bovine, feline, rodent and human species, *J Comp Pathol* 80:299–306, 1970.
27. Clemente M, Perez-Alenza MD, Pena L: Metastasis of canine inflammatory versus non-inflammatory mammary tumours, *J Comp Pathol* 143:157–163, 2010.
28. Sato T, Hontake S, Shibuya H, et al: A solid mature teratoma of a feline ovary, *J Feline Med Surg* 5:349–351, 2003.
29. Olsen J, Komtebedde J, Lackner A, et al: Cytoreductive treatment of ovarian carcinoma in a dog, *J Vet Intern Med* 8:133–135, 1994.

30. McEntee MC: Reproductive oncology, *Clin Tech Small Anim Pract* 17:133–149, 2002.
31. Hori Y, Uechi M, Kanakubo K, et al: Canine ovarian serous papillary adenocarcinoma with neoplastic hypercalcemia, *J Vet Med Sci* 68:979–982, 2006.
32. McCandlish IA, Munro CD, Breeze RG, et al: Hormone producing ovarian tumours in the dog, *Vet Rec* 105:9–11, 1979.
33. Yamini B, VanDenBrink PL, Refsal KR: Ovarian steroid cell tumor resembling luteoma associated with hyperadrenocorticism (Cushing's disease) in a dog, *Vet Pathol* 34:57–60, 1997.
34. Cellio LM, Degner DA: Testosterone-producing thecoma in a female cat, *J Am Anim Hosp Assoc* 36:323–325, 2000.
35. Diez-Bru N, Garcia-Real I, Martinez EM, et al: Ultrasonographic appearance of ovarian tumors in 10 dogs, *Vet Radiol Ultrasound* 39:226–233, 1998.
36. Moore AS, Kirk C, Cardona A: Intracavitary cisplatin chemotherapy experience with six dogs, *J Vet Intern Med* 5:227–231, 1991.
37. Knapp DW, Richardson RC, DeNicola DB, et al: Cisplatin toxicity in cats, *J Vet Intern Med* 1:29–35, 1987.
38. Cannistra SA, Gershenson DM, Recht A: Ovarian cancer, fallopian tube carcinoma, and peritoneal carcinoma. In DeVita VT, Lawrence TS, Rosenberg SA, editors: *Cancer: principles & practice of oncology*, ed 8, Philadelphia, 2008, Lippincott Williams & Wilkins.
39. Miller MA, Ramos-Vara JA, Dickerson MF, et al: Uterine neoplasia in 13 cats, *J Vet Diagn Invest* 15:515–522, 2003.
40. Cave TA, Hine R, Howie F, et al: Uterine carcinoma in a 10-month-old golden retriever, *J Small Anim Pract* 43:133–135, 2002.
41. McEntee K, Nielsen SW: Tumours of the female genital tract, *Bull World Health Organ* 53:217–226, 1976.
42. Cotchin E: Spontaneous uterine cancer in animals, *Br J Cancer* 18:209–227, 1964.
43. Brodey RS, Roszel JF: Neoplasms of the canine uterus, vagina, and vulva: a clinicopathologic survey of 90 cases, *J Am Vet Med Assoc* 151:1294–1307, 1967.
44. Wenzlow N, Tivers MS, Selmic LE, et al: Haemangiosarcoma in the uterine remnant of a spayed female dog, *J Small Anim Pract* 50:488–491, 2009.
45. Murphy ST, Kruger JM, Watson GL: Uterine adenocarcinoma in the dog: a case report and review, *J Am Anim Hosp Assoc* 30:440–444, 1994.
46. Marino G, Quartuccio M, Cristarella S, et al: Adenoma of the uterine tube in the bitch: two case reports, *Vet Res Commun* 31(Suppl 1): 173–175, 2007.
47. Lium B, Moe L: Hereditary multifocal renal cystadenocarcinomas and nodular dermatofibrosis in the German shepherd dog: macroscopic and histopathologic changes, *Vet Pathol* 22:447–455, 1985.
48. Moe L, Lium B: Hereditary multifocal renal cystadenocarcinomas and nodular dermatofibrosis in 51 German shepherd dogs, *J Small Anim Pract* 38:498–505, 1997.
49. Lingaas F, Comstock KE, Kirkness EF, et al: A mutation in the canine BHD gene is associated with hereditary multifocal renal cystadenocarcinoma and nodular dermatofibrosis in the German shepherd dog, *Hum Mol Genet* 12:3043–3053, 2003.
50. Anderson C, Pratschke K: Uterine adenocarcinoma with abdominal metastases in an ovariohysterectomised cat, *J Feline Med Surg* 13:44–47, 2011.
51. Gil da Costa RM, Santos M, Amorim I, et al: An immunohistochemical study of feline endometrial adenocarcinoma, *J Comp Pathol* 140:254–259, 2009.
52. Fukui K, Matsuda H: Uterine haemangioma in a cat, *Vet Rec* 113:375, 1983.
53. Cooper TK, Ronnett BM, Ruben DS, et al: Uterine myxoid leiomyosarcoma with widespread metastases in a cat, *Vet Pathol* 43:552–556, 2006.
54. Nicotina PA, Zanghi A, Catone G: Uterine malignant mixed Müllerian tumor (metaplasic carcinoma) in the cat: clinicopathologic features and proliferation indices, *Vet Pathol* 39:158–160, 2002.
55. Papparella S, Roperto F: Spontaneous uterine tumors in three cats, *Vet Pathol* 21:257–258, 1984.
56. Bae IH, Kim Y, Pakhrin B, et al: Genitourinary rhabdomyosarcoma with systemic metastasis in a young dog, *Vet Pathol* 44:518–520, 2007.
57. Gilmore CE: Tumors of the female reproductive tract, *Calif Vet* 19:12–15, 1965.
58. O'Rourke MD, Geib LW: Endometrial adenocarcinoma in a cat, *Cornell Vet* 60:598–604, 1970.
59. Schmidt RE, Langham RF: A survey of feline neoplasms, *J Am Vet Med Assoc* 151:1325–1328, 1967.
60. Thacher C, Bradley RL: Vulvar and vaginal tumors in the dog: a retrospective study, *J Am Vet Med Assoc* 183:690–692, 1983.
61. Wolke RE: Vaginal leiomyoma as a cause of chronic constipation in the cat, *J Am Vet Med Assoc* 143:1103–1105, 1963.
62. Hill TP, Lobetti RG, Schulman ML: Vulvovaginectomy and neo-urethrostomy for treatment of haemangiosarcoma of the vulva and vagina, *J S Afr Vet Assoc* 71:256–259, 2000.

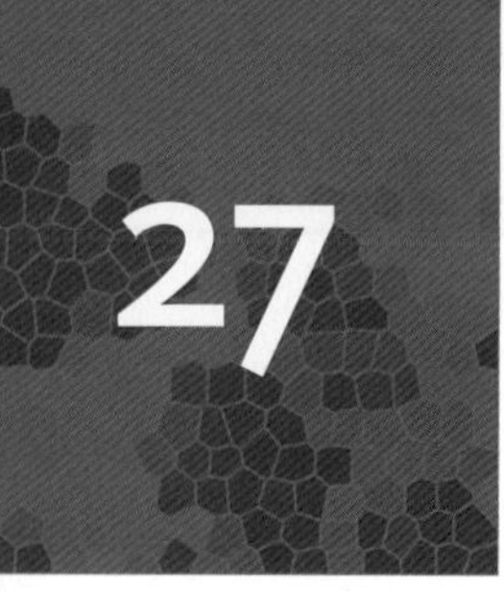

27 Tumors of the Mammary Gland

KARIN U. SORENMO, DEANNA R. WORLEY, AND MICHAEL H. GOLDSCHMIDT

Mammary Gland Tumors in Dogs

Epidemiology and Risk Factors

Epidemiology

Mammary gland tumors are common in dogs and represent the most common neoplasms in sexually intact female dogs.[1-6] The incidence rates reported vary, depending on the origin of the studies and characteristics of the source population. The current incidence of mammary tumors in the United States is lower than in many other countries due to the common practice of performing ovariohysterectomy (OHE) at a young age. Data from several European national or regional canine cancer registries, including Norway, Denmark, and Italy, provide information regarding tumor incidence in general, as well as details regarding the relative frequency of various tumors according to site, age, and breed. These registries consist of a population of predominantly sexually intact dogs and thus provide insight into the natural or true mammary tumor risk in unaltered dogs. Results from these registries show that mammary tumors are the most common tumors in female dogs and represent 50% to 70% of all tumors in this subset of the population.[2,6] In general, open population-based and insurance-based studies may underestimate the true incidence of disease, especially if the diagnosis and subsequent registration require a surgical biopsy. Furthermore, the insured dog population may be skewed toward younger animals because of age restriction and may be void after the tenth year of age, which coincides with the peak incidence age of mammary tumor diagnosis.[3,4] Early data from the surveys of Alameda and Contra Costa counties reported an estimated annual incidence rate of 257.7 malignant mammary tumors per 100,000 in intact female dogs.[1] A more recent large Swedish study based on 80,000 insured female dogs, most of which were sexually intact, reported a rate of 111 mammary tumors (including both benign and malignant) per 10,000 dog-years at risk.[3] This study also reported an increasing risk for tumors with advancing age; 6% of all 8-year-old dogs and 13% of all 10-year-old dogs were diagnosed with at least one mammary tumor. Another large insurance-based study from the United Kingdom reported an annual incidence rate of 205 mammary tumors per 100,000 dogs. This study included all mammary tumors regardless of histology.[4]

In addition to these open and more heterogeneous population-based studies, closed population studies provide another source of incidence and natural progression data. Longitudinal studies may provide a more accurate estimate of the total lifetime risk of mammary tumors because dogs are monitored closely and all tumors are noted, biopsied, and reported. In a large beagle colony morbidity and mortality study, 71% of female dogs developed at least one mammary gland neoplasm in their lifetime.[7] However, this may not accurately represent the incidence in other breeds. Many of the various tumor registries have reported significant breed variations in mammary tumor incidence, suggesting that, in addition to age and hormonal factors, hereditary breed-associated genetic susceptibility also contributes to mammary tumor risk.

Risk Factors

As noted, the incidence of mammary tumors varies, depending on where the studies are performed and the specific characteristics of the population in terms of spay status, age, and breed distribution. Thus, in addition to providing data regarding incidence, the epidemiologic studies also help identify risk factors for mammary tumors. Three main factors have been identified that play important roles in mammary tumor risk: age, hormonal exposure, and breed. To a lesser degree, diet and body weight or obesity may also contribute to risk.

Age

Mammary tumors affect middle-aged and older dogs.[1,8-11] Mammary tumors, especially malignant tumors, are extremely rare in dogs younger than 5 years old.[1,8,12] The tumor risk increases with age and becomes significant when dogs turn 7 or 8 years old and continues to increase until the age of 11 to 13 years.[8,12] Dogs with malignant tumors have been found to be significantly older than dogs with benign tumors: mean age of dogs with malignant tumors is 9 to 11 years and 7 to 9 years with benign tumors.[13,14] The peak incidence age also depends on the lifespan of various breeds. In general, larger breeds have a naturally shorter lifespan and therefore tend to be younger than smaller breeds when they are diagnosed. These differences may be further exaggerated in high-risk breeds such as the English Springer spaniels.[3,15]

Hormonal Exposure

Many mammary tumors in dogs are preventable. Dogs spayed prior to their first estrus have only a 0.5 % risk of developing mammary tumors in their lifetime.[16] The protective effect of OHE decreases quickly over the first few estrus cycles, and most studies have not found significant benefit after 4 years of age. According to Schneider's original study, the risk increases and the benefit diminishes with each estrus cycle, as illustrated by an increasing risk of 8% and 26%, depending on whether the OHE was performed prior to the second or third heat cycle.[16] This study found no significant risk reduction in dogs spayed after the second heat cycle, although other researchers have found some modest benefit in dogs spayed later.[12,17,18] There is general agreement that the greatest benefit on mammary tumor prevention is seen if the dog is not allowed to go through any heat cycles, suggesting that the pivotal and irreversible effects of ovarian hormones on the mammary glands in terms of cancer risk occur early in life, likely during puberty when the mammary gland develops and matures. These findings may also explain why other factors resulting in physiologic variation in hormonal influence on the mammary tissues such as pseudopregnancy, pregnancy, or parity, which typically occur after a few estrus cycles, have not been found to significantly influence the tumor risk.[12,16,19] Exposure to exogenous or pharmacologic doses of hormones (both progestins and estrogens), however, has been found to increase the risk for developing mammary tumors in dogs. Dogs treated with progestins are more likely to develop tumors and are younger when they do. According to the Norwegian Canine Cancer Registry, dogs treated with progestins to prevent estrus had a 2.3 times higher risk for mammary tumors when compared to dogs not receiving such treatment.[20] Similarly, a Dutch study found that privately owned dogs with mammary tumors were significantly more likely to have received progestins.[18] Numerous studies have investigated the effect of dose, duration, and type of hormones (progestins, estrogens, or combination of both) on mammary tumor development in laboratory dogs. Although some discordance exists, most conclude that low-dose progestins alone increase the risk for predominantly benign tumors, whereas a combination of estrogens and progestins tends to induce malignant tumors.[21-25]

Breeds and Genetic Susceptibility

In general, mammary tumors tend to be more common in the smaller breeds. Purebred dogs are more commonly affected[1]; poodles, Chihuahuas, dachshunds, Yorkshire terriers, Maltese, and cocker spaniels are frequently listed as high-risk breeds in the small-breed category.[1,2,14,26] However, some of the larger breeds are also at increased risk, including the English Springer spaniel, English setters, Brittany spaniels, German shepherds, Pointers, Dobermans, and Boxers.[1-3,14,26] Some noteworthy discrepancies exist, specifically between the U.S. and the European reports. Boxers are noted to have a decreased risk for mammary tumors according to data from the University of Pennsylvania, whereas Scandinavian studies reflect an increased risk in Boxers.[2,3,14] A closed population beagle study also has shown that two different lines or families of beagles have very different mammary tumor risk.[27] These results collectively support a genetic influence on mammary cancer development. Familial or inherited germline mutations in *BRCA1* and *BRCA2* account for 5% to 10 % of all human breast cancers and are associated with an 85% cumulative lifetime risk of breast cancer in affected individuals.[28-31] Studies of *BRCA* mutations in canine mammary tumors have so far been limited to tumor gene expression studies and the results have varied; some found underexpression of *BRCA1* in malignant tumors and others have documented overexpression of *BRCA2* in metastatic tumors.[32,33] Germline mutations in both *BRCA1* and *BRCA2* were found to be associated with significantly increased risk in English Springer spaniels in a large Swedish study.[3,15]

Other Risk Factors

Body weight, specifically during puberty (9 to 12 months), is found to have a significant effect on later mammary tumor risk; being underweight during this time period provides significant protection against later tumor development.[17] This study did not find an increased risk for tumors in dogs fed a high-fat diet or dogs that were obese around the time of tumor detection. However, a subsequent case-control study did document an association between diet and mammary cancer in which obesity early in life and a diet high in red meat were found to increase risk.[34] Obesity has also been recognized as a risk factor for developing postmenopausal breast cancer in women.[35,36] One of the proposed mechanisms by which diet/obesity may be linked to breast carcinogenesis is via its effect on serum estrogen levels. Obesity is associated with decreased concentration of sex hormone–binding globulin and thus results in elevated serum free estrogen levels.[37-41] In addition, adipose tissues may be a source of increased estrogen production via aromatase-mediated conversion of androgens. Interestingly, the mammary cancer–sparing influence of being underweight is most significant during the first year of life when the effects of the endogenous hormones are the greatest.

Tumor Biology: Development, Hormones, Growth Factors, and Clinical Implications

Based on the previous discussion of risk factors, it is clear that exposure to ovarian hormones is important in the development of mammary tumors in dogs. Both estrogens and progesterone are necessary for normal mammary gland development and maturation. The mammary glands undergo distinct clinical and histopathologic changes as hormone levels fluctuate according to the phases of the estrus cycle.[42,43] Estrogens and progesterone are mitogens of breast epithelium and induce proliferation of intralobular ductal epithelium and development of ducts and lobules, resulting in expansion of the mammary glands. Historically, the tumorigenic effects of estrogen in human breast cancer were thought to be mediated via their receptor binding and enhanced production of growth factors resulting in increased cellular proliferation.[44] However, more recent research shows that estrogen and its metabolites also have direct genotoxic effects by increasing mutations and induction of aneuploidy independent of the estrogen receptors.[45-47] The tumorigenic effects of progesterone are in part thought to be mediated via a progesterone-induced increased mammary gland production of growth hormone (GH) and growth hormone receptors (GHR).[48-50] GH has direct stimulatory effects on mammary tissues, as well as indirect effects via increasing insulin-like growth factor-1 (IGF-1).[51] The GH/IGF-1 axis has been implicated in human breast carcinogenesis. IGF-1 is both a proliferative and a survival factor for breast epithelial cells and regulates the expression of numerous genes involved in breast cancer development.[52-57] The complex dysregulation of growth factors and hormones that precedes, initiates, and potentially drives canine mammary tumorigenesis is far from understood; evidence exists indicating that both growth factors and steroid hormones are intrinsically implicated and contribute in an autocrine/paracrine manner. Malignant tumors have significantly higher tissue concentrations of GH, IGF-1, progesterone, and 17β-estradiol than benign tumors, and moreover, levels correspond with important clinicopathologic parameters, such as growth rate, size, and specific histopathologic type.[58,59] A complete review of the biologic and molecular aspects of mammary tumor carcinogenesis is beyond the scope of this chapter, but recent reviews provide more complete information.[60,61]

The entire mammary chains are exposed to growth factors and sex hormones, resulting in a field carcinogenesis effect. Consequently, most dogs develop tumors in multiple glands.[7,12,13,62-64] Histologic progression with increasing tumor size is often noted in dogs with multiple tumors and areas of transitions such as carcinoma in situ can be seen in benign tumors.[13,62] This provides direct evidence that benign and malignant mammary tumors are not separate entities—instead, they are part of a biologic and histopathologic continuum in which the malignant invasive carcinomas are the endstage of the process. Earlier publications support this hypothesis and document associations between tumors of benign and malignant histology. For instance, dogs with carcinomas often had concurrent benign tumors of the same cell type and dogs with benign mammary tumors were at increased risk for developing subsequent malignant tumors.[63] Furthermore, risk was even higher in dogs diagnosed with carcinomas or carcinoma in situ.[13,62,64] Evidence of histologic progression has also been reported in which a high incidence of carcinoma in situ and intraepithelial lesions with atypia was noted adjacent to invasive carcinomas.[62,65] These studies provide support for the hypothesis that mammary tumors develop initially from benign lesions and progress to invasive malignant lesions as part of a continuum influenced by hormonal field effects on mammary tissues. There are likely regional variations in terms of exposure, resulting in a range of histopathologic and clinical changes. Some tumors may never change and remain small and benign, whereas others progress and become malignant and many develop new tumors in other glands. This suggests that canine mammary tumors provide unique comparative opportunities to study mammary carcinogenesis and progression with direct applications to human breast cancer research.

Tumor Hormone Receptors: Prognostic, Clinical, and Therapeutic Implications

Hormonal exposure plays an important role in mammary tumor development, and many tumors, specifically tumors of epithelial origin, express hormone receptors (HRs), suggesting continued hormonal influence and dependence. Benign tumors are more likely than malignant tumors to retain HRs—both estrogen receptors (ER) and progesterone receptors (PR).[66-70] The HR status is also influenced by age and hormonal status: dogs that are intact, younger, and in estrus are more likely to have receptor-positive tumors than dogs that are spayed, older, and anestrous.[70,71] Furthermore, the HR expression is inversely correlated with tumor size and histopathologic differentiation; larger tumors and undifferentiated or anaplastic tumors are less likely to express receptors than tumors with more differentiated histology, reflecting a biologic drift toward hormone independence and corresponding with aggressive histology and clinical behavior.[71-73] HR expression analysis is most commonly performed by immunohistochemistry (IHC). Results from various studies are quite disparate, especially in terms of ER-alpha positivity in malignant tumors, and range from 10% to 92%.[66-74] These variations may in part be due to differences between study populations (tumor size, castration status, tumor types) and the fact that IHC methods vary and are neither standardized nor validated. This makes it difficult to consider HR expression results when making treatment decisions. Despite these discrepancies, several studies have documented that tumor expression of ER and PR is associated with a more favorable outcome.[71-73] Endocrine therapy is recommended to all women with ER-positive tumors, regardless of intensity of staining, and results in significant improvement in the adjuvant setting.[75-80] Currently, there are no published prospective studies on the predictive value of HR status and the effect or benefit of hormonal therapy in dogs with mammary tumors. Until results from such studies are available and found to be predictive, routine IHC for HRs is not likely to influence treatment decisions. In addition to the presence of HRs, the overexpression of human epidermal growth factor receptor-2 (HER2/erb-2), a member of the epidermal growth factor receptor (EGFR) family involved in signal transduction pathways that regulate cell growth and differentiation, may also provide clinical and prognostic insight, as well as therapeutic opportunities in mammary tumors. Overexpression or amplification of HER2 is found in 20% to 25% of all human breast cancer patients and is associated with aggressive behavior, resistance to hormonal therapy, and a poor prognosis.[81-83] HER2 overexpression has also been documented in canine mammary tumors using the same HercepTest scoring systems used in human breast cancer and documented positive staining ranging from 17% to 29% in malignant tumors.[84,85] HER2 staining was associated with negative histologic features and short survival according to one of these studies,[84] but contrary to the human studies, HER2 expression was associated with an increased survival in two other independent studies.[85,86]

History and Clinical Presentation

Mammary tumors are usually easy to detect through routine physical examinations. However, high-risk dogs, specifically older intact female dogs, should undergo a thorough examination of the mammary glands. Mammary tumors typically affect the two caudal pairs, where the mammary glands or tissues are naturally larger; thus careful palpation may be necessary to detect small tumors.[7,12,63,64] The mammary glands should be palpated again under general anesthesia to ensure that all tumors are found and included in the surgical planning, and both chains should be carefully evaluated. A recent study documented that 70% of intact females had more than one tumor at diagnosis.[13] The size of the tumor(s), stage of disease, and presence of systemic signs of illness vary widely. Inflammatory mammary carcinomas represent a rare but clinically important subset of mammary tumors in dogs. Affected dogs may easily be misdiagnosed as having mastitis or severe dermatitis because, rather than presenting with discrete well-circumscribed tumors, the entire mammary chain may appear edematous, swollen, warm, and painful (Figure 27-1).[87,88] In addition to the extensive locoregional involvement, most dogs with inflammatory carcinomas have distant metastatic disease and signs of systemic illness.[87,88] These dogs are therefore poor surgical candidates. The majority of dogs with mammary tumors are systemically healthy, and the tumors are confined to the mammary glands when they are diagnosed.

Clinical Assessment, Diagnosis, Work-Up, and Staging

Due to the risk of metastasis associated with mammary tumors, staging prior to initiating therapy is strongly recommended, especially if benign disease cannot be histologically confirmed. Minimal staging can include complete blood count (CBC), serum

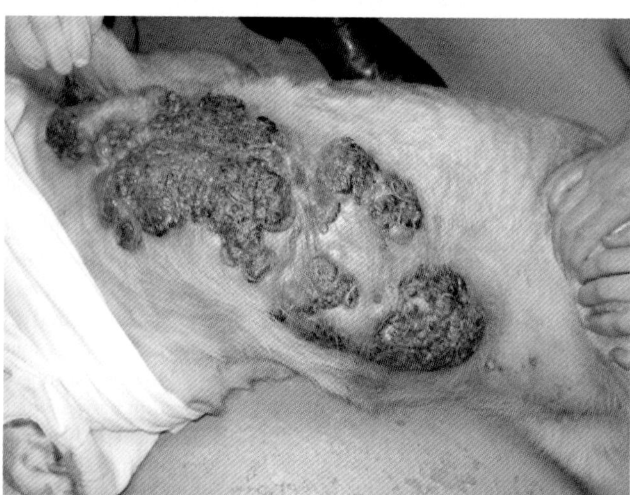

FIGURE 27-1 Inflammatory mammary carcinoma in a dog. *(Courtesy Dr. Nicholas Bacon, University of Florida, Gainesville, Florida.)*

biochemistry, three-view thoracic radiographs, and fine-needle aspiration (FNA) of regional lymph nodes, even if palpably normal. Abdominal ultrasound may be indicated in dogs with suspected regional lymph node involvement or changes on preoperative blood work suggesting tumor-related or non–tumor-related serum biochemistry changes. Even though osseous metaplasia occurs occasionally with mammary adenocarcinoma and the mammary glands are a common site for extraskeletal osteosarcoma, there has been no prognostic value found for serum alkaline phosphatase activity.[89,90] There may be value in performing mammary tumor cytology to help rule out nonmammary dermal and subcutaneous tumors (e.g., mast cell tumors, lipomas). Additionally, correlations between cytopathology and ex vivo histopathology have been reported to be between 67.5% and 93%,[91,92] and the reported cytologic sensitivity and specificity for a malignant mammary tumor diagnosis were 88% and 96%, respectively.[93] Computed tomography (CT) imaging of the thoracic cavity provides more sensitive detection of pulmonary nodules than does thoracic radiography, but this may not be applicable for every patient due to a need for general anesthesia, the increased expense, and decreased availability.[93,94] Distant metastatic sites can include lymph nodes, liver, lungs, and bone.[95]

Lymphatic drainage of normal mammary glands is very complex, with documented drainage occurring to multiple ipsilateral lymph nodes and even to contralateral lymph nodes.[96-98] The amount of variation in lymphatic drainage increases in the neoplastic mammary gland.[96] Tumor-induced lymphangiogenesis, well documented in human breast cancer, may be responsible for the unpredictable and erratic location of susceptible or "at-risk" lymph nodes in dogs having malignant mammary tumors.[99] Thus exclusive anatomic sampling of nearby lymph nodes is not sufficient for accurate lymph node staging and may miss the presence of locoregional disease.[100]

Staging System

Mammary tumors are staged according to the T (tumor), N (lymph node), and M (metastasis) system. A modified version of the original staging system published by Owens[101] is currently used by most oncologists and stage advances from I to II to III as the size of the primary tumor increases from smaller than 3 cm, to between 3 and 5 cm, to larger than 5 cm.[102] These size categories capture important changes in prognosis and outcome. Lymph node metastasis represents stage IV disease, regardless of tumor size, and distant metastasis constitutes stage V disease. This staging system should be used for dogs with epithelial tumors (noninflammatory) and not sarcomas (Table 27-1).

TABLE 27-1 Staging of Canine Mammary Tumors

STAGE	TUMOR SIZE	LYMPH NODE STATUS	METASTASIS
Stage 1	T1 <3 cm	N0	M0
Stage 2	T2 3-5 cm	N0	M0
Stage 3	T3 >5 cm	N0	M0
Stage 4	Any	N1 (positive)	M0
Stage 5	Any	Any	M1(metastasis)

Data from Rutteman G, Withrow S, MacEwen E: Tumors of the mammary gland. In Withrow S, MacEwen E, editors: *Small animal clinical oncology*, ed 3, Philadelphia, 2001, WB Saunders.

Histopathology

The normal mammary gland is a complex branching structure and the histologic and immunohistochemical characteristics are equally complex—the interested reader is referred to a thorough review on the subject.[103]

Classification Systems

Two early classifications of canine and feline mammary tumors were published in 1974[104] and 1999,[105] and a revised system for the dog was published in 2011.[106] In dogs, although there may be histopathologic evidence of malignancy, only a small percentage of cases will have lymphatic and vascular invasion and metastatic disease, whereas in cats the majority are malignant and metastasis to local lymph nodes is more common. The classification used in this text is based on both morphology[106] and prognosis.[107] When discussing the classification of mammary neoplasms the terms *simple* and *complex* are commonly used. *Simple* denotes that the neoplasm is composed of *one* cell type resembling either luminal epithelial cells or myoepithelial cells, whereas *complex* neoplasms are composed of *two* cell types, both luminal and myoepithelial cells.[106]

Canine Mammary Hyperplasia and Dysplasia

Several hyperplastic and dysplastic lesions are considered precursor lesions to the development of mammary neoplasms.[106] These include duct ectasis, lobular hyperplasia (with or without secretory activity), lobular hyperplasia with fibrosis, epitheliosis, papillomatosis, fibroses (fibrosclerosis), and fibroadenomatous change (fibroepithelial hyperplasia, fibroepithelial hypertrophy, mammary hypertrophy).

Benign Mammary Neoplasms

Several types of benign mammary neoplasms exist in the dog and include adenoma, intraductal papillary adenoma (duct papilloma), ductal adenoma, fibroadenoma, myoepithelioma, complex adenoma (adenomyoepithelioma), and benign mixed tumors. A histologic description of these various entities is beyond the scope of this chapter, and interested readers are directed to a more thorough review.[106]

Malignant Canine Mammary Neoplasms

Malignant Epithelial Tumors

Several types of malignant epithelial tumors (Table 27-2) exist, including carcinoma in situ (well-demarcated, noninfiltrative nodule[s] that have not extended through the basement membrane) and a variety of carcinomas. In addition, several less common subtypes of malignant epithelial neoplasms are squamous cell carcinomas, adenosquamous carcinomas, mucinous carcinomas, lipid-rich carcinomas, and spindle cell carcinomas (including malignant myoepithelioma, squamous cell carcinoma–spindle cell variant, and carcinoma–spindle cell variant).[106]

Malignant Mesenchymal Neoplasms: Sarcomas

Malignant mesenchymal neoplasms include osteosarcoma, chondrosarcoma, fibrosarcoma, hemangiosarcoma, and carcinosarcoma (malignant mixed mammary tumor).[106]

Osteosarcoma is the most common mesenchymal neoplasm of the canine mammary gland, and there is often a history of recent rapid growth of a mammary mass that might have been present for some time. A proliferation of cells varies from fusiform to stellate to ovoid, and there is an association with islands of tumor

TABLE 27-2 Classification of Malignant Epithelial Mammary Tumors

CLASSIFICATION	HISTOLOGIC CHARACTERISTICS
Carcinoma in situ	▪ Well-demarcated, noninfiltrative nodule(s) of closely packed cells arranged in irregular tubules or nests that have not extended through the basement membrane. ▪ Loss of normal architecture, cell and nuclear polarity with anisocytosis, anisokaryosis, and increased numbers of mitotic figures.
Carcinomas: Simple	1. Tubular carcinoma • Cells arranged in tubules and intertubular stroma consists of vessels and fibroblast. • Neoplastic cells can infiltrate the surrounding mammary tissue and evoke a stromal response. 2. Tubulopapillary • Papillae extend into tubular lumina and are supported by a fine fibrovascular connective tissue stroma. 3. Cystic-papillary • Papillae extending into cystic tubular lumina. 4. Cribriform • Proliferation of neoplastic cells forming a sieve-like arrangement. • Lumina formed are very small and surrounded by bridges of neoplastic cells.
Carcinoma: Micropapillary invasive	▪ Intraductal neoplastic population forms small intraluminal irregular aggregates and small papillae that do not have a supporting fibrovascular stalk.
Carcinoma: Solid	▪ Closely packed cells arranged in nests and cords form dense, irregularly sized lobules surrounded by fine fibrovascular stroma.
Comedocarcinoma	▪ Necrotic areas within the center of neoplastic cell aggregates. ▪ Necrotic areas characterized by abundant amorphous eosinophilic material admixed with cell debris.
Carcinoma: Anaplastic	▪ Most malignant of the carcinomas. ▪ Neoplastic cells individualized or in small nests. ▪ Invading cells often evoke a desmoplastic host response. ▪ Inflammatory carcinoma is a clinical diagnosis. ▪ Anaplastic histology characterized by extensive histologic invasion with neoplastic emboli in the overlying dermal lymphatic vessels.
Carcinoma arising in a complex adenoma/mixed tumor	▪ Benign counterpart detectable with areas of more pleomorphic epithelial cells has increased numbers of mitoses when compared to the preexisting benign epithelial component.
Carcinomas: Complex	▪ Malignant epithelial component, but myoepithelium is benign. ▪ Only the epithelial cells exhibit considerable anisokaryosis and anisocytosis.
Ductal carcinoma	▪ Cells arranged in cords and tubules that surround slitlike lumina lined by a double layer of epithelial cells. ▪ Exhibit anisokaryosis, anisocytosis, and increased mitotic figures.
Intraductal papillary carcinoma	▪ Proliferation of multilayered epithelial cells. ▪ Fibrous connective tissue and normal myoepithelial cells are retained as the supporting stroma for the papillae.

osteoid and/or bone formation. Mitoses are frequently found. Metastasis occurs via the hematogenous route, mainly to the lungs.

Carcinosarcoma (malignant mixed mammary tumor) is composed partly of cells morphologically resembling the epithelial component and partly of cells morphologically resembling connective tissue elements, both types of which are malignant. It is an uncommon mammary neoplasm, but it most often presents as a carcinoma and osteosarcoma (see previous paragraph). The epithelial component metastasizes via lymphatic vessels to regional lymph nodes and the lungs, and the mesenchymal component metastasizes via the hematogenous route to the lungs.

Hyperplasia/Dysplasia/Neoplasia of the Nipple

Ductal adenoma and carcinoma are rare and involve only the nipple, with no neoplastic tissue in the underlying mammary gland. The nipple is enlarged and firm. The histopathology mimics that of ductal adenomas and carcinomas. Carcinoma with epidermal infiltration (Paget-like disease) is a neoplasm occasionally seen in the dog that mimics Paget's disease of the nipple in women. The carcinoma is present within the mammary gland, and carcinoma cells, either as individual cells or small aggregates, are present within the epidermis of the nipple.

Histopathologic Prognostic Factors and Grading

The epithelial tumors are also graded according to specific histopathologic criteria. Several systems for both canine and feline tumors exist, most of which are based on the Elston and Ellis grading system,[108] which incorporates information regarding (1)

TABLE 27-3 Criteria Used for Histologic Grading of Malignancy in Feline and Canine Mammary Carcinomas

TUBULE FORMATION	NUCLEAR PLEOMORPHISM	MITOSES/10 HPF	
		CANINE	FELINE
Tubule formation >75% of the specimen: **1 point**	Uniform or regular small nucleus and occasional nucleoli: **1 point**	0-9: **1 point**	0-7: **1 point**
Moderate formation of tubular arrangements (10%-75% of the specimen) admixed with areas of solid tumor growth: **2 points**	Moderate degree of variation in nuclear size and shape, hyperchromatic nucleus, and presence of nucleoli (some of which can be prominent): **2 points**	10-19: **2 points**	8-14: **2 points**
Minimal or no tubule formation (<10%): **3 points**	Marked variation in nuclear size and hyperchromatic nucleus, often with one or more prominent nucleoli: **3 points**	>20: **3 points**	>15: **3 points**

TABLE 27-4 Tumor Grade Based on Histologic Score in Felines and Canines

TOTAL SCORE	GRADE OF MALIGNANCY
3 to 5	I (low) Well differentiated
6 to 7	II (intermediate) Moderately differentiated
8 to 9	III (high) Poorly differentiated

Data from Misdorp W: Tumors of the mammary gland. In Meuten DJ, editor: *Tumors in domestic animals,* ed 4, Ames, Iowa, 2002, Iowa State Press; Clemente M, Perez-Alenza MD, Illera JC, et al: Histological, immunohistological, and ultrastructural description of vasculogenic mimicry in canine mammary cancer, *Vet Pathol* 47:265-274, 2010; and Castagnaro M, Casalone C, Bozzetta E, et al: Tumour grading and the one-year post-surgical prognosis in feline mammary carcinomas, *J Comp Pathol* 119:263-275, 1998.

tubule formation, (2) nuclear pleomorphism, and (3) mitosis per 10 HPF (Table 27-3).[109-111] Based on the total score derived from this system, the grade of the tumor will be determined: grade 1 (low score) is a well-differentiated tumor, grade 2 (intermediate score) is moderately differentiated, and grade 3 (high total score) is poorly differentiated (Table 27-4). Tumor grade has been found to provide consistent and reliable prognostic information.[71,106-111] In addition to the grading system, information regarding vascular/lymphatic invasion, surrounding stromal invasion, lymph node involvement, and tumor type may also predict behavior.* Sarcomas are typically not graded according to this system, but the majority tend to be biologically aggressive tumors and associated with a very poor long-term survival.[111,112]

Mammary tumors in dogs represent a wide histologic spectrum with both benign and malignant lesions originating from different tissue types or a combination of tissues. Many dogs present with several different tumors and tumors of different types and can as such represent a rather daunting histopathologic picture; prognosis is determined by the most aggressive tumor, and decisions regarding adjuvant treatments should be based on the largest or the most aggressive histology. In many cases, the most aggressive tumor is the largest.[13]

*References 11, 26, 62, 107, 111-113.

Clinical Prognostic Factors

The three prognostic factors that are most consistently reported to be associated with prognosis include tumor size, lymph node involvement, and World Health Organization (WHO) stage (modified and original). These are the only factors that will be discussed here.

Tumor Size

According to MacEwen et al, dogs with tumor volume larger than 40 cc (approximately 3.4 cm in diameter) have a statistically significant worse outcome than smaller tumors, both in terms of remission and survival.[114] Other investigators have classified tumors as stage I, smaller than 3 cm; stage II, between 3 cm and 5 cm; and stage III, larger than 5 cm.[101,114] Dogs with tumors smaller than 3 cm were reported to have a significantly longer survival.[11,71,115] Others, however, have found that a change in prognosis only becomes significant when tumors are larger than 5 cm.[26,116] The change in prognosis is likely gradual as tumors increase in size. The modified WHO staging system has incorporated these three size categories representing stage I, stage II, and stage III, respectively.[102] These stages are commonly used in mammary tumor staging. Importantly, however, the size of the tumor becomes irrelevant if the local lymph node is involved; according to Kurzman et al, the size of the primary tumor was not significant in dogs with local lymph node involvement.[11] A positive lymph node constitutes stage IV disease according to the revised WHO system, attributing a worse prognosis to lymph node involvement rather than tumor size.

Lymph Node

A large retrospective study, including only dogs with carcinomas, all of which had the local or draining lymph node removed and biopsied, found that the status of the local lymph nodes was highly prognostic.[11] Others have confirmed these findings.* Therefore information regarding the status of the local lymph node is extremely important when considering the need for adjuvant or systemic therapy in dogs with mammary tumors.

WHO Staging System

Both the original and the revised WHO staging system provide prognostic information. When performing a side-by-side comparison of the two systems, the revised system appears to better reflect the stronger impact of lymph node status on prognosis.[103]

*References 26, 71, 73, 111, 112, 117.

Nevertheless, the original staging system also provides useful prognostic information as illustrated in two larger separate retrospective studies in which dogs with higher WHO stage disease had a significantly worse prognosis than dogs with lower stage disease.[26,117]

Therapy

Surgical Treatment

The challenge in preparing surgical recommendations is the lack of uniform, robust prospective clinical trials that clarify the extent or "dose" of surgical excision: simple lumpectomy, mastectomy, regional mastectomy, chain mastectomy, or staged bilateral mastectomies. The goal of the surgery must be defined through staging and counseling with the owner. Is the goal to remove the current tumor(s) with clean margins or remove the current tumor(s) with clean margins *and* prevent new tumors in the remaining glands? The latter option would require prophylactic mastectomies of clinically normal glands in addition to affected glands.

Several studies have evaluated the effect of surgical dose in canine mammary tumors. A prospective randomized trial of 144 dogs with naïve malignant tumors comparing the overall survival benefit and disease-free interval (DFI) relative to either chain mastectomy or simple mastectomy found no differences.[114] Similarly, a retrospective case series of 79 dogs treated at a single institution found no difference in overall survival or DFI comparable to the type of surgical procedure performed, whether lumpectomy, mastectomy, regional mastectomy with en bloc lymph node excision, or chain mastectomy with en bloc lymph node excision.[117] However, the relative hazard for death within the first 2 years after surgery was slightly higher for dogs receiving a regional mastectomy over a chain mastectomy.[117] Interestingly, in the study by MacEwen et al, the hazard curves for DFI and survival were quite similar, suggesting that most dogs that experienced recurrence developed metastasis and not new tumors. However, the rate of new tumors was not reported in this study.[114] A differing study indicates that surgical "dose" is important. In this case series of 99 dogs, all intact female dogs underwent either a regional or chain mastectomy for a single mammary gland tumor with unknown histology.[118] Of these, 58% of dogs developed a new tumor in the remaining ipsilateral mammary gland tissue following a regional mastectomy and those whose initial tumor was subsequently determined to be malignant were more likely to develop an ipsilateral tumor. The authors advocated for an initial unilateral chain mastectomy for female intact dogs with a single mammary tumor, although, in their population, 42% of dogs did not develop a subsequent tumor and would have experienced a larger surgical dose than needed.[118] Unfortunately, other large useful studies investigating the association between OHE and survival did not report on the completeness or extent of mammary tumor removal.[18,119,120] Development of second mammary tumors is well documented and has been reported in over 70% of dogs with malignant mammary tumors following lumpectomy, although the impact of second mammary tumor development on survival is not clear.[16,114,118] It seems intuitive that a single standardized guideline for surgical treatment omits consideration of factors such as the dog's age, tumor size, tumor number, previous mammary tumors, and stage and may not provide the optimal outcome. Future carefully constructed clinical trials may offer more tailored recommendations based on the individual patient's risk.

Current recommendations based on available data suggest that for dogs with a single mammary tumor of known or unknown histotype, surgical excision wide enough to completely remove the mammary gland tumor is adequate. Incomplete excision or cytoreductive procedures are not endorsed.[95] Tumors that are fixed or have skin ulceration and are less than 1 cm in diameter may be sufficiently managed with a mammectomy (Figure 27-2).[95] "Wide excision" has not been well defined, but for larger tumors, this may be generalized to a 2-cm lateral margin and modified according to the size of the patient and tumor.[95] The deep margin may need to include the abdominal muscular fascia and/or portions of the abdominal wall to be excised en bloc with the mammary tumor, depending on size and fixation.[95] If abdominal surgery is to be performed simultaneously for OHE, penetration of the tumor prior to abdominal entry is to be avoided to prevent direct spread of tumor cells; rather, tumor removal should follow abdominal closure. For animals with multiple mammary tumors, more extensive resections such as a regional mastectomy or unilateral chain mastectomy may need to be pursued. As with other tumor resections, surgical margin assessment is critical for malignant mammary tumors, and additional surgery should be pursued if incompletely excised. Elective unilateral or bilateral chain mastectomies may be reasonable for young intact bitches with multiple tumors because there is a suggestion for development of additional tumors (Figure 27-3).[95] In spite of the evidence for recurrent mammary gland tumor development, there is no sufficiently compelling evidence at this time for routine recommendation of complete, unilateral or bilateral chain mastectomies.

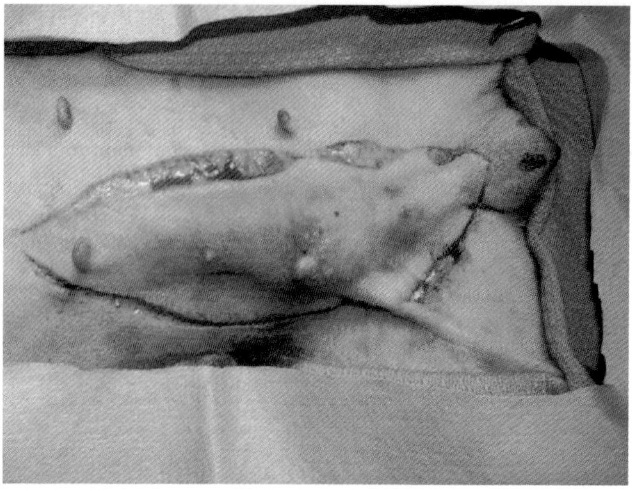

FIGURE 27-2 Regional mastectomy in a dog. *(Courtesy Dr. Julius Liptak, Alta Vista Animal Hospital, Ottawa, Canada.)*

Surgical excision is questionable as an adjuvant treatment for dogs presenting with inflammatory carcinoma due to the profound diffuse microscopic extent of cutaneous disease, the significant metastatic rate, and the local tissue coagulopathy that may be present. In 43 dogs with inflammatory carcinoma, only three dogs were considered suitable for unilateral chain mastectomy based on physical examination, yet all three had residual neoplastic cells at the surgical margins.[88] Interestingly, two of the dogs also received adjuvant chemotherapy and were among the longer survivors in that study.[88]

In women, the use of sentinel lymph node mapping has dramatically altered the surgical treatment of breast cancer. As canine mammary carcinoma has been demonstrated as a relevant model for human disease,[121,122] incorporation of human lymph node staging techniques should be reconsidered for the dog.[100] Sentinel lymph node mapping is a means of detecting which nodes are receiving draining tumor lymph and thus most at risk for

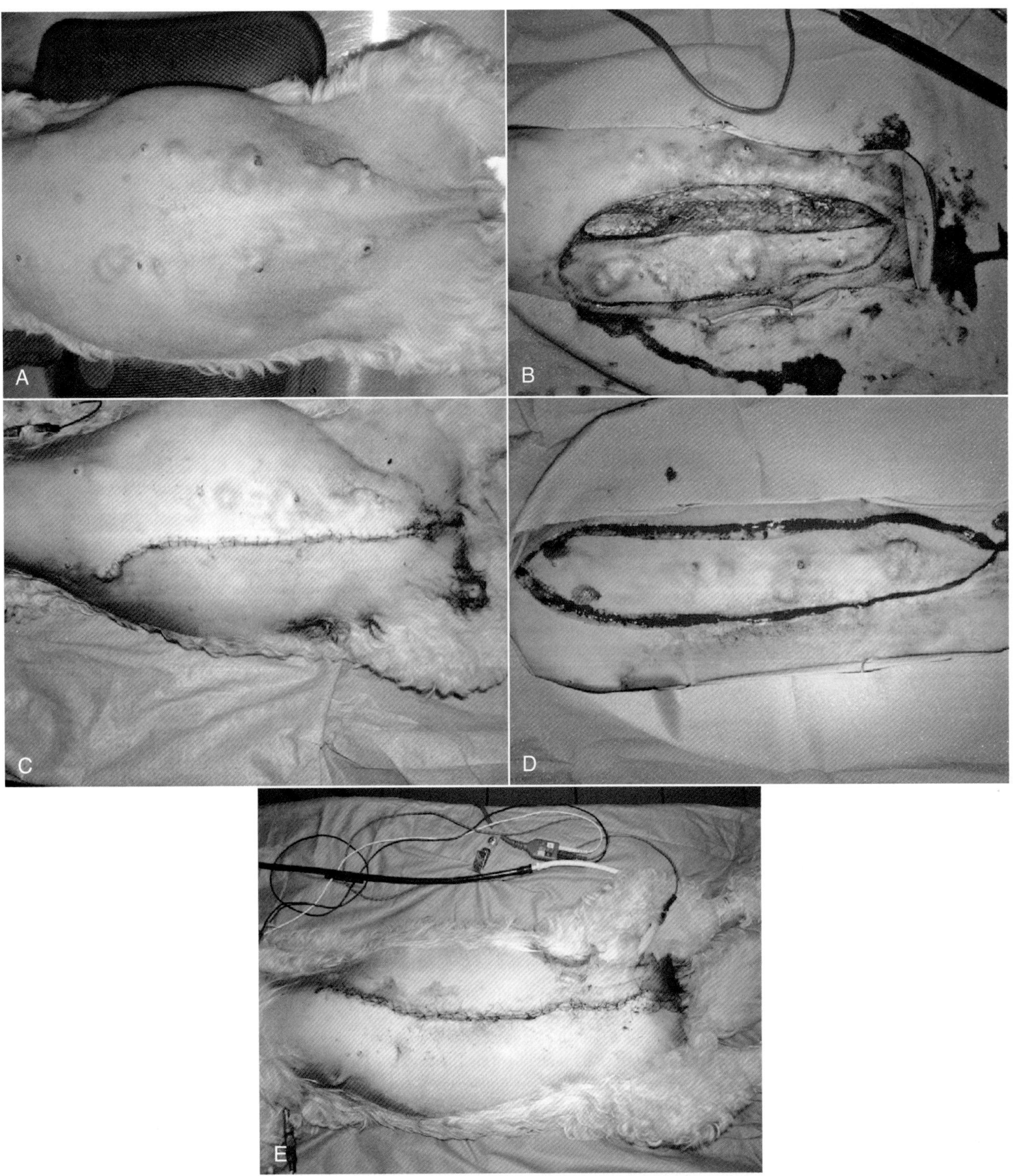

FIGURE 27-3 **A,** Multiple bilateral mammary tumors in a dog with taut abdominal tissue. **B,** A staged left chain mastectomy was performed initially of the side with the larger tumors. **C,** Immediate postsurgical appearance following the staged unilateral chain mastectomy without undue tension. **D,** The staged right chain mastectomy was performed 6 weeks later. **E,** Immediate postsurgical appearance following completed resection of all mammary tumors in this dog. *(Courtesy Dr. Julius Liptak, Alta Vista Animal Hospital, Ottawa, Canada.)*

lymph node metastasis. Some techniques described for sentinel lymph node mapping in the dog include lymphoscintigraphy using technetium, contrast-enhanced ultrasonography, autogenous hemosiderin, and intraoperative dyes (Figure 27-4).[97,100,123-125] The first description of sentinel lymph node mapping in any animal was done in cats 20 years ago.[126] Benefits include greater ease in identifying the at-risk lymph nodes intraoperatively with minimal surgical incisions and with efficiency, especially for the rarely assessed axillary nodes. The prognostic value of sentinel lymph node mapping is currently unknown for the dog as is the presence of mammary carcinoma lymph node micrometastasis.[127]

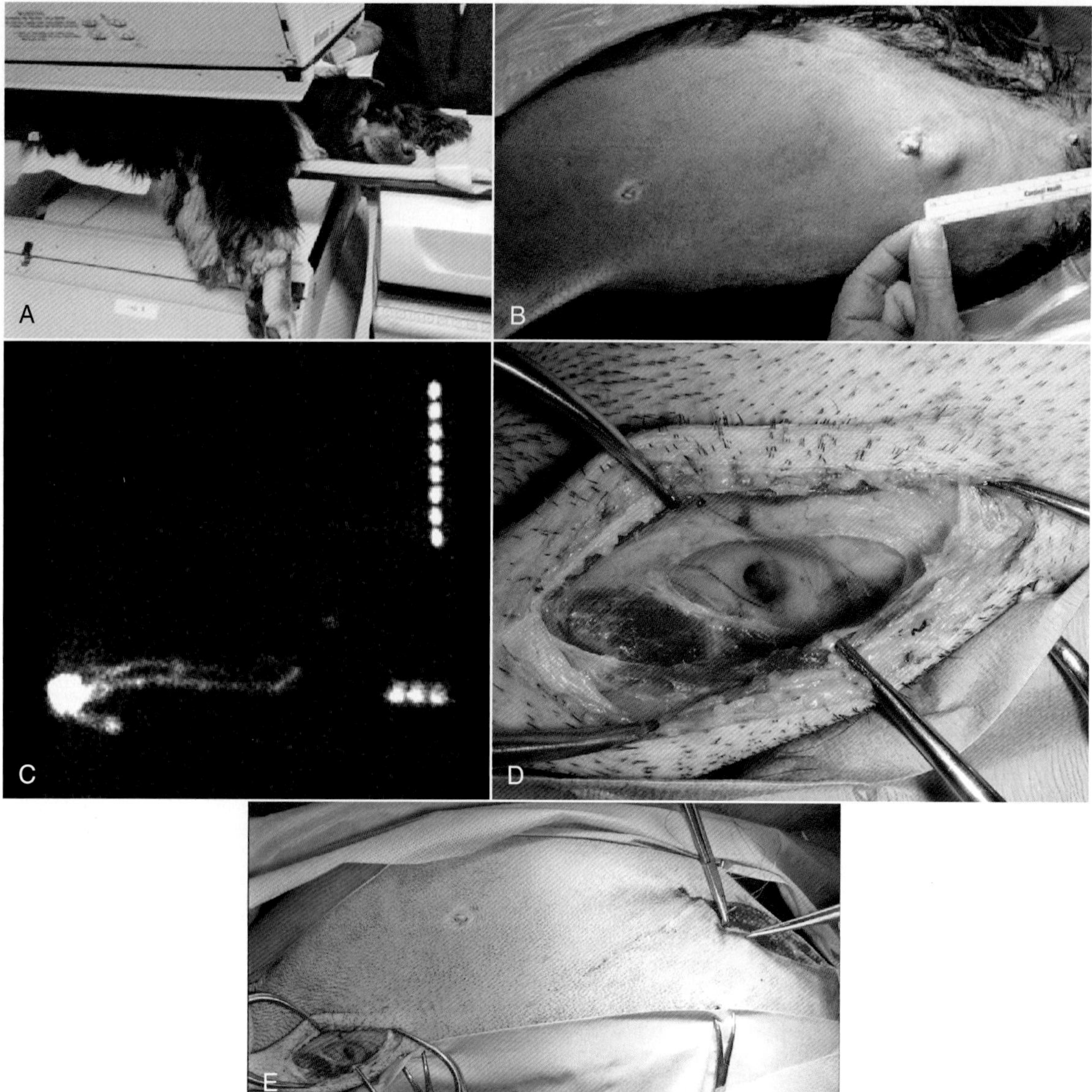

FIGURE 27-4 **A,** Regional lymphoscintigraphy being performed in a dog with a single mammary carcinoma. Technetium was injected in four quadrants around the primary tumor in the cranial abdominal mammary gland. **B,** Gross image of the same tumor in vivo. **C,** Regional lymphoscintigram of the patient highlighting radiopharmaceutical uptake in the mammary tumor and in the sentinel ipsilateral axillary lymph nodes. **D,** Close-up surgical appearance of a "hot" and "blue" sentinel accessory axillary lymph node visualized on the lymphoscintigram enhanced with intraoperative methylene blue dye mapping. **E,** Surgical field highlighting the distance between the mammary tumor and the same sentinel lymph node. *(Courtesy Dr. Deanna Worley, Colorado State University, Fort Collins, Colorado.)*

Systemic Treatment

Few clinical studies investigate systemic therapy for mammary tumors, and its efficacy has not been evaluated and confirmed according to the highest evidence-based standards. Despite this uncertainty, systemic therapy is routinely recommended and administered in dogs with high-risk tumors. This practice is based on the recognition that dogs with large tumors, positive lymph nodes, and aggressive histology are not treated effectively with surgery alone. The use of hormonal therapy in canine mammary tumors is based on tumor hormone dependence (tumor risk and HRs), as well as the potential to significantly reduce recurrence and prolong survival in HR-positive cancers similar to human hormonal therapy. This can be achieved by surgical means (ovariectomy [OVE] or OHE) or medical means, including specific ER modulators (SERMs) and suppression of estrogen synthesis by aromatase inhibitors or luteinizing hormone-releasing hormone (LHRH) agonists. Tamoxifen, an ER antagonist commonly used in women with ER-positive breast cancer, has been evaluated in dogs both with and without mammary tumors. Due to the side effects, mostly from proestrogenic signs, this strategy may not be tolerable or feasible in dogs.[128,129] Surgical ovarian ablation, specifically OVE/OHE, is a more practical solution in the dog. The results are in discordance, however. The majority of earlier publications did not report survival benefit in ovariohysterectomized dogs compared to intact dogs.[16,114,115,128,130]

Despite some study flaws, it is also possible that hormonal therapy is not effective. Dogs with large primary tumors, lymph node involvement, and undifferentiated histology have a poor

TABLE 27-5 Prognostic Factors and Indication for Adjuvant Chemotherapy with Supporting Level of Evidence in Dogs with Malignant Mammary Tumors

Tumor Size	Lymph Node Involvement	Histopathologic Type	Indication for Chemotherapy – (No) or + (Yes)	Evidence Level 1-5*
<3 cm/40 cc	Negative	Carcinoma	–†	1[114]
>3 cm/40 cc	Negative	Carcinoma	+‡	1,[114] 2,[131] 4,[142] 5[75]
Any	Positive	Carcinoma	+	3,[11,26,71,73,111,112,117] 2,[131] 5[75]
Any	Any	Osteosarcoma	+	3[112,138]
Any	Any	Inflammatory carcinoma	+	3[87,88,137]

*Evidence level 1: Prospective randomized trial (PRT); level 2: Prospective, nonrandomized trial (PT); level 3: Retrospective (RT); level 4: Case report(s) (CR); level 5: Extrapolation from human breast cancer studies (EH).

†Chemotherapy may be considered if unfavorable histology (vascular invasion or high grade).[110-113]

‡Dogs with stage III disease according to the original WHO staging system were included.[131] Stage III disease includes dogs with tumors >5 cm. with or without lymph node metastasis.[101]

prognosis and are less likely to have HR-positive tumors; thus they are less likely to benefit from hormonal ablation. A few studies have found that OHE significantly improves survival in dogs with mammary carcinomas or complex carcinomas. One study found the timing of OHE in relation to tumor surgery was important because only dogs with OHE within 2 years prior to or concurrently with tumor removal benefited. Dogs with OHE more than 2 years prior to surgery had a similar survival to dogs that remained intact.[120] Another study found that the benefit of OHE was only significant in dogs with complex carcinomas.[117] It is clear that only an adequately powered prospective randomized trial in which the effect of OHE is analyzed in context of HR status can answer questions regarding hormonal therapy in dogs with mammary tumors.

Chemotherapy is often administered to dogs with mammary tumors considered to be at risk for metastasis or recurrence. Most of the evidence regarding the efficacy of adjuvant chemotherapy is weak. A prospective nonrandomized study on dogs with high-risk mammary tumors (stage III or IV) did show a significant survival benefit in dogs receiving a combination of 5-fluorouracil and cyclophosphamide adjuvant to surgery compared to dogs treated with surgery alone.[131] Today, anthracycline or taxane combinations are considered part of first-line protocols in human breast cancer therapy in women requiring adjuvant therapy[75,132-134]; however, only inadequately powered studies on the efficacy of doxorubicin or docetaxel in dogs with mammary tumors exist and they did not establish benefit.[135] Similarly underpowered investigations of adjuvant gemcitabine in dogs with advanced stage (IV or V) mammary carcinoma did not establish benefit.[136] Adequately powered, randomized prospective trials are needed to determine the future role of adjuvant chemotherapy in dogs with high-risk mammary tumors. Systemic treatment, including nonsteroidal antiinflammatory drugs (NSAIDs), with or without chemotherapy, was found to be effective in prolonging survival in dogs with inflammatory carcinomas according to two independent retrospective case series.[88,137] Chemotherapy may also have a role in the treatment of primary mammary gland osteosarcoma. The mammary gland is one of the most common sites for extraskeletal osteosarcoma and according to a small retrospective case series (including primary mammary gland osteosarcoma, as well as other extraskeletal sites), dogs treated with adjuvant chemotherapy were significantly less likely to die from tumor-related causes than dogs treated with surgery alone.[138] More recently, a prospective randomized trial documented significant improvement in survival in dogs with histologic grade 2 or 3 carcinoma treated with perioperative desmopressin.[139] The antimetastatic properties of desmopressin are not fully understood, but it is hypothesized that they in part are mediated through improving hemostasis and preventing cancer cells from gaining access to the vasculature during surgical manipulation.[140,141] The results are intriguing, and further confirmatory studies are warranted. As illustrated previously, there is currently a paucity of high-quality trial evidence from which to draw information and guidance for treating dogs with malignant high-risk mammary tumors. Table 27-5 provides general guidance and treatment consideration/options and the level of supporting evidence.

Mammary Tumors in Cats

Epidemiology and Risk Factors

Epidemiology

There are fewer epidemiologic studies regarding the incidence of mammary neoplasia in cats compared to dogs. Furthermore, due to differences in veterinary care for cats, the available data likely underestimate the true incidence of disease. According to data from one of the largest Swedish insurance companies, approximately 40% to 50 % of all dogs had insurance to cover veterinary expenses, whereas only 20% of cats had such coverage.[143,144] Another study from the United States also reported that a significantly lower percentage of cats than dogs receives regular veterinary care.[145]

The overall mammary tumor incidence is lower in cats than in dogs. According to the California Animal Neoplasia Registry (CANR), mammary tumors represent the third most common tumor type in female cats (after skin tumors and lymphoma), with an annual incidence rate of 25.4/100,000 (compared to 198/100,000 in female dogs), and 12% of tumors in cats regardless of sex.[1] Data from an animal tumor registry from two provinces in northern Italy reported that mammary tumors represented 16% of all tumors in cats and 25% in female cats.[146] Data from the Swedish insurance company indicate that mammary tumors were the most common cancer, representing 40% of all tumor-related claims in cats.[143] It is unclear whether the higher relative incidence of mammary tumors in the latter studies is due to differences in neutering practices or use of progestins in the source population because no information regarding spay status was provided.

Risk Factors

Three main risk factors in cats have been identified: age, breed, and hormonal influence.

Age As in the dog, mammary neoplasia is a disease seen predominantly in middle-aged to older cats. The mean age of diagnosis is between 10 and 12 years of age.[1,147-150] Risk increases incrementally with age but does not become significant until 7 to 9 years, according to the age-specific incidence curves from the CANR, and continues to increase up until 12 to 14 years.[1]

Breed Siamese cats are significantly younger when diagnosed with mammary tumors, and risk plateaus at 9 years of age.[151] In general, genetic predisposition for a disease is often associated with a younger age of diagnosis. Siamese cats appear overrepresented when compared to other breeds.[151,152] However, Siamese cats have an increased risk for many tumor types, not only mammary tumors.[153-157] It is therefore possible that the increased incidence in Siamese cats is due to breed-associated germline alterations in common tumor susceptibility genes or defective tumor suppressor gene function that confers increased risk for many different malignancies.

Hormonal Association Exposure to ovarian hormones is also strongly implicated in mammary tumorigenesis in the cat. According to Dorn et al, sexually intact cats have a sevenfold higher risk than spayed cats.[1] The increased risk in intact cats has been confirmed by others.[148,151,158] Similar to findings in dogs, exposure from ovarian hormones in cats at an early age appears crucial. The protective effect of OHE diminishes quickly over the first few years; risk reductions of 91%, 86%, and 11% are seen in cats that are ovariohysterectomized before 6 months, between 7 and 12 months, or 13 and 24 months, respectively. No benefit was found after 24 months.[158] According to the same study, parity did not influence risk for mammary tumors.

In addition to endogenous ovarian hormonal influence, exposure to exogenous progestins also increases risk. Cats treated with progestins have an overall relative risk of 3.4 compared to those not receiving such treatments, although benign tumors arise more commonly than malignant tumors (relative risk 5.28 versus 2.8).[148] Unlike in dogs, progestin-treated cats were not younger than non-treated cats when they developed tumors.[148] The tumorigenic effects of oral progestins in cats are supported by reports of male cats with mammary tumors. Mammary tumors are rare in males, but in a report of 22 cases, 8 (36%) had a history of progestin use.[159] In a recent case series of three male cats with mammary tumors, all had received multiple injections of a long-lasting (depot) progestin over 5 to 6 years prior to tumor development. All had malignant tumors and all developed subsequent malignant tumors in other glands after initial surgery.[160] Shorter duration of treatment or inconsistent administration is less likely to result in malignant tumors but nevertheless induce changes in the mammary glands.[161] Fibroepithelial hyperplasia is the most common histopathologic change in cats treated for shorter periods of time and can occur relatively quickly, even after one injection. However, studies show that regular and prolonged administration is needed for malignant tumors to develop.[148]

Tumor Biology: Development, Hormones, Growth Factors, and Prognostic Implications

The risk for mammary tumor development in cats is determined by exposure to ovarian hormones early in life, but the latency period appears long because most cats are older when diagnosed. In many species, ovarian hormones are necessary for normal mammary gland development and maturation, but few studies have examined hormonal effects on mammary tumorigenesis in cats. The complex interactions between sex hormones, growth hormones, and IGF have been discussed in more detail in the section on canine mammary tumors, but progestin-induced mammary production of growth hormone has been documented in the cat.[162,163] It is, however, biologically plausible that the tumorigenic effects on mammary tissues are similar across species and that the same general mechanisms are involved, specifically sex hormones and growth hormones. Despite ER and PR expression being implicated in the initial stages of mammary tumor development, many investigators have reported that most feline mammary carcinomas are ER and PR negative, although slightly more than one-third are PR positive.[69,164-167] The percentage of ER/PR expression varies between studies and is likely the result of differences in case selection, methods, and interpretation of the results. The biochemical method, the dextran-coated charcoal (DCC) method, may be more sensitive than IHC when analyzing ER in cats.[166] Standardized IHC methods have high concordance with DCC methods; 38.5% of the malignant tumors and 66.7% of the benign lesions expressed PR according to IHC.[166] In this particular study, sexually intact cats were more likely to have PR-positive tumors. Lower concordance was found between ER analysis by DCC and IHC, with IHC being less sensitive than DCC; only 20% of the malignant tumors expressed ER according to IHC compared to 44% according to the DCC assay.[166] These results are consistent with other publications showing a relatively low ER expression in feline mammary tumors when using IHC.

The low HR-positivity in the tumors is consistent with the higher rate of malignancy and a more aggressive clinical behavior in feline mammary tumors. In contrast to malignant tumors, normal mammary tissue and dysplastic lesions in the mammary gland express both ER and PR.[69,164,165] However, this hormone dependence appears to wane with histologic progression from benign to malignant. None of the intermediate- or high-grade ductal carcinomas in situ were ER or PR positive, whereas the normal and hyperplastic adjacent mammary tissue expressed receptors.[69,164,165] Fibroepithelial hyperplasia, a progesterone-induced change, has been reported to have high PR expression[161] and can be effectively treated by OHE or antiprogesterones (Figure 27-5).[168]

In human breast cancer, an inverse relationship between the HR status and HER-2/neu expression is documented. HER-2/neu expression tends to be higher in cats than in dogs and humans; however, a wide range (5.5% to 90%) of HER-2/neu-positive tumors is reported.[169-172] Although the clinical and histologic association with HER-2/neu expression varies, cats with spontaneous mammary carcinomas may be good models for HER-2/neu-positive, hormone refractory breast cancer in women.

History and Clinical Presentation

Cats with mammary tumors are often older and may be sexually intact or spayed after they were 2 years old. Tumors are easy to detect on physical examination and appear as firm discrete mass(es) in the mammary gland(s). One study reported that all glands are equally susceptible to tumor development, but a later study showed that the anterior glands were less commonly affected.[173,174] Multiple tumors are common; 60% of cats had more than one tumor at diagnosis in one report.[149] Careful examination of the remaining mammary glands is important when evaluating a cat with a prior history of mammary tumors, especially if treated with simple mastectomy, because new primary tumors are common. Tumor(s) size

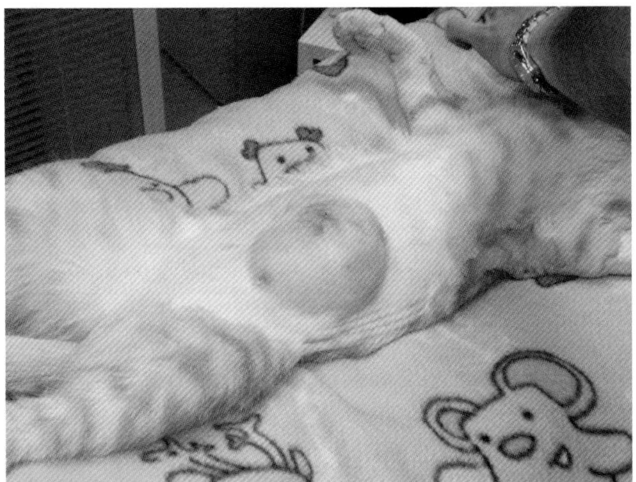

FIGURE 27-5 Fibroepithelial hyperplasia in a cat. *(Courtesy Dr. Lisa Mestrinho, Faculdade de Medicina Veterinária, Universidade Lusofona de Humanidades e Tecnologias, Lisboa, Portugal.)*

at diagnosis depends on how early it is detected and how aggressive the tumor behaves. Larger tumors may become ulcerated, inflamed, and infected. Local lymph nodes may or may not appear enlarged. Inflammatory mammary carcinomas are rare in cats, and the clinical picture and outcome are similar to those described in the dog.[175]

Clinical Assessment, Diagnosis, Work-Up, and Staging

Cats with mammary masses tend to be older and their tumors are commonly malignant; therefore, a thorough work-up is recommended to ascertain any comorbidity as well as advanced disease. This may include at a minimum a CBC, serum biochemistry, serum T_4 concentration, three-view thoracic radiographs, abdominal ultrasound, and urinalysis, in addition to FNA of any mammary masses and any palpable (including normal-sized) regional lymph nodes.

Staging System

Feline mammary tumors are staged similar to canine tumors using a modification of the original system published by Owens.[101,176] In the modified system, stage advances from I to II to III as the size increases from smaller than 2 cm, to between 2 and 3 cm, to larger than 3 cm.[102] Unlike the canine system, stage III disease also includes T1 or T2 tumors with concurrent lymph node metastasis and lymph node metastasis does not need to be present with T3 tumors. Stage IV disease is any tumor with any lymph node metastasis and distant metastasis.[176] This staging system should not be used with mammary gland sarcomas (Table 27-6).

Histopathology

The vast majority of feline mammary tumors are malignant (85% to 95%), with an aggressive biologic behavior, and lymphatic invasion and lymph node metastasis are more common at the time of initial diagnosis than in dogs. Early classifications of feline mammary tumors were simpler than that used for canine tumors[105]; however, several new tumor types have subsequently been reported.

TABLE 27-6 Staging of Feline Mammary Tumors

Stage	Tumor Size	Lymph Node Status	Metastasis
Stage 1	T1 <2 cm	N0	M0
Stage 2	T2 2-3 cm	N0	M0
Stage 3	T1 or T2	N1 (positive)	M0
	T3 >3 cm	N0 or N1	M0
Stage 4	Any	Any	M1

Data from McNeill CJ, Sorenmo KU, Shofer FS, et al: Evaluation of adjuvant doxorubicin-based chemotherapy for the treatment of feline mammary carcinoma, *J Vet Intern Med* 23:123-129, 2009.

Hyperplasia and Dysplasia[105]

The various hyperplastic and dysplastic lesions included in this group include duct ectasia, lobular hyperplasia, lobular hyperplasia with secretory (lactational) activity, lobular hyperplasia with fibrosis (interlobular fibrous connective tissue), epitheliosis (intralobular ducts), papillomatosis (interlobular ducts), and fibroadenomatous change.[177] Fibroadenomatous change (fibroepithelial hyperplasia, fibroepithelial hypertrophy, mammary hypertrophy) is more common in the cat than the dog and is characterized by the proliferation of interlobular ducts and periductal stromal cells. The stroma is often edematous or myxomatous, and both the ductal and stromal cell nuclei exhibit some pleomorphism with mitoses. This lesion is hormonally induced and occurs in progestin-treated female and male cats, as well as being associated with pregnancy. Most cases regress at the end of pregnancy or cessation of progestin treatment.

Benign Feline Mammary Neoplasms[105]

Benign tumors in cats are uncommon and include adenoma, ductal adenoma, fibroadenoma, and intraductal papillary adenoma (duct papilloma).

Malignant Feline Mammary Neoplasms[105,172,175,177-183]

The predominant malignant tumor types in cats are simple and epithelial in origin and as such represent carcinomas of various types. Adenocarcinomas, tubular carcinomas, or a combination of tubular, papillary, and solid carcinomas are most common. Other variants include cystic papillary carcinoma, cribriform carcinoma, micropapillary invasive carcinoma, comedocarcinoma, and less commonly, squamous cell carcinoma, mucinous carcinoma, and lipid-rich carcinoma.

Histopathologic Prognostic Factors and Grading

Grading was initially thought not to be prognostic in cats; therefore the classification of mammary tumors was based on morphologic criteria only. More recently, grading, using a system similar to that in dogs (based on the Elston and Ellis scoring system; see Tables 27-3 and 27-4), has been shown to be prognostic in cats. In addition to grade, lymphovascular invasion and lymph node metastasis are independent prognostic factors.[178,184] Thus the histopathologic criteria used in dogs (i.e., grade, vascular invasion, lymph node status) can be used in cats when assessing risk for metastasis and prognosis and should be incorporated into decisions regarding the need for systemic treatment in cats with mammary tumors (Table 27-7).

Clinical Prognostic Factors

Few studies reporting prognostic factors in cats with mammary tumors are prospective, only one is randomized, and most are

TABLE 27-7 Prognostic Factors and Indications for Adjuvant Chemotherapy with Level of Supporting Evidence in Cats with Malignant Mammary Tumors

TUMOR SIZE	LYMPH NODE INVOLVEMENT	HISTOPATHOLOGIC PARAMETERS	INDICATION FOR CHEMOTHERAPY −(NO) OR +(YES)	EVIDENCE LEVEL*
<2 cm/8 cm^3	Negative	Carcinoma	−	−1[185]
			+†	+3[178,184,186]
2-3 cm/8-27 cm^3	Negative	Carcinoma	−	−3[187]
			+†	+3[178,184,186]
>3 cm/27 cm^3	Negative	Carcinoma	+	1,[185] 2,[174] 3[187]
Any	Positive	Carcinoma	+	2,[174] 3,[184] 5[75]

*Evidence level 1: Prospective randomized trial (PRT); level 2: Prospective, nonrandomized trial (PT); level 3: Retrospective (RT); level 5: Extrapolation from human breast cancer studies (EH).

†Vascular invasion and high grade were found to be independent negative prognostic factors in multivariate analysis.

underpowered or not stratified according to treatment. Therefore the results vary and may be significantly affected by bias. Tumor size has, however, consistently been reported to have prognostic significance, including the results of two large prospective studies.

Tumor Size and Prognosis

Three size categories have shown prognostic significance: (1) smaller than 8 cm^3 or smaller than 2 cm diameter; (2) larger than 8 to 27 cm^3 or larger than 2 to 3 cm diameter; and (3) larger than 27 cm^3 or larger than 3 cm diameter. Cats with small tumors (<2 cm) can be effectively treated with surgery alone with a median survival time (MST) of more than 3 years, whereas cats with tumors larger than 3 cm have a MST of only 6 months according to a large, high-quality retrospective study.[187] Cats with 2- to 3-cm diameter tumors survived an average of 2 years. Several other publications have confirmed this association between survival and tumor size.[150,152,174,185,186] Tumor size is one of the most important factors when assessing risk for metastasis and the need for adjuvant treatments.

Lymph Nodes and Prognosis

Surprisingly few studies have evaluated lymph node status and its prognostic significance in cats with mammary tumors. In a large prospective study of 202 cats, those with lymph node metastasis had a significantly shorter survival than cats with negative lymph nodes.[174] A recent retrospective study with 92 cats supported these findings; all cats with lymph node metastasis died within the first 9 months of diagnosis.[184]

Breed and Prognosis

Domestic shorthair cats had significantly better outcomes than purebred cats in a prospective randomized trial of cats with mammary carcinomas.[185] A recent retrospective case series reported that Siamese cats had a worse prognosis than domestic shorthairs.[188] These studies may in fact complement each other; however, the first study did not provide information regarding how many Siamese cats were included in the purebred group. Several other studies have not found breed to be prognostic when adjusted for other factors.

Age

The results regarding age and prognosis are conflicting. Several studies report that older cats have a worse prognosis; however, bias due to differences in treatments or differences in tumor size and stage may exist. Importantly, a prospective randomized trial found no difference according to age when comparing cats that were younger or older than 10 years.[185]

Surgical Treatment

The surgical dose recommended for treating feline mammary tumors is much clearer than in the dog. A chain mastectomy (unilateral for cats possessing a single tumor or a 2-staged bilateral chain mastectomy for cats with bilateral tumors) resulted in a favorable statistically significant DFI, as opposed to cats receiving conservative tumor excision in a series of 100 cats.[187] In that same case series, there was a trend for improved survival times for cats receiving chain mastectomies.[187] In a retrospective case series of 53 cats, while no significant relation was found between the type of surgical procedure performed, cats experienced longer DFIs following either unilateral or bilateral chain mastectomies.[152] In a multiinstitutional retrospective case series comparing patients receiving surgery versus surgery with adjuvant doxorubicin-based chemotherapy, the subset of cats having unilateral chain mastectomies followed with chemotherapy had significantly longer MSTs than cats having unilateral chain mastectomies performed without chemotherapy (1998 versus 414 days).[176] In that series, local recurrence developed in 50% of cats and, although not statistically significant, appears to support the use of chain mastectomies for feline mammary carcinomas.[176] In a report of male cats diagnosed with mammary carcinomas, a trend toward more frequent local recurrence correlated with more conservative resections.[159] Thus, for cats, a unilateral or staged bilateral chain mastectomy is recommended for treatment of mammary carcinoma. For some cats with excessively loose mammary tissue, a bilateral chain mastectomy can be performed during a single surgical session if minimal postsurgical tension can be achieved, but subjectively these cats may have a more difficult recovery (Figure 27-6). For tumors that are fixed, muscular fascia or portions of the body wall should be included with en bloc resections.

The high malignancy rate of mammary carcinoma and the poor prognosis associated with lymph node metastasis supports aggressive lymph node assessment. This could include ultrasound-guided FNA of difficult to palpate regional nodes and inguinal lymphadenectomy concurrent with chain mastectomy. Sentinel lymph node mapping has been described in the cat and was the original model for the procedure, which is common for human breast cancer patients.[126,189] Published techniques in the cat include CT evaluation following intramammary injection of iopamidol and radiographic imaging following intramammary ethiodized oil injections.[189]

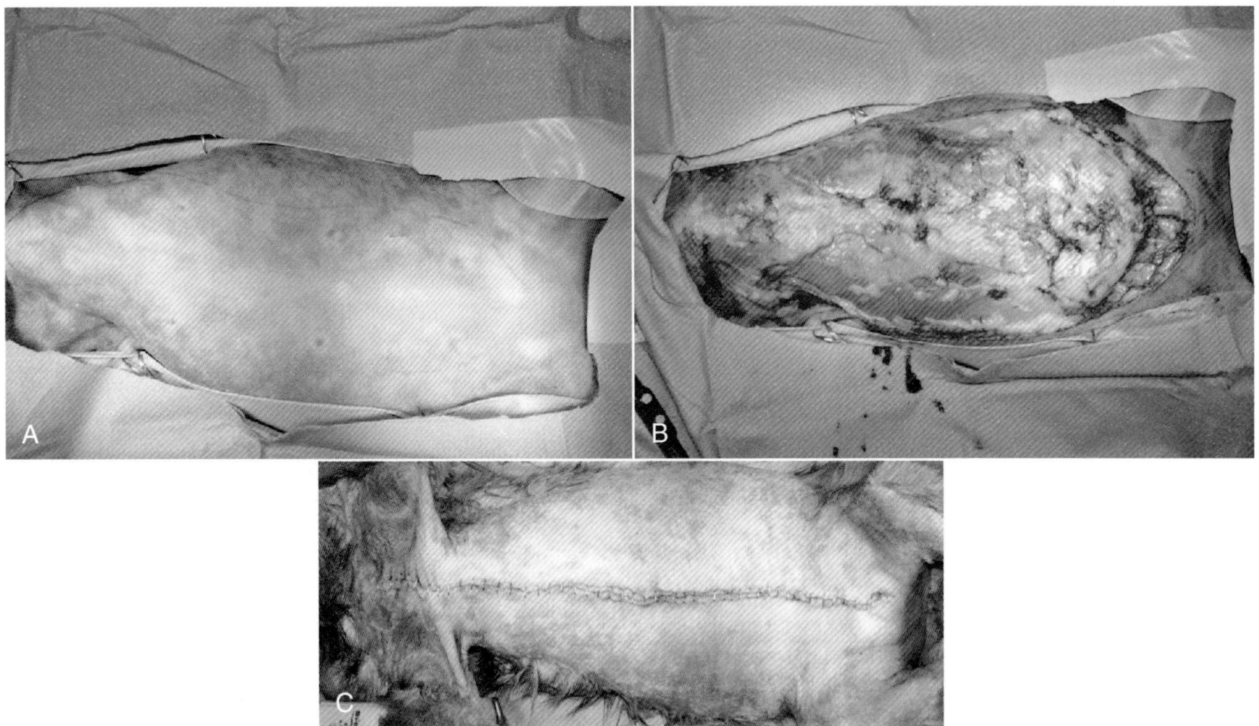

FIGURE 27-6 **A,** Cat having mammary adenocarcinoma prepared for bilateral simultaneous chain mastectomies. **B,** Intraoperative view following excision of all mammary tissue. **C,** Immediate postsurgical appearance following the bilateral chain mastectomies. *(Courtesy Dr. Julius Liptak, Alta Vista Animal Hospital, Ottawa, Canada.)*

There are no clinical reports utilizing nuclear lymphoscintigraphy in the cat. Use of blue dyes for node visualization is not recommended because their use may cause Heinz body anemia and methemoglobinemia in this species.

Fibroepithelial hyperplasia has a classic appearance that is very difficult to mistake for malignant mammary tumors. This condition is typically treated with either OHE or medical hormone therapy management. Inflammatory mammary carcinoma has very rarely been reported in cats; in a sole case series of three cats, the disease was described as occurring secondary to postsurgical mastectomy with nonhealing incisions, edema, and suture rejections.[175]

Systemic Treatment

Early detection and aggressive surgery (including prophylactic chain mastectomy) can result in long-term survival in cats with early stage mammary tumors. However, cats with delayed diagnosis, large primary tumors, or metastatic local lymph nodes are not treated effectively with surgery alone. The incidence of distant metastasis, primarily to the lungs and pleura, is high, although other organs are also frequently involved.[174] Despite the high rate of metastasis after surgery, very few advances have been made in identifying effective adjuvant systemic treatments.

Due to low HR expression in feline mammary carcinoma, hormonal therapy is not likely to be effective; however, randomized trials have not been performed to confirm this.

Several studies, all retrospective, have evaluated the use of chemotherapy in cats with mammary cancer. Two case series of cats with macroscopic primary and/or metastatic tumors documented objective responses in 40% to 50% of the cats treated with a combination of doxorubicin and cyclophosphamide.[190,191] The relatively high response rate in the macroscopic setting suggests that this may be an effective protocol in patients with microscopic minimal residual disease (i.e., following surgical cytoreduction). However, results from adjuvant studies do not reflect this, albeit none of the studies were prospective or randomized. A multiinstitutional retrospective study describing outcome in cats treated with adjuvant single-agent doxorubicin reported a median survival of 450 days in cats with tumors less than 2 cm in diameter.[176] This is shorter than survival times reported in cats treated with surgery alone (3 years). Interestingly, another study evaluating the combination of a doxorubicin-based chemotherapy protocol and an NSAID (meloxicam) reported similar MSTs of 460 days.[188] No control arm consisting of cats treated with surgery alone was included; thus the additive benefit of chemotherapy was not possible to determine. A more recent retrospective, nonrandomized study also compared outcome in cats treated with surgery alone to cats treated with surgery and adjuvant chemotherapy.[176] No significant differences in terms of surgical procedure, tumor size, stage, or histopathologic parameters existed between the groups. No difference in overall survival was found between treatment groups. Further subgroup analysis failed to reveal differences in survival between the groups when comparing cats with tumors less than 2 cm (611 days with surgery alone versus 729 with surgery and chemotherapy). However, cats treated with chain mastectomy and adjuvant chemotherapy survived significantly longer than cats treated with chain mastectomy alone (1998 days versus 414 days). These results support the use of adjuvant chemotherapy in this setting. It is interesting that none of these retrospective studies reported survival times as long as earlier studies using surgery alone, especially in the subset of cats with small tumors. This further illustrates the difficulty in comparing outcomes between retrospective studies, especially noncontemporaneous ones. Ultimately, prospective, randomized trials will be necessary to determine the appropriate use of chemotherapy in cats with mammary tumors. Despite the lack of quality evidence in the literature to support it, veterinary oncologists continue to make decisions regarding the use of chemotherapy in cats with mammary tumors. Table 27-7 summarizes the most important prognostic factors, general guidelines for systemic treatments, and the strength of supporting evidence.

REFERENCES

1. Dorn CR, Taylor DO, Schneider R, et al: Survey of animal neoplasms in Alameda and Contra Costa Counties, California. II. Cancer morbidity in dogs and cats from Alameda County, *J Natl Cancer Inst* 40:307–318, 1968.
2. Moe L: Population-based incidence of mammary tumours in some dog breeds, *J Reprod Fertil Suppl* 57:439–443, 2001.
3. Egenvall A, Bonnett BN, Ohagen P, et al: Incidence of and survival after mammary tumors in a population of over 80,000 insured female dogs in Sweden from 1995 to 2002, *Prev Vet Med* 69:109–127, 2005.
4. Dobson JM, Samuel S, Milstein H, et al: Canine neoplasia in the UK: estimates of incidence rates from a population of insured dogs, *J Small Anim Pract* 43:240–246, 2002.
5. Bronden LB, Nielsen SS, Toft N, et al: Data from the Danish veterinary cancer registry on the occurrence and distribution of neoplasms in dogs in Denmark, *Vet Rec* 166:586–590, 2010.
6. Merlo DF, Rossi L, Pellegrino C, et al: Cancer incidence in pet dogs: findings of the Animal Tumor Registry of Genoa, Italy, *J Vet Intern Med* 22:976–984, 2008.
7. Benjamin SA, Lee AC, Saunders WJ: Classification and behavior of canine mammary epithelial neoplasms based on life-span observations in beagles, *Vet Pathol* 36:423–436, 1999.
8. Schneider R: Comparison of age, sex, and incidence rates in human and canine breast cancer, *Cancer* 26:419–426, 1970.
9. Priester WA, Mantel N: Occurrence of tumors in domestic animals: data from 12 United States and Canadian colleges of veterinary medicine, *J Natl Cancer Inst* 47:1333–1344, 1971.
10. Brodey RS, Goldschmidt MH, Roszel JR: Canine mammary gland neoplasms, *J Am Anim Hosp Assoc* 19:61–90, 1983.
11. Kurzman ID, Gilbertson SR: Prognostic factors in canine mammary tumors, *Semin Vet Med Surg (Small Anim)* 1:25–32, 1986.
12. Taylor GN, Shabestari L, Williams J, et al: Mammary neoplasia in a closed beagle colony, *Cancer Res* 36:2740–2743, 1976.
13. Sorenmo KU, Kristiansen VM, Cofone MA, et al: Canine mammary gland tumours: a histological continuum from benign to malignant; clinical and histopathological evidence, *Vet Comp Oncol* 7:162–172, 2009.
14. Goldschmidt M, Shofer FS, Smelstoys JA: Neoplastic lesions of the mammary gland. In Mohr U, Carlton WW, Dungworth DL, et al, editors: *Pathobiology of the aging dog*, Ames, Iowa, 2001, Iowa State University Press.
15. Rivera P, Melin M, Biagi T, et al: Mammary tumor development in dogs is associated with BRCA1 and BRCA2, *Cancer Res* 69:8770–8774, 2009.
16. Schneider R, Dorn CR, Taylor DO: Factors influencing canine mammary cancer development and postsurgical survival, *J Natl Cancer Inst* 43:1249–1261, 1969.
17. Sonnenschein EG, Glickman LT, Goldschmidt MH, et al: Body conformation, diet, and risk of breast cancer in pet dogs: a case-control study, *Am J Epidemiol* 133:694–703, 1991.
18. Misdorp W: Canine mammary tumours: protective effect of late ovariectomy and stimulating effect of progestins, *Vet Q* 10:26–33, 1988.
19. Brodey RS, Fidler IJ, Howson AE: The relationship of estrous irregularity, pseudopregnancy, and pregnancy to the development of canine mammary neoplasms, *J Am Vet Med Assoc* 149:1047–1049, 1966.
20. Stovring M, Moe L, Glattre E: A population-based case-control study of canine mammary tumours and clinical use of medroxyprogesterone acetate, *APMIS* 105:590–596, 1997.
21. Concannon PW, Spraker TR, Casey HW, et al: Gross and histopathologic effects of medroxyprogesterone acetate and progesterone on the mammary glands of adult beagle bitches, *Fertil Steril* 36:373–387, 1981.
22. Giles RC, Kwapien RP, Geil RG, et al: Mammary nodules in beagle dogs administered investigational oral contraceptive steroids, *J Natl Cancer Inst* 60:1351–1364, 1978.
23. Kwapien RP, Giles RC, Geil RG, et al: Malignant mammary tumors in beagle dogs dosed with investigational oral contraceptive steroids, *J Natl Cancer Inst* 65:137–144, 1980.
24. Selman PJ, van Garderen E, Mol JA, et al: Comparison of the histological changes in the dog after treatment with the progestins medroxyprogesterone acetate and proligestone, *Vet Q* 17:128–133, 1995.
25. Geil RG, Lamar JK: FDA studies of estrogen, progestogens, and estrogen/progestogen combinations in the dog and monkey, *J Toxicol Environ Health* 3:179–193, 1977.
26. Yamagami T, Kobayashi T, Takahashi K, et al: Prognosis for canine malignant mammary tumors based on TNM and histologic classification, *J Vet Med Sci* 58:1079–1083, 1996.
27. Schafer KA, Kelly G, Schrader R, et al: A canine model of familial mammary gland neoplasia, *Vet Pathol* 35:168–177, 1998.
28. Ford D, Easton DF, Stratton M, et al: Genetic heterogeneity and penetrance analysis of the BRCA1 and BRCA2 genes in breast cancer families. The Breast Cancer Linkage Consortium, *Am J Hum Genet* 62:676–689, 1998.
29. King MC, Marks JH, Mandell JB: Breast and ovarian cancer risks due to inherited mutations in BRCA1 and BRCA2, *Science* 302:643–646, 2003.
30. Easton DF, Ford D, Bishop DT: Breast and ovarian cancer incidence in BRCA1-mutation carriers. Breast Cancer Linkage Consortium, *Am J Hum Genet* 56:265–271, 1995.
31. Fackenthal JD, Olopade OI: Breast cancer risk associated with BRCA1 and BRCA2 in diverse populations, *Nat Rev Cancer* 7:937–948, 2007.
32. Klopfleisch R, Gruber AD: Increased expression of BRCA2 and RAD51 in lymph node metastases of canine mammary adenocarcinomas, *Vet Pathol* 46:416–422, 2009.
33. Nieto A, Perez-Alenza MD, Del Castillo N, et al: BRCA1 expression in canine mammary dysplasias and tumours: relationship with prognostic variables, *J Comp Pathol* 128:260–268, 2003.
34. Perez Alenza D, Rutteman GR, Pena L, et al: Relation between habitual diet and canine mammary tumors in a case-control study, *J Vet Intern Med* 12:132–139, 1998.
35. Calle EE, Kaaks R: Overweight, obesity and cancer: epidemiological evidence and proposed mechanisms, *Nat Rev Cancer* 4:579–591, 2004.
36. Carmichael AR, Bates T: Obesity and breast cancer: a review of the literature, *Breast* 13:85–92, 2004.
37. Tymchuk CN, Tessler SB, Barnard RJ: Changes in sex hormone-binding globulin, insulin, and serum lipids in postmenopausal women on a low-fat, high-fiber diet combined with exercise, *Nutr Cancer* 38:158–162, 2000.
38. Wu AH, Pike MC, Stram DO: Meta-analysis: dietary fat intake, serum estrogen levels, and the risk of breast cancer, *J Natl Cancer Inst* 91:529–534, 1999.
39. Hankinson SE, Willett WC, Manson JE, et al: Plasma sex steroid hormone levels and risk of breast cancer in postmenopausal women, *J Natl Cancer Inst* 90:1292–1299, 1998.
40. Cleary MP, Grossmann ME: Minireview: Obesity and breast cancer: the estrogen connection, *Endocrinology* 150:2537–2542, 2009.
41. Cleary MP, Grossmann ME, Ray A: Effect of obesity on breast cancer development, *Vet Pathol* 47:202–213, 2010.
42. Rehm S, Stanislaus DJ, Williams AM: Estrous cycle-dependent histology and review of sex steroid receptor expression in dog reproductive tissues and mammary gland and associated hormone levels, *Birth Defects Res B Dev Reprod Toxicol* 80:233–245, 2007.

43. Santos M, Marcos R, Faustino AM: Histological study of canine mammary gland during the oestrous cycle. *Reprod Domest Anim* 45:e146–e154, 2010.
44. Pike MC, Spicer DV, Dahmoush L, et al: Estrogens, progestogens, normal breast cell proliferation, and breast cancer risk, *Epidemiol Rev* 15:17–35, 1993.
45. Russo J, Russo IH: The role of estrogen in the initiation of breast cancer, *J Steroid Biochem Mol Biol* 102:89–96, 2006.
46. Okoh V, Deoraj A, Roy D: Estrogen-induced reactive oxygen species-mediated signalings contribute to breast cancer, *Biochim Biophys Acta* 1815:115–133, 2011.
47. Dickson RB, Lippman ME, Slamon D: UCLA colloquium. New insights into breast cancer: the molecular biochemical and cellular biology of breast cancer, *Cancer Res* 50:4446–4447, 1990.
48. Mol JA, Lantinga-van Leeuwen IS, van Garderen E, et al: Mammary growth hormone and tumorigenesis–lessons from the dog, *Vet Q* 21:111–115, 1999.
49. Selman PJ, Mol JA, Rutteman GR, et al: Progestin-induced growth hormone excess in the dog originates in the mammary gland, *Endocrinology* 134:287–292, 1994.
50. van Garderen E, Schalken JA: Morphogenic and tumorigenic potentials of the mammary growth hormone/growth hormone receptor system, *Mol Cell Endocrinol* 197:153–165, 2002.
51. Mol JA, Selman PJ, Sprang EP, et al: The role of progestins, insulin-like growth factor (IGF) and IGF-binding proteins in the normal and neoplastic mammary gland of the bitch: a review, *J Reprod Fertil Suppl* 51:339–344, 1997.
52. Hamelers IH, van Schaik RF, van Teeffelen HA, et al: Synergistic proliferative action of insulin-like growth factor I and 17 beta-estradiol in MCF-7S breast tumor cells, *Exp Cell Res* 273:107–117, 2002.
53. Thorne C, Lee AV: Cross talk between estrogen receptor and IGF signaling in normal mammary gland development and breast cancer, *Breast Dis* 17:105–114, 2003.
54. Laban C, Bustin SA, Jenkins PJ: The GH-IGF-I axis and breast cancer, *Trends Endocrinol Metab* 14:28–34, 2003.
55. van der Burg B, Rutteman GR, Blankenstein MA, et al: Mitogenic stimulation of human breast cancer cells in a growth factor-defined medium: synergistic action of insulin and estrogen, *J Cell Physiol* 134:101–108, 1988.
56. Osborne CK, Clemmons DR, Arteaga CL: Regulation of breast cancer growth by insulin-like growth factors, *J Steroid Biochem Mol Biol* 37:805–809, 1990.
57. Dupont J, Le Roith D: Insulin-like growth factor 1 and oestradiol promote cell proliferation of MCF-7 breast cancer cells: new insights into their synergistic effects, *Mol Pathol* 54:149–154, 2001.
58. Queiroga FL, Perez-Alenza D, Silvan G, et al: Serum and intratumoural GH and IGF-I concentrations: prognostic factors in the outcome of canine mammary cancer, *Res Vet Sci* 89:396–403, 2010.
59. Queiroga FL, Perez-Alenza MD, Silvan G, et al: Crosstalk between GH/IGF-I axis and steroid hormones (progesterone, 17beta-estradiol) in canine mammary tumours, *J Steroid Biochem Mol Biol* 110:76–82, 2008.
60. Klopfleisch R, von Euler H, Sarli G, et al: Molecular carcinogenesis of canine mammary tumors: news from an old disease, *Vet Pathol* 48:98–116, 2011.
61. Rivera P, von Euler H: Molecular biological aspects on canine and human mammary tumors, *Vet Pathol* 48:132–146, 2011.
62. Gilbertson SR, Kurzman ID, Zachrau RE, et al: Canine mammary epithelial neoplasms: biologic implications of morphologic characteristics assessed in 232 dogs, *Vet Pathol* 20:127–142, 1983.
63. Moulton JE, Rosenblatt LS, Goldman M: Mammary tumors in a colony of beagle dogs, *Vet Pathol* 23:741–749, 1986.
64. Bender AP, Dorn CR, Schneider R: An epidemiologic study of canine multiple primary neoplasma involving the female and male reproductive systems, *Prev Vet Med* 2:715–731, 1984.
65. Antuofermo E, Miller MA, Pirino S, et al: Spontaneous mammary intraepithelial lesions in dogs—a model of breast cancer, *Cancer Epidemiol Biomarkers Prev* 16:2247–2256, 2007.
66. MacEwen EG, Patnaik AK, Harvey HJ, et al: Estrogen receptors in canine mammary tumors, *Cancer Res* 42:2255–2259, 1982.
67. Rutteman GR, Misdorp W, Blankenstein MA, et al: Oestrogen (ER) and progestin receptors (PR) in mammary tissue of the female dog: different receptor profile in non-malignant and malignant states, *Br J Cancer* 58:594–599, 1988.
68. Illera JC, Perez-Alenza MD, Nieto A, et al: Steroids and receptors in canine mammary cancer, *Steroids* 71:541–548, 2006.
69. Millanta F, Calandrella M, Bari G, et al: Comparison of steroid receptor expression in normal, dysplastic, and neoplastic canine and feline mammary tissues, *Res Vet Sci* 79:225–232, 2005.
70. Donnay I, Rauis J, Devleeschouwer N, et al: Comparison of estrogen and progesterone receptor expression in normal and tumor mammary tissues from dogs, *Am J Vet Res* 56:1188–1194, 1995.
71. de Las Mulas JM, Millan Y, Dios R: A prospective analysis of immunohistochemically determined estrogen receptor alpha and progesterone receptor expression and host and tumor factors as predictors of disease-free period in mammary tumors of the dog, *Vet Pathol* 42:200–212, 2005.
72. Chang CC, Tsai MH, Liao JW, et al: Evaluation of hormone receptor expression for use in predicting survival of female dogs with malignant mammary gland tumors, *J Am Vet Med Assoc* 235:391–396, 2009.
73. Nieto A, Pena L, Perez-Alenza MD, et al: Immunohistologic detection of estrogen receptor alpha in canine mammary tumors: clinical and pathologic associations and prognostic significance, *Vet Pathol* 37:239–247, 2000.
74. Geraldes M, Gartner F, Schmitt F: Immunohistochemical study of hormonal receptors and cell proliferation in normal canine mammary glands and spontaneous mammary tumours, *Vet Rec* 146:403–406, 2000.
75. Effects of chemotherapy and hormonal therapy for early breast cancer on recurrence and 15-year survival: an overview of the randomised trials, *Lancet* 365:1687–1717, 2005.
76. Winer EP, Hudis C, Burstein HJ, et al: American Society of Clinical Oncology technology assessment on the use of aromatase inhibitors as adjuvant therapy for postmenopausal women with hormone receptor-positive breast cancer: status report 2004, *J Clin Oncol* 23:619–629, 2005.
77. Network NCC: *Clinical practice guidelines in oncology-version 2.2006*, 2005, National Comprehensive Cancer Network, Inc.
78. Tamoxifen for early breast cancer: an overview of the randomised trials. Early Breast Cancer Trialists' Collaborative Group, *Lancet* 351:1451–1467, 1998.
79. Thuerlimann B, Koeberle D, Senn HJ: Guidelines for the adjuvant treatment of postmenopausal women with endocrine-responsive breast cancer: past, present and future recommendations, *Eur J Cancer* 43:46–52, 2007.
80. Fisher B, Costantino JP, Wickerham DL, et al: Tamoxifen for prevention of breast cancer: report of the National Surgical Adjuvant Breast and Bowel Project P-1 Study, *J Natl Cancer Inst* 90:1371–1388, 1998.
81. Sjogren S, Inganas M, Lindgren A, et al: Prognostic and predictive value of c-erbB-2 overexpression in primary breast cancer, alone and in combination with other prognostic markers, *J Clin Oncol* 16:462–469, 1998.
82. Slamon DJ, Clark GM, Wong SG, et al: Human breast cancer: correlation of relapse and survival with amplification of the HER-2/neu oncogene, *Science* 235:177–182, 1987.
83. Slamon DJ, Leyland-Jones B, Shak S, et al: Use of chemotherapy plus a monoclonal antibody against HER2 for metastatic breast cancer that overexpresses HER2, *N Engl J Med* 344:783–792, 2001.
84. Martin de las Mulas J, Ordas J, Millan Y, et al: Oncogene HER-2 in canine mammary gland carcinomas: an immunohistochemical and

chromogenic in situ hybridization study, *Breast Cancer Res Treat* 80:363–367, 2003.
85. Hsu WL, Huang HM, Liao JW, et al: Increased survival in dogs with malignant mammary tumours overexpressing HER-2 protein and detection of a silent single nucleotide polymorphism in the canine HER-2 gene, *Vet J* 180:116–123, 2009.
86. Gama A, Alves A, Schmitt F: Identification of molecular phenotypes in canine mammary carcinomas with clinical implications: application of the human classification, *Virchows Arch* 453:123–132, 2008.
87. Perez Alenza MD, Tabanera E, Pena L: Inflammatory mammary carcinoma in dogs: 33 cases (1995-1999), *J Am Vet Med Assoc* 219:1110–1114, 2001.
88. Marconato L, Romanelli G, Stefanello D, et al: Prognostic factors for dogs with mammary inflammatory carcinoma: 43 cases (2003-2008), *J Am Vet Med Assoc* 235:967–972, 2009.
89. Karayannopoulou M, Koutinas AF, Polizopoulou ZS, et al: Total serum alkaline phosphatase activity in dogs with mammary neoplasms: a prospective study on 79 natural cases, *J Vet Med A Physiol Pathol Clin Med* 50:501–505, 2003.
90. Karayannopoulou M, Polizopoulou ZS, Koutinas AF, et al: Serum alkaline phosphatase isoenzyme activities in canine malignant mammary neoplasms with and without osseous transformation, *Vet Clin Pathol* 35:287 290, 2006.
91. Cassali GD, Gobbi H, Malm C, et al: Evaluation of accuracy of fine needle aspiration cytology for diagnosis of canine mammary tumours: comparative features with human tumours, *Cytopathology* 18:191–196, 2007.
92. Simon D, Schoenrock D, Nolte I, et al: Cytologic examination of fine-needle aspirates from mammary gland tumors in the dog: diagnostic accuracy with comparison to histopathology and association with postoperative outcome, *Vet Clin Pathol* 38:521–528, 2009.
93. Eberle N, Fork M, von Babo V, et al: Comparison of examination of thoracic radiographs and thoracic computed tomography in dogs with appendicular osteosarcoma, *Vet Comp Oncol* 9:131–140, 2011.
94. Otoni CC, Rahal SC, Vulcano LC, et al: Survey radiography and computerized tomography imaging of the thorax in female dogs with mammary tumors, *Acta Vet Scand* 52:20, 2010.
95. Lana SE, Rutteman GR, Withrow SJ: Tumors of the mammary gland. In Withrow SJ,Vail DM, editors: *Withrow & MacEwen's small animal clinical oncology*, ed 4, St. Louis, 2007, Saunders Elsevier.
96. Pereira CT, Rahal SC, de Carvalho Balieiro JC, et al: Lymphatic drainage on healthy and neoplastic mammary glands in female dogs: can it really be altered? *Anat Histol Embryol* 32:282–290, 2003.
97. Pereira CT, Luiz Navarro Marques F, Williams J, et al: 99mTc-labeled dextran for mammary lymphoscintigraphy in dogs, *Vet Radiol Ultrasound* 49:487–491, 2008.
98. Patsikas MN, Dessiris A: The lymph drainage of the mammary glands in the bitch: a lymphographic study. Part II: The 3rd mammary gland, *Anat Histol Embryol* 25:139–143, 1996.
99. Ran S, Volk L, Hall K, et al: Lymphangiogenesis and lymphatic metastasis in breast cancer, *Pathophysiology* 17(4):229–251, 2009.
100. Tuohy JL, Milgram J, Worley DR, et al: A review of sentinel lymph node evaluation and the need for its incorporation into veterinary oncology, *Vet Comp Oncol* 7:81–91, 2009.
101. Owens L: *Classification of tumors in domestic animals*, Geneva, 1980, World Health Organization.
102. Rutteman G, Withrow S, MacEwen E: Tumors of the mammary gland. In Withrow S, MacEwen E, editors: *Small animal clinical oncology*, ed 3, Philadelphia, 2001, WB Saunders.
103. Sorenmo KU, Rasotto R, Zappulli V, et al: Development, anatomy, histology, lymphatic drainage, clinical features, and cell differentiation markers of canine mammary gland neoplasms, *Vet Pathol* 48:85–97, 2011.
104. Hampe JF, Misdorp W: Tumours and dysplasias of the mammary gland, *Bull World Health Organ* 50:111–133, 1974.
105. Misdorp W, Else R, Hellmen E, et al: *Histological classification of mammary tumors of the dog and the cat*, Washington, DC, 1999, American Registry of Pathology.
106. Goldschmidt M, Pena L, Rasotto R, et al: Classification and grading of canine mammary tumors, *Vet Pathol* 48:117–131, 2011.
107. Rasotto R, Zappulli V, Castagnaro M, et al: A retrospective study of those histopathologic parameters predictive of invasion of the lymphatic system by canine mammary carcinomas, *Vet Pathol* 49(2):330–340, 2012.
108. Elston CW, Ellis IO: Pathological prognostic factors in breast cancer. I. The value of histological grade in breast cancer: experience from a large study with long-term follow-up, *Histopathology* 19:403–410, 1991.
109. Misdorp W: Tumors of the mammary gland. In Meuten DJ, editor: *Tumors in domestic animals*, ed 4, Ames, Iowa, 2002, Iowa State Press.
110. Clemente M, Perez-Alenza MD, Illera JC, et al: Histological, immunohistological, and ultrastructural description of vasculogenic mimicry in canine mammary cancer, *Vet Pathol* 47:265–274, 2010.
111. Karayannopoulou M, Kaldrymidou E, Constantinidis TC, et al: Histological grading and prognosis in dogs with mammary carcinomas: application of a human grading method, *J Comp Pathol* 133:246–252, 2005.
112. Hellmen E, Bergstrom R, Holmberg L, et al: Prognostic factors in canine mammary tumors: a multivariate study of 202 consecutive cases, *Vet Pathol* 30:20–27, 1993.
113. Perez Alenza MD, Pena L, Nieto AI, et al: Clinical and pathological prognostic factors in canine mammary tumors, *Ann Ist Super Sanita* 33:581–585, 1997.
114. MacEwen EG, Harvey HJ, Patnaik AK, et al: Evaluation of effects of levamisole and surgery on canine mammary cancer, *J Biol Response Mod* 4:418–426, 1985.
115. Philibert JC, Snyder PW, Glickman N, et al: Influence of host factors on survival in dogs with malignant mammary gland tumors, *J Vet Intern Med* 17:102–106, 2003.
116. Morris JS, Dobson JM, Bostock DE: Use of tamoxifen in the control of canine mammary neoplasia, *Vet Rec* 133:539–542, 1993.
117. Chang SC, Chang CC, Chang TJ, et al: Prognostic factors associated with survival two years after surgery in dogs with malignant mammary tumors: 79 cases (1998-2002), *J Am Vet Med Assoc* 227:1625–1629, 2005.
118. Stratmann N, Failing K, Richter A, et al: Mammary tumor recurrence in bitches after regional mastectomy, *Vet Surg* 37:82–86, 2008.
119. Morris JS, Dobson JM, Bostock DE, et al: Effect of ovariohysterectomy in bitches with mammary neoplasms, *Vet Rec* 142:656–658, 1998.
120. Sorenmo KU, Shofer FS, Goldschmidt MH: Effect of spaying and timing of spaying on survival of dogs with mammary carcinoma, *J Vet Intern Med* 14:266–270, 2000.
121. MacEwen EG: Spontaneous tumors in dogs and cats: models for the study of cancer biology and treatment, *Cancer Metastasis Rev* 9:125–136, 1990.
122. Vail DM, MacEwen EG: Spontaneously occurring tumors of companion animals as models for human cancer, *Cancer Invest* 18:781–792, 2000.
123. Gelb HR, Freeman LJ, Rohleder JJ, et al: Feasibility of contrast-enhanced ultrasound-guided biopsy of sentinel lymph nodes in dogs, *Vet Radiol Ultrasound* 51:628–633, 2010.
124. Pinheiro LG, Oliveira Filho RS, Vasques PH, et al: Hemosiderin: a new marker for sentinel lymph node identification, *Acta Cir Bras* 24:432–436, 2009.
125. Balogh L, Thuroczy J, Andocs G, et al: Sentinel lymph node detection in canine oncological patients, *Nucl Med Rev Cent East Eur* 5:139–144, 2002.
126. Wong JH, Cagle LA, Morton DL: Lymphatic drainage of skin to a sentinel lymph node in a feline model, *Ann Surg* 214:637–641, 1991.

127. Szczubiał M, Łopuszynski W: Prognostic value of regional lymph node status in canine mammary carcinomas, *Vet Comp Oncol* 9:296–303, 2011.
128. Allen S, Mahaffey E: Canine mammary neoplasia: prognostic indicators and response to surgical therapy, *J Amer Anim Hosp Assoc* 25:504–546, 1989.
129. Tavares WL, Lavalle GE, Figueiredo MS, et al: Evaluation of adverse effects in tamoxifen exposed healthy female dogs, *Acta Vet Scand* 52:67, 2010.
130. Yamagami T, Kobayashi T, Takahashi K, et al: Influence of ovariectomy at the time of mastectomy on the prognosis for canine malignant mammary tumours, *J Small Anim Pract* 37:462–464, 1996.
131. Karayannopoulou M, Kaldrymidou E, Constantinidis TC, et al: Adjuvant post-operative chemotherapy in bitches with mammary cancer. *J Vet Med A Physiol Pathol Clin Med* 48:85–96, 2001.
132. Nabholtz JM, Senn HJ, Bezwoda WR, et al: Prospective randomized trial of docetaxel versus mitomycin plus vinblastine in patients with metastatic breast cancer progressing despite previous anthracycline-containing chemotherapy. 304 Study Group, *J Clin Oncol* 17:1413–1424, 1999.
133. Sjostrom J, Blomqvist C, Mouridsen H, et al: Docetaxel compared with sequential methotrexate and 5-fluorouracil in patients with advanced breast cancer after anthracycline failure: a randomised phase III study with crossover on progression by the Scandinavian Breast Group, *Eur J Cancer* 35:1194–1201, 1999.
134. Morabito A, Piccirillo MC, Monaco K, et al: First-line chemotherapy for HER-2 negative metastatic breast cancer patients who received anthracyclines as adjuvant treatment, *Oncologist* 12:1288–1298, 2007.
135. Simon D, Schoenrock D, Baumgartner W, et al: Postoperative adjuvant treatment of invasive malignant mammary gland tumors in dogs with doxorubicin and docetaxel, *J Vet Intern Med* 20:1184–1190, 2006.
136. Marconato L, Lorenzo RM, Abramo F, et al: Adjuvant gemcitabine after surgical removal of aggressive malignant mammary tumours in dogs, *Vet Comp Oncol* 6:90–101, 2008.
137. de MSCH, Toledo-Piza E, Amorin R, et al: Inflammatory mammary carcinoma in 12 dogs: clinical features, cyclooxygenase-2 expression, and response to piroxicam treatment, *Can Vet J* 50:506–510, 2009.
138. Kuntz CA, Dernell WS, Powers BE, et al: Extraskeletal osteosarcomas in dogs: 14 cases, *J Am Anim Hosp Assoc* 34:26–30, 1998.
139. Hermo GA, Turic E, Angelico D, et al: Effect of adjuvant perioperative desmopressin in locally advanced canine mammary carcinoma and its relation to histologic grade, *J Am Anim Hosp Assoc* 47:21–27, 2011.
140. Terraube V, Marx I, Denis CV: Role of von Willebrand factor in tumor metastasis, *Thromb Res* 120(Suppl 2):S64–S70, 2007.
141. Ripoll GV, Giron S, Krzymuski MJ, et al: Antitumor effects of desmopressin in combination with chemotherapeutic agents in a mouse model of breast cancer, *Anticancer Res* 28:2607–2611, 2008.
142. Hahn K, Richardson R, Knapp D: Canine malignant mammary neoplasia: biological behavior, diagnosis, and treatment alternatives, *J Am Anim Hosp Assoc* 28:251–256, 1992.
143. Egenvall A, Bonnett BN, Haggstrom J, et al: Morbidity of insured Swedish cats during 1999-2006 by age, breed, sex, and diagnosis, *J Feline Med Surg* 12:948–959, 2010.
144. Bonnett BN, Egenvall A: Age patterns of disease and death in insured Swedish dogs, cats and horses, *J Comp Pathol* 142(Suppl 1):S33–S38, 2010.
145. Teclaw R, Mendlein J, Garbe P, et al: Characteristics of pet populations and households in the Purdue Comparative Oncology Program catchment area, 1988, *J Am Vet Med Assoc* 201:1725–1729, 1992.
146. Vascellari M, Baioni E, Ru G, et al: Animal tumour registry of two provinces in northern Italy: incidence of spontaneous tumours in dogs and cats, *BMC Vet Res* 5:39, 2009.
147. Hayden DW, Nielsen SW: Feline mammary tumours, *J Small Anim Pract* 12:687–698, 1971.
148. Misdorp W, Romijn A, Hart AA: Feline mammary tumors: a case-control study of hormonal factors, *Anticancer Res* 11:1793–1797, 1991.
149. Hayes AA, Mooney S: Feline mammary tumors, *Vet Clin North Am Small Anim Pract* 15:513–520, 1985.
150. Weijer K, Head KW, Misdorp W, et al: Feline malignant mammary tumors. I. Morphology and biology: some comparisons with human and canine mammary carcinomas, *J Natl Cancer Inst* 49:1697–1704, 1972.
151. Hayes HM Jr, Milne KL, Mandell CP: Epidemiological features of feline mammary carcinoma, *Vet Rec* 108:476–479, 1981.
152. Ito T, Kadosawa T, Mochizuki M, et al: Prognosis of malignant mammary tumor in 53 cats, *J Vet Med Sci* 58:723–726, 1996.
153. Patnaik AK, Liu SK, Hurvitz AI, et al: Nonhematopoietic neoplasms in cats, *J Natl Cancer Inst* 54:855–860, 1975.
154. Rissetto K, Villamil JA, Selting KA, et al: Recent trends in feline intestinal neoplasia: an epidemiologic study of 1,129 cases in the veterinary medical database from 1964 to 2004, *J Am Anim Hosp Assoc* 47:28–36, 2011.
155. Louwerens M, London CA, Pedersen NC, et al: Feline lymphoma in the post-feline leukemia virus era, *J Vet Intern Med* 19:329–335, 2005.
156. Gabor LJ, Malik R, Canfield PJ: Clinical and anatomical features of lymphosarcoma in 118 cats, *Aust Vet J* 76:725–732, 1998.
157. Miller MA, Nelson SL, Turk JR, et al: Cutaneous neoplasia in 340 cats, *Vet Pathol* 28:389–395, 1991.
158. Overley B, Shofer FS, Goldschmidt MH, et al: Association between ovarihysterectomy and feline mammary carcinoma, *J Vet Intern Med* 19:560–563, 2005.
159. Skorupski KA, Overley B, Shofer FS, et al: Clinical characteristics of mammary carcinoma in male cats, *J Vet Intern Med* 19:52–55, 2005.
160. Jacobs TM, Hoppe BR, Poehlmann CE, et al: Mammary adenocarcinomas in three male cats exposed to medroxyprogesterone acetate (1990-2006), *J Feline Med Surg* 12:169–174, 2010.
161. Loretti AP, Ilha MR, Ordas J, et al: Clinical, pathological and immunohistochemical study of feline mammary fibroepithelial hyperplasia following a single injection of depot medroxyprogesterone acetate, *J Feline Med Surg* 7:43–52, 2005.
162. Mol JA, van Garderen E, Rutteman GR, et al: New insights in the molecular mechanism of progestin-induced proliferation of mammary epithelium: induction of the local biosynthesis of growth hormone (GH) in the mammary glands of dogs, cats and humans, *J Steroid Biochem Mol Biol* 57:67–71, 1996.
163. Mol JA, van Garderen E, Selman PJ, et al: Growth hormone mRNA in mammary gland tumors of dogs and cats, *J Clin Invest* 95:2028–2034, 1995.
164. Burrai GP, Mohammed SI, Miller MA, et al: Spontaneous feline mammary intraepithelial lesions as a model for human estrogen receptor- and progesterone receptor-negative breast lesions, *BMC Cancer* 10:156, 2010.
165. Millanta F, Calandrella M, Vannozzi I, et al: Steroid hormone receptors in normal, dysplastic and neoplastic feline mammary tissues and their prognostic significance, *Vet Rec* 158:821–824, 2006.
166. de las Mulas JM, van Niel M, Millan Y, et al: Immunohistochemical analysis of estrogen receptors in feline mammary gland benign and malignant lesions: comparison with biochemical assay, *Domest Anim Endocrinol* 18:111–125, 2000.
167. Martin de las Mulas J, Van Niel M, Millan Y, et al: Progesterone receptors in normal, dysplastic and tumourous feline mammary glands. Comparison with oestrogen receptors status, *Res Vet Sci* 72:153–161, 2002.
168. Meisl D, Hubler M, Arnold S: [Treatment of fibroepithelial hyperplasia (FEH) of the mammary gland in the cat with the progesterone antagonist Aglepristone (Alizine)], *Schweiz Arch Tierheilkd* 145:130–136, 2003.

169. Ordas J, Millan Y, Dios R, et al: Proto-oncogene HER-2 in normal, dysplastic and tumorous feline mammary glands: an immunohistochemical and chromogenic in situ hybridization study, *BMC Cancer* 7:179, 2007.
170. Millanta F, Calandrella M, Citi S, et al: Overexpression of HER-2 in feline invasive mammary carcinomas: an immunohistochemical survey and evaluation of its prognostic potential, *Vet Pathol* 42:30–34, 2005.
171. Winston J, Craft DM, Scase TJ, et al: Immunohistochemical detection of HER-2/neu expression in spontaneous feline mammary tumours, *Vet Comp Oncol* 3:8–15, 2005.
172. Rasotto R, Caliari D, Castagnaro M, et al: An immunohistochemical study of HER-2 expression in feline mammary tumours, *J Comp Pathol* 144:170–179, 2011.
173. Brodey RS: Canine and feline neoplasms, *Adv Vet Sci* 24:434, 1957.
174. Weijer K, Hart AA: Prognostic factors in feline mammary carcinoma, *J Natl Cancer Inst* 70:709–716, 1983.
175. Perez-Alenza MD, Jimenez A, Nieto AI, et al: First description of feline inflammatory mammary carcinoma: clinicopathological and immunohistochemical characteristics of three cases, *Breast Cancer Res* 6:R300–R307, 2004.
176. McNeill CJ, Sorenmo KU, Shofer FS, et al: Evaluation of adjuvant doxorubicin-based chemotherapy for the treatment of feline mammary carcinoma, *J Vet Intern Med* 23:123–129, 2009.
177. Hayden DW, Barnes DM, Johnson KH: Morphologic changes in the mammary gland of megestrol acetate-treated and untreated cats: a retrospective study, *Vet Pathol* 26:104–113, 1989.
178. Castagnaro M, Casalone C, Bozzetta E, et al: Tumour grading and the one-year post-surgical prognosis in feline mammary carcinomas, *J Comp Pathol* 119:263–275, 1998.
179. Seixas F, Palmeira C, Pires MA, et al: Mammary invasive micropapillary carcinoma in cats: clinicopathologic features and nuclear DNA content, *Vet Pathol* 44:842–848, 2007.
180. Seixas F, Pires MA, Lopes CA: Complex carcinomas of the mammary gland in cats: pathological and immunohistochemical features, *Vet J* 176:210–215, 2008.
181. Sarli G, Brunetti B, Benazzi C: Mammary mucinous carcinoma in the cat, *Vet Pathol* 43:667–673, 2006.
182. Kamstock DA, Fredrickson R, Ehrhart EJ: Lipid-rich carcinoma of the mammary gland in a cat, *Vet Pathol* 42:360–362, 2005.
183. Matsuda K, Kobayashi S, Yamashita M, et al: Tubulopapillary carcinoma with spindle cell metaplasia of the mammary gland in a cat, *J Vet Med Sci* 70:479–481, 2008.
184. Seixas F, Palmeira C, Pires MA, et al: Grade is an independent prognostic factor for feline mammary carcinomas: a clinicopathological and survival analysis, *Vet J* 187:65–71, 2011.
185. MacEwen EG, Hayes AA, Mooney S, et al: Evaluation of effect of levamisole on feline mammary cancer, *J Biol Response Mod* 3:541–546, 1984.
186. Viste JR, Myers SL, Singh B, et al: Feline mammary adenocarcinoma: tumor size as a prognostic indicator, *Can Vet J* 43:33–37, 2002.
187. MacEwen EG, Hayes AA, Harvey HJ, et al: Prognostic factors for feline mammary tumors, *J Am Vet Med Assoc* 185:201–204, 1984.
188. Borrego JF, Cartagena JC, Engel J: Treatment of feline mammary tumours using chemotherapy, surgery and a COX-2 inhibitor drug (meloxicam): a retrospective study of 23 cases (2002-2007)*, *Vet Comp Oncol* 7:213–221, 2009.
189. Patsikas MN, Papadopoulou PL, Charitanti A, et al: Computed tomography and radiographic indirect lymphography for visualization of mammary lymphatic vessels and the sentinel lymph node in normal cats, *Vet Radiol Ultrasound* 51:299–304, 2010.
190. Jeglum KA, deGuzman E, Young KM: Chemotherapy of advanced mammary adenocarcinoma in 14 cats, *J Am Vet Med Assoc* 187:157–160, 1985.
191. Mauldin GN, Matus RE, Patnaik AK, et al: Efficacy and toxicity of doxorubicin and cyclophosphamide used in the treatment of selected malignant tumors in 23 cats, *J Vet Intern Med* 2:60–65, 1988.

Tumors of the Male Reproductive System

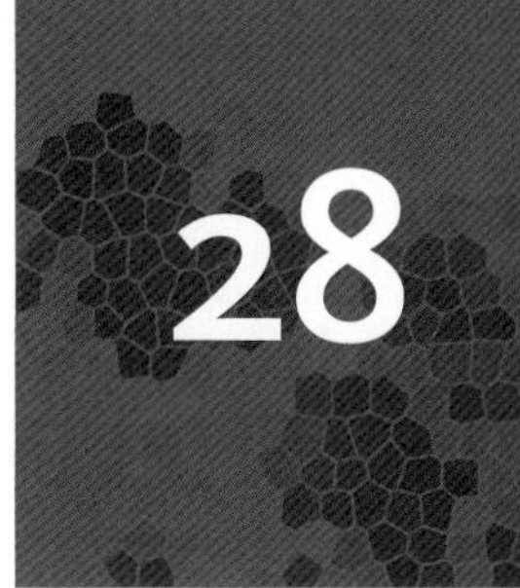

JESSICA A. LAWRENCE AND COREY F. SABA

Canine Testicular Tumors

Prevalence/Incidence

Testicular tumors are the most common tumors of the canine male genitalia and account for approximately 90% of all cancers in the male reproductive tract.[1-4] In the intact male dog, the testis is overall the second most common anatomic site for tumor development, with an overall prevalence ranging between 6% and 27%.[1,3-7] Many of these reports are case series and involve dogs submitted for routine necropsy and/or castration for cryptorchidism, making comparisons between study prevalence data difficult. However, a recent population-based study conducted in Norway, where elective castration is rare, reported a similar prevalence of 7% for testicular tumors.[8]

The rate of development of testicular cancer in humans has increased in some populations over time and across successive birth cohorts, and a similar phenomenon has been suggested in dogs.[7,9-13] A recent population-based study did not find increased rates of testicular tumors among intact dogs; however, only an 8-year period was evaluated.[8] Testicular tumors are most often diagnosed in geriatric male dogs with a median age of approximately 10 years.[1,3,4,14,15]

The three most common testicular tumors arise from distinct testicular subsets: sustentacular cells of Sertoli, the spermatic germinal epithelium, and the interstitial cells of Leydig, giving rise to Sertoli cell tumors, seminomas, and interstitial cell tumors, respectively (Table 28-1).[2] The World Health Organization (WHO) classification of tumors of domestic animals differentiates the major types of testicular tumors in dogs as sex cord stromal tumors (Sertoli cell tumors, interstitial cell tumors), germ cell tumors (seminoma, teratoma), and mixed germ cell sex cord stromal tumors.[16] Sertoli cell tumors, interstitial cell tumors, and seminomas have historically developed with equal frequency, although recent studies have suggested that the prevalence of Sertoli cell tumors is lower (8% to 16%).* In one study evaluating lifetime occurrence of neoplasia in German shepherds and Belgian Malinois, seminoma occurred most frequently.[17] Human testicular tumors are often divided into seminoma and nonseminoma, with the former further subdivided as classical seminoma (SE), atypical seminoma, and spermatocytic seminoma (SS) according to WHO, and some effort has been made to apply this to canine tumors.[9,13,19-23] Sertoli cell tumors and seminomas occur with higher frequency in cryptorchid testes.[3,24,25]

Rarely, other cell lineages can give rise to testicular tumors such as hemangiomas, granulosa cell tumors, teratomas, sarcomas, embryonal carcinomas, gonadoblastomas, lymphomas, schwannoma, mesothelioma, and rete testis mucinous adenocarcinomas.[26-30] Many dogs diagnosed with testicular cancer have more than one primary tumor.[3,6,18,31] In three separate studies evaluating relatively large numbers of dogs with testicular tumors, between 4% and 20% of dogs had more than one type of testicular tumor.[3,8,32]

*References 1, 3, 4, 7, 17, 18.

Risk Factors

Several factors may influence the development of testicular tumors in the dog, including cryptorchidism, age, breed, and carcinogen exposure. There is a significant association between cryptorchidism and the development of Sertoli cell tumors and seminomas but not interstitial cell tumors.[4,15,25] An early prospective epidemiologic study compared the incidence of testicular tumors in cryptorchid dogs to age- and breed-matched control dogs.[15] None of the control dogs developed testicular tumors during the study, in which the average duration of monitoring was 2 years. The incidence of testicular neoplasia in the cryptorchid dogs was 12.7 per 1000 dog-years at risk, whereas for cryptorchid dogs older than 6 years, the incidence increased to 68.1 per 1000 dog-years at risk. Inguinal cryptorchidism may further increase the risk of testicular tumor development compared to abdominal cryptorchidism (Figure 28-1).[4,15,25] In cryptorchid dogs, tumors more frequently develop in the right testicle; however, this is probably due to the fact that the right testicle is more likely to be retained.[4,15,32] One study of cryptorchid dogs found that chronologic age was a risk factor for development of a primary testicular tumor and dogs older than 10 years were more likely to develop tumors compared to dogs younger than 6 years.[15] A recent study indicated that the detection rate of testicular tumors in dogs younger than 10 years was significantly associated with cryptorchidism, with over 60% of cryptorchid testicular tumors identified in middle-aged dogs (6 to 10 years).[4]

Several breeds have been reported to have increased risk of developing primary testicular tumors, including the Boxer, German shepherd, Afghan hound, Weimaraner, Shetland sheepdog, Collie, and Maltese.* The flat-coated retriever, Rottweiler, Bouvier de Flandres, and Leonbergers may have a reduced risk of developing testicular tumors, although low numbers of the latter two breeds were evaluated.[8]

Two studies evaluating military working dogs suggested evidence of environmental carcinogen exposure during the Vietnam War.[35,36] Pathologic changes in the testicles such as hemorrhage, epididymitis, orchitis, sperm granuloma, testicular degeneration, and seminoma were noted, although the causative factor of these could not be definitively determined. These epidemiologic studies postulated that exposure to phenoxy herbicide, dioxin, or tetracycline may have promoted the development of testicular tumors.[35,36]

*References 3, 8, 14, 25, 32-34.

TABLE 28-1 Characteristics of the Three Most Common Testicular Tumors in the Dog

Tumor Type	Incidence (% of All Testicular Tumors)	Origin	Hormone Production	Clinical Findings	Gross Appearance	Biologic Behavior and Potential for Metastasis
Sertoli cell tumor	8-33	Sustentacular cells of seminiferous tubules	≥50% Estrogen	Feminization syndrome Pancytopenia	Firm Lobulated White-gray "Greasy"	<15% regional or distant metastasis
Interstitial cell tumor (Leydig cell tumor)	33-50	Leydig cells between seminiferous tubules	Rarely estrogen Testosterone	Often incidental finding Perianal gland hyperplasia/adenomas	Soft Expansive Yellow-orange Often cystic	Rarely metastasize
Seminomas	33-52	Germinal epithelium of seminiferous tubules	Rarely estrogen	Often incidental finding Metastasis may cause lethargy	Soft Homogeneous May be lobulated Ivory	<15% regional or distant metastasis

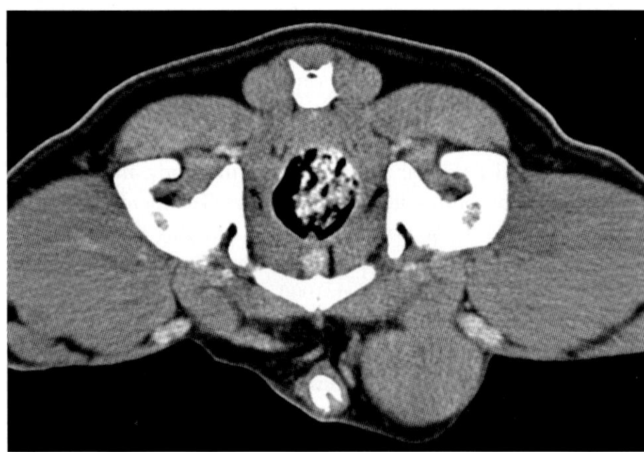

FIGURE 28-1 Cross-sectional CT image demonstrating an enlarged, minimally rim-enhancing Sertoli cell tumor in a dog with inguinal cryptorchidism. *(Courtesy Dr. T. Schwarz, University of Edinburgh.)*

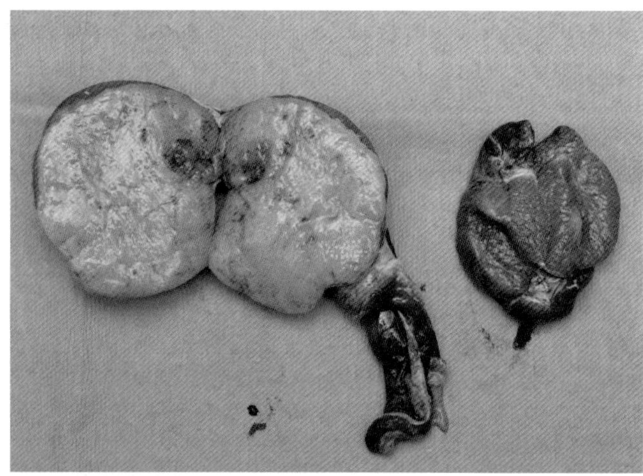

FIGURE 28-2 Sectioned seminoma in a dog demonstrating its ivory, homogenous appearance in comparison to a mildly atrophied contralateral testicle.

Pathology and Pathogenesis

Sertoli cell tumors arise from the sustentacular cells of seminiferous tubules, and seminomas arise from the germinal epithelium of seminiferous tubules. Interstitial cell tumors arise from Leydig cells located between seminiferous tubules. All three tumors have relatively distinct gross appearance but require histopathology for definitive diagnosis. Sertoli cell tumors are firm, lobulated, white-to-gray in appearance, and characterized as "greasy" on palpation.[37] Seminomas tend to be homogeneous, soft, and occasionally lobulated and have an ivory appearance when sectioned (Figure 28-2).[37] Interstitial cell tumors are soft, expansive, and yellow-to-orange in color when sectioned and often contain cysts with serous or serosanguineous fluid.[37]

The molecular and cellular biology of primary testicular tumors has been investigated. Proliferation markers (proliferating-cell nuclear antigen [PCNA], Ki67, and argyrophilic nucleolar organizer regions [AgNORs]) and TERT expression (the catalytic reverse transcriptase subunit of telomerase) have been interrogated as indicators of degree of malignancy, local progression, and metastasis with discordant results.[38-43] Investigators sought to relate TERT to proliferation indices and p53 expression; however, due to the fact that PCNA and TERT were expressed in all testicular tumors, this limited their prognostic potential.[40] However, aggressive testicular tumors did tend to express high levels of all markers examined: TERT, p53, PCNA, and Ki67.[40] Proliferative activity in seminomas was assessed using AgNORs in a separate study, in which mean AgNOR scores were higher in invasive or diffuse tumors compared to well-differentiated intraductal seminomas.[43] Results suggest that testicular tumors develop a proliferative advantage as they become less differentiated, although larger studies should be performed before proliferative indices can be definitively relied on for prognostication in canine testicular tumors. Cyclins, which are intracellular proteins that form complexes with cyclin-dependent kinases to regulate cell-cycle checkpoints, have also been evaluated in normal and neoplastic testes; however, their significance is yet to be determined.[44]

The neoplastic and stromal cellular environment plays an important role in tumor invasion and progression, and a few studies have attempted to investigate changes in canine testicular tumors. Laminin is an extracellular matrix protein that plays a role in anchoring cells to the basement membrane. As tumors became more invasive, laminin expression became fragmented or lost in Sertoli cell tumors and seminomas and correlated to increasing proliferative activity as assessed by PCNA scoring, Ki67 index, and mitotic index.[38] Connexin 43 is the predominant gap junction protein of the testis that plays a role in phenotypic differentiation, cell pattern formation, and morphogenesis, and altered expression patterns may contribute to tumorigenesis and progression.[45-49] Similar to other work, differential alterations in connexin 34 expression occur in canine testicular tumors, and its expression may aid in differentiating neoplastic Sertoli cells from seminomas.[50]

Mutations of the p53 tumor suppressor gene are a common genetic alteration in both human and canine malignancies, and increased p53 expression has been associated with tumor progression.[51-55] A recent evaluation of testicular tumors indicated that nuclear p53 immunoreactivity was detected in 15 of 20 seminomas (75%), 6 of 12 Sertoli cell tumors, and all 3 interstitial cell tumors evaluated.[40] Interestingly, expression intensity was stronger in diffuse type Sertoli cell tumors and seminomas.[40,54] Results suggest that p53 may be an indicator of tumor aggression; however, further studies should be done to corroborate this.

Similar to p53 and proliferation indices, angiogenesis plays an important role in cancer progression and metastasis. Vascular endothelial growth factor (VEGF) expression and microvessel density (MVD) were higher in seminomas compared to normal testes in one study.[56] Additionally, both VEGF expression and MVD were higher in diffuse seminomas compared to more well-differentiated intratubular seminomas, potentially providing a histologic indicator of malignant behavior.[56]

The KIT protein or CD117 is a transmembrane protein for a tyrosine kinase receptor encoded by the proto-oncogene *c-kit,* which, when bound to its ligand stem cell factor (SCF), is essential to the development, proliferation, and maturation of several cell types, including germ cells.[57-59] Primordial germinal cells express KIT and migrate to interact with Sertoli cells that express SCF to guide the differentiation of the primordial cells into gonocytes.[60] Interstitial cells of Leydig also express KIT and, when stimulated by SCF, are stimulated by Sertoli cells to produce testosterone.[57,60,61] The expression of KIT is maintained by spermatogonia until differentiation into spermatocytes, making it a useful marker to define primordial germinal cells and early germinal cells.[60,62] In human seminomas, immunohistochemical labeling for KIT and placental alkaline phosphatase (PLAP) is used to distinguish SE and SS because SE should express both and SS should be negative.[63,64] Normal and neoplastic canine testes were recently characterized for KIT expression, and results were consistent with humans and rodents in that spermatogonia and Leydig cells were KIT positive, whereas Sertoli cells were negative.[62] Interestingly, canine testicular tumors in this study maintained the same KIT expression as their cell of origin, with interstitial tumors consistently expressing KIT, similar to human tumors. Similar to human seminomas, canine seminomas appeared to be differentiated into SE and SS on the basis of KIT and PLAP staining.[22,62] Further studies investigating the behavior of SE and SS may support the dog as a relevant model for human disease, permitting investigation into additional roles of KIT-inhibitors.[65-67]

Natural Behavior

Most primary testicular tumors in the dog are characterized by local invasion and rarely metastasize. Regional or distant metastasis occurs in less than 15% of dogs diagnosed with Sertoli cell tumors or seminomas.[6,32,68-74] Due to the malignant histologic appearance but low malignant behavior, canine seminoma has been compared to human spermatocytic seminoma, thereby spawning interest in using canine seminoma as a relevant comparative model.[21] Recent work has tried to further classify canine seminoma into classic and spermatocytic seminomas in an attempt to help determine metastatic potential, but no clinical conclusions may be drawn as yet.[19,21,22] Interstitial cell tumors very rarely metastasize.[6] Sites of metastasis may include regional lymph nodes, eyes, brain, lungs, kidney, spleen, liver, adrenal glands, pancreas, skin, and peritoneum.[6,32,68-74]

Primary testicular tumors can also cause imbalances in hormone levels, regardless of the degree of local invasion and presence or absence of metastasis. Sertoli cell tumors can cause signs of feminization, and over 50% of affected dogs display signs of estrogen production.[14,25,32,69] Seminomas and interstitial cell tumors are rarely associated with feminization.[75-77] Excess estrogen can cause signs such as bilateral symmetric alopecia, cutaneous hyperpigmentation, epidermal thinning, squamous metaplasia of the prostatic epithelium, gynecomastia, galactorrhea, attraction of other males, preputial atrophy, atrophy of the nonneoplastic testicle, and bone marrow suppression.[32] Sertoli cell tumors that develop in retained testicles are more likely to produce signs of hyperestrogenism; however, 17% of dogs with scrotal Sertoli cell tumors developed feminization.[14,25,32,69] Plasma hormone concentrations from dogs with primary testicular tumors have been investigated in order to better understand their contribution to tumor type and clinical signs.[77-80] Estradiol-17β concentrations were higher in dogs with Sertoli cell tumors compared to normal and were significantly higher in dogs with feminization syndrome secondary to Sertoli cell tumors. Testosterone and testosterone/estradiol ratios are lower in dogs with Sertoli cell tumors when compared to healthy control dogs.[76] Plasma estradiol concentrations were lower in seminomas compared to normal dogs in one study but were not significantly altered from normal in another study.[76,77] It has been suggested that clinical signs of feminization due to Sertoli cell tumors best correlated to testosterone/estradiol ratio reductions rather than to absolute increases in estradiol.[76] Expression of inhibins (inhibins α, β, βα), 3β-hydroxysteroid dehydrogenases, and insulin-like growth factors (IGF-1 and IGF-2) has also been assessed, and further study may shed light on their utility as diagnostic or prognostic markers.[77-80] A recent study suggested IGF gene expression was altered in canine testicular tumors compared to normal testicular tissue. A unique pattern of expression, as determined by reverse-transcriptase polymerase chain reaction (RT-PCR) of IGFs, their receptors, and their binding proteins, was observed in interstitial cell tumors compared to Sertoli cell tumors and seminomas.[80] The overall changes in gene expression were small, however, and it remains unclear how significant the IGF signaling system is in canine testicular neoplasia.

History and Clinical Signs

Most dogs with testicular tumors are asymptomatic, and a testicular mass is discovered as an incidental finding. However, clinical signs may be attributable to the primary tumor, to the presence of metastasis, or to paraneoplastic syndromes such as hyperestrogenism. Additionally, breeding dogs may present with fertility problems. Diagnosis is usually made via palpation of an enlarged testicle or a testicular mass during routine physical examination, abdominal ultrasound, or necropsy. Atrophy of the remaining normal testicle is common (Figure 28-3). Tumors in cryptorchid dogs may cause

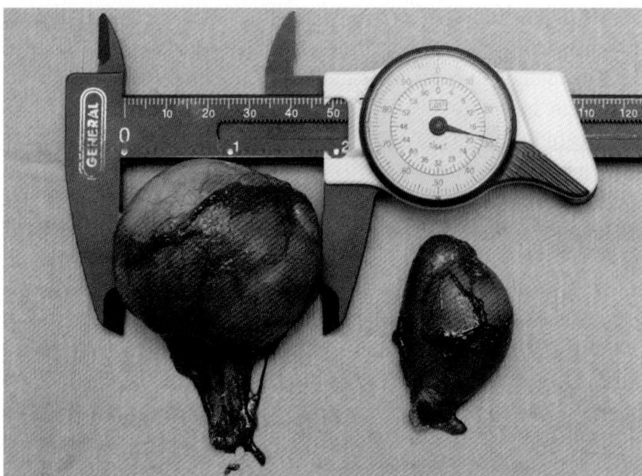

FIGURE 28-3 Large left seminoma with mild atrophy of the right normal testicle identified as an incidental finding on physical examination.

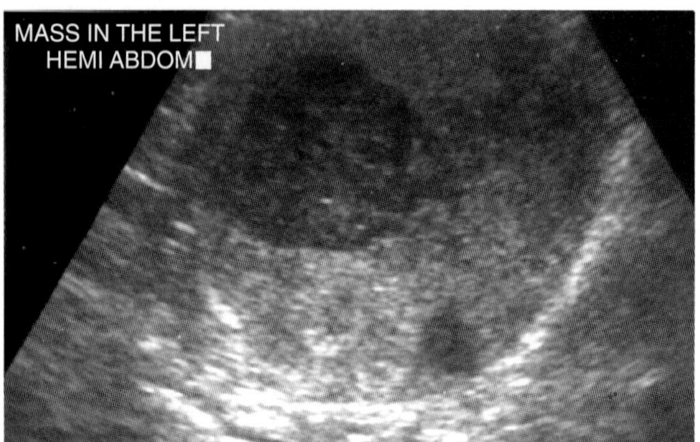

FIGURE 28-4 Large mixed echogenic and cavitated testicle within the left midabdomen on abdominal ultrasound in a cryptorchid dog. *(Courtesy Dr. T. Schwarz, University of Edinburgh.)*

a regional mass effect within the caudal abdominal cavity or inguinal region (Figure 28-4).

Excess estrogen may cause signs of feminization and is the most common paraneoplastic syndrome associated with canine testicular tumors. As stated previously, seminomas and interstitial cell tumors are rarely associated with feminization, whereas over 50% of dogs with Sertoli cell tumors show signs of hyperestrogenism.[14,32,69,75-77] Common clinical signs include bilateral symmetric alopecia and hyperpigmentation, pendulous prepuce, gynecomastia, galactorrhea, atrophy of the penis, and squamous metaplasia of the prostate.[32] The most deleterious effect of hyperestrogenism is bone marrow suppression, which may be irreversible and life threatening. Early effects of estrogen on the bone marrow include a transient increase in granulopoiesis with peripheral neutrophilia followed by progressive neutropenia, thrombocytopenia, and nonregenerative anemia.[75,81] Severe pancytopenia from bone marrow hypoplasia and blood dyscrasias can be fatal, and clinical signs can range from hemorrhage secondary to thrombocytopenia, anemia, and febrile neutropenia.[75,81] Less common reported signs associated with testicular neoplasia include lethargy (Sertoli cell tumors), presence of concurrent prostatic cyst or abscess, hematuria, hemoperitoneum, spermatic cord torsion, hypertrophic osteopathy, and perianal

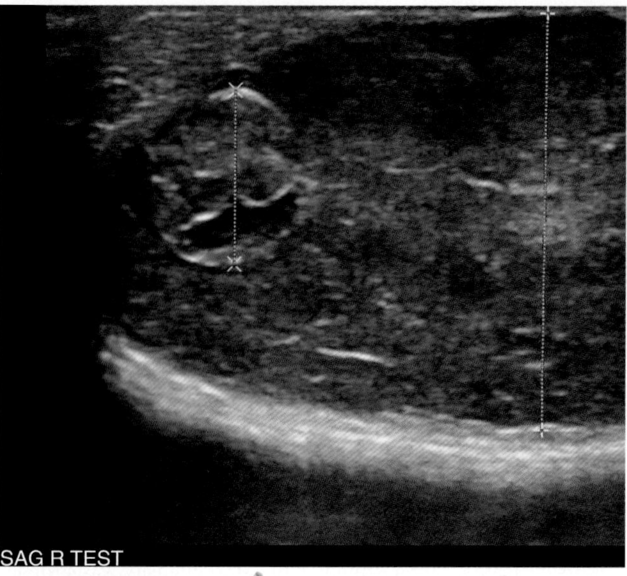

FIGURE 28-5 Sagittal ultrasound image of the testicle of a dog demonstrating a mixed echogenic neoplastic nodule. *(Courtesy Dr. D. Jimenez, University of Georgia.)*

gland hyperplasia/adenomas (interstitial cell tumors).[3,32,69,82-85] There are several reports of a syndrome in middle-aged miniature Schnauzers of Sertoli cell tumors occurring in cryptorchid male pseudohermaphrodites.[86-88] A recent report also described the presence of both a Sertoli cell tumor and an interstitial cell tumor in a mixed breed male pseudohermaphrodite dog.[89]

Diagnostic Techniques and Staging

Physical examination of intact male dogs, particularly older dogs, should always include palpation of the testicles for masses and/or asymmetry. A thorough rectal palpation should be performed to evaluate the prostate gland, regional lymph nodes, and perianal region. In dogs with clinical signs of hormone imbalance, serum testosterone and estradiol-17β can be measured along with testosterone : estradiol ratio.[76,77] It is important to note that not all dogs with signs of feminization have absolute increases in estradiol-17β, and clinical signs may be more closely linked to altered androgen : estrogen ratios.[76]

Definitive diagnosis is achieved by histopathologic evaluation, although the presence of a testicular mass and cytology may be supportive of testicular neoplasia. Because most dogs with testicular tumors are older and therefore have a high likelihood of another primary tumor (up to 50%) or concurrent diseases, complete staging prior to surgery is generally recommended. Preoperative staging typically includes a complete blood count (CBC) to evaluate for hematologic abnormalities, chemistry profile, urinalysis, abdominal ultrasound, and three-view thoracic radiographs. A coagulation profile may be warranted in dogs with anemia and signs of hemorrhage. Abdominal ultrasound may serve multiple purposes: it can aid in identification of undescended testicles in the abdominal cavity or inguinal canal, assessment of regional lymph nodes, assessment of prostatic changes, and evaluation of common sites of metastasis such as spleen and liver (Figure 28-5). Testicular ultrasonography may aid in differentiating neoplastic processes from orchitis, testicular torsion, and epididymitis; however, changes are not specific enough to identify tumor type.[90-92] Ultrasound-guided fine-needle aspiration (FNA) may support a suspicion of neoplasia prior to orchiectomy, particularly in breeding animals.[90,93] For owners with financial constraints, minimum staging should consist of a CBC, chemistry profile, and urinalysis. Castration may be performed prior to full staging for some cases, with the decision to do a full work-up following histopathologic evaluation because it is appropriate therapy for most testicular tumors. Histopathologic diagnosis is generally straightforward; however, occasionally, immunohistochemistry (IHC) using vimentin, cytokeratin, desmin, and possibly KIT and inhibin may be indicated to identify the underlying cell of origin.[26,78,94-97]

Treatment and Prognosis

As most primary canine testicular tumors are characterized by local infiltration with low potential for metastasis, orchiectomy with scrotal ablation is the treatment of choice and is often curative. Bilateral orchiectomy is the treatment of choice for testicular tumors, given that up to 50% of dogs have bilateral tumors and only 12% are clinically detectable in the contralateral testicle.[15] In valuable breeding dogs, unilateral orchiectomy can be considered with continued monitoring afterward.[98,99] Exploratory laparotomy is indicated in cryptorchid dogs, in which case the regional lymph nodes can be visually assessed and biopsied if indicated. In dogs with signs of hyperestrogenism secondary to the primary tumor, clinical signs typically resolve within 1 to 3 months following castration, unless metastatic lesions provide persistent estrogen release.[68,69,74] Recurrence of feminization following castration may be associated with the presence of metastasis.[69] Serum hormone levels may be monitored following castration and may correlate to resolution of clinical signs.[76,100] Dogs with bone marrow hypoplasia secondary to estrogen toxicity require close monitoring perioperatively and postoperatively for complications requiring medical intervention with blood products and/or antibiotics. These dogs carry a guarded prognosis due to the high morbidity and mortality associated with neutropenia and hemorrhage.[75,81] Dogs with aplastic anemia warrant a poor prognosis.[75]

Primary testicular tumors occasionally metastasize to regional lymph nodes and other distant sites, and therapy other than surgery may be warranted in these dogs. Optimal management employing chemotherapy, radiation therapy (RT), and novel targeted therapies is currently unknown. Cisplatin, actinomycin-D, chlorambucil, mithramycin, and bleomycin have been used; however, too few dogs were treated and evaluated to formulate conclusions regarding efficacy.[70,71,73,101] Cisplatin was evaluated in three dogs with aggressive testicular tumors, with survival ranging from 5 months to greater than 31 months.[70] RT was successfully used in four dogs with metastatic seminoma confined to the regional lymph nodes using total doses ranging from 17 to 40 Gy with ^{137}Cesium teletherapy.[102] In all four cases, tumors regressed and survival times ranged from 6 to 37 months; importantly, none of the dogs died of seminoma. Numbers were small, and further studies are warranted to evaluate the role of external-beam RT in managing metastatic seminomas because seminomas are considered extremely radioresponsive.[103]

Comparative Aspects

In the United States, testicular cancer is the most common cancer in men 15 to 44 years old but is one of the most curable cancers with early diagnosis.[104] Recent studies have shown an increase in testicular cancer over the past 40 years, suggesting that an individual's risk is a function of the era in which he was born.[104,105] Causal factors such as genetic predisposition, maternal estrogen exposure, occupational hazards, dietary factors, smoking habits, and birthplace have been evaluated, but, to date, the most established risk factor remains cryptorchidism.[23,104,106-114] Most cancers in men are germ cell tumors and are divided into seminomas and nonseminomas, with the former comprising 50% of tumors in this group.[13,20,23] Seminomas are further classified into classical, atypical, or spermatocytic seminoma, although management does not vary considerably between types.[20] Standard staging in human seminomas consists of physical examination;, radiographic studies; determination of serum markers, including alpha-fetoprotein (AFP), human chorionic gonadotropin (hCG), and lactate dehydrogenase; and histopathologic assessment. Spermatocytic seminoma is a rare variant of germ cell neoplasia that is most commonly seen in older men and carries a low risk of metastasis, suggesting similar behavior to most canine seminomas.[21,23] Treatment generally includes surgery for stage I seminomas, and/or RT and chemotherapy for individuals with advanced stage disease.[23,103,115-117] Cisplatin-based chemotherapy protocols are generally employed for patients with greater than stage I disease, with cure rates in the range of 70% to 80% despite advanced tumor burdens.[23,103,118] The dog has been proposed as a model for studies evaluating the development of testicular tumors.[18,21,22] Further interrogation of the molecular pathogenesis, classification system, and behavior of canine tumors may yield further support for use of spontaneously occurring testicular tumors as good comparative models for human disease.

Feline Testicular Tumors

Feline testicular tumors are rare, although Sertoli cell tumor, seminoma, interstitial cell tumor, and teratoma have been reported.[34,119-125] The biologic behavior of testicular neoplasia in the cat is unclear due to the sparse literature available. Metastasis of a Sertoli cell tumor to the liver and spleen has been reported, and teratoma metastasis to the omentum was observed in another report.[122,125] Optimal therapy other than orchiectomy is not known.

Canine Prostate Tumors

Incidence/Prevalence

Prostatic tumors are relatively uncommon in dogs and have a low prevalence at less than 1% (0.2% to 0.6%).[126-130] In a collection of over 17,000 confirmed neoplasms of the dog collected from veterinary schools in North America, only 11 prostate carcinomas were identified (0.06%).[33] In a separate study that evaluated lifetime occurrence of neoplasia in predominantly intact German shepherd and Belgian Malinois working dogs, over 30% developed at least one cancer; however, only 2 of the 104 primary tumors were prostate adenocarcinomas.[17] Despite this low incidence, the dog is one of the few domestic species to develop spontaneous prostate cancer, thus sparking interest in the dog as a comparative model for prostate cancer in men.[129,131,132] In three retrospective reviews of dogs with prostatic disease, between 7% and 16% were diagnosed with prostatic adenocarcinoma.[133-135] One study of 177 dogs found that prostatic adenocarcinoma was the most common disease in neutered dogs, whereas bacterial prostatitis and prostatic cysts were more common in intact male dogs.[134] Elderly dogs are more commonly diagnosed with prostatic carcinoma, with a median age at diagnosis of 10 years.[129,135,136] The underlying etiology of canine prostatic cancer is unknown; however, high-grade prostatic intraepithelial neoplasia (PIN or HGPIN), which is believed to be a precursor of human prostate carcinoma, has been detected in dogs without evidence of prostatic disease and in those with existing prostatic carcinoma.[137-139] The occurrence of PIN in dogs with concurrent carcinoma varies from 7% to 72%, although in two large studies of dogs without histologic evidence of prostatic carcinoma, the occurrence was low at 0% to 3%.[128,137-139]

Most tumors of the canine prostate are carcinomas, and the majority are adenocarcinomas. It is believed that prostate tumors in the dog arise from a urothelial or ductular origin rather than acinar because most canine tumors are androgen independent.[140-145] Other types of carcinomas, including transitional cell carcinoma (TCC) arising from the prostatic ducts, mixed carcinomas, and squamous cell carcinomas, can occur. Classifying carcinomas on the basis of subtype is somewhat subjective, and there is no standard for definitive diagnosis of canine prostate tumors as there is with humans.[139,146,147] Fibrosarcoma, leiomyosarcoma, osteosarcoma, lymphoma, and hemangiosarcoma have also been reported to affect the prostate.[128,148-153] Benign tumors of the prostate are rare, although there is a single case report of a dog with a benign prostatic adenoma or nodular hyperplasia.[154] TCC of the prostatic urethra will frequently invade the prostate, and it may be difficult to distinguish primary TCC from secondary invasion of a urethral tumor.

Risk Factors

Both intact and castrated dogs develop prostate carcinomas, although multiple studies have suggested there is an increased risk of prostatic adenocarcinoma in castrated male dogs compared to intact male dogs with an odds ratio of approximately 2.3 : 4.3.[126,135,136,140,143] More aggressive tumors may develop in castrated males with a higher risk of metastasis.[136] The reason for this difference is unclear, although it is possible that castrated dogs live longer than intact dogs and are thus predisposed to developing age-related cancers.[135,143] It is also possible that androgens provide a protective effect on prostatic tissue or that, on castration, the relative estrogen effect aids in neoplastic transformation.[143,155-157] A recent study observed that prostatic adenocarcinoma may occur relatively more frequently in intact male dogs, further complicating this issue.[128,139,143] Although several studies have suggested that androgens may not be required for initiation or progression of adenocarcinoma of the canine prostate, further controlled studies should be done to definitively determine the role of androgens and the impact of early or late castration.[140,142-145,158]

Breeds that may be at increased risk of developing prostate carcinomas include the Bouvier des Flandres, Doberman Pinscher, Shetland sheepdog, Scottish terrier, beagle, miniature poodle, German shorthaired pointer, Airedale terrier, and Norwegian elkhound.[135,143] The Shetland sheepdog and Scottish terrier remained at increased risk even when TCC was excluded in one study.[143] Mixed breed dogs have also been reported as at increased risk for prostate carcinoma, regardless of neutering status, suggesting environmental influences may play a significant role in tumor development.[143] The American cocker spaniel, miniature poodle, and dachshund may be at decreased risk for developing prostate cancer.[143]

Natural Behavior

At the time of diagnosis, most canine prostatic tumors are characterized by local invasion with a high propensity for regional and distant metastasis. In one postmortem study that retrospectively evaluated 76 dogs, 80% of those with prostate carcinoma had evidence of measurable metastatic disease, with lung and lymph node being the most common sites.[128] Importantly, similar to high-grade prostatic carcinoma in men, canine prostatic carcinomas have a tendency to metastasize to bone and 22% to 42% of canine patients develop skeletal metastasis, predominantly to the lumbar vertebrae and pelvis.[128,144,159,160] Younger dogs may be at increased risk for metastasis, although the role of castration status in this group is unclear.[128,161] Longitudinal studies in dogs with evidence of PIN are not available, and it is unclear if prostate carcinoma can behave in a slowly progressive fashion in early phases of development. It is presumed that most dogs are diagnosed at an advanced stage of disease due to the high metastatic rate; however, the true behavior from time of onset is not definitively known and prostate carcinoma may behave differently in intact and castrated dogs.[135,136]

Pathology/Pathogenesis

The underlying cause of prostate tumors is unknown, and it is possible that both genetic and environmental factors contribute to tumor development. As previously mentioned, HGPIN is considered a precursor of human prostate carcinoma and occurs under the influence of androgenic stimulation in those patients at risk for carcinoma.[162] Although PIN has been detected in dogs with existing prostatic carcinoma, it has also been detected in dogs without evidence of prostatic disease, making its role in the dog less clear.[137-139] HGPIN as a predictor of carcinoma occurrence is likely not as reliable in the dog as it is in men.[138,155] It is not known with certainty if low- and intermediate-grade PIN occurs in dogs, although a recent immunohistochemical study suggested the presence of low-grade PIN.[163] Investigators evaluated five prostates from middle-aged to older intact dogs containing lesions of PIN and compared nuclear protein p63 (marker of prostatic basal cells), androgen receptor expression, and PCNA to normal prostatic tissue from intact dogs. PIN foci had higher p63 expression, higher PCNA index, and heterogenous androgen receptor expression, suggesting similarities to human low grade PIN.[163]

The role of hormones in prostate development and tumor progression is also unclear in the dog. Castration does not provide a protective effect and, in fact, may contribute to tumor development and/or progression, although prostatic carcinoma may behave differently in the intact male compared to the neutered male.[135,136] Normal prostate development and regulation is androgen dependent in both humans and dogs; however, neoplastic human prostate remains androgen dependent unlike in the dog. Androgen receptor expression within the nuclei can be identified in 90% to 95% of normal noncastrated prostatic secretory epithelial cells and in the majority of acinar basal cells.[144,145,164,165] In neutered dogs and dogs with prostatic carcinoma, nuclear androgen expression decreases and is usually lost.[144,145] The role of estrogen and progesterone has yet to be fully defined, although nuclear estrogen receptor expression appears to be decreased in prostatic carcinoma tissue compared to normal and hyperplastic prostate tissue.[141,165]

Chromosomal abnormalities of the neoplastic prostate have only recently been studied, and preliminary data suggest abnormalities such as aneuploidy, centromeric fusions, polysomy of chromosome 13, and hyperdiploidy may occur in the dog.[166-168]

Because of its aggressive behavior at the time of diagnosis, some investigators have considered mechanisms that may contribute to prostate carcinoma progression and metastasis. The role of cyclooxygenase (COX) has received considerable attention in the human and veterinary literature and inhibition of COX-2 may play a role in the management of prostate tumors. Expression of COX-2 was noted in 75% of prostate carcinomas in one study, whereas none of the normal prostate tissue had expression.[169] Two other studies support the notion that COX-2 and its downstream prostaglandin E2 production play a role in prostate carcinomas.[170,171] Indeed, a clinical study identified COX-2 protein expression in 88% of 16 prostate carcinomas examined and further showed a survival benefit in dogs treated with either piroxicam or carprofen.[172] As stated earlier, prostatic carcinoma has a predilection for bone, which may be mediated in part by transforming growth factor-β (TGF-β), parathyroid hormone–related protein (PTHrP), and endothelin.[173-175] PTHrP mediates pathologic bone resorption in many different tumors, including prostate carcinomas, which may encourage release of TGF-β into the microenvironment. In a positive feedback loop, canine prostatic carcinoma cells can increase gene transcription for PTHrP in response to exogenous TGF-β.[174] Although PTHrP and TGF-β may be important in establishing skeletal metastases, it is interesting to note that prostate metastases are more commonly osteoblastic in nature. In a rat model, osteoblast activation was increased following incubation with normal canine prostate protein homogenates through an endothelin-dependent pathway, suggesting a possible contribution to bone metastasis formation.[175]

History and Clinical Signs

Clinical signs in dogs with prostate cancer are variable and may be reflective of local and/or metastatic disease. Common historic and clinical examination signs include hematuria, dysuria, stranguria, dyschezia, tenesmus, bacteriuria, and altered stool shape (flattened or ribbonlike stools).[128,136,160,176,177] If complete obstruction of urinary outflow results from prostatic compression or direct tumor extension into the urethra, hydroureter, hydronephrosis, and renal failure may occur. Local invasion into the lumbar vertebrae or nerve roots may cause signs of pain, gait abnormalities, lameness, and/or constipation. Nonspecific systemic illness, including lethargy, exercise intolerance, tachypnea or dyspnea, inappetence, and weight loss, can occur with advanced disease. Dogs with skeletal metastasis may present with signs of severe bone pain, pathologic fracture, or rarely with a palpable mass.[128,160,178] Dogs may present with a history of clinical signs that partially improved with empiric therapy for prostatitis.

Diagnostic Techniques and Staging

Dogs with suspected prostatic carcinoma should be fully staged in order to determine extent of disease and to rule out other causes of prostatic disease, such as benign prostatic hypertrophy (BPH), prostatitis, and prostatic cysts or abscesses.[177,179,180] Physical examination, including a thorough rectal examination, should be performed on every patient. Rectal palpation often reveals a large, firm, and asymmetric or irregular prostate that may be painful. Sublumbar lymphadenopathy may be detected on rectal or abdominal palpation. A normal-sized prostate on rectal examination in a castrated dog is considered abnormal, even if symmetric and nonpainful. CBC and serum chemistry profile may demonstrate anemia, leukocytosis, hypercalcemia, elevated bone alkaline phosphatase activity, or signs of concurrent disease. Urinalysis and culture may show pyuria, bacteriuria, dysplastic urinary epithelial cells, and secondary urinary bacterial infection. Three-view thoracic radiographs may show evidence of pulmonary metastatic disease, sternal lymphadenopathy, or rarely metastasis to the extrathoracic skeletal structures (ribs, scapula).[160] Abdominal radiographs may reveal evidence of an enlarged prostate, with or without evidence of mineralization; periosteal reactions on the vertebrae, femur, or pelvic bones; or sublumbar or retroperitoneal lymphadenopathy (Figure 28-6).[136,160,181,182] It is important to note that the presence of mineralization, particularly in intact dogs, is not pathognomonic for neoplasia and can occur in dogs with prostatitis, BPH, or prostatic cysts.[182-184] However, neutered dogs with prostatic mineralization

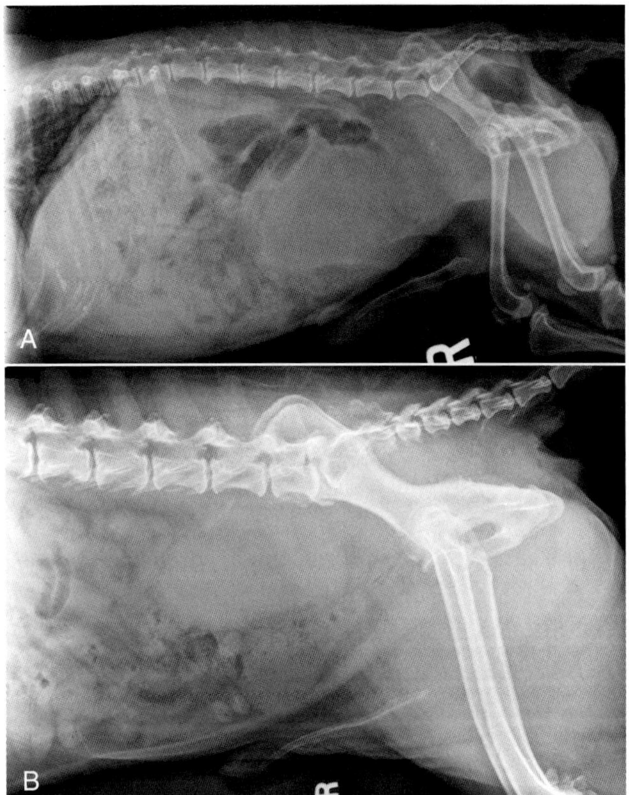

FIGURE 28-6 **A,** Right lateral abdominal radiograph demonstrating prostatic mineralization, which may be a feature of benign and malignant disease in intact dogs. **B,** Right lateral abdominal radiograph of a dog with prostatic carcinoma with metastasis to the sublumbar lymph nodes and local invasion along the sacrum and ventral aspect of the seventh lumbar vertebral body. *(**A** courtesy Dr. S. Holmes, University of Georgia; **B** courtesy Dr. D. Jimenez, University of Georgia.)*

are highly likely to have prostatic neoplasia and should undergo further diagnostics.[182] If a clinical suspicion of skeletal metastasis exists, survey radiographs or bone scintigraphy may be useful for localization.[178] Prostate carcinoma metastases to bone most commonly have an osteoproductive component but may be osteolytic, osteoproductive, or mixed. Contrast studies such as retrograde urethrography may be useful to evaluate irregularities in the prostatic urethra or reflux of contrast into a prostatic mass; however, they are not specific enough to differentiate neoplasia from inflammatory or infectious processes.[181,185] Abdominal ultrasound can be useful to further evaluate the prostate, urethra, bladder, locoregional lymph nodes, and cranial abdominal organs. Lymphadenopathy, echogenicity changes, and mineralization may be visualized on ultrasound, although they can also be features of nonneoplastic diseases (Figure 28-7).[181,182]

Obtaining tissue samples is considered the gold standard of diagnosis of canine prostatic neoplasia; however, a definitive diagnosis of prostatic neoplasia may be garnered from cytology samples as well.[177,186] A number of methods may provide adequate samples for diagnosis, including ejaculation, traumatic catheterization, prostatic massage, prostatic wash, ultrasound-guided FNA cytology, impression smears during surgery, or biopsy via percutaneous, perineal transrectal, or surgical routes. Risks of percutaneous biopsies, ultrasound-guided aspirates or biopsies, and transrectal aspirates may include hemorrhage, urethral trauma, and tumor seeding.[179,187-190] Cytology or histology of suspected metastatic lesions (e.g., lymph node) may also aid with diagnosis and offer an easier approach at diagnosis (Figure 28-8). Histologic grading of prostate cancers is not routinely performed because there is no support for its impact on prognostication.[128,191] Cytologic evaluation of samples collected via traumatic catheterization or prostatic wash may prove challenging as it can be difficult to differentiate dysplastic epithelial cells from neoplasia.[186,192] In one study, discordant results between cytology and histology in prostatic disorders occurred in 20% of cases but were not considered a flaw of aspiration techniques but rather of the pathologic process.[186] Multiple techniques were employed, including ultrasound-guided FNA, prostatic massage and wash, and impression smears of biopsies. Other factors such as serum and seminal plasma concentrations of acid phosphatase (AP), prostate-specific antigen (PSA), and canine prostate-specific esterase have not been useful in the definitive diagnosis of prostate carcinoma in the dog.[127,193] Although significantly higher serum total AP, prostatic AP, and nonprostatic AP concentrations were noted in dogs with prostatic carcinoma compared to healthy dogs or dogs with BPH, they were neither sensitive nor specific enough to warrant definitive diagnosis.[193]

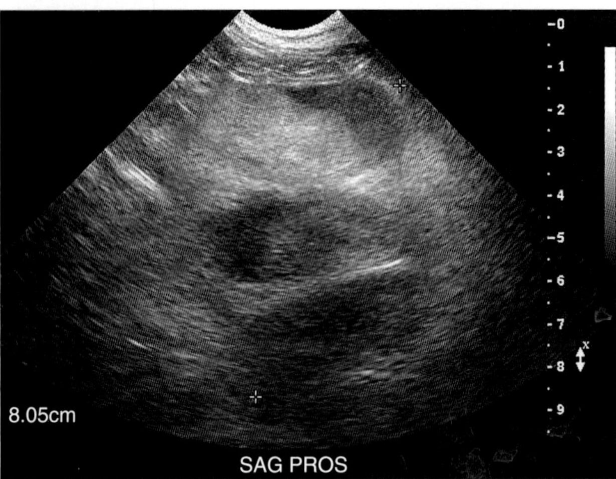

FIGURE 28-7 Ultrasound image of a symmetrically but severely enlarged prostate of heterogeneous echogenicity in a dog diagnosed with Rocky Mountain spotted fever and bacterial prostatitis. *(Courtesy Dr. D. Jimenez, University of Georgia.)*

Treatment and Prognosis

Because prostate cancer in dogs is characterized by insidious local progression and a high rate of metastasis, most dogs are diagnosed with advanced disease and the overall prognosis is poor. Median survival times (MSTs) for dogs without therapy are often less than 30 days, and in one report of 76 dogs, most dogs were euthanized at the time of diagnosis.[128,172] If therapy is attempted, effort is generally made to control local disease, as well as locoregional and distant metastases, although therapy is considered largely palliative. There is currently no standard-of-care consensus therapy for canine prostate tumors, although use of nonsteroidal antiinflammatory drugs (NSAIDs) is often recommended as minimal therapy.

Therapeutic options for managing local disease include prostatectomy, electrosurgical transurethral resection (TUR), photodynamic therapy (PDT), RT, laser therapy, and medical management. Surgery is generally considered to be a palliative procedure; surgical goals are to minimize clinical signs secondary to the primary tumor while maintaining normal urethral function. Prostatectomy is generally recommended for dogs with early stage disease that is still confined within the capsule (intracapsular disease). Total prostatectomy can be performed, although it is associated with a high rate of postoperative morbidity and a survival benefit has not been definitively demonstrated.[194-199] Subtotal intracapsular prostatectomy may be a useful alternative in dogs. In one study that compared 10 dogs that underwent total prostatectomy to 11 dogs that underwent subtotal intracapsular prostatectomy, the latter

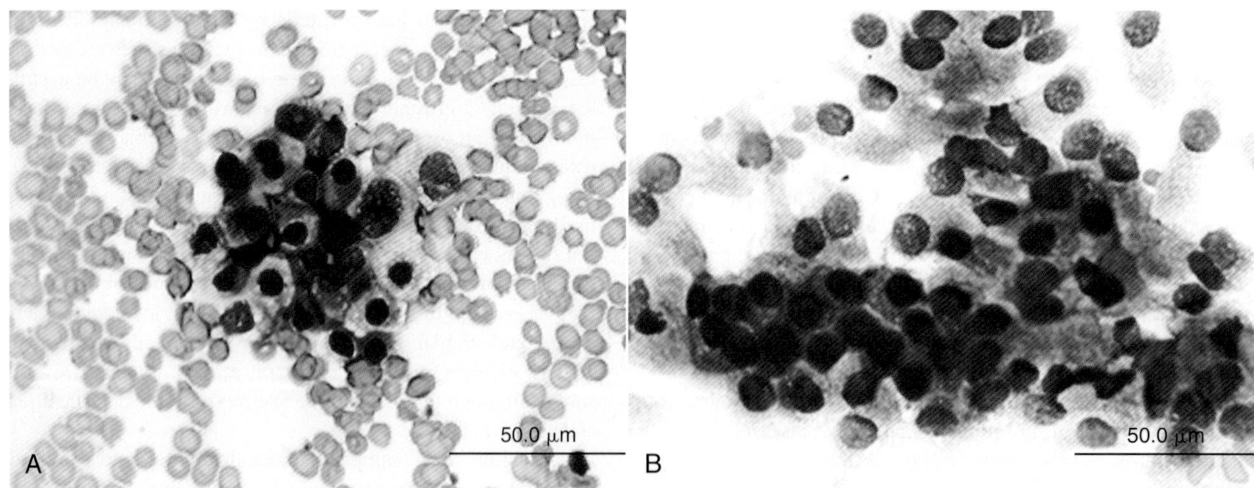

FIGURE 28-8 **A,** Prostatic carcinoma showing a cluster of variably sized polygonal epithelial cells with a moderate amount of basophilic cytoplasm, which often contains clear, nonstaining vacuoles. These cells have round-to-ovoid nuclei with coarsely granular chromatin pattern and occasional distinct nucleoli. A single binucleated cell is seen. Nuclear to cytoplasmic (N:C) ratios are moderate, and there is mild-to-moderate anisocytosis and anisokaryosis. **B,** Normal prostate composed of loosely cohesive clusters of polygonal to columnar epithelial cells with a moderate amount of basophilic cytoplasm that often appears stippled with both eosinophilic granules and tiny, crisp, nonstaining vacuoles. Nuclei are round to ovoid and are often eccentrically located. Chromatin is condensed, and there is minimal anisocytosis and anisokaryosis. *(Courtesy Dr. M. Camus, University of Georgia.)*

procedure was associated with longer mean survival time (112 days versus 20 days) and a decreased rate of postoperative complications.[196] Importantly, 7 of the 10 dogs that underwent total prostatectomy were euthanized within 2 weeks of surgery compared to only 2 dogs in the subtotal intracapsular group.[196] Urinary incontinence is a common sequela to prostatectomy and attempts have been made to reduce trauma to the prostatic urethra, including use of a neodymium:yttrium-aluminum-garnet (Nd:YAG) laser; however, there is still a risk of significant postoperative complications.[195,198,199] In one recent report, TUR using an electrocautery cutting loop was performed with or without intraoperative RT in three dogs with prostatic TCC or undifferentiated carcinoma.[200] All dogs experienced rapid palliation of dysuria but complications, including urinary tract infection, tumor seeding, and urethral perforation, occurred and survival for all dogs was short.[200] Although dogs with prostatic carcinomas may be palliated early with surgical intervention, TUR and total prostatectomy are associated with a high risk of complications and cases should be selected carefully.

In dogs with urethral obstruction due to a prostatic tumor, palliative measures may be attempted to alleviate the obstruction. Placement of a cystostomy tube permits urinary diversion and bladder emptying, but owners should be aware that it generally does not resolve incontinence and stranguria and secondary urinary tract infections are common.[201-203] Palliative stenting of the urethra in the obstructed area is a reasonable alternative to cystostomy tubes. The extent and location of the obstruction is determined using fluoroscopy, and stents are typically selected to extend approximately 1 cm proximal and distal to the obstruction.[148] Stents can be ordered in various diameters and are recommended to be 10% greater than the diameter of healthy appearing urethra. Of eight dogs with prostatic tumors stented in one study, the severe complication rate was low (two dogs) and the procedure immediately alleviated the obstruction in all dogs.[148] Median survival time in this study involving 12 dogs with bladder TCC or prostate tumors was short (20 days) despite stenting and therapy with a COX-2 inhibitor; however, further experience and evaluation of this technique may demonstrate improved quality of life. PDT may be an option, particularly for dogs with minimally invasive prostate cancer. There is one case report describing the resolution of macroscopic hematuria and sanguineous preputial discharge with stable disease for at least 6 months in a dog with prostatic carcinoma.[204] PDT remains predominantly investigational, although several recent reports have suggested that the dog provides a good model to investigate novel treatments for prostatic carcinoma that may benefit both dogs and humans.[205-208] Challenges in delivering a homogenous dose may limit the utility of PDT in advanced tumors; however, further evaluation may indicate a role in the management of prostatic carcinomas.

RT may be useful in the palliation of clinical signs related to local prostatic carcinoma as well as to palliate painful skeletal metastases, although optimal dose and fractionation are unknown. In one study, 10 dogs with prostatic carcinoma were treated with intraoperative orthovoltage therapy.[209] Nine were prescribed 20 to 30 Gy to the prostate, with an MST of 114 days, although the range extended to 750 days.[209] It is probable that with advances in 3-dimensional (3D) imaging and intensity-modulated RT (IMRT) planning and delivery, local disease may be better targeted and controlled. However, metastatic disease will remain a challenge unless early prostatic carcinoma can be detected.

The benefit of systemic therapy to manage canine prostatic tumors is unclear, although a pivotal study demonstrated a clear survival benefit in dogs with prostate carcinomas treated with piroxicam or carprofen compared to those untreated (6.9 months versus 0.7 month).[172] The role of chemotherapy is less clear, although prospective studies are warranted for further investigation of NSAIDs alone and in combination with chemotherapy.

For dogs with skeletal metastasis, palliative options include systemic analgesics, RT, aminobisphosphonate administration, and ^{153}samarium ethylenediamine-tetramethylene phosphonate (^{153}SM-EDTMP).[210,211] Standardized protocols have not been determined, although RT and pamidronate are both widely available options and relatively easy to administer.[210,212,213]

Comparative Aspects

Prostate cancer is the second most frequently diagnosed cancer and the sixth most common fatal cancer among men worldwide, and its incidence is increasing.[214,215] The only well-established and consistent risk factors for prostate cancer in men are race/ethnicity, family history, and age, although other factors such as diet and lifestyle may contribute as well.[214-221] As in dogs, most prostatic tumors in men are carcinomas; however, the incidence of disease is considerably higher in men. Geriatric men have a high rate of asymptomatic prostate cancer, in part due to the increased occurrence of PSA-driven biopsies. Serum PSA is a readily detectable serine protease produced by both malignant and benign prostate tissues. The dog is one of the few domestic species to develop spontaneous prostate cancer, resulting in considerable interest in the dog as a model for prostatic carcinoma in men.[129,131,132] A similar canine PSA is not detectable with commercially available human antibodies, thus limiting comparisons made between diagnosis of human PSA-driven and canine prostate cancer.[127,222] Another important challenge in using the dog as a model is that most early-stage prostate carcinomas in men are highly androgen dependent and disease progression can be manipulated through androgen deprivation.[214,223] Prostate carcinoma in men typically initiates as PIN, which is often seen as multifocal premalignant lesions that progress to neoplasia; the role of PIN in the development of canine prostatic diseases in either the intact or castrated dog is unclear. High-grade prostate cancer in men behaves similarly to the disease in dogs, with significant local invasion and a propensity to metastasize to the skeleton. While high-grade aggressive prostate carcinoma is less common in the elderly man, the dog may serve as a model for interventional strategies in this setting. Therapy in humans varies from active surveillance to prostatectomy to RT (external beam and brachytherapy) and is highly dependent on the stage of disease at presentation and partially on risks versus benefits of intervention.[214,215,223] Treatment strategies, including chemotherapy, vascular targeting, RT approaches, and management of skeletal metastasis, may be investigated in canine models and ultimately benefit both species.

Feline Prostate Tumors

Prostate tumors in the cat are rare and reports in the veterinary literature are sparse.[224-229] Of the few case reports, most tumors are adenocarcinomas and affect older castrated cats. Definitive risk factors have not been identified due to the lack of frequent cases and epidemiologic data. Clinical signs often include lower urinary tract signs, as well as obstipation or constipation, tenesmus, and dyschezia. Rectal palpation can reveal the presence of a mass, which may be further characterized with abdominal ultrasound. There is no standard-of-care therapy, and it is difficult to state overall prognosis. Metastasis appears common, and sites of spread include pancreas, lung, and lymph nodes; most cats died within 3 months of diagnosis.[224-228] A recent report described the use of prostatectomy for a low-grade prostatic sarcomatoid carcinoma, with no evidence of local or metastatic disease at 2 years.[229] One report described the use of prostatectomy followed by doxorubicin and cyclophosphamide to yield a survival time of 10 months.[225]

Canine Penile, Preputial, and Scrotal Tumors

Multiple tumor types can affect the soft tissues of the canine penis, prepuce, and scrotum, including transmissible venereal tumor (TVT), squamous cell carcinoma, sebaceous gland adenoma, mesothelioma, papilloma, lymphoma, plasma cell tumor, mast cell tumor, hemangioma, melanoma, and fibrosarcoma.[37,230-237] Overall, TVT and squamous cell carcinomas are the most common neoplasms of the canine penis. Ossifying fibroma, benign mesenchymoma, multilobular osteochondrosarcoma, and osteosarcoma can arise from the penile bone (os penis).[238-243] Osteosarcoma of the os penis may behave similarly to other axial skeleton sites, with a potential to develop local recurrence following narrow excision and distant metastasis.[238,240]

Clinical signs are often associated with local disease, and many dogs present with hematuria, stranguria, or dysuria. Occasionally, dogs may present with a visible mass and the absence of urinary signs; this is likely more common in scrotal tumors compared to other tumor sites. It is also possible for clinical signs to be secondary to locoregional or distant metastasis. It is recommended to fully stage dogs with penile tumors prior to definitive therapy. Surgical excision is generally recommended and often involves partial or complete penile amputation and perineal urethrostomy. TVT is an obvious exception because it is a chemoresponsive and radiation-responsive tumor, although surgery may be used for refractory cases.[244,245] For dogs with scrotal tumors, castration (if intact) with scrotal ablation is recommended. Depending on the underlying tumor type, adjuvant therapy such as RT or chemotherapy may be indicated. Prognosis is heavily dependent on underlying histology, as well as the ability to obtain adequate local control.

Feline Penile, Preputial, and Scrotal Tumors

Little information exists on tumors that affect the feline penis, prepuce, and scrotum. There is a report of fibroma affecting the scrotum of a cat; however, it is probable that clinical signs would be similar to those in dogs.[246]

Comparative Aspects

Penile tumors in the United States are rare, although they remain a problem in a number of countries in Asia, Africa, and South America, where up to 10% of cancer may arise in the penis.[247] The incidence of penile cancer has been declining in part due to increased personal hygiene and circumcision.[248-250] Indeed, neonatal circumcision, as practiced by a number of groups, virtually eliminates penile carcinoma from the population.[249] Poor local hygiene, phimosis, tobacco, chronic inflammation, lack of circumcision, infection with human papilloma virus, and having multiple sexual partners are associated with the development of malignant penile lesions.[249,251-253] Most penile tumors are carcinomas and over 95% of carcinomas are squamous cell in origin. Clinical signs in men are varied and range from a subtle erythematous local lesion to an ulcerated, infected mass lesion. Full staging is important in men who present with penile cancer because nodal status is one of the most significant prognostic variables for survival.[247] The prognosis is generally excellent for patients with early stage disease and treatment typically consists of surgery. Occasionally, RT is used for primary treatment of early stage disease, but local recurrence rates are higher than with surgery.[247,254-256] In advanced cases, aggressive surgery may include emasculation procedures or hemipelvectomy followed by RT. The role of chemotherapy is still evolving in human penile carcinoma management, but agents such as cisplatin, methotrexate, and bleomycin appear to have modest activity.

REFERENCES

1. Cotchin E: Testicular neoplasms in dogs, *J Comp Pathol* 70:232, 1960.
2. von-Bomhard D, Pukkavesa C, Haenichen T: The ultrastructure of testicular tumours in the dog. I. Germina cells and seminomas, *J Comp Pathol* 88:49, 1978.
3. Hayes HM, Pendergrass TW: Canine testicular tumors: epidemiologic features of 410 dogs, *Int J Cancer* 18:482, 1976.
4. Liao AT, Chu PY, Yeh LS, et al: A 12-year retrospective study of canine testicular tumors, *Theriogenology* 71:919, 2009.
5. Cohen D, Reif J, Brodey R, et al: Epidemiologic analysis of the most prevalent sites and types of canine neoplasia observed in a veterinary hospital, *Cancer Res* 34:2859, 1974.
6. Dow C: Testicular tumours in the dog, *J Comp Pathol* 72:247, 1962.
7. Grieco V, Riccardi E, Greppi GF, et al: Canine testicular tumours: a study on 232 dogs, *J Comp Pathol* 138:86, 2008.
8. Nodtvedt A, Gamlem H, Gunnes G, et al: Breed differences in the proportional morbidity of testicular tumours and distribution of histopathologic types in a population-based canine cancer registry, *Vet Comp Oncol* 9:45, 2011.
9. Bray F, Ferlay J, Devesa SS, et al: Interpreting the international trends in testicular seminoma and nonseminoma incidence, *Nat Clin Pract Urol* 3:532, 2006.
10. Chia VM, Quraishi SM, Devesa SS, et al: International trends in the incidence of testicular cancer, 1973-2002, *Cancer Epidemiol Biomarkers Prev* 19:1151, 2010.
11. Shah MN, Devesa SS, McGlynn KA: Trends in testicular germ cell tumours by ethnic group in the United States, *Int J Androl* 30:206, 2007.
12. Townsend JS, Richardson LC, German RR: Incidence of testicular cancer in the United States, 1999-2004, *Am J Mens Health* 4:353, 2010.
13. Bray F, Richiardi L, Ekbom A, et al: Do testicular seminoma and nonseminoma share the same etiology? Evidence from an age-period-cohort analysis of incidence trends in eight European countries, *Cancer Epidemiol Biomarkers Prev* 15:652, 2006.
14. Weaver AD: Survey with follow-up of 67 dogs with testicular Sertoli cell tumours, *Vet Rec* 113:105, 1983.
15. Reif JS, Maguire TG, Kenney RM, et al: A cohort study of canine testicular neoplasia, *J Am Vet Med Assoc* 175:719, 1979.
16. Kennedy PC, Cullen JM, Edwards JF, et al: Histological classifications of tumors of the genital system of domestic animals. *World Health Organization international histological classification of tumors of domestic animals*, ed 2, Washington, DC, 1998, American Registry of Pathology.
17. Peterson JR, Frommelt RA, Dunn DG: A study of the lifetime occurrence of neoplasia and breed differences in a cohort of German shepherd dogs and Belgian Malinois military working dogs that died in 1992, *J Vet Int Med* 14:140, 2000.
18. Peters MA, DeRooij DG, Teerds KJ, et al: Spermatogenesis and testicular tumours in ageing dogs, *J Reprod Fertil* 120:443, 2000.
19. Maiolino P, Restucci B, Papparella S, et al: Correlation of nuclear morphometric features with animal and human World Health Organization international histological classifications of canine spontaneous seminomas, *Vet Pathol* 41:608, 2004.

20. Mostofi FK, Sesterhenn IA: Histologic typing of testis tumors. *World Health Organization international histological classification of tumors*, ed 2, Geneva, 1998, Springer.
21. Kim JH, Yu CH, Yhee JY, et al: Canine classical seminoma: a specific malignant type with human classifications is highly correlated with tumor angiogenesis, *BMC Cancer* 10:243, 2010.
22. Grieco V, Riccardi E, Rondena M, et al: Classical and spermatocytic seminoma in the dog: histochemical and immunohistochemical findings, *J Comp Pathol* 137:41, 2007.
23. Bosl GJ, Bajorin DF, Sheinfeld J, et al: Cancer of the testis. In DeVita VT, Lawrence TS, Rosenberg SA, editors: *Cancer: principles and practice of oncology*, Philadelphia, 2008, Lippincott Williams and Wilkins.
24. Ortega-Pacheco A, Rodriguez-Buenfil JC, Segura-Correa JC, et al: Pathological conditions of the reproductive organs of male stray dogs in the tropics: prevalence, risk factors, morphological findings and testosterone concentrations, *Reprod Domest Anim* 41:429, 2006.
25. Reif JS, Brodey RS: The relationship between cryptorchidism and canine testicular neoplasia, *J Am Vet Med Assoc* 155:2005, 1969.
26. Patnaik AK, Mostofi FK: A clinicopathologic, histologic, and immunohistochemical study of mixed germ cell-stromal tumors of the testis in 16 dogs, *Vet Pathol* 30:287, 1993.
27. Radi ZA, Miller DL, Hines ME: Rete testis mucinous adenocarcinoma in a dog, *Vet Pathol* 41:75, 2004.
28. Turk JR, Turk MA, Gallina AM: A canine testicular tumor resembling gonadoblastoma, *Vet Pathol* 18:201, 1981.
29. Rothwell TLW, Papdimitriou JM, Zu FN, et al: Schwannoma in the testis of a dog, *Vet Pathol* 23:629, 1986.
30. Vascellari M, Carminato A, Camall G, et al: Malignant mesothelioma of the tunica vaginalis testis in a dog: histological and immunohistochemical characterization, *J Vet Diagn Invest* 23:135, 2011.
31. Scully RE, Coffin DL: Canine testicular tumors with special reference to their histogenesis, comparative morphology, and endocrinology, *Cancer Epidemiol Biomarkers Prev* 5:592, 1952.
32. Lipowitz AJ, Schwartz A, Wilson GP, et al: Testicular neoplasms and concomitant clinical changes in the dog, *J Am Vet Med Assoc* 163:1364, 1973.
33. Priester WA, McKay FW: The occurrence of tumors in domestic animals, *Natl Cancer Inst Monogr* 54:1, 1980.
34. Sapierzynski R, Malicka E, Bielecki W, et al: Tumors of the urogenital system in dogs and cats. Retrospective review of 138 cases, *Pol J Vet Sci* 10:97, 2007.
35. Hayes HM, Tarone RE, Casey HW: A cohort study of the effects of Vietnam service on testicular pathology of US military working dogs, *Mil Med* 160:248, 1995.
36. Hayes HM, Tarone RE, Casey HW, et al: Excess of seminomas observed in Vietnam service U.S. military working dogs, *J Natl Cancer Inst* 82:1042, 1990.
37. McEntee MC: Reproductive oncology, *Clin Tech Small Anim Pract* 17:133, 2002.
38. Benazzi C, Sarli G, Preziosi R, et al: Laminin expression in testicular tumours of the dog, *J Comp Pathol* 112:141, 1995.
39. Sarli G, Benazzi C, Preziosi R, et al: Proliferative activity assessed by anti-PCNA and Ki67 MAbs in canine testicular tumours, *J Comp Pathol* 110:357, 1994.
40. Papaioannou N, Psalla D, Zavlaris M, et al: Immunohistochemical expression of dog TERT in canine testicular tumours in relation to PCNA, ki67 and p53 expression, *Vet Res Commun* 33:905, 2009.
41. Nasir L: Telomeres and telomerase: biological and clinical importance in dogs, *Vet J* 175:155, 2008.
42. Nasir L, Devlin P, McKevitt T, et al: Telomere lengths and telomerase activity in dog tissues: a potential model system to study human telomere and telomerase biology, *Neoplasia* 3:351, 2001.
43. DeVico G, Papparella S, DiGuardo G: Number and size of silver-stained nucleoli (Ag-NOR clusters) in canine seminomas: correlation with histological features and tumour behaviour, *J Comp Pathol* 110:267, 1994.
44. Murakami Y, Tateyama S, Uchida K, et al: Immunohistochemical analysis of cyclins in canine normal testes and testicular tumors, *J Vet Med Sci* 63:909, 2001.
45. Brehm R, Ruttinger C, Fischer P, et al: Transition from preinvasive carcinoma in situ to seminoma is accompanied by a reduction of connexin 43 expression in Sertoli cells and germ cells, *Neoplasia* 8:499, 2006.
46. Lin JH, Takano T, Cotrina ML, et al: Connexin 43 enhances the adhesivity and mediates the invasion of malignant glioma cells, *J Neurosci* 22:4302, 2002.
47. Risley MS, Tan IP, Roy C, et al: Cell-, age-, and stage-dependent distribution of connexin43 gap junctions in testes, *J Cell Sci* 103:81, 1992.
48. Steger K, Tetens F, Bergmann M: Expression of connexin43 in human testis, *Histochem Cell Biol* 112:215, 1999.
49. Zhang W, Nwagwu C, Le DM, et al: Increased invasive capacity of connexin43-overexpressing malignant glioma cells, *J NeuroSci* 99:1039, 2003.
50. Ruttinger C, Bergmann M, Fink L, et al: Expression of connexin 43 in normal canine testes and canine testicular tumors, *Histochem Cell Biol* 130:537, 2008.
51. Lee CH, Kim WH, Lim JH, et al: Mutation and overexpression of p53 as a prognostic factor in canine mammary tumors, *J Vet Sci* 5:63, 2004.
52. Lee CH, Kweon OK: Mutations of p53 tumor suppressor gene in spontaneous canine mammary tumors, *J Vet Sci* 3:321, 2002.
53. Queiroga FL, Raposo T, Carvalho MI, et al: Canine mammary tumours as a model to study human breast cancer: most recent findings, *In Vivo* 25:455, 2011.
54. Inoue M, Wada N: Immunohistochemical detection of p53 and p21 proteins in canine testicular tumours, *Vet Rec* 146:370, 2000.
55. Vitellozzi G, Mariotti F, Ricci G: Immunohistochemical expression of the p53 protein in testicular tumours in the dog, *Eur J Vet Pathol* 4:61, 1998.
56. Restucci B, Maiolino P, Paciello O, et al: Evaluation of angiogenesis in canine seminomas by quantitative immunohistochemistry, *J Comp Pathol* 128:252, 2003.
57. Yoshinaga K, Nishikawa S, Ogawa M, et al: Role of c-kit in mouse spermatogenesis: identification of spermatogonia as a specific site of c-kit expression and function, *Development* 113:689, 1991.
58. Sattler M, Salgia R: Targeting c-kit mutation: basic science to novel therapies, *Leuk Res* 28S1:S11, 2004.
59. Goddard NC, McIntyre A, Summersgill B, et al: KIT and RAS signalling pathways in testicular germ cell tumours: new data and a review of the literature, *Int J Androl* 30:337, 2007.
60. Mauduit C, Hamamah S, Benahmed M: Stem cell factor/c-kit system in spermatogenesis, *Hum Reprod Update* 5:535, 1999.
61. Rothschild G, Sottas CM, Kissel H, et al: A role for kit receptor signaling in Leydig cell steroidogenesis, *Biol Reprod* 69:925, 2003.
62. Grieco V, Banco B, Giudice C, et al: Immunohistochemical expression of the KIT protein (CD117) in normal and neoplastic canine testes, *J Comp Pathol* 142:213, 2010.
63. Stoop H, Honecker F, vandeGeijn GJ, et al: Stem cell factor as a novel diagnostic marker for early malignant germ cells, *J Pathol* 216:43, 2008.
64. Cummings OW, Ulbright TM, Eble JN, et al: Spermatocytic seminoma: an immunohistochemical study, *Hum Pathol* 25:54, 1994.
65. Nurmio M, Toppari J, Zaman F, et al: Inhibition of tyrosine kinases PDGFR and c-kit by imatinib mesylate interferes with postnatal testicular development in the rat, *Int J Androl* 30:366, 2007.
66. Nurmio M, Kallio J, Toppari J, et al: Adult reproductive functions after early postnatal inhibition of the two receptor tyrosine kinases, c-kit and PDGFR, in the rat testis, *Reprod Toxicol* 25:442, 2008.
67. Basciani S, Brama M, Mariani S, et al: Imatinib mesylate inhibits Leydig cell tumor growth: evidence for in vitro and in vivo activity, *Cancer Res* 65:1897, 2005.

68. Hogenesch H, Whitely HE, Vicini DS, et al: Seminoma with metastases in the eyes and the brain in a dog, *Vet Pathol* 24:278, 1987.
69. Brodey RS, Martin JE: Sertoli cell neoplasms in the dog: the clinicopathological and endocrinological findings in thirty-seven dogs, *J Am Vet Med Assoc* 133:249, 1958.
70. Dhaliwal RS, Kitchell BE, Knight BL, et al: Treatment of aggressive testicular tumors in four dogs, *J Am Anim Hosp Assoc* 35:311, 1999.
71. Spugnini EP, Bartolazzi A, Ruslander D: Seminoma with cutaneous metastases in a dog, *J Am Anim Hosp Assoc* 36:253, 2000.
72. Takiguchi M, Iida T, Kudo T, et al: Malignant seminoma with systemic metastases in a dog, *J Small Anim Pract* 42:360, 2001.
73. Weller RE, Palmer B: Metastatic seminoma in a dog, *Mod Vet Pract* 64:275, 1983.
74. Gopinath D, Draffan D, Philbey AW, et al: Use of intralesional oestradiol concentration to identify a functional pulmonary metastasis of canine Sertoli cell tumor, *J Small Anim Pract* 50:198, 2009.
75. Morgan RV: Blood dyscrasias associated with testicular tumors in the dog, *J Am Anim Hosp Assoc* 18:970, 1982.
76. Mischke R, Meurer D, Hoppen HO, et al: Blood plasma concentrations of oestradiol-17B, testosterone and testosterone/oestradiol ratio in dogs with neoplastic and degenerative testicular diseases, *Res Vet Sci* 73:267, 2002.
77. Peters MAJ, Jong FS, Teerds KJ, et al: Ageing, testicular tumours and the pituitary-testis axis in dogs, *J Endocrinol* 166:153, 2000.
78. Taniyama H, Hirayama K, Nakada K, et al: Immunohistochemical detection of inhibin-alpha, -beta B, and –beta A chains and 3beta-hydroxysteroid dehydrogenase in canine testicular tumors and normal testes, *Vet Pathol* 38:661, 2001.
79. Grootenhuis AJ vanSluijs FJ, Klaij IA, et al: Inhibin, gonadotrophins and sex steroids in dogs with Sertoli cell tumours, *J Endocrinol* 127:235, 1990.
80. Peters MA, Mol JA, vanWolferen ME, et al: Expression of the insulin-like growth factor (IGF) system and steroidogenic enzymes in canine testis tumors, *Reprod Biol Endocrinol* 14:22, 2003.
81. Sherding RG, Wilson GP, Kociba GJ: Bone marrow hypoplasia in eight dogs with Sertoli cell tumor, *J Am Vet Med Assoc* 178:497, 1981.
82. Scott DW, Reimers TJ: Tail gland and perianal gland hyperplasia associated with testicular neoplasia and hypertestosteronemia in a dog, *Canine Pract* 13:15, 1986.
83. Laing EJ, Harari J, Smith CW: Spermatic cord torsion and Sertoli cell tumor in a dog, *J Am Vet Med Assoc* 183:879, 1983.
84. Spackman CJ, Roth L: Prostatic cyst and concurrent Sertoli cell tumor in a dog, *J Am Vet Med Assoc* 192:1096, 1988.
85. Barrand KR, Scudamore CL: Canine hypertrophic osteoarthropathy associated with a malignant Sertoli cell tumour, *J Small Anim Pract* 42:143, 2001.
86. Brown TT, Burek JD, McEntee K: Male pseudohermaphroditism, cryptorchism, and Sertoli cell neoplasia in three miniature Schnauzers, *J Am Vet Med Assoc* 169:821, 1976.
87. Norrdin RW, Baum AC: A male pseudohermaphrodite dog with a Sertoli's cell tumor, mucometra, and vaginal glands, *J Am Vet Med Assoc* 156:204, 1970.
88. Frey DC, Tyler DE, Ramsey FK: Pyometra associated with bilateral cryptorchidism and Sertoli's cell tumor in a male pseudohermaphroditic dog, *J Am Vet Med Assoc* 146:723, 1965.
89. Bigliardi E, Parma P, Peressotti P, et al: Clinical, genetic, and pathological features of male pseudohermaphroditism in dog, *Reprod Biol Endocrinol* 9:12, 2011.
90. Johnston GR, Feeney DA, Johnston SD, et al: Ultrasonographic features of testicular neoplasia in dogs: 16 cases (1980-1988), *J Am Vet Med Assoc* 198:1779, 1991.
91. Pugh CR, Konde LJ: Sonographic evaluation of canine testicular and scrotal abnormalities: a review of 26 case histories, *Vet Radiol* 32:243, 1991.
92. Eilts BE, Pechman RD, Hedlund CS, et al: Use of ultrasonography to diagnose Sertoli cell neoplasia and cryptorchidism in a dog, *J Am Vet Med Assoc* 192:533, 1988.
93. Masserdotti C, DeLorenzi D, Gasparotto L: Cytologic detection of Call-Exner bodies in Sertoli cell tumors from 2 dogs, *Vet Clin Pathol* 37:112, 2008.
94. Banco B, Giudice C, Veronesi MC, et al: An immunohistochemical study of normal and neoplastic canine Sertoli cells, *J Comp Pathol* 143:239, 2010.
95. Peters MA, Teerds KJ, vanderGaag I, et al: Use of antibodies against LH receptor, 3beta-hydroxysteroid dehydrogenase and vimentin to characterize different types of testicular tumour in dogs, *Reproduction* 121:287, 2001.
96. Yu CH, Hwang DN, Kim JH, et al: Comparative immunohistochemical characterization of canine seminomas and Sertoli cell tumors, *J Vet Sci* 10:1, 2009.
97. Doxsee AL, Yager JA, Best SJ, et al: Extratesticular interstitial and Sertoli cell tumors in previously neutered dogs and cats: a report of 17 cases, *Can Vet J* 47:763, 2006.
98. Archbald LI, Waldow D, Gelatt K: Interstitial cell tumor, *J Am Vet Med Assoc* 210:1423, 1997.
99. England GC: Ultrasonographic diagnosis of non-palpable Sertoli cell tumours in infertile dogs, *J Small Anim Pract* 36:476, 1995.
100. Metzger FL, Hattel AL: Hematuria, hyperestrogenemia, and hyperprogesteronemia due to a Sertoli-cell tumor in a bilaterally cryptorchid dog, *Canine Pract* 18:32, 1993.
101. Madewell BR, Theilen GH: Tumors of the genital tract. In Theilen GH, Madewell BR, editors: *Veterinary cancer medicine*, Philadelphia, 1987, Lea & Febiger.
102. McDonald RK, Walker M, Legendre A, et al: Radiotherapy of metastatic seminoma in the dog. Case reports, *J Vet Intern Med* 2:103, 1988.
103. Albers P, Albrecht W, Algaba F, et al: EAU Guidelines on testicular cancer: 2011 update, *Eur Urol* 60:304, 2011.
104. Rosen A, Jayram G, Drazer M, et al: Global trends in testicular cancer incidence and mortality, *Eur Urol* 60:374, 2011.
105. Jacobsen R, Moller H, Thoresen S, et al: Trends in testicular cancer incidence in the Nordic countries, focusing on the recent decrease in Denmark, *Int J Androl* 29:199, 2006.
106. Myrup C, Wohlfahrt J, Oudin A, et al: Risk of testicular cancer according to birthplace and birth cohort in Denmark, *Int J Cancer* 126:217, 2010.
107. Henderson BE, Benton B, Jing J, et al: Risk factors for cancer of the testis in young men, *Int J Cancer* 23:598, 1979.
108. Weir HK, Marrett LD, Kreiger N, et al: Pre-natal and peri-natal exposures and risk of testicular germ-cell cancer, *Int J Cancer* 87:438, 2000.
109. Garner MJ, Birkett NJ, Johnson KC, et al: Dietary risk factors for testicular carcinoma, *Int J Cancer* 106:934, 2003.
110. Hu J, LaVecchia C, Morrison H, et al: Salt, processed meat and the risk of cancer, *Eur J Cancer Prev* 20:132, 2011.
111. Kratz CP, Mai PL, Greene MH: Familial testicular germ cell tumours, *Best Pract Res Clin Endocrinol Metab* 24:503, 2010.
112. VandenEeden SK, Weiss NS, Strader CH, et al: Occupation and the occurrence of testicular cancer, *Am J Ind Med* 19:327, 1991.
113. Garner MJ, Turner MC, Ghadirian P, et al: Epidemiology of testicular cancer: an overview, *Int J Cancer* 116:331, 2005.
114. Pinczowski D, McLaughlin JK, Lackgren G, et al: Occurrence of testicular cancer in patients operated on for cryptorchidism and inguinal hernia, *J Urol* 146:1291, 1991.
115. Tandstad T, Smaaland R, Solberg A, et al: Management of seminomatous testicular cancer: a binational prospective population-based study from the Swedish Norwegian testicular cancer study group, *J Clin Oncol* 29:719, 2011.
116. Aparicio J, delMuro G, Maroto P, et al: Multicenter study evaluating a dual policy of postorchiectomy surveillance and selective adjuvant single-agent carboplatin for patients with clinical stage I seminoma, *Ann Oncol* 14:867, 2003.

117. Oliver RT, Mead GM, Rustin GJ, et al: Randomized trial of carboplatin versus radiotherapy for stage I seminoma: mature results on relapse and contralateral testis cancer rates in MRC TE19/ EORTC 30982 study (ISRCTN27163214), *J Clin Oncol* 29:957, 2011.
118. Motzer RJ, Nichols CJ, Margolin KA, et al: Phase III randomized trial of conventional-dose chemotherapy with or without high-dose chemotherapy and autologous hematopoietic stem-cell rescue as first-line treatment for patients with poor-prognosis metastatic germ cell tumors, *J Clin Oncol* 25:247, 2007.
119. Rosen DK, Carpenter JL: Functional ectopic interstitial cell tumor in a castrated male cat, *J Am Vet Med Assoc* 202:1865, 1993.
120. Cotchin E: Neoplasia. In Wilkinson GT, editor: *Diseases of the cat and their management*, Oxford, 1984, Blackwell.
121. Miller MA, Hartnett SE, Ramos-Vara JA: Interstitial cell tumor and Sertoli cell tumor in the testis of a cat, *Vet Pathol* 44:394, 2007.
122. Miyoshi N, Yasuda N, Kamimura Y, et al: Teratoma in a feline unilateral cryptorchid testis, *Vet Pathol* 38:729, 2001.
123. Ferreira-da-Silva J: Teratoma in a feline unilateral cryptorchid testis (letter to the editor), *Vet Pathol* 39:516, 2002.
124. Benazzi C, Sarli G, Brunetti B: Sertoli cell tumour in a cat, *J Vet Med A Physiol Pathol Clin Med* 51:124, 2004.
125. Meier H: Sertoli-cell tumor in the cat: report of two cases, *North Am Vet* 37:979, 1956.
126. Obradovich J, Walshaw R, Goullaud E: The influence of castration on the development of prostatic carcinoma in the dog: 43 cases, *J Vet Intern Med* 1:183, 1987.
127. Bell FW, Klausner JS, Hayden DW, et al: Evaluation of serum and seminal plasma markers in the diagnosis of canine prostatic disorders, *J Vet Intern Med* 9:149, 1995.
128. Cornell KK, Bostwick DG, Cooley DM, et al: Clinical and pathological aspects of spontaneous canine prostate carcinoma: a retrospective analysis of 76 cases, *Prostate* 45:173, 2000.
129. Waters DJ, Sakr WA, Hayden DW, et al: Workgroup 5: spontaneous prostate cancer in dogs and non-human primates, *Prostate* 36:64, 1998.
130. Weaver AD: Fifteen cases of prostatic carcinoma in the dog, *Vet Rec* 109:71, 1981.
131. Waters DJ, Shen S, Glickman LT, et al: Prostate cancer risk and DNA damage: translational significance of selenium supplementation in a canine model, *Carcinogenesis* 26:1256, 2005.
132. Maini A, Archer C, Wang CY, et al: Comparative pathology of benign prostatic hyperplasia and prostate cancer, *In Vivo* 11:293, 1997.
133. Hornbuckle WE, MacCoy DM, Allan GS, et al: Prostatic disease in the dog, *Cornell Vet* 68:284, 1978.
134. Krawiec DR, Heflin D: Study of prostatic disease in dogs: 177 cases (1981-1986), *J Am Vet Med Assoc* 200:1119, 1992.
135. Teske E, Naan EC, vanDijk EM, et al: Canine prostate carcinoma: epidemiological evidence of an increased risk in castrated dogs, *Mol Cell Endocrinol* 197:251, 2002.
136. Bell FW, Klausner JS, Hayden DW, et al: Clinical and pathologic features of prostatic adenocarcinoma in sexually intact and castrated dogs: 31 cases (1970-1987), *J Am Vet Med Assoc* 199:623, 1991.
137. Waters DJ, Bostwick DG: Prostatic intraepithelial neoplasia occurs spontaneously in the canine prostate, *J Urol* 157(2):713–716, 1997.
138. Madewell BR, Gandour-Edwards R, DeVere-White RW: Canine prostatic intraepithelial neoplasia: is the comparative model relevant? *Prostate* 58:314, 2004.
139. Aquilina JW, McKinney L, Pacelli A, et al: High grade prostatic intraepithelial neoplasia in military working dogs with and without prostate cancer, *Prostate* 36:189, 1998.
140. Sorenmo KU, Goldschmidt M, Shofer F, et al: Immunohistochemical characterization of canine prostatic carcinoma and correlation with castration status and castration time, *Vet Comp Oncol* 1:48, 2003.
141. Grieco V, Riccardi E, Rondena M, et al: The distribution of oestrogen receptors in normal, hyperplastic and neoplastic canine prostate, as demonstrated immunohistochemically, *J Comp Pathol* 135:11, 2006.
142. LeRoy BE, Nadella MV, Toribio RE, et al: Canine prostate carcinomas express markers of urothelial and prostatic differentiation, *Vet Pathol* 41:131, 2004.
143. Bryan JN, Keeler MR, Henry CJ, et al: A population study of neutering status as a risk factor for canine prostate cancer, *Prostate* 67:1174, 2007.
144. Leav I, Schelling KH, Adams JY, et al: Role of canine basal cells in postnatal prostatic development, induction of hyperplasia, and sex hormone-stimulated growth; and the ductal origin of carcinoma, *Prostate* 48:210, 2001.
145. Lai CL, vandenHam R, Mol J, et al: Immunostaining of the androgen receptor and sequence analysis of its DNA-binding domain in canine prostate cancer, *Vet J* 181:256, 2009.
146. Humphrey PA: Gleason grading and prognostic factors in carcinoma of the prostate, *Modern Pathol* 17:292, 2004.
147. Young RH, Srigley JR, Amin MB, et al: *Tumors of the prostate gland, seminal vesicles, male urethra, and penis. Atlas of Tumor Pathology: Third Series, Fascicle 28*, Washington, DC, 2000, Armed Forces Institute of Pathology.
148. Weisse C, Berent A, Todd K, et al: Evaluation of palliative stenting for management of malignant urethral obstructions in dogs, *J Am Vet Med Assoc* 229:226, 2006.
149. Mainwaring CJ: Primary lymphoma of the prostate in a dog, *J Small Anim Pract* 31:617, 1990.
150. Winter MD, Locke JE, Penninck DG: Imaging diagnosis: urinary obstruction secondary to prostatic lymphoma in a young dog, *Vet Radiol Ultrasound* 47:597, 2006.
151. Hayden DW, Klausner JS, Waters DJ: Prostatic leiomyosarcoma in a dog, *J Vet Diagn Invest* 11:283, 1999.
152. Bacci B, Vignoli M, Rossi F, et al: Primary prostatic leiomyosarcoma with pulmonary metastases in a dog, *J Am Anim Hosp Assoc* 46:103, 2010.
153. Hayden DW, Bartges JW, Bell FW, et al: Prostatic hemangiosarcoma in a dog: clinical and pathologic findings, *J Vet Diagn Invest* 4:2009, 1992.
154. Gilson SD, Miller RT, Hardie EM, et al: Unusual prostatic mass in a dog, *J Am Vet Med Assoc* 200:702, 1992.
155. LeRoy BE, Northrup N: Prostate cancer in dogs: comparative and clinical aspects, *Vet J* 180:149, 2009.
156. Dore M, Chevalier S, Sirois J: Estrogen-dependent induction of cyclooxygenase-2 in the canine prostate in vivo, *Vet Pathol* 42:100, 2005.
157. Shidaifat F, Daradka M, Al-Omari R: Effect of androgen ablation on prostatic cell differentiation in dogs, *Endocr Res* 30:327, 2004.
158. Grieco V, Patton V, Romussi S, et al: Cytokeratin and vimentin expression in normal and neoplastic canine prostate, *J Comp Pathol* 129:78, 2003.
159. Cooley DM, Waters DJ: Skeletal metastasis as the initial clinical manifestation of metastatic carcinoma in 19 dogs, *J Vet Intern Med* 12:288, 1998.
160. Durham SK, Dietze AE: Prostatic adenocarcinoma with and without metastasis to bone in dogs, *J Am Vet Med Assoc* 188:1432, 1986.
161. Waters DJ, Cooley DM, Allen DK, et al: Host age influences the biological behavior of cancer: studies in pet dogs with naturally occurring malignancies, *Gerontologist* 38:110, 1998.
162. Ross RK, Pike MC, Coetzee GA, et al: Androgen metabolism and prostate cancer: establishing a model of genetic susceptibility, *Cancer Res* 58:4497, 1998.
163. Matsuzaki P, Cogliati B, Sanches DS, et al: Immunohistochemical characterization of canine prostatic intraepithelial neoplasia, *J Comp Pathol* 142:84, 2010.
164. Gallardo F, Lloreta J, Garcia F, et al: Immunolocalization of androgen receptors, estrogen alpha receptors, and estrogen beta receptors in experimentally induced canine prostatic hyperplasia, *J Androl* 30:240, 2009.
165. Gallardo F, Mogas T, Baro T, et al: Expression of androgen, oestrogen alpha and beta, and progesterone receptors in the canine

prostate: differences between normal, inflamed hyperplastic and neoplastic glands, *J Comp Pathol* 136:1, 2007.

166. Winkler S, Reimann-Berg N, Murua-Escobar H, et al: Polysomy 13 in a canine prostate carcinoma underlining its significance in the development of prostate cancer, *Cancer Genet Cytogenet* 169:154, 2006.
167. Winkler S, Murua-Escobar H, Eberle N, et al: Establishment of a cell line derived from a canine prostate carcinoma with a highly rearranged karyotype, *J Hered* 96:782, 2005.
168. Madewell BR, Deitch AD, Higgins RJ, et al: DNA flow cytometric study of the hyperplastic and neoplastic canine prostate, *Prostate* 18:173, 1991.
169. Tremblay C, Dore M, Bochsler PN, et al: Induction of prostaglandin G/H synthase-2 in a canine model of spontaneous prostatic adenocarcinoma, *J Natl Cancer Inst* 91:1398, 1999.
170. Mohammed SI, Coffman K, Glickman NW, et al: Prostaglandin E2 concentrations in naturally occurring canine cancer, *Prostaglandins Leukot Essent Fatty Acids* 64:1, 2001.
171. Mohammed SI, Khan KN, Sellers RS, et al: Expression of cyclooxygenase-1 and 2 in naturally-occurring canine cancer, *Prostaglandins Leukot Essent Fatty Acids* 70:479, 2004.
172. Sorenmo KU, Goldschmidt MH, Shofer FS, et al: Evaluation of cyclooxygenase-1 and cyclooxygenase-2 expression and the effect of cyclooxygenase inhibitors in canine prostatic carcinoma, *Vet Comp Oncol* 2:13, 2004.
173. Keller ET, Zhang J, Cooper CR, et al: Prostate carcinoma skeletal metastases: cross-talk between tumor and bone, *Cancer Metastasis Rev* 20:333, 2001.
174. Sellers RS, LeRoy BE, Blomme EA, et al: Effects of transforming growth factor-beta1 on parathyroid hormone-related protein mRNA expression and protein secretion in canine prostate epithelial, stromal, and carcinoma cells, *Prostate* 58:366, 2004.
175. LeRoy BE, Sellers RS, Rosol TJ: Canine prostate stimulates osteoblast function using the endothelin receptors, *Prostate* 59:148, 2004.
176. Leav I, Ling GV: Adenocarcinoma of the canine prostate, *Cancer* 22:1329, 1968.
177. Smith J: Canine prostatic disease: a review of anatomy, pathology, diagnosis, and treatment, *Theriogenology* 70:375, 2008.
178. Lee-Parritz DE, Lamb CR: Prostatic adenocarcinoma with osseous metastases in a dog, *J Am Vet Med Assoc* 192:1569, 1988.
179. Barsanti JA, Finco DR: Canine prostatic disease, *Vet Clin North Am* 16:587, 1986.
180. Johnston SD, Kamolpatana K, Root-Kustritz MV, et al: Prostatic disorders in the dog, *Anim Reprod Sci* 61:405, 2000.
181. Feeney DA, Johnston GR, Klausner JS, et al: Canine prostatic disease–comparison of radiographic appearance with morphologic and microbiologic findings: 30 cases (1981-1985), *J Am Vet Med Assoc* 190:1018, 1987.
182. Bradbury CA, Westropp JL, Pollard RE: Relationship between prostatomegaly, prostatic mineralization, and cytologic diagnosis, *Vet Radiol Ultrasound* 50:167, 2009.
183. Head LL, Francis DA: Mineralized paraprostatic cyst as a potential contributing factor in the development of perineal hernias in a dog, *J Am Vet Med Assoc* 221:533, 2002.
184. Zekas LJ, Forrest LJ, Swainson S, et al: Radiographic diagnosis: mineralized paraprostatic cyst in a dog, *Vet Radiol Ultrasound* 45:310, 2004.
185. Ackerman N: Prostatic reflux during positive contrast retrograde urethrography in the dog, *Vet Radiol* 24:251–259, 1983.
186. Powe JR, Canfield PJ, Martin PA: Evaluation of the cytologic diagnosis of canine prostatic disorders, *Vet Clin Pathol* 33:150, 2004.
187. Barsanti JA, Shotts EB, Prasse K, et al: Evaluation of diagnostic techniques for canine prostatic diseases, *J Am Vet Med Assoc* 177:160, 1980.
188. Barsanti JA, Finco DR: Evaluation of techniques for diagnosis of canine prostatic diseases, *J Am Vet Med Assoc* 185:198, 1984.
189. Leeds EB, Leav I: Perineal punch biopsy of the canine prostate gland, *J Am Vet Med Assoc* 154:925, 1969.
190. Nyland TG, Wallack ST, Wisner ER: Needle-tract implantation following US-guided fine-needle aspiration biopsy of transitional cell carcinoma of the bladder, urethra, and prostate, *Vet Radiol Ultrasound* 43:50, 2002.
191. MacLachan NJ, Kennedy PC: Tumors of the genital systems. In Mueten DJ, editor: *Tumors in domestic animals*, Ames, Iowa, 2002, Iowa State University Press.
192. Thrall MA, Olsen PN, Freemyer FG: Cytologic diagnosis of canine prostatic disease, *J Am Anim Hosp Assoc* 21:95, 1985.
193. Corazza M, Guidi G, Romagnoli S, et al: Serum total prostatic and non-prostatic acid phosphatases in healthy dogs and in dogs with prostatic diseases, *J Small Anim Pract* 35:307, 1994.
194. Hardie EM, Barsanti JA, Rawlings CA: Complications of prostatic surgery, *J Am Anim Hosp Assoc* 20:50, 1984.
195. Hardie EM, Stone EA, Spaulding KA, et al: Subtotal canine prostatectomy with the neodymium:yttrium-aluminum-garnet laser, *Vet Surg* 19:348, 1990.
196. Vlasin M, Rauser P, Fichtel T, et al: Subtotal intracapsular prostatectomy as a useful treatment for advanced-stage prostatic malignancies, *J Small Anim Pract* 47:512, 2006.
197. Basinger RR, Rawlings CA, Barsanti JA, et al: Urodynamic alterations associated with clinical prostatic diseases and prostate surgery in 23 dogs, *J Am Anim Hosp Assoc* 25:385, 1989.
198. Goldsmid SE, Bellenger CR: Urinary incontinence after prostatectomy in dogs, *Vet Surg* 20:253, 1991.
199. L'Epplattenier HF, Klem B, Teske E, et al: Partial prostatectomy using Nd:YAG laser for management of canine prostate carcinoma, *Vet Surg* 35:406, 2006.
200. Liptak JM, Brutscher SP, Monnet E, et al: Transurethral resection in the management of urethral and prostatic neoplasia in 6 dogs, *Vet Surg* 33:505, 2004.
201. Williams JM, White RAS: Tube cystostomy in the dog and cat, *J Small Anim Pract* 32:598, 2007.
202. Smith JD, Stone EA, Gilson SD: Placement of a permanent cystostomy catheter to relieve urine outflow obstruction in dogs with transitional cell carcinoma, *J Am Vet Med Assoc* 206:496, 1995.
203. Mann FA, Barrett RJ, Henderson RA: Use of a retained urethral catheter in three dogs with prostatic neoplasia, *Vet Surg* 21:342, 1992.
204. Lucroy MD, Bowles MH, Higbee RG, et al: Photodynamic therapy for prostatic carcinoma in a dog, *J Vet Intern Med* 19:235, 2003.
205. Chevalier S, Anidjar M, Scarlata E, et al: Preclinical study of the novel vascular occluding agent, WST11, for photodynamic therapy of the canine prostate, *J Urol* 186:302, 2011.
206. Xiao Z, Owen RJ, Liu W, et al: Lipophilic photosensitizer administration via the prostate arteries for photodynamic therapy of the canine prostate, *Photodiagnosis Photodyn Ther* 7:106, 2010.
207. Du KL, Mick R, Busch TM, et al: Preliminary results of interstitial motexafin lutetium-mediated PDT for prostate cancer, *Lasers Surg Med* 38:427, 2006.
208. Huang Z, Chen Q, Luck D, et al: Studies of a vascular-acting photosensitizer, Pd-bacteriopheophorbide (Tookad), in normal canine prostate and spontaneous canine prostate cancer, *Lasers Surg Med* 36:390, 2005.
209. Turrel JM: Intraoperative radiotherapy of carcinoma of the prostate gland in ten dogs, *J Am Vet Med Assoc* 190:48, 1987.
210. Fan TM, deLorimier LP, Charney SC, et al: Evaluation of intravenous pamidronate administration in 33 cancer-bearing dogs with primary or secondary bone involvement, *J Vet Intern Med* 19:74, 2005.
211. Lattimer JC Jr, Corwin LA, Stapleton J, et al: Clinical and clinicopathologic response of canine bone tumor patients to treatment with samarium-153-EDTMP, *J Nucl Med* 31:1316, 1990.
212. Fan TM, Charney SC, deLorimier LP, et al: Double-blind placebo-controlled trial of adjuvant pamidronate with palliative radiotherapy and intravenous doxorubicin for canine appendicular osteosarcoma bone pain, *J Vet Intern Med* 23:152, 2009.

213. Klausner JS, Johnston SD, Bell FW: Canine prostatic diseases. In Kirk RW, editor: *Current veterinary therapy XII*, Philadelphia, 1995, WB Saunders.
214. Zelefsky MJ, Eastham JA, Sartor OA, et al: Cancer of the prostate. In DeVita VT, Lawrence TS, Rosenberg SA, editors: *Cancer: principles and practice of oncology*, Philadelphia, 2008, Lippincott Williams and Wilkins.
215. Damber JE, Aus G: Prostate cancer, *Lancet* 371:1710, 2008.
216. Walsh PC, Partin AW: Family history facilitates the early diagnosis of prostate carcinoma, *Cancer* 80:1871, 1997.
217. Lichtenstein P, Holm NV, Verkasalo PK, et al: Environmental and heritable factors in the causation of cancer: analyses of cohorts of twins from Sweden, Denmark, and Finland, *N Engl J Med* 343:78, 2000.
218. Boyle P, Severi G, Giles GG: The epidemiology of prostate cancer, *Urol Clin North Am* 30:209, 2003.
219. Severi G, Morris HA, MacInnis RJ, et al: Circulating steroid hormones and the risk of prostate cancer, *Cancer Epidemiol Biomarker Prev* 15:86, 2006.
220. Wolk A: Diet, lifestyle and risk of prostate cancer, *Acta Oncol* 44:277, 2005.
221. Gronberg H: Prostate cancer epidemiology, *Lancet* 361(9360):859–864, 2003.
222. Anidjar M, Villette JM, Devauchelle P, et al: In vivo model mimicking natural history of dog prostate cancer using DPC-1, a new canine prostate carcinoma cell line, *Prostate* 46:2, 2001.
223. Lin AM, Small EJ: Prostate cancer update: 2007, *Curr Opin Oncol* 20:294, 2007.
224. Hawe JS: What is your diagnosis? Prostatic adenocarcinoma in a cat, *J Am Vet Med Assoc* 182:1257, 1983.
225. Hubbard BS, Vulgamott JC, Liska WD: Prostatic adenocarcinoma in a cat, *J Am Vet Med Assoc* 197:1493, 1990.
226. Caney SM, Hold PE, Day MJ, et al: Prostatic carcinoma in two cats, *J Small Anim Pract* 39:140, 1998.
227. LeRoy BE, Lech ME: Prostatic carcinoma causing urethral obstruction and obstipation in a cat, *J Feline Med Surg* 6:397, 2004.
228. Tursi M, Costa T, Valenza F, et al: Adenocarcinoma of the disseminated prostate in a cat, *J Feline Med Surg* 10:600, 2008.
229. Zambelli D, Cunto M, Raccagni R, et al: Successful surgical treatment of a prostatic biphasic tumour (sarcomatoid carcinoma) in a cat, *J Feline Med Surg* 12:161, 2010.
230. Michels GM, Knapp DW, David M, et al: Penile prolapse and urethral obstruction secondary to lymphosarcoma of the penis in a dog, *J Am Anim Hosp Assoc* 37:474, 2001.
231. Cornegliani L, Vercelli A, Abramo F: Idiopathic mucosal penile squamous papillomas in dogs, *Vet Dermatol* 18:439, 2007.
232. Ndiritu CG: Lesions of the canine penis and prepuce, *Mod Vet Pract* 60:712, 1979.
233. Patnaik AK, Matthiesen DT, Zawie DA: Two cases of canine penile neoplasm: squamous cell carcinoma and mesenchymal chondrosarcoma, *J Am Anim Hosp Assoc* 24:403, 1988.
234. Hall WC, Nielsen SW, McEntee K: Tumours of the prostate and penis, *Bull World Health Organ* 53:247, 1976.
235. Bloom F: *Pathology of the dog and cat: the genitourinary system with clinical considerations*, Evanston, 1954, American Veterinary Publications.
236. Vascellari M, Carminato A, Camali G, et al: Malignant mesothelioma of the tunica vaginalis testis in a dog: histological and immunohistochemical characterization, *J Vet Diagn Invest* 23:135, 2011.
237. Cihak RW, Roen DR, Klaassen J: Malignant mesothelioma of the tunica vaginalis in a dog, *J Comp Pathol* 96:459, 1986.
238. Peppler C, Weissert D, Kappe E, et al: Osteosarcoma of the penile bone (os penis) in a dog, *Aust Vet J* 87:52, 2009.
239. Webb JA, Liptak JM, Hewitt SA, et al: Multilobular osteochondrosarcoma of the os penis in a dog, *Can Vet J* 50:81, 2009.
240. Bleier T, Lewitschek HP, Reinacher M: Canine osteosarcoma of the penile bone, *J Vet Med A Physiol Pathol Clin Med* 50:397, 2003.
241. Mirkovic TK, Shmon CL, Allen AL: Urinary obstruction secondary to an ossifying fibroma of the os penis in a dog, *J Am Anim Hosp Assoc* 40:152, 2004.
242. Root-Kustritz MV, Fick JL, American College of Theriogenologists: Theriogenology question of the month: neoplasia of the os penis, *J Am Vet Med Assoc* 230:197, 2007.
243. Patnaik AK: Canine extraskeletal osteosarcoma and chondrosarcoma: a clinicopathologic study of 14 cases, *Vet Pathol* 27:46, 1990.
244. Rogers KS, Walker MA, Dillon HB: Transmissible venereal tumor: a retrospective study of 29 cases, *J Am Anim Hosp Assoc* 34:463, 1998.
245. Thrall DE: Orthovoltage radiotherapy of canine transmissible venereal tumors, *Vet Radiol* 23:217, 1982.
246. Milks HJ: Some diseases of the genito-urinary system. *Cornell Vet* 29:105, 1939.
247. Trabulsi EJ, Gomella LG: Cancer of the urethra and penis. In DeVita VT, Lawrence TS, Rosenberg SA, editors: *Cancer: principles and practice of oncology*, Philadelphia, 2008, Lippincott Williams and Wilkins.
248. Yeole BB, Jussawalla DJ: Descriptive epidemiology of the cancers of male genital organs in greater Bombay, *Indian J Cancer* 34:30, 1997.
249. Maden C, Sherman KJ, Beckman AM, et al: History of circumcision, medical conditions, and sexual activity and risk of penile cancer, *J Natl Cancer Inst* 85:19, 1993.
250. Hanash KA, Furlow WL, Utz DC, et al: Carcinoma of the penis: a clinicopathologic study, *J Urol* 104:291, 1970.
251. Shabbir M, Minhas S, Muneer A: Diagnosis and management of premalignant penile lesions, *Ther Adv Urol* 3:151, 2011.
252. Harish K, Ravi R: The role of tobacco in penile carcinoma, *Br J Urol* 75:375, 1995.
253. Backes DM, Kurman RJ, Pimenta JM, et al: Systematic review of human papillomavirus prevalence in invasive penile cancer, *Cancer Causes Control* 20:449, 2009.
254. Shapiro D, Shasha D, Tareen M, et al: Contemporary management of localized penile cancer, *Expert Rev Anticancer Ther* 11:29, 2011.
255. Stancik I, Holtl W: Penile cancer: review of the recent literature, *Curr Opin Urol* 13:467, 2003.
256. Lawindy SM, Rodriguez AR, Horenblas S, et al: Current and future strategies in the diagnosis and management of penile cancer, *Adv Urol* Epub 30 May 2011.

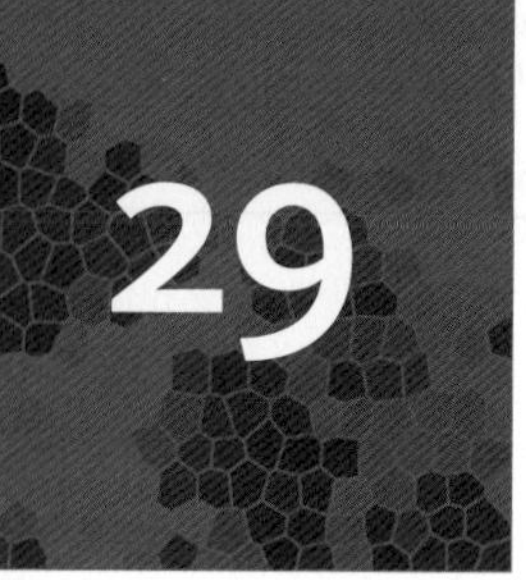

29 Tumors of the Urinary System

Deborah W. Knapp and Sarah K. McMillan

Canine Urinary Bladder Tumors

Urinary bladder cancer accounts for approximately 2% of all reported malignancies in the dog.[1-4] With more than 70 million dogs in the United States, even uncommon forms of cancer affect thousands of dogs each year.[2,3] The hospital prevalence or proportionate morbidity of bladder cancer at university-based veterinary hospitals is increasing.[2] Invasive transitional cell carcinoma (TCC) is the most common form of canine urinary bladder cancer.[1-4] Most TCCs are intermediate- to high-grade papillary infiltrative tumors.[2-4] Other types of bladder tumors reported less frequently include squamous cell carcinoma, adenocarcinoma, undifferentiated carcinoma, rhabdomyosarcoma, lymphoma, hemangiosarcoma, fibroma, and other mesenchymal tumors.[4-10]

TCC is most often located in the trigone region of the bladder. Papillary lesions and a thickened bladder wall (Figure 29-1) are common features and can lead to partial or complete urinary tract obstruction. In a series of 102 dogs with TCC of the bladder, the cancer also involved the urethra in 56% of dogs and involved the prostate in 29% of male dogs.[2] Nodal and distant metastases were present in 16% and 14% of dogs, respectively, at diagnosis.[2] At the time of death, distant metastases were detected in 50% of the dogs.[2] Following World Health Organization (WHO) criteria for staging canine bladder tumors[11] (Box 29-1), 78% of dogs had T2 tumors and 20% had T3 tumors.[2]

Etiology and Prevention

The etiology of canine bladder cancer is multifactorial. Risk factors include exposure to older-generation flea control products and lawn chemicals, obesity, possibly cyclophosphamide exposure, female sex, and a very strong breed-associated risk (Table 29-1).[1,2,12-15] The female : male ratio of dogs with TCC has been reported to range from 1.71 : 1 to 1.95 : 1.[1-3] TCC risk is higher in neutered dogs than in intact dogs of both sexes, although the reason for this has not been determined.[2,13]

Two case control studies have implicated chemical exposure in TCC risk in dogs. In a case control study of dogs of several breeds, an association between TCC and exposure to topical flea and tick dips was noted.[12] In the highest risk group (overweight female dogs), the risk of TCC was 28 times that of normal-weight male dogs not exposed to the insecticides.[12] The authors speculated that the "inert" ingredients (solvents and petroleum distillates), which accounted for more than 95% of the product, were the probable carcinogens. Newer, spot-on type flea control products appear safer. In a case control study in Scottish terriers, spot-on products containing fipronil were not associated with increased risk of TCC.[14]

In a case control study in Scottish terriers (STs), exposure to lawn herbicides and pesticides was compared between STs with TCC (n = 83) and a control group of STs (n = 83, ≥6 years of age, no history of urinary tract disease in the previous 2 years).[15] TCC risk was significantly higher in STs that had been exposed to lawn herbicides alone (odds ratio [OR], 3.62; 95% confidence interval [CI] 1.17 to 11.19; p <0.03) or herbicides and insecticides (OR, 7.19; 95% CI 2.15 to 24.07; p <0.001) than in dogs not exposed.[15]

A positive finding in the STs study was that dogs that ate vegetables at least three times a week, along with their normal diet, had a reduced risk of TCC (OR, 0.30; 95% CI 0.01 to 0.97; p <0.001).[16] The specific type of vegetable with the most benefit could not be determined, but carrots, given as treats, were the most frequently fed vegetable in the study.

Although prospective prevention studies have not yet been performed, it would appear appropriate to limit exposure to lawn chemicals and older types of flea control products and to feed vegetables at least three times per week, especially in dogs in breeds with high risk for TCC. The owners of dogs in high-risk breeds should be informed of the TCC risk and encouraged to take note of urinary tract signs should they occur and to pursue veterinary care in a timely fashion. Prospective studies to determine the value of TCC screening and early detection have not yet been reported.

Diagnosis and Differential Diagnoses

Many conditions can mimic TCC in regards to clinical signs, abnormal epithelial cells in urine, and mass lesions within the urinary tract (Figures 29-2 and 29-3; Table 29-2). Differential diagnoses include other neoplasia, chronic cystitis, polypoid cystitis, fibroepithelial polyps, granulomatous cystitis/urethritis, gossypiboma, calculi, and inflammatory pseudotumor.[4-10,17-21] It is important to distinguish non-TCC conditions from TCC because the treatment and prognosis differ considerably and depend on the condition present.

A diagnosis of TCC requires histopathologic confirmation. Although neoplastic cells may be present in the urine of 30% of dogs with TCC,[4] neoplastic cells often are indistinguishable from reactive epithelial cells associated with inflammation. Urine antigen tests for TCC have been found to be sensitive,[22] but a high number of false-positive results limits the value of these tests. A bladder or urethral mass may raise suspicion for TCC, but as discussed previously, other conditions can cause bladder and urethral masses (see Figures 29-2 and 29-3 and Table 29-2). Therefore histopathologic examination of the abnormal tissues is essential to determine whether TCC is present. In addition, different pathologic types of TCC can be identified with histopathology.[4,21]

Methods for obtaining tissue for histopathologic diagnosis include cystotomy, cystoscopy (see Figure 29-2), and traumatic catheterization.[2,23-25] Cystoscopy provides the opportunity to visually inspect the urethra and bladder and to obtain biopsies in a noninvasive method. With the small size of cystoscopic biopsies, the operator must be diligent to collect sufficient tissue for

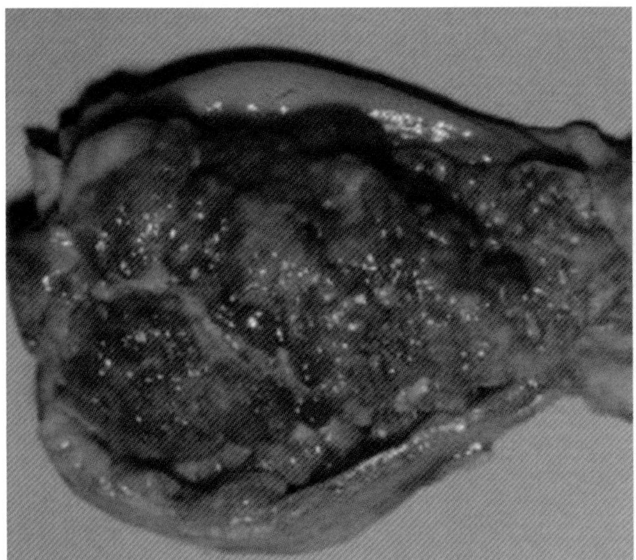

FIGURE 29-1 Papillary invasive transitional cell carcinoma observed in the urinary bladder of a dog during postmortem examination. *(Courtesy T. Lin, Purdue University.)*

Box 29-1 TNM Clinical Staging System for Canine Bladder Cancer

T—Primary Tumor

- Tis Carcinoma in situ
- T0 No evidence of a primary tumor
- T1 Superficial papillary tumor
- T2 Tumor invading the bladder wall, with induration
- T3 Tumor invading neighboring organs (prostate, uterus, vagina, and pelvic canal)

N—Regional Lymph Node (Internal and External Iliac Lymph Node)

- N0 No regional lymph node involvement
- N1 Regional lymph node involved
- N2 Regional lymph node and juxtaregional lymph node involved

M—Distant Metastases

- M0 No evidence of metastasis
- M1 Distant metastasis present

Modified from Owen LN: *TNM classification of tumours in domestic animals,* Geneva, 1980, World Health Organization.

diagnosis. Placing tissue samples in a histology cassette prior to processing helps prevent loss of small samples (see Figure 29-2, *F*). In a recent report of 92 dogs, diagnostic samples were obtained by cystoscopy in 96% of female dogs and 65% of male dogs that ultimately had hisotopathologically diagnosed TCC.[25] The more recent use of a wire basket designed to capture stones during cystoscopy (see Figure 29-2, *D* and *E*) allows collection of larger samples and is expected to increase the yield of diagnostic biopsy samples. Traumatic catheterization to collect tissues for diagnosis can also be performed, although samples collected by this method are usually small and the diagnostic quality varies considerably from case to case. Percutaneous biopsy methods can lead to tumor seeding and are best avoided.[26,27]

TABLE 29-1 Breed and Risk of Transitional Cell Carcinoma (TCC) in Pet Dogs*

Breed	Odds Ratio	95% Confidence Interval
Mixed breed	1.0†	—
All purebreds	0.74	0.62-0.88
Scottish terrier	18.09	7.30-44.86
Shetland sheepdog	4.46	2.48-8.03
Beagle	4.15	2.14-8.05
Wire-haired fox terrier	3.20	1.19-8.63
West Highland white terrier	3.02	1.43-6.40
Miniature schnauzer	0.92	0.54-1.57
Miniature poodle	0.86	0.55-1.35
Doberman pinscher	0.51	0.30-0.87
Labrador retriever	0.46	0.30-0.69
Golden retriever	0.46	0.30-0.69
German shepherd	0.40	0.26-0.63

Modified from previous report by Knapp DW, Glickman NW, DeNicola DB, et al: Naturally-occurring canine transitional cell carcinoma of the urinary bladder: a relevant model of human invasive bladder cancer, *Urol Oncol* 5:47–59, 2000.

*This table represents a summary of data from 1290 dogs with TCC and 1290 institution and age-matched control dogs without TCC in the Veterinary Medical Data Base.

†Reference category.

In poorly differentiated carcinomas, immunohistochemistry for uroplakin III (UPIII) can be helpful in distinguishing TCC from other carcinomas. UPIII, a transmembrane protein expressed in superficial transitional epithelial cells in the urinary tract, is expressed in more than 90% of canine TCC and has been considered a specific marker for TCC.[28] Recently, UPIII expression has also been reported in canine prostate cancer,[29] although it is not known if the immunoreactive cells originated from the transitional epithelium of the prostatic ducts or elsewhere in the gland.

Presentation and Clinical Staging

Common clinical signs in dogs with TCC include hematuria, dysuria, pollakiuria, and, less commonly, lameness caused by bone metastasis or hypertrophic osteopathy.[1] Urinary tract signs may be present for weeks to months and may resolve temporarily with antibiotic therapy.

In dogs with TCC, a physical examination, which includes a rectal examination, may reveal thickening of the urethra and trigone region of the bladder, enlargement of iliac lymph nodes, and sometimes a mass in the bladder or a distended bladder. However, normal findings on a physical examination do not rule out TCC.

In dogs with confirmed or suspected TCC, evaluation should include an assessment of overall health (complete blood count [CBC], serum biochemistry profile, urinalysis, ± urine culture) and staging of the cancer (thoracic radiography, abdominal ultrasonography, and urinary tract imaging). To avoid the risk of seeding TCC through cystocentesis, urine may be collected by free catch or

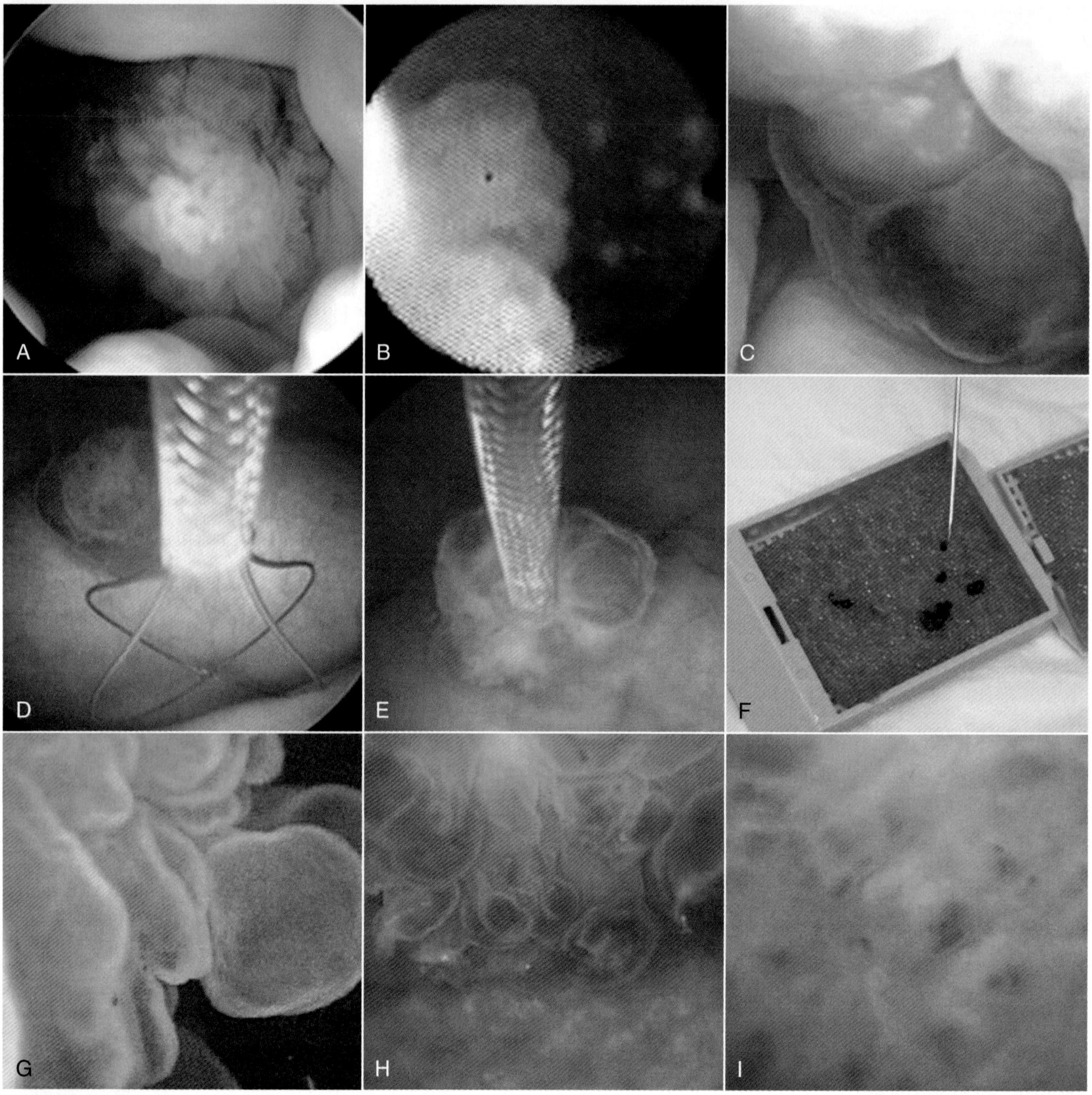

FIGURE 29-2 **A** to **E,** Images from cystoscopy of dogs with transitional cell carcinoma (TCC) and biopsy material obtained **(F)**, and images of dogs with polypoid cystitis (**G** to **I**). TCC can appear as a ruffled frond-like mass or less commonly as polyp-like lesions. The images obtained with rigid cystoscopes typically used in female dogs (**A** and **C** to **E**) are usually better than those obtained with smaller diameter flexible scopes used in male dogs (**B,** image from a male Scottish terrier), although both types of cystoscopes allow adequate visualization for biopsy. The use of a cystoscopic wire stone basket (**D** and **E**) allows collection of larger biopsies. Regardless of the biopsy instrument used, however, cystoscopic biopsies are relatively small, and placing the samples in a tissue cassette **(F)** may facilitate processing. Polypoid cystitis (**G** to **I**) appears very similar to TCC, but it is treated differently and has a better prognosis than TCC. Dog with polypoid cystitis before **(H)** and after **(I)** a month of clavamox treatment alone with no other therapy. The polpys had regressed by >80% **(I)** at the time of rescoping. Cases such as this one emphasize the importance of histopathology in the diagnosis of urinary tract masses, especially when selecting therapy, and even more so when dogs are participating in clinical trials. *(Courtesy L.G. Adams, Purdue University.)*

catheterization. If a catheter is to be passed, care must be taken to avoid penetrating the diseased bladder or urethral wall. Common sites of metastases detected with thoracic radiography and abdominal ultrasonography include lymph nodes, liver, and lungs, although metastases can occur in other areas as well.[1-3] TCC infrequently metastasizes to bone. Side-by-side comparison of radiographs and a nuclear bone scan may help detect possible bone metastases in dogs with unexplained lameness or bone pain.

Urinary tract imaging is used to assess the TCC location for potential surgical intervention and to map and measure TCC

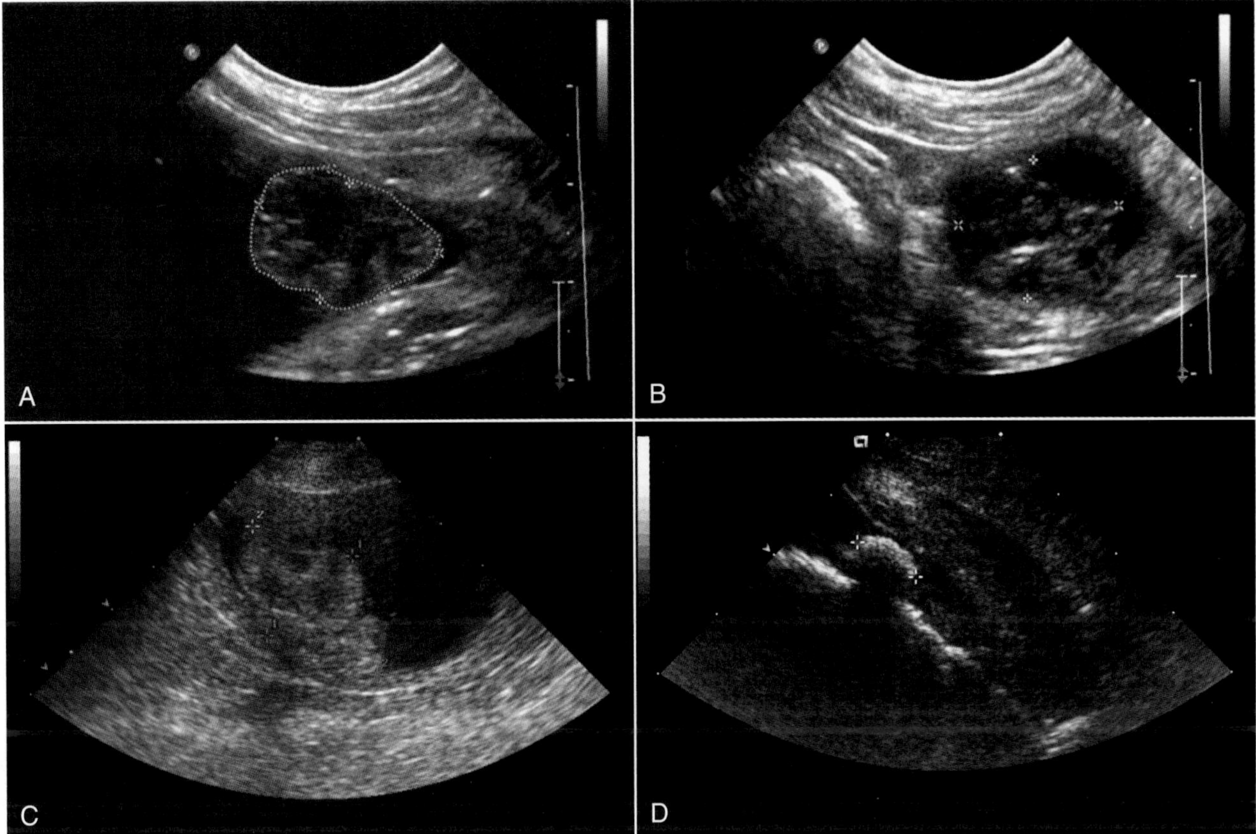

FIGURE 29-3 Cystosonography images from dogs with bladder masses. Note images made in the sagittal **(A)** and transverse **(B)** planes (5 mL/kg fluid distension of the bladder) of an 11-year-old neutered male Shih Tzu with transitional cell carcinoma (TCC). To measure bladder masses over multiple time points, it is important to follow a consistent protocol in regards to level of bladder distension, and patient and probe positioning; and to have the same operator perform the ultrasonography on each visit. Polypoid cystitis **(C** and **D)**, which can appear very similar to TCC, can occur in any part of the bladder, including the mid/apex **(C)** and trigone **(D)**. The dog imaged in **D** was a 13-year-old spayed female Bichon Frise with history of previous urinary tract infection, current hematuria, stranguria, atypical epithelial cells in urine, and masses in the mid/apex and trigone areas of the bladder. Surgical biopsies of the masses confirmed polyps. *(Courtesy J.F. Naughton, Purdue University.)*

masses in order to subsequently determine response to medical therapy. Mapping TCC in the bladder, proximal urethra, and prostate can be accomplished by cystosonography (see Figure 29-3), cystography, or computed tomography (CT).[30,31] Regardless of the imaging technique used, to accurately track response to therapy, it is important to follow a consistent protocol from visit to visit for bladder distension and patient positioning. In addition, when using cystosonography to monitor therapy response, it is critical to have the same operator perform the examinations over multiple visits.

Treatment

Surgery and Nonsurgical Procedures

In dogs with TCC, surgery may be indicated for one or more of the following reasons: (1) to obtain tissue for a diagnosis, (2) to attempt to remove the TCC within the bladder if lesions are away from the trigone, and (3) to maintain or restore urine flow. The potential value of cytoreductive surgery to enhance the activity of adjuvant therapy requires further study. If surgery is performed, it is crucial to take measures to avoid seeding the cancer.

Complete surgical excision of TCC is not usually possible because of the typical trigonal location, urethral involvement, and metastases in some cases. Although techniques for trigone resection[32] or cystectomy[33,34] and the use of grafting materials to replace bladder tissues[35,36] have been reported in the dog, these approaches are associated with substantial morbidity and expense and in most cases are not feasible. In addition, many dogs develop multifocal TCC in the bladder, consistent with the "field effect" proposed in humans in which the entire bladder lining is thought to undergo malignant change in response to carcinogens in the urine. In a series of 67 dogs with TCC that underwent surgery for biopsy or for therapeutic intent, complete surgical excision of the tumor with tumor-free margins was possible in only two dogs.[2] One of the two dogs had a relapse in the bladder 8 months later, and the second dog developed metastatic disease.

Although surgery is rarely curative in dogs with TCC, surgery can be important in restoring or maintaining urine flow. Ureteral stents, when indicated, have traditionally been placed surgically, although less invasive techniques to place stents have recently been described.[37] Previously described ureterocolonic anastomosis is not recommended due to the high complication rate and limited survival.[38] Prepubic cystostomy catheters that bypass urethral obstruction can be very effective.[39,40] More recently, the placement of urethral stents has gained favor over cystotomy tubes in some cases because external tubes are avoided and the pet owner does not have to drain the bladder.[41] The survival following stent placement can

TABLE 29-2 Characteristics of 21 Dogs Presented to the Purdue University Veterinary Teaching Hospital (PUVTH) in Recent Years With Bladder/Urethral Masses Caused by Conditions Other Than Transitional Cell Carcinoma (TCC)*

Histopathologic Diagnosis	Dogs (No.)	Age (Years)	Sex	Breed	Location of Bladder Lesions
Polypoid cystitis	7	Median 10, range 5-13	4 FS, 3 MN	6 pure bred† and 1 mixed breed	Multiple masses; involved trigone area in 4 cases
Cystitis/urethritis	7	Median 8, range 4-12	7 FS	6 pure bred‡ and 1 mixed breed	Lesions involved the trigone in 6 cases
Hyperplasia in absence of inflammation§	2	9, 9	1 FS, 1 MN	1 beagle, 1 Scottish terrier	Thick, irregular wall, involved trigone in both dogs
Inflammatory pseudotumor‖	1	12	M	German shepherd	Entire bladder wall
Hydronephrosis¶	1	8	MN	Scottish terrier mix	Outside bladder¶
Leiomyosarcoma	1	12	FS	Greyhound	Trigone
Plasma cell tumor	1	11	FS	Miniature dachshund	Trigone and urethra
Fibroblastic proliferation and stromal polyp	1	8	FS	Golden retriever	Midbody

FS, Female spayed; *MN*, male neutered; *M*, male.

*Excludes dogs with prostatic carcinoma or other prostatic disease and dogs with cystic calculi.

†One each of the following: Australian shepherd, Jack Russell terrier, Bichon Frise, Swiss mountain dog, golden retriever, Rhodesian ridgeback.

‡One each of the following: German shepherd, Great Dane, Cocker spaniel, English Springer spaniel, West Highland white terrier, Chesapeake Bay retriever.

§One dog had surgical biopsies. The other dog had cystoscopic biopsies and no evidence of progression to TCC >2 years later.

‖The dog was presented for urinary obstruction and bladder mass. Prior to presentation at the PUVTH, surgery had been performed to remove a testicle from the abdomen. The testicle and spermatic cord were noted to be wrapped around the urethra. The mesenchymal changes were thought to be due to the bladder response to chronic urethral obstruction.

¶The dog was referred to the PUVTH for inappropriate urination and abdominal mass. Based on signalment and history, TCC was included on the differential list. Ultrasonography and computed tomography (CT) demonstrated a large cystic mass associated with the right kidney. A 15 × 10 × 10 cm mass containing 500 mL of fluid was removed surgically. Histopathology of the mass revealed renal atrophy, fibrosis, and moderate hydronephrosis, most likely due to a urinary obstruction event. No cause for urinary obstruction was found, and the dog was normal at last follow-up 7 months post op.

vary considerably from dog to dog. In preliminary findings from Purdue University, survival following stent placement in dogs ranged from a few days to a year.[42] Urethral stents can be placed nonsurgically with fluoroscopic guidance. Although there has been interest in the potential use of laser ablation of tumor tissue to relieve urethral obstruction, in published work to date this has not been successful due to advanced local disease, complications of the procedure, and local disease recurrence.[43] One of the challenges in transurethral resection is the difficulty in judging the deeper tumor margin and the risk of cutting too deep and perforating the urinary tract.

Radiation Therapy

Information on the use of radiation therapy (RT) in TCC and other bladder tumors is limited.[44,45] In one report, one of seven dogs treated with intraoperative radiation was alive at 1 year.[45] In another report of 13 dogs, the 1- and 2-year survival rates following intraoperative RT were 69% and 23%, respectively, but complications of therapy (i.e., urinary incontinence and cystitis with accompanying pollakiuria and stranguria) detracted from the dogs' quality of life.[44] Other studies have confirmed complications associated with pelvic irradiation.[46] A laparoscopically implanted tissue expander to reduce exposure to surrounding organs during RT of the bladder has been described, but this approach requires more study before routine use.[47] In a report of 10 dogs, weekly coarse fraction external-beam RT combined with mitoxantrone and piroxicam was tolerated, but results were no better than those with medical therapy alone.[48] Studies of intensity-modulated RT (IMRT) for TCC are ongoing.

Medical Therapy

Systemic Medical Therapy Systemic medical therapy is the mainstay of TCC treatment in dogs and usually consists of chemotherapy, cyclooxygenase (COX) inhibitors (nonselective COX inhibitors and COX-2 inhibitors), and combinations of these (Table 29-3).* Although medical therapy is not usually curative, several different drugs can lead to remission or stable disease of TCC, and most therapies are well tolerated. Resistance to one drug does not necessarily imply resistance to other drugs. Some of the best results are seen in dogs that sequentially receive multiple different treatment protocols over the course of their disease. The approach used at the Purdue University Veterinary Teaching Hospital (PUVTH) is to obtain baseline measurements of the TCC masses, to initiate a starting treatment, to monitor the response to that treatment at 4- to 8-week intervals, and to continue that treatment as long as the TCC is controlled, side effects are acceptable, and quality of life is good. If cancer progression or unacceptable toxicity occurs, then a different treatment is instituted. Subsequent treatment changes are based on tumor response and treatment tolerability. By following this approach, TCC growth can be controlled in approximately 75% of dogs, the dogs' quality of life is usually very good, and median survival times (MSTs) can extend well beyond a year. Although it could be tempting to simultaneously combine multiple chemotherapy agents in dogs with TCC, the benefit of this has not been determined and the potential development of resistance to multiple drugs at the same time could limit the options for subsequent therapy.

*References 1-3, 30, 49-51, 53-56, 58-60.

TABLE 29-3 Study Results Reported for the Medical Therapy of Transitional Cell Carcinoma (TCC) in Dogs*

Drug	Dogs (No.)†	N1 or N2/ M1/Any Metastasis (% of Total Dogs)	CR (%)	PR (%)	SD (%)	PD (%)	PFI (Days)	Median Survival From Start of Drug (Days)	Reference
Single-Arm Trials									
Piroxicam‡	34	20/15/23	6	12	53	29	NA	181	49
Deracoxib‡	26/24	4/11/15	0	17	71	12	133	323	50
Mitoxantrone/piroxicam§	55/48	NA/NA/11	2	33	46	19	194	291	51
Vinblastine‡‖	28/28	11/21/28	0	36	50	14	122	147‖	52
Cisplatin (60 mg/m^2)‡	18/16	NA/28/33	0	19	25	56	75	130	53
Cisplatin (50 mg/m^2)‡	15/12	27/33/40	0	25	50	25	NA	105	54
Cisplatin (40-50 mg/m^2)‡	14	7/7/7	0	7	36	57	78	307	55
Cisplatin (60 mg/m^2)/ piroxicam‡	14/12	14/14/28	0	50	17	33	NA	329	55
Carboplatin‡	14 /12	21/14/28	0	0	8	92	41	132	30
Carboplatin/piroxicam‡	31/29	13/13/19	0	38	45	17	NA	161	56
Mitomycin C—intravesical‡	13/12	0/0/0	0	42	58	0	120	223	57
Gemcitabine/piroxicam§	38/37	11/3/11	5	22	51	22	NA	230	58
Randomized Trials									
Cisplatin (60 mg/m^2)‡	8	12/12/12	0	0	50	50	84	300¶	59
Cisplatin (60 mg/m^2)/ piroxicam‡**	14	28/14/43	14	57	28	0	124	246	59

CR, Complete remission; *PR,* partial remission; *SD,* stable disease; *PD,* progressive disease; *PFI,* progression-free interval; *NA,* information not available.

*More advanced TNM stage is associated with a poorer prognosis; the percentages of dogs with metastasis for each study are included.

†Total/evaluable for tumor response.

‡Diagnosis based on histopathology.

§Study included dogs with cytologic evidence of TCC and dogs with biopsy-proved TCC.

‖The majority of dogs had failed prior therapy before receiving vinblastine. The dosage of vinblastine used in this trial was 3 mg/m^2 every 2 weeks. In most dogs in the trial, however, subsequent dose reduction was necessary because of myelosuppression. Currently, at our institution, the starting dosage of vinblastine for dogs with TCC is 2.5 mg/m^2 every 2 weeks for medium to large dogs and 2.25 mg/m^2 every 2 weeks for small dogs.

¶Dogs that initially received cisplatin alone and had tumor progression were then treated with piroxicam alone; two dogs had PR, and five dogs had SD with piroxicam treatment. This may have contributed to the favorable survival in that treatment arm.

**Despite favorable tumor response, the combination of cisplatin and piroxicam is not recommended for routine use due to frequent renal toxicity.

Two treatment approaches that have been used most commonly in dogs with TCC are (1) a single-agent COX inhibitor and (2) mitoxantrone combined with a COX inhibitor. As a single agent, the nonselective COX inhibitor, piroxicam, is a useful palliative treatment for dogs with TCC.[1-3,49] The quality of life in dogs that receive piroxicam has been excellent. Responses in 62 dogs with TCC that received piroxicam as a single agent included two complete remissions (CR), nine partial remissions (PR, ≥50% decrease in tumor volume), 35 stable diseases (SD, <50% change in tumor volume), and 16 progressive diseases (PD, ≥50% increase in tumor volume or new tumor masses). The two dogs that had CR died of non–tumor-related causes more than 2 years after beginning piroxicam therapy and were free of tumor at necropsy. The survival time (median 195 days) compared favorably to that of 55 dogs in the Purdue Comparative Oncology Program Tumor Registry that were treated with cytoreductive surgery alone (median survival 109 days).[2] Piroxicam is administered at a dosage of 0.3 mg/kg PO once daily in dogs. Although most dogs tolerate the drug well, care must be taken to watch for gastrointestinal (GI) toxicity, particularly ulceration. If vomiting, melena, and anorexia occur, the drug must be withdrawn and supportive care provided as needed until the toxicity resolves. In these cases, it may be safest to switch to a COX-2 inhibitor if further COX inhibitor treatment is indicated.

A COX-2 inhibitor, deracoxib (Dermaxx, Novartis), has been evaluated as a single agent at a dosage of 3 mg/kg PO daily in 26 dogs with TCC.[50] Tumor responses included four (17%) PR, 17 (71%) SD, and three (12%) PD. The median survival following deracoxib and subsequent therapies was 323 days. Mild GI toxicity occurred in 20% of dogs, and 4% of dogs had renal or hepatic side effects. The 17% remission rate with deracoxib appears comparable to the remission rate with piroxicam; however, occasional CRs occur in dogs receiving piroxicam, whereas CR was not noted in dogs treated with deracoxib.

In a pilot study at the PUVTH, adjuvant deracoxib was given to nine dogs (four spayed female, three neutered male, and two intact male dogs) following surgical removal of TCC.[61] Three dogs had tumor-free margins, and six dogs had microscopic TCC present in surgical margins. Deracoxib (3 mg/kg PO daily) was instituted postoperatively. Of three dogs with tumor-free margins, recurrence (consistent with the field effect) was noted in two dogs at 210 and 332 days, respectively. The third dog died with no relapse detected at 1437 days. Of six dogs with microscopic residual TCC after surgery, recurrence was noted in two dogs at 140 and 231 days, respectively. One of the six dogs is alive, tumor free, and still receiving deracoxib at 2057 days. Three dogs with microscopic residual TCC have died with no relapse detected at 345, 749, and 963 days. The median survival of the nine dogs was 749 days (range 231 to 2581 days). Without a randomized trial comparing deracoxib to placebo, it is not possible to know the extent to which deracoxib may have prolonged the disease-free interval in these dogs. The findings, however, of no relapse in four dogs with residual microscopic TCC following surgery at 345, 749, 963, and 2057 days are encouraging.

In unpublished work, another COX-2 inhibitor, firocoxib (Previcox, Merial) has also had antitumor activity against canine TCC.[62]. It is not yet known if nonselective COX inhibitors and COX-2 inhibitors are equally effective in treating TCC. COX-2 inhibitors, however, offer an advantage of less GI toxicity.

The most commonly used chemotherapy protocol in dogs with TCC is mitoxantrone combined with piroxicam.[51] In a study of 55 dogs, 35% of dogs had remission with minimal toxicity, and the median survival was 291 days (n = 55).[51] Although a higher remission rate (50% to 70%) has been noted with cisplatin combined with piroxicam, this protocol is limited by frequent renal damage.[55,59,60] Lowering the cisplatin dose did not reduce the renal toxicity of this combination.[55] Carboplatin, a platinum drug with less renal toxicity, was combined with piroxicam. Remission occurred in 38% of dogs with TCC, but the median remission duration and survival were relatively short.[56]

In a recent study, gemcitabine (800 mg/m^2) and piroxicam were given to dogs with cytologic evidence of TCC or biopsy-confirmed TCC.[58] The reported tumor responses included two (5%) CR, eight (21%) PR, and 19 (50%) SD. The median survival was 230 days. Other emerging therapies that have shown promise include single-agent vinblastine[52] and metronomic chlorambucil.[63] Thirty-six percent of dogs with TCC receiving vinblastine had partial remission.[52]

Localized Therapy Localized therapies studied in dogs with TCC include intravesical mitomycin C (MMC) and photodynamic therapy (PDT). Intravesical therapy is commonly used in humans with superficial TCC, and there has been interest in this approach to potentially treat the higher grade invasive TCC that occurs in dogs. A phase I clinical trial and pharmacokinetic (PK) study of intravesical MMC (1-hour dwell time/day, 2 consecutive days each month, escalating concentrations) was performed in dogs with TCC.[57] Tumor response was assessed in 12 of 13 dogs, and responses included five PR and seven SD. The treatment was well tolerated in most dogs, and the maximum tolerated dose based on local toxicity (bladder irritation of 1 to 2 days duration) was 700 μg/mL (1-hour dwell time/day, 2 consecutive days/month). It was noted that care should be taken to prevent the drug from pooling in the prepuce as this could cause more severe irritation. Unfortunately, a much more serious toxicosis emerged. Marked myelosuppression and severe GI upset were noted in two dogs, suggesting that the drug had been absorbed systemically. This occurred after the first treatment cycle in one dog and the fourth cycle in another dog. Serum MMC concentrations were minimal in dogs that provided samples for PK analyses, but neither of the two dogs with severe toxicity had blood sampled for PK analyses. Although both dogs with severe toxicity recovered with supportive care, systemic exposure is of great concern. The amount of drug being instilled in the bladder is great enough that, if a substantial proportion of the drug were to be systemically absorbed, it could be lethal. Therefore intravesical therapy is not recommended for initial management in dogs with TCC. If other drugs have failed and a given patient does not have other options, then the clinician and pet owner would need to carefully consider the risk versus potential benefit before deciding to use intravesical therapy. In the future, other intravesical therapies may emerge. Experimentally, paclitaxel gelatin nanoparticles have been delivered intravesically to dogs with TCC, but this approach is not in routine use.[64]

Another localized therapy studied in dogs with TCC is PDT.[65-67] PDT with 5-aminolevulinic acid (ALA) had potent antiproliferative effects in canine TCC cells in vitro.[65] ALA was given to healthy dogs, and induction of the photoactive metabolite, protoporphyrin IX (Pp IX), was confined to the bladder mucosa.[66] In five dogs with TCC treated with ALA-based PDT, the progression-free interval ranged from 4 to 34 weeks (median was 6 weeks). ALA-based PDT was used in a male dog with urethral TCC, and this dog was still disease free 1 year after treatment.[67]

Supportive Care

Dogs with TCC are at high risk for secondary bacterial infections. Urine samples collected by free catch or catheter (to avoid potential seeding from cystocentesis) should be submitted for urinalyses and culture regularly and antibiotics prescribed as indicated. Urination should be monitored closely. If urinary tract obstruction occurs, catheterization, definitive anticancer therapy, antibiotics to reduce inflammation associated with secondary bacterial infection, or placement of stents or prepubic cystotomy tube may be pursued.

Prognosis

The progress being made to help dogs with TCC is encouraging. Multiple different treatments have been identified that result in remission or SD for several months, and the quality of life can be excellent. Unfortunately, most dogs with TCC still ultimately die of the disease. Survival has been strongly associated with the TNM stage at the time of diagnosis (Table 29-4). Factors associated with a more advanced TNM stage at diagnosis include younger age (increased risk of nodal metastasis), prostate involvement (increased risk of distant metastasis), and higher T stage (increased risk of nodal and distant metastasis).[2] Information on the treatment and prognosis of other types of bladder cancer has been limited. Remission has been reported in a dog with bladder lymphoma treated with radiation and chemotherapy.[6]

TABLE 29-4 TNM Stage at Diagnosis and Survival of 102 Dogs with Urinary Bladder Transitional Cell Carcinoma (TCC)

Tumor Stage	Dogs (No.)	Median Survival (Days)	Wilcoxon 2-Sample Test (P Value)
T1 or T2	82	218	0.0167
T3	20	118	
N0	86	234	0.0001
N1	16	70	
M0	88	203	0.0163
M1	14	105	

Modified from previous report by Knapp DW, Glickman NW, DeNicola DB, et al: Naturally-occurring canine transitional cell carcinoma of the urinary bladder: a relevant model of human invasive bladder cancer, *Urol Oncol* 5:47–59, 2000.

Feline Urinary Bladder Tumors

Bladder cancer is rarely reported in cats. A series of 27 feline bladder tumors included 15 carcinomas, 5 benign mesenchymal tumors, 5 malignant mesenchymal tumors, and 2 lymphomas.[68] There were 20 male and 7 female cats, and most were elderly. Partial cystectomy was performed in 9 cats, and 4 cats (2 with leiomyoma, 1 with hemangiosarcoma, and 1 with leiomyosarcoma) survived longer than 6 months.[68]

A series of 20 cats with TCC has been reported, including 13 neutered male and 7 spayed female cats (median age 15.2 years).[69] A series of 15 cats with TCC examined at the PUVTH in recent years included 6 neutered male and 9 spayed female cats (median age 13 years, range 4 to 18 years).[70] Clinical signs in cats with TCC include hematuria, stranguria, and pollakiuria. Concurrent urinary tract infection is common, being reported in 75% of cats in the published study[69] and 67% of cats at the PUVTH.[70] Regional and distant metastasis of feline TCC is clearly possible, but the metastatic rate has not been defined.

Of 20 cats with TCC in the published series, treatment was given to 14 cats and included surgery alone (2), surgery plus other therapy (8), piroxicam (3), and chemotherapy (1).[69] The MST was 261 days.[69] Due to the limited number of cats receiving each treatment, the value of specific treatments cannot be determined. In a case report, one cat with urethral TCC had surgical debulking, and recurrence was noted 316 days postoperative.[71] This cat subsequently was treated with RT and died 70 days later.

Urethral Tumors

Most urethral tumors are malignant epithelial tumors (TCC or squamous cell carcinoma), with smooth muscle tumors reported less frequently. It is important to distinguish urethral tumors from granulomatous urethritis because the treatment and prognosis differ. Although most urethral tumors are not resectable, long-term survival has been reported in a dog with multiple chondrosarcomas in the urethra following surgery.[72] Urinary diversion techniques described under "surgery and nonsurgical procedures" of urinary bladder TCC could be considered. The response of urethral TCC to chemotherapy or piroxicam appears similar to that of TCC of the urinary bladder.[49,59]

Renal Tumors

Tumors that have metastasized to the kidneys from other locations are more common than primary renal tumors, which comprise fewer than 2% of all canine cancers.[73] Most primary renal tumors are malignant, and more than half of these are epithelial in origin. The most common renal tumor in dogs is renal cell carcinoma (RCC), accounting for 49% to 65% of primary tumors. Other tumors that can occur in the kidney include TCC, nephroblastoma, hemangiosarcoma, other sarcomas, and lymphomas (see Chapter 32, Section A).[73-75] Lymphoma and RCC often occur bilaterally. RCC can be highly invasive into adjacent structures and may invade the vena cava.

An unusual syndrome in German shepherd dogs consists of slow-growing dermal fibrosis and fibromas, concomitant renal cystadenocarcinoma, and uterine tumors in affected females.[76] This syndrome results from a dominantly inherited missense mutation in folliculin, a putative tumor suppressor gene.[77,78] This condition in dogs is thought to be similar to Birt-Hogg-Dubé syndrome in humans.[77,78]

Diagnosis and Clinical Staging

Most RCCs and sarcomas occur in older dogs (mean age 8 years), but nephroblastoma may occur at any age. The male : female ratio of dogs with epithelial renal tumors has been reported to be 1.2 : 1 to 1.6 : 1.[73,74] Clinical signs in dogs with renal tumors are often nonspecific and may include anorexia, weight loss, polyuria, lethargy, or hematuria. Gross hematuria is not a consistent finding. Physical examination may reveal a palpable abdominal mass or, in some cases, pain in the region of the kidneys. Bone metastases or hypertrophic osteopathy is uncommon.

Laboratory findings in dogs with renal tumors may include mild-to-moderate anemia or polycythemia from a suspected increased production of erythropoietin. Serum biochemical changes are nonspecific and can include azotemia, elevation in alkaline phosphatase, or hypoalbuminemia.

Clinical staging of renal cancer should include radiography of the thorax and abdominal ultrasonography. Excretory urography, CT, and evaluation of glomerular filtration rate (GFR) via scintigraphy may also be useful, especially for surgical planning. Evaluation of possible tumor extension into the vena cava is important if surgery is considered. Histopathologic examination is required for diagnosis. Tumor tissue can be obtained by ultrasound-guided percutaneous biopsy or at surgery. Immunoreactivity to uromodulin, c-Kit, and vimentin has been reported in canine RCC.[79] Immunohistochemical findings vary across subtypes of RCC. Papillary and tubulopapillary RCCs appear to express cytokeratins more often than solid RCCs.[79]

Treatment and Prognosis

Nephrectomy is the treatment of choice for dogs with unilateral renal tumors that have not metastasized. Surgery should include removal of the ureter and possibly retroperitoneal muscle and tissue if the tumor has extended through the capsule and invaded surrounding tissues. In 68 dogs with various renal tumors that underwent nephrectomy, the MST was 16 months.[74] Renal lymphoma is generally treated with chemotherapy (see the section on Lymphoma in Chapter 32, Section A). Successful chemotherapy protocols for other forms of renal cancer have not been identified, and surgery remains the mainstay of treatment.

Pulmonary metastases have been detected radiographically in 16% to 34% of dogs with primary renal tumors at the time of diagnosis.[73,74] At death, metastases were detected in 69% of dogs with carcinomas, 88% of dogs with sarcomas, and 75% of dogs with nephroblastomas. Although the survival time for dogs with malignant renal tumors can be short, long-term survival (up to 5 years) in individual dogs has been observed. The median survival in a series of dogs with renal hemangiosarcoma was 278 days.[80]

Feline Renal Tumors

Primary renal tumors in cats are rare.[81] Of 19 cats with primary renal tumors, excluding lymphoma, the median age at diagnosis was 11 years, with similar numbers of male and female cats.[81] The tumors were typically unilateral and included 11 tubular renal carcinoma, 2 tubulopapillary renal carcinomas, 3 TCCs, and 1 each of nephroblastoma, hemangiosarcoma, and adenoma. One cat had polycythemia. The majority of cats had metastases. In a case report involving two cats with renal adenocarcinoma and secondary polycythemia, the polycythemia resolved in both cats following nephrectomy.[82]

Comparative Aspects

Transitional Cell Carcinoma

Urinary bladder cancer is newly diagnosed in more than 65,000 humans each year in the United States.[83] Cigarette smoking is by far the most common known cause of human bladder cancer. In humans, more than two-thirds of bladder tumors are superficial low-grade tumors in the bladder mucosa.[83] These tumors generally respond well to transurethral resection and intravesical therapy, although recurrence is common, and progression to invasive TCC is a risk. Approximately 20% of human bladder cancers are higher grade invasive TCC at the time of diagnosis. Metastasis to the regional lymph nodes, lungs, and other organs occurs in approximately 50% of cases of invasive TCC.[83] More than 14,000 people die of bladder cancer each year in the United States, and most deaths are due to invasive, metastatic TCC.[83] TCC in dogs is extremely similar to invasive TCC in humans in histopathologic characteristics; cellular and molecular features studied to date; biologic behavior, including metastasis; and response to therapy.[1-3,21,84-90] Canine TCC has emerged as a highly relevant model for human invasive bladder cancer.[2,3] Successful therapies in dogs have been translated into human clinical trials, and similar effects have been observed between both species.[91]

Renal Cancer

Major types of renal cancer in humans include RCC, TCC of the renal pelvis, and Wilms' tumor (nephroblastoma), which is most commonly diagnosed in children.[92,93] Renal cancer is newly diagnosed in 58,000 people and results in approximately 13,000 deaths each year in the United States. RCC accounts for 90% of adult renal carcinomas. Risk factors for RCC include cigarette smoking, obesity, and hypertension.[92] Multiple subtypes of RCC exist, including clear cell, papillary, and chromophobe types. The clear cell type is associated with von Hippel-Lindau (VHL) disease in which mutations occur in the VHL gene. A small number of canine RCC samples have been studied for VHL gene mutations.[94] Mutations were not identified, but this does not rule out mutations in other dogs.[94] Metastases (lymph nodes, lung, bone, liver, others) are present at diagnosis in 30% of people with RCC. RCC in humans has been treated with surgery, radiation, chemotherapy, and biologic therapy (interferon and interleukin-2). Further study would be indicated to more fully examine the similarities and differences between canine and human RCC.

REFERENCES

1. Mutsaers AJ, Widmer WR, Knapp DW: Canine transitional cell carcinoma, *J Vet Intern Med* 17:136–144, 2003.
2. Knapp DW, Glickman NW, DeNicola DB, et al: Naturally-occurring canine transitional cell carcinoma of the urinary bladder: a relevant model of human invasive bladder cancer, *Urol Oncol* 5:47–59, 2000.
3. Knapp DW: Animal models: naturally occurring canine urinary bladder cancer. In Lerner SP, Schoenberg MP, Sternberg CN, editors: *Textbook of bladder cancer*, Oxon, United Kingdom, 2006, Taylor and Francis.
4. Valli VE, Norris A, Jacobs RM, et al: Pathology of canine bladder and urethral cancer and correlation with tumour progression and survival, *J Comp Pathol* 113:113–130, 1995.
5. Gelberg HB: Urinary bladder mass in a dog, *Vet Pathol* 47:181–184, 2010.
6. Kessler M, Kandel-Tschiederer B, Pfleghaar S, et al: Primary malignant lymphoma of the urinary bladder in a dog: long term remission following treatment with radiation and chemotherapy, *Schweiz Arch Tierheilkd* 150:565–569, 2008.
7. Bae IH, Kim Y, Pakhrin B, et al: Genitourinary rhabdomyosarcoma with systemic metastasis in a young dog, *Vet Pathol* 44:518–520, 2007.
8. Benigni L, Lamb CR, Corzo-Menendez N, et al: Lymphoma affecting the urinary bladder in three dogs and a cat, *Vet Radiol Ultrasound* 47:592–596, 2006.
9. Heng HG, Lowry JE, Boston S, et al: Smooth muscle neoplasia of the urinary bladder wall in three dogs, *Vet Radiol Ultrasound* 47:83–86, 2006.
10. Liptak JM, Dernell WS, Withrow SJ: Haemangiosarcoma of the urinary bladder in a dog, *Aust Vet J* 82:215–217, 2004.
11. Owen LN: *TNM classification of tumours in domestic animals*, Geneva, 1980, World Health Organization.
12. Glickman LT, Schofer FS, McKee LJ: Epidemiologic study of insecticide exposures, obesity, and risk of bladder cancer in household dogs, *J Toxicol Environ Health* 28:407–414, 1989.
13. Bryan JN, Keeler MR, Henry CJ, et al: A population study of neutering status as a risk factor for canine prostate cancer, *Prostate* 67:1174–1181, 2007.
14. Raghavan M, Knapp DW, Dawson MH, et al: Topical spot-on flea and tick products and the risk of transitional cell carcinoma of the urinary bladder in Scottish terrier dogs, *J Am Vet Med Assoc* 225:389–394, 2004.
15. Glickman LT, Raghavan M, Knapp DW, et al: Herbicide exposure and the risk of transitional cell carcinoma of the urinary bladder in Scottish terrier dogs, *J Am Vet Med Assoc* 224:1290–1297, 2004.
16. Raghavan M, Knapp DW, Bonney PL, et al: Evaluation of the effect of dietary vegetable consumption on reducing risk of transitional cell carcinoma of the urinary bladder in Scottish terriers, *J Am Vet Med Assoc* 227:94–100, 2005.
17. Gelberg HB: Urinary bladder mass in a dog, *Vet Pathol* 47:181–184, 2010.
18. Deschamps JY, Roux FA: Extravesical textiloma (gossypiboma) mimicking a bladder tumor in a dog, *J Am Anim Hosp Assoc* 45:89–92, 2009.
19. Böhme B, Ngendahayo P, Hamaide A, et al: Inflammatory pseudotumours of the urinary bladder in dogs resembling human myofibroblastic tumours: a report of eight cases and comparative pathology, *Vet J* 183:89–94, 2010.
20. Martinez I, Mattoon JS, Eaton KA, et al: Polypoid cystitis in 17 dogs (1978-2001), *J Vet Intern Med* 17:499–509, 2003.
21. Patrick DJ, Fitzgerald SD, Sesterhenn IA, et al: Classification of canine urinary bladder urothelial tumours based on the World Health Organization/International Society of Urological Pathology Consensus Classification, *J Comp Pathol* 135:190–199, 2006.
22. Henry CJ, Tyler JW, McEntee MC, et al: Evaluation of a bladder tumor antigen test as a screening test for transitional cell carcinoma of the lower urinary tract in dogs, *Am J Vet Res* 64:1017–1020, 2003.
23. Holak P, Nowicki M, Adamiak Z, et al: Applicability of endoscopic examination as a diagnostic approach in urinary tract ailments in dogs, *Pol J Vet Sci* 10:233–238, 2007.
24. Messer JS, Chew DJ, McLoughlin MA: Cystoscopy: techniques and clinical applications, *Clin Tech Small Anim Pract* 20:52–64, 2005.
25. Childress MO, Adams LG, Ramos-Vara J, et al: Results of biopsy via transurethral cystoscopy vs cystotomy for diagnosis of transitional cell carcinoma of the urinary bladder and urethra in dogs: 92 cases (2003-2008), *J Am Vet Med Assoc* 239:350–356, 2011.
26. Vignoli M, Rossi F, Chierici C, et al: Needle tract implantation after fine needle aspiration biopsy (FNAB) of transitional cell carcinoma of the urinary bladder and adenocarcinoma of the lung, *Schweiz Arch Tierheilkd* 149:314–318, 2007.
27. Nyland TG, Wallack ST, Wisner ER: Needle tract implantation following US-guided fine-needle aspiration biopsy of transitional cell carcinoma of the bladder, urethra, and prostate, *Vet Radiol Ultrasound* 43:50–53, 2002.
28. Ramos-Vara JA, Miller MA, Boucher M, et al: Immunohistochemical detection of uroplakin III, cytokeratin 7, and cytokeratin 20 in canine urothelial tumors, *Vet Pathol* 40:55–62, 2003.

29. Lai CL, van den Ham R, van Leenders G, et al: Histopathological and immunohistochemical characterization of canine prostate cancer, *Prostate* 68:477–488, 2008.
30. Chun R, Knapp DW, Widmer WR, et al: Phase II clinical trial of carboplatin in canine transitional cell carcinoma of the urinary bladder, *J Vet Intern Med* 11:279–283, 1997.
31. Hume C, Seiler G, Porat-Mosenco Y, et al: Cystosonographic measurements of canine bladder tumours, *Vet Comp Oncol* 8:122–126, 2010.
32. Saulnier-Troff FG, Busoni V, Hamaide A: A technique for resection of invasive tumors involving the trigone area of the bladder in dogs: preliminary results in two dogs, *Vet Surg* 37:427–437, 2008.
33. Hautmann RE: Ileal bladder substitute, *Urologe A* 47:33–40, 2008.
34. Stratmann N, Wehrend A: Unilateral ovariectomy and cystectomy due to multiple ovarian cysts with subsequent pregnancy in a Belgian shepherd dog, *Vet Rec* 160:740–741, 2007.
35. Wongsetthachai P, Pramatwinai C, Banlunara W, et al: Urinary bladder wall substitution using autologous tunica vaginalis in male dogs, *Res Vet Sci* 90:156–159, 2011.
36. Zhang Y, Frimberger D, Cheng EY, et al: Challenges in a larger bladder replacement with cell-seeded and unseeded small intestinal submucosa grafts in a subtotal cystectomy model, *BJU Int* 98:1100–1105, 2006.
37. Berent AC: Ureteral obstructions in dogs and cats: a review of traditional and new interventional diagnostic and therapeutic options, *J Vet Emerg Crit Care* 21:86–103, 2011.
38. Stone EA, Withrow SJ, Page RL, et al: Ureterocolonic anastomosis in ten dogs with transitional cell carcinoma, *Vet Surg* 17:147–153, 1988.
39. Smith JD, Stone EA, Gilson SD: Placement of a permanent cystostomy catheter to relieve urine outflow obstruction in dogs with transitional cell carcinoma, *J Am Vet Med Assoc* 206:496–499, 1995.
40. Salinardi BJ, Marks SL, Davidson JR, et al: The use of a low-profile cystostomy tube to relieve urethral obstruction in a dog, *J Am Anim Hosp Assoc* 39:403–405, 2003.
41. Weisse C, Berent A, Todd K, et al: Evaluation of palliative stenting for management of malignant urethral obstructions in dogs, *J Am Vet Med Assoc* 229:226–234, 2006.
42. Adams L, McMillan S: Personal communication.
43. Liptak JM, Brutscher SP, Monnet E, et al: Transurethral resection in the management of urethral and prostatic neoplasia in 6 dogs, *Vet Surg* 33:505–516, 2004.
44. Walker M, Breider M: Intraoperative radiotherapy of canine bladder cancer, *Vet Radiol* 28:200–204, 1987.
45. Withrow SJ, Gillette EL, Hoopes PJ, et al: Intraoperative irradiation of 16 spontaneously occurring canine neoplasms, *Vet Surg* 18:7–11, 1989.
46. Anderson CR, McNiel EA, Gillette EL, et al: Late complications of pelvic irradiation in 16 dogs, *Vet Radiol Ultrasound* 43:187–192, 2002.
47. Murphy S, Gutiérrez A, Lawrence J, et al: Laparoscopically implanted tissue expander radiotherapy in canine transitional cell carcinoma, *Vet Radiol Ultrasound* 49:400–405, 2008.
48. Poirier VJ, Forrest LJ, Adams WM, et al: Piroxicam, mitoxantrone, and coarse fraction radiotherapy for the treatment of transitional cell carcinoma of the bladder in 10 dogs: a pilot study, *J Am Anim Hosp Assoc* 40:131–136, 2004.
49. Knapp DW, Richardson RC, Chan TCK, et al: Piroxicam therapy in 34 dogs with transitional cell carcinoma of the urinary bladder, *J Vet Intern Med* 8:273–278, 1994.
50. McMillan SK, Boria P, Moore GE, et al: Antitumor effects of deracoxib treatment in 26 dogs with transitional cell carcinoma of the urinary bladder, *J Am Vet Med Assoc* 239:1084–1089, 2011.
51. Henry CJ, McCaw DL, Turnquist SE, et al: Clinical evaluation of mitoxantrone and piroxicam in a canine model of human invasive urinary bladder carcinoma, *Clin Cancer Res* 9:906–911, 2003.
52. Arnold EJ, Childress MO, Fourez LM, et al: Clinical trial of vinblastine in dogs with transitional cell carcinoma of the urinary bladder, *J Vet Intern Med* 25(6):1385–1390, 2011.
53. Chun R, Knapp DW, Widmer WR, et al: Cisplatin treatment of transitional cell carcinoma of the urinary bladder in dogs: 18 cases (1983-1993), *J Am Vet Med Assoc* 209:1588–1591, 1996.
54. Moore AS, Cardona A, Shapiro W, et al: Cisplatin (cis-diamminedichloroplatinum) for treatment of transitional cell carcinoma of the urinary bladder or urethra: a retrospective study of 15 dogs, *J Vet Intern Med* 4:148–152, 1990.
55. Greene SN, Lucroy MD, Greenberg CB, et al: Evaluation of cisplatin administered with piroxicam in dogs with transitional cell carcinoma of the urinary bladder, *J Am Vet Med Assoc* 231:1056–1060, 2007.
56. Boria PA, Glickman NW, Schmidt BR, et al: Carboplatin and piroxicam in 31 dogs with transitional cell carcinoma of the urinary bladder, *Vet Comp Oncol* 3:73–78, 2005.
57. Abbo AH, Jones DR, Masters AR, et al: Phase 1 clinical trial and pharmacokinetics of intravesical Mitomycin C in dogs with localized transitional cell carcinoma of the urinary bladder, *J Vet Intern Med* 24:1124–1130, 2010.
58. Marconato L, Zini E, Lindner D, et al: Toxic effects and antitumor response of gemcitabine in combination with piroxicam treatment in dogs with transitional cell carcinoma of the urinary bladder, *J Am Vet Med Assoc* 238:1004–1010, 2011.
59. Knapp DW, Glickman NW, Widmer WR, et al: Cisplatin versus cisplatin combined with piroxicam in a canine model of human invasive urinary bladder cancer, *Cancer Chemother Pharmacol* 46:221–226, 2000.
60. Mohammed SI, Craig BA, Mutsaers AJ, et al: Effects of the cyclooxygenase inhibitor piroxicam in combination with chemotherapy on tumor response, apoptosis, and angiogenesis in a canine model of human invasive urinary bladder cancer, *Mol Cancer Ther* 2:183–188, 2003.
61. Knapp D, McMillan S: Personal communication.
62. Knapp D, Henry C: Personal communication.
63. Knapp D, Schrempp D, Leach T: Personal communication.
64. Lu Z, Yeh TK, Wang J, et al: Paclitaxel gelatin nanoparticles for intravesical bladder cancer therapy, *J Urol* 185:1478–1483, 2011.
65. Ridgway TD, Lucroy MD: Phototoxic effects of 635-nm light on canine transitional cell carcinoma cells incubated with 5-aminolevulinic acid, *Am J Vet Res* 64:131–136, 2003.
66. Lucroy MD, Ridgway TD, Peavy GM, et al: Preclinical evaluation of 5-aminolevulinic acid–based photodynamic therapy for canine transitional cell carcinoma, *Vet Comp Oncol* 1:76–85, 2003.
67. Lucroy M: Personal communication.
68. Schwarz PD, Greene RW, Patnaik AK: Urinary bladder tumors in the cat: a review of 27 cases, *J Am Anim Hosp Assoc* 21:237–245, 1985.
69. Wilson HM, Chun R, Larson VS, et al: Clinical signs, treatments, and outcome in cats with transitional cell carcinoma of the urinary bladder: 20 cases (1990-2004), *J Am Vet Med Assoc* 231:101–106, 2007.
70. Knapp D, McMillan S: Personal communication.
71. Takagi S, Kadosawa T, Ishiguro T, et al: Urethral transitional cell carcinoma in a cat, *J Small Anim Pract* 46:504–506, 2005.
72. Davis GJ, Holt D: Two chondrosarcomas in the urethra of a German shepherd dog, *J Small Anim Pract* 44:169–171, 2003.
73. Klein MK, Cockerell GL, Withrow SJ, et al: Canine primary renal neoplasms: a retrospective review of 54 cases, *J Am Anim Hosp Assoc* 24:443–452, 1988.
74. Bryan JN, Henry CJ, Turnquist SE, et al: Primary renal neoplasia of dogs, *J Vet Intern Med* 20:1155–1160, 2006.
75. Grillo TP, Brandão CV, Mamprim MJ, et al: Hypertrophic osteopathy associated with renal pelvis transitional cell carcinoma in a dog, *Can Vet J* 48:745–747, 2007.
76. Lingaas F, Comstock KE, Kirkness EF, et al: A mutation in the canine BHD gene is associated with hereditary multifocal renal

cystadenocarcinoma and nodular dermatofibrosis in the German shepherd dog, *Hum Mol Genet* 12:3043–3053, 2003.
77. Bonsdorff TB, Jansen JH, Lingaas F: Second hits in the FLCN gene in a hereditary renal cancer syndrome in dogs, *Mamm Genome* 19:121–126, 2008.
78. Bonsdorff TB, Jansen JH, Thomassen RF, et al: Loss of heterozygosity at the FLCN locus in early renal cystic lesions in dogs with renal cystadenocarcinoma and nodular dermatofibrosis, *Mamm Genome* 20:315–320, 2009.
79. Gil da Costa RM, Oliveira JP, Saraiva AL, et al: Immunohistochemical characterization of 13 canine renal cell carcinomas, *Vet Pathol* 48:427–432, 2011.
80. Locke JE, Barber LG: Comparative aspects and clinical outcomes of canine renal hemangiosarcoma, *J Vet Intern Med* 20:962–967, 2006.
81. Henry CJ, Turnquist SE, Smith A, et al: Primary renal tumours in cats: 19 cases (1992-1998), *J Feline Med Surg* 1:165–170, 1999.
82. Klainbart S, Segev G, Loeb E, et al: Resolution of renal adenocarcinoma-induced secondary inappropriate polycythaemia after nephrectomy in two cats, *J Feline Med Surg* 10:264–268, 2008.
83. Lerner SP, Schoenberg MP, Sternberg CN: *Textbook of bladder cancer*, Oxon, UK, 2006, Taylor and Francis.
84. Lin TY, Zhang H, Wang S, et al: Targeting canine bladder transitional cell carcinoma with a human bladder cancer-specific ligand, *Mol Cancer* 10:9, 2011.
85. McCleary-Wheeler AL, Williams LE, Hess PR, et al: Evaluation of an in vitro telomeric repeat amplification protocol assay to detect telomerase activity in canine urine, *Am J Vet Res* 71:1468–1474, 2010.
86. Lee JY, Tanabe S, Shimohira H, et al: Expression of cyclooxygenase-2, P-glycoprotein and multi-drug resistance-associated protein in canine transitional cell carcinoma, *Res Vet Sci* 83:210–216, 2007.
87. Rankin WV, Henry CJ, Turnquist SE, et al: Identification of survivin, an inhibitor of apoptosis, in canine urinary bladder transitional cell carcinoma, *Vet Comp Oncol* 6:141–150, 2008.
88. Rankin WV, Henry CJ, Turnquist SE, et al: Comparison of distributions of survivin among tissues from urinary bladders of dogs with cystitis, transitional cell carcinoma, or histologically normal urinary bladders, *Am J Vet Res* 69:1073–1078, 2008.
89. Dill AL, Ifa DR, Manicke NE, et al: Lipid profiles of canine invasive transitional cell carcinoma of the urinary bladder and adjacent normal tissue by desorption electrospray ionization imaging mass spectrometry, *Anal Chem* 81:8758–8764, 2009.
90. Wilson CR, Regnier FE, Knapp DW, et al: Glycoproteomic profiling of serum peptides in canine lymphoma and transitional cell carcinoma, *Vet Comp Oncol* 6:171–181, 2008.
91. Dhawan D, Craig BA, Cheng L, et al: Effects of short-term celecoxib treatment in patients with invasive transitional cell carcinoma of the urinary bladder, *Mol Cancer Ther* 9:1371–1377, 2010.
92. Chow WH, Dong LM, Devesa SS: Epidemiology and risk factors for kidney cancer, *Nat Rev Urol* 7:245–257, 2010.
93. Jemal A, Siegel R, Xu J, et al: Cancer statistics, 2010, *CA Cancer J Clin* 60:277–300, 2010.
94. Pressler BM, Williams LE, Ramos-Vara JA, et al: Sequencing of the von Hippel-Lindau gene in canine renal carcinoma, *J Vet Intern Med* 23:592–597, 2009.

Tumors of the Nervous System

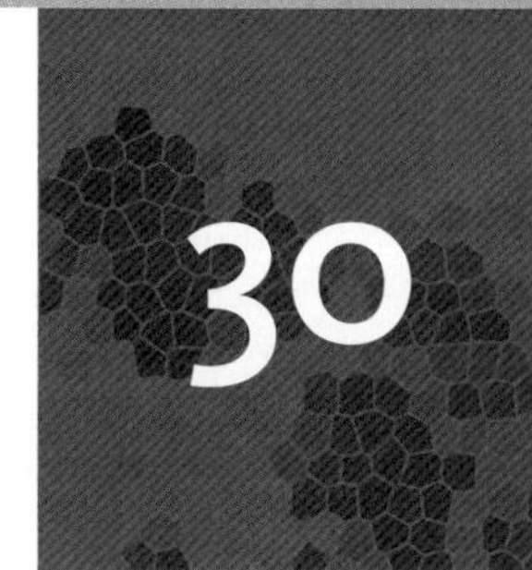

MARGARET C. MCENTEE AND CURTIS W. DEWEY

Brain Tumors

Incidence and Risk Factors

Brain tumors are frequently encountered in dogs and cats, with reported incidence rates of 14.5 dogs and 3.5 cats per 100,000 pets at risk, respectively.[1,2] In addition to being more common in dogs than in cats, there is a wider variety of canine brain tumors than reported in cats; in addition, there is a wider range of histologic subtypes of canine meningioma reported compared with feline meningiomas.[3,4]

Most brain tumors encountered in clinical practice are primary tumors originating from brain parenchyma (e.g., glial cells and neurons, cells that line the interior and exterior brain surfaces [such as meningeal and ependymal cells]) or cells from vascular structures (e.g., choroid plexus). Meningioma is the most frequently reported primary brain tumor in dogs and cats, although gliomas are also frequently encountered in dogs.[2,5-7] More than 50% of reported feline brain tumors are meningiomas.[2,5,6] Gliomas are occasionally reported in cats.[2,5] Other primary brain tumors less commonly reported in dogs include choroid plexus tumors; primary central nervous system (CNS) lymphosarcomas; primitive neuroectodermal tumors (PNETs), which typically includes neuroblastoma; primary CNS histiocytic sarcomas (also termed *malignant histiocytosis*); ependymomas; and vascular hamartomas. Other primary brain tumors occasionally encountered in cats include (in addition to gliomas): ependymomas, olfactory neuroblastomas, and choroid plexus tumors.[2,5,7] In both dogs and cats, there are case reports of medulloblastomas, usually involving the cerebellum. Microglial tumors are considered rare in dogs and cats.[1-3] Primary brain tumors in dogs and cats are typically solitary. Approximately 17% of cats with intracranial meningioma have more than one tumor.[8,9] Multiple masses of the same primary brain tumor type in dogs are typically associated with choroid plexus tumors; in this scenario, tumor cells are disseminated or "dropped" via cerebrospinal fluid (CSF) flow in the ventricular system ("drop" metastases).[5] The authors have encountered a number of Boxers with multiple intracranial gliomas. In one study, 10% of cats were found to have two different types of intracranial neoplasia concurrently.[2] The occurrence of more than one histologic tumor type in dogs is considered rare.

Secondary brain tumors include metastatic neoplasia, as well as tumors that affect the brain by local extension. Examples of metastatic neoplasia include mammary, pulmonary, and prostatic carcinoma; hemangiosarcoma; malignant melanoma; and lymphosarcoma. Tumors that may extend into the brain from the periphery include nasal and frontal sinus carcinoma (adenocarcinoma, squamous cell carcinoma), calvarial tumors (e.g., osteosarcoma, chondrosarcoma, multilobular osteochondrosarcoma), pituitary tumors (e.g., pituitary macroadenomas in hyperadrenocorticism), and nerve sheath tumors (e.g., cranial nerve [CN] V tumors). In one large retrospective study of secondary brain tumors in dogs,[10] the most common secondary brain tumor was hemangiosarcoma (29%), followed by pituitary tumors (25%), lymphosarcoma (12%), metastatic carcinoma (11%), and invasive nasal tumors (6%). In one report,[2] secondary (multicentric) lymphoma and pituitary tumors were the second and third most common intracranial neoplasms found in cats. Lymphoma/lymphosarcoma is considered the most common secondary brain tumor type encountered in cats.

Brain tumors in dogs and cats can occur at any age, in either sex, and in any breed. However, brain tumors occur most commonly in older patients, with a median age of 9 years for dogs and older than 10 years for cats.[2,5,6] Compared with other tumor types, dogs and cats with meningioma tend to be diagnosed at older ages.[2,5-7] Male cats are more likely to develop intracranial meningioma than female cats.[5,6] Golden retrievers and Boxers are considered to be predisposed to developing primary brain tumors.[5-7] In general, dolichocephalic dog breeds are prone to develop meningiomas, whereas brachycephalic dog breeds are more likely to be afflicted with gliomas.[5-7] There is no known breed predilection for cats to develop primary brain tumors.[2,5,6] Cerebral tumors are more commonly encountered than tumors in the brainstem or cerebellum. Gliomas have a tendency to occur in the diencephalon and cerebellum, however.[5,6]

Pathology

As mentioned previously, brain tumors are broadly classified as primary (neoplastic cells originating from tissues intrinsic to the brain, its vasculature, and meninges/ependyma) or secondary (neoplastic cells originating from tissues extrinsic to those comprising primary brain tumors).[5] Brain tumors exert their pathologic effects both by directly encroaching on and/or invading brain tissue and by secondary effects, such as peritumoral edema, inflammation, obstructive hydrocephalus, and hemorrhage.

The terms *benign* and *malignant* have different connotations when used in the context of intracranial neoplasia compared with tumors in other locations. Even slow-growing, readily removable brain tumors are not benign when considering the potential effect on the patient if therapy is not aggressively pursued in a timely fashion. Cytologic features of tumors are used to assess potential benignity or malignancy and include invasiveness, number of mitotic figures, and nuclear pleomorphism. Meningiomas are often regarded as benign. Considering the aggressive cytologic nature of many canine meningiomas (in comparison with human and feline meningiomas), this is probably an overstatement for this tumor type—especially in dogs.[6,11]

There are multiple histologic subtypes of meningiomas frequently encountered in dogs, including meningothelial, transitional, fibroblastic, psammomatous, angiomatous, microcystic, papillary, granular cell, myxoid, and anaplastic.[3,4,6,11] In addition to these histologic subtypes, a grading system used in humans to predict the biologic behavior of intracranial meningiomas has recently been adapted to dogs; this grading system includes grade I (benign), grade II (atypical), and grade III (malignant).[11] The repertoire of feline meningioma histologic subtypes is comparatively limited; the majority of feline meningiomas are meningothelial or psammomatous.[2-4,6]

Gliomas in dogs and cats include astrocytomas, oligodendrogliomas, and glioblastoma multiforme, in addition to undifferentiated gliomas. Gliomas as a group are considered to be malignant because these tumors tend to invade tissue and are typically resistant to all forms of definitive therapy.[2,4,5,7,12]

Clinicopathologic features of choroid plexus tumors in dogs have recently been reviewed.[13] Choroid plexus tumors comprise choroid plexus papillomas (CPP) and choroid plexus carcinomas (CPC). Choroid plexus tumors in general tended to occur in the fourth ventricle in one report, and only CPCs occurred in the lateral ventricles.[14] The two tumor subtypes are differentiated based on the presence or absence of local or distant metastases, as well as on histopathologic features.

In one large study,[7] it was found that half of canine primary brain tumors occupy more than one anatomic region of the brain; this could lead to the false conclusion based on neurologic examination that a patient with a solitary brain mass has multifocal disease. Also in that study, it was found that 23% of dogs with primary brain tumors had concurrent, unrelated neoplasia (e.g., pulmonary carcinoma, hemangiosarcoma), most of which involved the thoracic or abdominal cavity; this finding underscores the importance of screening for concurrent unrelated neoplasia (via thoracic radiography and abdominal ultrasonography) prior to pursuing advanced diagnostics and definitive therapy for the brain tumor.

History and Clinical Signs

The diagnosis of brain tumor should be highly suspected in an elderly dog or cat with slowly progressive signs of brain dysfunction. A brain tumor should also be suspected in animals that experience a recent onset of seizure activity after 5 years of age, especially in certain breeds (e.g., golden retrievers, Boxers). Depending on the location and size of the tumor, such patients may appear neurologically normal interictally. Historic and presenting clinical signs for dogs and cats with brain tumors are variable and reflect both the location and the secondary effects (e.g., edema, hemorrhage) of the tumor. Seizures represent the most common presenting clinical sign of neurologic dysfunction in dogs with brain tumors, occurring in approximately half of the patients.[5,6,15] In one study of feline brain tumors, the overall incidence of seizure activity was 23%, occurring more commonly with glioma (26.7%) and lymphoma (26.3%), in comparison with meningioma (15%).[16] Cats with brain tumors are commonly presented to the veterinarian with a complaint of behavior change. In cats with primary brain tumors, nonspecific presenting clinical signs (i.e., signs not obviously referable to neurologic dysfunction) are fairly common, occurring in over 20% of cats in one large study.[2] These clinical signs included lethargy, inappetence, and anorexia. Also in that study, it was found that approximately 19% of feline brain tumors were considered an incidental finding. Cerebral tumors are more common than tumors of the brainstem or cerebellum. Cerebral and diencephalic tumors tend to cause clinical signs of dysfunction such as seizure activity, behavior changes, circling, head-pressing, visual deficits, and hemi-inattention (hemineglect) syndrome (ignoring environmental cues from the side opposite the tumor). Proprioceptive placing deficits and neck pain are often appreciable on neurologic examination. Tumors of the brainstem from midbrain through medulla often cause alterations of consciousness, dysfunction of cranial nerves (other than CN I and CN II), and obvious gait/proprioceptive abnormalities. Cerebellar tumors may result in clinical signs of dysfunction such as ataxia, dysmetria, intention tremors, vestibular abnormalities, and menace reaction deficits with normal vision.[5,6]

In most cases, clinical signs of neurologic dysfunction occur slowly and insidiously over time, especially with meningiomas. Owners of pets with meningiomas will often retrospectively realize that their pet had a behavior change for months to over a year prior to diagnosis. The subtle behavior changes are often attributed to "old age." However, brain tumor patients can have subacute to acute development of neurologic dysfunction. These patients may experience sudden exhaustion of brain compensatory mechanisms or may suffer hemorrhage or acute obstructive hydrocephalus due to the tumor.[5,6]

Diagnostic Techniques and Work-Up

Signalment, history, and neurologic examination findings often provide a strong index of suspicion of a brain tumor as the cause of neurologic dysfunction in a dog or cat. However, there are a number of disorders (e.g., inflammatory/infectious, congenital, degenerative) that can produce similar signs of neurologic dysfunction in patients at risk for developing brain tumors. It is imperative therefore to follow an ordered diagnostic work-up in patients suspected of having brain tumors.

Minimum Database

Before pursuing advanced imaging, basic blood work (complete blood count [CBC] and chemistry profile) and a urinalysis should be performed. Thoracic radiographs should be taken to help rule out the possibility of metastatic cancer or a second unrelated neoplastic process. Considering the likelihood of concurrent neoplasia in dogs with brain tumors, performing abdominal ultrasound examination is also often advisable.

Imaging

Radiographs of the skull typically do not provide useful clinical information in cases of brain tumor. Computed tomography (CT) and magnetic resonance imaging (MRI) are commonly used in the diagnosis of brain tumors, with MRI being the preferred imaging modality. Although specific types of brain tumors can vary in their appearance with these imaging modalities, there are some characteristic features that help distinguish meningiomas from gliomas. Meningiomas tend to have a broad-based, extraaxial attachment (they arise from the periphery of the brain and move inward, or axially), exhibit distinct tumor margins, and uniformly contrast enhance (Figure 30-1). Meningiomas tend to displace, rather than invade, parenchymal tissue; as discussed previously, however, many canine meningiomas do display some degree of invasiveness. Some meningiomas will calcify, which can be appreciated on a noncontrast CT image (Figure 30-2). The "dural tail" sign is an MRI feature typically associated with meningiomas, in which a contrast-enhancing meningeal-associated "tail" is seen extending from the main tumor mass (Figure 30-3). Meningiomas also may occasionally have a cystic component (cystic meningioma) extending from the main tumor mass (Figure 30-4). Gliomas tend to arise from an intraaxial location (from within the substance of the brain, moving outward), often lack distinct tumor margins (they tend to infiltrate, rather than displace normal tissue), and typically contrast enhance

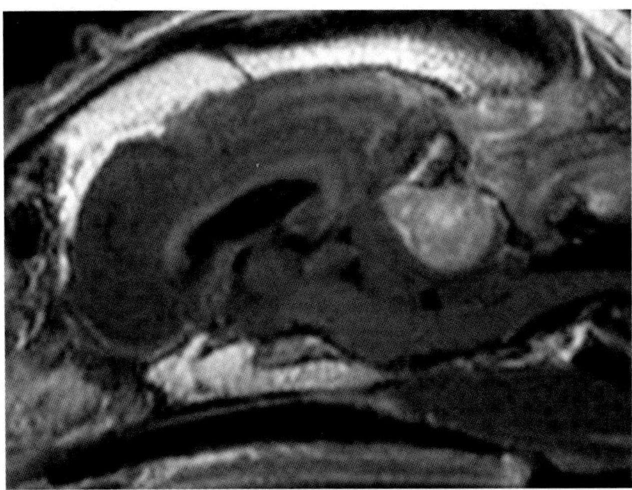

FIGURE 30-1 Postcontrast MRI of a cerebellar meningioma.

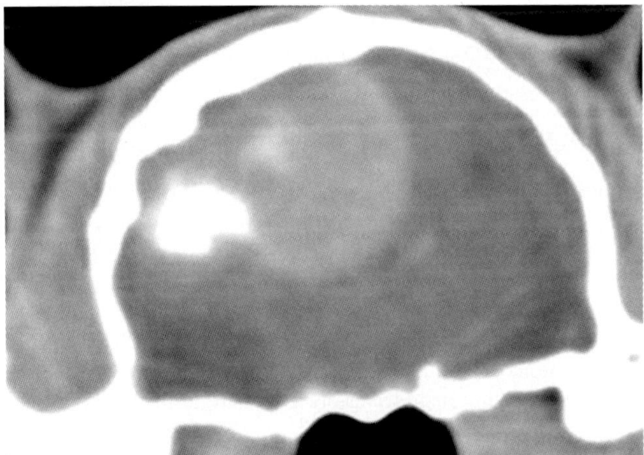

FIGURE 30-2 Precontrast CT image of feline meningioma with calcification.

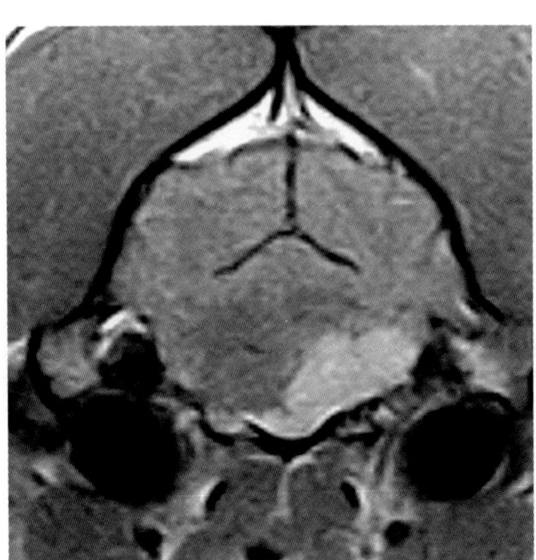

FIGURE 30-3 Postcontrast MRI of canine meningioma at the cerebellomedullary angle demonstrating a meningeal tail.

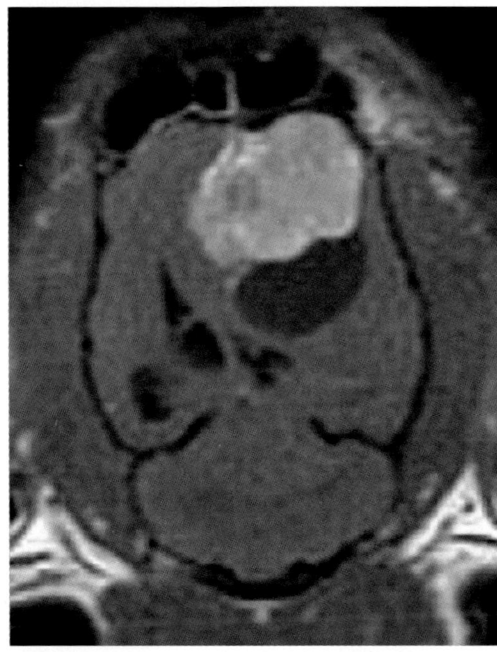

FIGURE 30-4 Feline meningioma with cystic component.

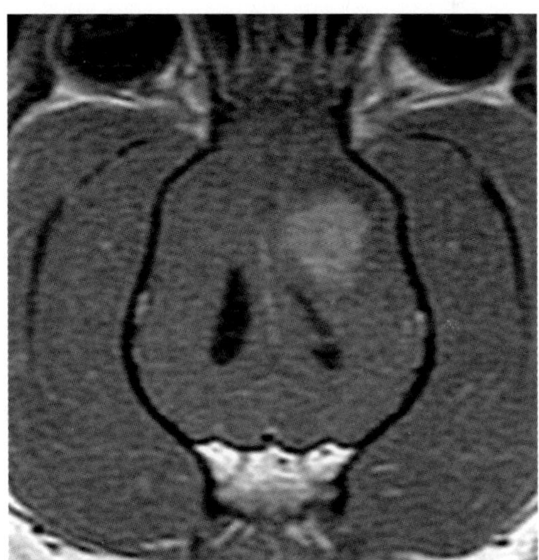

FIGURE 30-5 Postcontrast CT of canine glioma.

poorly and nonuniformly (Figure 30-5). Choroid plexus tumors and ependymomas tend to be intraventricular in location and often uniformly contrast enhance (Figure 30-6). The phenomenon of "ring enhancement," in which a circular ring of contrast enhancement surrounds nonenhancing tissue, is nonspecific and has been associated with several neoplastic and nonneoplastic brain diseases. However, ring enhancement is often associated with gliomas (see Chapter 6). Meningeal contrast enhancement evident on MR images of the brain has been described but is not specific for brain tumors. These typical imaging features are guidelines only. Meningiomas can arise from the falx cerebri or the choroid plexus and appear intraaxial. Gliomas can be peripherally located and contrast enhancing. In a recent study, the accuracy of predicting primary brain tumor type based on MR images of 40 dogs was 70%.[17] Stereotactic biopsy of brain tumors using MRI or CT images is now

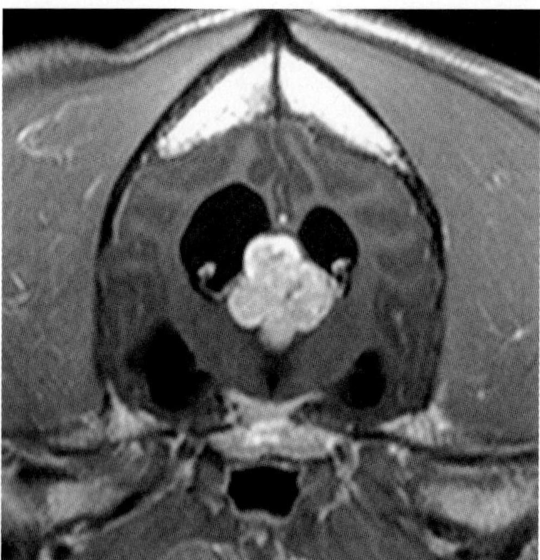

FIGURE 30-6 Postcontrast MRI of a canine choroid plexus tumor.

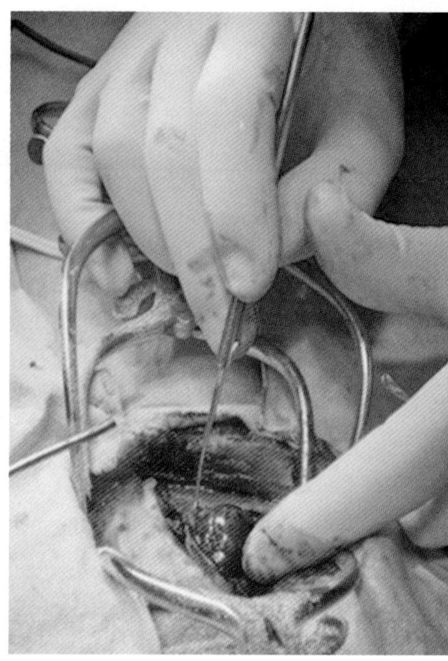

FIGURE 30-7 Surgical removal of cerebral cortical meningioma.

available at several veterinary referral centers.[5] With this new technology, a definitive diagnosis can be obtained at the time of imaging without the need for major intracranial surgery.

Cerebrospinal Fluid Analysis

The utility of CSF evaluation for the suspected brain tumor patient is controversial. CSF is often abnormal in patients with brain tumors, but the white blood cell (WBC) counts and protein levels are variable and nonspecific for neoplasia. In fact, dogs and cats with meningiomas tend to have CSF with predominantly polymorphonuclear (neutrophilic) WBC counts. The authors often do not pursue CSF analysis if the CT or MR image strongly suggests a brain neoplasm. Although the risk of CSF procurement in the face of elevated intracranial pressure (ICP) in a brain tumor patient is often not great, the potential benefit of a nonspecific CSF result may not outweigh even a small danger of harming the patient with the procedure. Although CSF analysis tends to yield fairly nonspecific information in brain tumor cases, it may be helpful in distinguishing whether a choroid plexus tumor is a CPP or CPC. In one study,[13] the more malignant CPC was significantly more likely to be associated with a CSF protein concentration greater than 100 mg/dL than the less malignant CPP tumor subtype. Regardless of whether CSF analysis is performed, imaging should always precede CSF analysis when a focal neoplasm is highly suspected. Anesthetizing a patient who is most likely to have a brain tumor solely for the purpose of obtaining CSF is generally contraindicated because the resultant information is unlikely to assist in either planning treatment or estimating prognosis.

Therapy

Surgery

In addition to removing neoplastic tissue, surgical debulking/removal allows for a histologic diagnosis, as well as potentially providing an immediate decompressive effect (decreasing ICP). Feline meningiomas are typically located over the cerebral convexities and tend to "peel away" from normal brain tissue at surgery. In most cases, feline meningiomas can be relatively easily removed en masse. The authors have had considerable experience dealing with recurrent or repeat feline intracranial meningiomas; overall, these tumors are also typically readily removable. Surgical removal is the primary mode of definitive therapy for feline intracranial meningiomas.[2,5,6,9] Canine meningiomas are also often located over the cerebral cortical surface and are thus surgically accessible (Figure 30-7). However, meningiomas in the cerebellar and brainstem regions are frequently encountered in dogs. Cerebellar meningiomas are often surgically accessible; meningiomas in the brainstem may not be accessible. Meningiomas in dogs are much less predictable than those in cats in terms of ease of surgical removal. Unlike cats, there are multiple histologic subtypes of canine meningiomas, and nearly one-third of these tumors are invasive.[3-6,11] The authors have successfully used intraoperative ultrasound to assist in locating brain tumors and in judging completeness of removal (Figure 30-8). The authors do not recommend pursuing surgical removal of canine meningiomas if adjunctive therapy (e.g., radiation) is not planned to be used following removal. Some gliomas are surgically accessible, but surgical removal/debulking of gliomas is considerably more difficult than meningiomas. Gliomas tend to infiltrate normal brain parenchyma, and it is often difficult to discern tumor margin from brain tissue at surgery. Surgical removal of intracranial glioma is seldom attempted in dogs and cats because of the invasive nature of these neoplasms. Removal of other brain tumor types (e.g., choroid plexus tumor, ependymoma) is also uncommonly performed because of the intraaxial location of these masses. Surgical removal of secondary brain tumors is also not commonly performed because many of these tumors are invasive as are their extraneural source neoplasms. However, some calvarial tumors (e.g., multilobular osteochondrosarcoma [MLO]) are surgically resectable with good outcomes (see Chapter 24).[5,18] On rare occasions, metastatic brain tumors are removed surgically.

Radiation Therapy

Radiation therapy (RT) is used in the treatment of primary brain tumors, as well as secondary brain tumors that arise by local extension or from metastasis from a distant site. Treatment options have advanced from early reports of the use of orthovoltage RT to

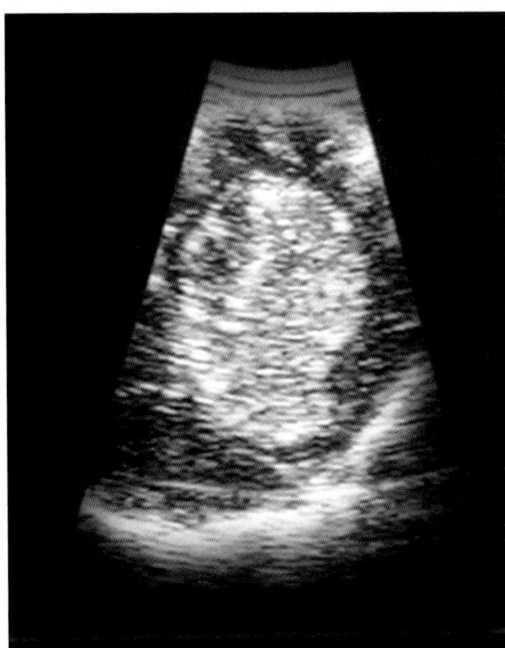

FIGURE 30-8 Intraoperative ultrasound evaluation of canine meningioma.

current options, including intensity-modulated RT (IMRT) and stereotactic RT (SRT).[19,20] Fractionated radiation protocols have largely transitioned from alternate day treatments to daily therapy (Monday through Friday), although there are reports on the application of hypofractionated protocols.[21-23] Radiation dose per fraction, total dose of radiation, and the volume of the brain irradiated are important considerations when irradiating brain tumors.[24,25] In one report of hypofractionated brain irradiation, 14.5% (12/83) of dogs died or were euthanized due to suspected delayed radiation side effects caused by delivery of a high dose per fraction.[22] There are reports on the results of RT alone or in combination with surgery for canine primary brain tumors.[19,24,26-29] RT improves survival over surgery alone or medical management alone.[26,28] Median overall survival for 29 dogs (presumptive diagnosis of meningioma in 22 dogs, glioma in 4 dogs, and choroid plexus tumor in 3 dogs) that were treated with RT alone was 250 days, with 76% dying of presumptive recurrence or tumor progression.[27] In another report of 46 dogs irradiated only for a range of different tumor types the median survival time (MST) was 699 days.[24] It is a well-accepted principle that postoperative RT in the microscopic disease setting is generally more efficacious than treating macroscopic disease, including brain tumors. However, it may be difficult to determine if there are postoperative changes versus residual macroscopic disease when CT imaging is done for radiation treatment planning postoperatively.[30] With no therapy or only supportive therapy, survival is reported to be 0.2 months in comparison to dogs irradiated with Cobalt-60 external-beam RT alone or in combination with other modalities with a median survival of 4.9 months.[26] In another report comparing surgery alone to surgery plus RT, the median survival was 7 months (surgery alone and survival >1 week) compared to 16.5 months (combination therapy).[28] In a report of 20 dogs with meningioma that had RT after incomplete resection, the median progression-free survival time was 35 months.[29] In a retrospective study of endoscopic-assisted tumor removal in dogs (n = 33) and cats (n = 6), 44% were alive after more than 2 years, only 4 were irradiated postoperatively, and the MST for dogs with meningiomas was 2104 days.[31]

An alternative to conventional fractionated RT is stereotactic radiosurgery for the management of CNS tumors, which entails the precise delivery of a larger dose per fraction to the tumor in 1 to a few fractions for a total dose of 10 to 15 Gy.[20] Limited information is available in the literature, but there are a number of veterinary facilities that now have equipment with this capability.

RT has also been used successfully to irradiate a calvarial allograft used in the repair of a calvarial defect in a cat with an intracranial meningioma.[32] It is important to consider the potential impact on radiation dose distribution in patients that have undergone surgery and require reconstruction that may include the use of metal implants.[33-36] This is potentially of more concern when larger metal implants (e.g., plates, rods, screws) are used to stabilize the spine.[37]

Chemotherapy

There are a limited number of reports on the use and efficacy of chemotherapy in the management of brain tumors in companion animals, including individual case reports and small case series.[21,38-44] Lomustine, carmustine, and hydroxyurea have been utilized in the treatment of canine brain tumors, but there are limited data to provide validation of the utility of chemotherapy. Based on a retrospective study of oral hydroxyurea in combination with glucocorticoids, 33 dogs with MRI-diagnosed meningioma had a significantly longer survival time than observed in 10 dogs treated with glucocorticoids alone.[45] The MST for the combination therapy group was 28 weeks versus 14 weeks for dogs treated with glucocorticoids alone.[45] A report on the use of 1-(2-chloroethyl)-3-cyclohexyl-1-nitrosourea (CCNU) in 206 dogs with a number of different tumor types, including 11 dogs with brain tumors, documented toxicity of this chemotherapeutic agent but did not provide response data.[38] Chemotherapy (carmustine, lomustine) alone or in combination with RT or cytoreductive surgery in dogs with astrocytomas has resulted in survival times of 3 to 8 months.[21,40]

Other Therapies

There is limited information on other therapeutic approaches to the management of canine brain tumors, including the use of whole body hyperthermia in conjunction with RT and/or chemotherapy, radioactive iodine-125 implants in combination with other therapeutic approaches, gene therapy, and convection-enhanced delivery of liposomal nanoparticles containing topoisomerase inhibitor CPT-11, which is still being developed.[26,46-52] The use of whole body hyperthermia in conjunction with external-beam irradiation did not alter survival.[46] Dogs with meningiomas that were irradiated had a mean survival of 314 days versus 288 days for dogs treated with RT plus whole body hyperthermia.[46] Gene therapy strategies in dogs have included the delivery of an adeno-associated viral vector containing prodrug activating genes that confer sensitivity to toxic metabolites and cytokine-based gene therapy using an intravenously delivered cationic DNA lipid complex containing murine endostatin gene in a DNA plasmid to perturb tumor angiogenesis.[47,48] There is limited information on the application of brachytherapy in conjunction with excisional biopsy, but it may represent another potential avenue of treatment.[26,53]

Based on the association between vascular endothelial growth factor (VEGF) expression and survival in dogs with intracranial meningiomas, administration of antiangiogenic agents may have future therapeutic potential.[54,55]

There is information available that indicates that dynamic contrast-enhanced CT may have utility in evaluating and classifying intracranial lesions and for determining response to therapy.[56]

Prognosis

Prognosis is poor with no therapy or only supportive therapy or palliative therapy in dogs with a MST of 0.2, or less than 2 months.[23,26] Results of RT based on a subset of the reports in the literature are difficult to interpret because a definitive histopathologic diagnosis is not always obtained and tumor types are grouped together (including pituitary tumors).[19,24,26,27] A presumptive diagnosis may be made based on either CT or MRI findings.[27,57] However, this may not be a reliable means of arriving at a presumptive diagnosis.[58] The interpretation of results is improving with the advent of minimally invasive techniques for brain tumor biopsies or cytology, as well as advancements in surgical techniques and tumor extirpation for histopathologic analysis, including endoscopic-assisted intracranial tumor removal.[31,59-64] The ability to definitively diagnose the specific histopathologic type of brain tumor prior to surgery may aid both clinicians and clients in deciding on a course of treatment and in understanding the potential prognosis.[48] Additional potential positive prognostic factors that have been identified include solitary versus multiple lesions, limited neurologic dysfunction, and treatment with RT or a combination of surgery and RT.[26,28] Tumor location may also impact survival; MST for forebrain versus caudal brain meningiomas was 2104 days and 702 days, respectively.[31] Pneumonia can develop due to aspiration postoperatively and may have a negative impact on survival.[65]

Meningiomas are the most common intracranial tumor in dogs, but attempts to correlate tumor grade or histologic subtype and MRI features largely have not identified any significant associations that would allow preoperative prognostication.[11] In a study of 112 dogs with intracranial meningiomas using criteria of the human WHO international histologic classification system 56% were classified as benign, 43% were atypical, and 1% were malignant meningiomas; the atypical and malignant meningiomas were noted to behave more aggressively with a higher potential for recurrence.[11] In one report of 17 dogs treated surgically for meningioma, survival was correlated with histologic tumor type: anaplastic 0 days, fibroblastic 10 days, psammomatous more than 313 days, meningothelial more than 523 days, and transitional 1254 days.[44] Of interest is that use of a surgical aspirator to resect intracranial meningiomas resulted in a MST of 1254 days.[44] None of the dogs were irradiated, and only 2 of 17 received postoperative chemotherapy (hydroxyurea) when there were MRI findings suggestive of recurrence.[44] In a study of 17 dogs with benign meningiomas treated with surgery and postoperative hypofractionated RT, significantly shorter survival times were associated with greater VEGF expression.[54] The MST was 748 days for dogs with tumors with 75% or fewer cells staining for VEGF compared with 442.5 days for dogs with tumors with more than 75% of cell staining for VEGF.[54] Furthermore, dogs with more intense staining had a significantly shorter survival time.[54] In a more recent study, tumor proliferation defined by reactivity of the monoclonal antibody MIB-1 to the Ki67 antigen was not associated with survival, and there was no association between VEGF and tumor proliferation.[66] In this study, 70 dogs underwent surgery and postoperative hypofractionated RT, and the overall MST from the date of diagnosis was 514 days.[66] Progesterone and estrogen receptor expression has been evaluated in meningiomas in dogs and cats; further investigation will be necessary to determine if there is prognostic significance or a role for targeted intervention.[29,67] In one study, progesterone receptor expression was inversely related to tumor proliferative fraction measured by immunohistochemical detection of proliferating cell nuclear antigen (PF_{PCNA} index), which was predictive of survival in dogs with meningiomas after surgery and postoperative RT.[29] The 2-year progression-free survival was 43% for tumors with a high PF_{PCNA} index and 91% for tumors with a low PF_{PCNA} index. Furthermore, tumors with a high PF_{PCNA} index were 9.1 times more likely to recur.[29] Cyclooxygenase-2 (COX-2) expression has been demonstrated in the majority of intracranial meningiomas (21/24 or 87%), but the role in tumorigenesis and the potential for therapeutic intervention with COX-2 inhibitors have not been elucidated.[68] Conversely, in a study of 20 canine gliomas, none of the tumors expressed COX-2.[69] In this same study that also evaluated c-kit overexpression, the authors speculated that c-kit inhibitors may have an antiangiogenic effect in high-grade tumors due to presence of intramural vascular expression.[69]

Stereotactic radiosurgery may provide comparable or improved tumor control with a fewer number of anesthetic episodes but is limited in its application due to a limited number of facilities with this capability.[20] Two dogs with meningiomas survived 227 and 56 weeks after radiosurgery; a dog with an oligodendroglioma survived 66 weeks.[20] Additional information should be forthcoming with increased availability of RT units with advanced capability to deliver radiation.

In dogs with choroid plexus tumors, it should be noted that local spread of the tumor within the ventricular system can occur and distant metastasis via the subarachnoid space occurs in approximately 50% of dogs.[13] Additionally, at necropsy in one study of 56 dogs with choroid plexus tumors, 19% had evidence of gross and/or microscopic spinal cord metastases that should impact considerations of diagnostics, approaches to treatment, and prognosis.[13]

There are descriptive reports but limited prognostic information available for other specific tumor types, such as for astrocytomas.[12,70,71] In a report of 86 dogs treated for brain tumors that included 27 meningiomas, 7 astrocytomas, and 6 choroid plexus tumors, survival based on tumor type was evaluated as meningioma versus other; dogs with meningiomas lived significantly longer.[26] In a study of dogs irradiated with a hypofractionated protocol, the MST for 34 dogs with intraaxial tumors (presumably gliomas) was 40.4 weeks versus 49.7 weeks for 41 dogs with extraaxial tumors (presumably meningioma, including schwannoma and choroid plexus tumor).[22]

Histiocytic sarcoma can affect the CNS in dogs with systemic disease, but there are a limited number of reports of localized CNS histiocytic sarcoma, with one report with necropsy information that confirmed the localized nature.[72-76] Rapid disease progression and euthanasia was the outcome for two dogs: one with primary spinal cord involvement and the other with brain involvement.[76] Surgical intervention has been reported in 12 dogs with subdural histiocytic sarcomas, although no follow-up information was provided.[75]

There are a number of studies that have been conducted to further elucidate the mechanisms of tumorigenesis and determination of the immunohistochemical profiles of brain tumors.[77-83] Such efforts may ultimately lead to a better understanding and ability to prognosticate for individual patients based on identification of specific markers and for determination of appropriate targeted therapy. However, to date, targeted therapies in humans with meningiomas have only realized modest success and are associated with toxicity.[84]

It should be noted that multiple meningiomas, multifocal oligodendroglioma, and synchronous brain tumors (oligodendroglioma and meningioma) have been reported, as well as synchronous primary and metastatic tumors in dogs.[43,85-89] Based on one small case series, survival may be comparable for dogs with multiple meningiomas as seen for dogs treated for a solitary meningioma.[43] Additionally, dogs with a primary brain tumor may have another primary tumor that may affect prognosis.[7] In a report of 170 dogs with primary intracranial neoplasia, 38/170 (23%) had another tumor unrelated to the brain tumor.[7] In a study of 28 dogs with meningiomas 7 (25%) had another tumor in addition to the meningioma.[87] Although rare, pulmonary metastasis in three dogs with intracranial meningioma has been reported.[90] Cats are also reported to have multiple or two different types of intracranial tumors and, in fact, more commonly have multiple meningiomas (17%) than dogs.[2,8,91,92] It has been questioned whether multiple meningiomas represent multicentric disease or metastasis. Dogs with metastatic intracranial neoplasms most commonly have metastatic hemangiosarcoma or carcinomas, representing 50% and 20% of metastatic tumors, respectively, with an anticipated poor prognosis.[10,93] Meningeal carcinomatosis results from spread of a solid tumor that can be an intracranial primary tumor or of distant origin (e.g., mammary gland carcinoma) and is associated with a very poor prognosis.[94-96] Metastatic disease is usually recognized as multiple mass lesions, but a solitary lesion may represent metastasis. Full staging is necessary to rule out other disease because secondary intracranial neoplasia may be more common than primary intracranial neoplasia.[10]

Cats respond well to surgery alone for intracranial meningiomas, which is the most common primary intracranial tumor in cats, and have a MST of approximately 2 years.[2,9,97,98] In one report, the MST for cats treated surgically was 685 days compared to 18 days for cats that did not have surgery.[2] Recurrence is documented to occur; 20.6% in one report had a median postoperative time to recurrence of 285 days (range 123 to 683 days; n = 6 cats); second surgeries are feasible in cats.[2,9] Cats with multiple meningiomas based on one report have long-term survival when treated surgically with follow-up chemotherapy (hydroxyurea) for 2 (n = 3 cats) or 4 (n = 1 cat) meningiomas.[91]

Cats with intracranial lymphoma more commonly have multicentric disease; fewer cats have primary intracranial lymphoma.[2] In cats treated palliatively with systemic corticosteroids, the MST was 21 days (range 9 to 270 days in nine cats).[2]

Two cats with oligodendrogliomas were euthanized at the time of diagnosis or 6 weeks after diagnosis due to their poor neurologic status.[99] Of six cats with oligodendrogliomas, three had surgery (n = 2) and/or received corticosteroids (n = 1), with survival times of 1 day, 5 days, and one cat that had surgery was lost to follow-up at 1 month.[2] Four cats with cerebral astrocytomas (three of which were managed medically) lived for 1 to 3 years with anticonvulsant therapy.[100] Two of six cats with astrocytomas had surgery, followed by RT in one cat with survival times of 1 day and 179 days; a third cat treated with only corticosteroids survived 35 days.[2] One cat with an ependymoma that had two surgeries ultimately survived for 667 days; another cat treated with corticosteroids was euthanized at 685 days.[2]

Comparative Aspects

Humans are afflicted with the same overall cadre of brain tumor types that are reported in dogs and cats. Overall, the incidence of brain tumors in people is approximately 19 per 100,000 person-years, with about 60% of these being benign tumors; the most common benign brain tumor in people is meningioma and the most common malignant brain tumor in people is glioblastoma multiforme (also called grade IV astrocytoma).[101,102] Intracranial meningiomas in humans are often classified based on three histologic grades (benign, atypical, malignant) that predict biologic behavior. Approximately 80% of human meningiomas are considered benign according to this scheme, with atypical and malignant grades accounting for 8% and less than 3%, respectively. Although the specific histologic subtypes (e.g., transitional, psammomatous) of canine and human meningiomas are very similar, the percentage of atypical tumors is much higher in dogs at 43%.[11,103] Treatment modalities used for human brain tumors are similar to those used for canine and feline brain tumors. Surgical removal is the primary treatment method used for human meningiomas, and survival is linked to the completeness of surgical removal. Adjunctive RT improves survival rates in people for incompletely resected meningiomas.[11,101,102,104] Oral hydroxyurea therapy may be an effective treatment for human meningioma as well, although this is not as well established as RT.[104] The prognosis for long-term control or cure of human intracranial meningioma is good.[11,104] The morbidity and mortality for human gliomas is poor overall, with survival times often ranging from 7 to 24 months, even with combination (surgery, radiation, chemotherapy) therapy.[102]

Spinal Tumors

Incidence and Risk Factors

The actual incidence of spinal tumors in dogs and cats is unknown but appears to be considerably less than that of brain tumors. As with brain tumors, spinal tumors are broadly classified as primary or secondary. Spinal tumors are usually also classified in terms of their anatomic location: extradural, intradural/extramedullary, intramedullary, or mixed compartment. The most common primary spinal cord tumor in dogs is meningioma, and in cats the most common primary spinal cord tumor is lymphoma.[6,105-109] Hemangiosarcoma is the most commonly reported secondary spinal cord tumor in dogs, and osteosarcoma is the most commonly reported secondary spinal cord tumor in cats.[105,106] In one large retrospective study of 399 histopathologically confirmed spinal cord tumors in dogs, 48% were extradural, 13% were intradural/extramedullary, 6% were intramedullary, and 33% were mixed compartment.[110]

Canine spinal tumors tend to occur in large breeds, typically at an older age (e.g., 9 to 10 years).[105,106] Meningiomas and malignant nerve sheath tumors (MNSTs) arise most frequently in the cervical spinal cord, and MNSTs are especially prominent in the cervical intumescence area.[105,106] Boxers may be predisposed to spinal meningiomas.[109] More aggressive meningiomas (grade II versus grade I) are likely to occur in the thoracolumbar region and in younger dogs.[109] Spinal nephroblastoma typically occurs in young dogs (between 6 months and 3 years of age); this tumor also has a predilection for golden retrievers and German shepherd dogs and is usually located between the T10 and L2 spinal cord segments.[105,106,111,112] Spinal lymphoma often affects young cats, is often associated with the feline leukemia virus (FeLV), tends to occur in the thoracic and lumbar spine, and is usually present in multiple extraneural locations.[105-108] Vertebral osteosarcoma in cats is usually reported in older patients (e.g., >8 years).[107,108]

Pathology

The category of extradural tumors includes primary and secondary (metastatic or local invasion) vertebral and soft tissue tumors. Primary vertebral tumors such as osteosarcoma, chondrosarcoma, myeloma (plasma cell tumor), fibrosarcoma, and hemangiosarcoma are common extradural tumors encountered in dogs.[105,106] In one study, vertebral tumors were slightly less prevalent than lymphosarcoma in cats, with osteosarcoma being the most common.[107] Other vertebral tumors reported in cats include fibrosarcoma, undifferentiated sarcoma, and plasma cell tumors. The most common primary vertebral body tumor in dogs is also osteosarcoma.[105,110] It may be difficult in some cases to ascertain whether a vertebral tumor is primary or metastatic. Other tumors may occur in the epidural space, without directly involving the vertebrae. Common among these are sarcomas—most frequently osteosarcoma and hemangiosarcoma. Lymphosarcoma can be primary or metastatic and is often located in the extradural space, particularly in cats. Meningioma and MNSTs usually are typically located intradurally but occasionally will exhibit an extradural pattern on imaging. Metastatic carcinomas (e.g., mammary carcinoma, prostatic carcinoma) may localize to the extradural space. A number of fatty tumors have been reported to affect the spinal cord in dogs, including lipoma, myelolipoma, infiltrative lipoma, and liposarcoma. These all generally occur in an extradural location.[105,106,110,113-115]

Meningiomas and MNSTs are the two most common neoplasms in the intradural/extramedullary location category, with meningiomas predominating. An uncommon blast cell tumor of young dogs called *nephroblastoma* also typically displays an intradural/extramedullary pattern on spinal imaging.*

Intramedullary tumors are infrequently encountered and include primary spinal parenchymal tumors (e.g., astrocytoma, oligodendroglioma, ependymoma) and intramedullary metastases. The most common intramedullary metastases in dogs are thought to be hemangiosarcoma and lymphosarcoma.[105,106] In one study, hemangiosarcoma was the most common tumor type in the intramedullary category.[110]

History and Clinical Signs

Spinal tumors typically cause progressive signs of a myelopathy, but acute or subacute development of spinal cord dysfunction often occurs, especially with feline lymphosarcoma and intramedullary neoplasms. Rapid onset of clinical signs may be due to factors such as pathologic fracture of a cancerous vertebra, acute hemorrhage or necrosis of a tumor, or rapid growth of a neoplasm with subsequent damage to spinal cord parenchyma (more likely with intramedullary tumors). Spinal cord tumors are typically solitary and can occur anywhere along the length of the spine. As with brain tumors, the specific neurologic deficits associated with a spinal tumor will depend on the specific neuroanatomic location of that tumor.

A prominent feature of extradural and intradural/extramedullary spinal neoplasia is spinal hyperesthesia, which often precedes the onset of proprioceptive and voluntary motor deficits. Spinal hyperesthesia is often not a prominent early clinical feature in patients with intramedullary spinal tumors, probably due to the lack of meningeal involvement. In MNSTs of the cervical intumescence, a history of unilateral thoracic limb lameness (on the side of the tumor) preceding the development of clinical signs of myelopathy is common.[6,105,106]

Diagnostic Techniques and Work-Up

Minimum Database

The minimum database for a patient with a suspected spinal neoplasm is similar to that for a patient with a suspected brain tumor. Blood work (CBC and chemistry profile) and urinalysis should be performed, and survey radiographs should be procured to help rule out metastatic disease or a secondary neoplastic process.

Imaging

Survey spinal radiographs are generally recommended to identify the presence or absence of any obvious bony lesions (e.g., bone lysis and/or proliferation). In the majority of soft tissue spinal neoplasms, plain radiographs of the spine are normal. In some cases, however, the expanding neoplasm leads to expansion of either the vertebral canal or the intervertebral foramen, with or without obvious thinning of the surrounding bone. As with brain tumors, the preferred imaging modality for investigation of suspected spinal neoplasia is MRI (Figure 30-9). CT, alone or in combination with myelography, can also be used to diagnose spinal cord tumors but is considered to be inferior to MRI in most cases. Lesions that are difficult to distinguish as being either intradural/extramedullary or intramedullary on myelographic images may be better delineated on MRI or CT/myelography; however, some spinal tumors have enough associated spinal cord swelling that this distinction may be difficult to make, even on MR images. Also, intradural/extramedullary spinal tumors will occasionally infiltrate the spinal cord parenchyma (mixed compartment mass), which may contribute to the development of an intramedullary imaging pattern (Figure 30-10).[105,106,110]

Cerebrospinal Fluid Analysis

CSF analysis is often pursued in combination with spinal imaging. As with brain tumors, CSF analysis is likely to be abnormal but usually does not provide specific information about the disease process. With the possible exception of spinal lymphosarcoma, CSF evaluation rarely reveals neoplastic cells and may reveal increased protein levels, with or without elevated cell counts (more likely with tumors with meningeal involvement).[6,105,106]

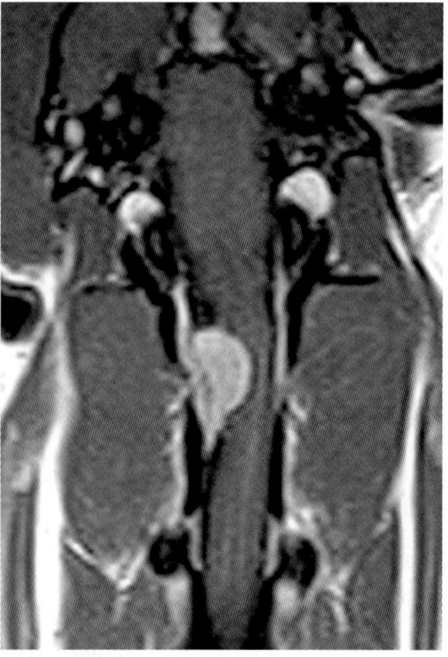

FIGURE 30-9 Postcontrast MRI of spinal meningioma.

*References 6, 105, 106, 110, 112, 113.

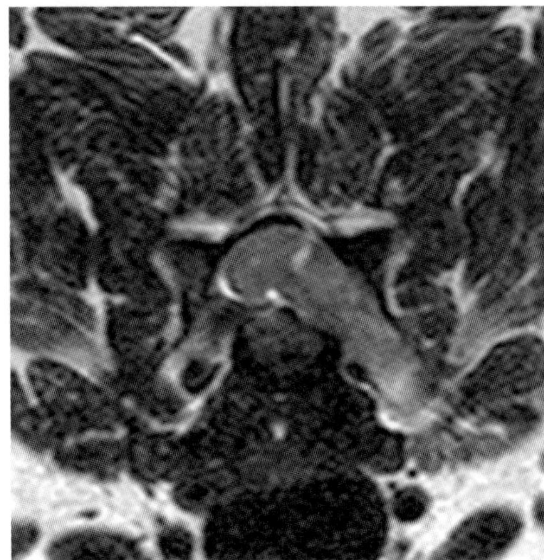

FIGURE 30-10 Postcontrast MRI of cervical axial nerve sheath tumor.

Therapy

Therapeutic options for spinal cord tumors are similar to those available for brain tumor management. Surgical removal may be advisable for those neoplasms that have not infiltrated spinal cord parenchyma.

Meningioma is reported to be the most common intraspinal tumor in dogs and can be treated effectively with surgery with or without postoperative external-beam RT.[109,116-118] RT results in an improved outcome and can contribute to prevention of or delay in local recurrence.[109,116] With surgery alone for intraspinal meningioma, the mean survival time has been reported to be 19 months for 8 of 10 dogs that had evidence of postoperative recurrence.[109] In a report of the results of surgery in nine dogs with spinal meningioma, five were alive longer than 6 months postoperatively.[119] In two dogs treated surgically for spinal meningiomas, the survival time was 1410 and 1440 days.[118] In seven dogs that underwent a combination of surgery and postoperative RT, survival times ranged from 18 to 78 months.[109] Six dogs that had postoperative RT for spinal meningioma had a MST of 13.5 months (range 8 to 25 months).[116] One dog that had recurrence of an intraspinal meningioma 15 months postoperatively was irradiated with almost complete resolution of neurologic deficits and was ultimately euthanized for recurrence 19 months after RT.[117] As with RT for intracranial tumors, the trend has been to reduce the dose per fraction and increase the total dose. The goal is to maximize the dose of radiation that can be delivered while minimizing the risk of radiation myelopathy. Also, there is a dose-volume relationship, and the length of the spinal cord irradiated has to be considered when prescribing the dose.[120]

Dogs with spinal nephroblastomas can be treated effectively with a combination of surgery and RT.[111,112,121] The results reported for surgery alone are widely variable with MSTs of 70.5 days and 380.5 days.[111,112,122] It should be noted that since this is a tumor that develops in young dogs, RT carries the risk for the development of radiation-induced tumors.[121] There is one report of possible intraspinal metastasis of a canine spinal cord nephroblastoma, which alternatively may have represented multifocal disease.[123]

A report of two dogs with intramedullary spinal cord hemangioma included information on one dog treated with lomustine (no specific details); this dog was euthanized 15 months after the initial diagnosis.[124]

Three dogs treated for spinal lymphoma had a MST of 560 days (range = 560 to 1030 days).[118] Two of the dogs were treated with RT and chemotherapy in addition to surgery.

There is limited information on results of treatment of spinal meningiomas in cats.[107,125] In one report, a cat that underwent decompressive surgery for a spinal meningioma was doing well but was lost to follow-up 7 months postoperatively.[107] The MST for 16 cats that underwent surgery for spinal meningiomas was 518 days.[125]

There are reports on spinal lymphoma in cats, although there is limited information on the results of treatment.[107,126,127] Lymphoma is the most common tumor affecting the spinal cord in cats and often affects multiple regions of the spinal cord and brain.[107,128] Treatment options include surgery, RT, and/or chemotherapy.

Spinal nerve sheath tumors treated surgically in seven dogs (with one dog also treated with radiation and chemotherapy) had a MST of 180 days (range of 21 to 300 days).[118] One dog irradiated postoperatively for a spinal nerve sheath tumor was alive but lost to follow-up at 25 months.[116] Spinal nerve sheath tumors in three cats treated surgically resulted in survival times of 67 days (failed to improve), 112 days, and 275 days (both had local recurrence).[125]

Outcomes for other types of spinal cord tumors in cats are relatively unknown because of the limited number of cases, the tendency to euthanize due to a presumed poor prognosis, or a poor neurologic condition. A tetraparetic cat with a spinal cord glioma at cervical spinal cord segments C3-C4 was euthanized at the time of diagnosis.[129]

Prognosis

The majority of dogs (17/21, 81%) with intraspinal meningiomas improve neurologically postoperatively.[109] Some reports provide histopathologic grade for meningiomas, although this is not done consistently.[109,116,130] Based on relatively small numbers of dogs, there does not appear to be a correlation between grade and long-term outcome.[109] Perioperative complications are more commonly encountered for lesions in the cranial cervical region. It should be noted that outcome in dogs that decline neurologically after RT may represent either local tumor recurrence or late radiation damage to the spinal cord, and without necropsy examination it is difficult to discern the cause of neurologic impairment.[116] Nine dogs (meningioma in six dogs, and one each nerve sheath tumor, ependymoma, and neuroepithelioma) treated postoperatively with RT had MSTs of 17 months (range 6.5 to 70 months).[116] There is overall limited information on the results of treatment of spinal cord tumors in dogs or cats.

In cats with lymphoma of the spinal cord, it is important to note that in one study of 26 cats that had necropsy examination, lymphoma was identified in extraneural locations in 22 (84.6%), with the most common locations bone marrow, kidneys, liver, skeletal muscle, and spleen.[107] This is important in considering treatment options, as well as prognosis, in cats with spinal lymphoma. Six cats treated with a combination of vincristine, cyclophosphamide, and prednisone had a complete remission rate of 50%; median duration of remission was 14 weeks.[127] Another cat treated with decompressive surgery in combination with chemotherapy had a remission of 62 weeks.[127] In another report of four cats with spinal lymphoma, three were treated with L-asparaginase, vincristine, and prednisone after RT and one cat had surgery; three cats were euthanized or died within 20 weeks and one cat was alive at 13 months.[126]

There are limited reports on the outcome of surgery in cats with spinal meningioma.[125,131] Of five cats with spinal cord meningioma, one cat was alive 1400 days postoperatively, and the MST for the other four cats was 180 days (range = 30 to 600 days).[131] A MST of 426 days (range 211 to 842 days) was reported for 16 cats treated surgically for spinal cord meningioma.[125] One cat with a spinal cord nerve sheath tumor treated surgically was alive 2190 days postoperatively.[131]

Comparative Aspects

In humans, primary spinal cord tumors are approximately 10 to 15 times less common than primary brain tumors, comprising 2% to 4% of all primary tumors of the CNS.[132] Primary spinal tumors are typically intradural (intradural extramedullary and intramedullary); extradural spinal tumors in humans are most often metastatic.[132-134] The most common intramedullary spinal tumors in people are ependymoma and low-grade astrocytoma. Ependymomas are typically readily resectable as are some astrocytomas. These tumors carry a fair-to-good prognosis, with surgical resection often combined with radiation and chemotherapy.[132] The most common intradural extramedullary spinal tumors in people are meningiomas and nerve sheath tumors (schwannoma, neurofibroma, and malignant peripheral nerve sheath tumor [MPNST]); with the exception of MPNST, the prognosis for patients with these tumors is favorable with surgical removal.[132]

Extradural spinal metastases generally portend a poor prognosis in humans. In addition to histologic features of the specific tumor, neurologic status at the time of diagnosis influences the likelihood of treatment response. Treatment of metastatic extradural spinal metastases in people typically involves RT and chemotherapy, with or without surgical intervention.[133,134]

Peripheral Nerve Tumors

Incidence and Risk Factors

In general, peripheral nerve tumors (also called *peripheral nerve sheath tumors* [PNSTs]) are infrequently reported in dogs and rarely in cats. Peripheral nerve tumors arise in the cranial nerves, spinal nerve roots, and peripheral nerves. These tumors occur most commonly in middle-aged to older dogs of medium and large breeds. The most common cranial nerve affected is the trigeminal (CN V), and the most common spinal nerve roots affected are in the region of the brachial plexus (C6-T2).[106,135-137] Tumors of the thoracic and lumbar spinal nerve roots also occur with some frequency and tend to cause signs of spinal cord compression as an early clinical sign of disease. Secondary peripheral nerve tumors (lymphoma, malignant sarcomas, hamartomas) can occasionally involve peripheral nerves as well.[106,135]

Pathology

Peripheral nerve tumors occur mainly in the cranial, spinal, and associated peripheral nerves and less commonly in the autonomic nervous system (e.g., sympathetic nerves and ganglia). These tumors arise from Schwann cells, perineurial fibroblasts, or a combination of these two cell types.[135-138] The traditional nomenclature for these neoplasms is confusing and of limited clinical use. These neoplasms have been classified as schwannomas, neurofibromas and neurofibrosarcomas. They have also been more broadly classified as benign peripheral nerve sheath tumors (BPNSTs) and malignant peripheral nerve sheath tumors (MPNSTs).[135-138] This latter terminology is more useful from a clinical standpoint, especially considering that the majority of reported PNSTs in dogs are histologically and biologically aggressive masses.[138,139] PNSTs in cats are uncommon, but the proportion of benign tumor types may be higher than that reported for dogs.[140]

History and Clinical Signs

As with brain and spinal tumors, the clinical signs of peripheral nerve tumors reflect the anatomic location of the tumor. The majority of reported canine peripheral nerve tumors involve the nerve roots and/or nerves of the brachial plexus region; in such cases, the typical scenario is a chronic progressive unilateral thoracic limb lameness that often eludes diagnosis for months. These dogs are often evaluated for possible orthopedic conditions prior to evaluation for a potential peripheral nerve tumor. A palpable mass may be found in the axillary region in some of these dogs (37% in one report),[137] and pain is usually easily elicited when palpating this region on the lame side. If the mass invades the vertebral canal and causes spinal cord compression, clinical signs of an asymmetric C6-T2 myelopathy may be apparent.[106,135-138] Less commonly, a peripheral nerve tumor will involve the thoracolumbar region of the spine; in these cases, a more rapidly progressive development of a T3-L3 myelopathy is common.[106,135] Peripheral nerve tumors also will occasionally affect nerve roots of the cauda equina, leading to clinical signs of progressive unilateral pelvic limb lameness (similar to the situation described for brachial plexus tumors).[106,135]

As mentioned previously, the cranial nerve typically affected by peripheral nerve tumor is the trigeminal nerve (CN V). Dogs afflicted by CN V nerve sheath tumors typically develop unilateral atrophy of the muscles of mastication (e.g., temporalis and masseter muscles) over weeks to months. Other clinical features associated with CN V involvement may include decreased-to-absent facial sensation and Horner's syndrome. If the intracranial portion of CN V becomes compressive, clinical signs of brainstem compression (e.g., hemiparesis, dysphagia) may develop.[135,141,142]

Diagnostic Techniques and Work-Up

Peripheral nerve tumors, especially those involving the brachial plexus region, can be challenging to diagnose. There should be a high index of suspicion for dogs with chronic thoracic limb lameness for which an obvious musculoskeletal cause cannot be found. The most useful imaging tool for diagnosing peripheral nerve tumors is MRI, whether the tumor involves a plexus, the spinal cord, or a cranial nerve. It is important in cases of brachial plexus nerve sheath tumors to image the axillary region, as well as the cervical spinal cord. Small brachial plexus tumors may be difficult to impossible to see on MR images; in some cases, subtle asymmetry in the suspected abnormal region is appreciated without an obvious mass being apparent.[106,135,141-143] Some dogs may have axillary masses that are visible via ultrasonography, in which case a needle aspirate may be obtained.[144,145] In the authors' opinion, CT is a poor second choice for imaging patients with suspected nerve sheath tumors. Myelography is unlikely to provide adequate information in such cases and should be avoided if possible. Electrodiagnostics may be useful in cases of suspected nerve sheath tumor. Abnormal electromyographic (EMG) findings may distinguish atrophied muscles from a primary neurogenic or myopathic disorder from atrophy due to musculoskeletal disease. Nerve conduction studies performed on peripheral nerves of limbs may also indicate abnormalities. In cases for which a peripheral nerve tumor is highly suspected but diagnostic tests are all negative or equivocal, exploratory surgery (e.g., brachial plexus exploratory) may be an option.[106,135,146]

Therapy

Surgery is the reported approach for the treatment of PNSTs in dogs and cats, although complete resection is difficult to achieve.[137,140,141,147] Amputation may be necessary alone or in conjunction with laminectomy to accomplish tumor resection as high up as possible for nerve root tumors.[137,147] Adjunctive RT is a postoperative option for residual microscopic disease, but there are only anecdotal reports regarding the success of treatment. Historically, dogs have been reportedly euthanized intraoperatively due to the recognition of the extent of disease during surgical exploration.[147] Preoperative cross-sectional imaging is recommended to define the extent of disease and for preplanning, particularly when considering combination therapy. Chemotherapy and/or RT is an option for lymphoma involving peripheral nerves.

Prognosis

The prognosis for PNSTs in dogs depends in part on tumor location and whether or not the tumor is amenable to surgery (amputation, laminectomy, or combination), with very limited information available on the results of adjunctive therapy.[137,141,147,148] The prognosis for dogs treated surgically has been reported to be guarded to poor, although earlier detection after the onset of clinical signs may improve outcome.[137] Long-term survival has been reported (>18 months, >27 months, >42 months).[141,147,148] Of seven dogs with trigeminal nerve sheath tumors that were not treated, the survival time was up to 21 months after onset of clinical signs, although several died or were euthanized at the time of presentation.[141] Postoperative RT is feasible, but there is limited information on results of treatment. There is no information available on the use of chemotherapy for the treatment of PNSTs. Failure is typically due to neurologic signs associated with local recurrence. Although usually solitary, multicentric disease involving multiple cranial nerve roots has been reported.[149] Additionally, metastasis of PNSTs can occur but is relatively rare.[141]The prognosis for cats is more favorable than what has been reported for dogs. In a report of 53 cats with 59 PNSTs, follow-up information was available for 45 cats that had surgical excision and/or amputation.[140] Of the 45 cats, 9 (20%) had local recurrence with histologically malignant tumors more likely to recur than histologically benign tumors, and 3 recurred locally twice. The median follow-up period was 21 months; 13 cats were euthanized at 2 weeks to 52 months (median 21.5 months; mean 22.6 months) after surgery.[140] Although PNSTs in cats can recur postoperatively, metastasis has not been documented to occur; euthanasia when disease related is due to local disease.[140]

Comparative Aspects

People are affected by peripheral nerve tumors of the same cellular origins as those that affect dogs. However, the vast majority of peripheral nerve tumors in humans are biologically benign (most are schwannomas and neurofibromas). These tumors are usually readily excised and rarely recur.[150,151] In comparison, most peripheral nerve tumors in dogs are aggressive and tend to recur following surgical excision.[135-138]

REFERENCES

1. Vandevelde M: Brain tumors in domestic animals: an overview. *Proceedings of the Conference on Brain Tumors in Man and Animals*. Research Triangle Park, NC, September 5-6, 1984.
2. Troxel MT, Vite CH, Van Winkle TJ, et al: Feline intracranial meningioma: a retrospective review of 160 cases (1985-2001), *J Vet Intern Med* 17:850–859, 2003.
3. Koestner A, Bilzer T, Fatzer R, et al: *Histological classification of tumors of the nervous system of domestic animals*, Washington, DC, 1999, Armed Forces Institute of Pathology.
4. Summers BA, Cummings JF, deLahunta A: Tumors of the central nervous system. In Summers BA, Cummings JF, deLahunta A, editors: *Veterinary neuropathology*, St Louis, 1995, Mosby.
5. Dewey CW: Encephalopathies: disorders of the brain. In Dewey CW, editor: *A practical guide to canine and feline neurology*, ed 2, Ames, Iowa, 2008, Wiley-Blackwell.
6. Adamo PF, Forrest L, Dubielzig R: Canine and feline meningiomas: diagnosis, treatment and prognosis, *Compend Contin Educ Pract Vet* 27:951–966, 2004.
7. Snyder JM, Shofer FS, Van Winkle TJ, et al: Canine intracranial primary neoplasia: 173 cases (1986-2003), *J Vet Intern Med* 20:669–675, 2006.
8. Nafe LA: Meningiomas in cats: a retrospective clinical study of 36 cases, *J Am Vet Med Assoc* 174:1224–1227, 1979.
9. Gordon LE, Thacher C, Matthiesen DT, et al: Results of craniotomy for the treatment of cerebral meningioma in 42 cats, *Vet Surg* 23:94–100, 1994.
10. Snyder JM, Lipitz L, Skorupski KA, et al: Secondary intracranial neoplasia in the dog: 177 cases (1986-2003), *J Vet Intern Med* 22:172–177, 2008.
11. Sturges BK, Dickinson PJ, Bollen AW, et al: Magnetic resonance imaging and histological classification of intracranial meningiomas in 112 dogs, *J Vet Intern Med* 22:586–595, 2008.
12. Lipsitz D, Higgins RJ, Kortz GD, et al: Glioblastoma multiforme: clinical findings, magnetic resonance imaging, and pathology in five dogs, *Vet Pathol* 40:659–669, 2003.
13. Westworth DR, Dickinson PJ, Vernau W, et al: Choroid plexus tumors in 56 dogs (1985-2007), *J Vet Intern Med* 22:1157–1165, 2008.
14. Thankey K, Faissler A, Kavirayani A, et al: Clinical presentation and outcome in dogs with histologically confirmed choroid plexus papillomas, *J Vet Intern Med* 20:782–783 (abstract), 2006.
15. Bagley RS, Gavin PR, Moore MP, et al: Clinical signs associated with brain tumors in dogs: 97 cases (1992-1997), *J Am Vet Med Assoc* 215:818–819, 1999.
16. Tomek A, Cizinauskas S, Doherr M, et al: Intracranial neoplasia in 61 cats: localization, tumour types and seizure patterns, *J Feline Med Surg* 8:243–253, 2006.
17. Rodenas S, Pumarola M, Gaitero L, et al: Magnetic resonance imaging findings in 40 dogs with histologically confirmed intracranial tumours, *Vet J* 187:85–91, 2011.
18. Dernell WS, Straw RC, Cooper MF, et al: Multilobular osteochondrosarcoma in 39 dogs: 1979-1993, *J Am Anim Hosp Assoc* 34:11–18, 1998.
19. Evans SM, Dayrell-Hart B, Powlis W, et al: Radiation therapy of canine brain masses, *J Vet Intern Med* 7:216–219, 1993.
20. Lester NV, Hopkins AL, Bova FJ, et al: Radiosurgery using a stereotactic headframe system for irradiation of brain tumors in dogs, *J Am Vet Med Assoc* 219:1562–1567, 2001.
21. Jeffrey N, Brearley MJ: Brain tumours in the dog: treatment of 10 cases and review of recent literature, *J Small Anim Pract* 34:367–372, 1993.
22. Brearley MJ, Jeffery ND, Phillips SM, et al: Hypofractionated radiation therapy of brain masses in dogs: A retrospective analysis of survival of 83 cases (1991-1996), *J Vet Intern Med* 13:408–412, 1999.
23. Turrel JM, Fike JR, LeCouteur RA, et al: Radiotherapy of brain tumors in dogs, *J Am Vet Med Assoc* 184:82–86, 1984.
24. Bley CR, Sumova A, Roos M, et al: Irradiation of brain tumors in dogs with neurologic disease, *J Vet Intern Med* 19:849–854, 2005.
25. Schultheiss TE, Kun LE, Ang KK, et al: Radiation response of the central nervous system, *Int J Radiation Oncology Biol Phys* 31:1093–1112, 1995.
26. Heidner GL, Kornegay JN, Page RL, et al: Analysis of survival in a retrospective study of 86 dogs with brain tumors, *J Vet Intern Med* 5:219–226, 1991.

27. Spugnini EP, Thrall DE, Price GS, et al: Primary irradiation of canine intracranial masses, *Vet Radiol Ultrasound* 41:377–380, 2000.
28. Axlund TW, McGlasson ML, Smith AN: Surgery alone or in combination with radiation therapy for treatment of intracranial meningiomas in dogs: 31 cases (1989-2002), *J Am Vet Med Assoc* 221:1597–1600, 2002.
29. Théon AP, LeCouteur RA, Carr EA, et al: Influence of tumor cell proliferation and sex-hormone receptors on effectiveness of radiation therapy for dogs with incompletely resected meningiomas, *J Am Vet Med Assoc* 216:701–707, 2000.
30. Bergman R, Jones J, Lanz O, et al: Post-operative computed tomography in two dogs with cerebral meningioma, *Vet Radiol Ultrasound* 41:425–432, 2000.
31. Klopp LS, Rao S: Endoscopic-assisted intracranial tumor removal in dogs and cats: long-term outcome of 39 cases, *J Vet Intern Med* 23:108–115, 2009.
32. O'Brien CS, Bagley RS, Hicks DG, et al: Gamma-irradiated calvarium allograft cranioplasty in a cat following brain tumor removal, *J Am Anim Hosp Assoc* 46:268–273, 2010.
33. Bordelon JT, Rochat MC: Use of a titanium mesh for cranioplasty following radical rostrotentorial craniectomy to remove an ossifying fibroma in a dog, *J Am Vet Med Assoc* 231:1692–1695, 2007.
34. Gordon PN, Kornegay JN, Lattimer JC, et al: Use of a rivet-like titanium clamp closure system to replace an external frontal bone flap after transfrontal craniotomy in a dog, *J Am Vet Med Assoc* 226:752–755, 2005.
35. Bryant KJ, Steinberg H, McAnulty JF: Cranioplasty by means of molded polymethylmethacrylate prosthetic reconstruction after radical excision of neoplasms of the skull in two dogs, *J Am Vet Med Assoc* 223:67–72, 2003.
36. Son SH, Kang YN, Ryu MR: The effect of metallic implants on radiation therapy in spinal tumor patients with metallic spinal implants, *Med Dosim* 37(1):98–107, 2011.
37. Pekmezci M, Dirican B, Yapici B, et al: Spinal implants and radiation therapy: the effect of various configurations of titanium implant systems in a single-level vertebral metastasis model, *J Bone Joint Surg* 88:1093–1100, 2006.
38. Heading KL, Brockley LK, Bennett PF: CCNU (lomustine) toxicity in dogs: a retrospective study (2002-07), *Aust Vet J* 89:109–116, 2011.
39. Fulton LM, Steinberg HS: Preliminary study of lomustine in the treatment of intracranial masses in dogs following localization by imaging techniques, *Sem Vet Med Surg* (Sm Anim) 5:241–245, 1990.
40. Dimski DS, Cook JR: Carmustine-induced partial remission of an astrocytoma in a dog, *J Am Anim Hosp Assoc* 26:179–182, 1990.
41. Tamura S, Tamura Y, Ohoka A, et al: A canine case of skull base meningioma treated with hydroxyurea, *J Vet Med Sci* 69:1313–1315, 2007.
42. Jung D, Kim H, Park C, et al: Long-term chemotherapy with lomustine of intracranial meningioma occurring in a miniature schnauzer, *J Vet Med Sci* 68:383–386, 2006.
43. McDonnell JJ, Kalbko K, Keating JH, et al: Multiple meningiomas in three dogs, *J Am Anim Hosp Assoc* 43:201–208, 2007.
44. Greco JJ, Aiken SA, Berg JM, et al: Evaluation of intracranial meningioma resection with a surgical aspirator in dogs: 17 cases (1996-2004), *J Am Vet Med Assoc* 229:394–400, 2006.
45. Cautela MA, Dewey CW, Cerda-Gonzalez S, et al: Oral hydroxyurea therapy for dogs with suspected intracranial meningioma: a retrospective cohort study (2004-2009), *J Vet Intern Med* 23:737, 2009.
46. Thrall DE, LaRue SM, Powers BE, et al: Use of whole body hyperthermia as a method to heat inaccessible tumours uniformly: a phase III trial in canine brain masses, *Int J Hyperthermia* 15:383–398, 1999.
47. Chauvet AE, Kesava PP, Goh CS, et al: Selective intraarterial gene delivery into a canine meningioma, *J Neurosurg* 88:870–873, 1998.
48. LeCouteur RA: Current concepts in the diagnosis and treatment of brain tumors in dogs and cats, *J Small Anim Pract* 40:411–416, 1999.
49. Candolfi M, Pluhar GE, Kroeger K, et al: Optimization of adenoviral vector-mediated transgene expression in the canine brain in vivo, and in canine glioma cells in vitro, *Neuro Oncol* 9:245–258, 2007.
50. Oh S, Pluhar GE, McNeil EA, et al: Efficacy of nonviral gene transfer in the canine brain, *J Neurosurg* 107:136–144, 2007.
51. Dickinson PJ, LeCouteur RA, Higgins RJ, et al: Canine spontaneous glioma: a translational model system for convection-enhanced delivery, *Neuro Oncol* 12:928–940, 2010.
52. Dickinson PJ, LeCouteur RA, Higgins RJ, et al: Canine model of convection-enhanced delivery of liposomes containing CPT-11 monitored with real-time magnetic resonance imaging, *J Neurosurg* 108:989–998, 2008.
53. Packer RA, Freeman LJ, Miller MA, et al: Evaluation of minimally invasive excisional brain biopsy and intracranial brachytherapy catheter placement in dogs, *Am J Vet Res* 72:109–121, 2011.
54. Platt SR, Scase TJ, Adams V, et al: Vascular endothelial growth factor expression in canine intracranial meningiomas and association with patient survival, *J Vet Intern Med* 20:663–668, 2006.
55. Platt SR: Angiogenesis and cerebral neoplasia, *Vet Comp Oncol* 3:123–138, 2005.
56. MacLeod AG, Dickinson PJ, LeCouteur RA, et al: Quantitative assessment of blood volume and permeability in cerebral mass lesions using dynamic contrast-enhanced computed tomography in the dog, *Acad Radiol* 16:1187–1195, 2009.
57. Wisner ER, Dickinson PJ, Higgins RJ: Magnetic resonance imaging features of canine intracranial neoplasia, *Vet Radiol Ultrasound* 52:S52–S61, 2011.
58. Singh JB, Oevermann A, Lang J, et al: Contrast media enhancement of intracranial lesions in magnetic resonance imaging does not reflect histopathologic findings consistently, *Vet Radiol Ultrasound* 52:619–626, 2011.
59. Vernau KM, Higgins RJ, Bollen AW, et al: Primary canine and feline nervous system tumors: intraoperative diagnosis using the smear technique, *Vet Pathol* 38:47–57, 2001.
60. Koblik PD, LeCouteur RA, Higgins RJ, et al: CT-guided brain biopsy using a modified Pelorus mark III stereotactic system: experience with 50 dogs, *Vet Radiol Ultrasound* 40:434–440, 1999.
61. Koblik PD, LeCouteur RA, Higgins RJ, et al: Modification and application of a Pelorus mark II stereotactic system for CT-guided brain biopsy in 50 dogs, *Vet Radiol Ultrasound* 40:424–433, 1999.
62. Moissonnier P, Blot S, Devauchelle P, et al: Stereotactic CT-guided brain biopsy in the dog, *J Small Anim Pract* 43:115–123, 2002.
63. De Lorenzi D, Mandara MT, Tranquillo M, et al: Squash-prep cytology in the diagnosis of canine and feline nervous system lesions: a study of 42 cases, *Vet Clin Pathol* 35:208–214, 2006.
64. Klopp LS, Ridgway M: Use of an endoscope in minimally invasive lesion biopsy and removal within the skull and cranial vault in two dogs and one cat, *J Am Vet Med Assoc* 234:1573–1577, 2009.
65. Fransson BA, Bagley RS, Gay JM, et al: Pneumonia after intracranial surgery in dogs, *Vet Surg* 30:432–439, 2001.
66. Matiasek LA, Platt SR, Adams V, et al: Ki-67 and vascular endothelial growth factor expression in intracranial meningiomas in dogs, *J Vet Intern Med* 23:146–151, 2009.
67. Adamo PF, Cantile C, Steinberg H: Evaluation of progesterone and estrogen receptor expression in 15 meningiomas of dogs and cats, *Am J Vet Res* 64:1310–1318, 2003.
68. Rossmeisl JH, Robertson JL, Zimmerman KL, et al: Cyclooxygenase-2 (COX-2) expression in canine intracranial meningiomas, *Vet Comp Oncol* 7:173–180, 2009.
69. Jankovsky JM, Newkirk KM, Ilha MR, et al: COX-2 and c-kit expression in canine gliomas, *Vet Comp Oncol* 23 Nov 2011 Epub.
70. Stoica G, Levine J, Wolff J, et al: Canine astrocytic tumors: a comparative review, *Vet Pathol* 48:266–275, 2011.
71. Frenier SL, Kraft SL, Moore MP, et al: Canine intracranial astrocytomas and comparison with the human counterpart, *Comp Cont Educ Small Anim* 12:1422–1433, 1990.
72. Chandra AM, Ginn PE: Primary malignant histiocytosis of the brain in a dog, *J Comp Pathol* 121:77–82, 1999.

73. Uchida K, Morozumi M, Yamaguchi R, et al: Diffuse leptomeningeal malignant histiocytosis in the brain and spinal cord of a Tibetan terrier, *Vet Pathol* 38:219–222, 2001.
74. Zimmerman K, Almy F, Carter L, et al: Cerebrospinal fluid from a 10-year-old dog with a single seizure episode, *Vet Clin Pathol* 35:127–131, 2006.
75. Ide T, Uchida K, Kagawa Y, et al: Pathological and immunohistochemical features of subdural histiocytic sarcomas in 15 dogs, *J Vet Diagn Invest* 23:127–132, 2011.
76. Tzipory L, Vernau KM, Sturges BK, et al: Antemortem diagnosis of localized central nervous system histiocytic sarcoma in 2 dogs, *J Vet Intern Med* 23:369–374, 2009.
77. Courtay-Cahen C, Platt SR, De Risio L, et al: Preliminary analysis of genomic abnormalities in canine meningiomas, *Vet Comp Oncol* 6:182–192, 2008.
78. Dickinson PJ, Roberts BN, Higgins RJ, et al: Expression of receptor tyrosine kinases VEGFR-1 (FLT-1), VEGFR-2 (KDR), EGFR-1, PDGFRα and c-Met in canine primary brain tumours, *Vet Comp Oncol* 4:132–140, 2006.
79. Dickinson PJ, Surace EI, Campbell M, et al: Expression of the tumor suppressor genes NF2, 4.1B, and TSLC1 in canine meningiomas, *Vet Pathol* 46:884–892, 2009.
80. Dickinson PJ, Sturges BK, Higgins RJ, et al: Vascular endothelial growth factor mRNA expression and peritumoral edema in canine primary central nervous system tumors, *Vet Pathol* 45:131–139, 2008.
81. Higgins RJ, Dickinson PJ, LeCouteur RA, et al: Spontaneous canine gliomas: overexpression of EGFR PDGFRα and IGFBP2 demonstrated b tissue microarray immunophenotyping, *J Neurooncol* 98:49–55, 2010.
82. Thomson SAM, Kennerly E, Olby N, et al: Microarray analysis of differentially expressed genes of primary tumors in the canine central nervous system, *Vet Pathol* 42:550–558, 2005.
83. York D, Higgins RJ, LeCouteur RA, et al: TP53 mutations in canine brain tumors, *Vet Pathol* Epub 2012 March 12.
84. Chamberlain MC, Barnholtz-Sloan JS: Medical treatment of recurrent meningiomas, *Expert Rev Neurother* 11:1425–1432, 2011.
85. Stacy BA, Stevenson TL, Lipsitz D, et al: Simultaneously occurring oligodendroglioma and meningioma in a dog, *J Vet Intern Med* 17:357–359, 2003.
86. Lobetti RG, Nesbit JW, Miller DB: Multiple malignant meningiomas in a young cat, *J S Afr Vet Assoc* 68:62–65, 1997.
87. Patnaik AK, Kay WJ, Hurvitz AI: Intracranial meningioma: a comparative pathologic study of 28 dogs, *Vet Pathol* 23:369–373, 1986.
88. Koch MW, Sánchez MD, Long S: Multifocal oligodendroglioma in three dogs, *J Am Anim Hosp Assoc* 47:77–85, 2011.
89. Alves A, Prada J, Almeida JM, et al: Primary and secondary tumours occurring simultaneously in the brain of a dog, *J Small Anim Pract* 47:607–610, 2006.
90. Schulman FY, Ribas JL, Carpenter JL, et al: Intracranial meningioma with pulmonary metastasis in three dogs, *Vet Pathol* 29:196–202, 1992.
91. Forterre F, Tomek A, Konar M, et al: Multiple meningiomas: clinical, radiological, surgical and pathological findings with outcome in four cats, *J Feline Med Surg* 9:36–43, 2007.
92. Zaki FA, Hurvitz AI: Spontaneous neoplasms of the central nervous system of the cat, *J Small Anim Pract* 17:773–782, 1976.
93. Waters DJ, Hayden DW, Walter PA: Intracranial lesions in dogs with hemangiosarcoma, *J Vet Intern Med* 3:222–230, 1989.
94. Mandara MT, Rossi F, Lepri E, et al: Cerebellar leptomeningeal carcinomatosis in a dog, *J Small Anim Pract* 48:504–507, 2007.
95. Mateo I, Lorenzo V, Munoz A, et al: Meningeal carcinomatosis in a dog: magnetic resonance imaging features and pathological correlation, *J Small Anim Pract* 51:43–48, 2010.
96. Patnaik AK, Erlandson RA, Lieberman PH, et al: Choroid plexus carcinoma with meningeal carcinomatosis in a dog, *Vet Pathol* 17:381–385, 1980.
97. Gallagher JG, Berg J, Knowles KE, et al: Prognosis after surgical excision of cerebral meningiomas in cats: 17 cases (1986-1992), *J Am Vet Med Assoc* 203:1437–1440, 1993.
98. Lawson DC, Burk RL, Prata RG: Cerebral meningioma in the cat: diagnosis and surgical treatment of ten cases, *J Am Anim Hosp Assoc* 20:333–342, 1984.
99. Dickinson PJ, Keel MK, Higgins RJ, et al: Clinical and pathologic features of oligodendrogliomas in two cats, *Vet Pathol* 37:160–167, 2000.
100. Sarfaty D, Carrillo JM, Patnaik AK: Cerebral astrocytoma in four cats: clinical and pathological findings, *J Am Vet Med Assoc* 191:976–978, 1987.
101. Ostrum QT, Barnholtz-Sloan JS: Current state of our knowledge on brain tumor epidemiology, *Curr Neurol Neurosci Rep* 11:329–335, 2011.
102. Preusser M, deRibaupierre S, Wohrer A, et al: Current concepts and management of glioblastoma, *Ann Neurol* 70:9–21, 2011.
103. Mawrin C, Perry A: Pathological classification and molecular genetics of meningiomas, *J Neurooncol* 99:379–391, 2010.
104. Wen PY, Quant E, Drappatz J, et al: Medical therapies for meningiomas, *J Neurooncol* 99:365–378, 2010.
105. Dewey CW: Myelopathies: disorders of the spinal cord. In Dewey CW, editor: *A practical guide to canine and feline neurology*, ed 2, Ames, Iowa, 2008, Wiley-Blackwell.
106. Bagley RS: Spinal neoplasms in small animals, *Vet Clin Small Anim* 40:915–927, 2010.
107. Marioni-Henry K, Van Winkle TJ, Smith SH, et al: Tumors affecting the spinal cord of cats: 85 cases (1980-2005), *J Am Vet Med Assoc* 232:237–243, 2008.
108. Marioni-Henry K: Feline spinal cord diseases, *Vet Clin Small Anim* 40:1011–1028, 2010.
109. Petersen SA, Sturges BK, Dickinson PJ, et al: Canine intraspinal meningiomas: imaging features, histopathologic classification, and long-term outcome in 34 dogs, *J Vet Intern Med* 22:946–953, 2008.
110. Johnson KB, Manhart K, Vite C, et al: 399 spinal tumors in dogs (abstract), *J Vet Intern Med* 21:639–640, 2007.
111. Brewer DM, Cerda-Gonzalez S, Dewey CW, et al: Spinal cord nephroblastoma in dogs: 11 cases (1985-2007), *J Am Vet Med Assoc* 238:618–624, 2011.
112. Liebel FX, Rossmeisl JH, Lanz OI, et al: Canine spinal nephroblastoma: long-term outcomes associated with treatment of 10 cases (1996-2009), *Vet Surg* 40:244–252, 2011.
113. Ueno H, Miyake T, Kobayashi Y, et al: Epidural spinal myelolipoma in a dog, *J Am Anim Hosp Assoc* 43:132–135, 2007.
114. Rodenas S, Valin I, Devauchelle P, et al: Combined use of surgery and radiation in the treatment of an intradural myxoid liposarcoma in a dog, *J Am Anim Hosp Assoc* 42:386–391, 2006.
115. Morgan LW, Toal R, Siemering G, et al: Imaging diagnosis-infiltrative lipoma causing spinal cord compression in a dog, *Vet Rad Ultrasound* 48:35–37, 2007.
116. Siegel S, Kornegay JN, Thrall DE: Postoperative irradiation of spinal cord tumors in 9 dogs, *Vet Radiol Ultrasound* 37:150–153, 1996.
117. Bell FW, Feeney DA, O'Brien TJ, et al: External beam radiation therapy for recurrent intraspinal meningioma in a dog, *J Am Anim Hosp Assoc* 28:318–322, 1992.
118. Levy MS, Kapatkin AS, Patnaik AK, et al: Spinal tumors in 37 dogs: clinical outcome and long-term survival (1987-1994), *J Am Anim Hosp Assoc* 33:307–312, 1997.
119. Fingeroth JM, Prata RG, Patnaik AK: Spinal meningiomas in dogs: 13 cases (1972-1987), *J Am Vet Med Assoc* 191:720–726, 1987.
120. Powers BE, Beck ER, Gillette EL, et al: Pathology of radiation injury to the canine spinal cord, *Int J Radiation Oncology Biol Phys* 23:539–549, 1992.
121. Dickinson PJ, McEntee MC, Lipsitz D, et al: Radiation induced vertebral osteosarcoma following treatment of an intradural extramedullary spinal cord tumor in a dog, *Vet Radiol Ultrasound* 42:463–470, 2001.

122. Macri NP, Van Alstine W, Coolman RA: Canine spinal nephroblastoma, *J Am Anim Hosp Assoc* 33:302–306, 1997.
123. Terrell SP, Platt SR, Chrisman CL, et al: Possible intraspinal metastasis of a canine spinal cord nephroblastoma, *Vet Pathol* 37:94–97, 2000.
124. Jull P, Walmsley GL, Benigni L, et al: Imaging diagnosis – spinal cord hemangioma in two dogs, *Vet Radiol Ultrasound* 52:653–657, 2011.
125. Rossmeisl JH, Lanz OI, Waldron DR, et al: Surgical cytoreduction for the treatment of non-lymphoid vertebral and spinal cord neoplasms in cats: retrospective evaluation of 26 cases (1990-2005), *Vet Com Oncol* 4:411–450, 2006.
126. Lane SB, Kornegay JN, Duncan JR, et al: Feline spinal lymphosarcoma: a retrospective evaluation of 23 cats, *J Vet Intern Med* 8:99–104, 1994.
127. Spodnick GJ, Berg J, Moore FM, et al: Spinal lymphoma in cats: 21 cases (1976-1989), *J Am Vet Med Assoc* 200:373–376, 1992.
128. Marioni-Henry K, Vite CH, Newton AL, et al: Prevalence of disease of the spinal cord of cats, *J Vet Intern Med* 18:851–858, 2004.
129. Haynes JS, Leininger JR: A glioma in the spinal cord of a cat, *Vet Pathol* 19:713–715, 1982.
130. Barnhart KF, Wojcieszyn J, Storts RW: Immunohistochemical staining patterns of canine meningiomas and correlation with published immunophenotypes, *Vet Pathol* 39:311–321, 2002.
131. Levy MS, Mauldin G, Kapatkin AS, et al: Nonlymphoid vertebral canal tumors in cats: 11 cases (1987-1995), *J Am Vet Med Assoc* 210:663–664, 1997.
132. Chamberlain MC, Tredway TL: Adult primary intradural spinal cord tumors: a review, *Curr Neurol Neurosci Rep* 11:320–328, 2011.
133. Taylor JW, Schiff D: Metastatic epidural spinal cord compression, *Semin Neurol* 30:245–253, 2010.
134. Quraishi NA, Gokaslan ZL, Boriani S: The surgical management of metastatic epidural compression of the spinal cord, *J Bone Joint Surg* 92B:1054–1060, 2010.
135. Dewey CW: Disorders of the peripheral nervous system: mononeuropathies and polyneuropathies. In Dewey CW, editor: *A practical guide to canine and feline neurology*, ed 2, Ames, Iowa, 2008, Wiley-Blackwell.
136. Targett MP, Dyce J, Houlton JEF: Tumours involving the nerve sheaths of the forelimb in dogs, *J Small Anim Pract* 34:221–225, 1993.
137. Brehm DM, Vite CH, Steinberg HS, et al: A retrospective evaluation of 51 cases of peripheral nerve sheath tumors in the dog, *J Am Anim Hosp Assoc* 31:349–359, 1995.
138. Summers BA, Cummings JF, deLahunta A: Diseases of the peripheral nervous system. In Summers BA, Cummings JF, deLahunta A, editors: *Veterinary neuropathology*, St Louis, 1995, Mosby.
139. Chijiwa K, Uchida K, Tateyama S: Immunohistochemical evaluation of canine peripheral nerve sheath tumors and other soft tissue sarcomas, *Vet Pathol* 41:307–318, 2004.
140. Schulman FY, Johnson TO, Facemire PR, et al: Feline peripheral nerve sheath tumors: histologic, immunohistochemical, and clinicopathologic correlation (59 tumors in 53 cats), *Vet Pathol* 46:1166–1180, 2009.
141. Bagley RS, Wheeler SJ, Klopp L, et al: Clinical features of trigeminal nerve-sheath tumor in 10 dogs, *J Am Anim Hosp Assoc* 34:19–25, 1998.
142. Schultz RM, Tucker RL, Gavin PR, et al: Magnetic resonance imaging of acquired trigeminal nerve disorders in six dogs, *Vet Rad Ultrasound* 48:101–104, 2007.
143. Kraft S, Ehrhart EJ, Gall D, et al: Magnetic resonance imaging characteristics of peripheral nerve sheath tumors of the canine brachial plexus in 18 dogs, *Vet Rad Ultrasound* 48:1–7, 2007.
144. Rose S, Long C, Knipe M, et al: Ultrasonographic evaluation of brachial plexus tumors in five dogs, *Vet Rad Ultrasound* 46:514–517, 2005.
145. daCosta RC, Parent JM, Dobson H, et al: Ultrasound-guided fine needle aspiration in the diagnosis of peripheral nerve sheath tumors in 4 dogs, *Can Vet J* 49:77–81, 2008.
146. Sharp NJH: Craniolateral approach to the canine brachial plexus, *Vet Surg* 17:18–21, 1988.
147. Bradley RL, Withrow SJ, Snyder SP: Nerve sheath tumors in the dog, *J Am Anim Hosp Assoc* 18:915–921, 1982.
148. Bailey CS: Long-term survival after surgical excision of a schwannoma of the sixth cervical spinal nerve in a dog, *J Am Vet Med Assoc* 196:754–756, 1990.
149. Zachary JF, O'Brien DP, Ingles BW, et al: Multicentric nerve sheath fibrosarcomas of multiple cranial nerve roots in two dogs, *J Am Vet Med Assoc* 188:723–726, 1986.
150. Woertler K: Tumors and tumor-like lesions of peripheral nerves, *Semin Musculoskel Radiol* 14:547–558, 2010.
151. Clarke SE, Kaufman RA: Nerve tumors, *J Hand Surg Am* 2010:1520–1522, 2010.

Ocular Tumors 31

PAUL E. MILLER AND RICHARD R. DUBIELZIG

Tumors of the eye, orbit, or adnexa can have devastating consequences for an animal's vision, appearance, and comfort and may be harbingers of potentially life-threatening disease elsewhere in the body. By virtue of their location, even benign ocular tumors may cause blindness and loss of the eye. Although these tumors reportedly affected only 0.87% of all dogs and 0.34% of all cats recorded in the Veterinary Medical Data Base (VMDB) over a 10-year period, their actual frequency is undoubtedly greater because many presumably benign ocular tumors are not histologically examined. Additional insights into the relative frequency of ocular tumors can also be gained by reviewing submissions over several decades to the large ophthalmic pathology database compiled by the Comparative Ocular Pathology Laboratory of Wisconsin (COPLOW) (Figure 31-1). This chapter describes the more common ocular tumors in small animals and also uses the database of the COPLOW laboratory to estimate the relative frequency of various ocular tumors.

Tumors of the Eyelids, Third Eyelid, Conjunctiva, and Ocular Surface

Incidence and Risk Factors

Benign adenomas and melanomas of the haired skin or eyelid margin make up 81% of eyelid tumors in the COPLOW database and tend to affect old dogs. One study suggests Boxers, collies, Weimaraners, cocker spaniels, and springer spaniels are at greater risk for eyelid neoplasia than the general hospital population,[1] and another study suggests that beagles, Siberian huskies, and English setters are at greater risk than mixed-breed dogs.[2] Canine juvenile histiocytomas affect the eyelid skin of young to middle-aged dogs[1,2] but are relatively uncommon, comprising only 2% of eyelid biopsy samples submitted to COPLOW. Squamous cell carcinoma (SCC) comprises up to two-thirds of feline eyelid and third eyelid tumors and has a predilection for the lower eyelid and medial canthus of white cats.[3] Ocular SCC is less frequent in dogs, but in both cats and dogs increased exposure to solar radiation, lack of adnexal pigmentation, and possibly chronic ocular surface irritation are believed to be predisposing factors (Figure 31-2).[1,4,5]

Vascular endothelial cell tumors of the lateral limbus or the leading edge of the third eyelid constitute 27% of conjunctival tumors in dogs and tend to occur in the nonpigmented conjunctiva in Bassett hounds, springer spaniels and beagles. Melanomas often occur in dogs with a pigmented conjunctiva and are the most common malignant tumor of the canine conjunctiva, making up 17% of conjunctival tumor biopsies. Older (mean = 11 years), female, Weimaraner, and possibly German shepherd/large-breed dogs may be predisposed to conjunctival melanomas.[6] Melanomas also have a propensity for the nictitating membrane and superior palpebral conjunctiva.[6,7] Ocular viral papillomas compose about 3% of conjunctival tumors and tend to occur in young dogs and are believed to have a papillomavirus etiology (perhaps canine oral papillomavirus).[8] Canine squamous papilloma is a benign papillary tumor of unknown etiology and makes up 9% of conjunctival tumor biopsies. Reactive papilloma is seen secondary to other conditions such as meibomian tumors, but they make up 18% of conjunctival tumor biopsies. Corneal tumors have a predilection for the limbus.

Pathology and Natural Behavior

Sebaceous or meibomian gland adenomas and epitheliomas, papillomas, and melanomas comprise more than 85% of canine eyelid and conjunctival neoplasms, and a substantial majority of these tumors are histologically benign.[1,2] Even histologically malignant eyelid tumors in dogs rarely metastasize, although they are more likely to be locally invasive and recur following surgery.[1,2] In contrast, most feline eyelid and ocular surface tumors such as SCC are malignant.[3]

Viral papillomas tend to be well demarcated and superficial, minimally altering deeper tissues. Surgical manipulation has occasionally been associated with dispersal of papillomas throughout the ocular surface.[9,10] Papillomas, like histiocytomas, often spontaneously resolve in young dogs, although they may persist in the older dog. SCC may also develop superficially, but following malignant transformation the preinvasive actinic plaque can invade deeper tissues. SCC may spread to regional lymph nodes late in the course of the disease and uncommonly distantly metastasize. SCC of the third eyelid may more readily invade the orbit than corneal or eyelid SCC.

Adenocarcinomas of the gland of the third eyelid constitute 13% of conjunctival tumors in dogs. They are variable in morphology and often show moderate infiltrative growth.[11] They may mimic prolapse of the gland of the nictitans ("cherry eye") by appearing as localized, firm, smooth, pink swellings on the posterior surface of the nictitans, but a key differentiating feature is their occurrence in much older dogs (10 to 16 years). Although excision of the grossly visible tumor may initially appear adequate, recurrence is common if the entire gland is not removed, and metastasis, especially to the regional lymph nodes and orbit, is possible.[11,12]

The natural behavior of conjunctival vascular, melanocytic, and mast cell tumors is poorly understood, in part because they are uncommon. Conjunctival hemangiomas and hemangiosarcomas tend to remain relatively superficial but may recur following simple excision.[13-17] Hemangiosarcomas may exhibit a more aggressive course and a primary ocular hemangiosarcoma must be differentiated from a metastatic lesion. However, metastasis of primary conjunctival vascular tumors, even when classified as hemangiosarcomas, appears to be rare.[13-17]

Feline conjunctival melanomas originate on the bulbar conjunctiva and invade the eyelid.[18,19] Melanoma of the conjunctiva in dogs is most often morphologically malignant, but metastatic disease is not common. As in cats, canine conjunctival melanomas have been reported to recur locally following surgical excision in 55% of cases, and at least 17% of the dogs experienced orbital invasion or spread to the regional lymph nodes or lungs.[6] Melanomas originating from the palpebral conjunctiva may have greater metastatic potential.[6] Mitotic index, cell type, and degree of pigmentation are not useful predictors of malignancy for canine conjunctival melanomas.[6] Subconjunctival mast cell tumors make up 4% of conjunctival tumors, but their natural history is poorly understood in part because they are uncommon. Nevertheless, they have been suggested to have a relatively benign course in dogs.[20]

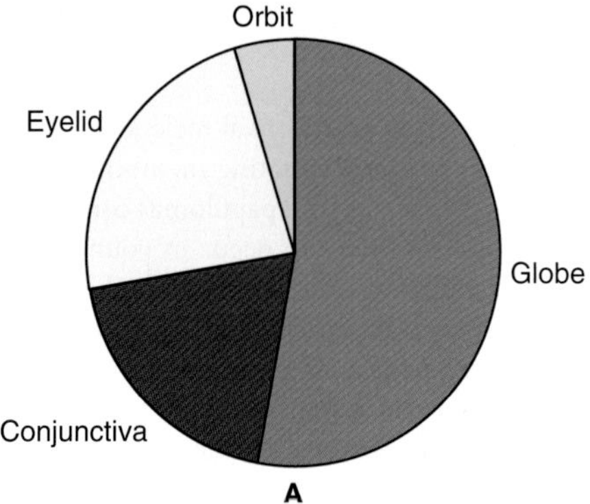

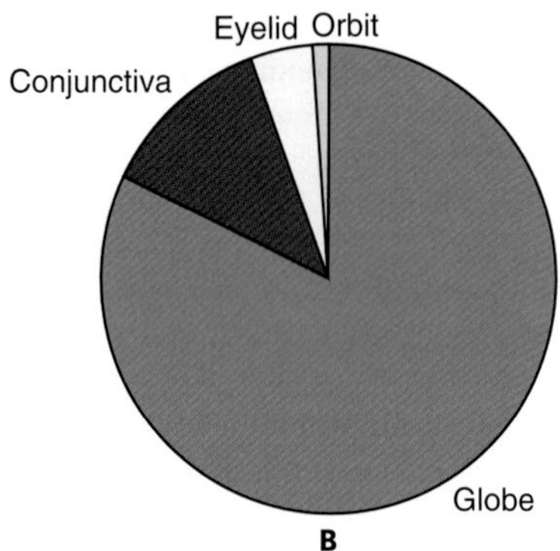

FIGURE 31-1 The distribution of canine **(A)** and feline **(B)** ocular tumors submitted to the Comparative Ocular Pathology Laboratory of Wisconsin.

History and Clinical Signs

Vascular tumors are often focal, raised, soft, red masses with visible feeder vessels arising from the surface of the conjunctiva or third eyelid.[13-17] SCC of the eyelid, third eyelid, or ocular surface may appear as a focally thickened, roughened, and usually pink-to-red lesion in older animals or, more commonly, as an ulcerated lesion with a protracted course.[3-5] In contrast, papillomas in young dogs appear verrucous and usually progress rapidly over weeks to a few months. Nonneoplastic conditions such as nodular granulomatous episcleritis can be mistaken for neoplasia.

In addition to a mass lesion, other clinical signs of eyelid or ocular surface tumors may include epiphora, conjunctival vascular injection, mucopurulent ocular discharge, protrusion of the third eyelid, conjunctival/corneal roughening or ulceration, and corneal neovascularization or pigmentation. Occasionally, palpebral conjunctival masses protrude only when their bulk no longer can be accommodated by the space between the eyelid and globe, and very advanced tumors may create exophthalmia or enophthalmia if the orbit is invaded. Large tumors and sebaceous adenomas often have a substantial inflammatory component and may be secondarily infected. Mesenchymal hamartoma appears to have a predisposition for the skin of lateral canthus.[21]

Diagnostic Techniques and Work-Up

In addition to fluorescein staining and examination of the ocular surface with a cobalt filter or black light, the extent of involvement of the bulbar and palpebral conjunctiva should be determined by everting the eyelid (and third eyelid if affected). Careful palpation of the lesion by inserting a lubricated finger in the conjunctival cul-de-sac can be invaluable for determining the full extent of the tumor and whether bony involvement has occurred. Nasolacrimal

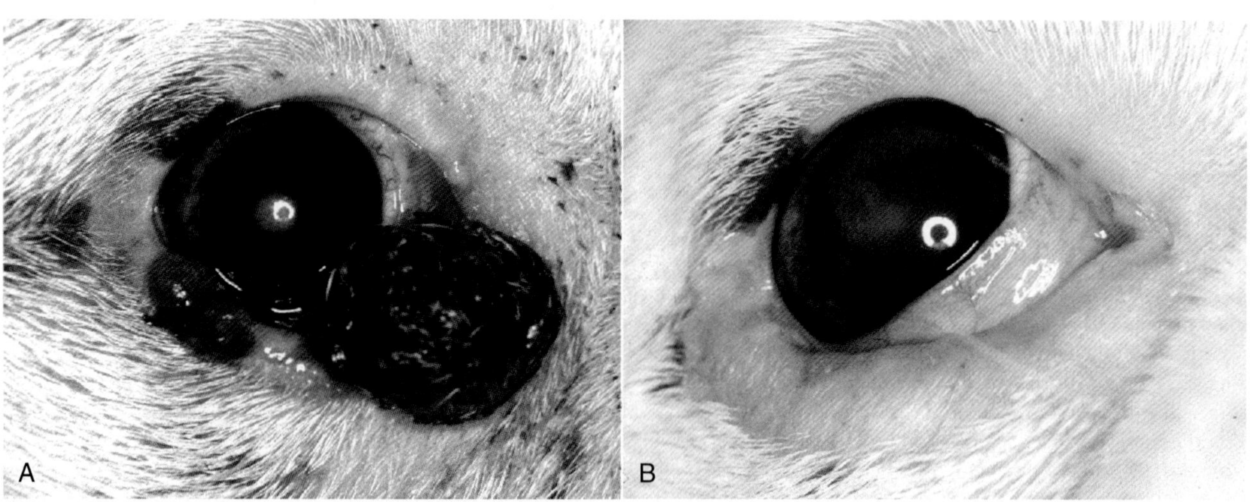

FIGURE 31-2 **A,** Squamous cell carcinoma affecting the lower eyelids of a Boxer. **B,** Same dog after cryosurgical ablation of the tumor. Lid function is spared.

lavage and possibly positive contrast dacryocystorhinography may help characterize medial canthal masses. In general, small eyelid and ocular surface tumors are best diagnosed and treated by excisional biopsy. Fine-needle aspiration (FNA) or incisional biopsies of larger tumors aid in determining prognosis and planning definitive therapy. Occasionally, orbital ultrasound, skull radiographs, computed tomography (CT), magnetic resonance imaging (MRI), regional lymph node cytology, and thoracic radiographs are required to localize or clinically stage potentially malignant tumors such as SCC, mast cell tumors, adenocarcinomas of the third eyelid, and conjunctival melanomas.

Therapy

Specific therapy varies with the type of tumor; its location, size, and extent; whether the eye still has useful vision; the animal's expected lifespan; the degree of discomfort the mass is creating; and the owner's financial limitations. All eyelid tumors, whether benign or malignant, have the potential to affect vision or ocular comfort. Indications for tumor removal include any eyelid tumor in a cat, rapid growth, ocular surface irritation, impaired eyelid function, owner concern, or an unappealing appearance. In young dogs, observation of nonirritating papillomas or histiocytomas, even if quite large, may be appropriate as spontaneous regression is common.

Tumors involving less than one-fourth to one-third of the length of the eyelid are best treated by a V-plasty (wedge) or four-sided excision.[22] The latter technique affords superior apposition of the eyelid margins and wound stability, especially in tumors approaching the one-fourth to one-third limit, because the initial incision is made perpendicular to the eyelid margin rather than obliquely. In general, only one-third to one-fourth of the eyelid in dogs and one-fourth of the eyelid in cats can be removed with these techniques. Antibiotic or antiinflammatory therapy may reduce the size of large tumors that are infected or inflamed so that a wedge or four-sided excision becomes possible. Electrosurgical excision should be avoided because it may result in substantial scarring of the eyelids. Carbon dioxide (CO_2) laser ablation may be appropriate for some tumors.

Tumors greater than one-fourth to one-third of the eyelid typically require more advanced reconstructive blepharoplasty or utilization of other therapeutic modalities. Some tumors may be responsive to systemic chemotherapy (e.g., lymphoma, mast cell tumors), local infiltration with chemotherapeutic agents such as cisplatin (e.g., SCC),[23] and/or local radiation therapy (RT; e.g., SCC). In some cases, these modalities will completely eliminate the tumor or shrink it to the point in which a less extensive surgical procedure can be performed. Reconstructive blepharoplasty, however, is the procedure of choice if surgical cure is a possibility and these other modalities have failed or are unlikely to substantially impact the tumor or if the nature of the tumor indicates extensive margins are required.

Cryosurgery is an attractive alternative to extensive blepharoplasty and has been reported to be effective in several canine eyelid tumor types (see Figure 31-2, see also Chapter 10).[2,24] It is quick, less technically demanding than reconstructive blepharoplasty, and usually permits preservation of the nasolacrimal puncta and canaliculus. In many old or debilitated patients, cryosurgery can be accomplished with only sedation or local/topical anesthesia. Following pretreatment with dexamethasone (0.1 mg/kg intravenous [IV]), the mass is isolated with a chalazion forceps (if possible) and debulked flush with the lid margin. Using liquid nitrogen and a closed probe that approximates the diameter of the mass as much as possible, a double freeze-thaw is performed so that the iceball extends 3 to 5 mm beyond the visible margins of the mass. Iceballs should overlap in large tumors. Freezing may be repeated a second or third time if complete regression is not achieved following the first session. Substantial postoperative swelling and usually transient depigmentation of the frozen tissue are to be expected.

Tumors involving the conjunctiva and third eyelid (especially conjunctival hemangiosarcomas, melanomas, and nictitans adenocarcinomas) are most effectively treated by wide surgical excision—perhaps to the point of exenterating the orbit. If the globe is to be spared, however, excision of the entire nictitans should not be taken lightly because undesirable sequelae such as ocular drying and chronic keratitis frequently result. Bulbar conjunctival tumors move freely and, if small, are generally amenable to excision under only topical anesthesia and perhaps sedation. Cryosurgery may permit the nictitans to be spared in the cases of papillomas and early SCC, or it can be used as an adjunct to excision in advanced canine conjunctival melanomas and SCC.[6,24]

Superficial keratectomy/sclerectomy is preferred for many corneal and scleral tumors, although some tumors require a full-thickness resection of the cornea or sclera. In the latter case, corneal or scleral allografts or autologous tissue grafts should be used to maintain ocular structural integrity. Limbal SCC and epibulbar melanoma may also be amenable to cryosurgery, although the iceball should be carefully monitored to avoid unnecessary freezing of intraocular structures.

Prognosis

The prognosis for most canine primary eyelid tumors is excellent, whether treated by excision or cryosurgery. Metastasis is rare, even in histologically malignant primary lid tumors, and recurrence rates are low (approximately 10% to 15%).[2] New primary eyelid tumors are not uncommon and must be distinguished from recurrence. Because most eyelid tumors in cats are malignant, the prognosis is not as good as that for dogs, but it is unclear how prognosis correlates with the histologic features. Conjunctival melanomas and nictitans adenocarcinomas frequently recur following partial excision of the nictitans, even if all of the clinically visible tumor was removed.[6] Conjunctival hemangiosarcomas appear to have a good prognosis because total excision may be curative, although recurrence and loss of the eye is still possible.[13-17]

Limbal (Epibulbar) Melanomas

Limbal melanomas are typically benign, slightly raised, heavily pigmented masses originating from melanocytes in the sclera or subconjunctival connective tissue (Figure 31-3).[25-30] They comprise 3.5% of all canine ocular tumors and 1% of feline ocular tumor submissions to COPLOW. The majority of these slow-growing tumors originate in the superior limbal region, suggesting exposure to solar radiation may be a risk factor.[13] Affected dogs average 5 to 6 years old (cats 8+ years), and a female sex and German shepherd, golden retriever and Labrador retriever breed predilection has been inconsistently reported.[25-29] Confirmed metastasis has not been reported in dogs or cats and mitotic figures are rarely encountered; although in one study, two of four cats also had feline leukemia virus (FeLV)-associated lymphoma or leukemia, and a third cat had a second intraocular pigmented mass unassociated with the limbal tumor.[29] Lightly pigmented spindle cells capable of division are seen histologically, but the dominant cell is presumably a hypermature spindle cell that is large, round, pigment laden, and benign.[26] These masses are often only incidentally noted and the clinical signs

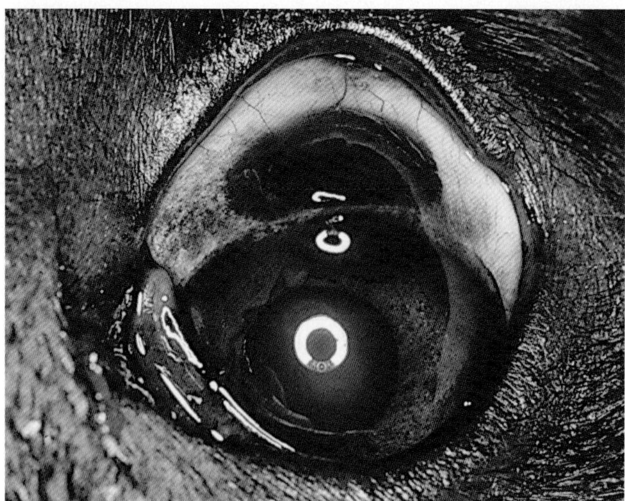

FIGURE 31-3 Epibulbar melanomas typically originate from the superior limbal region of the globe.

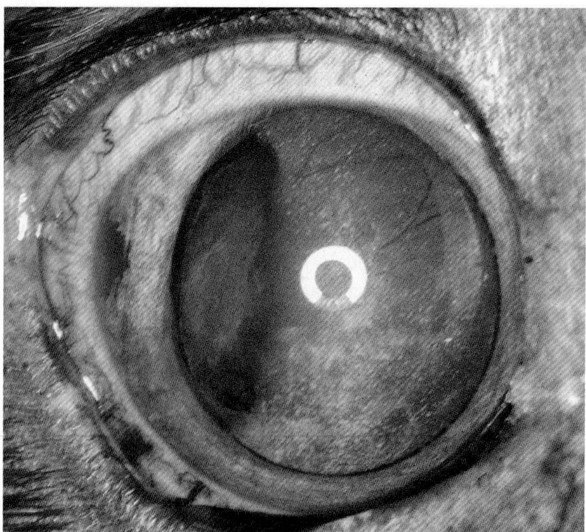

FIGURE 31-4 Most anterior uveal melanomas originate from the iris or ciliary body and are benign.

are typically minimal, although local corneal invasion, epiphora, and mild conjunctival irritation may be seen.[27,28] Differential diagnoses include conjunctival melanoma, invasive uveal melanoma, metastatic melanoma, and staphyloma or coloboma. Gonioscopy aids in differentiating invasive intraocular tumors from limbal melanomas.

Therapy should be considered if the tumor has invaded the eye or if growth is rapid. Given its benign nature and usually slow growth rate (imperceptible growth over 18 months has been described), observation alone may be appropriate in older dogs. If intervention is required, lamellar keratectomy/sclerectomy with graft placement is often curative.[31] Beta-irradiation and cryosurgery have been used as adjuncts to surgery.[31,32] Cryosurgery alone or laser photocoagulation[30] has also been described as effective means of treatment. Regrowth following local surgical excision occurs in approximately 30% of patients, but 2 to 3 years may pass before the anterior chamber is invaded and enucleation is required.[26-28] The addition of adjunctive therapy such as cryotherapy or beta-irradiation substantially reduces the risk of recurrence following local excision.[31,32] Enucleation is curative and indicated if painful intraocular disease is present.[26]

Primary Ocular Tumors

Canine Anterior Uveal Melanomas

Incidence and Risk Factors

In the Armed Forces Institute of Pathology collection of tumors from the canine eye, orbit, and adnexa, intraocular melanomas constitute 12%, other primary intraocular tumors 14%, and metastatic intraocular neoplasms 9%.[33] In the COPLOW archive, uveal melanocytic tumors make up 27% of all ocular tumor submissions. Any age is at risk, but most affected dogs are older than 7 years of age, and breed or sex predilections are inconsistent.[26]

Pathology and Natural Behavior

Approximately 78% of canine intraocular melanomas are benign, and 93% arise from the iris or ciliary body (Figure 31-4).[26,27,34] The most clinically useful classification scheme classifies these tumors simply as melanocytoma (benign) and melanoma (potentially malignant) based on nuclear features of the tumor cells—with mitotic rate being the most important.[26] Benign tumors have fewer than 2 mitotic figures/10 HPF (mitotic index), and malignant tumors demonstrate nuclear pleomorphism and a mitotic index of at least 4 and often more than 30. Destruction of the eye is not by itself sufficient for a diagnosis of malignancy.[26] The overall rate of metastasis of intraocular melanomas is approximately 4%[34] and usually occurs via the hematogenous route. Local spread along ocular vessels and nerves or via direct penetration of the sclera or cornea also occurs. Benign tumors tend to be more darkly pigmented than malignant tumors.[26]

Circumscribed, nevus-like pigmented iridal growths have been described in young dogs (7 months to 2 years old).[27] The natural history of these lesions is variable because enlargement may not occur over several years.[27,33] Some, however, are capable of rapid growth, but to date all are clinically and histologically benign.

Ocular melanosis of Cairn terriers resembles feline diffuse iris melanoma in some respects.[35] This disorder is probably an autosomal-dominant condition with a variable age of onset and rate of progression. It results in a thickening and pigmentation of the iris, release of pigment into the aqueous, pigment deposition in the sclera/episclera, and to a lesser extent posterior segment pigment deposition. Secondary glaucoma is common, and overt uveal melanocytic neoplasia occurs in a small percentage of dogs.[35]

History and Clinical Signs

Common presentations of intraocular tumors include a visible intraocular or scleral mass, glaucoma, hyphema, anterior uveitis, or extrabulbar spread, or they can be an incidental finding during an ophthalmic examination.[26,34] Because glaucoma or hyphema are often the only overtly visible clinical signs,[26,34] intraocular neoplasia should always be considered in animals with hyphema, glaucoma, or both when there is no history of trauma or coagulopathy. Small masses frequently create few symptoms other than pupillary distortion. Pigmentation is variable and not a reliable indicator of tumor type.

Diagnostic Techniques and Work-Up

Usually, the clinical or ultrasonographic appearance (if the media are opaque) is strongly suggestive of intraocular neoplasia, although it may be difficult to arrive at a definitive diagnosis without invading the eye or removing it because organizing blood clots are not always distinguishable from neoplastic mass lesions. Because most anterior uveal brown or black masses are cystic and not neoplastic, transillumination should be attempted before more invasive procedures. Uveal cysts typically permit bright light to pass through them, are roughly spherical, and may be attached to the ciliary body or free-floating in the anterior chamber. Once suspected, most primary canine intraocular tumors are observed for progression, although occasionally FNA (with its risks of inflammation, infection, and hemorrhage) or attempts at intraocular resection or enucleation are used for diagnostic purposes. The possibility of metastasis from another primary site (i.e., oral cavity or nail bed) to the eye or from the eye to other organs should be eliminated.

Therapy

Canine primary intraocular tumors are generally carefully observed. Digital photographs are a valuable aid in assessing progression. Enucleation is advised if there is concern about malignancy or if complications such as intractable uveitis or secondary glaucoma occur.[36] In the COPLOW collection, 14% of canine globes with glaucoma that are removed also had melanoma. The low risk of metastasis and unproved efficacy of enucleation at preventing metastasis in the few malignant tumors that have been reported, however, make it difficult to automatically advise enucleation of normotensive, noninflamed, visual eyes.[26] Isolated primary masses involving only the iris or a portion of the ciliary body may be amenable to local resection by sector iridectomy/cyclectomy in order to preserve the eye and vision.[27,33] These intraocular procedures, however, require an accomplished ophthalmic surgeon and often have unsatisfactory long-term results. Transscleral and transcorneal Nd:YAG or diode laser therapy has induced remission in some small- to moderate-sized primary intraocular tumors.[36,37] Specialized goniolens may also allow laser treatment of masses that have invaded into the iridocorneal angle. Although the results were variable, perhaps because these tumors varied histologically in nature, laser therapy holds promise for the palliation or potential cure of a number of intraocular tumor types while also preserving vision. Metastasis was not observed following this procedure, although this obviously remains a risk when the tumor is malignant.[36]

Prognosis

Although the data in most studies are heavily "censored," the prognosis for histologically benign melanomas appears to be excellent. Enucleation is curative, but attempts at local excision or laser photoablation may be only palliative, especially if the ciliary body or trabecular meshwork is involved. The presence of black, nonsolid material within the orbit following the enucleation of benign melanomas with scleral invasion apparently does not affect prognosis because these cells appear incapable of continued growth.[27] In one study, approximately 25% of histologically malignant melanomas demonstrated metastasis, typically within 3 months of enucleation, and most dogs with metastasis are euthanatized within 6 months of enucleation.[26] This surprisingly poor prognosis has not been the experience of cases followed recently in the COPLOW data set, and in a larger study, dogs with tumors classified as malignant were reported to have only a somewhat decreased survival time compared to dogs with melanocytoma and dogs from a control population.[38]

Choroidal Melanomas

Choroidal melanomas are rare intraocular melanocytic tumors, comprising only 4% to 7% of canine uveal melanomas, with no clear breed or sex predisposition.[39] Middle-aged (6 to 7 years), medium- to large-breed dogs predominate.[39] Generally, these tumors are well-delineated, raised subretinal pigmented masses with tapering margins, bulging centers, and a propensity for the peripapillary region and optic nerve.[39,40] In some cases, the tumor may remain virtually static for many years, whereas others exhibit infiltration into the overlying retina, through the sclera, up the optic nerve, and into the orbit.[39] Nuclear anaplasia is minimal and generally mitotic figures are absent.[40] Despite these benign cytologic features, metastasis has been described in one dog 21 months after exenteration, and follow-up in most studies is incomplete.[41] In general, however, these tumors appear to be benign in the vast majority of dogs. Most dogs with tumors involving a limited portion of the choroid are asymptomatic, and the mass is noted incidentally on ophthalmoscopy. Larger tumors frequently present with chronic uveitis, secondary glaucoma, retinal detachment, intraocular hemorrhage, or blindness.[39,40] Extension into the orbit can occur, and documentation of this is important in planning for enucleation surgery. Ocular ultrasonography may demonstrate mass lesions if anterior segment changes or retinal detachment obscures an underlying mass. Therapy usually consists of enucleation once progression has been documented or if the eye is painful. Diode laser ablation may offer an alternative to enucleation if the lesion is small and does not involve the optic nerve. Optic nerve or scleral invasion may warrant a more cautious prognosis.

Feline Primary Intraocular Melanomas (Feline Diffuse Iris Melanoma)

Incidence and Risk Factors

Anterior uveal melanomas are the most common primary intraocular tumor in cats (Figure 31-5).[42] They account for 49% of all neoplastic submissions to the COPLOW in cats. There appears to be no breed or sex predisposition, and most cats are more than 9 years of age at the time of diagnosis,[42,43] although the prodromal period for many of these tumors may be quite long.

Pathology and Natural Behavior

In the malignant form of uveal melanoma, the rate of metastasis (frequently to the liver and lungs) has been reported to vary from

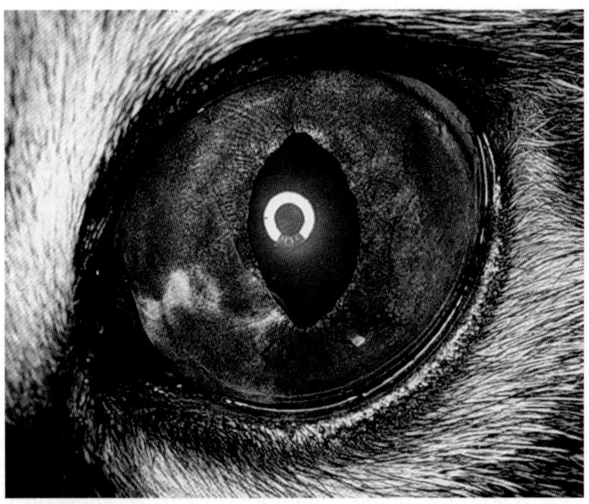

FIGURE 31-5 Diffuse iris melanomas may first appear as multifocal to diffuse pigmentary changes, as seen in the coalescing darker regions of the iris in this cat.

55% to 66% or higher.[42-45] Iridal hyperpigmentation, however, frequently takes months to years to progress to the extent to which the eye must be enucleated, and an additional 1 to 3 years after enucleation are required before metastatic disease may become evident.[42,43,45,46] No single morphologic feature is predictive of outcome, but metastasis has been linked to a greater mitotic index, larger tumors, and extension through the iris into the ciliary body stroma and involvement of the scleral venous plexus.[42,43]

Most ophthalmologists have noted unilateral or occasionally bilateral slowly progressive iridal pigmentary changes (especially in older orange cats) over many years to a decade or more that apparently do not lead to disease beyond the pigmentation, although eventual removal of these eyes can show melanoma. It is possible in some cats that these initially benign-appearing accumulations of small, angular pigmented cells on the anterior iridal surface undergo transformation to the larger, rounded cells typical of the potentially malignant diffuse iris melanoma. Of concern to the clinician waiting to document progression before advising treatment, however, is that malignant transformation is not readily observable clinically and that these cells, once transformed, appear to be capable of quickly dropping off into the anterior chamber and entering the drainage apparatus and vasculature.[43]

History, Clinical Signs, Diagnostic Techniques, and Work-Up

Slowly progressive, diffuse iridal hyperpigmentation is the most common clinical sign, although occasionally a pigmented iridal nodule or amelanotic mass is seen. Secondary glaucoma will eventually occur, and the diffuse form may be mistaken for chronic anterior uveitis with iridal hyperpigmentation.

The diagnosis of melanoma, generally made clinically, requires demonstration of progression and iridal thickening or irregularity of the iris surface or pupil. The prognostic and diagnostic value of fine-needle aspirates of the iridal surface or iridal biopsies is unclear and worthy of further study.

Therapy

The treatment of feline uveal melanomas is controversial. Ideally, enucleation would be delayed until just *prior* to malignant transformation, invasion into other ocular structures, secondary glaucoma, or metastasis. Such precise timing, however, is seldom attainable in a clinical setting, and enucleation is commonly performed if iridal pigment changes have been demonstrated to progressively increase to the point that virtually the entire iridal surface is involved, pigmented cells are present in the trabecular meshwork, the pupil is distorted (indicating iridal invasion), ciliary body or scleral invasion is threatened, uveitis is present, or glaucoma is impending. Although it would seem logical that early enucleation would optimize survival, this is unproved. In one study, enucleation has been shown to markedly enhance the rate of metastasis in cats with feline sarcoma virus–induced uveal melanomas.[47] The applicability of this experimental model to spontaneous disease, however, is unclear and neither feline sarcoma virus nor FeLV were found in a study of 10 eyes with spontaneous diffuse iris melanoma.[48] Recently, some ophthalmologists have attempted to ablate small, focal, hyperpigmented foci on the iris of cats with a diode laser, thereby preserving vision and the eye. The long-term success rate and side effects of this procedure, however, are not known. Finally, most slowly progressing lesions are simply monitored, ideally by comparison to baseline photographs. This option is particularly suitable for older cats with other diseases that limit their expected lifespan. In many cats, progression may be so slow as to permit the patient to be followed for many years to a decade or more without apparent metastasis.

Prognosis

In one study, the metastatic potential of feline uveal melanomas has been correlated with the extent of ocular involvement seen histologically.[43] Because the tumor is relatively slow-growing, however, the period until metastatic disease becomes apparent may be measured in years, and even then substantial additional time may be required before the metastasis is life threatening. Cats with tumors confined to iris stroma and trabecular meshwork at the time of enucleation have survival times comparable to those of age-matched controls. Enucleation after the tumor has invaded into the ciliary body but not the sclera warrants a poorer prognosis, but median survival time (MST) is still approximately 5 years.[43] Enucleation after the tumor has invaded into the ciliary body and the sclera merits an even poorer prognosis, with a MST of approximately 1.5 years.[43] MST is also reduced if secondary glaucoma has occurred.[43]

Feline Ocular Posttraumatic Sarcoma

Sarcomas following ocular trauma, although uncommon, are second only to melanomas in frequency as a primary ocular tumor of cats.[49-52] In the COPLOW collection, 8% of feline ocular tumors are posttraumatic sarcoma. These tumors are subdivided into three morphologic subtypes: spindle cell sarcoma (the most common), round cell sarcoma, and osteosarcoma/chondrosarcoma. All three have similar histories leading up to tumor presentation. Cats that are 7 to 15 years of age are most commonly affected, the latency period following trauma averages 5 years,[50] and 67% of affected cats are males or neutered males. Damage to the lens and chronic uveitis may be risk factors.[49-51] Because of the risk of posttraumatic sarcoma, many clinicians are cautious about cataract surgery or the use of an intrascleral prosthesis in cats. The cell of origin in the three subtypes is not definitively known, but it is likely that the released lens epithelial cell is the cell of origin in the spindle cell variant and the round cell variant likely represents a form of lymphoma.[53] Chronic inflammation may support neoplastic transformation of a pluripotent cell.[49-51] These tumors, often within the same eye, exhibit a spectrum of changes ranging from granulation tissue to fibrosarcoma, osteosarcoma, and anaplastic spindle cell sarcoma.[50,51] All of these tumors tend to circumferentially line the choroid and quickly infiltrate the retina and optic nerve.[50,51] The round cell variant tends to infiltrate the retina early.[53,54] White or pinkish discoloration of the affected eye or change in the shape or consistency of the globe are the most common presenting signs. Skull radiographs may demonstrate bone involvement or metallic foreign bodies.[52]

Because this tumor is uncommon, many ophthalmologists will not remove a comfortable phthisical feline eye unless it changes appearance. The advanced stage at which many of these tumors are first identified, however, and the propensity for early optic nerve involvement indicate that enucleation at this point may be only palliative and not prolong life. This has led some authors to advocate prophylactic enucleation of phthisical feline eyes or of feline eyes that are blind and have been severely traumatized or are chronically inflamed.[49,52] Further support for this approach comes from the observation that approximately 8% of globes removed prophylactically in the COPLOW collection already have tumors. Extension beyond the sclera or into the optic nerve may occur and are poor prognostic indicators, further supporting the concept of early enucleation. As much of the optic nerve as possible should be removed during enucleation for confirmed or suspected ocular sarcoma so that the extent of infiltrative disease and prognosis may be accurately determined. There is reason to believe that the prognosis is considerably better if enucleation is performed before the tumor invades the optic nerve or extends beyond the sclera.[55] To date, there have been no reports of treatment by radiation or chemotherapy.

Extraocular extension is common, as is recurrence following orbital exenteration.[49,52] Continued growth up the remainder of the optic nerve into the chiasm and brain, with vision loss or other neurologic signs, involvement of regional lymph nodes, and distant metastasis, has been reported.[40,50] The vast majority of animals die from local invasion and recurrence, typically within several months of enucleation.[49,52]

Spindle Cell Tumors of Blue-Eyed Dogs

Dogs with a blue, or partially blue, iris appear to be at risk of developing a spindle cell sarcoma in the uvea.[56] These tumors usually involve the iris but can originate or extend into the ciliary body, choroid, and even the vitreous. Breeds that commonly have blue irides are more likely to develop an iridal spindle cell sarcoma, but any dog with any blue in its iris appears to be at risk. The origin of these tumors is thought to be Schwann cells of nonmyelinated peripheral nerves.[57] The cells stain positive with glial fibrillary acidic protein (GFAP), as do the Schwann cells of nonmyelinating nerves. In a case series involving 11 dogs, more than half of the tumors were not clinically recognized and the diagnosis of neoplasia was not made until histopathology was performed. Metastatic disease has not been seen; however, local recurrence within the scleral shell was seen in a dog that had been treated by evisceration and placement of an intrascleral prosthesis.[56]

Iridociliary Epithelial Tumors

Primary iridociliary epithelial tumors (ciliary body adenomas, adenocarcinomas, pleomorphic adenocarcinoma, and less commonly, medulloepitheliomas) are infrequent in dogs and rare in cats.[58] The two main histologic forms that have been described are papillary (57% of cases in one study) and solid tumors (43%).[58] In the authors' experience, these tumors often appear nonpigmented clinically, but histologically at least some pigmented cells are present in approximately one-half of cases. Pigmented tumors of the ciliary body may be grossly indistinguishable from anterior uveal melanomas. Middle-aged to older dogs are the most commonly affected and golden and Labrador retrievers may be predisposed, for they comprised 27% of dogs with iridociliary epithelial tumors in one survey.[58] Most of these tumors appear to be benign, fairly well-delineated, sometimes pedunculated, slow-growing masses that originate in the pars plicata of the ciliary body or the iris epithelium.[58,59] Although approximately 60% invade the uveal tract, only 21% invade the sclera.[58] Tumors that invade the sclera are typically classified as adenocarcinomas and have anaplastic features, but metastasis is uncommon and occurs late in the course of the disease, if at all.[58-61] A small series of truly malignant pleomorphic adenocarcinomas with potentially fatal metastasis has been described in dogs.[62] Dogs affected with this rare form usually have long-standing disease thought to be inflammatory or traumatic, and 4 of 25 cases have a prior history of an intravitreous gentamicin injection for the treatment of glaucoma.[62]

Clinical signs include a retro-iridal mass that may displace the iris or lens by expansive growth, and if the tumor is large, secondary glaucoma, ocular pain, and intraocular hemorrhage may be noted.[60] The diagnostic work-up and differential diagnosis are similar to that of anterior uveal melanomas. Given the high frequency of ciliary body cysts in some predisposed breeds (especially the golden retriever), it is essential to differentiate ciliary body tumors from a benign cystic lesion prior to enucleation. Cystic lesions, which rarely require any intervention, are usually seen as lightly pigmented, ovoid, retro-iridal masses that can be shown to be hollow by transillumination or hypoechoic by ultrasonography. Early enucleation of ciliary body tumors has been recommended, although benign adenomas may remain static for years, making enucleation controversial for small tumors unassociated with secondary ocular disease. Local intraocular resection or laser photoablation may permit vision and ocular comfort to be maintained.[36] Systemic administration of 5-fluorouracil (5-FU) has been described as an adjunct to local resection of ciliary body tumors, but the efficacy of this therapy is unknown.[61]

Secondary Uveal Neoplasms

Numerous malignant tumors, especially adenocarcinomas, have been reported to metastasize to the highly vascular uveal tract. Lymphoma is the most common secondary intraocular tumor in the dog and cat, and ocular lesions are present in approximately one-third of dogs with the disease.[60,63-65] Common presentations include severe uveitis, glaucoma, retinal hemorrhages, hyphema, conjunctivitis, and keratitis characterized by corneal infiltrates, edema, vascularization, and intrastromal hemorrhage.[60,63-65] Exophthalmia resulting from orbital invasion by the tumor and vision loss due to optic nerve or central nervous system (CNS) disease may also be present. Posterior segment lesions may include retinal vascular tortuosity, papilledema, multiple intraretinal hemorrhages, and retinal detachment. In one study, the lifespan of dogs with intraocular lymphoma was only 60% to 70% as long as dogs without ocular involvement when treated with cyclophosphamide, vincristine, and prednisolone (COP), or with doxorubincin.[64] Topical or systemic corticosteroid therapy or enucleation is palliative. (See Chapter 32 for the definitive therapy of lymphoma.) Ophthalmic disease, especially intraocular or retinal hemorrhage, may also be the presenting complaint in animals with multiple myeloma.[66]

Tumors of the Orbit and Optic Nerve

Incidence and Risk Factors

Risk factors other than middle to old age, possibly large-breed dogs,[67] and possibly sex (female dogs, male cats) have not been described.[67-75] Tumors involving the optic nerve are rare, although secondary invasion occurs in feline posttraumatic sarcomas, feline SCC, and canine choroidal melanomas. Canine orbital meningioma is the most common tumor of the optic nerve but comprises only 3% of all meningiomas in dogs (Figure 31-6).[71,73] Lobular adenomas of unspecified glandular origin have been recently reported to involve the anterior orbit in dogs.[72]

Pathology and Natural Behavior

Orbital neoplasia may be primary (most common in dogs), secondary to extension of adjacent tumors into the orbit (most common in cats), or the result of distant metastasis. In cats and dogs, more than 90% of orbital tumors are malignant, and regional infiltration (including into the CNS) or distant metastasis is common.[67-70] At least 26 types of orbital tumors, roughly equally divided among connective tissue, bone, epithelial, and hemolymphatic origins, have been reported in dogs.[70] Osteosarcomas, mast cell tumors, reticulum cell sarcomas, fibrosarcomas, and neurofibrosarcomas are the most common canine primary orbital tumors.[70] More than two-thirds of feline orbital tumors are epithelial in origin, with SCC

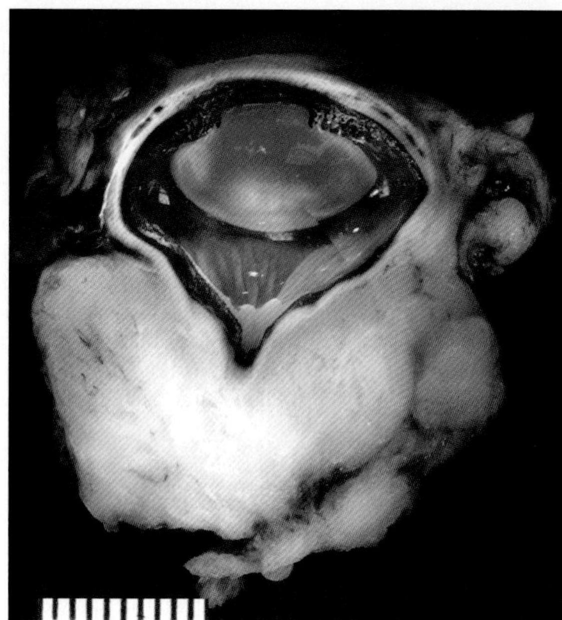

FIGURE 31-6 Orbital meningioma in a dog.

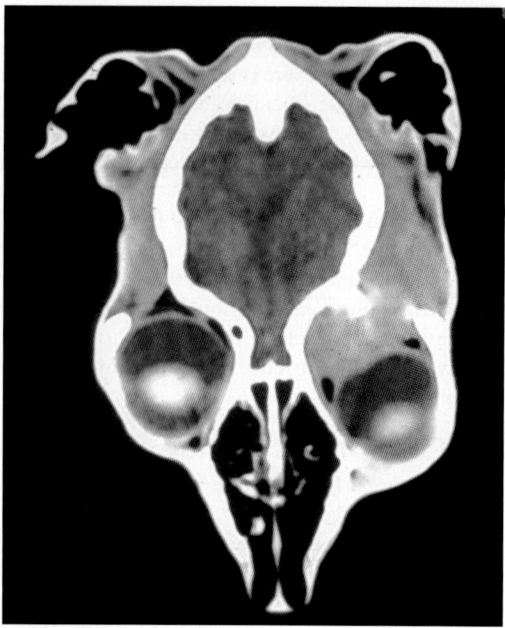

FIGURE 31-7 CT (dorsal view) provides detailed information about the location and extent of orbital tumors, as in this 17-year-old cat with orbital osteosarcoma.

being the most common,[69] but at least 15 other tumor types have been described in cats.

Canine orbital meningiomas exhibit predictable biologic behavior. They are slowly progressive and rarely metastasize; they may be osteolytic and invade surrounding tissues, including the CNS via the optic foramen.[70,72,73] Primary optic nerve tumors in dogs include glioma and meningioma.[70,71,73,74] Retinal and optic nerve gliomas may be considered as differential diagnoses of intraocular and orbital masses. The metastatic potential of gliomas appears to be low, but ascending invasion into the ventral aspect of the brain is possible.[75] Lobular orbital adenomas are made up of multiple friable lobules in the anterior orbit, making complete surgical excision difficult.[72]

History and Clinical Signs

Slowly progressive exophthalmia, absent to minimal pain on opening the mouth, difficulty in retropulsing the eye, and deviation of the globe typify orbital neoplasia. Sudden erosion of nasal or sinus tumors into the orbit occasionally results in acute exophthalmia and substantial orbital pain. Enophthalmia may occur if the mass is anterior to the equator of the globe. Lobular adenomas may present as soft, raised, subconjunctival masses and create either enophthalmia or exophthalmia. Chronic epiphora secondary to obstruction of the nasolacrimal duct, exposure keratoconjunctivitis, palpable orbital masses following enucleation, or unexplained orbital pain also suggests orbital neoplasia.[67-70] Measurement of corneal diameters and intraocular pressure (IOP) aids in differentiating glaucomatous ocular enlargement (large corneal diameter, high IOP) from exophthalmia (normal corneal diameter and IOP).

Optic nerve lesions may result in unilateral or bilateral blindness (the latter if the optic chiasm is affected), optic nerve head pallor, papilledema, or marked protrusion and congestion of the optic disc on ophthalmoscopy. A relatively mild degree of exophthalmia with vision loss suggests optic nerve neoplasia because tumors of other orbital tissues typically cause profound exophthalmos before visual loss. Tumors affecting the retrobulbar, intracanalicular, or chiasmal portions of the optic nerve may not result in exophthalmia or a visible change in the optic nerve head.

Diagnostic Techniques and Work-Up

It is essential to differentiate nonneoplastic orbital inflammatory diseases (granulomas, cellulitis, abscesses, myositis of the extraocular and masticatory muscles) from neoplasia. Animals with inflammatory disease typically exhibit significant pain on opening the mouth. The location of an orbital mass can usually be determined by careful physical examination, including retropulsion of the globe, oral examination caudal to the last molar, and determination of the direction of malposition of the eye.

In addition to physical examination, cytology of regional lymph nodes, orbital ultrasound, and skull and thoracic radiographs should be performed. In one study of cats with orbital neoplasia, 59% had radiographic signs of orbital bone lesions and 15% had evidence of metastasis on thoracic radiographs.[69] CT or MRI offer superior depictions of the orbit and facilitate planning of either radiation or surgical therapy (Figure 31-7). Histologic characterization by FNA or needle core biopsies (performed via the mouth or through the orbital skin), with ultrasound guidance if necessary, are helpful in arriving at a definitive diagnosis. The globe, major orbital blood vessels, and optic nerve should be avoided. Because 50% of orbital tumors may have a nondiagnostic FNA, especially in cases of SCC,[69] exploratory orbitotomy via a number of approaches[76-80] or exenteration may be required to characterize the mass and resect it if possible. Cerebrospinal fluid taps may aid in distinguishing optic nerve neoplasia from optic neuritis.

Therapy

Primary orbital and optic nerve tumors that lack metastasis or regional lymph node involvement may be amenable to surgical excision. If bony involvement is not present, orbital exenteration by widely dissecting around the mass (stripping periorbita if necessary) is usually the preferred procedure, as the advanced stage of the tumor at the time of diagnosis typically makes it impossible to excise the mass completely and preserve a functional or comfortable eye. If periorbital bones are involved, radical "orbitectomy," which resects the affected orbital tissues and surrounding bones, should be considered.[78] When treating optic nerve tumors, as much of the ipsilateral optic nerve as possible should be removed in an attempt to obtain complete excision.[70]

If preservation of a comfortable eye and vision appears possible, a variety of orbitotomy techniques, ranging from small incisions through the eyelid or mouth to reflection of the zygomatic arch, temporalis muscle elevation, and zygomatic process osteotomy, have been described.[76-80] Postoperative complications are common and may include secondary enophthalmia with entropion and possibly diplopia (double vision). Surgical debulking can be palliative, and some dogs may survive a year or more with minimal therapy.

The role of chemotherapy and RT, either alone or as an adjunct to surgery, is yet to be defined in the treatment of orbital tumors, although chemotherapy for orbital lymphoma may be effective. Systemic corticosteroids may permit some patients with optic nerve meningioma to maintain vision for several weeks to months. RT may be helpful in the case of nasal tumors with orbital extension, in subtotally excised or recurrent meningiomas, and in other select cases.

Prognosis

With conservative treatment the prognosis for most tumors involving the orbit and optic nerve is poor,[69,70] especially if there is bony involvement on skull radiographs. Recurrence at the primary site and involvement of adjacent or distant sites are common, often occurring within weeks to a few months. Even benign-appearing tumors such as lobular orbital adenomas and orbital meningiomas may be locally invasive and have a propensity for recurrence following wide excison.[67-73,78] In one study, however, radical orbitectomy (with or without chemotherapy or RT) provided a local disease-free interval of more than 1 year in more than 50% of patients and a 70% survival rate for the first year.[78] In another study, the mean survival time for cats with orbital tumors treated by RT, chemotherapy, or surgery that included resection of affected orbital bones was only 4.3 months.[69] In a study of 23 dogs with orbital tumors, most of whom were treated by exenteration with or without adjunct therapy, only 3 survived 3 years or longer.[70] The majority of these animals died as a direct result of the tumor or were euthanatized at the time of diagnosis.[67-70]

Ocular Effects of Cancer Therapeutic Modalities

The ocular effect of external-beam RT for nasal and periocular tumors can have a substantial impact on an animal's quality of life. Common complications include chronic keratoconjunctivitis, corneal ulceration, "dry eye," enophthalmia, entropion, cataracts, retinal hemorrhages, retinal detachments, and blindness.[81,82] Many of these conditions respond poorly to treatment, and vigorous attempts at prevention should be made in order to avoid chronic ocular pain and blindness. Recently, intensity-modulated RT (IMRT), which uses conformal avoidance, has been shown to significantly decrease the ocular toxicity seen in dogs treated by RT for spontaneous sinonasal tumors (Figure 31-8).[83,84]

In humans, blurred vision, partial visual field defects, loss of color vision, and diplopia have been associated with several antineoplastic drugs.[85] Similar effects probably occur in animals but

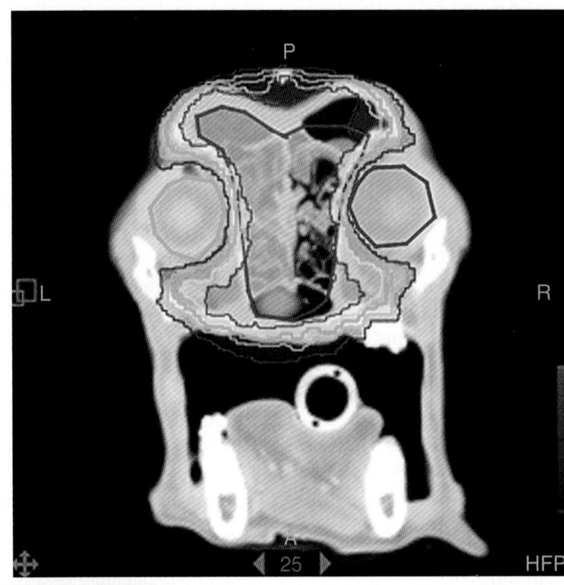

FIGURE 31-8 Intensity-modulated radiation therapy (IMRT), which uses conformal avoidance, can spare the eyes (*green* and *blue circles*) and has been shown to significantly decrease the ocular toxicity of radiation therapy for sinonasal tumors.

would be difficult to detect. Additionally, in humans, the bacillus Calmette-Guérin (BCG) has been associated with uveitis; cyclophosphamide has been associated with dry eye; cisplatin has been associated with neuroretinal toxicity; doxorubicin has been associated with excessive lacrimation and conjunctivitis; 5-FU has been associated with blurred vision, excessive lacrimation, blepharitis, conjunctivitis, and keratitis; and vincristine has been associated with cranial nerve palsies, optic neuropathy, and cortical and night blindness.[85] Monoclonal antibodies directed at the vasculature supporting the tumor also have been associated with uveitis.[86]

Comparative Aspects

Malignant melanoma of the choroid is the most common primary ocular malignancy in adult humans. Initially, it was believed that enucleation of these patients may enhance the risk of metastasis; thus a large, randomized clinical trial (the Collaborative Ocular Melanoma Study) was conducted comparing enucleation to iodine-125 brachytherapy, which left the globe intact.[87,88] Both treatment modalities were found to yield similar results, although many patients still died from metastatic melanoma, and it appears that significant improvement in survival rates will depend on developing effective systemic therapeutic modalities for melanoma.[87,88] Retinoblastoma is the most common malignant intraocular tumor of children and has a genetic basis. No cases of retinoblastoma have been described in nonhuman primates, and only one case of retinoblastoma has been described in a dog.[89] With therapy, long-term survival in children is over 85%, but many patients develop second tumors, especially osteosarcoma.[90] Cancer-associated retinopathy is an uncommon, immune-mediated paraneoplastic phenomenon in humans in which antibodies are directed against specific retinal autoantigens, such as recoverin.[91-93] In this condition, patients with small-cell lung carcinoma and other tumors may develop blurred vision, impaired color vision, substantial visual field defects, or complete blindness as tumor antigens cross-react with specific retinal components.[91-93] Treatment with IV immunoglobulin has been reported to return vision to some patients.[91] Although cancer-associated retinopathy has been suggested to occur in dogs, especially those with sudden acquired retinal degeneration syndrome (SARDS), definitive proof is lacking and one study did not identify antibody activity against retinal proteins or evidence of neoplasia in dogs with SARDS.[94]

REFERENCES

1. Krehbiel JD, Langham RF: Eyelid neoplasms in dogs, *Am J Vet Res* 36:115–119, 1975.
2. Roberts SM, Severin GA, Lavach JD: Prevalence and treatment of palpebral neoplasms in the dog: 200 cases (1975-1983), *J Am Vet Med Assoc* 189:1355–1359, 1986.
3. McLaughlin SA, Whitley RD, Gilger BC, et al: Eyelid neoplasms in cats: A review of demographic data (1979 to 1989), *J Am Anim Hosp Assoc* 29:63–67, 1983.
4. Barrie KP, Gelatt KN, Parshall CP: Eyelid squamous cell carcinoma in four dogs, *J Am Anim Hosp Assoc* 18:123–127, 1982.
5. Bernays ME, Flemming D, Peiffer RL: Primary corneal papilloma and squamous cell carcinoma associated with pigmentary keratitis in four dogs, *J Am Vet Med Assoc* 214:215–217, 1999.
6. Collins BK, Collier LL, Miller MA, et al: Biologic behavior and histologic characteristics of canine conjunctival melanoma, *Prog Vet Comp Ophthalmol* 3:135–140, 1993.
7. Roels S, Ducatelle R: Malignant melanoma of the nictitating membrane in a cat (Felix vulgaris), *J Comp Pathol* 119:189–193, 1998.
8. Brandes K, Fritsche J, Mueller N, et al: Detection of canine oral papillomavirus DNA in conjunctival epithelial hyperplastic lesions of three dogs, *Vet Pathol* 46:34–38, 2009.
9. Bonney CH, Koch SA, Dice PF, et al: Papillomatosis of conjunctiva and adnexa in dogs, *J Am Vet Med Assoc* 176:48–51, 1980.
10. Collier LL, Collins BK: Excision and cryosurgical ablation of severe periocular papillomatosis in a dog, *J Am Vet Med Assoc* 204:881–885, 1994.
11. Wilcock B, Peiffer R: Adenocarcinoma of the gland of the third eyelid in seven dogs, *J Am Vet Med Assoc* 193:1549–1550, 1988.
12. Schäffer EH, Pfleghaar S, Gordon S, et al: Malignant nictitating membrane tumors in dogs and cats, *Tierarztliche Praxis* 22:382–389, 1994.
13. Hargis AM, Lee AC, Thomassen RW: Tumor and tumor-like lesions of perilimbal conjunctiva in laboratory dogs, *J Am Vet Med Assoc* 173:1185–1190, 1978.
14. Mughannam AJ, Hacker DV, Spangler WL: Conjunctival vascular tumors in six dogs, *Vet Comp Ophthalmol* 7:56–59, 1997.
15. Multari D, Vascellari M, Mutinelli F: Hemangiosarcoma of the third eyelid in a cat, *Vet Ophthalmol* 5:273–276, 2002.
16. Pirie CG, Knollinger AM, Thomas CB, et al: Canine conjunctival hemangioma and hemangiosarcoma: a retrospective evaluation of 108 cases (1989-2004), *Vet Ophthalmol* 9:215–226, 2006.
17. Pirie CG, Dubielzig RR: Feline conjunctival hemangioma and hemangiosarcoma: a retrospective evaluation of eight cases (1993-2004), *Vet Ophthalmol* 9:227–231, 2006.
18. Patnaik AK, Mooney S: Feline melanoma: a comparative study of ocular, oral and dermal neoplasms, *Vet Pathol* 25:105–112, 1988.
19. Schobert CS, Labelle P, Dubielzig RR: Feline conjunctival melanoma: histopathological characteristics and clinical outcomes, *Vet Ophthalmol* 13:43–46, 2010.
20. Johnson BW, Brightman, Whiteley HE: Conjunctival mast cell tumor in two dogs, *J Am Anim Hosp Assoc* 24:439–442, 1988.
21. Kafarnik C, Calvarese S, Dubielzig RR: Canine mesenchymal hamartoma of the eyelid, *Vet Ophthalmol* 13:94–98, 2010.
22. Maggs DJ: Eyelids. In Maggs DJ, Miller PE, Ofri R, editors: *Slatter's fundamentals of veterinary ophthalmology*, ed 4, St. Louis, 2008, Elsevier.
23. Guiliano EA: Equine ocular adnexal and nasolacrimal disease. In Gilger BC, editor: *Equine ophthalmology*, ed 2, St. Louis, 2011, Elsevier.
24. Holmberg DL, Withrow SJ: Cryosurgical treatment of palpebral neoplasms: clinical and experimental results, *Vet Surg* 8:68–73, 1979.
25. Donaldson D, Sansom J, Scase T, et al: Canine limbal melanoma: 30 cases (1992-2004). Part 1. Signalment, clinical and histological features and pedigree analysis, *Vet Ophthalmol* 9:115–119, 2006.
26. Wilcock BP, Peiffer RL: Morphology and behavior of primary ocular melanomas in 91 dogs, *Vet Pathol* 23:418–424, 1986.
27. Diters RW, Dubielzig RR, Aquirre GD, et al: Primary ocular melanoma in dogs, *Vet Pathol* 20:379–395, 1983.
28. Diters RW, Ryan AM: Canine limbal melanoma, *Vet Med Small Anim Clin* 78:1529–1534, 1983.
29. Harling DE, Peiffer RL, Cook CS, et al: Feline limbal melanoma: four cases, *J Am Anim Hosp Assoc* 22:795–802, 1986.
30. Sullivan TC, Nasisse MP, Davidson MG, et al: Photocoagulation of limbal melanoma in dogs and cats: 15 cases (1989-1993), *J Am Vet Med Assoc* 208:891–894, 1996.
31. Featherstone HJ, Renwick P, Heinrich CL, et al: Efficacy of lamellar resection, cryotherapy, and adjunctive grafting for the treatment of canine limbal melanoma, *Vet Ophthalmol* 12(Suppl 1):65–72, 2009.
32. Donaldson D, Sansom J, Scase T, et al: Canine limbal melanoma: 30 cases (1992-2004). Part 2. Treatment with lamellar resection and adjunctive strontium-90 beta plesiotherapy—efficacy and morbidity, *Vet Ophthalmol* 9:179–185, 2006.
33. Gelatt KN, Johnson KA, Peiffer RL: Primary iridal pigmented masses in three dogs, *J Am Anim Hosp Assoc* 15:339–344, 1979.
34. Bussanich NM, Dolman PJ, Rootman J, et al: Canine uveal melanomas: series and literature review, *J Am Anim Hosp Assoc* 23:415–422, 1987.
35. Petersen-Jones SM, Forcier J, Mentzer AL: Ocular melanosis in the Cairn Terrier: clinical description and investigation of mode of inheritance, *Vet Ophthalmol* 10(Suppl 1):63–69, 2007.
36. Nasisse MP, Davidson MG, Olivero DK, et al: Neodymium:YAG laser treatment of primary canine intraocular tumors, *Prog Vet Comp Ophthalmol* 3:152–157, 1993.
37. Cook CS, Wilkie DA: Treatment of presumed iris melanoma in dogs by diode laser photocoagulation: 23 cases, *Vet Ophthalmol* 2:217–225, 1999.
38. Giuliano EA, Chappell R, Fischer B, et al: A matched observational study of canine survival with primary melanocytic neoplasia, *Vet Ophthalmol* 2:185–190, 1999.
39. Collinson PN, Peiffer RL: Clinical presentation, morphology, and behavior of primary choroidal melanomas in eight dogs, *Prog Vet Comp Ophthalmol* 3:158–164, 1993.
40. Dubielzig RR, Aquirre GD, Gross SL, et al: Choroidal melanomas in dogs, *Vet Pathol* 22:582–585, 1985.
41. Hyman JA, Koch SA, Wilcock BP: Canine choroidal melanoma with metastases, *Vet Ophthalmol* 5:113–117, 2002.
42. Duncan DE, Peiffer RL: Morphology and prognostic indicators of anterior uveal melanomas in cats, *Prog Vet Comp Ophthalmol* 1:25–32, 1991.
43. Kalishman JB, Chappell R, Flood LA, et al: A matched observational study of survival in cats with enucleation due to diffuse iris melanoma, *Vet Ophthalmol* 1:21–24, 1998.
44. Bellhorn RW, Henkind P: Intraocular malignant melanomas in domestic cats, *J Small Anim Pract* 10:631–637, 1970.
45. Patnaik AK, Mooney S: Feline melanoma: A comparative study of ocular, oral and dermal neoplasms, *Vet Pathol* 25:105–112, 1988.
46. Acland GM, McLean IW, Aquirre GD, et al: Diffuse iris melanoma in cats, *J Am Vet Med Assoc* 176:52–56, 1980.
47. Niederkorn JY, Shadduck JA, Albert DM: Enucleation and the appearance of second primary tumors in cats bearing virally induced intraocular tumors, *Invest Ophthalmol Vis Sci* 23:719–725, 1982.
48. Cullen CL, Haines DM, Jackson ML, et al: Lack of detection of feline leukemia and feline sarcoma viruses in diffuse iris melanomas of

cats by immunohistochemistry and polymerase chain reaction, *J Vet Diagn Invest* 14:340–343, 2002.
49. Peiffer RL, Monticello T, Bouldin TW: Primary ocular sarcomas in the cat, *J Small Anim Pract* 29:105–116, 1988.
50. Dubielzig RR, Everitt J, Shadduck JA, et al: Clinical and morphologic features of post-traumatic ocular sarcomas in cats, *Vet Pathol* 27:62–65, 1990.
51. Dubielzig RR, Hawkins KL, Toy KA, et al: Morphologic features of feline ocular sarcomas in 10 cats: Light microscopy, ultrastructure, and immunohistochemistry, *Vet Comp Ophthalmol* 4:7–12, 1994.
52. Håkansson N, Shively JN, Reed RE, et al: Intraocular spindle cell sarcoma following ocular trauma in a cat: case report and literature review, *J Am Anim Hosp Assoc* 26:63–66, 1990.
53. Naranjo C, Schobert CS, Dubielzig RR: Round cell variant of feline ocular posttraumatic sarcoma: a retrospective study (abstract), *Vet Ophthalmol* 10:399, 2007.
54. Dubielzig RR, Zeiss C: Feline post-traumatic ocular sarcoma: Three morphologic variants and evidence that some are derived from lens epithelial cells. *Proceedings of the Association for Research in Vision and Ophthalmology,* Fort Lauderdale, 2004.
55. Dubielzig RR: Feline post-traumatic ocular sarcoma: a review of 110 cases. Proceedings American College of Veterinary Pathologists, New Orleans, *Vet Pathol* 39:619, 2002.
56. Klauss G, Dubielzig RR: Characteristics of primary spindle cell neoplasm of the anterior uveal tract: 11 dogs. Proceedings American College of Veterinary Pathologists, Salt Lake City, *Vet Pathol* 38:574, 2001.
57. Zarfoss MK, Klauss G, Newkirk K, et al: Uveal spindle cell tumor of blue-eyed dogs: an immunohistochemical study, *Vet Pathol* 44:276–284, 2007.
58. Dubielzig RR, Steinberg H, Garvin H, et al: Iridociliary epithelial tumors in 100 dogs and 17 cats: a morphological study, *Vet Ophthalmol* 1:223–231, 1998.
59. Peiffer RL: Ciliary body epithelial tumors in the dog and cat: a report of thirteen cases, *J Small Anim Pract* 24:347–370, 1983.
60. Gwin RM, Gelatt KN, Williams LW: Ophthalmic neoplasms in the dog, *J Am Anim Hosp Assoc* 18:853–866, 1982.
61. Clerc B: Surgery and chemotherapy for the treatment of adenocarcinoma of the iris and ciliary body in five dogs, *Vet Comp Ophthalmol* 6:265–270, 1996.
62. Bell CM, Dubielzig RR: Canine iridociliary epithelial tumors: a morphologic review of 702 cases (abstract), *Vet Pathol* 46:1064, 2009.
63. Williams LW, Gelatt KN, Gwin RM: Ophthalmic neoplasms in the cat, *J Am Anim Hosp Assoc* 17:999–1008, 1981.
64. Krohne SG, Henderson NM, Richardson RC, et al: Prevalence of ocular involvement in dogs with multicentric lymphoma: prospective evaluation of 94 cases, *Vet Comp Ophthalmol* 4:127–135, 1994.
65. Corcoran KA, Peiffer RL, Koch SA: Histopathologic features of feline ocular lymphosarcoma: 49 cases (1978-1992), *Vet Comp Ophthalmol* 5:35–41, 1995.
66. Hendrix DV, Gelatt KN, Smith PJ, et al: Ophthalmic disease as the presenting complaint in five dogs with multiple myeloma, *J Am Anim Hosp Assoc* 34:121–128, 1998.
67. Attali-Soussay K, Jegou JP, Clerc B: Retrobulbar tumors in dogs and cats: 25 cases, *Vet Ophthalmol* 4:19–27, 2001.
68. Mauldin EA, Deehr AJ, Hertzke D, et al: Canine orbital meningiomas: a review of 22 cases, *Vet Ophthalmol* 3:11–16, 2000.
69. Gilger BC, McLaughlin SA, Whitley RD, et al: Orbital neoplasms in cats: 21 cases (1974-1990), *J Am Vet Med Assoc* 201:1083–1086, 1992.
70. Kern TJ: Orbital neoplasia in 23 dogs, *J Am Vet Med Assoc* 186:489–491, 1985.
71. Braund KG, Ribas JL: Central nervous system meningiomas, *Compend Contin Educ Pract Vet* 8:241–248, 1986.
72. Headrick JK, Bentley E, Dubielzig RR: Canine lobular orbital adenoma: a report of 15 cases with distinctive features, *Vet Ophthalmol* 7:47–51, 2004.
73. Dugan SJ, Schwarz PD, Roberts SM, et al: Primary optic nerve meningioma and pulmonary metastasis in a dog, *J Am Anim Hosp Assoc* 29:11–16, 1993.
74. Spiess BM, Wilcock BP: Glioma of the optic nerve with intraocular and intracranial involvement in a dog, *J Comp Pathol* 97:79–84, 1987.
75. Naranjo C, Schobert C, Dubielzig RR: Canine ocular gliomas: a retrospective study, *Vet Ophthalmol* 11:356–362, 2008.
76. Slatter DH, Abdelbaki Y: Lateral orbitotomy by zygomatic arch resection in the dog, *J Am Vet Med Assoc* 175:1179–1182, 1979.
77. Gilger BC, Whitely RD, McLaughlin SA: Modified lateral orbitotomy for removal of orbital neoplasms in two dogs, *Vet Surg* 23:53–58, 1994.
78. O'Brien MG, Withrow SJ, Straw RC, et al: Total and partial orbitectomy for the treatment of periorbital tumors in 24 dogs and 6 cats: a retrospective study, *Vet Surg* 25:471–479, 1996.
79. Håkansson NW, Håkansson BW: Transfrontal orbitotomy in the dog: an adaptable three-step approach to the orbit, *Vet Ophthalmol* 13:377–383, 2010.
80. Bartoe JT, Brightman AH, Davidson HJ: Modified lateral orbitotomy for vision-sparing excision of a zygomatic mucocele in a dog, *Vet Ophthalmol* 10:127–131, 2007.
81. Adams WM, Miller PE, Vail DM, et al: An accelerated technique for irradiation of malignant canine nasal and paranasal sinus tumors, *Vet Radiol Ultrasound* 5:475–481, 1998.
82. Roberts SM, Lavach JD, Severin GA, et al: Ophthalmic complications following megavoltage irradiation of the nasal and paranasal cavities in dogs, *J Am Vet Med Assoc* 190:43–47, 1987.
83. Miller PE, Turek MM, Forrest LJ, et al: Ocular sparing using intensity modulated radiation therapy (IMRT) in a canine model of spontaneous sinonasal cancer: Proof of principle of conformal avoidance. *Proceedings of the Association for Research in Vision and Ophthalmology,* Fort Lauderdale, Florida, 2005.
84. Lawrence JA, Forrest LJ, Turek MM, et al: Proof of principle of ocular sparing in dogs with sinonasal tumors treated with intensity-modulated radiation therapy, *Vet Radiol Ultrasound* 51:561–570, 2010.
85. Imperia PS, Lazarus HM, Lass JH: Ocular complications of systemic cancer chemotherapy, *Surg Ophthalmol* 34:209–230, 1989.
86. Martin PL, Miller PE, Mata M, et al: Ocular inflammation in cynomolgus macaques following intravenous administration of a human monoclonal antibody, *J Toxicol* 28:5–16, 2009.
87. Robertson DM: Changing concepts in the management of choroidal melanoma, *Am J Ophthalmol* 136:161–170, 2003.
88. Diener-West M, Earle JD, Fine SL, et al: The COMS randomized trial of iodine 125 brachytherapy for choroidal melanoma, III: Initial mortality findings. COMS Report No. 18, *Arch Ophthalmol* 119:969–982, 2001.
89. Syed NA, Nork TM, Poulsen GL, et al: Retinoblastoma in a dog, *Arch Ophthalmol* 115:758–763, 1997.
90. Shields CL, Meadows AT, Leahey AM, et al: Continuing challenges in the management of retinoblastoma with chemotherapy, *Retina* 24:849–862, 2004.
91. Guy J, Aptiauri N: Treatment of paraneoplastic visual loss with intravenous immunoglobulin: report of 3 cases, *Arch Ophthalmol* 117:471–477, 1999.
92. Subramanian L, Polan AS: Cancer-related diseases of the eye: The role of calcium-binding proteins, *Biochem Biophys Res Commun* 322:1153–1165, 2004.
93. Ohgura H, Yokoi Y, Ohguro I, et al: Clinical and immunologic aspects of cancer-associated retinopathy, *Am J Ophthalmol* 137:1117–1119, 2004.
94. Gilmour MA, Cardenas MR, Blaik MA, et al: Evaluation of a comparative pathogenesis between cancer-associated retinopathy in humans and sudden acquired retinal degeneration syndrome in dogs via diagnostic imaging and western blot analysis, *Am J Vet Res* 67:877–881, 2006.

32 Hematopoietic Tumors

SECTION A
Canine Lymphoma and Lymphoid Leukemias

DAVID M. VAIL, MARIE E. PINKERTON, AND KAREN M. YOUNG

Lymphoma

The lymphomas (malignant lymphoma or lymphosarcoma) are a diverse group of neoplasms that have in common their origin from lymphoreticular cells. They usually arise in lymphoid tissues such as lymph nodes, spleen, and bone marrow; however, they may arise in almost any tissue in the body. Although the annual incidence of lymphoma is difficult to predict in the absence of a national canine tumor registry, it is clear that it represents one of the most common neoplasms seen in the dog. The annual incidence has been estimated to range between 13 to 24 per 100,000 dogs at risk.[1-3] The annual incidence rates at specific ages are estimated to be 1.5 per 100,000 for dogs less than 1.0 year of age and 84 per 100,000 in the 10- to 11-year-old group. Lymphoma comprises approximately 7% to 24% of all canine neoplasia and 83% of all canine hematopoietic malignancies.[4,5] In a review of the Veterinary Medical Data Base Program (VMDP) at Purdue University from 1987 to 1997, the frequency of canine lymphoma patients presented to 20 veterinary institutions increased from 0.75% of total case load to 2.0%, and it appears the frequency is continuing to increase. A similar trend is present in physician-based oncology; non-Hodgkin's lymphoma (NHL) represents 5% of all new cancer cases, the fifth leading cause of cancer death, and the second fastest growing cancer in terms of mortality in humans.[6] Middle-aged to older (median age of 6 to 9 years) dogs are primarily affected. A decreased risk for lymphoma is reported for intact females.[7] Breeds reported to have a higher incidence include Boxers, bull mastiffs, basset hounds, St. Bernards, Scottish terriers, Airedales, and bulldogs; breeds at lower risk include dachshunds and Pomeranians.[8,9]

Etiology

The etiology of canine lymphoma is likely multifactorial and largely unknown; however, investigations are currently shedding significant light on the subject.

Genetic and Molecular Factors

Recent advances in molecular cytogenetics (see Chapter 1, Section A), including gene microarray techniques, have been and are currently being applied to investigations of chromosomal aberrations in dogs with lymphoma.[10-16] The publication of the canine genome and the commercial availability of canine gene microarrays (GeneChip Canine Genome 2.0 Array, Affymetrix, Inc.) have led to advances in our understanding of genetic events occurring in lymphoma.[17] Breen's group has documented gain of dog chromosomes 13 and 31 and loss of chromosome 14 as the most common aberrations in a group of 25 cases analyzed.[11] Chromosomal aberrations have also been associated with prognosis in dogs with lymphoma. A study of 61 dogs with lymphoma demonstrated a prognostic advantage in dogs with trisomy of chromosome 13 (25% of the dogs studied) as evidenced by increase in duration of first remission and overall survival time.[18] Germline and somatic genetic mutations and altered oncogene/tumor suppressor gene expression, epigenetic changes (e.g., DNA hypomethylation), signal transduction, and death-pathway alterations (e.g., *Bcl-2* family) are common in human lymphomas and have been reported in the dog as well (see Chapter 1, Section A, and Chapter 14, Section B). These include *N-ras, p53, Rb,* and p16 cyclin-dependent kinase aberrations.[19-24] Additionally, differences in the prevalence of immunophenotypic subtypes of lymphoma among different breeds indicate heritable risks.[25] Additionally, telomerase activity (see Chapter 2) has been documented in canine lymphoma tissues.[26-28]

Infectious Factors

The hypothesis that a retrovirus may be involved in the pathogenesis of canine lymphoma has not been confirmed. However, serologic detection of Epstein-Barr virus infection, linked to some forms of lymphoma in humans, has been documented in dogs with lymphoma and is currently being investigated.[29]

In humans, a direct association between *Helicobacter* sp. infections and development of gastric lymphoma has been made.[30] Although this has not been definitively shown in dogs, there is evidence of *Helicobacter* sp. infection in laboratory beagle dogs resulting in gastric lymphoid follicle formation that is considered a precursor of mucosa-associated lymphoid tissue (MALT) lymphoma in humans.[31]

Environmental Factors

In humans, evidence has accumulated implicating phenoxyacetic acid herbicides, in particular 2, 4-dichlorophenoxyacetic acid (2, 4-D), in the development of NHL. A published hospital-based case-control study of dogs indicated that owners in households with dogs that develop malignant lymphoma applied 2, 4-D herbicides to their lawn and/or employed commercial lawn care companies to treat their yard more frequently than owners of dogs without lymphoma.[32] The risk of canine lymphoma was reported to rise twofold (odds ratio [OR] = 1.3) with four or more yearly owner applications of 2, 4-D. The results of this study have come under criticism, and three additional follow-up investigations have not validated assertions of increased risk.[33-35] In another study, dogs exposed to lawn treatment within 7 days of application were greater than 50 times more likely to have urine levels of 2, 4-D at 50 µg/L or higher.[36] The highest concentration was noted 2 days after application. In an environmental case-control study performed in Europe, two variables, residency in industrial areas and use of chemicals (defined as paints or solvents) by owners, modestly increased the risk of developing lymphoma; however, no link was found with pesticide use.[37]

A weak association between lymphoma in dogs and exposure to strong magnetic fields was observed in a preliminary epidemiologic study.[38] In this hospital-based case-control study, the risk of developing lymphoma categorized into high or very high exposure was increased (odds ratio = 1.8). More thorough studies are necessary to evaluate this association further. Proximity to environmental waste was implicated in two European studies; however, it was felt to be a risk indicator rather than a risk factor and would require further case-control investigations.[39,40]

Immunologic Factors

Impaired immune function has also been implicated in dogs with lymphoma. Immune system alterations in the dog such as immune-mediated thrombocytopenia, independent of age and sex, have been associated with a higher risk of subsequently developing lymphoma when compared to the normal population.[41,42] Additional evidence comes from observations in human and feline transplantation patients. In a case-control study of cats undergoing renal transplant, 24% of cases developed cancer (36% of those were lymphoma) while on cyclosporine immunosuppressive therapy compared to 5.1% of control cats, none of which developed lymphoma (OR, 6.1; $p = 0.001$).[43] A case of lymphoma developing in a dog following treatment with cyclosporine also exists.[44] One report suggests an association between the immunodysregulation observed in dogs with atopic dermatitis and the risk of developing epitheliotropic T-cell lymphoma; whether this is associated with the disease or the immunomodulatory treatments commonly applied is unknown.[45]

Classification and Pathology

Classification of malignant lymphoma in dogs is based on anatomic location, histologic criteria, and immunophenotypic characteristics. The most common anatomic forms of lymphoma, in order of decreasing prevalence, are multicentric, gastrointestinal (GI), mediastinal, and cutaneous forms.[46] Primary extranodal forms, which can occur in any location outside the lymphatic system, include the eyes, central nervous system (CNS), bone marrow, bladder, heart, and nasal cavity. The pathologic characteristics of the various anatomic classifications will be discussed in this section and clinical characteristics will be described in subsequent sections.

Eighty-four percent of dogs with lymphoma develop the multicentric form, which is usually characterized by the presence of superficial lymphadenopathy (Figure 32-1).[46] The alimentary form of lymphoma is much less common, accounting for 5% to 7% of all canine lymphomas. This form is reported to be more common in male dogs than female dogs.[6] Primary GI lymphoma in dogs may occur focally but more often affects multiple segments, with thickening of the wall, narrowing of the lumen, and frequently mucosal ulceration.[47,48] Histologically, there is infiltration of neoplastic lymphocytes throughout the mucosa and submucosa, with occasional transmural infiltration. Liver and local lymph nodes are often secondarily involved. Lymphocytic-plasmacytic enteritis (LPE) can be seen adjacent to or distant from the primary tumor. Pathologically, some of these neoplasms may resemble plasma cell tumors, and aberrant production of immunoglobulins may occur.

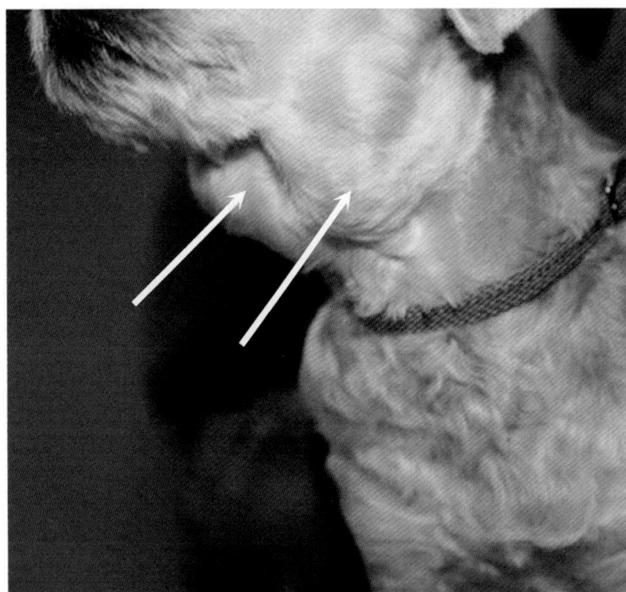

FIGURE 32-1 A dog with obvious mandibular lymphadenopathy resulting from multicentric lymphoma.

Histopathologically, distinguishing between GI lymphoma and LPE can be difficult. Some have suggested that LPE may be a prelymphomatous change in the GI tract. A syndrome of immunoproliferative intestinal disease characterized by LPE has been described in Basenjis, which subsequently develop GI lymphoma.[49] In addition, plasma cell–rich areas with heterogeneous lymphomatous infiltration may resemble lesions of LPE. Only a few reports specifically identify the immunophenotype of the lymphocyte subpopulations in alimentary lymphoma in dogs. Historically, it was presumed that they most likely originate from B cells; however, recent evidence suggests that most GI lymphomas in dogs arise from T cells and often exhibit epitheliotropism.[48,50] The Boxer and Shar-pei breeds may be overrepresented in cases of alimentary lymphoma.[50,51]

The mediastinal form of the disease occurs in approximately 5% of cases.[46] This form is characterized by enlargement of the cranial mediastinal lymph nodes, thymus, or both (Figure 32-2). Hypercalcemia is reported to occur in 10% to 40% of dogs with lymphoma and is most common with the mediastinal form. In a study of 37 dogs with lymphoma and hypercalcemia, 16 (43%) had mediastinal lymphoma.[52] The mediastinal form in dogs is most commonly associated with a T-cell phenotype.[53,54]

Cutaneous lymphoma can be solitary or more generalized and usually is classified as epitheliotropic (mycosis fungoides) or nonepitheliotropic.[55] Canine epitheliotropic cutaneous lymphoma originates from T-cells,[55-60] similar to its development in humans. In dogs, these more commonly represent $CD8^+$ cells, whereas in humans they are typically $CD4^+$ cells. A rare form of cutaneous T-cell lymphoma, characterized by skin involvement with evidence of peripherally circulating large (15 to 20 µm in diameter) malignant T-cells with folded, grooved nuclei, has been described. In humans, this is referred to as Sézary syndrome and has been reported in both dogs and cats.[61-63] Nonepitheliotropic cutaneous lymphomas form single or multiple dermal or subcutaneous nodules or plaques; histologically, they spare the epidermis and papillary dermis and affect the middle and deep portions of the dermis and subcutis.[55]

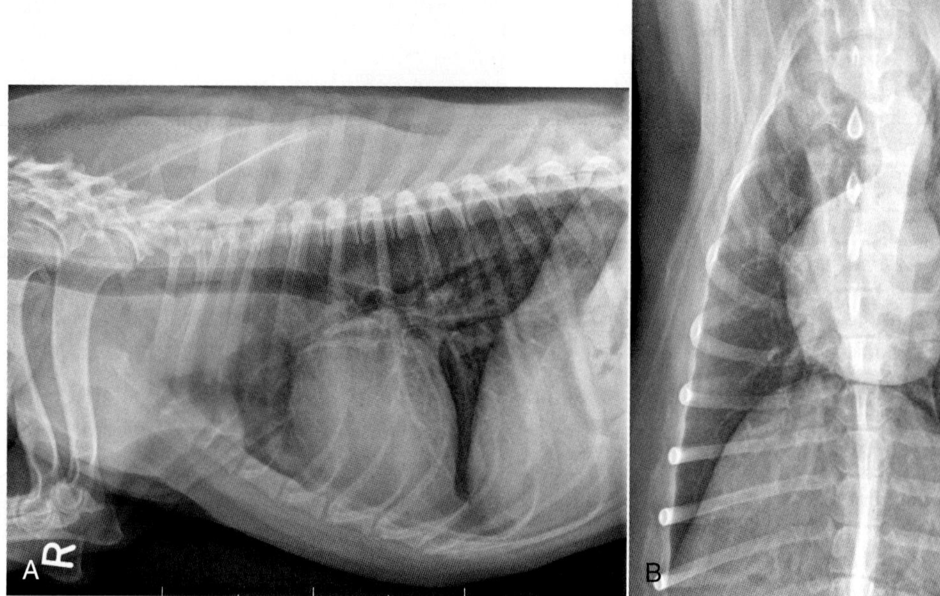

FIGURE 32-2 **A,** Lateral radiographic projection of a dog with mediastinal lymphoma. **B,** Ventrodorsal projection of the same dog.

Atypical Anatomic Forms of Lymphoma

Hepatosplenic lymphoma is a relatively uncommon, distinct presentation in the dog marked by a lack of significant peripheral lymphadenopathy in the face of hepatic, splenic, and bone marrow infiltration with malignant lymphocytes, usually of T-cell origin.[64,65] Biologically, this form of lymphoma is extremely aggressive and poorly responsive to therapy. In humans the tumor usually is composed of γδT-cells (i.e., T-cells that express the γδT-cell receptor), and this immunophenotype has been confirmed in at least one dog in the veterinary literature.[65]

Intravascular (angiotropic, angioendotheliomatosis) lymphoma is a distinct form of lymphoma defined as proliferations of neoplastic lymphocytes within the lumen and wall of blood vessels in the absence of a primary extravascular mass or leukemia. It has been reported several times in the veterinary literature, and in most cases it involves the CNS and peripheral nervous system (PNS), including the eye.[66-71] The B-cell immunophenotype is most common in humans; however, in most reported cases in dogs, the origin is either T-cell or null cell (neither B- nor T-cell), although one case of a B-cell phenotype has been reported.

Pulmonary lymphomatoid granulomatosis (PLG) is a rare pulmonary infiltrative and/or nodular disorder characterized by a heterogenous accumulation of lymphocytes (both B and T, although some evidence suggests primarily a T-cell origin), neutrophils, plasma cells, and macrophages, often arranged angiocentrically.[72-75] Whether this syndrome is a true lymphoma or a prelymphoma state is debatable. Clinical signs are related to respiratory compromise, and various chemotherapeutic protocols have been used with reported results varying from rapid progression to long-term clinical remissions.

Histologic Classification Systems

Lymphomas arise from clonal expansion of lymphoid cells with distinctive morphologic and immunophenotypic features. Many histologic systems have been used to classify NHL in humans, and some of these have been applied to lymphoma in the dog and other species. The National Cancer Institute (NCI) Working Formulation[76] and the updated Kiel system[77] have been adapted to canine tumors with some success. The World Health Organization (WHO) also publishes a histologic classification scheme, which uses the revised European American lymphoma (REAL) system as a basis for defining histologic categories of hematopoietic and lymphoid tumors in domestic animals.[78] This system incorporates anatomic, histologic, and immunophenotypic criteria (B- and T-cell immunophenotype), with the goal of enabling accurate and reproducible diagnosis of specific neoplastic disease entities. This theoretically should assist in better tailoring of treatment protocols, better correlation of prognosis, and better comparative capabilities. Table 32-1 shows some of the WHO categories in three different surveys, including a 2-year survey (2008-2009) of canine necropsy and biopsy cases at the University of Wisconsin-Madison Veterinary Medical Teaching Hospital pathology service[79,80]; some of the less common categories in the WHO system were not represented and are not listed. The WHO system provides accurate and consistent reproducible diagnostic results similar to the system used in human pathology; accuracy among a group of pathologists examining 300 cases was at 83% agreement, and accuracy in evaluating the six most common diagnoses (80% of the cases) was 87%.[81] Clinical studies are needed to correlate the various categories of disease with biologic behavior, response to treatment, and prognosis. Preliminary results indicate dogs with indolent lymphoma (e.g., marginal zone lymphoma, follicular lymphoma, B- or T-cell small cell lymphoma, T-cell–rich B-cell lymphoma, and T zone lymphoma) maintain normal activity and appetite levels even during advanced stages of disease and experience long-term survival even with limited or no therapy.[81-84]

The Working Formulation (WF) was developed to allow investigators to "translate" among the numerous classification systems so that clinical trials could be compared in humans. Most of the larger compilations agree that most canine lymphomas are intermediate or high grade; however, diffuse immunoblastic forms appear to predominate in the United States, whereas the follicular

TABLE 32-1 World Health Organization Classification System for Canine Lymphoma

CATEGORY	PERCENTAGE		
	SUEIRO ET AL (N = 55)	VEZZALI ET AL (N = 123)	UNIVERSITY OF WISCONSIN (N = 122)
B-cell neoplasms	72.7	78.9	59.0
Precursor B lymphoblastic leukemia/lymphoma	—	2.4	8.2
B-cell chronic lymphocytic leukemia/small lymphocytic lymphoma	1.8	2.4	0.8
Lymphocytic lymphoma—intermediate type	—	0.8	—
Lymphoplasmacytic lymphoma	10.9	3.3	0.8
Mantle cell lymphoma	—	1.6	—
Follicular center cell lymphomas	1.8	2.4	—
Marginal zone lymphoma (splenic, nodal, mucosa-associated lymphoid tissue)	—	3.3	2.5
Plasma cell myeloma/plasmacytoma	—	16.3	9.8
Diffuse large cell lymphoma	56.3	33.3	24.6
T-cell–rich, B-cell lymphoma	—	0.8	—
Large cell immunoblastic lymphoma	—	10.6	10.7
Mediastinal (thymic) large B-cell lymphoma	—	0.8	—
Burkitt's lymphoma/leukemia	—	0.8	1.6
T-cell and natural killer (NK) cell lymphomas	21.8, 5.4*	21.1	41.0
Precursor T lymphoblastic lymphoma/leukemia	—	6.5	9.8
T-cell chronic lymphocytic leukemia (CLL)	—	3.3	0.8
Intestinal T-cell lymphoma	—	4.1	4.1
Mycosis fungoides/Sézary syndrome	—	1.6	11.5
Cutaneous nonepitheliotropic lymphoma	12.7†	3.3	—
Anaplastic large cell lymphoma	1.8	—	0.8
Peripheral T-cell lymphoma, unspecified	20.0	2.4	13.1‡

*Non-B, non-T lymphomas.

†Three B-cell and four T-cell cutaneous lymphomas, not specified as epitheliotropic/nonepitheliotropic.

‡Includes one T-zone lymphoma.

Modified from Sueiro FAR, Alessi AC, Vassallo J: Canine lymphomas: A morphological and immunohistochemical study of 55 cases, with observations on p53 immunoexpression, *J Comp Pathol* 131:207–213, 2004; and Vezzali E, Parodi AL, Marcato PS, et al: Histopathological classification of 171 cases of canine and feline non-Hodgkin lymphoma according to the WHO, *Vet Comp Oncol* 8:36–49, 2009.

large cell variations predominate in Europe. A comparison of European and American classifications is warranted based on this discrepancy. The WF categorizes tumors according to pattern (diffuse or follicular) and cell type (e.g., small cleaved cell, large cell, immunoblastic), but it does not include information about the immunophenotype of the tumor.[76] The WF subtypes are related to the biology of the tumor and patient survival. The updated Kiel classification includes the architectural pattern, morphology (centroblastic, centrocytic, or immunoblastic), and immunophenotype (B-cell or T-cell) of the tumor cells.[77] In both systems, the tumors can then be categorized as low-grade, intermediate grade, or high-grade malignancies. Low-grade lymphomas composed of small cells with a low mitotic rate typically progress slowly and are associated with long survival times but are ultimately incurable. High-grade lymphomas with a high mitotic rate progress rapidly but are more likely to respond initially to chemotherapy and, in humans, are potentially curable.

Several features of canine lymphomas become apparent when these classification systems are applied. The most striking difference between canine and human lymphomas is the scarcity of follicular lymphomas in the dog.[79,80] Some diffuse lymphomas in the dog may initially be follicular, but these may progress to the more aggressive, diffuse form by the time of diagnostic biopsy. The most common form of canine lymphoma is diffuse large-cell lymphoma, a high-grade tumor most commonly of B-cell origin.[80,81,85] Only a small percentage of canine lymphomas (5.3% to 29%) are considered low-grade tumors.

High-grade lymphomas occur frequently if diffuse large-cell lymphomas, classified as intermediate grade in the WF, are considered high-grade, as in the updated Kiel classification (in which they are labeled as diffuse centroblastic lymphomas). A documented difference exists in the prevalence of the various immunophenotypes based on breed.[25] For example, cocker spaniels and Doberman pinschers are more likely to develop B-cell lymphoma, Boxers are more likely to have T-cell lymphoma, and golden retrievers appear to have an equal likelihood of B- and T-cell tumors.

To be clinically useful, these classification systems in the end must yield information about response to therapy, maintenance of remission, and survival. Some studies suggest that the subtypes in the WF can be correlated with survival, and the Kiel system may be useful for predicting relapse.[86,87] In most studies, high-grade lymphomas achieve a complete response (CR) to chemotherapy significantly more often than low-grade tumors. However, dogs with low-grade tumors may live a long time without aggressive chemotherapy.[83,84] Dogs with T-cell lymphomas have shown a lower rate of CR to chemotherapy and shorter remission and survival times than dogs with B-cell tumors (with the exception of low-grade T-cell subtypes).[53,54,86,88] Furthermore, T-cell lymphomas tend to be associated with hypercalcemia.[89,90]

In the veterinary literature, 60% to 80% of canine lymphomas are of B-cell origin; T-cell lymphomas account for 10% to 38%; mixed B- and T-cell lymphomas account for as many as 22%; and null cell tumors (i.e., neither B-cell nor T-cell immunoreactive) represent fewer than 5%.[53,54,91-93] The development of monoclonal antibodies to detect specific markers on canine lymphocytes has made immunophenotyping of tumors in dogs routinely available in many commercial laboratories. Such techniques can be performed on paraffin-embedded samples, from tissue microarrays, on cytologic specimens obtained by fine-needle aspiration (FNA) of lesions, or by flow cytometric analysis of cellular fluid samples (e.g., peripheral blood, effusions) and lesion aspirates.

The Rappaport classification system, proposed in 1956 for human NHL, describes the architectural pattern (follicular or diffuse) and the cytologic features (well differentiated, poorly differentiated, or histiocytic) of lymphoma.[94,95] This system has not proved useful in providing prognostic information or in guiding therapy in dogs with lymphoma because of the low number of follicular lymphomas in dogs, the problematic "histiocytic" subgroup, and the failure to account for different morphologic and immunologic cell types.

One criticism of the Rappaport, Kiel, and WF classification systems is that they fail to include extranodal lymphomas as a separate category. The WHO system does include anatomic location as a factor in determining certain categories. Although differences between nodal and extranodal tumors in biologic behavior and prognosis are well recognized, comparative information about the histogenesis of these tumors is lacking. For example, in humans small-cell lymphomas arising from MALT are composed of cells with a different immunophenotype than that of other small-cell lymphomas (i.e., MALT lymphomas typically are negative for both CD5 and CD10). Except for cutaneous lymphoid neoplasms, detailed characterization of extranodal lymphomas in dogs has not been done. Although cutaneous lymphoma is a heterogeneous group of neoplasms that includes an epitheliotropic form resembling mycosis fungoides and a nonepitheliotropic form, most cutaneous lymphomas have a T-cell phenotype.[64,96]

To summarize, it is important to determine the histologic grade of canine lymphomas as low (small lymphocytic or centrocytic lymphomas) or intermediate to high (diffuse large cell, centroblastic, and immunoblastic lymphomas) and the architecture as diffuse or follicular. Furthermore, determining the immunophenotype of the tumor provides useful information. Response rates to chemotherapy are, in general, better in animals with B-cell tumors and intermediate- to high-grade lymphomas. Dogs with low-grade lymphomas can have long survival times without aggressive therapy.

History and Clinical Signs

The clinical signs associated with canine lymphoma are variable and depend on the extent and location of the tumor. Multicentric lymphoma, the most common form, is usually distinguished by the presence of generalized painless lymphadenopathy (see Figure 32-1). Enlarged lymph nodes are usually painless, rubbery, and discrete and may initially include the mandibular and prescapular nodes. In addition, hepatosplenomegaly and bone marrow involvement occur commonly. Most dogs with multicentric lymphoma present without dramatic signs of systemic illness (WHO substage *a*) (Box 32-1); however, a large array of nonspecific signs such as anorexia, weight loss, vomiting, diarrhea, emaciation, ascites, dyspnea, polydipsia, polyuria, and fever can occur (WHO substage *b*). Dogs presented with T-cell lymphoma are more likely to have constitutional (i.e., substage *b*) signs. Polydipsia and polyuria are particularly evident in dogs with hypercalcemia of malignancy. Dogs may also be presented with clinical signs related to blood dyscrasias secondary to marked tumor infiltration of bone marrow (myelophthisis) or paraneoplastic anemia, thrombocytopenia, or neutropenia. These could include fever, sepsis, anemia, and hemorrhage. Diffuse pulmonary infiltration is seen in 27% to 34% of dogs with the multicentric form, as detected by radiographic changes (Figure 32-3).[97,98] Based on bronchoalveolar lavage, the actual incidence of lung involvement may be higher.[99,100]

Box 32-1 World Health Organization's Clinical Staging System for Lymphoma in Domestic Animals

Anatomic Site

- A Generalized
- B Alimentary
- C Thymic
- D Skin
- E Leukemia (true)*
- F Others (including solitary renal)

Stage (to include anatomic site)

- I Involvement limited to a single node or lymphoid tissue in a single organ.†
- II Involvement of many lymph nodes in a regional area (±tonsils).
- III Generalized lymph node involvement.
- IV Liver and/or spleen involvement (±stage III).
- V Manifestation in the blood and involvement of bone marrow and/or other organ systems (±stage I-IV).

Each stage is subclassified into:

- a Without systemic signs
- b With systemic signs

*Only blood and bone marrow involved.

†Excluding bone marrow.

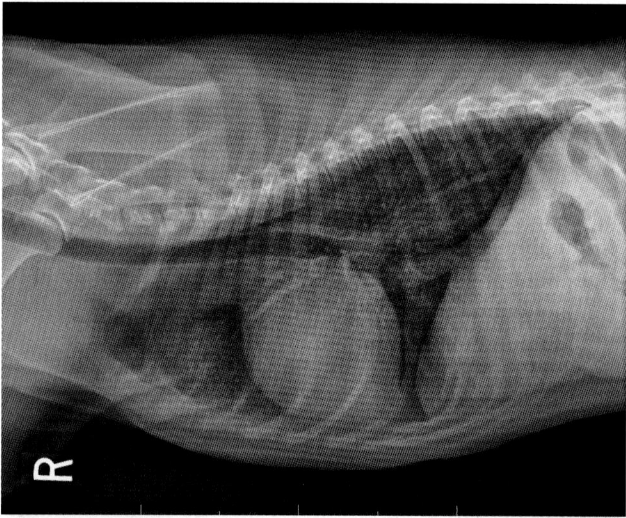

FIGURE 32-3 Lateral projection of a thoracic radiograph of a dog with diffuse interstitial infiltration with lymphoma secondary to multicentric lymphoma.

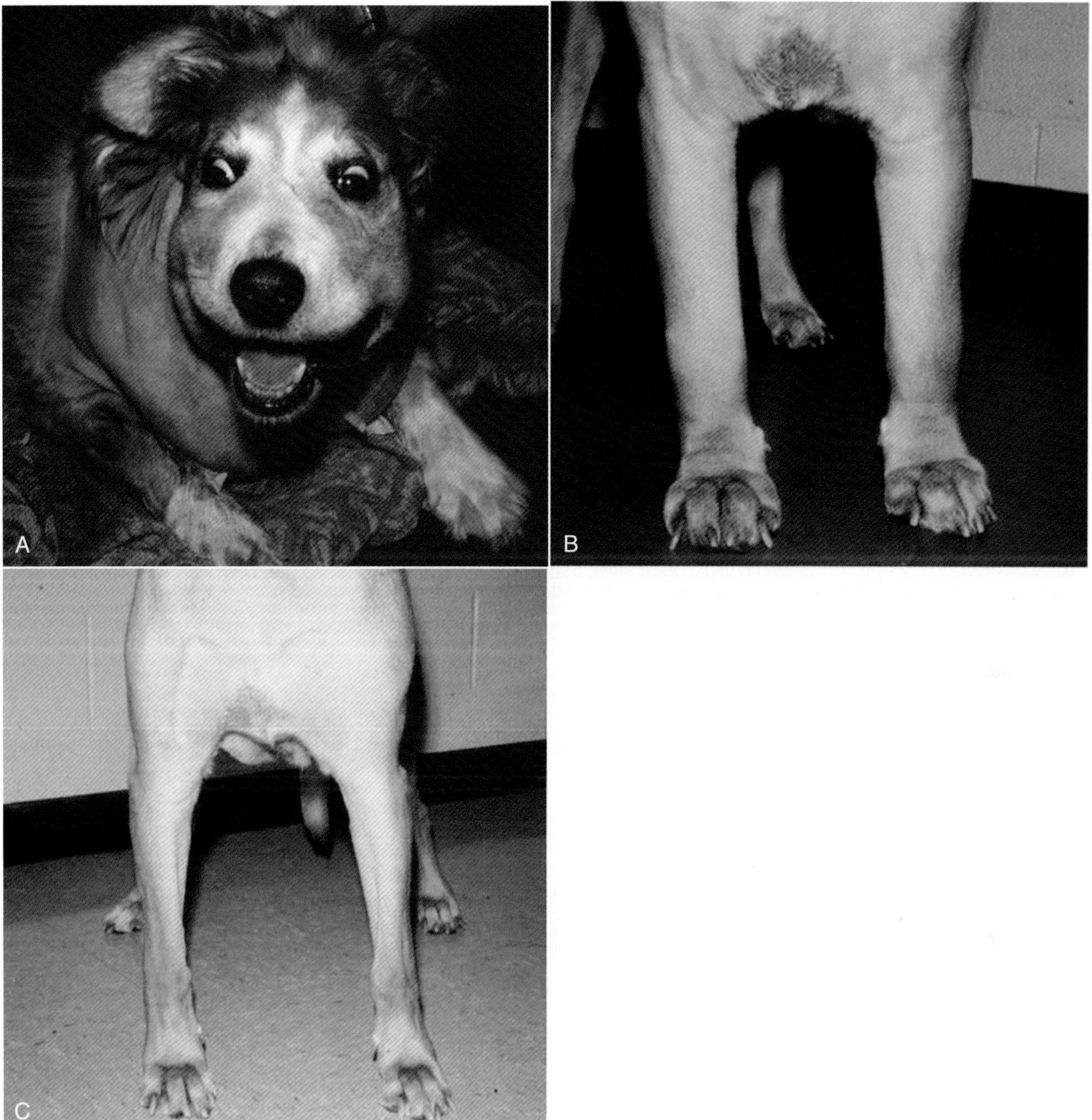

FIGURE 32-4 **A,** Facial edema in a dog with precaval syndrome secondary to mediastinal lymphoma. **B,** Forelimb edema in a dog with precaval syndrome secondary to mediastinal lymphoma. **C,** The dog in **B** 24 hours after radiation therapy to the cranial mediastinal mass, showing resolution of pitting edema.

Dogs with GI or alimentary lymphoma are usually presented with nonspecific GI signs, such as vomiting, diarrhea, weight loss, and malabsorption.[47,101,102] Mesenteric lymph nodes, spleen, and liver may be involved.

The mediastinal form of lymphoma is characterized by enlargement of the cranial mediastinal structures and/or thymus (see Figure 32-2), and clinical signs are associated with the extent of disease with resulting respiratory compromise or polydipsia/polyuria from hypercalcemia. Commonly, dogs are presented with respiratory distress caused by a space-occupying mass and pleural effusion, exercise intolerance, and possibly regurgitation. Additionally, dogs with mediastinal lymphoma may present with precaval syndrome, characterized by pitting edema of the head, neck, and forelimbs secondary to tumor compression or invasion of the cranial vena cava (Figure 32-4).

Signs in dogs with extranodal lymphoma depend on the specific organ involved. Cutaneous lymphoma is usually generalized or multifocal.[55-57] Tumors occur as nodules, plaques, ulcers, and erythemic or exfoliative dermatitis with focal hypopigmentation and alopecia. Epitheliotropic T-cell lymphoma (e.g., mycosis fungoides) typically has a clinical course with three apparent clinical stages. Initially, there will be scaling, alopecia, and pruritus (Figure 32-5, *A*), which can mimic a variety of other skin conditions. As the disease progresses, the skin becomes more erythematous,

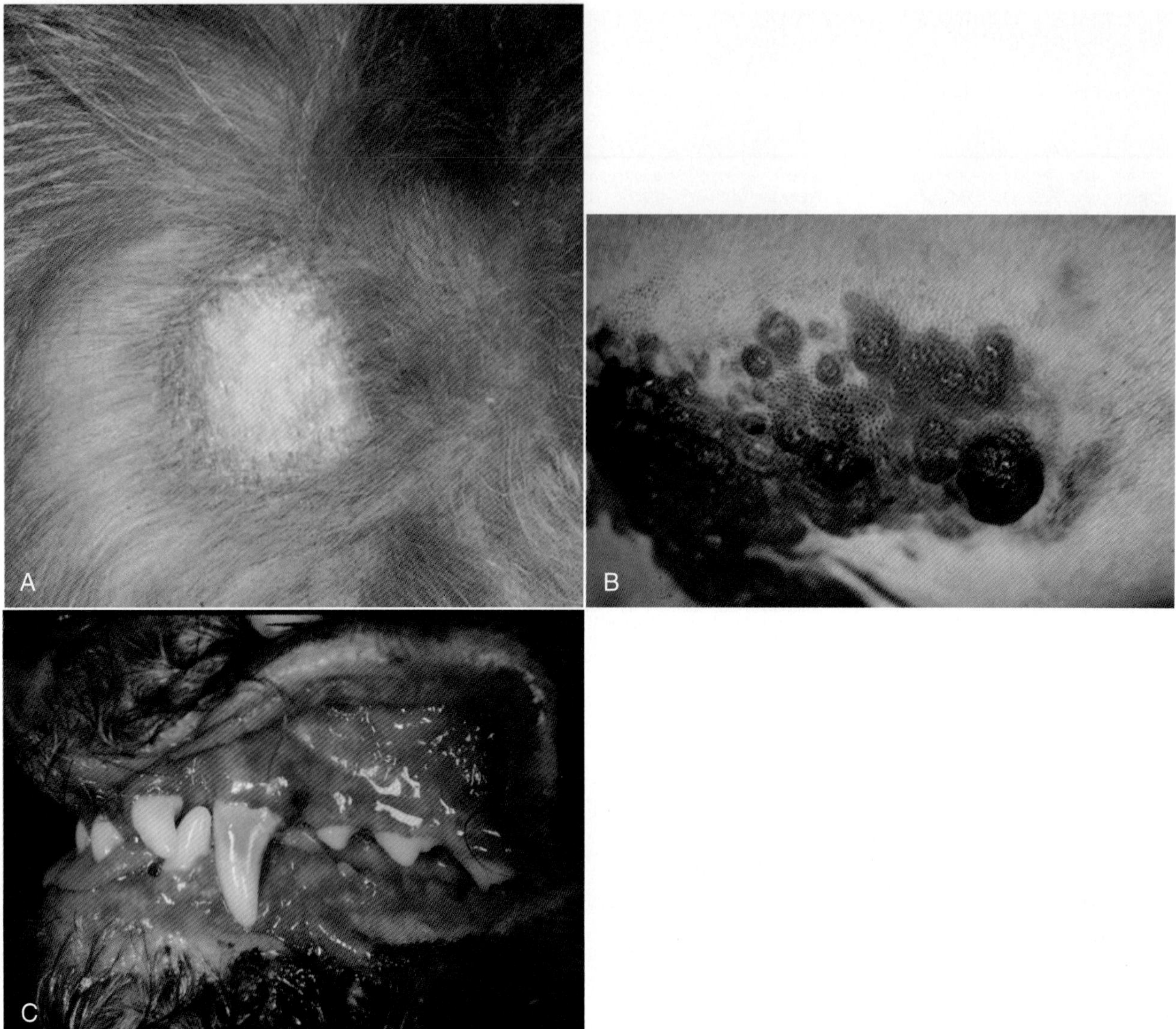

FIGURE 32-5 **A,** Early epitheliotropic cutaneous lymphoma in the scaly, plaque stage in a dog. **B,** Advanced epitheliotropic cutaneous lymphoma in the nodular stage in a dog. **C,** Oral mucosal epitheliotropic cutaneous lymphoma in a dog.

thickened, ulcerated, and exudative. The final stage is characterized by proliferative plaques and nodules with progressive ulceration (Figure 32-5, *B*). Oral involvement may also occur and this can appear as multicentric erythematous plaque-like lesions or nodules associated with the gum and lips (Figure 32-5, *C*). Extracutaneous involvement can also occur, most often in the lymph nodes, spleen, liver, and bone marrow. Nonepitheliotropic cutaneous lymphomas form single or multiple dermal or subcutaneous nodules or plaques; histologically, they spare the epidermis and papillary dermis and affect the middle and deep portions of the dermis and subcutis.[55]

Dogs with primary CNS lymphoma may be presented with either multifocal or solitary involvement.[103-105] Seizures, paralysis, and paresis may be noted. Ocular lymphoma is characterized by infiltration and thickening of the iris, uveitis, hypopyon, hyphema, posterior synechia, and glaucoma.[106,107] In one study of 94 cases of canine multicentric lymphoma, 37% had ocular changes consistent with lymphoma, and in a series of 102 cases of uveitis in dogs, 17% were secondary to lymphoma.[107] Anterior uveitis was most commonly seen in advanced stage of disease (stage V). Dogs with intravascular lymphoma usually present with signs relative to CNS, PNS, or ocular involvement.[66-71] These include paraparesis, ataxia, hyperesthesia, seizures, blindness, lethargy, anorexia, weight loss, diarrhea, polyuria, polydipsia, and intermittent fever. Finally, dogs with pure hepatosplenic lymphoma usually are presented with nonspecific signs of lethargy, inappetence, and weakness and often are icteric.[64,65]

The differential diagnosis of lymphadenopathy depends on the dog's travel history (i.e., relative to infectious disease) and the size, consistency, and location of affected lymph nodes. Other causes of lymphadenopathy include infections caused by bacteria, viruses, parasites (*Toxoplasma* sp., *Leishmania* sp.), rickettsial organisms (Salmon-poisoning, *Ehrlichia* sp.), and fungal agents (*Blastomyces* and *Histoplasma* sp.). The potential for hypercalcemia to accompany systemic fungal diseases may further complicate differentiation from lymphoma. Discrete, hard, asymmetric lymph nodes, particularly if they are fixed to underlying tissues, may indicate metastatic tumors such as mast cell tumor or carcinoma. Immune-mediated diseases (e.g., pemphigus, systemic lupus erythematosus) also may result in mild-to-moderately enlarged lymph nodes. The

TABLE 32-2 Differential Diseases or Conditions That Can Resemble Canine Lymphoma

FORM OF LYMPHOMA	OTHER DISORDERS
Multicentric	Disseminated infections: Bacterial, viral, rickettsial, parasitic, fungal Immune-mediated disorders: Dermatopathies, vasculitis, polyarthritis, lupus erythematosus Tumors metastatic to nodes Other hematopoietic tumors: Leukemia, multiple myeloma, malignant or systemic histiocytosis
Mediastinal	Other tumors: Thymoma, chemodectoma, ultimobranchial cyst, ectopic thyroid carcinoma, pleural carcinomatosis, pulmonary lymphomatoid granulomatosis* Infectious disease: Granulomatous disease, pyothorax Miscellaneous: Congestive heart failure, chylothorax, hemothorax
Alimentary	Other gastrointestinal tumors, foreign body, lymphangiectasia, lymphocytic-plasmacytic enteritis, systemic mycosis, gastroduodenal ulceration
Cutaneous	Infectious dermatitis: Advanced pyoderma Immune-mediated dermatitis: Pemphigus Other cutaneous neoplasms (in particular histiocytic disorders)
Extranodal	Variable, depending on organ/system involved

*The existence of this disease is controversial; in most cases, the disease has been reclassified as a lymphoid neoplasm.

various differential diseases or conditions that can resemble canine lymphoma are listed in Table 32-2.

Canine lymphoma also may be associated with paraneoplastic syndromes (see Chapter 5). Anemia is the most common lymphoma-related paraneoplastic syndrome.[108] Paraneoplastic hypercalcemia is also common and is characterized clinically by anorexia, weight loss, muscle weakness, lethargy, polyuria, polydipsia, and rarely CNS depression and coma. Lymphoma-induced hypercalcemia in most cases results from parathyroid hormone–related peptide (PTHrP), elaborated by neoplastic cells; however, it can also be related to the production of several other humoral factors, including interleukin-1 (IL-1), tumor necrosis factor-α (TNF-α), transforming growth factor-β (TGF-β), and vitamin D analogs (e.g., 1,25-dihydroxyvitamin D).[89,109,110] As previously discussed, hypercalcemia is most commonly associated with the T-cell immunophenotype. Other paraneoplastic syndromes that may be encountered include monoclonal gammopathies, neuropathies, and cancer cachexia.

Diagnostics and Clinical Staging

For dogs suspected of having lymphoma, the diagnostic evaluation should include a thorough physical examination; complete blood count (CBC), with a differential cell count, including a platelet count; a serum biochemical profile; and urinalysis. Optimally, ionized calcium should be measured. Ultimately, obtaining tissue or cytologic specimens for a definitive diagnosis is essential.

Physical Examination

A thorough physical examination should include palpation of all assessable lymph nodes, including a rectal examination; in the authors' experience, a significant proportion of dogs will have rectal polyps consisting of aggregates of neoplastic lymphocytes. Inspection of mucous membranes for pallor, icterus, petechiae, and ulceration should be undertaken as these signs may indicate anemia or thrombocytopenia secondary to myelophthisis or immune-mediated disease or may be evidence of major organ failure or uremia. Abdominal palpation may reveal organomegaly, intestinal wall thickening, or mesenteric lymphadenopathy. The presence of a mediastinal mass and/or pleural effusion can be suspected following thoracic auscultation. An ocular examination, including funduscopic assessment, may reveal abnormalities (e.g., uveitis, retinal hemorrhage, ocular infiltration) in approximately one-third to one-half of dogs with lymphoma.[107,111]

Complete Blood Count, Biochemistry Profile, and Urinalysis

Anemia, the most common lymphoma-related hematologic abnormality, is usually normochromic and normocytic (nonregenerative), consistent with anemia of chronic disease.[108] However, hemorrhagic and hemolytic anemias may also occur, and regenerative anemias may reflect concomitant blood loss or hemolysis. Additionally, if significant myelophthisis is present, anemia may be accompanied by thrombocytopenia and leukopenia.[112,113] In animals with anemia or evidence of bleeding, in addition to a platelet count, a reticulocyte count and coagulation testing may be indicated. Thrombocytopenia may be seen in 30% to 50% of cases, but bleeding is seldom a clinical problem. Neutrophilia can be seen in 25% to 40% of dogs and lymphocytosis occurs in approximately 20% of affected dogs.[108] Circulating atypical lymphocytes may be indicative of bone marrow involvement and leukemia. It is important to differentiate multicentric lymphoma with bone marrow involvement (i.e., stage V disease) from primary lymphoblastic leukemia (see later), as the prognosis for each is entirely different. Hypoproteinemia is observed more frequently in animals with alimentary lymphoma. In dogs with a high total protein or evidence of an increased globulin fraction on a chemistry profile, serum proteins may be evaluated by serum electrophoresis. Monoclonal gammopathies have been reported to occur in approximately 6% of dogs with lymphoma.[114]

Serum biochemical abnormalities often reflect the anatomic site involved, as well as paraneoplastic syndromes such as hypercalcemia. In cases of hypercalcemia of unknown origin, lymphoma should always be considered high on the differential disease list, and diagnostic testing directed at this possibility should be undertaken (see Chapter 5). In addition, the presence of hypercalcemia can serve as a biomarker for response to therapy and early recurrence. Increased urea nitrogen and creatinine concentrations can occur secondary to renal infiltration with tumor, hypercalcemic nephrosis, or prerenal azotemia from dehydration. Increases in liver-specific enzyme activities or bilirubin concentrations may result from hepatic parenchymal infiltration. Increased serum globulin concentrations, usually monoclonal, occur infrequently with B-cell lymphoma.

Urinalysis is part of the minimum database used to assess renal function and the urinary tract. For example, isosthenuria and proteinuria in the absence of an active sediment may indicate renal disease, and hematuria may result from a hemostatic abnormality. It is important to remember that isosthenuria in azotemic dogs with hypercalcemia is not necessarily indicative of renal disease as the high calcium levels interfere with tubular concentration capabilities through disruption of antidiuretic hormone (ADH) control.

Several abnormalities in serum have been explored as biomarkers of lymphoma in the dog. Examples include alpha-fetoprotein, alpha-1 glycoprotein levels, zinc, chromium, iron, endostatin, vascular endothelial growth factor (VEGF), lactate dehydrogenase, C-reactive protein haptoglobin, and antioxidants/oxidative stress markers.[115-122] The clinical, biologic, and prognostic significance of these alterations is yet to be definitively characterized.

Histologic and Cytologic Evaluation of Lymph Nodes

Morphologic examination of the tissue and cells that constitute the tumor is essential to the diagnosis of lymphoma. Care should be taken to avoid lymph nodes from reactive areas (e.g., mandibular lymph nodes), unless those nodes are the only ones enlarged; the prescapular or popliteal lymph nodes are preferable if also involved. Also, lymphoid cells are fragile, and in preparing smears of aspirated material only gentle pressure should be applied in spreading material on the slides. In most cases, a diagnosis of lymphoma can be made on evaluation of fine-needle aspirates of affected lymph nodes or other tissues. Typically, most of the cells are large lymphoid cells (>2 times the diameter of a red blood cell [RBC] or larger than neutrophils), and they may have visible nucleoli and basophilic cytoplasm (Figure 32-6, *A*) or fine chromatin with indistinct nucleoli. Because tissue architecture is not maintained in cytologic specimens, effacement of the node or capsular disruption cannot be detected. Therefore marked reactive hyperplasia characterized by increased numbers of large lymphoid cells may be difficult to distinguish from lymphoma, and small cell lymphomas may have few cytologic clues that point to malignancy. Also, classification of lymphoma, which has been attempted using cytologic appearance and immunophenotypic analysis,[123] into subcategories that make up the low-, intermediate-, and high-grade forms is performed most accurately on histologic sections (discussed previously).

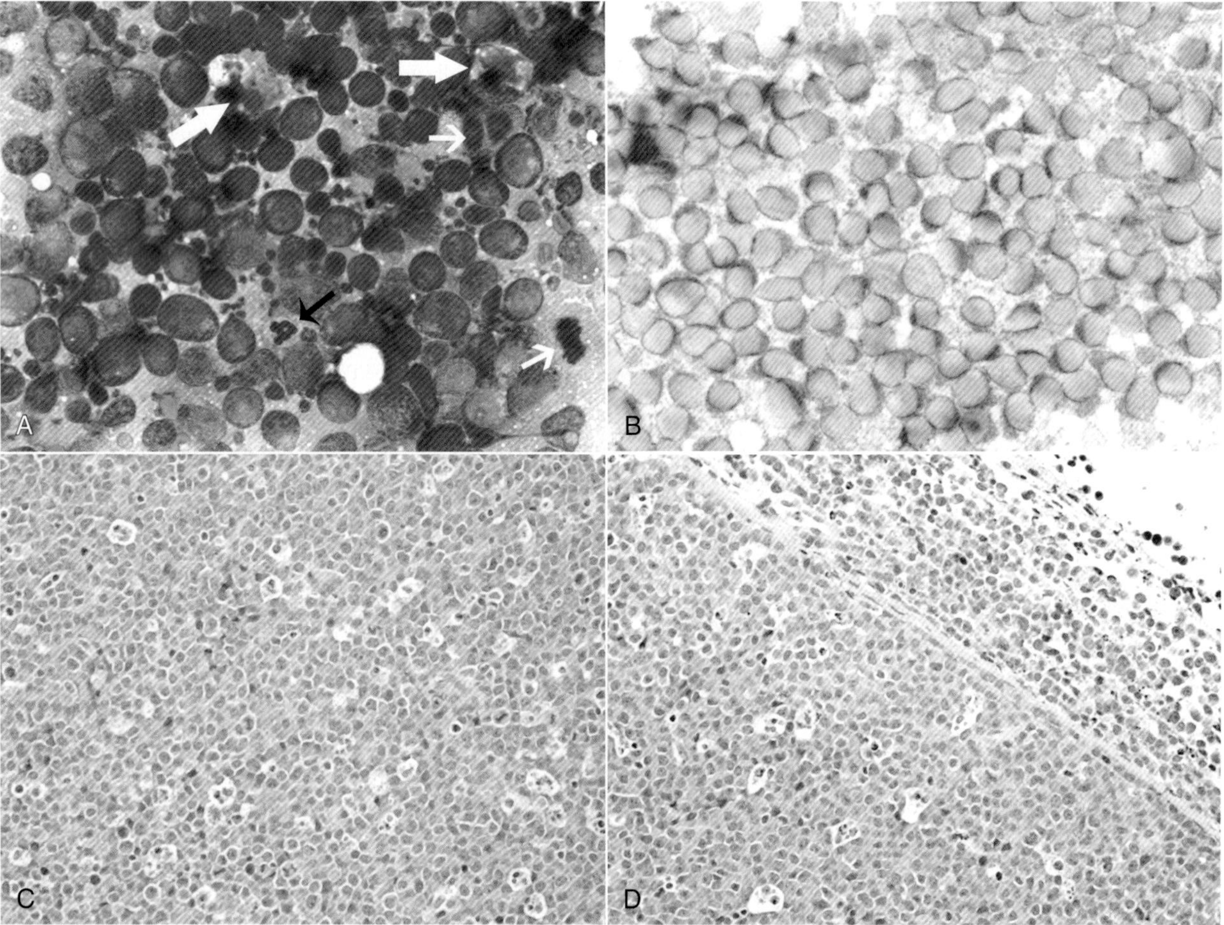

FIGURE 32-6 Lymph nodes from dogs with lymphoma. **A,** Fine-needle aspirate. Note the homogenous population of large lymphoid cells with prominent nucleoli and basophilic cytoplasm. These cells are larger than the neutrophil *(black arrow)* in the field. Mitotic figures *(thin white arrows)* and tingible body macrophages *(thick white arrows)* also are present. (Wright's stain, ×60 objective.) **B,** Fine-needle aspirate stained for immunoreactivity for CD79a. Note that nearly all of the lymphocytes express CD79A. The diagnosis was B-cell lymphoma. (Alkaline phosphatase/fast red, ×60 objective.) **C,** Histologic section. Note effacement of normal architecture. The white spaces are macrophages, giving a "starry sky" appearance to the lymph node. (H&E, ×20 objective.) **D,** Histologic section. Note the presence of tumor cells outside the capsule of the lymph node. (H&E, ×20 objective.)

For accurate histopathologic evaluation, an entire lymph node, including the capsule, should be removed, placed in buffered formalin, and submitted to a pathologist. Although needle core biopsies may be satisfactory, it is important to avoid crush artifact or inadequate sample size. Most pathologists prefer whole node biopsies because they provide the maximal amount of information. Effacement of normal nodal architecture by neoplastic lymphocytes and capsular disruption are characteristic findings (Figure 32-6, *C* and *D*). Diagnostic ultrasonography and ultrasound-guided FNA or needle biopsy have been useful for evaluation of involvement of the liver, spleen, or abdominal lymph nodes.[124-126] Aspiration of ultrasonographically normal splenic tissue is rarely contributory to a diagnosis.[124] If possible, the diagnosis should be made by sampling peripheral nodes, avoiding percutaneous biopsies of the liver and spleen. However, if there is no peripheral node involvement, it is appropriate to biopsy affected tissues in the abdominal cavity.

Histologic and Cytologic Evaluation of Extranodal Sites

When GI lymphoma is suspected, an open surgical wedge biopsy of the intestine is preferred in most cases to differentiate lymphoma from lymphocytic enteritis. If associated abdominal lymph nodes also appear involved, image-guided biopsies may be associated with less morbidity than intestinal biopsies. Multiple samples may be necessary to accurately diagnose segmental disease. Endoscopic biopsies may be inadequate as only a superficial specimen is obtained; however, more aggressive endoscopic biopsy techniques combined with more accurate histopathologic, immunophenotypic, and molecular assessments are improving the diagnostic yield of these less invasive techniques.[127-130] In many dogs with primary GI lymphoma, an inflammatory nonneoplastic infiltrate (i.e., LPE) may be misdiagnosed on biopsy specimens that are too superficial. The application of assays for clonal expansion (e.g., PARR—see next section on molecular diagnostic techniques) does not appear as yet to be as accurate for endoscopically derived intestinal biopsies as with other solid lymphoid tumors in dogs.

Cytologic examination of cerebrospinal fluid (CSF), thoracic fluid, or mass aspirates is indicated in animals with CNS disease, pleural effusion, or an intrathoracic mass, respectively. In one study of dogs with CNS involvement, CSF analysis was diagnostic in seven of eight dogs.[103] Characteristics of the CSF included an increased nucleated cell count in the seven dogs, and 95% to 100% of the cells were atypical lymphocytes. The CSF protein concentration was increased in five of the dogs, ranging from 34 to 310 mg/dL (reference interval: <25 mg/dL).

For cutaneous lymphoma, punch biopsies (4 to 8 mm) should be taken from the most representative and infiltrative, but not secondarily infected, skin lesions. Application of immunophenotypic and clonality assessments of cutaneous biopsies can aid in differentiating lymphoma from benign lymphocytic lesions.[58,131,132]

Molecular Diagnostic Techniques

Molecular techniques can be used to establish a diagnosis of lymphoma or to further characterize the tumor after the initial diagnosis is made. Tissues and cells from peripheral blood, lymph nodes, nonlymphoid sites, and effusions can be analyzed by various molecular means to aid in cases that represent a more difficult diagnostic challenge, particularly in cases where reactive lymphocytosis and lymphoma are both possible based on standard histologic or cytologic assessment. These include histochemical and cytochemical, immunohistochemical and immunocytochemical, flow cytometric, and polymerase chain reaction (PCR) techniques. For example, the immunophenotype (B-cell versus T-cell),[93,133-140] proliferation rate (e.g., expression of Ki67, proliferating cell nuclear antigen [PCNA] expression, argyrophilic nucleolar organizer regions [AgNOR]),[53,133,141-145] and clonality (PCR for antigen receptor gene rearrangement [PARR])[146-154] of the tumor can be determined. The availability of such analyses is increasing; however, at present, only immunophenotype and PARR clonality assays are routinely used in dogs to inform clinical decision making.

Immunophenotyping

Immunophenotyping is used to determine the type of cells that comprise the tumor, but this technique also can be helpful for making the initial diagnosis.[133-140,155] When a heterogenous population of lymphocytes is expected in a tissue, documentation of a homogeneous population of the same immunophenotype is supportive of a neoplastic process. The immunophenotype of a lymphocyte is identified by determining the expression of molecules specific for B-cells (e.g., CD79a, CD20) and T-cells (e.g., CD3). Although tumor cells sometimes have morphologic characteristics that typify a particular immunophenotype, exceptions occur, and morphologic appearance cannot be used as the sole determinant of immunophenotype. For example, in a series of nine high-grade T-cell lymphomas and leukemias in dogs, the cells had a plasmacytoid appearance, typically associated with B-cell lymphoma.[156] Similarly, anatomic location does not always predict the immunophenotype.

For accurate determination of immunophenotype, antibodies against lymphocyte markers are applied to tissue sections (immunohistochemistry), cytologic specimens (immunocytochemistry), or individual cells in a fluid medium (flow cytometry). Flow cytometric evaluation of cells obtained by needle aspiration is also feasible. For T-cells, markers include CD3 (pan T), CD4 (helper T), and CD8 (cytotoxic T); for B-cells, the markers are CD79a (Figure 32-6, *B*), CD20, and CD21. Increasingly, aberrant expression of CD molecules has been reported in canine lymphoma. In a study of 59 dogs with lymphoma, tumor cells from six dogs were positive for both T- and B-cell markers; however, a clonality assay (see later) revealed clonality either of the T-cell or the immunoglobulin receptor but not both. This indicates that in some cases, the malignant cells may co-express B- and T-cell markers.[93] Antibodies against these molecules are used to determine the immunophenotype; however, they also have potential utility as a therapeutic modality if tumor cells could be targeted using these antibodies.

Other Immunohistochemical and Immunocytochemical Assessments

Assessments of markers of multidrug resistance and apoptotic pathways (e.g., P-glycoprotein, p53, Bcl-2 proteins) have been evaluated in dogs with lymphoma.[19,79,142,156a,156b] However, their clinical significance and utility await further evaluation.

Clonality Assays

Occasionally, diagnosis of lymphoma and differentiation of malignant versus benign proliferation of lymphocytes are not possible based on standard histologic and cytologic criteria. In these cases, advanced molecular analyses may be helpful to confirm a diagnosis. Clonality is the hallmark of malignancy; that is, the malignant cell population theoretically should be derived from expansion of a single malignant clone characterized by a particular DNA region unique to that tumor. For example, in a dog with T-cell lymphoma, all the malignant cells theoretically should have the same DNA sequence for the variable region of the T-cell receptor gene.

Likewise, in a dog with B-cell lymphoma, the tumor cells should have identical DNA sequences in the variable region of the immunoglobulin (Ig) receptor gene. Conversely, in reactive lymphocytosis, the cells are polyclonal for their antigen receptors. Using this knowledge, investigators have used PCR technology to amplify the variable regions of the T-cell and immunoglobulin receptor genes to detect the presence of clonal lymphocyte populations in dogs (see Figure 8-4 of Chapter 8). These techniques are reviewed in Chapter 8 and elsewhere.[150] In physician-based medicine, such assays of clonality are approximately 70% to 90% sensitive and have a false-positive rate of approximately 5%, and recent studies report similar rates in dogs. False-negative and false-positive results can occur with clonality assays. For example, cells from a dog with lymphoma may be negative for clonality if the clonal segment of DNA is not detected with the primers used, if the malignant cells are natural killer (NK) cells (rare), or if the malignant cells are present in too low a frequency to be detected. False positives occur rarely in some infectious diseases (e.g., ehrlichiosis and Lyme disease). In these cases, a diagnosis should be made only after considering the results of all the diagnostic tests, including histologic/cytologic evaluation, immunophenotyping, and clonality studies in conjunction with signalment and physical examination findings. These molecular techniques, although helpful for diagnosis, could also have utility in detecting early recurrence and in determining more accurate clinical stage and so-called "molecular remission rates" because they are more sensitive than standard cytologic assessment of peripheral blood, bone marrow, or lymph nodes (covered subsequently in section on treatment response).

Proteomics

Proteomics comprises, simplistically, methodologies that analyze the entire protein component or protein signature of cells (the proteome). Protein components of a cell (normal or malignant) change over time with upregulation and downregulation of gene expression in response to varied stimuli (e.g., growth factors, environmental cues). It may therefore be possible to use the field of proteomics to identify serum biomarkers of malignancy (i.e., cancer-specific protein markers) and to further analyze response to therapy or even to predict which therapies are appropriate for an individual patient's tumor. Although in its infancy in veterinary oncology, preliminary investigations of the proteome of dogs with lymphoma have been reported[157-160]; however, they have yet to reach the level of sophistication in which useful output would have an impact on clinical decision making.

Staging

After a diagnosis has been established, the extent of disease should be determined and categorized by the clinical stage of disease. The WHO staging system routinely used to stage dogs with lymphoma is presented in Box 32-1. Most dogs (>80%) are presented in advanced stages (III to IV). Diagnostic imaging and assessment of bone marrow involvement may be indicated for staging. The degree to which thorough staging is implemented depends on whether the result will alter the treatment plan, whether relevant prognostic information is gleamed, and whether the clients need to know the stage prior to initiating (or declining) a treatment plan. Additionally, when comparing different treatment protocols with respect to efficacy, consistent and similar staging diagnostics should be used to avoid so-called "stage migration," which results when one staging methodology is more accurate than another.[161] The impact of stage migration on prognosis should be considered when comparing different published outcomes.

Bone Marrow Evaluation

A bone marrow aspirate or biopsy (from proximal humerus or iliac crest) is recommended for complete staging and prognostication and is indicated in dogs with anemia, lymphocytosis, peripheral lymphocyte atypia, or other peripheral cytopenias. In one study of 53 dogs with lymphoma, 28% had circulating malignant cells and were considered leukemic, whereas bone marrow examination indicated involvement in 57% of the dogs.[162] The presence of a few prolymphocytes and large lymphocytes with nucleoli in the circulation of dogs with lymphoma may indicate bone marrow involvement. It is important to remember these cells also can be seen with GI parasitism, immune-mediated hemolytic anemia, and other immune-mediated and infectious diseases. As discussed previously, tumor cells within the peripheral and bone marrow compartments can also be identified using clonality assays (PARR) that are more sensitive than routine microscopic examination in detecting malignant cells; however, the prognostic significance of the knowledge gained with more sensitive staging methodologies is yet to be determined. Although bone marrow evaluation may offer prognostically valuable information, it is not necessary to perform the procedure if the client is committed to treat regardless of stage.

Imaging

Evaluation of thoracic and abdominal radiographs may be important in determining the extent of internal involvement (Figure 32-7). Approximately 60% to 75% of dogs with multicentric lymphoma have abnormalities on thoracic radiographs, with one-third having evidence of pulmonary infiltrates (see Figure 32-3) and two-thirds having thoracic lymphadenopathy (sternal and tracheobronchial lymph nodes [see Figure 32-7]) and widening of the cranial mediastinum (see Figure 32-2).[97,98] Pulmonary infiltrates usually are represented by an interstitial and/or alveolar pattern; however, nodules (rarely) and bronchial infiltrates can also occur.[163] Pleural effusion may also be present. Cranial mediastinal lymphadenopathy is detected in 20% of dogs with lymphoma.[97,163] Abdominal radiographs reveal evidence of involvement of medial iliac (sublumbar) and/or mesenteric lymph node, spleen, or liver in approximately 50% of cases. In the authors' practice, for the typical cases of canine multicentric lymphoma, imaging is limited to thoracic

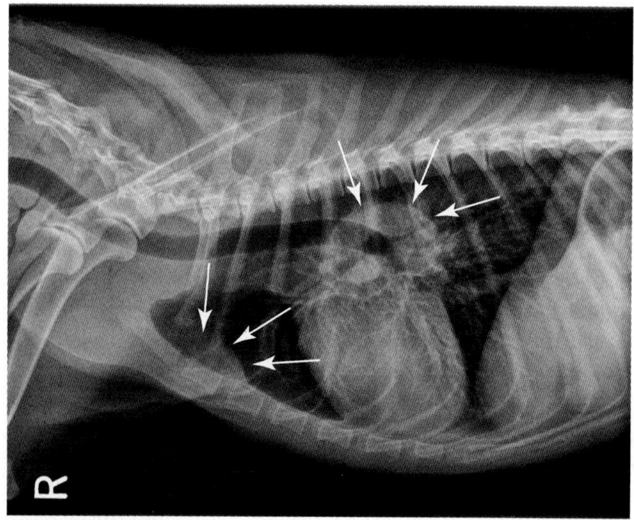

FIGURE 32-7 Lateral radiographic projection of a dog with sternal and hilar lymphadenopathy due to lymphoma.

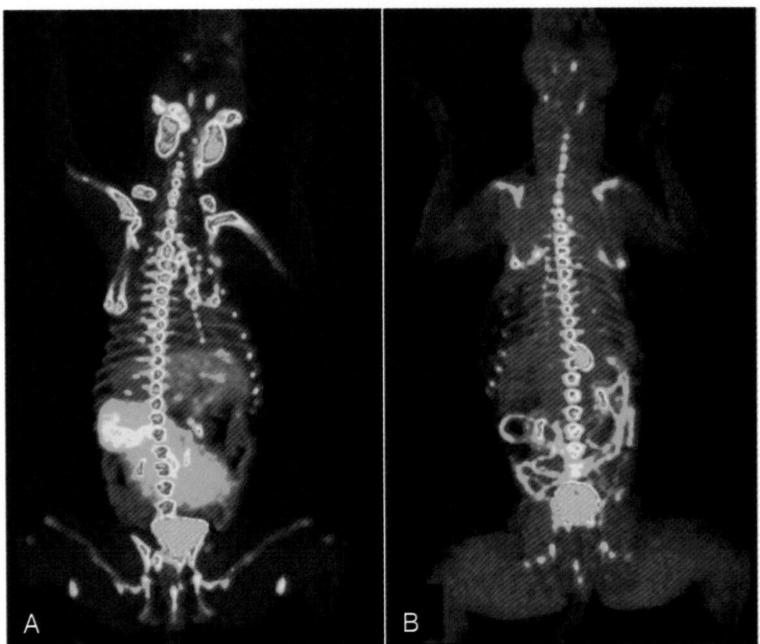

FIGURE 32-8 **A,** FLT-PET/CT image of a 3-year-old MN Hound cross illustrating FLT uptake in the peripheral nodes, bone marrow, kidneys, bladder, and spleen. **B,** FLT-PET/CT image of the same dog 3 weeks after his final dose of chemotherapy. The lymph nodes were small on CT with minimal FLT uptake on PET images. Note the persistent uptake in the bone marrow, kidneys, and bladder. *(Reprinted with permission from Lawrence J, Vanderhoek M, Barbee D, et al: Use of 3′-deoxy-3′-[18F]fluorothymidine PET/CT for evaluating response to cytotoxic chemotherapy in dogs with non-Hodgkin's lymphoma,* Vet Radiol Ultrasound *50:660–668, 2009.)*

radiographs as there is no prognostic difference between dogs with stage III and IV disease (i.e., liver/spleen involvement), whereas the presence of cranial mediastinal lymphadenopathy is of prognostic significance (see prognosis section). However, if there are clinical signs attributable to abdominal disease or if complete staging is necessary (e.g., for clinical trial inclusion), further imaging of the abdomen is warranted. Abdominal ultrasonography can be important for obtaining ultrasound-guided intraabdominal samples for diagnosis. It may also be useful for the diagnosis of GI, abdominal nodal, and hepatosplenic lymphoma.[125] Ultrasonographic (including Doppler ultrasound) assessment of peripheral lymph nodes has also been explored[126]; however, its clinical applicability is questionable because cytologic assessment of peripheral nodes is easy, inexpensive, and of higher diagnostic utility.

Advanced imaging modalities, including computed tomography (CT), magnetic resonance imaging (MRI), positron emission tomography (PET), or PET/CT imaging, are becoming more commonplace in veterinary practice and their utility is only now being determined.[164-169] PET/CT imaging is the current standard of care for following and indeed predicting durability of treatment response in human patients with lymphoma, and both [18F]fluorothymidine (18FLT) PET/CT and [18F]fluoro-D-glucose (18FDG) PET imaging have been reported in dogs with lymphoma.[164-166] 18FLT-PET/CT functional and anatomic imaging shows promise for the evaluation of response to cytotoxic chemotherapy in dogs with lymphoma and for predicting relapse before standard clinical and clinicopathologic confirmation (Figure 32-8).

Treatment of Multicentric Lymphoma

The therapeutic approach to a particular patient with lymphoma is determined by the stage and substage of disease, the presence or absence of paraneoplastic disease, the overall physiologic status of the patient, financial and time commitment of the clients, and their level of comfort with respect to likelihood of treatment-related success and/or side effects.

Without treatment, most dogs with lymphoma will die of their disease in 4 to 6 weeks after diagnosis, although significant variability exists.[114] With few exceptions, canine lymphoma is considered a systemic disease and therefore requires systemic therapy in order to achieve remission and prolong survival. The majority of canine multicentric lymphomas are intermediate to high grade, and, currently, histopathologic and immunophenotypic characterization has not played a significant role in determining the initial treatment protocol. It is hoped that in the near future, sufficient data will emerge to better tailor treatment protocols chosen for dogs with lymphoma based on these and other yet to be characterized parameters. That being said, systemic multiagent chemotherapy continues to be the therapy of choice for canine lymphoma. In general, combination chemotherapy protocols are superior in efficacy to single-agent protocols. Single-agent protocols result in lower response rates that are not as durable as combination chemotherapy, which is summarized in Table 11-2 in Chapter 11. In rare cases in which lymphoma is limited to one site (especially an extranodal site), the animal can be treated with a local modality such as surgery or radiation therapy (RT) as long as the client and clinician are committed to diligent reevaluation to document subsequent progression to systemic involvement, should it occur.

Multidrug Combination Protocols

Many chemotherapeutic protocols for dogs with lymphoma have been developed over the past 15 to 20 years (Table 32-3).[91,170-190] Significant limitations arise when comparing efficacy studies in the

TABLE 32-3 Summary of First Remission Outcomes of Combination or Single-Agent Doxorubicin Lymphoma Chemotherapy Protocols (Minimum of 30 Cases Required for Inclusion)*

PROTOCOL	DOGS (NO)	REMISSION RATE (%)	MEDIAN REMISSION (MONTHS)	1-YEAR SURVIVAL (%)	REFERENCES
COP	77	75	6.0	19	170
A	37	59	4.4	NR	171
A[†]	121	85	4.3	NR	172
A	42	74	4.9	NR	173
A + piroxicam	33	79	4.3	NR	173
VMC-L	59	90	4.4	25	174
VMC-L	147	77	4.7	25	175
VCA-L	112	73	7.9	50	91
L-COPA	41	76	11.0[‡]	48	176
L-COPA (II)	68	75	9.0[‡]	27 (13 at 2 years)	177
COPLA/LVP	75	92 (80[‡])	5.8	17	178
VELCAP-SC	94	70	5.6	44	179
VLCAP-Long	98	69	12.5[‡]	NR	180
L-VCAMP (UW-Madison)	55	84	8.4	50 (24% at 2 years)	181
L-VCAMP	96	79 (CR)	9	NR	182
(continuous maintenance)	86	90	6.8[‡]	35[‡]	183
L-VCAMP (± intensification)	130	94.6	7.3§	NR	184
L-VCAP (25 weeks)	51	94	9.1	NR	185
L-VCAP-Mx[‖]	65	94	10	NR	186
L-VCAP	71	88	9.7[‡]	32 (13% at 2 years)	187
L-VCAP (12 weeks)	77	89	8.1[‡]	28[‡]	188
L-VCAP/CCNU/MOPrP	66	94	10.6[‡]	46 (35% at 2 years)	187
COArP	71	92	3	NR	189
L-VCADP	39	100	11[§]	NR	190

L, L-Asparaginase; *V*, vincristine; *C*, cyclophosphamide; *M*, methotrexate; *Mx*, mitoxantrone; *O*, Oncovin (vincristine); *P*, prednisone; *A*, Adriamycin (doxorubicin); *D*, dactinomycin; *Pr*, procarbazine; *Ar*, cytosine arabinoside; *NR*, not reported; *CR*, complete response.

*Few of these protocols include sufficient numbers for adequate statistical power and fewer compare treatment protocols in a randomized prospective fashion. In addition, staging, inclusion, and response criteria vary considerably between protocols presented. Therefore evaluations of efficacy between the various protocols are subject to bias, making direct comparisons difficult and indeed precarious.

[†]With COP rescue.

[‡]Only durations of cases achieving CR reported.

[§]Time to progression.

[‖]Questionable (only one-third reportedly finished).

veterinary literature for the various published protocols. Few of these studies include sufficient numbers for adequate statistical power and even fewer compare treatment protocols in a randomized prospective fashion. In addition, staging, inclusion, and response criteria vary considerably between reports. Therefore evaluations of efficacy among various protocols are subject to substantial bias, making direct comparisons difficult and indeed precarious. A recurring theme in the concluding statement in most of these published protocols is some variation of "prospective randomized trials will be required to confirm these suggestive findings." In an attempt to better standardize response criteria and outcome reporting of future trials, the Veterinary Cooperative Oncology Group (VCOG) has recently published response evaluation criteria (v1.0)[169] (see subsequent response evaluation section). The greatest obstacle to the performance of prospective randomized comparative lymphoma trials in veterinary oncology is financial; that is, clinical trials are inherently costly, and because most of the known effective drugs are unregistered off-label human generic (i.e., off patent) drugs, the incentive for pharmaceutical-funded, sufficiently powered, randomized field trials is low, resulting in a general lack of comparative data.

Despite the plethora of available combination protocols, most are modifications of CHOP protocols initially designed for human oncologic use, and currently randomized prospective evidence does not exist to clearly recommend one over the other as long as the basic "CHOP" components are present. CHOP represents combinations of cyclophosphamide (C), doxorubicin (H, hydroxydaunorubicin), vincristine (O, Oncovin), and prednisone (P). Conventional CHOP-based chemotherapy induces remission in approximately 80% to 95% of dogs, with overall median survival times (MSTs) of 10 to 12 months. Approximately 20% to 25% of treated dogs will be alive 2 years after initiation of these protocols (Figure 32-9).

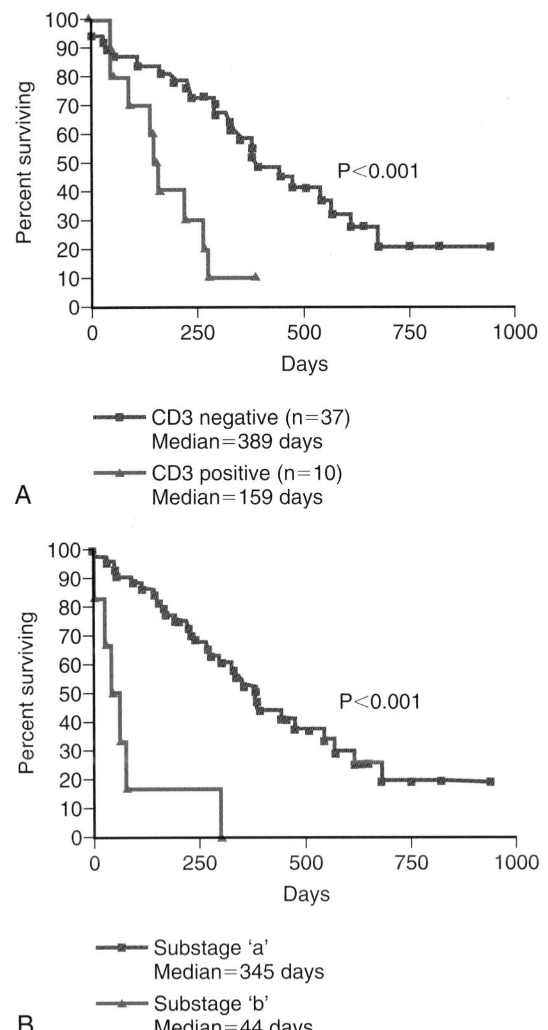

FIGURE 32-9 **A,** Kaplan-Meier survival duration estimates for a group of 55 dogs with lymphoma treated with an identical CHOP-based combination chemotherapy protocol. Dogs with CD3 immunoreactive (T-cell) lymphoma had significantly shorter survival durations. **B,** Kaplan-Meier survival duration estimates for a group of 55 dogs with lymphoma treated with an identical CHOP-based combination chemotherapy protocol at the University of Wisconsin. Dogs with substage *b* disease (i.e., clinically ill) had significantly shorter survival durations. *(From Vail DM: Hematopoietic tumors. In Ettinger SJ, Feldman EC, editors:* Textbook of veterinary internal medicine, *ed 6, St. Louis, 2005, Elsevier.)*

Response rates and duration of response vary according to the presence or absence of prognostic factors discussed subsequently in the section on prognosis in this chapter. The relative cost of the various protocols to the client depends on the drug(s) selected, the size of the animal, the frequency of administration, and the laboratory tests required to monitor adverse events and response.

Dogs responding to chemotherapy and undergoing complete remission are usually free of clinical signs associated with lymphoma and subsequently return to a very good quality of life. Treating dogs with lymphoma is initially gratifying because a high percentage enjoy a complete response. Most dogs tolerate chemotherapy well, and although dose reductions and treatment breaks ("treatment holidays") are not uncommonly required in individual cases, only a minority of dogs develop significant adverse events requiring hospitalization.[191,192] Studies assessing client perceptions of medical treatment for cancer in general and lymphoma in particular report a positive experience; most owners feel treatment was worthwhile, that it resulted in improvement in the well-being of their pet, and that quality of life during treatment was good.[193,194] Very few clients express regret about treating lymphoma using a multidrug protocol.

With lymphoma, the fundamental goals of chemotherapy are to induce a complete durable (>6 months) first remission (termed *induction*), to reinduce a remission when the tumor recrudesces (or the patient relapses) following achievement of a remission (termed *reinduction*), and, finally, to induce remissions when the cancer fails to respond to induction or reinduction using drugs not present in the initial protocols (termed *rescue*).

An unanswered question in the treatment of lymphoma has been whether long-term maintenance chemotherapy is useful following an initial course of aggressive induction chemotherapy lasting 6 months or less. Long-term maintenance chemotherapy has not been shown to be of significant value in humans with most forms of NHL; however, in humans, the initial induction course of chemotherapy is much more aggressive than that used in veterinary patients. Although no randomized prospective studies have been performed to address the therapeutic benefit of long-term maintenance chemotherapy in dogs, most comparisons of dogs treated with CHOP-based protocols do not show any clear advantage for a maintenance or consolidation phase after induction therapy.* Indeed, in most reports, dogs receiving shorter, less costly protocols that do not include a prolonged maintenance phase have comparable remission and progression-free survival (PFS) durations and appear to more readily achieve second remissions when they relapse following completion of chemotherapy than their counterparts receiving long-term maintenance. These data, taken together, suggest that maintenance therapy is not beneficial for most dogs with lymphoma. Until well-designed randomized prospective trials indicate otherwise, the author (DMV) prefers protocols that utilize an aggressive induction without maintenance.

Single-Agent Chemotherapy with Known Activity for Dogs with Lymphoma

The most effective, currently available chemotherapeutic agents for canine lymphoma include doxorubicin, L-asparaginase, vincristine, cyclophosphamide, and prednisone—most of which are represented to one degree or another in most first-line multiagent chemotherapy protocols. Other drugs that have documented activity are often considered second-line agents and include lomustine, vinblastine, actinomycin-D, mitoxantrone, mustargen, chlorambucil, methotrexate, dacarbazine (DTIC), 9-aminocamptothecin, ifosfamide, cytosine arabinoside, and gemcitabine. Of these, cytosine arabinoside,[199] ifosfamide,[200] and gemcitabine[201] appear to have only minimal activity. With the exception of doxorubicin, induction therapy with single-agent chemotherapy does not typically result in durable remission durations when compared with standard combination protocols (see Table 11-2, Chapter 11). Incorporation of other standard cytotoxic drugs with single-agent activity into standard CHOP-based protocols has not resulted in significant gains, and most are reserved for subsequent rescue settings.

*References 53, 177, 180, 182-186, 188, 190, 195-198.

Overall Chemotherapy Recommendations for Multicentric Lymphoma (Author Preference)

Several factors should be considered and discussed with caregivers on a case-by-case basis when choosing the protocol to be used. These factors include cost, time commitment involved, efficacy, adverse event profiles, and experience of the clinician with the protocols under consideration.

Induction in Treatment-Naïve Patients

It is now clearly established that "standard of care" combination protocols used in dogs with lymphoma are essentially variations of "CHOP" protocols (see Table 32-3). Specific details regarding dose and timing of the CHOP protocol currently preferred by the author (DMV) are outlined in Box 32-2. This protocol does not have a maintenance therapy arm, and all treatments cease at 19 weeks, provided the animal is in complete remission. Although several other CHOP-based protocols include L-asparaginase either at initiation or at varying times throughout the protocol, several studies suggest this does not result in clinically relevant increases in remission rate, speed of attaining remission, or first-remission duration, and therefore the author reserves its use for rescue situations.[172,195,202,203]

If client or other considerations preclude a CHOP-based protocol, single-agent doxorubicin (30 mg/m^2, intravenous [IV], every 3 weeks for 5 total treatments) is offered along with a 4-week tapering oral prednisone regimen (same prednisone regimen in Box 32-2) as a less aggressive and less costly approach. The expected CR rate will range from 50% to 75%, with an anticipated median survival of 6 to 8 months.[171,172,204,205] The addition of oral cyclophosphamide (50 mg/m^2 daily for 3 days starting on the same day as doxorubicin) to single-agent doxorubicin resulted in a numerically but not statistically superior outcome in a recent randomized trial[205] comparing doxorubicin/prednisone with doxorubicin/cyclophosphamide/prednisone (PFS of 5.6 months versus 8.2 months, respectively). This trial was only powered to detect a threefold difference in PFS; therefore larger trials should be undertaken to confirm any benefit.

If clients are reticent to include IV medications, the author often recommends a protocol of oral lomustine (CCNU; 70 mg/m^2 by mouth [PO] every 3 weeks for 5 treatments) and prednisone. This protocol has been associated with short median remissions (40 days) in only one small case series[206]; however, in the author's experience, a subset of dogs have remained in remission for several months on this protocol when clients decline IV medication.

If financial or other client concerns preclude the use of systemic chemotherapy, prednisone alone (2 mg/kg PO, daily) will often result in short-lived remissions of approximately 1 to 2 months. In these cases, it is important to educate clients that, should they decide to pursue more aggressive therapy at a later date, dogs receiving single-agent prednisone therapy are more likely to develop multidrug resistance (MDR) and experience shorter remission and survival durations with subsequent combination protocols.[207-209] This is especially true following long-term prednisone use or in dogs that have experienced a recurrence while receiving prednisone. Therefore the earlier that clients opt for more aggressive therapy, the more likely a durable response will result.

A CBC should be performed prior to each chemotherapy treatment. A minimum of 1500 neutrophils/μL (some oncologists use a cut-off of 2000 neutrophils/μL) and 50,000 platelets/μL should be present prior to the administration of myelosuppressive chemotherapy. If the neutrophil count is lower than 1500/μL, it is best to wait 5 to 7 days and repeat the CBC; if the neutrophil count has increased to more than 1500 cells/μL, the drug can be safely administered. A caveat to these restrictions is that for dogs presented prior to initiation of chemotherapy with low neutrophil and platelet counts due to bone marrow effacement, myelosuppressive chemotherapy is instituted in the face of cytopenias in order to clear the bone marrow of neoplastic cells and allow hematopoiesis to normalize.

In those breeds likely to have *MDR1* gene mutations (e.g., collies; see Chapter 11) and therefore to be at risk for serious chemotherapeutic toxicity,[210] the author will initiate a CHOP protocol out of sequence, beginning with non-MDR1–associated drugs, such as cyclophosphamide. This ensures treatment of the lymphoma while allowing sufficient time for analysis of *MDR1* gene mutations prior to initiating MDR1 substrate drugs. No specific protocols have been scrutinized for treating dogs that are double-mutant for MDR1; however, if using MDR1 substrate drugs, the author initiates at a 40% dose reduction. Subsequent dose modifications (increased or decreased dosage) can be implemented,

Box 32-2 Current Canine Lymphoma Protocol (UW-Madison-Short)

Week 1: Vincristine 0.7 mg/m^2 IV
Prednisone 2 mg/kg PO, q24hr
Week 2: Cyclophosphamide* 250 mg/m^2 IV
Prednisone 1.5 mg/kg PO, q24hr
Week 3: Vincristine 0.7 mg/m^2 IV
Prednisone 1.0 mg/kg PO, q24hr
Week 4: Doxorubicin† 30 mg/m^2 IV
Prednisone 0.5 mg/kg PO, q24hr
Week 6: Vincristine 0.7 mg/m^2 IV
Week 7: Cyclophosphamide* 250 mg/m^2 IV
Week 8: Vincristine 0.7 mg/m^2 IV
Week 9: Doxorubicin† 30 mg/m^2 IV
Week 11: Vincristine 0.7 mg/m^2 IV
Week 12: Cyclophosphamide* 250 mg/m^2 IV
Week 13: Vincristine 0.7 mg/m^2 IV
Week 14: Doxorubicin† 30 mg/m^2 IV
Week 16: Vincristine 0.7 mg/m^2 IV
Week 17: Cyclophosphamide* 250 mg/m^2 IV
Week 18: Vincristine 0.7 mg/m^2 IV
Week 19: Doxorubicin† 30 mg/m^2 IV

IV, Intravenous; *PO*, by mouth.

*Furosemide (1 mg/kg) is given IV, concurrent with cyclophosphamide to reduce incidence of sterile hemorrhagic cystitis.

†In dogs <15 kg in body weight, a doxorubicin dose of 1 mg/kg is substituted for 30 mg/m^2.

1. All treatments discontinued after week 19 if in complete remission (CR).
2. A complete blood count (CBC) should be performed prior to each chemotherapy. If neutrophil count <1500 (some use 2000), wait 5-7 days and repeat CBC.
3. If sterile hemorrhagic cystitis occurs on cyclophosphamide, discontinue and substitute chlorambucil (1.4 mg/kg PO) for subsequently scheduled cyclophosphamide injections.
4. For acute lymphoblastic leukemia (ALL): Administer L-asparaginase 400 IU/kg subcutaneously (SQ) with each vincristine injection, until a CR is achieved.

depending on adverse event levels observed, particularly neutrophil counts at nadir.

The Case for Treating T-Cell Lymphoma Differently

With some exceptions, multicentric T-cell lymphoma, when compared with multicentric B-cell lymphoma, is associated with similar initial response rates, but significantly lower response durability (e.g., PFS) following chemotherapy (including CHOP-based protocols).* Additionally, the effectiveness of a single treatment of doxorubicin in the treatment of naïve dogs with lymphoma in one retrospective case series suggested a lower initial response rate for T-cell, compared with B-cell, immunophenotypes.[213] This has led many to question whether dogs diagnosed with T-cell lymphoma should be treated with standard CHOP-based protocols or with alternative protocols. This is a valid question; however, the answer remains elusive because adequately powered randomized controlled trials do not currently exist in the literature to show superiority for an alternate protocol in this scenario. A retrospective study of an L-asparaginase and MOPP (*M,* mechlorethamine; *O,* Oncovin; *P,* procarbazine; *P,* prednisone) protocol suggested improvement in PFS in dogs with either confirmed T-cell lymphoma or lymphoma with hypercalcemia and no immunophenotypic classification.[214] However, differences in determining PFS, response evaluation, and study population in this retrospective study did not definitively confirm superiority.[211] Further, some have advocated early inclusion of lomustine (CCNU) into protocols for treating multicentric T-cell lymphoma based on moderate success of lomustine-based rescue protocols in dogs failing CHOP. As yet, no randomized trials have documented superiority with this approach. Ultimately, superior protocol development for T-cell lymphoma awaits careful, randomized, prospective trial assessment. Until such time, the author prefers to initiate CHOP-based induction and switch to lomustine-based rescue at the first sign of progression.

Treatment Response Evaluation for Lymphoma

VCOG has recently published response evaluation criteria (v1.0)[169] to standardize reporting of outcome results and comparisons among protocols for peripheral nodal disease. The most important of these outcome measures and the preferred temporal outcome criterion for assessing protocol activity is now considered to be PFS, which is defined as being from the time of treatment initiation until tumor progression or death from any cause. This brings veterinary outcome reporting more in line with human standards. Because the majority of dogs with lymphoma eventually experience recurrence following chemotherapy-induced remissions and because methodology for differentiating complete and partial responses is analysis dependent, PFS removes many sources of bias. Further, overall survival in published reports invariably includes patients who go on to receive varied rescue protocols that bias the overall result, making it a less comparable outcome. Widespread application of these standardized criteria should allow more suitable comparisons in the future.

Superior methods of detection of minimal residual disease (MRD) or early recurrence have been investigated in dogs with lymphoma and include advanced imaging and detection of molecular and biologic markers of minimal disease. Advanced functional and anatomic imaging (i.e., PET/CT) are the current standard for assessing treatment response and early relapse of lymphoma in humans and have also been investigated in dogs (see Figure 32-8).[164-166,168] As this technology becomes available to a broader veterinary population, its clinical application will surely increase. Molecular detection of MRD applies clonality and PCR techniques previously discussed in this chapter. Beyond diagnostic applications, these techniques have been applied to determine cytoreductive efficacy of various chemotherapeutic drugs and to document and predict early relapse in patients prior to more conventional methods.[215-219] Regarding biomarkers of MRD, preliminary investigations have suggested serum lactate dehydrogenase activity,[120] thymidine kinase 1 activity,[220] and serum C-reactive protein[221] may be candidates in the dog.

As we become more proficient at defining MRD, the pressing clinical question becomes how we use this information. Theoretically, such information could suggest when more aggressive therapy or alternative therapy should be instituted in patients who have not achieved a "molecular remission" or who are undergoing early relapse; however, until we determine what these interventions should be, their clinical utility remains theoretical.

Reinduction and Rescue Chemotherapy

Eventually, the majority of dogs that achieve a remission will relapse or experience recrudescence of lymphoma. This usually represents the emergence of tumor clones or tumor stem cells[222] (see Chapter 2) that are inherently more resistant to chemotherapy than the original tumor, the so-called MDR clones that either were initially drug resistant or became so following exposure to selected chemotherapy agents. Evidence suggests that in dogs with recurrent lymphoma, tumor cells are more likely to express the *MDR1* gene that encodes the protein transmembrane drug pump often associated with MDR.[156a,156b,225] *MDR1* represents only one of the plethora of mechanisms that lead to drug-resistant disease (see Chapter 11). Other causes for relapse following chemotherapy include inadequate dosing and frequency of administration of chemotherapy, failure to achieve high concentrations of chemotherapeutic drugs in certain sites such as the CNS, and initial treatment with prednisone alone.

At the first recurrence of lymphoma, it is recommended that reinduction be attempted first by reintroducing the induction protocol that was initially successful, provided the recurrence occurred temporally far enough from the conclusion of the initial protocol (e.g., ≥2 months) to make reinduction likely. Attention must be given to the cumulative dose of doxorubicin that will result from reinduction, and baseline cardiac assessment, the use of cardioprotectants, alternative drug choices, and client education should all be considered. In general, the length of the reinduction will be half that encountered in the initial therapy; however, a subset of animals will enjoy long-term reinductions, especially if the dog completed the initial induction treatment protocol and was currently not receiving chemotherapy for several months when relapse occurred. Nearly 80% to 90% reinduction rates can be expected in dogs that have completed CHOP-based protocols and then relapse while not receiving therapy.[185,226] The duration of a second CHOP-based remission in one report was predicted by the duration of the interval between protocols and the duration of the first remission.[226]

If reinduction fails or the dog does not respond to the initial induction, the use of so-called "rescue" agents or "rescue" protocols may be attempted. These are single drugs or drug combinations that are typically not found in standard CHOP protocols and are

*References 53, 86, 88, 91, 166, 188, 190, 209, 211-213.

TABLE 32-4 Summary of Response for Rescue Protocols (Minimum 25 Cases)*

PROTOCOL	ANIMALS (NO)	OVERALL RESPONSE (%)	COMPLETE RESPONSE (%)	MEDIAN RESPONSE DURATION† (DAYS)	MEDIAN DURATION OF COMPLETE RESPONSE (DAYS)	REFERENCE
Actinomycin-D	25	0	0	0	0	227
Actinomycin-D	49‡	41	41	129	129	228
Dacarbazine	40	35	3	43	144	229
Dacarbazine or temozolomide-anthracycline	63	71	55	45	NR	230
DMAC (dexamethasone, melphalan, actinomycin-D, cytosine arabinoside)	54	72	44	61	112	231
Lomustine (CCNU)	43	27	7	86	110	232
Lomustine-L-asparaginase-prednisone	48	77	65	70	90	233
Lomustine-L-asparaginase-prednisone	31	87	52	63	111	234
Lomustine-DTIC	57	35	23	62	83	235
Mitoxantrone	44	41	30	NR	127	236
MOPP (mechlorethamine, vincristine, procarbazine, prednisone)	117	65	31	61	63	237
MPP (mechlorethamine, procarbazine, prednisone)	41	34	17	56	238	238

NR, Not reported.

*Few of these protocols include sufficient numbers for adequate statistical power and fewer compare treatment protocols in a randomized prospective fashion. In addition, staging, inclusion, and response criteria vary considerably between protocols presented. Therefore evaluations of efficacy between the various protocols are subject to bias, making direct comparisons difficult and indeed precarious.

†Various temporal response endpoints were used, including disease-free interval, time to progression, and progression-free survival.

‡Prednisone often used concurrently.

withheld for use in the drug-resistant setting. The most common rescue protocols used in dogs include single-agent use or a combination of actinomycin D, mitoxantrone, doxorubicin (if doxorubicin was not part of the original induction protocol), dacarbazine (DTIC), temozolomide, lomustine (CCNU), L-asparaginase, mechlorethamine, vincristine, vinblastine, procarbazine, prednisone, and etoposide. Some rescue protocols are easy and convenient single-agent treatments, whereas others are more complicated (and expensive) multiagent protocols, such as MOPP. Overall rescue response rates of 40% to 90% are reported; however, responses are usually not durable, with median responses of 1.5 to 2.5 months being typical, regardless of the complexity of the protocol. A small (<20%) subset of animals will enjoy longer rescue durations. Table 32-4 provides a summary of canine rescue protocols and published results.[227-238] Current published data from rescue protocols do not include sufficient numbers for adequate statistical power nor do they compare protocols in a randomized prospective fashion. Therefore evaluations of efficacy among various protocols are subject to substantial bias, making direct comparisons difficult and indeed precarious. Choice of a particular rescue protocol should depend on several factors, including cost, time commitment required, efficacy, toxicity, and experience of the clinician with the protocols in question. As the complexity of rescue protocols does not yet appear to be associated with significant gains in rescue durability, the author tends to choose simpler and less costly protocols (e.g., CCNU/L-asparaginase/prednisone) (Table 32-5). However, the use of multiple varied rescue protocols, switching as needed based on response, continues as long as clients are comfortable with their dog's quality of life. This sequential application of several different rescue protocols can result in several months of extended survival with acceptable quality of life.

Strategies to Enhance Effectiveness of Therapy in Lymphoma

Despite the plethora of published chemotherapeutic protocols for dogs with lymphoma, it appears we have achieved as much as we can from currently available chemotherapeutics in standard settings. The 12-month median survival "wall" and the 20% to 25% 2-year survival rates have not improved dramatically. Further advances in remission and survival durations await the development of new methods of delivering or targeting traditional chemotherapeutic drugs, new generations of chemotherapeutic drugs, or novel nonchemotherapeutic treatment modalities. Mechanisms of avoiding or abrogating MDR, enhancing tumor apoptosis (programmed cell death), tumor ablation, and immune-system reconstitution, as well as novel immunomodulatory therapies for lymphoma, are all active areas of investigation in both human and veterinary medicine.

Mechanisms of Drug Resistance

Drug resistance can be inherent in cancer cells or develop following exposure to selected chemotherapeutic agents and often is associated with increased expression of members of the adenosine triphosphate (ATP)-binding cassette (ABC) transporter superfamily (e.g., P-glycoprotein pump), many of which efflux various

TABLE 32-5 First-Line Rescue Protocol*

CYCLE 1	
Week 1	**Baseline ALT ________ U/L** L-Asparaginase 400 U/kg SQ CCNU 70 mg/m^2 PO Prednisone 2mg/kg PO, once daily
Week 2	Prednisone 1.5 mg/kg PO, once daily
Week 3	Prednisone 1.0 mg/kg PO, once daily
CYCLE 2	
Week 1	**Optional ALT/ ________ U/L** L-asparaginase 400 U/kg SQ CCNU 70 mg/m^2 PO Prednisone 1.0 mg/kg PO, EOD
Week 2	Prednisone 1.0 mg/kg PO, EOD
Week 3	Prednisone 1.0 mg/kg PO, EOD
CYCLE 3 TO 5	
Week 1	**Mandatory ALT ________ U/L** CCNU 70 mg/m^2 PO Prednisone 1.0 mg/kg PO, EOD
Week 2	Prednisone 1.0 mg/kg PO, EOD
Week 3	Prednisone 1.0 mg/kg PO, EOD

ALT, Alanine aminotransferase; *SQ,* subcutaneous; *PO,* by mouth; *EOD,* every other day.

*Treatment discontinuation criteria:

1. After completion of protocol, two treatments beyond complete response (CR).
2. Progressive disease.
3. Increase in ALT activity >2× upper limit of normal (or 2× baseline if higher than upper limit of normal at initiation)—institute drug discontinuation and reinstitution/dose reduction depending on normalization of ALT.

chemotherapeutic compounds from cells (see Chapter 11).[239] P-glycoprotein is under the control of the *MDR1* gene. MDR has been reported in canine lymphoma following exposure to chemotherapy.[156a,225,240] Expression levels of mRNA encoding the canine *MDR1* gene have been characterized in canine cell lines and lymphomas. Although expression of MDR1 mRNA correlated with in vitro drug sensitivity, it did not correlate with in vivo doxorubicin sensitivity in dogs with lymphoma in this study. Additionally, quantitative analysis of mRNA for 10 different drug-resistance factors was performed in 23 dogs with lymphoma.[241] These dogs were divided into drug "sensitive" and "resistant" categories based on response to a CHOP-based protocol; however, significant differences in expression were not observed in this small study.

Altering Drug Pharmacokinetics

Methods of increasing the time that tumor cells are exposed to chemotherapeutics should theoretically enhance tumor killing. These methods could include long-term continuous infusions (impractical in many veterinary situations), increasing the frequency of treatments, or enhancing the circulation time of drugs used. In one study, dogs with lymphoma received lower dose doxorubicin weekly rather than a higher dose every 3 weeks (thereby decreasing C_{max}, which is associated with cardiotoxicity) in order to potentially increase the time of drug exposure.[242] No benefit was noted, and, in fact, remission rates were inferior. Studies evaluating pegylated long-circulating doxorubicin-containing liposome drug delivery systems in dogs with lymphoma have also been performed.[243,244] Although efficacy was established, enhancement of remission or survival durations over equivalent doses of native doxorubicin was not observed.

Treatment Approaches Using Immunologic or Biologic Agents

Monoclonal Antibody Approaches

In the past decade, enhanced durability of first remissions in humans with non-Hodgkin's B-cell lymphoma has been achieved primarily through the institution of monoclonal antibody (MAb)-based therapies (so-called R-CHOP protocols); the "R" refers to rituximab, a recombinant chimeric murine/human antibody directed against the CD20 antigen, a hydrophobic transmembrane protein located on normal pre-B and mature B lymphocytes. Following binding, rituximab triggers a host cytotoxic immune response against CD20-positive cells. Unfortunately, rituximab does not have therapeutic activity in dogs due to a lack of external recognition of a similar antigen on canine lymphoma cells and the inherent antigenicity of human-derived antibodies in dogs.[245,246] Another immunotherapy approach involved MAb-231, a murine-derived anticanine MAb (IgG2a). It mediates antibody-dependent cellular cytotoxicity (ADDC) and complement-mediated cellular cytotoxicity (CMCC).[247-249] It also prevented outgrowth of canine lymphoma xenografts in nude mice. In a noncontrolled clinical study of 215 dogs treated with CHOP-based chemotherapy and MAb-231, enhanced overall survival was observed; however, the antibody was removed from the commercial market in the mid-1990s without definitive randomized trials being performed. Several laboratories throughout the world are currently working to characterize and develop effective MAb therapies for use in dogs.

Antitumor Vaccine Approaches

Several antitumor vaccine approaches have been applied in dogs with lymphoma. A tumor vaccine extract using killed lymphoma cells combined with Freund's adjuvant was administered to a small number of dogs after remission induction with combination chemotherapy.[250] Prolongation of median survival was noted in the treatment group; however, a subsequent study revealed that prolongation was likely due to the Freund's adjuvant.[251] An autologous killed lymphoma tumor cell vaccine has been intralymphatically administered to dogs placed in remission using a combination chemotherapy protocol, and, although modest gains were reported in remission times, no survival advantage was found.[252] An exploratory vaccine study targeting telomerase[253] (see Chapter 14, Section D) and one using RNA-loaded CD40-activated B cells[254] in dogs with lymphoma have also been conducted. These studies involved small numbers of nonrandomized patients and lacked controlled populations for comparison. In a randomized study of 60 dogs with lymphoma comparing CHOP-based chemotherapy with CHOP-based chemotherapy and a human granulocyte-macrophage colony-stimulating factor (GM-CSF) DNA cationic-lipid complexed autologous whole tumor cell vaccine, a small measure of immunomodulation was documented by delayed-type hypersensitivity; however, significant improvement in clinical outcome was not noted.[255] Although little well-supported activity is reported to date with these immunomodulatory approaches, our basic understanding of methodologies is expanding.

Surgery

Most dogs with lymphoma have multicentric disease and therefore require systemic chemotherapy to effectively treat their disease.

However, surgery has been used to treat solitary lymphoma (early stage I) or solitary extranodal disease. Careful staging is necessary in such cases to rule out multicentric involvement prior to treating local disease.

The benefit of surgical removal of the spleen in dogs with massive splenomegaly remains unclear.[82,83,256] In an older report, 16 dogs with lymphoma underwent splenectomy to remove a massively enlarged spleen and were subsequently treated with chemotherapy.[256] Within 6 weeks of splenectomy, 5 of the 16 dogs died of disseminated intravascular coagulation (DIC) and sepsis. The remaining 11 dogs (66%) had a CR, and 7 dogs had a MST of 14 months. No staging or histologic information was provided, so the information appears of limited usefulness, although those with follow-up lived approximately 1 year. In two reports of indolent nodular lymphoma of the spleen (marginal zone lymphoma [MZL] and mantle cell lymphoma [MCL]), outcome was available on seven MZL cases, including three cases that did not receive adjuvant chemotherapy after surgery,[82,83] and only one died of lymphoma following splenectomy. In a recent report of indolent lymphomas, four splenic lymphomas (three MZL and one MCL) underwent splenectomy alone and all survived greater than 1 year with none dying of their primary disease.[84] Splenectomy should be considered if the lymphoma is not documented in other sites following thorough staging, if lymphoma is an indolent form histologically, or if splenic rupture has occurred. Of note, no control population consisting of dogs that did not undergo splenectomy exists, so the natural history of indolent splenic lymphoma remains uncertain.

Radiation Therapy

Radiation therapy, although its use is limited in the treatment of lymphoma, may be indicated in selected cases.[257] Indications are as follows:

1. Curative intent therapy for stage I lymph node and solitary extranodal disease (i.e., nasal, cutaneous, spinal lymphoma).
2. Palliation for local disease (e.g., mandibular lymphadenopathy, rectal lymphoma, mediastinal lymphoma where precaval syndrome is present, localized bone involvement).
3. Total body radiation combined with bone marrow or stem cell transplantation.
4. Whole or staged half-body RT following chemotherapy-induced remissions.

In the latter case, staged half-body irradiation sandwiched between chemotherapy cycles or following the attainment of remission by induction chemotherapy has been preliminarily investigated as a form of consolidation or maintenance.[198,258-262] Radiation therapy was delivered to either the cranial or the caudal half of the dog's body in 4 to 8 Gy fractions, and following a 2- or 4-week rest the other half of the body was irradiated in a similar fashion. Although these preliminary investigations were not randomized, they suggest that RT applied when dogs are in either complete or partial remission is safe and warrants further investigation to determine if a significant therapeutic gain can be realized. A pilot study of low-dose (1 Gy) single-fraction total body irradiation in seven dogs with relapsed drug-resistant lymphoma, although safely applied, resulted in only partial nondurable (1 to 4 week) remissions.[263]

Total body irradiation (and/or ablative chemotherapy) for complete or partial bone marrow ablation followed by reconstitution with bone marrow or stem-cell transplant in dogs, although a recognized model in comparative research settings,[264,265] is still in its early phases of development and application in clinical veterinary practice.[266,267] Because of the high cost, limited accessibility to relatively sophisticated equipment, and management requirements, these types of procedures are limited to preliminary investigations at a few centers. Currently, long-term results in significant numbers of treated cases have yet to be presented.

Treatment of Extranodal Lymphoma

In general, the veterinary literature suffers from a paucity of information on treating various extranodal forms of lymphoma in dogs, and our ability to predict outcome is thus limited. In general, it is recommended that, following extensive staging, in those cases where disease is shown to be localized to a solitary site, local therapies (e.g., surgery, local RT) can be used. In contrast, if multiple extranodal sites are involved or they are part of a more generalized process, systemic chemotherapy should be chosen.

Alimentary Lymphoma

Most dogs with alimentary lymphoma are presented with diffuse involvement of the intestinal tract, and involvement of local lymph nodes and liver is common. Chemotherapy in dogs with diffuse disease has been reported to be unrewarding for the most part[47,268,269]; however, more aggressive CHOP-based protocols used extensively for multicentric lymphoma in dogs have resulted in durable remissions in a small subset of cases. Solitary alimentary lymphoma is rare in the dog; however, if the tumor is localized and can be surgically removed, results (with or without follow-up chemotherapy) can be encouraging.

Primary Central Nervous System Lymphoma

CNS lymphoma in dogs usually results from extension of multicentric lymphoma. However, primary CNS lymphoma (PCNSL) has been reported.[103-105] If tumors are localized, local RT should be considered. Few studies have reported the use of chemotherapy. In one study, cytosine arabinoside (Ara-C) at a dosage of 20 mg/m^2 was given intrathecally; this treatment was combined with systemic chemotherapy and CNS radiation.[103] Overall, the response rates are low and of short duration (several weeks to months).

Cutaneous Lymphoma

Treatment of cutaneous lymphoma depends on the extent of disease. Solitary lesions may be treated with surgical excision or RT. Fractionated RT (to a total dose of 30 to 45 Gy) has been associated with long-term control.[270] Diffuse cutaneous lymphoma is best managed with combination chemotherapy, although the rate and durability of response is generally less than in multicentric lymphoma. The most widely used protocols for epitheliotropic cutaneous T-cell lymphoma include CCNU (60 to 70 mg/m^2 PO, every 3 weeks) along with prednisone.[271,272] Although response rates approach 80%, median remission is approximately 3 months; occasionally, durable remissions are encountered. The author has added L-asparaginase to this protocol (see Table 32-5), and although anecdotally it appears to improve response, comparative data are not available. Sporadic reports of other therapies for cutaneous lymphoma in small numbers of cases include the use of COAP (cyclophosphamide, vincristine [Oncovin], Ara-C, and prednisone),[273] retinoic acid analogs (e.g., Accutane, etretinate),[274] L-asparaginase and pegylated L-asparaginase,[275] topical mechlorethamine (Mustargen),[276] and recombinant human α-interferon.[277] All of these reports involved small numbers of cases and resulted in limited response rates with short durations.

A form of cutaneous lymphocytic infiltration has recently been characterized as an indolent T-cell lymphoma based on clonality.[131]

It is associated with slow progression and long-term survival following corticosteroid management; however, it does have the potential to progress to high-grade lymphoma.

Prognosis

The prognosis for dogs with lymphoma is highly variable and depends on a wide variety of factors documented or presumed to affect response to therapy. Although rarely curable (<10% of cases), CRs and a good quality of life during extended remissions and survival are typical. Factors that have been shown to influence treatment response and survival are summarized in Tables 32-6* and 32-7.† The two prognostic factors most consistently identified are immunophenotype and WHO substage (see Figure 32-9). Many reports have confirmed that dogs with CD3-immunoreactive tumors (i.e., T-cell derivation) are associated with significantly shorter remission and survival durations.‡ This holds true primarily for dogs with multicentric lymphoma because the immunophenotype of solitary or extranodal forms of lymphoma has not been thoroughly investigated with respect to prognosis. Additionally, it has been shown that dogs with B-cell lymphomas that express lower than normal levels of B5 antigen (expressed in 95% of nonneoplastic lymphocytes) also experience shorter remission and survival durations.[54] Recently, low levels of class II MHC expression on B-cell lymphoma predicted poor outcomes.[279] Dogs presented with WHO substage *b* disease (i.e., clinically ill) also do poorly when compared with dogs with substage *a* disease.[53,86,91,181,278] Dogs with stage I and II disease have a better prognosis than those dogs in more advanced stages (stage III, IV, and V).

Histologic grade (subtype) has been found to influence prognosis in some studies; however, our ability to predict outcome based on subtype is still quite limited. Dogs with lymphoma classified as intermediate or high grade (large cell, centroblastic, and immunoblastic) tend to respond to chemotherapy but can relapse early. Dogs with low-grade lymphomas (small lymphocytic or centrocytic) have a poorer response rate to chemotherapy, yet have a survival advantage over dogs with intermediate- and high-grade lymphomas (Figure 32-10) in that the disease may be more indolent. Several case compilations have documented that dogs with indolent lymphoma (e.g., MZL, MCL, T-zone) experience prolonged survivals, often in the absence of any or aggressive chemotherapy.[82-84] Proliferative assays such as analysis of bromodeoxyuridine (BrdU) uptake, Ki67 antibody reactivity, and argyrophilic nucleolar organizer region (AgNOR) indices to measure proliferative activity of tumor cells have been shown to provide prognostic information in dogs treated with combination chemotherapy. Results of different studies are contradictory, however. In two trials, dogs having tumors with short doubling times, high AgNOR frequencies, or high Ki67 immunoreactivity had a better prognosis than those with tumors with long doubling times or low AgNOR frequencies.[53,142] In other trials, the low-proliferating tumor groups were associated with a better prognosis.[283,284] Additionally, in one trial, the proportion of tumor cells undergoing apoptosis was modestly predictive of remission duration.[142]

The anatomic site of disease is also of considerable prognostic importance. Primary diffuse cutaneous, diffuse GI, hepatosplenic, and primary CNS lymphomas tend to be associated with a poor prognosis. Dogs with indolent cutaneous T-cell lymphocytic infiltration experience long-term survivals.[131] Sex has been shown to influence prognosis in some studies.[175, 181] Neutered females tend to have a better prognosis; male dogs may have a higher incidence of the T-cell phenotype, which may account for the poorer prognosis.

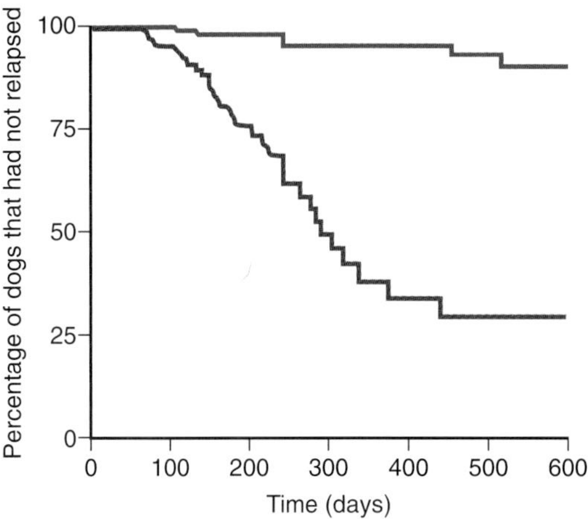

FIGURE 32-10 Kaplan-Meier curves illustrating time to relapse adjusted for clinical stage and immunophenotype among dogs treated for low-grade (n = 17) *(blue line)* or high-grade (n = 51) *(red line)* Kiel classification lymphoma. *(From Teske E, van Heerde P, Rutteman GR, et al: Prognostic factors for treatment of malignant lymphoma in dogs,* J Am Vet Med Assoc *205:1722–1728, 1994.)*

Reported biomarkers of prognosis, summarized in Table 32-7, include circulating levels of glutathione-S-transferase, thymidine kinase, lactate dehydrogenase, serum C-reactive proteins, and VEGF. Finally, one report suggests that a history of chronic inflammatory disease of several types predicts likelihood of early relapse.[291] These putative prognostic indicators require further confirmation in larger trials.

Lymphocytic Leukemia

Lymphocytic leukemia is typically defined as proliferation of neoplastic lymphocytes in bone marrow. Neoplastic cells usually originate in the bone marrow, but occasionally in the spleen, and may or may not be circulating in the peripheral blood. Although our ability to diagnose lymphocytic leukemias using flow cytometric and molecular diagnostic techniques has increased significantly in the past decade, little information on treatment and prognosis is available except for chronic lymphocytic leukemia (CLL). Differentiating between true leukemia and stage V lymphoma can be difficult and arbitrary and is often based on lack of significant lymphadenopathy, degree of blood and bone marrow involvement, and immunophenotypic characteristics.

Incidence, Risk Factors, and Etiology

Lymphocytic leukemia is more common than acute myeloid leukemia and myeloproliferative disorders (MPD), but the true incidence is unknown. German shepherd dogs and golden retrievers may be overrepresented.[137,292] Lymphocytic leukemia can occur in dogs of any age but typically occurs in middle-aged to older dogs (mean of 7 to 10 years); CLL usually occurs in older dogs (mean of 10 years).[137,280,292,293] A significant sex predilection is not reported. As with lymphoma, the etiology of lymphocytic leukemia is for the

*References 53, 82-84, 89, 91, 97, 107, 142, 156a, 156b, 170, 175, 181, 204, 207-209, 217-219, 225, 278-285.

†References 91, 119, 120, 209, 220, 221, 286-290.

‡References 53, 54, 86, 88, 91, 209, 279.

TABLE 32-6 Prognostic Factors for Lymphoma in Dogs

FACTOR	STRONG ASSOCIATION	MODEST ASSOCIATION REQUIRING FURTHER INVESTIGATION	COMMENTS	REFERENCES
WHO clinical stage		X	Stage I/II—favorable. Stage V with significant bone marrow involvement—unfavorable.	170, 204, 278
WHO clinical substage	X		Substage b (clinically ill)—associated with decreased survival.	53, 86, 91, 181, 278
Histopathology	X		High-grade/medium-grade—associated with high response rate but reduced survival. The indolent lymphomas generally experience prolonged survivals, often in the absence of systemic therapy.	82-84, 86, 87, 209
Immunophenotype	X		T-cell phenotype associated with reduced survival. Low MHC II expression on B-cell associated with reduced survival.	53, 54, 86, 88, 91, 209, 279
Flow cytometric characteristics of peripheral blood	X		Includes combined size and immunophenotypic analysis.	280
Sex		X	Some studies suggest females have a favorable prognosis.	175, 181
Anemia	X		Presence of anemia diminishes prognosis.	209, 281, 282
Molecular assessment of minimal residual disease (e.g., PARR)		X	Likely to become much more important when more "curative" therapeutic approaches are developed and instituted.	217-219
Measures of proliferation		X	Contradictory reports exist.	53, 142, 283, 284
Prolonged steroid pretreatment	X		Most reports suggest previous steroid use shortens response durations; however, length of exposure necessary is unknown.	207, 208
P-glycoprotein expression (drug resistance factors add)		X	May be associated with poor response rates and shortened remissions	223-225
Cranial mediastinal lymphadenopathy	X		Large compilation of cases reports shorter remission and survival durations.	97
Anatomic location	X		Leukemia, diffuse cutaneous and alimentary, hepatosplenic forms associated with unfavorable prognosis	See text for extra nodal sites
Chemotherapy-induced hematologic toxicity		X	Dogs experiencing grade III/IV neutropenia have prolonged first remission durations.	285

PARR, PCR for antigen receptor gene rearrangement.

TABLE 32-7 Circulating (Serum/Plasma) Biomarkers as Prognostic Indices in Dogs with Lymphoma

BIOMARKER	COMMENTS	REFERENCES
Lactate dehydrogenase activity	Increased activity predicted early recurrence.	120
Thymidine kinase activity	Increases associated with diminished prognosis.	220, 286
Serum VEGF levels	Small study suggests pretreatment levels predictive of remission duration.	119, 287
Glutathione-S-transferase	Increases associated with diminished prognosis.	288
Hypercalcemia	Negative factor if associated with T-cell subtype and reduced renal function.	91, 289, 290
Serum cobalamine	Hypocobalaminemia associated with poor outcome.	290
Serum C-reactive protein	Although it may be used to characterize remission status, variable levels preclude utility.	221

VEGF, Vascular endothelial growth factor.

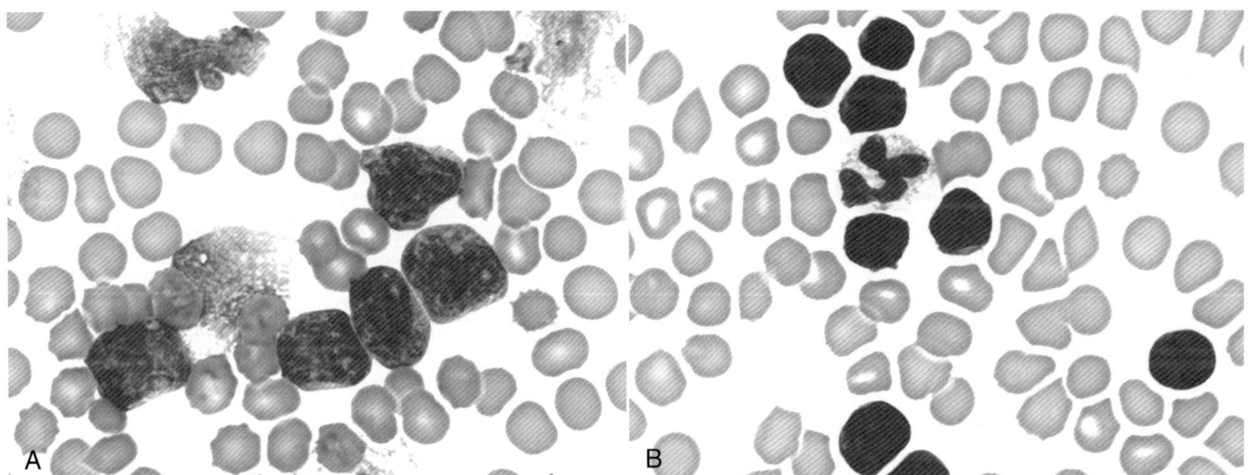

FIGURE 32-11 **A,** Peripheral blood from a dog with acute lymphoblastic leukemia (ALL). Note the large lymphoid cells with visible nucleoli. Chromatin from disintegrated cells also is visible. (Wright's stain, ×60 objective.) **B,** Peripheral blood from a dog with chronic lymphocytic leukemia (CLL). Note the small lymphocytes of normal morphology (smaller than the neutrophil). (Wright's stain, ×60 objective.)

most part unknown. Genetic factors likely play a role and have been compared between dogs and humans.[16] Retroviruses have been implicated in diverse animal species such as cats, cattle, fish, snakes, birds, rodents, nonhuman primates, and humans; however, there is no proven evidence implicating a retroviral cause in dogs. In humans, acute lymphocytic leukemia (ALL) has been associated with genetic factors and exposure to radiation, benzene, phenylbutazone, and antineoplastic agents. Extrapolation of predisposing factors across species is not warranted; in fact, etiologic factors in dogs may be quite different from those for humans given the difference in the predominant immunophenotype of the neoplastic cells (see later).

Pathology and Classification

Lymphocytic leukemias can be subdivided based on cell size, maturity, genetic aberrations, microRNA expression, and immunophenotype.* The simplest classification divides leukemia into two groups: chronic (small cells with a mature cytologic phenotype) and acute (large cells with an immature cytologic phenotype). Immunophenotypic assessment using flow cytometric and molecular assays can further characterize these two major subtypes; however, some discordance exists in the veterinary literature.

Three primary subtypes of CLL are reported in dogs, based primarily on immunophenotyping[137,280,293]: (1) T-CLL, which is the most common form, with cells in the majority of cases being $CD8^+$ granular lymphocytes; (2) B-CLL, which is the next most common subtype; and (3) atypical CLL, which represents a combination of immunophenotypes ($CD3^-$, $CD8^+$; $CD3^+$, $CD4^-$, $CD8^-$; $CD3^+$, $CD4^+$, $CD8^+$; and $CD3^+$ + $CD21^{+}$*). This is in contrast to CLL in humans, which is primarily a disease of B-cells. In CLL, lymphocytes often are indistinguishable morphologically from normal small lymphocytes (Figure 32-11) and have a low rate of proliferation; accumulation of lymphocytes likely results from their prolonged lifespan.

The immunophenotype of ALL typically is B-cell ($CD21^+$, $CD3^-$, $CD4^-$, $CD8^-$), although a smaller percentage (<10%) are of T-cell

*References 16, 137, 150, 280, 292-294.

*Note that either CD21 or CD79 can be used for assessing B-cell lineage in this context.

origin ($CD3^+$,$CD4^-$, $CD8^-$, $CD21^-$).[137] In general, these cells tend to be intermediate-sized or large cells with moderate amounts of basophilic cytoplasm. Perhaps the most distinguishing feature of lymphoblasts is the nuclear chromatin pattern, which typically is more condensed than the chromatin in myeloblasts. Lymphoblasts are larger than neutrophils, have a high nuclear:cytoplasmic ratio, and contain blue cytoplasm that in some cases is intensely basophilic (see Figure 32-11). Nucleoli, although present, are less prominent in lymphoblasts than in myeloblasts. Nevertheless, these cells cannot be distinguished easily from blast cells of other hematopoietic lineages, and identification of lineage-specific markers by immunocytochemical or flow cytometric analysis is required to ascertain the lineage. If the cells express CD34, a stem cell marker, an acute phenotype is implied[137,280]; however, both myeloid and lymphoid lineages express CD34, and our ability to differentiate ALL from acute myeloid leukemia (AML) relies on detection of other markers, including T- and B-cell markers and myeloperoxidase, a myeloid marker.

History and Clinical Signs

Dogs with CLL are often asymptomatic, but some owners report lethargy and decreased appetite. Mild lymphadenopathy and splenomegaly may be present, although late in the disease splenomegaly may be marked.[295] The white blood cell (WBC) count is usually greater than 30,000 cells/μL but can vary from normal to greater than 100,000 cells/μL because of an increase in circulating mature lymphocytes. Lymphocytosis is persistent and granulocytes are usually present in normal numbers. Other than lymphocytosis, hemograms of dogs with CLL tend to have few abnormalities when lymphocytes are less than 30,000/μL.[137,280,293] In some dogs, the disease is identified incidentally when the animal is undergoing evaluation for an unrelated problem. Mild anemia, neutropenia, and thrombocytopenia are common but may become marked as the disease progresses and lymphocyte counts increase above 30,000/μL. Despite the well-differentiated appearance of the lymphocytes in CLL, these cells may function abnormally. Paraneoplastic syndromes include monoclonal gammopathies, immune-mediated hemolytic anemia, pure red cell aplasia, and, rarely, hypercalcemia.[296,297] In one report of 22 dogs with CLL, 68% had monoclonal gammopathies (usually IgM or IgA).[296] The immunophenotypes were not reported, but a monoclonal gammopathy would be more likely to occur in B-CLL.

Dogs with ALL usually are presented with clinical signs of anorexia, weight loss, and lethargy. Splenomegaly is typical and other physical abnormalities may include hemorrhage, lymphadenopathy, and hepatomegaly.[298] Infiltration of bone marrow by neoplastic lymphoblasts may be extensive, resulting in significant depression of normal hematopoietic elements or myelophthisis.[137,280,292,298,299] Anemia, neutropenia, and thrombocytopenia are typically much more severe than with CLL and may become life threatening. Infiltration of extramedullary sites such as the CNS, bone, and GI tract may also occur and can result in neuropathies, bone pain, and GI signs, respectively.

Diagnostics and Clinical Staging

Consideration of signalment, history, physical findings, and morphologic appearance and immunophenotype of cells is essential in making an accurate diagnosis. It is helpful to know the profile of lymphocyte subsets in the peripheral blood of normal dogs to determine if a particular subset has expanded. Approximately 80% of circulating lymphocytes in normal dogs are T-cells, and about 15% are B-cells. NK cells and double-negative ($CD4^-$, $CD8^-$) T-cells constitute the remaining fraction. In the T-cell fraction, helper T-cells ($CD4^+$) outnumber cytotoxic T-cells ($CD8^+$).[296] Lymphocytic leukemia should be a consideration if atypical lymphocytes are in circulation, the immunophenotype of the lymphocytes in circulation is homogenous as determined by flow cytometric analysis, a phenotype typically present in low frequency has increased, or if clonality is documented (e.g., by PARR analysis). Other differential diagnoses for lymphocytosis include infectious diseases, such as chronic ehrlichiosis, postvaccinal responses in young dogs, IL-2 administration, and transient physiologic or epinephrine-induced lymphocytosis. In some cases, reactive and neoplastic lymphocytosis are difficult to distinguish.

Expansion of neoplastic lymphocytes in bone marrow is the hallmark of ALL and, in most cases, CLL. Careful examination of peripheral blood and bone marrow by an experienced cytopathologist is important in establishing a diagnosis of lymphoid leukemia; in cases of marked lymphocytosis with atypia, peripheral blood can be used for analysis of immunophenotype and clonality, and examination of bone marrow is not essential. If diagnostic bone marrow cannot be adequately obtained by aspiration, bone marrow core biopsy should be performed. In ALL, lymphoblasts predominate in the bone marrow and are also present in peripheral blood, and other lineages are decreased. In B- and T-cell CLL, the lymphocytes are small mature cells that occur in excessive numbers in bone marrow (≥30% of all nucleated cells) early in the disease.[295] In T-CLL, lymphocytes may contain pink granules. Infiltration becomes more extensive as the disease slowly progresses, and eventually the neoplastic cells replace normal marrow.

A separate clinical staging system has not been developed for lymphoid leukemia. Currently, all dogs with leukemia are classified as stage V based on the WHO Staging System for lymphoma as presented in Table 32-2.

Treatment of Chronic Lymphocytic Leukemia

Because of the indolent and often asymptomatic nature of CLL, the decision to treat is often based on the clinical and laboratory findings in the individual dog. Most oncologists recommend active surveillance (monthly or bimonthly physical examination and CBC) over active therapy for patients when CLL is identified incidentally, there are no accompanying clinical signs, and other significant hematologic abnormalities are not identified. If the animal is significantly anemic or thrombocytopenic, is showing evidence of significant lymphadenopathy or hepatosplenomegaly, or has an excessively high lymphocyte count (e.g., >60,000/μL), therapy should be instituted. The definition of "excessively high" varies among oncologists, and a standard has not been established in veterinary medicine. The author (DMV) prefers to base treatment decisions on the presence of significant constitutional signs and peripheral cytopenias. Currently, the most effective drug available for treatment of CLL is chlorambucil.[295] Chlorambucil is given orally at a dose of 0.2 mg/kg or 6 mg/m^2 PO once daily for 7 to 14 days; the dose can then be reduced to 0.1 mg/kg or 3 mg/m^2 PO daily. For long-term maintenance, a dose of 2.0 mg/m^2 every other day can be used. The dose is adjusted based on clinical response and bone marrow tolerance. Oral prednisone is used concurrently with chlorambucil at doses of 1 mg/kg daily for 1 to 2 weeks, then 0.5 mg/kg every other day thereafter. The addition of vincristine or the substitution of cyclophosphamide for chlorambucil has been advocated in animals that do not respond to chlorambucil.

Treatment of CLL is primarily palliative with rare complete remissions. Owing to the indolent nature of this disease, however, survival times have been in the range of 1 to 3 years with a good quality of life.[295,300] The phenotypic expression of CLL is usually stable over months to years. However, the disease may evolve into an acute phase, and some dogs will develop a form of lymphoma that is rapidly progressive and characterized by the presence of pleomorphic immunoblasts; in humans, this is termed *Richter's syndrome.*[301] The prognosis for response to treatment is poor for this form of lymphoma.

Treatment of Acute Lymphoblastic Leukemia

Much of the morbidity in dogs with ALL results from effacement of bone marrow (myelophthisis) and subsequent life-threatening peripheral cytopenias. Neutropenia, thrombocytopenia, and anemia may be severe. Patients often require supportive therapy, such as fresh whole-blood transfusions, broad-spectrum antibiotics, fluid therapy, and nutritional support. Careful monitoring for sepsis, hemorrhage, and DIC is important. Specific treatment of ALL requires aggressive chemotherapy. Consistently efficacious protocols for ALL have not been developed in veterinary medicine, and there are few published reports. CHOP-based protocols, similar to those used for lymphoma (see Table 32-4), have been used by the author (DMV) for dogs with ALL; however, responses and durability of response are generally disappointing. The standard of care in humans with acute leukemia generally involves bone marrow ablative treatments with stem cell or marrow replacement, a protocol not generally available in veterinary oncology.

Prognosis

In general, CLL is a slowly progressive disease, and some animals will not require therapy for some time after diagnosis; one dog was reported to survive almost 2 years without treatment.[302] For those dogs that are treated, normalization of lymphocyte counts can be expected in 70% of cases. In one report of 17 dogs treated with vincristine, chlorambucil, and prednisone, MST was approximately 12 months with an expected 30% survival at 2 years.[295] In larger compilations of cases that include immunophenotypic analysis, treatment protocols were poorly documented, although most received chlorambucil and prednisone; in 43 dogs with follow-up, for dogs with T-CLL, B-CLL, and atypical CLL, median survival was 930, 480, and only 22 days, respectively.[293] In this group of dogs, young age and anemia were also associated with a poor prognosis. In another series with limited treatment information, dogs with CLL of a $CD8^+$ immunophenotype that presented with less than 30,000 lymphocytes/μL or greater than 30,000 lymphocytes/μL had median survivals of 1098 and 131 days, respectively.

Prognosis for dogs with ALL is generally very poor. In a study of 21 dogs treated with vincristine and prednisone, the dogs achieving complete or partial remission (29%) had a MST of 120 days, and few dogs survived longer than 8 months with that protocol.[298] In one report of 46 cases of ALL with a $CD34^+$ phenotype, dogs had a median survival of 16 days (ranged from 3 to 128 days), even though the majority received a CHOP-based treatment protocol.[280] Additionally, dogs with B-cell ALL ($CD21^+$) in which the lymphocytes were large cells (forward scatter lymphocyte/forward scatter neutrophil ratio of >0.58 by flow cytometric analysis) had a median survival of only 129 days, independent of treatment protocol.[280]

REFERENCES

1. Dorn CR, Taylor DON, Schneider R, et al: Survey of animal neoplasms in Alameda Contra Costa counties, California. II. Cancer morbidity in dogs and cats from Alameda County, *J Natl Cancer Inst* 40:307–318, 1968.
2. Dorn CR, Taylor DON, Schneider R: The epidemiology of canine leukemia and lymphoma. In Dutcher RM, editor: Comparative Leukemia Research Proceedings. 4th International Symposium in Comparative Leukemia Research, Cherry Hill, NJ, *Bibl Haematol* 36:403–415, 1970.
3. Merlo DF, Rossi L, Pellegrino C, et al: Cancer incidence in pet dogs: findings of the Animal Tumor Registry of Genoa, Italy, *J Vet Intern Med* 22:976–984, 2008.
4. Kaiser HE: Animal neoplasia: a systemic review. In Kaiser HE, editor: *Neoplasms-comparative pathology in animals, plants and man*, Baltimore, 1981, Williams & Wilkins.
5. Moulton JE, Harvey JW: Tumors of lymphoid and hematopoietic tissue. In Moulton JE, editor: *Tumors of domestic animals*, ed 3, 1990, University of California Press.
6. Jemal A, Tiwari RC, Murray T, et al: Cancer statistics, 2004, *CA Cancer J Clin* 54:8, 2004.
7. Villamil JA, Henry CJ, Hahn AW, et al: Hormonal and sex impact on the epidemiology of canine lymphoma, *J Cancer Epidemiol* 2009:591753. Epub 2010 Mar 14.
8. Priester WA, McKay FW: The occurrence of tumors in domestic animal, *Nat Cancer Inst Monogr* 54:1–210, 1980.
9. Edwards DS, Henley WE, Harding EF, et al: Breed incidence of lymphoma in a UK population of insured dogs, *Vet Comp Oncol* 1:200–206,2003.
10. Thomas R, Smith KC, Bould R, et al: Molecular cytogenetic analysis of a novel high-grade T-lymphoblastic lymphoma demonstrating co-expression of CD3 and CD79a cell markers, *Chromosome Res* 9:649–657, 2001.
11. Thomas R, Smith KC, Ostrander EA, et al: Chromosome aberrations in canine multicentric lymphomas detected with comparative genomic hybridisation and a panel of single locus probes, *Br J Canc* 89:1530–1537, 2003.
12. Thomas R, Fiegler H, Ostrander EA, et al: A canine acner-gene microarray for CGH analysis of tumors, *Cytogenet Genome Res* 102:254–260, 2003.
13. Thomas R, Seiser EL, Motsinger-Reif A, et al: Refining tumor-associated aneuploidy through "genomic recording" of recurrent DNA copy number aberrations in 150 canine non-Hodgkin's lymphomas, *Leuk Lymphoma* 52:1321–1335, 2011.
14. Starky MP, Murphy S: Using lymph node fine needle aspirates for gene expression profiling of canine lymphoma, *Vet Comp Oncol* 8:56–71, 2010.
15. Devitt JJ, Maranon DG, Ehrhart EJ, et al: Correlations between numerical chromosomal aberrations in the tumor and peripheral blood in canine lymphoma, *Cytogenet Genome Res* 124:12–18, 2009.
16. Breen M, Modiano JF: Evolutionarily conserved cytogenetic changes in hematological malignancies of dogs and humans—man and his best friend share more than companionship, *Chromosome Res* 16:145–154, 2008.
17. Lindblad-Toh K, Wade CM, Mikkelsen TS, et al: Genome sequence, comparative analysis and haplotype structure of the domestic dog, *Nature* 438:803–819, 2005.
18. Hahn KA, Richardson RC, Hahn EA, et al: Diagnostic and prognostic importance of chromosomal aberrations identified in 61 dogs with lymphosarcoma, *Vet Pathol* 31:528–540, 1994.
19. Veldhoen N, Stewart J, Brown R, et al: Mutations of the p53 gene in canine lymphoma and evidence for germ line p53 mutations in the dog, *Oncogene* 16:249–255, 1998.
20. Nasir L, Argyle DJ: Mutational analysis of the tumour suppressor gene p53 in lymphosarcoma in two bull mastiffs, *Vet Rec* 145:23–24, 1999.
21. Sokolowski J, Cywinska A, Malicka E: p53 expression in canine lymphoma, *J Vet Med A Physiol Pathol Clin Med* 52:172–175, 2005.

22. Setoguchi A, Sakai T, Okuda M, et al: Aberrations of the p53 suppressor gene in various tumors in dogs, *Am J Vet Res* 62:433–439, 2001.
23. Sueiro FAR, Alessi AC, Vassallo J: Canine lymphomas: a morphological and immunohistochemical study of 55 cases, with observations on p53 immunoexpression, *J Comp Pathol* 131:207–213, 2004.
24. Pelham JT, Irwin PJ, Kay PH: Genetic hypomethylation in neoplastic cells from dogs with malignant lymphoproliferative disorders, *Res Vet Sci* 74:101–104, 2003.
25. Modiano JF, Breen M, Burnett RC, et al: Distinct B-cell and T-cell lymphoproliferative disease prevalence among dog breeds indicates heritable risk, *Cancer Res* 65:5654–5661, 2005.
26. Nasir L, Devlin P, McKevitt T, et al: Telomere lengths and telomerase activity in dog tissues, *Neoplasia* 3(4):351–359, 2001.
27. Carioto LM, Kruth SA, Betts DH, et al: Telomerase activity in clinically normal dogs and dogs with malignant lymphoma, *Am J Vet Res* 62:1442–1446 ,2001.
28. Yazawa M, Okuda M, Kanaya N, et al: Molecular cloning of the canine telomerase reverse transcriptase gene and its expression in neoplastic and non-neoplastic cells, *Am J Vet Res* 64:1395–1400, 2003.
29. Milman G, Smith KC, Erles K: Serological detection of Epstein-Barr virus infection in dogs and cats, *Vet Microbiol* 150:15–20, 2011.
30. Farinha P, Gascoyne D: Helicobacter pylori and MALT lymphoma, *Gastroenterology* 128:1579–1605, 2005.
31. Rossi G, Ross M, Vitali CG, et al: A conventional beagle dog model for acute and chronic infection with Helicobacter pylori, *Infect Immun* 67:3112–3120, 1999.
32. Hayes HM, Tarone RE, Cantor KP, et al: Case-control study of canine malignant lymphoma: Positive association with dog owner's use of 2, 4-dichlorophenoxyacetic acid herbicides, *J Natl Cancer Inst* 83:1226–1231, 1991.
33. Carlo GL, Cole P, Miller AB, et al: Review of a study reporting an association between 2, 4-dichlorophenoxyacetic acid and canine malignant lymphoma: report of an expert panel, *Regul Toxicol Pharmacol* 16:245–252, 1992.
34. Garabrant DH, Philbert MA: Review of 2,4-dichlorophenoxyacetic acid (2,4-D) epidemiology and toxicology, *Crit Rev Toxicol* 32:233–257, 2002.
35. Kaneene JB, Miller R: Re-analysis of 2,4-D use and the occurrence of canine malignant lymphoma, *Vet Hum Toxicol* 41:164–170, 1999.
36. Reynolds PM, Reif JS, Ramsdell HS: Canine exposure to herbicide treated lawns and urinary excretion of 2, 4-dichlorophenoxyacetic acid, *Cancer Epidemiol Biomarkers Prev* 3:233–237, 1994.
37. Gavazza A, Presciuttini S, Barale R, et al: Association between canine malignant lymphoma, living in industrial areas, and use of chemicals by dog owners, *J Vet Intern Med* 15:190–195, 2001.
38. Reif JS, Lower KS, Ogilvie GK: Residential exposure to magnetic fields and risk of canine lymphoma, *Am J Epidemiol* 141:352–359, 1995.
39. Marconato L, Leo C, Girelli R, et al: Association between waste management and cancer in companion animals, *J Vet Intern Med* 23:564–569, 2009.
40. Pastor M, Chalvet-Monfray K, Marchal T, et al: Genetic and environmental risk indicators in canine non-Hodgkin's lymphomas: breed associations and geographic distribution of 608 cases diagnosed throughout France over 1 year, *J Vet Intern Med* 23:301–310, 2009.
41. Keller ET: Immune-mediated disease as a risk factor for canine lymphoma, *Cancer* 70:2334–2337, 1992.
42. Foster AP, Sturgess CP, Gould DJ, et al: Pemphigus foliaceus in association with systemic lupus erythematosus and subsequent lymphoma in a cocker spaniel, *J Small Anim Pract* 41:266–270, 2000.
43. Schmiedt CW, Grimes JA, Holzman G, et al: Incidence and risk factors for development of malignant neoplasia after feline renal transplantation and cyclosporine-based immunosuppression, *Vet Comp Oncol* 7:45–53, 2009.
44. Blackwood L, German AJ, Stell AJ, et al: Multicentric lymphoma in a dog after cyclosporine therapy, *J Small Anim Pract* 45:259–262, 2004.
45. Santoro D, Marsella R, Hernandez J: Investigation on the association between atopic dermatitis and the development of mycosis fungoides in dogs: a retrospective case-control study, *Vet Dermatol* 18:101–106, 2007.
46. Madewell BR, Theilen GH: Hematopoietic neoplasms, sarcomas and related conditions. In Theilen GH, Madewell BR, editors: *Veterinary cancer medicine*, ed 2, Philadelphia, 1987, Lea and Febiger.
47. Couto CG, Rutgers HC, Sherding RG, et al: Gastrointestinal lymphoma in 20 dogs: a retrospective study, *J Vet Intern Med* 3:73–78, 1989.
48. Ozaki K, Yamagami T, Nomura K, et al: T-cell lymphoma with eosinophilic infiltration involving the intestinal tract in 11 dogs, *Vet Pathol* 43:339–344, 2006.
49. Breitschwerdt EB, Waltman C, Hagastad HV, et al: Clinical and epidemiological characterization of a diarrheal syndrome in Basenji dog, *J Am Vet Med Assoc* 180:914–920, 1982.
50. Coyle KA, Steinberg H: Characterization of lymphocytes in canine gastrointestinal lymphoma, *Vet Pathol* 41:141–146, 2004.
51. Steinberg H, Dubielzig, RR, Thomson J, et al: Primary gastrointestinal lymphosarcoma with epitheliotropism in three Shar-Pei and one Boxer dog, *Vet Pathol* 32:423–426, 1995.
52. Rosenberg MP, Matus RE, Patnaik AK: Prognostic factors in dogs with lymphoma and associated hypercalcemia, *J Vet Intern Med* 5:268–271, 1991
53. Vail DM, Kisseberth WC, Obradovich JE, et al: Assessment of potential doubling time (T_{pot}), argyrophilic nucleolar organizer regions (AgNOR), and proliferating cell nuclear antigen (PCNA) as predictors of therapy response in canine non-Hodgkin's lymphoma, *Experim Hematol* 24:807–815, 1996.
54. Ruslander DA, Gebhard DH, Tompkins MG, et al: Immunophenotypic characterization of canine lymphoproliferative disorders, *In Vivo* 11:169–172, 1997.
55. Gross TL, Ihrke PJ, Walder EJ, et al: Lymphocytic neoplasms. In *Skin diseases of the dog and cat*, ed 2, Oxford, 2005, Blackwell.
56. Fontaine J, Heimann M, Day MJ: Canine cutaneous epitheliotropic T-cell lymphoma: a review of 30 cases, *Vet Dermatol* 21:267–275, 2010.
57. Fontaine J, Bovens C, Bettenay S, et al: Canine cutaneous epitheliotropic T-cell lymphoma: a review, *Vet Comp Oncol* 7:1–14, 2009.
58. Moore PF, Affolter VK, Graham PS, et al: Canine epitheliotropic cutaneous T-cell lymphoma: an investigation of T-cell receptor immunophenotype, lesion topography and molecular clonality, *Vet Dermatol* 20:569–576, 2009.
59. Broder S, Muul L, Marshall S, et al: Neoplasms of immunoregulatory T-cells in clinical investigation, *J Invest Dermatol* 74:267–271, 1980.
60. Moore PF, Olivry T, Naydan D: Canine cutaneous epitheliotrophic lymphoma (mycosis fungoides) is a proliferative disorder of CD+8 T-cells, *Am J Pathol* 144:421–429, 1994.
61. Thrall MA, Macy DW, Snyder SP, et al: Cutaneous lymphosarcoma and leukemia in a dog resembling Sézary's syndrome in man, *Vet Pathol* 21:182–186, 1984.
62. Schick RO, Murphy GF, Goldschmidt MH: Cutaneous lymphosarcoma and leukemia in a cat, *J Am Vet Med Assoc* 203:1155–1158, 1993.
63. Foster AP, Evans E, Kerlin RL, et al: Cutaneous T-cell lymphoma with Sézary syndrome in a dog, *Vet Clin Pathol* 26:188–192, 1997.
64. Fry MM, Vernau W, Pesavento PA, et al: Hepatosplenic lymphoma in a dog, *Vet Pathol* 40:556–562, 2003.
65. Cienava EA, Barnhart KF, Brown R, et al: Morphologic, immunohistochemical, and molecular characterization of hepatosplenic T-cell lymphoma in a dog, *Vet Clin Pathol* 33:105–110, 2004.
66. Bush WW, Throop JL, McManus PM, et al: Intravascular lymphoma involving the central and peripheral nervous systems in a dog, *J Am Anim Hosp Assoc* 39:90–96, 2003.

67. Dargent FJ, Fox LE, Anderson WI: Neoplastic angioendotheliomatosis in a dog: an angiotropic lymphoma, *Cornell Vet* 78:253–262, 1988.
68. Summers BA, deLahunta A: Cerebral angioendotheliomatosis in a dog, *Acta Neuropathol* 68:10–14, 1985.
69. Cullen CL, Caswell JL, Grahn BH: Intravascular lymphoma presenting as bilateral panophthalmitis and retinal detachment in a dog, *J Am Anim Hosp Assoc* 36:337–342, 2000.
70. McDonough SP, Van Winkle TJ, Balentine BA, et al: Clinicopathological and immunophenotypical features of canine intravascular lymphoma (malignant angioendotheliomatosis), *J Comp Path* 126:277–288, 2002.
71. Ridge L, Swinney G: Angiotrophic intravascular lymphosarcoma presenting as bi-cavity effusion in a dog, *Aust Vet J* 82:616–618, 2004.
72. Hatoya S, Kumagai D, Takeda S, et al: Successful management with CHOP for pulmonary lymphomatoid granulomatosis in a dog, *J Vet Med Sci* 73:527–530, 2011.
73. Berry CR, Moore PF, Thomas WP, et al: Pulmonary lymphomatoid granulomatosis in seven dogs (1976-1987), *J Vet Intern Med* 4:157–166, 1990.
74. Park HM, Hwang DN, Kang BT, et al: Pulmonary lymphomatoid granulomatosis in a dog: Evidence of immunophenotypic diversity and relationship to human pulmonary lymphomatoid granulomatosis and pulmonary Hodgkin's disease, *Vet Pathol* 44:921–923, 2007.
75. Fitzgerald SD, Wolf DC, Carlton WW: Eight cases of canine lymphomatoid granulomatosis, *Vet Pathol* 28:241–245, 1991.
76. National Cancer Institute sponsored study of classifications of non-Hodgkin's lymphomas: summary and description of a working formulation for clinical usage. The Non-Hodgkin's Lymphoma Pathologic Classification Project, *Cancer* 49:2112–2135, 1982.
77. Lennert K, Feller A: *Histopathology of non-Hodgkin's lymphomas (based on the Updated Kiel Classification)*, ed 2, Berlin, 1990, Springer-Verlag.
78. Valli VE, Jacobs RM, Parodi AL, et al: *Histological classification of hematopoietic tumors of domestic animals*, Washington, DC, 2002, Armed Forces Institute of Pathology and The World Health Organization.
79. Sueiro FA, Alessi AC, Vassallo J: Canine lymphomas: a morphological and immunohistochemical study of 55 cases, with observations on p53 immunoexpression, *J Comp Pathol* 131:207–213, 2004.
80. Vezzali E, Parodi AL, Marcato PS, et al: Histopathological classification of 171 cases of canine and feline non-Hodgkin lymphoma according to the WHO, *Vet Comp Oncol* 8:38–49, 2009.
81. Valli VE, Myint MS, Barthel A, et al: Classification of canine malignant lymphomas according to the World Health Organization criteria, *Vet Pathol* 48:198–211, 2011.
82. Stefanello D, Valenti P, Zini E, et al: Splenic marginal zone lymphoma in 5 dogs (2001-2008), *J Vet Intern Med* 25:90–93, 2011.
83. Valli VE, Vernau W, de Lorimier P, et al: Canine indolent nodular lymphoma, *Vet Pathol* 43:241–256, 2006.
84. Flood-Knapik KE, Durham AC, Gregor TP, et al: Clinical, histopathological, and immunohistochemical characterization of canine indolent lymphoma, *Vet Comp Oncol* 2012. Epub ahead of print.
85. Carter RF, Valli VE, Lumsden JH: The cytology, histology and prevalence of cell types in canine lymphoma classified according to the National Cancer Institute Working Formulation, *Can J Vet Res* 50:154–164, 1986.
86. Teske E, van Heerde P, Rutteman GR, et al: Prognostic factors for treatment of malignant lymphoma in dogs, *J Am Vet Med Assoc* 205:1722–1728, 1994.
87. Ponce F, Magnol JP, Ledieu D, et al: Prognostic significance of morphological subtypes in canine malignant lymphomas during chemotherapy, *Vet J* 167:158–166, 2004.
88. Appelbaum FR, Sale GE, Storb R, et al: Phenotyping of canine lymphoma with monoclonal antibodies directed at cell surface antigens: classification, morphology, clinical presentation and response to chemotherapy, *Hematol Oncol* 2:151–168, 1984.
89. Rosol TJ, Capen CC: Biology of disease: Mechanisms of cancer-induced hypercalcemia, *Lab Invest* 67:680–702, 1992.
90. Weir EC, Greelee P, Matus R, et al: Hypercalcemia in canine lymphosarcoma is associated with the T-cell subtype and with secretion of a PTH-like factor, *J Bone Miner Res* 3:S106 (abstract), 1988.
91. Greenlee PG, Filippa DA, Quimby FW, et al: Lymphoma in dogs: A morphologic, immunologic, and clinical study, *Cancer* 66:480–490, 1990.
92. Fournel-Fleury C, Ponce F, Felman P, et al: Canine T-cell lymphomas: A morphological, immunological and clinical study of 46 new cases, *Vet Pathol* 39:92–109, 2002.
93. Wilkerson MJ, Dolce K, Koopman T, et al: Lineage differentiation of canine lymphoma/leukemias and aberrant expression of CD molecules, *Vet Immunol Immunopathol* 106:179–196, 2005.
94. Rappaport H, Winter WJ, Hicks EB: Follicular lymphoma: A re-evaluation of its position in the scheme of malignant lymphoma, based on a survey of 253 cases, *Cancer* 9:792–821, 1956.
95. Rappaport H: Tumors of the hematopoietic system. In *Atlas of tumor pathology*, Section 3, Fasicle 8. Washington DC, 1966, Armed Forces Institute of Pathology.
96. Day MJ: Immunophenotypic characterization of cutaneous lymphoid neoplasia in the dog and cat, *J Comp Pathol* 112:79–96, 1995.
97. Starrak GS, Berry CR, Page RL, et al: Correlation between thoracic radiographic changes and remission/survival duration in 270 dogs with lymphosarcoma, *Vet Radiol Ultrasound* 38:411–418, 1997
98. Blackwood L, Sullivan M, Lawson H: Radiographic abnormalities in canine multicentric lymphoma: A review of 84 cases, *J Small Anim Pract* 38:62–69, 1997.
99. Hawkins EG, Morrison WB, DeNicola DB, et al: Cytologic analysis of bronchoalveolar lavage fluid from 47 dogs with multicentric malignant lymphoma, *J Am Vet Med Assoc* 203:1418–1425, 1993
100. Yohn SE, Hawkins EC, Morrison WB, et al: Confirmation of a pulmonary component of multicentric lymphosarcoma with bronchoalveolar lavage in two dogs, *J Am Vet Med Assoc* 204:97–101, 1994.
101. Leib MS, Bradley RL: Alimentary lymphosarcoma in a dog, *Compend Pract Vet Contin Educ* 9:809–815, 1987.
102. Gieger T: Alimentary lymphoma in cats and dogs, *Vet Clin North Am Small Anim Pract* 41:419–432, 2011.
103. Couto CG, Cullen J, Pedroia V, et al: Central nervous system lymphosarcoma in the dog, *J Am Vet Med Assoc* 184:809–813, 1984.
104. Dallman MJ, Saunders GK: Primary spinal cord lymphosarcoma in a dog, *J Am Vet Med Assoc* 189:1348–1349, 1986.
105. Rosin A: Neurologic diseases associated with lymphosarcoma in ten dogs, *J Am Vet Med Assoc* 181:50–53, 1982.
106. Swanson JF: Ocular manifestations of systemic disease in the dog and cat: recent development, *Vet Clin North Am (Small Anim Pract)* 20:849–867, 1990.
107. Krohne SDG, Vestre WA, Richardson RC, et al: Ocular involvement in canine lymphosarcoma: A retrospective study of 94 cases, *Am College Vet Ophth Proc* 68–84, 1987.
108. Madewell BR, Feldman BF: Characterization of anemias associated with neoplasia in small animals, *J Am Vet Med Assoc* 176:419–425, 1980.
109. Kubota A, Kano R, Mizuno T, et al: Parathyroid hormone-related protein (PTHrP) produced by dog lymphoma cells, *J Vet Med Sci* 64:835–837, 2002.
110. Gerger B, Hauser B, Reusch CE: Serum levels of 25-hydroxycholecalciferol and 1,25-dihydroxycholecalciferol in dogs with hypercalcemia, *Vet Res Commun* 28:669–680, 2004.
111. Massa KL, Gilger BC, Miller TL, et al: Causes of uveitis in dogs: 102 cases (1989-2000), *Vet Ophthalmol* 5:9–98, 2002.

112. Madewell BR: Hematological and bone marrow cytological abnormalities in 75 dogs with malignant lymphoma, *J Am Anim Hosp Assoc* 22:235–240, 1986.
113. Grindem CB, Breitschwadt, EB, Corbett WT, et al: Thrombocytopenia associated with neoplasia in dogs, *J Vet Intern Med* 8:400–405, 1994.
114. MacEwen, EG, Patnaik AK, Wilkins RJ: Diagnosis and treatment of canine hematopoietic neoplasms, *Vet Clin North Am (Small Anim Pract)* 7:105–118, 1977.
115. Lechowski R, Jagielski D, Hoffmann-Jagielska M, et al: Alpha-fetoprotein in canine multicentric lymphoma, *Vet Res Commun* 26:285–296, 2002.
116. Hahn KA, Freeman KP, Barnhill MA, et al: Serum alpha 1-acid glycoprotein concentrations before and after relapse in dogs with lymphoma treated with doxorubicin, *J Am Vet Med Assoc* 214: 1023–1025, 1999.
117. Kazmeirski KJ, Ogilvie GK, Fettman MJ, et al: Serum zinc, chromium, and iron concentrations in dogs with lymphoma and osteosarcoma, *J Vet Intern Med* 15:585–588, 2001.
118. Rossmeisl JH, Bright P, Tamarkin L, et al: Endostatin concentrations in healthy dogs and dogs with selected neoplasms, *J Vet Intern Med* 16:565–569, 2002.
119. Zizzo N, Patruno R, Zito FA, et al: Vascular endothelial growth factor concentrations from platelets correlate with tumor angiogenesis and grading in a spontaneous canine non-Hodgkin's lymphoma model, *Leuk Lymphoma* 51:291–296, 2010.
120. Marconato L, Crispino G, Finotello R, et al: Clinical relevance of serial determinations of lactate dehydrogenase activity used to predict recurrence in dogs with lymphoma, *J Am Vet Med Assoc* 236:969–974, 2010.
121. Winter JL, Freeman LG, Barber LG, et al: Antioxidant status and biomarkers of oxidative stress in dogs with lymphoma, *J Vet Intern Med* 23:311–316, 2009.
122. Mischke R, Waterston M, Eckersall PD: Changes in C-reactive protein and haptoglobin in dogs with lymphatic neoplasia, *Vet J* 174:188–192, 2007.
123. Sozmen M, Tasca S, Carli E, et al: Use of fine needle aspirates and flow cytometry for the diagnosis, classification, and immunophenotyping of canine lymphomas, *J Vet Diagn Invest* 17:323–330, 2005
124. Crabtree AC, Spangler E, Beard D, et al: Diagnostic accuracy of gray-scale ultrasonography for the detection of hepatic and splenic lymphoma in dogs, *Vet Radiol Ultrasound* 51:661–664, 2010.
125. Kinns J, Mai W: Association between malignancy and sonographic heterogeneity in canine and feline abdominal lymph nodes, *Vet Radiol Ultrasound* 48:565–569, 2007.
126. Nyman HT, Lee MH, McEvoy FJ, et al: Comparison of B-mode and Doppler ultrasonographic findings with histologic features of benign and malignant superficial lymph nodes in dogs, *Am J Vet Res* 67:978–984, 2006.
127. Miura T, Maruyama H, Sakai M, et al: Endoscopic finding on alimentary lymphoma in 7 dogs, *J Vet Med Sci* 66:577–580, 2004.
128. Fukushima K, Ohno K, Koshino-Goto Y, et al: Sensitivity for the detection of a clonally rearranged antigen receptor gene in endoscopically obtained biopsy specimens from canine alimentary lymphoma, *J Vet Med Sci* 71:1673–1676, 2009.
129. Kaneko N, Yamamoto Y, Wada Y, et al: Application of polymerase chain reaction to analysis of antigen receptor rearrangements to support endoscopic diagnosis of canine alimentary lymphoma, *J Vet Med Sci* 71:555–559, 2009.
130. Kleinschmidt S, Meneses F, Noltel I, et al: Retrospective study on the diagnostic value of full-thickness biopsies from the stomach and intestines of dogs with chronic gastrointestinal disease symptoms, *Vet Pathol* 43:1000–1003, 2006.
131. Affolter VK, Gross TL, Moore PF: Indolent cutaneous T-cell lymphoma presenting as cutaneous lymphocytosis in dogs, *Vet Dermatol* 20:577–585, 2009.
132. Chaubert P, Baur-Chaubert AS, Sattler U, et al: Improved polymerase chain reaction-based method to detect early-stage epitheliotropic T-cell lymphoma (mycosis fungoides) in formalin-fixed, paraffin-embedded skin biopsy specimens of the dog, *J Vet Diagn Invest* 22:20–29, 2010.
133. Vail DM, Kravis LD, Kisseberth WC, et al: Application of rapid CD3 immunophenotype analysis and argyrophilic nucleolar organizer region (AgNOR) frequency to fine needle aspirate specimens from dogs with lymphoma, *Vet Clin Pathol* 26:66–69, 1997
134. Fisher DJ, Naydan D, Werner LL, et al: Immunophenotyping lymphomas in dogs: A comparison of results from fine needle aspirate and needle biopsy samples, *Vet Clin Pathol* 24:118–123, 1995.
135. Culmsee K, Simon D, Mischke R, et al: Possibilities of flow cytometric analysis for immunophenotypic characterization of canine lymphoma, *J Vet Med A Physiol Pathol Clin Med* 48:199–204, 2001.
136. Comazzi S, Gelain ME: Use of flow cytometric immunophenotyping to refine the cytological diagnosis of canine lymphoma, *Vet J* 188:149–155,2011.
137. Tasca S, Carli E, Caldin M, et al: Hematologic abnormalities and flow cytometric immunophenotyping results in dogs with hematopoietic neoplasia: 210 cases (2002-2006), *Vet Clin Pathol* 38:2–12, 2009.
138. Gelain ME, Mazzilli M, Riondato F, et al: Aberrant phenotypes and quantitative antigen expression in different subtypes of canine lymphoma by flow cytometry, *Vet Immunol Immunopathol* 121:179–188, 2008.
139. Lana S, Plaza S, Hampe K, et al: Diagnosis of mediastinal masses in dogs by flow cytometry, *J Vet Intern Med* 20:1161–1165, 2006.
140. Gibson D, Aubert I, Woods JP, et al: Flow cytometric immunophenotype of canine lymph node aspirates, *J Vet Intern Med* 18:710–717, 2004.
141. Fournel-Fleury C, Magnol JP, Chabanne L, et al: Growth fractions in canine non-Hodgkin's lymphomas as determined in situ by the expression of the Ki-67 antigen, *J Comp Pathol* 117:61–72, 1997.
142. Phillips BS, Kass PH, Naydan DK, et al: Apoptotic and proliferation indexes in canine lymphoma, *J Vet Diagn Invest* 12:111–117, 2000.
143. Hung LC, Pong VF, Cheng CR, et al: An improved system for quantifying AgNOR and PCNA in canine tumors, *Anticancer Res* 20:3273–3280, 2000.
144. Vajdovich P, Psader R, Toth ZA, et al: Use of the argyrophilic nucleolar region method for cytologic and histologic examination of the lymph nodes in dogs, *Vet Pathol* 41:338–345, 2004.
145. Bauer NB, Zervos D, Moritz A: Argyrophilic nucleolar organizing regions and Ki67 equally reflect proliferation in fine needle aspirates of normal, hyperplastic, inflamed and neoplastic canine lymph nodes (n = 101), *J Vet Intern Med* 21:928–935, 2007.
146. Burnett RC, Vernau W, Modiano JF, et al: Diagnosis of canine lymphoid neoplasia using clonal rearrangements of antigen receptor genes, *Vet Pathol* 40:32–41, 2003.
147. Keller RL, Avery AC, Burnett RC, et al: Detection of neoplastic lymphocytes in peripheral blood of dogs with lymphoma by polymerase chain reaction for antigen receptor gene rearrangement, *Vet Clin Pathol* 33:145–149, 2004.
148. Avery PR, Avery AC: Molecular methods to distinguish reactive and neoplastic lymphocyte expansions and their importance in transitional neoplastic states, *Vet Clin Pathol* 33:196–207, 2004.
149. Drietz MJ, Ogilvie G, Sim GK: Rearranged T lymphocyte antigen receptor genes as markers of malignant T cells, *Vet Immunol Immunopathol* 69:113–119, 1999.
150. Avery A: Molecular diagnostics of hematologic malignancies, *Top Companion Anim Med* 24:144–150, 2009.
151. Kaneko N, Tanimoto T, Morimoto M, et al: Use of formalin-fixed paraffin-embedded tissue and single-strand conformation

polymorphism analysis for polymerase chain reaction of antigen receptor rearrangements in dogs, *J Vet Med Sci* 71:535–538, 2009.

152. Gentilini F, Calzolari C, Turba ME, et al: Gene scanning analysis of Ig/TCR gene rearrangements to detect clonality in canine lymphomas, *Vet Immunol Immunopathol* 127:47–56,2009.
153. Yagihara H, Tamura K, Isotani M, et al: Genomic organization of the T-cell receptor gamma gene and PCR detection of its clonal rearrangement in canine T-cell lymphoma/leukemia, *Vet Immunol Immunopathol* 115:375–382, 2007.
154. Tamura K, Yagihara H, Isotani M, et al: Development of the polymerase chain reaction assay based on the canine genome database for detection of monoclonality in B cell lymphoma, *Vet Immunol Immunopathol* 110:163–167, 2006.
155. Fournel-Fleury C, Magnol JP, Bricaire P, et al: Cystohistological and immunological classification of canine malignant lymphomas: comparison with human non-Hodgkin's lymphomas, *J Comp Pathol* 117:35–59, 1997.
156. Ponce F, Magnol JP, Marchal T, et al: High-grade T-cell lymphoma/leukemia with plasmacytoid morphology: a clinical pathological study of nine case, *J Vet Diagn Invest* 15:330–337, 2003.

156a. Bergman PJ, Ogilvie GK, Powers BE: Monoclonal antibody C219 immunohistochemistry against P-glycoprotein: sequential analysis and predictive ability in dogs with lymphoma, *J Vet Intern Med* 10:354–359, 1996.

156b. Moore AS, Leveille CT, Reimann KA, et al: The expression of P-glycoprotein in canine lymphoma and its association with multidrug resistance, *Cancer Invest* 13:475–479, 1995.

157. Ratcliffe L, Mian S, Slater K, et al: Proteomic identification and profiling of canine lymphoma patients, *Vet Comp Oncol* 7:92–105, 2009.
158. Wilson CR, Regnier FE, Knapp DW, et al: Glycoproteomic profiling of serum peptides in canine lymphoma and transitional cell carcinoma, *Vet Comp Oncol* 6:171–181, 2008.
159. McCaw DL, Chan AS, Stegner AL, et al: Proteomics of canine lymphoma identifies potential cancer-specific protein markers, *Clin Cancer Res* 13:2496–2503, 2007.
160. Gaines PJ, Powell TD, Walmsley SJ, et al: Identification of serum biomarkers for canine B-cell lymphoma by use of surface-enhanced laser desorption-ionization time-of-flight spectrometry, *Am J Vet Res* 68:405–410, 2007.
161. Flory AB, Rassnick KM, Stokol T, et al: Stage migration in dogs with lymphoma, *J Vet Intern Med* 21:1041–1047, 2007.
162. Raskin RE, Krehbiel JD: Prevalence of leukemic blood and bone marrow in dogs with multicentric lymphoma, *J Am Vet Med Assoc* 194:1427–1429, 1989.
163. Geyer NE, Reichie JK, Valdes-Martinez A, et al: Radiographic appearance of confirmed pulmonary lymphoma in cats and dogs, *Vet Radiol Ultrasound* 51:386–390, 2010.
164. Lawrence J, Vanderhoek M, Barbee D, et al: Use of 3′-deoxy-3′-[18F] fluorothymidine PET/CT for evaluating response to cytotoxic chemotherapy in dogs with non-Hodgkin's lymphoma, *Vet Radiol Ultrasound* 50:660–668, 2009.
165. LeBlanc AK, Jakoby BW, Townsend DW, et al: 18FDG-PET imaging in canine lymphoma and cutaneous mast cell tumor, *Vet Radiol Ultrasound* 50(2):215–223, 2009.
166. Vail DM, Thamm DH, Tumas DB, et al: Assessment of GS-9219 in a pet dog model of non-Hodgkin's lymphoma, *Clin Cancer Res* 15:3503–3510, 2009.
167. Yoon J, Feeney DA, Cronk DE, et al: Computed tomographic evaluation of canine and feline mediastinal masses in 14 patients, *Vet Radiol Ultrasound* 45:542–546, 2004.
168. Bassett CL, Daneil GB, Legendre AM, et al: Characterization of uptake of 2-deoxy-2-[18F] fluoro-D-glucose by fungal-associated inflammation: the standardized uptake value is greater for lesions of blastomycosis than for lymphoma in dogs with naturally occurring disease, *Mol Imaging Biol* 4:201–207, 2002.
169. Vail DM, Michels GM, Khanna C, et al and the Veterinary Co-operative Oncology Group: Response evaluation criteria for peripheral nodal lymphoma in dogs (v1.0): A Veterinary Co-operative Oncology Group (VCOG) Consensus Document, *Vet Comp Oncol* 8(1):28–37, 2010.
170. Cotter SM, Goldstein MA: Treatment of lymphoma and leukemia with cyclophosphamide, vincristine, and prednisone: I. Treatment of dog, *J Am Anim Hosp Assoc* 19:159–165, 1983.
171. Postorino NC, Susaneck SJ, Withrow SJ, et al: Single agent therapy with Adriamycin for canine lymphosarcoma, *J Am Anim Hosp Assoc* 25:221–225, 1989.
172. Valerius KD, Ogilvie GK, Mallinckrodt CH, et al: Doxorubicin alone or in combination with asparaginase, followed by cyclophosphamide, vincristine, and prednisone for treatment of multicentric lymphoma in dogs: 121 cases (1987-1995), *J Am Vet Med Assoc* 210:512–516, 1997.
173. Mutsaers AJ, Blickman NW, DeNicola DB, et al: Evaluation of treatment with doxorubicin and piroxicam or doxorubicin alone for multicentric lymphoma in dogs, *J Am Vet Med Assoc* 220:1813–1817, 2002.
174. MacEwen EG, Brown NO, Patnaik AK, et al: Cyclic combination chemotherapy of canine lymphosarcoma, *J Am Vet Med Assoc* 178:1178–1181, 1981.
175. MacEwen EG, Hayes AA, Matus RE, et al: Evaluation of some prognostic factors for advanced multicentric lymphosarcoma in the dog: 147 cases (1978-1981), *J Am Vet Med Assoc* 190:564–568, 1987.
176. Stone MS, Goldstein MA, Cotter SM: Comparison of two protocols for induction of remission in dogs with lymphoma, *J Am Anim Hosp Assoc* 27:315–321, 1991.
177. Myers NC, Moore AS, Rand WM, et al: Evaluation of a multidrug chemotherapy protocol (ACOPA II) in dogs with lymphoma, *J Vet Intern Med* 11:333–339, 1997.
178. Boyce KL, Kitchell BE: Treatment of canine lymphoma with COPLA/LVP, *J Am Anim Hosp Assoc* 36:395–403, 2000.
179. Morrison-Collister KE, Rassnick KM, Northrup NC, et al: A combination chemotherapy protocol with MOPP and CCNU consolidation (Tufts VELCAP-SC) for the treatment of canine lymphoma, *Vet Comp Oncol* 1:180–190, 2003.
180. Zemann BI, Moore AS, Rand WM, et al: A combination chemotherapy protocol (VELCAP-L) for dogs with lymphoma, *J Vet Intern Med* 12:465–470, 1998.
181. Keller ET, MacEwen EG, Rosenthal RC: Evaluation of prognostic factors and sequential combination chemotherapy with doxorubicin for canine lymphoma, *J Vet Intern Med* 7:289–295, 1993.
182. Kaiser CI, Fidel JL, Roos M, et al: Reevaluation of the University of Wisconsin 2-year protocol for treating canine lymphosarcoma, *J Am Anim Hosp Assoc* 43:85–92, 2007.
183. Simon D, Moreno SN, Hirschberger J, et al: Efficacy of a continuous, multiagent chemotherapeutic protocol versus a short-term single-agent protocol in dogs with lymphoma, *J Am Vet Med Assoc* 232:879–885, 2008.
184. Sorenmo K, Overley B, Krick E, et al: Outcome and toxicity associated with a dose-intensified, maintenance-free CHOP-based chemotherapy protocol in canine lymphoma: 130 cases, *Vet Comp Oncol* 8:196–208, 2010.
185. Garrett LD, Thamm DH, Chun R, et al: Evaluation of a 6-month chemotherapy protocol with no maintenance therapy for dogs with lymphoma, *J Vet Intern Med* 16:704–709, 2002.
186. Daters AT, Mauldin GE, Mauldin GN, et al: Evaluation of a multidrug chemotherapy protocol with mitoxantrone based maintenance (CHOP-MA) for the treatment of canine lymphoma, *Vet Comp Oncol* 8:11–22, 2010.
187. Rassnick KM, Bailey DB, Malone EK, et al: Comparison between L-CHOP and an L-CHOP protocol with interposed treatments of CCNU and MOPP (L-CHOP-CCNU-MOPP) for lymphoma in dogs, *Vet Comp Oncol* 8:243–253, 2010.
188. Simon D, Nolte I, Everle N, et al: Treatment of dogs with lymphoma using a 12-week, maintenance-free combination chemotherapy protocol, *J Vet Intern Med* 20:948–954, 2006.

189. Hosoya K, Kisseberth WC, Lord LK, et al: Comparison of COAP and UW-19 protocols for dogs with multicentric lymphoma, *J Vet Intern Med* 21:1355–1363, 2007.
190. Siedlecki CT, Kass PH, Jakubiak MJ, et al: Evaluation of an actinomycin-D-containing combination chemotherapy protocol with extended maintenance therapy for canine lymphoma, *Can Vet J* 47:52–59, 2006.
191. Vail DM: Cytotoxic chemotherapy agents, *Clin Brief* 8(4):18–22, 2010.
192. Tomiyasu H, Takahashi M, Fujino Y, et al: Gastrointestinal and hematologic adverse events after administration of vincristine, cyclophosphamide, and doxorubicin in dogs with lymphoma that underwent a combination multidrug chemotherapy protocol, *J Vet Med Sci* 72:1391–1397, 2010.
193. Mellanby RJ, Herrtage ME, Dobson JM: Owners' assessments of their dog's quality of life during palliative chemotherapy for lymphoma, *J Small Anim Prac* 44:100–103, 2003.
194. Bronden LB, Rutteman GR, Flagstad A, et al: Study of dog and cat owners' perceptions of medical treatment for cancer, *Vet Rec* 152:77–80, 2003.
195. Piek CJ, Rutteman GR, Teske E: Evaluation of the results of a L-asparaginase-based continuous chemotherapy protocol in dogs with malignant lymphoma, *Vet Q* 21:44–49, 1999.
196. Moore AS, Cotter SM, Rand WM, et al: Evaluation of discontinuous treatment protocol (VELCAP-s) for canine lymphoma, *J Vet Intern Med* 15:348–354, 2001.
197. Zenker I, Meichner K, Steinle K, et al: Thirteen-week dose-intensifying simultaneous combination chemotherapy protocol for malignant lymphoma in dogs, *Vet Rec* 167:744–748, 2010.
198. Rassnick KM, McEnteee MC, Erb HN, et al: Comparison of 3 protocols for treatment after induction of remission in dogs with lymphoma, *J Vet Intern Med* 21:1364–1373, 2007.
199. Ruslander D, Moore AS, Gliatto JM, et al: Cytosine arabinoside as a single agent for the induction of remission in canine lymphoma, *J Vet Intern Med* 8:299–301, 1994.
200. Rassnick KM, Frimberger AE, Wood CA, et al: Evaluation of ifosfamide for treatment of various canine neoplasms, *J Vet Intern Med* 14:271–276, 2000.
201. Turner AI, Hahn KA, Rusk A, et al: Single agent gemcitabine chemotherapy in dogs with spontaneously occurring lymphoma, *J Vet Intern Med* 20:1384–1388, 2006.
202. MacDonald VS, Thamm DH, Kurzman ID, et al: Does L-asparaginase influence efficacy or toxicity when added to a standard CHOP protocol for dogs with lymphoma? *J Vet Intern Med* 19:732–736, 2005.
203. Jeffreys AB, Knapp DW, Carlton WW, et al: Influence of asparaginase on a combination chemotherapy protocol for canine multicentric lymphoma, *J Am Anim Hosp Assoc* 41:221–226, 2005.
204. Carter RF, Harris CK, Withrow SJ, et al: Chemotherapy of canine lymphoma with histopathological correlation: Doxorubicin alone compared to COP as first treatment regimen, *J Am Anim Hosp Assoc* 23:587–596, 1987.
205. Lon JC, Stein TJ, Thamm DH: Doxorubicin and cyclophosphamide for the treatment of canine lymphoma: a randomized, placebo-controlled study, *Vet Comp Oncol* 8:188–195, 2010.
206. Sauerbry ML, Mullins MN, Bannink EO, et al: Lomustine and prednisone as a first-line treatment for dogs with multicentric lymphoma: 17 Cases (2004-2005), *J Am Vet Med Assoc* 230:1866–1869, 2007.
207. Khanna C, Lund EM, Redic KA, et al: Randomized controlled trial of doxorubicin versus dactinomycin in a multiagent protocol for treatment of dogs with malignant lymphoma, *J Am Vet Med Assoc* 213:985–990, 1998.
208. Price SG, Page RL, Fischer BM, et al: Efficacy and toxicity of doxorubicin/cyclophosphamide maintenance therapy in dogs with multicentric lymphosarcoma, *J Vet Intern Med* 5:259–262, 1991.
209. Marconato L, Stefanello D, Valenti P, et al: Predictors of long-term survival in dogs with high-grade multicentric lymphoma, *J Am Vet Med Assoc* 238:480–485, 2011.
210. Mealey KL, Fidel JM, Gay JA, et al: ABCB1-1Δ polymorphism can predict hematologic toxicity in dogs treated with vincristine, *J Vet Intern Med* 22:996–1000, 2008.
211. Rebhun RB, Kent MS, Borrofka SA, et al: CHOP chemotherapy for the treatment of canine multicentric T-cell lymphoma, *Vet Comp Oncol* 9:38–44, 2011.
212. Dobson JM, Blackwood LB, McInnes EF, et al: Prognostic variables in canine multicentric lymphosarcoma, *J Small Anim Pract* 42:377–384, 2001.
213. Beaver LM, Strottner G, Klein MK: Response rate after administration of a single dose of doxorubicin in dogs with B-cell or T-cell lymphoma:41 cases (2006-2008), *J Am Vet Med Assoc* 237:1052–1055, 2010.
214. Brodsky EM, Mauldin GN, Lachowicz JL, et al: Asparaginase and MOPP treatment of dogs with lymphoma, *J Vet Intern Med* 23:578–584, 2009.
215. Sato M, Yamazaki J, Goto-Koshino Y, et al: Evaluation of cytoreductive efficacy of vincristine, cyclophosphamide, and Doxorubicin in dogs with lymphoma by measuring the number of neoplastic lymphoid cells with real-time polymerase chain reaction, *J Vet Intern Med* 25:285–291, 2011.
216. Sato M, Yamazaki J, Goto-Koshino Y, et al: Increase in minimal residual disease in peripheral blood before clinical relapse in dogs with lymphoma that achieved complete remission after chemotherapy, *J Vet Intern Med* 25:292–296, 2011.
217. Yamazaki J, Takahashi M, Setoguchi A, et al: Monitoring of minimal residual disease (MRD) after multidrug chemotherapy and its correlation to outcome in dogs with lymphoma: a proof-of-concept pilot study, *J Vet Intern Med* 24:897–903, 2010.
218. Thilakaratne DN, Mayer MN, MacDonald VS, et al: Clonality and phenotyping of canine lymphomas before chemotherapy and during remission using polymerase chain reaction (PCR) on lymph node cytologic smears and peripheral blood, *Can Vet J* 51:79–84, 2010.
219. Yamazaki J, Baba K, Goto-Koshino Y, et al: Quantitative assessment of minimal residual disease (MRD) in canine lymphoma by using real-time polymerase chain reaction, *Vet Immunol Immunopathol* 126:321–331, 2008.
220. Von Euler HP, Rivera P, Aronsson AC, et al: Monitoring therapy in canine malignant lymphoma and leukemia with serum thymidine kinase 1 activity—evaluation of a new, fully automated non-radiometric assay, *Int J Oncol* 34:505–510, 2009.
221. Nielsen L, Toft N, Eckersall PD, et al: Serum C-reactive protein concentration as an indicator of remission status in dogs with multicentric lymphoma, *J Vet Intern Med* 21:1231–1236, 2007.
222. Ito D, Endicott MM, Jubala CM, et al: A tumor-related lymphoid progenitor population supports hierarchical tumor organization in canine B-cell lymphoma, *J Vet Intern Med* 25:890–896, 2011.
223. Reference deleted in pages.
224. Reference deleted in pages.
225. Lee JJ, Hughes CS, Fine RL, et al: P-glycoprotein expression in canine lymphoma, *Cancer* 77:1892–1898, 1986.
226. Flory AB, Rassnick KM, Erb HN, et al: Evaluation of factors associated with second remission in dogs with lymphoma undergoing retreatment with a cyclophosphamide, doxorubicin, vincristine and prednisone chemotherapy protocol: 95 cases (2000-2007), *J Am Vet Med Assoc* 238:501–506, 2011.
227. Moore AS, Ogilvie GK, Vail DM: Actinomycin D for reinduction of remission in dogs with resistant lymphoma, *J Vet Intern Med* 8:343–344, 1994.
228. Bannink EO, Sauerbrey ML, Mullins MN, et al: Actinomycin D as rescue therapy in dogs with relapsed or resistant lymphoma: 49 cases (1999-2006), *J Am Vet Med Assoc* 233:446–451, 2008.
229. Griessmayr PB, Payne SE, Winger JE, et al: Dacarbazine as single-agent therapy for relapsed lymphoma in dogs, *J Vet Intern Med* 23:1227–1231, 2009.

230. Dervisis NG, Dominguez PA, Sarbu L, et al: Efficacy of temozolomide or dacarbazine in combination with an anthracycline for rescue chemotherapy in dogs with lymphoma, *J Am Vet Med Assoc* 231:563–569, 2007.
231. Alvarez FJ, Kisseberth WC, Gallant SL, et al: Dexamethasone, melphalan, actinomycin D, cytosine arabinoside (DMAC) protocol for dogs with relapsed lymphoma, *J Vet Intern Med* 20:1178–1183, 2006.
232. Moore AS, London CA, Wood CA, et al: Lomustine (CCNU) for the treatment of resistant lymphoma in dogs, *J Vet Intern Med,* 13:395–398, 1999.
233. Saba CF, Hafeman SD, Vail DM, et al: Combination chemotherapy with continuous L-asparaginase, lomustine and prednisone for relapsed canine lymphoma, *J Vet Intern Med* 23:1058–1063, 2009.
234. Saba CF, Thamm DH, Vail DM: Combination chemotherapy with L-asparaginase, lomustine, and prednisone for relapsed or refractory canine lymphoma, *J Vet Intern Med* 21:127–132, 2007.
235. Flory AB, Rassnick KM, Al-Sarraf R, et al: Combination of CCNU and DTIC chemotherapy for treatment of resistant lymphoma in dogs, *J Vet Intern Med* 22:164–171, 2008.
236. Moore AS, Ogilvie GK, Ruslander D, et al: Evaluation of mitoxantrone for the treatment of lymphoma in dogs, *J Am Vet Med Assoc* 204:1903–1905, 1994.
237. Rassnick KM, Mauldin GE, Al-Sarraf R, et al: MOPP chemotherapy for treatment of resistant lymphoma in dogs: A retrospective study of 117 cases (1989-2000), *J Vet Intern Med* 16:576–580, 2002.
238. Northrup NC, Gieger TL, Kosarek CE, et al: Mechlorethamine, procarbazine and prednisone for the treatment of resistant lymphoma in dogs, *Vet Comp Oncol* 7:38–44, 2009.
239. Fletcher JL, Haber M, Henderson MJ, et al: ABC transporters in cancer: more than just efflux pumps, *Nature Rev Canc* 10:147–156, 2010.
240. Steingold SF, Sharp NJ, McGahan MC, et al: Characterization of canine MDR1 mRNA: its abundance in drug resistant cell lines and in vivo, *Anticancer Res* 18:393–400, 1998.
241. Tomiyasu H, Goto-Koshino Y, Takahashi M, et al: Quantitative analysis of mRNA for 10 different drug resistance factors in dogs with lymphoma, *J Vet Med Sci* 72:1165–1172, 2010.
242. Ogilvie GK, Vail DM, Klein MK, et al: Weekly administration of low-dose doxorubicin for treatment of malignant lymphoma in dogs, *J Am Vet Med Assoc* 198:1762–1764, 1991.
243. Vail DM, Kravis LD, Cooley AJ, et al: Preclinical trial of doxorubicin entrapped in sterically stabilized liposomes in dogs with spontaneously arising malignant tumors, *Cancer Chemother Pharmacol* 39:410–416, 1997.
244. Vail DM, Chun R, Thamm DH, et al: Efficacy of pyridoxine to ameliorate the cutaneous toxicity associated with doxorubicin containing pegylated (stealth) liposomes: a randomized, double-blind clinical trial using a canine model, *Clin Canc Res* 4:1567–1571, 1998.
245. Jubala CM, Wojcieszyn JW, Valli VE, et al: CD20 expression in normal canine B cells and in canine non-Hodgkin's lymphoma, *Vet Pathol* 42:468–476, 2005.
246. Impellizeri JA, Howell K, McKeever KP, et al: The role of rituximab in the treatment of canine lymphoma: an ex vivo evaluation, *Vet J* 171:556–558, 2006.
247. Steplewski Z, Jeglum KA, Rosales C, et al: Canine lymphoma-associated antigens defined by murine monoclonal antibodies, *Cancer Immunol Immunother* 24:197–201, 1987.
248. Rosales C, Jeglum KA, Obrocka M, et al: Cytolytic activity of murine anti-dog lymphoma monoclonal antibodies with canine effector cells and complement, *Cell Immunol* 115:420–428, 1988.
249. Steplewski Z, Rosales C, Jeglum KA, et al: In vivo destruction of canine lymphoma mediated by murine monoclonal antibodies, *In Vivo* 4:231–234, 1990.
250. Crow SE, Theilen GH, Benjaminini E, et al: Chemoimmunotherapy for canine lymphosarcoma, *Cancer* 40:2102–2108, 1977.
251. Weller RE, Theilen GH, Madewell BR, et al: Chemoimmunotherapy for canine lymphosarcoma: A prospective evaluation of specific and nonspecific immunomodulation, *Am J Vet Res* 41:516–521, 1980.
252. Jeglum KA, Young KM, Barnsley K, et al: Chemotherapy versus chemotherapy with intralymphatic tumor cell vaccine in canine lymphoma, *Cancer* 61:2042–2050, 1988.
253. Peruzzi D, Gavazza A, Mesiti G, et al: A vaccine targeting telomerase enhances survival of dogs affected by B-cell lymphoma, *Mol Ther* 18:1559–1567, 2010.
254. Mason NJ, Coughlin CM, Overley B, et al: RNA-loaded CD40-activated B cells stimulate antigen-specific T-cell responses in dogs with spontaneous lymphoma, *Gene Ther* 15:955–965, 2008.
255. Turek MM, Thamm DH, Mitzey A, et al: hGM-CSF DNA Cationic-lipid complexed autologous tumor cell vaccination in the treatment of canine b-cell multicentric lymphoma, *Vet Comp Oncol* 5(4):219–231, 2007.
256. Brooks MB, Matus RE, Leifer CE, et al: Use of splenectomy in the management of lymphoma in dogs: 16 cases (1976-1985), *J Am Vet Med Assoc* 191:1008–1010, 1987.
257. Meleo KA: The role of radiotherapy in the treatment of lymphoma and thymoma, *Vet Clin North Am (Small Anim Pract),* 27:115–129, 1997.
258. Williams LE, Johnson JL, Hauck ML, et al: Chemotherapy followed by half-body radiation therapy for canine lymphoma, *J Vet Intern Med* 18:703–709, 2004.
259. Gustavson NR, Lana SE, Mayer MN, et al: A preliminary assessment of whole-body radiotherapy interposed within a chemotherapy protocol for canine lymphoma, *Vet Comp Oncol* 2:125–131, 2004.
260. Lurie DM, Gordon IK, Theon AP, et al: Sequential low-dose rate half-body irradiation and chemotherapy for the treatment of canine multicentric lymphoma, *J Vet Intern Med* 23:1064–1070, 2009.
261. Lurie DM, Kent MS, Fry MM, et al: A toxicity study of low-dose rate half-body irradiation and chemotherapy in dogs with lymphoma, *Vet Comp Oncol* 6:257–267, 2008.
262. Axiak SM, Carreras JK, Hahn KA, et al: Hematologic changes associated with half-body irradiation in dogs with lymphoma, *J Vet Intern Med* 20:1398–1401, 2006.
263. Brown EM, Ruslander DM, Azuma C, et al: A feasibility study of low-dose total body irradiation for relapsed canine lymphoma, *Vet Comp Oncol* 4:75–83, 2006.
264. Gyurkocza B, Rezvani A, Storb RF: Allogeneic hematopoietic cell transplantation: the state of the art, *Expert Rev Hematol* 3:285–299, 2010.
265. Appelbaum FR, Deeg HJ, Storb R, et al: Marrow transplant studies in dogs with malignant lymphoma, *Transplant* 39:499–504, 1985.
266. Escobar C, Grindem C, Neel JA, et al: Hematologic changes after total body irradiation and autologous transplantation of hematopoietic peripheral blood progenitor cells in dogs with lymphoma, *Vet Pathol* 2011. [Epub ahead of print]
267. Frimberger AE, Moore AS, Rassnick KM, et al: A combination chemotherapy protocol with dose intensification and autologous bone marrow transplant (VELCAP-HDC) for canine lymphoma, *J Vet Intern Med* 20:355–364, 2006.
268. Rassnick KM, Moore AS, Collister KE, et al: Efficacy of combination chemotherapy for treatment of gastrointestinal lymphoma in dogs, *J Vet Intern Med* 23:317–322, 2009.
269. Frank JD, Reimer SB, Kass PH, et al: Clinical outcomes of 30 cases (1997-2004) of canine gastrointestinal lymphoma, *J Am Anim Hosp Assoc* 43:313–321, 2007.
270. DeBoer DJ, Turrel JM, Moore PF: Mycosis fungoides in a dog: Demonstration of T-cell specificity and response to radiotherapy, *J Am Anim Hosp Assoc,* 26:566–572, 1990.
271. Risbon RE, de Lorimier LP, Skorupski K, et al: Response of canine cutaneous epitheliotropic lymphoma to lomustine (CCNU):

a retrospective study of 46 cases (1999-2004), *J Vet Intern Med* 20:1389–1397, 2006.
272. Williams LE, Rassnick KM, Power HT, et al: CCNU in the treatment of canine epitheliotropic lymphoma, *J Vet Intern Med* 20:136–143, 2006.
273. Couto CG: Cutaneous lymphosarcoma, *Proceed Kal Kan Symp* 11:17–77, 1987.
274. White SD, Rosychuk RAW, Scott KV, et al: Use of isotretinoin and etretinate for the treatment of benign cutaneous neoplasia and cutaneous lymphoma in dogs, *J Am Vet Med Assoc* 202:387–391, 1993.
275. Moriello KA, MacEwen EG, Schultz KT: PEG-asparaginase in the treatment of canine epitheliotrophic lymphoma and histiocytic proliferative dermatitis. In Ihrke PJ, Mason IS, White SD, editors: *Advances in veterinary dermatology*, New York, 1993, Pergamon Press.
276. McKeever PJ, Grindem CB, Stevens JB, et al: Canine cutaneous lymphoma, *J Am Vet Med Assoc* 180:531–536, 1982.
277. Tzannes S, Ibarrola P, Batchelor DJ, et al: Use of recombinant human interferon alpha-2a in the management of a dog with epitheliotropic lymphoma, *J Am Anim Hosp Assoc* 44:276–282, 2008.
278. Jagielski D, Lechowski R, Hoffmann-Jagielska M, et al: A retrospective study of the incidence and prognostic factors of multicentric lymphoma in dogs (1998-2000), *J Vet Med A Physiol Pathol Clin Med* 49:419, 2002.
279. Rao S, Lana S, Eickhoff J, et al: Class II major histocompatibility complex expression and cell size independently predict survival in canine B-cell lymphoma, *J Vet Intern Med* 25:1097–1105, 2011.
280. Williams MJ, Avery AC, Lana SE, et al: Canine lymphoproliferative disease characterized by lymphocytosis: immunophenotypic markers of prognosis, *J Vet Intern Med* 22:596–601, 2008.
281. Miller AG, Morley PS, Rao S, et al: Anemia is associated with decreased survival time in dogs with lymphoma, *J Vet Intern Med* 23:116–122, 2009.
282. Abbo AH, Lucroy MD: Assessment of anemia as an independent predictor of response to chemotherapy and survival in dogs with lymphoma: 96 cases (1993-2006), *J Am Vet Med Assoc* 231:1836–1842, 2007.
283. Kiupel M, Bostock D, Bergmann V: The prognostic significance of AgNOR counts and PCNA-positive cell counts in canine malignant lymphomas, *J Comp Pathol* 119:407–418, 1998.
284. Larue SM, Fox MH, Ogilvie GK, et al: Tumour cell kinetics as predictors of response in canine lymphoma treated with chemotherapy alone or combined with whole body hyperthermia, *Int J Hyperthermia* 15:475–486, 1999.
285. Vaughan A, Johnson JL, Williams LE: Impact of chemotherapeutic dose intensity and hematologic toxicity on first remission duration in dogs with lymphoma treated with a chemoradiotherapy protocol, *J Vet Intern Med* 21:1332–1339, 2007.
286. von Euler H, Einarsson R, Olsson U, et al: Serum thymidine kinase activity in dogs with malignant lymphoma: a potent marker for prognosis and monitoring the disease, *J Vet Intern Med* 18:595–596, 2004.
287. Gentilini F, Calzolari C, Turba ME, et al: Prognostic value of serum vascular endothelial growth factor (VEGF) and plasma activity of matrix metalloproteinase (MMP) 2 & 9 in lymphoma-affected dogs, *Leukemia Res* 29:1263–1269, 2005.
288. Hahn KA, Barnhill MA, Freeman KP, et al: Detection and clinical significance of plasma glutathione-S-transferases in dogs with lymphoma, *In Vivo* 13:173–175, 1999.
289. Weller RE, Holmberg CA, Theilen GH, et al: Canine lymphosarcoma and hypercalcemia: clinical, laboratory and pathologic evaluation of twenty-four cases, *J Small Anim Pract* 23:649–658, 1982.
290. Cook AK, Wright ZM, Suchodolski JS, et al: Prevalence and prognostic impact of hypocobalaminemia in dogs with lymphoma, *J Am Vet Med Assoc* 235:1437–1441, 2009.
291. Baskin GR, Couto CG, Wittum TE: Factors influencing first remission and survival in 145 dogs with lymphoma: A retrospective study, *J Am Anim Hosp Assoc* 36:404–409, 2000.
292. Adam F, Villiers E, Watson S, et al: Clinical pathological and epidemiological assessment of morphologically and immunologically confirmed canine leukaemia, *Vet Comp Oncol* 7:181–195, 2009.
293. Comazzi S, Gelain ME, Martini V, et al: Immunophenotype predicts survival time in dogs with chronic lymphocytic leukemia, *J Vet Intern Med* 25:100–106, 2011.
294. Gioia G, Mortarino M, Gelain ME, et al: Immunophenotype-related microRNA expression in canine chronic lymphocytic leukemia, *Vet Immunol Immunopathol* 142:228–235, 2011.
295. Leifer CE, Matus RE: Chronic lymphocytic leukemia in the dog: 22 cases (1974-1984), *J Am Vet Med Assoc* 189:214–217, 1986.
296. Workman HC, Vernau W: Chronic lymphocytic leukemia in dogs and cats: the veterinary perspective, *Vet Clin North Am (Small Anim Pract)* 33:1397–1399, 2003.
297. Kleiter M, Hirt R, Kirtz G, et al: Hypercalcaemia associated with chronic lymphocytic leukaemia in Giant Schnauzer, *Aust Vet J* 79:335–338, 2001.
298. Matus RE, Leifer CE, MacEwen EG: Acute lymphoblastic leukemia in the dog: A review of 30 cases, *J Am Vet Med Assoc* 183:859–862, 1983.
299. Adams J, Mellanby RJ, Viliers E, et al: Acute B cell lymphoblastic leukemia in a 12-week-old greyhound, *J Small Anim Pract* 45:553–557, 2004.
300. Hodgkins EM, Zinkl JG, Madewell BR: Chronic lymphocytic leukemia in the dog, *J Am Vet Med Assoc* 117:704–707, 1980.
301. Januszewicz E, Cooper IA, Pelkington G, et al: Blastic transformation of chronic lymphocytic leukemia, *Am J Hematol* 15:399–402, 1983.
302. Harvey JW, Terrell TG, Hyde DM, et al: Well-differentiated lymphocytic leukemia in a dog: long-term survival without therapy, *Vet Pathol* 18:37–47, 1981.

SECTION B
Feline Lymphoma and Leukemia

DAVID M. VAIL

Lymphoma

The lymphomas (malignant lymphoma or lymphosarcoma) are a diverse group of neoplasms that have in common their origin from lymphoreticular cells. They usually arise in lymphoid tissues such as lymph nodes, spleen, and bone marrow; however, they may arise in almost any tissue in the body. Lymphoma is one of the most common neoplasms seen in the cat.

Incidence

Epidemiologic reports prior to 1990 suggested that lymphoma accounted for 50% to 90% of all hematopoietic tumors in the cat,[1,2] and since hematopoietic tumors (lymphoid and myeloid) represent approximately one-third of all feline tumors, it was estimated lymphoid neoplasia accounted for an incidence of 200 per 100,000 cats at risk.[3] In one series of 400 cats with hematopoietic tumors, 61% had lymphoma and 39% had leukemias and MPDs, of which 21% were categorized as undifferentiated leukemias, most likely myeloid in origin.[4] However, a significant change in the epidemiology and characteristics of lymphoma in cats coincides with the widespread integration of clinically relevant feline leukemia virus (FeLV) diagnostic assays and affected animal elimination regimens of the late 1970s and 1980s and was further enhanced by the commercially available FeLV vaccines appearing in the late 1980s (see the later section on viral etiology). The decline in FeLV-associated lymphoma was mirrored by a decline in the overall prevalence per year of FeLV positivity in cats tested as characterized by reports, including the Tufts Veterinary Diagnostic Laboratory from 1989 to 1997,[5,6] and by the Louwerens group, who reported a decline in FeLV association in over 500 cases of lymphoma in cats presenting to the University of California at Davis veterinary teaching hospital.[7] In these reports, FeLV antigenicity declined to represent only 14% to 25% of cats presenting with lymphoma. Importantly, Louwerens' study revealed that despite a sharp drop in FeLV-associated lymphoma, the overall prevalence of lymphoma in cats is increasing. The increased prevalence appears due to an increase in the number and relative frequency of the alimentary (and in particular the intestinal) anatomic form of lymphoma in the species. This is supported by an epidemiologic survey of 619 cases of feline intestinal lymphoma; 534 (86%) were from the 20 years following 1985 and only 14% were from cases diagnosed in the 20 years prior to 1985.[8] The true annual incidence rate for lymphoma in cats is currently unknown. With respect to feline pediatric tumors, a study in the United Kingdom (n = 233 pathology specimens) found that 73 (31%) represented hematopoietic tumors, of which 51 (70%) were lymphoma—note that FeLV status was unavailable for this compilation of cases.[9]

The typical signalment for cats with lymphoma cannot be uniformly stated as it varies widely based on anatomic site and FeLV status and therefore will be discussed individually under site-specific discussions. In general, based on two large compilations (n = 700) of cases in North America,[5,7] Siamese cats appear overrepresented and although a 1.5 : 1 male to female ratio was observed in one, no association with sex or neutering status was observed in the other. In a large compilation of Australian cases, male cats and the Siamese/oriental breeds were overrepresented,[10] and similar breed findings have been observed in North America, although similar sex predilections have not been found. Within the Siamese/oriental breeds, there appears to be a predisposition for a mediastinal form that is not FeLV associated and represents a younger population (median of 2 years).

Etiology

Viral Factors

FeLV was the most common cause of hematopoietic tumors in the cat in the so-called "FeLV era" of the 1960s through the 1980s when approximately two-thirds of lymphoma cases were associated with FeLV antigenemia. Several studies have documented the potential molecular means by which FeLV can result in lymphoid neoplasia (see Chapter 1, Section C). As one would predict, along with a shift away from FeLV-associated tumors came a shift away from traditional signalment and relative frequency of anatomic sites. This is also supported outside of North America by similar signalment and anatomic frequency data observed in Australia where FeLV infection is quite rare.[10,11] The median age of approximately 11 years now reported in North America is considerably higher than the median ages of 4 to 6 years reported in the FeLV era.[1,2,5-7] The median age of cats within various anatomic tumor groupings has not changed, and anatomic forms traditionally associated with FeLV such as the mediastinal form still occur in younger, FeLV antigenemic cats. Similarly, the alimentary form occurs most often in older, FeLV-negative cats. Table 32-8 presents an overview of the characteristics, including FeLV antigenemic status, of the various anatomic sites of lymphoma in cats. As our ability to interrogate FeLV associations on a molecular basis has improved (e.g., PCR amplification and fluorescent in-situ hybridization), several reports exist defining the role or potential role of FeLV in cats with and without FeLV antigenemia.[12-17] Collectively, these studies indicate FeLV proviral insertion exists in a significant proportion of feline lymphoma tissues and is more common in those of T-cell origin, particularly the thymic and peripheral lymph node anatomic forms. They also suggest that several common FeLV integration sites exist.

There is also evidence that feline immunodeficiency virus (FIV) infection can increase the incidence of lymphoma in cats.[18-27] In contrast to the direct role of FeLV in tumorigenesis, most evidence

TABLE 32-8 General Characteristics of the Most Commonly Encountered Anatomic Forms of Lymphoma in Cats*

Anatomic Form†	Relative Frequency	Median Age (Years)	FeLV Antigenemic	B-Cell	T-Cell	General Prognosis
Alimentary/Gastrointestinal‡						
Small cell/low grade	Common	13	Rare	Rare	Common	Good
Large cell/intermediate grade	Moderate	10	Rare	Common	Rare	Poor
Nasal	Uncommon	9.5	Rare	Common	Uncommon	Good
Mediastinal	Uncommon	2-4	Common	Uncommon	Common	Poor to fair
Peripheral nodal	Uncommon	7	Uncommon	Moderate	Moderate	Fair to poor
Laryngeal/tracheal	Rare	9	Rare	ID	ID	Good to fair
Renal	Rare	9	Rare	Common	Uncommon	Poor to fair
CNS	Rare	4-10	Rare	ID	ID	Poor
Cutaneous	Rare	10-13	Rare	Rare	Common	Fair
Hepatic (pure)	Rare	12	Rare	Uncommon	Common	Poor

FeLV, Feline leukemia virus; *ID,* insufficient data; *CNS,* central nervous system.

Common = >50% of clinical presentations; moderate = 20%-50% of clinical presentations; uncommon = 5%-20% of clinical presentation; rare = <5% of clinical presentations.

*Data may include overlap or mixing of sites and represents the post-FeLV era.

†As the primary site of presentation, rather than extension or progression.

‡Includes those reported as "intraabdominal" in which intestinal is a documented component.

points toward an indirect role for FIV secondary to the immunosuppressive effects of the virus. Shelton[18] determined that FIV infection alone in cats was associated with a fivefold increased risk for development of lymphoma. Coinfection with FeLV will further potentiate the development of lymphoproliferative disorders. Experimentally, cats infected with FIV have developed lymphoma in the kidney, alimentary tract, liver, and multicentric sites. FIV-associated lymphoma is more likely that of the B-cell immunophenotype rather than the T-cell predominance associated with FeLV. It has been suggested that FIV infection may be associated more commonly with alimentary lymphoma of B-cell origin,[28,29] and this may be related to chronic dysregulation of the immune system or the activation of oncogenic pathways; however, FIV antigenemia was only rarely associated with alimentary lymphoma in other large compilations of cases.[5,30-33]

Genetic and Molecular Factors

As discussed earlier in Section A, recent advances in molecular cytogenetics (see Chapter 1, Section A, and Chapter 8), including gene microarray techniques, have and are currently being applied to investigations of chromosomal aberrations in veterinary species with lymphoma. Indeed a predisposition of the oriental cat breeds to develop lymphoma suggests a genetic predisposition and indicates heritable risk.[7,10] Altered oncogene/tumor suppressor gene expression, epigenetic changes, signal transduction, and cell death-pathway alterations are common in lymphomas of humans and are likely also involved in the cat. Several genetic factors have already been discussed as they relate to FeLV associations. Additionally, N-*ras* aberrations have been implicated, although they are rare in cats.[34] Furthermore, telomerase activity (see Chapter 2) has been documented in feline lymphoma tissues.[35,36] Alterations in cellular proliferation and in cell-cycle and death (apoptosis) pathways, in particular the cyclin-dependent kinase cell-cycle regulators and the Bcl-2 family of proapoptotic and antiapoptotic governing molecules, have also been implicated in feline lymphoma.[37-39]

Environmental Factors

Evidence for exposure to environmental tobacco smoke (ETS) as a risk factor for lymphoma in humans has prompted investigations in cats. In one report, the relative risk of developing lymphoma in cats with any exposure to ETS and with 5 or more years of exposure to ETS was 2.4 and 3.2, respectively.[40] A large European study documenting an association between proximity of waste management and cancer in dogs failed to show increased risk in cats.[41]

Immunosuppression

Immune system alterations in the cat such as those accompanying FIV infection has been implicated in the development of lymphoma.[18-20,25] As is the case in immunosuppressed human organ transplantation patients, two reports of immunosuppressed feline renal transplant recipients document increased risk of lymphoma following transplant and associated immunosuppressive therapy.[42,43] In both studies, nearly 10% of transplanted cats developed de novo malignant lymphoma.

Chronic Inflammation

Although definitive proof is lacking, there is a growing body of indirect evidence to suggest that lymphoma can be associated with the presence of chronic inflammation, which theoretically could be the case with intestinal and nasal lymphoma. In particular, an association has been suggested between intestinal lymphoma and inflammatory bowel disease[7,44-46]; however, others have not found support for this concept.[47] Additionally, an association between gastric *Helicobacter* infection and gastric MALT lymphoma in cats is suggested in one study, and because this is a recognized syndrome in humans, it warrants further investigation.[47a]

Diet and Intestinal Lymphoma

Although no direct evidence exists, a link between diet and the development of intestinal lymphoma in cats has been suggested.[7] Support is offered by the relative and absolute increase in the alimentary form of lymphoma in the past 20 years and the fact that several dietary modifications in cat food have occurred in a similar timeframe in response to diseases, such as urinary tract disease. Further investigation is warranted to prove or disprove such assertions.

Pathology and Natural Behavior

Lymphoma can be classified based on anatomic location and histologic and immunophenotypic criteria; often, the two are intimately associated because certain histologic and immunophenotypic types are commonly associated with specific anatomic locations necessitating discussions within the individual anatomic categories that follow. The largest compilation of feline cases subjected to rigorous histologic classification was reported by Valli and others[48] using the NCI WF. WHO has also published a histologic classification system that uses the REAL system as a basis for defining histologic categories of hematopoietic tumors of domestic animals.[49] This system incorporates both histologic criteria and immunohistologic criteria (e.g., B- and T-cell immunophenotype). Regarding anatomic location, as discussed previously, a profound change in presentation, signalment, FeLV antigenemia, immunophenotype, and frequency of anatomic sites has occurred in cats with lymphoma in the "post-FeLV" era (see Table 32-8). Because of this shift, characteristics of feline lymphoma discussed in this chapter will be primarily limited to reports collected from cases presenting after 1995.

Several anatomic classifications exist for lymphoma in the cat, and some categorize the disease as mediastinal, alimentary, multicentric, nodal, leukemic, and individual extranodal forms. Others have combined various nodal and extranodal forms into categories of atypical, unclassified, and mixed, and others have combined intestinal, splenic, hepatic, and mesenteric nodal forms into one category termed *intraabdominal.* Some discrepancies in the discussion of frequency will inevitably result from the variations in classification used in the literature. The relative frequency of anatomic forms and their associated immunophenotype may also vary with geographic distribution and may be related to genetic and FeLV strain differences, as well as prevalence of FeLV vaccine use.

Alimentary/Gastrointestinal Lymphoma

Alimentary/GI lymphoma can present as a purely intestinal infiltration or a combination of intestinal, mesenteric lymph nodes and liver involvement. The tumors can be solitary but more commonly diffuse throughout the intestines. Some reports limit the alimentary form to GI involvement with or without extension to the liver. Lymphoma is the most common tumor type found in the intestines of cats, representing 55% of cases in an epidemiologic survey of 1129 intestinal tumors in the species.[8] The Siamese breed is reported at increased risk.[7,8] While lymphoma may occur in cats of any age, it is primarily a disease of aged cats with a mean age of approximately 13 years for T-cell alimentary lymphoma and 12 years for B-cell lymphoma.[7,8,50-52] No consistent sex bias is noted. Anatomically, alimentary lymphoma is nearly 4 times more likely to occur in the small intestine than the large intestine.[52] In a series of colonic neoplasia in cats, lymphoma was the second most common malignancy (41%), second only to adenocarcinoma.[33]

There is some discordance in the literature regarding the histologic type (primarily cell size: small versus large), immunophenotype, and architecture involved with GI lymphoma. While studies (often older or smaller reports) suggest a majority of B-cell immunophenotypes,[5,53] larger, more recent reports[51,54,55] indicate the majority represent mucosal low-grade T-cell immunophenotypes. Conversely, the vast majority of B-cell GI lymphomas in cats are large cells and intermediate or high grade.[51,53] The largest compilation to date (n = 120), by Moore and others,[51] classified GI lymphomas based on immunophenotype, then as either mucosal (infiltrate confined to mucosa and lamina propria with minimal submucosal extension) or transmural (significant extension into submucosa and muscularis propria). They then compared infiltration patterns with the WHO classification scheme,[56] as well as documenting anatomic location, cell size, presence of epitheliotropism, clonality, and outcome data. This information is summarized in Table 32-9. Of the 120 cases, none tested serologically positive for FeLV and only 3 for FIV. Four cats had concurrent large B-cell lymphoma (stomach, cecum, or colon) and small T-cell lymphoma of the small intestine. Topographically, T-cell variants are much more likely to occur in the small intestine (94%) and rarely in the stomach or large intestine. Conversely, B-cell variants were often multiple and often occurred simultaneously within the stomach, small intestine, and ileocecocolic junction. The vast majority of T-cell variants were mucosal (equivalent to WHO enteropathy-associated T-cell lymphoma [WHO EATCL] type II), and the vast majority of B-cell tumors were transmural (equivalent to WHO EATCL type I classification). Regarding cell size, nearly all mucosal T-cell tumors were composed of small lymphocytes, and slightly more than half of transmural T-cell and all B-cell variants were composed of larger cells. Epitheliotropism is present in approximately 40% of T-cell tumors but is rare in B-cell tumors. Other abdominal organ involvement is common, and in one report of 29 cases of low-grade T-cell intestinal lymphoma, liver and mesenteric involvement was documented in 53% and 33% of cases, respectively.[57] Hepatic lymphoma can occur concurrently with GI lymphoma or be confined solely to the liver.[52,58] Most are T-cell and clonal or oligoclonal based on PCR analysis.

A less common, distinct form of alimentary lymphoma, large granular lymphoma (LGL), also occurs in older (median age 9 to 10 years) cats.[51,53,59-61] These granulated round cell tumors have been termed *globule leukocyte tumors*, although they are likely variations of the same disease. LGL is characterized by lymphoblasts described as 12 to 20 μm in diameter with a round, clefted, or cerebriform nucleus; variably distinct nucleoli; finely granular to lacey chromatin; and a moderate amount of basophilic granular cytoplasm that was occasionally vacuolated.[59] Prominent magenta or azurophilic granules are characteristic (see Figure 7-34, Chapter 7). They are granzyme B positive by immunohistochemistry.[51] This population of cells includes cytotoxic T-cells and occasionally NK cell immunophenotypes—most are $CD3^+$, $CD8^+$, and $CD20^-$ and have T-cell receptor gene rearrangement.[51,60] In one report, nearly 60% expressed CD103 (integrin).[60] Approximately 10% express neither B- or T-cell markers and are thus classified as NK cells. These NK tumors commonly originate in the small intestine, especially the jejunum, are transmural, often exhibit epitheliotropism, and at least two-thirds present with other organs involved—most with mesenteric lymph node involvement and many with liver, spleen, kidney, peritoneal malignant effusions, and bone marrow infiltration. Also, thoracic involvement may occur with malignant pleural effusion and a mediastinal mass present. Peripheral blood involvement was present in 10% of cases in one report[59] and 86% in another.[60] Affected cats are generally FeLV/FIV negative.

Mediastinal Form

The mediastinal form can involve the thymus, mediastinal, and sternal lymph nodes. Pleural effusion is common. In two large compilations, 63% of cats with thymic disease and 17% of cats with pleural effusion were documented as having lymphoma.[62,63] Hypercalcemia occurs frequently with mediastinal lymphoma in dogs but is rare in cats. The majority of cats with mediastinal lymphoma are young (median age 2 to 4 years), FeLV positive, and the T-cell immunophenotype.[5,7,9-11] The disease is confined to the mediastinum in most cases.[7] There also exists a form of mediastinal lymphoma occurring primarily in young, FeLV-negative Siamese cats that appears to be less biologically aggressive and more responsive to chemotherapy than FeLV-associated forms.[64]

Nodal Lymphoma

Involvement limited to peripheral lymph nodes is unusual in cats with lymphoma, representing approximately 4% to 10% of cases.[5,7] In contrast, approximately one-quarter of all other anatomic forms of lymphoma have some component of lymph node involvement. One-third of cats with nodal lymphoma are T-cell immunophenotype and FeLV antigenemic; however, complete categorizations have not occurred in the post-FeLV era and this may no longer be true.[5,7,11,55] Peripheral nodal lymphoma was the most common anatomic form of lymphoma reported in a recent compilation of cases in cats under the age of 1 year, representing a full third of cases in this age group.[9] As lymphoma progresses, bone marrow and hepatic infiltration may develop.

An uncommon and distinct form of nodal lymphoma in cats referred to as "Hodgkin's-like" lymphoma has been reported.[65,66] This form typically involves solitary or regional nodes of the head and neck (Figure 32-12) and histologically resembles Hodgkin's lymphoma in humans. Affected cats generally present with enlargement of one or two mandibular or cervical nodes initially, and tumors are immunophenotypically classified as T-cell–rich, B-cell lymphoma. One case each of inguinal node, multicentric nodal, and

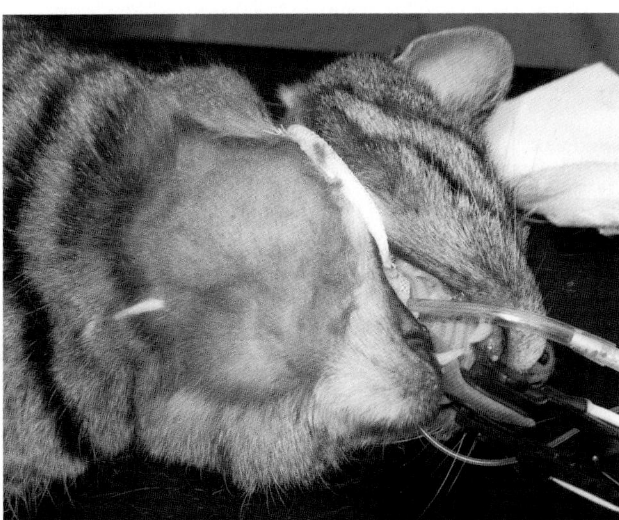

FIGURE 32-12 A cat presented with mandibular lymphadenopathy that was confirmed to be Hodgkin's-like lymphoma following histologic assessment.

TABLE 32-9 Characteristics of Feline Gastrointestinal Lymphoma

Major Characteristic	%*	Cell Size	Epitheliotropism	Median Survival	Clonal or Oligoclonal	Topography
T-cell	**83%**				**90%**	
Mucosal	81%		62%	29 months	91%	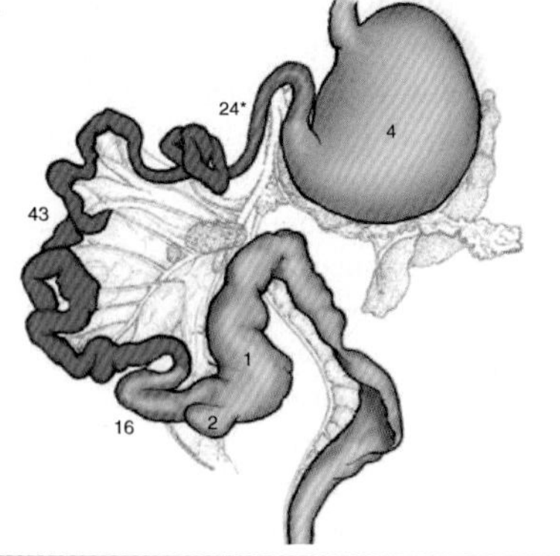
WHO EATCL type II		Small (95%) Large (5%)		NR NR		
Transmural	19%		58%	1.5 months	90%	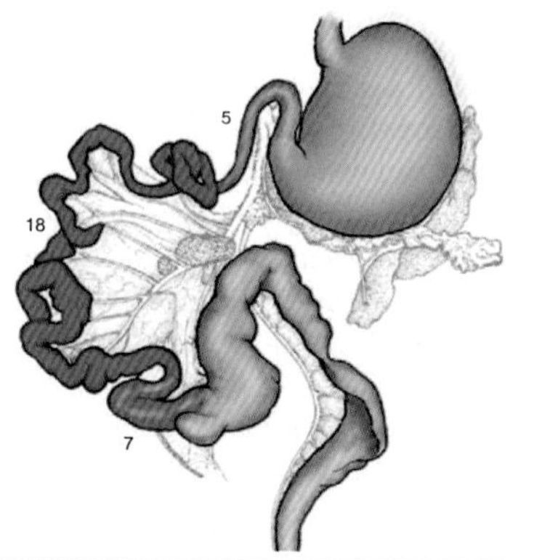
WHO EATCL type I		Small (42%) Large[†] 58%)		NR NR		
B-cell	**17%**				**50%[‡]**	
Mucosal	5%	All				
Transmural	95%	Large (100%)	<5%	3.5 months		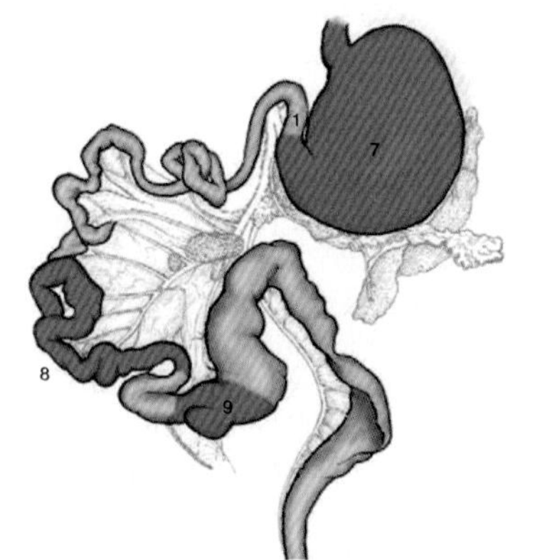

Data modified from Moore PF, Rodriguez-Bertos A, Kass PH: Feline gastrointestinal lymphoma: Mucosal architecture, immunophenotype and molecular clonality, *Vet Pathol* April 19, 2011. Epub ahead of print.

WHO EATCL, World Health Organization enteropathy-associated T-cell lymphoma; *NR*, not report

Numbers in figures indicate case incidence out of 103 reported cases.

*3% of cats had both B- and T-cell immunophenotypes within the gastrointestinal tract.

[†]82% of transmural large T-cell lymphomas are large granular lymphoma subtype.

[‡]39% pseudo-clonal.

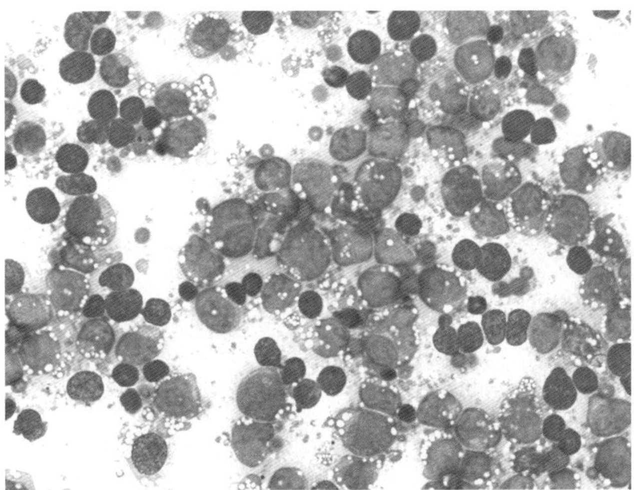

FIGURE 32-13 Fine-needle aspirate of a lymph node in a cat with Hodgkin's-like lymphoma. The large lymphocytes have prominent nucleoli and smooth basophilic cytoplasm. Several binucleate lymphocytes are present.

conjunctival involvement have been reported.[66,67] Histologically, lymph nodes can be effaced by either nodular or diffuse small to blastic lymphocytes with characteristic bizarre or multinucleated cells (Reed-Sternberg–like cells) (Figure 32-13). No association with FeLV or FIV has been documented.

Extranodal Lymphoma

The most common extranodal sites for lymphoma in cats include nasal (including nasopharyngeal and sinonasal), kidney, CNS, laryngeal and tracheal, ocular, retrobulbar, and skin.

Nasal lymphoma is the most common extranodal lymphoma in cats.[68] It is usually a localized disease; however, 20% have local extension or distant metastasis at necropsy.[69] The majority of nonviral nasal/paranasal disease in cats are neoplasias, and lymphoma represents nearly one-third to half of these cases.[70-72] It occurs primarily in older (median age 9 to 10 years; range 3 to 17 years) FeLV/FIV-negative cats and at least three-quarters are B-cell in origin, although T-cell and mixed B-cell/T-cell immunophenotypes can be seen in approximately 10% to 15% of cases.[5,68,69,73] Siamese cats appear overrepresented, and one report[73] observed a 2 : 1 male-to-female ratio. Most are of intermediate- or high-grade histology.[69,73] Epitheliotropism is common if the epithelium is present in the biopsy.

Renal lymphoma is the second most common form of extranodal lymphoma after the nasal form, occurring in approximately one-third of cases.[68] It can present as primary to kidney lymphoma or occur concurrent with alimentary lymphoma. In more contemporary reports, the median age at presentation is 9 years, although 6% occurred in cats under 1 year of age.[68,69] The vast majority of cases are not associated with either FeLV or FIV. The greater median age and lack of FeLV/FIV association are in contrast to reports compiled prior to the post-FeLV era; in earlier studies, the median age was approximately 7.5 years, 25% of cases were FeLV antigenemic, and the majority constituted a B-cell immunophenotype. Little contemporary information exists on the immunohistologic classification of renal lymphoma; however, in Australia where FeLV is not a significant problem, most renal lymphoma is B-cell and intermediate to high grade.[11] Extension to the CNS is a frequent sequela to renal lymphoma and occurs in 40% to 50% of treated cats.[74]

CNS lymphoma can be intracranial, spinal, or both. CNS lymphoma made up 14% of 110 reported cases of extranodal lymphoma,[68] 15% to 31% of intracranial tumors,[75,76] and 39% of spinal cord tumors,[77] making it one of the most common malignancies encountered in the CNS in cats. Although some discordance exists in the literature, cats with CNS lymphoma are younger (median ages of 4 to 10.5 years reported), and 17% to 50% of cases are FeLV antigenemic.[76-78] Approximately two-thirds of intracranial cases are part of a multicentric, extracranial process, and approximately 40% of spinal lymphoma cases occur in multiple spinal cord sites with one-third also involving intracranial locations.[76-78] In a compilation of 160 cases of intracranial tumors in cats, diffuse cerebral and diffuse brainstem involvement was most common for lymphoid malignancies.[76] Spinal lesions are usually both extradural and intradural, although they can be limited to one or the other compartment.[77] Feline CNS lymphoma may be primary but more commonly (approximately 80%) represents a multicentric process (especially renal or bone marrow).[76,78] A paucity of information exists on the immunophenotype of CNS lymphoma.

Laryngeal lymphoma made up 10% of 110 cases of extranodal forms in one report and represented 11% of all laryngeal disease in the species.[68,79] It occurs in older cats (median age 9 years), is not associated with FeLV, and may be a solitary lesion or occur in the presence of other multicentric sites. No information on immunophenotype is available.

Cutaneous lymphoma is a rarely encountered anatomic form in the cat. It is usually seen in older cats (median age 10 to 13.5 years), with no sex or breed predominance, and is not associated with FeLV/FIV.[80,81] It can be solitary or generalized, often affecting the head and face and is generally a slow chronic disease. Two forms of cutaneous lymphoma have been distinguished histologically and immunohistochemically. Most reports in the cat are epitheliotropic and consist of T-cells, although unlike the disease in dogs, adnexal structures are often spared. A report of nonepitheliotropic cutaneous lymphoma in cats also found five of six cases to be of T-cell derivation.[82] Cutaneous "lymphocytosis," an uncommon disease histologically resembling well-differentiated lymphoma, was characterized in 23 cats.[83] Solitary lesions were most common, and all were composed primarily of T-cells, with two-thirds having some B-cell aggregates. Cutaneous lymphocytosis was characterized as a slowly progressive disorder; however, a few cases went on to develop internal organ infiltration. Two case reports exist of cats with cutaneous T-cell lymphoma and circulating atypical lymphocytes.[84,85] The circulating cells were lymphocytes with large, hyperchromatic, grooved nuclei, and one case was immunophenotyped as a CD3/CD8 population. In humans, cutaneous T-cell lymphoma with circulating malignant cells is termed *Sézary syndrome.*

Ocular lymphoma was identified in 5 of 110 cases of extranodal lymphoma in one report.[68] In a compilation of 75 cases of intraocular tumors, 15 (20%) were lymphoma (7 B-cell and 4 T-cell).[86] It was presumed but not proved that the majority were part of a systemic multicentric process.

History, Clinical Signs, and Physical Examination Findings

The clinical signs associated with feline lymphoma are variable and depend on anatomic location and extent of disease.

The alimentary form is most commonly associated with nonspecific signs associated with the intestinal tract. In the more

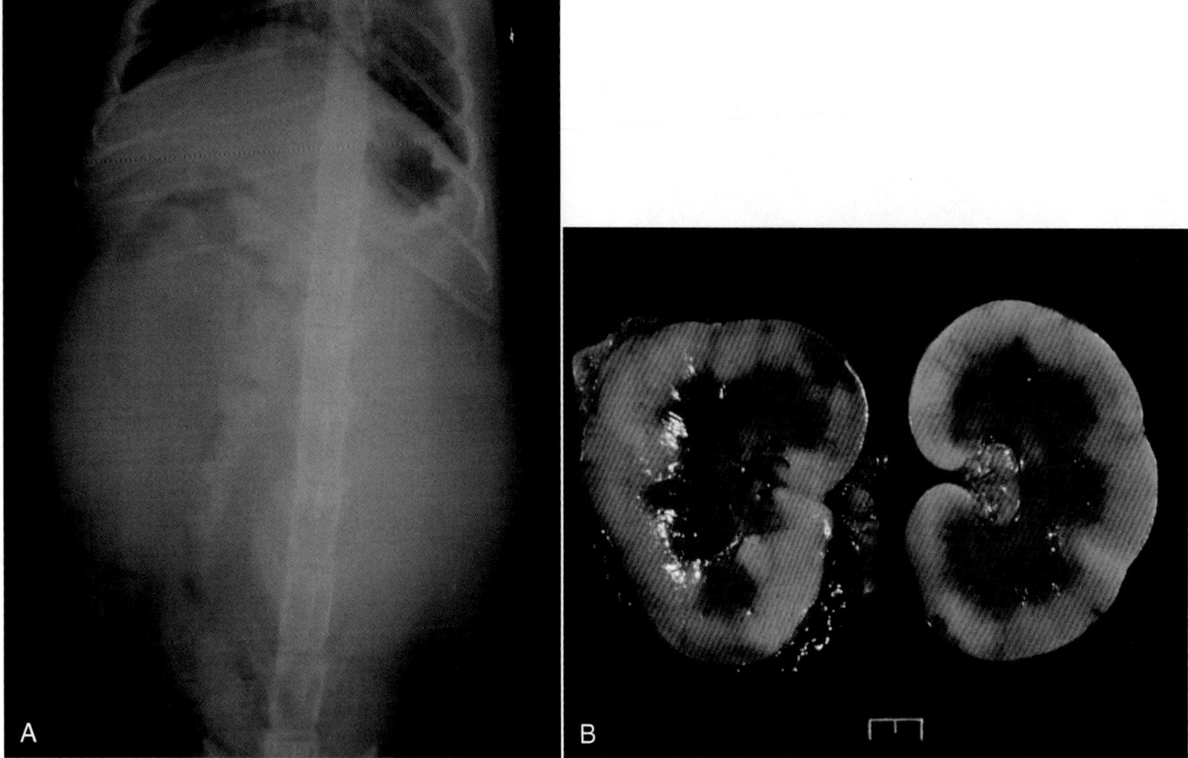

FIGURE 32-14 **A,** Ventrodorsal projection of a cat with renal lymphoma. Massive, bilateral renomegaly is observed. **B,** Necropsy specimens of a cat with bilateral renal lymphoma illustrating the diffuse cortical nature of the disease that is most common.

common low-grade small cell forms, weight loss (83% to 100%), vomiting and/or diarrhea (73% to 88%), and anorexia (66%) are the most common findings, and icterus is uncommon (7%).[50,52,87] Abdominal palpation is abnormal in approximately 70% of cases, with half consisting of intestinal wall thickening and one-third having a palpable mass. Clinical signs are usually present for several months (median: 6 months).[87] In contrast, although the lymphoblastic high-grade forms tend to cause similar clinical signs, they progress more rapidly with signs present for days or weeks and are more likely to present with a palpable abdominal mass originating from the GI tract, enlarged mesenteric lymph nodes, or liver.[31,50,88] Icterus is also more common in large cell forms. Hematochezia and tenesmus may also be present if the colon is involved.[33] Rarely, cats may present with signs consistent with an acute abdomen due to intestinal obstruction or perforation and concurrent peritonitis. Cats with intestinal LGL are presented with anorexia, weight loss, lethargy, and vomiting.[59,60] A palpable abdominal mass is present in approximately half of LGL cases, and hepatomegaly, splenomegaly, and renomegaly are common. Abdominal effusions, pleural effusions, and icterus are observed in less than 10% of cases.

The clinical signs associated with the mediastinal form of lymphoma include dyspnea, tachypnea, and a noncompressible anterior mediastinum with dull heart and lung sounds.[89] Rarely, a Horner's syndrome and precaval syndrome may be observed. Pleural effusion is common and characterized by serohemorrhagic to chylous effusion, and in most cases, neoplastic cells (lymphoblasts) are identified.[63,90]

Cats with the nodal form of lymphoma present with variable clinical signs depending on the extent of disease; however, they are often depressed and lethargic. Peripheral lymphadenopathy, as the only physical finding, is an uncommon presentation. Cats with Hodgkin's-like nodal lymphoma usually present without overt clinical signs.[65,66]

Cats with nasal lymphoma are typically presented with nasal discharge (60% to 85%), sneezing (20% to 70%), upper respiratory noise (stridor, stertor, wheezing; 20% to 60%), facial deformity (0% to 20%), anorexia (10% to 60%), epiphora (10% to 30%), and occasionally increased respiratory effort and coughing.[68,69,73] The nasal discharge is usually mucopurulent, although epistaxis is present in up to one-third of cases. Regional lymphadenopathy can also occur. The median duration of clinical signs prior to diagnosis is 2 months (range of 1 to 1800 days).

Cats with renal lymphoma present with signs consistent with renal insufficiency: inappetence, weight loss, and polyuria/polydipsia.[68,74] On physical examination, renomegaly (usually bilateral, lumpy, and irregular) is palpated in the majority of cases (Figure 32-14).

Cats with CNS lymphoma can present with constitutional signs (anorexia, lethargy) and signs referring to intracranial lesions, spinal lesions, or both.[68,75-77,91,92] Intracranial signs may include ataxia, altered consciousness, aggression, central blindness, and vestibular abnormalities. In a study of cats with seizures, of those diagnosed with intracranial lesions, 8% were due to lymphoma.[75] Clinical signs referring to spinal cord involvement may include paresis or paraplegia (>80%; tetraparesis in 20%), ataxia, pain, and constipation, and nonspecific constitutional signs (e.g., anorexia, lethargy, weight loss) are also common.[77,92] In cats with spinal cord involvement, neurologic examination may further reveal tetraparesis, lower or upper motor neuron bladder, tail flaccidity, and absent deep pain; approximately one-third of signs will be asymmetric and most refer to thoracolumbar involvement. The neurologic dysfunction may be insidious or progress rapidly.

Signs associated with laryngeal lymphoma in cats most commonly include dyspnea, dysphonia, stridor, gagging or retching, and rarely, coughing.[68,79]

Cutaneous lymphoma may be solitary or diffuse with a varied presentation.[80,83] In decreasing order of likelihood, lesions may include erythematous patches, alopecia, scaling, dermal nodules, or ulcerative plaques. Nasal hypopigmentation, miliary dermatitis, and mucosal lesions are rarely observed. Peripheral lymphadenopathy may also be present. In most cats, the duration of signs will be prolonged, lasting several months.

Cats with ocular lymphoma are presented with uveitis or iridial masses, as well as signs related to systemic involvement of disease.[68]

Nonspecific Signs

All cats with lymphoma, regardless of site, may be presented with nonspecific constitutional signs that may include anorexia, weight loss, lethargy, or depression. Secondary bone marrow infiltration may lead to anemia—at least 50% of affected cats have moderate-to-severe nonregenerative anemia. Signs related to paraneoplastic hypercalcemia (PU/PD) can occur in cats, however, much less commonly than in the dog. In one survey of hypercalcemia in cats, approximately 10% were diagnosed with lymphoma of various anatomic types.[93]

Diagnosis and Clinical Staging

For most cats with suspect lymphoma, the diagnostic evaluation should include a baseline assessment consisting of a CBC with differential cell count, platelet count, serum chemistry profile, urinalysis, and retroviral (FeLV/FIV) screen. Serum chemistry profiles can help establish the overall health of the animal, as well as, in some cases, suggest site-specific tumor involvement; for example, increased activities of liver enzymes may indicate hepatic infiltration and increased blood urea nitrogen (BUN) and creatinine may indicate renal lymphoma. For cats with alimentary lymphoma, hypoproteinemia and anemia are reported to occur in up to 23% and 76% of cases, respectively.[31,52,94] Hypercalcemia is rarely seen in cats but has been reported in cats with lymphoma at various anatomic sites. Hypoglycemia was reported in approximately one-third of cats with lymphoma in one Australian study.[94] In a series of cats with various anatomic forms of lymphoma, serum albumin concentrations were significantly lower and β-globulin concentrations (as measured by protein electrophoresis) were significantly higher than a healthy control population.[95]

The use of various imaging modalities in cats with lymphoma depends on the anatomic site and will be discussed in site-specific discussions to follow.

Cytopathologic or histopathologic evaluation of lymph node or involved organ tissue, procured via needle aspirate cytology (see Chapter 7), surgical, endoscopic, or needle-core biopsy (see Chapter 9) is required for a definitive diagnosis. FNA cytology alone may not be sufficient in some cases, owing to difficulties encountered in distinguishing lymphoma from benign hyperplastic or reactive lymphoid conditions. In such cases, whole lymph node excision and/or involved organ biopsy is preferred because orientation and information regarding invasiveness and architectural abnormalities may be necessary for diagnosis. Additionally, involved tissue, needle aspirate, and fluid samples can be further interrogated by various histochemical, immunohistochemical, flow cytometric analysis (e.g., size and immunophenotypic assessment), and molecular techniques (e.g., PARR to assess clonality) to further characterize the disease process and refine the diagnosis in equivocal cases.

The reader is referred to Chapter 8 for a general discussion of flow cytometric analysis and molecular diagnostic techniques, as well as the molecular diagnostic techniques section in Section A of this chapter for specific applications to lymphoma. PARR applications in cats have been described as being approximately 80% sensitive for the diagnosis of feline lymphoma[96]; however, assessment of specificity has not been clearly established. Clonality assessment tools (e.g., primers) for both Ig and T-cell receptor variable region genes have been developed in cats.[97-100]

Assessments of tumor proliferation rates (e.g., Ki67, PCNA, AgNOR), telomerase activity, and serum protein electrophoresis can also be performed on involved tissues in cats; however, consistent prognostic value across the anatomic, histopathologic, and immunophenotypic variants of lymphoma in cats is not well characterized. If these ancillary assays are helpful with respect to prognosis or diagnosis, they will be discussed in site-specific discussions to follow.

Thorough staging, including a bone marrow aspiration or biopsy, peripheral lymph node assessment (clinically normal or abnormal nodes), and thoracic and/or abdominal imaging, is indicated when (1) solitary site disease is suspected (in particular, extranodal sites) and a decision between locoregional therapy (i.e., surgery and/or RT) versus systemic therapy (i.e., chemotherapy) is being considered; (2) it provides prognostic information that will help a caregiver make treatment decisions; and (3) complete staging of the extent of disease is required as part of a clinical trial. Bone marrow evaluation may be of particular interest if anemia, cellular atypia, and leukopenia are present. A WHO staging system exists for the cat that is similar to that used in the dog (see Box 32-1); however, because of the high incidence of visceral/extranodal involvement in the feline species, a separate staging system has been evaluated and is often used (Box 32-3).[101] Because lymphoma in cats is more varied with respect to anatomic locations, staging systems are generally less helpful for predicting response.

Anatomic Site-Specific Diagnostics

Alimentary/Gastrointestinal Lymphoma The diagnosis of large cell, high-grade alimentary/GI lymphoma is generally less complicated than for the more common low-grade GI type. The former (including LGL) is often diagnosed with physical examination, abdominal imaging (e.g., ultrasound), and cytologic or histologic assessment of needle aspirate or needle biopsy samples from intestinal masses, enlarged mesenteric lymph nodes, or liver because mass lesions and gross lymphadenopathy are more commonly present. If obvious abdominal masses are present on physical examination, transabdominal needle aspiration may be possible without the aid of abdominal imaging. Less commonly, abdominal exploration is necessary if lesions are more subtle or not amenable to transabdominal sampling. Further staging via thoracic imaging, peripheral lymph node aspiration, and bone marrow assessment may be performed, but rarely contributes prognostic information or alters treatment decisions because the disease is already widespread and systemic therapy is required.

In contrast, low-grade, small cell GI lymphoma is more commonly associated with modest (or palpably absent) intestinal thickening without mass effect and is clinically similar if not identical in presentation to benign inflammatory bowel disease (IBD). Cytologic assessment alone is often not sufficient for diagnosis; in one study, eight of nine cases in which mesenteric lymph nodes were confirmed histologically as lymphoma, cytologic assessment incorrectly indicated benign lymphoid hyperplasia.[52] The key elements necessary for the diagnosis of low-grade, small cell GI lymphoma

Box 32-3 Clinical Staging System for Feline Lymphoma

Stage 1

- A single tumor (extranodal) or single anatomic area (nodal)
- Includes primary intrathoracic tumors

Stage 2

- A single tumor (extranodal) with regional lymph node involvement
- Two or more nodal areas on the same side of the diaphragm
- Two single (extranodal) tumors with or without regional lymph node involvement on the same side of the diaphragm
- A resectable primary gastrointestinal tract tumor, usually in the ileocecal area, with or without involvement of associated mesenteric nodes only

Stage 3

- Two single tumors (extranodal) on opposite sides of the diaphragm
- Two or more nodal areas above and below the diaphragm
- All extensive primary unresectable intraabdominal disease
- All paraspinal or epidural tumors, regardless of other tumor site or sites

Stage 4

- Stages 1-3 with liver and/or spleen involvement

Stage 5

- Stages 1-4 with initial involvement of CNS or bone marrow or both

Data from Terry A, Callanan JJ, Fulton R, et al: Molecular analysis of tumours from feline immunodeficiency virus (FIV)-infected cats: An indirect role for FIV, *Int J Cancer* 61:227–232, 1995.

(and differentiation from IBD) include abdominal imaging (usually ultrasound), procurement of tissue for histopathology, and if necessary, assessment of immunophenotype and clonality.

Abdominal ultrasound will be abnormal in approximately 60% to 90% of cats with low-grade, small cell GI lymphoma.[31,52,102,103] Diffuse small intestinal wall thickening is the most common finding; 50% to 70% of cats with lymphoma will have ultrasonic evidence of wall thickening, which predominantly involves the muscularis propria, and submucosa, although mucosal thickening can also occur. Focal mural masses are uncommon. Mesenteric lymphadenopathy is also common and reported in 45% to 80% of affected cats. These ultrasonographic findings are by no means pathognomonic for lymphoma, however, because 10% to 50% and 15% to 20% of cats with IBD also have ultrasonographic evidence of intestinal wall thickening and lymphadenopathy, respectively.[102,103] Mucosal thickening is more common, and muscularis propria thickening is less common in IBD than lymphoma. Less commonly, cats with low-grade intestinal lymphoma will have ultrasonographic abnormalities in other abdominal organs such as the stomach, liver, spleen, colon, and pancreas, and occasionally, mild effusions are observed.

As mentioned previously, although aspirate cytology may be sufficient for diagnosis of large cell intermediate- or high-grade alimentary lymphoma in cats, it is rarely diagnostic for low-grade, small cell intestinal lymphoma, and tissue procurement for histologic and ancillary assessment is required for diagnosis (and differentiation from IBD). The debate still rages as to whether endoscopically obtained tissue is sufficient for diagnosis or if full-thickness tissue procured during laparotomy or laparoscopy is necessary in light of similarities with IBD.[51,54,103,104] As previously discussed, histologic features that help differentiate intestinal lymphoma from IBD include lymphoid infiltration of the intestinal wall beyond the mucosa, epitheliotropism (especially intraepithelial nests and plaques), heterogeneity, and nuclear size of lymphocytes.[51,54] Although the presence of transmural involvement is highly suggestive of lymphoma, the lack of transmural infiltration is not pathognomonic for IBD; transmural infiltration is common with B-cell and large T-cell (including LGL) intestinal lymphoma but is observed in the minority of low-grade T-cell intestinal lymphomas that represent the largest group in cats (see Table 32-9).[51] For these reasons, if the differentiation of lymphoma and IBD is equivocal after standard histopathologic assessment, the addition of immunophenotypic and PARR analysis in a stepwise fashion, as proposed by Kiupel and others,[54] may be ultimately necessary for a definitive diagnosis. Their study of 63 cats with either lymphoma or IBD found that, although standard histopathology was highly specific for diagnosis of lymphoma (99% specific, 72% sensitive), sensitivity was enhanced by the addition of immunophenotypic analysis (99% specific, 78% sensitive) and further enhanced by PARR analysis (99% specific, 83% sensitive).

Mediastinal Lymphoma For cats with mediastinal lymphoma, diagnostic suspicion may begin with a noncompressible cranial thorax on physical examination and confirmation of a mediastinal mass/pleural effusion on thoracic radiograph. FNA of the mass or cytologic evaluation of pleural fluid may be sufficient to establish a diagnosis. In most cats, the finding of a monotonous population of intermediate- or high-grade cells will establish a diagnosis. However, definitive diagnosis of lymphoma in cats with a mediastinal mass and concurrent chylothorax can be challenging. CT appearance may be helpful but generally does not contribute to a definitive diagnosis. If lymphoblasts are not identified in the pleural chylous effusion, then cholesterol and triglyceride concentrations can be measured.[105] In chylous effusions, the pleural fluid triglyceride concentration will be greater than in the serum; however, anorectic cats will have lower triglyceride levels in the pleural fluid. A major differential for mediastinal lymphoma is thymoma. The cytologic features of thymoma can be distinct from lymphoma in many cases, but the diagnosis can be challenging because of a preponderance of small lymphocytes in thymoma. Mast cells can also be seen in up to 50% of aspirations from thymomas. The addition of immunophenotypic and clonality assessment may be helpful in equivocal cases.

Nasal Lymphoma If nasal lymphoma is suspected, advanced imaging (CT, MRI), rhinoscopy, and biopsy are usually necessary for diagnosis (see Chapter 23, Section B). CT or MRI is useful to determine the extent of involvement and to help plan biopsy procurement and RT if that treatment option is pursued. CT characteristics associated with sinonasal tumors in cats include the presence of a unilateral or bilateral nasal/sinus mass or fluid, bulla

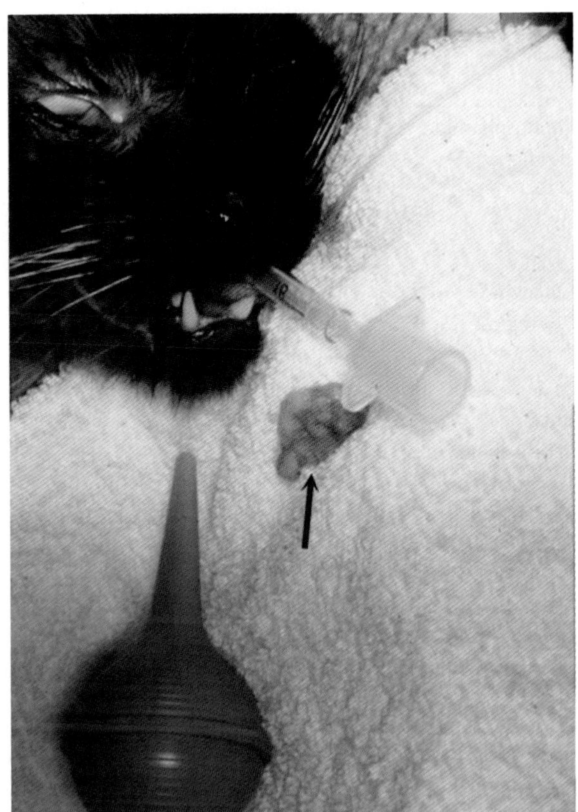

FIGURE 32-15 Flush biopsy of nasal lymphoma. Note the large sample *(arrow)* procured by retrograde flushing of saline through one nares while occluding the contralateral nares. The sample is flushed through the pharynx and out the mouth.

effusion, and lysis of associated bony structures.[106,107] A biopsy can be procured either by intranasal procurement (with or without rhinoscopy) or by flushing one hemicavity with a bulb syringe and saline while occluding the contralateral cavity and collecting samples flushed out of the nasopharynx (Figure 32-15). Thorough staging (i.e., regional node assessment, thoracic and abdominal staging, and bone marrow assessment) to ensure the disease is confined to the nasal passages is recommended, if local RT without systemic chemotherapy is being considered.

Renal Lymphoma In the case of renal lymphoma, physical examination findings of massive and often bilateral renomegaly will raise the index of suspicion. Radiographic appearance is smooth-to-irregular renomegaly (see Figure 32-14, *A*). Ultrasonographic imaging usually reveals bilateral (>80%), irregular renomegaly with hypoechoic subcapsular thickening.[108] Approximately one-third of cases will have ultrasonographic evidence of other abdominal organ involvement. The disease is usually diffuse throughout the renal cortex (see Figure 32-14, *B*) and transabdominal needle aspirate or core biopsy is diagnostic in most cases.

Central Nervous System Lymphoma In cats with suspected spinal lymphoma, survey radiographs of the spine will rarely reveal osseous lesions. Myelograms, CT, or MRI are indicated, and in approximately 75% of the cases, an extradural or intradural mass will be detected.[76,77,91,92] Most lesions occur at a thoracolumbar or lumbosacral location, and they are often found in more than one location. Image-guided needle aspiration of epidural lesions may yield enough tissue for a cytologic diagnosis. CT or MR also reveals multifocal disease in the majority of cats with intracranial lymphoma.[75,76] CSF analysis may be helpful but is rarely definitive for lymphoma. One of 11 cats with confirmed spinal lymphoma in one study[77] and 6 of 17 with confirmed intracranial lymphoma in another[76] had evidence of lymphoblasts in the CNS, and an increased protein content was commonly found. In cats suspected of CNS lymphoma, bone marrow and renal involvement are often present, and cytologic assessment of these or other more accessible organs is generally more easily attainable than from spinal sites.

For cats suspected of cutaneous lymphoma, punch biopsies (4 to 8 mm) should be taken from the most representative and infiltrative sites, while avoiding overtly infected skin lesions. Immunophenotypic and PARR analysis often are helpful in definitive diagnosis. Complete staging to rule out systemic disease is also recommended for cats with cutaneous lymphoma because local therapies can be applied in cases of solitary disease.

Treatment and Prognosis

Our knowledge base for treating cats with lymphoma is less well established, and outcomes are less predictable than that in dogs, primarily due to the greater variation in histologic type and anatomic location observed in the species. This is further complicated by the plethora of papers that "lump" very small numbers of cases representing multiple anatomic/immunophenotypic and histologic subtypes (e.g., small cell versus large cell variants) together when reporting survival analysis following chemotherapy. This provides only general observations rather than important specific outcome information (i.e., response rate and durability of response) that can vary significantly with respect to anatomic and histologic subtype. In general, canine lymphoma is most commonly intermediate-high grade and nodal, whereas cats more commonly present with GI or extranodal (±nodal extension), small cell, low-grade, and/or indolent forms. As will be discussed subsequently, the author bases most treatment decisions on assessment of whether the individual case represents a low-grade (e.g., indolent, small cell variants) versus an intermediate- or high-grade (e.g., large cell) lymphoma. Finally, much of the early work on chemotherapy protocol development for cats with lymphoma occurred during the FeLV era, and care should be exercised when applying this information in the post-FeLV era.

In general, cats tolerate chemotherapy for lymphoma quite well, most clients are happy with their choice to initiate treatment, and quality of life generally improves following commencement of therapy.[109,110] The chemotherapeutic agents used most commonly to treat intermediate- or high-grade lymphoma in cats are similar to those used for dogs and humans with lymphoma (see Section A in this chapter) and include doxorubicin, vincristine, cyclophosphamide, methotrexate, L-asparaginase, CCNU (lomustine), and prednisone. Most combination induction protocols currently employed in cats are modifications of CHOP protocols initially designed for human oncologic use.[5,110-116] CHOP represents combinations of cyclophosphamide (C), doxorubicin (H, hydroxydaunorubicin), vincristine (O, Oncovin) and prednisone (P). In general, CHOP-based protocols are appropriate for cats with large cell, intermediate- and high-grade lymphoma involving any anatomic site (e.g., peripheral nodal, mediastinal, and renal forms) but should not be first-line therapy for small cell, low-grade variants. As in the dog (see Section A in this chapter), a plethora of modifications are used with CHOP-based protocols, although virtually no quality comparative data exist to compare outcomes, and as such, the protocol used should be based on cost, ease, client/veterinarian preference, and level of comfort. The current CHOP-based protocol in use by

TABLE 32-10 The CHOP-Based Chemotherapy Protocol for Cats with Lymphoma Employed by the Author

TREATMENT WEEK	DRUG, DOSAGE, AND ROUTE
1	Vincristine 0.5-0.7 mg/m² IV L-Asparaginase 400 Units/kg SQ Prednisone 2.0 mg/kg PO, q24hr
2	Cyclophosphamide 200 mg/m² IV Prednisone 2.0 mg/kg PO, q24hr
3	Vincristine 0.5-0.7 mg/m² IV Prednisone 1.0 mg/kg PO, q24hr
4	Doxorubicin 25 mg/m² IV Prednisone 1.0 mg/kg PO*
6	Vincristine 0.5-0.7 mg/m² IV
7†	Cyclophosphamide 200 mg/m² IV
8	Vincristine 0.5-0.7 mg/m² IV
9‡	Doxorubicin 25 mg/m² IV
11	Vincristine 0.5-0.7 mg/m² IV
13†	Cyclophosphamide 200 mg/m² IV
15	Vincristine 0.5-0.7 mg/m² IV
17	Doxorubicin 25 mg/m² IV
19	Vincristine 0.5-0.7 mg/m² IV
21†	Cyclophosphamide 200 mg/m² IV
23	Vincristine 0.5-0.7 mg/m² IV
25§	Doxorubicin 25 mg/m² IV

IV, Intravenous; *SQ,* subcutaneous; *PO,* by mouth.

*Prednisone is continued (1 mg/kg PO) every other day from this point on.

†If renal lymphoma or central nervous system (CNS) lymphoma is present, substitute cytosine arabinoside (Ara-C) at 600 mg/m² divided SQ twice a day (BID) over 2 days at these treatments.

‡If in complete remission at week 9, continue to week 11.

§If in complete remission at week 25, therapy is discontinued and cat is rechecked monthly for recurrence.

NOTE: A complete blood count (CBC) should be performed prior to each chemotherapy. If neutrophils are <1500 cells/UL, wait 5 to 7 days, repeat CBC, then administer the drug if neutrophils have risen above the 1500 cell/UL cutoff.

TABLE 32-11 COP Protocol for Lymphoma in Cats

DRUG	FREQUENCY OF DRUG DELIVERY
Cyclophosphamide 300 mg/m² IV	Given every 3 weeks on the day after vincristine. Discontinued if animal is in complete remission at 1 year.
Vincristine (Oncovin) 0.75 mg/m² IV	Given weekly on weeks 1, 2, 3, and 4, then given every 3 weeks thereafter on the day before cyclophosphamide, Discontinued if animal is in complete remission at 1 year.
Prednisone/ prednisolone 50 mg/m² orally	Given daily for 1 year.

NOTE: A complete blood count (CBC) should be performed prior to each treatment. If neutrophils are $<1.5 \times 10^9$/L, wait 5 to 7 days and repeat the CBC. Treat if neutrophils are $\geq 1.5 \times 10^9$/L.

the author is presented in Table 32-10. This protocol has been used in many cats with various forms of intermediate- and high-grade lymphoma and is generally well tolerated. At present, most canine lymphoma protocols (see Section A in this chapter) discontinue chemotherapy by the 25th week, and we have sufficient data to show shorter, maintenance-free protocols are as good if not superior to longer maintenance protocols; however, similar comparative data do not exist in the cat. Until such time as evidence to the contrary exists, the author presently recommends discontinuation of chemotherapy at week 25 in cats who have attained a complete remission. Doxorubicin alone (25 mg/m², every 3 weeks for 5 total treatments) or palliative prednisone therapy is offered if clients decline more aggressive CHOP-based therapy. Cats are generally less tolerant of doxorubicin than are dogs; therefore a lower dosage (25 mg/m² IV or 1 mg/kg IV) is used (see Chapter 11). Cardiac toxicity does not appear to be a clinically significant problem in cats, although renal toxicity is more commonly encountered in the species[117] and renal function should be monitored (i.e., serial BUN, creatinine, and urine specific gravity) closely prior to and during therapy. The use of COP (i.e., CHOP without the addition of doxorubicin) is often used in cats in Europe, and one compilation reported similar results to CHOP.[64] A COP protocol commonly employed in cats is presented in Table 32-11. Some studies with relatively few case entries have reported limited activity for doxorubicin as a single agent in cats with lymphoma[118,119]; however, larger studies using combination protocols have more consistently reported the addition of doxorubicin as necessary for the attainment of more durable responses.[5,114] Interestingly, in a report of 23 cats having relapsed following COP-based protocols (without doxorubicin), only 22% responded subsequently to doxorubicin-containing rescue therapy.[120] A small number of cats with lymphoma have been treated with single-agent oral CCNU (lomustine) at a dosage range of 30 to 60 mg/m² every 3 to 6 weeks.[121,122] Whereas activity was noted, only partial responses were reported. L-asparaginase, which is often included in protocols for lymphoma in cats, has a much shorter asparagine-depleting effect in cats (lost by 7 days) than in dogs and in one study in 13 cats with lymphoma resulted in only a 30% response rate.[123]

In general, cats with intermediate- and high-grade lymphoma treated with CHOP-based or COP protocols do not enjoy the same level of success as dogs. Bearing in mind that these reports group together a wide variety of subtypes having dissimilar prognoses (see subsequent site-specific treatment sections), the overall response rates tend to be in the 50% to 80% range with median remission and survival durations of 4 and 6 months, respectively.[5,64,110-116,124]

Anatomic Site-Specific Treatment

Alimentary/Gastrointestinal Lymphoma Representing the most common presentation for cats with lymphoma, the large majority have the small cell, mucosal, T-cell variant that carries a good prognosis, often with less aggressive chemotherapy protocols (e.g., oral chlorambucil and prednisone).[51,52,87,125] Chlorambucil (20 mg/m² PO, every 2 weeks [preferred by the author] or 2 mg PO every other day) and prednisone or prednisolone (initially 1 to 2 mg/kg PO daily, reduced to 0.5 to 1.0 mg/kg every other day over several weeks) results in response rates (i.e., resolution of clinical signs) of greater than 90% and median survivals of approximately 2 years or longer.[52,87,125] Cats who relapse with this protocol often will subsequently respond to alternative alkylators, such as cyclophosphamide or lomustine.[125] Anecdotally, many will also respond to vinblastine chemotherapy if they no longer are responsive to alkylators.

In contrast, cats with B-cell or large T-cell (including LGL) or small T-cell lymphoma that is transmural typically do not enjoy a durable response to therapy and survivals are much shorter.[31,51,59,60] Median survivals range from 45 to 100 days, even in cats treated with more aggressive COP-based protocols. In the author's experience, these variants are more likely to respond to CHOP-based protocols than chlorambucil/prednisone; however, durable responses occur only in a minority of cases. In particular, LGL appears to carry a grave prognosis[59,60]; in 2 compilations of 66 cats with LGL, median survivals of approximately 2 months were reported, including 23 cats receiving either COP or CHOP-based protocols, which resulted in only a 30% response rate.

Nutritional support is especially important for cats with GI lymphomas. It may be necessary to place a feeding tube in cats undergoing chemotherapy, particularly if prolonged anorexia is present (see Chapter 15, Section B).

Recently, two preliminary studies evaluated RT, either as rescue following recurrence or in addition to chemotherapy for the treatment of intestinal lymphoma in cats.[126,127] Eleven cats (6 small cell, 4 large cell, and 1 LGL) that progressed following chemotherapy received abdominal radiation (8 Gy in 2 fractions over 2 days) and resulted in a median survival of 7 months, although numbers were small and 40% were lost to follow-up.[127] A second report of eight cats (seven with large cell lymphoma) underwent 6 weeks of CHOP-based combination chemotherapy, followed 2 weeks later by whole abdomen radiation consisting of 10 daily 1.5 Gy fractions.[126] Although three cats died within 3 weeks of RT, five enjoyed durable remissions. These preliminary promising outcomes warrant further investigation.

Mediastinal Lymphoma Mediastinal lymphoma in young FeLV-positive cats is generally associated with a poor prognosis, and survival times of approximately 2 to 3 months are expected following CHOP- or COP-based protocols .[5,116] In contrast, young FeLV-negative Siamese cats with mediastinal lymphoma experience remission rates approaching 90%, and responses tend to be more durable (median ≈9 months).[64]

Nodal Lymphoma The treatment choice for peripheral nodal lymphoma in cats depends on whether the individual case represents a low-grade (e.g., indolent, small cell variants) versus an intermediate- or high-grade (e.g., large cell) lymphoma; the latter are best treated with CHOP- or COP-based protocols and carry a less favorable prognosis, whereas the former generally respond to less aggressive chlorambucil/corticosteroid protocols and enjoy durable responses. Less is known regarding the treatment of Hodgkin's-like lymphoma involving solitary or regional nodes of the head and neck.[65,66] Clinical outcome following surgical extirpation of the affected node (or nodes if a reasonable number) is often associated with long-term, disease-free intervals and survivals of approximately 1 year, suggesting it is a more indolent form of lymphoma. Eventual recurrence in distal nodes following surgical excision is common, and the author currently offers clients the option of adjuvant chlorambucil/corticosteroids following surgery—this theoretically may have benefit; however, insufficient data exist to document a survival advantage with this approach.

Nasal Lymphoma Cats with nasal lymphoma generally enjoy durable remissions following therapy and lengthy overall survival durations.[5,68,73,128,129] If disease is documented as confined to the nasal cavity following thorough staging (node cytology, thoracic and abdominal imaging, bone marrow aspiration), then RT is the treatment of choice. CRs in the order of 75% to 95% are reported, with reports of median survivals following RT of 1.5 to 3 years.[73,129] Cats that do not achieve a CR with RT have a median survival of approximately 4.5 months. Total radiation dosage does affect survival durations, and a total dose greater than 32 Gy is recommended.[73] The addition of chemotherapy has not been shown to enhance survival for cats with locally confined disease; combinations of RT and chemotherapy result in similar response rates and survival times.[73,128,129] Chemotherapy (COP- or CHOP-based protocols) used in the absence of RT is a reasonable alternative, with complete response rates of approximately 75% and median survivals of approximately 2 years reported for cats achieving CR.[68] The author's preference is to initiate systemic chemotherapy only for (1) cases that have confirmed disease beyond the nasal passage, (2) cases that relapsed following RT, or (3) cases in which RT is unavailable or declined.

Central Nervous System Lymphoma Very few cases involving treatment for CNS lymphoma exist, and although an occasional case experienced durable response to systemic chemotherapy, generally less than 50% will respond and median survivals of 1 to 2 months can be expected.[68,76,77]

Laryngeal/Tracheal Lymphoma The vast majority of cats with laryngeal or tracheal lymphoma respond to either RT (if localized) or systemic chemotherapy (90% CR to COP- or CHOP-based protocols) (Figure 32-16).[68] Whereas the authors experience is that most have durable responses and survival durations typically approach or exceed 1 year, the only case series (n = 8) reported a median survival of 5.5 months following achievement of a CR.

Cutaneous Lymphoma Very little has been published regarding the treatment of cutaneous lymphoma or mycosis fungoides in cats[80]; however, a report of a CR to lomustine exists.[130] Cats with a solitary disease could theoretically be treated with surgical excision

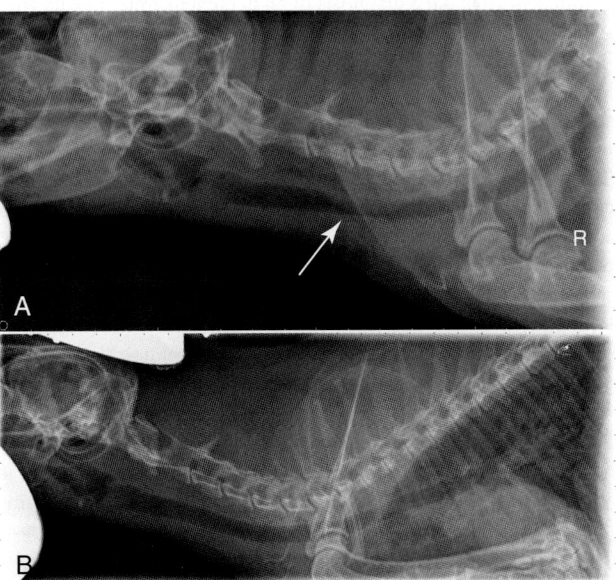

FIGURE 32-16 **A,** Lateral radiographic projection of a cat with tracheal lymphoma prior to treatment. **B,** The same cat 6 weeks following initiation of CHOP-based chemotherapy protocol.

or RT, although clinical staging is necessary to rule out possible further systemic involvement. For multiple sites, combination chemotherapy may be considered.

General Summary of Prognosis for Cats with Lymphoma

As previously discussed, the prediction of outcomes in cats with lymphoma is not generalizable due to the wide spectrum of histologic and anatomic subtypes encountered. Much has been mentioned in the previous treatment sections, and Tables 32-8 and Table 32-9 summarize prognostic parameters for lymphoma in cats.

Feline Leukemias, Myeloproliferative Disorders, and Myelodysplasia

For a complete discussion of leukemias and MPDs, including a general discussion of hematopoiesis, etiologies, lineage classification and descriptions, see Section C of this chapter. The classification of leukemias in cats is difficult because of the similarity of clinical and pathologic features and the transition, overlap, or mixture of cell types involved.[131-135] Most case-series reports are from the FeLV era and generally only single case reports exist from the more contemporary post-FeLV era, which further confuses our understanding of the biology and outcome. For this reason, only a simplistic discussion, primarily relating to the lymphoid leukemias will be presented here and the interested reader is again referred to Section C for a general discussion of nonlymphoid leukemia.

For cats with suspected leukemia, peripheral blood assessment (e.g., CBC with differential, flow cytometric analysis for size and immunophenotype, and PARR [for lymphoid leukemias]), and bone marrow aspiration or biopsy may contribute to a diagnosis. The preferred sites for bone marrow aspiration are the proximal humerus or iliac crest. Cats with acute leukemia are likely to have malignant cellular infiltrates in organs other than bone marrow.[134] A bone marrow aspirate with greater than 30% abnormal blast cells is sufficient to make a diagnosis of an acute leukemia. In cats with suspected CLL, infiltration of the bone marrow with more than 20% mature lymphocytes helps confirm the diagnosis. All cats with leukemia should be tested for FeLV/FIV. Determining the lineage of some leukemias can be challenging; most can be distinguished from one another by histologic appearance, histochemical stains, or immunohistochemical or flow cytometric analysis of the leukemic cells for cellular antigens that identify their lineage (see Chapter 8 and Section C in this chapter).[131,133,136] In addition, examination of blast cells by electron microscopy may reveal characteristic ultrastructural features. The French-American-British (FAB) classification system is considered useful in cats with myelodysplastic syndromes and almost all will be FeLV antigenemic.[136,137]

Lymphoid Leukemia

ALL was the most commonly encountered type of leukemia in cats in the FeLV era; however, it is much less common today. ALL is characterized by poorly differentiated lymphoblasts and prolymphocytes in blood and bone marrow. Approximately 60% to 80% of cats with ALL were FeLV positive, and most malignant cells have T-cell immunophenotypes[138]; however, little information is available in the contemporary literature.

CLL is rarely reported in cats and is characterized by well-differentiated, small, mature lymphocytes in peripheral blood and bone marrow. Whereas most are of the T-cell lineage, B-cell CLL has also been reported.[136,139,140] Most cats have increased WBC counts greater than 50,000/μl, and most are FeLV negative.

Treatment of Leukemias

The use of chemotherapy to treat ALL has been disappointing. Using COP-based protocols, Cotter[124] reported a 27% CR rate. CLL can be treated with chlorambucil (0.2 mg/kg PO or 2 mg/cat QOD) and prednisone (1 mg/kg PO daily); however, little information exists regarding outcome. As in humans and dogs, if significant clinical signs or profound cytopenias are not present, treatment can be withheld—one cat with CLL remained stable without chemotherapy for over a year.[140] The prognoses for acute nonlymphoblastic leukemias are generally very poor, although some exceptions exist in case report form in the historic literature.

REFERENCES

1. Couto CG: Oncology. In Sherding RG, editor: *The cat: diseases and clinical management*, New York, 1989, Churchill Livingstone.
2. Hardy WD Jr: Hematopoietic tumors of cats, *J Am Anim Hosp Assoc* 17:921–940, 1981.
3. Essex M, Francis DP: The risk to humans from malignant diseases of their pets: An unsettled issue, *J Am Anim Hosp Assoc* 12:386–390, 1976.
4. Theilen GH, Madewell BR: Feline hematopoietic neoplasms. In Theilen GH, Madewell BR, editors: *Veterinary cancer medicine*, ed 2, Philadelphia, 1987, Lea & Febiger.
5. Vail DM, Moore AS, Ogilvie GK, et al: Feline lymphoma (145 cases): Proliferation indices, CD3 immunoreactivity and their association with prognosis in 90 cats receiving therapy, *J Vet Intern Med* 12:349–354, 1998.
6. Cotter SM: Feline viral neoplasia. In Greene CE, editor: *Infectious diseases of the dog and cat*, ed 3, Philadelphia, 1998, WB Saunders.
7. Louwerens M, London CA, Pedersen NC, et al: Feline lymphoma in the post-feline leukemia virus era, *J Vet Intern Med* 19:329–335, 2005.
8. Rissetto K, Villamil JA, Selting KA, et al: Recent trends in feline intestinal neoplasia: an epidemiologic study of 1,129 cases in the veterinary medical database from 1964 to 2004, *J Am Anim Hosp Assoc* 47:28–36, 2011.
9. Schmidt JM, North SM, Freeman KP, et al: Feline paediatric oncology: retrospective assessment of 233 tumours from cats up to one year (1993 to 2008), *J Small Anim Pract* 51:306–311, 2010.
10. Gabor LJ, Malik R, Canfield PJ: Clinical and anatomical features of lymphosarcoma in 118 cats, *Aust Vet J* 76:725–732, 1998.
11. Gabor LJ, Canfield PJ, Malik R: Immunophenotypic and histological characterization of 109 cases of feline lymphosarcoma, *Aust Vet J* 77:436–441, 1999.
12. Stutzer B, Simon K, Lutz H, et al: Incidence of persistent viraemia and latent feline leukaemia virus infection in cats with lymphoma, *J Feline Med Surg* 13:81–87, 2011.
13. Weiss AT, Klopfleisch R, Gruber AD: Prevalence of feline leukaemia provirus DNA in feline lymphomas, *J Feline Med Surg* 12:929–935, 2010.
14. Ahmad S, Levy LS: The frequency of occurrence and nature of recombinant feline leukemia viruses in the induction of multicentric lymphoma by infection of the domestic cat with FeLV-945, *Virology* 403:103–111, 2010.
15. Fuhino Y, Satoh H, Ohno K, et al: Molecular cytogenetic analysis of feline leukemia virus insertions in cat lymphoid tumor cells, *J Virol Methods* 163:344–352, 2010.
16. Fujino Y, Liao CP, Zhao YS, et al: Identification of a novel common proviral integration site, flit-1, in feline leukemia virus induced thymic lymphoma, *Virology* 30:16–22, 2009.

17. Fujino Y, Ohno K, Tsujimoto H: Molecular pathogenesis of feline leukemia virus-induced malignancies: insertional mutagenesis, *Vet Immunol Immunopathol* 123:138–143, 2008.
18. Shelton GH, Grant CK, Cotter SM, et al: Feline immunodeficiency virus (FIV) and feline leukemia virus (FeLV) infections and their relationship to lymphoid malignancies in cats: a retrospective study (1968-1988), *J Acquir Immune Def Synd* 3:623–630, 1990.
19. Hutson CA, Rideout BA, Pederson NC: Neoplasia associated with feline immunodeficiency virus infection in cats of southern California, *J Am Vet Med Assoc.* 199:1357–1362, 1991.
20. Endo Y, Cho KW, Nishigaki K, et al: Molecular characteristics of malignant lymphomas in cats naturally infected feline immunodeficiency virus, *Vet Immun Immunopath* 57:153–167, 1997.
21. Terry A, Callanan JJ, Fulton R, et al: Molecular analysis of tumours from feline immunodeficiency virus (FIV)-infected cats: an indirect role for FIV, *Int J Cancer* 61:227–232, 1995.
22. Wang J, Kyaw-Tanner M, Lee C, et al: Characterisation of lymphosarcomas in Australian cats using polymerase chain reaction and immunohistochemical examination, *Aust Vet J* 79:41–46, 2001.
23. Beatty JA, Lawrence CE, Callanan JJ, et al: Feline immunodeficiency virus (FIV)-associated lymphoma: a potential role for immune dysfunction in tumourigenesis, *Vet Immunol Immunopathol* 23:309–322, 1998.
24. Gabor LJ, Love DN, Malik R, et al: Feline immunodeficiency virus status of Australian cats with lymphosarcoma, *Aust Vet J* 79:540–545, 2001.
25. Beatty J, Terry A, MacDonald J, et al: Feline immunodeficiency virus integration in B-cell lymphoma identifies a candidate tumor suppressor gene on human chromosome 15q15, *Cancer Res* 62:7175–7180, 2002.
26. Poli A, Abramo F, Baldinotti F, et al: Malignant lymphoma associated with experimentally induced feline immunodeficiency virus infection, *J Comp Pathol* 110:319–328, 1994.
27. Callanan JJ, McCandlish IA, O'Neil B, et al: Lymphosarcoma in experimentally induced feline immunodeficiency virus infection, *Vet Rec* 130:293–295, 1992.
28. Rosenberg MP, Hohenhaus AE, Matus RE: Monoclonal gammopathy and lymphoma in a cat infected with feline immunodeficiency virus, *J Am Anim Hosp Assoc* 27:335–337, 1991.
29. Buracco P, Guglielmino R, Abate O, et al: Large granular lymphoma in a FIV-positive and FeLV-negative cat, *J Small Anim Pract* 33:279–284, 1992.
30. Zwahlen CH, Lucroy MD, Kraegel SA, et al: Results of chemotherapy for cats with alimentary malignant lymphoma: 21 cases (1993-1997), *J Am Vet Med Assoc* 213:1144–1149, 1998.
31. Mahony OM, Moore AS, Cotter SM, et al: Alimentary lymphoma in cats: 28 cases (1988-1993), *J Am Vet Med Assoc* 207:1593–1598, 1995.
32. Rassnick KM, Mauldin GN, Moroff SD, et al: Prognostic value of argyrophilic nucleolar organizer region (AgNOR) staining in feline intestinal lymphoma, *J Vet Intern Med* 13:187–190, 1999.
33. Slawienski MJ, Mauldin GE, Mauldin GN, et al: Malignant colonic neoplasia in cats: 46 cases (1990-1996), *J Am Vet Med Assoc* 211:878–881, 1997.
34. Mayr B, Winkler G, Schaffner G, et al: N-ras mutations in a feline lymphoma: Low frequency of N-ras mutations in a series of feline, canine and bovine lymphomas, *Vet J* 163:326–328, 2002.
35. Cadile CD, Kitchell BE, Biller BJ, et al: Telomerase activity as a marker for malignancy in feline tissues, *Am J Vet Res* 62:1578–1581, 2001.
36. Yazawa M, Okuda M, Uyama R, et al: Molecular cloning of the feline telomerase reverse transcriptase (TERT) gene and its expression in cell lines and normal tissues, *J Vet Med Sci* 65:573–577, 2003.
37. Kano R, Sato E, Okamura T, et al: Expression of Bcl-2 in feline lymphoma cell lines, *Vet Clin Pathol* 37:57–60, 2008.
38. Madewell B, Griffey S, Walls J, et al: Reduced expression of cyclin-dependent kinase inhibitor p27^{Kip1} in feline lymphoma, *Vet Pathol* 38:698–702, 2001.
39. Dank G, Lucroy MD, Griffey SM, et al: Bcl-2 and MIB-1 labeling indexes in cats with lymphoma, *J Vet Intern Med* 16:720–725, 2002.
40. Bertone ER, Snyder LA, Moore AS: Environmental tobacco smoke and risk of malignant lymphoma in pet cats, *Am J Epidemiol* 156:268–273, 2002.
41. Marconato L, Leo C, Girelli R, et al: Association between waste management and cancer in companion animals, *J Vet Intern Med* 23:564–569, 2009.
42. Schmiedt CW, Grimes JA, Holzman G, et al: Incidence and risk factors for development of malignant neoplasia after feline renal transplantation and cyclosporine-based immunosuppression, *Vet Comp Oncol* 7:45–53, 2009.
43. Wooldridge JD, Gregory CR, Mathews KG, et al: The prevalence of malignant neoplasia in feline renal-transplant recipients, *Vet Surg* 31:94–97, 2002.
44. Carreas JK, Goldschmidt M, Lamb M, et al: Feline epitheliotropic intestinal malignant lymphoma: 10 cases(1997-2000), *J Vet Intern Med* 17:326–331, 2003.
45. Ragaini L, Aste G, Cavicchioli L, et al: Inflammatory bowel disease mimicking alimentary lymphosarcoma in a cat, *Vet Res Commun* 27(Suppl 1):791–793, 2003.
46. Tams TR: *Inflammatory bowel disease*, Philadelphia, 1991, WB Saunders, pp 409–414.
47. Hart JF, Shaker E, Patnaik AK, et al: Lymphocytic-plasmacytic enterocolitis in cats: 60 cases (1988-1990), *J Am Anim Hosp Assoc* 30:505–514, 1994.

47a. Bridgeford ED, Marini RP, Feng Y, et al: Gastric helicobacter species as a cause of feline gastric lymphoma: a viable hypothesis, *Vet Immunol Immunopathol* 1123:106–113, 2008.

48. Valli VE, Jacobs RM, Norris A, et al: The histologic classification of 602 cases of feline lymphoproliferative disease using the National Cancer Institute working formulation, *J Vet Diagn Invest* 12:295–306, 2000.
49. Valli VE, Jacobs RM, Parodi AL, et al: *Histological classification of hematopoietic tumors of domestic animals*, Washington, DC, 2002, Armed Forces Institute of Pathology and The World Health Organization.
50. Gieger T: Alimentary lymphoma in cats and dogs, *Vet Clin North Am Small Anim Pract* 41:419–432, 2011.
51. Moore PF, Rodriguez-Bertos A, Kass PH: Feline gastrointestinal lymphoma: Mucosal architecture, immunophenotype and molecular clonality, *Vet Pathol* 2011. [Epub ahead of print]
52. Lingard AE, Briscoe K, Beatty JA, et al: Low-grade alimentary lymphoma: clinicopathological findings and response to treatment in 17 cases, *J Feline Med Surg* 11:692–700, 2009.
53. Pohlman LM, Higginbotham ML, Welles EG, et al: Immunophenotypic and histologic classification of 50 cases of feline gastrointestinal lymphoma, *Vet Pathol* 46:259–268, 2009.
54. Kiupel M, Scedley RC, Pfent C, et al: Diagnostic algorithm to differentiate lymphoma from inflammation in feline small intestinal biopsy samples, *Vet Pathol* 48:212–222, 2011.
55. Vezzali E, Parodi AL, Marcato PS, et al: Histopathologic classification of 171 cases of canine and feline non-Hodgkin lymphoma according to the WHO, *Vet Comp Oncol* 8:38–49, 2010.
56. Swerdlow SH, Campo E, Harris NL, et al: *WHO classification of tumors of the haematopoietic and lymphoid tissues*, ed 4, Lyon, France, 2008, International Agency for Research on Cancer (IARC).
57. Briscoe KA, Krockenberger M, Beatty JA, et al: Histopathological and immunohistochemical evaluation of 53 cases of feline lymphoplasmacytic enteritis and low-grade alimentary lymphoma, *J Comp Pathol* 145:187–198, 2011.
58. Warren A, Center S, McDonough S, et al: Histopathologic features, immunophenotyping, clonality, and eubacterial fluorescence in situ hybridization in cats with lymphocytic cholangitis/cholangiohepatitis, *Vet Pathol* 48:627–641, 2011.

59. Krick EL, Little L, Patel R, et al: Description of clinical and pathological findings, treatment and outcome of feline large granular lymphocyte lymphoma (1996-2004), *Vet Comp Oncol* 6:102–111, 2008.
60. Roccabianca P, Vernau W, Caniatti M, et al: Feline large granular lymphocyte (LGL) lymphoma with secondary leukemia: primary intestinal origin with predominance of a CD3/CD8(alpha)(alpha) phenotype, *Vet Pathol* 43:15–28, 2006.
61. Ezura K, Nomura I, Takahashi T, et al: Natural killer-like T cell lymphoma in a cat, *Vet Rec* 28:268–270, 2004.
62. Day MJ: Review of thymic pathology in 30 cats and 36 dogs, *J Small Anim Prac* 38:393–403, 1997.
63. Davies C, Forrester SD: Pleural effusion in cats: 82 cases (1987 to 1995), *J Small Anim Prac* 37:217–224, 1996.
64. Teske E, Sraten GV, van Noort R, et al: Chemotherapy with cyclophosphamide, vincristine and prednisolone (COP) in cats with malignant lymphoma: New results with an old protocol, *J Vet Intern Med* 16:179–186, 2002.
65. Day MJ, Kyaw-Tanner M, Silkstone MA, et al: T-cell-rich B-cell lymphoma in the cat, *J Comp Pathol* 120:155–167, 1999.
66. Walton RM, Hendrick MJ: Feline Hodgkin's-like lymphoma: 20 cases (1992-1999), *Vet Pathol* 38:504–511, 2001.
67. Holt E, Goldschmidt MH, Skorupski K: Extranodal conjunctival Hodgkin's-like lymphoma in a cat, *Vet Ophthalmol* 9:141–144, 2006.
68. Taylor SS, Goodfellow MR, Browne WJ, et al: Feline extranodal lymphoma: response to chemotherapy and survival in 110 cats, *J Small Anim Pract* 50:584–592, 2009.
69. Little L, Patel R, Goldschmidt M: Nasal and nasopharyngeal lymphoma in cats: 50 cases (1989-2005), *Vet Pathol* 44:885–892, 2007.
70. Henderson SM, Bradley K, Day MJ, et al: Investigation of nasal disease in the cat- a retrospective study of 77 cases, *J Feline Med Surg* 6:245–257, 2004.
71. Mukaratirwa S, van der Linde-Sipman JS, Gruys E, et al: Feline nasal and paranasal sinus tumours: clinicopathological study, histomorphological description and diagnostic immunohistochemistry of 123 cases, *J Feline Med Surg* 3:235–245, 2001.
72. Demko JL, Cohn LA: Chronic nasal discharge in cats: 75 cases (1993-2004), *J Am Vet Med Assoc* 230:1032–1037, 2007.
73. Haney SM, Beaver L, Turrel J, et al: Survival analysis of 97 cats with nasal lymphoma: a multi-institutional retrospective study (1986-2006), *J Vet Intern Med* 23:287–294, 2009.
74. Mooney SC, Hayes AA, Matus RE, et al: Renal lymphoma in cats: 28 cases (1977-1984), *J Am Vet Med Assoc* 191:1473–1477, 1987.
75. Tomek A, Cizinauskas S, Doherr M, et al: Intracranial neoplasia in 61 cats: localization, tumour types and seizure patterns, *J Feline Med Surg* 8:243–253, 2006.
76. Troxel MT, Vite CH, Van Winkle TJ, et al: Feline intracranial neoplasia: retrospective review of 160 cases (1985-2001), *J Vet Intern Med* 17:850–859, 2003.
77. Marioni-Henry K, Van Winckle TJ, Smith SH, et al: Tumors affecting the spinal cord of cats: 85 cases (1980-2005), *J Am Vet Med Assoc* 232:237–243, 2008.
78. Marioni-Henry K, Vite CH, Newton AL, et al: Prevalence of diseases of the spinal cord of cats, *J Vet Intern Med* 18:851–858, 2004.
79. Taylor SS, Harvey AM, Bar FJ, et al: Laryngeal disease in cats: a retrospective study of 35 cases, *J Feline Med Surg* 11:954–962, 2009.
80. Fontaine J, Heimann M, Day MJ: Cutaneous epitheliotropic T-cell lymphoma in the cat: a review of the literature and five new cases, *Vet Dermatol* 22:454–461, 2011.
81. Caciolo PL, Nesbitt GH, Patnaik AK, et al: Cutaneous lymphosarcoma in the cat: a report of nine cases, *J Am Anim Hosp Assoc* 20:491–496, 1984.
82. May MJ: Immunophenotypic characterization of cutaneous lymphoid neoplasia in the dog and cat, *J Comp Pathol* 112:79–96, 1995.
83. Gilbert S, Affolter VK, Gross TL, et al: Clinical, morphological and immunohistochemical characterization of cutaneous lymphocytosis in 23 cats, *Vet Dermatol* 15:3–12, 2004
84. Wood C, Almes K, Bagladi-Swanson M, et al: Sézary syndrome in a cat, *J Am Anim Hosp Assoc* 44:144–148, 2008.
85. Schick RO, Murphy GF, Goldschmidt MH: Cutaneous lymphosarcoma and leukemia in a cat, *J Am Vet Med Assoc* 203:1155–1158, 1993.
86. Grahn BH, Peiffer RL, Cullen CL, et al: Classification of feline intraocular neoplasms based on morphology, histochemical staining and immunohistochemical labeling, *Vet Ophthalmol* 9:395–403, 2006.
87. Kiselow MA, Rassnick KM, McDonough SP, et al: Outcome of cats with low-grade lymphocytic lymphoma: 41 cases (1995-2005), *J Am Vet Med Assoc* 232:405–410, 2008.
88. Fondacaro JV, Richter KP, Carpenter JL, et al: Feline gastrointestinal lymphoma:67 cases (1988-1996), *Eur J Comp Gastroenterol* 4:1999.
89. Court EA, Watson ADJ, Peaston AE: Retrospective study of 60 cases of feline lymphosarcoma, *Aust Vet J* 75:424–427, 1997.
90. Forrester SD, Fossum TW, Rogers KS, et al: Diagnosis and treatment of chylothorax associated with lymphoblastic lymphosarcoma in four cats, *J Am Vet Med Assoc* 198:291–294, 1991.
91. Spodnick GJ, Berg J, Moore FM, et al: Spinal lymphoma in cats: 21 cases (1976-1989), *J Am Vet Med Assoc* 200:373–376, 1992.
92. Lane SB, Kornegay JN, Duncan JR, et al: Feline spinal lymphosarcoma: a retrospective evaluation of 23 cats, *J Vet Intern Med* 8:99–104, 1994.
93. Savary KCM, Price GS, Vaden SL: Hypercalcemia in cats: A retrospective study of 71 cases (1991-1997), *J Vet Intern Med* 14:184–189, 2000.
94. Gabor LJ, Canfield PJ, Malik R: Haematological and biochemical findings in cats in Australia with lymphosarcoma, *Aust Vet J* 78:456–461, 2000.
95. Gerou-Ferriani M, McBrearty AR, Burchmore RJ, et al: Agarose gel serum protein electophoresis in cats with and without lymphoma and preliminary results of tandem mass fingerprinting analysis, *Vet Clin Pathol* 40:159–173, 2011.
96. Avery A: Molecular diagnostics of hematologic malignancies, *Top Companion Anim Med* 24:144–150, 2009.
97. Werner JA, Woo JC, Vernau W, et al: Characterization of feline immunoglobulin heavy chain variable region genes for the molecular diagnosis of B-cell neoplasia, *Vet Pathol* 42:596–607, 2005.
98. Moore PF, Woo JC, Vernau W, et al: Characterization of feline T cell receptor gamma (TCRG) variable region genes for the molecular diagnosis of feline intestinal T cell lymphoma, *Vet Immunol Immunopathol* 106:167–178, 2005.
99. Weiss AT, Klopfleisch R, Gruber AD: T-cell receptor γ chain variable and joining region genes of subgroup 1 are clonally rearranged in feline B- and T-cell lymphoma, *J Comp Pathol* 144:123–134, 2011.
100. Henrich M, Hecht W, Weiss AT, et al: A new subgroup of immunoglobulin heavy chain variable region genes for the assessment of clonality in feline B-cell lymphomas, *Vet Immunol Immunopathol* 130:59–69, 2009.
101. Mooney SC, Hayes AA: Lymphoma in the cat: An approach to diagnosis and management, *Sem Vet Med Surg (Small Anim)* 1:51–57, 1986.
102. Zwingenberger AL, Marks SL, Baker TW, et al: Ultrasonographic evaluation of the muscularis propria in cats with diffuse small intestinal lymphoma or inflammatory bowel disease, *J Vet Intern Med* 24:289–292, 2010.
103. Evans SE, Bonczynski JJ, Broussard JD, et al: Comparison of endoscopic and full-thickness biopsy specimens for diagnosis of inflammatory bowel disease and alimentary tract lymphoma in cats, *J Am Vet Med Assoc* 229:1447–1450, 2006.
104. Kleinschmidt S, Harder J, Nolte I, et al: Chronic inflammatory and non-inflammatory diseases of the gastrointestinal tract in cats: diagnostic advantage of full-thickness intestinal and extraintestinal biopsies, *J Feline Med Surg* 12:97–103, 2010.

105. Fossum TW, Jacobs RM, Birchard SJ: Evaluation of cholesterol and triglyceride concentrations in differentiating chylous and nonchylous pleural effusions in dogs and cats, *J Am Vet Med Assoc* 188:49–51, 1986.
106. Tromblee TC, Jones JC, Etue AE, et al: Association between clinical characteristics, computed tomography characteristics, and histologic diagnosis for cats with sinonasal disease, *Vet Radiol Ultrasound* 47:241–248, 2006.
107. Detweiler DA, Johnson LR, Kass PH, et al: Computed tomographic evidence of bulla effusions in cats with sinonasal diseases: 2001-2004, *J Vet Intern Med* 20:1080–1084, 2006.
108. Valdes-Martinez A, Cianciolo R, Mai W: Association between renal hypoechoic subcapsular thickening and lymphosarcoma in cats, *Vet Radiol Ultrasound* 48:357–360, 2007.
109. Tzannes S, Hammond MF, Murphy S, et al: Owners' perception of their cats' quality of life during COP chemotherapy for lymphoma, *J Feline Med Surg* 10:73–81, 2008.
110. Malik R, Gabor LJ, Foster SF, et al: Therapy for Australian cats with lymphosarcoma, *Aust Vet J* 79:808–817, 2001.
111. Hadden AG, Cotter SM, Rand W, et al: Efficacy and toxicosis of VECAP-C treatment of lymphoma in cats, *J Vet Intern Med* 22:153–157, 2008.
112. Simon D, Eberle N, Laacke-Singer L, et al: Combination chemotherapy in feline lymphoma: Treatment, outcome, tolerability and duration in 23 cats, *J Vet Intern Med* 22:394–400, 2008.
113. Milner RJ, Peyton J, Cooke K, et al: Response rates and survival times for cats with lymphoma treated with the University of Wisconsin-Madison chemotherapy protocol: 38 cases (1996-2003), *J Am Vet Med Assoc* 227:1118–1122, 2005.
114. Moore AS, Cotter SM, Frimberger AE, et al: A comparison of doxorubicin and COP for maintenance of remission in cats with lymphoma, *J Vet Intern Med* 10:372–375, 1996.
115. Mooney SC, Hayes AA, MacEwen EG, et al: Treatment and prognostic factors in lymphoma in cats: 103 cases (1977-1981), *J Am Vet Med Assoc* 194:696–699, 1989.
116. Jeglum KA, Whereat A, Young K: Chemotherapy of lymphoma in 75 cats, *J Am Vet Med Assoc* 190:174–178, 1987.
117. Poirier VJ, Thamm DH, Kurzman ID, et al: Liposome-encapsulated doxorubicin (Doxil) and doxorubicin in the treatment of vaccine-associated sarcoma in cats, *J Vet Intern Med* 16:726–731, 2002.
118. Peaston AE, Maddison JE: Efficacy of doxorubicin as an induction agent for cats with lymphosarcoma, *Aust Vet J* 77:442–444, 1999.
119. Kristal O, Lana SE, Ogilvie GK, et al: Single agent chemotherapy with doxorubicin for feline lymphoma: a retrospective study of 19 cases (1994-1997), *J Vet Intern Med* 15:125–130, 2001.
120. Oberthaler KT, Mauldin E, McManus PM, et al: Rescue therapy with doxorubicin-based chemotherapy for relapsing or refractory feline lymphoma: a retrospective study of 23 cases, *J Feline Med Surg* 11:259–265, 2009.
121. Fan TM, Kitchell BE, Dhaliwal RS, et al: Hematological toxicity and therapeutic efficacy of lomustine in 20 tumor-bearing cats: critical assessment of a practical dosing regimen, *J Am Anim Hosp Assoc* 38:357–363, 2002.
122. Rassnick KM, Gieger TL, Williams LE, et al: Phase I evaluation of CCNU (lomustine) in tumor-bearing cats, *J Vet Intern Med* 15:196–199, 2001.
123. LeBlanc AK, Cox SK, Kirk CA, et al: Effects of L-asparaginase on plasma amino acid profiles and tumor burden in cats with lymphoma, *J Vet Intern Med* 21:760–763, 2007.
124. Cotter SM: Treatment of lymphoma and leukemia with cyclophosphamide, vincristine, and prednisone: II. Treatment of cats, *J Am Anim Hosp Assoc* 19:166–172, 1983.
125. Stein TJ, Pellin M, Steinberg H, et al: Treatment of feline gastrointestinal small-cell lymphoma with chlorambucil and glucocorticoids, *J Am Anim Hosp Assoc* 46:413–417, 2010.
126. Williams LE, Pruitt AF, Thrall DE: Chemotherapy followed by abdominal cavity irradiation for feline lymphoblastic lymphoma, *Vet Radiol Ultrasound* 51:681–687, 2010.
127. Parshley DL, LaRue SM, Kitchell B, et al: Abdominal irradiation as a rescue therapy for feline gastrointestinal lymphoma: a retrospective study of 11 cats (2001-2008), *J Feline Med Surg* 13:63–68, 2011.
128. Sfiligoi GA, Theon AP, Kent MS: Response of 19 cats with nasal lymphoma to radiation therapy and chemotherapy, *Vet Rad Ultrasound* 48:388–392, 2007.
129. Elmslie RE, Ogilvie GK, Gillette EL, et al: Radiotherapy with and without chemotherapy for localized lymphoma in 10 cats, *Vet Radiol* 32:277–280, 1991.
130. Komori S, Nakamura S, Takahashi K, et al: Use of lomustine to treat cutaneous nonepitheliotropic lymphoma in a cat, *J Am Vet Med Assoc* 226:237–239, 2005.
131. Grindem CB: Ultrastructural morphology of leukemia cells in the cat, *Vet Pathol* 22(2):147–155, 1988.
132. Gorman NT, Evans RJ: Myeloproliferative disease in the dog and cat: clinical presentations, diagnosis and treatment, *Vet Rec* 121:490–496, 1987.
133. Grindem CB, Perman V, Stevens JB: Morphological and clinical and pathological characteristics of spontaneous leukemia in 10 cats, *J Am Anim Hosp Assoc* 21:227, 1985.
134. Blue JT, French TW, Scarlett-Kranz J: Non-lymphoid hematopoietic neoplasia in cats: a retrospective study of 60 cases, *Cornell Vet* 78:21–42, 1988.
135. Facklam NR, Kociba GJ: Cytochemical characterization of feline leukemic cells, *Vet Pathol* 23:155–161, 1986.
136. Weiss DJ: Differentiating benign and malignant causes of lymphocytosis in feline bone marrow, *J Vet Intern Med* 19:855–859, 2005.
137. Hisasue M, Okayama H, Okayama T, et al: Hematologic abnormalities and outcome of 16 cats with myelodysplastic syndromes, *J Vet Intern Med* 15:471–477, 2001.
138. Essex ME: Feline leukemia: a naturally occurring cancer of infectious origin, *Epidemiol Rev* 4:189–203, 1982.
139. Workman HC, Vernau W: Chronic lymphocytic leukemia in dogs and cats: the veterinary perspective, *Vet Clin North Am Small Anim Pract* 33:1379–1399, 2003.
140. Tebb A, Cave T, Barron R, et al: Diagnosis and management of B cell chronic lymphocytic leukaemia in a cat, *Vet Rec* 154:430–433, 2004.

SECTION C

Canine Acute Myeloid Leukemia, Myeloproliferative Neoplasms, and Myelodysplasia

Karen M. Young and David M. Vail

Myeloproliferative disorders (MPDs) are a group of neoplastic diseases of bone marrow in which there are clonal disorders of hematopoietic stem cells.[1] Aberrant proliferation of cells with defective maturation and function leads to reduction of normal hematopoiesis and invasion of other tissues. These disorders have been classified based on biologic behavior, degree of cellular differentiation, and lineage of the neoplastic cells (granulocytic, monocytic, erythroid, megakaryocytic, or mixed). Newer classification systems in humans have incorporated genetics and molecular genetic analysis; these are currently areas of active investigation in the study of animal leukemias.[2] In 1991 the Animal Leukemia Study Group made recommendations for classifying nonlymphoid leukemias in dogs and cats.[3] More recently, the Oncology Committee of the American College of Veterinary Pathologists (ACVP) has been reexamining criteria for a classification system and spearheading large multiinstitutional studies to validate the criteria. Long-term objectives of these studies are to define molecular lesions, establish prognostic markers, and target effective therapeutic approaches.[4]

Incidence and Risk Factors

Myeloid neoplasms are uncommon or rare in the dog and occur 10 times less frequently than lymphoproliferative disorders.[5] Accurate information about incidence and other epidemiologic information await consistent use of a uniform classification system (see later discussion). There is no known age, breed, or sex predisposition, although in some retrospective studies, large-breed dogs have been overrepresented.[6-14] In dogs, the etiology of spontaneously occurring leukemia is unknown. It is likely that genetic and environmental factors (including exposure to radiation, drugs, or toxic chemicals) play a role. In humans, acquired chromosomal derangements lead to clonal overgrowth with arrested development.[15] At the end of the last century, chromosomal abnormalities were reported in dogs with AML, chronic myelogenous leukemia (CML), and lymphoid leukemia.[16,17] However, because karyotyping is difficult to perform in dogs because of the large number and morphologic similarity of their chromosomes and their resistance to banding, defining genetic factors in canine myeloid neoplasms has awaited application of molecular technologies and use of the canine genome map.[2,18-21] Certain forms of leukemia in dogs have been produced experimentally following irradiation.[22-24] In contrast to MPDs in cats, no causative viral agent has been demonstrated in dogs, although retrovirus-like budding particles were observed in the neoplastic cells of a dog with granulocytic leukemia.[25]

Pathology and Natural Behavior

A review of normal hematopoiesis will aid in understanding the various manifestations of MPDs. Hematopoiesis is the process of proliferation, differentiation, and maturation of stem cells into terminally differentiated blood cells. A simplified scheme is presented in Figure 32-17. Pluripotent stem cells differentiate into either lymphopoietic or hematopoietic multipotent stem cells.[26] Under the influence of specific regulatory and microenvironmental factors, multipotent stem cells in bone marrow differentiate into progenitor cells committed to a specific hematopoietic cell line, for example, erythroid, granulocytic-monocytic, or megakaryocytic. Maturation results in the production of terminally differentiated blood cells—erythrocytes, granulocytes, monocytes, and platelets—that are delivered to the circulation. In some cases, as in the maturation of reticulocytes to erythrocytes, final development may occur in the spleen.

Proliferation and differentiation of hematopoietic cells are controlled by a group of regulatory growth factors.[26,27] Of these,

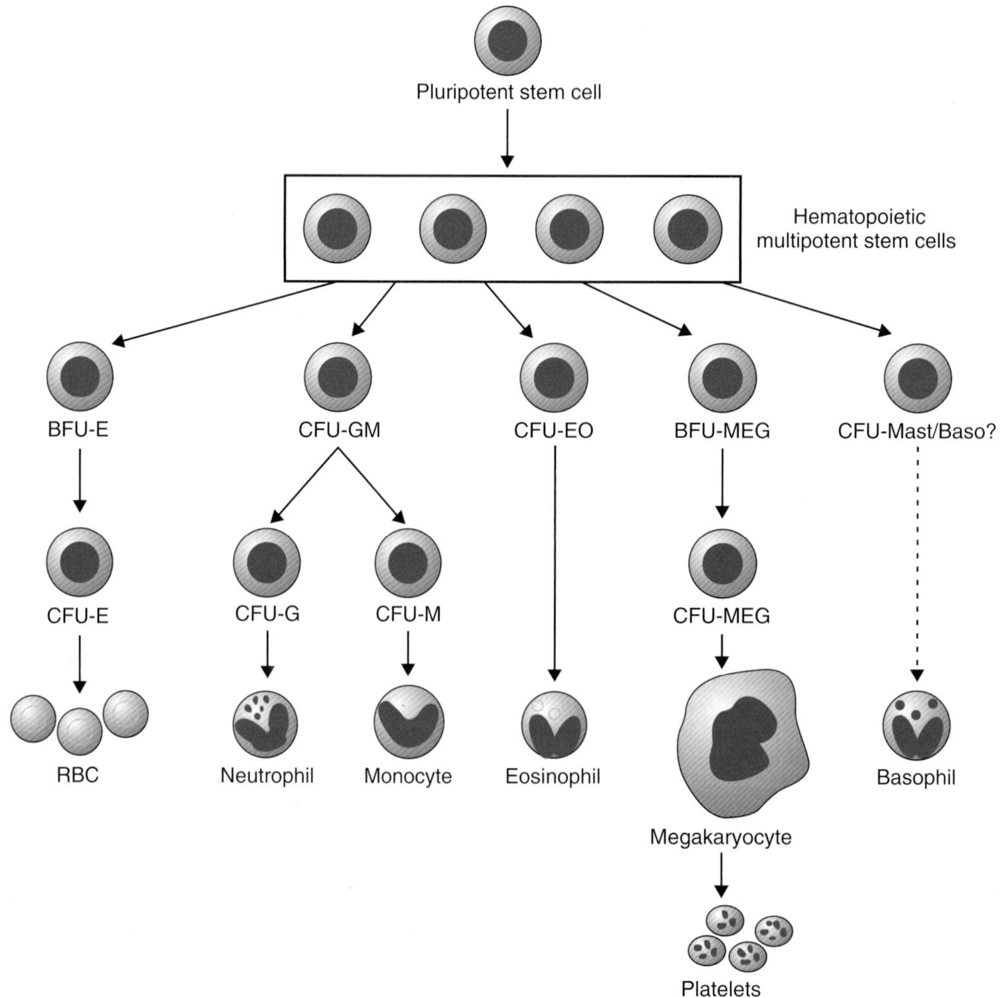

FIGURE 32-17 A simplified scheme of hematopoiesis. *BFU*, Blast-forming units; *CFU*, colony-forming units; *E*, erythroid; *GM*, granulocytic-monocytic; *EO*, eosinophil; *MEG*, megakaryocyte.

erythropoietin is the best characterized; it regulates erythroid proliferation and differentiation and is produced in the kidney, where changes in oxygen tension are detected. The myeloid compartment depends on a group of factors, collectively referred to as *colony-stimulating factors* (CSFs). These factors act at the level of the committed progenitor cells but also influence the functional capabilities of mature cells. Some of these factors have a broad spectrum of activity; others are more restricted in their target cells and actions. CSFs are produced in vitro by a multitude of cell types, including monocytes, macrophages, lymphocytes, and endothelial cells, and these cells likely play a role in the production and regulation of these factors in vivo. The gene for thrombopoietin also has been cloned, and it appears that this hormone alone can induce differentiation of megakaryocytes and platelet production.[28] Recombinant forms of many of these hormones are increasingly available.

Clonal disorders of bone marrow include myeloaplasia (usually referred to as *aplastic anemia*), myelodysplasia, and myeloproliferation. A preleukemic syndrome, characterized by peripheral pancytopenia and bone marrow hyperplasia with maturation arrest, is more correctly termed *myelodysplasia* because the syndrome does not always progress to overt leukemia. This syndrome has been described in cats, usually in association with FeLV infection but has only rarely been recognized in dogs.[29-32] These clonal disorders may be manifested by abnormalities in any or all lineages because hematopoietic cells share a common stem cell. In addition, transformation from one form to another may occur.[33]

Myeloid neoplasms are classified in several ways. The terms *acute* and *chronic* refer to the degree of cellular differentiation of the leukemic cells, but these terms also correlate with the biologic behavior of the neoplasm.[34] Disorders resulting from uncontrolled proliferation or decreased apoptosis of cells incapable of maturation lead to the accumulation of poorly differentiated or "blast" cells. These disorders are included under the umbrella term, *acute myeloid leukemia* (AML). Disorders resulting from unregulated proliferation of cells that exhibit progressive, albeit incomplete and defective, maturation lead to the accumulation of differentiated cells. These disorders are termed *myeloproliferative neoplasms* (MPN) and include polycythemia vera, CML and its variants, essential thrombocythemia, and possibly primary myelofibrosis. Myeloid neoplasms are further classified by the lineage of the dominant cell type(s), defined by Romanowsky stains, special cytochemical stains, ultrastructural features, flow cytometric analysis, and immunologic cell markers, and they have been classified into subtypes (see later discussion).

AML has a more sudden onset and is more aggressive. In both acute and chronic disorders, however, abnormalities in proliferation, maturation, and functional characteristics can occur in any hematopoietic cell line.[1] In addition, normal hematopoiesis is adversely affected. Animals with leukemia usually have decreased numbers of circulating normal cells. The pathogenesis of the cytopenias is complex and may result in part from production of inhibitory factors. Eventually, neoplastic cells displace normal hematopoietic cells, and this is termed *myelophthisis.* Anemia and thrombocytopenia are particularly common. Neutropenia and thrombocytopenia result in infection and hemorrhage, which may be more deleterious to the animal than the primary disease process.

Acute Myeloid Leukemia

AML is rare and is characterized by aberrant proliferation and/or decreased apoptosis of a clone of cells without maturation. This results in accumulation of immature blast cells in bone marrow and peripheral blood (Figure 32-18, *A* to *E*). The WBC count is variable and ranges from leukopenia to counts up to 150,000/μL. Spleen, liver, and lymph nodes are frequently involved, and other tissues, including tonsils, kidney, heart, and the CNS, may be infiltrated as well. There is no characteristic age, and even very young dogs may be affected.[35] The clinical course of these disorders tends to be rapid. Production of normal peripheral blood cells is usually diminished or absent, and anemia, neutropenia, and thrombocytopenia are common with infection and hemorrhage occurring as frequent sequelae. Occasionally, neoplastic blasts are present in bone marrow but not in peripheral blood. This is termed *aleukemic* leukemia, whereas *subleukemic* suggests a normal or decreased WBC count with some neoplastic cells in circulation.

In 1985 the Animal Leukemia Study Group was formed under the auspices of the American Society for Veterinary Clinical Pathology to develop specific morphologic and cytochemical criteria for classifying acute nonlymphocytic leukemias. Recognition of specific subtypes of leukemia is required to compile accurate and useful information about prognosis and response to treatment, as well as to compare studies from different sites. In 1991, this group proposed a classification system following adaptation of the French-American-British (FAB) system and criteria established by the NCI Workshop.[3] Group members examined blood and bone marrow from 49 dogs and cats with myeloid neoplasms. Romanowsky-stained specimens were examined first to identify blast cells and their percentages. Lineage specificity was then determined using cytochemical markers. The percentage of blasts and the information about lineage specificity were used in combination to classify disorders as acute undifferentiated leukemia (AUL), acute myeloid leukemia (AML, subtypes M1 to M5 and M7), and erythroleukemia with or without erythroid predominance (M6 and M6Er). A description of these subtypes is presented in Table 32-12.

Canine karyotyping is difficult, but with advancements in molecular cytogenetic analysis, chromosome painting, and genomic hybridization, AML in dogs can now be analyzed at the base-pair level,[18,19] and missense mutations in *FLT3*, *C-KIT*, and *RAS* sequences have been identified in dogs with AML, similar to what has been found for human AML.[36] In addition to serving as diagnostic and prognostic markers, cytogenetic lesions may be therapeutic targets. As cytogenetic abnormalities continue to be identified, this information will need to be incorporated into classification schemes.

With the exception of acute promyelocytic leukemia or M3, all of these subtypes have been described in dogs. However, because this modified FAB system has been adopted only recently, the names given to these disorders in the literature vary considerably. In addition, in the absence of cytochemical staining, immunophenotyping, or electron microscopic evaluation, the specific subtype of leukemia has often been uncertain, making retrospective analysis of epidemiologic information, prognosis, and response to therapy confusing at best. Although defining specific subtypes may seem to be an academic exercise owing to the uniformly poor prognosis of acute leukemias, this information is critical to improving the management of these diseases. Because of the low incidence of AML, national and international cooperative efforts will be required to accumulate information on the pathogenesis and response to different treatment modalities of specific subtypes. Utilization of a uniform classification system is an essential first step.

Different forms of AML are demonstrated in Figure 32-18, *A* to *E*. The most frequently reported forms of AML in the dog are acute myeloblastic leukemia (M1 and M2) and acute myelomonocytic

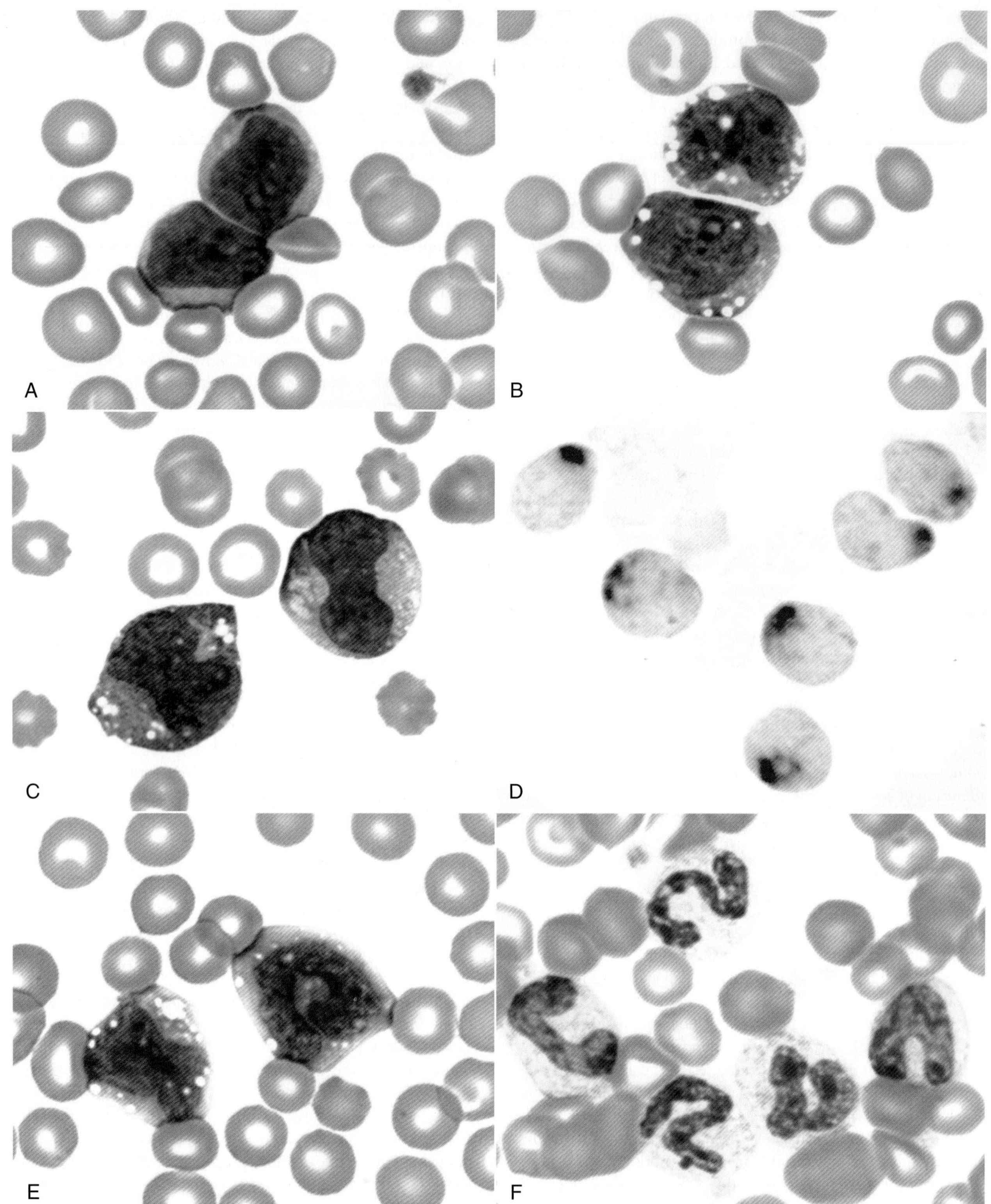

FIGURE 32-18 Peripheral blood from dogs with myeloid neoplasms. All diagnoses were confirmed by cytochemical staining. Note how similar the blast cells appear in **A** to **C**. **A,** Acute myeloblastic leukemia (M1). (Wright's stain, ×100 objective.) **B,** Acute myelomonocytic leukemia (M4). (Wright's stain, ×100 objective.) **C,** Acute monocytic leukemia (M5a); Wright's stain. **D,** Acute monocytic leukemia (M5a). (Cytochemical stain: a-naphthyl butyrate esterase [nonspecific esterase] with red reaction product.) **E,** Acute monocytic leukemia with some differentiation (M5b). (Wright's stain, ×100 objective.) **F,** Chronic myelogenous leukemia (CML). (Wright's stain, ×100 objective.)

TABLE 32-12 Subtypes of Leukemias and Dysplasias Adapting the FAB System

SUBTYPE	DESCRIPTION
Acute Leukemias	
AUL	Acute undifferentiated leukemia (formerly called *reticuloendotheliosis*)
M1	Myeloblastic leukemia, without differentiation
M2	Myeloblastic leukemia, with some neutrophilic differentiation
M3	Promyelocytic leukemia (not recognized in animals)
M4	Myelomonocytic leukemia
M5a	Monocytic leukemia, without differentiation
M5b	Monocytic leukemia, with some monocytic differentiation
M6	Erythroleukemia
M6Er	Variant of M6, with erythroblasts constituting the erythroid component
M7	Megakaryoblastic leukemia
Chronic Myeloid Leukemias	
CML	Chronic myelogenous leukemia
CMML	Chronic myelomonocytic leukemia
CMoL	Chronic monocytic leukemia
Hematopoietic Dysplasia	
MDS	Myelodysplastic syndrome
MDS-Er	Myelodysplastic syndrome with erythroid predominance

leukemia (M4).* Megakaryoblastic leukemia (M7) also is well recognized in dogs[10,47-58] and may be associated with platelet dysfunction.[51] Monocytic leukemias have likely included those with and without monocytic differentiation (M5a and M5b),[11,59] but in some cases the diagnosis may have been chronic myelomonocytic or chronic monocytic leukemia (see later discussion). There are few reports in dogs of spontaneously occurring erythroleukemia (M6) in which the leukemic cells include myeloblasts, monoblasts, and erythroid elements.[60-62] AULs have uncertain lineages because they are negative for all cytochemical markers. These leukemias should be distinguished from lymphoid leukemias by flow cytometric analysis of the leukemic cells for cellular antigens that identify their lineage.[63] In addition, examination of blast cells by electron microscopy may reveal characteristic ultrastructural features.

Myeloproliferative Neoplasms

MPNs, previously termed *chronic myeloproliferative disorders,* are characterized by excessive production of differentiated bone marrow cells, resulting in the accumulation of erythrocytes (polycythemia vera), granulocytes and/or monocytes (CML and its variants), or platelets (essential thrombocythemia). Primary myelofibrosis as a clonal disorder of marrow stromal cells, characterized by proliferation of megakaryocytes and granulocytic precursors with accumulation of collagen in bone marrow, has been recognized only rarely in animals. Myelofibrosis is considered a response to injury and may occur secondary to other neoplasms, systemic inflammation, drug exposure, or FeLV infection in cats.

Polycythemia Vera

Polycythemia vera (PV) is a clonal disorder of stem cells, although whether the defect is in the pluripotent stem cell or the hematopoietic multipotent stem cell is still not clear. In humans, progenitor cells have an increased sensitivity to insulin-like growth factor 1, which stimulates hematopoiesis.[64] It is not known whether this hypersensitivity is the primary defect or is secondary to another gene mutation. In any case, the result is overproduction of red blood cells (RBCs). The disease is rare and must be distinguished from more common causes of polycythemia, including relative and secondary absolute polycythemia (see later discussion). In PV, there is neoplastic proliferation of the erythroid series with terminal differentiation to RBCs. The disease has been reported in dogs that tend to be middle-aged with no breed or sex predilection[65-73] and is characterized by an increased RBC mass evidenced by an increased packed cell volume (PCV), RBC count, and hemoglobin concentration. The PCV is typically in the range of 65% to 85%. The bone marrow is hyperplastic, although the myeloid : erythroid (M : E) ratio tends to be normal. In contrast to the disease in humans, other cell lines do not appear to be involved, and transformation to other MPNs has not been reported. The disease in dogs may be more appropriately termed *primary erythrocytosis.* In humans, acquired *JAK2* gene mutations are identified in 90% of patients with primary polycythemia, and recently an identical mutation in the *JAK2* gene of one of five dogs with primary polycythemia was reported.[74]

Chronic Myelogenous Leukemia

In dogs, CML is more similar to chronic neutrophilic leukemia, a rare form of MPN in humans, than to CML in humans because it is a neoplastic proliferation of the neutrophil series, although concurrent eosinophilic and basophilic differentiation can occur. CML can occur in dogs of any age.[35,75-79] Neutrophils and neutrophilic precursors accumulate in bone marrow and peripheral blood as well as in other organs. The peripheral WBC count is usually, but not always, greater than 100,000/μL. Both immature and mature neutrophils are present, as demonstrated in Figure 32-18, *F.* Mature forms are usually more numerous, but sometimes an "uneven" left shift is present. Signs of dysplasia may be evident, including hypersegmentation, ringed nuclei, and giant forms. Eosinophils and basophils may also be increased. The bone marrow is characterized by granulocytic hyperplasia, and morphologic abnormalities may not be present. Erythroid and megakaryocytic lines may be affected, resulting in anemia, thrombocytopenia, or less commonly, thrombocytosis. This disorder must be distinguished from severe neutrophilic leukocytosis and "leukemoid reactions" caused by inflammation or immune-mediated diseases. Leukemoid reactions can also occur as a paraneoplastic syndrome. In humans with CML, characteristic cytogenetic abnormalities are present in all bone marrow cells, signifying a lesion at the level of an early multipotent stem cell. Typically, these individuals have a chromosomal translocation, resulting in the Philadelphia chromosome or BCR-ABL translocation between chromosomes 9 and 22.[80] The analogous chromosomes in dogs are chromosomes 9 and 26, and BCR-ABL mutations have now been reported in three cases of CML in dogs.[2] Variants of CML are chronic myelomonocytic leukemia (CMML) and chronic monocytic leukemia (CMoL).[81-83] These diagnoses are made based on the percentage of monocytes in the leukemic cell

*References 5-9, 23-34, 37-46.

population. BCR-ABL translocation has also been reported in a dog with CMoL.[45]

In addition to accumulating in bone marrow and peripheral blood, leukemic cells also are found in the red pulp of the spleen, the periportal and sinusoidal areas of the liver, and sometimes lymph nodes. Other organs such as the kidney, heart, and lung are less commonly affected. In addition, extramedullary hematopoiesis may be present in the liver and spleen. Death is usually due to complications of infection or hemorrhage secondary to neutrophil dysfunction and thrombocytopenia. In some cases, CML may terminate in "blast crisis," in which there is a transformation from a predominance of well-differentiated granulocytes to excessive numbers of poorly differentiated blast cells in peripheral blood and bone marrow. This phenomenon is well documented in the dog.[75,76,78]

Basophilic and Eosinophilic Leukemia

Basophilic leukemia, although rare, has been reported in dogs and is characterized by an increased WBC count with a high proportion of basophils in peripheral blood and bone marrow.[84-86] Hepatosplenomegaly, lymphadenopathy, and thrombocytosis may be present. All the dogs have been anemic. Basophilic leukemia should be distinguished from mast cell leukemia (mastocytosis). Whether dogs develop eosinophilic leukemia remains in question. Reported cases have had high blood eosinophil counts and eosinophilic infiltrates in organs.[87,88] One dog responded well to treatment with corticosteroids. The distinction between neoplastic proliferation of eosinophils and idiopathic hypereosinophilic syndrome remains elusive. Disorders associated with eosinophilia such as parasitism, skin diseases, or diseases of the respiratory and GI tracts should be considered first in an animal with eosinophilia. One distinguishing feature should be clonality, with reactive eosinophilia comprising polyclonal cells and the neoplastic condition arising from a single clone. As clonality assays become more available, this discrepancy may be resolved.

Essential Thrombocythemia

In humans, essential thrombocythemia, or primary thrombocytosis, is characterized by platelet counts that are persistently greater than 600,000/μL. There are no blast cells in circulation, and marked megakaryocytic hyperplasia of the bone marrow without myelofibrosis is present. Thrombosis and bleeding are the most common sequelae, and most patients have splenomegaly. Other MPDs, especially PV, should be ruled out, and importantly, there should be no primary disorders associated with reactive thrombocytosis.[89] These include inflammation, hemolytic anemia, iron deficiency anemia, malignancies, recovery from severe hemorrhage, rebound from immune-mediated thrombocytopenia, and splenectomy. In addition, certain drugs such as vincristine can induce thrombocytosis. Essential thrombocythemia has been recognized in dogs.[33,90-93] In one dog, the platelet count exceeded 4 million/μL and bizarre giant forms with abnormal granulation were present. The bone marrow contained increased numbers of megakaryocytes and megakaryoblasts, but circulating blast cells were not seen. Other findings included splenomegaly, GI bleeding, and increased numbers of circulating basophils. Causes of secondary or reactive thrombocytosis were ruled out.[90] Basophilia was also reported in a more recent case.[92] In another dog, primary thrombocytosis was diagnosed and then progressed to CML.[33] In some cases reported in the literature as essential thrombocythemia, the dogs had microcytic hypochromic anemias. Because iron deficiency anemia is associated with reactive or secondary thrombocytosis, care must be taken to rule out this disorder. However, spurious microcytosis may be reported if a dog has many giant platelets that are counted by an analyzer as small RBCs.[93] Microscopic review of the blood film may be helpful in these cases.

Other Bone Marrow Disorders

Myelofibrosis

Primary myelofibrosis has been reported only rarely in dogs and is usually a secondary, or reactive, process.[94,95] In humans, myelofibrosis is characterized by collagen deposition in bone marrow and increased numbers of megakaryocytes and granulocytic precursors, many of which exhibit morphologic abnormalities. In fact, breakdown of intramedullary megakaryocytes and subsequent release of factors that promote fibroblast proliferation or inhibit collagen breakdown may be the underlying pathogenesis of the fibrosis.[96] Focal osteosclerosis is sometimes present. Anemia, thrombocytopenia, splenomegaly, and myeloid metaplasia (production of hematopoietic cells outside the bone marrow) are consistent features.

In dogs, myelofibrosis occurs secondary to MPDs, radiation damage, and congenital hemolytic anemias.[97-100] In some cases, the inciting cause is unknown (idiopathic myelofibrosis). There may be concurrent marrow necrosis in cases of ehrlichiosis, septicemia, or drug toxicity (estrogens, cephalosporins), and there is speculation that fibroblasts proliferate in response to release of inflammatory mediators associated with the necrosis.[94] Myeloid metaplasia has been reported to occur in the liver, spleen, and lung.[100] Extramedullary hematopoiesis is ineffective in preventing or correcting the pancytopenia that eventually develops.

Myelodysplastic Syndrome

Dysfunction of the hematopoietic system can be manifested by a variety of abnormalities that constitute myelodysplastic syndrome (MDS). In dogs, in which the syndrome is rare, there usually are cytopenias in two or three lines in the peripheral blood (anemia, neutropenia, and/or thrombocytopenia). Other blood abnormalities can include macrocytic erythrocytes and metarubricytosis. The bone marrow is typically normocellular or hypercellular, and dysplastic changes are evident in several cell lines. If blast cells are present, they make up less than 30% of all nucleated cells,[2] although this threshold is being changed to less than 20%.[4,20] Myelodysplasia is sometimes referred to as *preleukemia* because, in some cases, it may progress to acute leukemia.[29-31] Based on reported cases, poor prognostic indices include increased percentage of blast cells, cytopenias involving more than one lineage, and cellular atypia. Primary MDSs are clonal disorders and are considered neoplastic. Complex classification schemes for human MDS, based on percentages of blasts in bone marrow, cytogenetic analysis, cytopenias, need for transfusions, and other variables, comprise at least nine subtypes; their applicability to veterinary medicine is unknown.[5] Three subtypes are proposed for dogs and cats and include MDS with excessive blasts (MDS-EB), in which blast percentages are greater than 5% and less than 20%, and progression to AML may occur; MDS with refractory cytopenia (MDS-RC) with blast percentages less than 5% and cytopenias in one or more lineages; and MDS with erythroid predominance (MDS-ER) in which the M:E ratio is less than 1 and prognosis is poor.[4] Larger studies are needed to determine the utility of this classification scheme and other potential prognostic indices, such as sex, age, and FeLV positivity. In addition to accumulating enough cases, another confounding factor to studying and classifying MDS is the presence of reversible MDSs that occur secondary to immune-mediated, infectious, and other diseases in both dogs and cats.

History and Clinical Signs

Dogs with myeloid neoplasms have similar presentations regardless of the specific disease entity, although animals with AML have a more acute onset of illness and a more rapid clinical course. A history of lethargy, inappetence, and weight loss is common. Clinical signs include emaciation, persistent fever, pallor, petechiation, hepatosplenomegaly, and, less commonly, lymphadenopathy and enlarged tonsils. Shifting leg lameness, ocular lesions, and recurrent infections are also seen. Vomiting, diarrhea, dyspnea, and neurologic signs are variable features. Serum biochemical analytes may be within the reference intervals but can change if significant organ infiltration occurs. Animals with MDS may be lethargic and anorectic and have pallor, fever, and hepatosplenomegaly. In PV, dogs often have erythema of mucous membranes owing to the increase in RBC mass. Some dogs are polydipsic. In addition, neurologic signs such as disorientation, ataxia, or seizures may be present and are thought to be the result of hyperviscosity or hypervolemia.[69] Hepatosplenomegaly is usually absent.

Peripheral blood abnormalities are consistently found. In addition to the presence of neoplastic cells, other abnormalities, including cytopenias of any lineage, may be present. Low numbers of nucleated RBCs are present in the blood of about half the dogs with acute nonlymphocytic leukemia.[3] Nonregenerative anemia and thrombocytopenia are present in most cases. Anemia is usually normocytic and normochromic, although macrocytic anemia is sometimes present. Pathogenic mechanisms include effects of inhibitory factors leading to ineffective hematopoiesis, myelophthisis, immune-mediated anemia secondary to neoplasia, and hemorrhage secondary to thrombocytopenia, platelet dysfunction, or DIC. Anemia is most severe in AML, although both anemia and thrombocytopenia may be milder in animals with the M5 subtype (acute monocytic leukemia). In myelofibrosis, the anemia is characterized by anisocytosis and poikilocytosis. In addition, pancytopenia and leukoerythroblastosis, in which immature erythroid and myeloid cells are in circulation, may be present. These phenomena probably result from replacement of marrow by fibrous tissue with resultant shearing of red cells and escape of immature cells normally confined to bone marrow. In PV, the PCV is increased, usually in the range of 65% to 85%. The bone marrow is hyperplastic, and the M:E ratio is usually in the normal range.

Neoplastic cells are often defective functionally. Platelet dysfunction has been reported in a dog with acute megakaryoblastic leukemia (M7),[51] and in CML, neutrophils have decreased phagocytic capacity and other abnormalities. One exception to this was a report of CML in a dog in which the neutrophils had enhanced phagocytic capacity and superoxide production.[101] The authors hypothesized that increased synthesis of GM-CSF resulted from a lactoferrin deficiency in the neoplastic neutrophils and mediated the enhanced function of these cells.

Diagnostic Techniques and Work-Up

In all cases of myeloid neoplasms, diagnosis depends on examination of peripheral blood and bone marrow. AML is diagnosed on the basis of finding blast cells with clearly visible nucleoli in blood and bone marrow. Most dogs with acute leukemia have circulating blasts. These cells may be present in low numbers in peripheral blood, and a careful search of the smear, especially at the feathered edge, should be made. Even if blasts are not detected in circulation, indications of bone marrow disease such as nonregenerative anemia or thrombocytopenia are usually present. Occasionally, neoplastic cells can be found in cerebrospinal fluid in animals with invasion of the CNS. Smears of aspirates from tissues such as the lymph nodes, spleen, or liver may contain blasts but usually contribute little to the diagnostic work-up.

Examination of blasts stained with standard Romanowsky stains may give clues as to the lineage of the cells (Figure 32-18, *A* to *C* and *E*). In myelomonocytic leukemia, the nuclei of the blasts are usually pleomorphic, with round to lobulated forms. In some cells, the cytoplasm may contain large azurophilic granules or vacuoles. Blasts in megakaryocytic leukemia may contain vacuoles and have cytoplasmic blebs. In addition, bizarre macroplatelets may be present. Although these distinguishing morphologic features may suggest a definitive diagnosis, cytochemical staining or immunophenotyping are usually required to define the lineage of the blasts. Several investigators have reported modification of diagnoses following cytochemical staining.[102,103] It is especially important to distinguish AML from lymphocytic leukemia in order to provide accurate prognostic information to the owner and institute appropriate therapy.

The Animal Leukemia Group has recommended the following diagnostic criteria, summarized in Figure 32-19.[3] Using well-prepared Romanowsky-stained blood and bone marrow films, a minimum of 200 cells are counted to determine the leukocyte differential in blood and the percentage of blast cells in bone marrow and/or blood. In bone marrow, blast cells are calculated both as a percentage of all nucleated cells (ANC) and nonerythroid cells (NEC) and are further characterized using cytochemical markers.[102-104] Neutrophil differentiation is identified by positive staining of blasts for peroxidase, Sudan Black B, and chloracetate esterase. Nonspecific esterases (alpha-naphthyl acetate esterase or alpha-naphthyl butyrate esterase), especially if they are inhibited by sodium fluoride, mark monocytes. Canine monocytes may also contain a few peroxidase-positive granules. Acetylcholinesterase is a marker for megakaryocytes in dogs and cats. In addition, positive immunostaining for von Willebrand's factor (factor VIII-related antigen) and platelet glycoproteins on the surface of blasts identifies them as megakaryocyte precursors.[10,49-53] Alkaline phosphatase (AP) only rarely marks normal cells in dogs and cats but is present in blasts cells in acute myeloblastic and myelomonocytic leukemias. However, owing to reports of AP activity in lymphoid leukemias in dogs, its specificity as a marker for myeloid cells is not certain. Omega exonuclease is a specific marker for basophils, which are also positive for chloracetate esterase activity.[86]

Blood and bone marrow differential counts and cytochemical staining should be performed and interpreted by experienced veterinary cytopathologists. If erythroid cells are less than 50% of ANC and the blast cells are greater than 30%, a diagnosis of AML or AUL is made. If erythroid cells are greater than 50% of ANC and the blast cells are greater than 30%, a diagnosis of erythroleukemia (M6) is made. If rubriblasts are a significant proportion of the blast cells, a diagnosis of M6Er, or erythroleukemia with erythroid predominance, can be made. It should be noted that in the human AML classification system, the blast threshold has been lowered to 20% and similar recommendations are being made for AML in dogs and cats.

In some cases, electron microscopy is required to identify the lineage of the blast cells. For example, megakaryocyte precursors are positive for platelet peroxidase activity and contain demarcation membranes and alpha granules.[49,53] Both of these features are detected at the ultrastructural level. Immunophenotyping, used to identify cell lineages in human patients, awaits development of

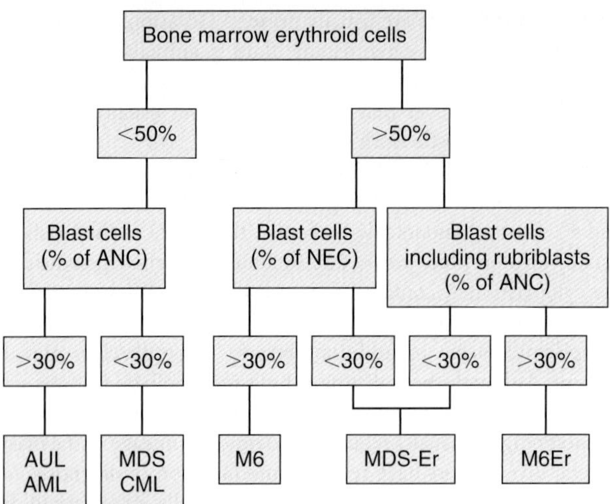

FIGURE 32-19 A scheme to classify myeloid neoplasms and myelodysplastic syndromes in dogs and cats. (*Blast cells,* Myeloblasts, monoblasts, and megakaryoblasts; *ANC,* all nucleated cells in bone marrow, including lymphocytes, plasma cells, macrophages, and mast cells; *NEC,* nonerythroid cells in bone marrow; *AUL,* acute undifferentiated leukemia; *AML,* acute myeloid leukemias M1 to M5 and M7; *CML,* chronic myeloid leukemias, including chronic myelogenous, chronic myelomonocytic, and chronic monocytic leukemias; *MDS,* myelodysplastic syndrome; *MDS-Er,* myelodysplastic syndrome with erythroid predominance; *M6,* erythroleukemia; *M6Er,* erythroleukemia with erythroid predominance.) *(From Jain NC, Blue JT, Grindem CB, et al: Proposed criteria for classification of acute myeloid leukemia in dogs and cats,* Vet Clin Pathol *20(3):63–82, 1991.)*

appropriate markers for animal species (see later). Increasingly, cytogenetic abnormalities are being identified in animal leukemias; cytogenetic analysis may yield important diagnostic and prognostic information and become a valuable tool for identifying targeted therapeutic approaches.

Although morphologic and cytochemical analyses have formed the mainstay of cell identification, newer technologies now are routinely used to classify leukemias by using monoclonal antibodies to detect antigens associated with certain cell types. Cells can be immunophenotyped using flow cytometric analysis or immunocytochemistry.[20,63,105-108] Cells from both acute lymphoid leukemia and AML are positive for CD34. Many lymphocyte markers, including CD3, CD4, CD8, CD18, CD21, CD45, CD79, and IgG, are available for dogs and can be used to rule out lymphoblastic leukemia in dogs with acute leukemias.[63,105] Other markers include myeloperoxidase (MPO) and CD11b for myeloid cells and CD41 for megakaryoblasts. There is some overlap in expression of these cellular antigens. For example, canine (but not human) granulocytes express CD4. It is best to use a panel of antibodies (similar to using a battery of cytochemical stains) because antigens are often expressed on multiple lineages, and lineage infidelity can occur. These tests have become more valuable with the availability of canine reagents. Currently, the ACVP Oncology Committee recommends that the following immunophenotyping panel be done on bone marrow and/or blood smears to characterize animal leukemias: for B lymphocytes, CD79a; for T lymphocytes, CD3; for myeloid cells, MPO and CD11b; for megakaryoblasts, CD41; for dendritic cells, CD1c; and for acute leukemias, CD34.[20]

Because of the degree of differentiation of cells in MPN, these disorders must be distinguished from nonneoplastic causes of increases in these cell types. In order to make a diagnosis of PV, it must first be established that the polycythemia is absolute rather than relative. In relative polycythemias, plasma volume is decreased from hemoconcentration, dehydration, or hypovolemia, and the absolute RBC mass is not increased. Splenic contraction can also result in relative polycythemia. Absolute polycythemia, in which RBC mass is increased, is usually secondary to tissue hypoxia, causing appropriate increased production of erythropoietin. Rarely, erythropoietin may be produced inappropriately by a tumor (e.g., renal cell carcinoma) or in renal disease (pyelonephritis) or localized renal hypoxia.[109-111] These causes of polycythemia should be eliminated by appropriate laboratory work, thoracic radiographs, arterial blood gas analysis, and renal ultrasonography. In humans with PV, plasma erythropoietin (EPO) levels are low. EPO levels in dogs with PV tend to be low or low-normal, whereas in animals with secondary absolute polycythemia, the levels are high.[112,113] Samples for determination of EPO concentrations should be taken prior to therapeutic phlebotomy used to treat hyperviscosity and, owing to fluctuations in EPO levels, should be repeated if results are incongruous with other information.

There are no pathognomonic features of CML in dogs, and other common causes for marked leukocytosis with a left shift ("leukemoid reaction") and granulocytic hyperplasia of bone marrow must be eliminated. These include infections, especially pyogenic ones; immune-mediated diseases; and other malignant neoplasms. In CML, maturation sometimes appears disorderly, and there may be variation in the size and shape of neutrophils at the same level of maturation. In addition, neoplastic leukocytes may disintegrate more rapidly and appear vacuolated.[35] Because of the invasive nature of CML, biopsy of liver or spleen may also help to distinguish true leukemia from a leukemoid reaction, assuming the animal can tolerate the procedure. If characteristic cytogenetic abnormalities can be found in dogs with CML, this analysis may be helpful.

Basophilic leukemia is diagnosed by finding excessive numbers of basophils in circulation and in bone marrow. Basophilic leukemia must be differentiated from mastocytosis based on the morphology of the cell type present. Basophils have a segmented nucleus and variably sized granules, whereas mast cells have a round-to-oval nucleus that may be partially or totally obscured by small, round, metachromatic-staining granules. This distinction is usually easy to make; however, in basophilic leukemia, changes in the morphology of the nucleus and granules make the distinction less clear.[85]

Essential thrombocythemia has been diagnosed based on finding persistent and excessive thrombocytosis (>600,000/μL) without circulating blast cells and in the absence of another MPD (e.g., PV), myelofibrosis, or disorders known to cause secondary thrombocytosis.[89] These include iron deficiency anemia, chronic inflammatory diseases, recovery from severe hemorrhage, rebound from immune-mediated thrombocytopenia, and absence of a spleen. Thrombocytosis is transient in these disorders or abates with resolution of the primary disease. In essential thrombocythemia, platelet morphology may be abnormal, with bizarre giant forms and abnormal granulation.[90] In the bone marrow, megakaryocytic hyperplasia is a consistent feature, and dysplastic changes may be evident in megakaryocytes.[93] Spurious hyperkalemia may be present in serum samples from dogs with thrombocytosis from any cause due to the release of potassium from platelets during clot formation.[114] Measuring potassium in plasma is recommended in these cases and usually demonstrates a potassium concentration within reference interval. Platelet aggregability has been variably reported as impaired[90] or enhanced.[93] In the one dog in which it was measured, the plasma thrombopoietin (TPO) concentration was normal.[92] It is unclear whether TPO plays a role in essential thrombocythemia or is suppressed by the high platelet mass. Elucidation of the pathogenesis of this disorder should be aided by the recent cloning of the genes for thrombopoietin and its receptor, the proto-oncogene *mpl.*[115]

In MDS, abnormalities in two or three cell lines are usually manifested in peripheral blood as neutropenia with or without a left shift, nonregenerative anemia, or thrombocytopenia. Other changes include macrocytosis and metarubricytosis. The bone marrow is typically normocellular or hypercellular with an increased M:E ratio, and blasts cells, although increased, constitute less than 20% of nucleated cells; in a report of 13 dogs with primary or secondary MDS, in all but one dog the blast cell percentage was less than 20%.[116] Dysplastic changes can be detected in any cell line. Dyserythropoiesis is characterized by asynchronous maturation of erythroid cells typified by large hemoglobinized cells with immature nuclei (megaloblastic change). If the erythroid component is dominant, the MDS is called *MDS-Er* (see Table 32-12).[3,32] In dysgranulopoiesis, giant neutrophil precursors and abnormalities in nuclear segmentation and cytoplasmic granulation can be seen. Finally, dysthrombopoiesis is characterized by giant platelets and micromegakaryocytes.

Myelofibrosis should be suspected in animals with nonregenerative anemia or pancytopenia, abnormalities in erythrocyte morphology (especially shape), and leukoerythroblastosis. Bone marrow aspiration is usually unsuccessful, resulting in a "dry tap." This necessitates a bone marrow biopsy taken with a Jamshidi needle.[117] The specimen is processed for routine histopathologic examination, and if necessary, special stains for fibrous tissue can be used. Because myelofibrosis occurs secondary to other diseases of bone marrow such as chronic hemolytic anemia or bone marrow necrosis, the clinician should look for a primary disease process.

Treatment

Acute Myeloid Leukemia

Treatment of acute nonlymphocytic leukemias has been unrewarding to date. However, we have little information on the response of specific subtypes of leukemia to uniform chemotherapeutic protocols, in part due to the rarity of these disease processes and the paucity of cases in the literature. The veterinarian is advised to contact a veterinary oncologist for advice on new protocols and appropriate management of these cases.

The therapeutic goal is to eradicate leukemic cells and reestablish normal hematopoiesis. Currently, this is best accomplished by cytoreductive chemotherapy, and the agents most commonly utilized include a combination of Ara-C plus an anthracycline, such as doxorubicin or cyclophosphamide, vincristine, and prednisone.* In humans, the introduction of cytosine arabinoside has been the single most important development in the therapy of acute nonlymphocytic leukemia.[120] In dogs, Ara-C, 100 to 200 mg/m^2, given by slow infusion (12 to 24 hrs) daily for 3 days and repeated weekly, has been used, as well as several other variations using subcutaneous injections of cytosine (see Chapter 11). Doxorubicin, 30 mg/m^2 IV every 2 to 3 weeks, can be administered at intervals alternating with Ara-C. If remission is achieved, as evidenced by normalization of the hemogram, the COAP protocol (cyclophosphamide, vincristine (Oncovin), Ara-C, and prednisone), as described for canine lymphoma, could be used as maintenance therapy.[9,118] Another protocol that has been used in treating acute myeloblastic leukemia is presented in Table 32-13.

TABLE 32-13 Protocol for the Treatment of Acute Myeloproliferative Disorders

DRUG	DOSAGE	ROUTE
Remission Induction		
Cytosine arabinoside (Ara-C)	100 mg/m^2/day	IV over 60 minutes every 12 hours
6-Thioguanine	40 mg/m^2	PO for 4 days
Doxorubicin	10-15 mg/m^2	IV daily for 3 days
Maintenance		
Ara-C	100 mg/m2/day	SQ or IV once or twice/week
6-Thioguanine	40 mg/m^2	PO twice weekly
Doxorubicin	30 mg/m^2	IV every 3 weeks

Data from Mears EA, Raskin RE, Legendre AM: Basophilic leukemia in a dog, *J Vet Intern Med* 11(2):92–94, 1997.

IV, Intravenous; *PO,* by mouth; *SQ,* subcutaneous.

Regardless of the chemotherapy protocol used, significant bone marrow suppression will develop, and intensive supportive care will be necessary. Transfusions of whole blood or platelet-rich plasma may be required to treat anemia and thrombocytopenia, and infection should be managed with aggressive antibiotic therapy. Because of the generally poor response, the major thrust of therapy may be to provide palliative supportive care.

Polycythemia Vera

In treating PV, therapy is directed at reducing RBC mass. The PCV should be reduced to 50% to 60% or by one-sixth of its starting value; phlebotomies should be performed as needed, administering appropriate colloid and crystalloid solutions to replace lost electrolytes; 20 mL of whole blood/kg of body weight can be removed at regular intervals.[67] In humans, phlebotomy continues to be the therapeutic approach used most frequently.

Radiophosphorus (^{32}P) has been shown to provide long-term control but can only be used in specialized centers.[121] The chemotherapeutic drug of choice is hydroxyurea, an inhibitor of DNA synthesis. This drug should be administered at an initial dose of 30 mg/kg for 10 days and then reduced to 15 mg/kg PO daily.[69] The major goal of treatment is to maintain the PCV as close to normal as possible.

Chronic Myelogenous Leukemia

CML is best managed with chemotherapy to control the proliferation of the abnormal cell line and improve the quality of life. Hydroxyurea is the most effective agent for treating CML during the chronic phase.[75,122] The initial dosage is 20 to 25 mg/kg twice daily. Treatment with hydroxyurea should continue until the leukocyte count falls to 15,000 to 20,000 cells/μL.[75,79,84] Then the dosage of hydroxyurea can be reduced by 50% on a daily basis or to 50 mg/kg given biweekly or triweekly. In humans, the alkylating agent busulfan can be used as an alternative.[123] An effective dosage has not been established in the dog, but following human protocols, 0.1 mg/kg/day PO is given until the leukocyte count is reduced to 15,000 to 20,000 cells/μL.

*References 9, 12, 29, 39, 118, 119.

Despite response to chemotherapy and control for many months, most dogs with CML will eventually enter a terminal phase of their disease. In one study of seven dogs with CML, four underwent terminal phase blast crisis.[75] In humans, blast crisis may be lymphoid or myeloid.[124] In dogs, it is usually difficult to determine the cell of origin. These dogs have a poor prognosis, and the best treatment to consider, if any, would be that listed in Table 32-13.

It has now been documented that a subset of CML in dogs may be associated with a BCR-ABL chromosomal abnormality (the so-called "Raleigh chromosome") similar to the "Philadelphia chromosome" translocation responsible for a large majority of CML in humans.[2] While imatinib mesylate (Gleevec) is known to be an effective therapy for CML in humans, BCR-ABL kinase inhibitors have, as yet, not been investigated for this subset of CML in dogs.

Essential Thrombocythemia

Few cases have been reported, but one dog was treated successfully with a combination chemotherapy protocol that included vincristine, Ara-C, cyclophosphamide, and prednisone.[91] Treatment is controversial in humans because of the lack of evidence that asymptomatic patients benefit from chemotherapy. Patients with thrombosis or bleeding are given cytoreductive therapy. Hydroxyurea is the drug of choice for initially controlling the thrombocytosis.[89]

Myelodysplastic Syndrome

There is no standard therapeutic regime for MDS. Often, humans receive no treatment if the cytopenias do not cause clinical signs. Transfusions are given when necessary, and patients with fever are evaluated aggressively to detect infections. Growth factors, such as EPO, GM-CSF, G-CSF, and IL-3, are sometimes used in patients who require frequent transfusions to increase their blood cell counts and enhance neutrophil function.[125,126] In one case report, human EPO was administered (100 U/kg SQ, every 48 hours) to a dog with MDS because of profound anemia. The rationale for use of EPO was to promote terminal differentiation of dysplastic erythrocytes. The PCV increased from 12% to 34% by day 19 of EPO treatment. This dog remained in remission for more than 30 months.[32] Other factors that induce differentiation of hematopoietic cells include retinoic acid analogs,[127] 1,25 dihydroxyvitamin D3,[128] interferon-α, and conventional chemotherapeutic agents, such as 6-thioguanine and Ara-C.[129] The propensity of these factors to enhance progression to leukemia is not known in many cases, but the potential risk exists.

Prognosis

In general, the prognosis for animals with MPN is better than for dogs with AML, in which it is grave. The prognosis for PV and CML is guarded, but significant remissions have been achieved with certain therapeutic regimes and careful monitoring. Animals commonly survive a year or more.[75,84] Development of blast crisis portends a grave prognosis.

Comparative Aspects

The pathophysiology and therapy of nonlymphocytic leukemia in humans are being studied intensively. Myeloid neoplasms have been demonstrated to be clonal, with abnormalities evident in all hematopoietic cell lines. Leukemogenesis is likely caused by mutation or amplification of proto-oncogenes in a two-step process that initially involves a single cell and is followed by additional chromosomal alterations that may involve oncogenes.[1,15] These alterations are manifested as cytogenetic abnormalities. Environmental factors known to cause leukemia are exposure to high-dose radiation, benzene (chronic exposure), and alkylating agents.[130] New classification systems have incorporated genetic mutations, more accurately reflect prognoses, and facilitate use of consistent categorization among institutions.[131]

Therapeutic modalities under investigation or development include combination chemotherapy, immunotherapy, cytokine therapy, drug-resistance modulators, proapoptotic agents, antiangiogenic factors, signal transduction-active agents, and bone marrow transplantation. The prognosis for MPN is better than for AML. For acute nonlymphocytic leukemias, the prognosis is better for children than adults, with only 10% of adults receiving chemotherapy maintaining remissions for more than 5 years.[130] The spontaneous canine diseases probably occur too infrequently to serve as useful models. Myeloid neoplasms have been induced experimentally in the dog by irradiation and transplantation in an attempt to create models for study. Many similarities between human and canine myeloid neoplasms exist, and veterinary medicine may benefit from any therapeutic advances made in the human field.

REFERENCES

1. Lichtman MA: Classification and clinical manifestations of the clonal myeloid disorders. In: Lichtman MA, Kipps TJ, Seligsohn U, et al, editors: *Williams hematology*, ed 8, New York, 2010, McGraw-Hill. http://www.accessmedicine.com/content.aspx?aID=6121127. Accessed December 23, 2011.
2. Breen M, Modiano JF: Evolutionarily conserved cytogenetic changes in hematologic malignancies of dogs and humans—man and his best friend share more than companionship, *Chromosome Res* 16(1):145–154, 2008.
3. Jain NC, Blue JT, Grindem CB, et al: A report of the animal leukemia study group. Proposed criteria for classification of acute myeloid leukemia in dogs and cats, *Vet Clin Pathol* 20(3):63–82, 1991.
4. Juopperi TA, Bienzle D, Bernreuter DC, et al: Prognostic markers for myeloid neoplasms: a comparative review of the literature and goals for future investigation, *Vet Pathol* 48(1):182–197, 2011.
5. Nielsen SW: Myeloproliferative disorders in animals. In Clarke WJ, Howard EB, Hackett PL, editors: *Myeloproliferative disorders in animals and man*, Oak Ridge, Tenn, 1970, USAEC Division of Technical Information Extension.
6. Christopher MM, Metz AL, Klausner J, et al: Acute myelomonocytic leukemia with neurologic manifestations in the dog, *Vet Pathol* 23(2):140–147, 1986.
7. Keller P, Sager P, Freudiger U, et al: Acute myeloblastic leukemia in a dog, *J Comp Pathol* 95(4):619–632, 1985.
8. Clark P, Swenson CL, Drenen CM: A 6-year-old Rottweiler with weight loss, *Aust Vet J* 75(10):709, 714–715, 1997.
9. Graves TK, Swenson CL, Scott MA: A potentially misleading presentation and course of acute myelomonocytic leukemia in a dog, *J Am Anim Hosp Assoc* 33:37–41, 1997.
10. Colbatzy F, Hermanns W: Acute megakaryoblastic leukemia in one cat and two dogs, *Vet Pathol* 30(2):186–194, 1993.
11. Latimer KS, Dykstra MJ: Acute monocytic leukemia in a dog, *J Am Vet Med Assoc* 184:852–854, 1984.
12. Hamlin RH, Duncan RC: Acute nonlymphocytic leukemia in a dog, *J Am Vet Med Assoc* 196:110–112, 1990.
13. Grindem CB, Stevens JB, Perman V: Morphologic classification and clinical and pathological characteristics of spontaneous leukemia in 17 dogs, *J Am Anim Hosp Assoc* 21:219–226, 1985.
14. Modiano JF, Smith R III, Wojcieszyn J, et al: The use of cytochemistry, immunophenotyping, flow cytometry, and in vitro differentiation to determine the ontogeny of a canine monoblastic leukemia, *Vet Clin Pathol* 27:40–49, 1998
15. Jandl JH: Hematopoietic malignancies. In *Blood: pathophysiology*, Boston, 1991, Blackwell Scientific Publications.

16. Grindem CB, Buoen LC: Cytogenetic analysis of leukemic cells in the dog: A report of 10 cases and a review of the literature, *J Comp Pathol* 96:623–635, 1986.
17. Reimann N, Bartnitzke S, Bullerdiek J, et al: Trisomy 1 in a canine acute leukemia indicating the pathogenetic importance of polysomy 1 in leukemias of the dog, *Cancer Genet Cytogenet* 101:49–52, 1997.
18. Breen M: Canine cytogenetics—from band to base pair, *Cytogenet Genome Res* 120(1-2):50–60, 2008.
19. Breen M: Update on genomics in veterinary oncology, *Top Companion Anim Med* 24(3):113–121, 2009.
20. McManus PM: Classification of myeloid neoplasms: a comparative review, *Vet Clin Pathol* 34:189–212, 2005.
21. Reimann N, Bartnitzke S, Nolte I, et al: Working with canine chromosomes: current recommendations for karyotype description, *J Hered* 90:31–34, 1999.
22. Anderson AC, Johnson RM: Erythroblastic malignancy in a beagle, *J Am Vet Med Assoc* 141:944–946, 1962.
23. Seed TM, Tolle DV, Fritz TE, et al: Irradiation-induced erythroleukemia and myelogenous leukemia in the beagle dog: Hematology and ultrastructure, *Blood* 50:1061–1079, 1977.
24. Tolle DV, Seed TM, Fritz TE, et al: Acute monocytic leukemia in an irradiated beagle, *Vet Pathol* 16:243–254, 1979.
25. Sykes GP, King JM, Cooper BC: Retrovirus-like particles associated with myeloproliferative disease in the dog, *J Comp Pathol* 95(4):559–564, 1985.
26. Quesenberry PJ: Hemopoietic stem cells, progenitor cells, and cytokines. In Beutler E, Lichtman MA, Coller BS, et al, editors: *Williams hematology*, ed 5, New York, 1995, McGraw-Hill.
27. Metcalf D: *The hemopoietic colony stimulating factors*, New York, 1984, Elsevier.
28. Lok S, Kaushansky K, Holly RD, et al: Cloning and expression of murine thrombopoietin cDNA and stimulation of platelet production in vivo, *Nature* 369:565–568, 1994.
29. Couto CG, Kallet AJ: Preleukemic syndrome in a dog, *J Am Vet Med Assoc* 184:1389–1392, 1984.
30. Couto CG: Clinicopathologic aspects of acute leukemias in the dog, *J Am Vet Med Assoc* 186(7):681–685, 1985.
31. Weiss DJ, Raskin R, Zerbe C: Myelodysplastic syndrome in two dogs, *J Am Vet Med Assoc* 187(10):1038–1040, 1985.
32. Boone LI, Knauer KW, Rapp SW, et al: Use of human recombinant erythropoietin and prednisone for treatment of myelodysplastic syndrome with erythroid predominance in a dog, *J Am Vet Med Assoc* 213(7):999–1001, 1998.
33. Degen MA, Feldman BF, Turrel JM, et al: Thrombocytosis associated with a myeloproliferative disorder in a dog, *J Am Vet Med Assoc* 194(10):1457–1459, 1989.
34. Evans JR, Gorman NT: Myeloproliferative disease in the dog and cat: Definition, aetiology and classification, *Vet Rec* 121:437–443, 1987.
35. Jain NC: The leukemia complex. In *Schalm's veterinary hematology*, ed 4, Philadelphia, 1986, Lea & Febiger.
36. Usher SG, Radford AD, Villiers EJ, et al: RAS, FLT3, and C-KIT mutations in immunophenotyped canine leukemias, *Exp Hematol* 37(1):65–77, 2009.
37. Barthel CH: Acute myelomonocytic leukemia in a dog, *Vet Pathol* 11:79–86, 1974.
38. Green RA, Barton CL: Acute myelomonocytic leukemia in a dog, *J Am Anim Hosp Assoc* 13:708- 712, 1977.
39. Jain NC, Madewell BR, Weller RE, et al: Clinical-pathological findings and cytochemical characterizations of myelomonocytic leukaemia in 5 dogs, *J Comp Pathol* 91:17–31, 1981.
40. Linnabary RD, Holscher MA, Glick AD, et al: Acute myelomonocytic leukemia in a dog, *J Am Anim Hosp Assoc* 14:71–75, 1978.
41. Moulton JE, Dungworth DL: Tumors of the lymphoid and hemopoietic tissues. In Moulton JE, editor:: *Tumors in domestic animals*, ed 2, Berkeley, 1978, University of California Press.
42. Ragan HA, Hackett PL, Dagle GE: Acute myelomonocytic leukemia manifested as myelophthistic anemia in a dog, *J Am Vet Med Assoc* 169:421–425, 1976.
43. Rohrig KE: Acute myelomonocytic leukemia in a dog, *J Am Vet Med Assoc* 182:137–141, 1983.
44. Madewell BR, Jain NC, Munn RJ: Unusual cytochemical reactivity in canine acute myeloblastic leukemia, *Comp Haematol Int* 1(2):117–120, 1991.
45. Hayashi A, Tanaka H, Kitamura M, et al: Acute myelomonocytic leukemia (AML-M4) in a dog with the extradural lesion, *J Vet Med Sci* 73:419–422, 2011.
46. Hisasue M, Nishimura T, Neo S, et al: A dog with acute myelomonocytic leukemia, *J Vet Med Sci* 70:619–621, 2008.
47. Holscher MA, Collins RD, Glick AD, et al: Megakaryocytic leukemia in a dog, *Vet Pathol* 15:562–565, 1978.
48. Canfield PJ, Church DB, Russ IG: Myeloproliferative disorder involving the megakaryocytic line, *J Small Anim Pract* 34(6):296–301, 1993.
49. Bolon B, Buergelt CD, Harvey JW, et al: Megakaryoblastic leukemia in a dog, *Vet Clin Pathol* 18(3):69–72, 1989.
50. Shull RM, DeNovo RC, McCracken MD: Megakaryoblastic leukemia in a dog, *Vet Pathol* 23(4):533–536, 1986.
51. Cain GR, Feldman BF, Kawakami TG, et al: Platelet dysplasia associated with megakaryoblastic leukemia in a dog, *J Am Vet Med Assoc* 188(5): 529–530, 1986.
52. Cain GR, Kawakami TG, Jain NC: Radiation-induced megakaryoblastic leukemia in a dog, *Vet Pathol* 22(6):641–643, 1985.
53. Mesick J, Carothers M, Wellman M: Identification and characterization of megakaryoblasts in acute megakaryoblastic leukemia in a dog, *Vet Pathol* 27(3):212–214, 1990.
54. Comazzi S, Gelain ME, Belfanti U, et al: Acute megakaryoblastic leukemia in a dog : a report of 3 cases and review of the literature, *J Am Anim Hosp Assoc* 46:327–335, 2010.
55. Willan M, Mulaire L, Schwendenwein I, et al: Chemotherapy in canine acute megakaryoblastic leukemia: a case report and review of the literature, *In Vivo* 23:911–918, 2009.
56. Ferreira HM, Smith SH, Schwartz AM, et al: Myeloperoxidase-positive acute megakaryoblastic leukemia in a dog, *Vet Clin Pathol* 40:530–537, 2011.
57. Suter SE, Vernau W, Fry MM, et al: CD34+, CD41+ acute megakaryoblastic leukemia in a dog, *Vet Clin Pathol* 36:288–292, 2007.
58. Park HM, Doster AR, Tashbaeva RE, et al: Clinical, histopathological and immunohistochemical findings in a case of megakaryoblastic leukemia in a dog, *J Vet Diagn Invest* 18:287–291, 2006.
59. Mackey LJ, Jarrett WFH, Lauder IM: Monocytic leukaemia in the dog, *Vet Rec* 96:27–30, 1975.
60. Capelli JL: Erythroleukemia in a dog, *Pratique Medicale and Chirurgicale de l'Animal de Compagnie* 26(4):337–340, 1990.
61. Hejlasz Z: Three cases of erythroleukemia in dogs, *Medycyna Weterynaryjna* 42(6):346–349, 1986.
62. Tomiyasu H, Fujino Y, Takahashi M, et al: Spontaneous erythroblastic leukaemia (AML-M6Er) in a dog, *J Small Anim Pract* 52:445–457, 2011.
63. Grindem CB: Blood cell markers, *Vet Clin North Am* 26(5):1043–1064, 1996.
64. Prchal J: Primary polycythemias. In Adamson JW, editor: *Current opinion in hematology*, Philadelphia, 1995, Current Science.
65. Bush BM, Fankhauser R: Polycythaemia vera in a bitch, *J Small Anim Pract* 13:75–89, 1972.
66. Carb AV: Polycythemia vera in a dog, *J Am Vet Med Assoc* 154:289–297, 1969.
67. McGrath CJ: Polycythemia vera in dogs, *J Am Vet Med Assoc* 164:1117–1122, 1974.
68. Miller RM: Polycythemia vera in a dog, *Vet Med/Small Anim Clin* 63:222–223, 1968.
69. Peterson ME, Randolph JK: Diagnosis of canine primary polycythemia and management with hydroxy-urea, *J Am Vet Med Assoc* 180:415–418, 1982.

70. Quesnal AD, Kruth SA: Polycythemia vera and glomerulonephritis in a dog, *Can Vet J* 33(10):671–672, 1992.
71. Meyer HP, Slappendel RJ, Greydanus-van-der-Putten SWM: Polycythaemia vera in a dog treated by repeated phlebotomies, *Vet Q* 15(3):108–111, 1993.
72. Wysoke JM, Van Heerden J: Polycythaemia vera in a dog, *J S Afr Vet Assoc* 61(4):182–183, 1990.
73. Holden AR: Polycythaemia vera in a dog, *Vet Rec* 120(20):473–475, 1987.
74. Beurlet S, Krief P, Sansonetti A, et al: identification of JAK2 mutations in canine primary polycythemia, *Exp Hematol* 39:542–545, 2011.
75. Leifer CE, Matus RE, Patnaik AK, et al: Chronic myelogenous leukemia in the dog, *J Am Vet Med Assoc* 183:686–689, 1983.
76. Pollet L, Van Hove W, Matheeuws D: Blastic crisis in chronic myelogenous leukaemia in a dog, *J Small Anim Pract* 19:469–475, 1978.
77. Grindem CB, Stevens JB, Brost DR, et al: Chronic myelogenous leukaemia with meningeal infiltration in a dog, *Comp Haematol Int* 2(3):170–174, 1992.
78. Dunn JK, Jeffries AR, Evans RJ, et al: Chronic granulocytic leukaemia in a dog with associated bacterial endocarditis, thrombocytopenia and preretinal and retinal hemorrhages, *J Small Anim Pract* 28(11):1079–1086, 1987.
79. Fine DM, Tvedten HW: Chronic granulocytic leukemia in a dog, *J Am Vet Med Assoc* 214(2):1809–1812, 1999.
80. Liesveld JL, Lichtman MA: Chronic myelogenous leukemia and related disorders. In Lichtman MA, Kipps TJ, Seligsohn U, et al, editors. *Williams hematology*, ed 8, New York, 2010, McGraw-Hill.
81. Cruz Cardona JA, Milner R, Alleman AR: BCR-ABL translocation in a dog with chronic monocytic leukemia, *Vet Clin Pathol* 40(1):40–47, 2011.
82. Rossi G, Gelain ME, Foroni S, et al: Extreme monocytosis in a dog with chronic monocytic leukaemia, *Vet Rec* 165:54–56, 2009.
83. Hiraoka H, Hisasue M, Nagashima N, et al: A dog with myelodysplastic syndrome: chronic myelomonocytic leukemia, *J Vet Med Sci* 69:665–668, 2007.
84. MacEwen EG, Drazner FH, McClellan AJ, et al: Treatment of basophilic leukemia in a dog, *J Am Vet Med Assoc* 166:376–380, 1975.
85. Mahaffey EA, Brown TP, Duncan JR, et al: Basophilic leukemia in a dog, *J Comp Pathol* 97(4):393–399, 1987.
86. Mears EA, Raskin RE, Legendre AM: Basophilic leukemia in a dog, *J Vet Intern Med* 11(2):92–94, 1997.
87. Jensen AL, Nielsen OL: Eosinophilic leukemoid reaction in a dog, *J Small Anim Pract* 33(7):337–340, 1992.
88. Ndikuwera J, Smith DA, Obwolo MJ, et al: Chronic granulocytic leukaemia/eosinophilic leukaemia in a dog, *J Small Anim Pract* 33(11):553–557, 1992.
89. Beer PA, Green AR: Essential thrombocythemia. In Lichtman MA, Kipps TJ, Seligsohn U, et al, editors. *Williams hematology*, ed 8, New York, 2010, McGraw-Hill. http://www.accessmedicine.com/content.aspx?aID=6136261. Accessed December 23, 2011.
90. Hopper PE, Mandell CP, Turrel JM, et al: Probable essential thrombocythemia in a dog, *J Vet Intern Med* 3(2):79–85, 1989.
91. Simpson JW, Else RW, Honeyman P: Successful treatment of suspected essential thrombocythemia in the dog, *J Small Anim Pract* 31(7):345–348, 1990.
92. Bass MC, Schultze AE: Essential thrombocythemia in a dog: Case report and literature review, *J Am Anim Hosp Assoc* 34:197–203, 1998.
93. Dunn JK, Heath MF, Jeffries AR, et al: Diagnostic and hematologic features of probable essential thrombocythemia in two dogs, *Vet Clin Pathol* 28(4):131–138, 1999.
94. Reagan WJ: A review of myelofibrosis in dogs, *Toxicol Pathol* 21(2):164–169, 1993.
95. Weiss DJ: A retrospective study of the incidence and the classification of bone marrow disorders in the dog at a veterinary teaching hospital (1996-2004), *J Vet Intern Med* 20(4):955–961, 2006.
96. Castro-Malaspina H: Pathogenesis of myelofibrosis: Role of ineffective megakaryopoiesis and megakaryocyte components. In Berk PD, Castro-Malaspina H, Wasserman LR, editors: *Myelofibrosis and the biology of connective tissue*, New York, 1984, Alan R. Liss.
97. Rudolph R, Huebner C: Megakaryozytenleukose beim hund, *Kleintier-Praxis* 17:9–13, 1972.
98. Dungworth DL, Goldman M, Switzer JW, et al: Development of a myeloproliferative disorder in beagles continuously exposed to ^{90}Sr, *Blood* 34:610–632, 1969.
99. Prasse KW, Crouser D, Beutler E, et al: Pyruvate kinase deficiency anemia with terminal myelofibrosis and osteosclerosis in a beagle, *J Am Vet Med Assoc* 166:1170–1175, 1975.
100. Thompson JC, Johnstone AC: Myelofibrosis in the dog: Three case reports, *J Small Anim Pract* 24(9):589–601, 1983.
101. Thomsen MK, Jensen AL, Skak-Nielsen T, et al: Enhanced granulocyte function in a case of chronic granulocytic leukemia in a dog, *Vet Immunol Immunopathol* 28(2):143–165, 1991.
102. Grindem CB, Stevens JB, Perman V: Cytochemical reactions in cells from leukemic dogs, *Vet Pathol* 23:103–109, 1986.
103. Facklam NR, Kociba GJ: Cytochemical characterization of leukemic cells from 20 dogs, *Vet Pathol* 22:363–369, 1986.
104. Goldman EE, Graham JC: Clinical diagnosis and management of acute nonlymphoid leukemias and chronic myeloproliferative disorders. In Feldman BF, Zinkl JG, Jain NC, editors: *Schalm's veterinary hematology*, ed 5, Philadelphia, 2000, Lippincott Williams & Wilkins.
105. Cobbold S, Metcalfe S: Monoclonal antibodies that define canine homologues of human CD antigens: Summary of the First International Canine Leukocyte Antigen Workshop (CLAW), *Tissue Antigens* 43(3):137–154, 1994.
106. Tasca S, Carli E, Caldin M, et al: Hematologic abnormalities and flow cytometric immunophenotyping results in dogs with hematopoietic neoplasia: 210 cases (2002-2006), *Vet Clin Pathol* 38:2–12, 2009.
107. Villiers E, Baines S, Law AM, et al: Identification of acute myeloid leukemia in dogs using flow cytometry with myeloperoxidase, MAC387, and a canine neutrophil-specific antibody, *Vet Clin Pathol* 35:55–71, 2006.
108. Comazzi S, Gelain ME, Spagnolo V, et al: Flow cytometric patterns in blood from dogs with non-neoplastic and neoplastic hematologic diseases using double labeling for CD18 and CD45, *Vet Clin Pathol* 35:47–54, 2006.
109. Peterson ME, Zanjani ED: Inappropriate erythropoietin production from a renal carcinoma in a dog with polycythemia, *J Am Vet Med Assoc* 179:995–996, 1981.
110. Scott RC, Patnaik AK: Renal carcinoma associated with secondary polycythemia in a dog, *J Am Anim Hosp Assoc* 8:275–283, 1972.
111. Waters DJ, Prueter JC: Secondary polycythemia associated with renal disease in the dog: Two case reports and review of literature, *J Am Anim Hosp Assoc* 24:109–114, 1988.
112. Cook SM, Lothrop CD: Serum erythropoietin concentrations measured by radioimmunoassay in normal, polycythemic, and anemic dogs and cats, *J Vet Intern Med* 8(1):18–25, 1994.
113. Giger U: Serum erythropoietin concentrations in polycythemic and anemic dogs. *Proceedings of the 9th Annual Vet Med Forum (ACVIM)*, 1991, pp. 143–145.
114. Reimann KA, Knowlen CG, Tvedten HW: Factitious hyperkalemia in dogs with thrombocytosis, *J Vet Intern Med* 3:47–52, 1989.
115. Kaushansky K: Thrombopoietin: The primary regulator of platelet production, *Blood* 86(2):419–431, 1995.
116. Weiss DJ, Aird B: Cytologic evaluation of primary and secondary myelodysplastic syndromes in the dog, *Vet Clin Pathol* 30:67–75, 2001.
117. Friedrichs KR, Young KM: How to collect diagnostic bone marrow samples, *Vet Med* 8:578–588, 2005.
118. Theilen GH, Madewell BR, Gardner MB: Hematopoietic neoplasms, sarcomas and related conditions. In Theilen GH, Madewell BR,

editors: *Veterinary cancer medicine*, ed 2, Philadelphia, 1987, Lea & Febiger.
119. Gorman NT, Evans RJ: Myeloproliferative disease in the dog and cat: Clinical presentations, diagnosis and treatment, *Vet Rec* 121:490–496, 1987.
120. Mayer RJ: Current chemotherapeutic treatment approaches to the management of previously untreated adults with de novo acute myelogenous leukemia, *Semin Oncol* 14:384–396, 1987.
121. Smith M, Turrel JM: Radiophosphorus (^{32}P) treatment of bone marrow disorders in dogs: 11 cases (1970-1987), *J Am Vet Med Assoc* 194:98–102, 1982.
122. Lyss AP: Enzymes and random synthetics. In Perry MC, editor: *The chemotherapy source book*, Baltimore, 1992, Williams & Wilkins, pp. 398- 412.
123. Bolin RW, Robinson WA, Sutherland J, et al: Busulfan versus hydroxyurea in long-term therapy of chronic myelogenous leukemia, *Cancer* 50:1683–1686, 1982.
124. Rosenthal S, Canellos GP, Whang-Pang J, et al: Blast crisis of chronic granulocytic leukemia: Morphologic variants and therapeutic implications, *Am J Med* 63:542–547, 1977.
125. Liesveld JL, Lichtman MA: Myelodysplastic syndromes (clonal cytopenias and oligoblastic myelogenous leukemia). In Lichtman MA, Kipps TJ, Seligsohn U, et al, editors. *Williams hematology*, ed 8, New York, 2010, McGraw-Hill. http://www.accessmedicine.com/content.aspx?aID=6139818. Accessed December 23, 2011.
126. Ganser A, Hoelzer D: Treatment of myelodysplastic syndromes with hematopoietic growth factors, *Hematol Oncol Clin North Am* 6:633–653, 1992.
127. Ohno R, Noe T, Hirano M, et al: Treatment of myelodysplastic syndromes with all-trans retinoic acid, *Blood* 81:1152–1154, 1993.
128. Kelsey SM, Newland AC, Cunningham J, et al: Sustained haematological response to high dose oral alfacalcidol in patients with myelodysplastic syndrome [Letter], *Lancet* 340:316, 1992.
129. Jacobs A: Treatment for the myelodysplastic syndromes, *Hematologica* 72:477–480, 1987.
130. Liesveld JL, Lichtman MA: Acute myelogenous leukemia. In Lichtman MA, Kipps TJ, Seligsohn U, et al, editors. *Williams hematology*, ed 8, New York, 2010, McGraw-Hill. http://www.accessmedicine.com/content.aspx?aID=6140629. Accessed December 23, 2011.
131. Vardiman JW, Thiele J, Arber DA, et al: The 2008 revision of the World Health Organization (WHO) classification of the myeloid neoplasms and acute leukemia: rationale and important changes, *Blood* 114(5):937–951, 2009.

SECTION D
Myeloma-Related Disorders

DAVID M. VAIL

Myeloma-related disorders (MRDs) arise when a cell of the plasma cell or immunoglobulin-producing B-lymphocyte precursor lineage transforms and proliferates to form a neoplastic population of similar cells. This population is believed in most instances to be monoclonal (i.e., derived from a single cell) because they typically produce homogenous immunoglobulin, although some examples of biclonal and polyclonal MRD neoplasms exist. A wide variety of clinical syndromes are represented by MRDs, including multiple myeloma (MM), extramedullary plasmacytoma (EMP [both cutaneous and noncutaneous]), IgM (Waldenström's) macroglobulinemia, solitary osseous plasmacytoma (SOP), and Ig-secreting lymphomas and leukemias (including plasma cell leukemia). MM is the most important MRD based on clinical incidence and severity. There appears to be some discordance and blurring of the distinction between MM and multicentric noncutaneous EMP in cats and these two MRDs will be discussed together in this species.

Multiple Myeloma

Incidence and Etiology

Although MM represents less than 1% of all malignant tumors in animals, it is responsible for approximately 8% of all hematopoietic tumors and 3.6% of all primary and secondary tumors affecting bone in dogs.[1,2] In a compilation of bone marrow disorders in dogs (n = 717), MM represented 4.4% and 19.8% of all abnormal samples and neoplastic processes, respectively.[3] Further, in a compilation of serum protein electrophoretic samples (n = 147 dogs), MM accounted for 4.3% of abnormal and 28.5% of neoplastic processes encountered, respectively.[4] Early studies suggested a male predisposition,[5] although subsequent reports have not supported this.[1,6] Older dogs are affected with an average age of between 8 and 9 years.[1,5,6] In one large case series, German shepherd dogs were overrepresented based on the hospital population.[1] The true incidence of MM in the cat is unknown; however, it is a more rare diagnosis than in the dog, representing only 1 of 395 and 4 of 3248 tumors in two large compilations of feline malignancies and 0.9% of all malignancies and 1.9% of hematologic malignancies in another report.[7-9] MM represented 1.4% and 14% of abnormal and malignant serum protein electrophoretic samples, respectively, in a compilation of 155 feline samples.[10] MM occurs in aged cats (median age 12 to 14 years), most commonly in domestic short hairs and no sex predilection has been consistently reported, although a male preponderance may exist.[6,9,11,12] MM has not been associated with corona virus or FeLV or FIV infections.

The etiology of MM is for the most part unknown. Genetic predispositions, molecular aberrations (e.g., c-Kit), viral infections, chronic immune stimulation, and exposure to carcinogen stimulation have all been suggested as contributing factors.[6,13-18] Suggestion of a familial association in cats follows cases reported among siblings.[12] Evidence exists that molecular mechanisms of cellular control, including overexpression of cell cycle control components like cyclin D1 (see Chapter 2) and receptor tyrosine kinase dysregulation may be involved in canine myeloma and plasma cell tumors.[17,18] In rodent models, chronic immune stimulation and exposure to implanted silicone gel have been associated with development of MM,[13,14] as have chronic infections and prolonged hyposensitization therapy in humans.[15] Viral Aleutian disease of mink results in monoclonal gammopathies in a small percentage of cases.[16] Exposure to the agricultural industry, petroleum products, and irradiation are known risk factors for development in humans.[19-21] Additionally, progression of solitary plasma cell tumors to MM has been reported in both dogs and cats, and a single case of a B-cell lymphoma progressing to MM exists in the dog.[22,23]

Pathology and Natural Behavior

Multiple myeloma is a systemic proliferation of malignant plasma cells or their precursors arising as a clone of a single cell that usually involves multiple bone marrow sites in dogs. In cats, as previously stated, a blurring of the distinction of MM and multicentric noncutaneous EMP within the MRD occurs because widespread abdominal organ involvement without significant bone marrow infiltration has been described in a significant proportion of cases in European compilations.[11,24] Because both MM and multicentric noncutaneous EMP have a similar clinical course and widespread systemic involvement with hyperglobulinemia in cats, they will be

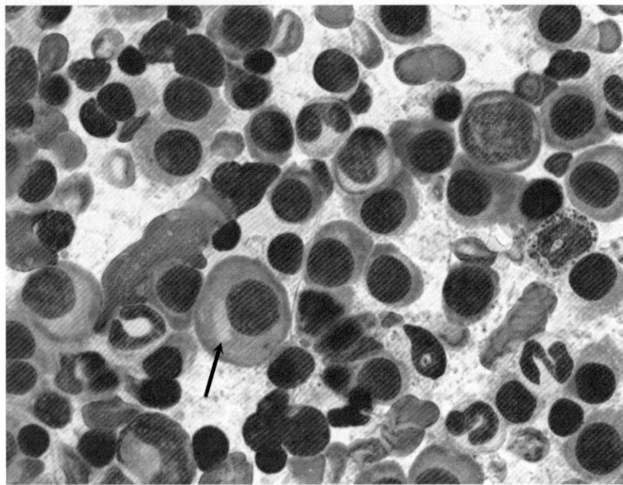

FIGURE 32-20 Bone marrow aspirate from a dog with multiple myeloma showing an overabundance of large neoplastic plasma cells with characteristic paranuclear clear zone representing the Golgi apparatus *(arrow)*. (Dif-quick stain, ×100 objective.)

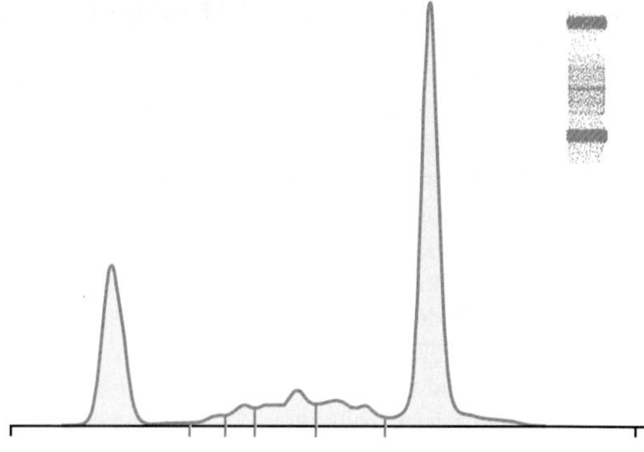

Animal protein electrophoresis

T.P.: 10.4 g/dl A/G 0.32

Fractions	%	Conc.	Ref. Conc.
Albumin	24.4	2.54 L	2.60 - 4.00
Alpha 1	1.6	0.17	0.11 - 0.35
Alpha 2	3.0	0.31 L	0.92 - 1.66
Beta 1	8.7	0.90 H	0.22 - 0.61
Beta 2	7.8	0.81 H	0.08 - 0.50
Gamma	54.5	5.67 H	0.66 - 2.48

FIGURE 32-21 Serum protein electrophoresis from a cat with multiple myeloma. Stained cellulose acetate electrophoretic strip *(upper right corner)* with accompanying densitogram. Note large M-component spike (representing an IgG monoclonal gammopathy) present in the gamma region. *(Courtesy Dr. Frances Moore, Marshfield Laboratories, Marshfield, WI.)*

discussed as MM in this chapter. Malignant plasma cells can have a varied appearance on histologic sections and cytologic preparations. The degree of differentiation ranges from those resembling normal plasma cells in late stages of differentiation (Figure 32-20) to very large anaplastic round cells (often referred to as *plasmablasts*), with a high mitotic index representing early stages of differentiation.[5,6,9,24,25] Binucleate and multinucleate cells are often present (see Figure 7-32, Chapter 7). In 16 cats with MM in a North American case series, the majority (83%) of plasma cells were immature and had marked atypia, including increased size, multiple nuclei, clefted nuclei, anisocytosis, anisokaryosis, variable N:C ratios, decreased chromatin density, and variable nucleoli; nearly one-quarter had "flame cell" morphology characterized by peripheral eosinophilic cytoplasmic processes.[9] However, in a European compilation of feline multicentric noncutaneous MRD cases (n = 17), 78% had well-differentiated morphologies.[24] The authors of this latter case series developed a grading system dependent on the percentage of plasmablasts within the neoplastic cells in which well-differentiated, intermediate-grade, and poorly differentiated have less than 15%, 15% to 49%, and 50% or more plasmablasts, respectively. Malignant plasma cells typically produce an overabundance of a single type of or component of immunoglobulin, which is referred to as the *M component* (Figure 32-21). The M component can be represented by any class of the entire immunoglobulin or only a portion of the molecule, such as the light chain (Bence Jones protein) or heavy chain (heavy chain disease) of the molecule. In the dog, the M component is usually represented by either IgA or IgG immunoglobulin types in nearly equal incidence, whereas the ratio of IgG:IgA in cats is approximately 5:1 in some reports and approximately 1:1 in others.[1,5-9,24,26] That being said, in the author's (DMV) experience, the vast majority of canine cases are of the IgA type. If the M component is the IgM type, the term *macroglobulinemia* (Waldenström's) is often applied. Several cases of biclonal gammopathy in dogs and cats have been reported.[9,11,12,27-32] Several cases of nonsecretory MM have been reported in dogs.[33,34] Rarely, cryoglobulinemia occurs in dogs with MM and IgM macroglobulinemia and has been reported in a cat with IgG myeloma.[6,35-37] Cryoglobulins are paraproteins that are insoluble at temperatures below 37° C and require blood collection and clotting to be performed at 37° C prior to serum separation. If whole blood is allowed to clot at temperatures below this, the protein precipitates in the clot and is lost. Pure light-chain M component is rare but has been reported in both dogs and cats.[38,39]

The pathology associated with MM is a result of either high levels of circulating M component, organ or bone infiltration with neoplastic cells, or both. Associated pathologic conditions include bone disease, bleeding diathesis, hyperviscosity syndrome, renal disease, hypercalcemia, immunodeficiency (and subsequent susceptibility to infections), cytopenias secondary to myelophthisis, and cardiac failure.

Bone lesions can be isolated, discrete osteolytic lesions (including pathologic fractures) (Figure 32-22, *A*) or diffuse osteopenias, or both (Figure 32-23). Approximately one-quarter to two-thirds of dogs with MM have radiographic evidence of bony lysis or diffuse osteoporosis.[1,5,6] The incidence of radiographic skeletal lesions in cats varies tremendously within reports, from as few as 8% in European case series to as high as 65% in North American case series.[8,9,11,12,26] Those bones engaged in active hematopoiesis are more commonly affected and include the vertebrae, ribs, pelvis, skull, and proximal or distal long bones. Skeletal lesions are rare with IgM (Waldenström's) macrogammaglobulinemia, in which malignant cells often infiltrate the spleen, liver, and lymph tissue rather than bone.[6,40-42]

Bleeding diathesis can result from one or a combination of events. M components may interfere with coagulation by (1) inhibiting platelet aggregation and the release of platelet factor-3; (2) causing adsorption of minor clotting proteins; (3) generating abnormal fibrin polymerization; and (4) producing a functional decrease in calcium.[6,43,44] Approximately one-third of dogs and

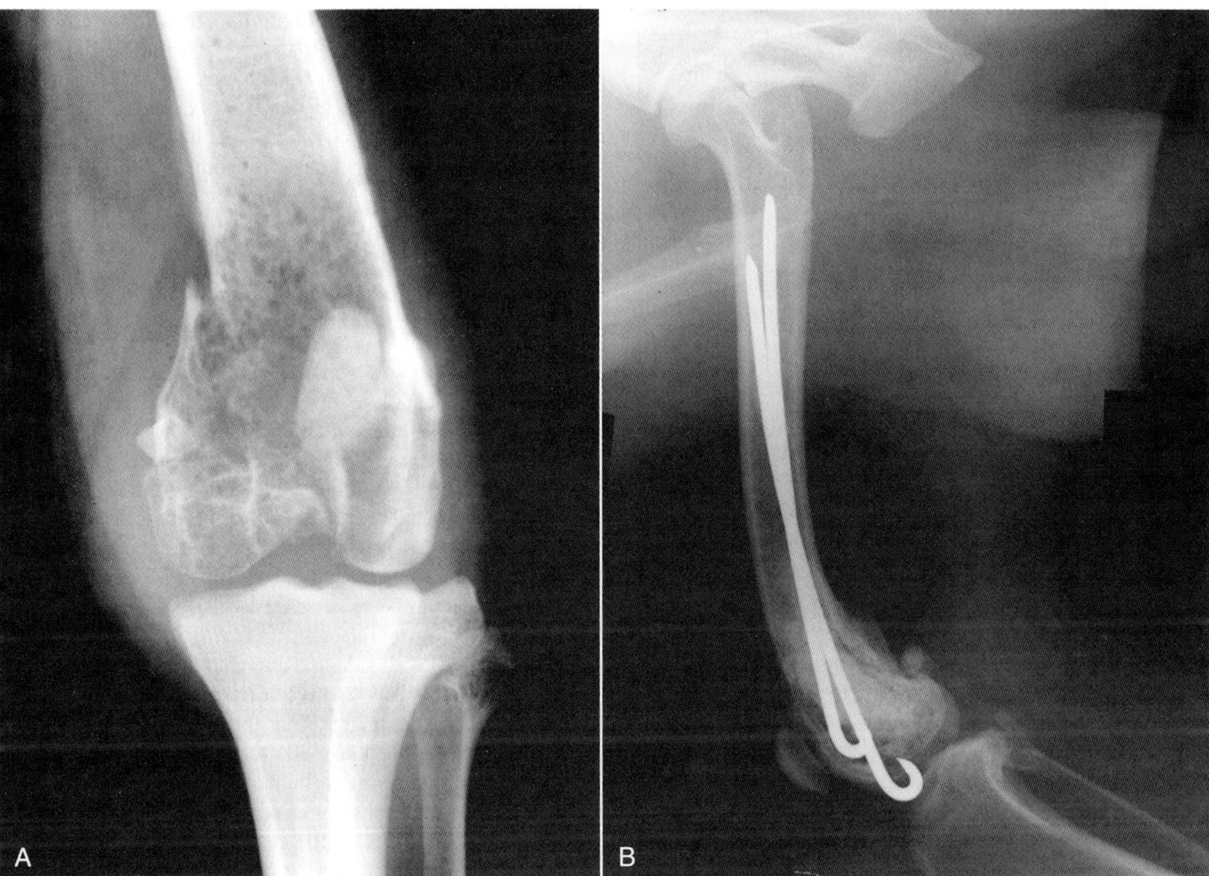

FIGURE 32-22 **A,** Radiograph of a distal femur in a dog demonstrating severe osteolysis and a pathologic fracture secondary to a plasma cell tumor. **B,** Radiograph of the same pathologic fracture after surgical repair with Rush rods and bone cement. Local site was treated with adjuvant radiation. The dog was continued on chemotherapy for 2 more years and did well.

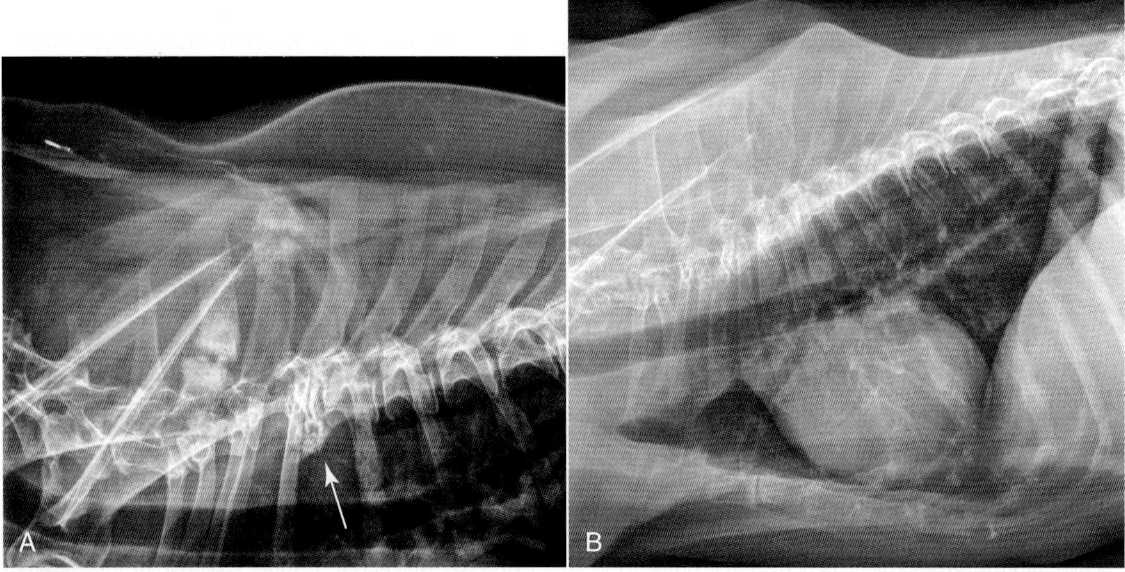

FIGURE 32-23 **A,** Lateral thoracic radiographs of a dog showing multiple expansile lytic lesions and pathologic fractures of the dorsal spinous processes and collapse fracture *(arrow)* of the third thoracic vertebral body. **B,** Lateral thoracic radiographs of a dog with diffuse osteopenia secondary to multiple myeloma. Note the overall decreased opacity of the lumbar vertebrae and dorsal spinous processes secondary to diffuse marrow involvement causing loss of bone trabeculae and thinning of the cortices.

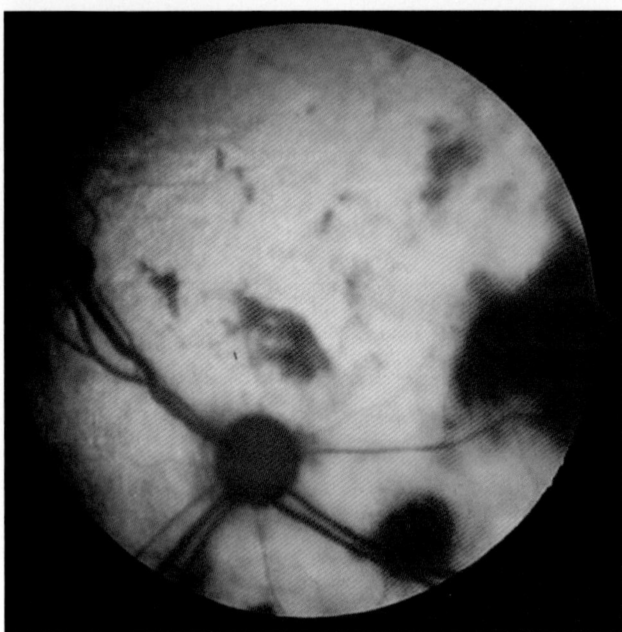

FIGURE 32-24 Multiple retinal hemorrhages on the fundus in a cat with hyperviscosity syndrome secondary to multiple myeloma.

one-quarter of cats have clinical evidence of hemorrhage.[1,9,11,12] In dogs, nearly half have abnormal prothrombin (PT) and partial thromboplastin (PTT) times. Thrombocytopenia may also play a role if bone marrow infiltration is significant (i.e., myelophthisis).

Hyperviscosity syndrome (HVS) represents one of a constellation of clinicopathologic abnormalities resulting from greatly increased serum viscosity. The magnitude of viscosity changes is related to the type, size, shape, and concentration of the M component in the blood. HVS is more common with IgM macroglobulinemias due to the high molecular weight of this class of immunoglobulin. IgA-secreting myelomas (usually present as a dimer in the dog), may undergo polymerization resulting in increased serum viscosity.[1,6,45] IgG-associated HVS can also occur, albeit less frequently. High serum viscosity occurs in approximately 20% of dogs with MM and can result in bleeding diathesis, neurologic signs (e.g., dementia, depression, seizure activity, coma), ophthalmic abnormalities (e.g., dilated and tortuous retinal vessels, retinal hemorrhage [Figure 32-24], retinal detachment), and increased cardiac workload with the potential for subsequent development of cardiomyopathy.* These consequences are thought to be a result of sludging of blood in small vessels, ineffective delivery of oxygen and nutrients, and coagulation abnormalities. HVS has been reported in cats with IgG-, IgA-, and IgM-secreting tumors.[6,8,49-53] In several of these cases, relative serum viscosity was increased above control ranges.

Renal disease is present in approximately one-third to one-half of dogs with MM, and azotemia was observed in one-third of cats in one report.[1,5,9,11] The pathogenesis of renal failure is often multifactorial and can ensue as a result of Bence Jones (light-chain) proteinuria, tumor infiltration into renal tissue, hypercalcemia, amyloidosis, diminished perfusion secondary to hyperviscosity syndrome, dehydration, or ascending urinary tract infections.[1,6,43,44] Normally, heavy- and light-chain synthesis is well balanced in nonneoplastic immunoglobulin production. In the case of MM, an unbalanced excess of light-chain products may be produced. Light chains are of low molecular weight and are normally filtered by the renal glomerulus, and their presence in urine can result in protein precipitates and subsequent renal tubular injury. The presence of light chains in urine without a concomitant monoclonal spike in serum, although rare, is indicative of pure light-chain disease.[38] Tubules become obstructed by large laminated casts containing albumin, immunoglobulin, and light chains.[6,38,43,44] Bence Jones proteinuria occurs in approximately 25% to 40% of dogs with MM.[1,5,6] Bence Jones proteinuria is reported to occur in approximately 40% of cats with MM/MRD.[9,11] Hypercalcemia is reported in 15% to 20% of dogs with MM and is thought to result primarily from the production of osteoclast-activating factor by neoplastic cells.[1,6,54] Other factors, including increased levels of various cytokines, TNF, IL-1, and IL-6 have been implicated in human MM. In two dogs with MM and hypercalcemia, serum elevations in circulating N-terminal PTHrP were noted.[55] Hypercalcemia may also be exacerbated by associated renal disease. Hypercalcemia, initially thought to be a rare event in cats with MM, occurred in 10% to 25% of recently reported cases.[9,11,12,56]

Susceptibility to infection and immunodeficiency have long been associated with MM and are often the ultimate cause of death in affected animals.[1,6,26] Infection rates in humans with MM are fifteen times higher than normal and usually represent pneumonia or urinary tract infections.[57] Response to vaccination has also been shown to be suppressed in humans with MM.[57] Immunoglobulin levels are often severely depressed in affected animals.[6] In addition, leukopenias may be present secondary to myelophthisis.

Variable cytopenias may be observed in association with MM. A normocytic, normochromic, nonregenerative anemia is encountered in approximately two-thirds of dogs with MM.[1,5,6] This can result from marrow infiltration (myelophthisis), blood loss from coagulation disorders, anemia of chronic disease, or increased erythrocyte destruction secondary to high serum viscosity. Rare erythrophagocytic forms of MM have also been reported in both dogs and cats and may contribute to anemia.[58,59] Similar factors lead to thrombocytopenia and leukopenia in nearly one-third and one-quarter of dogs with MM, respectively. In cats, approximately two-thirds, half, and one-third will be anemic, thrombocytopenic, and neutropenic, respectively.[9,11,12]

Cardiac disease if present is usually a result of excessive cardiac workload and myocardial hypoxia secondary to hyperviscosity.[43,45,53] Myocardial infiltration with amyloid and anemia may be complicating factors. Nearly half of cats with MM in one report presented with a cardiac murmur, the etiology of which was not established.[9] Three cats with HVS presented with congestive heart failure, murmurs, and echocardiographic signs consistent with hypertrophic cardiomyopathy.[53]

History and Clinical Signs

Clinical signs of MM may be present up to a year prior to diagnosis with a median duration of one month reported in dogs.[1,9] In one cat, M-component elevations were detected 9 years prior to clinical presentation. In this latter case, the M-component elevation was consistent with monoclonal gammopathy of unknown significance (MGUS). MGUS (i.e., benign, essential, or idiopathic monoclonal gammopathy) is a benign monoclonal gammopathy that is not associated with osteolysis, bone marrow infiltration, or Bence Jones proteinuria. MGUS has also been reported in dogs.[60,61] Signs of MM can be variable based on the wide range of pathologic effects

*References 1, 6, 40, 42, 45-48.

TABLE 32-14 Frequency of Clinical Signs Reported for Dogs with Multiple Myeloma (n = 60)

CLINICAL SIGN	FREQUENCY REPORTED (%)
Lethargy and weakness	62
Lameness	47
Bleeding diathesis	37
Funduscopic abnormalities	35
Polyuria/polydipsia	25
CNS deficits	12

Data from Matus RE, Leifer CE, MacEwen EG, et al: Prognostic factors for multiple myeloma in the dog, *J Am Vet Med Assoc* 188:1288–1291, 1986.
CNS, Central nervous system.

possible. Tables 32-14 and 32-15 list the relative frequencies of clinical signs observed in the dog and cat, respectively, based on a compilation of several reports.* Bleeding diathesis is usually represented by epistaxis and gingival bleeding. Funduscopic abnormalities may include retinal hemorrhage (see Figure 32-24), venous dilatation with sacculation and tortuosity, retinal detachment, and blindness.† CNS signs may include dementia, seizure activity, tremors, and deficiencies in midbrain or brain-stem localizing reflexes secondary to HVS or extreme hypercalcemia. Signs reflective of transverse myelopathies secondary to vertebral column infiltration, pathologic fracture, or extradural mass compression can also occur.[1,6,35,62,63] One case of ataxia and seizure activity in a dog with EMP secondary to tumor-associated hypoglycemia has been reported.[64] Additionally, paraneoplastic polyneuropathy has been reported in a dog with MM.[65] A history of chronic respiratory infections and persistent fever may also be present in cats. Hepatosplenomegaly and renomegaly can occur due to organ infiltration. Bleeding diathesis due to HVS is less common in the cat; however, epistaxis, pleural and peritoneal hemorrhagic effusions, retinal hemorrhage, and central neurologic signs have been reported.[6,8,49-53] Polydipsia and polyuria can occur secondary to renal disease or hypercalcemia, and dehydration may develop. Hindlimb paresis secondary to osteolysis of lumbar vertebral bodies or extradural compression has been reported in cats.[12,66]

Diagnosis and Staging

The diagnosis of MM in dogs usually follows the demonstration of bone marrow plasmacytosis (see Figure 32-20), the presence of osteolytic bone lesions (see Figures 32-22 and 32-23), and the demonstration of serum or urine myeloma proteins (M component) (see Figure 32-21). In the absence of osteolytic bone lesions, a diagnosis can also be made if marrow plasmacytosis is associated with a progressive increase in the M component. In the cat, because the degree of bone marrow infiltration may not be as marked, it has been suggested that consideration of plasma cell morphology and visceral organ infiltration (Figure 32-25) be given in cases with demonstrable M-component disease in the absence of marked (<20%) marrow plasmacytosis.[9,11,24]

All animals suspected of plasma cell tumors should receive a minimal diagnostic evaluation including a CBC, platelet count, serum biochemistry profile, and urinalysis. Particular attention should be paid to renal function and serum calcium levels. If clinical hemorrhage is present, a coagulation assessment (e.g., platelet count, PT, PTT) and serum viscosity measurements are indicated. All animals should undergo a careful funduscopic examination. Serum electrophoresis and immunoelectrophoresis are performed to determine the presence of a monoclonal M component (see Figure 32-21) and to categorize the immunoglobulin class involved. Heat precipitation and electrophoresis of urine may be performed to determine presence of Bence Jones proteinuria

*References 1, 6, 9, 11, 12, 26.

†References 1, 6, 11, 45, 46-48.

TABLE 32-15 Approximate Frequency of Clinical Signs Reported for Cats with Myeloma-Related Disorders (n = 53)

CLINICAL SIGN	FREQUENCY RANGE REPORTED (%)
Lethargy and weakness	40-100
Anorexia	33-100
Pallor	30-100
Polyuria/polydipsia	13-40
Vomiting/diarrhea	20-30
Dehydration	20-30
Palpable organomegaly	20-25
Lameness	10-25
Heart murmur	0-45
Hind limb paresis/paralysis	0-45
Bleeding diathesis	0-40
CNS signs	13-30
Concurrent cutaneous plasma cell tumor	0-30
Fundic changes	13
Lymphadenopathy	0-10

Data from MacEwen EG, Hurvitz AI: Diagnosis and management of monoclonal gammopathies, *Vet Clin N Am Small Anim Pract* 7:119–132, 1977; Patel RT, Caceres A, French AF, et al: Multiple myeloma in 16 cats: a retrospective study, *Vet Clin Pathol* 34:341–352, 2005; Mellor PJ, Haugland S, Murphy S, et al: Myeloma-related disorders in cats commonly present as extramedullary neoplasms in contrast to myeloma in human patients: 24 cases with clinical follow-up, *J Vet Intern Med* 20:1376–1383. 2006; Hanna F: Multiple myelomas in cats, *J Feline Med Surg* 7:275–287, 2005; and Drazner FH: Multiple myeloma in the cat, *Comp Cont Ed Pract Vet* 4:206–216, 1982.
CNS, Central nervous system.

FIGURE 32-25 Necropsy specimen of a spleen from a cat with multiple myeloma showing diffuse plasma cell infiltration.

because commercial urine dipstick methods are not capable of this determination. Definitive diagnosis usually follows the performance of a bone marrow aspiration in the dog. A bone marrow core biopsy or multiple aspirations may be necessary due to the possibility of uneven clustering or infiltration of plasma cells in the bone marrow. Normal marrow contains less than 5% plasma cells, whereas myelomatous marrow often greatly exceeds this level. Current recommendations require more than 20% marrow plasmacytosis to be present, although a 10% cutoff in cats has been recently recommended with special attention to cellular atypia.[9] Even the 10% threshold is problematic in cats, and cellular atypia and visceral organ involvement (assessed through needle aspiration cytology or tissue biopsy) should be considered equally important in the species.[9,11,24] Rarely, biopsy of osteolytic lesions (i.e., Jamshidi core biopsy; see Chapter 24) is necessary for diagnosis in the dog. In one case of MM in a dog, splenic aspirates were diagnostically helpful.[67] Overall frequencies of clinical diagnostic abnormalities for dogs and cats with MM are compiled from published series having at least five cases each and are listed in Table 32-16.

Immunohistochemical and Molecular Diagnostics

Histochemical and immunohistochemical analyses of cells or tissues suspected of MRD are more often applied in the case of solitary plasmacytomas or where EMP is suspected in the absence of marrow involvement and will be discussed in subsequent sections; however, they have been occasionally useful in the diagnosis of MM. Molecular diagnostic techniques for MM have received limited use thus far in veterinary oncology; however, determining clonality of the immunoglobulin heavy chain variable region gene has been performed in feline plasmacytoma and myeloma using PARR techniques (see Chapter 8),[68] and use of this technology in cases where diagnosis is not straightforward awaits further investigation. The author has used PARR analysis both before treatment and after clinical remission in a small number of dogs with MM involved in clinical trials and documented its utility (1) for initial diagnosis and (2) to characterize molecular remission.

Imaging

Routine thoracic and abdominal radiographs are recommended in suspected cases. Occasionally, bony lesions can be observed in skeletal areas on these standard films, and organomegaly (liver, spleen, kidney) is observed in the majority of cats.[9,11] Abdominal ultrasound is recommended in all cats suspected of MM because this modality reveals involvement of one or more abdominal organs in the majority of cases.[9,11] These include splenomegaly with or without nodules, diffuse hyperechoic hepatomegaly with or without nodules, renomegaly, and iliac lymph node enlargement. In one case series in cats, 85% of organs with ultrasonographic abnormalities were subsequently confirmed to have plasma cell infiltration.[11] Skeletal survey radiographs are recommended to determine presence and extent of osteolytic lesions, which may have diagnostic, prognostic, and therapeutic implications. Although nuclear scintigraphy (bone scan) for clinical staging of dogs with MM has been performed, due to the predominant osteolytic activity with osteoblastic inactivity present, scans seldom give positive results and are therefore not useful for routine diagnosis.[69] In physician-based oncology, bone mineral density analysis (dual-energy x-ray absorptiometry [DEXA] scan) to document osteoporosis, MRI scan of bone marrow, and PET/CT are commonly used for staging; however, these modalities have not been applied consistently in the veterinary literature. A clinical staging system for canine MM has been suggested[1]; however, at present, no prognostic significance has been attributed to it.

TABLE 32-16 Approximate Frequency of Clinical Diagnostic Abnormalities for Dogs and Cats* with Multiple Myeloma (n = 53 cats, 82 dogs)

	Frequency Range Reported (%)	
Abnormality	**Dogs**	**Cats**
Increased M component	100	94
Monoclonal	100	77-83
Biclonal	<5%†	16-23
IgG	46	84
IgA	54	16
Noncutaneous extramedullary extension	NR	65-100‡
Marrow plasmacytosis (>10%)	100	50-97
CBC abnormalities		
Anemia (nonregenerative)	68	50-64
Thrombocytopenia	33	50
Neutropenia	25	37
Circulating plasma cells (leukemia)	10	5-25
Hypoalbuminemia	65	36
Hypocholesterolemia	NR	68
Proteinuria	35	71
Bence Jones proteinuria	38	40-59
Bone lysis	51	5-45
Serum hyperviscosity	32	35-44
Azotemia	33	22-40
Hypercalcemia	16	10-25
Increased activities of liver enzymes	NR	43-50

NR, Not reported; *CBC*, complete blood count.

*Includes noncutaneous extramedullary plasmacytoma (EMP) cases from Mellor.[11]

†Several single case reports exist for biclonal gammopathy in dogs with MM.

‡11 of 11 in one report had evidence of infiltration in either spleen, lymph node, or liver.

Data from Matus RE, Leifer CE, MacEwen EG, et al: Prognostic factors for multiple myeloma in the dog. *J Am Vet Med Assoc* 188:1288–1291, 1986; MacEwen EG, Hurvitz AI: Diagnosis and management of monoclonal gammopathies, *Vet Clin N Am Small Anim Pract* 7:119–132, 1977; Patel RT, Caceres A, French AF, et al: Multiple myeloma in 16 cats: a retrospective study, *Vet Clin Pathol* 34:341–352, 2005; Mellor PJ, Haugland S, Murphy S, et al: Myeloma-related disorders in cats commonly present as extramedullary neoplasms in contrast to myeloma in human patients: 24 cases with clinical follow-up, *J Vet Intern Med* 20:1376–1383, 2006; Hanna F: Multiple myelomas in cats, *J Feline Med Surg* 7:275–287, 2005; and Drazner FH: Multiple myeloma in the cat, *Comp Cont Ed Pract Vet* 4:206–216, 1982.

Differential Diagnosis of MM

Disease syndromes other than plasma cell tumors can be associated with monoclonal gammopathies and should be considered in any list of differentials. These include other lymphoreticular tumors (B-cell lymphoma, extramedullary plasmacytoma, chronic and acute B-lymphocytic leukemia), chronic infections (e.g., ehrlichiosis, leishmaniasis, FIP), and MGUS.*

*References 5, 9, 60, 61, 70-73.

Treatment

Initial Therapy of Multiple Myeloma

Therapy for MM is directed at both the tumor cell mass and the secondary systemic effects they elicit. All diagnostic procedures should be completed before initiating primary therapy to ensure a diagnosis is complete and baseline values are procured for monitoring response. Chemotherapy is effective at reducing myeloma cell burden, relieving bone pain, allowing for skeletal healing, and reducing levels of serum immunoglobulins in the majority of dogs with MM and will greatly extend both the quality and quantity of most patients' lives. MM in dogs is initially a gratifying disease to treat for both the clinician and the companion animal owner, although complete elimination of neoplastic myeloma cells is rarely achieved and eventual relapse is to be expected. Unlike dogs, only one-half of cats with MM will respond to chemotherapy and most responses will be short-lived; however, several long-term responses (i.e., >1 year) have been reported and treatment should be attempted when educated clients decide on a therapeutic option.*

Melphalan, an alkylating agent, is the chemotherapeutic of choice for the treatment of multiple myeloma.[1,6] In the dog, an initial starting dose of 0.1 mg/kg PO, once daily for 10 days, is then reduced to 0.05 mg/kg PO, once daily continuously. The addition of prednisone therapy is thought to increase the efficacy of melphalan therapy. Prednisone is initiated at a dosage of 0.5 mg/kg PO, once daily for 10 days, then reduced to 0.5 mg/kg every other day prior to discontinuation after 60 days of therapy. Melphalan, however, is continued at 0.05 mg/kg/day until clinical relapse occurs or myelosuppression necessitates a dose reduction. The vast majority of dogs on melphalan and prednisone combination therapy tolerate the regimen well. The most clinically significant toxicity of melphalan is myelosuppression, in particular a delayed thrombocytopenia. CBCs, including platelet counts, should be performed biweekly for 2 months of therapy and monthly thereafter. If significant myelosuppression occurs (usually thrombocytopenia or neutropenia), reduction of the dosage or treatment frequency may be necessary. An alternative pulse-dosing regimen for melphalan (7 mg/m^2 PO, daily for 5 consecutive days every 3 weeks) has been used successfully by the author in a small number of cases in which myelosuppression was limiting more conventional continuous low-dose therapy. This pulse-dose regimen is now being used first-line by the author with the caveat that long-term response data are currently lacking.

Melphalan and prednisone therapy can also be used in cats with multiple myeloma; however, it appears this protocol is more myelosuppressive than in the dog and careful monitoring is required. In the cat, a dosing schedule similar to the dog has been reported[12,26]; 0.1 mg/kg (approximately 0.5 mg, or one-quarter of a 2 mg tablet) once daily for 10 to 14 days, then every other day until clinical improvement or leukopenia develop. Long-term continuous maintenance (0.1 mg/kg, once every 7 days) has been advocated.[12] An alternative protocol advocated in the cat uses melphalan at 2 mg/m^2, once every 4 days continuously, and appears to be well tolerated.[11]

Cyclophosphamide has been used as an alternative alkylating agent or in combination with melphalan in dogs and cats with MM.[1,6,11] There is no evidence to suggest it is superior to melphalan therapy. In the author's practice, cyclophosphamide is limited to those cases presenting with severe hypercalcemia or with widespread systemic involvement in which a faster acting alkylating agent may more quickly alleviate systemic effects of the disease. Cyclophosphamide is initiated at a dosage of 200 mg/m^2 IV, once, at the same time oral melphalan therapy is started. Because cyclophosphamide is less likely to affect thrombocytes, it may be substituted in those patients in which thrombocytopenia has developed secondary to long-term melphalan use.

Chlorambucil, another alkylating agent, has been used successfully for the treatment of IgM macroglobulinemia in dogs at a dosage of 0.2 mg/kg PO, once daily.[6,40] Little or no clinical signs of toxicity result from this dosing schedule. Chlorambucil has also been used in cats with MRD.[11]

Lomustine (CCNU), yet another alkylating agent, has been used in a limited number of cats with MM and a partial response has been reported following dosing at 50 mg/m^2 PO, every 21 days.[74]

*References 6, 9, 11, 12, 31, 26.

Evaluation of Response to Therapy

Evaluation of response to systemic therapy for multiple myeloma is based on improvement in clinical signs, clinicopathologic parameters, and radiographic improvement of skeletal lesions or ultrasonographic improvement of organ involvement.[1,6,11] Subjective improvement in clinical signs of bone pain, lameness, lethargy, and anorexia should be evident within 3 to 4 weeks following initiation of therapy. Objective laboratory improvement, including reduction in serum globulin, immunoglobulin, and calcium, along with normalization of the hemogram, is usually noted within 3 to 6 weeks (Figure 32-26). Radiographic improvement in osteolytic bone lesions may take months and resolution may only be partial. Ophthalmic complications (including long-standing retinal detachments) and paraneoplastic neuropathies can be expected to resolve along with tumor mass.[48,65] In cats responding to chemotherapy, clinical improvement is noted in 2 to 4 weeks and serum protein and radiographic bone abnormalities were greatly improved by 8 weeks.[11,12]

As previously discussed, complete resolution of MM does not generally occur and a good response is defined as a reduction in measured M component (i.e., immunoglobulin or Bence Jones proteins) of at least 50% of pretreatment values.[6] Reduction in serum immunoglobulin levels may lag behind reductions in Bence Jones proteinuria because the half-lives are 15 to 20 days and 8 to 12 hours, respectively.[75] For routine follow-up, quantification of the increased serum globulin, immunoglobulin, or urine Bence Jones protein is performed monthly until a good response is noted and then every 2 to 3 months thereafter. Repeat bone marrow aspiration or imaging (in the case of visceral disease) for evaluation of plasma cell infiltration may be occasionally necessary. Bone marrow reevaluation is particularly prudent when cytopenias develop during chemotherapy, and drug-induced myelosuppression must be differentiated from myelophthisis due to neoplastic marrow recurrence.

Therapy Directed at Complications of Multiple Myeloma

The long-term control of complications, including hypercalcemia, HVS, bleeding diathesis, renal disease, immunosuppression, ophthalmic complications, and pathologic skeletal fractures, depend on controlling the primary tumor mass. Therapy directed more specifically at these complications may, however, be indicated in the short term.

If hypercalcemia is marked and significant clinical signs exist, standard therapies, including fluid diureses, with or without pharmacologic agents (e.g., calcitonin), may be indicated (see Chapter 5). Moderate hypercalcemia will typically resolve within 2 to 3 days following initiation of melphalan/prednisone chemotherapy.

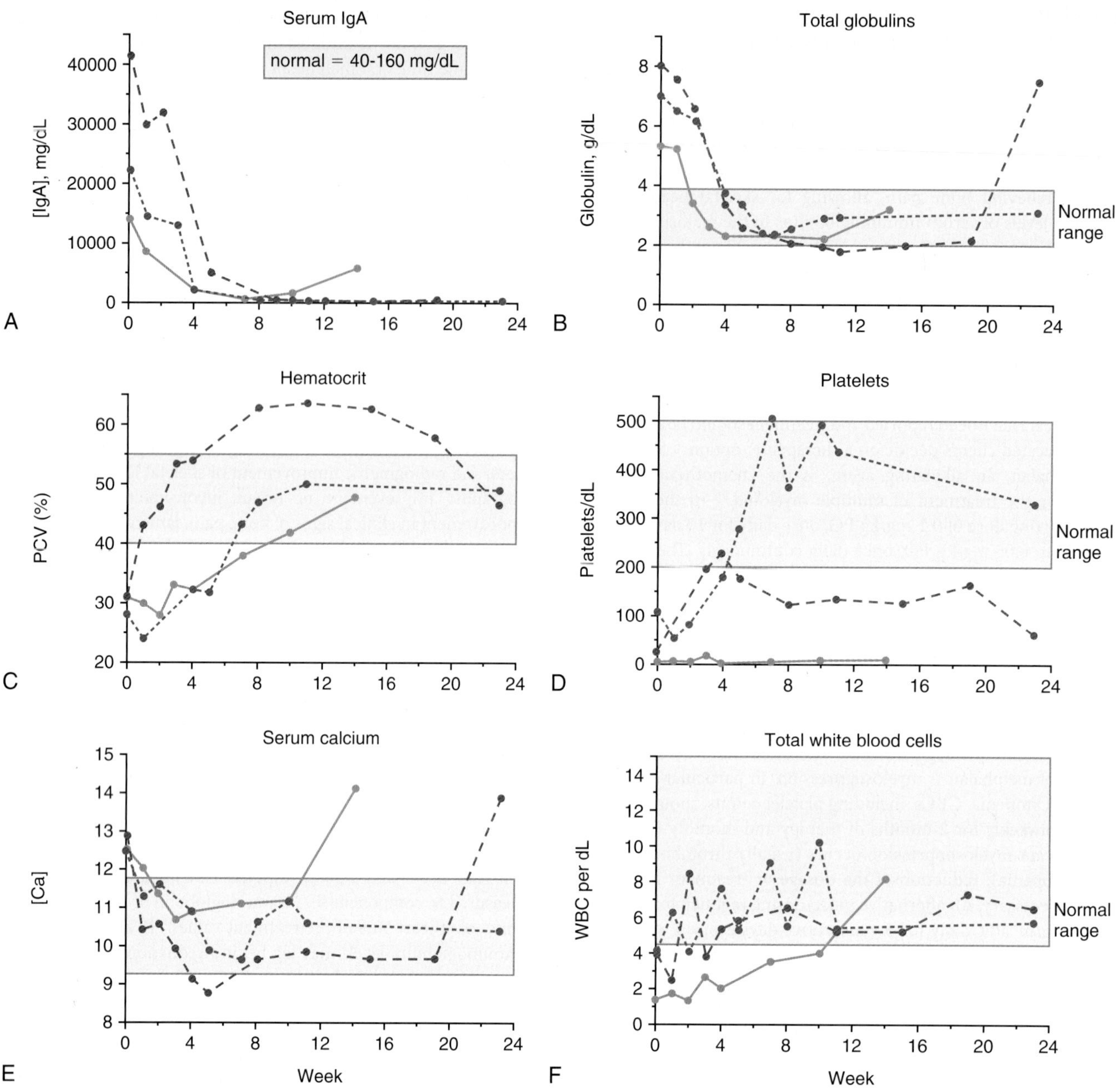

FIGURE 32-26 Clinicopathologic data changes over time (weeks) after initiation of cytotoxic chemotherapy in three dogs with IgA multiple myeloma. *Light blue area,* Normal reference range. **A,** Serum IgA (mg/dL); **B,** total globulins (g/dL); **C,** hematocrit (%); **D,** platelets/dL; **E,** serum calcium (mg/dL); **F,** total white blood cells/dL.

HVS is best treated in the short term by plasmapheresis.* Whole blood is collected from the patient and centrifuged to separate plasma from packed cells. Packed red cells are resuspended in normal saline or other crystalloid and reinfused into the patient. Bleeding diathesis will usually resolve along with HVS; however, platelet-rich plasma transfusions may be necessary in the face of thrombocytopenia.

Renal impairment may necessitate aggressive fluid therapy in the short term and maintenance of adequate hydration in the long term. Careful attention to secondary urinary tract infections and appropriate antimicrobial therapy is indicated. Ensuring adequate water intake at home is important, and occasionally, educating owners in subcutaneous fluid administration is indicated. Continued monitoring of renal function is recommended along with follow-up directed at tumor response.

Patients with MM can be thought of as immunologically impaired. Some have recommended prophylactic antibiotic therapy in dogs with MM[6]; however, in humans, no benefit for this approach over diligent monitoring and aggressive antimicrobial management when indicated has been observed.[43] Cidal antimicrobials are preferred over static drugs, and avoidance of nephrotoxic antimicrobials is recommended.

Pathologic fractures of weight-bearing long bones and vertebrae resulting in spinal cord compression may require immediate surgical intervention in conjunction with systemic chemotherapy.

*References 6, 45, 53, 72, 76, 77.

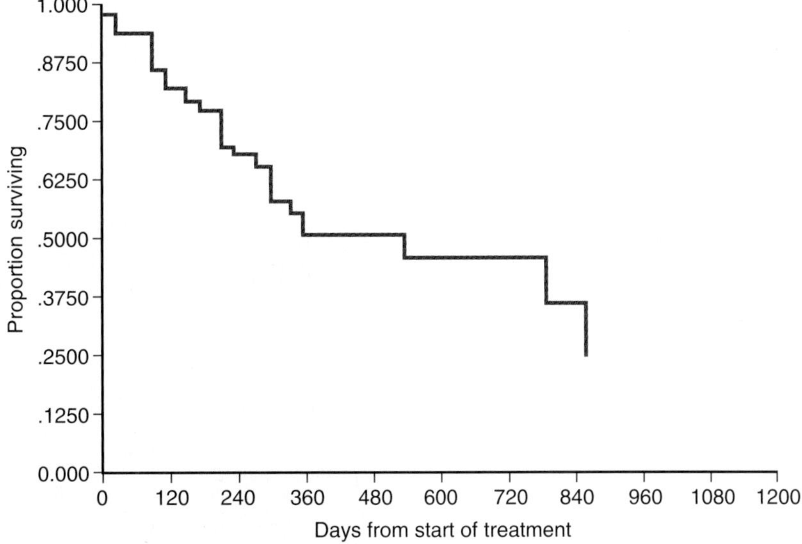

FIGURE 32-27 Survival curve of 37 dogs with multiple myeloma treated with chemotherapy. The median survival time (MST) is 540 days. *(From Matus RE, Leifer CE, MacEwen EG, et al: Prognostic factors for multiple myeloma in the dog,* J Am Vet Med Assoc *188:1288–1292, 1986.)*

Orthopedic stabilization of fractures should be undertaken and may be followed with external-beam RT (see Figure 32-22). Recently, inhibition of osteoclast activity by bisphosphonate drugs has been shown to reduce the incidence and severity of skeletal complications of MM in humans.[69] This class of drugs may hold promise for use in dogs and cats with various skeletal tumors; however, they have not been adequately evaluated in MRD.[78]

Rescue Therapy

When MM eventually relapses in dogs and cats undergoing melphalan therapy or in the uncommon case that is initially resistant to alkylating agents, rescue therapy may be attempted. The author has had success with VAD, which is a combination of doxorubicin (30 mg/m^2 IV, every 21 days), vincristine (0.7 mg/m^2 IV, days 8 and 15), and dexamethasone sodium phosphate (1.0 mg/kg IV, once a week on days 1, 8, and 15), given in 21-day cycles. Whereas most dogs initially respond to this rescue protocol, the duration of response tends to be short, lasting only a few months. High-dose cyclophosphamide (300 mg/m^2 IV, every 7 days) has also been used with limited success as a rescue agent. Liposomal doxorubicin has produced a long-term remission in a dog with MM previously resistant to native doxorubicin.[79]

Investigational Therapies

MM is ultimately a uniformly fatal disease in most species, including humans, and thus significant effort is being placed on investigational therapies for this disease. Currently, bone marrow ablative therapy and marrow or stem cell rescue, thalidomide (and other antiangiogenic therapies), bortezomib (a proteasome inhibitor), arsenic trioxide, the bisphosphonates, and several molecular targeting therapies are under investigation; however, their use in veterinary species is limited or completely absent at present. The promise of molecular targeted therapies is, however, foreshadowed by a case of a dog with MM that was resistant to melphalan, prednisone, and doxorubicin that subsequently achieved a partial response to tyrosine kinase inhibitor therapy (toceranib; see Chapter 14, Section B) that was maintained for 6 months.[18]

Prognosis

The prognosis for dogs with MM is good for initial control of tumor and a return to good quality of life. In a group of 60 dogs with MM, approximately 43% achieved a complete remission (i.e., serum immunoglobulins normalized), 49% achieved a partial remission (i.e., immunoglobulins <50% pretreatment values), and only 8% did not respond to melphalan and prednisone chemotherapy.[1] Long-term survival is the norm, with a median of 540 days reported (Figure 32-27). The presence of hypercalcemia, Bence Jones proteinuria, and extensive bony lysis are known negative prognostic indices in the dog.[1] The long-term prognosis for dogs with MM is poor because recurrence of tumor mass and associated clinical signs is expected. Eventually, the tumor is no longer responsive to available chemotherapeutics and death follows from renal failure, sepsis, or euthanasia for intractable bone or spinal pain.[1,6]

The prognosis for MM in the cat is not as favorable in the short term as it is in the dog.[6,9,11,12,26] Whereas most cats (approximately 60%) transiently respond to melphalan/prednisone or COP-based protocols, most responses are partial and not durable. Typically, cats with MM succumb to their disease within 4 months.[8,9,12,26] However, long-term survivors (>1 year) have been occasionally reported.* In one European case series, seven cats undergoing melphalan or COP-based therapy had a median survival of 9.5 months.[11] One investigator grouped MM in cats into two prognostic categories (Table 32-17) based on criteria known to predict behavior in dogs.[12] Although no rigorous statistical analysis was performed on this small group of nine cats, the median survival for cats in "aggressive" and "nonaggressive" categories was 5 days and 387 days, respectively.

Experience in dogs with IgM macroglobulinemia is limited.[6,40-42] Response to chlorambucil is to be expected, and in nine treated dogs, 77% achieved remission with a median survival of 11 months.[6]

*References 9, 11, 12, 26, 31, 56.

TABLE 32-17 Classification of Multiple Myeloma in Cats Based on Clinical and Diagnostic Criteria Suspected of Predicting Prognosis

BEHAVIOR CATEGORY	CRITERIA
Aggressive	Hypocalcemia, presence of bony lesions with pathological fracture, low packed cell volume (PCV), presence of light-chain Bence Jones protein in urine, azotemia, hypercreatinemia, persistence of high serum protein level after 8 weeks of treatment, little or no clinical improvement.
Less aggressive	Normal serum calcium, normal creatinine, blood urea nitrogen (BUN), PCV levels, presence of bony lesions without pathologic fractures, absence of light-chain Bence Jones protein, normalization of serum protein level after 8 weeks of treatment.

Data from Hanna F: Multiple myelomas in cats, *J Feline Med Surg* 7:275–287, 2005.

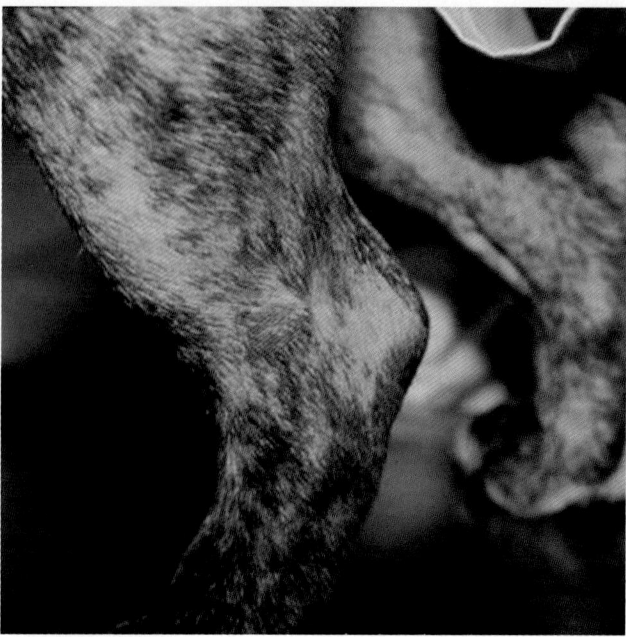

FIGURE 32-28 A cutaneous plasmacytoma on the limb of a dog.

Solitary and Extramedullary Plasmacytic Tumors

Solitary collections of monoclonal plasmacytic tumors can originate in soft tissues or bone and are referred to as *extramedullary plasmacytoma* (EMP) and *solitary osseous plasmacytoma* (SOP), respectively. The systemic, multicentric, biologically aggressive EMP syndrome encountered in cats[11,24] has been discussed in the MM section and will not be included in this discussion. A number of large case compilations of cutaneous plasmacytoma have been reported in the dog.[17,80-86] The most common locations for EMP in the dog are cutaneous (86%; Figure 32-28), the mucous membranes of the oral cavity and lips (9%; Figure 32-29), and the rectum and colon (4%). The skin of the limbs and head (including the ears) are most frequently reported cutaneous sites. Other sites accounted for only 1% of the remaining cases and can include stomach, spleen, genitalia, eye, uterus, liver, larynx, trachea, third eyelid, sinonasal cavity, and intracranial sites.[87-94] The American cocker spaniel, English cocker spaniel, and West Highland white terrier (and perhaps Yorkshire terriers, Boxers, German shepherds, and Airedale terriers) are at increased risk for developing plasmacytomas and the median age of affected dogs is 9 to 10 years of age.[86]

Cutaneous and oral EMP in dogs are typically benign tumors that are highly amenable to local therapy. There exists, however, a rare form of multiple cutaneous plasmacytomas in dogs that is part of a more generalized biologically aggressive MM process.[95,96] The natural behavior of noncutaneous/nonoral EMP appears to be somewhat more aggressive in the dog. GI EMP have been reported on a number of occasions in the veterinary literature, including the esophagus,[91] stomach,[97,98] and small[99] and large intestine.[98-101] Metastasis to associated lymph nodes is more common in these cases; however, bone marrow involvement and monoclonal gammopathies are less commonly encountered. Colorectal EMPs tend to be of low biologic aggressiveness, and most do not recur following surgical excision.[100] Conversely, the majority of SOPs eventually progress to systemic MM; however, the time course from local tumor development to systemic MM may be many months to years.[33,102] SOPs have been reported in the dog involving the appendicular skeleton, as well as the zygomatic arch, and ribs.[33]

SOPs are less common in cats, and fewer reports exist in the literature.[11,22,103-107] They occur in older cats (mean ages 9 to 14 years), with no significant sex predilection. The skin is the most common site; however, other sites include the oral cavity, eye, GI tract, liver, subcutaneous tissues, and brain. Reports exist of cutaneous EMP in cats that progressed to systemic MRD.[11,22,105]

Clinical Signs

Clinical signs associated with SOPs relate to the location of involvement, or in those rare cases with high levels of M component, HVS may occur. Most cutaneous plasmacytomas are solitary, smooth, raised pink nodules from 1 to 2 cm in diameter (see Figure 32-28), although tumors as large as 10 cm have been reported. Combining large series, greater than 95% occur as solitary masses and less than 1% occur as part of a systemic MM process.[17,80-86,95,96] Cutaneous and oral EMPs usually have a benign course with no related clinical signs. GI EMP, however, typically presents with relatively nonspecific signs, which may suggest alimentary involvement. Colorectal plasmacytomas usually present with rectal bleeding, hematochezia, tenesmus, and rectal prolapse.[100] One case of ataxia and seizure activity in a dog with EMP secondary to tumor-associated hypoglycemia has been reported.[64] SOP is usually associated with pain and lameness if the appendicular skeleton is affected or neurologic signs if vertebral bodies are involved.

Diagnosis for Solitary Plasmacytic Tumors

The diagnosis of SOP and EMP usually requires tissue biopsy or FNA for diagnosis. Cells making up solitary plasmacytic tumors in both cats and dogs have been histologically classified into mature, hyaline, cleaved, asynchronous, monomorphous blastic and

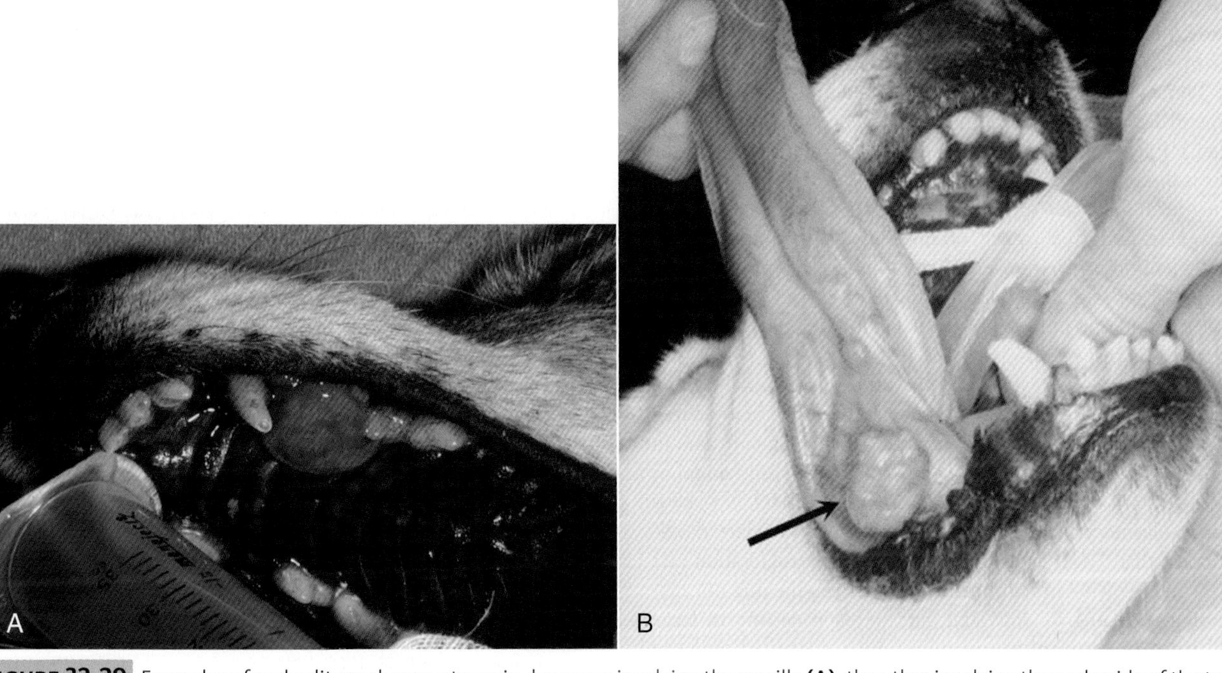

FIGURE 32-29 Examples of oral solitary plasmacytoma in dogs; one involving the maxilla **(A),** the other involving the underside of the tongue **(B).** Both dogs were cured following surgical excision.

polymorphous blastic cell types; however, no prognostic significance has been observed following classification, although it has been suggested that the polymorphous-blastic type may act more aggressively in the dog.[17,86,103] A different classification was proposed for EMP in cats based on percentage of plasmablasts (see previous section), and some prognostic importance has been documented.[24] In the case of poorly differentiated plasmacytic tumors, immunohistochemical studies, directed at detecting immunoglobulin, light- and heavy-chains, MM-1/interferon regulatory factor-4 (MUM1/IRF4), and thioflavin T, may be helpful in differentiation from other round cell tumors.[33,85,86,106-110] Immunoreactivity has been demonstrated for canine IgG F(ab)$_2$ and vimentin.[82] A variant characterized by an IgG-reactive amyloid interspersed with the neoplastic cells has also been described.[83] A panel of MAbs (recognizing tryptase, chymase, serotonin, CD1a, CD3, CD79a, CD18, MHC class II) in association with a histochemical stain (naphthol AS-D chloroacetate) has been advocated for use on formalin-fixed, paraffin-embedded sections of cutaneous round cell tumors to help classify poorly differentiated round cell tumors (mast cell tumors, histiocytomas, lymphomas, and plasmacytomas).[109] Additionally, clonality of the immunoglobulin heavy chain variable region gene can be performed in plasmacytomas and myelomas using PCR technology, and this may have some diagnostic utility in difficult cases.

It is important to thoroughly stage dogs and cats with plasmacytomas that are at higher risk for systemic spread if contemplating local or locoregional therapy without systemic therapy. This should include bone marrow aspiration, serum electrophoresis, abdominal ultrasound, and skeletal survey radiographs to ensure the disease is confined to a local site prior to initiation of therapy. This is most important in cases of SOP and GI EMP due to their relatively high metastatic rate and less important for cutaneous, oral, and colorectal plasmacytomas because of their more typical benign behavior. For GI EMP (including colorectal EMP), endoscopic evaluation of the entire GI tract is recommended. A single case report of the use of PET/CT imaging for extramedullary splenic plasmacytoma in a dog exists; however, its utility remains unknown.[111]

Therapy for Solitary Plasmacytic Tumors

Cutaneous and oral plasma cell tumors in the dog are almost always benign and carry an excellent prognosis following conservative surgical excision.[17,81-86,100,112] EMPs of the trachea, liver, and uterus have also been reported in dogs, and all had a benign course following local resection.[92-94] Successful therapy with melphalan and prednisone has been rarely applied for a local recurrence or incomplete margins in dogs and cats. RT has been used infrequently for cases that are nonsurgical, including the application of strontium-90 plesiotherapy for lingual plasmacytoma in a dog.[113] Surgery is recommended in combination with radiotherapy for those cases of SOP in which the lesion results in an unstable, long bone fracture (see Figure 32-22), or the patient is nonambulatory from neurologic compromise resulting from a vertebral body SOP. In the latter case, spinal cord decompression, mass excision, and possibly spinal stabilization may be necessary.[63] Radiotherapy can be used alone (i.e., without surgery) in those cases where fractures are stable, as a palliative measure for bone pain, or in the case of vertebral SOP if the patient is ambulatory and stable. Good local control is usually achieved; however, most go on to develop systemic multiple myeloma.[33,63,102] SOP of the axial skeleton can be managed by excision or radiotherapy alone. There is controversy as to whether systemic chemotherapy should be initiated at the time of local therapy for SOP when systemic involvement is not documented. Systemic spread may not occur for many months to even years beyond primary SOP diagnosis in humans and dogs, and studies in humans reveal no benefit derived from initiation of systemic chemotherapy prior to documentation of subsequent systemic spread.[44,63] Two cases of SOP in cats were recently reported; one was treated with external-beam RT and one managed with melphalan chemotherapy and both enjoyed durable remissions of greater than 4 years.[114] Similarly, EMP of the GI tract in humans are treated most commonly by surgical excision and thorough staging of disease. Systemic therapy is not initiated unless systemic involvement is documented. Systemic chemotherapy has been used following gastric EMP in a cat; however, the utility of adjuvant therapy in the species is unknown.[115]

Long-term follow-up of patients with SOP is indicated in order to recognize both recurrence of disease and systemic spread. Careful attention is given to serum globulin levels, bone pain, and radiographic appearance of bone healing in cases of SOP. Restaging of disease, including bone marrow evaluation, is indicated if systemic spread is suspected.

Prognosis for solitary plasma cell tumors is generally good. Cutaneous and mucocutaneous plasmacytomas are usually cured following surgical excision.[17,86,112] In large compilations of cases in dogs, the local recurrence rate was approximately 5%, and nodal or distant metastasis occurred in only 7 of 349 cases (2%).[17,80-82,86] New cutaneous plasmacytomas at sites distant from the primary developed in less than 2% of cases. Neither tumor cell proliferation rate (as measured by Ki67 immunohistochemistry) in the dog nor histopathologic grading in dogs and cats were prognostic in large compilations of cases, although it has been suggested that the polymorphous-blastic and plasmablastic type may act more aggressively in the dog and cat.[17,24,86] The presence of amyloid and overexpression of cyclin D1 (prognostic in human plasmacytomas) were not shown to be of prognostic value in dogs.[17] Dogs with EMP of the alimentary tract and other abdominal organs (e.g., liver, uterus) treated by surgical excision alone or in combination with systemic chemotherapy (if metastasis is present) can enjoy long-term survival in the majority of cases.* In a compilation of nine dogs with colorectal plasmacytoma, two dogs had local recurrence at 5 and 8 months following surgery, and the overall median survival was 15 months following surgery alone.[100] DNA ploidy and c-myc oncoprotein expression in biopsy samples were determined to be prognostic for EMPs in dogs; however, those that were malignant were all from noncutaneous sites (i.e., lymph node, colon, spleen). Therefore location appears to be as predictive.[116] As previously discussed, the majority of cases of SOP will eventually develop systemic disease; however, long disease-free periods usually precede the event.

The prognosis in cats is less well-defined because of the paucity of reported cases. If disease is confined to a local site and/or regional nodes, surgical excision and chemotherapy can result in long-term control; however, early, widespread metastasis and progression to MM is also reported in cats.†

REFERENCES

1. Matus RE, Leifer CE, MacEwen EG, et al: Prognostic factors for multiple myeloma in the dog, *J Am Vet Med Assoc* 188:1288–1291, 1986.
2. Liu S-K, Dorfman HD, Hurvitz AI, et al: Primary and secondary bone tumors in the dog, *J Small Anim Pract* 18:313–326, 1977.
3. Weiss DJ: A retrospective study of the incidence and the classification of bone marrow disorders in the dog at a veterinary teaching hospital (1996-2004), *J Vet Intern Med* 20:955–961, 2006.

*References 33, 91-94, 97-99, 101.

†References 11, 22, 84, 103, 104, 107, 115.

4. Tappin SW, Taylor SS, Tasker S, et al: Serum protein electrophoresis in 147 dogs, *Vet Rec* 168:456, 2011.
5. Osborne CA, Perman V, Sautter JH, et al: Multiple myeloma in the dog, *J Am Vet Med Assoc* 153:1300–1319, 1968.
6. MacEwen EG, Hurvitz AI: Diagnosis and management of monoclonal gammopathies, *Vet Clin North Am Small Anim Pract* 7:119–132, 1977.
7. Engle GC, Brodey RS: A retrospective study of 395 feline neoplasms, *J Am Anim Hosp Assoc* 5:21–31, 1969.
8. Carpenter JL, Andrews LK, Holzworth J: Tumors and tumor like lesions. In Holzworth J, editor: *Diseases of the cat: medicine and surgery*, Philadelphia, 1987, WB Saunders.
9. Patel RT, Caceres A, French AF, et al: Multiple myeloma in 16 cats: a retrospective study, *Vet Clin Pathol* 34:341–352, 2005.
10. Taylor SS, Tappin SW, Dodkin SJ, et al: Serum protein electrophoresis in 155 cats, *J Feline Med Surg* 12:643–653, 2010.
11. Mellor PJ, Haugland S, Murphy S, et al: Myeloma-related disorders in cats commonly present as extramedullary neoplasms in contrast to myeloma in human patients: 24 cases with clinical follow-up, *J Vet Intern Med* 20:1376–1383, 2006.
12. Hanna F: Multiple myelomas in cats, *J Feline Med Surg* 7:275–287, 2005.
13. Potter M: A resume of the current status of the development of plasma cell tumors in mice, *Cancer Res* 28:1891–1896, 1968.
14. Potter M, Morrison S, Weiner F, et al: Induction of plasmacytomas with silicone gel in genetically susceptible strains of mice, *J Natl Cancer Inst* 86:1058–1065, 1994.
15. Imahori S, Moore GE: Multiple myeloma and prolonged stimulation of RES, *N Y State J Med* 72:1625–1628, 1972.
16. Porter DD: The development of myeloma-like condition in mink with Aleutian disease, *Blood* 25:736–741, 1967.
17. Cangul IT, Wunen M, van Garderen E, et al: Clinico-pathological aspects of canine cutaneous and mucocutaneous plasmacytomas, *J Vet Med A Physiol Pathol Clin Med* 49:307–312, 2002.
18. London CA, Hannah AL, Zadovoskaya R, et al: Phase I dose-escalating study of SU11654, a small molecule receptor tyrosine kinase inhibitor, in dogs with spontaneous malignancies, *Clin Cancer Res* 9:2755–2768, 2003.
19. Bourget CC, Grufferman S, Delzell E, et al: Multiple myeloma and family history of cancer, *Cancer* 56:2133–2139, 1985.
20. Cuzick J, DeStavola B: Multiple myeloma: A case control study, *Br J Cancer* 57:516–520, 1988.
21. Linet MS, Sioban DH, McLaughlin JK: A case-control study of multiple myeloma in whites: chronic antigenic stimulation, occupation and drug use, *Cancer Res* 47:2978–2981, 1987.
22. Radhakrishnan A, Risbon RE, Patel RT, et al: Progression of a solitary, malignant cutaneous plasma-cell tumour to multiple myeloma in a cat, *Vet Comp Oncol* 2:36–42, 2004.
23. Burnett RC, Blake MK, Thompson LJ, et al: Evolution of a B-cell lymphoma to multiple myeloma after chemotherapy, *J Vet Intern Med* 18:768–771, 2004.
24. Mellor PJ, Haugland S, Smith KC, et al: Histopathologic, immunohistochemical, and cytologic analysis of feline myeloma-related disorders: further evidence for primary extramedullary development in the cat, *Vet Pathol* 45:159–173, 2008.
25. Valli VE, Jacobs RM, Parodi AL, et al: *Histological classification of hematopoietic tumors of domestic animals*, Washington, DC, 2002, Armed Forces Institute of Pathology and The World Health Organization.
26. Drazner FH: Multiple myeloma in the cat, *Comp Cont Ed Pract Vet* 4:206–216, 1982.
27. Jacobs RM, Couto CG, Wellman ML: Biclonal gammopathy in a dog with myeloma and cutaneous lymphoma, *Vet Pathol* 23:211–213, 1986.
28. Peterson EN, Neininger AC: Immunoglobulin A and immunoglobulin G biclonal gammopathy in a dog with multiple myeloma, *J Am Anim Hosp Assoc* 33:45–47, 1997.

29. Ramaiah SK, Sequin MA, Carwile HF, et al: Biclonal gammopathy associated with immunoglobulin A in a dog with multiple myeloma, *Vet Clin Pathol* 31:83–89, 2002.
30. Giraudel JM, Pages JP, Guelfi JF: Monoclonal gammopathies in the dog: A retrospective study of 18 cases (1986-1999) and literature review, *J Am Anim Hosp Assoc* 38:135–147, 2002.
31. Bienzle D, Silverstein DC, Chaffin K: Multiple myeloma in cats: Variable presentation with different immunoglobulin isotypes in two cats, *Vet Pathol* 37:364–369, 2000.
32. Facchini RV, Bertazzolo W, Zuliani D, et al: Detection of biclonal gammopathy by capillary zone electrophoresis in a cat and a dog with plasma cell neoplasia, *Vet Clin Pathol* 39:440–446, 2010.
33. MacEwen EG, Patnaik AK, Hurvitz AI, et al: Nonsecretory multiple myeloma in two dogs, *J Am Vet Med Assoc* 184:1283–1286, 1984.
34. Seelig DM, Perry JA, Avery AC, et al: Monoclonal gammopathy without hyperglobulinemia in 2 dogs with IgA secretory neoplasm, *Vet Clin Pathol* 39:447–453, 2010.
35. Braund KG, Everett RM, Bartels JE, et al: Neurologic complications of IgA multiple myeloma associated with cryoglobulinemia in a dog, *J Am Vet Med Assoc* 174:1321–1325, 1979.
36. Hurvitz AI, MacEwen EG, Middaugh CR, et al: Monoclonal cryoglobulinemia with macroglobulinemia in a dog, *J Am Vet Med Assoc* 170:511–516, 1977.
37. Hickford FH, Stokol T, vanGessel YA, et al: Monoclonal immunoglobulin G cryoglobulinemia and multiple myeloma in a domestic shorthair cat, *J Am Vet Med Assoc* 217:1029–1033, 2000.
38. Cowgill ES, Meel JA, Ruslander D: Light-chain myeloma in a dog, *J Vet Intern Med* 18:119–121, 2004.
39. Yamada O, Tamura K, Yagihara H, et al: Light-chain multiple myeloma in a cat. *J Vet Diagn Invest* 19:443–447, 2007.
40. Gentilini F, Calzolari C, Buonacucina A, et al: Different biological behaviour of Waldenstrom macroglobulinemia in two dogs, *Vet Comp Oncol* 3:87–97, 2005.
41. Hill RR, Clatworthy RH: Macroglobulinemia in the dog, the canine analogue of gamma M monoclonal gammopathy, *J S Afr Vet Med Assoc* 42:309–313, 1971.
42. Hurvitz AI, Haskins SC, Fischer CA: Macroglobulinemia with hyperviscosity syndrome in a dog, *J Am Vet Med Assoc* 157:455–460, 1970.
43. Anderson K: Plasma cell tumors. In Holland JF, Frei E, Bast RC, et al, editors: *Cancer medicine*, ed 3, Philadelphia, 1993, Lea & Febiger.
44. Salmon SE, Cassady JR: Plasma cell neoplasms. In DeVita VT, Hellman S, Rosenberg SA, editors: *Cancer: principles and practice of oncology*, ed 5, Philadelphia, 1997, JB Lippincott.
45. Shull RM, Osborne CA, Barrett RE, et al: Serum hyperviscosity syndrome associated with IgA multiple myeloma in two dogs, *J Am Anim Hosp Assoc* 14:58–70, 1978.
46. Center SA, Smith JF: Ocular lesions in a dog with hyperviscosity secondary to an IgA myeloma, *J Am Vet Med Assoc* 181:811–813, 1982.
47. Kirschner SE, Niyo Y, Hill BL, et al: Blindness in a dog with IgA-forming myeloma, *J Am Vet Med Assoc* 193:349–350, 1988.
48. Hendrix DV, Gelatt KN, Smith PJ, et al: Ophthalmic disease as the presenting complaint in five dogs with multiple myeloma, *J Am Anim Hosp Assoc* 34:121–128, 1998.
49. Hawkins EC, Feldman BF, Blanchard PC: Immunoglobulin A myeloma in a cat with pleural effusion and serum hyperviscosity, *J Am Vet Med Assoc* 188:876–878, 1986.
50. Williams DA, Goldschmidt MH: Hyperviscosity syndrome with IgM monoclonal gammopathy and hepatic plasmacytoid lymphosarcoma in a cat, *J Small Anim Pract* 23:311–323, 1982.
51. Forrester SD, Greco DS, Relford RL: Serum hyperviscosity syndrome associated with multiple myeloma in two cats, *J Am Vet Med Assoc* 200:79–82, 1992.
52. Hribernik TN, Barta O, Gaunt SD, et al: Serum hyperviscosity syndrome associated with IgG myeloma in a cat, *J Am Vet Med Assoc* 181:169–170, 1982.
53. Boyle TE, Holowaychuk MK, Adams AK, et al: Treatment of three cats with hyperviscosity syndrome and congestive heart failure using plasmapheresis, *J Am Anim Hosp Assoc* 47:50–55, 2011.
54. Mundy GR, Bertolini DR: Bone destruction and hypercalcemia in plasma cell myeloma, *Semin Oncol* 13:291–297, 1986.
55. Rosol TJ, Nagode LA, Couto CG, et al: Parathyroid hormone (PTH)-related protein, PTH, and 1,25-dihydroxyvitamin D in dogs with cancer associated hypercalcemia, *Endocrinology* 131:1157–1164, 1992.
56. Sheafor SE, Gamblin RM, Couto CG: Hypercalcemia in two cats with multiple myeloma, *J Am Animal Hosp Assoc* 32:503–508, 1996.
57. Twomey JJ: Infections complicating multiple myeloma and chronic lymphocytic leukemia, *Arch Intern Med* 132:562–565, 1973.
58. Webb J, Chary P, Northrup N, et al: Erythrophagocytic multiple myeloma in a cat, *Vet Clin Pathol* 37:302–307, 2008.
59. Yearly JH, Stanton C, Olivry T, et al: Phagocytic plasmacytoma in a dog, *Vet Clin Pathol* 36:293–296, 2007.
60. Hoenig M, O'Brien JA: A benign hypergammaglobulinemia mimicking plasma cell myeloma, *J Am Anim Hosp Assoc* 24:688–690, 1988.
61. Dewhirst MW, Stamp GL, Hurvitz AI: Idiopathic monoclonal (IgA) gammopathy in a dog, *J Am Vet Med Assoc* 170:1313–1316, 1977.
62. Van Bree H, Pollet L, Cousemont W, et al: Cervical cord compression as a neurologic complication in an IgG multiple myeloma in a dog, *J Am Anim Hosp Assoc* 19:317–323, 1983.
63. Rusbridge C, Wheeler SJ, Lamb CR, et al: Vertebral plasma cell tumors in 8 dogs, *J Vet Intern Med* 13:126–133, 1999.
64. DiBartola SP: Hypoglycemia and polyclonal gammopathy in a dog with plasma cell dyscrasia, *J Am Vet Med Assoc* 180:1345–1348, 1982.
65. Villiers E, Dobson J: Multiple myeloma with associated polyneuropathy in a German shepherd dog, *J Small Anim Pract* 39:249–251, 1998.
66. Mitcham SA, McGillivray SR, Haines DM: Plasma cell sarcoma in a cat, *Can Vet J* 26:98–100, 1985.
67. O'Keefe DA, Couto CG: Fine-needle aspiration of the spleen as an aid in the diagnosis of splenomegaly, *J Vet Intern Med* 1:102–109, 1987.
68. Werner JA, Woo JC, Vernau W, et al: Characterization of feline immunoglobulin heavy chain variable region genes for the molecular diagnosis of B-cell neoplasia, *Vet Pathol* 42:596–607, 2005.
69. Munshi NC, Anderson KC: Plasma cell neoplasms. In DeVita VT, Hellman S, Rosneberg SA, editors: *Cancer principles & practice of oncology*, ed 7, Philadelphia, 2005, Lippincott Williams & Wilkins.
70. Matus RE, Leifer CE, Jurvitz AI: Use of plasmapheresis and chemotherapy for treatment of monoclonal gammopathy associated with *Ehrlichia canis* infection in a dog, *J Am Vet Med Assoc* 190:1302–1304, 1987.
71. Breitschwerdt EB, Woody BJ, Zerbe CA, et al: Monoclonal gammopathy associated with naturally occurring canine ehrlichiosis, *J Vet Intern Med* 1:2–9, 1987.
72. MacEwen EG, Hurvitz AI, Hayes A: Hyperviscosity syndrome associated with lymphocytic leukemia in three dogs, *J Am Vet Med Assoc* 170:1309–1312, 1977.
73. Font A, Closa JM, Mascort J: Monoclonal gammopathy in a dog with visceral leishmaniasis, *J Vet Intern Med* 8:233–235, 1994.
74. Fan TM, Kitchell BE, Dhaliwal RS, et al: Hematological toxicity and therapeutic efficacy of lomustine in 20 tumor-bearing cats: critical assessment of a practical dosing regimen, *J Am Anim Hosp Assoc* 38:357–363, 2002.
75. Ferhangi M, Osserman EF: The treatment of multiple myeloma, *Sem Hematol* 10:149–161, 1973.
76. Bartges JW: Therapeutic plasmapheresis, *Sem Vet Med Surg* 12:170–177, 1997.
77. Farrow BRH, Penny R: Multiple myeloma in a cat, *J Am Vet Med Assoc* 158:606–611, 1971.
78. Milner RJ, Farese J, Henry CJ, et al: Bisphosphonates and cancer, *J Vet Intern Med* 18:597–604, 2004.

79. Kisseberth WC, MacEwen EG, et al: Response to liposome-encapsulated doxorubicin (TLC D-99) in a dog with myeloma, *J Am Vet Med Assoc* 9:425–428, 1995.
80. Clark GN, Berg J, Engler SJ, et al: Extramedullary plasmacytomas in dogs: results of surgical excision in 131 cases, *J Am Anim Hosp Assoc* 28:105–111, 1992.
81. Rakich PM, Latimer KS, Weiss R, et al: Mucocutaneous plasmacytomas in dogs: 75 cases (1980-1987), *J Am Vet Med Assoc* 194:803–810, 1989.
82. Baer KE, Patnaik AK, Gilbertson SR, et al: Cutaneous plasmacytomas in dogs: A morphologic and immunohistochemical study, *Vet Pathol* 26:216–221, 1989.
83. Rowland PH, Valentine BA, Stebbins KE, et al: Cutaneous plasmacytomas with amyloid in six dogs, *Vet Pathol* 28:125–130, 1991.
84. Lucke VM: Primary cutaneous plasmacytomas in the dog and cat, *J Small Anim Pract* 28:49–55, 1987.
85. Kyriazidou A, Brown PJ, Lucke VM: An immunohistochemical study of canine extramedullary plasma cell tumours, *J Comp Pathol* 100:259–266, 1989.
86. Platz SJ, Breuer W, Pfleghaar S, et al: Prognostic value of histopathological grading in canine extramedullary plasmacytomas, *Vet Pathol* 36:23–27, 1999.
87. Witham A, French A, Hill K: Extramedullary laryngeal plasmacytoma in a dog, *N Z Vet J* 60:61–64, 2012.
88. Hayes AM, Gregory SP, Murphy S, et al: Solitary extramedullary plasmacytoma of the canine larynx, *J Small Anim Pract* 48:288–291, 2007.
89. Perlmann E, Dagli ML, Martins MC, et al: Extramedullary plasmacytoma of the third eyelid gland in a dog, *Vet Ophthalmol* 12:102–105, 2009.
90. Schoniger S, Bridger N, Allenspach K, et al: Sinonasal plasmacytoma in a cat, *J Vet Diagn Invest* 19:573–577, 2007.
91. Van Wettere AJ, Linder KE, Suter SE, et al: Solitary intracerebral plasmacytoma in a dog: microscopic, immunohistochemical, and molecular features, *Vet Pathol* 46:949–951, 2009.
92. Chaffin K, Cross AR, Allen SW, et al: Extramedullary plasmacytoma in the trachea of a dog, *J Am Vet Med Assoc* 212:1579–1581, 1998.
93. Choi YK, Lee JY, Park JI, et al: Uterine extramedullary plasmacytoma in a dog, *Vet Rec* 154:699–700, 2004.
94. Aoki M, Kim T, Shimada T, et al: A primary hepatic plasma cell tumor in a dog, *J Vet Med Sci* 66:445–447, 2004.
95. Fukumoto S, Hanazono K, Kawasaki N, et al: Anaplastic atypical myeloma with extensive cutaneous involvement in a dog, *J Vet Med Sci* 2011. Epub ahead of print.
96. Mayer MN, Kerr ME, Grier CK, et al: Immunoglobulin A multiple myeloma with cutaneous involvement in a dog, *Can Vet J* 49:694–702, 2008.
97. Hamilton TA, Carpenter JL: Esophageal plasmacytoma in a dog, *J Am Vet Med Assoc* 204:1210–1211, 1994.
98. MacEwen EG, Patnaik AK, Johnson GF, et al: Extramedullary plasmacytoma of the gastrointestinal tract in two dogs, *J Am Vet Med Assoc* 184:1396–1398, 1984.
99. Jackson MW, Helfand SC, Smedes SL, et al: Primary IgG secreting plasma cell tumor in the gastrointestinal tract of a dog, *J Am Vet Med Assoc* 204:404–406, 1994.
100. Kupanoff PA, Popovitch CA, Goldschmidt MH: Colorectal plasmacytomas: A retrospective study of nine dogs, *J Am Anim Hosp Assoc* 42:37–43, 2006.
101. Trevor PB, Saunders GK, Waldron DR, et al: Metastatic extramedullary plasmacytoma of the colon and rectum in a dog, *J Am Vet Med Assoc* 203:406–409, 1993.
102. Meis JM, Butler JJ, Osborne BM, et al: Solitary plasmacytomas of bone and extramedullary plasmacytomas, *Cancer* 59:1475–1485, 1987.
103. Majzoub M, Breuer W, Platz SJ, et al: Histopathologic and immunophenotypic characterization of extramedullary plasmacytomas in nine cats, *Vet Pathol* 40:249–253, 2003.
104. Michau TM, Proulx DR, Rushton SD, et al: Intraocular extramedullary plasmacytoma in a cat, *Vet Ophthalmol* 6:177–181, 2003.
105. Carothers MA, Johnson GC, DiBartola SP, et al: Extramedullary plasmacytoma and immunoglobulin-associated amyloidosis in a cat, *J Am Vet Med Assoc* 195:1593–1597, 1989.
106. Kryriazidou A, Brown PJ, Lucke VM: Immunohistochemical staining of neoplastic and inflammatory plasma cell lesions in feline tissues, *J Comp Pathol* 100:337–341, 1989.
107. Breuer W, Colbatzky F, Platz S, et al: Immunoglobulin-producing tumours in dogs and cats, *J Comp Pathol* 109:203–216, 1993.
108. Brunnert SR, Altman NH: Identification of immunoglobulin light chains in canine extramedullary plasmacytomas by thioflavine T and immunohistochemistry, *J Vet Diagn Invest* 3:245–251, 1991.
109. Fernandez NJ, West KH, Jackson ML, et al: Immunohistochemical and histochemical stains for differentiating canine cutaneous round cell tumors, *Vet Pathol* 42:437–445, 2005.
110. Ramos-Vara JA, Miller MA, Valli VE: Immunohistochemical detection of multiple myeloma 1/interferon regulatory factor 4 (MUM1/IRF-4) in canine plasmacytoma: comparison with CD79a and CD20, *Vet Pathol* 44:875–884, 2007.
111. Lee AR, Lee MS, Jung IS, et al: Imaging diagnosis—FDG-PET/CT of a canine splenic plasma cell tumor, *Vet Radiol Ultrasound* 51:145–147, 2010.
112. Wright ZM, Rogers KS, Mansell J: Survival data for canine oral extramedullary plasmacytoma: a retrospective analysis (1996-2006), *J Am Anim Hosp Assoc* 44:75–81, 2008.
113. Ware K, Gieger T: Use of strontium-90 plesiotherapy for the treatment of a lingual plasmacytoma in a dog, *J Small Anim Pract* 52:220–223, 2011.
114. Mellor PJ, Polton GA, Brearley M, et al: Solitary plasmacytoma of bone in two successfully treated cats, *J Feline Med Surg* 9:72–77, 2007.
115. Zikes C, Spielman B, Shapiro W, et al: Gastric extramedullary plasmacytoma in a cat, *J Vet Intern Med* 12:381–383, 1998.
116. Frazier KS, Hines ME, Hurvitz AI, et al: Analysis of DNA aneuploidy and c-myc oncoprotein content of canine plasma cell tumors using flow cytometry, *Vet Pathol* 30:505–511, 1993.

Miscellaneous Tumors

33

SECTION A
Hemangiosarcoma

DOUGLAS H. THAMM

Incidence and Risk Factors

Hemangiosarcoma (HSA), also known as *malignant hemangioendothelioma* or *angiosarcoma,* is a malignant neoplasm of vascular endothelial origin. HSA occurs more frequently in dogs than in any other species.[1,2] It represents about 5% of all noncutaneous primary malignant neoplasms and 12% to 21% of all mesenchymal neoplasms in the dog.[3-5] HSA accounts for 2.3% to 3.6% of skin tumors in dogs[1,6] and 45% to 51% of splenic malignancies.[2,7,8] It is less common in the cat, occurring in approximately 0.5% of cats examined at necropsy in one study and accounting for 2% of all neoplasms in another.[9,10]

HSA is seen mostly in middle-aged to older animals, although there are reports in dogs less than 3 years of age.[7,10-14] German shepherds, golden retrievers, and Labrador retrievers are overrepresented in many case series.[7,11,14-16] There may be a slight male predisposition in dogs.[11,12,14,15,17]

Although the etiology is unknown, reports in humans have been related to exposure to thorium dioxide, arsenicals, vinyl chloride, and androgens.[18] It is reported as a rare late sequela to breast-conserving irradiation in humans with breast cancer.[19] The human vascular neoplasm Kaposi's sarcoma is causally associated with human herpesvirus 8, and although some studies have demonstrated herpesviral elements in human angiosarcoma as well, the majority have not.[20-23] There is a documented increase in HSA development in dogs exposed to ionizing radiation prenatally or postnatally.[24] Cutaneous HSAs are found more frequently in dogs with minimal pigmentation and thin hair coats[25] and have been associated with ultraviolet light exposure in laboratory dogs.[26]

There is increasing evidence that dysregulation of molecular pathways governing angiogenesis may be important in the pathogenesis of HSA. Studies in humans and dogs have demonstrated abundant expression of angiogenic growth factors such as vascular endothelial growth factor (VEGF), basic fibroblast growth factor (bFGF), and angiopoietins-1 and -2 (Ang-1 and -2) in HSA cells and tissues and concomitant expression of the cellular receptors for VEGF, bFGF, and Ang-1.[27-36] This suggests the potential for autocrine stimulation of one or more of these receptors leading to dysregulated proliferation and survival. Indeed, enforced overexpression of VEGF is sufficient to transform immortalized murine endothelial cells into HSA,[37] and in vivo overexpression of VEGF has led to vascular tumor formation in mice.[38]

Mutations in tumor suppressor genes such as *p53,*[39,40] *Ras,*[41-43] and *Tsc2*[44] have likewise been implicated in the pathogenesis of HSA, based on murine or human studies. Recent studies suggest that *p53* and *Ras* mutations are infrequent in canine HSA[45-47]; however, *PTEN* inactivation was demonstrated in greater than 50% of evaluated canine HSA samples in one study.[48] Key growth- and apoptosis-regulating proteins such as pRB, cyclin D1, BCL2, and survivin appear overexpressed in HSA when compared with hemangiomas or normal tissues.[46,49] Gene expression profiling studies indicate an enrichment for genes involved in inflammation and angiogenesis.[47]

Pathology and Natural Behavior

In the dog, the most common primary site for HSA is the spleen.[1,11,12,14,15] Other frequent sites include the right atrium, skin and subcutis, and liver.[11,14,25,50-53] Occurrence has also been reported in the lung, kidney, oral cavity, muscle, bone, urinary bladder, left ventricle, uterus, tongue, digit, and retroperitoneum.[12,14,54-60] In the cat, cutaneous and visceral (e.g., spleen, liver, intestine) locations are evenly distributed.[10,61] Other reported sites in the cat include the heart, thoracic cavity, eyelid, and nasal cavity.[10,53,61-64] HSA is the most common splenic neoplasm encountered but is by no means the only differential for splenomegaly or splenic masses in dogs. The "double two-thirds rule" has been applied to canine splenic masses: approximately two-thirds of dogs with splenic masses will have a malignant tumor, and approximately two-thirds of those malignancies will be HSA[2,8,17,65]; however, recent studies have found that 63% to 70% of dogs with splenic masses presenting with nontraumatic hemoabdomen were HSA.[66-68] Several splenic mass lesions (e.g., HSA, hematoma, hemangioma) can have a similar gross and ultrasonographic appearance, and large masses do not necessarily denote malignancy.[69] Histopathology is necessary to establish a definitive diagnosis in these cases.

HSA may be solitary, multifocal within an organ, or widely disseminated at presentation. Grossly, they are of variable size, pale gray to dark red or purple, and soft or gelatinous, often containing blood-filled or necrotic areas on cut surface (Figure 33-1). They are poorly circumscribed, nonencapsulated, and often adhered to adjacent organs. They are extremely friable, and complications associated with rupture and hemorrhage are frequent presenting complaints. Histologically, HSA consists of immature, pleomorphic endothelial cells forming vascular spaces containing variable amounts of blood and/or thrombi.[70,71] When such features are minimal but HSA is suspected, immunohistochemistry for von Willebrand's factor (factor VIII–related antigen) or CD31/platelet endothelial cell-adhesion molecule (PECAM) can be used to demonstrate endothelial derivation and support the diagnosis of

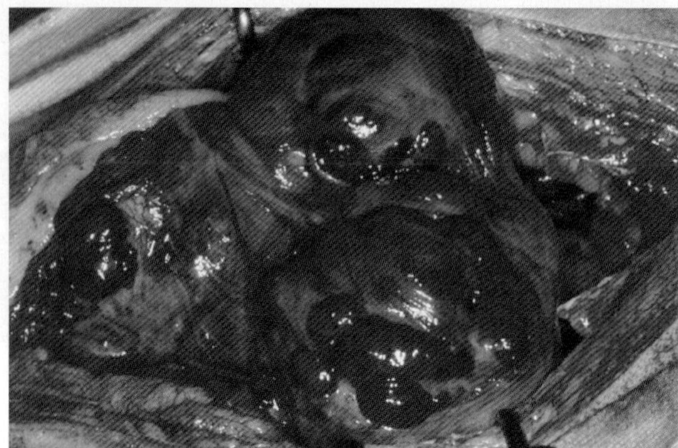

FIGURE 33-1 Intraoperative image of multifocal hemangiosarcoma (HAS) within the spleen of a dog. *(Courtesy M.G. O'Brien, Madison, Wisconsin.)*

HSA.[71-74] Recently, claudin-5 and CD117 (KIT) have also been identified as potentially useful immunohistochemical markers for distinguishing canine tumors of vascular endothelial origin.[75,76]

Perhaps owing to its intimate association with the vasculature, facilitating extravasation and angiogenesis of metastatic clones, canine HSA is typified by very aggressive biologic behavior, with rapid and wide metastasis occurring frequently. An exception to this rule is pure cutaneous or dermal HSA, without any clinical or histologic evidence of subdermal infiltration.[51] Metastasis is typically hematogenous or through transabdominal implantation following rupture. The most frequent metastatic sites are the liver, omentum, mesentery, and lungs.[14,77] One study suggested that approximately, 25% of dogs with splenic HSA will also have right atrial involvement.[77] However, the experience of the author suggests that this percentage at initial presentation is significantly lower (5% or less). Other reported sites of metastasis are the kidney, muscle, peritoneum, lymph nodes, adrenal gland, brain, and diaphragm. In dogs, HSA is considered the most common metastatic tumor to the brain.[78,79]

HSA in cats is considered to be a less aggressive disease. Cutaneous or subcutaneous HSA often behaves in a fashion similar to other soft tissue sarcomas, and local recurrence is the major concern.[72,80,81] Reports do exist of more aggressive biologic behavior in a subset of cats with cutaneous HSA, however.[80-82] Visceral HSAs have a higher metastatic rate, similar to that in dogs, and the common sites include the liver, omentum, diaphragm, pancreas, and lung.[10,61,81,83,84]

History and Clinical Signs

Presenting complaints vary, depending on the location of the primary tumor, and can range from vague, nonspecific signs of illness, to asymptomatic abdominal swelling, to acute collapse and death secondary to hemorrhagic/hypotensive shock. Common presenting complaints for visceral HSA are acute weakness or collapse. This may have been preceded by similar transient episodes occurring over a period of weeks or days, which resolved spontaneously in 12 to 36 hours. In such cases, it is theorized that HSA rupture leads to hemoperitoneum, followed by subsequent reabsorption (i.e., autotransfusion) of red blood cells. For those dogs that present asymptomatically or with vague signs (lethargy, inappetence, weight loss, abdominal distension), an abdominal mass may be palpated during examination. Dogs with cardiac HSA typically present with signs related to pericardial tamponade and associated right-sided heart failure, such as exercise intolerance, dyspnea, and ascites.

Common physical examination findings for visceral HSA include pale mucous membranes with delayed capillary refill, tachycardia with poor pulse quality, and a palpable fluid wave in the abdomen, with or without a palpable abdominal mass. Dogs with cardiac HSA may display ascites, muffled heart sounds, and/or pulsus paradoxus (variation in pulse quality associated with respiration).

In the cat, signs will depend on location and extent of tumor. Cats with visceral tumors usually have a history of lethargy, anorexia, vomiting, sudden collapse, dyspnea, or a distended abdomen.[61,81,83] On physical examination, pallor, pleural or peritoneal fluid, and a palpable abdominal mass may be detected.

Diagnostic Techniques and Work-Up

Complete staging for an HSA suspect typically includes hematology and serum biochemistry, coagulation testing, thoracoabdominal imaging, ±abdominocentesis, and/or echocardiography.

In both dogs and cats, anemia is often seen, usually characterized by the presence of schistocytes (associated with microangiopathic hemolysis) and acanthocytes in the peripheral blood.* Anemia may be regenerative or nonregenerative, depending on duration. Blood typing and/or crossmatching may be indicated if surgery is planned in a severely anemic patient. In addition, a neutrophilic leukocytosis may be seen.[61,66] Thrombocytopenia is observed in 75% to 97% of cases, ranging from mild to severe.[66,67,86,87] Serum biochemistry changes are typically nonspecific and can include hypoalbuminemia, hypoglobulinemia, and mild elevations in liver enzymes.[66,83]

A coagulogram is very useful in animals with suspected HSA. Perturbations in some aspect of the coagulation cascade (prothrombin time [PT], activated partial thromboplastin time [APTT], platelet count, activated clotting time, fibrinogen concentration, fibrin degradation products) are seen in the majority of patients (Table 33-1)[66,86-91] and approximately 50% have coagulation abnormalities that meet the criteria for disseminated intravascular coagulation (DIC).[86,88] Tumor vasculature, especially in the case of HSA, differs significantly from normal vasculature, commonly containing blind-ended or irregular tortuous vessels, incomplete endothelial lining, arteriovenous shunts, exposed subendothelial collagen, and platelet-tumor aggregates.[92] HSA-derived endothelial cells may also have an "activated" phenotype, further promoting initiation of the coagulation cascade.

HSA effusions are serosanguineous (or frank blood) and usually do not clot. Cytology of effusions is rarely diagnostic; although tumor cells are likely present, they are heavily diluted with peripheral blood.

Screening for metastasis is mandatory prior to definitive surgery for HSA. Dogs with gross evidence of metastasis have a grave prognosis, and surgery is purely palliative. Thoracic radiographs should be obtained in all cases. One study reported a 78% sensitivity and 74% negative predictive value for detecting pulmonary manifestations of HSA, and obtaining three views significantly decreased the

*References 12, 14, 61, 66, 83, 85.

false-negative rate.[93] Dogs with hemopericardium secondary to cardiac HSA will typically have a globoid cardiac silhouette, with or without distension of the caudal vena cava.[94] Abdominal radiographs may reveal a cranial abdominal mass in many cases; however, abdominal ultrasound is a superior modality for imaging the abdomen. Many animals with visceral HSA will have ascites, which diminishes abdominal detail with radiographs but not ultrasound. Ultrasound also allows for the more thorough evaluation of the rest of the abdomen for evidence of metastatic disease. HSA typically has a heteroechoic appearance, ranging from anechoic/cavitated to hyperechoic, or a targetoid appearance (Figure 33-2).[95,96]

Typical electrocardiographic signs consistent with pericardial effusion (decreased amplitude QRS complex, electrical alternans) can be seen in dogs with cardiac HSA and hemopericardium. Echocardiography can be useful in dogs with suspected pericardial effusion, and a right atrial mass may be visible in 65% to 90% of cases (Figure 33-3)[97-100]; however, some dogs may develop blood clots within the pericardium that can have a mass effect. Thus the absence of a mass does not rule out HSA, and the presence of a mass is not pathognomonic. Despite this, detection of a mass on echocardiography is strongly associated with a worse prognosis in dogs with pericardial effusion.[94,99] Other negative prognostic factors include

TABLE 33-1 Coagulation Abnormalities in Dogs with Hemangiosarcoma

COAGULATION PARAMETER	% ABNORMAL
Prolonged PT	12.5
Prolonged APTT	46
Thrombocytopenia	75-97
Increased fibrin degradation products	46-93
Hypofibrinogenemia	8-46
Criteria for DIC	47-50

PT, Prothrombin time; *APTT,* activated partial thromboplastin time; *DIC,* disseminated intravascular coagulation.

Data from Pintar J, Breitschwerdt EB, Hardie EM, et al: Acute nontraumatic hemoabdomen in the dog: a retrospective analysis of 39 cases (1987-2001), *J Am Anim Hosp Assoc* 39:518–522, 2003; Hammer AS, Couto CG, Swardson C, et al: Hemostatic abnormalities in dogs with hemangiosarcoma, *J Vet Intern Med* 5:11–14, 1991; Hargis AM, Feldman BF: Evaluation of hemostatic defects secondary to vascular tumors in dogs: 11 cases, *J Am Vet Med Assoc* 198:891–894, 1991; Maruyama H, Miura T, Sakai M, et al: The incidence of disseminated intravascular coagulation in dogs with malignant tumor, *J Vet Med Sci* 66:573–575, 2004; Mischke R, Wohlsein P, Schoon HA: Detection of fibrin generation alterations in dogs with haemangiosarcoma using resonance thrombography, *Thromb Res* 115:229–238, 2005; Rishniw M, Lewis DC: Localized consumptive coagulopathy associated with cutaneous hemangiosarcoma in a dog, *J Am Anim Hosp Assoc* 30:261–264, 1994; Maruyama H, Watari T, Miura T, et al: Plasma thrombin-antithrombin complex concentrations in dogs with malignant tumours, *Vet Rec* 156: 839–840, 2005.

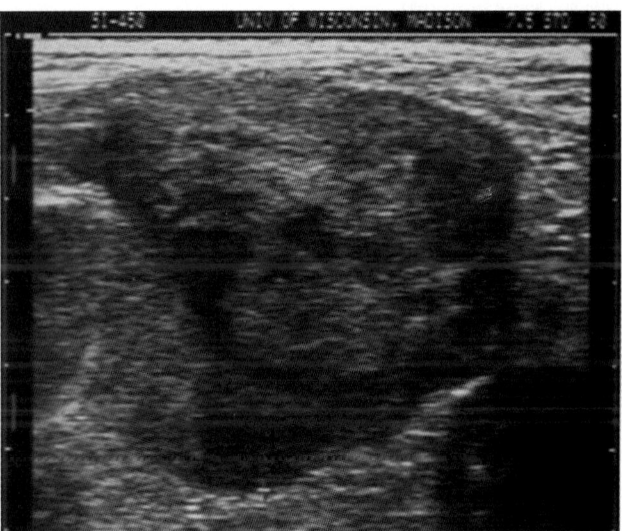

FIGURE 33-2 Ultrasound image of canine splenic hemangiosarcoma (HSA). *(Courtesy R.T. O'Brien, University of Illinois, College of Veterinary Medicine.)*

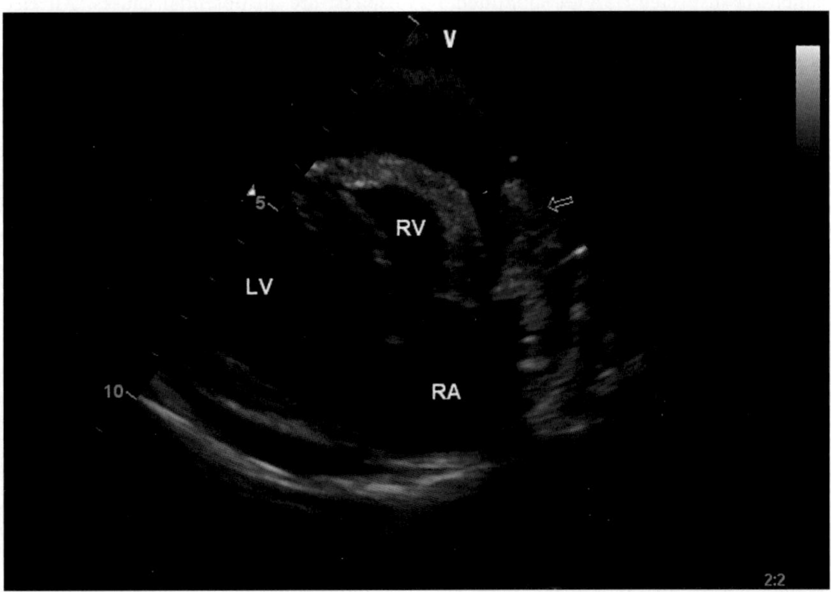

FIGURE 33-3 Echocardiographic image of right atrial hemangiosarcoma (HSA) with pericardial effusion. *LV,* Left ventricle; *RV,* right ventricle; *RA,* right atrium. Arrow indicates mass in region of right atrial appendage. *(Courtesy J Boon, Colorado State University, Veterinary Teaching Hospital.)*

TABLE 33-2 Clinical Staging System for Canine Hemangiosarcoma

Primary Tumor (T)	
T0	No evidence of tumor
T1	Tumor less than 5 cm diameter and confined to primary site
T2	Tumor 5 cm or greater or ruptured: invading subcutaneous tissues
T3	Tumor invading adjacent structures, including muscle
Regional Lymph Nodes (N)	
N0	No regional lymph node involvement
N1	Regional lymph node involvement
N2	Distant lymph node involvement
Distant Metastasis (M)	
M0	No evidence of distant metastasis
M1	Distant metastasis
Stages	
I	T0 or T1, N0, M0
II	T1 or T2, N0 or N1, M0
III	T2 or T3, N0, N1 or N2, M1

history of collapse and presence of ascites.[94] Routine evaluation of the heart for metastatic disease in a dog with subcutaneous or visceral HSA without evidence of other metastasis is rarely rewarding.

A clinical staging system for HSA is given in Table 33-2.

Ultimately, a definitive diagnosis of HSA usually requires a surgical biopsy. Needle aspiration cytology of suspicious masses, although simple and cost-effective, is of low diagnostic utility due to the hemodilution that usually accompanies sampling.[101] Needle core biopsies can be obtained of cutaneous or subcutaneous lesions but should not be performed on suspect visceral lesions due to the risk of induction of hemorrhage and subsequent seeding of the peritoneum. If only small samples of suspected HSA are submitted, histopathology may only reveal blood clots or other nonspecific findings. Submission of large samples of suspected HSA is preferred to maximize the likelihood of capturing a true tumor if present. This includes submission of entire spleens whenever possible or, at the very least, numerous parts of the mass.

Several investigators are evaluating additional tests, which may allow more accurate presurgical diagnosis. Pericardial fluid pH was suggested to correlate with presence or absence of neoplasia in one study[102]; however, subsequent studies have shown pericardial fluid analysis to be of little diagnostic benefit.[103,104] Recent studies have found a significant difference in concentrations of troponin I, an indicator of myocardial damage, between dogs with cardiac HSA and dogs with idiopathic pericardial effusions.[105,106] Plasma concentrations of VEGF and urine concentrations of bFGF are elevated in dogs with HSA versus normal controls[27,28]; however, neither was found to correlate with remission status, disease stage, or outcome. Advanced imaging techniques such as contrast-enhanced ultrasound,[107-113] contrast-enhanced computed tomography (CT),[114] and magnetic resonance imaging (MRI)[115] have been useful in discriminating malignant versus benign lesions in preliminary studies. Additional blood-based biomarkers showing early promise include measurement of serum alpha-1 acid glycoprotein,[116] lipocalin region of collagen XXVII alpha 1,[117] and thymidine kinase activity,[118,119] as well as multiparameter flow cytometry of peripheral blood utilizing a variety of endothelial and primitive hematopoietic cell markers.[120]

Treatment

Surgery

Surgery remains the primary method of treatment for almost all dogs and cats with HSA. Prior to surgery, appropriate treatment for shock (e.g., crystalloids, colloids) and correction of severe hematologic or coagulation abnormalities should be addressed with blood products as necessary. Surgery should be as aggressive as possible to remove all locally affected tissue.

For cutaneous or subcutaneous HSA, surgical considerations are similar to those for other soft-tissue sarcomas (see Chapter 21). Dermal HSA is usually discrete, and surgical margins of 1 to 2 cm are often adequate. Intramuscular HSA will often present with a large blood clot admixed with actual tumor. Wide margins can be difficult to achieve, short of limb amputation when possible. Debulking may provide short-term relief.

For splenic HSA, splenectomy is required and can be performed with sutures, staples, or electrothermal vessel sealant devices (e.g., LigaSure Force Triad, Covidien, Mansfield, MA).[121] The spleen should be carefully delivered from the abdomen to avoid iatrogenic rupture. Attached omentum should be removed en bloc. Intraoperative autotransfusion of blood has been described but requires specialized equipment and personnel and still remains controversial.[122] At the time of splenectomy, the abdomen should be thoroughly explored and any suspicious lesions in the liver or omentum, especially if actively bleeding, should be excised and submitted for histopathology. Biopsy of grossly normal livers is probably not useful. The abdomen should be thoroughly lavaged and instruments changed prior to closure to minimize the risk of abdominal/wound bed or suture line seeding. Dogs undergoing splenectomy are prone to develop ventricular arrhythmias following surgery. In one study of 59 dogs, 24% developed arrhythmias.[123] Poor myocardial perfusion secondary to hypoxia, hypovolemia, or anemia or a neurohormonal response associated with manipulation of the spleen are all potential causes. An electrocardiogram should be monitored intraoperatively and in the postoperative period, and arrhythmias treated as they arise. Arrhythmias usually resolve within 24 to 48 hours.

Surgery can be performed for primary cardiac HSA. An open or thoracoscopic pericardiectomy can be used as a palliative procedure, allowing effusion to escape into the thorax rather than accumulating in the pericardium, where a small volume can readily restrict function. Right atrial appendage masses can be resected with a stapling device or hand stitching,[124,125] and reconstructive procedures have been described in cases where extensive resection is required.[126,127] A recent retrospective study suggests that dogs surviving the perioperative period have a prognosis similar to dogs with HSA of other visceral sites.[125]

Chemotherapy

Given the very high metastatic rate of most canine HSA and the poor outcome associated with surgery alone (see later), adjuvant chemotherapy is indicated in all cases, with the exception of pure cutaneous tumors. Single-agent and combination doxorubicin (DOX)-based chemotherapy protocols are most frequently used (Box 33-1).[128-134] Other combinations such as vincristine, cyclophosphamide, and methotrexate (VCM) have yielded only modest improvements in survival time.[14] Recently, ifosfamide was shown

Box 33-1 Doxorubicin-Based Chemotherapy Protocols for Canine Hemangiosarcoma

1. VAC*

Day 1	Doxorubicin† 30 mg/m² IV Cyclophosphamide 100-150 mg/m² IV OR Cyclophosphamide 150-200 mg/m² PO, divided over 3-4 days
Days 8 and 15	Vincristine 0.75 mg/m² IV
Day 22	Repeat cycle for a total of 4-6 cycles

2. AC*

Day 1	Doxorubicin† 30 mg/m² IV Cyclophosphamide 100-150 mg/m² IV OR Cyclophosphamide 150-200 mg/m² PO, divided over 3-4 days
Day 22	Repeat cycle for a total of 4-6 cycles

3. DOX*	Doxorubicin† 30 mg/m² IV Repeat every 2-3 weeks for 5 treatments

VAC, Vincristine, doxorubicin, cyclophosphamide; *IV*, Intravenous; *PO*, by mouth; *AC*, doxorubicin, cyclophosphamide; *DOX*, doxorubicin.

*Perform complete blood count (CBC) prior to each chemotherapy treatment—delay treatment for 5-7 days if neutrophils <2000/uL or platelets <75,000/uL.

†Doxorubicin is given at 25 mg/m² or 1 mg/kg in dogs weighing less than 10 kg.

to also have some modest antitumor activity in canine HSA.[134,135] Both epirubicin and liposome-encapsulated DOX appear to have roughly equivalent activity to conventional DOX.[136,137] In cats, similar DOX-based protocols are employed, although reports of systematic evaluations are lacking. For cases in which surgery is declined or impossible due to size/location or presence of metastasis, DOX-based chemotherapy induces meaningful tumor regression in a large minority of animals[138-140]; however, remissions are typically incomplete and brief in duration. Isolated reports of antitumor activity have been reported with carboplatin as well.[141]

Immunotherapy

Very few studies have been conducted to evaluate biologic therapy for HSA (see Chapter 13). One study used a mixed killed bacterial vaccine following surgery and showed some improvement in survival time in dogs with splenic HSA.[14] More recently, a surgical adjuvant study was conducted in dogs with splenic HSA to compare chemotherapy (DOX and cyclophosphamide) to the same chemotherapy combined with immunotherapy using liposome-encapsulated muramyl tripeptide-phosphatidylethanolamine (L-MTP-PE). The median survival time (MST) for those dogs treated with chemotherapy alone was 5.7 months versus 9.1 months (p = 0.03) for those treated with L-MTP-PE and chemotherapy, with 40% of dogs in the L-MTP-PE group experiencing long-term survival.[133] L-MTP-PE is currently unavailable in the United States but has been granted orphan drug status for the treatment of pediatric osteosarcoma in the European Union. Investigations of allogeneic tumor cell vaccine approaches in combination with chemotherapy have shown initial promise in small numbers of dogs.[142]

Radiation Therapy

Radiation therapy (RT) is rarely utilized for HSA due to the anatomic sites involved and high metastatic rate. Coarsely fractionated (palliative) RT for peripheral masses (e.g., cutaneous and subcutaneous lesions) may dramatically decrease local disease but may not significantly impact overall survival.[143-145] It is conceivable that a combination of palliative RT and chemotherapy may provide better control, but this awaits further investigation. Full-course (definitive) RT may be reasonable for dogs with incompletely resected, solitary dermal HSA or feline nonvisceral HSA due to their reduced potential for metastasis.

Novel Therapies

Given the endothelial derivation of HSA, therapy directed against angiogenesis is a logical avenue of exploration, and murine HSA has been used as a model for the evaluation of novel antiangiogenic strategies. Antitumor activity has been seen in a murine HSA model to a variety of antiangiogenic treatments, such as VEGF receptor kinase inhibitors,[146] TNP-470,[147] and several others,[148-150] and objective responses have been observed with several angiogenic receptor tyrosine kinase inhibitors in human reports.[151,152] Interleukin-12 (IL-12) has been shown to retard tumor growth in a canine HSA xenograft as well.[33]

A small pilot study recently reported the outcome following treatment of dogs with splenic HSA with a combination of splenectomy, a nonsteroidal antiinflammatory drug (NSAID), and low-dose continuous (metronomic) chemotherapy with alternating courses of cyclophosphamide and etoposide. Outcome was similar to what has been reported following DOX-based injectable chemotherapy.[153]

Current studies are focusing on whether combinations of conventional DOX-based chemotherapy followed by "maintenance" therapy with low-dose continuous chemotherapy or VEGF receptor kinase inhibitors such as toceranib may improve postsurgical outcome in patients with HSA; the results of these studies are eagerly anticipated.

In humans with various vascular tumors, antitumor activity has been observed following the local administration of IL-2,[154,155] and the local or systemic administration of interferon-α (IFNα) in combination with traditional cytotoxics.[156-159] Additionally, paclitaxel, docetaxel, and gemcitabine appear to have activity against human HSA.[157,160-162]

Prognosis

Canine

A summary of the results of several reports on the treatment of splenic HSA is presented in Table 33-3. Overall, the prognosis for dogs with splenic HSA treated by surgery alone is extremely poor. MSTs for splenic HSA range from 19 to 86 days, and less than 10% survive to 12 months.[2,8,14,163,164] Primary hepatic HSA is thought to carry an equally poor prognosis. In contrast, one study suggests that dogs with primary renal HSA may have a more favorable outcome than those with HSA of other visceral sites.[60]

Surgery plus anthracycline-based chemotherapy following surgery will increase median survival times to 141 to 179 days.* Even with the addition of chemotherapy, the 12-month survival percentage is 10% or less. In one report, the addition of immunotherapy (L-MTP-PE) to standard chemotherapy increased median

*References 128, 129, 131, 132, 134, 136, 137.

TABLE 33-3 Comparison of Survival Times in Dogs with Splenic Hemangiosarcoma

TREATMENT	DOGS (NO)	MEDIAN SURVIVAL TIME (DAYS)	REFERENCES
Splenectomy	Various	19-86	2, 8, 14, 136, 137, 163
Splenectomy + MBV	10	91	14
Splenectomy + MBV + VMC	10	117	14
Splenectomy + LDCC	9	178	153
Splenectomy + Ifosfamide	6	142	135
Splenectomy + Ifosfamide/DOX	13	123	134
Splenectomy + Epirubicin	59	144	136
Splenectomy + Doxil	14	132	137
Splenectomy + VAC	6	145	128
Splenectomy + AC	Various	141-179	132, 133
Splenectomy + AC + L-MTP-PE	16	273	133

MBV, Mixed bacterial vaccine; *VMC,* vincristine, methotrexate, cyclophosphamide; *LDCC,* Low-dose, continuous chemotherapy; *DOX,* doxorubicin; *VAC,* vincristine, doxorubicin, cyclophosphamide; *AC,* doxorubicin, cyclophosphamide; *L-MTP-PE,* liposome muramyl tripeptide phosphatidylethanolamine.

survival time to 273 days.[133] In splenic HSA, stage I (nonruptured) tumors may have a more favorable outcome than stage II (ruptured) tumors when postoperative chemotherapy is used.[14,130,133] One study employed a histologic grading scheme, and demonstrated that dogs with low-grade tumors had a better prognosis than dogs with intermediate- or high-grade tumors.[129]

In a study of surgically treated cutaneous HSA, tumors involving the dermis (without subdermal invasion) had a MST of 780 days (n = 10).[51] Tumors with invasion into the subcutaneous tissues or muscle generally have worse outcomes than those confined to the dermis.[11,51,165,166] Therefore adjuvant medical therapy should be offered for subcutaneous or intramuscular HSA, although reports regarding efficacy are divergent.[165,166]

Overall, the prognosis is poor for cardiac HSA. In dogs undergoing surgery for right atrial HSA, the average survival time ranges from 1 to 4 months.[99,124] A recent study reported an outcome following surgery and chemotherapy roughly equivalent to that reported for HSA of the spleen.[125]

Feline

In cats, the prognosis for visceral HSA is poor. Most cats die from recurrence of the primary tumor or metastasis, and MSTs are generally short, owing to metastasis.[61,84] HSAs located in cutaneous and subcutaneous sites have recurrence rates of 60% to 80%,[61,72] although one recent case series reported a favorable outcome following aggressive surgery, and complete excision is associated with improvement in outcome.[80,81] Metastasis can develop following surgical resection in some cases, although the frequency is unknown.[82]

In summary, surgery still offers the best approach to diagnose and treat HSA even though it is generally only palliative. Novel avenues for adjuvant chemotherapy need evaluation. New approaches to treatment such as immunotherapy or antiangiogenic therapy may provide alternatives, and additional investigation into the biology of canine HSA, hopefully leading to clinical trials, is desperately needed.

Comparative Aspects

In humans, a spectrum of endothelial tumors, including hemangioma, hemangioblastoma, Kaposi's sarcoma, hemangioendothelioma, and angiosarcoma, is seen. Angiosarcoma is extremely rare in humans and can be a late sequela to RT in women treated for breast cancer.[167] With this exception, it has a lesion distribution and behavior similar to canine HSA. As in dogs, metastasis is frequent and adjuvant chemotherapy provides minimal benefit.

REFERENCES

1. Priester W, McKay F: *The occurrence of tumors in domestic animals,* Washington, DC, 1980, National Cancer Institute Monograph.
2. Spangler WL, Culbertson MR: Prevalence, type, and importance of splenic diseases in dogs: 1,480 cases (1985-1989), *J Am Vet Med Assoc* 200:829–834, 1992.
3. Bastianello SS: A survey on neoplasia in domestic species over a 40-year period from 1935 to 1974 in the republic of South Africa. VI. Tumors occurring in dogs, *Onderspoort J Vet Res* 50:199–220, 1983.
4. Dorn CR, Taylor DON, Schneider R, et al: Survey of animal neoplasms in Alameda and Contra Costa Counties. Cancer morbidity in dogs and cats from Alameda County, *J Natl Cancer Inst* 40:307–318, 1968.
5. MacVean DW, Monlux AW, Anderson PS, et al: Frequency of canine and feline tumors in a defined population, *Vet Pathol* 145:700–715, 1978.
6. Rostami M, Tateyama S, Uchida K, et al: Tumor in domestic animals examined during a ten-year period (1980 to 1989) at Miyazaki University, *J Vet Med Sci* 56:403–405, 1991.
7. Day MJ, Lucke VM, Pearson H: A review of pathological diagnoses made from 87 canine splenic biopsies, *J Small Anim Pract* 36: 426–433, 1995.
8. Spangler WL, Kass PH: Pathologic factors affecting postsplenectomy survival in dogs, *J Vet Intern Med* 11:166–171, 1997.
9. Carpenter JL, Andrews LK, Holzworth J: Tumors and tumor-like lesions. In Holzworth J, editor: *Diseases of the cat: medicine and surgery,* Philadelphia, 1987, WB Saunders.
10. Patnaik AK, Liu SK: Angiosarcoma in cats, *J Small Anim Pract* 18:191–198, 1977.
11. Schultheiss PC: A retrospective study of visceral and nonvisceral hemangiosarcoma and hemangiomas in domestic animals, *J Vet Diagn Invest* 16:522–526, 2004.
12. Oksanen A: Haemangiosarcoma in dogs, *J Comp Pathol* 88:585–595, 1978.
13. Arp LH, Grier RL: Disseminated cutaneous hemangiosarcoma in a young dog, *J Am Vet Med Assoc* 185:671–673, 1984.
14. Brown NO, Patnaik AK, MacEwen EG: Canine hemangiosarcoma: retrospective analysis of 104 cases, *J Am Vet Med Assoc* 186:56–58, 1985.
15. Srebernik N, Appleby EC: Breed prevalence and sites of haemangioma and haemangiosarcoma in dogs, *Vet Rec* 129:408–409, 1991.
16. Moe L, Gamlem H, Dahl K, et al: Canine neoplasia–population-based incidence of vascular tumours, *APMIS* Suppl:63–68, 2008.
17. Gamlem H, Nordstoga K, Arnesen K: Canine vascular neoplasia–a population-based clinicopathologic study of 439 tumours and tumour-like lesions in 420 dogs, *APMIS* Suppl:41–54, 2008.

18. Falk H, Herbert J, Crowley S, et al: Epidemiology of hepatic angiosarcoma in the United States: 1964-1974, *Environ Health Perspect* 41:107–113, 1981.
19. Weaver J, Billings SD: Postradiation cutaneous vascular tumors of the breast: a review, *Semin Diagn Pathol* 26:141–149, 2009.
20. Gessi M, Cattani P, Maggiano N, et al: Demonstration of human herpesvirus 8 in a case of primary vaginal epithelioid angiosarcoma by in situ hybridization, electron microscopy, and polymerase chain reaction, *Diagn Mol Pathol* 11:146–151, 2002.
21. Remick SC, Patnaik M, Ziran NM, et al: Human herpesvirus-8-associated disseminated angiosarcoma in an HIV-seronegative woman: report of a case and limited case-control virologic study in vascular tumors, *Am J Med* 108:660–664, 2000.
22. Fink-Puches R, Zochling N, Wolf P, et al: No detection of human herpesvirus 8 in different types of cutaneous angiosarcoma, *Arch Dermatol* 138:131–132, 2002.
23. Palacios I, Umbert I, Celada A: Absence of human herpesvirus-8 DNA in angiosarcoma, *Br J Dermatol* 140:170–171, 1999.
24. Benjamin SA, Lee AC, Angleton GM, et al: Mortality in beagles irradiated during prenatal and postnatal development. II. Contribution of benign and malignant neoplasia, *Radiat Res* 150:330–348, 1998.
25. Hargis AM, Ihrke PJ, Spangler WL, et al: A retrospective clinicopathologic study of 212 dogs with cutaneous hemangiomas and hemangiosarcomas, *Vet Pathol* 29:316–328, 1992.
26. Nikula KJ, Benjamin SA, Angleton GM, et al: Ultraviolet radiation, solar dermatosis, and cutaneous neoplasia in beagle dogs, *Radiat Res* 129:11–18, 1992.
27. Clifford CA, Hughes D, Beal MW, et al: Plasma vascular endothelial growth factor concentrations in healthy dogs and dogs with hemangiosarcoma, *J Vet Intern Med* 15:131–135, 2001.
28. Duda LE, Sorenmo KU: Urine basic fibroblast growth factor in canine hemangiosarcoma. In *Proceedings of the Veterinary Cancer Society Annual Conference*, 73, Chicago, 1997.
29. Amo Y, Masuzawa M, Hamada Y, et al: Observations on angiopoietin 2 in patients with angiosarcoma, *Br J Dermatol* 150:1028–1029, 2004.
30. Brown LF, Tognazzi K, Dvorak HF, et al: Strong expression of kinase insert domain-containing receptor, a vascular permeability factor/vascular endothelial growth factor receptor in AIDS-associated Kaposi's sarcoma and cutaneous angiosarcoma, *Am J Pathol* 148:1065–1074, 1996.
31. Hashimoto M, Oshawa N, Ohnishi A, et al: Expression of vascular endothelial growth factor and its receptor mRNA in angiosarcoma, *Lab Invest* 73:859–863, 1995.
32. Yamamoto T, Umeda T, Yokozeki H, et al: Expression of basic fibroblast growth factor and its receptor in angiosarcoma, *J Am Acad Dermatol* 41:127–129, 1999.
33. Akhtar N, Padilla ML, Dickerson EB, et al: Interleukin-12 inhibits tumor growth in a novel angiogenesis canine hemangiosarcoma xenograft model, *Neoplasia* 6:106–116, 2004.
34. Fosmire SP, Dickerson EB, Scott AM, et al: Canine malignant hemangiosarcoma as a model of primitive angiogenic endothelium, *Lab Invest* 84:562–572, 2004.
35. Yonemaru K, Sakai H, Murakami M, et al: Expression of vascular endothelial growth factor, basic fibroblast growth factor, and their receptors (flt-1, flk-1, and flg-1) in canine vascular tumors, *Vet Pathol* 43:971–980, 2006.
36. Kodama A, Sakai H, Matsuura S, et al: Establishment of canine hemangiosarcoma xenograft models expressing endothelial growth factors, their receptors, and angiogenesis-associated homeobox genes, *BMC Cancer* 9:363, 2009.
37. Arbiser JL, Larsson H, Claesson-Welsh L, et al: Overexpression of VEGF 121 in immortalized endothelial cells causes conversion to slowly growing angiosarcoma and high level expression of the VEGF receptors VEGFR-1 and VEGFR-2 in vivo, *Am J Pathol* 156:1469–1476, 2000.
38. Lee RJ, Springer ML, Blanco-Bose WE, et al: VEGF gene delivery to myocardium: deleterious effects of unregulated expression, *Circulation* 102:898–901, 2000.
39. Donehower LA, Harvey M, Slagle BL, et al: Mice deficient for p53 are developmentally normal but susceptible to spontaneous tumours, *Nature* 356:215–221, 1992.
40. Naka N, Tomita Y, Nakanashi H, et al: Mutations of *p53* tumor-suppressor gene in angiosarcoma, *Int J Cancer* 71:952–955, 1997.
41. Arbiser JL, Moses MA, Fernandez CA, et al: Oncogenic H-ras stimulates tumor angiogenesis by two distinct pathways, *Proc Natl Acad Sci USA* 94:861–866, 1997.
42. DeVivo I, Marion MJ, Smith SJ, et al: Mutant c-Ki-*ras* p21 protein in chemical carcinogenesis in humans exposed to vinyl chloride, *Cancer Causes Control* 5:273–278, 1994.
43. Garcia JM, Gonzalez R, Silva JM, et al: Mutational status of K-*ras* and *TP53* genes in primary sarcomas of the heart, *Br J Cancer* 82:1183–1185, 2000.
44. Onda H, Lueck A, Marks PW, et al: Tsc2(+/−) mice develop tumors in multiple sites that express gelsolin and are influenced by genetic background, *J Clin Invest* 104:687–695, 1999.
45. Mayr B, Zwetkoff S, Schaffner G, et al: Tumour suppressor gene p53 mutation in a case of haemangiosarcoma of a dog, *Acta Vet Hung* 50:157–160, 2002.
46. Yonemaru K, Sakai H, Murakami M, et al: The significance of p53 and retinoblastoma pathways in canine hemangiosarcoma, *J Vet Med Sci* 69:271–278, 2007.
47. Tamburini BA, Phang TL, Fosmire SP, et al: Gene expression profiling identifies inflammation and angiogenesis as distinguishing features of canine hemangiosarcoma, *BMC Cancer* 10:619, 2010.
48. Dickerson EB, Thomas R, Fosmire SP, et al: Mutations of phosphatase and tensin homolog deleted from chromosome 10 in canine hemangiosarcoma, *Vet Pathol* 42:618–632, 2005.
49. Murakami M, Sakai H, Kodama A, et al: Expression of the anti-apoptotic factors Bcl-2 and survivin in canine vascular tumours, *J Comp Pathol* 139:1–7, 2008.
50. Priester WA: Hepatic angiosarcomas in dogs: an excessive frequency as compared with man, *J Natl Cancer Inst* 57:451–454, 1976.
51. Ward H, Fox LE, Calderwood-Mays MB, et al: Cutaneous hemangiosarcoma in 25 dogs: a retrospective study, *J Vet Intern Med* 8:345–348, 1994.
52. Ware WA, Hopper DL: Cardiac tumors in dogs: 1982-1995, *J Vet Intern Med* 13:95–103, 1999.
53. Aupperle H, Marz I, Ellenberger C, et al: Primary and secondary heart tumours in dogs and cats, *J Comp Pathol* 136:18–26, 2007.
54. Erdem V, Pead J: Haemangiosarcoma of the scapula in three dogs, *J Small Anim Pract* 41:461–464, 2000.
55. Liptak JM, Dernell WS, Ehrhart EJ, et al: Retroperitoneal sarcomas in dogs: 14 cases (1992-2002), *J Am Vet Med Assoc* 224:1471–1477, 2004.
56. Liptak JM, Dernell WS, Withrow SJ: Haemangiosarcoma of the urinary bladder in a dog, *Aust Vet J* 82:215–217, 2004.
57. Pirkey-Ehrhart N, Withrow SJ, Straw RC, et al: Primary rib tumors in 54 dogs, *J Am Anim Hosp Assoc* 31:65–69, 1995.
58. Wobeser BK, Kidney BA, Powers BE, et al: Diagnoses and clinical outcomes associated with surgically amputated feline digits submitted to multiple veterinary diagnostic laboratories, *Vet Pathol* 44:362–365, 2007.
59. Dennis MM, Ehrhart N, Duncan CG, et al: Frequency of and risk factors associated with lingual lesions in dogs: 1,196 cases (1995-2004), *J Am Vet Med Assoc* 228:1533–1537, 2006.
60. Locke JE, Barber LG: Comparative aspects and clinical outcomes of canine renal hemangiosarcoma, *J Vet Intern Med* 20:962–967, 2006.
61. Scavelli TD, Patnaik AK, Mehlhaff CJ, et al: Hemangiosarcoma in the cat: retrospective evaluation of 31 surgical cases, *J Am Vet Med Assoc* 187:817–819, 1985.
62. Merlo M, Bo S, Ratto A: Primary right atrium haemangiosarcoma in a cat, *J Feline Med Surg* 4:61–64, 2002.

63. Pirie CG, Dubielzig RR: Feline conjunctival hemangioma and hemangiosarcoma: a retrospective evaluation of eight cases (1993-2004), *Vet Ophthalmol* 9:227–231, 2006.
64. Newkirk KM, Rohrbach BW: A retrospective study of eyelid tumors from 43 cats, *Vet Pathol* 46:916–927, 2009.
65. Johnson KA, Powers BE, Withrow SJ, et al: Splenomegaly in dogs: predictors of neoplasia and survival after splenectomy, *J Vet Intern Med* 3:160–166, 1989.
66. Pintar J, Breitschwerdt EB, Hardie EM, et al: Acute nontraumatic hemoabdomen in the dog: a retrospective analysis of 39 cases (1987-2001), *J Am Anim Hosp Assoc* 39:518–522, 2003.
67. Hammond TN, Pesillo-Crosby SA: Prevalence of hemangiosarcoma in anemic dogs with a splenic mass and hemoperitoneum requiring a transfusion: 71 cases (2003-2005), *J Am Vet Med Assoc* 232: 553–558, 2008.
68. Aronsohn MG, Dubiel B, Roberts B, et al: Prognosis for acute nontraumatic hemoperitoneum in the dog: a retrospective analysis of 60 cases (2003-2006), *J Am Anim Hosp Assoc* 45:72–77, 2009.
69. Mallinckrodt MJ, Gottfried SD: Mass-to-splenic volume ratio and splenic weight as a percentage of body weight in dogs with malignant and benign splenic masses: 65 cases (2007-2008), *J Am Vet Med Assoc* 239:1325–1327, 2011.
70. Pulley LT, Stannard AA: Tumors of the skin and subcutaneous tissues. In Moulton JE, editor: *Tumors in domestic animals*, ed 3, Berkeley, 1990, University of California Press.
71. Gamlem H, Nordstoga K: Canine vascular neoplasia–histologic classification and inmunohistochemical analysis of 221 tumours and tumour-like lesions, *APMIS* Suppl:19–40, 2008.
72. Miller MA, Ramos JA, Kreeger JM: Cutaneous vascular neoplasia in 15 cats: clinical, morphologic, and immunohistochemical studies, *Vet Pathol* 29:329–336, 1992.
73. von Beust BR, Suter MM, Summers BA: Factor VIII-related antigen in canine endothelial neoplasms: An immunohistochemical study, *Vet Pathol* 25:251–255, 1988.
74. Ferrer L, Fondevila D, Rabanal RM, et al: Immunohistochemical detection of CD31 antigen in normal and neoplastic canine endothelial cells, *J Comp Pathol* 112:319–326, 1995.
75. Jakab C, Halasz J, Kiss A, et al: Claudin-5 protein is a new differential marker for histopathological differential diagnosis of canine hemangiosarcoma, *Histol Histopathol* 24:801–813, 2009.
76. Sabattini S, Bettini G: An immunohistochemical analysis of canine haemangioma and haemangiosarcoma, *J Comp Pathol* 140:158–168, 2009.
77. Waters D, Caywood D, Hayden D, et al: Metastatic pattern in dogs with splenic hemangiosarcoma, *J Small Anim Pract* 29:805–814, 1988.
78. Waters D, Hayden D, Walter P: Intracranial lesions in dogs with hemangiosarcoma, *J Vet Intern Med* 3:222–230, 1989.
79. Snyder JM, Lipitz L, Skorupski KA, et al: Secondary intracranial neoplasia in the dog: 177 cases (1986-2003), *J Vet Intern Med* 22:172–177, 2008.
80. McAbee KP, Ludwig LL, Bergman PJ, et al: Feline cutaneous hemangiosarcoma: a retrospective study of 18 cases (1998-2003), *J Am Anim Hosp Assoc* 41:110–116, 2005.
81. Johannes CM, Henry CJ, Turnquist SE, et al: Hemangiosarcoma in cats: 53 cases (1992-2002), *J Am Vet Med Assoc* 231:1851–1856, 2007.
82. Kraje AC, Mears EA, Hahn KA, et al: Unusual metastatic behavior and clinicopathologic findings in eight cats with cutaneous or visceral hemangiosarcoma, *J Am Vet Med Assoc* 214:670–672, 1999.
83. Culp WT, Drobatz KJ, Glassman MM, et al: Feline visceral hemangiosarcoma, *J Vet Intern Med* 22:148–152, 2008.
84. Gordon SS, McClaran JK, Bergman PJ, et al: Outcome following splenectomy in cats, *J Feline Med Surg* 12:256–261, 2010.
85. Hirsch V, Jacobsen J, Mills J: A retrospective study of canine hemangiosarcoma and its association with acanthocytosis, *Can Vet J* 22:152–155, 1981.
86. Hammer AS, Couto CG, Swardson C, et al: Hemostatic abnormalities in dogs with hemangiosarcoma, *J Vet Intern Med* 5:11–14, 1991.
87. Hargis AM, Feldman BF: Evaluation of hemostatic defects secondary to vascular tumors in dogs: 11 cases, *J Am Vet Med Assoc* 198: 891–894, 1991.
88. Maruyama H, Miura T, Sakai M, et al: The incidence of disseminated intravascular coagulation in dogs with malignant tumor, *J Vet Med Sci* 66:573–575, 2004.
89. Mischke R, Wohlsein P, Schoon HA: Detection of fibrin generation alterations in dogs with haemangiosarcoma using resonance thrombography, *Thromb Res* 115:229–238, 2005.
90. Rishniw M, Lewis DC: Localized consumptive coagulopathy associated with cutaneous hemangiosarcoma in a dog, *J Am Anim Hosp Assoc* 30:261–264, 1994.
91. Maruyama H, Watari T, Miura T, et al: Plasma thrombin-antithrombin complex concentrations in dogs with malignant tumours, *Vet Rec* 156:839–840, 2005.
92. Thamm DH, Helfand SC: Acquired coagulopathy III: neoplasia. In Feldman BF, Zinkl JG, Jain NC, editors: *Schalm's veterinary hematology*, ed 5, Philadelphia, 2000, Lippincott Williams & Wilkins.
93. Holt D, Van Winkle T, Schelling C, et al: Correlation between thoracic radiographs and postmortem findings in dogs with hemangiosarcoma: 77 cases (1984-1989), *J Am Vet Med Assoc* 200:1535–1539, 1992.
94. Stafford Johnson M, Martin M, Binns S, et al: A retrospective study of clinical findings, treatment and outcome in 143 dogs with pericardial effusion, *J Small Anim Pract* 45:546–552, 2004.
95. Cuccovillo A, Lamb CR: Cellular features of sonographic target lesions of the liver and spleen in 21 dogs and a cat, *Vet Radiol Ultrasound* 43:275–278, 2002.
96. Wrigley RH, Park RD, Konde LJ, et al: Ultrasonographic features of splenic hemangiosarcoma in dogs: 18 cases (1980-1986), *J Am Vet Med Assoc* 192:1113–1117, 1988.
97. Thomas W, Sisson D, Bauer T, et al: Detection of cardiac masses in two-dimensional echocardiography, *Vet Radiol* 25:65–71, 1984.
98. Berg RJ, Wingfield W: Pericardial effusion in the dog: a review of 42 cases, *J Am Anim Hosp Assoc* 20:721–730, 1984.
99. Dunning D, Monnet E, Orton EC, et al: Analysis of prognostic indicators for dogs with pericardial effusion: 46 cases (1985-1996), *J Am Vet Med Assoc* 212:1276–1280, 1998.
100. Fruchter A, Miller C, O'Grady M: Echocardiographic results and clinical considerations in dogs with right atrial/auricular masses, *Can Vet J* 33:171–174, 1992.
101. Bertazzolo W, Dell'Orco M, Bonfanti U, et al: Canine angiosarcoma: cytologic, histologic, and immunohistochemical correlations, *Vet Clin Pathol* 34:28–34, 2005.
102. Edwards NJ: The diagnostic value of pericardial fluid pH determination, *J Am Anim Hosp Assoc* 32:63–67, 1996.
103. Fine DM, Tobias AH, Jacob KA: Use of pericardial fluid pH to distinguish between idiopathic and neoplastic effusions, *J Vet Intern Med* 17:525–529, 2003.
104. Sisson D, Thomas WP, Ruehl WW, et al: Diagnostic value of pericardial fluid analysis in the dog, *J Am Vet Med Assoc* 184:51–55, 1984.
105. Shaw SP, Rozanski EA, Rush JE: Cardiac troponins I and T in dogs with pericardial effusion, *J Vet Intern Med* 18:322–324, 2004.
106. Chun R, Kellihan HB, Henik RA, et al: Comparison of plasma cardiac troponin I concentrations among dogs with cardiac hemangiosarcoma, noncardiac hemangiosarcoma, other neoplasms, and pericardial effusion of nonhemangiosarcoma origin, *J Am Vet Med Assoc* 237:806–811, 2010.
107. O'Brien RT, Iani M, Matheson J, et al: Contrast harmonic ultrasound of spontaneous liver nodules in 32 dogs, *Vet Radiol Ultrasound* 45:547–553, 2004.
108. Kutara K, Asano K, Kito A, et al: Contrast harmonic imaging of canine hepatic tumors, *J Vet Med Sci* 68:433–438, 2006.
109. O'Brien RT: Improved detection of metastatic hepatic hemangiosarcoma nodules with contrast ultrasound in three dogs, *Vet Radiol Ultrasound* 48:146–148, 2007.

110. Ohlerth S, Dennler M, Ruefli E, et al: Contrast harmonic imaging characterization of canine splenic lesions, *J Vet Intern Med* 22:1095–1102, 2008.
111. Webster N, Holloway A: Use of contrast ultrasonography in the diagnosis of metastatic feline visceral haemangiosarcoma, *J Feline Med Surg* 10:388–394, 2008.
112. Ivancic M, Long F, Seiler GS: Contrast harmonic ultrasonography of splenic masses and associated liver nodules in dogs, *J Am Vet Med Assoc* 234:88–94, 2009.
113. Nakamura K, Takagi S, Sasaki N, et al: Contrast-enhanced ultrasonography for characterization of canine focal liver lesions, *Vet Radiol Ultrasound* 51:79–85, 2010.
114. Fife WD, Samii VF, Drost WT, et al: Comparison between malignant and nonmalignant splenic masses in dogs using contrast-enhanced computed tomography, *Vet Radiol Ultrasound* 45:289–297, 2004.
115. Clifford CA, Pretorius ES, Weisse C, et al: Magnetic resonance imaging of focal splenic and hepatic lesions in the dog, *J Vet Intern Med* 18:330–338, 2004.
116. Yuki M, Machida N, Sawano T, et al: Investigation of serum concentrations and immunohistochemical localization of alpha1-acid glycoprotein in tumor dogs, *Vet Res Commun* 35:1–11, 2010.
117. Kirby GM, Mackay A, Grant A, et al: Concentration of lipocalin region of collagen XXVII alpha 1 in the serum of dogs with hemangiosarcoma, *J Vet Intern Med* 25:497–503, 2011.
118. von Euler HP, Rivera P, Aronsson AC, et al: Monitoring therapy in canine malignant lymphoma and leukemia with serum thymidine kinase 1 activity—evaluation of a new, fully automated non-radiometric assay, *Int J Oncol* 34:505–510, 2008.
119. Thamm DH, Kamstock DS, Sharp CR, et al: Elevated serum thymidine kinase activity in canine splenic hemangiosarcoma, *Vet Comp Oncol* Epub ahead of print 2011.
120. Lamerato-Kozicki AR, Helm KM, Jubala CM, et al: Canine hemangiosarcoma originates from hematopoietic precursors with potential for endothelial differentiation, *Exp Hematol* 34:870–878, 2006.
121. Rivier P, Monnet E: Use of a vessel sealant device for splenectomy in dogs, *Vet Surg* 40:102–105, 2011.
122. Bower MR, Ellis SF, Scoggins CR, et al: Phase II comparison study of intraoperative autotransfusion for major oncologic procedures, *Ann Surg Oncol* 18:166–173, 2011.
123. Keyes M, Rush J: Ventricular arrhythmias in dogs with splenic masses, *Vet Emerg Crit Care* 3:33–38, 1994.
124. Aronsohn M: Cardiac hemangiosarcoma in the dog: a review of 38 cases, *J Am Vet Med Assoc* 187:922–926, 1985.
125. Weisse C, Soares N, Beal MW, et al: Survival times in dogs with right atrial hemangiosarcoma treated by means of surgical resection with or without adjuvant chemotherapy: 23 cases (1986-2000), *J Am Vet Med Assoc* 226:575–579, 2005.
126. Brisson BA, Holmberg DL: Use of pericardial patch graft reconstruction of the right atrium for treatment of hemangiosarcoma in a dog, *J Am Vet Med Assoc* 218:723–725, 2001.
127. Morges M, Worley DR, Withrow SJ, et al: Pericardial free patch grafting as a rescue technique in surgical management of right atrial HSA, *J Am Anim Hosp Assoc* 47:224–228, 2011.
128. Hammer AS, Couto CG, Filppi J, et al: Efficacy and toxicity of VAC chemotherapy (vincristine, doxorubicin, and cyclophosphamide) in dogs with hemangiosarcoma, *J Vet Intern Med* 5:160–166, 1991.
129. Ogilvie GK, Powers BE, Mallinckrodt CH, et al: Surgery and doxorubicin in dogs with hemangiosarcoma, *J Vet Intern Med* 10:379–384, 1996.
130. Sorenmo K, Duda L, Barber L, et al: Canine hemangiosarcoma treated with standard chemotherapy and minocycline, *J Vet Intern Med* 14:395–398, 2000.
131. Sorenmo KU, Baez JL, Clifford CA, et al: Efficacy and toxicity of a dose-intensified doxorubicin protocol in canine hemangiosarcoma, *J Vet Intern Med* 18:209–213, 2004.
132. Sorenmo KU, Jeglum KA, Helfand SC: Chemotherapy of canine splenic hemangiosarcoma with doxorubicin and cyclophosphamide, *J Vet Intern Med* 7:370–376, 1993.
133. Vail DM, MacEwen EG, Kurzman ID, et al: Liposome-encapsulated muramyl tripeptide phosphatidylethanolamine adjuvant immunotherapy for splenic hemangiosarcoma in the dog: A randomized multi-institutional clinical trial, *Clin Cancer Res* 1:1165–1170, 1995.
134. Payne SE, Rassnick KM, Northrup NC, et al: Treatment of vascular and soft-tissue sarcomas in dogs using an alternating protocol of ifosfamide and doxorubicin, *Vet Comp Oncol* 1:171–179, 2003.
135. Rassnick KM, Frimberger AE, Wood CA, et al: Evaluation of ifosfamide for treatment of various canine neoplasms, *J Vet Intern Med* 14:271–276, 2000.
136. Kim SE, Liptak JM, Gall TT, et al: Epirubicin in the adjuvant treatment of splenic hemangiosarcoma in dogs: 59 cases (1997-2004), *J Am Vet Med Assoc* 231:1550–1557, 2007.
137. Sorenmo K, Samluk M, Clifford C, et al: Clinical and pharmacokinetic characteristics of intracavitary administration of pegylated liposomal encapsulated doxorubicin in dogs with splenic hemangiosarcoma, *J Vet Intern Med* 21:1347–1354, 2007.
138. Ogilvie GK, Reynolds HA, Richardson RC, et al: Phase II evaluation of doxorubicin for treatment of various canine neoplasms, *J Am Vet Med Assoc* 195:1580–1583, 1989.
139. Wiley JL, Rook KA, Clifford CA, et al: Efficacy of doxorubicin-based chemotherapy for non-resectable canine subcutaneous haemangiosarcoma, *Vet Comp Oncol* 8:221–233, 2010.
140. Dervisis NG, Dominguez PA, Newman RG, et al: Treatment with DAV for advanced-stage hemangiosarcoma in dogs, *J Am Anim Hosp Assoc* 47:170–178, 2011.
141. Kisseberth WC, Vail DM, Yaissle J, et al: Phase I clinical evaluation of carboplatin in tumor-bearing cats: a Veterinary Cooperative Oncology Group study, *J Vet Intern Med* 22:83–88, 2008.
142. U'Ren LW, Biller BJ, Elmslie RE, et al: Evaluation of a novel tumor vaccine in dogs with hemangiosarcoma, *J Vet Intern Med* 21:113–120, 2007.
143. Blake MK, LaRue S, Withrow SJ: *Palliative radiation therapy of solid soft tissue malignancies.* In Proceedings of the Veterinary Cancer Society, Estes Park, CO, 20, 1988.
144. Lawrence JA, Thamm DH, Adams WM, et al: *Soft tissue sarcomas: a retrospective analysis of 16 dogs treated with palliative radiotherapy (1996-2001).* In Proceedings of the Veterinary Cancer Society, Kansas City, MO, 19, 2004.
145. Hillers KR, Lana SE, Fuller CR, et al: Effects of palliative radiation therapy on nonsplenic hemangiosarcoma in dogs, *J Am Anim Hosp Assoc* 43:187–192, 2007.
146. Gingrich DE, Reddy DR, Iqbal MA, et al: A new class of potent vascular endothelial growth factor receptor tyrosine kinase inhibitors: structure-activity relationships for a series of 9-alkoxymethyl-12-(3-hydroxypropyl)indeno[2, 1-a]pyrrolo[3,4-c] carbazole-5-ones and the identification of CEP-5214 and its dimethylglycine ester prodrug clinical candidate CEP-7055, *J Med Chem* 46:5375–5388, 2003.
147. Ma G, Masuzawa M, Hamada Y, et al: Treatment of murine angiosarcoma with etoposide, TNP-470 and prednisolone, *J Dermatol Sci* 24:126–133, 2000.
148. Liekens S, Verbeken E, De Clercq E, et al: Potent inhibition of hemangiosarcoma development in mice by cidofovir, *Int J Cancer* 92:161–167, 2001.
149. Bai X, Cerimele F, Ushio-Fukai M, et al: Honokiol, a small molecular weight natural product, inhibits angiogenesis in vitro and tumor growth in vivo, *J Biol Chem* 278:35501–35507, 2003.
150. Ruggeri BA, Robinson C, Angeles T, et al: The chemopreventive agent oltipraz possesses potent antiangiogenic activity in vitro, ex vivo, and in vivo and inhibits tumor xenograft growth, *Clin Cancer Res* 8:267–274, 2002.

151. Maki RG, D'Adamo DR, Keohan ML, et al: Phase II study of sorafenib in patients with metastatic or recurrent sarcomas, *J Clin Oncol* 27:3133–3140, 2009.
152. Kiesel H, Muller AM, Schmitt-Graeff A, et al: Dramatic and durable efficacy of imatinib in an advanced angiosarcoma without detectable KIT and PDGFRA mutations, *Cancer Biol Ther* 8:319–321, 2009.
153. Lana S, U'Ren L, Plaza S, et al: Continuous low-dose oral chemotherapy for adjuvant therapy of splenic hemangiosarcoma in dogs, *J Vet Intern Med* 21:764–769, 2007.
154. Masuzawa M, Ohkawa T, Inamura K, et al: Effects of intralesional injective recombinant interleukin-2 immunotherapy on malignant hemangioendothelioma, *Jpn J Dermatol* 99:1459–1466, 1989.
155. Takano M, Suzuki Y, Asai T, et al: A dramatic effect of continuous intra-arterial injective recombinant interleukin-2 immunotherapy on malignant hemangioendothelioma, *Jpn J Dermatol* 101:719–725, 1991.
156. Abdullah JM, Mutum SS, Nasuha NA, et al: Intramedullary spindle cell hemangioendothelioma of the thoracic spinal cord–case report, *Neurol Med Chir (Tokyo)* 42:259–263, 2002.
157. Jackel A, Deichmann M, Waldmann V, et al: Regression of metastatic angiosarcoma of the skin after systemic treatment with liposome-encapsulated doxorubicin and interferon-alpha, *Br J Dermatol* 140:1187–1188, 1999.
158. Spieth K, Gille J, Kaufmann R: Therapeutic efficacy of interferon alfa-2a and 13-cis-retinoic acid in recurrent angiosarcoma of the head, *Arch Dermatol* 135:1035–1037, 1999.
159. Durie BG, Clouse L, Braich T, et al: Interferon alfa-2b-cyclophosphamide combination studies: in vitro and phase I-II clinical results, *Semin Oncol* 13:84–88, 1986.
160. Fata F, O'Reilly E, Ilson D, et al: Paclitaxel in the treatment of patients with angiosarcoma of the scalp or face, *Cancer* 86: 2034–2037, 1999.
161. Isogai R, Kawada A, Aragane Y, et al: Successful treatment of pulmonary metastasis and local recurrence of angiosarcoma with docetaxel, *J Dermatol* 31:335–341, 2004.
162. Stacchiotti S, Palassini E, Sanfilippo R, et al: Gemcitabine in advanced angiosarcoma: a retrospective case series analysis from the Italian Rare Cancer Network, *Ann Oncol* 23(2):501–508, 2011.
163. Prymak C, McKee LJ, Goldschmidt MH, et al: Epidemiologic, clinical, pathologic, and prognostic characteristics of splenic hemangiosarcoma and splenic hematoma in dogs: 217 cases (1985), *J Am Vet Med Assoc* 193:706–712, 1988.
164. Wood CA, Moore AS, Gliatto JM, et al: Prognosis for dogs with stage I or II splenic hemangiosarcoma treated by splenectomy alone: 32 cases (1991-1993), *J Am Anim Hosp Assoc* 34:417–421, 1998.
165. Bulakowski EJ, Philibert JC, Siegel S, et al: Evaluation of outcome associated with subcutaneous and intramuscular hemangiosarcoma treated with adjuvant doxorubicin in dogs: 21 cases (2001-2006), *J Am Vet Med Assoc* 233:122–128, 2008.
166. Shiu KB, Flory AB, Anderson CL, et al: Predictors of outcome in dogs with subcutaneous or intramuscular hemangiosarcoma, *J Am Vet Med Assoc* 238:472–479, 2011.
167. Simonart T, Heenen M: Radiation-induced angiosarcomas, *Dermatology* 209:175–176, 2004.

SECTION B
Thymoma

CARLOS HENRIQUE DE MELLO SOUZA

Incidence and Risk Factors

Thymomas are one of the most common tumors of the cranial mediastinum, second only to lymphoma, yet they are uncommon in both dogs and cats. Thymomas can occur at any age but usually affect older patients. The reported peak age for presentation is 9 and 10 years in dogs and cats, respectively.[1,2] Breed predisposition has not been reported, and most studies do not show a sex predisposition.[1,2] Risk factors predisposing animals to thymoma have not been identified.

Pathology and Natural Behavior

Thymomas are neoplasms of thymic epithelial cells.[1] Different histologic types of thymoma have been described and include differentiated epithelial, lymphocyte-rich, and clear-cell type. The degree of lymphocyte infiltration within thymomas in dogs and cats has been shown to correlate positively with survival.[1,3] In cats, cystic thymomas seem to be the most common form, although squamous cell carcinoma variants and a thymolipoma have been reported.[1,4-8] The terms *benign* or *malignant thymoma* are commonly used and are based on clinical criteria of invasiveness and resectability rather than on histologic features of malignancy. Distant metastasis has been rarely reported in dogs.[5,9-11] The same is probably true in cats, although one study revealed a 20% metastatic rate in cystic thymomas in the species.[6] The differential diagnoses for mediastinal masses should include lymphoma, ectopic thyroid tumor, branchial cysts, rare sarcomas, and metastatic neoplasms. Tumors extending from the ribs or sternum into the mediastinum may sometimes resemble a mediastinal mass.[12]

History and Clinical Signs

Clinical signs are usually related to organ displacement due to the presence of a mediastinal mass and include lethargy, coughing, tachypnea, and dyspnea. Less commonly, cranial vena cava syndrome (edema of the head, neck, and front limbs) may occur and is related to obstruction of vessels draining the cranial part of the body.[3-7,10-12] Paraneoplastic syndromes are common in dogs and cats and may occur in as many as 67% of dogs with thymoma.[3,4] Reported paraneoplastic syndromes include myasthenia gravis (MG), exfoliative dermatitis, erythema multiforme, hypercalcemia, T-cell lymphocytosis, anemia, and polymyositis. Myasthenia gravis may occur in up to 40% of dogs with thymoma and has also been reported in cats.[3,10,11] Concurrent megaesophagus and aspiration pneumonia has been reported in as many as 40% of canine patients.[3] Paraneoplastic syndromes may occur at presentation, later in the course of the disease, or after tumor removal.*

Diagnostic Techniques and Work-Up

Physical examination findings may include edema of the head, cervical area, or front limbs, secondary to cranial vena cava syndrome. The jugular veins may be dilated and tortuous. Auscultation of the thoracic cavity may reveal decreased or absent lung sounds in the cranial mediastinum related to displacement by the mass or pleural effusion. Cardiac displacement may also occur, and the heart sounds may be heard either more dorsally, caudally, or both. In small dogs and cats, decreased compressibility of the anterior thorax may also be detected.[3-6,10-11,22]

Complete blood count (CBC) is usually normal, but anemia, thrombocytopenia (secondary to immune-mediated destruction),

*References 3, 5, 10, 11, 13-21.

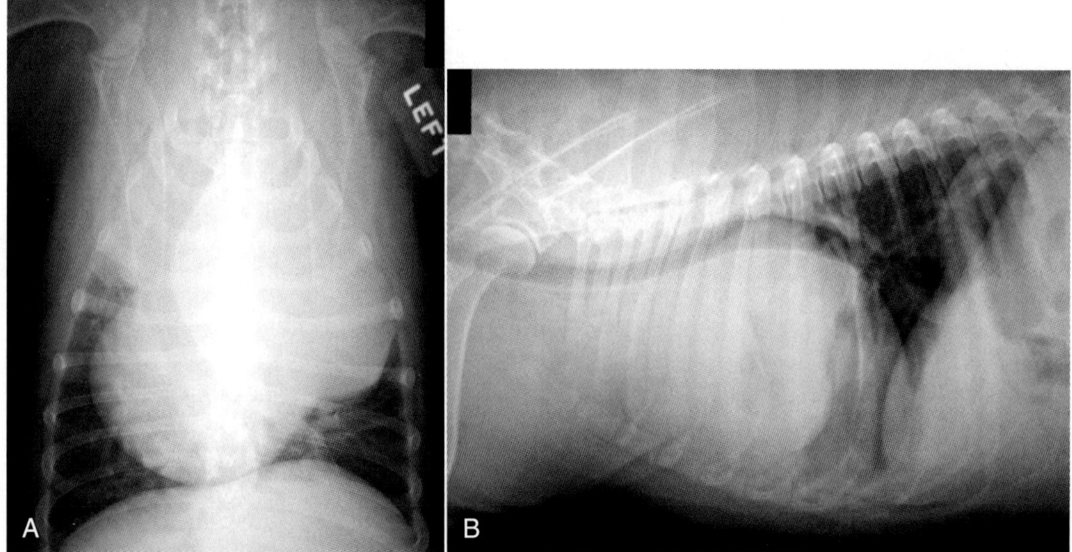

FIGURE 33-4 **A,** Ventrodorsal thoracic radiograph of a large left-sided cranial mediastinal mass that severely displaces the trachea and the heart. **B,** Lateral view of the same mass showing dorsal displacement of the trachea and caudal displacement of the heart. A small amount of pleural effusion can also be observed. *(Courtesy Dr. Christine Warzee, College of Veterinary Medicine, Michigan State University.)*

and lymphocytosis may occur. Hypercalcemia, although uncommon, has been reported in association with thymomas but is much more common in cases of mediastinal lymphoma.[5,11,23] In both tumors, hypercalcemia is usually the result of excessive production of parathyroid hormone–related peptide (PTHrP). The presence of hypercalcemia in an animal with a mediastinal mass should not be used as the sole means to differentiate thymoma from lymphoma.[22-26]

Thoracic radiographs may reveal the presence of a cranial mediastinal mass, pleural effusion, and cardiac displacement (Figure 33-4). Dilatation of the esophagus in the presence of megaesophagus secondary to MG and an increase in alveolar or interstitial lung pattern suggestive of aspiration pneumonia may also be detected. When MG is suspected, demonstration of serum antibodies against acetylcholine receptor is indicated. The Tensilon test (edrophonium chloride, which is an ultrashort anticholinesterase agent) can be used in cases suspected of having MG, in which muscle weakness and fatigue are observed. A marked short-lived improvement in muscle strength is considered a positive response.[18-21] In cases presenting with pleural effusion, fluid analysis after thoracocentesis usually reveals a modified transudate and numerous small mature lymphocytes or a mixed lymphocyte population.[3-5,10,22] Thoracic ultrasonography can be used to determine a presumptive diagnosis of thoracic masses, including thymomas. In addition ultrasound can guide biopsy needles for sampling of the mass.[27,28] More recently, endoscopic thoracic ultrasound has been described in dogs with the reported advantage of a decrease in artifacts caused by the lungs.[29] Transthoracic ultrasound-guided fine-needle aspiration (FNA) of the mediastinum can be easily and safely performed after deep sedation and analgesia or general anesthesia. The diagnosis of thymoma is made when the presence of neoplastic epithelial cells interspersed between large numbers of small mature lymphocytes (and occasional mast cells) is observed.[30,31] Unfortunately, nondiagnostic samples are common due to either a small percentage of epithelial cells, the presence of only small mature lymphocytes in the samples, or the presence of cysts within the mass. The diagnosis is further complicated due to the fact that both lymphoma and thymoma may be composed primarily of small lymphocytes. In three studies, a presumptive diagnosis of thymoma was achieved in approximately 20%, 40%, and 77% of mediastinal masses after FNA and cytology. In addition, Hassall's corpuscles, cytoplasmic structures present in thymocytes, are not usually visualized in Wright-Giemsa preparations in comparison to hematoxylin-eosin (H&E) used for formalin-fixed samples.[3,10,30,31]

Flow cytometry has been recently reported to aid in the specific diagnosis of mediastinal tumors. Flow cytometry of the thymus is based on the fact that thymic lymphocytes can be differentiated from peripheral lymphocytes by simultaneous expression of CD4 and CD8. In that study, all cases of thymoma expressed 10% lymphocytes co-expressing CD4 and CD8, whereas six of seven lymphomas contained less than 2% of $CD4^+CD8^+$ lymphocytes. The additional case of lymphoma was readily differentiated from thymoma by flow cytometric scatter plot analysis.[32]

Advanced imaging modalities such as CT are now used to help the surgeon evaluate the possibility of resection. Three-dimensional (3D) CT reconstructions can estimate the size and volume of the mass, in addition to identifying neighboring structures and whether invasion of these structures has occurred. If the tumor is deemed inoperable, CT will still be helpful if radiotherapy is to be employed (Figure 33-5). Furthermore, CT-guided biopsies can be obtained during the process. Despite these advantages, nonangiographic CT has been shown to have limitations, which were outlined by a recent study. In that study, nonangiographic CT scanning significantly underestimated vascular invasion when compared to surgical exploration. These limitations can be potentially overcome by the use of CT angiography.[33-36]

Therapy

A variety of different modalities have been described for the treatment of thymomas in dogs and cats, including surgery, RT, and chemotherapy and multimodality treatments. Unfortunately, there are no available studies comparing outcomes of animals treated

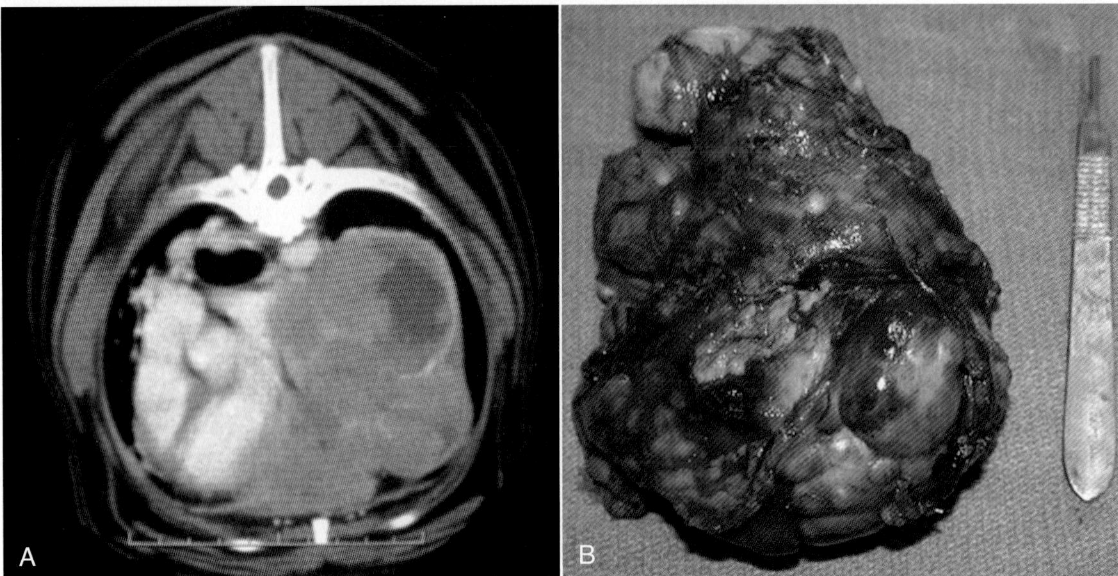

FIGURE 33-5 **A,** CT view of the mass. The mass occupies most of the lateral aspect of the thoracic cavity, and despite significant organ displacement, no evidence of vascular invasion is detected. **B,** Surgical specimen of the large mass after sternotomy and complete resection. *(Courtesy Dr. Christine Warzee, College of Veterinary Medicine, Michigan State University.)*

with these different modalities. In addition, in many studies, animals were treated by a combination of different methods.* In a recent retrospective study that evaluated 11 dogs and 9 cats with invasive and noninvasive thymomas treated by surgery alone, the median survival was 790 days and 1825 days, respectively. The 1- and 3-year survival rates were 64% and 42% for dogs and 89% and 74% for cats, respectively.[3] The successful resection of noninvasive thymomas in two dogs by video-assisted thoracoscopy has also been reported.[38]

In another retrospective study, 17 dogs and 7 cats with thymoma were treated with RT alone or as an adjunctive therapy. Twenty cases were available for follow-up, and a response rate of 75% (11 partial responses [PRs]; 4 complete responses [CRs]) was observed. MSTs for dogs and cats were 248 days and 720 days, respectively. In that study, the total radiation dose (15 to 54 Gy) and treatment interval (from daily to once weekly) varied markedly among animals. To further confound the effects of RT in thymomas, the same study reported that many animals received concurrent chemotherapy.[37]

The effects of chemotherapy for the treatment of thymomas have not been well evaluated in veterinary patients. Long-term remission and stable disease after treatment of thymomas in humans and dogs have been reported (single-case reports) with the use of high-dose prednisone. In one report a cat with thymoma achieved partial remission after treatment with DOX. Likely, the effects of chemotherapy and RT against thymomas reflect, at least in part, a greater reduction in the nonneoplastic lymphocyte population in the thymus, rather than in the primary carcinoma cells.[3-5,10,39]

Prognosis

Surgically resectable thymomas in dogs without megaesophagus and aspiration pneumonia are thought to carry a good prognosis.[3,5,10] The definition of surgical resectability will depend on the experience and ability of the surgeon. Vascular invasion, which could potentially limit resection in the past, may be managed with a jugular vein autograft for reconstruction of the cranial vena cava in a dog with invasive thymoma.[40]

As mentioned previously, thymomas with a significant lymphocytic infiltrate demonstrate improved survival. Age of the dog or cat, invasiveness of the tumor, and mitotic index had no effect on prognosis.[3]

In cats, cystic thymomas are commonly reported and they have been associated with better prognosis, although no other possible prognostic factors such as surgical resectability were critically evaluated.[3,41]

In conclusion, long-term survival should be expected for dogs and cats with thymomas that can be completely resected. Vascular invasion may increase surgical complexity but not necessarily exclude surgery as an option.

Comparative Aspects

Thymic neoplasms in humans constitute 30% of anterior mediastinal masses in adults and less than 15% in children. The majority will occur in elderly patients, 60 years or older, and no sex or race predilection is thought to occur.[42,43] A clinicopathologic classification has been adopted by the World Health Organization (WHO) and correlates well with behavior. In the WHO system, cells are classified as spindle (predominant in the medullary), oval and epithelioid (predominant in the cortex), or dendritic. The tumors are then further divided into medullary, mixed, predominantly cortical and cortical thymomas, and well-differentiated and high-grade thymic carcinoma. Medullary and mixed thymomas are considered benign tumors even in the face of capsular invasion. Predominantly cortical and cortical thymomas display intermediate aggressiveness and have a low risk of relapse independent of their invasiveness. Well-differentiated and high-grade thymomas are considered to be highly invasive and are associated with a high frequency of relapse and death. A staging system that employs both surgical and

*References 3-6, 10, 14, 21, 37.

histologic signs of invasiveness to describe five different stages correlates well with prognosis.[42,44]

MG is the most common paraneoplastic syndrome associated with thymomas, occurring in 30% to 50% of patients. Red cell aplasia and hypogammaglobulinemia are reported to occur in 5% to 10% of patients.

Complete surgical resection is considered the best predictor for long-term survival for humans with thymomas and is the standard of care in patients with resectable tumors. RT is indicated most commonly for extensive or recurrent disease. A variety of chemotherapy drugs have been used to treat inoperable thymomas or in cases in which gross residual disease is present after surgery. Cisplatin, ifosfamide, and prednisone are considered the most effective agents. In addition neoadjuvant chemotherapy has been shown to influence long-term survival for thymomas of Masaoka stages III and IVa.[45]

REFERENCES

1. Parker GA, Casey HW: Thymomas in domestic animals, *Vet Pathol* 13:353–364, 1976.
2. Aronsohn M: Canine thymomas, *Vet Clin North Am* 15:755–767, 1985.
3. Zitz JC, Birchard SJ, Couto GC, et al: Results of excision of thymomas in cats and dogs: 20 cases (1984-2005), *J Am Vet Med Assoc* 232(8):1186–1192, 2008.
4. Aronsohn MG, Schunk KL, Carpenter JL, et al: Clinical and pathologic features of thymomas in 15 dogs, *J Am Vet Med Assoc* 184:1355–1362, 1984.
5. Atwater SW, Powers BE, Park RD, et al: Canine thymomas: 23 cases (1980-1991), *J Am Vet Med Assoc* 205:1007–1013, 1994.
6. Patnaik AK, Lieberman PH, Erlandson RA, et al: Feline Cystic thymomas: a clinicopathologic, immunohistologic, and electron microscopic study of 14 cases, *J Feline Med Surg* 5:27–35, 2003.
7. Carpenter JL, Valentine BA: Brief communications and case reports: squamous cell carcinoma arising in two feline thymomas, *Vet Pathol* 29:541–543, 1992.
8. Vilafranca M, Font A: Thymolipoma in a cat, *J Feline Med Surg* 7:125–127, 2005.
9. Robinson WC, Cantwell HD, Crawley RR, et al: Invasive thymoma in a dog: a case report, *J Am Anim Hosp Assoc* 13:95–97, 1977.
10. Bella JR, Stiff ME, Russel RG: Thymoma in the dog: two case reports and review of 20 additional cases, *J Am Vet Med Assoc* 183:306–311, 1983.
11. Day MJ: Review of thymic pathology in 30 cats and 36 dogs, *J Small Anim Pract* 38:393–403, 1997.
12. Bell FW: Neoplastic diseases of the thorax, *Vet Clin North Am Small Anim Pract* 17:387, 1987.
13. Darke PG: Myasthenia gravis, thymoma, and myositis in a dog, *Vet Rec* 97:392–395, 1975.
14. Carpenter JL, Holzworth J: Thymoma in 11 cats, *J Am Vet Med Assoc* 181:248–251, 1982.
15. Turek MM: Cutaneous paraneoplastic syndromes in dogs and cats: A review of the literature, *Vet Dermatol* 14:279–296, 2003.
16. Rottenberg S, von Tscharner C, Roosje PJ: Thymoma-associated exfoliative dermatitis in cats, *Vet Pathol* 41:429–433, 2004.
17. Uchida K, Awamura Y, Nakamura T, et al: Thymoma and multiple thymic cysts in a dog with acquired myasthenia gravis, *J Vet Med Sci* 64:637–640, 2002.
18. Stenner VJ, Parry BW, Holloway SA: Acquired myasthenia gravis associated with a non-invasive thymic carcinoma in a dog, *Aust Vet J* 81:543–546, 2003.
19. Paciello O, Maiolino P, Navas L, et al: Acquired canine myasthenia gravis associated with thymoma: histological features and immunolocalization of HLA type II and IgG, *Vet Res Commun* 27(Suppl 1):715–718, 2003.
20. Moffet AC: Metastatic thymomas and acquired generalized myasthenia gravis in a beagle, *Can Vet J* 48:91–93, 2007.
21. Singh A, Boston SE, Poma R: Thymoma-associated exfoliative dermatitis with post-thymectomy myasthenia gravis in a cat, *Can Vet J* 51:757–760, 2010.
22. Theilen GH, Madewell BR: Tumors of the respiratory tract and thorax. In *Veterinary cancer medicine*, Philadelphia, 1979, Lea & Febiger.
23. Foley P, Shaw D, Runyon C: Serum parathyroid hormone-related protein concentration in a dog with thymomas and persistent hypercalcemia, *Can Vet J* 41:867–870, 2000.
24. Harris CL, Klausner JS, Caywood DD, et al: Hypercalcemia in a dog with thymomas, *J Am Anim Hosp Assoc* 27:281–284, 1991.
25. Bolliger AP, Graham PA, Richard V, et al: Detection of parathyroid hormone-related protein in cats with humoral hypercalcemia of malignancy, *Vet Clin Pathol* 31:3–8, 2002.
26. Marconato L, Stefanello D, Valenti P, et al: Predictors of long-term survival in dogs with high-grade multicentric lymphoma, *J Am Vet Med Assoc* 238:480–485, 2011.
27. Reickle JK, Wisner ER: Non-cardiac thoracic ultrasound in 75 feline and canine patients, *Vet Radiol Ultrasound* 41:154–162, 2000.
28. Larson MM: Ultrasound of the thorax (non-cardiac), *Vet Clin North Am* 39:733–745, 2009.
29. Gashen L, Kircher P, Hoffman G, et al: Endoscopic ultrasound for the diagnosis of intrathoracic lesions in two dogs, *Vet Radiol Ultrasound* 44:292–299, 2003
30. Rae CA, Jacobs RM, Couto CG: A comparison between the cytological and histological characteristics in thirteen canine and feline thymomas, *Can Vet J* 30:497–500, 1989.
31. Cowell RL, Tyler RD, Meinkoth JH: The lung parenchyma. In *Diagnostic cytology of the dog and cat*, ed 2, St Louis, 1999, Mosby.
32. Lana S, Plaza S, Hampe K, et al: Diagnosis of mediastinal masses in dogs by flow cytometry, *J Vet Intern Med* 20:1161–1165, 2006.
33. Yoon J, Feeney DA, Cronk DE, et al: Computed tomographic evaluation of canine and feline mediastinal masses in 14 patients, *Vet Radiol Ultrasound* 45:524–526, 2004.
34. Zekas LJ, Crawford JT, O'Brien RT: Computed tomographic-guided biopsy of intrathoracic lesions in 50 dogs and cats, *Vet Radiol Ultrasound* 46:200–204, 2005.
35. Hylands R: Veterinary diagnostic imaging. Thymoma, *Can Vet J* 47:593–596, 2006.
36. Scherrer W, Kyles A, Samii V, et al: Computed tomographic assessment of vascular invasion and resectability of mediastinal masses in dogs and cats, *NZ Vet J* 56:330–333, 2008.
37. Smith AN, Wright JC, Brawner WR Jr, et al: Radiation therapy in the treatment of canine and feline thymomas: a retrospective study (1985-1999), *J Am Anim Hosp Assoc* 37:489–496, 2001.
38. Mayhew PD, Friedberg JS: Video assisted thoracoscopic resection of noninvasive thymomas using one-lung ventilation in two dogs, *Vet Surg* 37:756–762, 2008
39. Moore AS: Chemotherapy for intrathoracic cancer in dogs and cats, *Prob Vet Med* 4:351–364, 1992.
40. Holsworth IG, Kyles AE, Bailiff NL: Use of a jugular vein autograft for reconstruction of the vena cava in a dog with invasive thymoma and cranial vena cava syndrome, *J Am Vet Med Assoc* 225:1205–1210, 2004.
41. Gores BR, Berg J, Carpenter JL: Surgical treatment of thymomas in cats: 12 cases (1987-1992), *J Am Vet Med Assoc* 204:1782–1785, 1994.
42. Tomaszek S, Wigle DA, Keshavjee S, et al: Thymomas: review of current clinical practice, *Ann Thorac Surg* 87:1973–1980, 2009.
43. Masaoka A, Monden W, Nakahara K, et al: Follow-up study of thymomas with special reference to their clinical stages, *Cancer* 48:2485–2492, 1981.
44. Ried M, Guth H, Potzger T, et al: Surgical resection of thymomas still represents the first choice of treatment, *Thorac Cardiovasc Surg* 60(2):145–149, 2011.
45. Cardillo G, Carleo F, Giunti R, et al: Predictors of survival in patients with locally advanced thymomas and thymic carcinoma (Masaoka stages III and IVa), *Eur J Cardiothorac Surg* 37:819–823, 2010.

SECTION C
Canine Transmissible Venereal Tumor

J. Paul Woods

Incidence and Risk factors

Canine transmissible venereal tumor (TVT), also known as transmissible venereal sarcoma and Sticker's sarcoma, is a naturally occurring, horizontally transmitted infectious histiocytic tumor of dogs usually spread by coitus, but it may also be spread by licking, biting, and sniffing tumor-affected areas.[1-5] It has been observed occasionally in other canids, such as foxes, coyotes, and jackals.[1,2] It has also been known as infectious sarcoma, venereal granuloma, canine condyloma, transmissible sarcoma, and transmissible lymphosarcoma.[6,7]

Although TVT has a worldwide distribution, its prevalence is highest in tropical and subtropical areas, particularly in the southern United States, Central and South America, southeast Europe, Ireland, Japan, China, the Far East, the Middle East, and parts of Africa.[1,2] In enzootic areas, where breeding is poorly controlled and there are high numbers of free-roaming sexually active dogs, TVT is the most common canine tumor.[1-3,8] In North America, prevalence of TVT is correlated with increased rainfall and mean annual temperature.[9] Occasional cases occur in regions otherwise free of TVT following travel to endemic areas as a result of tourism.[10] Pets travelling abroad can be exposed to TVT and carry it back home to nonendemic areas; therefore veterinarians may act as the first line of defense against the introduction of TVT as an emerging disease in nonendemic areas.

Because TVT is primarily spread by coitus, free-roaming, sexually intact mature dogs are at greatest risk.[2] Dogs of any breed, age, or sex are susceptible.[1,2,6] No heritable breed-related predisposition has been found.[2,6] In endemic areas, although dogs over 1 year of age are at high risk, TVT is most common in dogs 2 to 5 years of age.[2] The physical exertions associated with coitus in the dog with extensive abrasions and bleeding make both sexes susceptible to injury to the genital mucosa, which facilitates the exfoliation and implantation of tumor cells.[2,6] Transmission can occur efficiently in either direction between the dog and the bitch. The most common sites of involvement are the external genitalia, but other sites that can be affected through licking or sniffing include the nasal and oral cavities, subcutaneous tissues, and the eyes.[1-4,6,11-14] Spontaneous regressions occur and have been associated with immune responses against the tumor. Hence immunosuppression from any cause may be a risk factor for the development and maintenance of TVT and may predispose to widespread dissemination. When spontaneous regressions occurs, it usually starts within 3 months after implantation but rarely after 9 months of tumor.[6]

TVT is a transmissible allograft spread directly from dog to dog across major histocompatibility complex (MHC) barriers through transplantation of viable tumor cells on damaged mucosa through coitus or sniffing and licking.[15] TVT and Tasmanian devil facial tumor disease (DFTD) are the only known naturally occurring clonally transmissible cancers that behave like an infectious parasitic neoplastic tissue graft.[16] These cancers have overcome the limitations of existing within the single host, which gave rise to the tumors by gaining the ability to spread between individuals and thus survive long after the original hosts have died.

Pathology and Natural Behavior

TVT was initially recognized in 1876 and was utilized for the first successful experimental transmission of a tumor.[6] A number of characteristics of TVT suggest that the tumor originated in inbred wolves or dogs about 10,000 to 15,000 years ago around the time that the dog was domesticated and subsequently the tumor has been spread worldwide.[17] TVT has evolved into a transmissible parasite representing the oldest known colony of cloned somatic mammalian cells in continuous propagation.

Tumor growth generally appears on the external genitalia or nasal or oral mucosa within 2 to 6 months of mating and can either grow slowly and unpredictably for years or grow invasively and eventually become malignant and metastasize.[1,2,6] Extragenital lesions can occur both alone (in isolation) and in association with genital lesions; however, it has been suggested that in most cases neoplastic foci can be detected on the genitalia.

TVT usually remains localized, but metastasis occurs in up to 5% to 17% of cases to draining regional lymph nodes (i.e., inguinal, iliac, tonsils), subcutaneous tissue, skin, eyes, oral mucosa, liver, spleen, peritoneum, hypophysis, brain, and bone marrow.[2,11,18-20] Because TVT is also transmitted by licking, sniffing, and biting, many cases of reported metastases may instead actually be spread of the growth by mechanical extension or autotransplantation or heterotransplantation. Spontaneous regression can occur within 3 to 6 months of implantation, but the chance of self-regression is remote if the tumor is present for over 9 months.[2]

TVT is commonly described as a round (or discrete) cell tumor and suggested to be of histiocytic origin.[6] This is supported by immunohistochemical (IHC) expression of vimentin, lysozyme, alpha-1-antitrypsin (AAT), and macrophage-specific ACM1, as well as negative IHC staining specific for other cell types.[4,6,21,22] Immunohistochemistry has been helpful in confirming metastatic TVT in various anatomic locations.[18-20] Furthermore, there have been reports describing TVT cells with intracellular *Leishmania* organisms also suggesting a histiocytic origin.[14,23]

Cytogenetic and genetic analyses have provided robust evidence of clonality. Whereas normal canine cell chromosomes consist of 76 acrocentric autosomes plus submetacentric X and Y sex chromosomes, TVT cells have a vastly rearranged karyotype consisting of 57 to 59 chromosomes, including 15 to 17 submetacentric chromosomes as a result of multiple centric fusions.[4,17] However, the total number of chromosome arms in TVT is grossly comparable to the normal dog, so it appears the karyotypic rearrangement is not associated with significant change in DNA content.[15,17] Although TVT cells are aneuploid, they exhibit remarkably stable and similar karyotypes in samples obtained from widely separate geographic regions (i.e., different continents).[15] Likewise, molecular genetic studies of globally distributed TVT tumors provide evidence of a monophyletic origin, which has diverged into two subclades.[15,24]

In addition, TVT cells all share an insertion of a long interspersed nuclear element (LINE-1) upstream of the *c-myc* oncogene that is not found in normal dog genomes.[25-29] This insertion has the potential to disrupt transcriptional regulation of downstream genes, possibly initiating oncogenic activity, and may have been causally involved in the origin of the tumor.[30] This unique rearranged LINE-*c-myc* gene sequence has been used with polymerase chain reaction (PCR) as a diagnostic marker of TVT to confirm diagnosis.[31,32] TVT cells have also demonstrated point mutations in the tumor suppressor gene *p53*, which is responsible for protecting the integrity of the DNA.[29,33,34] Mutations of such a key regulator of the cell cycle, apoptosis, and senescence may be another factor in the oncogenesis of TVT.

TVT is an immunogenic tumor and the immunologic response of the host appears to play a critical role in determining the natural behavior of the disease. The course of disease is divided into a progressive phase (P) in which the tumor grows for 3 to 6 months, then a short stationary phase (S), which is followed by a regressive phase (R) in most dogs, unless the dog is elderly, in poor general condition, or immunologically compromised.[6,8,35-44]

Initially, in the P phase, the tumor downregulates its MHC class I β2-microglobulin and class II expression, which allows it to evade the host's histocompatibility barrier, particularly T-cell cytotoxicity.[45] Some cell-surface MHC class I expression remains, likely to prevent recognition and killing by natural killer (NK) cells. This immunoevasion is partly due to the high concentration of tumor-secreted transforming growth factor-β1 (TGF-β1), which inhibits tumor MHC antigen expression and NK cell activity.[40] TVT also targets and damages dendritic cells (DCs).[45] It has been suggested that TVT has evolved under survival pressures to escape host immunosurveillance.[46]

Tumor-infiltrating lymphocytes (TILs) produce IFNγ but fail to promote tumor MHC expression due to inhibition of IFNγ effects by tumor-derived TGF-β1, which also suppresses the cytotoxicity of the NK cells that migrate to the tumor site because of low tumor-antigen expression.[36,39,40] However, late in the P phase, TILs produce high concentrations of the proinflammatory cytokine IL-6, which acts synergistically with host-derived IFNγ to antagonize the immunoinhibitory activity of TGF-β1 and results in MHC expression in up to 40% of tumor cells and restores NK cytotoxicity.[37,47] A critical threshold level of IL-6 secreted by TILs has to be reached to trigger TVT into R phase.[40,47] Therefore, after progressive growth for 3 to 4 months, the tumor spontaneously regresses with upregulation of MHC antigen expression possibly under epigenetic control.[46]

In addition to cell-mediated immunity, TVT also elicits a humoral immune response demonstrable by antibodies against TVT antigens.[35,48] Experimentally, immunocompromised dogs do not demonstrate regression but rather continued progression of TVT and widespread metastatic disease.[6] Conversely, dogs recovered from TVT have serum-transferable immunity to reinfection and puppies born to bitches exposed to TVT are less susceptible to the disease.[49] In addition to the host immune response, during TVT regression stromal cells and extracellular matrix (ECM) react comparably to wound repair with collapse of the tumor parenchyma and replacement by fibrous stroma.[43]

History and Clinical Signs

The archetypical TVT patient is a sexually intact young adult dog either living in or having travelled to an area endemic for TVT, with a history of contact (coitus, sniffing, licking, or biting) with dogs of similar signalment.[1,2,6,7] The primary lesions are usually on the external genitalia. In the male, the tumor is usually located on the caudal part of the penis, requiring caudal retraction of the penile sheath for visualization (Figure 33-6).[2,6] Occasionally, it is on the prepuce. In the bitch, the tumor is usually in the posterior vagina or vestibule.[2,6] Tumors appear initially as small 1 to 3 mm hyperemic papules that progress by fusing together into nodular, papillary, multilobulated cauliflower-like or pedunculated proliferations up to 10 to 15 cm in diameter. The mass is firm but friable, with an ulcerated inflamed surface. The tumor often oozes a serosanguineous or hemorrhagic fluid. Examples of extragenital sites are illustrated in Figure 33-7.

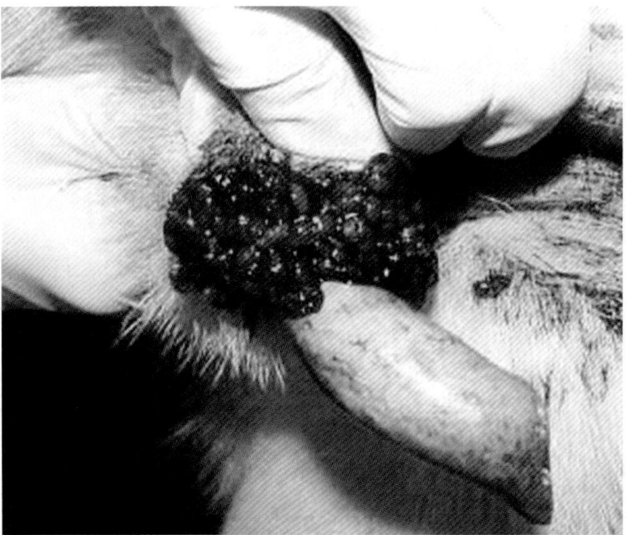

FIGURE 33-6 Typical appearance of a transmissible venereal tumor (TVT) in a male dog. The tumor is located at the base of the penis, has a cauliflower-like appearance, is very friable, and bleeds easily.

Clinical signs vary according to the location of the lesions. Genital lesions often manifest with chronic signs of discomfort or hemorrhagic discharge from the penile sheath or vulva for weeks to months prior to diagnosis, which can result in anemia.[2,6,7] Lesions can predispose to ascending bacterial urinary tract infections but rarely interfere with micturition.[50] Extragenital lesions cause a variety of signs, depending on anatomic location, such as sneezing, epistaxis, epiphora, halitosis, tooth loss, exophthalmos, skin masses, facial deformation, and regional lymph node enlargement.

Diagnostic Techniques and Work-Up

A presumptive diagnosis of TVT can be obtained based on history (including travel), signalment, clinical signs, and physical findings in dogs with the classic presentation. Definitive diagnosis is based on cytologic examination of cells obtained by swabs, FNAs, or imprints of the tumors or histologic examination of a biopsy from the mass. TVT is described as a discrete (or round) cell tumor. TVT has a characteristic morphologic appearance on cytopathology and is often diagnosed without need for histopathology (see Figure 7-37). Exfoliative cytology demonstrates uniform discrete round to polyhedral-shaped cells with moderately abundant pale blue cytoplasm and an eccentrically located nucleus, with occasional binucleation and mitotic figures.[4,6] Single or multiple nucleoli are often observed, surrounded by clumped chromatin. The most characteristic feature is the presence of numerous discrete clear cytoplasmic vacuoles. In R phase, TVTs contain a higher number of infiltrating lymphocytes. Other round cell tumors, including lymphomas, mast cell tumors, plasma cell tumors, histiocytomas, and amelanotic melanomas, are important differential diagnoses but are generally not confused with TVT on cytopathology.

Histopathology of TVT reveals compact masses of round or polyhedral cells with slightly granular, vacuolated, eosinophilic cytoplasm.[4,6] The neoplastic cells are arranged in a diffuse pattern and supported by a thin trabecula of fibrovascular tissue.

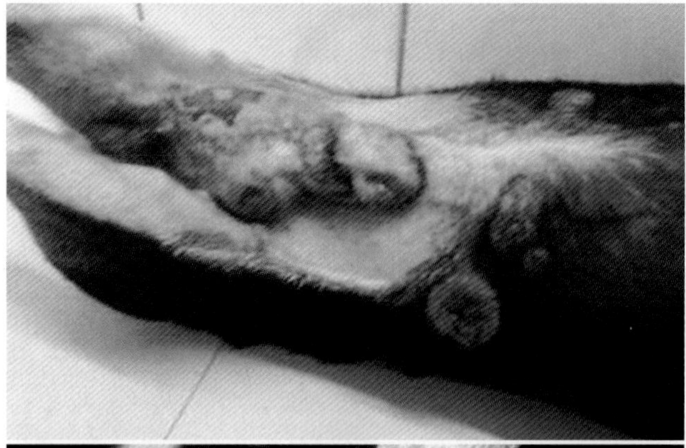

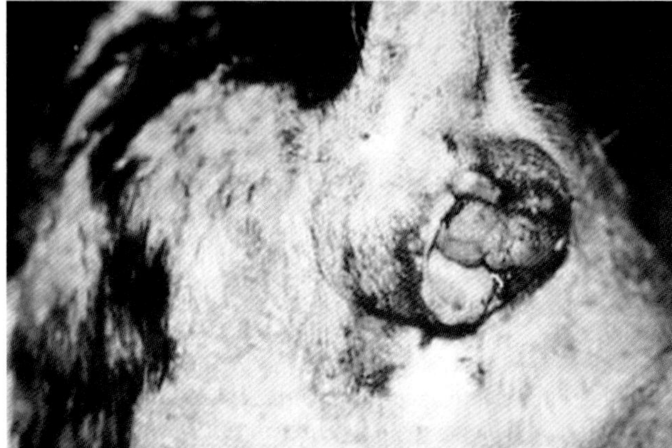

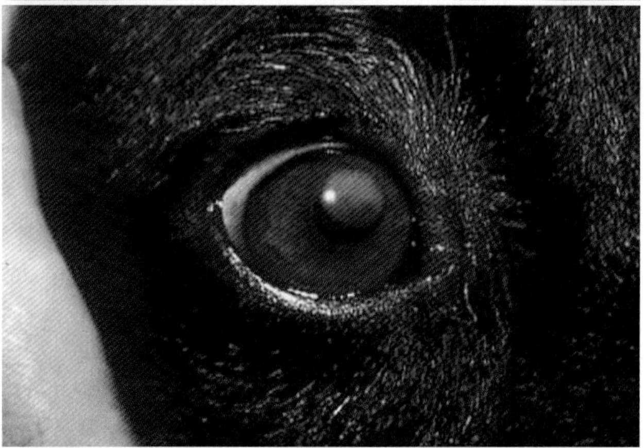

FIGURE 33-7 Other primary tumor sites. **A,** Male dog with cutaneous dissemination of transmissible venereal tumor (TVT) on the ventral abdomen. **B,** Mucocutaneous TVT of the anal area in a dog. **C,** Corneal involvement with TVT in a dog. *(Courtesy Pr. Noeme S. Rocha.)*

Regressing tumors are infiltrated by lymphocytes, plasma cells, and macrophages.[6] For atypical TVTs, if there is doubt about the diagnosis, specific molecular techniques can be utilized (e.g., in situ PCR of the rearranged LINE-*c-myc* gene sequence).[31]

The incidence of metastatic spread of TVT has been reported as less than 15%. However, in most cases of TVT, tumor staging is not performed. Therefore the metastatic rate might be higher. Regional lymph nodes should always be evaluated for metastasis by palpation and cytopathology. A thorough physical examination is essential to rule out other possible sites of involvement (i.e., skin, subcutis, nasal and oral cavities, the eye, the orbit). Diagnostic imaging is usually not required except with invasive TVT of the nasal cavity, orbit, or unusual locations. However, abdominal ultrasound may be used to image regional lymph nodes. CBC, serum biochemistry profile, and urinalysis do not reveal specific changes. Dogs bearing a large tumor burden of TVT have been associated with a paraneoplastic erythrocytosis that may require temporary symptomatic therapy.[6]

Therapy

TVTs will respond to many forms of therapy; however, chemotherapy is the most effective. Single-agent vincristine (0.5 to 0.7 mg/m^2 intravenous [IV], once weekly for 3 to 6 treatments) obtains a complete and durable response in 90% to 95% of treated dogs.* Other single-agent and combination multiagent protocols employing cyclophosphamide, vinblastine, methotrexate, and prednisolone have not demonstrated superiority to vincristine alone.[52,53,56] Resistant cases can be treated with DOX (25 to 30 mg/m^2 IV, every 21 days for 3 treatments).[1]

RT has demonstrated efficacy against TVT. In a study using orthovoltage radiation at 1000 to 3000 cGy, all 18 dogs treated responded with a complete and durable response.[57] Seven dogs were cured with a single coarse fraction of 1000 cGy. The other 11 dogs required 2 or 3 fractions to achieve complete response. Three of the 18 dogs were presented after recurrence following chemotherapy. Another study using megavoltage radiation from a Cobalt-60 unit reported all 15 dogs achieved complete and durable responses with 3 fractions administered over 1 week, for an average dose of 1500 cGy.[11]

Four of the 15 dogs had been resistant to vincristine. Therefore RT can be considered an effective treatment for TVT, particularly for lesions showing resistance to chemotherapy or located in sanctuary sites from chemotherapy (i.e., brain, testicle, eye).

Surgery can be an effective treatment for small localized TVT; however, surgery has an overall recurrence rate of 30% to 75%.[58,59] Marginal surgical excision is not effective, and it can be difficult to obtain wide surgical margins in the areas in which TVT typically appears.[58,59] In addition, tumor transplantation into the surgical wound by contamination from instruments or gloves may also cause postoperative tumor recurrence.

Other therapies described in spontaneous and experimentally induced cases include biologic-response modifiers, piroxicam, cryosurgery, radiofrequency ablation, laser ablation, and electrochemotherapy.[60-64]

Reduction of the incidence of TVT is possible by having dog owners and breeders carefully examine all males and females before mating to avoid breeding from affected animals.[2] In addition, stray dogs can act as a TVT reservoir; therefore the mingling of breeding dogs with strays should be prevented. In some areas, the control of ownerless, free-roaming dogs can drastically reduce the incidence of TVT. TVT can enter the wild canid population through physical contact (licking, biting, or mating), and it is not known whether TVT could pose a threat to endangered wild canids.[65]

Prognosis

In most cases, TVT remains localized and rarely becomes disseminated in an immunocompetent host. In fact, a number of dogs will have their TVT spontaneously regress. For those dogs requiring

*References 1, 2, 11-13, 42, 51-55.

treatment with vincristine or radiation, the prognosis for complete and durable clinical remission is excellent. Therefore the overall prognosis of canine TVT is generally very good to excellent. In stark contrast, the other naturally occurring transmissible tumor allograft, the Tasmanian DFTD, is highly virulent and kills most affected animals within 6 months by obstructing their ability to feed or breathe. It is speculated that the difference in virulence between the two allografts is due to the loss of MHC diversity in the Tasmanian devils, and perhaps one reason for MHC diversity in vertebrates is to ensure that cancer is not communicable between hosts like an infectious disease.[15,17,46]

REFERENCES

1. Rogers KS: Transmissible venereal tumor, *Compend Contin Educ Pract Vet* 19:1036–1045, 1997.
2. Das U, Das AK: Review of canine transmissible venereal sarcoma, *Vet Res Comm* 24:545–556, 2000.
3. Gurel A, Kuscu B, Gulanber EG, et al: Transmissible venereal tumors detected in the extragenital organs of dogs, *Israel J Vet Med* 57:23–26, 2002.
4. Mukaratirwa S, Gruys E: Canine transmissible venereal tumour: cytogenetic origin, immunophenotype, and immunobiology: a review, *Vet Q* 25:101–111, 2003.
5. Nielsen SW, Kennedy PC: Tumors of the genital systems. In Moulton JE, editor: *Tumors in domestic animals*, Berkeley, 1990, University of California Press.
6. Cohen D: The canine transmissible venereal tumor: a unique result of tumor progression, *Adv Cancer Res* 43:75–112, 1985.
7. de Lorimier LP, Fan TM: Canine transmissible venereal tumor. In Withrow SJ, Vail DM, editors: *Small animal clinical oncology*, ed 4, Philadelphia, 2007, WB Saunders Elsevier.
8. Higgins DA: Observations on the canine transmissible venereal tumour as seen in the Bahamas, *Vet Rec* 79:67 71, 1966.
9. Hayes HM, Biggar RJ, Pickle LW, et al: Canine transmissible venereal tumor: a model for Kaposi's sarcoma? *Am J Epidemiol* 117:108–109, 1983.
10. Mikaelian I, Girard C, Ivascu I: Transmissible venereal tumor: a consequence of sex tourism in a dog, *Can Vet J* 39:591, 1998.
11. Rogers KS, Walker MA, Dillon HB: Transmissible venereal tumor: a retrospective study of 29 cases, *J Am Anim Hosp Assoc* 34:463–470, 1998.
12. Papazoglou LG, Koutinas AF, Plevraki AG, et al: Primary intranasal transmissible venereal tumour in the dog: a retrospective study of six spontaneous cases, *J Vet Med A Physiol Pathol Clin Med* 48:391–400, 2001.
13. Brandao CV, Borges AG, Ranzani JJ, et al: Transmissible venereal tumour in dogs: a retrospective study of 127 cases (1998-2000), *Rev Educ Contin* 5:25–31, 2002.
14. Albanese E, Poli A, Millanta F, et al: Primary cutaneous extragenital canine transmissible venereal tumor with *Leishmania*-laden neoplastic cells: a further suggestion of histiocytic origin? *Vet Dermatol* 13:243–246, 2002.
15. Murgia C, Pritchard JK, Kim SY, et al: Clonal origin and evolution of a transmissible cancer, *Cell* 126:477–487, 2006.
16. Murchison EP: Clonally transmissible cancers in dogs and Tasmanian devils, *Oncogene* 27, S19–S30, 2009.
17. Rebbeck CA, Thomas R, Breen M, et al: Origins and evolution of a transmissible cancer, *Evolution* 63(9):2340–2349, 2009.
18. Pereira JS, Silva AB, Martins AL, et al: Immunohistochemical characterization of intraocular metastasis of a canine transmissible venereal tumor, *Vet Ophthalmol* 3:43–47, 2000.
19. Ferreira AT, Jaggy A, Varejao AP, et al: Brain and ocular metastases from a transmissible venereal tumour in a dog, *J Small Anim Pract* 41:165–168, 2000.
20. Kang MS, Park MS, Kim DY: Malignant transmissible venereal tumor with multiorgan metastases in a mastiff, *Vet Pathol* 41:560, 2004.
21. Mozos E, Méndez A, Gómez-Villamandos JC, et al: Immunohistochemical characterization of canine transmissible venereal tumor, *Vet Path* 33:257–263, 1996.
22. Marchal T, Chabanne L, Kaplanski C, et al: Immunophenotype of the canine transmissible venereal tumour, *Vet Immunol Immunopathol* 57:1–11, 1997.
23. Catone G, Marino G, Poglayen G, et al: Canine transmissible venereal tumor parasitized by *Leishmania infantum*, *Vet Res Comm* 27: 549–553, 2003.
24. Rebbeck CA, Leroi AM, Burt A: Mitochondrial capture by a transmissible cancer, *Science* 331(21):303, 2011.
25. Katzir N, Rechavi G, Cohen JB, et al: "Retroposon" insertion into the cellular oncogene *c-myc* in canine transmissible venereal tumor, *Proc Natl Acad Sci* 82: 1054–1058, 1985.
26. Katzir N, Arman E, Cohen D, et al: Common origin of transmissible venereal tumors (TVT) in dogs, *Oncogene* 1:445–448, 1987.
27. Amariglio EN, Hakim I, Brok-Simoni F, et al: Identity of rearranged LINE/*c-MYC* junction sequences specific for the canine transmissible venereal tumor, *Proc Natl Acad Sci* 88:8136–8139, 1991.
28. Choi Y, Ishiguro N, Shinagawa M, et al: Molecular structure of canine LINE-l elements in canine transmissible venereal tumor, *Anim Genet* 30:51–53, 1999.
29. Choi YK, Kim CJ: Sequence analysis of canine LINE-l elements and *p53* gene in canine transmissible venereal tumor, *J Vet Sci* 3:285–292, 2002.
30. vonHoldt BM, Ostrander EA: The singular history of a canine transmissible tumor, *Cell* 126:445–447, 2006.
31. Liao KW, Lin ZY, Pao HN, et al: Identification of canine transmissible venereal tumor cells using *in situ* polymerase chain reaction and the stable sequence of the long interspersed nuclear element, *J Vet Diagn Invest* 15:399–406, 2003.
32. Portela RF, Spim JS, Castelli EC, et al: The use of molecular approaches in the diagnosis of canine transmissible venereal tumor in Brazil, *Vet Pathol* 41:560, 2004.
33. Sánchez-Servín A, Martínez S, Cárdova-Alarcon E, et al: TP53 polymorphisms allow for genetic sub-grouping of the canine transmissible venereal tumor, *J Vet Sci* 10(4):353–355, 2009.
34. Stockman D, Ferrari HF, Andrade AL, et al: Detection of the tumour suppressor gene TP53 and expression of p53, Bcl-2 and p63 proteins in canine transmissible venereal tumour, *Vet Comp Oncol* 9(4): 251–259, 2011.
35. Fenton MA, Yang TJ: Role of humoral immunity in progressive and regressive and metastatic growth of the canine transmissible venereal sarcoma, *Oncology* 45:210–213, 1988.
36. Perez J, Day MJ, Mozos E: Immunohistochemical study of the local inflammatory infiltrate in spontaneous canine transmissible venereal tumour at different stages of growth, *Vet Immunol Immunopathol* 64:133–147, 1998.
37. Hsiao YW, Liao KW, Hung SW, et al: Effect of tumor infiltrating lymphocytes on the expression of MHC molecules in canine transmissible venereal tumor cells, *Vet Immunol Immunopathol* 87:19–27, 2002.
38. Chu RM, Sun TJ, Yang HY, et al: Heat shock proteins in canine transmissible venereal tumor, *Vet Immunol Immunopathol* 82:9–21, 2001.
39. Liao KW, Hung SW, Hsiao YW, et al: Canine transmissible venereal tumor cell depletion of B lymphocytes: molecule(s) specifically toxic for B cells, *Vet Immunol Immunopathol* 92:149–162, 2003.
40. Hsiao YW, Liao KW, Hung SW, et al: Tumor-infiltrating lymphocyte secretion of IL-6 antagonizes tumor-derived TGF-βl and restores the lymphokine-activated killing activity, *J Immunol* 172:1508–1514, 2004.
41. Yang TJ: Immunobiology of a spontaneously regressive tumor, the canine transmissible venereal sarcoma (review), *Anticancer Res* 8:93–95, 1988.
42. Gonzalez CM, Griffey SM, Naydan DK, et al: Canine transmissible venereal tumour: a morphological and immunohistochemical study

of 11 tumours in growth phase and during regression after chemotherapy, *J Comp Path* 122:241–248, 2000.
43. Mukaratirwa S, Chimonyo M, Obwolo M, et al: Stromal cells and extracellular matrix components in spontaneous canine transmissible venereal tumour at different stages of growth, *Histol Histopathol* 9:1117–1123, 2004.
44. Chu RM, Lin CY, Liu CC, et al: Proliferation characteristics of canine transmissible venereal tumor, *Anticancer Res* 21:4017–4024, 2001.
45. Liu CC, Wang YS, Lin CY, et al: Transient downregulation of monocyte-derived dendritic-cell differentiation, function, and survival during tumoral progression and regression in an *in vivo* canine model of transmissible venereal tumor, *Cancer Immunol Immunother* 57:479–491, 2008.
46. Fassati A, Mitchison NA: Testing the theory of immune selection in cancers that break the rules of transplantation, *Cancer Immunol Immunother* 59:643–651, 2010.
47. Hsiao YW, Liao KW, Chung TF, et al: Interactions of host IL-6 and IFN-γ and cancer-derived TGF-ß1 on MHC molecule expression during tumor spontaneous regression, *Cancer Immunol Immunother* 57:1091–1104, 2008.
48. Cohen D: Detection of humoral antibody to the transmissible venereal tumour of the dog, *Int J Cancer* 10:207–212, 1972.
49. Yang TJ, Palker TJ, Harding MW: Tumor size, leukocyte adherence inhibition and serum level of tumor antigen in dogs with the canine transmissible venereal sarcoma, *Cancer Immunol Immunother* 33:255–262, 1991.
50. Batamuzi EK, Kristensen F: Urinary tract infection: the role of canine transmissible venereal tumour, *J Small Anim Pract* 37:276–279, 1996.
51. Calvert CA, Leifer CE, MacEwen EG: Vincristine for treatment of transmissible venereal tumor in the dog, *J Am Vet Med Assoc* 181:163–164, 1982.
52. Amber EI, Henderson RA, Adeyanju JB, et al: Single-drug chemotherapy of canine transmissible venereal tumor with cyclophosphamide, methotrexate, or vincristine, *J Vet Intern Med* 4:144–147, 1990.
53. Singh J, Rana JS, Sood N, et al: Clinico-pathological studies on the effect of different anti-neoplastic chemotherapy regimens on transmissible venereal tumours in dogs, *Vet Res Comm* 20:71–81, 1996.
54. Nak D, Nak Y, Cangul IT, et al: A clinico-pathological study on the effect of vincristine on transmissible venereal tumour in dogs, *J Vet Med A* 52:366–370, 2005.
55. Scarpelli KC, Valladão ML, Metze K: Predictive factors for the regression of canine transmissible venereal tumor during vincristine therapy, *Vet J* 183:362–363, 2010.
56. Brown NO, Calvert C, MacEwen EG: Chemotherapeutic management of transmissible venereal tumors in 30 dogs, *J Am Vet Med Assoc* 176:983–986, 1980.
57. Thrall DE: Orthovoltage radiotherapy of canine transmissible venereal tumors, *Vet Radiol* 23:217–219, 1982.
58. Idowu AL: A retrospective evaluation of four surgical methods of treating canine transmissible venereal tumour, *J Small Anim Pract* 25:193–198, 1984.
59. Amber EI, Henderson RA: Canine transmissible venereal tumor evaluation of surgical excision of primary and metastatic lesions in Zaria-Nigeria, *J Am Anim Hosp Assoc* 18:350–352, 1982.
60. Knapp DW, Richardson RC, Bottoms GD, et al: Phase I trial of piroxicam in 62 dogs bearing naturally occurring tumors, *Chemother Pharmacol* 29:214–218, 1992.
61. Ahmed M, Liu Z, Afzal KS, et al: Radiofrequency ablation: effect of surrounding tissue composition on coagulation necrosis in a canine tumor model, *Radiology* 230:761–767, 2004.
62. Spugnini EP, Dotsinsky I, Mudrov N, et al: Biphasic pulses enhance bleomycin efficacy in a spontaneous canine genital tumor model of chemoresistance: sticker sarcoma, *J Exp Clin Cancer Res* 27:58, 2008.
63. Chou PC, Chuang TF, Jan TR, et al: Effects of immunotherapy of IL-6 and IL-15 plasmids on transmissible venereal tumor in beagles, *Vet Immunol Immunopathol* 130:25–34, 2009.
64. Pai CC, Kuo TF, Mao SJT, et al: Immunopathogenic behaviors of canine transmissible venereal tumor in dogs following an immunotherapy using dendritic/tumor cell hybrid, *Vet Immunol Immunopathol* 139:187–199, 2011.
65. Belov K: The role of the major histocompatibility complex in the spread of contagious cancers, *Mamm Genome* 22:83–90, 2011.

SECTION D
Mesothelioma

LAURA D. GARRETT

Incidence and Risk Factors

Mesothelioma is a rare neoplasm of dogs and cats affecting the cells lining the coelomic cavities of the body. In 1962, Gerb et al cited reports of one case of mesothelioma in 1000 dogs and three cases in 5315 dogs.[1] In dogs, primary mesothelial tumors affecting the thoracic cavity, abdominal cavity, pericardial sac, and vaginal tunics of the scrotum have been reported.[2-6] In the cat, primary mesotheliomas have been reported in the pericardium, pleura, and peritoneum, as well as throughout the abdomen with lung and mediastinal lymph node metastases.[7-12] Exposure to asbestos may be an important contributory factor to mesothelioma development in pet dog populations. Affected dogs often live with owners who have occupations or hobbies for which exposure to asbestos is a known risk.[13] The level of asbestos fibers in lung tissues of affected dogs has been documented to be greater than controls.[13,14] Asbestos refers to a family of silicate minerals that crystallize into long, flexible fibers. The fibers are categorized into two groups: thin rodlike amphibole and long curly serpentine, the main type being chrysotile. In humans, much greater risk has been related to amphibole asbestos compared to chrysotile exposure.[15] Chrysotile now accounts for 90% of asbestos used worldwide.[15]

The underlying mechanisms of the neoplastic transformation of mesothelial cells, despite its association with asbestos, are not completely understood. Asbestos interacts with mesothelial cells via direct and indirect mechanisms and is associated with both phenotypic and genotypic changes in the affected cells. Chromosomal missegregation, aneuploidy, and deletions are reported.[15,16] Loss of tumor suppressor gene products is thought to contribute to the transformation of mesothelial cells.[16] Also, reactive oxygen and nitrogen species generated by macrophages as the cellular response to asbestos fiber phagocytosis and by the fibers themselves add to the genetic damage in the tumor precursor cells.[15] Numerous growth factors (e.g., insulin-like growth factor-1 [IGF-1], platelet-derived growth factor [PDGF], and VEGF) produced by stimulated macrophages or mesothelial cells, as well as tumor suppressor genes, are likely important in the pathogenesis of mesothelioma.[16-18] A recent report of five golden retrievers that developed pericardial mesothelioma after a long-term (30 to 54 months) history of idiopathic hemorrhagic pericardial effusion (IHPE) supports the concept that chronic inflammation may lead to neoplastic transformation in canine mesothelial cells.[19]

Mesothelial tumors occur most often in older animals; however, in cattle and sheep, newborn or young animals may be affected.[20] Juvenile mesothelioma has been reported in two mixed-breed dogs under 1 year of age; no underlying etiology was identified.[21,22] A report of a 7-week-old puppy with mesothelioma suggests a congenital form may exist.[23]

Pathology and Natural Behavior

The normal mesothelium is a monolayer of flattened mesothelial cells. These cells are distinguished by the presence of microvilli, desmosomes, and evidence of phagocytic potential. Disease conditions associated with inflammation or irritation of the lining of body cavities commonly result in a marked physiologic proliferation of mesothelial cells. Fluid accumulation in a body cavity promotes exfoliation and implantation of mesothelial cells. Mesotheliomas are considered malignant due to their ability to seed the body cavity, resulting in multiple tumor growths. Distant metastasis is rare.

Mesothelial cells appear morphologically as epithelial cells; however, their derivation is from mesoderm. Mesothelioma can appear histologically as epithelial, mesenchymal, or biphasic, which is a combination of the two.[24] The epithelial form, which resembles carcinoma or adenocarcinoma, is by far the most common form in small animals. There are also several reports of a variation of the mesenchymal form, which resembles sarcoma and is referred to as *sclerosing mesothelioma*.[4,25,26] The biphasic form of mesothelioma has been reported in two dogs.[27,28] A cystic peritoneal mesothelioma has also been reported in the dog. This is a rare, benign, slowly progressive form of mesothelioma in humans, which is treated with surgical excision when the disease is localized.[29]

History and Clinical Signs

Classic mesotheliomas occur as a diffuse nodular mass or multifocal masses covering the surfaces of the body cavity (Figure 33-8). Extensive effusions occur due to exudation from the tumor surface or from tumor-obstructed lymphatics; therefore the most common presenting sign is dyspnea from pleural effusion or a distended abdomen from peritoneal effusion. Dogs with pericardial or heart-base mesotheliomas can present with acute tamponade and right-sided heart failure.[30-32]

Sclerosing mesothelioma is a variation of mesothelial tumor seen primarily in male dogs, with German shepherd dogs being overrepresented.[4,25,26,33] These tumors present as thick fibrous linings in the abdominal and/or pleural cavities. Restriction occurs around organs in the affected area, and in the abdomen such changes can impinge on organs and lead to vomiting and urinary tract signs.

Diagnostic Techniques and Work-Up

Mesothelioma should be suspected in adult dogs presenting with a history of chronic, nonspecific disease and fluid accumulation in any of the body cavities. Routine echocardiography and abdominal ultrasound are not typically helpful because the tumor cells cling to epithelial surfaces and a mass lesion is rarely noted.[34] In a recent study of echocardiography of dogs with pericardial effusion, only 5 of 15 dogs with pericardial effusion due to mesothelioma had a discrete cardiac mass identified.[32] Thoracic CT may be of benefit in identification of nodular lesions and in assessment of lung parenchyma in the face of pleural effusion[35,36] (Figure 33-9).

Cytologic evaluation of fluid can be diagnostic for other disease processes such as infection or lymphoma but will not conclusively diagnose mesothelioma. Mesothelial cells proliferate under any circumstance associated with fluid accumulation in the body cavity, making the distinction between physiologic mesothelial proliferation and neoplasia difficult. Although malignant mesothelial cells easily exfoliate into effusion fluid, they are hard to distinguish from reactive hypertrophic mesothelial cells cytologically. Reactive mesothelial cells display many cytologic features of malignancy, making a definitive diagnosis of neoplasia via cytology impossible in most cases. Although one study found pericardial fluid pH analysis to be a discriminatory test to differentiate benign from malignant effusions, subsequent studies found too much overlap in the pH values for the test to be of benefit.[37-39] Fibronectin concentrations have also been evaluated in pleural effusions in dogs and cats and were found to differentiate malignant or inflammatory causes from cardiogenic effusions. Elevation in fibronectin levels is a sensitive but nonspecific test for malignant effusions, and mesothelioma can be ruled out if fibronectin levels are not increased.[40]

Establishing a definitive diagnosis of malignant mesothelioma may be difficult, particularly early in the disease. The diagnosis of mesothelioma requires adequate tissue sampling, preferably from an open, visually directed biopsy. Increasing availability of thoracoscopy and laparoscopy for small animals provides a less invasive

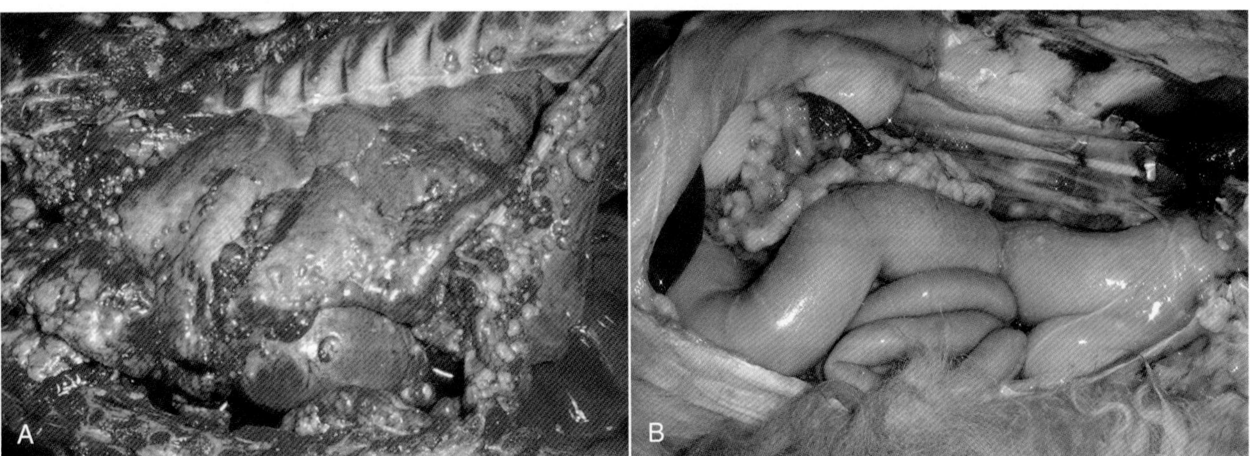

FIGURE 33-8 **A,** Pleural, parietal, and pericardial surfaces of a dog at necropsy illustrating nodular lesions histologically confirmed as mesothelioma. **B,** Mesothelioma involving the peritoneal surfaces of a cat at necropsy.

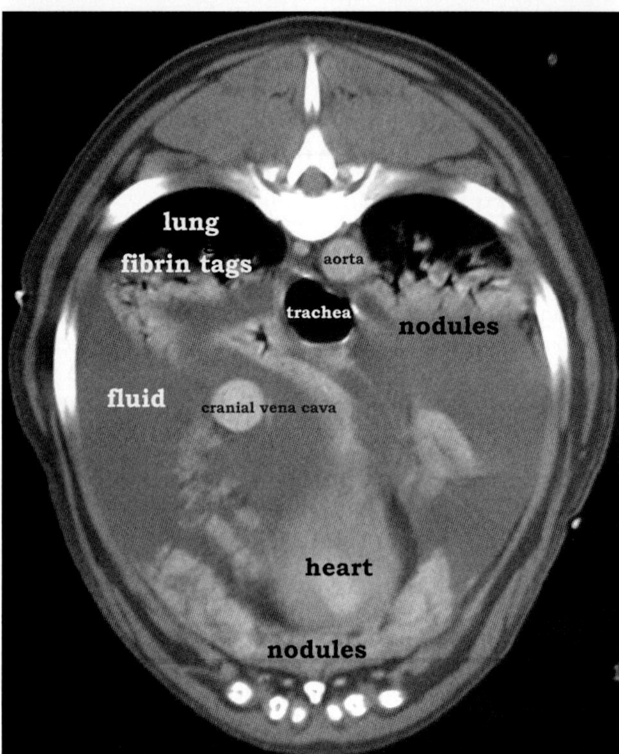

FIGURE 33-9 Thoracic CT (with contrast) from a dog with histologically confirmed mesothelioma. The effusion resolved following the first of five doxorubicin chemotherapy (30 mg/m^2 every 3 weeks, IV) treatments.

means to evaluate these cases.[41] In either procedure, the clinician is encouraged to biopsy any body cavity lining when an obvious cause for fluid accumulation is not found. Sclerosing mesothelioma must be distinguished from chronic inflammatory diseases of the body cavity, such as chronic peritonitis, and histologic examination of biopsy material is essential to establish the diagnosis. Additionally, embolized, nonneoplastic mesothelial cells within lymph nodes is a rare finding in humans with cavity effusions and has been reported in dogs affected with idiopathic hemorrhagic pericardial effusion; therefore care must be taken so as not to overinterpret these cells as indicative of a metastatic process.[42]

The most useful criteria in establishing a diagnosis of mesothelioma is to demonstrate that the tumor is primarily a neoplasm of the coelomic cavity lining and that the method of tumor spread is by transcoelomic implantation. Therefore mesothelioma should be considered when the bulk of the neoplastic tissue exists on the coelomic surface. Histologically, mesotheliomas need to be differentiated from carcinomas, adenocarcinomas, or sarcomas, depending on the morphologic type of the mesothelioma. Unfortunately, there are no cellular markers that conclusively define the mesothelial cell. Recent advances in IHC staining have provided additional ways to examine neoplastic cells to help differentiate mesothelioma from other epithelial or mesenchymal tumors in humans. Podoplanin and D2-40 were found to be highly sensitive IHC markers for sarcomatoid mesotheliomas.[43] Differentiation of malignant epithelial mesotheliomas from adenocarcinomas can be aided by application of a panel of different immunohistochemical stains, including calretinin, Wilms' tumor-1, and cytokeratin 5/6 for which mesotheliomas, but not adenocarcinomas, are strongly positive.[44]

Treatment and Prognosis

No satisfactory treatment exists for mesothelioma. Radical excision may benefit some animals, but usually the tumors are too advanced locally and have spread by implantation early in the course of disease. In one case report, a 2-year-old Siberian Husky with a solitary sclerosing mesothelioma affecting the left thoracic diaphragmatic surface with pericardial and mediastinal adhesions was treated with aggressive surgical resection and diaphragmatic reconstruction using the transversus abdominis muscle.[45] The dog recovered well, but subcutaneous masses at the surgery site, as well as hepatic and renal masses, were noted 54 days postoperatively, leading to euthanasia. Pericardiectomy may palliate mesothelioma patients that present with cardiac tamponade; two dogs treated with surgery alone survived 4 and 9 months in one study.[46] In another report, the median survival in five dogs treated with pericardiectomy was 13.6 months; three of these dogs received adjuvant IV chemotherapy (two DOX, one mitoxantrone).[47] A dog treated with pericardiectomy, intrathoracic and IV cisplatin, and IV DOX remained free of disease at 27 months.[48] In a report of eight dogs with pericardial mesothelioma, the MST was 60 days(range 15 to 300 days) following partial pericardiectomy. The one dog that survived 300 days was treated with DOX and intracavitary cisplatin for the 4 months preceding death.[34] Thoracoscopic partial pericardiectomy is a less invasive procedure than open thoracic surgical pericardiectomy and has been successfully performed in dogs with malignant pericardial effusions, including four dogs with mesotheliomas.[49] Portal site seeding with the mesothelioma is a potential complication of this procedure.[50] Median survival for animals with untreated mesotheliomas in any location is difficult to assess from reports because the tumors are rare and animals frequently are euthanized at the time of diagnosis.

Intracavitary cisplatin has shown palliative potential in the dog; it was well tolerated and greatly decreased mesothelioma-associated thoracic fluid accumulation in three dogs in one study.[51] The treatments also appeared to arrest tumor growth for a limited time. Two doses of intracavitary carboplatin were safely administered to a cat with suspected pleural mesothelioma and resulted in transient resolution of clinical signs for a total of 54 days, at which point the owners discontinued therapy.[52] Unfortunately, local penetration of intracavitary chemotherapy only occurs to a limited depth (2 to 3 mm); thus large masses will not be affected significantly, other than from ultimate exposure to the systemically absorbed intracavitary drug. In such cases, combining debulking surgery or systemic chemotherapy such as DOX or mitoxantrone with intracavitary cisplatin may be beneficial. For peritoneal mesothelioma, four doses of intracavitary cisplatin in two dogs and carboplatin in one cat, combined with piroxicam administration, resolved the effusion in all cases.[53] One of the dogs had debulking surgery first; this dog was still in remission at 2 years, whereas the other dog and the cat lived 8 and 6 months, respectively. IV chemotherapy may provide benefit in some patients; single-agent IV cisplatin administered every 3 weeks was reported to improve clinical signs in a dog with bicavitary epithelial mesothelioma, until sudden death occurred 5 months after treatment initiation.[54]

Comparative Aspects

In humans, mesothelioma is closely linked to exposure to aerosolized asbestos fibers. Approximately 70% to 80% of cases have a history of occupational exposure, with the type of employment significantly affecting relative risk.[17,55,56] Occupations such as construction work, ship building, heating trades, asbestos mining, and insulation work are strong risk factors in the development of mesothelioma in humans.[17] Family members of exposed industrial workers are at risk due to asbestos fiber exposure from the workers' clothing. Affected individuals routinely have greatly increased counts of asbestos fibers in parenchymal lung tissue.[55] The latency period from time of exposure to tumor development is long, with reports ranging from 12 to 50 years.[17] Other risk factors discussed in the development of mesotheliomas include past radiation, exposure to certain chemicals or nonasbestos fibers, and genetic tendency.[15,17] In addition, the DNA tumor virus Simian 40 (SV40) is suspected to act as a cocarcinogen with asbestos in causing mesotheliomas.[16,57,58] SV40 was introduced into a large percentage of humans through contaminated polio vaccines between 1955 and 1963. SV40 can transform cells and experimentally leads to mesothelioma development in laboratory animals. However, there is strong evidence against the proposed connection between SV40 and mesothelioma and data support that the high prevalence of SV40 found in human mesotheliomas in previous studies was likely due to false-positive molecular assays.[59,60]

In humans, the median survival is approximately 1 year from symptom onset. A prognostic index, based on a combination of prognostic factors and gene expression testing, allows for the determination of high- and low-risk patients with respective median survivals of 6.9 versus 31.9 months.[56] There is no consensus in the literature regarding surgery and RT for treatment, although recently several chemotherapy options have been shown to improve survival time and quality of life.[56] The current gold standard drugs are antifolates, specifically pemetrexed and raltitrexed, often combined with cisplatin or carboplatin.[56] Gemcitabine and vinorelbine have also shown some efficacy in humans with mesothelioma. Several novel therapies are also under investigation. Unfortunately, some therapies (e.g., epidermal growth factor receptor [EGFR] inhibitors) performing well in preclinical models did not show activity in clinical mesothelioma patients.[61] Trials of other novel therapies, including anti-VEGF antibody, cyclin-dependent kinase (CDK) inhibitor, antimesothelin antibody, and proteasome inhibitors, are ongoing. Multimodality therapy, including novel agents, will hopefully improve survival time in the future.[57,61]

REFERENCES

1. Geib LW, DeNarvaez F, Eby CH: Pleural mesothelioma in a dog, *J Am Vet Med Assoc* 140:1317–1319, 1962.
2. Cihak RW, Roen DR, Klaassen J: Malignant mesothelioma of the tunica vaginalis in a dog, *J Comp Pathol* 96:459–462, 1986.
3. Vascellari M, Carminato A, Camali G, et al: Malignant mesothelioma of the tunica vaginalis testis in a dog: histological and immunohistochemical characterization, *J Vet Diagn Invest* 23: 135–139, 2011.
4. Dubielzig RR: Sclerosing mesothelioma in five dogs, *J Am Anim Hosp Assoc* 15:745–748, 1979.
5. Thrall DE, Goldschmidt MH: Mesothelioma in the dog: six case reports, *J Am Vet Radial Soc* 19:107–115, 1978.
6. Morini M, Bettini G, Morandi F, et al: Deciduoid peritoneal mesothelioma in a dog, *Vet Pathol* 43:198–201, 2006.
7. Schaer M, Meyer D: Benign peritoneal mesothelioma, hyperthyroidism, nonsuppurative hepatitis, and chronic disseminated intravascular coagulation in a cat: a case report, *J Am Anim Hosp Assoc* 24:195–202, 1988.
8. Kobayashi Y, Usuda H, Ochiai K, et al: Malignant mesothelioma with metastases and mast cell leukaemia in a cat, *J Comp Path* 111: 453–458, 1994.
9. Carpenter JL, Andrews LK, Holzworth J: *Tumors and tumor-like lesions*, Philadelphia, 1987, WB Saunders.
10. Tilley LP, Owens JM, Wilkins RJ, et al: Pericardial mesothelioma with effusion in a cat, *J Am Anim Hosp Assoc* 60–65, 1975.
11. Umphlet RC, Bertoy RW: Abdominal mesothelioma in a cat, *Mod Vet Pract* 69:71–73, 1988.
12. Bacci B, Morandi F, De Meo M, et al: Ten cases of feline mesothelioma: an immunohistochemical and ultrastructural study, *J Comp Pathol* 134:347–354, 2006.
13. Glickman LT, Domanski LM, Maguire TG, et al: Mesothelioma in pet dogs associated with exposure of their owners to asbestos, *Environ Res* 32:305–313, 1983.
14. Harbison ML, Godleski JJ: Malignant mesothelioma in urban dogs, *Vet Pathol* 20:531–540, 1983.
15. Hughes RS: Malignant pleural mesothelioma, *Am J Med Sci* 329:29–44, 2005.
16. Jaurand MC, Fleury-Feith J: Pathogenesis of malignant pleural mesothelioma, *Respirology* 10:2–8, 2005.
17. Pistolesi M, Rusthoven J: Malignant pleural mesothelioma: update, current management, and newer therapeutic strategies, *Chest* 126:1318–1329, 2004.
18. Belli C, Anand S, Tassi G, et al: Translational therapies for malignant pleural mesothelioma, *Expert Rev Respir Med* 4:249–260, 2010.
19. Machida N, Tanaka R, Takemura N, et al: Development of pericardial mesothelioma in golden retrievers with a long-term history of idiopathic haemorrhagic pericardial effusion, *J Comp Pathol* 131:166–175, 2004.
20. Head KW: *Tumors of the alimentary tract*, ed 3, Berkeley, 1990, University of Calif Press.
21. Kim JH, Choi YK, Yoon HY, et al: Juvenile malignant mesothelioma in a dog, *J Vet Med Sci* 64:269–271, 2002.
22. Vural SA, Ozyildiz Z, Ozsoy SY: Pleural mesothelioma in a nine-month-old dog, *Ir Vet J* 60:30–33, 2007.
23. Leisewitz AL, Nesbit JW: Malignant mesothelioma in a seven-week-old puppy, *J S Afr Vet Assoc* 63:70–73, 1992.
24. Corson JM: Pathology of mesothelioma, *Thorac Surg Clin* 14:447–460, 2004.
25. Geninet C, Bernex F, Rakotovao F, et al: Sclerosing peritoneal mesothelioma in a dog - a case report, *J Vet Med A Physiol Pathol Clin Med* 50:402–405, 2003.
26. Schoning P, Layton CE, Fortney WD, et al: Sclerosing peritoneal mesothelioma in a dog evaluated by electron microscopy and immunoperoxidase techniques, *J Vet Diagn Invest* 4:217–220, 1992.
27. Dias Pereira P, Azevedo M, Gartner F: Case of malignant biphasic mesothelioma in a dog, *Vet Rec* 149:680–681, 2001.
28. Sato T, Miyoshi T, Shibuya H, et al: Peritoneal biphasic mesothelioma in a dog, *J Vet Med A Physiol Pathol Clin Med* 52:22–25, 2005.
29. DiPinto MN, Dunstan RW, Lee C: Cystic, peritoneal mesothelioma in a dog, *J Am Anim Hosp Assoc* 31:385–389, 1995.
30. Cobb MA, Brownlie SE: Intrapericardial neoplasia in 14 dogs, *J Small Anim Pract* 33:309–316, 1992.
31. McDonough SP, MacLachlan NJ, Tobias AH: Canine pericardial mesothelioma, *Vet Pathol* 29:256–260, 1992.
32. MacDonald KA, Cagney O, Magne ML: Echocardiographic and clinicopathologic characterization of pericardial effusion in dogs: 107 cases (1985-2006), *J Am Vet Med Assoc* 235:1456–1461, 2009.
33. Gumber S, Fowlkes N, Cho DY: Disseminated sclerosing peritoneal mesothelioma in a dog, *J Vet Diagn Invest* 23:1046–1050, 2011.
34. Stepien RL, Whitley NT, Dubielzig RR: Idiopathic or mesothelioma-related pericardial effusion: clinical findings and survival in 17 dogs studied retrospectively, *J Small Anim Pract* 41:342–347, 2000.
35. Echandi RL, Morandi F, Newman SJ, et al: Imaging diagnosis—canine thoracic mesothelioma, *Vet Radiol Ultrasound* 48:243–245, 2007.
36. Reetz JA, Buza EL, Krick EL: CT features of pleural masses and nodules, *Vet Radiol Ultrasound* 2011 November 18. Epub ahead of print.
37. Edwards NJ: The diagnostic value of pericardial fluid pH determination, *J Am Anim Hosp Assoc* 32:63–67, 1996.

38. Fine DM, Tobias AH, Jacob KA: Use of pericardial fluid pH to distinguish between idiopathic and neoplastic effusions, *J Vet Intern Med* 17:525–529, 2003.
39. de Laforcade AM, Freeman LM, Rozanski EA, et al: Biochemical analysis of pericardial fluid and whole blood in dogs with pericardial effusion, *J Vet Intern Med* 19:833–836, 2005.
40. Hirschberger J, Pusch S: Fibronectin concentrations in pleural and abdominal effusions in dogs and cats, *J Vet Intern Med* 10:321–325, 1996.
41. Reggeti F, Brisson B, Ruotsalo K, et al: Invasive epithelial mesothelioma in a dog, *Vet Pathol* 42:77–81, 2005.
42. Peters M, Tenhundfeld J, Stephan I, et al: Embolized mesothelial cells within mediastinal lymph nodes of three dogs with idiopathic haemorrhagic pericardial effusion, *J Comp Pathol* 128:107–112, 2003.
43. Chirieac LR, Pinkus GS, Pinkus JL, et al: The immunohistochemical characterization of sarcomatoid malignant mesothelioma of the pleura, *Am J Cancer Res* 1:14–24, 2011.
44. Chirieac LR, Corson JM: Pathologic evaluation of malignant pleural mesothelioma, *Semin Thorac Cardiovasc Surg* 21:121–124, 2009.
45. Liptak JM, Brebner NS: Hemidiaphragmatic reconstruction with a transversus abdominis muscle flap after resection of a solitary diaphragmatic mesothelioma in a dog, *J Am Vet Med Assoc* 228:1204–1208, 2006.
46. Kerstetter KK, Krahwinkel DJ, Millis DL, et al: Pericardiectomy in dogs: 22 cases (1978-1994), *J Am Vet Med Assoc* 211:736–740, 1997.
47. Dunning D, Monnet E, Orton EC, et al: Analysis of prognostic indicators for dogs with pericardial effusion: 46 cases (1985-1996), *J Am Vet Med Assoc* 212:1276–1280, 1998.
48. Closa JM, Font A, Mascort J: Pericardial mesothelioma in a dog: long-term survival after pericardiectomy in combination with chemotherapy, *J Small Anim Pract* 40:383–386, 1999.
49. Jackson J, Richter K, Launer D: Thoracoscopic partial pericardiectomy in 13 dogs, *J Vet Intern Med* 13:529–533, 1999.
50. Brisson BA, Reggeti F, Bienzle D: Portal site metastasis of invasive mesothelioma after diagnostic thoracoscopy in a dog, *J Am Vet Med Assoc* 229:980–983, 2006.
51. Moore AS, Kirk C, Cardona A: Intracavitary cisplatin chemotherapy experience with six dogs, *J Vet Intern Med* 5:227–231, 1991.
52. Sparkes A, Murphy S, McConnell F, et al: Palliative intracavitary carboplatin therapy in a cat with suspected pleural mesothelioma, *J Feline Med Surg* 7:313–316, 2005.
53. Spugnini EP, Crispi S, Scarabello A, et al: Piroxicam and intracavitary platinum-based chemotherapy for the treatment of advanced mesothelioma in pets: preliminary observations, *J Exp Clin Cancer Res* 27:6, 2008.
54. Seo KW, Choi US, Jung YC, et al: Palliative intravenous cisplatin treatment for concurrent peritoneal and pleural mesothelioma in a dog, *J Vet Med Sci* 69:201–204, 2007.
55. Zellos L, Christiani DC: Epidemiology, biologic behavior, and natural history of mesothelioma, *Thorac Surg Clin* 14:469–477, viii, 2004.
56. Campbell NP, Kindler HL: Update on malignant pleural mesothelioma, *Semin Respir Crit Care Med* 32:102–110, 2011.
57. Carbone M, Fisher S, Powers A, et al: New molecular and epidemiological issues in mesothelioma: role of SV40, *J Cell Physiol* 180:167–172, 1999.
58. Fisher SG, Weber L, Carbone M: Cancer risk associated with simian virus 40 contaminated polio vaccine, *Anticancer Res* 19:2173–2180, 1999.
59. Lopez-Rios F, Illei PB, Rusch V, et al: Evidence against a role for SV40 infection in human mesotheliomas and high risk of false-positive PCR results owing to presence of SV40 sequences in common laboratory plasmids, *Lancet* 364:1157–1166, 2004.
60. Gee GV, Stanifer ML, Christensen BC, et al: SV40 associated miRNAs are not detectable in mesotheliomas, *Br J Cancer* 103: 885–888, 2010.
61. Raja S, Murthy SC, Mason DP: Malignant pleural mesothelioma, *Curr Oncol Rep* 13:259–264, 2011.

SECTION E

Neoplasia of the Heart

WILLIAM C. KISSEBERTH

Incidence and Risk Factors

Neoplasia of the heart and pericardium is rare in the dog and even less common in the cat. The proportional morbidity of canine heart tumors was 0.19% in a Veterinary Medical Data Base (VMDB) search.[1] In two necropsy series, the overall frequency of primary or metastatic cardiac tumors was 0.12% to 5.73%[2-9] and 11.74% to 28.3% of neoplasms involving intrapericardial tissues, respectively.[2,3] Cardiac tumors (excluding lymphoma) occur most frequently in middle-aged to older (7 to 15 years) dogs.[1] Overwhelmingly, HSA is the most common primary cardiac tumor in the dog, followed by aortic body tumors (chemodectoma, paraganglioma) and then miscellaneous other tumors.[1] HSA represented 69% and aortic body tumor 8% of the histologically diagnosed cardiac tumors in the VMDB.[1] Breeds reported to be at increased risk or predisposed for cardiac HSA include the German shepherd dog and golden retriever.[3,10,11] Aortic body tumors occur most commonly in older brachycephalic dogs,[3,12-15] including Boxers, Boston terriers, English bulldogs, and also German shepherd dogs.[1] It has been suggested that chronic hypoxia may stimulate development of chemoreceptor tumors in both dogs and humans[12,13] and that this factor could explain the increased occurrence of aortic body chemodectomas in brachycephalic breeds; however, not all dogs diagnosed with aortic body tumors are brachycephalic nor do all brachycephalic breeds appear to be at increased risk, and thus other factors (e.g., genetic) presumably contribute to pathogenesis. Based on the VMDB study, 12 breeds were identified as having a significantly higher cardiac tumor incidence compared to all other breeds. Many of the breeds previously reported to be at increased risk for cardiac tumors were identified; however, other breeds were also identified with a relatively high incidence. Most notably, the golden retriever had a high incidence of cardiac tumors (primarily HSA) and total number of recorded tumors.[1]

A similar VMDB search determined an overall incidence of 0.0275% for feline cardiac tumors.[16] The only primary tumors of the cardiovascular system found in a series of 4933 feline necropsies were one case of mesothelioma of the pericardium and two cases of chemodectoma.[17] Overall, the most common primary or metastatic cardiac tumor in cats is lymphoma.[16]

Pathology and Natural Behavior

Neoplasms affecting the heart may occur in intracavitary, intramural, or pericardial locations or at the heart base. Primary tumors may be benign or malignant, with most in the dog occurring in the right atrium and auricle. The most common primary cardiac tumor in the dog is HSA (Figure 33-10, *A*), followed by aortic body tumor (Figure 33-10, *B*).[1-15] Cardiac HSAs often are associated with hemorrhagic pericardial effusion, cardiac tamponade, and metastatic disease.[10,11,18,19] Aortic body tumors arise from chemoreceptor cells at the heart base. Most frequently, they present as a single mass at the base of the heart; however, occasionally they present as a localized collection of focal masses or are infiltrative into the myocardium. Aortic body tumors are primarily locally invasive but occasionally metastasize. Functional tumors have not been found in domestic animals but have been reported in

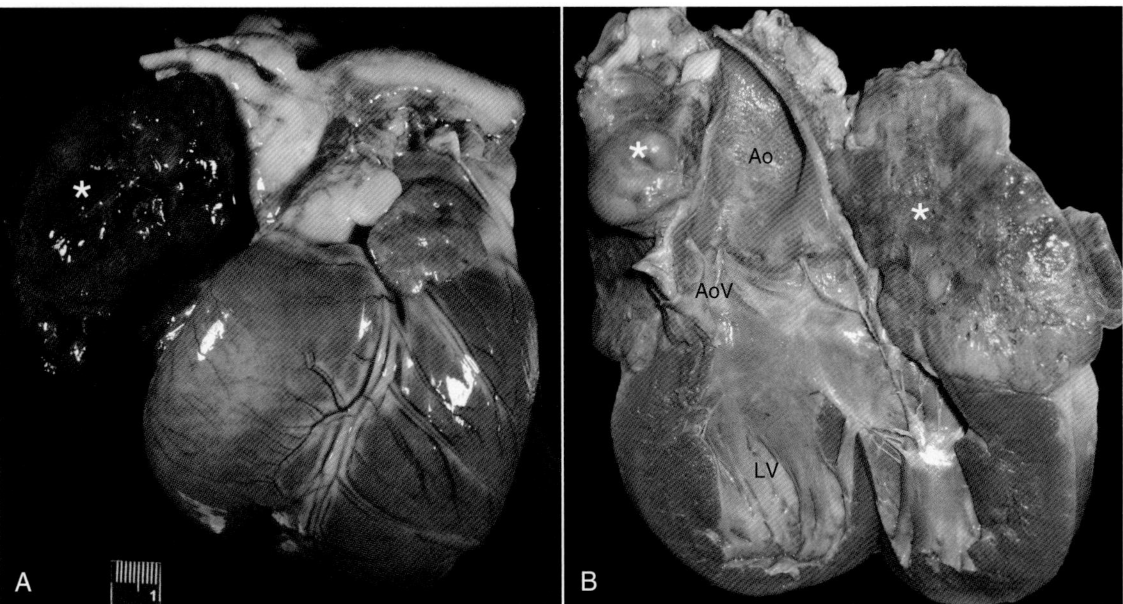

FIGURE 33-10 **A,** Gross postmortem specimen from a dog with right auricular HSA. Note the large, hemorrhagic mass effacing the right auricle *(*)*. **B,** Gross postmortem specimen from a dog with an aortic body tumor (chemodectoma). Note the large, multilobulated mass *(*)* surrounding the aorta and compressing the atria. *LV,* Left ventricle; *AoV,* aortic valve; *Ao,* ascending aorta. *(Courtesy Brian A. Scansen, DVM, MS, DACVIM [Cardiology], the Ohio State University, College of Veterinary Medicine.)*

humans.[20] Other primary cardiac tumors reported in the dog include lymphoma, undifferentiated sarcoma, myxoma, ectopic thyroid carcinoma, fibroma, fibrosarcoma, rhabdomyosarcoma, chondrosarcoma, mesothelioma, granular cell tumor, osteosarcoma, myxosarcoma, leiomyoma, thyroid adenoma, thyroid carcinosarcoma, leiomyosarcoma, lipoma, peripheral nerve sheath tumor, and mixed mesenchymal tumor.[21-48] In contrast to humans, primary cardiac tumors are more common than metastatic tumors in the dog.[1] This is due largely to the high incidence of HSA in dogs. HSA accounts for 40% to 69% of cardiac neoplasms in the dog.[1-3] In most studies, cardiac HSA is considered a primary site, although dogs often have evidence of disease at other locations at the time of diagnosis, and it usually is impossible to determine which is the primary site and which are the metastatic sites. In a recent necropsy case series, 24 of 66 dogs (36%) with extracardiac malignant tumors had metastases found in the heart (15 carcinomas, 6 lymphomas, 3 HSAs), suggesting that cardiac metastases may be underdiagnosed in dogs with malignant, especially advanced, cancers.[49] In individual reports, metastatic mammary carcinoma, melanoma, malignant histiocytosis, pheochromocytoma, granulosa cell tumor, gastric adenocarcinoma, lymphoma, and liposarcoma have been reported to occur in the heart of the dog.[50-58] Primary cardiac HSA, aortic body tumors, myxoma, and rhabdomyosarcoma have been reported in the cat[16,59-64]; however, metastatic tumors are more common—lymphoma (Figure 33-11), mammary gland carcinoma, pulmonary carcinoma, salivary gland adenocarcinoma, oral melanoma, rhabdomyosarcoma, sweat gland adenocarcinoma, squamous cell carcinoma, and mast cell tumor have been reported.[16,17,49,65-70]

History and Clinical Signs

Tumors involving the heart cause varied clinical signs. Cardiac tumors disrupt the normal function of the tissues from which they arise, leading to altered cardiovascular function. In general, signs result from (1) the physical presence of the mass causing obstruction of blood flow into or out of the heart, (2) external compression of the heart that impedes filling (e.g., pericardial effusion) and resulting cardiac tamponade, and (3) disruption of normal heart rhythm or contractility if myocardial infiltration occurs or ischemia develops. Clinical signs produced by cardiac tumors are more closely related to their precise anatomic location than their histologic type. Specific clinical signs observed in an individual patient are influenced by the tumor's size and location and the presence of pericardial effusion. Acute death from rupture of a tumor with subsequent blood loss, with or without cardiac tamponade, is a common sequela of cardiac HSA. Sudden death due to cardiac arrhythmias may also occur. Cardiac HSAs, as well as the majority of reported primary sarcomas of the right heart in dogs, often produce signs of right heart failure due to the presence of cardiac tamponade and inflow obstruction. These signs include ascites, pleural effusion, jugular venous distension, abnormal jugular pulsations, exercise intolerance, dyspnea, pulse deficits, muffled heart sounds, and syncope. Tumors that cause pericardial effusion and cardiac tamponade have been reported the most often.[1] Cardiac or pericardial tumors are responsible for approximately 60% of cases of pericardial effusion in dogs.[71] The most common tumors to cause pericardial effusion are right atrial HSA, aortic body tumors, and mesothelioma.[71] Associated clinical signs resulting from cardiac tamponade include restricted ventricular filling secondary to external cardiac compression, venous congestion, and poor cardiac output. Heart base tumors are most often associated with pericardial involvement of the tumor and accompanying pericardial effusion.[16] Edema, ascites, cough, dyspnea, weight loss, and vomiting are the signs most commonly reported with aortic body tumors in dogs.[14,16,72] Heart base masses are a common cause for cranial vena cava syndrome (edema of the head, neck, and forelimbs) due to tumor pressure on the cranial vena cava. Sometimes, these tumors may be present without causing clinical signs or are incidental findings at necropsy. Cardiac tumors that do not cause pericardial

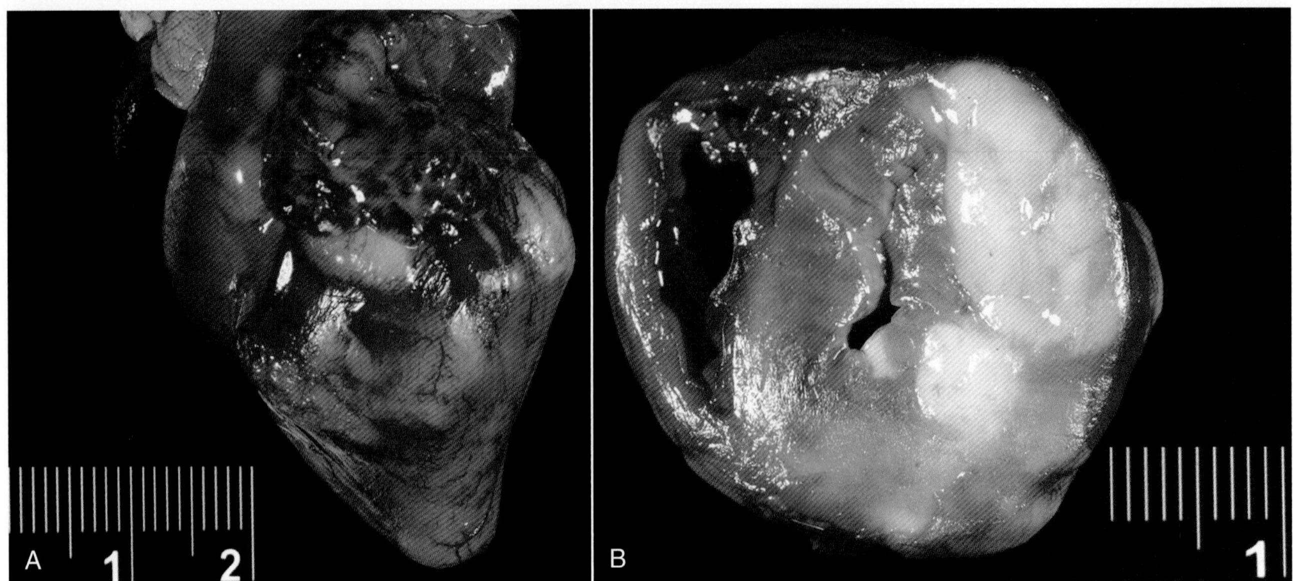

FIGURE 33-11 Gross postmortem specimen from a cat with cardiac lymphoma. **A,** The external surface of the heart shows several raised, white masses. **B,** A cross-section of the ventricles shows a large expansile infiltrate determined to be lymphoma by histopathology. *(Courtesy Paul C. Stromberg DVM, PhD, DACVP, the Ohio State University, College of Veterinary Medicine.)*

effusion can cause signs of congestive heart failure or low cardiac output by obstructing blood flow within the heart or great vessels and by inducing arrhythmias. Syncope and weakness with exertion or excitement are common signs in animals with cardiac tumors. These signs of low cardiac output can result from cardiac tamponade, blood flow obstruction, arrhythmias, impaired myocardial function, and hemorrhage.[1] Clinical signs may be absent if the tumor is small or in a location that does not affect cardiac function.

Diagnostic Techniques and Work-Up

The diagnosis of cardiac neoplasia in the dog and cat is usually based on clinical history, physical examination, and radiographic and echocardiographic findings. Occasionally, tumors, especially aortic body tumors, are an incidental finding at necropsy. In many instances, cytologic or histologic confirmation of neoplasia is not obtained antemortem; however, FNA or tissue biopsy should be obtained when indicated and technically feasible. An electrocardiogram may be normal in patients with cardiac tumors or may show any of a variety of arrhythmias, which may correlate with the underlying site of the primary or metastatic tumor or may be secondary to myocardial ischemia or hypoxia. Low-amplitude QRS complexes and electrical alternans may be seen in animals with pericardial effusion.[73] Sinus tachycardia is common with cardiac tamponade. Conduction and rhythm abnormalities are especially common with infiltrative tumors of the myocardium. Animals with a large volume of pericardial effusion may have a rounded ("globoid") cardiac silhouette (Figure 33-12). Smaller fluid accumulations may allow visualization of atrial and tumor shadows.[16] Thoracic radiographs may reveal cardiomegaly or effusions associated with cardiac tamponade. Mass lesions, if seen, are most common in the areas of the right atrium and heart base. Lung metastases may also be seen.

Echocardiography is the most valuable diagnostic procedure for identifying tumors of the heart in cats and dogs (Figure 33-13).[74-76] In a recent study of 107 dogs with pericardial effusion, the sensitivity and specificity of echocardiography were 82% and 100%, respectively, for detection of a cardiac mass; 82% and 99%, respectively, for detection of a right atrial mass; and 74% and 98%, respectively, for detection of a heart base mass.[77] The positive and negative predictive values of echocardiography were 100% and 75%, respectively, for detection of a cardiac mass; 100% and 87%, respectively, for the detection of a right atrial mass; and 89% and 93%, respectively, for detection of a heart base mass.[77] In another study of histologically confirmed HSA of the right atrium/auricle, echocardiography had a positive predictive value of 92% (11/12) and a negative predictive value of 64% (9/14) in dogs.[76] Tumor location (extrapericardial, noncavitary pericardial, and small auricular masses) and size appear to be the most important factors for false-negative results with echocardiography.[76] Pericardial effusions are a common finding associated with cardiac tumors in both cats and dogs.[36,76-78] Echocardiographic diagnosis of mesothelioma is difficult. Results of echocardiographic examination may be negative unless there are discrete mass lesions associated with the pericardium. Advanced imaging modalities, including CT, MRI, positron emission tomography (PET), and PET/CT, may be useful for selected cases.[79-82]

Other clinical diagnostic methods for the evaluation of cardiac or pericardial masses include pneumopericardiography, selective and nonselective angiography, gated radionuclide imaging, and endomyocardial biopsy in selected patients.[71,83,84] Cytologic evaluation of pericardial fluid and pericardial fluid pH has proved to be of limited usefulness in diagnosing or discriminating between neoplastic and nonneoplastic causes of pericardial effusion.[85-87]

Cardiac troponin I (cTnI) appears to be useful for diagnosing cardiac HSA in dogs.[88,89] cTnI and cardiac troponin T (cTnT) are sensitive and specific markers for myocardial ischemia and necrosis. In one study, dogs with pericardial effusion had

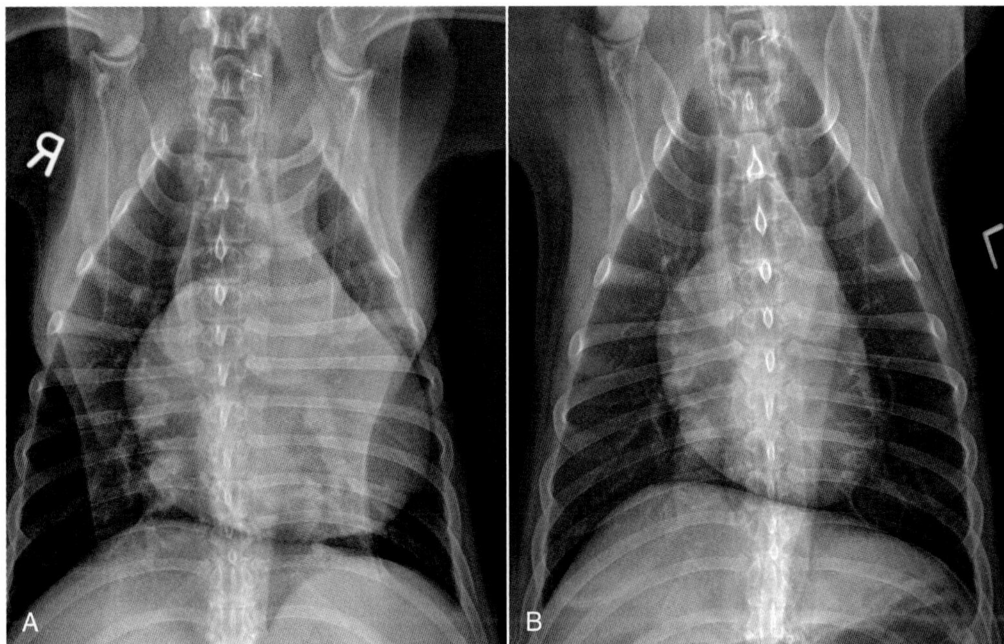

Figure 33-12 Thoracic radiographs from an 8-year-old golden retriever with moderate pericardial effusion before **(A)** and 5 days after pericardiocentesis **(B)**. Note the globoid cardiac silhouette prior to pericardiocentesis, compared to the normal cardiac silhouette seen after the pericardial fluid is removed. *(Courtesy Brian A Scansen, DVM, MS, DACVIM [Cardiology], the Ohio State University, College of Veterinary Medicine.)*

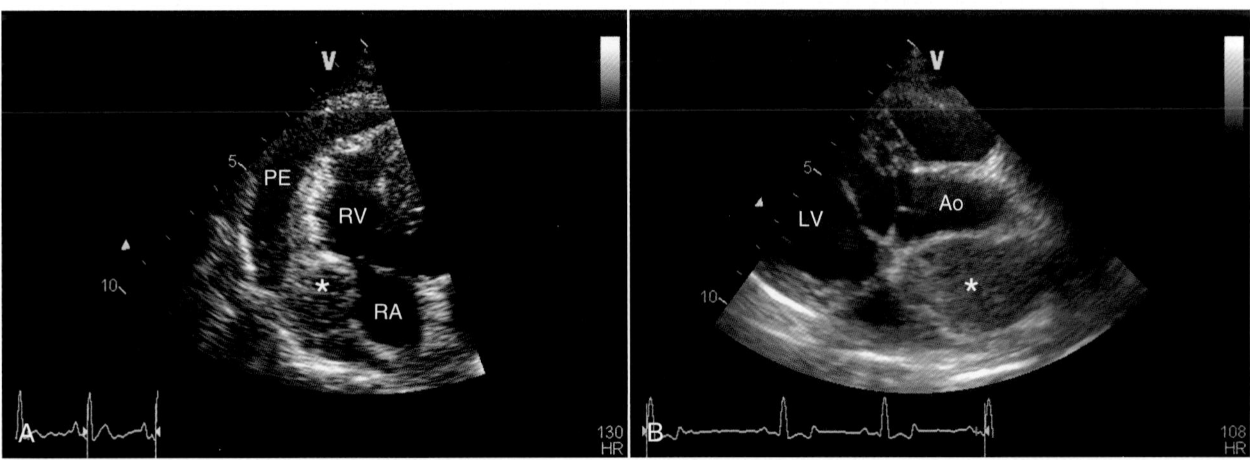

Figure 33-13 **A,** Echocardiographic image from a 12-year-old golden retriever presented for acute collapse. There is mild pericardial effusion *(PE)* and a circular mass of mixed echogenicity at the right atrioventricular groove *(*)* consistent with HSA. *RA,* Right atrium, *RV,* right ventricle. **B,** Echocardiographic image from an 8-year-old Boxer. A large mass *(*)* of mixed echogenicity is seen adjacent to the ascending aorta *(Ao)* consistent with an aortic body tumor. *LV,* Left ventricle. *(Courtesy Brian A Scansen, DVM, MS, DACVIM [Cardiology], the Ohio State University, College of Veterinary Medicine.)*

significantly higher serum concentrations of cTnI but not cTnT than normal dogs.[88] Furthermore, dogs with cardiac HSA had significantly higher concentrations of cTnI than did dogs with idiopathic pericardial effusion.[88] In another study, the median plasma cTnI concentration was higher in dogs with cardiac HSA compared with the median concentration in dogs with HSA at other sites, dogs with other neoplasms, and dogs with pericardial effusion not caused by HSA. Furthermore, dogs with cTnI concentrations higher than 0.25 ng/mL were found likely to have cardiac HSA, and a plasma cTnI higher than 2.45 ng/mL indicated that cardiac involvement is likely in dogs with HSA.[89]

For dogs and cats with a cardiac mass and suspected neoplasia, every effort should be made to determine the extent of disease and the existence of primary or metastatic sites elsewhere in the patient. In addition to echocardiography and possibly other advanced imaging, a minimum database, including a CBC, serum biochemical profile, coagulation profile, thoracic radiographs, and abdominal ultrasound or radiographs, should be obtained. A pathologic diagnosis may be obtained by FNA cytology, endomyocardial biopsy, or open surgical or thoracoscopic biopsy, although many animals are treated based on anatomic location of the mass (e.g., right auricle HSA).

Therapy

Initially, treatment of patients with cardiac tumors consists of treating existing arrhythmias and clinical signs of heart failure, if present. Unfortunately, without effective antitumor treatment, the hemodynamic consequences of the mass often are refractory to medical management. Surgical resection may be indicated for some primary cardiac tumors, especially those of the right auricular appendage.[10,19,26,90-94] However, surgical resection of right auricular masses in dogs with cardiac HSA must be considered a palliative procedure due to the high probability of metastatic disease, although a pericardiectomy may improve signs. Dogs with aortic body tumors generally benefit from pericardiectomy, independent of the presence or absence of pericardial effusion at the time of surgery.[14,72] Thoracoscopy has been recommended as an alternative to open thoracotomy for biopsy and pericardiectomy because almost all aortic body tumors and many (≈50%) right auricular masses are unresectable. Thoracoscopy requires advanced training and special instrumentation if it is to attain the goals of tissue diagnosis, decreased operative time, and decreased morbidity.[93,95-97] DOX-based chemotherapy protocols, including DOX alone, DOX and cyclophosphamide, and DOX-cyclophosphamide-vincristine have been used alone[98,99] and in combination with surgery[19] for the treatment of cardiac HSA.

Prognosis

The prognosis for primary cardiac tumors generally is poor. Most reported cases responded poorly to medical management. Mean survival of dogs with cardiac HSA treated with surgical resection alone is reported to be 46 days to 5 months.[10,19,90] Survival time was significantly longer in dogs treated with tumor resection and adjuvant chemotherapy, with a reported mean of 164 days,[19] comparable to dogs with splenic HSA treated with splenectomy and adjuvant chemotherapy.[99] Complete surgical resection of aortic body tumors usually is not possible; however, dogs that receive a pericardiectomy survive longer (median survival 730 days) than those that do not have a pericardiectomy (median survival 42 days).[72] Other cardiac tumors found during exploratory thoracotomy commonly are judged to be unresectable; however, a few cases with longer disease-free intervals following resection of tumors other than HSA have been reported.[26,28] In one study, dogs with HSA involving the pericardium survived a median of 16 days, whereas those with mesothelioma survived a median of 15.3 months following surgery.[100]

Comparative Aspects

In humans, primary tumors of the heart and pericardium are rare. The vast majority of such tumors are metastatic.[101] Primary cardiac tumors occur with a frequency of approximately 0.02% in pooled autopsy series.[102] Primary tumors are usually cavitary, and 75% are benign.[103] Familial cardiac myxomas occur and appear to have an autosomal dominant transmission and are caused by mutations in the *PRKAR1alpha* gene that encodes a regulatory subunit of protein kinase A.[104] Myxomas constitute nearly 50% of all histologically benign tumors of the heart in humans. Seventy-five percent of myxomas occur in the left atrium. Systemic tumor embolization occurs with high frequency. Surgical resection of myxoma is the treatment of choice, with recurrence of sporadic atrial myxomas being rare following excision. Rhabdomyoma is the most common cardiac tumor of infants and children.[103] Other benign primary cardiac tumors that have been reported in humans include fibroma, papillary fibroelastoma, lipoma, cystic tumors of the atrioventricular node, hemangioma, lymphangioma, and intrapericardial paraganglioma.[102,103]

Almost all primary malignant cardiac tumors are sarcomas, most frequently angiosarcomas.[103,105,106] As is the case with HSA in the dog, angiosarcoma of the heart in humans most commonly originates in the right atrium or pericardium.[103] Rhabdomyosarcoma and mesothelioma rank second and third, respectively, in frequency among primary malignant tumors of the heart and pericardium in humans. Palliative and local control of malignant primary tumors can be achieved with extensive resection. Adjuvant chemotherapy and RT have been used; however, their routine use for primary cardiac sarcomas has been questioned.[107] Cardiac transplantation has been utilized on occasion.

Metastatic tumors involving the heart and pericardium occur up to 100 times more frequently than primary tumors.[108] Incidence rates ranging from 2.3% and 18.3% are reported in autopsy studies of patients who died of cancer.[109] Malignant melanoma metastasizes most frequently to the myocardium, occurring in 46% of autopsies of cancer patients.[108] Cardiac metastasis also frequently occurs with bronchogenic carcinoma and carcinoma of the breast.[109]

REFERENCES

1. Ware WA, Hopper DL: Cardiac tumors in dogs: 1982-1995, *J Vet Intern Med* 13:95–103, 1999.
2. Girard C, Helie P, Odin M: Intrapericardial neoplasia in dogs, *J Vet Diagn Invest* 11:73–78, 1999.
3. Walter JH, Rudolph R: Systemic, metastatic, eu- and heterotope tumours of the heart in necropsied dogs, *Zentralbl Veterinarmed An* 43:31–45, 1996.
4. Prange H, Falk-Junge G, Katenkamp D, et al: Zur Verbreitung, Epizootiologie und Röntgendiagnostik intrathorakaler Geschwülste beim Hund, *Arch Exper Vet Med* 42:637–649, 1988.
5. Cammarata G, Caramelli M, Cavazzini E, et al: Neoplasie cardiache e della base del cuore nel cane: Contributo casistico e studio istologico, *Clinica Veterinaria* 110:97–110, 1987.
6. Priester WA, McKay FW: *The occurrence of tumors in domestic animals, National Cancer Institute Monograph 54*, Bethesda, 1980, National Institutes of Health.
7. Detweiler DK, Patterson DF: The prevalence and types of cardiovascular disease in dogs, *Ann N Y Acad Sci* 127:481–516, 1965.
8. Luginbuhl H, Detweiler K: Cardiovascular lesions in dogs, *Ann N Y Acad Sci* 127:517–540, 1965.
9. Detweiler DK: Wesen und Häufigkeit von Herzkrankheiten bei Hunden, *Zentralbl Veterinärmed [A]* 9:317–357, 1962.
10. Arosohn M: Cardiac hemangiosarcoma in the dog: A review of 38 cases, *J Am Vet Med Assoc* 187:922–926, 1985.
11. Kleine W, Zook BC, Munson TO: Primary cardiac hemangiosarcoma in dogs, *J Am Vet Med Assoc* 157:326–337, 1970.
12. Hayes HM Jr: A hypothesis for the aetiology of canine chemoreceptor neoplasms, based upon an epidemiological study of 73 cases among hospital patients, *J Small Anim Pract* 16:337–343, 1975.
13. Patnaik AK, Liu SK, Hurvitz AI, et al: Canine chemodectoma (extra-adrenal paragangliomas)-a comparative study, *J Small Anim Pract* 16:785–801, 1975.
14. Vicari ED, Brown DC, Holt DE, et al: Survival times of and prognostic indicators for dogs with heart base masses: 25 cases (1986-1999), *J Am Vet Med Assoc* 219:485–487, 2001.
15. Noszczyk-Nowak A, Nowak M, Paslawska U, et al: Cases with manifestation of chemodectoma diagnosed in dogs in Department of Internal Diseases with Horses, Dogs and Cats Clinic, Veterinary

Medicine Faculty, University of Environmental and Life Sciences, Wroclaw, Poland, *Acta Vet Scand* 52:35, 2010.
16. Ware WA: Cardiac neoplasia. In Bonagura JD, editor: *Kirk's current veterinary therapy XII*, Philadelphia, 1995, WB Saunders.
17. Tilley LP, Bond B, Patnaik AK, et al: Cardiovascular tumors in the cat, *J Am Anim Hosp Assoc* 17:1009–1021, 1981.
18. Berg J: Pericardial disease and cardiac neoplasia, *Semin Vet Med Surg (Small Anim)* 9:185–191, 1994.
19. Weisse C, Soares N, Beal MW, et al: Survival times in dogs with right atrial hemangiosarcoma treated by means of surgical resection with or without adjuvant chemotherapy: 23 cases (1986-2000), *J Am Vet Med Assoc* 226:575–579, 2005.
20. Yates WD, Lester SJ, Mills JH: Chemoreceptor tumors diagnosed at the Western College of Veterinary Medicine 1967-1979, *Can Vet J* 21:124–129, 1980.
21. Swartout MS, Ware WA, Bonagura JD: Intracardiac tumors in two dogs, *J Am Anim Hosp Assoc* 23:533–538, 1987.
22. Machida N, Hoshi K, Kobayashi M, et al: Cardiac myxoma of the tricuspid valve in a dog, *J Comp Pathol* 129:320–324, 2003.
23. Roberts SR: Myxoma of the heart in a dog, *J Am Vet Med Assoc* 134:185–188, 1959.
24. Bright JM, Toal RL, Blackford LM: Right ventricular outflow obstruction caused by primary cardiac neoplasia, *J Vet Intern Med* 4:12–16, 1990.
25. Sims CS, Tobias AH, Hayden DW, et al: Pericardial effusion due to primary cardiac lymphosarcoma in a dog, *J Vet Intern Med* 17:923–927, 2003.
26. Ware WA, Merkley DF, Riedesel DH: Intracardiac thyroid tumor in a dog: diagnosis and surgical removal, *J Am Anim Hosp Assoc* 30:20–23, 1994.
27. Madarame H, Sato K, Ogihara K, et al: Primary cardiac fibrosarcoma in a dog, *J Vet Med Sci* 66:979–982, 2004.
28. Lombard CW, Goldschmidt MH: Primary fibroma in the right atrium of a dog, *J Small Anim Pract* 21:439 448, 1980.
29. Atkins CE, Badertscher II RR, Greenlee P, et al: Diagnosis of an intracardiac fibrosarcoma using two-dimensional echocardiography, *J Am Anim Hosp Assoc* 20:131–137, 1984.
30. Vicini DS, Didier PJ, Ogilvie GK: Cardiac fibrosarcoma in a dog, *J Am Vet Med Assoc* 189:1486–1488, 1986.
31. Perez J, Perez-Rivero A, Montoya A, et al: Right-sided heart failure in a dog with primary cardiac rhabdomyosarcoma, *J Am Anim Hosp Assoc* 34:208–211, 1998.
32. Krotje LJ, Ware WA, Niyo Y: Intracardiac rhabdomyosarcoma in a dog, *J Am Vet Med Assoc* 197:368–371, 1990.
33. Caro-Vadillo A, Pizarro-Diaz M, Martinez-Merlo E, et al: Clinical and pathological features of a cardiac chondrosarcoma in a dog, *Vet Rec* 155:678–680, 2004.
34. Southerland EM, Miller RT, Jones CL: Primary right atrial chondrosarcoma in a dog, *J Am Vet Med Assoc* 203:1697–1698, 1993.
35. Greenlee PG, Liu SK: Chondrosarcoma of the mitral leaflet in a dog, *Vet Pathol* 21:540–542, 1984.
36. Cobb MA, Brownlie SE: Intrapericardial neoplasia in 14 dogs, *J Small Anim Pract* 33:309–316, 1992.
37. Sanford SE, Hoover DM, Miller RB: Primary cardiac granular cell tumor in a dog, *Vet Pathol* 21:489–494, 1984.
38. Schelling SH, Moses BL: Primary intracardiac osteosarcoma in a dog, *J Vet Diagn Invest* 6:396–398, 1994.
39. Sato T, Koie H, Shibuya H, et al: Extraskeletal osteosarcoma in the pericardium of a dog, *Vet Rec* 155:780–781, 2004.
40. Foale RD, White RA, Harley R, et al: Left ventricular myxosarcoma in a dog, *J Small Anim Pract* 44:503–507, 2003.
41. Gallay J, Bélanger MC, Hélie P, et al: Cardiac leiomyoma associated with advanced atrioventricular block in a young dog, *J Vet Cardiol* 13:71–77, 2011.
42. Di Palma S, Lombard C, Kappeler A, et al: Intracardiac ectopic thyroid adenoma in a dog, *Vet Rec* 167:709–710, 2010.
43. Almes KM, Heaney AM, Andrews GA: Intracardiac ectopic thyroid carcinosarcoma in a dog, *Vet Pathol* 45:500–504, 2008.
44. Fews D, Scase TJ, Battersby IA: Leiomyosarcoma of the pericardium, with epicardial metastases and peripheral eosinophilia in a dog, *J Comp Pathol* 138:224–228, 2008.
45. Ben-Amotz R, Ellison GW, Thompson MS, et al: Pericardial lipoma in a geriatric dog with an incidentally discovered thoracic mass, *J Small Anim Pract* 48:596–599, 2007.
46. Brambilla PG, Roccabianca P, Locatelli C, et al: Primary cardiac lipoma in a dog, *J Vet Intern Med* 20:691–693, 2006.
47. Wohlsein P, Cichowski S, Baumgartner W: Primary endocardial malignant spindle-cell sarcoma in the right atrium of a dog resembling a malignant peripheral nerve sheath tumour, *J Comp Pathol* 132:340–345, 2005.
48. Machida N, Kobayashi M, Tanaka R, et al: Primary malignant mixed mesenchymal tumour of the heart in a dog, *J Comp Pathol* 128:71–74, 2003.
49. Aupperle H, März I, Ellenberger C, et al: Primary and secondary heart tumours in dogs and cats, *J Comp Pathol* 136:18–26, 2007.
50. Wilkerson MJ, Dolce K, DeBey BM, et al: Metastatic balloon cell melanoma in a dog, *Vet Clin Pathol* 32:31–36, 2003.
51. Hilbe M, Hauser B, Zlinszky K, et al: Haemangiosarcoma with a metastasis of a malignant mixed mammary gland tumour in a dog, *J Vet Med A Physiol Pathol Clin Med* 49:443–444, 2002.
52. Sako T, Kitamura N, Kagawa Y, et al: Immunohistochemical evaluation of a malignant pheochromocytoma in a wolf dog, *Vet Pathol* 38:447–450, 2001.
53. Sabocanec R, Culjak K, Vrbanac L, et al: A case of metastasizing ovarian granulosa cell tumour in the myocardium of a bitch, *Acta Vet Hung* 44:189–194, 1996.
54. Uno Y, Momoi Y, Watari T, et al: Malignant histiocytosis with multiple skin lesions in a dog, *J Vet Med Sci* 55:1059–1061, 1993.
55. Guglielmini C, Civitella C, Malatesta D, et al: Metastatic pericardial tumors in a dog with equivocal pericardial cytological findings, *J Am Anim Hosp Assoc* 43:284–287, 2007.
56. Lowe AD: Alimentary lymphosarcoma in a 4-year-old Labrador retriever, *Can Vet J* 45:610–612, 2004.
57. Ogilvie GK, Brunkow CS, Daniel GB, et al: Malignant lymphoma with cardiac and bone involvement in a dog, *J Am Vet Med Assoc* 194:793–796, 1989.
58. Wang FI, Liang SL, Eng HL, et al: Disseminated liposarcoma in a dog, *J Vet Diagn Invest* 17:291–294, 2005.
59. Merlo M, Bo S, Ratto A: Primary right atrium haemangiosarcoma in a cat, *J Feline Med Surg* 4:61–64, 2002.
60. Campbell MD, Gelberg HB: Endocardial ossifying myxoma of the right atrium in a cat, *Vet Pathol* 37:460–462, 2000.
61. Paltrinieri S, Riccaboni P, Rondena M, et al: Pathologic and immunohistochemical findings in a feline aortic body tumor, *Vet Pathol* 41:195–198, 2004.
62. Venco L, Kramer L, Sola LB, et al: Primary cardiac rhabdomyosarcoma in a cat, *J Am Anim Hosp Assoc* 37:159–163, 2001.
63. Willis R, Williams AE, Schwarz T, et al: Aortic body chemodectoma causing pulmonary oedema in a cat, *J Small Anim Pract* 42:20–23, 2001.
64. George C, Steinberg H: An aortic body carcinoma with multifocal thoracic metastases in a cat, *J Comp Pathol* 101:467–469, 1989.
65. Klausner JS, Bell FW, Hayden DW, et al: Hypercalcemia in two cats with squamous cell carcinomas, *J Am Vet Med Assoc* 196:103–105, 1990.
66. Bortnowski HB, Rosenthal RC: Gastrointestinal mast cell tumors in two cats, *J Am Anim Hosp Assoc* 28:271–275, 1992.
67. Venco L, Kramer L, Sola LB, et al: Primary cardiac rhabdomyosarcoma in a cat, *J Am Anim Hosp Assoc* 37:159–163, 2001.

68. Meschter CL: Disseminated sweat gland adenocarcinoma with acronecrosis in a cat, *Cornell Vet* 81:195–203, 1991.
69. Wilkinson GT: Lymphosarcoma of the heart of a cat, *Vet Rec* 80:381–382, 1967.
70. Carter TD, Pariaut R, Snook E, et al: Multicentric lymphoma mimicking decompensated hypertrophic cardiomyopathy in a cat, *J Vet Intern Med* 22:1345–1347, 2008.
71. Berg RJ, Wingfield W: Pericardial effusion in the dog: a review of 42 cases, *J Am Anim Hosp Assoc* 20:131–137, 1984.
72. Ehrhart N, Ehrhart EJ, Willis J, et al: Analysis of factors affecting survival in dogs with aortic body tumors, *Vet Surg* 31:44–48, 2002.
73. Bonagura JD: Electrical alternans associated with pericardial effusion in the dog, *J Am Vet Med Assoc* 178:574–579, 1981.
74. Gidlewski J, Petrie JP: Pericardiocentesis and principles of echocardiographic imaging in the patient with cardiac neoplasia, *Clin Tech Small Anim Pract* 18:131–134, 2003.
75. Thomas WP, Sisson D, Bauer TG, et al: Detection of cardiac masses in dogs by two-dimensional echocardiography, *Vet Radiol* 25:65–71, 1984.
76. Fruchter AM, Miller CW, O'Grady MR: Echocardiographic results and clinical considerations in dogs with right atrial/auricular masses, *Can Vet J* 33:171–174, 1992.
77. MacDonald KA, Cagney O, Magne ML: Echocardiographic and clinicopathologic characterization of pericardial effusion in dogs: 107 cases (1985-2006), *J Am Vet Med Assoc* 235:1456–1461, 2009.
78. Rush JE, Keene BW, Fox PR: Pericardial disease in the cat: a retrospective evaluation of 66 cases, *J Am Anim Hosp Assoc* 26:39–46, 1990.
79. De Rycke LM, Gielen IM, Simoens PJ, et al: Computed tomography and cross-sectional anatomy of the thorax in clinically normal dogs, *Am J Vet Res* 66:512–524, 2005.
80. Mai W, Weisse C, Sleeper MM: Cardiac magnetic resonance imaging in normal dogs and two dogs with heart base tumor, *Vet Radiol Ultrasound* 51:428–435, 2010.
81. Hansen AE, McEvoy F, Engelholm SA, et al: FDG PET/CT imaging in canine cancer patients, *Vet Radiol Ultrasound* 52:201–206, 2011.
82. Naudé SH, Miller DB: Magnetic resonance imaging findings of a metastatic chemodectoma in a dog, *J S Afr Vet Assoc* 77:155–159, 2006.
83. Ogilvie GK, Brunkow CS, Daniel GB, et al: Malignant lymphoma with cardiac and bone involvement in a dog, *J Am Vet Med Assoc* 194:793–796, 1989.
84. Keene BW, Rush JE, Cooley AJ, et al: Primary left ventricular hemangiosarcoma diagnosed by endomyocardial biopsy in a dog, *J Am Vet Med Assoc* 197:1501–1503, 1990.
85. Sisson D, Thomas WP, Ruehl WW, et al: Diagnostic value of pericardial fluid analysis in the dog, *J Am Vet Med Assoc* 184:51–55, 1984.
86. Fine DM, Tobias AH, Jacob KA: Use of pericardial fluid pH to distinguish between idiopathic and neoplastic effusions, *J Vet Intern Med* 17:525–529, 2003.
87. de Laforcade AM, Freeman LM, Rozanski EA, et al: Biochemical analysis of pericardial fluid and whole blood in dogs with pericardial effusion, *J Vet Intern Med* 19:833–836, 2005.
88. Shaw SP, Rozanski EA, Rush JE: Cardiac troponin I and T in dogs with pericardial effusion, *J Vet Intern Med* 18:322–324, 2004.
89. Chun R, Kellihan HB, Henik RA, et al: Comparison of plasma cardiac troponin I concentrations among dogs with cardiac hemangiosarcoma, noncardiac hemangiosarcoma, other neoplasms, and pericardial effusion of nonhemangiosarcoma origin, *J Am Vet Med Assoc* 237:806–811, 2010.
90. Wykes PM, Rouse GP, Orton C: Removal of five canine cardiac tumors using a stapling instrument, *Vet Surg* 15:103–106, 1986.
91. Brisson BA, Holmberg DL: Use of pericardial patch graft reconstruction of the right atrium for treatment of hemangiosarcoma in a dog, *J Am Vet Med Assoc* 218:723–725, 2001.
92. Morges M, Worley DR, Withrow SJ, et al: Pericardial free patch grafting as a rescue technique in surgical management of right atrial HSA, *J Am Anim Hosp Assoc* 47:224–228, 2011.
93. Crumbaker DM, Rooney MB, Case JB: Thoracoscopic subtotal pericardiectomy and right atrial mass resection in a dog, *J Am Vet Med Assoc* 237:551–554, 2010.
94. Rioja E, Beaulieu K, Holmberg DL: Anesthetic management of an off-pump open-heart surgery in a dog, *Vet Anaesth Analg* 36: 361–368, 2009.
95. Walsh PJ, Remedios AM, Ferguson JF, et al: Thoracoscopic versus open partial pericardectomy in dogs: comparison of postoperative pain and morbidity, *Vet Surg* 28:472–479, 1999.
96. Jackson J, Richter KP, Launer DP: Thoracoscopic partial pericardiectomy in 13 dogs, *J Vet Intern Med* 13:529–533, 1999.
97. Kovak JR, Ludwig LL, Bergman PJ, et al: Use of thoracoscopy to determine the etiology of pleural effusion in dogs and cats: 18 cases (1998-2001), *J Am Vet Med Assoc* 221:990–994, 2002.
98. de Madron E, Helfand SC, Stebbins KE: Use of chemotherapy for treatment of cardiac hemangiosarcoma in a dog, *J Am Vet Med Assoc* 190:887–891, 1987.
99. Clifford CA, Mackin AJ, Henry CJ: Treatment of canine hemangiosarcoma: 2000 and beyond, *J Vet Intern Med* 14:479–485, 2000.
100. Dunning D, Monnet E, Orton EC, et al: Analysis of prognostic indicators for dogs with pericardial effusion: 46 cases (1985-1996), *J Am Vet Med Assoc* 212:1276–1280, 1998.
101. Reynen K, Köckeritz U, Strasser RH: Metastases to the heart, *Ann Oncol* 15:375–381, 2004.
102. Reynen K: Frequency of primary tumors of the heart, *Am J Cardiol* 77:107, 1996.
103. McAllister HA Jr, Hall RJ, Cooley DA: Tumors of the heart and pericardium, *Curr Probl Cardiol* 24:57–116, 1999.
104. Casey M, Vaughan CJ, He J, et al: Mutations in the protein kinase A R1alpha regulatory subunit cause familial cardiac myxomas and Carney complex, *J Clin Invest* 106:R31–R38, 2000.
105. Raaf HN, Raaf JH: Sarcomas related to the heart and vasculature, *Semin Surg Oncol* 10:374–382, 1994.
106. Donsbeck AV, Ranchere D, Coindre JM, et al: Primary cardiac sarcomas: an immunohistochemical and grading study with long-term follow-up of 24 cases, *Histopathology* 34:295–304, 1999.
107. Llombart-Cussac A, Pivot X, Contesso G, et al: Adjuvant chemotherapy for primary cardiac sarcomas: the IGR experience, *Br J Cancer* 78:1624–1628, 1998.
108. Burke A, Virmani R: Tumors of the cardiovascular system. In *Atlas of tumor pathology, 3rd series, fascicle 16*, Washington DC, 1996, Armed Forces Institute of Pathology.
109. Bussani R, De-Giorgio F, Abbate A, et al: Cardiac metastases, *J Clin Pathol* 60:27–34, 2007.

SECTION F
Histiocytic Diseases

CRAIG A. CLIFFORD, KATHERINE A. SKORUPSKI, AND PETER F. MOORE

Background

There are at least four well-defined histiocytic proliferative diseases that have been recognized in dogs. The challenge in some instances is to differentiate them from granulomatous, reactive inflammatory diseases or from lymphoma by examination of routine stains on paraffin sections alone. The clinical presentation and behavior and responsiveness to therapy vary tremendously between the syndromes observed.

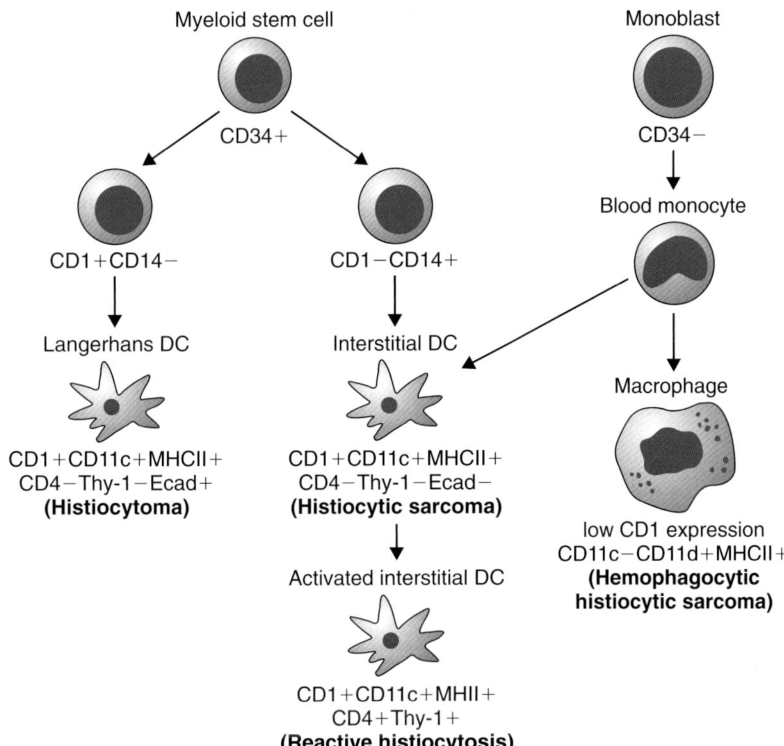

FIGURE 33-14 Lineage of histiocytic cells and the corresponding histiocytic disease syndromes.

Histiocytic Differentiation and Canine Histiocytosis

The development of canine-specific markers for differentiation molecules of macrophages and dendritic cells (DCs) has enabled the identification of the cell lineages involved in canine histiocytic diseases.[1-11] The majority of canine histiocytic diseases involve proliferations of cells of various DC lineages[1,2] (Figure 33-14).

The term *histiocyte* has been used to generically describe cells of DC or macrophage lineage. Histiocytes differentiate from $CD34^+$ stem cell precursors into macrophages and several DC lineages. Intraepithelial DCs are also known as *Langerhans cells* (LC). Interstitial DCs occur in perivascular locations in many organs except the brain, although they do occur in the meninges. Perhaps the most studied interstitial DCs are the dermal DCs. DCs that occur in T-cell domains in peripheral lymphoid organs (lymph node and spleen) are known as interdigitating DCs. Interdigitating DCs in lymph nodes are comprised of resident DCs and migratory DCs. The migratory DCs arrive in lymphatics from tissues and consist of LCs and interstitial DCs.[6] Cytokines and growth factors that influence DC development include FLT3 ligand, granulocyte-macrophage colony-stimulating factor (GM-CSF), tumor necrosis factor-α (TNF-α), IL-4, and TGF-β.[6,7] Macrophage development from $CD34^+$ precursors is influenced by GM-CSF and M-CSF. Blood monocytes can differentiate either into macrophages under the influence of M-CSF or into DCs under influence of GM-CSF and IL-4.[6-9]

DCs are the most potent antigen-presenting cells (APCs) for induction of immune responses in naïve T cells. The development of canine-specific monoclonal antibodies (MAbs) for functionally important molecules of DCs and macrophages has enabled their identification in canine tissues, especially skin.[1,10] DCs occur in two major locations: within the epidermis (LC) and within the dermis, especially adjacent to postcapillary venules (dermal interstitial DCs).[11] Canine DCs abundantly express CD1a molecules, which together with MHC class I and MHC class II molecules, are responsible for presentation of peptides, lipids, and glycolipids to T-cells.[1,3,12] Hence DCs are best defined by their abundant expression of molecules essential to their function as APCs. Of these, the family of CD1 proteins is largely restricted in expression to DCs in skin, whereas MHC class I and II are more broadly expressed.

The beta-2 integrins (CD11/CD18) are critically important adhesion molecules, which are differentially expressed by all leukocytes. CD11/CD18 expression is highly regulated in normal canine macrophages and DCs. CD11c is expressed by LCs and interstitial DCs, whereas macrophages predominately express CD11b (or CD11d in the splenic red pulp and bone marrow). A subset of dermal interstitial DCs also express CD11b.[13-15] In diseased tissues, these beta-2 integrin expression patterns may be broadened. LCs and dermal interstitial DCs are also distinguishable by their differential expression of E-cadherin (LC+) and Thy-1 (CD90) (dermal interstitial DC+). LCs localize within epithelia via E-cadherin homotypic adhesion with E-cadherin expressed by epithelial cells.[1]

Migration of DCs (as veiled cells) beyond the skin to the paracortex of lymph nodes, where they join forces with interdigitating DCs, occurs following contact with antigen. Successful interaction of DCs and T-cells in response to the antigenic challenge also involves the orderly appearance of co-stimulatory molecules (B7 family—CD80 and CD86) on DCs and their ligands (CD28 and CTLA-4) on T-cells.[16-18] In situ DCs have low expression of MHC II and co-stimulatory molecules and are more receptive to antigen uptake. Migratory DCs upregulate MHC class II and B7 family members and become more adept at antigen presentation to T-cells.[17,18]

TABLE 33-4 Cell Markers of Importance in the Diagnosis of Leukocytic Proliferative Diseases in Dogs

Marker	Description
CD3ε	Signaling component of the T-cell antigen receptor. Expressed by αβ T-cells and γδ T-cells. Cytoplasmic expression by natural killer (NK) cells is possible, especially if activated.
CD79a	Signaling component of the B-cell antigen receptor. Expressed by all stages of B-cell differentiation. Expression is less in plasma cells.
CD20	Surface molecule expressed at all stages of B-cell differentiation except for plasma cells. CD20 plays a role in regulation of B-cell activation and proliferation. CD20 is not lineage specific and has been observed uncommonly in T-cell lymphomas. Caution is advised in interpretation of diffuse cytoplasmic expression, which can occur in several cell types.
Pax5	Transcription factor essential for maintenance of B-cell differentiation. Useful B-cell marker.
MUM1/IRF4	Transcription factor essential for plasma cell differentiation. Useful plasma cell marker.
CD11d	αD subunit of beta-2 integrin (CD18) family. Expressed by macrophages and T-cells in hemopoietic environments, especially splenic red pulp. Bone marrow and lymph node medullary sinus macrophages express CD11d. CD11d is consistently expressed in diseases emanating from splenic red pulp (large granulated lymphoma [LGL] form of chronic lymphocytic leukemia [CLL], hepatosplenic lymphoma, and hemophagocytic histiocytic sarcoma).
CD18	β-subunit of the beta-2 integrin family of leukocyte adhesion molecules. Expressed as a heterodimer of CD11a, CD11b, CD11c, or CD11d with CD18. Leukocytes express at least one form of the heterodimer. Hence CD18 is expressed on all leukocytes—the expression level on myeloid cells is especially high compared to normal lymphocytes. CD18 has been used as a marker of histiocytes, but this depends on exclusion of lymphocyte differentiation by the use of other markers (CD3 and CD79a).
CD30	CD30 is an integral membrane glycoprotein and a member of the tumor necrosis factor receptor (TNFR) superfamily. It is not expressed by resting lymphocytes but is expressed by mitogen-activated T- and B-cells.
CD45	Surface molecule expressed by all leukocytes, formerly known as *leukocyte common antigen*. Antibodies to CD45 bind to the extracellular domain outside of the 3 variably spliced exons (A, B, and C).
CD45RA	Splice variant of CD45 in which the A exon is present. Expressed by B-cells and naïve T-cells. Not typically expressed by histiocytes.
CD90 (Thy-1)	Cell surface molecule with broad cell and tissue distribution. CD90 is expressed by interstitial-type dendritic cells (DC) but not by Langerhans cells (LC).
c-Kit	Surface molecule and member of the receptor tyrosine kinase family (type III). Expressed by most hemopoietic progenitor cells and by mast cells. Expression level is high in high-grade mast cell tumors.
E-cadherin	Adhesion molecule expressed by epithelia and by some leukocytes, especially useful in cutaneous round cell tumors to identify LC indicative of cutaneous histiocytoma.
Granzyme B (GrB)	Serine protease located in the granules of cytotoxic T-cells ($CD8^+$) and NK cells. GrB is expressed at high levels in activated cells and leads to rapid target cell death by apoptosis.
Myeloperoxidase (MPO)	MPO is a lysosomal protein stored in the azurophilic granules of neutrophils (and monocytes). MPO is an important marker of myeloid differentiation.
Ki67	Cell proliferation marker (nuclear) expressed in all phases of the cell cycle except G0 and early G1. Excellent marker for determining the growth fraction of a cell population.

Aspects of the developmental and migratory program of DCs are recapitulated in canine histiocytic diseases. Defective interaction of DCs and T-cells appears to contribute to the development of reactive histiocytoses (cutaneous and systemic histiocytosis), which are related interstitial DC disorders arising out of disordered immune regulation. The distant migratory potential of DCs is of immense clinical significance in the adverse prognosis of histiocytic sarcomas, which largely originate in interstitial DCs and rapidly disseminate via metastasis.

Immunophenotyping

To classify hematopoietic neoplasia according to the WHO system as applied to the canine, it is important to have access to markers for IHC analysis.[19,20] Table 33-4 lists the markers of value for determining cell lineages in leukocytic proliferations in dogs. These markers are suitable for use in formalin-fixed paraffin-embedded tissues with appropriate antigen retrieval protocols. Markers are available for the detection of B- and T-cells. However, markers for the unequivocal detection of NK cells are not available, so the existence of NK cell lymphomas in dogs is not easily assessable. Determination of T-cell receptor usage and major subsets of T-cells (CD4 or CD8), as well as dissecting the lineages of histiocytes (macrophages, interstitial type DCs, and LCs), is best done in unfixed cell smears or snap-frozen tissues or by flow cytometry. Important markers for the dissection of the histiocytic lineage that are only detectable in fresh smears or snap-frozen tissues include CD1a, CD11b, CD11c, MHC class II, CD80, and CD86. However, it is still possible to presumptively identify histiocytes in formalin-fixed tissues by using combinations of lymphoid markers coupled with CD18 staining (as indicated in Table 33-4) in an appropriate morphologic context.

Once IHC stains are performed, it may also be necessary to run molecular clonality analyses to rule out lymphoma. This is particularly so with inflamed T-cell lymphomas, which are readily mistaken for reactive histiocytoses when they arise in skin.

Cutaneous Histiocytoma

Cutaneous histiocytoma (CH) is a benign tumor that often occurs as a single lesion in young dogs (<3 years of age), although histiocytomas do occur in dogs of all ages. In a retrospective review from the United Kingdom of histopathologic diagnoses of neoplasia in dogs less than 1 year, of 20,280 submissions, CH was the most common diagnosis, representing 89%.[21] These tumors typically present as a solitary lesion often in the cranial portion of the body. The growth of the lesion can be quite rapid (1 to 4 weeks) and oftentimes will spontaneously regress within 1 to 2 months of presentation.[22-31] The regression is lymphocyte mediated.

Multiple tumors and metastatic histiocytomas have been reported, and the presence of multiple histiocytomas, especially in aged dogs, can present a diagnostic dilemma. Distinction from epitheliotropic and nonepitheliotropic cutaneous T-cell lymphoma may be challenging unless IHC stains for lymphoid and histiocytic markers are conducted. Definitive diagnosis of histiocytoma depends on IHC, which is best performed on frozen sections of tumor or cytologic preparations. Studies have demonstrated histiocytomas are of epidermal LC origin via expression of CD1a, CD11c, E-cadherin, and MHC class II molecules; inconsistent lysozyme immunoreactivity; and lack of expression of Thy-1 and CD4 (marker of activated DCs).[1,2,4,23,24] Among skin leukocytes, E-cadherin expression is largely restricted to LCs. LCs utilize E-cadherin to localize in the epidermis via homotypic interaction, with E-cadherin expressed by keratinocytes. E-cadherin expression has only rarely been observed in histocytic sarcoma (HS) in canine skin and subcutis, although a recent report challenges the specificity of E-cadherin for diagnosis of cutaneous round cell tumors.[32] The expression of E-cadherin is unique to histiocytomas, and negative expression of Thy-1 and CD4 helps to differentiate histiocytomas (CH) from reactive histiocytoses—systemic histiocytosis (SH) and cutaneous histiocytosis (CHS).[2,4] This differentiation can be made based on IHC or flow cytometry.[33] It is interesting to note that CH cells not only have the immunophenotypic characteristics of LCs but also the functional capability of being potent stimulators of the mixed leukocyte reaction.

The factors that determine the onset of regression in canine histiocytomas are unknown. Evidence of regression may be rapid (weeks), although regression can be delayed for many months. Regression is mediated by $CD8^+$ $\alpha\beta$ T-cells; only scant numbers of $CD4^+$T-cells are observed in histiocytoma lesions. Migration of tumor histiocytes and/or tumor-infiltrating reactive interstitial DCs to draining lymph nodes likely activate $CD4^+$ T-cells, which would assist in $CD8^+$ cytotoxic T-cell recruitment. Because massive $CD8^+$ T-cell infiltration is observed in all instances of histiocytoma regression, therapeutic intervention with the aim of immunosuppression should be avoided once a definitive diagnosis of histiocytoma has been reached to avoid interference with cytotoxic T-cell function. Recent evidence suggests E-cadherin staining correlates with the stage of regression. In more superficial regions of the tumor, membranous staining was noted versus deeper regions in which staining was decreased to nonexistent. The decrease in E-cadherin expression is associated with lymphoid infiltration and is linked to its spontaneous regression.

Cutaneous Langerhans Cell Histiocytosis

The presence of multiple histiocytomas is uncommon. Lesions may be limited to skin or involve skin and draining lymph nodes. Rarely, internal organ involvement also occurs. This spectrum of disease best fits under the umbrella of cutaneous Langerhans cell histiocytosis (LCH) because skin is invariably involved.

Cutaneous LCH limited to skin appears to be more common in Shar-Pei dogs (35% of cases) but can occur in any breed. Delayed regression of cutaneous LCH can occur, and lesions can persist for up to 10 months before onset of regression. In about 50% of instances, dogs with cutaneous LCH are euthanized due to lack of regression of lesions and complications in management of the extensive ulcerated lesions that are often present.

Cutaneous LCH with lymph node metastasis has an even poorer prognosis because spontaneous regression has not been encountered, and all of the dogs with this lesion distribution and stage have been euthanized. Cutaneous LCH may spread beyond skin and draining lymph nodes to involve internal organs. This is a more serious and rapidly progressive disease. This spectrum of disease manifestation and diverse clinical behavior is most like LCH of humans.[34,35] In veterinary medicine, anecdotal responses to this form have been noted with lomustine (CCNU) and the tyrosine kinase inhibitor masitinib (AB Science, Paris).

Reactive Histiocytosis

Reactive histiocytosis can be separated into CHS and SH. CHS represents a benign, diffuse aggregation of histiocytes that grows rapidly into infiltrating nodules, plaques, and crusts within the skin and subcutaneous tissue.[4,31,36] This disease tends to occur in younger dogs; however, one study noted a range of 2 to 11 years. A breed predisposition has yet to be identified, although, in one study of 32 dogs, golden retrievers, Great Danes, and Bouvier des Flandres were more common.[37] A study of 18 dogs with CHS noted a male predilection; however, in a second larger study, no sex predilection was identified.[4,37] Interestingly, a study of 32 dogs noted a previous history of dermatologic disease, with allergic dermatitis (n = 11) being most common. The duration from appearance of lesions to diagnosis via biopsy in one study was 1.75 months (range 0 to 30 months).[37]

This disease is limited to the skin and subcutis but can be multifocal. The head, pinna, limb, and scrotum are commonly reported sites.[4,31,36] Lesions may also be found on the nasal planum and within nasal mucosa, the gross appearance of which has been described as a "clown nose."[38] In a recent study, 10 of 32 dogs had nasal planum/nares involvement, which presented as swelling, erythema, depigmentation, and stertorous respiration. However, extension into the nasal mucosa would classify this disease as SH. Histologically, lesions contain a pleocellular histiocytic infiltrate, often perivascular within the dermis and subcutaneous tissue. Lymphoid infiltrates (T-cell predominance) and some neutrophils are common. Vascular invasion may be present. These histiocytes express CD1a, CD11c, MHC class II molecules, Thy-1, and CD4 but are negative for E-cadherin. The expression of Thy-1 and CD4 aids in differentiation of this disease, which appears to be of interstitial DC origin from CH, which is of epidermal LC origin.[4,31,36] Definitive diagnosis of CHS is typically based on history, clinical signs, histopathologic features, and ruling out infectious causes. Immunohistochemistry on fresh, snap-frozen tissue is required to differentiate between macrophages and DCs and to identify dermal DC origin.

CHS follows a benign course and is often responsive to immunosuppressive therapy, although spontaneous regressions have been reported. Surgical excision may be successful in a minority of cases as lesions typically recur in other locations. Antibiotics are generally ineffective in treating CHS. Systemic steroids are a standard of care, and PRs are seen in the majority of dogs.[4,36,38] However, recent findings and the author's impression are a 50% response rate with steroids. Many of these dogs require continuous therapy to prevent recurrence. A remission was reported in one dog receiving intralesional corticosteroids. Spontaneous regression occurred in 2 of 13 dogs and surgery was curative in another. In another study of 32 dogs, all had complete resolution of lesions within a median number of 45 days (range 10 to 162 days) from initial therapy.[37] Initial therapy included prednisone alone or in combination with antibiotics (n = 12), prednisone with tetracycline/doxycycline and niacinamide (n = 4), prednisone and azathioprine (n = 3), and tetracycline/niacinamide either alone or in combination with vitamin E and essential fatty acids (n = 6). Of the 19 dogs receiving prednisone, dosages ranged from 0.5 mg/kg to 2 mg/kg.[37]

Long-term maintenance therapies may be warranted to prevent recurrence; however, affected dogs may have a prolonged survival. In 32 dogs obtaining complete resolution of lesions, 17 were maintained on a variety of medications, including 12 with tetracycline/niacinamide, either alone (n = 7) or in various combinations with safflower oil, essential fatty acids, or vitamin E.[37] Other maintenance therapies included cyclosporine/ketoconazole, azathioprine alone, prednisone and azathioprine, or prednisone alone. Immunosuppressive agents such as leflunomide and cyclosporine A/ketoconazole and azathioprine have demonstrated efficacy in steroid refractory cases.

In a recent study with a median follow-up time of 25 months (mean 32 months, range 6 to 108 months), 26 of 32 dogs were alive with no lesions. Interestingly, 10 dogs were on a maintenance protocol, the majority of which entailed tetracycline/niacinamide alone or in combination with essential fatty acids, azathioprine, or vitamin E.

Systemic Histiocytosis

SH is a nonneoplastic disease of proliferative lymphocytes occurring in Bernese mountain dogs, Rottweilers, golden retrievers, and Irish wolfhounds.[4,31,38-42] In the Bernese mountain dog, this appears to be a familial disease, suggesting a genetic predisposition.[4,31,38,40] Earlier work also noted a male predilection in the Bernese breed.[3,38,40] The age of onset for SH is 3 to 9 years. Dermal lesions manifest in the skin with similar site predilection as CHS; however, other sites, including subcutaneous tissue, lymph node, bone marrow, spleen, liver, lung, and mucous membranes (nasal and ocular tissue), can be involved. Ocular involvement includes the conjunctiva, sclera, ciliary body, extraocular muscles, and retrobulbar tissue.[42] One distinguishing feature from CH is the presence of palpably enlarged peripheral lymph nodes and the presence of organ involvement.[4,31] Clinical signs vary, depending on the affected tissue and severity of disease; however, depression, anorexia, weight loss, conjunctivitis, and harsh respiration are common. In one study, 2 of 26 dogs were hypercalcemic at presentation.[4] This disease appears similar to some forms of the LC histiocytosis in humans, which are reactive disorders likely secondary to immune system dysregulation. Clinicopathologic features of SH are varied; however, anemia, monocytosis, and lymphopenia are consistently reported.[31,43]

Cytologically, SH lesions are similar to granulomatous inflammation or CHS, characterized by a predominance of benign histiocytes with occasional multinucleated giant cells.[43] Other inflammatory cells including lymphocytes, eosinophils, and neutrophils can be interspersed. Erythrophagia is reported but rare. Histiocytic cells are large, contain voluminous cytoplasm, and have indented nuclei with variable nucleoli.[43] Histologically, these lesions are characterized by multicentric, nodular, angiocentric histiocytic infiltrates within the deep dermis and panniculus. To a lesser degree, infiltration of lymphocytes, plasma cells, eosinophils, and neutrophils is present, with small lymphocytes making up the greatest proportion of nonhistiocytic cells.[1,4,31,38] Blood and lymphatic vessel invasion may also be noted. In some cases, vascular wall degeneration, thrombosis, and ischemic necrosis may be present.[4,31,38,40] The histologic appearance of lesions within other organs consists of nodular, perivascular accumulation of histiocytes, lymphocytes, and neutrophils.[4,31,38] With IHC, SH lesions express CD1a, CD11c, MHC class II, Thy-1, and CD4, similar to that of CHS.[3,4] This expression pattern suggests these cells are of activated interstitial DCs and not epidermal LCs (histiocytoma).[1,44] The majority of the small lymphocytes present within the lesions have been demonstrated to be of T-cell origin (CD3 and TCR$\alpha\beta$ positive) and 50% were CD8 positive.[3,4] Unlike cutaneous histiocytomas, the presence of T-cells is not associated with regression but likely secondary to cytokine-induced migration. Interestingly, ocular involvement appears similar to lesions described with fibrous histiocytoma.[42,43]

Lesions may have a waxing and waning presentation but generally do not spontaneously resolve and thus require long-term therapy. Corticosteroids alone appear ineffective in controlling this disease long term.[4,31,38,42] Experimentally, bovine thymosin fraction-5 demonstrated some efficacy in two dogs.[4,40] The use of azathioprine, cyclosporine A, or leflunomide (Hoechst Marion Roussel, Wiesbaden, Germany) has yielded long-term control in some cases.[4] Cyclosporine and leflunomide both have the ability to inhibit T-cells. The successful treatment with either agent suggests a significant role of T-cell lymphocytes in this disease. Two proposed mechanisms for immune dysregulation include an increase in proinflammatory cytokine (TNF-α, IL-6, IL-12, IFN-γ) production by T-cells due to persistent DC accumulation and inappropriate dendritic and T-cell interaction due to abnormal regulation of accessory ligands on both cell types.[4,11] These molecules are needed for induction of the immune response and the subsequent downregulation of the response. Without a proper interaction, the cells may remain within the area.[11] Although no infectious cause has been identified, it is important to rule out such etiologies with either a culture or immunohistochemistry of histopathology samples.[4,11] The clinical course of this disease is often prolonged but rarely results in death. Generally, there are episodic periods of response followed by recrudescence, with most dogs euthanized due to repeated relapses of the clinical condition or failure to respond to therapeutics.[4,31,40]

Histiocytic Sarcoma

Pathology and Natural Behavior

Malignant proliferations of histiocytic cells were first reported in the dog in the late 1970s. A predisposition in Bernese mountain dogs was reported in 1986 in a group of 11 dogs affected with the disease, 9 of which were related.[45] In that study group, a male predisposition was present (10 of 11 dogs) and the majority had pulmonary involvement. Histiocytic sarcoma (HS) has since been identified in a variety of breeds; however, flat-coated retrievers and Rottweilers also appear to be overrepresented.[46,47] Dogs are commonly middle aged or older, but HS has been reported in dogs as young as 3 years of age. HS may present with either localized organ involvement or disseminated, multiorgan involvement.

HS is the preferred term identifying malignant tumors of histiocytic origin and the older term *malignant histiocytosis* refers to the disseminated form of the disease. Reported anatomic sites include the lungs, lymph nodes, liver, spleen, stomach, pancreas, mediastinum, skin, skeletal muscle, central nervous system (CNS), bone, bone marrow, nasal cavity, and eyes.[46-53] In a clinical population, 5% of primary brain tumors were HS, as were 4.5% of secondary brain tumors in a necropsy population.[53,54] In a series of 26 dogs with ocular HS, ocular involvement was usually found in association with multisystem disease.[8] HS also appears to be the most common synovial tumor in dogs, with 18 of 35 tumors previously diagnosed as synovial cell sarcomas reclassified as HS based on IHC staining patterns.[47] Eleven of these 18 dogs with synovial HS were Rottweilers.

Hemophagocytic HS is a subtype of HS that arises from macrophages rather than DCs. The hemophagocytic HS variant can be definitively differentiated through confirmation of an IHC staining pattern consistent with macrophages.[5] Clinically, these tumors appear to behave more aggressively due to their cellular ability to phagocytose material, including host red blood cells.

History and Clinical Signs

Presenting complaints and clinical signs vary, depending on site(s) of tumor involvement, but nonspecific symptoms such as lethargy, inappetence, and weight loss are common. Other common signs include a visible mass, lameness, cough, vomiting, and lymphadenopathy.[51] Lymphadenopathy is sometimes the only clinical sign and can appear at a site distant to other tumor lesions. Patients may also present with clinical signs related to severe anemia or thrombocytopenia, especially in dogs with the hemophagocytic variant.[5,51]

Diagnosis and Staging

A diagnosis of HS can be obtained via cytologic or histologic examination of tumor tissue; however, definitive diagnosis can be challenging in pleomorphic tumors that have morphologic characteristics similar to carcinomas or round cell tumors. HS cells are large, discrete, mononuclear cells that often display marked anisocytosis and anisokaryosis. Nuclei are round, oval, or reniform with prominent nucleoli, and cytoplasm is moderate to abundant, lightly basophilic, and vacuolated. Mitotic figures are common, and some tumor cells may display erythrophagocytosis and/or multinucleated giant cells (Figure 33-15).[55] Evidence to support a diagnosis of HS may be acquired through immunocytochemistry or immunohistochemistry on formalin-fixed tissues using antibodies to CD18, CD3, and CD79a.[2] Macrophages and granulocytes express tenfold more CD18 than lymphocytes; thus for differentiation purposes, lymphomas express low or undetectable levels and usually express either CD3 or CD79a.[1] If fresh or frozen tissue is available, further confirmation and subclassification of the cell of origin can be performed using antibody staining for CD1 or the CD11 α subunits.[2]

Because the disease is multifocal or disseminated in most dogs, complete staging is recommended. CBC and biochemical screens are often abnormal. Anemia is common and usually regenerative when caused by erythrophagocytosis by neoplastic cells. Leukocytosis, thrombocytopenia, increased liver enzymes, hypoalbuminemia, and hypocholesterolemia are frequent findings, and hypercalcemia occurs occasionally.[5,51] HS was the second most common cause of pancytopenia in dogs in a retrospective study of 51 dogs at a veterinary teaching hospital.[56] Hyperferritinemia has also been documented in dogs with HS and is theorized to be the result of ferritin production by tumor cells.[57,58] Thoracic radiography and abdominal ultrasonography commonly reveal abnormalities. Pulmonary involvement may appear as a diffuse interstitial infiltrate, patchy consolidated areas, or focal or multifocal mass lesions (Figure 33-16). Radiographic evidence of sternal, cranial mediastinal, or tracheobronchial lymphadenopathy may also be noted. Hepatosplenomegaly, splenic or hepatic mottling, or discrete nodules or masses in these organs are the most common abdominal ultrasonographic abnormalities.[59]

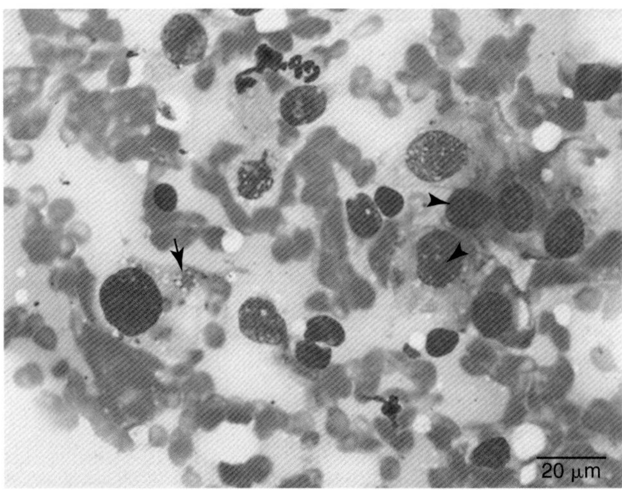

FIGURE 33-15 Cytology of histiocytic sarcoma in the liver of a dog. Note individualized and loosely cohesive moderately pleomorphic spindle cells with prominent nucleoli *(arrowheads)*. Some demonstrate phagocytic activity *(arrow)*. (Wright-Giemsa, 100× objective.) *(Courtesy Elizabeth Little, VMD, DACVP, IDEXX Laboratories, Langhorne, PA.)*

Bone marrow aspiration cytology may reveal tumor infiltrate, especially in patients with cytopenias. In addition, flow cytometry has been used to differentiate etiology of hemophagocytosis in bone marrow samples containing over 5% macrophages and cytologic evidence of hemophagocytosis (Figure 33-17).[60] Results suggested that cellular distribution in scatter plots and the number of histiocytes may help differentiate neoplastic from nonneoplastic causes of hemophagocytosis.

Treatment and Prognosis

The clinical course of disseminated HS, left untreated, is rapid and fatal, whereas the localized form may be more slowly progressive. Few reports documenting survival duration after surgical excision of localized HS exist. However, in a series of 18 synovial or periarticular HSs confirmed with CD18 staining, the MST for dogs undergoing amputation was 6 months and the metastatic rate was 91%.[47] The periarticular form of HS may be associated with a better prognosis than other locations. In one study, dogs with periarticular HS treated in a variety of ways had a MST of 391 days compared to 128 days in dogs with the nonperiarticular form.[61] Fewer dogs with periarticular HS had distant metastasis; however, it is not clear

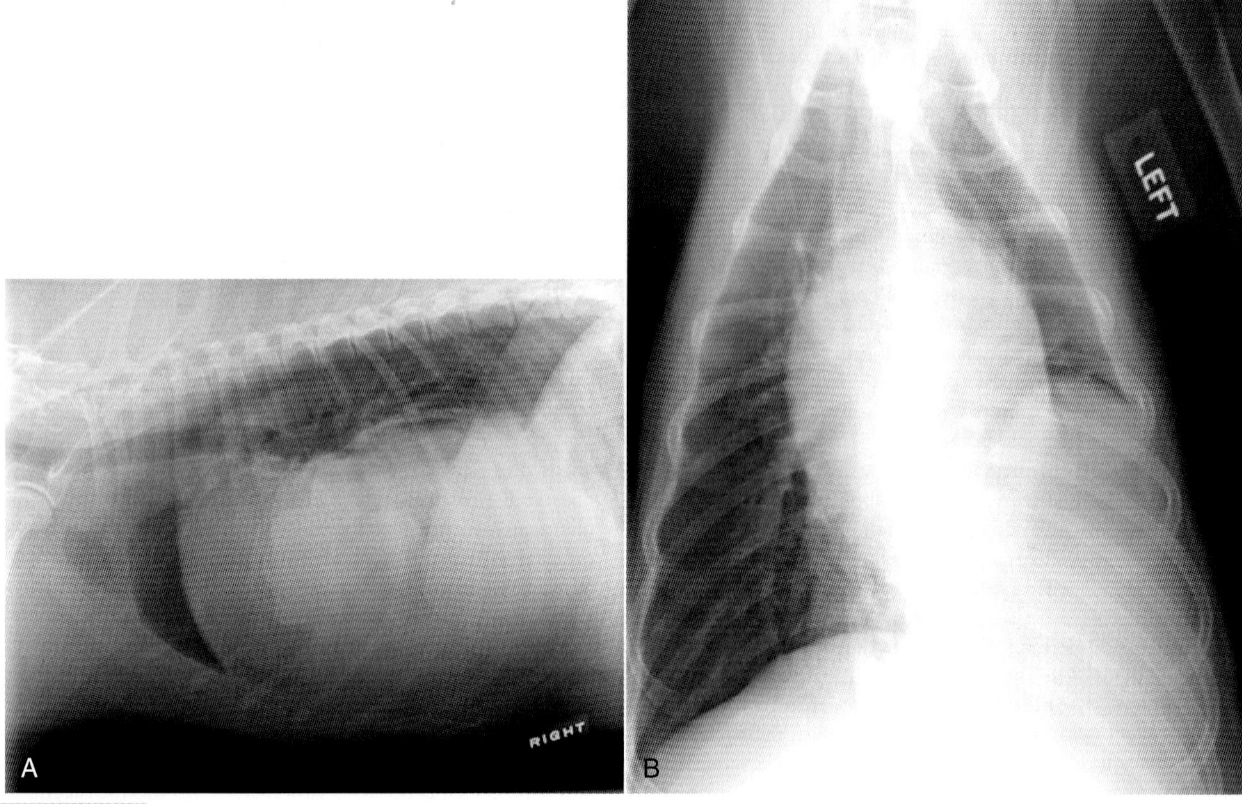

FIGURE 33-16 **A,** Right lateral radiograph of a 6-year-old female spayed German shepherd dog demonstrating a large, multilobular soft tissue mass and an adjacent yet separate smaller mass in the left caudal thorax. The mass displaces the caudal portion of the left lung bronchus and completely obscures the caudal bronchus. **B,** Ventrodorsal radiograph of the same patient demonstrating a soft tissue density in the left caudal thorax. Histopathology confirmed histiocytic sarcoma. *(Picture courtesy Dr. LP de Lorimier, Hôpital Vétérinaire Rive-Sud, Québec Canada; radiographic description courtesy Dr. Anthony Fischetti, the Animal Medical Center, New York City.)*

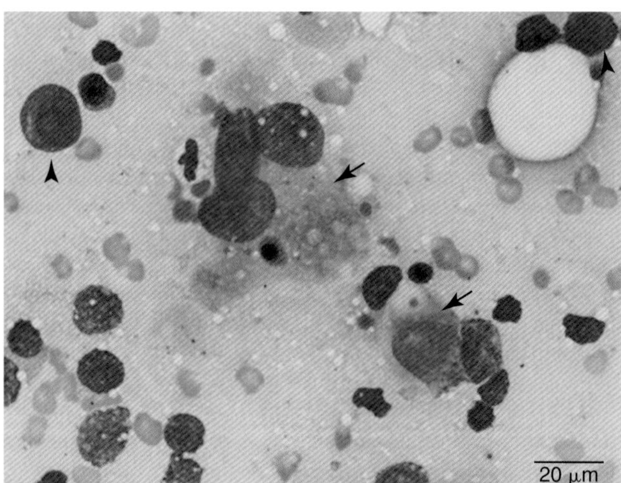

FIGURE 33-17 Cytology of histiocytic sarcoma in the bone marrow of a dog. Neoplastic cells *(arrows)* and erythroid progenitors *(arrowheads)* are visible. Note phagocytic activity of neoplastic cells. (Wright-Giemsa, 100× objective.) *(Courtesy Elizabeth Little, VMD, DACVP, IDEXX Laboratories, Langhorne, PA.)*

whether the improved survival may be due to primary tumor location or due to earlier stage of disease at diagnosis.[61]

CCNU appears to be the most effective chemotherapy agent against HS in dogs. One study reported a 46% response rate to CCNU in 56 dogs with gross measurable disease.[51] Median remission duration in dogs achieving CR or PR was 85 days, and the MST of responders was 172 days. In this study, anemia, thrombocytopenia, hypoalbuminemia, and splenic involvement, all factors associated with the hemophagocytic subtype of HS, were associated with a grave prognosis. Corticosteroids did not improve response to therapy in this study. In a prospective study of 21 dogs with HS treated with 90 mg/m^2 of CCNU, the response rate was lower at 29%, although 67% of dogs received only one dose of CCNU.[62] The median response duration was 96 days. CCNU therapy used as an adjuvant to surgery and/or RT may result in lengthy survival times in dogs with localized HS. One study documented a MST of 19 months in 16 dogs with localized HS treated with aggressive combination therapy.[63]

There is limited information in the literature regarding alternative chemotherapeutic options to treat HS, but reports of responses to liposomal DOX and paclitaxel chemotherapy exist.[64,65] In addition, a case report of a dog with cutaneous disseminated HS documented temporary remissions resulting from multiple protocols, including cyclophosphamide, vincristine, prednisone, mitoxantrone, dacarbazine, and etoposide.[66] The efficacy of the bisphosphonate, clodronate, has been recently studied in histiocytic cell lines and in five dogs with HS.[67] Two of the five dogs experienced tumor regression with this therapy, and further study is warranted. The efficacy of DOX against HS has not been published, but preliminary reports suggest that tumor responses can occur.[68] Additionally, the authors have observed responses to a nanoparticle formulation of paclitaxel in dogs with HS.

The efficacy of RT against HS has not been fully studied; however, preliminary evidence suggests that HS is radiosensitive. In a report of 37 flat-coated retrievers with mostly joint origin HS, dogs undergoing RT lived longer than those not having RT, with a MST of 182 days.[69] Dogs treated with a set combined protocol of a palliative radiation and CCNU had a MST of 208 days. Further study into the optimal radiation protocol for HS is necessary.

Hemophagocytic Histiocytic Sarcoma

Hemophagocytic HS is a variant of HS that originates from the tissue macrophage, not the DC.[5] This more aggressive form of HS invariably involves the spleen, but dogs may also have liver, bone marrow, lymph node, and/or lung involvement. Splenic involvement is usually diffuse, resulting in gross enlargement with diffuse infiltrates. In one study, common hematologic findings in dogs with the hemophagocytic variant of HS included a regenerative anemia (94%), thrombocytopenia (88%), hypoalbuminemia (94%), and hypocholesterolemia (69%).[5] A presumptive diagnosis of hemophagocytic HS may be obtained through splenic cytology, which shows infiltration with atypical to highly pleomorphic macrophages displaying phagocytosis of red blood cells, splenic origin red cell precursors, and white blood cells. However, definitive diagnosis and differentiation from nonhemophagocytic HS requires immunophenotyping. To date, effective treatment of hemophagocytic HS has not been described. Reported survival times are extremely short, ranging from days to 1 to 2 months.[5,51]

Feline Histiocytic Diseases

Histiocytic neoplasms are much rarer in cats than dogs, but three distinct forms have been documented in the species to date. These include HS, with features similar to the canine disease; feline progressive histiocytosis, a cutaneous form of histiocytic neoplasia with indolent but progressive behavior; and LC histiocytosis, with disease localized primarily to the lungs.

Feline Histiocytic Sarcoma

HS of DC origin and hemophagocytic HS of macrophage origin have both been documented in cats.[70-72] With both variants, cats usually present with multifocal or disseminated disease. Spleen, liver, and bone marrow involvement are most common, but lymph node, lung, trachea, mediastinum, kidney, bladder, and CNS involvement are also reported.[70-77] Bone marrow involvement appears commonly in cats, and all three cats in a case series were found to have positive bone marrow on postmortem evaluation.[71] Severe anemia and thrombocytopenia are also common findings and may indicate bone marrow involvement and/or hemophagocytic HS, which can be confirmed through immunophenotyping of tumor tissue samples.[70-72] The localized form of HS is extremely rare in cats but has been reported in the tarsus of a cat with local lymph node metastasis present at diagnosis.[78] An aggressive clinical course is typical of HS in cats, particularly in those with anemia and suspected hemophagocytic HS. Effective treatment options for feline HS have not been studied, although treatment with CCNU chemotherapy has been reported anecdotally.[72]

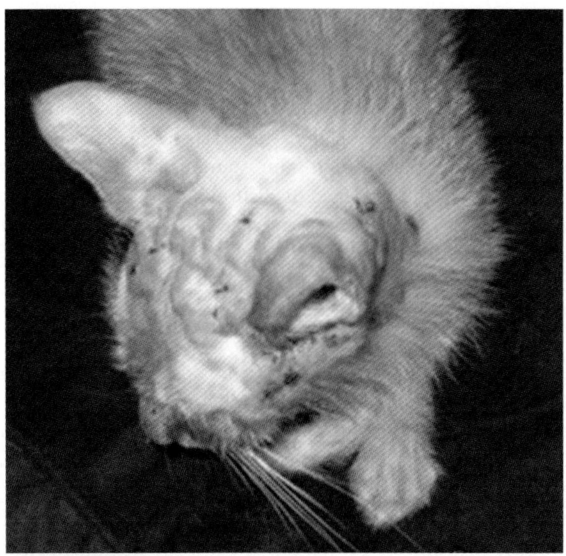

FIGURE 33-18 A cat with advanced feline progressive histiocytosis. The lesions consist of multiple coalescing hairless dermal nodules on the head, some of which have become ulcerated. *(Courtesy Emily Rothstein, DVM, DACVD, Animal Allergy and Dermatology Service of Connecticut, Plantsville, CT.)*

Feline Progressive Histiocytosis

Feline progressive histiocytosis is a recently described neoplasm of DCs that occurs initially on the skin and progresses over time to involve multiple organs. Lesions appear on the skin as multiple firm, haired or hairless, dermal papules or nodules with a predilection for the head, feet, and legs. The lesions may enlarge gradually and coalesce into plaques and can become ulcerated and painful over time. An example of a cat with advanced lesions is shown in Figure 33-18. The disease is usually progressive over months or years (median 13.4 months) with involvement of lymph nodes, lungs, and abdominal visceral organs. Females appear to be overrepresented.[79]

A diagnosis of feline progressive histiocytosis is made through biopsy and histopathologic evaluation of skin lesions. Lesions appear histologically as poorly circumscribed multinodular aggregates or masses of round cells with or without epitheliotropism in the dermis and, occasionally, invading subcutis. Cells have mild-to-moderate anisocytosis and anisokaryosis, and mitotic figures are rare. Immunohistochemistry may be necessary to confirm the diagnosis and rule out other round cell tumors.[79] Staging test results are usually negative for internal organ involvement early in the course of disease, but tumors may be found in lymph nodes, lung, and/or abdominal viscera as the disease progresses. Surgical excision may control solitary, superficial skin lesions early in the course of disease, but development of additional skin lesions is expected. Skin lesions do not appear to respond to corticosteroid therapy, and effective medical treatment of diffuse skin or visceral lesions has not yet been described.[79]

Langerhans Cell Histiocytosis

A single case series exists describing an aggressive neoplasm arising from LCs in three cats.[80] All three cats presented for respiratory compromise or distress, with symptom duration ranging from 5 days to 7 months. Thoracic radiographs showed a diffuse, severe bronchointerstitial lung pattern with diffuse miliary to nodular opacities in all lung fields. Symptomatic therapy was unsuccessful in all three cases and the diagnosis of LCH was made on necropsy through the use of extensive immunostaining and electron microscopy confirming the presence of Birbeck's granules. At necropsy, metastasis to pancreas, kidneys, liver, and/or visceral lymph nodes was noted in all three cats.

Malignant Fibrous Histiocytoma

The term *malignant fibrous histiocytoma* (MFH) refers to a group of tumors with histologic characteristics resembling both histiocytes and fibroblasts often displaying a storiform pattern with foam cells and multinucleated tumor giant cells.[81] In some cases, the term may be designated to poorly differentiated or pleomorphic forms of other soft tissue sarcomas.[82] With the widespread use of IHC techniques to delineate tumor cell lineage, the malignant fibrous histiocytomas have become separated from tumors of true histiocytic origin based on positive vimentin, desmin, and S100 staining but lack of CD18 and CD11 subunit staining.[82,83] Further discussion on the clinical behavior of soft tissue sarcomas such as MFH are located elsewhere in this text (see Chapter 21).

REFERENCES

1. Moore PF, Affolter V, Olivry T, et al: The use of immunological reagents in defining the pathogenesis of canine skin disease involving proliferation of leukocytes. In Kwochka KW, Wilemse T, von Tscharner C, editors: *Advances in veterinary dermatology*, Oxford, 1998, Butterworth-Heinemann.
2. Affolter VK, Moore PF: Localized and disseminated histiocytic sarcoma of dendritic cell origin in dogs, *Vet Pathol* 39:74–83, 2002.
3. Moore PF, Schrenzel MD, Affolter VK, et al: Canine cutaneous histiocytoma is an epidermotropic Langerhans cell histiocytosis that expresses CD1 and specific beta 2-integrin molecules, *Am J Pathol* 148:1699–1708, 1996.
4. Affolter VK, Moore PF: Canine cutaneous and systemic histiocytosis of dermal and dendritic origin, *Am J Dermatopathol* 22:40–48, 2000.
5. Moore PF, Affolter VK: Canine hemophagocytic histiocytic sarcoma: a proliferative disorder of CD11d+ macrophages, *Vet Pathol* 43:632–645, 2006.
6. Shortman, K, Naik SH: Steady-state and inflammatory dendritic-cell development, *Nat Rev Immunol* 7:19–30, 2007.
7. Larregina AT, Morelli AE: Dermal-resident CD14+ cells differentiate into Langerhans cells, *Nat Immunol* 2:1151–1158, 2001.
8. Shortman K, Caux C: Dendritic cell development: multiple pathways to nature's adjuvants, *Stem Cells* 15:409–419, 1997.
9. Shortman K, Liu YJ: Mouse and human dendritic cell subtypes, *Nat Rev Immunol* 2(3):151–161, 2002.
10. Ricklin ME, Roosje P: Characterization of canine dendritic cells in healthy, atopic, and non-allergic inflamed skin, *J Clin Immunol* 30:845–854, 2010.
11. Zaba LC, Krueger JG: Resident and inflammatory dendritic cells in human skin, *J Invest Dermatol* 129:302–308, 2009.
12. Looringh van Beeck FA, Zajonc DM: Two canine CD1a proteins are differentially expressed in skin, *Immunogenetics* 60:315–324, 2008.
13. Danilenko DM, Moore PF, Rossitto PV: Canine leukocyte cell adhesion molecules (LeuCAMS): characterization of the CD11/CD18 family, *Tissue Antigens* 40:13–21, 1992.
14. Danilenko DM, Rossitti PV, Van der Vieren M, et al: A novel canine leukointegrin, alpha d beta 2, is expressed by specific macrophage subpopulations in tissue and a minor CD8+ lymphocyte subpopulation in peripheral blood, *J Immunol* 155:35–44, 1995.
15. Ricklin ME, Roosje P: Characterization of canine dendritic cells in healthy, atopic, and non-allergic inflamed skin, *J Clin Immunol* 30:845–854, 2010.
16. Scalapino KJ, Daikh DI: CTLA-4: a key regulatory point in the control of autoimmune disease, *Immunol Rev* 223:143–155, 2008.
17. Banchereau J, Steinman RM: Dendritic cells and the control of immunity, *Nature* 392:245–252, 1998.
18. Banchereau J, Briere F, Caux C, et al: Immunology of dendritic cells, *Ann Rev Immunol* 18:767–811, 2000.
19. Swerdlow SH, Campo E: *WHO classification of tumors of the haematopoietic and lymphoid tissues*, Lyon, 2008, International Agency for Research on Cancer (IARC).
20. Valli VE, Jacobs RM: *Histological classification of hematopoietic tumors of domestic animals: World Health Organization international histological classification of tumors of domestic animals*, Washington, DC, 2002, Armed Forces Institute of Pathology, American Registry of Pathology.
21. Schmidt JM, North SM, Freeman KP, et al: Canine paediatric oncology: retrospective assessment of 9522 tumours in dogs up to 12 months (1993-2008), *Vet Comp Oncol* 8:283–292, 2010.
22. Glick AD, Holscher M, Campbell GR: Canine cutaneous histiocytoma: ultrastructural and cytochemical observations, *Vet Pathol* 13:374–380, 1976.
23. Kelly DF: Canine cutaneous histiocytoma: a light and microscopic study, *Vet Pathol* 7:12–27, 1970.
24. Moore PF, Schrenzel MD, Affolter VK, et al: Canine cutaneous histiocytoma is an epidermotropic Langerhans cell histiocytosis that expresses CD1 and specific beta 2-integrin molecules, *Am J Pathol* 148:1699–1708, 1996.
25. Bostock DE: Neoplasms of the skin and subcutaneous tissues in dogs and cats, *Br Vet J* 142:1–19, 1986.
26. Rothwell TLW, Howlett CR, Middleton DJ, et al: Skin neoplasms of dogs in Sydney, *Aust Vet J* 64:161–164, 1987.
27. Brodey RS: Canine and feline neoplasias, *Adv Vet Sci Comp Med* 14:309–354, 1970.
28. Gross TL, Affolter VK: Advances in skin oncology. In Kwochka KW, Willemse T, von Tscharner C, editors: *Advances in veterinary dermatology*, Oxford, UK, 1998, Butterworth-Heinemann.
29. Gross TL, Ihrke PJ, Walder EJ: *Veterinary dermatopathology; a macroscopic evaluation of canine and feline skin diseases*, St Louis, 1992, Mosby Year Book.
30. Yager JA, Wilcock BP: *Color atlas and text of surgical pathology of the dog and cat: dermatopathology and skin tumors*, London, 1994, M. Wolfe, p 320.
31. Angus JC, de Lorimier LP: Lymphohistiocytic neoplasms. In Campbell KL, editor: *Small animal dermatology secrets*, Philadelphia, 2004, Hanley and Belfus, pp 425–442.
32. Ramos-Vara JA, Miller MA: Immunohistochemical expression of E-cadherin does not distinguish canine cutaneous histiocytoma from other canine round cell tumors, *Vet Pathol* 48:758–763, 2011.
33. Baines SJ, McInnes EF, McConnell I: E-cadherin expression in canine cutaneous histiocytomas, *Vet Rec* 162:509–513, 2008.
34. Schmitz L, Favara BE: Nosology and pathology of Langerhans cell histiocytosis, *Hematol Oncol Clin North Am* 12:221–246, 1998.
35. Munn S, Chu AC: Langerhans cell histiocytosis of the skin, *Hematol Oncol Clin North Am* 12:269–286, 1998.
36. Mays MB, Bergeron JA: Cutaneous histiocytosis in dogs, *J Am Vet Med Assoc* 188:377–381, 1986.
37. Palmeiro BS, Morris DO, Goldschmidt MH, et al: Cutaneous reactive histiocytosis in dogs: a retrospective evaluation of 32 cases, *Vet Dermatol* 18:332–340, 2007.
38. Scott DW, Angurano DK, Suter MM: Systemic histiocytosis in 2 dogs, *Canine Pract* 14:7–12, 1987
39. Moore PF: Malignant histiocytosis of Bernese mountain dogs, *Vet Pathol* 23:1–10, 1986.
40. Moore PF: Systemic histiocytosis of Bernese mountain dogs, *Vet Pathol* 21:554–563, 1984.

41. Scott DW, Miller WH, Griffin CE: Lymphohistiocytic neoplasms. In *Muller and Kirk's small animal dermatology*, Philadelphia, 2000, WB Saunders, pp 1130–1357.
42. Scherlie PH, Smedes SL, Feltz T, et al: Ocular manifestations of systemic histiocytosis in a dog, *J Am Vet Med Assoc* 201:1229–1232, 1992.
43. DeHeer HL, Grindem CB: Histiocytic disorders. In Jain NC, editor: *Schalms veterinary hematology*, ed 4, Philadelphia, 1986, Lea & Febiger.
44. Pires I, Queiroga FL, Alves A, et al: Decrease of E-cadherin expression in canine cutaneous histiocytoma appears to be related to its spontaneous regression, *Anticancer Res* 29:2713–2717, 2009.
45. Rosin A, Moore P, Dubielzig R: Malignant histiocytosis in Bernese Mountain dogs, *J Am Vet Med Assoc* 188:1041–1045, 1986.
46. Dobson J, Hoather T, McKinley TJ, et al: Mortality in a cohort of flat-coated retrievers in the UK, *Vet Comp Oncol* 7:115–121, 2009.
47. Craig LE, Julian ME, Ferracone JD: The diagnosis and prognosis of synovial tumors in dogs: 35 cases, *Vet Pathol* 39:66–73, 2002.
48. Hayden DW, Waters DJ, Burke BA, et al: Disseminated malignant histiocytosis in a golden retriever: clinicopathologic, ultrastructural, and immunohistochemical findings, *Vet Pathol* 30:256–264, 1993.
49. Kohn B, Arnold P, Kaser-Hotz B, et al: Malignant histiocytosis of the dog: 26 cases (1989-1992), *Kleintierpraxis* 38:409–424, 1993.
50. Fant P, Caldin M, Furlanello T, et al: Primary gastric histiocytic sarcoma in a dog—a case report, *J Vet Med* 51:358–362, 2004.
51. Skorupski K, Clifford C, Paoloni M, et al: CCNU for the treatment of dogs with histiocytic sarcoma, *J Vet Intern Med* 21:121–126, 2007.
52. Naranjo C, Dubielzig R, Friedrichs K: Canine ocular histiocytic sarcoma, *Vet Ophthalmol* 10:179–185, 2007.
53. Vernau KM, Higgins RJ, Bollen AW, et al: Primary canine and feline nervous system tumors: intraoperative diagnosis using the smear technique, *Vet Pathol* 38:47–57, 2001.
54. Snyder J, Lipitz L, Skorupski K, et al: Secondary intracranial neoplasia in the dog: 177 cases (1986-2003), *J Vet Intern Med* 22:172–177, 2008.
55. Brown DE, Thrall MA, Getzy DM, et al: Cytology of canine malignant histiocytosis, *Vet Clin Pathol* 23:118–123, 1994.
56. Weiss DJ, Evanson OA, Sykes J: A retrospective study of canine pancytopenia, *Vet Clin Pathol* 28:83–88, 1999.
57. Newlands CE, Houston DM, Vasconcelos DY: Hyperferritinemia associated with malignant histiocytosis in a dog, *J Am Vet Med Assoc* 205:849–851, 1994.
58. Friedrichs K, Thomas C, Plier M, et al: Evaluation of serum ferritin as a tumor marker for canine histiocytic sarcoma, *J Vet Intern Med* 24:904–911, 2010.
59. Cruz-Arambulo R, Wrigley R, Powers B: Sonographic features of histiocytic neoplasms in the canine abdomen, *Vet Radiol Ultrasound* 45:554–558, 2004.
60. Weiss DJ: Flow cytometric evaluation of hemophagocytic disorders in canine, *Vet Clin Pathol* 31:36–41, 2002.
61. Klahn SL, Kitchell B, Dervisis N: Evaluation and comparison of outcomes in dogs with periarticular and nonperiarticular histiocytic sarcoma, *J Am Vet Med Assoc* 239:90–96, 2001.
62. Rassnick K, Moore A, Russell D, et al: Phase II, open-label trial of single-agent CCNU in dogs with previously untreated histiocytic sarcoma, *J Vet Intern Med* 24:1528–1531, 2010.
63. Skorupski K, Rodriguez C, Krick E, et al: Long-term survival in dogs with localized histiocytic sarcoma treated with CCNU as an adjuvant to local therapy, *Vet Comp Oncol* 7:139–144, 2009.
64. Vail DM, Kravis LD, Cooley AJ, et al: Preclinical trial of doxorubicin entrapped in sterically stabilized liposomes in dogs with spontaneously arising malignant tumors, *Cancer Chemother Pharmacol* 39:410–416, 1997.
65. Poirier VJ, Hershey AE, Burgess KE, et al: Efficacy and toxicity of paclitaxel (Taxol) for the treatment of canine malignant tumors, *J Vet Intern Med* 18:219–222, 2004.
66. Uno Y, Momio Y, Watari T, et al: Malignant histiocytosis with multiple skin lesions in a dog, *J Vet Med Sci* 55:1059–1061, 1993.
67. Hafeman S, London C, Elmslie R, et al: Evaluation of liposomal clodronate for treatment of malignant histiocytosis in dogs, *Cancer Immunol Immunother* 59:441–452, 2010.
68. Higuchi T, Dervisis N, Kitchell B: *Efficacy of doxorubicin for histiocytic sarcoma in dogs. 30th Annual Veterinary Cancer Society Meeting Conference*, San Diego, 2010.
69. Fidel J, Schiller I, Hauser Y, et al: Histiocytic sarcomas in flat-coated retrievers: a summary of 37 cases (November 1998-March 2005), *Vet Comp Oncol* 4:63–74, 2006.
70. Friedrichs K, Young K: Histiocytic sarcoma of macrophage origin in a cat: case report with a literature review of feline histiocytic malignancies and comparison with canine hemophagocytic histiocytic sarcoma, *Vet Clin Pathol* 37:121–128, 2008.
71. Walton RM, Brown DE, Burkhard MJ, et al: Malignant histiocytosis in a domestic cat: cytomorphologic and immunohistochemical features, *Vet Clin Pathol* 26:56–60, 1997.
72. Kraje AC, Patton CS, Edwards DF: Malignant histiocytosis in 3 cats, *J Vet Intern Med* 15:252–256, 2001.
73. Smoliga J, Schatzberg S, Peters J, et al: Myelopathy caused by a histiocytic sarcoma in a cat, *J Small Anim Pract* 46:34–38, 2005.
74. Bell R, Philbey A, Martineau H, et al: Dynamic tracheal collapse associated with disseminated histiocytic sarcoma in a cat, *J Small Anim Pract* 47:461–464, 2006.
75. Court E, Earnest-Koons K, Barr S, et al: Malignant histiocytosis in a cat, *J Am Vet Med Assoc* 203:1300–1302, 1993.
76. Ide T, Uchida K, Tamura S, et al: Histiocytic sarcoma in the brain of a cat, *J Vet Med Sci* 72:99–102, 2010.
77. Ide K, Setoguchi-Mukai A, Nakagawa T, et al: Disseminated histiocytic sarcoma with excessive hemophagocytosis in a cat, *J Vet Med Sci* 71:817–820, 2009.
78. Pinard J, Wagg C, Girard C, et al: Histiocytic sarcoma in the tarsus of a cat, *Vet Pathol* 43:1014–1017, 2006.
79. Affolter V, Moore P: Feline progressive histiocytosis, *Vet Pathol* 43:646–655, 2006.
80. Busch M, Reilly C, Luff J, et al: Feline pulmonary Langerhans cell histiocytosis with multiorgan involvement, *Vet Pathol* 45:816–824, 2008.
81. Pulley LT, Stannard AA: Tumors of the skin and soft tissues. In Moulton JE, editor: *Tumors in domestic animals*, ed 3, Los Angeles, 1990, University of California Press.
82. Morris JS, McInnes EF, Bostock DE, et al: Immunohistochemical and histopathologic features of 14 malignant fibrous histiocytomas from Flat-Coated Retrievers, *Vet Pathol* 39:473–479, 2002.
83. Thoolen RJ, Vos JH, van der Linde-Sipman JS, et al: Malignant fibrous histiocytomas in dogs and cats: an immunohistochemical study, *Res Vet Sci* 53:198–204, 1992.

Index

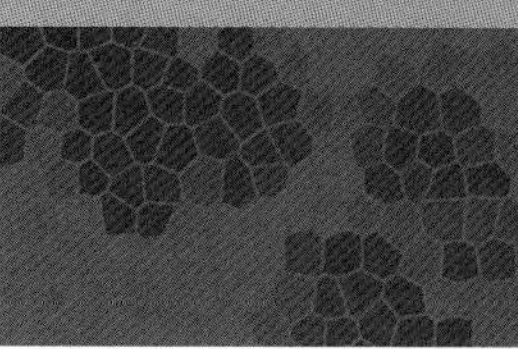

Page numbers followed by "f" indicate figures; "t" indicate tables; and "b" indicate boxes.

C

H

I